a Lange medical book

2005

CURRENT CONSULT

MEDICINE

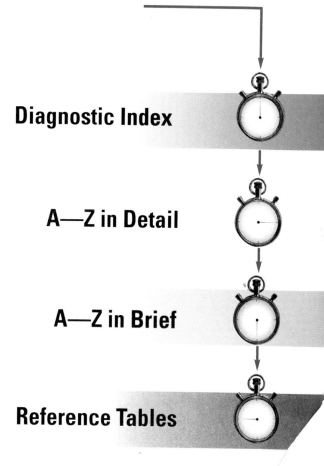

Diagnostic Index

A—Z in Detail

A—Z in Brief

Reference Tables

To James Ransom and Isabel Nogueira
for their uncompromising professionalism
and devotion to excellence
in medical education

a Lange medical book

2005
CURRENT CONSULT
MEDICINE

Edited by

Maxine A. Papadakis, MD
Professor of Clinical Medicine
Associate Dean for Student Affairs
School of Medicine
University of California, San Francisco

Stephen J. McPhee, MD
Professor of Medicine
Division of General Internal Medicine
Department of Medicine
University of California, San Francisco

Lange Medical Books/McGraw-Hill
Medical Publishing Division

New York   Chicago   San Francisco   Lisbon
London   Madrid   Mexico City   Milan   New Delhi
San Juan   Seoul   Singapore   Sydney   Toronto

Notice

Medicine is an ever-changing science. As new research and clinical experience broaden our knowledge, changes in treatment and drug therapy are required. The authors and the publisher of this work have checked with sources believed to be reliable in their efforts to provide information that is complete and generally in accord with the standards accepted at the time of publication. However, in view of the possibility of human error or changes in medical sciences, neither the authors nor the publisher nor any other party who has been involved in the preparation or publication of this work warrants that the information contained herein is in every respect accurate or complete, and they disclaim all responsibility for any errors or omissions or for the results obtained from use of the information contained in this work. Readers are encouraged to confirm the information contained herein with other sources. For example and in particular, readers are advised to check the product information sheet included in the package of each drug they plan to administer to be certain that the information contained in this work is accurate and that changes have not been made in the recommended dose or in the contraindications for administration. This recommendation is of particular importance in connection with new or infrequently used drugs.

This book was set in Adobe Garamond by Pine Tree Composition, Inc.
The editors were Isabel Nogueira, Harriet Lebowitz, and Peter J. Boyle.
The production supervisor was Philip Galea.
The art manager was Charissa Baker.
The text was designed by Eve Siegel.
The index was prepared by Kathrin Unger.

Quebecor Dubuque was printer and binder.

This book is printed on acid-free paper.

CURRENT CONSULT
Medicine: 4 Parts

1. Diagnostic Index 1

Differential diagnoses
and disease etiologies
for over 400 disorders
and symptoms

2. A-Z in Detail 65

Key diagnosis and treatment
information for 490
diseases and symptoms

3. A-Z in Brief 1047

Key diagnosis and treatment
information for 380
diseases and symptoms

4. Reference Tables 1191

Over 150 of the most popular
*Current Medical Diagnosis
& Treatment* tables, including
specific drug therapy
recommendations and essential
diagnosis information

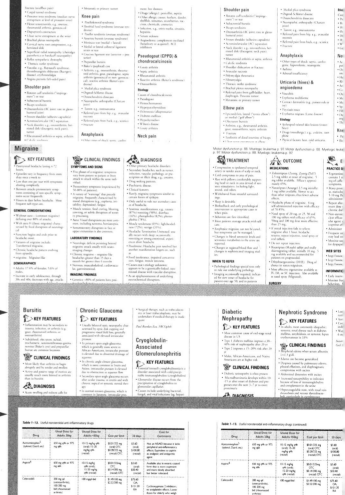

CONTENTS: Alphabetical

CONTENTS: Topical

CONTENTS: Reference Tables

Authors & Contributors

Associate Editor

Roni F. Zeiger, MD
Fellow in Medical Informatics, VA Palo Alto Health Care System, Palo Alto, California; Clinical Instructor of Medicine, Stanford University School of Medicine, Stanford, California

Authors

Daniel C. Adelman, MD
Adjunct Professor of Medicine, Division of Allergy and Immunology, University of California, San Francisco

Thomas M. Amidon, MD
Clinical Instructor, University of Washington, Bellevue

Michael J. Aminoff, MD, DSc, FRCP
Professor of Neurology, University of California, San Francisco; Attending Physician, University of California Medical Center, San Francisco

Robert B. Baron, MD, MS
Professor of Medicine; Associate Dean for Continuing Medical Education; Vice Chief and Director, Educational Programs, Division of General Internal Medicine; Director, Primary Care Internal Medicine Residency Program, University of California, San Francisco

Timothy G. Berger, MD
Professor of Clinical Dermatology, Department of Dermatology, University of California, San Francisco

Peter R. Carroll, MD
Professor and Chair, Department of Urology, Ken and Donna Derr-Chevron Endowed Chair in Prostate Cancer, University of California, San Francisco

Henry F. Chambers, MD
Professor of Medicine, University of California, San Francisco; Chief, Division of Infectious Diseases, San Francisco General Hospital

Mark S. Chesnutt, MD
Associate Professor of Medicine, Pulmonary & Critical Care Medicine; Director, Medical Critical Care, Oregon Health & Science University, Portland

Richard Cohen, MD, MPH
Clinical Professor, Division of Occupational and Environmental Medicine, University of California, San Francisco

Kenneth E. Covinsky, MD, MPH
Associate Professor of Medicine, University of California, San Francisco; Staff Physician, San Francisco Veterans Affairs Medical Center

William R. Crombleholme, MD
Chairman, Department of Obstetrics and Gynecology, The Stamford Hospital, Stamford, Connecticut

Stuart J. Eisendrath, MD
Professor of Clinical Psychiatry, University of California, San Francisco; Director, Clinical Services, Langley Porter Psychiatric Hospital and Clinics, San Francisco

Paul A. Fitzgerald, MD
Clinical Professor of Medicine, Department of Medicine, Division of Endocrinology, University of California, San Francisco

Lawrence S. Friedman, MD
Professor of Medicine, Harvard Medical School, Boston, Massachusetts; Chair, Department of Medicine, Newton-Wellesley Hospital, Newton, Massachusetts; Assistant Chief of Medicine, Massachusetts General Hospital, Boston, Massachusetts

Masafumi Fukagawa, MD, PhD, FJSIM
Associate Professor and Director, Division of Nephrology and Dialysis Center, Kobe University School of Medicine, Japan

Armando E. Giuliano, MD
Director, Joyce Eisenberg Keefer Breast Center; Clinical Professor of Surgery, University of California, Los Angeles; Chief of Surgical Oncology, John Wayne Cancer Institute, Santa Monica, California

Richard J. Hamill, MD
Professor, Departments of Medicine and Molecular Virology & Microbiology, Baylor College of Medicine; Staff Physician, Veterans Affairs Medical Center, Houston, Texas

David B. Hellmann, MD, FACP
Mary Betty Stevens Professor of Medicine; Chairman, Department of Medicine, Johns Hopkins Bayview Medical Center, Johns Hopkins University School of Medicine, Baltimore, Maryland

Harry Hollander, MD
Professor of Clinical Medicine and Director,
Categorical Medicine Residency Program, University
of California, San Francisco

Robert K. Jackler, MD
Sewall Professor and Chair, Department of
Otolaryngology-Head and Neck Surgery; Professor,
Neurosurgery and Surgery, Stanford University
School of Medicine, Stanford, California

Richard A. Jacobs, MD, PhD
Clinical Professor of Medicine and Clinical Pharmacy,
University of California, San Francisco

C. Bree Johnston, MD, MPH
Associate Professor of Clinical Medicine, Division of
Geriatrics, Department of Medicine, Veterans Affairs
Medical Center, University of California, San
Francisco

Michael J. Kaplan, MD
Professor, Department of Otolaryngology-Head and
Neck Surgery, Stanford University, Stanford,
California

Mitchell H. Katz, MD
Clinical Professor of Medicine, Epidemiology &
Biostatistics, University of California, San Francisco;
Director of Health, San Francisco Department of
Public Health

Jeffrey L. Kishiyama, MD
Assistant Clinical Professor of Medicine, University
of California, San Francisco

Kiyoshi Kurokawa, MD, MACP
President, Science Council of Japan, Tokyo, Japan;
Professor, Tokai University, Kanagawa, Japan

Jonathan E. Lichtmacher, MD
Assistant Clinical Professor of Psychiatry, University
of California, San Francisco; Associate Director, Adult
Psychiatry Clinic, Langley Porter Hospitals and
Clinics, University of California, San Francisco

Charles A. Linker, MD
Clinical Professor of Medicine and Director, Adult
Leukemia and Hematologic Malignancies Program,
University of California, San Francisco

William L. Lyons, MD
Assistant Professor, Section of Geriatrics and
Gerontology, Department of Internal Medicine,
Nebraska Medical Center, Omaha, Nebraska

H. Trent MacKay, MD, MPH
Associate Professor of Obstetrics and Gynecology,
Uniformed Services, University of the Health
Sciences, Bethesda, Maryland; Department Head,
Obstetrics and Gynecology, National Naval Medical
Center, Bethesda, Maryland

Umesh Masharani, MB, BS; MRCP(UK)
Associate Clinical Professor of Medicine, Division of
Endocrinology and Metabolism, University of
California, San Francisco

Barry M. Massie, MD
Professor of Medicine, University of California, San
Francisco; Chief, Cardiology Division, San Francisco
Veterans Affairs Medical Center

Stephen J. McPhee, MD
Professor of Medicine, Division of General Internal
Medicine, Department of Medicine, University of
California, San Francisco

Kenneth R. McQuaid, MD
Professor of Clinical Medicine, University of
California, San Francisco; Director of Gastrointestinal
Endoscopy, San Francisco Veterans Affairs Medicine
Center

Louis M. Messina, MD
Professor and Chief, Division of Vascular Surgery;
Vice Chair, Department of Surgery, University of
California, San Francisco

Brent R.W. Moelleken, MD, FACS
Plastic and Reconstructive Surgery; Assistant Clinical
Professor, Division of Plastic Surgery, Attending
Physician, University of California, Los Angeles
Medical Center; Private Practice, Beverly Hills,
California

Gail Morrison, MD, FACP
Vice Dean for Education, Director of Academic
Programs, and Professor of Medicine, School of
Medicine, University of Pennsylvania, Philadelphia

Kent R. Olson, MD
Clinical Professor of Medicine and Pharmacy,
University of California, San Francisco; Medical
Director, San Francisco Division, California Poison
Control System, University of California, San
Francisco

Laura K. Pak, MD
Vascular Surgeon, Cardiology Associates of Marin
and San Francisco; Director of Peripheral Vascular
Program Development, Marin General Hospital,
Greenbrae, California

Maxine A. Papadakis, MD
Professor of Clinical Medicine and Associate Dean for Student Affairs, School of Medicine, University of California, San Francisco

Thomas J. Prendergast, MD
Associate Professor of Medicine and Anesthesiology, Section of Pulmonary and Critical Care Medicine, Dartmouth-Hitchcock Medical Center, Lebanon, New Hampshire

Reed E. Pyeritz, MD, PhD
Professor of Medicine and Genetics; Chief, Division of Medical Genetics, University of Pennsylvania Health System and School of Medicine, Philadelphia

Paul Riordan-Eva, FRCS, FRCOphth
Consultant Ophthalmologist, King's College Hospital, London; Honorary Consultant Neuro-Ophthalmologist, National Hospital for Neurology and Neurosurgery, London, United Kingdom

Hope S. Rugo, MD
Clinical Professor of Medicine and Co-Director, Breast Oncology Clinical Trials Program, University of California, San Francisco Comprehensive Cancer Center

Wayne X. Shandera, MD
Assistant Professor of Internal Medicine, Baylor College of Medicine, Houston, Texas

Samuel A. Shelburne III, MD
Infectious Diseases Fellow, Department of Internal Medicine, Baylor College of Medicine, Houston, Texas

Marshall L. Stoller, MD
Professor of Urology and Chief of Urinary Stone Disease and Laparoscopy, University of California, San Francisco

John H. Stone, MD, MPH
Associate Professor of Medicine, Division of Rheumatology, Johns Hopkins University; Director, Johns Hopkins Vasculitis Center, Baltimore, Maryland

Lawrence M. Tierney, Jr., MD
Professor of Medicine, University of California, San Francisco; Associate Chief of Medical Service, San Francisco Veterans Affairs Medical Center

Suzanne Watnick, MD
Assistant Professor of Medicine, Division of Nephrology and Hypertension, Oregon Health & Science University, Portland; Director, Dialysis Unit, Portland VA Medical Center, Portland, Oregon

Contributors

Eva M. Aagaard, MD
Assistant Clinical Professor of Medicine, Division of General Internal Medicine, University of California, San Francisco

Thomas E. Baudendistel, MD
Associate Program Director, Internal Medicine, California-Pacific Medical Center; Adjunct Assistant Clinical Professor of Medicine, University of California, San Francisco

Thomas D. Denberg, MD, PhD
Assistant Professor, Division of General Internal Medicine, University of Colorado Health Sciences Center, Denver

Gurpreet Dhaliwal, MD
Assistant Clinical Professor of Medicine, University of California, San Francisco

Ashish K. Jha, MD
Assistant Professor of Medicine, Harvard Medical School, Boston, Massachusetts

Eric N. Swagel, MD
Clinical Instructor, University of California, San Francisco

Internet Resources

Jolaine Beal, MD, MPH
Resident Physician, Family Medicine, University of California, San Francisco, Santa Rosa

Janet Lee, MS
Medical Student / University of California, San Francisco

Guide to *Current Consult: Medicine*

To get practical, up-to-date information on diagnosis and treatment when you just have a few minutes, rely on *Current Consult: Medicine.* It is a single-source reference designed for quick-and-easy access to the information you need in the clinical setting. The four parts of the book, which are color-coded, include:

Diagnostic Index: THE DARK BLUE PAGES
A—Z in Detail: THE WHITE PAGES
A—Z in Brief: THE LIGHT BLUE PAGES
Reference Tables: THE GRAY PAGES

The **DIAGNOSTIC INDEX** provides a comprehensive outline of differential diagnoses and disease etiologies for over 400 disorders and symptoms. It is derived from Diagnosaurus, the PDA program that has become an extraordinarily popular differential diagnosis tool.

A—Z IN DETAIL and **A—Z IN BRIEF** present the right amount of information on each topic to give you the key diagnostic and treatment features of more than 860 diseases. To save you time, the disease entries are alphabetized. The bulleted form promotes rapid comprehension so that you can immediately apply what you learn from this quick consult on current medical practice. Each disease entry in the **A—Z IN DETAIL** includes:

- Key Features: essentials of diagnosis and general considerations
- Clinical Findings: symptoms and signs and differential diagnosis
- Diagnosis: laboratory tests, imaging studies, and diagnostic procedures
- Treatment: medications, surgery, and therapeutic procedures
- Outcome: complications, prognosis, when to refer, and when to admit
- Evidence: up-to-date clinical guidelines, targeted references, and Web sites for clinicians and patients.

The **REFERENCE TABLES** display specific diagnostic and treatment options to help you find the best solutions to immediate clinical problems. Using these tables, you can quickly pinpoint individual drugs and dosages.

The authors of *Current Consult: Medicine* are those you already know and trust from *Current Medical Diagnosis & Treatment,* the leading medicine textbook for both hospital and outpatient settings, now in its 44th annual edition. These authors provide the latest expert information on adult primary care topics that include gynecology, obstetrics, dermatology, otolaryngology, geriatrics and ophthalmology.

HOW TO USE *CURRENT CONSULT: MEDICINE*

If you know the diagnosis for which you need an immediate consult, go directly to that disorder in the WHITE PAGES: **A—Z IN DETAIL.** In addition to the disease entries in the white pages, you will see page numbers at the top of some of the white pages that direct you to specific disorders selected for the LIGHT BLUE PAGES: **A—Z IN BRIEF.**

If, instead, you are searching for a differential diagnosis, consult the DARK BLUE PAGES: **DIAGNOSTIC INDEX.** After identifying the most likely disorder(s), go to the WHITE PAGES: **A—Z IN DETAIL** to get diagnosis and treatment information.

If you want to find specifics about drugs and dosages, go to the GRAY PAGES: **REFERENCE TABLES.**

FEATURES

- Leaders in their medical subspecialties provide you with their expertise
- Content is organized into four, easy-to-use sections
- Bulleted clinical information and specific treatment options give you the current medical consult you need.

For electronic access, *Current Consult: Medicine* is also available as a PDA program (Palm and Pocket PC) and can be purchased at your local bookstore or ordered at www.accessmedbooks.com.

Maxine A. Papadakis, MD
Stephen J. McPhee, MD
San Francisco

Diagnostic
Index

Abdominal pain, generalized

- Gastritis
- Gastroenteritis
- Irritable bowel syndrome
- Pancreatitis
- Peritonitis
- Intestinal ischemia
- Constipation
- Urinary tract infection
- Intestinal obstruction
- Perforated viscus, eg, peptic ulcer, appendix, gallbladder, diverticulitis
- Physical or sexual abuse
- Abdominal abscess
- Ruptured ectopic pregnancy
- Ruptured spleen
- Inflammatory bowel disease
- Abdominal aortic aneurysm
- Diabetic ketoacidosis
- Hypercalcemia
- Uremia
- Parasitic infection, eg, giardiasis, strongyloidiasis, ascariasis, tapeworm
- Adrenal insufficiency
- Lead poisoning
- Iron poisoning
- Polyarteritis nodosa
- Henoch-Schönlein purpura
- Porphyria, eg, acute intermittent porphyria
- Familial Mediterranean fever
- Black widow spider bite

Abdominal pain, left lower quadrant

- Diverticulitis
- Gastroenteritis or colitis
- Constipation
- Irritable bowel syndrome
- Gynecologic: pelvic inflammatory disease, ovarian torsion, ruptured ovarian cyst, tubo-ovarian abscess, endometriosis, ectopic pregnancy, mittelschmerz
- Intestinal ischemia
- Cystitis
- Hernia, eg, femoral, inguinal, umbilical
- Testicular, eg, epididymitis, testicular torsion
- Prostatitis
- Urinary calculi
- Inflammatory bowel disease

- Colon cancer
- Intestinal obstruction
- Abdominal aortic aneurysm
- Herpes zoster
- Trauma or musculoskeletal pain
- Herniated disk
- Abdominal abscess
- Physical or sexual abuse

Abdominal pain, left upper quadrant

- Gastritis
- Gastroenteritis
- Pancreatitis
- Peptic ulcer disease (gastric)
- Splenomegaly, eg, leukemia, lymphoma
- Left lower lobe pneumonia
- Pyelonephritis
- Myocardial ischemia or pericarditis
- Ruptured spleen, eg, trauma, mononucleosis
- Splenic infarct, eg, endocarditis
- Urinary calculi
- Functional or nonulcer dyspepsia
- Gastric cancer
- Diverticulitis
- Herpes zoster
- Intestinal ischemia
- Trauma or musculoskeletal pain
- Herniated disk
- Abdominal abscess
- Physical or sexual abuse

Abdominal pain, right lower quadrant

- Appendicitis
- Gastroenteritis or colitis
- Irritable bowel syndrome
- Gynecologic: pelvic inflammatory disease, ovarian torsion, ruptured ovarian cyst, tubo-ovarian abscess, endometriosis, ectopic pregnancy, mittelschmerz
- Cystitis
- Hernia, eg, femoral, inguinal, umbilical
- Testicular, eg, epididymitis, testicular torsion
- Prostatitis
- Diverticulitis
- Colon cancer
- Urinary calculi
- Intestinal ischemia
- Intestinal obstruction

- Abdominal aortic aneurysm
- Inflammatory bowel disease
- Mesenteric adenitis, eg, *Yersinia,* tuberculosis
- Typhlitis (neutropenic colitis)
- Meckel's diverticulitis
- Herpes zoster
- Trauma or musculoskeletal pain
- Herniated disk
- Abdominal abscess
- Physical or sexual abuse

Abdominal pain, right upper quadrant

- Cholelithiasis
- Cholecystitis
- Hepatitis, eg, viral, alcoholic, toxic
- Cholangitis or choledocholithiasis
- Appendicitis (retrocecal)
- Peptic ulcer disease (duodenal)
- Pancreatitis
- Functional or nonulcer dyspepsia
- Liver abscess
- Liver, pancreatic, or biliary tract cancer
- Ischemic hepatopathy (shock liver)
- Hepatic vein obstruction (Budd-Chiari syndrome)
- Right lower lobe pneumonia
- Pyelonephritis
- Urinary calculi
- Fitz-Hugh-Curtis syndrome (with PID)
- Liver cell adenoma
- Herpes zoster
- Trauma or musculoskeletal pain
- Herniated disk
- Abdominal abscess
- Intestinal ischemia
- Physical or sexual abuse

Abdominal pain, upper or epigastric

- Functional or nonulcer dyspepsia (most common)
- Peptic ulcer disease
- Gastroesophageal reflux
- Gastritis, eg, NSAIDs, alcohol, stress, *Helicobacter pylori,* pernicious anemia
- Pancreatitis or pancreatic cancer
- "Indigestion" from overeating, high-fat foods, coffee
- Other drugs: aspirin, antibiotics (eg, macrolides, metronidazole), corticosteroids, digoxin, narcotics, theophylline

- Gastroparesis
- Lactase deficiency
- Malabsorption
- Gastric cancer
- Parasitic infection, eg, *Giardia, Strongyloides, Ascaris*
- Cholelithiasis, choledocholithiasis, or cholangitis
- *Helicobacter pylori* (controversial)
- Myocardial ischemia or pericarditis
- Pneumonia
- Abdominal hernia
- Pregnancy
- Intestinal ischemia
- Esophageal rupture
- Gastric volvulus
- Physical or sexual abuse

Abortion, recurrent

Etiology
- Luteal phase insufficiency (insufficient progesterone)
- Diabetes mellitus
- Hypothyroidism
- Congenital anatomic lesion, eg, septate uterus
- Acquired anatomic lesion, eg, incompetent cervix, intrauterine adhesions, submucous uterine leiomyoma (fibroid)
- Polycystic ovary syndrome
- Antiphospholipid antibody syndrome or other hypercoagulable state
- Balanced chromosomal translocation

Abortion, spontaneous
- Incompetent cervix
- Ectopic pregnancy
- Menses or menorrhagia
- Prolapsed uterine leiomyoma (fibroid)
- Hydatidiform mole
- Cervical neoplasm or lesion

Acanthosis nigricans
- Nevi
- Reticulated pigment anomaly (Dowling-Degos disease)
- Confluent and reticulated papillomatosis (of Gougerot and Carteaud)

Associated conditions
- Obesity
- Insulin resistance syndrome
- Diabetes mellitus

- Cushing's disease
- Acromegaly
- Hypothyroidism or hyperthyroidism
- Occult malignancy

Acute tubular necrosis
- Prerenal azotemia, eg, dehydration
- Postrenal azotemia, eg, benign prostatic hyperplasia
- Other renal causes of acute renal failure
  - Acute glomerulonephritis: immune complex (eg, IgA nephropathy), pauci-immune (eg, Wegener's granulomatosis), anti-GBM disease
  - Acute interstitial nephritis: drugs (eg, β-lactams), infections (eg, *Streptococcus*), immune (eg, systemic lupus erythematosus)

Etiology
- Toxins: NSAIDs, antibiotics, contrast, multiple myeloma, rhabdomyolysis, hemolysis, chemotherapy, hyperuricemia, cyclosporine
- Ischemia, eg, prolonged prerenal azotemia

Adrenal mass
- Nonfunctioning adrenal adenoma
- Metastatic cancer, eg, lung, breast, renal cell, lymphoma, melanoma
- Cortisol-producing adenoma
- Aldosterone-producing adenoma
- Adrenal carcinoma
- Pheochromocytoma
- Cyst or myelolipoma

Aggressive behavior
- Drugs, eg, PCP, alcohol, cocaine, amphetamines, anabolic steroids
- Impulse control disorder
- Psychiatric disease, eg, schizophrenia, personality disorder, mania
- Psychosis due to other causes

Airway obstruction, bronchi

Etiology
- Pulmonary secretions
- Aspiration
- Foreign body
- Bronchogenic carcinoma
- Extrinsic compression by mass
- Metastatic tumor

Airway obstruction, trachea

Etiology
- Tracheal stenosis, acquired (intubation, trauma)
- Tracheal stenosis, congenital
- Tracheal tumor (primary or metastatic)
- Extrinsic compression by tumor of lung, thyroid, thymus; lymphadenopathy; congenital vascular rings; aneurysms
- Foreign-body aspiration
- Tracheal granulomas or papillomas
- Tracheal trauma

Airway obstruction, upper

Etiology

Acute
- Foreign-body aspiration
- Laryngospasm
- Angioedema
- Laryngeal edema from airway burns
- Trauma to larynx or pharynx
- Epiglottitis
- Pharyngeal or retropharyngeal abscess
- Ludwig's angina
- Acute allergic laryngitis
- Vocal cord dysfunction

Chronic
- Carcinoma of larynx or pharynx
- Laryngeal or subglottic stenosis
- Laryngeal granulomas or webs
- Bilateral vocal cord paralysis
- Vocal cord dysfunction

Alcohol withdrawal
- Withdrawal from other sedatives, eg, benzodiazepines or opioids
- Drug intoxication, eg, cocaine, amphetamines
- Delirium due to medical illness, eg, hypoxia, hepatic encephalopathy, thiamine deficiency, bacteremia
- Anxiety disorder
- Hallucinosis due to other causes, eg, schizophrenia, amphetamine psychosis
- Seizure due to other causes, eg, hypoglycemia, epilepsy

Alkaline phosphatase increased

Etiology
- Obstructive hepatobiliary disease (GGT increased)

- Bone disease, eg, bone metastases, Paget's disease, osteomalacia, osteosarcoma, hyperparathyroidism (GGT normal)
- Pregnancy (third trimester)
- GI disease, eg, bowel infarction or perforated viscus
- Hepatitis, eg, viral, alcoholic, toxic
- Infiltrative liver disease, eg, tuberculosis, sarcoidosis, lymphoma, amyloidosis
- Hemochromatosis

Altered mental status

Drugs
- Opioids, alcohol, sedatives, antipsychotics, withdrawal, others

Metabolic
- Hypoxia, hypoglycemia, hyperglycemia, hypercalcemia, hypernatremia, hyponatremia, uremia, hepatic encephalopathy, hypothyroidism, hyperthyroidism, vitamin B$_{12}$ or thiamine deficiency, carbon monoxide poisoning, Wilson's disease

Infectious
- Meningitis, encephalitis, bacteremia, urinary tract infection, pneumonia, neurosyphilis

Structural
- Space-occupying lesion, eg, brain tumor, subdural hematoma, hydrocephalus

Vascular
- Stroke, subarachnoid hemorrhage, coronary ischemia, hypertensive encephalopathy, CNS vasculitis, thrombotic thrombocytopenic purpura, disseminated intravascular coagulation, hyperviscosity

Psychiatric
- Schizophrenia, depression

Other
- Seizure, hypothermia, heat stroke, ICU psychosis, "sundowning"

Altered mental status in a diabetic

- Hypoglycemia
- Diabetic ketoacidosis
- Hyperglycemic hyperosmolar state
- Lactic acidosis, eg, severe infection, metformin use
- Stroke
- Sepsis
- Uremia

Altered mental status in HIV/AIDS

- Mass lesion: toxoplasmosis, CNS lymphoma, brain abscess, metastatic tumor, cryptococcoma
- Other infections: bacterial meningitis, cryptococcal meningitis, herpes simplex virus encephalitis, neurosyphilis, tuberculous meningitis, bacteremia
- Other: AIDS dementia, progressive multifocal leukoencephalopathy, stroke, seizure, depression, metabolic, eg, hypoxia, hypoglycemia, uremic or hepatic encephalopathy

Alveolar hemorrhage, diffuse

Etiology

Immune causes
- Goodpasture's syndrome
- Systemic lupus erythematosus
- Wegener's granulomatosis
- Systemic necrotizing vasculitis
- Pulmonary capillaritis associated with idiopathic rapidly progressive glomerulonephritis

Nonimmune causes
- Coagulopathy
- Mitral stenosis
- Necrotizing pulmonary infection (eg, aspergillosis, cytomegalovirus, herpes simplex virus)
- Idiopathic pulmonary hemosiderosis
- Recent bone marrow transplant
- Drugs (penicillamine)
- Toxins (trimellitic anhydride)

Amaurosis fugax (fleeting blindness)

- Emboli from carotid
- Cardiac emboli
- Choroidal or retinal vascular spasm (especially younger patients)
- Severe occlusive carotid disease
- Aortic dissection
- Increased intracranial pressure (more transient, bilateral)
- Takayasu's arteritis
- Hyperviscosity, eg, polycythemia vera, leukemia, Waldenström's macroglobulinemia

Amenorrhea, primary

Etiology

Hypothalamic-pituitary causes (low-normal FSH)
- Idiopathic delayed puberty
- Pituitary tumor
- Hypothalamic amenorrhea, eg, stress, weight change, exercise
- Anorexia nervosa
- Hypothyroidism
- Cushing's syndrome
- GnRH or gonadotropin deficiency, eg, Kallmann syndrome
- Craniopharyngioma

Excess testosterone (low-normal FSH)
- Adrenal tumor or adrenal hyperplasia
- Polycystic ovary syndrome
- Ovarian tumor
- Androgenic steroids

Ovarian causes (high FSH)
- Gonadal dysgenesis, eg, Turner syndrome
- Autoimmune ovarian failure
- Rare ovarian enzyme deficiencies

Pseudohermaphroditism (high LH)
- Testosterone synthesis defect
- Complete androgen resistance (testicular feminization)

Anatomic defect (normal FSH)
- Vaginal agenesis, absent uterus, atrophic endometrium, imperforate hymen

Pregnancy (high hCG)

Amylase increased

Etiology

- Acute pancreatitis, pancreatic pseudocyst, or pancreatic duct obstruction (eg, cholecystitis, choledocholithiasis, pancreatic cancer)
- Intestinal obstruction or infarction
- Mumps (salivary amylase; may cause pancreatitis)
- Parotitis due to other causes, eg, sarcoidosis
- Diabetic ketoacidosis
- Penetrating duodenal ulcer
- Peritonitis
- Ruptured ectopic pregnancy
- Pelvic inflammatory disease
- Abdominal surgery
- Macroamylasemia
- Narcotic administration

Anal fissure

Etiology

- Trauma
- Crohn's disease
- Tuberculosis
- Leukemia

Anemia, general approach

Etiology

Macrocytic (MCV >100)

- Megaloblastic anemia: folic acid or vitamin B_{12} deficiency
- Liver disease (target cells)
- Alcoholism
- Reticulocytosis
- Hypothyroidism
- Myelodysplastic syndrome
- Antiretrovirals, eg, AZT

Microcytic (MCV <80)

- Iron deficiency
- Thalassemia
- Anemia of chronic disease
- Sideroblastic anemia
- Lead poisoning

Normocytic (MCV 80–100)

Low reticulocyte count

- Iron deficiency (especially early)
- Anemia of chronic disease
- Chronic renal disease (low erythropoietin)
- Hypothyroidism, adrenal insufficiency, or hypopituitarism
- Primary bone marrow disorder:
  - Aplastic anemia
  - Malignancy, eg, multiple myeloma, leukemia, metastases
  - Myelofibrosis
  - Myelodysplastic syndrome
  - Infection, eg, parvovirus B19 (causes red cell hypoplasia or aplastic anemia)

High reticulocyte count

- Blood loss
- Hemolysis
  - Coombs positive (immune): autoimmune, drugs, infection, lymphoproliferative disease, Rh or ABO incompatibility
  - Coombs negative
- Intrinsic red cell disease
- Abnormal hemoglobin: sickle cell disease, thalassemia, methemoglobinemia
- Membrane defect: hereditary spherocytosis, hereditary elliptocytosis, paroxysmal nocturnal hemoglobinuria
- Enzyme defect: G6PD deficiency, pyruvate kinase deficiency
- Extrinsic disease
- Microangiopathic hemolytic anemia, eg, thrombotic thrombocytopenic purpura, disseminated intravascular coagulation, prosthetic valve hemolysis
- Splenic sequestration
- Infection: malaria, *Clostridium, Borrelia*
- Burns

Anemia, hemolytic

Etiology

Coombs positive (immune)

- Autoimmune, drugs, infection, lymphoproliferative disease, Rh or ABO incompatibility

Coombs negative

- Intrinsic red cell disease
  - Abnormal hemoglobin: sickle cell disease, thalassemia, methemoglobinemia
  - Membrane defect: hereditary spherocytosis, hereditary elliptocytosis, paroxysmal nocturnal hemoglobinuria
  - Enzyme defect: G6PD deficiency, pyruvate kinase deficiency
- Extrinsic disease
  - Microangiopathic hemolytic anemia: thrombotic thrombocytopenic purpura, hemolytic uremic syndrome, disseminated intravascular coagulation, prosthetic valve hemolysis, metastatic adenocarcinoma, vasculitis, malignant hypertension, HELLP syndrome
  - Splenic sequestration
  - Infection: malaria, *Clostridium, Borrelia*
  - Burns

Anemia, iron deficiency

- Microcytic anemia due to other causes: thalassemia, anemic of chronic disease, sideroblastic anemia, lead poisoning

Etiology

- Blood loss: GI, menstrual, repeated blood donation
- Deficient diet
- Increased requirements: pregnancy, lactation

- Hemoglobinuria, eg, paroxysmal nocturnal hemoglobinuria
- Malabsorption, eg, gastric surgery, celiac disease
- Hemolysis
- Pulmonary hemosiderosis (iron sequestration)

Associated conditions

- Plummer-Vinson syndrome (iron deficiency and esophageal webs)

Anemia, macrocytic

Etiology

- Megaloblastic anemia: folic acid or vitamin B_{12} deficiency
- Liver disease (target cells)
- Alcoholism
- Reticulocytosis
- Hypothyroidism
- Myelodysplastic syndrome
- Antiretrovirals, eg, AZT

Anemia, microcytic

Etiology

- Iron deficiency
- Thalassemia
- Anemic of chronic disease (low-normal MCV)
- Sideroblastic anemia
- Lead poisoning

Anemia, normocytic

Etiology

Low reticulocyte count

- Iron deficiency (especially early)
- Anemia of chronic disease (low-normal MCV)
- Chronic renal disease (low erythropoietin)
- Hypothyroidism, adrenal insufficiency, or hypopituitarism
- Primary bone marrow disorder:
  - Aplastic anemia
  - Malignancy, eg, multiple myeloma, leukemia, metastases
  - Myelofibrosis
  - Myelodysplastic syndrome
  - Infection, eg, parvovirus B19 (causes red cell hypoplasia or aplastic anemia)

High reticulocyte count

- Blood loss
- Hemolysis

- Coombs positive (immune): autoimmune, drugs, infection, lymphoproliferative disease, Rh or ABO incompatibility
- Coombs negative
- Intrinsic red cell disease
- Abnormal hemoglobin: sickle cell disease, thalassemia, methemoglobinemia
- Membrane defect: hereditary spherocytosis, hereditary elliptocytosis, paroxysmal nocturnal hemoglobinuria
- Enzyme defect: G6PD deficiency, pyruvate kinase deficiency
- Extrinsic disease
- Microangiopathic hemolytic anemia, eg, thrombotic thrombocytopenic purpura, disseminated intravascular coagulation, prosthetic valve hemolysis
- Splenic sequestration
- Infection: malaria, *Clostridium*, *Borrelia*
- Burns

Angular cheilitis

- Candidiasis
- Iron deficiency
- Malnutrition
- Glucagonoma

Anion gap, decreased

Etiology

Decreased anion gap & metabolic acidosis

- Plasma cell dyscrasias, eg, multiple myeloma (cationic paraproteins accompanied by chloride and bicarbonate)
- Bromide or lithium intoxication

Decreased anion gap without acidosis

- Hypoalbuminemia (decreased unmeasured anion)
- Severe hyperlipidemia

Ankle pain

- Ankle sprain, eg, anterior talofibular ligament
- Fibular fracture
- Tibial avulsion fracture
- Arthritis, eg, gout, rheumatoid arthritis
- Posterior tibial tendinitis (pain posterior to medial malleolus)
- Peroneal tendonitis (pain at lateral malleolus)

- Arterial insufficiency ulcer with or without osteomyelitis
- Neuropathic arthropathy (Charcot joint)
- Avascular necrosis

Anorectal pain

- Hemorrhoids
- Perianal abscess
- Perianal fistula, eg, Crohn's disease
- Infectious proctitis, eg, gonorrhea, syphilis, chlamydia
- Rectal prolapse or intussusception
- Anal skin tag
- Anal fissure, eg, trauma, Crohn's disease, tuberculosis, leukemia
- Anorectal herpes simplex
- Anogenital warts (condyloma acuminata)
- Primary syphilis (chancre)
- Secondary syphilis (condyloma lata)
- Lymphogranuloma venereum (proctocolitis, perianal ulcer, anorectal strictures or fistulas)
- Pruritus ani
- Anal or rectal cancer
- Proctalgia fugax or levator ani syndrome
- Rectocele
- Solitary rectal ulcer syndrome

Anovulation in reproductive years

- Polycystic ovary syndrome
- Hypothalamic amenorrhea, eg, stress, weight change, exercise
- Obesity
- Hypothyroidism or hyperthyroidism
- Hyperprolactinemia
- Premature ovarian failure
- Discontinuation of oral contraceptives
- Cushing's syndrome
- Congenital adrenal hyperplasia
- Androgen-secreting tumor (adrenal, ovarian)
- Pregnancy

Anticholinergic poisoning

Etiology

- Atropine
- Scopolamine
- Tricyclic antidepressants

- Antihistamines
- Amantadine
- Phenothiazines (hypotension, small pupils)

Anxiety

- Generalized anxiety disorder
- Hyperthyroidism
- Medication or substance abuse, eg, caffeine, nicotine, cocaine, amphetamines, pseudoephedrine
- Medication or substance withdrawal, eg, alcohol, benzodiazepines
- Major depressive disorder
- Adjustment disorder
- Somatoform disorder (eg, somatization)
- Other anxiety disorder, eg, obsessive-compulsive disorder, panic disorder
- Pheochromocytoma

Aortic insufficiency

- Aortic dissection
- Graham Steell murmur (pulmonary insufficiency secondary to pulmonary hypertension)
- Mitral stenosis
- Tricuspid stenosis
- Dock's murmur of stenotic left anterior descending artery

Etiology

- Congenitally bicuspid aortic valve
- Hypertension
- Valvular calcification
- Infective endocarditis
- Rheumatic heart disease
- Aortic root (or arch) disease: Marfan syndrome, aortic dissection, temporal (giant cell) arteritis, Takayasu's arteritis, ankylosing spondylitis, syphilis, Reiter's syndrome (reactive arthritis), cystic medial necrosis, sinus of Valsalva aneurysm, relapsing polychondritis

Aortic stenosis

- Aortic sclerosis
- Mitral regurgitation
- Hypertrophic obstructive cardiomyopathy
- Supravalvular aortic stenosis
- Congenital subvalvular aortic stenosis

Etiology

- Valvular calcification, especially of congenitally bicuspid aortic valve
- Rheumatic heart disease

Arthritis & inflammatory bowel disease

- Reactive arthritis (Reiter's syndrome)
- Ankylosing spondylitis
- Psoriatic arthritis
- Whipple's disease

Arthritis and skin nodules

- Rheumatoid arthritis
- Tophaceous gout
- Sarcoidosis
- Systemic lupus erythematosus
- Palindromic rheumatism
- Rheumatic fever
- Multicentric reticular histiocytosis
- Endocarditis
- Hepatitis B with polyarteritis nodosa
- Coccidioidomycosis

Arthritis, acute, multijoint

- Reactive arthritis (Reiter's syndrome)
- Crystal-induced, eg, gout, pseudo-gout
- Infection, eg, gonococcal arthritis, endocarditis, hepatitis B, parvovirus B19, rubella or post-rubella vaccination
- Connective tissue disease, eg, rheumatoid arthritis, systemic lupus erythematosus, scleroderma, Sjögren's syndrome, adult Still's disease

Arthritis, acute, one joint

Inflammatory
- Infection, eg, *Staphylococcus aureus* septic arthritis, gonococcal arthritis, endocarditis, parvovirus B19
- Crystal-induced, eg, gout, pseudo-gout
- Reactive arthritis (Reiter's syndrome)
- Uncommon: other seronegative spondyloarthropathy, connective tissue disease

Noninflammatory
- Trauma
- Nontraumatic bleed, eg, coagulopathy
- Sickle cell crisis

Arthritis, chronic, multijoint

Inflammatory
- Connective tissue disease, eg, rheumatoid arthritis, systemic lupus erythematosus, scleroderma, Sjögren's syndrome, adult Still's disease
- Seronegative spondyloarthropathy, eg, reactive arthritis (Reiter's syndrome), psoriatic arthritis, ankylosing spondylitis, inflammatory bowel disease
- Crystal-induced, eg, gout, pseudo-gout
- Inflammatory osteoarthritis
- Lyme disease
- Paraneoplastic syndrome (especially in elderly, eg, hypertrophic pulmonary osteoarthropathy)

Noninflammatory
- Osteoarthritis (degenerative joint disease)

Arthritis, chronic, one joint

Noninflammatory
- Osteoarthritis (degenerative joint disease, DJD)
- Hemarthrosis (bleed)
- Sickle cell disease
- Repeated trauma (causing DJD)
- Charcot (neuropathic) joint, eg, diabetes mellitus, syphilis

Inflammatory
- Opportunistic infection, eg, tuberculosis of bone and joints, fungal, sporotrichosis

Arthritis, general

- Osteoarthritis (degenerative joint disease) or inflammatory osteoarthritis
- Connective tissue disease, eg, rheumatoid arthritis, systemic lupus erythematosus, scleroderma, Sjögren's syndrome, adult Still's disease
- Seronegative spondyloarthropathy, eg, reactive arthritis (Reiter's syndrome), psoriatic arthritis, ankylosing spondylitis, inflammatory bowel disease
- Infection, eg, *Staphylococcus aureus* septic arthritis, gonococcal arthritis, endocarditis, hepatitis B or hepatitis C, parvovirus B19, Lyme disease, rubella or post-rubella vaccination
- Crystal-induced, eg, gout, pseudo-gout
- Trauma

- Other joint disease, eg, Charcot (neuropathic) joint, sarcoidosis, tumor, paraneoplastic syndrome (eg, hypertrophic pulmonary osteoarthropathy, leukemia), avascular necrosis, amyloidosis, coagulopathy, sickle cell disease, Henoch-Schönlein purpura, relapsing polychondritis, Behçet's syndrome, Whipple's disease, palindromic rheumatism, ochronosis (alkaptonuria)
- Other non-joint disease, eg, tendonitis, bursitis, polymyalgia rheumatica, reflex sympathetic dystrophy

Arthritis, migratory

- Rheumatic fever
- Palindromic rheumatism
- Gonococcal arthritis
- Lyme disease
- Viral, eg, HIV, hepatitis B, hepatitis C
- Adult Still's disease
- Sarcoidosis
- Henoch-Schönlein purpura
- Relapsing polychondritis
- Whipple's disease

Ascites (common causes)

Etiology

- Cirrhosis (80–85%)
- Malignancy (10%)
- Congestive heart failure (3%)
- Tuberculous peritonitis
- Dialysis-related
- Bile or pancreatic ascites
- Lymphatic tear (chylous ascites)
- Nephrotic syndrome

Ascites (expanded list)

Etiology

Normal peritoneum

Portal hypertension (SAAG* ≥1.1 g/dL)
- Liver disease
  - Cirrhosis (most common)
  - "Mixed ascites" (portal hypertension with secondary process, eg, malignancy, infection)
  - Alcoholic hepatitis
  - Fulminant hepatic failure
  - Massive hepatic metastases
  - Hepatic fibrosis
  - Acute fatty liver of pregnancy

- Hepatic congestion (usually SAAG* ≥1.1 g/dL and ascites total protein >2.5 g/dL)
  - Congestive heart failure, constrictive pericarditis, tricuspid insufficiency
  - Budd-Chiari syndrome, veno-occlusive disease
- Portal vein occlusion

Hypoalbuminemia (SAAG* <1.1 g/dL)
- Nephrotic syndrome
- Protein-losing enteropathy
- Severe malnutrition with anasarca

Miscellaneous conditions (SAAG* <1.1 g/L)
- Chylous ascites
- Pancreatic ascites
- Bile ascites
- Nephrogenic ascites
- Urine ascites
- Myxedema (SAAG* ≥1.1 g/dL)
- Ovarian disease

Diseased peritoneum (SAAG* <1.1 g/dL except in "mixed ascites" with portal hypertension and secondary process, eg, infection, malignancy)

Infections
- Bacterial peritonitis
- Tuberculous peritonitis
- Fungal peritonitis
- HIV-associated peritonitis

Malignant conditions
- Peritoneal carcinomatosis
- Primary mesothelioma
- Pseudomyxoma peritonei
- Massive hepatic metastases
- Hepatocellular carcinoma

Other conditions
- Familial Mediterranean fever
- Vasculitis
- Granulomatous peritonitis
- Eosinophilic peritonitis

SAAG = serum-ascites albumin gradient

Ascites, chylous

Etiology

- Lymphatic obstruction, eg, lymphoma
- Postoperative trauma
- Cirrhosis
- Tuberculosis
- Pancreatitis
- Filariasis

Ascites, malignant

Etiology

- Peritoneal carcinomatosis: adenocarcinoma of ovary, uterus, pancreas, stomach, colon, lung, breast
- Hepatocellular carcinoma causing lymphatic obstruction or portal hypertension
- Diffuse hepatic metastases

Aspirated foreign body

- Asthma with mucus plugging
- Bronchiolitis
- Ludwig's angina
- Epiglottitis
- Laryngospasm, eg, anaphylaxis
- Lung cancer
- Substernal goiter
- Tracheal cystadenoma

Aspiration of gastric contents, chronic

Etiology

- Achalasia
- Esophageal stricture
- Scleroderma
- Esophageal carcinoma
- Esophagitis
- Gastroesophageal reflux disease
- Disorders of the larynx

Asplenia and infection risk

Etiology

- Encapsulated organisms: *Streptococcus pneumoniae, Haemophilus influenzae, Neisseria meningitidis*
- *Capnocytophaga canimorsus* (dog bites)
- Intraerythrocytic parasites, eg, malaria, babesiosis
- Others: *Salmonella typhi, Klebsiella*, herpes zoster, group B streptococci, enterococcus, *Bacteroides*

AST/ALT increased

Etiology

- Acute viral hepatitis (ALT > AST)
- Toxic hepatitis, eg, acetaminophen
- Alcoholic hepatitis (AST < ALT)
- Cirrhosis (AST > ALT)

- Vascular: right-sided congestive heart failure, shock liver, Budd-Chiari syndrome
- Biliary tract obstruction (followed by increased alkaline phosphatase and bilirubin)
- Nonalcoholic fatty liver disease (formerly NASH)
- Metabolic, eg, hemochromatosis, Wilson's disease
- Liver abscess
- Hepatocellular or metastatic cancer
- Drugs, eg, INH, statins
- Heart or skeletal muscle injury
- Celiac sprue (ALT)

AST/ALT 500–1000
- Acetaminophen, *Amanita* mushroom, other toxins
- Viral, especially hepatitis A
- Shock liver (ischemia)
- Budd-Chiari syndrome
- Right-sided heart failure

Ataxia

Etiology

- Intoxication, eg, alcohol, phenytoin
- Cerebellar infarct, mass, or hemorrhage
- Cerebellar degeneration, eg, alcoholism
- Parkinsonism
- Vascular (multi-infarct) dementia
- Multiple sclerosis
- Wernicke's encephalopathy
- Hydrocephalus
- Metabolic: hyponatremia, hypothyroidism, vitamin B_{12} deficiency
- Paraneoplastic syndrome, eg, breast, ovarian
- Progressive multifocal leukoencephalopathy in AIDS
- Lyme disease
- Neurosyphilis
- Inherited ataxia, eg, Friedreich's

Atrial fibrillation

- Frequent premature atrial contractions
- Atrial flutter (especially if variable block)
- Multifocal atrial tachycardia
- Sinus tachycardia
- Sinus arrhythmia
- Atrial tachycardia
- Supraventricular tachycardia
- Ventricular tachycardia

Etiology

- Rheumatic heart disease
- Dilated cardiomyopathy
- Pulmonary disease, eg, chronic obstructive pulmonary disease, pulmonary embolism
- Mitral stenosis
- Mitral regurgitation
- Mitral valve prolapse
- Coronary artery disease
- Atrial septal defect
- Atrial myxoma
- Hypertension
- Hypertrophic obstructive cardiomyopathy
- Thyrotoxicosis (hyperthyroidism)
- Pericarditis
- Chest trauma or chest surgery
- Medications: theophylline, beta-agonists
- Alcohol withdrawal
- Sepsis

Atrial flutter

- Sinus tachycardia
- Supraventricular tachycardia
- Atrial tachycardia
- Junctional tachycardia
- Atrial fibrillation

Etiology

- Chronic obstructive pulmonary disease
- Rheumatic heart disease
- Coronary artery disease
- Congestive heart failure
- Atrial septal defect

Atrial myxoma

- Infective endocarditis
- Systemic lupus erythematosus (with Libman-Sacks endocarditis)
- Lymphoma
- Mitral stenosis
- Cor triatriatum (congenital atrial anomaly)

Atrioventricular block (first, second, or third degree)

Etiology

- Increased vagal tone (first degree or Mobitz type I)

- Drugs: digitalis, calcium channel blockers, beta blockers, clonidine, other sympatholytics, amiodarone, other antiarrhythmics
- Age-related conduction system fibrosis or calcification (Lev's disease)
- Cardiac infiltrative disease (eg, amyloid, sarcoidosis, hemochromatosis)
- Myocardial ischemia or myocardial infarction
- Myocarditis
- Chagas' disease

Auricle diseases

- Skin cancer
- Traumatic auricular hematoma
- Cauliflower ear (cartilage dissolution post-trauma)
- Cellulitis
- Chondritis or perichondritis
- Relapsing polychondritis
- Chondrodermatitis nodularis helicis
- Cutaneous leishmaniasis

Autonomic insufficiency

Etiology

- Diabetes
- Adrenal insufficiency
- Spinal cord lesion
- Guillain-Barré syndrome
- Parkinsonism
- Chronic idiopathic orthostatic hypotension
- Shy-Drager syndrome (multiple system atrophy)

Bacteremia & sepsis

- Other types of shock: cardiogenic, hypovolemic, neurogenic, anaphylactic
- Toxic shock syndrome

Etiology

- Genitourinary system
- Hepatobiliary tract
- GI tract
- Lungs
- Indwelling catheter
- Surgical wound
- Decubitus ulcer

Belching

- Normal belching: air ingestion from rapid eating, carbonated beverages, gum chewing, smoking
- Excessive belching: aerophagia (air swallowing, often subconscious)

Bitemporal hemianopsia

- Pituitary tumor
- Craniopharyngioma
- Meningioma
- Aneurysm of circle of Willis
- Sarcoidosis
- Metastatic carcinoma

Bleeding, general approach

Etiology

Defect in platelet number or function (gum bleeding, petechiae, bruising)

- Thrombocytopenia, eg, idiopathic and thrombotic thrombocytopenic purpura, leukemia
- Acquired disorder, eg, aspirin-induced platelet dysfunction, uremia, myeloproliferative disorder, autoantibody
- Hereditary disorder, eg, von Willebrand's disease, Glanzmann's thrombasthenia

Defect in coagulation (skin and deep muscle bleeding)

- Acquired disorder, eg, liver disease, vitamin K deficiency, anticoagulants, disseminated intravascular coagulation, factor VIII antibodies
- Hereditary disorder, eg, hemophilia A

Blistering diseases (bullae)

- Pemphigus
- Bullous pemphigoid
- Drug eruption
- Erythema multiforme major or toxic epidermal necrolysis
- Bullous impetigo
- Contact dermatitis
- Dermatitis herpetiformis
- Cicatricial pemphigoid
- Paraneoplastic pemphigus
- Linear IgA dermatosis
- Pemphigus foliaceus
- Porphyria cutanea tarda
- Epidermolysis bullosa
- Staphylococcal scalded skin syndrome
- Herpes gestationis
- Graft-versus-host disease

- Disseminated *Vibrio vulnificus* (cirrhosis, seafood or seawater exposure)
- Ecthyma gangrenosum (neutropenic, pseudomonal)

Bone pain & pathologic fractures

- Osteoporosis (fracture)
- Malignancy, primary or metastatic (fracture)
- Hyperparathyroidism (bone pain)
- Hyperthyroidism (osteopenia)
- Cushing's syndrome (osteopenia)
- Osteogenesis imperfecta (fracture)
- Osteomalacia or rickets (bowing and pseudofractures)
- Multiple myeloma (bone pain, fracture)
- Paget's disease (bone pain)
- Leukemia (bone pain)
- Gaucher disease (fracture)
- Beta thalassemia (fracture)

Bone tumors

- Metastatic cancer
- Osteomyelitis
- Posttraumatic lesion
- Metabolic bone disease, eg, Paget's disease, hyperparathyroidism, osteoporosis
- Arthritis

Types
- Benign: osteoid osteoma, osteoblastoma, enchondroma, osteochondroma, chondroblastoma, chondromyxoid fibroma, giant cell tumor, hemangioma
- Malignant: multiple myeloma, osteosarcoma, chondrosarcoma, Ewing's sarcoma, malignant fibrous histiocytoma

Bradycardia

- Medications (eg, calcium channel blockers, beta blockers, digitalis, clonidine, other sympatholytics, amiodarone, other antiarrhythmics)
- Normal (especially athletes)
- Sick sinus syndrome
- Vasovagal response
- Atrioventricular block
- Hypothermia
- Hypothyroidism
- Myocardial ischemia involving right coronary artery
- Increased intracranial pressure (Cushing's reflex)

- Cardiac infiltrative disease (eg, amyloid, sarcoidosis, hemochromatosis)

Bradycardia, relative

- Typhoid fever (enteric fever)
- Legionnaire's disease
- Brucellosis
- Leptospirosis
- Psittacosis
- Q fever
- Viral hemorrhagic fever, eg, yellow fever
- Infections affecting cardiac conduction: acute rheumatic fever, viral myocarditis, Lyme disease, endocarditis
- Noninfectious causes: intrinsic cardiac conduction disease, beta blockers, calcium channel blockers, drug fever, neoplasm (eg, lymphoma), factitious fever, CNS lesion

Brain mass in HIV/AIDS

- Toxoplasmosis
- CNS lymphoma
- Bacterial brain abscess
- Fungal brain abscess, eg, *Aspergillus, Histoplasma*
- Cryptococcoma
- *Nocardia* brain abscess
- Tuberculoma
- Other primary or metastatic tumor

Brain tumors (brain mass)

- Primary brain tumor, eg, glioblastoma multiforme, meningioma, pituitary adenoma, neurofibroma, lymphoma
- Metastases, eg, lung, breast, renal, gastrointestinal, melanoma, lymphoma
- Brain abscess
- Cerebral infarction or intracerebral hemorrhage
- Subdural hematoma
- Multiple sclerosis
- Cryptococcoma
- Neurocysticercosis
- Tuberculoma

Breast lump or mass

- Fibrocystic breast disease or cyst
- Breast fibroadenoma
- Breast cancer
- Intraductal papilloma
- Lipoma
- Breast abscess (mastitis)

- Fat necrosis
- Phyllodes tumor

Breast pain

- Premenstrual syndrome or cyclic mastalgia
- Fibrocystic breast disease or cyst
- Pregnancy
- Breast-feeding
- Breast abscess (mastitis)
- Onset of menopause
- Breast cancer
- Breast fibroadenoma
- Trauma
- Estrogen replacement therapy
- Breast augmentation disorder (implants)
- Shingles
- Gynecomastia (men)

Bronchiectasis

- Chronic obstructive pulmonary disease
- Asthma
- Bronchiolitis
- Allergic bronchopulmonary aspergillosis

Etiology

- Cystic fibrosis
- Infection: tuberculosis, fungal, lung abscess, pneumonia, parasites
- Localized airway obstruction: retained foreign body, tumor, mucoid impaction
- Abnormal lung defense mechanisms
  – Hypogammaglobulinemia
  – Common variable immunodeficiency
  – Selective IgA, IgM, and IgG subclass deficiency
  – Acquired immunodeficiency from cytotoxic drugs, AIDS, lymphoma, leukemia, multiple myeloma, chronic renal disease, chronic liver disease
  – Alpha-1-antiprotease deficiency with cigarette smoking
  – Mucociliary clearance disorders (immotile cilia syndrome)
  – Rheumatic disease, eg, rheumatoid arthritis

Bruit

- Carotid stenosis (cervical bruit)
- Temporal (giant cell) arteritis (near clavicle)

- Renal artery bruit (epigastric)
- Peripheral vascular disease (femoral bruit)
- Abdominal aortic aneurysm
- Thoracic aortic aneurysm
- Takayasu's arteritis or "pulseless disease" (various bruits)

Budd-Chiari syndrome (hepatic vein obstruction)

- Cholecystitis
- Shock liver
- Cirrhosis
- Hepatic congestion from right-sided congestive heart failure
- Metastatic cancer involving the liver

Etiology

- Caval webs
- Myeloproliferative disease, eg, polycythemia vera
- Right-sided congestive heart failure or constrictive pericarditis
- Neoplasm compressing hepatic vein
- Paroxysmal nocturnal hemoglobinuria
- Behçet's syndrome
- Oral contraceptives or pregnancy
- Hypercoagulable state
- Post bone-marrow transplant
- "Bush teas" (pyrrolizidine alkaloids)

BUN increased with normal GFR

Etiology

- Prerenal azotemia
- Catabolic states
- High-protein diets
- Gastrointestinal bleeding
- Glucocorticoids
- Tetracycline

Café au lait spots

- Idiopathic
- Neurofibromatosis
- McCune-Albright syndrome

Calf pain

- Muscular strain
- Baker's (popliteal) cyst
- Deep vein thrombosis
- Claudication (arterial insufficiency)

- Superficial thrombophlebitis
- Varicose veins
- Achilles tendon rupture
- Myositis, eg, polymyositis, dermatomyositis
- Vasculitis, eg, polyarteritis nodosa, thromboangiitis obliterans (Buerger's disease)
- Spinal stenosis (pseudoclaudication; usually back and thigh pain)

Cancer of unknown primary

- Poorly differentiated: lymphoma, germ cell tumor, melanoma, neuroendocrine, prostate
- Adenocarcinoma: breast, prostate, pancreatic, hepatobiliary, lung, colorectal, ovarian
- Squamous cell (depending on location of adenopathy): head and neck, genital, anorectal, cervical, lung
- Others: melanoma, sarcoma, thyroid

Cardiac tamponade

- Tension pneumothorax
- Restrictive cardiomyopathy
- Constrictive pericarditis
- Right ventricular infarction
- Left ventricular failure

Etiology

- Malignancy
- Hemopericardium, eg, aortic dissection, iatrogenic cardiac perforation
- Uremia
- Less common: infection (viral, bacterial, tuberculous), radiation, myxedema, Dressler's syndrome, systemic lupus erythematosus

Cardiac tumors

Metastases (*most common*)

- Bronchogenic carcinoma
- Breast cancer
- Melanoma
- Lymphoma
- Renal cell carcinoma
- Kaposi's sarcoma (in AIDS)

Primary cardiac tumors

- Atrial myxoma (most common primary tumor)
- Rhabdomyoma
- Fibrous histiocytoma

- Hemangioma
- Sarcoma

Cardiomyopathy, primary dilated

- Hypertrophic obstructive cardiomyopathy
- Restrictive cardiomyopathy

Etiology

- Idiopathic
- Alcoholic
- Viral myocarditis
- Postpartum
- Cocaine
- Endocrinopathies: hyperthyroidism, acromegaly, pheochromocytoma
- Amyloidosis
- Sarcoidosis
- Hemochromatosis
- Diabetes mellitus
- Doxorubicin
- Genetic

Cardiomyopathy, restrictive

- Constrictive pericarditis
- Hypertrophic obstructive cardiomyopathy
- Hypertensive heart disease
- Ischemic heart disease
- Dilated cardiomyopathy

Etiology

- Amyloidosis
- Radiation-induced
- Fibrosis after open-heart surgery
- Sarcoidosis
- Hemochromatosis
- Carcinoid
- Scleroderma
- Diabetes mellitus
- Endomyocardial fibrosis

Carotid pulse, bisferiens

- Hypertrophic obstructive cardiomyopathy
- Mixed aortic stenosis and aortic insufficiency

Carotid upstroke, delayed

- Aortic stenosis

Cataract

- Corneal opacity, eg, scar, pterygium
- Refractive error
- Macular degeneration (atrophic)
- Diabetic retinopathy
- Glaucoma
- Anterior ischemic optic neuropathy, eg, temporal (giant cell) arteritis

Etiology

- Senile cataract
- Congenital, eg, rubella, cytomegalovirus, galactosemia
- Trauma
- Systemic disease, eg, diabetes mellitus, atopic dermatitis, myotonic dystrophy
- Corticosteroids (topical or systemic)
- Uveitis

Catatonia or stiffness

Severe stiffness or catatonia

- Catatonic schizophrenia
- Parkinson's disease
- Catatonic syndrome due to other CNS causes, eg, viral encephalitis, CNS bleed
- Neuroleptic-induced catatonia
- Seizure or status epilepticus
- Neuroleptic malignant syndrome
- Malignant hyperthermia
- Tetany, eg, hypocalcemia (usually distal muscles)
- Dystonic reaction to neuroleptics, eg, torticollis
- Huntington's disease
- Tetanus
- Strychnine poisoning
- Lethal catatonia
- Stiff-person syndrome
- Meningitis (stiff neck)

Mild stiffness

- Arthritis, eg, osteoarthritis, rheumatoid arthritis, pseudogout
- Early parkinsonism
- Fibromyalgia
- Polymyalgia rheumatica

Cervical (cervix) lesions

- Cervical polyp
- Nabothian cyst
- Cervical cancer or cervical intraepithelial neoplasia
- Cervical ectropion

- Cervical ectopy (columnar epithelium on face of os, common in adolescence)
- Cervicitis, eg, chlamydia, gonorrhea, herpes simplex virus, *Trichomonas* infection (severe)
- Genital warts (condyloma acuminata)
- Cervical ulcer: herpes simplex virus, syphilis, chancroid
- Granuloma inguinale
- Leiomyomas
- Endometriosis
- Deformity or hypoplasia due to DES exposure in utero

Cervical discharge

- Chlamydia
- Gonorrhea
- Herpes simplex virus
- *Trichomonas* infection (severe)
- Pelvic inflammatory disease
- Cervical polyp
- Cervical cancer
- Uterine cancer
- Reaction to douches, tampons, diaphragm

Cervical lymphadenopathy

- Upper respiratory tract infection
- Bacterial infection of upper extremities
- Metastasis from squamous cell carcinoma in mouth, pharynx, larynx, upper esophagus
- Lymphoma
- Tuberculous lymphadenitis (scrofula)
- Cat-scratch disease
- Sarcoidosis
- Lyme disease
- Toxoplasmosis
- Autoimmune adenopathy
- Kikuchi's disease (histiocytic necrotizing lymphadenitis)
- Tularemia
- Actinomycosis (cervicofacial)
- Drug-induced pseudolymphoma (classically phenytoin)

Cervicitis

Etiology

- Chlamydia
- Gonorrhea
- Herpes simplex virus
- *Trichomonas* infection (severe)
- Pelvic inflammatory disease

- Cervical inflammation due to vaginitis
- Cervical ectropion
- Cervical ectopy (columnar epithelium on face of os, common in adolescence)
- Cervical cancer
- Reaction to douches, tampons, diaphragm

Chest pain

Do not miss

- Myocardial ischemia, pericarditis, aortic dissection, pulmonary embolism, tension pneumothorax, esophageal rupture

Cardiovascular

- Myocardial ischemia (angina, myocardial infarction), pericarditis, aortic stenosis, aortic dissection, pulmonary embolism, cardiomyopathy, myocarditis, mitral valve prolapse, pulmonary hypertension, hypertrophic obstructive cardiomyopathy, carditis (eg, acute rheumatic fever), aortic insufficiency, right ventricular hypertrophy

Pulmonary

- Pneumonia, pleuritis, bronchitis, pneumothorax, tumor

Gastrointestinal

- Esophageal rupture, gastroesophageal reflux disease, esophageal spasm, Mallory-Weiss syndrome, peptic ulcer disease, biliary disease, pancreatitis, functional gastrointestinal pain

Musculoskeletal

- Cervical or thoracic disk disease or arthritis, shoulder arthritis, costochondritis (anterior chest wall syndrome or Tietze's syndrome), subacromial bursitis

Other

- Anxiety or panic attack, herpes zoster, breast disorders, chest wall tumors, thoracic outlet syndrome, mediastinitis

Chest pain, pleuritic

- Pneumonia
- Upper respiratory tract infection
- Rib fracture
- Pulmonary embolism
- Pneumothorax
- Pericarditis
- Aspiration pneumonia
- Myocarditis
- Mesothelioma
- Pleurodynia (coxsackievirus)

Cheyne-Stokes respiration

- Neurologic disease (coma, stroke, hemorrhage, tumor, meningitis)
- Severe congestive heart failure
- Hypoxia
- Normal at high altitude (especially during sleep)

Cholestasis

Etiology

Extrahepatic causes

- Choledocholithiasis or cholangitis
- Pancreatic tumor
- Biliary stricture
- Primary sclerosing cholangitis (intra- and extrahepatic)
- Carcinoma of the bile ducts
- Compression of common duct by metastatic cancer
- Gallbladder cancer extending to common duct
- Choledochal cyst
- Sepsis
- Parasites, eg, *Ascaris, Clonorchis, Fasciola hepatica,* hydatid disease

Intrahepatic causes

- Primary biliary cirrhosis
- Infiltrative disease, eg, tuberculosis, sarcoidosis, lymphoma, amyloidosis
- Drug-induced cholestasis, eg, chlorpromazine, estrogen
- Autoimmune cholangitis (like PBC but AMA negative)
- Idiopathic adulthood ductopenia

Cholesterol decreased

Etiology

- Malnutrition
- Malignancy or chronic infection, eg, AIDS
- Malabsorption
- Hyperthyroidism
- Cirrhosis

Cholesterol increased

Etiology

- Idiopathic
- Hypothyroidism
- Nephrotic syndrome
- Chronic renal insufficiency
- Obstructive liver disease
- Diabetes mellitus
- Anorexia nervosa
- Cushing's syndrome
- Familial, eg, familial hypercholesterolemia
- Drugs: oral contraceptives, thiazides (short-term effect), beta blockers (short-term effect), corticosteroids, cyclosporine

Cholinergic poisoning

Etiology

- Carbamate insecticide, eg, neostigmine, physostigmine
- Nicotine
- Organophosphates
- Poisonous mushrooms

Chorea

Etiology

- Huntington's disease
- Wilson's disease
- Sydenham's chorea
- Senile chorea
- Benign hereditary chorea
- Drugs, eg, antipsychotics, levodopa, anticholinergics, phenytoin, carbamazepine, lithium, amphetamines, oral contraceptives, bromocriptine

Cirrhosis

- Edema or ascites due to other causes, eg, congestive heart failure, nephrotic syndrome, myxedema
- Hepatomegaly due to other causes, eg, hepatitis, hepatocellular carcinoma
- Encephalopathy due to other causes, eg, uremia, thiamine deficiency
- Upper GI bleeding due to other causes, eg, peptic ulcer disease, Mallory-Weiss syndrome
- Noncirrhotic causes of portal hypertension, eg, portal or splenic vein thrombosis, schistosomiasis

Etiology

- Chronic hepatitis C or hepatitis B
- Alcoholism
- Nonalcoholic fatty liver disease
- Cryptogenic
- Metabolic, eg, hemochromatosis, Wilson's disease, alpha-1 antiprotease deficiency
- Primary biliary cirrhosis
- Secondary biliary cirrhosis (chronic obstruction due to stone, stricture, neoplasm)
- Congestive heart failure or constrictive pericarditis ("cardiac cirrhosis")
- Other: Budd-Chiari syndrome, cystic fibrosis, autoimmune hepatitis, *Clonorchis sinensis* infection, glycogen storage disease

Claudication, lower extremity

- Peripheral arterial disease
- Musculoskeletal pain
- Lumbar spinal stenosis (neurogenic or pseudoclaudication)
- Deep vein thrombosis
- Lumbar disk disease
- Peripheral neuropathy
- Nocturnal leg cramps
- Arterial embolism
- Thromboangiitis obliterans (Buerger's disease)
- Polyarteritis nodosa
- Unilateral claudication in young, athletic person: popliteal artery entrapment, trauma, compression by Baker's cyst, popliteal adventitial cystic disease

Claudication, upper extremity

- Thoracic outlet syndrome
- Takayasu's arteritis ("pulseless disease")
- Thromboangiitis obliterans (Buerger's disease)
- Hand-arm vibration syndrome or hypothenar hammer (jackhammer) syndrome

Clubbed digits

Etiology

- Chronic lung infection, eg, bronchiectasis, cystic fibrosis, lung abscess, tuberculosis, empyema
- Malignancy of lung or pleura, eg, hypertrophic pulmonary osteoarthropathy with bronchogenic carcinoma
- Chronic interstitial lung disease, eg, idiopathic pulmonary fibrosis
- Pulmonary atrioventricular malformations
- Cyanotic congenital heart disease
- Infective endocarditis
- Cirrhosis
- Inflammatory bowel disease
- Congenital or idiopathic

Coma

Etiology

Intracranial causes

- Anoxic brain injury or head trauma
- Ischemic stroke or intracerebral hemorrhage
- Subarachnoid hemorrhage
- Meningitis or encephalitis
- Brainstem hemorrhage, infarct, or mass
- Mass lesion causing brainstem compression
- Subdural hematoma
- Seizure

Metabolic causes

- Hypoglycemia
- Diabetic ketoacidosis
- Hyperglycemic hyperosmolar state
- Drugs, eg, alcohol, opioids, sedatives, antidepressants, salicylates
- Uremic or hepatic encephalopathy
- Hypernatremia or hyponatremia
- Hypercalcemia
- Hypothermia
- Heat stroke
- Myxedema
- Carbon monoxide poisoning

Congestive heart failure

- Chronic obstructive pulmonary disease
- Pneumonia
- Cirrhosis
- Peripheral venous insufficiency
- Nephrotic syndrome
- Myxedema (hypothyroidism)

Etiology

Left ventricular failure

- Ischemic cardiomyopathy (eg, myocardial infarction)
- Hypertension
- Cardiomyopathy (eg, idiopathic, alcoholic)
- Valvular disease (eg, aortic stenosis, aortic insufficiency, mitral regurgitation)
- Volume overload including thiazolidinediones, eg, rosiglitazone
- Arrhythmia, eg, atrial fibrillation
- High-output states
- Chagas' disease

Right ventricular failure

- Usually left ventricular failure (left-sided congestive heart failure)
- Cor pulmonale (right heart failure due to pulmonary disease)
- Chronic pulmonary embolism
- Right-sided valve disease

Diastolic dysfunction

- Left ventricular hypertrophy
- Hypertension
- Hypertrophic obstructive cardiomyopathy
- Restrictive cardiomyopathy
- Diabetes

High output heart failure

- Hyperthyroidism
- Severe anemia
- Arteriovenous shunting
- Paget's disease of the bone
- Beriberi
- Hepatic hemangiomatosis
- Sepsis
- Carcinoid

Congestive heart failure, right-sided

- Congestive heart failure, left-sided
- Cirrhosis
- Peripheral venous insufficiency
- Nephrotic syndrome

Etiology

- Usually left ventricular failure (left-sided congestive heart failure)
- Cor pulmonale (right heart failure due to pulmonary disease)
- Chronic pulmonary embolism
- Right-sided valve disease

Conjunctivitis

- Uveitis
- Acute glaucoma
- Foreign body or corneal abrasion
- Keratitis (corneal ulcer or inflammation), eg, herpes simplex
- Scleritis or episcleritis
- Dacryocystitis (lacrimal sac infection)

Etiology

- Viral infection, eg, adenovirus
- Bacterial infection, eg, *Staphylococcus, Streptococcus, Haemophilus, Pseudomonas, Moraxella, Chlamydia,* gonococci

- Allergic conjunctivitis
- Reactive arthritis (Reiter's syndrome)
- Keratoconjunctivitis sicca (dry eyes)
- Chemical irritants
- Systemic disease, eg, measles, Kawasaki syndrome, epidemic or scrub typhus, trichinosis

Constipation

Most common

- Inadequate fiber or fluid intake
- Poor bowel habits

Systemic disease

- Endocrine: hypothyroidism, hyperparathyroidism, diabetes mellitus
- Metabolic: hypercalcemia, hypokalemia, uremia, porphyria
- Neurologic: Parkinson's disease, multiple sclerosis, sacral nerve damage (pelvic surgery, tumor), paraplegia, autonomic neuropathy
- Rheumatologic: scleroderma, amyloidosis
- Medications: narcotics, diuretics, calcium channel blockers, anticholinergics, psychotropics, calcium, iron, NSAIDs, clonidine, sucralfate, cholestyramine
- Infectious: typhoid fever

Structural abnormalities

- Anorectal: rectal prolapse, rectocele, rectal intussusception, anorectal stricture, anal fissure, solitary rectal ulcer syndrome
- Pelvic floor dysfunction, eg, hysterectomy
- Obstructing colonic mass, eg, cancer
- Colonic stricture: radiation, ischemia, diverticulosis
- Hirschsprung's disease
- Chagas' disease
- Idiopathic megarectum

Slow colonic transit

- Idiopathic: isolated to colon
- Psychogenic
- Eating disorders
- Chronic intestinal pseudo-obstruction

Other

- Irritable bowel syndrome

Constricted pupil

- Opioids (pinpoint)
- Other causes of sympatholytic poisoning, eg, benzodiazepines, clonidine
- Horner's syndrome
- Myotic drugs, eg, pilocarpine

- Neurosyphilis (Argyll Robertson pupils)
- Pontine infarct
- Uveitis
- Inflammatory adhesions between iris and lens (posterior synechiae)
- Cholinergic poisoning, eg, organophosphates
- Physiologic anisocoria (unequal pupils, react normally)

Cough, acute

- Viral upper respiratory infection or postviral cough (most common)
- Bacterial upper respiratory infection
- Postnasal drip (allergic rhinitis)
- Pneumonia
- Pulmonary edema, eg, congestive heart failure
- Pulmonary embolism
- Aspiration pneumonia

Cough, chronic

- Top 3 causes: postnasal drip, asthma, gastroesophageal reflux disease

Pulmonary infection
- Postviral
- Bronchitis, especially in smokers
- Bronchiectasis
- Tuberculosis
- Cystic fibrosis
- *Mycobacterium avium* complex
- Pertussis
- *Mycoplasma*
- Chlamydia
- Respiratory syncytial virus
- Parasites, eg, ascariasis, paragonimiasis

Pulmonary noninfectious
- Asthma (cough-variant asthma)
- Beta blockers causing asthma
- Chronic obstructive pulmonary disease
- ACE inhibitors
- Irritant inhalation, eg, smoking
- Endobronchial lesion, eg, tumor
- Interstitial lung disease
- Sarcoidosis
- Chronic microaspiration

Nonpulmonary
- Gastroesophageal reflux disease
- Postnasal drip (allergic rhinitis)
- Sinusitis
- Congestive heart failure
- Laryngitis

- Ear canal or tympanic membrane irritation
- Psychogenic or habit cough

Cranial nerve 3 palsy

Etiology

- Microvascular infarction, eg, diabetes mellitus, hypertension
- Sarcoidosis
- Space-occupying lesion, especially posterior inferior cerebellar artery aneurysm
- Ophthalmoplegic migraine
- Brainstem infarct or vertebrobasilar insufficiency
- Temporal (giant cell) arteritis
- Uncal herniation

Cranial nerve 6 palsy

Etiology

- Microvascular infarction, eg, diabetes mellitus, hypertension
- Wernicke's encephalopathy
- Increased intracranial pressure, eg, pseudotumor cerebri
- Tuberculous meningitis
- Sphenoid sinusitis
- Cavernous sinus thrombosis
- Brainstem infarct or vertebrobasilar insufficiency
- Multiple sclerosis
- Temporal (giant cell) arteritis

Cranial nerve palsy

Etiology

- Microvascular infarction, eg, diabetes mellitus, hypertension
- Multiple sclerosis
- Acute or chronic otitis media
- Malignant otitis externa
- Infiltrating process at skull base: meningitis, sarcoidosis, intracranial metastases, lymphoma, nasopharyngeal cancer
- Brainstem infarct or vertebrobasilar insufficiency
- Arterial dissection, eg, internal carotid, vertebral
- Compression by aneurysm or tumor
- Neurosyphilis
- Systemic lupus erythematosus
- Neurofibromatosis
- Paget's disease

- Myasthenia gravis
- Guillain-Barré syndrome
- Diphtheria
- Glomus jugulare (middle ear tumor)
- Pituitary apoplexy
- Graves' ophthalmopathy (not a palsy, but affects extraocular movements)

Cyanosis

- Hypoxia, eg, pneumonia, pulmonary embolism, congestive heart failure, valvular heart disease, hypotension, shunt, severe anemia, high altitude
- Cold exposure
- Raynaud's syndrome
- Reflex sympathetic dystrophy
- Methemoglobinemia
- Thoracic outlet syndrome
- Polyarteritis nodosa

Decubitus ulcers

- Herpes simplex
- Skin cancer
- Pyoderma gangrenosum
- Ecthyma gangrenosum (neutropenic, pseudomonal)

Dementia

- Delirium
- Depression (pseudodementia)
- Vision or hearing impairment

Etiology

Reversible causes
- Hypothyroidism or hyperthyroidism
- Depression
- Drugs, eg, anticholinergics, sedatives, antipsychotics, opioids
- Vitamin B_{12} or thiamine deficiency
- Hypercalcemia
- Uremic or hepatic encephalopathy
- Space-occupying lesion, eg, brain tumor, subdural hematoma
- Neurosyphilis
- HIV
- Normal pressure hydrocephalus
- Wilson's disease
- Sleep apnea
- Chronic meningitis

Irreversible causes
- Alzheimer's disease
- Vascular (multi-infarct) dementia

- Parkinson's disease
- Dementia with Lewy bodies
- Huntington's disease
- Frontotemporal dementia, eg, Pick's disease
- Progressive supranuclear palsy
- Creutzfeldt-Jakob disease

Depression

- Normal grief response
- Bipolar disorder
- Alcohol, sedative, or opiate abuse
- Stimulant withdrawal, eg, cocaine, amphetamines
- Anxiety disorder, eg, generalized anxiety disorder, post-traumatic stress disorder
- Domestic violence
- Hypothyroidism
- Dementia, parkinsonism, or stroke
- Other chronic medical illness, eg, anemia, chronic infection, renal failure
- Drug-induced, eg, reserpine, corticosteroids, oral contraceptives, clonidine, levodopa
- Personality disorder, eg, borderline

Types
- Adjustment disorder with depressed mood
- Major depressive disorder
- Dysthymia (some depressive symptoms for >2 years)
- Seasonal affective disorder
- Postpartum depression
- Premenstrual dysphoric disorder

Dermatitis, exfoliative (exfoliative erythroderma)

- Psoriasis
- Seborrheic dermatitis
- Drug eruption
- Toxic shock syndrome (staphylococcal or streptococcal)
- Scarlet fever
- Staphylococcal scalded skin syndrome
- Erythema multiforme major or toxic epidermal necrolysis

Etiology
- Idiopathic
- Drug eruption
- Seborrheic dermatitis
- Contact dermatitis
- Atopic dermatitis
- Psoriasis

- Cancer (Sézary syndrome of cutaneous T cell lymphoma, Hodgkin's disease)
- Pityriasis rubra pilaris

Desquamative erythema

- Toxic shock syndrome (staphylococcal or streptococcal)
- Scarlet fever
- Kawasaki syndrome
- Staphylococcal scalded skin syndrome
- Exfoliative erythroderma syndrome (eg, underlying psoriasis, eczema, drug eruption)
- Erythema multiforme major or toxic epidermal necrolysis

Diarrhea in diabetes

- Sorbitol in dietetic foods
- Celiac sprue
- Pancreatic insufficiency
- Bacterial overgrowth
- Visceral autonomic neuropathy

Diarrhea in HIV/AIDS

- Viral: cytomegalovirus, adenovirus, HIV (AIDS enteropathy)
- Bacterial: *Campylobacter, Salmonella, Shigella, Clostridium difficile, Mycobacterium avium* complex, tuberculosis
- Protozoal: *Cryptosporidium, Entamoeba histolytica, Giardia, Isospora,* microsporidia
- HIV-associated malabsorption

Diarrhea, acute

Infectious: noninflammatory (nonbloody)
- Viruses: Norwalk virus, rotavirus, adenoviruses, astrovirus, coronavirus
- Preformed toxin (food poisoning): *Staphylococcus aureus, Bacillus cereus, Clostridium perfringens*
- Toxin production: enterotoxigenic *Escherichia coli, Vibrio cholerae, Vibrio parahaemolyticus*
- Protozoa: *Giardia lamblia, Cryptosporidium, Cyclospora, Isospora*

Infectious: invasive or inflammatory
- *Shigella, Salmonella, Campylobacter,* enteroinvasive *E. coli, E. coli* O157:H7, *Yersinia enterocolitica, Clostridium difficile* (eg, pseudomembranous colitis),

Entamoeba histolytica, Neisseria gonorrhoeae, Listeria monocytogenes

Associated with unprotected anal intercourse
- *Neisseria gonorrhoeae,* syphilis, lymphogranuloma venereum, herpes simplex

Noninfectious
- Drug reaction, especially antibiotics
- Ulcerative colitis, Crohn's disease (inflammatory)
- Ischemic colitis (inflammatory)
- Fecal impaction (stool may leak around impaction)
- Laxative abuse
- Radiation colitis (inflammatory)
- Emotional stress

Diarrhea, chronic

Common
- Irritable bowel syndrome, lactase deficiency, parasites, caffeine, alcohol, laxative abuse

Osmotic
- Lactase deficiency
- Medications: antacids, lactulose, sorbitol, Olestra
- Factitious: magnesium-containing antacids or laxatives

Secretory
- Hormonal: Zollinger-Ellison syndrome (gastrinoma), carcinoid, VIPoma, medullary thyroid carcinoma
- Laxative abuse: phenolphthalein, cascara, senna
- Villous adenoma
- Medications

Inflammatory conditions
- Inflammatory bowel disease
- Microscopic colitis (lymphocytic or collagenous)
- Cancer with obstruction and pseudodiarrhea
- Radiation colitis

Malabsorption
- Small bowel: celiac sprue, Whipple's disease, tropical sprue, eosinophilic gastroenteritis, small bowel resection, Crohn's disease
- Lymphatic obstruction: lymphoma, carcinoid, tuberculosis, *Mycobacterium avium* complex, Kaposi's sarcoma, sarcoidosis, retroperitoneal fibrosis
- Pancreatic insufficiency: chronic pancreatitis, cystic fibrosis, pancreatic cancer
- Bacterial overgrowth, eg, diabetes mellitus

- Reduced bile salts: ileal resection, Crohn's disease, postcholecystectomy

Motility disorders
- Irritable bowel syndrome
- Postsurgical: vagotomy, partial gastrectomy, blind loop with bacterial overgrowth
- Systemic disease: diabetes mellitus, hyperthyroidism, scleroderma
- Caffeine or alcohol use

Chronic infections
- Parasites: giardiasis, amebiasis, strongyloidiasis

Other
- Ischemic colitis
- Adrenal insufficiency

Dilated pupil

- Cranial nerve 3 palsy
- Iris damage due to acute glaucoma
- Mydriatic drugs, eg, atropine
- Sympathomimetic poisoning, eg, amphetamine or cocaine
- Anticholinergic poisoning, eg, atropine, tricyclic antidepressant
- Physiologic anisocoria (unequal pupils, react normally)

Diplopia or ophthalmoplegia

- Microvascular infarction, eg, diabetes mellitus, hypertension
- Wernicke's encephalopathy
- Multiple sclerosis
- Myasthenia gravis
- Graves' ophthalmopathy
- Botulism
- Internal carotid artery aneurysm or carotid dissection
- Posterior inferior cerebellar artery aneurysm
- Other mass compressing nerves to extraocular muscles
- Brainstem infarct
- Neurosyphilis
- Systemic lupus erythematosus
- Sarcoidosis
- Pseudotumor cerebri
- Muscle entrapment from orbital blowout fracture
- Orbital cellulitis
- Sphenoid sinusitis
- Cavernous sinus thrombosis
- Ophthalmoplegic migraine
- Temporal (giant cell) arteritis

- Tuberculous meningitis
- Diphtheria
- Progressive supranuclear palsy
- Progressive external ophthalmoplegia (mitochondrial myopathy)
- Other causes of cranial nerve palsy

Monocular diplopia (*with one eye closed*)
- Refractive error
- Early cataract
- Lens dislocation, eg, Marfan syndrome, homocystinuria
- Corneal opacity, eg, scar, pterygium

Drug eruption, fixed

- Bullous pemphigoid
- Erythema multiforme
- Sweet's syndrome (acute febrile neutrophilic dermatosis)
- Genital lesions: psoriasis, lichen planus, syphilis

Dry eyes (keratoconjunctivitis sicca)

- Allergic conjunctivitis
- Chronic blepharitis
- Age-related
- Dry environment
- Abnormal lipid component of tears, eg, blepharitis
- Autoimmune disease, eg, Sjögren's syndrome, systemic lupus erythematosus
- Xerophthalmia (vitamin A deficiency)
- Sarcoidosis
- Pemphigoid or Stevens-Johnson syndrome
- Impaired eyelid or lacrimal gland function
- Systemic or topical drugs

Dry mouth (xerostomia)

- Sjögren's syndrome
- Mumps
- Sarcoidosis
- Drugs: psychiatric, anticholinergic, antihypertensive
- Local irradiation
- Diabetes mellitus
- Lymphoma
- Psychogenic
- Idiopathic

Dysarthria

Etiology

- Painful oral ulcers, eg, herpes simplex, aphthous ulcers
- Cerebral stroke or subarachnoid hemorrhage
- Brainstem or cerebellar infarct, mass, or hemorrhage
- Multiple sclerosis
- Pseudobulbar palsy
- Amyotrophic lateral sclerosis
- Poliomyelitis
- Guillain-Barré syndrome
- Myasthenia gravis
- Botulism
- Parkinsonism
- Huntington's disease
- Wilson's disease
- Trauma to cranial nerve V or XII
- Diphtheria
- Macroglossia, eg, amyloidosis, hypothyroidism

Dysmenorrhea

Etiology

- Primary dysmenorrhea
- Endometriosis
- Adenomyosis (uterine endometriosis)
- Pelvic inflammatory disease
- Uterine leiomyomas (fibroids)
- Intrauterine device
- Pelvic pain syndrome
- Endometrial polyp
- Cervicitis
- Retroverted uterus
- Cervical stenosis
- Cystitis
- Interstitial cystitis

Dyspareunia

- Vulvodynia or vulvar vestibulitis
- Vaginismus
- Insufficient vaginal lubrication
- Atrophic vaginitis
- Vulvovaginitis, cervicitis, or pelvic inflammatory disease
- Endometriosis
- Lichen sclerosus
- Ovarian tumor
- Pelvic adhesions
- Remnants of the hymen

Dysphagia

Etiology

Esophageal dysphagia

Mechanical obstruction (solids worse than liquids)

- Esophageal web, ring (eg, Schatzki's), or diverticulum (intermittent dysphagia, not progressive)
- Peptic stricture (chronic heartburn, progressive dysphagia)
- Esophageal cancer (progressive dysphagia, age >50)

Motility disorder (solids and liquids)

- Achalasia (progressive dysphagia)
- Diffuse esophageal spasm (intermittent, not progressive)
- Scleroderma (chronic heartburn)

Oropharyngeal dysphagia

Neurologic disorders

- Brainstem stroke, mass lesion
- Amyotrophic lateral sclerosis, multiple sclerosis, pseudobulbar palsy, postpolio syndrome, Guillain-Barré syndrome
- Parkinson's disease, Huntington's disease, dementia
- Tardive dyskinesia

Muscular and rheumatologic disorders

- Myopathy, polymyositis
- Oculopharyngeal dystrophy
- Sjögren's syndrome

Metabolic disorders

- Thyrotoxicosis, amyloidosis, Cushing's disease, Wilson's disease
- Drugs: anticholinergics, phenothiazines

Infectious disease

- Polio, diphtheria, botulism, Lyme disease, syphilis, mucositis (**Candida**, herpes)

Structural disorders

- Zenker's diverticulum
- Cervical osteophytes, cricopharyngeal bar, proximal esophageal webs
- Oropharyngeal tumors
- Postsurgical or radiation changes
- Pill-induced injury

Motility disorders

- Upper esophageal sphincter dysfunction

Dyspnea

Acute

- Asthma, pneumonia, pulmonary edema, pneumothorax, pulmonary embolism, metabolic acidosis, acute respiratory distress syndrome, panic attack

Pulmonary

- Airflow obstruction (asthma, chronic obstructive pulmonary disease, upper airway obstruction), restrictive lung disease (interstitial lung disease, pleural thickening or effusion, respiratory muscle weakness, obesity), pneumonia, pneumothorax, pulmonary embolism, aspiration, acute respiratory distress syndrome

Cardiac

- Myocardial ischemia, congestive heart failure, valvular obstruction, arrhythmia, cardiac tamponade

Metabolic

- Acidosis, hypercapnia, sepsis

Hematologic

- Anemia, methemoglobinemia

Psychiatric

- Anxiety

Dyspnea, episodic

- Congestive heart failure
- Asthma
- Acute or chronic bronchitis
- Recurrent pulmonary emboli

Dystonia

Etiology

- Idiopathic torsion dystonia
- Focal torsion dystonia, eg, blepharospasm, torticollis, oromandibular dystonia, writer's cramp
- Perinatal anoxia or birth trauma
- Kernicterus
- Wilson's disease
- Huntington's disease
- Parkinsonism
- Encephalitis lethargica
- Drugs, eg, antipsychotics
- Tetanus

Dysuria

- Cystitis
- Urethritis, eg, gonorrhea, chlamydia
- Pyelonephritis
- Vaginitis
- Epididymitis
- Balanitis
- Prostatitis
- Interstitial cystitis
- Urethral syndrome
- Genital herpes
- Atrophic vaginitis
- Reactive arthritis (Reiter's syndrome)

Ear canal diseases

- Cerumen impaction (ear wax)
- Otitis externa (external otitis)
- Malignant otitis externa (osteomyelitis)
- Ear pruritus
- Osteoma
- Exostoses
- Squamous cell carcinoma
- Cholesteatoma
- Seborrheic dermatitis

Ear pain

- Acute otitis media
- Otitis externa
- Chronic otitis media
- Auditory (eustachian) tube dysfunction
- Mastoiditis
- Referred pain: sinusitis, tooth pain, cancer of upper aerodigestive tract
- Temporomandibular joint syndrome
- Trauma or barotrauma
- Foreign body
- Osteoma
- Cholesteatoma
- Ramsay-Hunt syndrome (herpes zoster oticus)
- Acoustic neuroma
- Bullous myringitis
- Glossopharyngeal neuralgia

Ear pruritus

- Otitis externa (external otitis)
- Seborrheic dermatitis
- Psoriasis
- Excoriation
- Excessive ear cleaning

Eczema, nummular or discoid

- Tinea corporis
- Psoriasis
- Xerosis (dry skin)
- Impetigo
- Contact dermatitis
- Lichen simplex chronicus
- Pityriasis rosea

Edema, lower extremity

Cardiovascular

- Congestive heart failure (right-sided)
- Pericardial effusion

- Pericarditis
- Tricuspid regurgitation
- Tricuspid stenosis
- Pulmonary stenosis
- Cor pulmonale
- Venous insufficiency (most common)
- Venous obstruction

Noncardiovascular
- Cirrhosis
- Low albumin (nephrotic syndrome, malnutrition, protein-losing enteropathy)
- Cellulitis
- Premenstrual fluid retention
- Drugs (vasodilators, eg, calcium channel blockers, salt-retaining medications, eg, NSAIDs, thiazolidinediones)
- Musculoskeletal (Baker's cyst, gastrocnemius tear, compartment syndrome)
- Lymphatic obstruction
- Preeclampsia-eclampsia
- Myxedema
- Lymphatic filariasis
- Eosinophilic fasciitis

Edema, unilateral

- Deep vein thrombosis
- Venous insufficiency
- Baker's cyst (rupture or obstruction of popliteal vein)
- Cellulitis
- Trauma
- Lymphatic obstruction, eg, obstruction by pelvic tumor
- Reflex sympathetic dystrophy
- Tumor or fibrosis obstructing iliac vein
- May-Thurner syndrome (left iliac vein compressed by right common iliac artery)
- Loiasis (*Loa loa* infection)

Edema, upper extremity

- SVC syndrome
- Upper extremity deep vein thrombosis
- Lymphatic obstruction
- Reflex sympathetic dystrophy
- Eosinophilic fasciitis

Electrocardiogram: electrical alternans

- Pericardial effusion
- Dilated cardiomyopathy
- Transient electrical alternans with supraventricular tachycardia

Electrocardiogram: left atrial enlargement

- Left ventricular hypertrophy
- Coronary artery disease
- Mitral valve disease
- Cardiomyopathy

Electrocardiogram: left axis deviation

- Left anterior fascicular block
- Inferior myocardial infarction
- Ventricular pre-excitation (Wolff-Parkinson-White pattern)
- Chronic obstructive pulmonary disease

Electrocardiogram: long QT

Etiology

Electrolyte abnormalities
- Hypokalemia
- Hypomagnesemia
- Hypocalcemia

Drugs (selected examples)
- Class Ia antiarrhythmics (quinidine, procainamide)
- Class Ic antiarrhythmics (propafenone)
- Class III antiarrhythmics (amiodarone, bretylium, sotalol)
- Tricyclic antidepressants
- Astemizole, terfenadine
- Antibiotics: erythromycin, trimethoprim-sulfamethoxazole, levofloxacin, ketoconazole, itraconazole
- Phenothiazines, haldol
- Prednisone

Miscellaneous
- Congenital long QT syndrome
- Third-degree A-V block
- Second-degree A-V block
- Left ventricular hypertrophy
- Myocardial ischemia
- Significant bradycardia
- Stroke or subarachnoid hemorrhage
- Hypothermia

Electrocardiogram: low voltage

Myocardial causes
- Multiple or massive myocardial infarctions
- Infiltrative disease (eg, amyloidosis, sarcoidosis, hemochromatosis)

Nonmyocardial causes
- Pericardial effusion
- Chronic obstructive pulmonary disease
- Pleural effusion
- Obesity
- Anasarca
- Myxedema (due to skin changes, pericardial effusion, and myocardial disease)
- Subcutaneous emphysema

Electrocardiogram: right atrial enlargement

- Right ventricular hypertrophy

Electrocardiogram: right axis deviation

- Right ventricular hypertrophy
- Anteroapical myocardial infarction
- Ventricular pre-excitation (Wolff-Parkinson-White pattern)
- Left posterior fascicular block

Electrocardiogram: short QT

- Hypercalcemia
- Digoxin
- Thyrotoxicosis
- Increased sympathetic tone

Electrocardiogram: ST depression or T wave inversion

- Subendocardial ischemia
- Right bundle branch block (V1)
- Left bundle branch block (V5–V6)
- Left ventricular hypertrophy with repolarization abnormality (V5–V6)
- Subarachnoid hemorrhage
- Right ventricular hypertrophy (V1–V3)
- Hypokalemia
- Digoxin

Electrocardiogram: ST elevation

- Acute myocardial infarction
- Vasospasm (Prinzmetal's angina)
- Pericarditis

- Left bundle branch block (V1–V3)
- Left ventricular hypertrophy with repolarization abnormality (V1–V3)
- Early repolarization (normal variant)
- Ventricular pacemaker
- Cocaine
- Myocarditis

Electrocardiogram: U waves

- Hypokalemia
- Bradycardia
- Digoxin
- Antiarrhythmic drugs

Electrocardiogram: wide QRS

- Bundle branch block or intraventricular conduction delay
- Ventricular ectopy
- Pacemaker
- Hyperkalemia
- Wolff-Parkinson-White syndrome
- Drugs: tricyclic antidepressants, class Ia antiarrhythmics (eg, quinidine), class Ic antiarrhythmics (eg, propafenone), phenothiazines

Elbow pain

- Epicondylitis, lateral ("tennis elbow") or medial ("golf elbow")
- Olecranon bursitis
- Arthritis, eg, rheumatoid arthritis, gout, osteoarthritis, septic arthritis
- Fracture
- Tendonitis of distal insertion of biceps
- Ulnar nerve entrapment at elbow
- Avascular necrosis
- Metastatic or primary tumor

Encephalitis, viral

- Aseptic or bacterial meningitis
- Lymphocytic choriomeningitis
- Encephalitis accompanying exanthematous diseases of childhood: measles, varicella, infectious mononucleosis, rubella
- Nonparalytic poliomyelitis
- Subarachnoid hemorrhage, stroke, brain tumor, brain abscess
- Lupus cerebritis
- Behçet's syndrome
- Lyme disease or neurosyphilis
- Toxoplasmosis or cryptococcosis
- Encephalitis following vaccination (for rabies, measles, pertussis)
- Reye's syndrome
- Toxic encephalitis, eg, drugs, poisons, Shiga toxin
- Amebic meningoencephalitis (*Naegleria fowleri*) or granulomatous amebic encephalitis (*Acanthamoeba*)
- African trypanosomiasis (sleeping sickness)

Etiology

- Herpes simplex, mumps, HIV, poliovirus, rabies, cytomegalovirus
- Viral and mosquito-borne (arboviruses): St. Louis, California, Japanese B, Western equine, Eastern equine, West Nile encephalitis

Eosinophilia

Etiology

- Drug hypersensitivity
- Allergic state, eg, asthma, urticaria, atopic dermatitis
- Tissue invasion by parasites, eg, ascariasis, visceral larva migrans
- Other skin disorder, eg, pemphigoid, dermatitis herpetiformis
- Malignancy, especially lymphoma
- Connective tissue disease, eg, Churg-Strauss syndrome, polyarteritis nodosa, eosinophilic fasciitis
- Eosinophilic pulmonary syndrome
- Fungal infection, eg, coccidioidomycosis
- Idiopathic
- Other: adrenal insufficiency, cholesterol emboli, eosinophilic leukemia

Eosinophilic pulmonary syndromes

Etiology

- Chronic eosinophilic pneumonia
- Acute eosinophilic pneumonia (Loeffler's syndrome)
- Drugs: nitrofurantoin, phenytoin, ampicillin, penicillin, sulfonamides, acetaminophen, ranitidine, methotrexate
- Helminth infection: ascariasis, hooworm, strongyloidiasis, paragonimiasis, toxocariasis (visceral larva migrans),

tropical pulmonary eosinophilia (*Wuchereria bancrofti, Brugia malayi*)
- Allergic bronchopulmonary aspergillosis
- Churg-Strauss syndrome
- Systemic hypereosinophilic syndromes
- Eosinophilic granuloma (Langerhans cell histiocytosis, histiocytosis X)
- Malignancy
- Numerous interstitial lung diseases
- Toxins: inhaled crack cocaine, heroin, Scotchguard, sulfite pesticides

Epistaxis

- Nasal trauma, eg, nose picking, forceful nose blowing, foreign body
- Allergic rhinitis or viral rhinitis
- Dry nasal mucosa
- Deviated septum
- Chronic sinusitis
- Inhaled steroids
- Cocaine use
- Alcohol use
- Antiplatelet drugs, eg, aspirin, clopidogrel
- Thrombocytopenia, eg, idiopathic thrombocytopenia purpura, thrombotic thrombocytopenia purpura
- Hemophilia
- Hereditary hemorrhagic telangiectasia (Osler-Weber-Rendu syndrome)
- Polycythemia vera
- Leukemia
- Wegener's granulomatosis
- Nasal tumor

Erectile dysfunction

- Diabetes mellitus
- Atherosclerosis (Leriche syndrome: impotence and claudication)
- Hypogonadism (primary or secondary testicular failure)
- Stroke
- Local trauma
- Hyperprolactinemia
- Hyperthyroidism
- Cushing's syndrome
- Addison's disease
- Acromegaly
- Multiple sclerosis
- Spinal cord trauma or tumor
- Psychogenic
- Drugs (selected): alcohol, tobacco, recreational drugs, SSRIs, clonidine, thi-

azides, spironolactone, tricyclic antidepressants, antihistamines, beta blockers
(uncommon)

Erythema, figurate (shaped)

- Urticaria
- Erythema multiforme
- Erythema migrans (Lyme disease)
- Erysipelas
- Cellulitis
- Erysipeloid
- Arthropod bites (insect bites)

Erythromelalgia

- Raynaud's phenomenon
- Venous insufficiency
- Arterial insufficiency
- Peripheral neuropathy

Etiology

- Idiopathic
- Polycythemia vera
- Essential thrombocytosis
- Drugs: bromocriptine, nifedipine, felodipine, desmopressin
- Hypertension
- Gout

Erythroplakia

- Usually dysplasia or carcinoma

Esophageal motility disorders

- Achalasia (idiopathic)
- Chagas' disease
- Pseudoachalasia (tumor invading gastroesophageal junction)
- Diffuse esophageal spasm
- Scleroderma
- Nutcracker esophagus

Esophagitis

Etiology

- Infectious: *Candida,* herpes simplex virus, cytomegalovirus
- Reflux esophagitis
- Pill-induced esophagitis: NSAIDs, KCl, AZT, alendronate, iron, antibiotics
- Caustic esophageal injury (alkali or acid ingestion)
- Radiation esophagitis

Eye pain

- Viral or bacterial conjunctivitis
- Foreign body or corneal abrasion
- Keratitis (corneal ulcer or inflammation), eg, herpes simplex
- Trauma
- Acute glaucoma
- Orbital or periorbital cellulitis
- Ultraviolet (actinic) keratitis
- Eyelid disorder, eg, hordeolum, chalazion, blepharitis
- Inverted eyelash (eg, entropion)
- Dacryocystitis (lacrimal sac infection)
- Decreased tearing, eg, age-related, Sjögren's syndrome, anticholinergics
- Sinusitis
- Migraine or cluster headache
- Temporal (giant cell) arteritis
- Ophthalmic zoster (pain may precede rash)
- Uveitis
- Scleritis or episcleritis
- Optic neuritis
- Intracranial mass

Eyelid disorders

- Blepharitis
- Hordeolum (sty)
- Chalazion
- Entropion or ectropion
- Xanthelasma (lipid disorder or idiopathic)
- Tumor, eg, verrucae, papilloma, basal or squamous cell carcinoma, melanoma
- Dacryocystitis (lacrimal sac infection)

Facial erythema

- Erysipelas
- Cellulitis
- Impetigo
- Acne rosacea
- Contact dermatitis
- Seborrheic dermatitis
- Systemic lupus erythematosus
- Herpes zoster (shingles)
- Tinea
- Angioedema
- Necrotizing fasciitis
- Erysipeloid
- Dermatomyositis (purplish rash on upper eyelids)

Facial palsy (Bell's palsy)

Etiology

- Bell's palsy (idiopathic)
- HIV
- Lyme disease
- Sarcoidosis
- Ramsay Hunt syndrome (herpes zoster of geniculate ganglion)
- Acoustic neuroma
- Acute or chronic otitis media
- Malignant otitis externa
- Guillain-Barré syndrome
- Tumor, eg, parotid, temporal bone tumor
- Brainstem infarct

Facial, tooth, or jaw pain

- Dental caries or abscess
- Sinusitis
- Temporal arteritis
- Trigeminal neuralgia
- TMJ syndrome
- Migraine
- Sialadenitis (eg, parotitis)
- Sialolithiasis (salivary gland calculi)
- Otitis media
- Orbital or periorbital cellulitis
- Peritonsillar abscess
- Ludwig's angina (retropharyngeal infection)
- Carotid dissection
- Glossopharyngeal neuralgia
- Atypical facial pain
- Postherpetic neuralgia
- Bruxism (teeth grinding)
- Dental misalignment
- Acoustic neuroma
- Trauma
- Glaucoma
- Dacryocystitis (lacrimal sac infection)
- Angina pectoris
- Numb chin syndrome (mental neuropathy) due to malignancy in mandible

Falls & gait disorders

- Visual impairment
- Gait impairment due to:
  - Podiatric disorder, eg, ingrown nail
  - Arthritis
  - Muscular weakness, eg, myopathy
  - Cerebellar ataxia, eg, alcoholism

- Sensory ataxia, eg, vitamin B_{12} deficiency, neurosyphilis
- Other neurologic disorder, eg, parkinsonism, Alzheimer's disease, spinal stenosis, multiple sclerosis, peripheral neuropathy
- Environmental hazards, eg, poor lighting, stairs, rugs, uneven floors
- Polypharmacy, eg, benzodiazepines, opioids, phenothiazines, vasodilators, diuretics
- Alcohol use
- Orthostatic or postprandial hypotension
- Vertigo, presyncope, syncope, or dysequilibrium
- Medical illness, eg, pneumonia, myocardial infarction, anemia, hyponatremia
- Other contributing factors: urinary urgency, peripheral edema, insomnia

Fatigue

- Hypothyroidism
- Anemia
- Depression
- Sleep apnea or insufficient sleep
- Infection, eg, tuberculosis, hepatitis, endocarditis, HIV, Lyme disease
- Diabetes mellitus
- Congestive heart failure, chronic obstructive pulmonary disease, or chronic renal failure
- Cancer
- Alcoholism
- Hypercalcemia
- Drugs, eg, sedatives, beta blockers
- Chronic fatigue syndrome
- Somatoform disorder (eg, somatization)
- Fibromyalgia
- Mononucleosis
- Autoimmune disease
- Adrenal insufficiency

Fecal incontinence

- Acute or chronic diarrhea
- Perianal fistula, eg, Crohn's disease
- Rectal prolapse

Etiology

- Hemorrhoids or anal skin tags (disrupt anal seal)
- Proctitis
- Irritable bowel syndrome
- Constipation with "overflow" incontinence
- Chronic diarrhea due to other causes

- Sphincter damage, eg, traumatic childbirth, episiotomy, rectal prolapse, surgery, cancer
- Neurologic, eg, pudendal nerve damage (obstetric trauma), diabetes mellitus, aging, dementia, multiple sclerosis, spinal cord injury, cauda equina syndrome

Fever

Common causes

- Infection
  - Bacterial, viral, rickettsial, fungal, parasitic
  - CNS, sinusitis, dental, endocarditis, pneumonia, liver, biliary system, GI, peritonitis, abdominal abscess, UTI, prostatitis, sexually transmitted disease, cellulitis, soft tissues, bone, joints
- Autoimmune disease
- CNS disease including head trauma, mass lesion
- Malignancy, especially lymphoma, leukemia, renal cell carcinoma, primary or metastatic liver cancer

Less common causes

- Cardiovascular disease, eg, myocardial infarction, deep vein thrombosis, pulmonary embolism
- Gastrointestinal disease, eg, inflammatory bowel disease, alcoholic hepatitis, granulomatous hepatitis
- Miscellaneous, eg, drug fever, sarcoidosis, familial Mediterranean fever, tissue injury, hematoma, factitious fever

Hyperthermia

- Heat stroke, neuroleptic malignant syndrome, malignant hyperthermia

Fever and rash

Diffuse maculopapular rash

- Viral exanthem: measles, rubella (German measles), erythema infectiosum ("slapped-cheek" disease), exanthem subitum (roseola), primary HIV infection, infectious mononucleosis, dengue
- Other infection: typhoid fever, secondary syphilis, Lyme disease, leptospirosis, rat bite fever, relapsing fever, ehrlichiosis, epidemic typhus, endemic typhus, scrub typhus, erythema marginatum (rheumatic fever)
- Noninfectious: drug rash (with drug fever or unrelated infection), systemic lupus erythematosus, adult Still's disease

---

Peripheral eruption

- Meningococcemia or gonococcemia
- Secondary syphilis
- Rocky Mountain spotted fever
- Erythema multiforme
- Bacterial endocarditis
- Hand, foot, and mouth disease

Desquamative erythema

- Toxic shock syndrome (staphylococcal or streptococcal)
- Scarlet fever
- Kawasaki syndrome
- Staphylococcal scalded skin syndrome
- Exfoliative erythroderma syndrome (eg, underlying psoriasis, eczema, drug eruption)
- Erythema multiforme major or toxic epidermal necrolysis

Vesicles or bullae

- Varicella (chickenpox)
- Staphylococcal scalded skin syndrome
- Erythema multiforme major or toxic epidermal necrolysis
- Hand, foot, and mouth disease
- Rickettsialpox
- Ecthyma gangrenosum (neutropenic, pseudomonal)
- Disseminated *Vibrio vulnificus* (cirrhosis, seafood or seawater exposure)

Purpura or petechiae

- Bacterial endocarditis
- Meningococcemia or gonococcemia
- Rocky Mountain spotted fever
- Purpura fulminans (severe disseminated intravascular coagulation)
- Thrombotic thrombocytopenic purpura
- Other: epidemic typhus, rat bite fever, enteroviral petechial rash, viral hemorrhagic fever

Other

- Urticarial vasculitis (serum sickness, connective tissue disease, infection, idiopathic)
- Nodules due to disseminated infection (eg, fungal), erythema nodosum, Sweet's syndrome (acute febrile neutrophilic dermatosis)
- Pustular psoriasis

Fever in immunocompromised

Neutropenia

- Gram-negative enteric organisms
- *Pseudomonas*

- Gram-positive cocci, eg, *S. aureus, S. epidermidis*
- *Candida*
- *Aspergillus* and other fungi

Cellular immune defect (HIV, lymphoma, immunosuppressive drugs)
- Bacteria: *Listeria, Legionella, Salmonella, Mycobacterium*
- Viruses: herpes simplex virus, varicella, cytomegalovirus
- Fungi: *Cryptococcus, Coccidioides, Histoplasma, Pneumocystis*
- Protozoa: *Toxoplasma*

Humoral immune defect (congenital, multiple myeloma, chronic lymphocyic leukemia)
- Encapsulated organisms: *Streptococcus pneumoniae, Haemophilus influenzae, Neisseria meningitidis*

Asplenia (functional or anatomic)
- Encapsulated organisms: *Streptococcus pneumoniae, Haemophilus influenzae, Neisseria meningitidis*

Noninfectious causes
- Transplant rejection
- Organ ischemia or necrosis
- Thrombophlebitis
- Lymphoma

Fever in parenteral drug user

- Community-acquired pneumonia
- Endocarditis
- Complications of endocarditis, eg, pulmonary septic emboli, epidural abscess, osteomyelitis
- Skin abscess, cellulitis, myositis, necrotizing fasciitis
- Pelvic inflammatory disease
- Urinary tract infection

Fever in returning traveler

- Malaria
- Typhoid fever (enteric fever)
- Prodrome of hepatitis A, B, or E
- Dengue
- Amebiasis or amebic liver abscess
- Rickettsial spotted fever, eg, Mediterranean spotted fever, rickettsialpox, Rocky Mountain spotted fever
- Tuberculosis
- Visceral leishmaniasis
- Acute HIV infection
- Leptospirosis

- Acute schistosomiasis
- Yellow fever
- Scrub typhus
- African trypanosomiasis
- Rabies

Fever of unknown origin

Infection
- Tuberculosis, endocarditis, osteomyelitis, UTI, sinusitis, occult abscess (intra-abdominal, dental, brain), cholangitis, primary HIV, Epstein-Barr virus, cytomegalovirus, systemic mycosis, toxoplasmosis, brucellosis, Q fever, cat-scratch disease, salmonellosis, malaria

Neoplasm
- Hodgkin's or non-Hodgkin's lymphoma, leukemia, primary or metastatic liver cancer, renal cell carcinoma, atrial myxoma, others

Autoimmune
- Adult Still's disease, systemic lupus erythematosus, cryoglobulinemia, polyarteritis nodosa, temporal (giant cell) arteritis, polymyalgia rheumatica, Wegener's granulomatosis

Other
- Drug fever, sarcoidosis, granulomatous or alcoholic hepatitis, Crohn's disease, ulcerative colitis, factitious fever, thyroiditis, hematoma, recurrent pulmonary emboli, hypersensitivity pneumonitis, familial Mediterranean fever, Whipple's disease

Fever, hospital-acquired

- Noninfectious: drug fever, postoperative atelectasis or tissue necrosis, hematoma, pancreatitis, pulmonary embolism, myocardial infarction, ischemic colitis
- Pneumonia
- Bacteremia, eg, indwelling catheter, wound, abscess, pneumonia, GU or GI tract
- Wound infection, eg, decubitus ulcer
- *Clostridium difficile* colitis

Fever, postoperative

- Wind: pneumonia, atelectasis
- Water: urinary tract infection
- Wound: wound infection
- Walking: deep vein thrombosis from immobilization
- Wonderdrugs: drug fever

Fever, postpartum

- Endometritis
- Urinary tract infection
- Pneumonia
- Septic pelvic vein thrombosis or pelvic abscess
- Retained products of conception
- Deep vein thrombosis or pulmonary embolism (including amniotic embolism)
- Wound infection
- Mastitis
- Thyroiditis

Fever, relapsing or recurrent

- Malaria
- Typhoid fever (enteric fever)
- Brucellosis
- Borreliosis
- Lymphoma (especially Hodgkin's disease)
- Tuberculosis
- Rat bite fever
- Occult abscess
- Trench fever (*Bartonella quintana*)
- Familial Mediterranean fever

Flatfoot

- Idiopathic
- Posterior tibial tendon rupture, eg, acute flatfoot after ankle sprain

Flatus (flatulence, gas)

- Carbohydrate-rich food
- Air swallowing
- Lactase deficiency
- Malabsorption, eg, celiac sprue
- Irritable bowel syndrome
- Parasites, eg, *Giardia, Strongyloides, Trichuris* (whipworm)
- Gas-producing foods: beans, peas, lentils, broccoli, Brussels sprouts, cauliflower, cabbage, parsnips, leeks, onions, beer, coffee

Flexor (volar) tenosynovitis

- Overuse
- Disseminated gonococcal infection
- Rheumatic fever
- Arthritis, eg, rheumatoid arthritis, psoriatic arthritis, osteoarthritis

- Sarcoidosis
- Fungal or atypical mycobacterial infection, eg, *Mycobacterium marinum*

Floaters

- Benign vitreous opacities
- Posterior vitreous detachment
- Vitreous hemorrhage
- Posterior uveitis
- Retinal detachment or tear (acute onset, especially with flashing lights)
- Cysticercosis

Focal segmental glomerulosclerosis

Etiology

- Heroin use
- Morbid obesity
- HIV
- Reflux nephropathy
- Idiopathic

Foot drop

Etiology

- Peroneal nerve compression
- L5 radiculopathy
- Diabetes mellitus
- Polyarteritis nodosa
- Charcot-Marie-Tooth disease
- Lyme disease

Foot pain

- Ingrown toenail
- Bunions, warts, calluses, corns
- Plantar fasciitis
- Morton's neuroma
- Metatarsalgia, eg, rheumatoid arthritis
- Pes planus (flatfoot)
- Bursitis of first MTP (inflamed bunion)
- Metatarsal stress fracture
- Arthritis, eg, gout, psoriatic arthritis, rheumatoid arthritis, osteoarthritis
- Poorly fitting shoes
- Lumbar disk herniation
- Achilles tendinitis
- Retrocalcaneal bursitis
- Tarsal tunnel syndrome
- Peripheral neuropathy, eg, diabetes mellitus, alcoholism
- Arterial insufficiency
- Diabetic or arterial insufficiency ulcer with or without osteomyelitis

- Polyarteritis nodosa, thromboangiitis obliterans (Buerger's disease), Raynaud's syndrome
- Erythromelalgia

Fever of unknown origin in HIV/AIDS

- Disseminated *Mycobacterium avium* complex
- *Pneumocystis* pneumonia (PCP)
- Cytomegalovirus infection
- Disseminated histoplasmosis
- Lymphoma
- Tuberculosis
- Cryptococcal meningitis
- Drug fever
- Sinusitis
- *Salmonella* infection
- Kaposi's sarcoma
- Neurosyphilis
- Visceral leishmaniasis

Galactorrhea

- Physiologic: pregnancy, postpartum
- Idiopathic (normal prolactin level in parous woman)
- Hyperprolactinemia, eg, medications, prolactinoma, hypothyroidism
- Benign or malignant neoplasm
- Nipple stimulation
- Mastitis
- Oral contraceptives or estrogen replacement therapy

Gastric tumor

Benign

- Gastric epithelial polyp
- Adenomatous polyp
- Submucosal: benign stromal tumor (leiomyoma), pancreatic rest

Malignant

- Gastric adenocarcinoma
- Gastric lymphoma (primary, eg, MALToma, or secondary)
- Gastric carcinoid
- Leiomyosarcoma
- Kaposi's sarcoma

Gastritis

- Peptic ulcer disease
- Functional or nonulcer dyspepsia
- Gastroesophageal reflux disease or hiatal hernia

- Biliary disease or pancreatitis
- Gastric or pancreatic cancer
- Viral gastroenteritis
- "Indigestion" from overeating, high-fat foods, coffee
- Angina pectoris
- Severe pain: esophageal rupture, gastric volvulus, ruptured aortic aneurysm

Etiology

- Erosive gastritis: NSAIDs, alcohol, stress, caustic ingestion, radiation
- Portal gastropathy
- *Helicobacter pylori* gastritis
- Pernicious anemia gastritis
- Uncommon infections: necrotizing gastritis; cytomegalovirus or *Candida* (common in immunosuppressed); *Anisakis marina* (raw fish)
- Chronic granulomatous inflammation: tuberculosis, syphilis, fungal infection, sarcoidosis, Crohn's disease
- Eosinophilic gastritis
- Lymphocytic gastritis

Gastroparesis

- Mechanical obstruction of stomach, small intestine, or colon

Etiology

- Endocrine: diabetes mellitus, hypothyroidism, cortisol insufficiency
- Postsurgical: vagotomy, partial gastric resection, fundoplication, gastric bypass, Whipple procedure
- Neurologic: Parkinson's disease, muscular and myotonic dystrophy, autonomic dysfunction, multiple sclerosis, postpolio syndrome, porphyria
- Rheumatologic: scleroderma
- Infection: postviral, Chagas' disease
- Other: amyloidosis, paraneoplastic, drugs, anorexia nervosa, idiopathic

GI bleeding, lower

Etiology

- Diverticulosis
- Vascular ectasias (angiodysplasias), eg, idiopathic atrioventricular malformation, CREST syndrome, hereditary hemorrhagic telangiectasias
- Colonic polyps
- Colorectal cancer
- Inflammatory bowel disease
- Hemorrhoids

- Anal fissure
- Ischemic colitis
- Infectious colitis
- Radiation colitis or proctitis
- Iron or bismuth subsalicylate ingestion (false melena)

Rare causes
- Aortoenteric fistula
- Vasculitis
- Solitary rectal ulcer
- NSAID-induced ulcers of small bowel or right colon
- Small bowel diverticula
- Colonic varices

GI bleeding, occult

Etiology
- Malignancy
- Vascular ectasias (angiodysplasias), eg, idiopathic atrioventricular malformation, CREST syndrome, hereditary hemorrhagic telangiectasias
- Portal hypertensive gastropathy
- Peptic ulcer disease
- Ulcerated polyp
- Infections, eg, hookworm, tuberculosis
- Drugs, eg, NSAIDs, aspirin
- Inflammatory bowel disease
- Malabsorption, especially celiac sprue
- Menstrual or pregnancy-associated iron loss
- Idiopathic

GI bleeding, upper

Etiology
- Hemoptysis
- Peptic ulcer disease
- Esophageal varices
- Gastric or duodenal varices (rare)
- Erosive gastritis, eg, NSAIDs, alcohol, stress
- Mallory-Weiss syndrome
- Portal hypertensive gastropathy
- Vascular ectasias (angiodysplasias), eg, idiopathic atrioventricular malformation, CREST syndrome, hereditary hemorrhagic telangiectasias
- Gastric cancer

Rare causes
- Erosive esophagitis
- Aortoenteric fistula
- Dieulafoy's lesion (aberrant gastric submucosal artery)

- Hemobilia (blood in biliary tree), eg, iatrogenic, malignancy
- Pancreatic cancer
- *Hemosuccus pancreaticus* (pancreatic pseudoaneurysm)

Gingival hyperplasia

- Gingivitis
- Leukemia
- Scurvy (vitamin C deficiency)
- Kaposi's sarcoma
- Drugs: phenytoin, cyclosporine, calcium channel blockers, ethosuximide, atropine/diphenoxylate (Lomotil)
- Familial gingival fibromatosis

Glomerulonephritis

Etiology
Immune complex
- IgA nephropathy
- Endocarditis
- Systemic lupus erythematosus
- Cryoglobulinemia
- Postinfectious glomerulonephritis
- Membranoproliferative
- Henoch-Schönlein purpura

Pauci-immune (ANCA+)
- Wegener's granulomatosis
- Churg-Strauss syndrome
- Microscopic polyarteritis

Anti-GBM
- Goodpasture's syndrome
- Anti-GBM glomerulonephritis

Other
- Malignant hypertension
- Thrombotic thrombocytopenic purpura

Glomerulonephropathies

- Nephritic syndrome or glomerulonephritis (hematuria, proteinuria, HTN, renal insufficiency)
- Nephrotic syndrome (heavy proteinuria, hypoalbuminemia, hyperlipidemia, edema)

Glossitis

- Nutritional deficiency, eg, niacin (pellagra), riboflavin, pyridoxine, vitamin B_{12}, folic acid, iron, vitamin E
- Drug reaction
- Dehydration
- Irritants

- Pernicious anemia
- Psoriasis
- Glucagonoma
- Median rhomboid glossitis

Glossodynia

- Diabetes mellitus
- Drugs, eg, diuretics
- Tobacco
- Dry mouth (xerostomia)
- Oral candidiasis

Glucosuria

Etiology
- Hyperglycemia, eg, diabetes mellitus, gestational diabetes, Cushing's syndrome
- Nondiabetic (benign) glycosuria: genetic, Fanconi's syndrome, chronic renal failure, pregnancy
- Lead toxicity

Goiter

- Benign multinodular goiter
- Iodine-deficient goiter
- Pregnancy (in areas of iodine deficiency)
- Graves' disease
- Hashimoto's thyroiditis
- Subacute (de Quervain's) thyroiditis
- Drugs causing hypothyroidism: lithium, amiodarone, propylthiouracil, methimazole, phenylbutazone, sulfonamides, interferon α, iodide
- Infiltrating disease, eg, malignancy, sarcoidosis
- Suppurative thyroiditis
- Riedel's thyroiditis

Etiology
- Iodine deficiency (most common)
- Foods: sorghum, millet, maize, cassava, turnip
- Mineral deficiency: selenium, iron
- Water pollutants

Gynecomastia

- Breast cancer
- Fatty breast enlargement of obesity
- Breast abscess (mastitis)
- Metastatic cancer, eg, prostate

Etiology
- Physiologic: neonatal, pubertal, aging, obesity

- Endocrine: hyperprolactinemia, hyperthyroidism, Klinefelter syndrome, hypogonadism
- Systemic disease: chronic liver or renal disease
- Neoplasms: adrenal, testicular, lung, liver, breast
- Drugs (selected): alcohol, amiodarone, anabolic steroids, cimetidine, diazepam, digoxin, estrogens, finasteride, flutamide, INH, ketoconazole, marijuana, omeprazole, opioids, progestins, protease inhibitors & antiretrovirals, spironolactone, testosterone, tricyclic antidepressants

Halitosis (bad breath)

- Gingivitis
- Dental caries
- Dental abscess
- Sinusitis
- Gastroesophageal reflux
- Cancer of upper aerodigestive tract
- Zenker's diverticulum

Hallucinations

- Schizophrenia
- Major depressive or manic episode with psychotic features
- Drugs or substance abuse, eg, steroids, cocaine, amphetamines, alcohol withdrawal
- Psychotic symptoms associated with dementia
- Delirium
- CNS disease, eg, complex partial seizures, brain tumor, neurosyphilis
- Nutritional deficiency, eg, thiamine, vitamin B_{12}
- Heavy metal poisoning, eg, mercury
- Endocrinopathy, eg, hypothyroidism, Cushing's syndrome
- Other psychotic disorder, eg, schizoaffective or schizophreniform disorder, delusional disorder (nonbizarre delusions, minimal impairment of daily functioning), brief psychotic disorder
- Personality disorder, eg, paranoid, schizotypal, schizoid

Hand pain

- Trauma or overuse, eg, fracture, dislocation, tendinitis
- Trigger finger
- Arthritis, eg, osteoarthritis (DIP and PIP joints), rheumatoid arthritis (MCPs, not DIPs), psoriatic arthritis, reactive arthritis (Reiter's syndrome), gout, septic arthritis
- Finger: felon (infected pad), paronychia, subungual hematoma
- Area of first CMC joint: osteoarthritis, de Quervain's tenosynovitis, scaphoid fracture (snuffbox pain)
- Carpal tunnel syndrome
- Pronator teres syndrome (median nerve entrapment at level of pronator teres)
- Flexor tenosynovitis, eg, overuse, rheumatoid arthritis, gonococcal
- Dupuytren's contracture
- Ulnar nerve entrapment at the wrist
- Brachial plexus neuropathy
- Cervical nerve root compression, eg, herniated disk
- Superficial radial neuropathy (cheiralgia paresthetica or handcuff neuropathy)
- Reflex sympathetic dystrophy
- Thoracic outlet syndrome
- Vascular, eg, Raynaud's syndrome, thromboangiitis obliterans (Buerger's disease), erythromelalgia
- Angina pectoris (left-sided pain)

HDL decreased

Etiology

- Obesity
- "Metabolic syndrome" (insulin resistance, hypertriglyceridemia)
- Malnutrition
- Sedentary lifestyle
- Cigarette smoking
- Familial
- Beta blockers (short-term effect)

Headache

Do not miss
- Subarachnoid hemorrhage
- Meningitis
- Temporal (giant cell) arteritis
- Glaucoma
- Hypertension
- Cerebral ischemia
- Arterial dissection (carotid or vertebral)
- Brain tumor

Intracranial
- Migraine
- Cluster headache
- Subarachnoid hemorrhage
- Meningitis
- Brain abscess
- Temporal (giant cell) arteritis
- Hypertension
- Caffeine, alcohol, or drug withdrawal
- Pseudotumor cerebri
- Subdural hemorrhage
- Cerebral ischemia
- Arterial dissection (carotid or vertebral)
- Arteriovenous malformation
- Head injury
- Neurocysticercosis
- Venous sinus thrombosis (intracranial venous thrombosis)
- Post-lumbar puncture
- Carbon monoxide poisoning

Extracranial
- Tension headache
- Sinusitis
- Cervical arthritis
- Glaucoma
- Refractive error
- Dental abscess
- Otitis media
- Temporomandibular joint syndrome
- Depression
- Somatoform disorder (eg, somatization)
- Trigeminal neuralgia
- Glossopharyngeal neuralgia

Headache, cough-associated

- Idiopathic
- Intracranial lesion, usually posterior fossa, eg, Arnold-Chiari malformation

Hearing loss

Conductive (external or middle ear)
- Cerumen impaction (ear wax)
- Transient auditory tube dysfunction (upper respiratory infection, allergies)
- Acute or chronic otitis media
- Mastoiditis
- Otosclerosis
- Disruption of ossicles
- Trauma or barotrauma
- Glomus tympanicum (middle ear tumor)
- Paget's disease

Sensory
- Presbycusis (age-related)
- Excessive noise exposure
- Ménière's disease (endolymphatic hydrops)

- Labyrinthitis
- Head trauma
- Ototoxicity, eg, salicylates, aminoglycosides, loop diuretics, cisplatin
- Occlusion of ipsilateral auditory artery (acute)
- Hereditary hearing loss
- Autoimmune: systemic lupus erythematosus, Wegener's granulomatosis, Cogan's syndrome
- Other systemic causes: diabetes mellitus, hypothyroidism, hyperlipidemia, renal failure, infections (eg, measles, mumps, syphilis)

Neural
- Acoustic neuroma
- Multiple sclerosis
- Cerebrovascular disease

Heart sound, fixed split S2

- Atrial septal defect

Heart sound, loud P2

- Pulmonary hypertension

Heart sound, loud S1

- Mitral stenosis
- Short PR interval

Heart sound, paradoxically split S2 (or no split)

- Aortic stenosis
- Left ventricular failure
- Left bundle branch block

Heart sound, S3

- Normal (eg, young or pregnant)
- Congestive heart failure
- Volume overload

Heart sound, S4

- Normal (especially athletes)
- Hypertensive
- Coronary artery disease
- Aortic stenosis
- Cardiomyopathy

Heart sound, widely split S2

- Right bundle branch block

Heartburn

- Gastroesophageal reflux disease (most common)
- Hiatal hernia (causing gastroesophageal reflux)
- Gastritis
- Peptic ulcer disease
- Functional or nonulcer dyspepsia
- Esophagitis, eg, candidiasis
- Angina pectoris
- Cholelithiasis
- Esophageal motility disorder

Heel pain

- Plantar fasciitis
- Enthesopathy due to seronegative spondyloarthropathy (eg, ankylosing spondylitis)
- Achilles tendinitis
- Metatarsal stress fracture
- Retrocalcaneal bursitis
- Tarsal tunnel syndrome
- Genital herpes simplex (referred pain from sacral ganglion)

Hematochezia

- Gastrointestinal (lower) bleeding
- Gastrointestinal (upper) bleeding (massive)

Hematuria

- Cystitis
- Urinary calculi
- Benign prostatic hyperplasia (usually microscopic hematuria)
- Renal cell carcinoma
- Transitional cell carcinoma (urethra, bladder, ureter, or renal pelvis)
- Glomerulonephritis, eg, IgA nephropathy
- Polycystic kidney disease
- Anticoagulant use
- Prostate cancer
- Papillary necrosis, eg, NSAID overuse, diabetes mellitus, sickle cell trait or disease
- Renal infarction
- Interstitial nephritis
- Medullary sponge kidney
- Radiation or chemical cystitis, eg, cyclophosphamide
- Atrophic vaginitis (usually microscopic hematuria)
- Schistosomiasis
- Menses

Hemoglobinuria

Etiology
- Hemolysis, eg, thrombotic thrombocytopenia purpura, prosthetic heart valve, march hemoglobinuria
- Paroxysmal nocturnal hemoglobinuria

Hemoptysis

Airways
- Bronchitis
- Bronchiectasis
- Bronchogenic carcinoma

Pulmonary vasculature
- Left-sided congestive heart failure
- Mitral stenosis
- Pulmonary embolism
- Arteriovenous malformation

Pulmonary parenchyma
- Pneumonia
- Lung abscess
- Tuberculosis
- Aspergilloma
- Parasites, eg, paragonimiasis, ascariasis, hookworm, strongyloidiasis
- Goodpasture's syndrome
- Wegener's granulomatosis
- Systemic lupus erythematosus
- Crack cocaine inhalation
- Idiopathic pulmonary hemosiderosis
- Leukemia

Iatrogenic
- Transbronchial lung biopsy
- Anticoagulation
- Pulmonary artery rupture by PA line

Hepatic failure, acute

Etiology
- Viral: hepatitis B (common), hepatitis A, hepatitis D (in presence of B), hepatitis E (especially in pregnancy), hepatitis C (rare), herpes virus simplex, cytomegalovirus, infectious mononucleosis, parvovirus B19
- Toxins (predictable): acetaminophen (common), *Amanita* mushrooms, tetracycline, valproic acid, carbon tetrachloride
- Toxins (idiosyncratic): INH, NSAIDs, halothane, ecstasy, kava
- Vascular: right-sided congestive heart failure, shock liver, portal vein thrombosis, Budd-Chiari syndrome
- Metabolic & other: Wilson's disease, acute fatty liver of pregnancy, HELLP

syndrome, Reye's syndrome, hyperthermia or hypothermia, lymphoma

Hepatitis, acute

Etiology

Causes of acute hepatitis

- Viral: hepatitis A, hepatitis B, hepatitis C, hepatitis D (in presence of B), hepatitis E, infectious mononucleosis, cytomegalovirus, herpes simplex virus, parvovirus B19
- Other infections, eg, leptospirosis, secondary syphilis, brucellosis, Q fever
- Alcoholic hepatitis
- Toxins (predictable): acetaminophen, *Amanita* mushrooms, tetracycline, valproic acid
- Toxins (idiosyncratic): INH, NSAIDs, statins, azole antifungals, halothane, ecstasy, kava
- Vascular: right-sided congestive heart failure, shock liver, portal vein thrombosis, Budd-Chiari syndrome
- Metabolic: Wilson's disease, acute fatty liver of pregnancy, Reye's syndrome
- Autoimmune hepatitis
- Lymphoma or metastatic cancer

Causes of cholestasis (selected)

- Extrahepatic: choledocholithiasis, pancreatic tumor, biliary stricture, primary sclerosing cholangitis (intra- and extra-hepatic)
- Intrahepatic: primary biliary cirrhosis, autoimmune cholangitis, infiltrative disease (eg, tuberculosis, sarcoidosis, lymphoma, amyloidosis), drugs

Hepatitis, chronic

Etiology

- Viral: hepatitis B, hepatitis C, hepatitis D (in presence of B)
- Alcoholic cirrhosis
- Genetic and metabolic: hemochromatosis, Wilson's disease, alpha-1-antiprotease deficiency
- Autoimmune hepatitis
- Chronic hepatitis due to drugs, eg, nitrofurantoin, methyldopa, INH

Hepatomegaly

- Viral, eg, hepatitis A, hepatitis B, hepatitis C, hepatitis E, infectious mononucleosis, cytomegalovirus
- Bacterial, eg, leptospirosis, brucellosis
- Protozoal and helminthic, eg, malaria, leishmaniasis, amebiasis, schistosomiasis, toxoplasmosis, fascioliasis, clonorchiasis, filariasis
- Alcoholic hepatitis
- Toxic hepatitis
- Fatty liver
- Cirrhosis
- Congestive heart failure
- Hepatocellular carcinoma or metastatic cancer
- Leukemia or myeloproliferative disease
- Hemochromatosis
- Primary biliary cirrhosis
- Budd-Chiari syndrome
- Autoimmune hepatitis
- Infiltrative disease, eg, sarcoidosis, amyloidosis
- Carcinoma of the biliary tract
- Normal variant, eg, Riedel's lobe
- Sickle cell disease
- Polycystic disease of the liver
- Glycogen storage disease

Hiccups (singultus)

Self-limited

- Idiopathic
- Gastric distension, eg, carbonated beverage, air swallowing, overeating
- Sudden temperature changes, eg, hot then cold beverage, hot then cold shower
- Alcohol ingestion
- Excitement, stress, or laughing

Recurrent or persistent

- CNS: neoplasm, infection, stroke, trauma
- Metabolic: uremia, hypocapnia (hyperventilation)
- Vagus or phrenic nerve irritation:
  - Head & neck: ear foreign body, goiter, neoplasm
  - Thorax: pneumonia, empyema, neoplasm, myocardial infarction, pericarditis, aneurysm, esophageal obstruction, reflux esophagitis
  - Abdomen: subphrenic abscess, hepatomegaly, hepatitis, cholecystitis, gastric distension, gastric neoplasm, pancreatitis, pancreatic malignancy
- Surgical: general anesthesia, postoperative
- Psychogenic
- Idiopathic

Hip pain

- Hip joint arthritis, eg, osteoarthritis, rheumatoid arthritis, septic arthritis, gout
- Trochanteric bursitis
- Hip fracture
- Sciatica
- Sacroiliitis, eg, ankylosing spondylitis
- Lumbar facet joint degenerative arthritis
- Lumbar disk herniation
- Ischial bursitis
- Piriformis syndrome
- Iliopsoas bursitis
- Claudication (arterial insufficiency)
- Polymyalgia rheumatica
- Fibromyalgia
- Meralgia paresthetica (compression of lateral femoral cutaneous nerve; anterolateral thigh pain)
- Avascular necrosis
- Hip dislocation

Hirsutism & virilization

- Idiopathic or familial
- Polycystic ovary syndrome
- Drugs, eg, minoxidil, cyclosporine, phenytoin, anabolic steroids, diazoxide, some progestins
- Congenital adrenal hyperplasia (may be late-onset)
- Ovarian tumor or adrenal tumor
- Adrenocorticotrophic hormone-induced Cushing's syndrome

Hoarseness

- Laryngitis
- Voice overuse
- Vocal cord nodules, polyps, or papillomas
- Laryngeal cancer
- Lung cancer (with paralysis of recurrent laryngeal nerve)
- Unilateral vocal cord paralysis
- Hypothyroidism
- Substernal goiter, thyroiditis, multinodular goiter, or thyroid cancer
- Gastroesophageal reflux
- Angioedema

Horner's syndrome

Etiology

- Pancoast tumor (lung cancer)
- Neck trauma or tumor
- Lung abscess or tuberculoma
- Internal carotid dissection
- Brainstem infarct (Wallenberg or lateral medullary syndrome)

- Demyelinating disease, eg, multiple sclerosis
- Syringomyelia
- Cluster headache
- Substernal goiter

Hyperacusis

- Idiopathic
- Hearing loss (recruitment causing sensitivity to loud sounds despite reduced sensitivity to softer ones)
- Bell's palsy
- Migraine
- Adrenal insufficiency

Hypercoagulable state

Etiology

Acquired

- Immobility or postoperative state
- Cancer
- Inflammatory disorders, eg, ulcerative colitis
- Myeloproliferative disorder, eg, polycythemia vera, essential thrombocytosis
- Estrogens, pregnancy
- Heparin-induced thrombocytopenia
- Lupus anticoagulant
- Anticardiolipin antibodies
- Nephrotic syndrome
- Paroxysmal nocturnal hemoglobinuria
- Disseminated intravascular coagulation
- Congestive heart failure

Congenital

- Factor V Leiden
- Prothrombin 20210 mutation
- Antithrombin III deficiency
- Protein C deficiency
- Protein S deficiency
- Hyperhomocysteinemia
- Dysfibrinogenemia
- Abnormal plasminogen

Hyperglycemia

Etiology

Endocrinopathies

- Diabetes mellitus, Cushing's syndrome, acromegaly, pheochromocytoma, glucagonoma, somatostatinoma

Drugs

- Glucocorticoids, thiazides, phenytoin, niacin, oral contraceptives, pentamidine

Pancreatic insufficiency

- Subtotal pancreatectomy, chronic pancreatitis, hemochromatosis ("bronze diabetes"), cystic fibrosis, hemosiderosis

Other

- Gestational diabetes, cirrhosis, Schmidt syndrome (polyglandular failure: Addison's disease, autoimmune thyroiditis, diabetes)

Hyperhidrosis

- Anxiety
- Idiopathic
- Hyperthyroidism
- Infection or malignancy
- Hypoglycemia
- Menopause
- Pheochromocytoma
- Reflex sympathetic dystrophy

Hyperpigmentation

- Pigmented nevi
- Ephelides (juvenile freckles)
- Lentigines (senile freckles, liver spots)
- Postinflammatory (eg, acne, atopic dermatitis)
- Chronic venous insufficiency
- Melasma (chloasma)
- Neurofibromatosis (café au lait spots, axillary freckling)
- Hemochromatosis
- Addison's disease
- Acanthosis nigricans
- Hyperbilirubinemia (eg, primary biliary cirrhosis)
- Ochronosis (alkaptonuria)
- Pellagra (niacin deficiency)
- Porphyria cutanea tarda
- Wilson's disease
- Whipple's disease
- Scleroderma
- Vitamin B_{12} deficiency
- Folic acid deficiency
- Medications: chloroquine, chlorpromazine, minocycline, amiodarone
- Topicals: benzoyl peroxide, tretinoin, fluorouracil
- Fixed drug eruption to laxatives (phenolphthalein), trimethoprim-sulfamethoxazole, NSAIDs, tetracyclines
- Exogenous pigment exposure: carotenemia, argyria, gold, tattooing, arsenic
- Berloque hyperpigmentation (phototoxicity form citrus or celery)

- Visceral leishmaniasis (kala azar)
- POEMS syndrome (polyneuropathy, organomegaly, endocrinopathy, monoclonal gammopathy, skin changes)

Hypersensitivity pneumonitis

- Sarcoidosis
- Asthma
- Atypical pneumonia
- Collagen vascular disease, eg, systemic lupus erythematosus
- Idiopathic pulmonary fibrosis
- Lymphoma

Etiology

- Farmer's lung (moldy hay)
- Humidifier lung (contaminated humidifier, heating, or air conditioning)
- Bird fancier's lung (pigeon breeder's disease)
- Bagassosis (moldy sugar cane fiber)
- Sequoiosis (moldy redwood sawdust)
- Maple bark stripper's disease
- Mushroom picker's disease (moldy compost)
- Suberosis (moldy cork dust)
- Detergent worker's lung (enzyme additives)

Hypersomnia

- Insomnia of any cause limiting nighttime sleep
- Inadequate sleep time (lifestyle)
- Sleep apnea
- Narcolepsy
- Primary insomnia (primary CNS hypersomnolence)
- Drugs, eg, sedatives, opiates
- Depression
- Hypothyroidism
- Kleine-Levin syndrome

Hypertension

- Essential hypertension
- "White-coat" hypertension
- Cuff too small

Secondary hypertension

Adrenal

- Primary hyperaldosteronism, Cushing's syndrome, pheochromocytoma

Renal

- Chronic renal disease, renal artery stenosis (atherosclerotic or fibromuscular dysplasia), polyarteritis nodosa

Other
- Oral contraceptives, alcohol, NSAIDs, pregnancy-associated, hypercalcemia, hyperthyroidism, obstructive sleep apnea, obesity, coarctation of the aorta, acromegaly, increased intracranial pressure

Hyperthermia

Etiology

- Heat stroke
- Neuroleptic malignant syndrome
- Malignant hyperthermia (anesthetic-associated)
- Serotonin syndrome, eg, SSRI used with monoamine oxidase inhibitor
- Other drugs: anticholinergics, antihistamines, tricyclic antidepressants, monoamine oxidase inhibitors, salicylates, amphetamines, cocaine, PCP, LSD
- Thyrotoxicosis
- Prolonged seizures

Hyperuricemia, endogenous

Etiology

Primary hyperuricemia
Increased production of purine
- Idiopathic
- Specific enzyme defects (eg, Lesch-Nyhan syndrome, glycogen storage diseases)

Decreased renal clearance of uric acid (idiopathic)

Secondary hyperuricemia
Increased purine catabolism and turnover
- Myeloproliferative disorders (eg, chronic myelogenous leukemia)
- Lymphoproliferative disorders (eg, non-Hodgkin's lymphoma)
- Carcinoma and sarcoma (disseminated)
- Chronic hemolytic anemias
- Cytotoxic drugs
- Psoriasis

Decreased renal clearance of uric acid
- Intrinsic kidney disease
- Functional impairment of tubular transport:
  - Drug-induced (eg, thiazides, probenecid)
  - Hyperlacticacidemia (eg, lactic acidosis, alcoholism)

- Hyperketoacidemia (eg, diabetic ketoacidosis, starvation)
- **Diabetes insipidus** (vasopressin-resistant)
- Bartter's syndrome

Hyperventilation

Etiology

- Anxiety
- Hypoxemia
- Acidemia
- Pregnancy
- Obstructive lung disease
- Interstitial lung disease
- Sepsis
- Hepatic failure
- Fever
- Pain
- Central neurogenic hyperventilation (in comatose)

Hypoglycemia

Etiology

- Surreptitious or excess use of insulin or sulfonylurea
- Liver failure
- Acute alcohol intoxication
- Renal failure
- Sepsis
- Hypopituitarism
- Adrenal insufficiency
- Myxedema
- Insulinoma (pancreatic B cell tumor)
- Postprandial (reactive) hypoglycemia: postgastrectomy, occult diabetes, idiopathic
- Drugs: pentamidine, sulfamethoxazole (eg, TMP-SMX), quinine
- Extrapancreatic tumors (rare): hepatocellular carcinoma, retroperitoneal sarcoma, adrenocortical carcinoma
- Anti-insulin antibodies or antibodies to insulin receptors (very rare)

Hypogonadism, male

Etiology

Hypogonadotropic (low or normal LH)
- Hypopituitarism, eg, pituitary adenoma
- Cushing's syndrome
- Hypothyroidism
- Hyperprolactinemia

- Hemochromatosis
- Estrogen-secreting tumor (testicular, adrenal)
- Idiopathic
- GnRH agonist therapy, eg, leuprolide
- Drugs: alcohol, ketoconazole, spironolactone, marijuana, prior androgens, phenytoin, cimetidine, intrathecal opioids
- Anorexia nervosa
- Cirrhosis
- Serious illness or malnutrition
- Kallmann syndrome
- Prader-Willi syndrome

Hypergonadotropic (primary testicular failure; high LH)
- Male climacteric (andropause or male menopause)
- Orchitis, eg, mumps, gonorrhea, tuberculosis, leprosy
- Radiation therapy
- Cancer chemotherapy
- Klinefelter syndrome
- Autoimmune
- Uremia
- Testicular trauma or torsion
- Lymphoma
- Myotonic dystrophy
- Androgen insensitivity
- Idiopathic

Hypopigmentation or depigmentation

- Postinflammatory (eg, acne, atopic dermatitis)
- Vitiligo
- Albinism
- Tinea versicolor (pityriasis versicolor)
- Pityriasis alba (pityriasis simplex)
- Seborrheic dermatitis
- Piebaldism (white forelock)
- Tuberous sclerosis
- Halo nevi or halo around melanoma
- Leukoderma
- Liquid nitrogen treatment
- Intralesional corticosteroids
- Morphea (localized scleroderma)
- Lichen sclerosis
- Hansen's disease (leprosy)

Hypopituitarism

- Anorexia nervosa (hypogonadotropic hypogonadism)

- Serious illness (hypogonadotropic hypogonadism, functional suppression of TSH and thyroxine)
- Severe malnutrition (hypogonadotropic hypogonadism)
- Hypothyroidism
- Addison's disease
- High-dose glucocorticoids (secondary adrenal insufficiency for months)
- Cachexia due to other causes (eg, carcinoma, tuberculosis)
- Empty sella syndrome

Etiology

Mass lesions
- Pituitary adenoma (prolactinoma, nonfunctioning, growth hormone-secreting)
- Granuloma
- Brain tumor (eg, craniopharyngioma, meningioma, germinoma, glioma, chondrosarcoma, chordoma of the clivus)
- Rathke's cleft cyst
- Intracranial aneurysm
- Pituitary apoplexy (hemorrhage in pituitary tumor)
- Metastatic carcinoma

Without mass lesion
- Idiopathic
- Trauma
- Cranial irradiation
- Hemochromatosis
- Sarcoidosis
- Surgery
- Encephalitis
- Autoimmune
- Stroke
- Status post–coronary artery bypass graft
- Postpartum pituitary necrosis (Sheehan's syndrome)
- Langerhans cell histiocytosis
- Eclampsia-preeclampsia
- Sickle cell disease
- African trypanosomiasis

Hypotension or shock

Low stroke volume
- Hypovolemia, eg, hemorrhage, vomiting, diarrhea, burns, "third spacing"
- Pneumothorax
- Pulmonary embolism
- Cardiac tamponade
- "Pump failure" due to myocardial ischemia or cardiomyopathy
- Aortic stenosis

- Aortic insufficiency
- Mitral regurgitation
- Aortic dissection
- Rupture of ventricular septum or free wall

Abnormal heart rate
- Bradycardia
- Tachycardia

Low systemic vascular resistance
- Sepsis
- Adrenal insufficiency
- Anaphylaxis
- Drugs, eg, vasodilators
- Neurogenic shock

Hypothermia

Etiology
- Cold exposure including drowning
- Infection
- Other causes of altered mental status, eg, hypoglycemia, drugs, stroke
- Hypothyroidism
- Anorexia or malnutrition (poor fat stores)
- Adrenal insufficiency
- Burns
- Spinal cord injury

Hypothermia of extremities

Etiology
- Cold exposure
- Raynaud's syndrome
- Polyarteritis nodosa
- Reflex sympathetic dystrophy
- Thoracic outlet syndrome
- Acrocyanosis (vasospastic disorder)
- Chilblain (erythema pernio)
- Chilblain lupus erythematosus

Hypoventilation, chronic

Etiology
- Obstructive or central sleep apnea
- Obesity-hypoventilation syndrome (Pickwickian syndrome)
- Central alveolar hypoventilation (brainstem disorder)
- Primary alveolar hypoventilation (Ondine's curse)
- Neuromuscular disorder, eg, myasthenia gravis, poliomyelitis, spinal cord trauma
- Chronic obstructive pulmonary disease

- Chronic hypnotic use

Hypoxia and normal CXR

- Asthma
- Pulmonary embolism
- Early pneumonia
- Early interstitial lung disease
- Early pneumocystis pneumonia
- Shunt, eg, atrial or ventricular septal defect, atrioventricular malformation, atelectasis
- Pulmonary hypertension
- Chronic alveolar hypoventilation

Immobility (especially in elderly)

- Weakness, eg, disuse, anemia, malnutrition, electrolyte abnormality, neurologic disorder, myopathy
- Stiffness, eg, arthritis, parkinsonism, polymyalgia rheumatica
- Bone pain, eg, vertebral fracture, metastases, Paget's disease
- Joint pain, eg, arthritis, hip fracture
- Bursa or muscle pain, eg, bursitis, polymyalgia rheumatica, claudication, pseudoclaudication (spinal stenosis)
- Foot pain, eg, ingrown nail, plantar warts, bunions, calluses & corns
- Imbalance (often multifactorial):
  - Neurologic disease, eg, stroke, cervical myelopathy, peripheral neuropathy, vestibular or cerebellar disorder
  - Orthostatic or postprandial hypotension
  - Drugs, eg, antihypertensives, diuretics, sedatives, neuroleptics, antidepressants
- Anxiety or depression

Infertility, female

- Male factor, eg, hypogonadism, varicocele, alcohol or drug use, immotile cilia syndrome
- Polycystic ovary syndrome
- Premature ovarian failure
- Hyperprolactinemia
- Hypothyroidism
- Inadequate luteal progesterone or short luteal phase
- Endometriosis
- Uterine leiomyomas (fibroids) or polyps
- Prior pelvic inflammatory disease

- Pelvic adhesions, eg, pelvic surgery, therapeutic abortion, ectopic pregnancy, septic abortion, intrauterine device use
- Cervical factors, eg, unfavorable mucus, antisperm antibodies

Infertility, male

- Female infertility
- Erectile dysfunction
- Hypogonadism (deficient testosterone from primary or secondary testicular failure)
- Spermicidal lubricants
- Cryptorchism
- Epididymitis
- Retrograde ejaculation, eg, diabetic neuropathy
- Varicocele
- Ejaculatory duct obstruction
- Vas deferens obstruction
- Absent seminal emission from sympathetic nerve injury, eg, pelvic or retroperitoneal surgery
- Hernia repair damaging vas deferens or testicular blood supply
- Drugs: sulfasalazine, nitrofurantoin affect sperm motility (see also drugs in Hypogonadism)

Insomnia

- Acute: emotional stress, physical discomfort, jet lag
- Alcohol abuse
- Stimulants, eg, caffeine, nicotine, cocaine, pseudoephedrine
- Depression
- Poor sleep hygiene, eg, daytime naps, TV in bed
- Mania or bipolar disorder
- Medical illness, eg, chronic obstructive pulmonary disease, uremia, hyperthyroidism, hepatic encephalopathy, gastroesophageal reflux disease
- Nocturia, eg, diuretics, benign prostatic hyperplasia, urinary incontinence, congestive heart failure
- Restless leg syndrome
- Menopause
- CNS disease, eg, complex partial seizures, brain tumor, neurosyphilis
- Medications, eg, corticosteroids, SSRIs, theophylline, benzodiazepine withdrawal
- Circadian rhythm disorder

Interstitial lung disease

Etiology

Drug-related

- Amiodarone
- Antibacterials (nitrofurantoin, sulfonamides)
- Antineoplastics (bleomycin, cyclophosphamide, methotrexate, nitrosoureas)
- Antirheumatics (gold salts, penicillamine)
- Phenytoin

Environmental & occupational

- Inorganic dust (asbestos, silica, hard metals, beryllium)
- Organic dust or hypersensitivity pneumonitis (thermophilic actinomycetes, avian antigens, *Aspergillus* spp.)
- Gases, fumes, vapors (chlorine, isocyanates, paraquat, sulfur dioxide)
- Ionizing radiation
- Talc (injection drug users)

Infections

- Disseminated fungus (coccidioidomycosis, blastomycosis, histoplasmosis)
- Disseminated mycobacteria
- *Pneumocystis* pneumonia
- Viruses

Primary pulmonary syndromes

- Idiopathic fibrosing interstitial pneumonia [idiopathic pulmonary fibrosis (IPF)]:
  - Acute interstitial pneumonitis
  - Desquamative interstitial pneumonia
  - Nonspecific interstitial pneumonitis
  - Usual interstitial pneumonia
  - Respiratory bronchiolitis-associated interstitial lung disease
- Bronchiolitis obliterans-organizing pneumonia

Systemic disorders

- Acute respiratory distress syndrome
- Amyloidosis
- Ankylosing spondylitis
- Autoimmune disease: dermatomyositis, polymyositis, rheumatoid arthritis, systemic sclerosis (scleroderma), systemic lupus erythematosus
- Chronic eosinophilic pneumonia
- Goodpasture's syndrome
- Idiopathic pulmonary hemosiderosis
- Inflammatory bowel disease
- Eosinophilic granuloma (Langerhans cell histiocytosis, histiocytosis X)
- Lymphangitic carcinomatosis

- Lymphangioleiomyomatosis
- Pulmonary edema
- Pulmonary venous hypertension
- Sarcoidosis
- Wegener's granulomatosis

Interstitial nephritis

- Acute tubular necrosis
- Acute glomerulonephritis
- Prerenal azotemia
- Chronic glomerulopathy, eg, diabetic nephropathy
- Hypertensive nephrosclerosis
- Obstructive uropathy

Etiology

Acute

- Antibiotics: β-lactams, sulfa, ciprofloxacin, erythromycin, tetracycline, vancomycin, rifampin, ethambutol
- NSAIDs
- Diuretics: thiazides, furosemide
- Other drugs: phenytoin, allopurinol, cimetidine
- Infections: *Streptococcus*, leptospirosis, cytomegalovirus, Epstein-Barr virus, histoplasmosis, Rocky Mountain spotted fever, *Legionella*, *Mycoplasma*, *Toxoplasma*
- Immune: Systemic lupus erythematosus, Sjögren's syndrome, sarcoidosis, cryoglobulinemia

Chronic

- Obstructive uropathy
- Vesicoureteral reflux (reflux nephropathy)
- Analgesic nephropathy
- Heavy metals: lead, cadmium, mercury, bismuth
- Multiple myeloma
- Gout

Intestinal ischemia, acute

- Diverticulitis
- Appendicitis
- Peptic ulcer disease or gastritis
- Acute pancreatitis or cholecystitis
- Myocardial infarction
- Vasculitis, eg, polyarteritis nodosa

Etiology

- Emboli, eg, atrial fibrillation

- Thrombosis of mesenteric vessel
- Low flow due to congestive heart failure or arterial spasm (eg, ergotamine or cocaine)
- Mesenteric vein occlusion
- Postcoarctectomy syndrome (mesenteric vasoconstriction after coarctation repair)

Intestinal ischemia, chronic

- Peptic ulcer disease
- Gastroesophageal reflux disease
- Chronic pancreatitis
- Irritable bowel syndrome
- Visceral malignancy
- Vasculitis, eg, polyarteritis nodosa

Etiology

- Atherosclerosis

Intracranial pressure, increased

Etiology

- Space-occupying lesion, eg, brain tumor, brain abscess
- Pseudotumor cerebri
- Subdural hematoma
- Meningitis
- Cerebral edema, eg, trauma, encephalitis, infarction
- Malignant hypertension
- Venous sinus thrombosis
- Dural arteriovenous malformation
- Hydrocephalus
- Neurocysticercosis

Intraocular pressure, increased

Etiology

- Acute (angle-closure) glaucoma
- Open-angle glaucoma (primary)
- Open-angle glaucoma secondary to uveitis, trauma
- Corticosteroids (topical or systemic)
- Ophthalmic zoster

Jaundice (icterus)

Hyperbilirubinemia

Unconjugated (indirect bilirubin)
- Increased production: hemolysis, hematoma, pulmonary infarction

- Impaired uptake and storage: posthepatitis hyperbilirubinemia, Gilbert's syndrome, Crigler-Najjar syndrome, drugs Conjugated (direct bilirubin)
- Biliary obstruction: choledocholithiasis, pancreatic tumor, biliary stricture, primary sclerosing cholangitis, biliary duct carcinoma
- Hepatocellular damage or intrahepatic cholestasis: hepatitis (eg, alcoholic, viral), hepatic cirrhosis, biliary cirrhosis, drugs, sepsis, cholangitis, liver abscess, Budd-Chiari syndrome, infectious mononucleosis, spirochetal infection, infiltrative disease (tuberculosis, sarcoidosis, lymphoma), industrial toxins
- Hereditary bilirubin excretion defect: Dubin-Johnson syndrome, Rotor's syndrome

Other causes of yellow skin

- Carotenemia (excessive beta-carotene ingestion, especially in hypothyroidism)

Jaundice in pregnancy

- Viral hepatitis (including herpes simplex virus-related)
- Acute fatty liver of pregnancy
- Choledocholithiasis
- Idiopathic cholestasis of pregnancy
- HELLP syndrome (hemolysis, elevated liver enzymes, low platelets)
- Primary biliary cirrhosis

Joint effusion by joint fluid type

Etiology

Group I: Noninflammatory (200–300 WBC, <25% PMNs)

- Osteoarthritis
- Trauma (may be hemorrhagic)
- Osteochondritis dissecans
- Osteochondromatosis
- Neuropathic arthropathy (may be hemorrhagic)
- Subsiding or early inflammation
- Hypertrophic osteoarthropathy (group I or II)
- Pigmented villonodular synovitis (may be hemorrhagic)

Group II: Inflammatory (3000–50,000 WBC, >50% PMNs)

- Rheumatoid arthritis
- Gout or pseudogout
- Reactive arthritis (Reiter's syndrome)

- Ankylosing spondylitis
- Psoriatic arthritis
- Arthritis accompanying inflammatory bowel disease
- Rheumatic fever (group I or II)
- Systemic lupus erythematosus (group I or II)
- Scleroderma (group I or II)
- Tuberculosis of bone and joints
- Mycotic infection

Group III: Purulent (>50,000 WBC, >75% PMNs)

- Pyogenic bacterial infection (septic arthritis)

Hemorrhagic

- Hemophilia or other bleeding disorder
- Trauma with or without fracture
- Neuropathic arthropathy
- Pigmented villonodular synovitis
- Synovioma
- Hemangioma and other benign neoplasms

Keratitis (corneal ulcer or inflammation)

- Corneal abrasion or foreign body
- Conjunctivitis
- Uveitis
- Acute glaucoma

Etiology

- Bacterial, eg, *Pseudomonas, Moraxella, Staphylococcus,* pneumococcus
- Herpes simplex keratitis
- Ophthalmic zoster
- Fungal keratitis
- *Acanthamoeba* keratitis
- Contact lenses (especially soft)
- Neurotrophic keratitis (lack of corneal sensation)
- Exposure keratitis (inadequate eyelid closure)
- Severe dry eyes
- Severe allergic eye disease
- Behçet's syndrome
- Topical steroids

Kidneys, large

- Diabetes mellitus
- Polycystic kidney disease
- HIV-associated nephropathy
- Amyloidosis

- Scleroderma
- Lymphoma
- Bilateral hydronephrosis

Knee effusion

Etiology

- Trauma, eg, fracture, ligament or meniscal injury, overuse syndrome
- Infection, eg, gonococcal arthritis, *Staphylococcus aureus* septic arthritis, Lyme disease, tuberculosis of bone and joints
- Gout or pseudogout
- Seronegative spondyloarthropathy, eg, reactive arthritis (Reiter's syndrome)
- Rheumatoid arthritis
- Osteoarthritis or inflammatory osteoarthritis
- Hemarthrosis due to bleeding disorder
- Malignant or benign tumor

Knee pain

- Patellofemoral syndrome
- Iliotibial band syndrome
- Patellar tendonitis
- Anserine bursitis
- Meniscus tear (medial > lateral)
- Medial or lateral collateral ligament strain or tear
- Cruciate ligament tear (anterior > posterior)
- Prepatellar bursitis
- Baker's (popliteal) cyst
- Arthritis, eg, osteoarthritis, rheumatoid arthritis, gout, pseudogout, septic arthritis, reactive arthritis (Reiter's syndrome)
- Medial plica syndrome
- Osgood-Schlatter disease
- Osteochondritis dissecans
- Neuropathic arthropathy (Charcot joint)
- Tumor, eg, osteosarcoma
- Referred pain from hip, eg, avascular necrosis
- Referred pain from back, eg, sciatica
- Fracture

Kussmaul's sign

- Constrictive pericarditis
- Restrictive cardiomyopathy

Laryngeal tumor

- Vocal cord nodules
- Vocal cord polyps
- Laryngeal papillomas
- Laryngeal granulomas
- Laryngeal leukoplakia
- Laryngeal squamous cell carcinoma

Leukoplakia (oral leukoplakia)

- Hyperkeratosis due to irritation, eg, dentures, tobacco, cheek biting
- Dysplasia or carcinoma
- Lichen planus
- Oral candidiasis
- Oral hairy leukoplakia
- White sponge nevus
- Secondary syphilis
- Necrotizing sialometaplasia
- Pseudoepitheliomatous hyperplasia

Lift, parasternal

- Right ventricular hypertrophy
- Cor pulmonale
- Pulmonary hypertension
- Left atrial enlargement
- Pulmonary stenosis

Limb ischemia, acute

- Lumbar spinal stenosis (neurogenic or pseudoclaudication)
- Musculoskeletal pain
- Peripheral neuropathy, eg, diabetes mellitus, alcoholism
- Osteomyelitis

Etiology

- Emboli, eg, atrial fibrillation, cholesterol emboli after aortic instrumentation
- Thrombosis
- Trauma
- Thromboangiitis obliterans (Buerger's disease)

Livedo reticularis

- Benign idiopathic
- Occult malignancy
- Polyarteritis nodosa
- Cholesterol emboli
- Antiphospholipid antibody syndrome
- Systemic lupus erythematosus

- Dermatomyositis
- Rheumatoid arthritis
- Thromboangiitis obliterans (Buerger's disease)

Liver mass

- Hepatocellular carcinoma
- Metastatic cancer
- Cavernous hemangioma
- Liver cell adenoma
- Cyst, eg, congenital, echinococcal (hydatid), associated with polycystic kidney disease
- Pyogenic liver abscess
- Amebic liver abscess
- Focal nodular hyperplasia

Low back pain

- Muscular strain
- Osteoarthritis
- Herniated disk
- Spinal stenosis
- Sciatica
- Sacroiliitis, eg, ankylosing spondylitis
- Rheumatoid arthritis
- Metastatic cancer
- Compression fracture, eg, osteoporosis, multiple myeloma
- Osteomyelitis or epidural abscess
- Cauda equina tumor
- Ischial bursitis
- Piriformis syndrome
- Fibromyalgia
- Polymyalgia rheumatica
- Aortic aneurysm
- Duodenal ulcer
- Urinary calculi or pyelonephritis
- Pancreatitis
- Prostatitis
- Hip osteoarthritis

Lung cavities, multiple

- Septic emboli
- Metastatic cancer
- Wegener's granulomatosis
- Tuberculosis
- Coccidioidomycosis

Lung cavity

- Lung abscess
- Tuberculosis

- Aspergilloma
- Mycetoma (eg, *Nocardia brasiliensis*)
- Lung cancer
- Lung infarction
- Wegener's granulomatosis
- Coccidioidomycosis
- Histoplasmosis

Lung disease, drug-induced

Etiology

- Asthma: beta blockers, aspirin, NSAIDs, histamine, methacholine, acetylcysteine, aerosolized pentamidine, any nebulized medication
- Chronic cough: ACE inhibitors
- Pulmonary infiltration:
  - with eosinophilia: amitriptyline, amiodarone
  - without eosinophilia: sulfonamides, penicillin, methotrexate, crack cocaine
- Drug-induced systemic lupus erythematosus: hydralazine, procainamide, isoniazid, chlorpromazine, phenytoin
- Interstitial pneumonitis/fibrosis: nitrofurantoin, cyclophosphamide, phenytoin
- Pulmonary edema: aspirin, chlordiazepoxide, cocaine, heroin
- Pleural effusion: bromocriptine, nitrofurantoin, any drug inducing systemic lupus erythematosus
- Mediastinal widening: phenytoin, corticosteroids, methotrexate
- Respiratory failure:
  - Neuromuscular blockade: aminoglycosides, succinylcholine
  - CNS depression: sedatives, opioids, alcohol, tricyclic antidepressants

Lung disease, lower lobe

- Alpha-1 antiprotease deficiency
- Asbestosis (parenchymal)
- Tuberculosis (primary)

Lung disease, upper lobe

- Silicosis
- Tuberculosis
- Ankylosing spondylitis
- Sarcoidosis
- Eosinophilic granuloma (Langerhans cell histiocytosis, histiocytosis X)
- Cystic fibrosis
- Hypersensitivity pneumonitis (extrinsic allergic alveolitis)
- Histoplasmosis

Lymphadenopathy, generalized

Infection

- Viral, eg, infectious mononucleosis (Epstein-Barr virus, cytomegalovirus), hepatitis, herpes simplex virus, varicella, rubella, acute HIV infection or AIDS
- Bacterial, eg, streptococci, staphylococci, cat-scratch disease, tuberculosis, syphilis, tularemia, chancroid, plague, leprosy
- Fungal, eg, histoplasmosis, coccidioidomycosis
- Chlamydial, eg, lymphogranuloma venereum
- Parasitic, eg, toxoplasmosis, leishmaniasis, trypanosomiasis, filariasis
- Rickettsial, eg, scrub typhus

Malignancy

- Hodgkin's or non-Hodgkin's lymphoma
- Leukemia
- Metastatic cancer
- Virchow's (left supraclavicular) node: GI (classically gastric) cancer
- Sister Mary Joseph (umbilical) node: GI cancer
- Right subclavian node: lung cancer

Immunologic disease

- Rheumatoid arthritis, systemic lupus erythematosus, dermatomyositis, Sjögren's syndrome
- Drug hypersensitivity
- Serum sickness

Other

- Sarcoidosis
- Amyloidosis
- Lipid storage disease, eg, Gaucher, Niemann-Pick
- Hyperthyroidism
- Castleman's disease (giant lymph node hyperplasia)
- Dermatopathic lymphadenitis
- Kikuchi's disease (histiocytic necrotizing lymphadenitis)
- Kawasaki syndrome
- Eosinophilic granuloma (Langerhans cell histiocytosis, histiocytosis X)
- Familial Mediterranean fever
- Drug-induced pseudolymphoma (classically phenytoin)

Lymphedema

Etiology

- Congenital
- Trauma
- Regional lymph node dissection
- Irradiation
- Bacterial or fungal infection
- Lymphoproliferative disease
- Filariasis

Lymphocytosis

Etiology

- Viral infection, eg, infectious mononucleosis
- Chronic lymphocytic leukemia
- Pertussis
- Lymphoma in leukemic phase

Macroglossia

- Amyloidosis
- Acromegaly
- Hypothyroidism
- Multiple myeloma
- Down syndrome
- Lymphoma
- Angioedema
- Hemangioma

Malabsorption

Etiology

- Small bowel: celiac sprue, Whipple's disease, tropical sprue, eosinophilic gastroenteritis, small bowel resection, Crohn's disease
- Lymphatic obstruction: lymphoma, carcinoid, tuberculosis, *Mycobacterium avium* complex, Kaposi's sarcoma, sarcoidosis, retroperitoneal fibrosis
- Pancreatic insufficiency: chronic pancreatitis, cystic fibrosis, pancreatic cancer
- Bacterial overgrowth, eg, diabetes
- Reduced bile salts: ileal resection, Crohn's disease, postcholecystectomy
- Strongyloidiasis

Malingering

- Factitious disorder (Munchausen syndrome)
- Somatoform disorder
- Organic disease producing symptoms

Mania

- Bipolar disorder (manic depression)
- Substance abuse, eg, cocaine, amphetamines

- Hypomania
- Cyclothymic disorder (depression and hypomania)
- Schizophrenia
- Hyperthyroidism
- Medications, eg, corticosteroids, thyroxine
- CNS disease, eg, complex partial seizures, brain tumor, neurosyphilis
- Personality disorder, eg, borderline, narcissistic

Mediastinal mass

Anterior
- Thymoma
- Teratoma
- Thyroid lesion
- Lymphoma
- Mesenchymal tumors (lipoma, fibroma)

Middle
- Lymphadenopathy
- Pulmonary artery enlargement
- Aneurysm of aorta or innominate artery
- Developmental cyst (bronchogenic, enteric, pleuropericardial)
- Dilated azygos or hemiazygos vein
- Foramen of Morgagni hernia

Posterior
- Hiatal hernia
- Neurogenic tumor (neurilemmoma, neurofibroma, neurosarcoma, ganglioneuroma, pheochromocytoma)
- Meningocele
- Esophageal tumor
- Foramen of Bochdalek hernia
- Thoracic spine disease
- Extramedullary hematopoiesis

Melena

- Gastrointestinal (upper or lower) bleeding
- Iron or bismuth subsalicylate ingestion (false melena)

Membranous nephropathy

Etiology
- Infections: Hepatitis B, endocarditis, syphilis, malaria
- Autoimmune: systemic lupus erythematosus, mixed connective tissue disease, thyroiditis
- Non-Hodgkin's lymphoma
- Carcinomas: colorectal, renal cell, bronchogenic, thyroid cancer
- Drugs: gold, penicillamine, captopril
- Idiopathic

Meningitis

- Subarachnoid hemorrhage
- Encephalitis
- "Neighborhood reaction" causing abnormal CSF, eg, brain abscess, epidural abscess, vertebral osteomyelitis, mastoiditis, sinusitis, brain tumor
- Dural sinus thrombosis
- Noninfectious meningeal irritation: carcinomatous meningitis, sarcoidosis, systemic lupus erythematosus, drugs (eg, NSAIDs, TMP-SMX), pneumonia, shigellosis
- If fever and rash: gonococcemia, infective endocarditis, thrombotic thrombocytopenic purpura, Rocky Mountain spotted fever, viral exanthem
- Seizure due to other causes, eg, febrile seizure
- Amebic meningoencephalitis (*Naegleria fowleri*)

Etiology

Purulent meningitis
- 18–50 years: *S. pneumoniae* (pneumococcal), *N. meningitidis* (meningococcal)
- >50 years: *S. pneumoniae* (pneumococcal), *N. meningitidis* (meningococcal), *Listeria*, gram-negative bacilli
- Impaired cellular immunity: *Listeria*, gram-negative bacilli, *S. pneumoniae* (pneumococcal)
- Postsurgical or posttraumatic: *S. aureus*, *S. pneumoniae* (pneumococcal), gram-negative bacilli

Aseptic meningitis
- Mumps, coxsackievirus, echoviruses
- Infectious mononucleosis
- Leptospirosis, syphilis, Lyme disease

Chronic meningitis
- Tuberculous meningitis or atypical mycobacteria
- Fungi: *Cryptococcus, Coccidioides, Histoplasma*
- Spirochetes: syphilis, Lyme disease, leptospirosis
- Other: brucellosis, HIV infection, neurocysticercosis

Menorrhagia

- Uterine leiomyomas (fibroids)
- Endometrial polyp
- Adenomyosis (uterine endometriosis)
- Bleeding disorder, eg, von Willebrand's disease, thrombocytopenia, leukemia
- Hypothyroidism

Metastases to bone

- Lung cancer
- Breast cancer
- Prostate cancer
- Multiple myeloma (not truly metastatic)
- Renal cell carcinoma
- Others: skin, oral, esophageal, cervical, gastric, colorectal, melanoma

Metastases to brain

- Parenchymal: lung cancer, breast cancer, renal cell carcinoma, gastrointestinal, melanoma, lymphoma
- Leptomeningeal: breast cancer, lymphoma, leukemia, prostate cancer

Metastases to kidney

- Cysts (simple, acquired, polycystic kidney disease, medullary sponge kidney, medullary cystic kidney)
- Renal cell carcinoma
- Metastases, eg, lung, breast, gastric, contralateral kidney
- Renal abscess
- Transitional cell carcinoma of renal pelvis
- Adrenal tumor
- Renal oncocytoma
- Renal angiomyolipoma
- Lymphoma
- Nephrolithiasis
- Renal infarction

Metastases to liver

- GI tract, eg, colorectal cancer
- Lung cancer
- Breast cancer
- Malignant melanoma
- Prostate cancer
- Thyroid cancer
- Skin cancer
- Carcinoid
- Most cancers can metastasize to liver

Metastases to lung

- Renal cell carcinoma
- Breast cancer
- Colon cancer

- Cervical cancer
- Malignant melanoma
- Almost every cancer can metastasize to lung

Metastases to meninges

- Leukemia or lymphoma
- Breast cancer
- Lung cancer
- Malignant melanoma
- Prostate cancer

Metastases to skin

- Metastatic melanoma
- Breast cancer
- Others: colorectal, lung, renal cell, bladder, ovarian, cervical, prostate

Methemoglobinemia

- Hypoxia, eg, congestive heart failure
- Right-to-left shunt, eg, arteriovenous fistula
- Cold exposure
- Sulfhemoglobinemia
- Carbon monoxide poisoning

Etiology

- Dapsone
- Benzocaine
- Pyridium
- Primaquine
- Sulfonamides
- Aniline
- Nitrites
- Nitrogen oxide gases
- Nitrobenzene

Microalbuminuria

Etiology

- Early proteinuria of any cause
- Acute hyperglycemia
- Urinary tract infection
- Marked hypertension
- Congestive heart failure
- Menses (false positive)

Microangiopathic hemolytic anemia

Etiology

- Thrombotic thrombocytopenic purpura

- Hemolytic uremic syndrome
- Disseminated intravascular coagulation
- Prosthetic valve hemolysis
- Metastatic adenocarcinoma
- Vasculitis
- Malignant hypertension
- HELLP syndrome (hemolysis, elevated liver enzymes, low platelets)

Midcycle spotting

- Ovulation bleeding (normal)
- Sexually transmitted disease
- Oral contraceptive pill (OCP) with low estrogen dose, first months of OCP use, or OCP not taken at same time each day
- Depo-Provera or intrauterine device use

Mitral regurgitation

- Aortic stenosis
- Aortic sclerosis
- Tricuspid regurgitation
- Hypertrophic obstructive cardiomyopathy
- Atrial septal defect
- Ventricular septal defect

Etiology

- Myxomatous degeneration (eg, mitral valve prolapse, Marfan syndrome)
- Infective endocarditis
- Subvalvular dysfunction (papillary muscle dysfunction or ruptured chordae tendinae)
- Rheumatic heart disease
- Dilated cardiomyopathy
- Congenital cleft mitral valve
- Left atrial myxoma (rare)

Mitral stenosis

- Mitral valve prolapse
- Atrial myxoma
- Cor triatriatum (congenital atrial anomaly)

Etiology

- Usually rheumatic heart disease
- Rarely: systemic lupus erythematosus, rheumatoid arthritis, mitral annular calcification, carcinoid, congenital

Murmur, diastolic

- Aortic regurgitation
- Mitral stenosis

- Tricuspid stenosis
- Patent ductus arteriosus (continuous murmur)
- Graham Steell murmur (pulmonary insufficiency secondary to pulmonary hypertension)

Murmur, systolic

- Aortic stenosis
- Aortic sclerosis
- Mitral regurgitation
- Mitral valve prolapse
- Flow murmur (anemia, pregnancy, hyperthyroidism, sepsis)
- Tricuspid regurgitation
- Hypertrophic obstructive cardiomyopathy (HOCM)
- Pulmonary stenosis
- Atrial septal defect
- Ventricular septal defect
- Coarctation of the aorta

Muscle cramps or tetany

Nocturnal leg cramps
- Idiopathic
- Diabetes
- Parkinson's disease
- CNS or spinal cord disease
- Peripheral neuropathy
- Hemodialysis
- Peripheral vascular disease
- Pregnancy
- Drugs: cisplatin, vincristine

Other causes of muscle cramps
- Muscle injury, eg, sports
- Dehydration
- Hypocalcemia, hypokalemia, hyponatremia, hypoglycemia, hyperkalemia, hypermagnesemia
- Alkalosis (eg, vomiting, hyperventilation)
- Arterial insufficiency (claudication)
- Restless leg syndrome
- Dystonia
- Hyperthyroidism
- Hypothyroidism
- Celiac disease
- Amyotrophic lateral sclerosis
- Black widow spider bite
- McArdle's disease (muscle fatigue, cramping, high CK)

Myelofibrosis

- Other myeloproliferative disorder, eg, chronic myelogenous leukemia
- Bone marrow infiltrative process, eg, metastatic cancer, tuberculosis, fungal infection
- Other causes of bone marrow fibrosis: Hodgkin's disease, hairy cell leukemia

Myocarditis, acute

- Angina or myocardial infarction
- Pneumonia
- Congestive heart failure

Etiology

Infectious myocarditis

- Viral, eg, coxsackie (most common), HIV
- Rickettsial, eg, scrub typhus, Rocky Mountain spotted fever, Q fever
- Diphtheria
- Chagas' disease
- Toxoplasmosis
- Trichinosis (*Trichinella* infection)

Drug-induced & toxic myocarditis

- Doxorubicin
- Emetine
- Catecholamines (eg, pheochromocytoma)
- Phenothiazines
- Lithium
- Chloroquine
- Disopyramide
- Antimony-containing compounds
- Arsenicals
- Hypersensitivity to sulfonamides, penicillins, aminosalicylic acid
- Radiation
- Cocaine

Myoclonus

Etiology

- Anoxic brain injury
- Epilepsy
- Uremic or hepatic encephalopathy
- Idiopathic
- Drugs, eg, levodopa, alcohol, drug withdrawal
- Lipid storage diseases
- Ramsay Hunt syndrome type II (rare degenerative disorder)
- Subacute sclerosing panencephalitis

- Creutzfeldt-Jakob disease
- Spinal cord lesion (segmental myoclonus)

Myopathy

Etiology

- Alcoholism
- Endocrine: hypothyroidism, hyperthyroidism, Cushing's syndrome
- Chronic hypokalemia
- Polymyositis
- Dermatomyositis
- HIV myopathy
- Hyperparathyroidism
- Muscular dystrophy, eg, Duchenne, Becker, limb-girdle, facioscapulohumeral
- Myotonic dystrophy
- Myotonia congenita
- Inclusion body myositis
- Mitochondrial myopathy
- Sarcoidosis
- Drugs: corticosteroids, statins, clofibrate, colchicine, chloroquine, zidovudine, emetine, aminocaproic acid, bretylium, penicillamine, drugs causing hypokalemia

Myositis

Muscle inflammation

- Polymyositis
- Dermatomyositis
- Systemic lupus erythematosus
- Scleroderma
- Sjögren's syndrome
- Inclusion body myositis
- Trichinosis (*Trichinella* infection)
- Sarcocystosis

Other causes of proximal muscle weakness

- Polymyalgia rheumatica
- Endocrine: hypothyroidism, hyperthyroidism, Cushing's syndrome
- Alcoholism
- Drugs: corticosteroids, statins, clofibrate, colchicine, chloroquine, emetine, aminocaproic acid, bretylium, penicillamine, drugs causing hypokalemia
- HIV myopathy
- Hyperparathyroidism
- Spinal stenosis
- Osteomalacia
- Mitochondrial myopathy

Nail disorders, miscellaneous

- Nail pitting: psoriasis, alopecia areata, hand eczema
- Beau's lines (transverse) after serious illness
- Longitudinal groove: genetic or trauma
- Nail atrophy: congenital, trauma, vascular or neuralgic disease
- Spoon nails: anemia
- Nail hyperpigmentation: zidovudine, doxorubicin, cyclophosphamide, bleomycin, daunorubicin, fluorouracil, hydroxyurea, melphalan, mechlorethamine, nitrosoureas

Nails, discolored or thick

- Onychomycosis (tinea unguium)
- Psoriasis
- Keratoderma blennorrhagica (with reactive arthritis or Reiter's syndrome)
- Crusted (Norwegian) scabies
- Lichen planus
- Allergy to nail polish or nail glue

Nails, distorted

- Chronic inflammation of nail matrix
- Warts, tumors, nevi, or cysts impinging on nail matrix
- Lichen planus
- Allergy to nail polish or nail glue
- Keratosis follicularis (Darier disease)

Nasal deformity or saddle nose

- Syphilis
- Wegener's granulomatosis
- Relapsing polychondritis
- Rhinophyma (rosacea)
- Trauma
- Nasopharyngeal carcinoma
- Polymorphic reticulosis (lethal midline granuloma)
- Mucocutaneous leishmaniasis
- Hansen's disease (leprosy)
- Paracoccidioidomycosis
- Sarcoidosis

Nasal polyps

- Idiopathic
- Cystic fibrosis

Nasal tumors

- Nasal polyps
- Inverted papilloma
- Juvenile angiofibroma
- Nasopharyngeal carcinoma (usually squamous cell, also adenocarcinoma, mucosal melanoma, sarcoma, non-Hodgkin's lymphoma)
- Wegener's granulomatosis
- Sarcoidosis
- Polymorphic reticulosis (lethal midline granuloma)

Nausea and vomiting

Infections
- Norwalk or rotavirus
- "Food poisoning" by toxins from *B. cereus, S. aureus, C. perfringens*
- Hepatitis A or B
- Meningitis or encephalitis
- Acute systemic infections

Hepatobiliary or pancreatic disease
- Acute pancreatitis
- Cholecystitis or cholelithiasis

Topical gastrointestinal irritants
- Alcohol, NSAIDs, oral antibiotics

Systemic drugs
- Antitumor chemotherapy
- Alcohol
- Calcium channel blockers
- Opioids

Mechanical obstruction
- Gastric outlet obstruction: peptic ulcer disease, malignancy, gastric volvulus
- Small intestine: adhesions, hernias, volvulus, Crohn's disease, carcinomatosis

Dysmotility
- Gastroparesis: diabetic, medications, postviral, postvagotomy
- Small intestine: scleroderma, amyloidosis, chronic intestinal pseudo-obstruction, familial myoneuropathies

Peritonitis
- Perforated viscus
- Appendicitis
- Spontaneous bacterial peritonitis

Vestibular disorders
- Labyrinthitis, Ménière's disease, motion sickness, migraine

Increased intracranial pressure
- CNS tumors
- Subdural or subarachnoid hemorrhage

Psychogenic
- Anticipatory vomiting
- Bulimia
- Psychiatric disorders

Other
- Myocardial infarction, hypercalcemia, kidney stones, pyelonephritis, diabetic ketoacidosis, uremia, pregnancy, radiation therapy, adrenal crisis, parathyroid disease, hypothyroidism, paraneoplastic syndrome

Neck mass

- Reactive lymphadenopathy, eg, pharyngitis, tuberculous lymphadenitis (scrofula), cat-scratch disease, Lyme disease
- Lymphoma
- Skin abscess
- Parotitis
- Goiter or thyroiditis
- Branchial cleft cyst
- Thyroglossal duct cyst
- Metastasis from squamous cell carcinoma in mouth, pharynx, larynx, upper esophagus
- Metastatic thyroid carcinoma
- Sarcoidosis
- Cervical rib
- Zenker's diverticulum
- Carotid artery aneurysm
- Carotid body tumor
- Autoimmune adenopathy
- Kikuchi's disease (histiocytic necrotizing lymphadenitis)
- Esophageal diverticulum

Neck pain

- Acute or chronic cervical strain, eg, poor sleeping posture, whiplash injury
- Osteoarthritis, eg, cervical spondylosis on x-ray
- Herniated disk (discogenic neck pain)
- Rheumatoid arthritis
- Ankylosing spondylitis
- Compression fracture
- Osteomyelitis
- Meningitis
- Metastatic cancer
- Spinal stenosis
- Fibromyalgia
- Deep neck infection, eg, Ludwig's angina
- Thyroiditis
- Shoulder disorder
- Subarachnoid hemorrhage
- Thoracic outlet syndrome
- Temporal (giant cell) arteritis
- Carotid artery aneurysm or carotid dissection
- If myelopathy (eg, bilateral upper extremity findings, lower extremity spasticity or weakness, bladder dysfunction): osteoarthritis, rheumatoid arthritis, ankylosing spondylitis, motor neuron disease, multiple sclerosis, spinal cord tumor, syringomyelia, tropical spastic paresis (HTLV-1)

Neck stiffness

- Meningitis
- Subarachnoid hemorrhage
- Cervical arthritis, eg, osteoarthritis, rheumatoid arthritis
- Cervical strain, eg, poor sleeping posture, whiplash injury
- Fibromyalgia
- Polymyalgia rheumatica
- Tetanus

Nephrotic syndrome

- Congestive heart failure
- Cirrhosis
- Venous insufficiency
- Protein-losing enteropathy
- Malnutrition
- Hypothyroidism

Etiology
- Diabetes mellitus
- Lupus nephritis
- Amyloidosis
- HIV-associated nephropathy
- Multiple myeloma
- Idiopathic
  - Membranous nephropathy
  - Minimal change disease
  - Focal segmental glomerulosclerosis
  - Membranoproliferative glomerulonephritis

Neurogenic bladder

- Stroke
- Multiple sclerosis
- Parkinson's disease
- Spinal cord lesion or injury
- Diabetes mellitus
- Pelvic surgery or trauma
- Tabes dorsalis (neurosyphilis)
- Herniated lumbar disk

Neutropenia

Etiology

Bone marrow disorders

- Aplastic anemia
- Drugs: sulfonamides, chlorpromazine, procainamide, penicillin, cephalosporins, cimetidine, methimazole, phenytoin, chlorpropamide, antiretrovirals
- Cyclic neutropenia
- Pure white cell aplasia
- "Chronic benign neutropenia" in African-American and other populations
- Congenital (rare)

Peripheral disorders

- Hypersplenism
- Sepsis
- Immune destruction, eg, systemic lupus erythematosus
- Felty's syndrome (with rheumatoid arthritis and splenomegaly)
- HIV infection
- Acute viral infection
- Large granular lymphocytosis

Neutrophilia

Etiology

- Bacterial infection
- Inflammation, eg, rheumatoid arthritis, inflammatory bowel disease
- Malignancy or myeloproliferative disorder, eg, chronic myelogenous leukemia
- Corticosteroid administration
- Physiologic stress

Nipple discharge

- Galactorrhea, eg, pregnancy, postpartum, hyperprolactinemia
- Mammary duct ectasia
- Intraductal papilloma
- Breast cancer
- Oral contraceptives or estrogen replacement
- Subareolar abscess
- Fibrocystic breast disease

Nipple or areolar lesions

- Atopic dermatitis (eczema)
- Contact or irritant dermatitis
- Trauma, eg, breast-feeding
- Breast abscess (mastitis)
- Candidiasis
- Seborrheic keratosis
- Fox-Fordyce spots (sebaceous glands)
- Breast cancer, especially Paget's disease
- Bowen's disease (squamous cell carcinoma in situ)

Nocturia

- Benign prostatic hyperplasia
- Congestive heart failure (fluid redistribution)
- Diabetes mellitus
- Diuretic use
- Cystitis
- Urinary incontinence
- Obstructive sleep apnea

Nodules, subcutaneous

- Rheumatoid nodules (rheumatoid arthritis or rheumatic fever)
- Erythema nodosum
- Gout
- Lipoma
- Coccidioidomycosis
- Endocarditis (Osler's nodes)
- Sarcoidosis
- Polyarteritis nodosa
- Foreign-body granuloma
- Sporotrichosis
- Subcutaneous granuloma annulare
- Lupus panniculitis
- Calcinosis cutis
- Parasites, eg, cysticercosis, loiasis, paragonimiasis, onchocerciasis

Nonalcoholic fatty liver disease

Etiology

- Obesity
- Diabetes mellitus
- Hypertriglyceridemia
- Corticosteroids
- Cushing's syndrome
- Starvation or rapid weight loss
- Hypobetalipoproteinemia
- Total parenteral nutrition
- Drugs: corticosteroids, amiodarone, tamoxifen
- Wilson's disease
- Jejunoileal bypass
- Poisons: carbon tetrachloride, yellow phosphorus
- Microvesicular steatosis (NAFLD usually macrovesicular): Reye's syndrome, valproic acid toxicity, tetracycline, acute fatty liver of pregnancy

Other causes of hepatomegaly

- Alcoholic fatty liver disease
- Hepatitis, eg, viral, alcoholic, toxic
- Cirrhosis
- Congestive heart failure
- Hepatocellular carcinoma or metastatic cancer

Obesity

- Increased caloric intake
- Fluid retention: congestive heart failure, cirrhosis, nephrotic syndrome
- Cushing's syndrome, eg, exogenous corticosteroids (central obesity)
- Hypothyroidism (edema and fat accumulation)
- Alcoholism (via hypercortisolism)
- Menopause (decreased metabolic rate)
- Polycystic ovary syndrome
- Syndrome X (obesity, diabetes, and hypertension)
- Insulinoma (hypoglycemia causing overeating)
- Insulin or thiazolidinedione therapy (worsen obesity)
- Other drugs, eg, antipsychotics, antidepressants
- Pregnancy
- Growth hormone deficiency
- Hypothalamic disorders
- Congenital leptin deficiency (morbid obesity)
- Defects in α-MSH (melanocortin 4) receptor (morbid obesity)
- Genetic syndromes of obesity and mental retardation
  - Prader-Willi syndrome (hypotonia, hypogonadism)
  - Laurence-Moon-Bardet-Biedl syndrome (polydactyly, renal anomalies, retinitis pigmentosa, hypogonadism)
  - Cohen's syndrome (microcephaly, hypotonia, short stature, ocular anomalies, neutropenia)
  - Biemond syndrome (diabetes mellitus, polydactyly, coloboma, facial anomalies, hypogonadism)

Obstruction of large intestine

Etiology

- Mechanical colonic obstruction, eg, malignancy, diverticulitis, volvulus, fecal impaction
- Toxic megacolon due to inflammatory bowel disease or *Clostridium difficile* colitis
- Megacolon due to Chagas' disease, Hirschsprung's disease (aganglionic), multiple sclerosis, sacral nerve damage, myxedema (hypothyroidism)
- Chronic intestinal pseudo-obstruction
- Acute colonic pseudo-obstruction (Ogilvie's syndrome), associated with:
  - Trauma, burns, or postoperative
  - Respiratory failure
  - Malignancy
  - Myocardial infarction or congestive heart failure
  - Pancreatitis
  - Stroke or subarachnoid hemorrhage
  - Intestinal ischemia
  - Drugs, eg, opioids, anticholinergics

Obstruction of small intestine

Etiology

- Mechanical obstruction of small intestine or proximal colon, eg, adhesions, volvulus, Crohn's disease
- Acute paralytic ileus due to:
  - GI or abdominal surgery
  - Peritoneal irritation, eg, peritonitis, pancreatitis, ruptured viscus
  - Severe medical illness, eg, sepsis, electrolyte abnormality
  - Drugs, eg, opioids, anticholinergics
  - Myxedema (hypothyroidism)
- Chronic intestinal pseudo-obstruction

Obstructive voiding symptoms

- Benign prostatic hyperplasia (especially with anticholinergics)
- Urethral stricture
- Neurogenic bladder
- Prostate cancer
- Bladder cancer

- Extrinsic compression, eg, pelvic or GI tumor, radiation-induced fibrosis
- Urethral carcinoma
- Meatal stenosis

Occupational pulmonary disease

Obstructive airway disorders
- Occupational asthma
- Industrial bronchitis
- Byssinosis (textile workers)

Toxic lung injury
- Smoke inhalation
- Toxic gas inhalation
- Silo-filler's disease

Lung cancer
- Asbestos, others

Pleural diseases
- Asbestos exposure
- Talc inhalation

Other
- Berylliosis

Odynophagia

- Infectious esophagitis: *Candida,* herpes simplex virus, cytomegalovirus
- Pill-induced esophagitis: NSAIDs, KCl, AZT, alendronate, iron, antibiotics
- Caustic esophageal injury (alkali or acid ingestion)
- Radiation esophagitis
- Reflux esophagitis

Olfactory dysfunction

- Anatomic blockage of nares, eg, polyps, septal deformity, nasal tumor
- Viral rhinitis
- Allergic rhinitis
- Idiopathic
- CNS tumor in olfactory groove (cribriform plate) or temporal lobe
- Head trauma
- Parkinson's disease
- Alzheimer's disease

Oligomenorrhea & amenorrhea

- Pregnancy
- Menopause or perimenopause
- Polycystic ovary syndrome

- Hypothalamic amenorrhea, eg, stress, weight change, exercise
- Hyperprolactinemia
- Hypothyroidism or hyperthyroidism
- Diabetes mellitus
- Premature ovarian failure
- Other endocrine causes: Cushing's syndrome, Addison's disease, hypopituitarism (pituitary tumor), androgen-secreting tumor (adrenal, ovarian), congenital adrenal hyperplasia, acromegaly, Turner syndrome
- Anorexia nervosa
- Endometrial scarring (Asherman's syndrome)
- Anabolic steroids

Onycholysis

- Excess water, soap, detergent, alkali
- Candidiasis
- Nail hardeners
- Photosensitive drug eruption
- Hyperthyroidism
- Hypothyroidism
- Keratoderma blennorrhagica (with reactive arthritis or Reiter's syndrome)
- Lichen planus
- Allergy to nail polish or nail glue

Opioid withdrawal

- Other drug withdrawal, eg, alcohol, benzodiazepines, amphetamines, cocaine
- Nausea or vomiting due to other causes
- Influenza or other viral syndrome

Optic disc swelling

- Glaucomatous cupping

Etiology

- Increased intracranial pressure (papilledema)
- Optic neuritis, eg, multiple sclerosis
- Anterior ischemic optic neuropathy, eg, temporal (giant cell) arteritis
- Severe hypertensive retinopathy
- Central retinal vein occlusion
- Posterior uveitis
- Posterior scleritis
- Optic disc drusen (pseudopapilledema)
- Optic nerve sheath meningioma
- Optic nerve infiltration by sarcoidosis, leukemia, or lymphoma

Optic neuritis

- Anterior ischemic optic neuropathy, eg, temporal (giant cell) arteritis
- Papilledema
- Retinal detachment
- Macular degeneration (exudative)
- Retinal artery or vein occlusion
- Vitreous hemorrhage
- Compressive lesion or intrinsic optic nerve tumor

Etiology

- Multiple sclerosis
- Viral infection, eg, measles, mumps, influenza, herpes zoster
- Autoimmune, eg, systemic lupus erythematosus
- Spread of inflammation from meninges, orbital tissues, paranasal sinuses

Oral lesions in HIV/AIDS

- Oral candidiasis
- Oral hairy leukoplakia
- Kaposi's sarcoma
- Necrotizing ulcerative periodontitis
- Oral ulcers: herpes simplex, aphthous ulcers, cytomegalovirus, histoplasmosis, herpes zoster, lymphoma

Oral ulcers

- Aphthous ulcer (canker sore, ulcerative stomatitis)
- Herpes simplex virus infection
- Erythema multiforme
- Drug reaction
- Pemphigus
- Bullous pemphigoid
- Systemic lupus erythematosus
- Lichen planus
- Coxsackievirus (herpangina, hand-foot-mouth disease)
- Acute HIV infection
- Parvovirus
- Varicella zoster
- Syphilis
- Oral candidiasis
- Behçet's syndrome
- Reactive arthritis
- Inflammatory bowel disease
- Squamous cell carcinoma
- Necrotizing ulcerative gingivostomatitis (Vincent's fusospirochetal disease)

Orthopnea or nocturnal dyspnea

- Congestive heart failure (left-sided)
- Asthma
- Gastroesophageal reflux disease
- Sleep apnea

Osmolar gap

Etiology

- Methanol
- Ethylene glycol
- Isopropyl alcohol
- Ethanol toxicity
- Acetone
- Propylene glycol
- Severe alcoholic or diabetic ketoacidosis
- Lactic acidosis

Otitis media, chronic

- Otitis externa
- Auditory (eustachian) tube dysfunction
- Mastoiditis
- Tympanosclerosis (scarred tympanic membrane)
- Referred pain: sinusitis, tooth pain
- Temporomandibular joint syndrome
- Foreign body
- Cholesteatoma
- Bullous myringitis
- Nasopharyngeal carcinoma

Ovarian tumor

- Benign ovarian tumor, eg, follicle cyst, corpus luteum cyst
- Malignant ovarian tumor
- Teratoma (usually benign)
- Tubo-ovarian abscess
- Endometriosis
- Colon cancer
- Ectopic pregnancy
- Metastases to ovary, eg, GI, breast
- Hydatidiform mole

Pain, chronic

- Major depressive disorder
- Somatoform disorder, eg, pain disorder associated with psychological factors
- Anxiety disorder, eg, general anxiety disorder, post-traumatic stress disorder
- Factitious disorder
- Malingering
- Organic disease producing symptoms

Palpitations

Cardiac

- Arrhythmia
- Valvular regurgitation

Noncardiac

- Exercise-associated
- Thyrotoxicosis
- Anemia
- Anxiety

Pancreatitis, acute

- Acute cholecystitis or cholangitis
- Penetrating duodenal ulcer
- Pancreatic pseudocyst
- Ischemic colitis
- Small bowel obstruction
- Abdominal aortic aneurysm
- Kidney stone
- Nonpancreatic causes of increased amylase

Etiology

- Gallstone
- Alcohol
- Hypertriglyceridemia
- Hypercalcemia
- Abdominal trauma or surgery
- Post-ERCP
- Drugs, eg, azathioprine, mercaptopurine, pentamidine, didanosine (ddI), valproic acid, tetracycline, estrogen, sulfonamides, thiazides, glucocorticoids
- Viral, eg, mumps, HIV
- Vasculitis
- Pregnancy
- Pancreas divisum
- Penetrating duodenal ulcer
- Pancreatic cancer
- Parasites, eg, *Clonorchis, Ascaris*
- Peritoneal dialysis
- Cardiopulmonary bypass

Pancreatitis, chronic

- Cholelithiasis
- Diabetes mellitus
- Malabsorption due to other causes
- Intractable duodenal ulcer
- Pancreatic cancer
- Irritable bowel syndrome

Etiology

- Alcoholism
- Chronic pancreatic obstruction by stricture, stone, or tumor
- Hyperparathyroidism
- Hereditary pancreatitis
- Abdominal trauma
- Tropical pancreatitis (tropical Africa & Asia)
- Autoimmune chronic pancreatitis
- Idiopathic

Pancytopenia

Etiology

Bone marrow disorders

- Aplastic anemia
- Myelodysplastic syndrome
- Acute leukemia
- Myelofibrosis
- Infiltrative disease: lymphoma, myeloma, carcinoma, hairy cell leukemia
- Megaloblastic anemia
- Paroxysmal nocturnal hemoglobinuria
- Bone marrow irradiation
- Genetic, eg, Fanconi's anemia

Nonmarrow disorders

- Hypersplenism
- Systemic lupus erythematosus
- Infection: tuberculosis, AIDS, leishmaniasis, brucellosis, histoplasmosis. (Viruses causing aplastic anemia: hepatitis, Epstein-Barr virus, HIV, parvovirus B19)

Panic

- Supraventricular tachycardia or angina pectoris
- Hyperthyroidism
- Pheochromocytoma
- Medication or substance abuse, eg, caffeine, nicotine, cocaine, amphetamines, pseudoephedrine
- Other anxiety disorder, eg, obsessive-compulsive disorder, post-traumatic stress disorder
- Somatoform disorder (eg, somatization)

Papillary necrosis

- Renal tuberculosis
- Medullary sponge kidney

Etiology

- Analgesic nephropathy

- Diabetes mellitus
- Sickle cell trait or disease
- Pyelonephritis
- Urinary tract obstruction
- Renal vein thrombosis
- Tuberculosis
- Cirrhosis

Papules and nodules

Skin-colored, *white*, *or yellow*

- Skin tag (acrochordon)
- Warts
- Basal cell carcinoma
- Squamous cell carcinoma
- Sebaceous (epidermal inclusion) cyst
- Lipoma
- Xanthoma
- Molluscum contagiosum
- Nevus (intradermal)
- Sebaceous hyperplasia
- Milia
- Keratosis pilaris
- Granuloma annulare
- Rheumatoid nodules
- Gout
- Sarcoidosis
- Calcinosis cutis
- Metastases (color variable)
- Calluses or corns
- Gummas (tertiary syphilis)
- Sporotrichosis
- Foreign-body granuloma

Brown

- Seborrheic keratosis
- Nevus (compound, intradermal)
- Melanoma
- Dermatofibroma
- Neurofibroma

Red

- Insect bites
- Acne vulgaris
- Cherry angioma
- Hemangioma
- Folliculitis
- Inflamed sebaceous (epidermal inclusion) cyst
- Furuncle
- Scabies
- Erythema nodosum
- Basal cell carcinoma
- Keratoacanthoma
- Prurigo nodularis
- Miliaria (heat rash)

- Urticaria
- Sporotrichosis

Blue, *violaceous*, *or purple*

- Vasculitis (palpable purpura)
- Lichen planus
- Melanoma
- Kaposi's sarcoma
- Blue nevus
- Venous lake
- Mycosis fungoides (cutaneous T cell lymphoma)
- Endocarditis (Osler's)

Parasites involving the lung

- Ascariasis
- Hookworm
- Strongyloidiasis
- Paragonimiasis
- Toxocariasis (visceral larva migrans)
- Tropical pulmonary eosinophilia (*Wuchereria bancrofti, Brugia malayi*)
- Echinococcosis (hydatid disease)
- Amebic abscess

Parasomnias

- Nightmares or sleep terrors
- Sleepwalking: idiopathic, dementia, drugs (marijuana, alcohol), partial complex seizures
- Enuresis (bedwetting)

Paresthesias

- Alcoholism
- Diabetes mellitus
- Entrapment neuropathy, eg, carpal tunnel syndrome, tarsal tunnel syndrome, meralgia paresthetica
- Hypocalcemia
- Multiple sclerosis
- Spinal cord lesion
- Nerve root compression
- Herpes zoster
- Transient ischemic attack
- Guillain-Barré syndrome
- Trigeminal neuralgia
- Migraine
- Partial seizure
- Reflex sympathetic dystrophy
- Thoracic outlet syndrome
- Brachial plexus neuropathy

Parkinsonism

Etiology

- Parkinson's disease (idiopathic)
- Vascular parkinsonism (due to stroke)
- Essential tremor
- Depression
- Wilson's disease
- Huntington's disease
- Normal pressure hydrocephalus
- Shy-Drager syndrome
- Progressive supranuclear palsy
- Cortical-basal ganglionic degeneration
- Creutzfeldt-Jakob disease
- Drugs causing parkinsonism: antipsychotics, reserpine, metoclopramide

Paronychia

- Bacterial
- Candidiasis
- Felon (finger pad infection)
- Associated conditions: hypoparathyroidism, celiac sprue, acrodermatitis enteropathica, reactive arthritis (Reiter's syndrome)

Pelvic pain, acute

- Pelvic inflammatory disease
- Ectopic pregnancy
- Appendicitis
- Urinary calculi
- Primary dysmenorrhea
- Septic abortion
- Ruptured ovarian cyst or tumor
- Ovarian torsion
- Tubo-ovarian abscess
- Degeneration of leiomyoma (fibroid)
- Endometriosis
- Diverticulitis
- Cystitis

Pelvic pain, chronic

Gynecologic

- Endometriosis, adenomyosis (uterine endometriosis), pelvic adhesions, prior or chronic pelvic inflammatory disease, uterine leiomyomas (fibroids), ovarian tumor

Gastrointestinal

- Irritable bowel syndrome, inflammatory bowel disease, diverticulosis, constipation, colon cancer, abdominal hernia

Urologic

- Detrusor overactivity, interstitial cystitis, urinary calculi, urethral syndrome, bladder cancer

Musculoskeletal

- Myofascial pain, low back pain, disk disease, nerve entrapment, muscle strain or spasm

Psychiatric

- Somatization, depression, physical or sexual abuse, anxiety

Penile pain

- Urethritis
- Herpes simplex
- Balanitis, eg, candidiasis
- Paraphimosis (in uncircumcised)
- Peyronie's disease
- Priapism
- Prostatitis
- Passage of a urinary calculus
- Trauma

Penile papules & other lesions

- Pearly penile papules (benign)
- Genital warts (condyloma)
- Molluscum contagiosum
- Syphilis
- Scabies
- Lice
- Herpes simplex (vesicles & ulcers)
- Lichen planus (lacy white patches)
- Psoriasis (plaques)
- Neoplasm
- Bowenoid papulosis
- Vitiligo (white patches)

Penile ulcer

- Herpes simplex
- Primary syphilis (chancre)
- Chancroid
- Lymphogranuloma venereum
- Granuloma inguinale
- Trauma
- Behçet's syndrome (usually glans)
- Systemic lupus erythematosus (usually glans)
- Neoplasm (usually glans)
- Lichen planus

Perianal fistula

Etiology

- Crohn's disease
- Lymphogranuloma venereum
- Cancer
- Rectal tuberculosis

Pericardial effusion

- Cardiac tamponade
- Restrictive cardiomyopathy
- Constrictive pericarditis
- Pericarditis
- Hemopericardium
- Congestive heart failure

Etiology

- Malignancy, eg, lung, breast, leukemia
- Infection, eg, viral, bacterial, mycobacterial, *Mycoplasma*
- Iatrogenic, eg, catheterization, pacemaker placement, postcardiotomy
- Idiopathic
- Uremia
- Radiation-induced
- Collagen vascular disease, eg, systemic lupus erythematosus
- Anticoagulation
- Aortic dissection
- Myxedema (hypothyroidism)

Pericarditis

- Myocardial infarction
- Aortic dissection
- Pneumothorax
- Pneumonia
- Pleurisy
- Costochondritis (anterior chest wall syndrome or Tietze's syndrome)
- Pericardial effusion
- Cholecystitis

Etiology

Infectious

- Viral (especially coxsackie and echovirus, also influenza, Epstein-Barr, varicella, hepatitis, mumps, HIV)
- Idiopathic (many likely viral)
- Tuberculous
- Bacterial, eg, extension from pulmonary infection, Lyme disease

Noninfectious

- Malignancy, eg, lung, breast, renal cell, lymphoma
- Uremia
- Dressler's syndrome (post-MI or postcardiotomy)
- Radiation
- Systemic lupus erythematosus (including drug-induced, eg, procainamide, hydralazine)
- Rheumatoid arthritis
- Scleroderma
- Mixed connective tissue disease
- Drugs: minoxidil, penicillins
- Myxedema

Periorbital edema or swelling

- Allergies (allergic rhinitis)
- Nephrotic syndrome
- Orbital or periorbital cellulitis
- Hypothyroidism (myxedema)
- Herniated fat (usually in elderly)
- Angioedema
- Dermatomyositis
- Cavernous sinus thrombosis
- Mononucleosis (early)
- Trichinosis (*Trichinella* infection)
- Otorhinolaryngeal tumor
- Chagas' disease
- Dacryocystitis (lacrimal sac infection)

Peripheral neuropathy (mononeuropathy)

Etiology
- Nerve entrapment or compression
- Less often systemic disease, eg, diabetes mellitus, amyloidosis, rheumatoid arthritis
- Peripheral nerve tumor (rare except in neurofibromatosis)

Examples
- Carpal tunnel syndrome
- Ulnar entrapment, eg, cubital tunnel syndrome
- Radial nerve palsy (wrist drop)
- Femoral neuropathy
- Meralgia paresthetica
- Sciatica
- Common peroneal nerve palsy
- Tarsal tunnel syndrome

Peripheral neuropathy (polyneuropathy)

Etiology
Metabolic & systemic
- Diabetes mellitus
- Alcoholism
- Uremia
- Thiamine deficiency
- Vitamin B_{12} deficiency
- Multiple myeloma
- Amyloidosis
- Cryoglobulinemia
- Hypothyroidism or hyperthyroidism
- Sarcoidosis
- Paraneoplastic syndrome, eg, lung cancer
- Neuropathy associated with critical illness

Infectious & inflammatory
- Hansen's disease (leprosy)
- HIV/AIDS
- Lyme disease
- Diphtheritic neuropathy
- Polyarteritis nodosa
- Rheumatoid arthritis
- Temporal (giant cell) arteritis

Toxic
- Metals: lead, mercury, arsenic, thallium
- Drugs: isoniazid, phenytoin, pyridoxine, nitrofurantoin, vincristine
- Industrial agents or pesticides: acrylamide, organophosphates, hexacarbon solvents, methyl bromide, carbon disulfide

Hereditary
- Charcot-Marie-Tooth disease (hereditary motor and sensory neuropathy, type I & II)
- Porphyria
- Friedrich's ataxia
- Dejerine-Sottas disease (HMSN type III)
- Refsum disease (HMSN type IV)

Mostly motor
- Guillain-Barré syndrome
- Chronic inflammatory demyelinating polyneuropathy (CIDP)
- Porphyria
- Diphtheritic neuropathy
- Toxic neuropathy
- Poliomyelitis
- Periodic paralysis syndrome

Pharyngitis

- Viral, eg, adenovirus, herpes simplex virus
- Group A streptococci
- Infectious mononucleosis
- Gonorrhea
- *Mycoplasma*
- *Chlamydia pneumoniae*
- Influenza
- Diphtheria
- Necrotizing gingivostomatitis (Vincent's angina, trench mouth)
- *Arcanobacterium haemolyticum*

Other causes of sore throat
- Peritonsillar abscess
- Oral candidiasis
- Epiglottitis
- Acute HIV infection
- Dry mouth (xerostomia)
- Nasopharyngeal carcinoma
- Glossopharyngeal neuralgia
- With rash: meningococcemia, toxic shock syndrome, drug eruption, viral exanthem

Photophobia

- Migraine
- Corneal abrasion
- Meningitis or encephalitis
- Uveitis
- Acute glaucoma
- Viral or bacterial conjunctivitis
- Keratitis (corneal ulcer or inflammation), eg, herpes simplex
- Systemic viral infection, eg, measles
- Severe dry eyes
- Ultraviolet (actinic) keratitis
- Aphakia (absence of lens)
- Albinism
- Eyestrain from refractive error
- Optic neuritis

Pigmented lesions

- Freckles (ephelides, juvenile freckles)
- Lentigo, eg, solar lentigo (liver spots, senile freckles)
- Seborrheic keratosis
- Acquired nevus (mole), eg, junctional nevus, compound nevus
- Congenital nevus
- Dysplastic (atypical) nevus
- Blue nevus

- Halo nevus
- Malignant melanoma
- Café au lait spots
- Pigmented basal cell carcinoma (uncommon)
- Diabetic dermopathy

Platelet disorders, qualitative

Etiology

Acquired disorders
- Drugs: aspirin, NSAIDs, antibiotics
- Uremia
- Myeloproliferative disorder, eg, polycythemia vera, essential thrombocytosis
- Autoantibody
- Paraproteins, eg, multiple myeloma
- Fibrin degradation products

Hereditary disorders
- von Willebrand's disease
- Glanzmann's thrombasthenia
- Bernard-Soulier syndrome
- Storage pool disease, eg, gray platelet syndrome

Platypnea

- Arteriovenous malformation at lung bases

Pleural effusion

- Atelectasis
- Chronic pleural thickening
- Lobar consolidation
- Subdiaphragmatic process

Etiology

Transudates
- Congestive heart failure (most common)
- Cirrhosis with ascites
- Nephrotic syndrome
- Peritoneal dialysis
- Myxedema
- Acute atelectasis
- Constrictive pericarditis
- Superior vena cava obstruction
- Pulmonary embolism

Exudates
- Pneumonia (parapneumonic effusion)
- Cancer
- Pulmonary embolism
- Empyema

- Tuberculosis
- Connective tissue disease (eg, rheumatoid arthritis)
- Viral infection
- Fungal infection
- Rickettsial infection
- Parasitic infection (eg, *Paragonimus*)
- Asbestosis
- Meigs' syndrome
- Pancreatic disease
- Uremia
- Chronic atelectasis
- Trapped lung
- Chylothorax
- Sarcoidosis
- Drug reaction
- Postmyocardial infarction syndrome
- Esophageal rupture

Pleural plaques (masses or thickening)

Malignant tumors
- Metastatic cancer
- Mesothelioma
- Bronchogenic carcinoma
- Lymphoma (subpleural tumor plaque)
- Thymoma

Benign tumors
- Lipoma
- Fibrous tumor
- Neurogenic

Other
- Asbestosis plaques
- Nonspecific response to: inflammation, trauma, neoplasm, radiation
- Talc inhalation
- Extramedullary hematopoiesis

Pleuritis (pleurisy)

Etiology
- Upper respiratory tract infection
- Pneumonia
- Rib fracture
- Pneumothorax
- Pulmonary embolism
- Pneumothorax
- Pericarditis
- Aspiration pneumonia
- Mesothelioma

Pneumaturia

- Fistula between bladder & GI tract, eg, diverticulitis, carcinoma, Crohn's disease, radiation enteritis
- Infection with gas-producing organisms (rare)

Pneumoconiosis

- Tuberculosis
- Sarcoidosis
- Histoplasmosis
- Coccidioidomycosis
- Idiopathic pulmonary fibrosis

Etiology

Metal dusts
- Siderosis (mining, welding)
- Stannosis (mining, tin-working, smelting)
- Baritosis (glass & insecticide manufacturing)

Coal dust
- Coal worker's pneumoconiosis (common)

Inorganic dusts
- Silicosis (rock mining, stonecutting; common)

Silicate dusts
- Asbestosis (mining, insulation, construction, shipbuilding; common)
- Talcosis (mining, insulation, construction, shipbuilding)
- Kaolin pneumoconiosis (pottery, cement work)
- Shaver's disease (corundum manufacture)

Pneumonia in immunocompromised

- Bacterial pneumonia
- Pneumocystis pneumonia
- Tuberculosis
- Fungal pneumonia, eg, coccidioidomycosis, histoplasmosis, cryptococcosis, aspergillosis, candidiasis
- Cytomegalovirus
- Lymphoma
- Kaposi's sarcoma

Pneumonia, anaerobic, & lung abscess

- Tuberculosis
- Bronchogenic carcinoma
- Fungal infection, eg, histoplasmosis

- Bronchiectasis
- Cavitary bacterial pneumonia
- Pulmonary vasculitis, eg, Wegener's granulomatosis

Etiology

- Usually polymicrobial
- *Prevotella melaninogenica*
- *Peptostreptococcus*
- *Fusobacterium nucleatum*
- *Bacteroides*

Pneumonia, community-acquired

- Bacterial pneumonia
- Viral pneumonia
- Aspiration pneumonia
- Pneumocystis pneumonia
- Bronchitis
- Lung abscess
- Tuberculosis
- Pulmonary embolism
- Myocardial infarction
- Sarcoidosis
- Lung cancer
- Hypersensitivity pneumonitis
- Bronchiolitis or BOOP

Etiology

Bacterial

- *Streptococcus pneumoniae* (most common)
- *Haemophilus influenzae*
- *Mycoplasma pneumoniae* (young adults, summer & fall)
- *Chlamydia pneumoniae* (young adults)
- *Staphylococcus aureus* (influenza epidemics, IV drug use, bronchiectasis)
- *Neisseria meningitidis*
- *Moraxella catarrhalis* (lung disease, elderly)
- *Klebsiella pneumoniae* (alcohol, diabetes)
- *Legionella* spp. (contaminated construction site, water source, or air conditioner)

Viral

- Influenza virus
- Respiratory syncytial virus
- Adenovirus
- Parainfluenza virus

Special risk factors

- *Chlamydia psittaci* (psittacosis)–birds
- *Coxiella burnetii* (Q fever)–cattle, sheep, goats; especially newborns or products of conception
- *Francisella tularensis* (tularemia)–tick or skinning rabbit
- Endemic fungi (*Blastomyces*–Ohio and Mississippi River valleys; *Coccidioides*–Southwest United States or Latin America; *Histoplasma*–Ohio & Mississippi River valleys)
- Sin nombre virus (hantavirus pulmonary syndrome)–rodent waste, Southwest United States

Pneumonia, hospital-acquired

- Bacterial pneumonia
- Viral pneumonia
- Aspiration pneumonia
- Pneumocystis pneumonia
- Bronchitis
- Lung abscess
- Tuberculosis
- Pulmonary embolism
- Myocardial infarction
- Sarcoidosis
- Lung cancer
- Hypersensitivity pneumonitis
- Bronchiolitis or BOOP

Etiology

More common

- *Pseudomonas aeruginosa*
- *Staphylococcus aureus*
- *Enterobacter*
- *Klebsiella pneumoniae*
- *Escherichia coli*

Less common

- *Proteus*
- *Serratia marcescens*
- *H. influenzae*
- Streptococci
- *Acinetobacter*

Pneumonia, recurrent or persistent

- Lung cancer (postobstructive pneumonia)
- Hypersensitivity pneumonitis
- Eosinophilic pneumonia
- BOOP

- *Mycobacterium avium* complex (MAC)
- Asplenism

Pneumothorax

- Myocardial infarction
- Pulmonary embolism
- Pneumonia
- Chronic obstructive pulmonary disease
- Asthma
- Pleural effusion
- Aortic dissection
- Pericarditis
- Aortic aneurysm rupture

Etiology

Primary pneumothorax

- Apical bleb rupture (tall, thin males age 10–30)

Secondary pneumothorax

- Chronic obstructive pulmonary disease (ruptured bleb or bulla)
- Asthma
- Cystic fibrosis
- Tuberculosis
- Pneumocystis pneumonia
- Menstruation (catamenial pneumothorax)
- Interstitial lung disease, eg, sarcoidosis, lymphangioleiomyomatosis (LAM), eosinophilic granuloma (Langerhans cell histiocytosis, histiocytosis X)

Tension pneumothorax

- Penetrating or blunt trauma
- Lung infection
- Cardiopulmonary resuscitation
- Positive-pressure mechanical ventilation

Traumatic or iatrogenic

- Penetrating or blunt trauma
- Thoracentesis
- Pleural biopsy
- Percutaneous or transbronchial lung
- Central line placement
- Positive-pressure mechanical ventilation

Podagra

- Gout
- Trauma
- Cellulitis
- Sarcoidosis
- Pseudogout
- Psoriatic arthritis
- Bursitis of first MTP joint (inflamed bunion)

Polycythemia

Etiology

- Relative ("spurious") polycythemia
- Polycythemia vera (primary polycythemia)
- Secondary polycythemia
  - Hypoxia: cardiac disease, pulmonary disease, high altitude
  - Carboxyhemoglobin (smoking)
  - Renal cyst or hydronephrosis
  - Erythropoietin-secreting tumors (rare): renal cell or hepatocellular carcinoma, adrenal tumor, cerebellar hemangioma, uterine leiomyoma
  - Abnormal hemoglobins (rare)

Polydipsia

- Diabetes mellitus
- Diabetes insipidus
- Hypercalcemia
- Psychogenic polydipsia (associated with schizophrenia)
- Sjögren's syndrome
- Anticholinergics
- Primary hyperaldosteronism

Polyps of colon and small intestine

Etiology

- Mucosal neoplastic: adenoma (tubular, villous, or tubulovillous)
  - Nonfamilial (sporadic) adenomatous polyps
  - Familial adenomatous polyposis
- Mucosal nonneoplastic: hyperplastic, juvenile, hamartoma, inflammatory
  - Hamartomatous polyposis syndromes, eg, Peutz-Jeghers syndrome, familial juvenile polyposis, Cowden's syndrome
- Submucosal: lipoma, lymphoid aggregates, carcinoid, pneumatosis cystoides intestinalis

Polyuria

- Osmotic diuresis: diabetes mellitus, mannitol infusion, radiocontrast media, high-protein tube feeds
- Drugs: diuretics, lithium, caffeine
- Diabetes insipidus
- Hypercalcemia, eg, hyperparathyroidism

- Psychogenic polydipsia (eg, schizophrenia)
- Excess IV fluids
- Chronic renal failure (early)
- Diuretic phase of acute tubular necrosis
- Hypokalemia
- Post transurethral resection of the prostate
- Cushing's syndrome
- Primary hyperaldosteronism
- Inability to concentrate urine: sickle cell trait or disease, chronic pyelonephritis, amyloidosis
- Anxiety

Portal hypertension

Etiology

- Cirrhosis (most common)
- Portal vein thrombosis
- Splenic vein thrombosis
- Schistosomiasis
- Noncirrhotic intrahepatic portal sclerosis
- Arterial-portal vein fistula

Postcholecystectomy pain

- Retained common bile duct stone
- Common bile duct stricture
- Dilated cystic duct remnant
- Sphincter of Oddi spasm or stenosis
- Foreign-body granuloma
- Traction on common duct by long cystic duct
- Functional pain
- Pain due to nonbiliary disease, eg, peptic ulcer disease

Premature ovarian failure

Etiology

- Surgical bilateral oophorectomy
- Autoimmune
- X chromosome mosaicism
- Pelvic irradiation or chemotherapy
- Hysterectomy (even without oophorectomy)
- Turner syndrome
- Myotonic dystrophy
- Galactosemia
- Mumps oophoritis
- Familial or idiopathic

Proptosis (exophthalmos)

- Graves' ophthalmopathy
- Orbital cellulitis
- Orbital pseudotumor
- Tumor, eg, hemangioma, optic nerve glioma
- Trauma or orbital hemorrhage
- Retracted eyelid (normal variant)
- Inflammatory disease, eg, Wegener's granulomatosis, sarcoidosis
- Carotid cavernous fistula, dural arteriovenous malformation, or cavernous sinus thrombosis
- Posterior scleritis
- Hand-Schuller-Christian disease (eosinophilic granuloma)

Prostatodynia

- Chronic bacterial prostatitis
- Nonbacterial prostatitis
- Urethritis
- Cystitis
- Interstitial cystitis
- Prostatic abscess
- Prostate cancer
- Perirectal abscess
- Proctitis
- Diverticulitis
- Anal fissure or fistula

Proteinuria

Etiology

- Functional (benign): acute illness, exercise, "orthostatic proteinuria"
- Overload: multiple myeloma, rhabdomyolysis, leukemia
- Glomerular: diabetes, postinfectious glomerulonephritis, HIV, systemic lupus erythematosus, amyloid, IgA nephropathy, membranous nephropathy
- Tubulointerstitial: acute tubular necrosis, aminoglycosides, interstitial nephritis, Wilson's disease, Fanconi's syndrome
- Other: polycystic kidney disease, preeclampsia-eclampsia

Pruritus (itching)

Skin diseases

- Xerosis (dry skin)
- Scabies
- Urticaria
- Atopic dermatitis
- Contact dermatitis

- Arthropod bites (insect bites)
- Pediculosis (lice)
- Dermatitis herpetiformis
- Anogenital pruritus
- Lichen simplex chronicus
- Drug reaction
- Urticarial eruptions of pregnancy
- Folliculitis

Non-skin diseases
- Uremia
- Hyperbilirubinemia or cholestasis
- Hepatitis C
- Amphetamine or cocaine use
- Hypothyroidism or hyperthyroidism
- Intestinal parasites
- Lymphoma, leukemia, other malignancy
- Polycythemia vera
- Iron deficiency anemia
- Psychiatric

Pseudogout & chondrocalcinosis

- Gouty arthritis
- Septic arthritis
- Rheumatoid arthritis
- Reactive arthritis (Reiter's syndrome)
- Osteoarthritis

Etiology
Causes of chondrocalcinosis
- Pseudogout
- Hemochromatosis
- Hyperparathyroidism
- Ochronosis (alkaptonuria)
- Diabetes mellitus
- Hypothyroidism
- Wilson's disease
- Gouty arthritis

Prothrombin time increased
Etiology
- Liver disease
- Warfarin therapy
- Vitamin K deficiency
- Factor VII deficiency or inhibitor
- Heparin therapy (PTT increased more than PT)
- Disseminated intravascular coagulation (PT & PTT increased)
- Rare isolated factor deficiencies (II, V, X, I)

Ptosis

- Cranial nerve 3 palsy (dilated or normal pupil), eg, diabetic neuropathy, posterior inferior cerebellar artery aneurysm
- Horner's syndrome (constricted pupil)
- Myasthenia gravis
- Botulism
- Age-related (sagging eyelid)
- Eyelid inflammation or deformity
- Congenital
- Progressive external ophthalmoplegia (mitochondrial myopathy)

PTT increased

Etiology
Congenital factor deficiencies
- Contact factors (no clinical bleeding)
- Factor XII (no clinical bleeding)
- Factor XI
- Factor IX (hemophilia B)
- Factor VIII (hemophilia A)
- Factor VIII (von Willebrand's disease)

Anticoagulants
- Factor VIII inhibitor
- Lupus anticoagulant (no clinical bleeding)
- Heparin
- Warfarin (PT increased more than PTT)

Other
- Disseminated intravascular coagulation (PT & PTT increased)
- Liver disease (PT increased more than PTT)
- Vitamin K deficiency (PT increased more than PTT)

Pulmonary edema, acute

Etiology
Cardiogenic
- Congestive heart failure
- Myocardial infarction
- Myocardial ischemia
- Volume overload of left ventricle: mitral regurgitation, aortic insufficiency, ventricular septal defect
- Mitral stenosis

Noncardiogenic
- Acute respiratory distress syndrome
- Sepsis
- Disseminated intravascular coagulation
- Increased intracerebral pressure (eg, intracerebral bleed or stroke)

- Aspiration pneumonia
- High altitude
- Drug reaction
- Transfusion reaction
- Salicylate intoxication
- Radiographic contrast allergy
- Inhaled toxins, eg, smoke inhalation

Pulmonary embolism

- Myocardial infarction
- Pneumonia
- Pericarditis
- Congestive heart failure
- Pleuritis (pleurisy)
- Pneumothorax
- Pericardial tamponade

Etiology
- Thromboembolism (most common)
- Fat embolism
- Air embolism
- Amniotic fluid embolism
- Septic embolism (eg, endocarditis)
- Tumor embolism (eg, renal cell carcinoma)
- Foreign-body embolism (eg, talc in IV drug use)
- Parasite egg embolism (schistosomiasis)

Pulmonary function test, DLCO (diffusion capacity) decreased

- Emphysema
- Interstitial lung disease
- Pulmonary embolism
- Pneumocystis pneumonia

Pulmonary function test, DLCO (diffusion capacity) increased

- Pulmonary hemorrhage
- Asthma
- Congestive heart failure (acute)
- Pregnancy

Pulmonary function test, obstructive disease

- Asthma
- Chronic obstructive pulmonary disease
- Bronchiectasis

- Bronchiolitis
- Upper airway obstruction

Pulmonary function test, restrictive disease

Decreased lung compliance
- Interstitial lung disease
- Pneumonia
- Sarcoidosis
- Adult respiratory distress syndrome

Decreased muscle strength
- Neuromuscular disease (eg, myasthenia gravis, Guillain-Barré)
- Diaphragm dysfunction
- Phrenic nerve injury

Extrapulmonic disease
- Pleural effusion
- Pleural thickening
- Obesity
- Kyphoscoliosis

Pulmonary hypertension

- Primary pulmonary hypertension
- Secondary pulmonary hypertension
- Cor pulmonale (right heart failure due to pulmonary disease)
- Congestive heart failure
- Right-sided valve disease
- Mitral stenosis

Etiology
- Primary pulmonary hypertension
- Chronic pulmonary embolism
- Chronic obstructive pulmonary disease
- Interstitial lung disease
- Sleep apnea
- Pickwickian syndrome (obesity-hypoventilation syndrome)
- Scleroderma or other connective tissue disease
- Left to right intracardiac shunt
- Drugs or toxins: fenfluramine, dexfenfluramine, phentermine, bleomycin, amiodarone, talc (via IV drug use)
- Radiation
- Pulmonary veno-occlusive disease
- Valve disease: mitral stenosis, mitral regurgitation, aortic stenosis
- Left-sided heart failure
- Atrial myxoma
- High altitude (chronic mountain sickness)
- Polycythemia vera

- Cirrhosis with portal hypertension
- HIV
- Schistosomiasis
- Sickle cell disease

Pulmonary insufficiency

Etiology
- Pulmonary hypertension (usually)
- Rare: congenital, rheumatic heart disease, endocarditis, carcinoid

Pulmonary nodule, solitary

- Bronchogenic carcinoma
- Granuloma (tuberculous, fungal)
- Lung abscess
- Hamartoma
- Metastatic cancer
- Arteriovenous malformation
- Resolving pneumonia
- Rheumatoid nodule
- Pulmonary infarction
- Carcinoid
- Pseudotumor (loculated fluid in a fissure)

Pulmonary nodules (multiple)

- Metastatic cancer
- Bronchogenic carcinoma
- Lymphoproliferative cancer
- Tuberculosis
- Lung abscess
- Granulomas (eg, tuberculous, fungal)
- Coccidioidomycosis
- Histoplasmosis
- Sarcoidosis
- Silicosis
- Coal worker's pneumoconiosis
- *Mycobacterium avium* complex (MAC)
- Arteriovenous malformations
- Rheumatoid nodules
- Hamartomas
- Wegener's granulomatosis
- Methotrexate-induced
- Eosinophilic granuloma (Langerhans cell histiocytosis, histiocytosis X)
- Congenital cysts
- Echinococcosis (hydatid disease)
- Paragonimiasis

Pulmonary-renal syndromes

- Goodpasture's syndrome
- Severe congestive heart failure (pulmonary edema and prerenal azotemia)
- Renal failure (with hypervolemia and pulmonary edema)
- Microscopic polyangiitis (polyarteritis nodosa)
- Systemic lupus erythematosus
- Henoch-Schönlein purpura
- Wegener's granulomatosis
- Churg-Strauss syndrome
- Legionnaire's disease
- Renal vein thrombosis with pulmonary embolism

Pulse pressure, wide

High output states
- Thyrotoxicosis
- Pregnancy
- Beriberi heart disease
- Vasodilating drugs

Increased run-off of LV outflow
- Aortic regurgitation
- Patent ductus arteriosus

Other
- Old age (rigid arteries)
- Severe bradycardia

Pulse, absent or decreased

- Peripheral vascular disease
- Takayasu's arteritis or "pulseless disease" (various pulses)
- Temporal (giant cell) arteritis (temporal artery)
- Thromboangiitis obliterans or Buerger's disease (distal pulses)
- Aortic dissection (decreased or unequal pulses)
- Coarctation of the aorta (femoral pulses)

Pulseless electrical activity (PEA)

- Cardiac tamponade
- Hypoxia, hypovolemia, hypothermia, hyperkalemia
- Embolism (massive pulmonary embolism)
- Acidosis
- Pneumothorax (tension pneumothorax)
- Myocardial infarction

- Drug overdose, eg, tricyclic antidepressant, digoxin, beta blocker, calcium channel blocker

Pulsus alternans

- Low ejection fraction
- Large pericardial effusion

Pulsus paradoxus

- Asthma
- Chronic obstructive pulmonary disease
- Pericardial effusion
- Cardiac tamponade
- Constrictive pericarditis (rarely)

Purpura, nonpalpable

- Trauma
- Senile or solar purpura
- Corticosteroid use
- Idiopathic (autoimmune) thrombocytopenic purpura
- Thrombotic thrombocytopenic purpura
- Disseminated intravascular coagulation
- Other thrombocytopenia or platelet dysfunction
- Clotting factor defect
- Vitamin K deficiency
- Warfarin necrosis
- Amyloidosis
- Waldenström's macroglobulinemia
- Scurvy
- Ehlers-Danlos syndrome

Purpura, palpable

Vasculitis
- Polyarteritis nodosa
- Rheumatoid arthritis
- Wegener's granulomatosis
- Churg-Strauss syndrome
- Henoch-Schönlein purpura
- Systemic lupus erythematosus
- Hypersensitivity (leukocytoclastic) vasculitis

Infection or emboli
- Meningococcemia
- Gonococcemia
- Endocarditis
- Rocky Mountain spotted fever
- *Aspergillus*
- Candidiasis
- Ecthyma gangrenosum (neutropenic, pseudomonal)

Other
- Sarcoidosis
- Cryoglobulinemia
- Ulcerative colitis
- Crohn's disease
- Medications

Pustules

- Acne vulgaris
- Acne rosacea
- Folliculitis
- Candidiasis
- Tinea
- Miliaria (heat rash)
- Gonococcemia
- Vesicles (can be pustular)
- Scabies
- Keratosis pilaris
- Hidradenitis suppurativa

.

Pyoderma gangrenosum

- Ulcer secondary to underlying infection (eg, mycobacterial, fungal, tertiary syphilis, amebiasis)
- Ulcer secondary to underlying neoplasm
- Folliculitis
- Arthropod bites (insect bites)
- Sweet's syndrome (acute febrile neutrophilic dermatosis)
- Vasculitis (eg, Wegener's granulomatosis)
- Warfarin necrosis

Associated conditions
- Ulcerative colitis
- Crohn's disease
- Rheumatoid arthritis
- Hepatitis B and hepatitis C
- HIV
- Systemic lupus erythematosus
- IgA gammopathy
- Leukemia

Pyuria

- Cystitis
- Urethritis
- Epididymitis
- Orchitis
- Prostatitis
- Pyelonephritis
- Perinephric abscess
- Renal tuberculosis (sterile pyuria)

Rash, annular

- Tinea corporis (body ringworm)
- Psoriasis
- Secondary syphilis
- Erythema multiforme
- Pityriasis rosea
- Nummular (discoid) eczema
- Discoid lupus erythematosus
- Erythema migrans (Lyme disease)
- Granuloma annulare
- Erythema nodosum (nodular)

Rash, intertriginous

- Tinea cruris (jock itch)
- Candidiasis
- Intertrigo
- Seborrheic dermatitis
- Cellulitis
- Psoriasis of body folds ("inverse psoriasis")
- Erythrasma
- Tinea versicolor (pityriasis versicolor) (rarely)
- Scratching due to lice
- Contact dermatitis

Rash, morbilliform

- Drug eruption
- Viral exanthem
- Secondary syphilis
- Early erythema multiforme major
- Scarlet fever
- Toxic shock syndrome
- Acute HIV infection
- Acute graft-versus-host disease

Rash, palms and soles

- Tinea
- Warts
- Dyshidrotic eczema (pompholyx, dyshidrosis)
- Secondary syphilis
- Dermatophytid reaction (allergy or sensitivity to fungi)
- Erythema multiforme
- Rocky Mountain spotted fever
- Drug eruption
- Janeway lesions or Osler's nodes (bacterial endocarditis)
- Cholesterol emboli
- Contact dermatitis (palms)

- Pitted keratolysis (soles)
- Keratoderma blennorrhagica (with reactive arthritis or Reiter's syndrome)
- Psoriasis
- Gonococcemia or meningococcemia
- Hand, foot, and mouth disease
- Toxic shock syndrome
- Lichen planus (ulcerative)
- Melanoma
- Calluses or corns
- Rat bite fever
- Arsenic poisoning

Raynaud's syndrome

- Raynaud's disease (idiopathic)
- Raynaud's phenomenon: associated with conditions listed under Associated Conditions
- Livedo reticularis
- Acrocyanosis
- Erythromelalgia

Associated conditions

- Autoimmune disease, eg, scleroderma, systemic lupus erythematosus, dermatomyositis, rheumatoid arthritis
- Arterial occlusive disease, eg, atherosclerosis, emboli, thromboangiitis obliterans (Buerger's disease)
- Cryoglobulinemia, myeloproliferative disorders, multiple myeloma, macroglobulinemia
- Thoracic outlet syndrome
- Carpal tunnel syndrome
- Myxedema (hypothyroidism)
- Chemotherapeutic agents, ergotamine, nicotine, estrogen, sympathomimetics, cocaine, polyvinyl chloride
- Frostbite
- Hand-arm vibration syndrome or hypothenar hammer (jackhammer) syndrome

Red eye

- Conjunctivitis (viral, bacterial, allergic)
- Uveitis
- Acute glaucoma
- Foreign body or corneal abrasion
- Keratitis (corneal ulcer or inflammation), eg, herpes simplex
- Scleritis or episcleritis
- Trauma
- Subconjunctival hemorrhage

- Eyelid disorder, eg, hordeolum, chalazion, blepharitis
- Cluster headache

Red eye, circumcorneal (ciliary injection)

- Corneal abrasion or keratitis
- Intraocular inflammation, eg, uveitis
- Acute glaucoma

Reflexes, delayed relaxation

Etiology

- Hypothyroidism
- Diabetes mellitus
- Pernicious anemia
- Hypothermia

Renal cysts

- Renal cell carcinoma
- Renal abscess
- Transitional cell carcinoma of renal pelvis
- Adrenal tumor
- Renal oncocytoma
- Renal angiomyolipoma
- Metastases, eg, lung, breast, stomach, contralateral kidney
- Lymphoma
- Nephrolithiasis
- Renal infarction

Types

- Simple cysts
- Acquired cysts (dialysis patients)
- Polycystic kidney disease
- Medullary sponge kidney
- Medullary cystic kidney

Renal failure in HIV/AIDS

Etiology

- Typical causes of acute renal failure
- HIV-associated nephropathy
- Acute tubular necrosis due to pentamidine, amphotericin, foscarnet, cidofovir, aminoglycosides, rifampin, acyclovir
- Interstitial nephritis due to TMP-SMX, sulfadiazine, acyclovir
- Nephrolithiasis due to indinavir
- Postinfectious glomerulonephritis

- Membranous nephropathy due to hepatitis B, syphilis
- Membranoproliferative glomerulonephritis due to hepatitis C, cryoglobulinemia
- Ureteral compression due to lymphoma, lymphadenopathy
- IgA immune-complex deposition
- Thrombotic thrombocytopenia purpura

Renal failure, acute

Etiology

Prerenal azotemia

- Dehydration
- Hemorrhage, eg, gastrointestinal bleeding
- Congestive heart failure
- Renal artery stenosis including fibromuscular dysplasia
- NSAIDs, ACE inhibitors

Postrenal azotemia

- Obstruction, eg, benign prostatic hypertrophy, bladder tumor, pelvic mass

Intrinsic renal disease

Acute tubular necrosis

- Toxins: NSAIDs, antibiotics, contrast, multiple myeloma, rhabdomyolysis, hemolysis, chemotherapy, hyperuricemia, cyclosporine
- Ischemia, eg, prolonged prerenal azotemia

Acute glomerulonephritis

- Immune complex: IgA nephropathy, endocarditis, systemic lupus erythematosus, cryoglobulinemia, postinfectious glomerulonephritis, membranoproliferative, Henoch-Schönlein purpura
- Pauci-immune (ANCA+): Wegener's granulomatosis, Churg-Strauss syndrome, microscopic polyarteritis
- Anti-GBM: Goodpasture's syndrome, anti-GBM glomerulonephritis
- Other: malignant hypertension, thrombotic thrombocytopenia purpura, scleroderma renal crisis, preeclampsia-eclampsia

Acute interstitial nephritis

- Drugs: beta-lactams, sulfa, diuretics, NSAIDs, rifampin, phenytoin, allopurinol
- Infections: *Streptococcus,* leptospirosis, cytomegalovirus, histoplasmosis, Rocky Mountain spotted fever
- Immune: systemic lupus erythematosus, Sjögren's syndrome, sarcoidosis, cryoglobulinemia

Renal failure, chronic

Etiology

Glomerulopathies
Primary glomerular diseases
- IgA nephropathy
- Focal segmental glomerulosclerosis
- Membranoproliferative glomerulonephritis
- Membranous nephropathy

Secondary glomerular diseases
- Diabetic nephropathy (very common)
- Hypertensive nephropathy
- Amyloidosis
- Postinfectious glomerulonephritis
- HIV-associated nephropathy
- Collagen vascular diseases, eg, systemic lupus erythematosus
- Sickle cell nephropathy

Tubulointerstitial nephritis
- Drug hypersensitivity
- Heavy metals
- Analgesic nephropathy
- Vesicoureteral reflux
- Idiopathic

Obstructive uropathy
- Prostatic disease
- Urinary calculi
- Retroperitoneal fibrosis or tumor

Vascular diseases
- Hypertensive nephrosclerosis (very common)
- Renal artery stenosis including fibromuscular dysplasia

Hereditary diseases
- Polycystic kidney disease
- Medullary cystic kidney disease
- Alport's syndrome

Renal tubular acidosis

Other causes of normal gap metabolic acidosis
- Gastrointestinal loss of HCO_3^-, eg, diarrhea, pancreatic ileostomy or ileal loop bladder
- Renal tubular acidosis
- Recovery from diabetic ketoacidosis
- Dilutional acidosis from rapid administration of 0.9% NaCl
- Carbonic anhydrase inhibitors
- Chloride retention or administration of HCl equivalent or NH_4Cl

Etiology
- Type I (distal H^+ secretion defect): low serum K^+, urine pH >5.5, associated with autoimmune disease, hypercalcemia
- Type II (proximal HCO_3^- reabsorption defect): low serum K^+, urine pH <5.5, associated with multiple myeloma, drugs (eg, sulfa)
- Type III (rare): normal serum K^+, urine pH <5.5, associated with renal insufficiency
- Type IV (hyporeninemic hypoaldosteronism): high serum K^+, urine pH <5.5, associated with diabetes mellitus, drugs (eg, NSAIDs)

Respiratory failure, acute

Airway disorders
- Asthma
- Chronic obstructive pulmonary disease exacerbation
- Airway obstruction

Pulmonary edema
- Left ventricular dysfunction
- Mitral regurgitation or mitral stenosis
- Volume overload states
- Acute respiratory distress syndrome
- Re-expansion

Parenchymal lung disorders
- Pneumonia or aspiration pneumonitis
- Interstitial lung disease
- Lung contusion

Pulmonary vascular disorders
- Pulmonary thromboembolism

Chest wall, diaphragm, & pleural disorders
- Flail chest
- Pneumothorax
- Pleural effusion
- Massive ascites

Neuromuscular & related disorders
- Guillain-Barré syndrome
- Myasthenia gravis
- Poliomyelitis
- Botulism
- Organophosphates or aminoglycosides
- Spinal cord injury
- Phrenic nerve injury or dysfunction
- Hypokalemia, hypophosphatemia
- Myxedema

CNS disorders
- Drugs: sedative, hypnotic, opioid, anesthetics
- Brainstem disorder
- Intracranial hypertension
- CNS infections

Increased CO_2 production
- Fever, infection, seizures, drugs

Respiratory tract infections, recurrent
- Seasonal allergies (allergic rhinitis)
- Selective IgA deficiency
- Common variable immunodeficiency
- Anatomic abnormalities

Retinal artery occlusion
- Ophthalmic artery occlusion
- Ophthalmic migraine
- Retinal detachment
- Retinal vein occlusion

Etiology
- Emboli from carotid or heart
- Vasculitis, eg, temporal (giant cell) arteritis
- Internal carotid dissection
- Thrombophilia

Retinal detachment
- Retinal artery or vein occlusion
- Vitreous hemorrhage
- Macular degeneration (exudative)
- Anterior ischemic optic neuropathy, eg, temporal (giant cell) arteritis
- Amaurosis fugax (transient ischemic attack)

Retinal vein occlusion
- Retinal artery occlusion
- Retinal detachment
- Anterior ischemic optic neuropathy, eg, temporal (giant cell) arteritis
- Papilledema
- Diabetic retinopathy
- Hypertensive retinopathy

Associated conditions
- Glaucoma
- Hypertension
- Diabetes mellitus
- Hyperlipidemia
- Hypercoagulable state
- Behçet's syndrome
- Systemic lupus erythematosus

- Hyperviscosity, eg, polycythemia vera, leukemia, Waldenström's macroglobulinemia

Retinopathy

Etiology

- Diabetic retinopathy
- Hypertensive retinopathy
- Radiation retinopathy
- Retinal vein occlusion
- Anterior ischemic optic neuropathy, eg, temporal (giant cell) arteritis
- Sickle cell retinopathy
- Retinopathy of severe anemia
- Retinopathy due to autoimmune disease, eg, systemic lupus erythematosus
- Emboli from IV drug use (talc retinopathy)
- Eales' disease (idiopathic retinal vasculitis)

Rhinitis (nasal congestion)

- Viral rhinitis (common cold)
- Allergic rhinitis
- Sinusitis (rhinosinusitis)
- Vasomotor rhinitis (eg, cold air- or irritant-induced)
- Nasal polyposis
- Rhinitis medicamentosa
- Foreign body
- Wegener's granulomatosis
- CSF leak

Rickettsial diseases

Etiology

- Typhus group: epidemic (louse-borne) typhus, scrub typhus, endemic typhus, California flea rickettsiosis
- Spotted fever group: Rocky Mountain spotted fever, rickettsialpox, RMSF-like, Boutonneuse fever, Kenya tick typhus, South African tick fever, Indian tick typhus, Queensland tick typhus, North Asian tick typhus
- Other: ehrlichiosis (human monocytic and human granulocytic), Q fever

Sacroiliitis

- Causes or mimics of sacroiliitis: ankylosing spondylitis, reactive arthritis (Reiter's syndrome), psoriatic arthritis, inflammatory bowel disease, osteitis condensans ilii, hyperparathyroidism, Whipple's disease

- Diffuse idiopathic skeletal hyperostosis (in elderly)
- Synovitis-acne-pustulosis-hyperostosis-osteitis syndrome
- Sciatica
- Lumbar disk herniation, spinal stenosis, or facet joint degenerative arthritis
- Ochronosis (alkaptonuria)

Salivary gland tumor

- Sialadenitis
- Sialolithiasis (salivary gland calculi)
- Lymphadenopathy (eg, from conjunctivitis, otitis media, sinusitis)
- Metastatic submandibular lymph node

Scaly lesions

- Atopic dermatitis (eczema)
- Seborrheic dermatitis
- Psoriasis
- Tinea, eg, tinea corporis, cruris, or pedis
- Contact dermatitis
- Stasis dermatitis (due to venous insufficiency)
- Xerosis (dry skin)
- Lichen simplex chronicus (circumscribed neurodermatitis)
- Tinea versicolor (pityriasis versicolor)
- Nummular eczema (discoid eczema, nummular dermatitis)
- Intertrigo
- Secondary syphilis
- Pityriasis rosea
- Discoid lupus erythematosus
- Exfoliative dermatitis (exfoliative erythroderma)
- Actinic keratoses
- Cutaneous T cell lymphoma (mycosis fungoides)
- Bowen's disease (squamous cell carcinoma in situ)
- Paget's disease

Scleritis or episcleritis

- Conjunctivitis
- Keratitis
- Uveitis
- Acute glaucoma
- Corneal abrasion

Etiology

- Autoimmune: rheumatoid arthritis, systemic lupus erythematosus, polyarteritis nodosa, Wegener's granulomatosis, re-

lapsing polychondritis, inflammatory bowel disease, sarcoidosis
- Infectious: ophthalmic zoster, herpes simplex, Lyme disease, HIV, syphilis, tuberculosis

Seizure

- Syncope
- Cardiac arrhythmia
- Stroke or transient ischemic attack
- Pseudoseizure
- Panic attack
- Migraine
- Narcolepsy

Etiology

- Idiopathic (epilepsy)
- Hypoglycemia
- Drugs: alcohol withdrawal, cocaine, amphetamines, benzodiazepine withdrawal, heroin withdrawal, SSRIs
- Electrolyte abnormality, eg, hyponatremia, hypocalcemia
- Infection: bacterial meningitis, herpes encephalitis, neurocysticercosis, neurosyphilis
- Space-occupying lesion, eg, brain tumor, arteriovenous malformation
- Trauma
- Stroke
- CNS vasculitis, eg, systemic lupus erythematosus
- Uremia
- Febrile seizures
- Congenital abnormality or perinatal injury
- Degenerative disease, eg, Alzheimer's disease

Seizure in HIV/AIDS

Etiology

- CNS toxoplasmosis
- Cryptococcal meningitis
- Herpes encephalitis
- Bacterial meningitis
- CNS lymphoma
- Neurosyphilis

Septal perforation

- Nose picking
- Prior surgery
- Cocaine use
- Wegener's granulomatosis

Seronegative spondyloarthropathy

Etiology

- Reactive arthritis (Reiter's syndrome)
- Psoriatic arthritis
- Ankylosing spondylitis
- Arthritis associated with inflammatory bowel disease
- Ochronosis (alkaptonuria; mimics ankylosing spondylitis)

Sexual dysfunction, women

- Depression
- Dyspareunia
- Chronic pelvic pain
- Menopause
- Oral contraceptive use
- Hypothyroidism
- Hyperprolactinemia
- Diabetes mellitus
- Cushing's syndrome
- Addison's disease
- Hypopituitarism
- Drugs: alcohol, recreational drugs, SSRIs, tricyclic antidepressants
- Physical or sexual abuse
- Anorexia nervosa
- Multiple sclerosis

Shoulder pain

- Rotator cuff tendonitis ("impingement") or tear
- Subacromial bursitis
- Biceps tendonitis
- Osteoarthritis (AC joint; rare in glenohumeral joint)
- Frozen shoulder (adhesive capsulitis)
- Acromioclavicular separation
- Neck disorder, eg, osteoarthritis, herniated disk (discogenic neck pain), tumor
- Rheumatoid arthritis or septic arthritis
- Calcific tendinitis
- Shoulder dislocation or fracture
- Avascular necrosis
- Polymyalgia rheumatica
- Fibromyalgia
- Thoracic outlet syndrome
- Brachial plexus neuropathy
- Referred pain from gallbladder, heart, diaphragm, Pancoast tumor
- Metastatic or primary tumor

Shunt (right to left, anatomic shunts)

Etiology

Pulmonary
- Arteriovenous fistula (eg, idiopathic arteriovenous malformation, Osler-Weber-Rendu, hepatopulmonary)
- Atelectasis
- Pulmonary edema
- Pneumonia
- Acute respiratory distress syndrome

Cardiac
- Atrial septal defect
- Ventricular septal defect
- Patent foramen ovale
- Patent ductus arteriosus

Sialolithiasis or sialadenitis

- Sialolithiasis (salivary gland calculi)
- Bacterial sialadenitis
- Salivary gland tumor
- Facial cellulitis
- Dental abscess
- TMJ syndrome
- Trigeminal neuralgia
- Lymphadenopathy (eg, from conjunctivitis, otitis media, sinusitis)
- Parotid enlargement due to starch ingestion

Etiology

- Viral: mumps, HIV, influenza, Epstein-Barr virus, cytomegalovirus, coxsackie
- Bacterial infection, eg, *S. aureus*
- Sjögren's syndrome
- Sarcoidosis
- Amyloidosis
- Alcohol
- Bulimia
- Dehydration
- Diabetes, cirrhosis, chronic pancreatitis
- Vitamin deficiency
- Acromegaly
- Drugs: antithyroid drugs, iodine, cholinergics, eg, phenothiazines

Sick sinus syndrome

- Sinus bradycardia
- Atrioventricular block
- Tachy-brady syndrome

Etiology

- Drugs: digitalis, calcium channel blockers, beta blockers, clonidine, other sympatholytics, amiodarone, other antiarrhythmics
- Age-related conduction system fibrosis or calcification (Lev's disease)
- Cardiac infiltrative disease (eg, amyloid, sarcoidosis, hemochromatosis)
- Chagas' disease

Sinopulmonary syndromes

Infection
- HIV
- Aspergillosis

Allergic
- Asthma and allergic rhinitis
- ABPA and allergic fungal sinusitis

Idiopathic
- Wegener's granulomatosis
- Churg-Strauss syndrome

Altered defenses
- Cystic fibrosis
- Immotile cilia syndrome
- Common variable immunodeficiency
- IgA deficiency
- IgG subclass deficiency
- Complement deficiency

Sinusitis, chronic

- Wegener's granulomatosis
- Neoplasm
- Cystic fibrosis
- Immotile cilia syndrome (eg, Kartagener's)
- Aspergillosis

Small intestinal tumor

Benign
- Adenomatous polyp
- Villous adenoma
- Lipoma
- Benign stromal tumor (leiomyoma)
- Crohn's disease (may mimic tumor)

Malignant
- Adenocarcinoma, especially in ampulla of Vater
- Lymphoma (primary or secondary)
- Carcinoid
- Leiomyosarcoma
- Kaposi's sarcoma

Sneezing

- Allergic rhinitis
- Upper respiratory tract infection
- Influenza
- Nasal polyp
- Deviated septum

Spasticity

Etiology

- Stroke
- Cerebral palsy
- Anoxic brain injury, head trauma, or space-occupying lesion
- Spinal cord tumor or injury
- Multiple sclerosis

Spells (nonspecific)

- Neurologic: syncope or presyncope, vertigo, transient ischemic attack, absence seizure, temporal lobe seizure, pseudoseizure, migraine, narcolepsy, multiple sclerosis, porphyria
- Psychiatric: anxiety, panic attack, conversion disorder, domestic violence
- Cardiac: arrhythmia, mitral valve prolapse
- Pulmonary: pulmonary embolism, pulmonary hypertension
- Endocrine: hypoglycemia, hypocalcemia, pheochromocytoma, carcinoid, hyperthyroidism, hypothyroidism, hot flashes (menopausal)
- Rheumatologic: CNS vasculitis
- Drugs, eg, alcohol, cocaine, withdrawal
- Infectious: Lyme disease, neurosyphilis

Spinal cord tumor

- Primary tumor, eg, ependymoma, meningioma, neurofibroma
- Lymphoma, leukemia, multiple myeloma
- Metastases: prostate cancer, breast cancer, lung cancer, renal cell carcinoma, colon cancer, melanoma
- Epidural abscess
- Multiple sclerosis
- Tuberculosis (Pott's disease)

Splenomegaly

- Infections, eg, mononucleosis (Epstein-Barr virus), cytomegalovirus, acute HIV, endocarditis, histoplasmosis, malaria, schistosomiasis, leishmaniasis, filariasis
- Chronic hemolytic anemia
- Leukemia
- Lymphoma
- Extramedullary hematopoiesis, eg, myelofibrosis, marrow toxin
- Polycythemia vera
- Essential thrombocytosis
- Cirrhosis or noncirrhotic portal hypertension
- Congestive heart failure
- Immune thrombocytopenias
- Splenic vein thrombosis
- Rheumatoid arthritis (Felty's syndrome)
- Systemic lupus erythematosus
- Sarcoidosis
- Wilson's disease
- Amyloidosis
- Budd-Chiari syndrome
- Gaucher disease
- Niemann-Pick disease
- Splenic cysts, hemangiomas, hamartomas, fibromas
- Metastases, eg, melanoma
- Eosinophilic granuloma (Langerhans cell histiocytosis, histiocytosis X)

Splinter hemorrhages

- Trauma
- Endocarditis
- Antiphospholipid antibody syndrome
- Rheumatoid vasculitis
- Trichinosis (*Trichinella* infection)
- Scurvy

Stroke

- Transient ischemic attack
- Ischemic stroke
- Intracerebral hemorrhage
- Subdural or epidural hematoma
- Space-occupying lesion, eg, brain tumor
- Seizure (Todd's paralysis)
- Migraine
- Peripheral causes of vertigo, eg, Ménière's disease
- Hypoglycemia
- Guillain-Barré syndrome
- Multiple sclerosis
- Aortic dissection

Etiology

- Embolic: atrial fibrillation, carotid atherosclerosis, left ventricular aneurysm, dilated cardiomyopathy, acute myocardial infarction, endocarditis, mechanical valve, mitral valve prolapse, aortic arch atherosclerosis, atrial myxoma, patent foramen ovale
- Thrombotic: atherosclerosis, small vessel ischemia, vasculitis, eg, systemic lupus erythematosus, polycythemia, thrombocytosis, sickle cell disease, meningovascular syphilis, arterial dissection or aneurysm, eg, intracerebral carotid or vertebral
- Hemorrhagic: hypertension, amyloidosis, conversion of ischemic stroke, cocaine

Sudden death

Cardiac causes

- Ventricular fibrillation
- Acute myocardial infarction
- Complete heart block
- Sinus node arrest
- Hypertrophic obstructive cardiomyopathy
- Congestive heart failure
- Long QT syndrome
- Atrial myxoma
- Mitral valve prolapse
- Pre-excitation syndrome (eg, Wolff-Parkinson-White)
- Chagas' disease
- Coronary anomalies
- Brugada syndrome
- Arrhythmogenic right ventricular dysplasia

Noncardiac causes & associated conditions

- Pulmonary embolism
- Asthma
- Aortic dissection
- Ruptured aortic aneurysm
- Intracerebral hemorrhage
- Tension pneumothorax
- Anaphylaxis
- Electrolyte abnormalities
- Cocaine or other drug use
- Primary pulmonary hypertension
- Aortic stenosis
- Pulmonary stenosis

Sympatholytic poisoning

Etiology

- Barbiturates
- Benzodiazepines, other sedatives
- Gamma-hydroxybutyrate

- Clonidine
- Ethanol
- Opioids

Sympathomimetic poisoning

Etiology

- Amphetamines
- Cocaine
- Ephedrine, pseudoephedrine
- PCP (pupils normal or small)
- Phenylpropanolamine (bradycardia common)
- Theophylline toxicity

Syncope

- Seizure
- Transient ischemic attack or stroke
- Hypoglycemia
- Narcolepsy
- Vertigo

Etiology

Cardiac

- Arrhythmia (ventricular tachycardia, supraventricular tachycardia, sick sinus syndrome, sinus bradycardia, sinus arrest, atrioventricular block)
- Aortic stenosis
- Myocardial infarction
- Hypertrophic obstructive cardiomyopathy
- Pulmonary hypertension, pulmonary embolism, pulmonary stenosis
- Atrial myxoma

Noncardiac

- Orthostatic or postural hypotension
  - Hypovolemia
  - Drugs, eg, beta blockers, calcium channel blockers, vasodilators, diuretics
  - Autonomic insufficiency, eg, diabetes, adrenal insufficiency, spinal cord lesion, Guillain-Barré syndrome, chronic idiopathic orthostatic hypotension
- Situational, eg, micturition, defecation, cough, swallow
- Carotid sinus hypersensitivity

Tachycardia

Narrow & regular

- Sinus tachycardia
- Atrial flutter
- AV node re-entry tachycardia
- Atrial ventricular re-entry tachycardia (AVRT)
- Wolff-Parkinson-White syndrome (subset of AVRT)
- Atrial tachycardia
- Junctional tachycardia

Narrow & irregular

- Atrial fibrillation
- Frequent premature atrial contractions
- Atrial flutter with variable block
- Multifocal atrial tachycardia
- Sinus arrhythmia

Wide & regular

- Ventricular tachycardia
- Supraventricular tachycardia with aberrancy (eg, pre-existing bundle branch block, rate-related bundle branch block, or WPW)

Wide & irregular

- Torsades de pointes
- Frequent PVCs

Tachycardia, multifocal atrial

- Atrial fibrillation
- Frequent premature atrial contractions
- Atrial flutter (especially if variable block)

Etiology

- Pulmonary disease, eg, chronic obstructive pulmonary disease
- Hypokalemia
- Hypomagnesemia

Tachycardia, paroxysmal supraventricular

Etiology

- Digitalis toxicity
- AV node re-entry tachycardia
- Atrial ventricular re-entry tachycardia (AVRT)
- Wolff-Parkinson-White syndrome (subset of AVRT)

Tachycardia, sinus

- Fever
- Exercise
- Emotion
- Pain
- Anemia
- Heart failure
- Shock
- Hyperthyroidism
- Drugs
- Alcohol withdrawal

Tachycardia, ventricular

- Supraventricular tachycardia with aberrancy (eg, pre-existing bundle branch block, rate-related bundle branch block, or WPW)
- Atrial flutter or atrial fibrillation with aberrancy
- Hyperkalemia (severe)
- Torsades de pointes
- Frequent PVCs

Etiology

- Myocardial infarction
- Dilated cardiomyopathy
- Coronary artery disease
- Hypertrophic obstructive cardiomyopathy
- Mitral valve prolapse
- Myocarditis
- Long QT

Telangiectasia

- Actinic (sun) damage
- Cirrhosis ("spiders")
- Acne rosacea
- Basal cell carcinoma
- Hereditary hemorrhagic telangiectasia (Osler-Weber-Rendu syndrome)
- Scleroderma or CREST syndrome
- Systemic lupus erythematosus
- Dermatomyositis
- Pregnancy
- Necrobiosis lipoidica diabeticorum

Testicular mass or swelling

- Inguinal hernia
- Hydrocele
- Testicular cancer
- Epididymitis
- Orchitis
- Testicular torsion
- Varicocele
- Testicular cyst (epidermoid cyst)
- Lymphoma
- Metastases (rare): prostate, lung, GI, melanoma, kidney

- Lymphedema, eg, filariasis (elephantiasis)

Testicular pain (scrotal pain, groin pain)

- Trauma
- Epididymitis
- Testicular torsion
- Inguinal hernia
- Hydrocele
- Varicocele
- Orchitis
- Torsion of appendix of testis or epididymis
- Testicular tumor
- Prostatitis
- Urinary calculi
- Renal disorder
- Hip joint arthritis, eg, osteoarthritis, septic arthritis
- Iliopsoas bursitis
- Ilioinguinal, iliohypogastric, or genitofemoral neuralgia
- Lumbosacral disk or cord disease

Thalassemias

- Iron deficiency anemia
- Other hemoglobinopathy, eg, sickle thalassemia, hemoglobin C disorders
- Sideroblastic anemia
- Anemia of chronic disease

Etiology

Alpha thalassemia syndromes

- Silent carrier (3 alpha globin genes, normal hematocrit)
- Alpha thalassemia minor or trait (2 genes, hematocrit 32–40%, MCV 60-75)
- Hemoglobin H disease (3 genes, hematocrit 22-32%, MCV 60–70)
- Hydrops fetalis (0 genes)

Beta thalassemia syndromes

- Beta thalassemia minor
- Beta thalassemia intermedia
- Beta thalassemia major

Thrombocytopenia

Etiology

Decreased production (bone marrow disorder)

- Aplastic anemia
- Hematologic malignancies
- Myelodysplastic syndrome

- Megaloblastic anemia
- Chronic alcoholism
- Other infiltrative process, eg, myelofibrosis, infection

Increased destruction

- Immune disorders
  - Idiopathic (autoimmune) thrombocytopenic purpura
  - Drug-induced, eg, heparin, sulfonamides, thiazides, quinine
  - Secondary (chronic lymphocytic leukemia, systemic lupus erythematosus)
  - Posttransfusion purpura
- Disseminated intravascular coagulation
- Thrombotic thrombocytopenic purpura
- Hemolytic uremic syndrome
- Sepsis
- Viral infections, AIDS
- Liver failure
- Preeclampsia-eclampsia

Splenic sequestration

Thrombocytosis

Etiology

Reactive thrombocytosis (usually platelets <1,000,000)

- Inflammatory disease, eg, rheumatoid arthritis, ulcerative colitis
- Chronic infection
- Iron deficiency anemia
- Postsplenectomy (transient)

Myeloproliferative disorder

- Essential thrombocytosis
- Polycythemia vera
- Chronic myelogenous leukemia
- Myelofibrosis

Thyroid nodules

- Adenoma, colloid nodule, or cyst
- Benign multinodular goiter
- Thyroid cancer
- Hashimoto's thyroiditis (may be nodular)
- Metastatic cancer

Tinnitus

- Idiopathic
- Excessive noise exposure
- Ménière's disease
- Labyrinthitis
- Acute otitis media
- Chronic otitis media

- Auditory (eustachian) tube dysfunction
- Ototoxicity, eg, salicylates, aminoglycosides, loop diuretics, cisplatin
- Glomus tumor
- Any cause of sensory hearing loss

Pulsatile tinnitus

- Glomus tumor
- Carotid stenosis or carotid dissection
- Arteriovenous malformation
- Aneurysm
- Pseudotumor cerebri

Toxidromes (poisoning syndromes)

Etiology

- Sympathomimetic poisoning
- Sympatholytic poisoning
- Cholinergic poisoning
- Anticholinergic poisoning
- Acetaminophen poisoning
- Amphetamines or cocaine intoxication
- Beta blocker overdose
- Carbon monoxide poisoning
- Chemical warfare agents (eg, cholinergic poisoning)
- Digitalis overdose
- Iron poisoning
- Isoniazid (INH) poisoning
- Lead poisoning
- Methanol and ethylene glycol poisoning
- Methemoglobinemia
- Opioid overdose
- Salicylate poisoning
- Tricyclic antidepressant overdose

Transient ischemic attack

- Stroke
- Hypoglycemia
- Seizure (Todd's paralysis)
- Syncope
- Migraine
- Peripheral causes of vertigo, eg, Ménière's disease

Etiology

- Embolic: atrial fibrillation, carotid atherosclerosis, left ventricular aneurysm, dilated cardiomyopathy, acute myocardial infarction, endocarditis, mechanical valve, mitral valve prolapse, aortic arch atherosclerosis, atrial myxoma, patent foramen ovale
- Thrombotic: atherosclerosis, small vessel ischemia, vasculitis, eg, systemic lupus

erythematosus, polycythemia, thrombocytosis, sickle cell disease, meningovascular syphilis, arterial dissection or aneurysm, eg, intracerebral carotid or vertebral
• Hemorrhagic: hypertension, amyloidosis, conversion of ischemic stroke, cocaine

Traveler's diarrhea

• Most common: Enterotoxigenic *E. coli, Shigella, Campylobacter*
• Less common: *Aeromonas, Salmonella,* noncholera vibrios, *Entamoeba histolytica, Giardia lamblia,* adenoviruses, rotavirus
• Chronic watery diarrhea: *Entamoeba histolytica, Giardia lamblia,* tropical sprue (rare)
• From unprotected anal intercourse: *Neisseria gonorrhoeae,* syphilis, lymphogranuloma venereum, herpes simplex virus

Tremor

Etiology

• Enhanced physiologic tremor, eg, anxiety
• Essential tremor
• Parkinson's disease
• Hyperthyroidism
• Hepatic encephalopathy
• Cerebellar tremor, eg, multiple sclerosis
• Adult-onset idiopathic dystonia
• Wilson's disease
• Drugs: caffeine, alcohol withdrawal, sympathomimetics, antipsychotics, theophylline, metoclopramide, lithium, levothyroxine, tricyclic antidepressants, valproic acid, reserpine
• Psychogenic tremor

Tricuspid regurgitation

• Mitral regurgitation
• Aortic stenosis
• Pulmonary stenosis
• Atrial septal defect
• Ventricular septal defect

Etiology

• Right ventricular overload due to left ventricular failure
• Infective endocarditis
• Pulmonary hypertension
• Right ventricular or inferior myocardial infarction
• Rheumatic heart disease

• Carcinoid syndrome
• Systemic lupus erythematosus
• Myxomatous degeneration or mitral valve prolapse
• Ebstein's anomaly

Triglycerides increased

Etiology

• Alcohol
• Obesity
• "Metabolic syndrome" (insulin resistance, low HDL)
• Diabetes mellitus
• Chronic renal insufficiency
• Lipodystrophy, eg, protease inhibitors
• Pregnancy
• Familial
• Drugs: oral contraceptives, isotretinoin, thiazides (short-term effect), beta blockers (short-term effect), corticosteroids, bile acid-binding resins

TSH decreased

Etiology

• Primary hyperthyroidism, eg, Graves' disease, toxic multinodular goiter, toxic thyroid nodule, subacute thyroiditis, early Hashimoto's disease
• Thyroid hormone administration
• Severe nonthyroidal illness
• Dopamine or dopamine agonists (levodopa, bromocriptine)
• Pregnancy
• hCG-secreting trophoblastic tumor
• Acute psychiatric illness
• Acute glucocorticoid administration
• Other drugs, eg, NSAIDs, amphetamines, octreotide, opioids, nifedipine, verapamil
• "Subclinical" hyperthyroidism: low TSH, clinically euthyroid, normal T4, common in elderly (10%), risk of atrial fibrillation and osteoporosis

TSH increased

Etiology

• Primary hypothyroidism
• "Subclinical" hypothyroidism: high TSH, clinically euthyroid, normal T4
• Autoimmune disease (assay interference)
• Recovery from nonthyroidal illness
• Acute psychiatric illness
• Drugs: dopamine antagonists (eg, metoclopramide), phenothiazines, atypical antipsychotics

• Rare cases of hyperthyroidism due to inappropriate pituitary TSH secretion, eg, neoplasm

Ulcer and eschar

• Cutaneous anthrax
• Warfarin necrosis
• Antiphospholipid antibody syndrome
• Aspergillosis
• Mucormycosis
• Brown recluse spider bite
• Cutaneous leishmaniasis
• Ecthyma gangrenosum (neutropenic, pseudomonal)
• Tularemia
• Rickettsialpox
• Plague

Ulcer, leg

• Venous stasis ulcers (due to venous insufficiency)
• Arterial insufficiency (arterial ulcer)
• Stasis dermatitis (due to venous insufficiency)
• Diabetic neuropathy
• Bacterial pyoderma (eg, infected wound or bite)
• Trauma
• Pressure ulcer
• Vasculitis, eg, thromboangiitis obliterans (Buerger's disease)
• Rheumatoid arthritis or Felty's syndrome
• Pyoderma gangrenosum
• Underlying skin cancer
• Sickle cell anemia
• Embolic disease (including cholesterol emboli)
• Cryoglobulinemia
• Erythema induratum (associated with tuberculosis)
• Other underlying infection (eg, fungal, tertiary syphilis, leishmaniasis, amebiasis, dracunculiasis)
• Calciphylaxis

Upper respiratory tract infection (URI)

• Allergic rhinitis
• Sinusitis (rhinosinusitis)
• Pharyngitis
• Bronchitis
• Otitis media

- Asthma
- Influenza
- Pneumonia
- Mononucleosis
- Laryngitis
- Pertussis
- Epiglottitis

Urethral discharge, men

- Gonorrhea
- Nongonococcal urethritis, eg, chlamydia, *Ureaplasma urealyticum,* trichomoniasis
- Balanitis, eg, candidiasis
- Reactive arthritis (Reiter's syndrome)
- Urethral carcinoma

Urethral discharge, women

- Gonorrhea
- Nongonococcal urethritis, eg, chlamydia, *Ureaplasma urealyticum*
- Trichomoniasis
- Candidiasis
- Cystitis
- Reactive arthritis (Reiter's syndrome)
- Urethral carcinoma

Urinary frequency

- Cystitis
- Urethritis
- Pyelonephritis
- Diabetes mellitus
- Diabetes insipidus
- Excess fluid intake
- Diuretics
- Caffeine, alcohol
- Chronic urinary retention
- Neurogenic bladder
- Interstitial cystitis
- Urethral syndrome
- Extrinsic bladder compression, eg, pelvic tumor, radiation-induced fibrosis
- Urinary calculi
- Anxiety

Urinary incontinence

- Cystitis
- Prostatitis
- Interstitial cystitis
- Medications, eg, diuretics, alcohol, caffeine, hypnotics

- Polyuria, eg, diabetes mellitus, diabetes insipidus, hypercalcemia
- Vesicovaginal or ureterovaginal fistula
- Dementia
- Normal pressure hydrocephalus

Etiology

Transient incontinence

- Delirium
- Infection
- Atrophic vaginitis or urethritis
- Pharmacology, eg, anticholinergics, diuretics, hypnotics
- Psychiatric disorders, eg, psychosis, depression
- Excess urine, eg, edema, hyperglycemia, hypercalcemia
- Restricted mobility
- Stool impaction

Established incontinence

- Detrusor overactivity (urge incontinence or "overactive" bladder)
- Urethral incompetence (stress incontinence, eg, multiparity, pelvic surgery)
- Urethral obstruction (eg, benign prostatic hyperplasia; can also present as urge or overflow)
- Detrusor underactivity (overflow incontinence, eg, neurogenic bladder, anticholinergics)
- Mixed incontinence (urge and stress)

Urinary tract infection

- Acute cystitis
- Pyelonephritis
- Acute bacterial prostatitis
- Chronic bacterial prostatitis

Urinary tract obstruction

- Benign prostatic hyperplasia (especially with anticholinergics or over-the-counter sympathomimetics)
- Bilateral ureteral calculi
- Urethral stricture
- Neurogenic bladder
- Prostate cancer
- Bladder cancer
- Extrinsic compression, eg, pelvic or GI tumor, radiation-induced fibrosis
- Urethral carcinoma
- Meatal stenosis

Urinary urgency

- Cystitis
- Urethritis

- Pyelonephritis
- Neurogenic bladder
- Interstitial cystitis
- Urethral syndrome
- Urinary calculi

Urine, cloudy

- Urinary tract infection
- Alkaline urinary pH
- Chyluria (lymph in urine) due to fistula with lymphatics, eg, filariasis, tuberculosis, retroperitoneal tumor

Urine, dark

- Hematuria
- Biliary tract obstruction
- Hepatitis
- Dehydration (concentrated urine)
- Hemolytic anemia
- Rhabdomyolysis
- Ingestion of beets
- Phenazopyridine (Pyridium) use
- Alkaptonuria (ochronosis)
- Acute intermittent porphyria

Urticaria & angioedema

- Vasculitis
- Erythema multiforme
- Contact dermatitis (eg, poison oak or ivy)
- Pityriasis rosea
- Erythema migrans (Lyme disease)

Etiology

- Arthropod-related skin lesions (insect bites)
- Drugs (nonallergic), eg, codeine, morphine
- Physical factors: heat, cold urticaria, solar, pressure, water, vibratory
- Cholinergic urticaria: exercise, excitement, hot showers
- Drugs (allergic): penicillin, aspirin
- Other allergic causes: feathers, dander, shellfish, tomatoes, strawberries, vaccines, chemicals, cosmetics
- Infection, eg, otitis media, sinusitis, hepatitis
- Serum sickness
- Angioedema: complement-mediated (hereditary or acquired), ACE inhibitors

Uveitis (iritis, cyclitis, choroiditis, retinitis)

- Acute glaucoma
- Keratitis (corneal ulcer or inflammation), eg, herpes simplex
- Conjunctivitis
- Scleritis or episcleritis
- Retinal detachment
- Intraocular tumor, eg, retinoblastoma, leukemia, melanoma
- CNS lymphoma
- Retained intraocular foreign body

Etiology

- HLA-B27–related conditions: ankylosing spondylitis, reactive arthritis (Reiter's syndrome), psoriasis, inflammatory bowel disease
- Behçet's syndrome
- Herpes simplex or zoster infection
- Sarcoidosis
- Tuberculosis, syphilis, toxoplasmosis
- AIDS: Cytomegalovirus, herpes simplex virus, herpes zoster, mycobacteria, *Cryptococcus, Toxoplasma, Candida*
- Vogt-Koyanagi-Harada syndrome (uveitis, alopecia, poliosis, vitiligo, hearing loss)
- Autoimmune retinal vasculitis

Vaginal bleeding, abnormal premenopausal (increased or irregular)

- Ovulation bleeding (spotting episode between menses)
- Anovulatory cycle (dysfunctional uterine bleeding)
- Polycystic ovary syndrome (type of anovulatory cycle)
- Pregnancy
- Ectopic pregnancy
- Spontaneous abortion
- Uterine leiomyomas (fibroids)
- Endometrial polyp
- Cervicitis or pelvic inflammatory disease
- Adenomyosis (uterine endometriosis)
- Cervical cancer
- Cervical polyp
- Endometrial hyperplasia
- Endometrial cancer
- Hypothyroidism
- Hyperprolactinemia
- Diabetes mellitus

- Bleeding disorder, eg, von Willebrand's disease
- Hydatidiform mole

Vaginal bleeding, postmenopausal

- Atrophic endometrium
- Endometrial hyperplasia or proliferation
- Endometrial cancer
- Atrophic vaginitis
- Perimenopausal bleeding
- Endometrial polyp
- Unopposed exogenous estrogen
- Cervical cancer
- Uterine leiomyomas (fibroids)
- Trauma
- Bleeding disorder
- Cervical polyp
- Cervical ulcer
- Vaginal cancer
- Vulvar cancer

Vaginal bleeding, third-trimester

- Placental causes: placenta previa, placental abruption, vasa previa
- Infection, eg, vaginitis, cervicitis
- Labor (blood or mucus plug)
- Ruptured cervical blood vessel (eg, by intercourse)
- Bleeding disorder
- Cervical cancer

Vaginal discharge

- Normal vaginal discharge
- Bacterial vaginosis
- *Trichomonas* vaginitis
- *Candida* vulvovaginitis
- Cervicitis
- Pelvic inflammatory disease
- Reaction to douches, tampons, condoms, soap
- Cervical cancer
- Uterine cancer

Vaginitis

Etiology

- Normal vaginal discharge
- Bacterial vaginosis
- *Trichomonas* vaginitis
- *Candida* vulvovaginitis
- Atrophic vaginitis

- Genital warts (condyloma acuminata)
- Friction from intercourse
- Reaction to douches, tampons, condoms, soap

Varicocele

Etiology

- Right-sided: retroperitoneal malignancy obstructing right spermatic vein
- Left-sided: left renal vein obstruction, eg, renal cell carcinoma

Vasculitis syndromes

- Polyarteritis nodosa: fever, hypertension, abdominal pain, often hepatitis B or C
- Microscopic polyangiitis: overlaps with PAN, glomerulonephritis, pulmonary hemorrhage
- Churg-Strauss syndrome: asthma, transient pulmonary infiltrates
- Wegener's granulomatosis: respiratory disease and glomerulonephritis
- Temporal (giant cell) arteritis: headache, jaw claudication, blindness, associated with polymyalgia rheumatica
- Takayasu's arteritis: young Asian women, aortic arch vasculitis
- Henoch-Schönlein purpura: children, palpable purpura, abdominal pain
- Hypersensitivity (leukocytoclastic) vasculitis: lower extremity palpable purpura; associated with drugs, neoplasms, connective tissue disease, viral or bacterial infection, cryoglobulinemia, serum sickness
- Thromboangiitis obliterans (Buerger's disease): smokers, extremity ischemia
- Behçet's syndrome: oral and genital ulcers, ocular lesions
- Kawasaki syndrome: children, fever, rash, conjunctivitis, cardiac disease

Vasculitis, hypersensitivity (leukocytoclastic)

- Polyarteritis nodosa
- Henoch-Schönlein purpura
- Meningococcemia
- Disseminated gonococcal infection
- Cryoglobulinemia

Vertigo

By episode duration

Auditory symptoms present
- Seconds: perilymphatic fistula

- Hours: endolymphatic hydrops (Ménière's disease, syphilis)
- Days: labyrinthitis, labyrinthine concussion (head trauma)
- Months: acoustic neuroma, ototoxicity

Auditory symptoms absent
- Seconds: positioning vertigo (cupulolithiasis), vertebrobasilar insufficiency, cervical vertigo (head-extension vertigo), diplopia
- Hours: recurrent vestibulopathy (Ménière's disease without auditory symptoms), vestibular migraine
- Days: vestibular neuronitis, head trauma
- Months: vertebrobasilar insufficiency, arteriovenous malformation, brainstem or cerebellar tumor, cerebellar degeneration, multiple sclerosis, vertebrobasilar migraine

Drugs
- Anticonvulsants (eg, phenytoin), antibiotics (eg, aminoglycosides, doxycycline, metronidazole), hypnotics (eg, diazepam), analgesics (eg, aspirin), alcohol

Vesicles

- Herpes simplex virus infection (cold sore, genital herpes)
- Varicella (chicken pox)
- Herpes zoster (shingles)
- Contact dermatitis
- Scabies
- Dyshidrotic eczema (pompholyx, dyshidrosis)
- Vesicular tinea
- Dermatitis herpetiformis
- Atopic dermatitis (eczema) (acute)
- Dermatophytid reaction (allergy or sensitivity to fungi)
- Miliaria (heat rash)
- Porphyria cutanea tarda
- Photodermatitis
- Smallpox
- Rickettsialpox
- Hand, foot, and mouth disease

Visual loss, acute

Inflamed (red) eye
- Acute glaucoma
- Uveitis
- Keratitis (corneal ulcer or inflammation), eg, herpes simplex
- Conjunctivitis (blurry)

Uninflamed eye
- Retinal detachment
- Central retinal vein occlusion
- Central retinal artery occlusion
- Vitreous hemorrhage
- Macular degeneration (exudative)
- Anterior ischemic optic neuropathy, eg, temporal (giant cell) arteritis
- Optic neuritis, eg, multiple sclerosis
- Papilledema
- Hyperglycemia (blurry; subacute)
- Polycythemia vera (blurry; subacute)
- Trauma
- Conversion disorder
- Episodic: amaurosis fugax (transient ischemic attack), ophthalmic migraine
- Diplopia

Visual loss, chronic

- Refractive error
- Cataract
- Macular degeneration (atrophic)
- Diabetic retinopathy
- Glaucoma
- Corneal opacity, eg, scar, pterygium
- Chronic uveitis
- Pituitary tumor (bitemporal)
- Other types of retinopathy, eg, hypertensive, sickle cell, severe anemia, radiation, systemic lupus erythematosus, talc (emboli from IV drug use)
- Cerebrovascular disease or brain tumor affecting visual pathways
- Intraorbital tumor
- Toxic optic neuropathy, eg, methanol
- Lens dislocation, eg, Marfan syndrome, homocystinuria
- Other worldwide causes: trachoma, Hansen's disease (leprosy), onchocerciasis, xerophthalmia (vitamin A deficiency)

Vitreous hemorrhage

Etiology
- Diabetic retinopathy
- Retinal tear (with or without retinal detachment)
- Retinal vein occlusion
- Macular degeneration (exudative)
- Blood dyscrasias
- Trauma
- Subarachnoid hemorrhage

Vocal cord paralysis

Etiology
- Recurrent laryngeal nerve damage: thyroid or other neck surgery, lung cancer, thyroid cancer
- Laryngeal cancer
- Esophageal cancer
- Intubation injury
- Cricoarytenoid arthritis (in rheumatoid arthritis)
- Glottic or subglottic stenosis
- Skull base tumor involving cranial nerves IX, X, and XI
- Idiopathic

Vulvar lesions

- Genital warts (condyloma acuminata)
- Contact dermatitis
- Vulvovaginal candidiasis
- Ulcer: herpes simplex virus, chancroid, syphilis, granuloma inguinale, lymphogranuloma venereum, Behçet's syndrome
- Vulvar cancer
- Vulvar intraepithelial neoplasia
- Vulvar vestibulitis
- Bartholin's cyst or abscess
- Epidermal cyst
- Epithelial polyp
- Lichen sclerosus
- Hypertrophic vulvar dystrophy
- Lichen planus
- Psoriasis
- Cicatricial pemphigoid
- Hidradenitis suppurativa
- Lichen simplex chronicus
- Papillary hidradenoma
- Paget's disease
- Melanoma
- Vitiligo
- Molluscum contagiosum
- Pediculosis (lice)

Weakness

General
- Disuse of muscles
- Anemia
- Malnutrition
- Electrolyte abnormality, eg, hypercalcemia, hypokalemia, hyponatremia
- Endocrine disease, eg, hypothyroidism, diabetes mellitus, Cushing's

syndrome, Addison's disease, hyperaldosteronism
- Chronic lung or heart disease
- Malingering

Upper motor neuron disease
- Stroke
- Space-occupying lesion, eg, brain tumor
- Spinal cord lesion
- Multiple sclerosis

Lower motor neuron disease
- Anterior horn cell, eg, poliomyelitis, amyotrophic lateral sclerosis, West Nile virus
- Motor nerve root, eg, disk protrusion
- Nerve plexus, eg, brachial plexus neuropathy
- Peripheral nerve, eg, diabetes mellitus, alcoholism, heavy metals, Guillain-Barré syndrome
- Neuromuscular junction, eg, myasthenia gravis, Eaton-Lambert syndrome, botulism, organophosphate poisoning, tick paralysis, drug-induced, eg, aminoglycoside
- Myopathy, eg, polymyositis, corticosteroids, hypothyroidism, alcohol
- Other: aortic dissection, periodic paralysis, eg, hypokalemic, hyperkalemic, thyrotoxic

Weakness, proximal muscle

Muscle inflammation
- Polymyositis
- Dermatomyositis
- Systemic lupus erythematosus
- Scleroderma
- Sjögren's syndrome
- Inclusion body myositis
- Trichinosis (*Trichinella* infection)
- Sarcocystosis

Other causes of proximal muscle weakness
- Polymyalgia rheumatica
- Endocrine: hypothyroidism, hyperthyroidism, Cushing's syndrome

- Alcoholism
- Drugs: corticosteroids, statins, clofibrate, colchicine, chloroquine, emetine, aminocaproic acid, bretylium, penicillamine, drugs causing hypokalemia
- HIV myopathy
- Hyperparathyroidism
- Spinal stenosis
- Osteomalacia
- Mitochondrial myopathy

Weeping or encrusted lesions

- Impetigo
- Contact dermatitis (acute)
- Any vesicular dermatitis can become crusted

Weight loss, involuntary

Medical
- Malignancy
- Gastrointestinal disorders, eg, malabsorption, pancreatic insufficiency, peptic ulcer
- Hyperthyroidism
- Chronic heart, lung, or renal disease
- Uncontrolled diabetes mellitus
- Intestinal ischemia
- Dysphagia
- Anorexia due to azotemia
- Hypercalcemia
- Tuberculosis
- Subacute bacterial endocarditis

Psychosocial
- Depression
- Dementia
- Alcoholism
- Anorexia nervosa
- Loss of teeth, poor denture fit
- Social isolation
- Poverty
- Inability to buy or prepare food

Drug related
- NSAIDs
- Antiepileptics

- Digoxin
- SSRIs

Wheezing

- Asthma
- Chronic obstructive pulmonary disease
- Congestive heart failure (cardiac asthma)
- Acute bronchitis
- Pneumonia
- Gastroesophageal reflux disease
- Airway obstruction (eg, tumor, goiter)
- Foreign-body aspiration
- Aspiration pneumonia
- Interstitial lung disease
- Pulmonary embolism
- Angioedema or anaphylaxis
- Carcinoid syndrome
- Vocal cord dysfunction
- Ascariasis

Wrist drop (radial nerve palsy)

Etiology
- Radial nerve compression
- Diabetes mellitus

Wrist pain

- Sprain
- Area of first CMC joint: osteoarthritis, de Quervain's tenosynovitis, scaphoid fracture (snuffbox pain)
- Carpal tunnel syndrome
- Pronator teres syndrome (median nerve entrapment at level of pronator teres)
- Lunate fracture or dislocation
- Colles (distal radius) fracture
- Triangular fibrocartilage complex injury
- Arthritis, eg, rheumatoid arthritis, osteoarthritis, reactive arthritis (Reiter's syndrome), psoriatic arthritis, gout or pseudogout, septic arthritis
- Dorsal ganglion (may be ventral)
- Superficial radial neuropathy (cheiralgia paresthetica or handcuff neuropathy)

A–Z
in Detail

Abdominal Aortic Aneurysm

 KEY FEATURES

ESSENTIALS OF DIAGNOSIS

- Defined as an aortic diameter exceeding 3 cm
- Most are asymptomatic, detected during a routine physical examination or imaging performed for another reason
- Severe back or abdominal pain and hypotension indicate rupture
- Concomitant atherosclerotic occlusive disease of lower extremities in 25%

GENERAL CONSIDERATIONS

- Over 90% of abdominal aneurysms originate below the renal arteries, many extend into the common iliac arteries
- Half are <5 cm in diameter
- On routine ultrasound surveillance, two-thirds will increase in size to require repair
- Yearly rupture risk is 2% for 4–5.4 cm aneurysms, 7% for 6–6.9 cm aneurysms, and 25% for 7 cm aneurysms
- Patients with chronic obstructive pulmonary disease are more likely to rupture smaller aneurysms
- More than one-third of patients with popliteal aneurysms have abdominal aortic aneurysms

DEMOGRAPHICS

- Aortic aneurysm is present in 5–8% of the population over the age of 65
- Incidence has tripled over the last 30 years

 CLINICAL FINDINGS

SYMPTOMS AND SIGNS

- Asymptomatic aneurysms: prominent aortic pulsation on routine physical examination and incidental finding on abdominal ultrasound or CT scan: coexisting renal or lower extremity arterial occlusive disease is present in 25%, popliteal artery aneurysms in 15%
- Symptomatic aneurysms: midabdominal or lower back pain (or both)
- Inflammatory aortic aneurysms: low-grade fever, elevated sedimentation rate, and recent upper respiratory tract infection
- Infected aneurysms (rare): fever of unknown origin, peripheral emboli, positive blood cultures, caused by septic emboli to a normal aorta or bacterial colonization of an existing aneurysm
- Ruptured aneurysms: severe back, abdominal, or flank pain and hypotension; 90% of patients die before reaching the hospital or in the perioperative period

DIFFERENTIAL DIAGNOSIS

- Asymptomatic abdominal aortic aneurysms: intraabdominal tumor, iliac aneurysm, or mesenteric artery
- Symptomatic/ruptured abdominal aortic aneurysms: acute myocardial infarction, aortic dissection, renal stones, gastroenteritis, bowel obstruction, and bowel infarction

 DIAGNOSIS

LABORATORY TESTS

- Preoperative evaluation: obtain electrocardiogram, serum creatinine, hematocrit and hemoglobin, and type and cross-match

IMAGING STUDIES

- Abdominal ultrasonography: indicated for screening and for following aneurysm growth (annually for aneurysms >3.5 cm in diameter)
- Abdominal radiograph: curvilinear calcifications are much less accurate
- Contrast-enhanced CT scanning: precisely sizes the aneurysm, defines its relationship to the renal arteries
- MRI is as sensitive and specific as CT and is useful if renal insufficiency precludes contrast-enhanced CT
- Aortography: indicated prior to elective aneurysm repair when arterial occlusive disease of the visceral or lower extremity arteries is suspected or when endograft repair is being considered
- Preoperative evaluation assessment of cardiac risk and examination of the carotid arteries

TREATMENT

MEDICATIONS

- β-Blockers and oral roxithromycin (300 mg daily for 30 days) decrease the expansion rate of small aneurysms

SURGERY

- In asymptomatic good-risk patients, surgery advised when aneurysm diameter exceeds 5 cm
- In poor-risk patients, surgery advised when aneurysm diameter exceeds 6 cm
- Urgent repair advised for symptomatic aneurysms irrespective of diameter
- Ruptured aneurysms require emergent surgery
- Open repair: surgical resection and synthetic graft replacement for most thoracic, abdominal, juxtarenal, and infrarenal aortic aneurysms with diameter >5 cm
- Endovascular repair: Uniiliac or bifurcated endovascular stent grafts, deployed via the common femoral arteries, can be considered for infrarenal aneurysms with favorable anatomy
- Endovascular repair involves bilateral inguinal incisions under epidural anesthesia, and thus has made repair of aortic aneurysms feasible in elderly high-risk patients
- Long-term durability of endovascular grafts needs to be established

THERAPEUTIC PROCEDURES

- Physical examination
- Ultrasound of abdominal aorta every 6 months

OUTCOME

FOLLOW-UP

- Open repair: yearly physical examination
- Endovascular repair: routine surveillance, CT abdomen, and physical examination

COMPLICATIONS

- Open repair: acute myocardial infarction, arrhythmia, bleeding, respiratory failure, limb ischemia, renal failure, stroke, ischemic colitis, bowel infarction, liver dysfunction, acalculous cholecystitis, graft infection, graft-enteric fistula
- Endovascular repair: persistent filling of the aneurysm (endoleak), graft migration, graft thrombosis, graft infection (rare), renal failure, conversion to open repair

PROGNOSIS

- Mortality following elective open or endovascular repair is 1–5%
- A patient with a >5-cm aortic aneurysm and life expectancy of more than 1 year, has a 3-fold greater chance of dying of rupture than of dying from surgical resection
- 5-year survival after surgical repair is 60–80%
- 5–10% will develop another aortic aneurysm adjacent to the graft or in the thoracic aorta

WHEN TO REFER

- Any patient with an aneurysm 4.0 cm or greater
- Any patient with a symptomatic or suspected ruptured abdominal aortic aneurysm

WHEN TO ADMIT

- All patients with symptomatic or suspected ruptured abdominal aortic aneurysms or suspected infected aneurysms

PREVENTION

- Blood pressure control
- Cardiovascular risk assessment and treatment
- Smoking cessation
- Screening of family members over 65

EVIDENCE

PRACTICE GUIDELINES

- Brewster DC et al: Guidelines for the treatment of abdominal aortic aneurysms. Report of a subcommittee of the Joint Council of the American Association for Vascular Surgery and Society for Vascular Surgery. J Vasc Surg 2003;37:1106. [PMID: 12756363]

WEB SITES

- MEDLINEplus—Abdominal aortic aneurysm http://www.nlm.nih.gov/medlineplus/ency/article/000162.htm
- NIH—Patient Education Institute: Abdominal Aortic Aneurysm http://www.nlm.nih.gov/medlineplus/tutorials/abdominalaorticaneurysm.html

INFORMATION FOR PATIENTS

- Cleveland Clinic—Abdominal aortic aneurysm http://www.clevelandclinic.org/health/health-info/docs/ 2400/2455.asp?index=9513

REFERENCES

- Ashton HA et al: The multicentre aneurysm screening study (MASS) into the effect of abdominal aortic aneurysm screening on mortality in men: a randomized controlled trial. Lancet 2002;360:1531. [PMID: 12443589]
- Ohki T et al: Increasing incidence of mid-term and long-term complications after endovascular graft repair of abdominal aortic aneurysms: a note of caution based on a 9-year experience. Ann Surg 2001;234:323. [PMID: 11524585]
- Vammen S et al: Randomized double-blind controlled trial of roxithromycin for prevention of abdominal aortic aneurysm expansion. Br J Surg 2001;88:1066. [PMID: 11488791]

Louis M. Messina, MD
Laura K. Pak, MD
Lawrence M. Tierney, Jr., MD

Abortion

 KEY FEATURES

ESSENTIALS OF DIAGNOSIS

- In the United States, 90% of abortions are performed before 12 weeks' gestation and only 3–4% after 17 weeks
- If abortion is chosen, every effort should be made to encourage an early procedure

GENERAL CONSIDERATIONS

- The abortion-related maternal mortality rate has fallen markedly since the legalization of abortion in the United States in 1973.
- Abortions are rarely performed after 20 weeks from the last menstrual period (LMP); it is believed that fetal viability is established at about 24 weeks
- The long-term sequelae of repeated induced abortions are uncertain regarding increased rates of fetal loss or premature labor
- Adverse sequelae can be minimized by performing early abortion with minimal cervical dilation or by the use of osmotic dilators to induce gradual cervical dilation

 CLINICAL FINDINGS

SYMPTOMS AND SIGNS

- Pregnancy that is less than 20 weeks from the LMP

 DIAGNOSIS

LABORATORY TESTS

- Determine if patient is Rh positive or negative

DIAGNOSTIC PROCEDURES

- Establish date of LMP

TREATMENT

MEDICATIONS

- An FDA-approved oral abortifacient, mifepristone (RU 486), 600 mg as a single dose followed in 36–48 h by a prostaglandin vaginally or orally, is 95% successful in terminating pregnancies of up to 9 weeks' duration with minimum complications
- Although not approved by the FDA for this indication, a combination of intramuscular methotrexate, 50 mg/m^2 of body surface area, followed 7 days later by vaginal misoprostol, 800 μg, is 98% successful in terminating pregnancy at 8 weeks or less; minor side effects of nausea, vomiting, and diarrhea are common. There is a 5–10% incidence of hemorrhage or incomplete abortion requiring curettage, but there are no known long-term complications

THERAPEUTIC PROCEDURES

- Abortion in the first trimester is performed by vacuum aspiration under local anesthesia
- A similar technique, dilation and evacuation, is often used in the second trimester, with general or local anesthesia
- Techniques utilizing intraamniotic instillation of hypertonic saline solution or prostaglandins are also occasionally used after 18 weeks from the LMP but are more difficult for the patient

 OUTCOME

COMPLICATIONS

- Retained products of conception (often associated with infection and heavy bleeding) and unrecognized ectopic pregnancy
- Immediate analysis of the removed tissue for placenta can exclude or corroborate the diagnosis of ectopic pregnancy
- Women presenting with fever, bleeding, or abdominal pain after abortion should be examined; use of broad-spectrum antibiotics and reaspiration of the uterus are frequently necessary

PROGNOSIS

- Legal abortion has a mortality rate of <1:100,000. Rates of morbidity and mortality rise with length of gestation

WHEN TO ADMIT

- Hospitalization is advisable if acute salpingitis requires intravenous administration of antibiotics
- Complications following illegal abortion often need emergency care for hemorrhage, septic shock, or uterine perforation

PREVENTION

- Contraception should be thoroughly discussed and contraception provided at the time of abortion
- In women with a past history of pelvic inflammatory disease, prophylactic antibiotics are indicated: a one-dose regimen is doxycycline, 200 mg orally 1 h before the procedure, or aqueous penicillin G, 1 million units intravenously 30 min before. In the second trimester, use cefazolin, 1 g intravenously 30 min before the procedure. Many prescribe tetracycline, 500 mg four times daily, for 5 days after the procedure for all patients
- Rh immune globulin should be given to all Rh-negative women following abortion

 EVIDENCE

PRACTICE GUIDELINES

- National Guideline Clearinghouse http://www.guideline.gov/summary/ summary.aspx?doc_id=3689&nbr=2915 &string=abortion

INFORMATION FOR PATIENTS

- American College of Obstetricians and Gynecologists http://www.medem.com/medlb/ article_detaillb.cfm?article_ID= ZZZ2K98T77C&sub_cat=2006 http://www.medem.com/search/ article_display.cfm?path=\\ TANQUERAY\M_ContentItem& mstr=/M_Content Item/ZZZHSWHG97C.html&soc= ACOG&srch_typ=NAV_SERCH

REFERENCES

- Grimes DA: A 26-year-old woman seeking an abortion. JAMA 1999;282:1169. [PMID: 10501121]
- Newhall EP et al: Abortion with mifepristone and misoprostol: regimens, efficacy, acceptability and future directions. Am J Obstet Gynecol 2000;183:S44. [PMID: 10944369]

H. Trent MacKay, MD, MPH

Abortion, Spontaneous

 ## KEY FEATURES

ESSENTIALS OF DIAGNOSIS

- Intrauterine pregnancy at less than 20 weeks
- Low or falling levels of human chorionic gonadotropin (hCG)
- Bleeding and/or midline cramping pain
- Open cervical os
- Complete or partial expulsion of products of conception

GENERAL CONSIDERATIONS

- Defined as termination of gestation prior to the 20th week of pregnancy
- 75% of cases occur before the 16th week, with 75% of these before the 8th week
- Almost 20% of clinically recognized pregnancies terminate in spontaneous abortion
- More than 60% of cases result from chromosomal defects
- About 15% of cases are associated with maternal trauma, infection, dietary deficiency, diabetes mellitus, hypothyroidism, or anatomic malformations
- There is no evidence that psychic stimuli such as severe fright, grief, anger, or anxiety can induce termination
- There is no evidence that electromagnetic fields are associated with an increased risk of termination
- It is important to distinguish women with incompetent cervix from more typical early abortion, premature labor, or rupture of the membranes

DEMOGRAPHICS

- Predisposing factors are a history of incompetent cervix, cervical conization or surgery, cervical injury, diethylstilbestrol exposure, and anatomical abnormalities of the cervix

 ## CLINICAL FINDINGS

SYMPTOMS AND SIGNS

- *Incompetent cervix* classically presents as "silent" cervical dilation (without contractions) between weeks 16 and 28
- *Threatened abortion*: bleeding or cramping without termination. The cervix is not dilated
- *Inevitable abortion*: the cervix is dilated and membranes may be ruptured; passage of products of conception has not occurred, but is considered inevitable
- *Complete abortion:* the fetus and placenta are completely expelled. Pain ceases, but spotting may persist
- *Incomplete abortion:* some portion of the products of conception remain in the uterus. Cramps are usually mild; bleeding is persistent and often excessive
- *Missed abortion*: the pregnancy has ceased to develop, but the conceptus has not been expelled. Symptoms of pregnancy disappear; there is brownish vaginal discharge but no free bleeding

DIFFERENTIAL DIAGNOSIS

- Ectopic pregnancy
- Hydatidiform mole
- Incompetent cervix
- Anovular bleeding in a nonpregnant women
- Menses or menorrhagia
- Cervical neoplasm or lesion

 ## DIAGNOSIS

LABORATORY TESTS

- Falling levels of hCG
- Complete blood count should be obtained if bleeding is heavy
- Rh type should be determined and Rho(D) Ig given if the type is Rh negative
- All recovered tissue should be preserved and assessed by a pathologist

IMAGING STUDIES

- Ultrasound can identify the gestational sac 5–6 weeks from the last menstrual period, a fetal pole at 6 weeks, and fetal cardiac activity at 6–7 weeks
- With accurate dating, a small, irregular sac without a fetal pole is diagnostic of an abnormal pregnancy

Abortion, Spontaneous

 ## TREATMENT

MEDICATIONS

- Antibiotics should be used only if there is evidence of infection
- Hormonal treatment is contraindicated in *threatened abortion*
- Prostaglandin vaginal suppositories may be used in termination for *missed* or *inevitable abortion*

SURGERY

- *Incomplete abortion* is treated with prompt removal of any remaining products of conception to stop bleeding and prevent infection

THERAPEUTIC PROCEDURES

- *Threatened abortion* can be treated with bed rest for 24–48 h with gradual resumption of activities, but abstinence from coitus and douching
- *Missed* or *inevitable abortion* requires evacuation. Dilation with laminaria insertion and aspiration is preferred for missed abortion, though prostaglandin suppositories are an alternative
- *Incompetent cervix* is treated with cerclage and restriction of activities. Cervical cultures for *Neisseria gonorrhoeae*, *Chlamydia*, and group B *Streptococcus* should be obtained before the procedure

 ## OUTCOME

FOLLOW-UP

- With recurrent first-trimester losses (3 or more) chromosomal analysis of tissue may be informative

COMPLICATIONS

- Retained tissue and prolonged bleeding can occur with prostaglandin use

WHEN TO REFER

- Missed abortion
- Inevitable or incomplete abortion

WHEN TO ADMIT

- Vital signs unstable from excessive bleeding
- When evacuation of uterine contents cannot be done as an outpatient

 ## EVIDENCE

PRACTICE GUIDELINES

- ACOG practice bulletin. American College of Obstetricians and Gynecologists. Management of recurrent pregnancy loss. Number 24, February 2001. (Replaces Technical Bulletin Number 212, September 1995.) American College of Obstetricians and Gynecologists. Int J Gynaecol Obstet 2002;78:179. [PMID: 12360906]

WEB SITE

- Guidelines, Recommendations, and Evidence-Based Medicine in Obstetrics http://matweb.hcuge.ch/matweb/endo/cours_4e_MREG/obstetrics_gynecology_ guidelines.htm

INFORMATION FOR PATIENTS

- JAMA patient page: Miscarriage. JAMA 2002;288:1936.
- American College of Obstetricians and Gynecologists http://www.medem.com/medlb/article_ detaillb.cfm?article_ID=ZZZANQ5H97C&sub_cat=2005

REFERENCES

- George L et al: Plasma folate levels and risk of spontaneous abortion. JAMA 2002; 288:1867. [PMID:12377085]
- Hurd WW et al: Expectant management versus elective curettage for the treatment of spontaneous abortion. Fertil Steril 1997;68:601. [PMID: 9341597]
- Ness RB et al: Cocaine and tobacco use and the risk of spontaneous abortion. N Engl J Med 1999;340:333. [PMID: 9929522]

William R. Crombleholme, MD

Acanthamoeba Infections

 KEY FEATURES

ESSENTIALS OF DIAGNOSIS

Syndromes

- Encephalitis
- Skin lesions
- Keratitis
- Granulomatous dissemination to many tissues

GENERAL CONSIDERATIONS

Granulomatous lesions

- Free-living amebas of the genus *Acanthamoeba*
- Found in soil and in fresh, brackish, and thermal water as trophozoites (15–45 μm) or cysts (10–25 μm)
- Several species, including *A castellanii* and *A culbertsoni*, cause a number of poorly defined syndromes, especially in debilitated or immunosuppressed patients: subacute and chronic multifocal granulomatous necrotizing encephalitis, skin lesions (ulcers or hard nodules in which ameba may be detected), and granulomatous dissemination to many tissues
- Portals of entry may include the skin, eyes, or respiratory tract
- A commensal nasal carrier state is established

Keratitis

- *Acanthamoeba* keratitis and uveitis occur; most are associated with wearing contact lenses, others with penetrating corneal trauma or exposure to contaminated water

 CLINICAL FINDINGS

SYMPTOMS AND SIGNS

Encephalitis

- Mental status abnormalities
- Meningismus
- Neurological features of a space-occupying lesion

Keratitis

- Waxing and waning clinical course over several months
- Severe ocular pain, photophobia, tearing, blurred vision, and conjunctival injection
- Partial or 360° paracentral stromal ring infiltrate on ophthalmological examination
- Recurrent corneal epithelial breakdown
- A corneal lesion refractory to the usual medications

DIFFERENTIAL DIAGNOSIS

- Many cases of *Acanthamoeba* keratitis are misdiagnosed as viral keratitis

 DIAGNOSIS

LABORATORY TESTS

Encephalitis

- Cerebrospinal fluid lymphocytosis may be present
- Brain biopsy, culture, or cerebrospinal fluid wet mounts using specific fluorescent stains

Keratitis

- The diagnosis can be confirmed by vigorously scraping the cornea with a swab or platinum-tipped scapula
- The material is microscopically examined as a wet preparation for cysts and motile trophozoites, after staining, by immunofluorescent techniques, and after being cultured using various media
- Isolates can be identified by isoenzyme analysis and DNA profiles and tested for drug sensitivity

IMAGING STUDIES

- Focal consolidation on chest films may be present in patients with encephalitis

TREATMENT

MEDICATIONS

Granulomatous lesions

- No treatment has been effective, but ketoconazole, miconazole, itraconazole, sulfonamides, clotrimazole, pentamidine, paromomycin, propamidine, neomycin, amphotericin B, or flucytosine can be tried

Keratitis

- Treat with topical propamidine isothionate (0.1%) with either chlorhexidine digluconate (0.02%), polyhexamethylene biguanide, or neomycin-polymyxin B-gramicidin
- Topical miconazole has also been used
- Oral itraconazole or ketoconazole can be added for deep keratitis
- Use of corticosteroid therapy is controversial

THERAEUTIC PROCEDURES

- In spite of medical treatment of keratitis, penetrating keratoplasty is often necessary to excise diseased tissue; corneal grafting can be done after the amebic infection has been eradicated

 OUTCOME

PROGNOSIS

- With early treatment, many patients can expect cure and a good visual result
- Untreated encephalitis can lead to death in weeks to months
- Untreated keratitis can progress slowly over months and can lead to blindness

WHEN TO REFER

- All patients with keratitis should be referred to an ophthalmologist

WHEN TO ADMIT

- All cases of encephalitis

PREVENTION

- Prevention of keratitis requires immersion of contact lenses in disinfectant solutions or heat sterilization. The lens should not be cleaned in homemade saline solutions nor be worn while swimming

 EVIDENCE

PRACTICE GUIDELINES

- National Guideline Clearinghouse http://www.guideline.gov/summary/ summary.aspx?doc_id=2603&nbr=1829 &string=acanthamoeba

INFORMATION FOR PATIENTS

- Centers for Disease Control http://www.cdc.gov/ncidod/dpd/ parasites/acanthomoeba/factsht_ acanthamoeba.htm

REFERENCES

- Kumar R et al: Recent advances in the treatment of *Acanthamoeba* keratitis. Clin Infect Dis 2002;35:434. [PMID: 12145728]
- McCulley JP et al: The diagnosis and management of *Acanthamoeba* keratitis. CLAO J 2000;26:47. [PMID: 10656311]
- Moshari A et al: Chorioretinitis after keratitis caused by *Acanthamoeba:* case report and review of the literature. Ophthalmology 2001;108:2232. [PMID: 11733264]

Achalasia

KEY FEATURES

ESSENTIALS OF DIAGNOSIS

- Gradual, progressive dysphagia for solids and liquids
- Regurgitation of undigested food
- Barium esophagogram shows "bird's beak" distal esophagus
- Esophageal manometry confirms diagnosis

GENERAL CONSIDERATIONS

- Idiopathic motility disorder characterized by loss of peristalsis in the distal two-thirds (smooth muscle) of the esophagus and impaired relaxation of the lower esophageal sphincter
- Cause unknown

DEMOGRAPHICS

- Increased incidence with advancing age

CLINICAL FINDINGS

SYMPTOMS AND SIGNS

- Gradual onset of dysphagia for solid foods and, in the majority, liquids also
- Symptoms persist for months to years
- Substernal chest pain, discomfort, or fullness
- Regurgitation of undigested food
- Nocturnal regurgitation
- Coughing or aspiration
- Weight loss is common
- Physical examination unhelpful

DIFFERENTIAL DIAGNOSIS

- Chagas' disease
- Primary or metastatic tumors at the gastroesophageal junction
- Diffuse esophageal spasm
- Scleroderma esophagus
- Peptic stricture

DIAGNOSIS

IMAGING STUDIES

- Chest x-ray: air-fluid level in an enlarged, fluid-filled esophagus
- Barium esophagography: esophageal dilation, loss of esophageal peristalsis, poor esophageal emptying, and a smooth, symmetric "bird's beak" tapering of the distal esophagus

DIAGNOSTIC PROCEDURES

- Endoscopy to exclude a distal stricture or carcinoma
- Esophageal manometry confirms the diagnosis: characteristic features include complete absence of peristalsis, elevated lower esophageal sphincter pressure with incomplete relaxation during swallowing

TREATMENT

MEDICATIONS

- Calcium channel blockers (nifedipine) may provide temporary symptomatic improvement

SURGERY

- Surgical myotomy: modified Heller cardiomyotomy of the lower esophageal sphincter and cardia plus an antireflux procedure (fundoplication) results in improvement in >85%; this is now routinely performed laparoscopically

THERAPEUTIC PROCEDURES

- Botulinum toxin injection: endoscopically guided injection of botulinum toxin directly into the lower esophageal sphincter results in improvement in 85%, but symptom relapse occurs in >50% within 6–9 months
- 75% of initial responders to botulinum toxin injection who relapse improve with repeated injections
- Pneumatic dilation: >60% experience relief of dysphagia after 1 or 2 sessions; goal is to disrupt lower esophageal sphincter; approximately 30% require second dilation

 OUTCOME

FOLLOW-UP

- No follow-up necessary unless symptoms recur

COMPLICATIONS

- Perforations occur in <3% of pneumatic dilations, may require operative repair
- Increased risk of squamous cell esophageal cancer

PROGNOSIS

- After successful dilation or myotomy, patients have near-normal swallowing, although esophageal peristalsis is absent

WHEN TO REFER

- Patients with achalasia should be evaluated by a gastrointestinal specialist

 EVIDENCE

PRACTICE GUIDELINES

- American College of Gastroenterology. Diagnosis and management of achalasia, 1999
  http://www-east.elsevier.com/ajg/issues/9412/ajg1639fla.htm
- American Gastroenterological Association medical position statement on treatment of patients with dysphagia caused by benign disorders of the distal esophagus. Reviewed 2001
  http://www2.gastrojournal.org/scripts/om.dll/serve?action=searchDB&searchDBfor=art&artType=fullfree&id=a0019900229
- Society for Surgery of the Alimentary Tract: Achalasia, 2002
  http://www.ssat.com//cgi-bin/achalasia.cgi

WEB SITES

- American College of Gastroenterology http://www.acg.gi.org/
- National Institute of Diabetes and Digestive and Kidney Diseases (NIDDK) NIH
  http://www.niddk.nih.gov

INFORMATION FOR PATIENTS

- MEDLINEplus
  http://www.nlm.nih.gov/medlineplus/ency/article/000267.htm
- Society of Thoracic Surgeons http://www.sts.org/doc/4120

REFERENCES

- Vaezi M et al: Diagnosis and management of achalasia. Am J Gastroenterol 1999;94:3406. [PMID: 10606295]
- West RL et al: Long term results of pneumatic dilation in achalasia followed for more than 5 years. Am J Gastroenterol 2002;97:1346. [PMID: 12094848]

Kenneth R. McQuaid, MD

Acidosis, Lactic

KEY FEATURES

ESSENTIALS OF DIAGNOSIS

- Severe acidosis with hyperventilation
- Blood pH below 7.30
- Serum bicarbonate <15 mEq/L
- Anion gap >15 mEq/L
- Absent serum ketones
- Serum lactate >5 mmol/L

GENERAL CONSIDERATIONS

- Characterized by overproduction of lactic acid (tissue hypoxia), deficient removal (hepatic failure), or both (circulatory collapse)
- Occurs often in severely ill patients suffering from cardiac decompensation, respiratory or hepatic failure, septicemia, or infarction of bowel or extremities
- With the discontinuance of phenformin therapy in the United States, lactic acidosis in diabetics is uncommon but occasionally occurs with use of metformin. It must be considered in the acidotic diabetic, especially if the patient is seriously ill

Etiology

- Tissue hypoxia, eg, cardiogenic, septic, or hemorrhagic shock; seizure; carbon monoxide or cyanide poisoning
- Hepatic failure
- Ischemic bowel
- Infarction of extremities
- Diabetes, especially with metformin use
- Ketoacidosis
- Renal failure
- Infection
- Leukemia or lymphoma
- Drugs: ethanol, methanol, salicylates, isoniazid
- AIDS
- Idiopathic

CLINICAL FINDINGS

SYMPTOMS AND SIGNS

- Main clinical feature is marked hyperventilation
- When lactic acidosis is secondary to tissue hypoxia or vascular collapse, the clinical presentation is variable, being that of the prevailing catastrophic illness
- In idiopathic, or spontaneous lactic acidosis, onset is rapid (usually over a few hours), blood pressure is normal, peripheral circulation is good, and there is no cyanosis

DIFFERENTIAL DIAGNOSIS

Other causes of metabolic acidosis

- Diabetic ketoacidosis
- Starvation ketoacidosis
- Alcoholic ketoacidosis
- Renal failure (acute or chronic)
- Ethylene glycol toxicity
- Methanol toxicity
- Salicylate toxicity
- Other: paraldehyde, metformin, isoniazid, iron, rhabdomyolysis

DIAGNOSIS

LABORATORY TESTS

- High anion gap [serum sodium minus the sum of chloride and bicarbonate anions (in meq/L) should be no greater than 15]. A higher value indicates the existence of an abnormal compartment of anions
- Plasma bicarbonate and blood pH are quite low, indicating the presence of severe metabolic acidosis
- Ketones are usually absent from plasma and urine or at least not prominent
- In the absence of azotemia, hyperphosphatemia may be a clue to the presence of lactic acidosis for reasons that are not clear
- The diagnosis is confirmed by demonstrating, in a sample of blood that is promptly chilled and separated, a plasma lactic acid concentration of 5 mmol/L or higher (values as high as 30 mmol/L have been reported)
- Normal plasma values average 1 mmol/L, with a normal lactate/pyruvate ratio of 10:1. This ratio is greatly exceeded in lactic acidosis

TREATMENT

- Empirical antibiotic coverage for sepsis should be given after culture samples are obtained if the etiology of lactic acidosis is unknown
- Alkalinization with intravenous sodium bicarbonate to keep the pH above 7.2 in the emergency treatment of lactic acidosis is controversial; as much as 2000 mEq in 24 h has been used. However, there is no evidence that the mortality rate is favorably affected by administering bicarbonate

THERAPEUTIC PROCEDURES

- Aggressive treatment of the precipitating cause is the main component of therapy, such as ensuring adequate oxygenation and vascular perfusion of tissues
- Hemodialysis may be useful in cases where large sodium loads are poorly tolerated

OUTCOME

PROGNOSIS

- The mortality rate of spontaneous lactic acidosis is high. The prognosis in most cases is that of the primary disorder that produced the lactic acidosis

WHEN TO ADMIT

- All patients because of the high mortality rate

EVIDENCE

PRACTICE GUIDELINES

- American Association of Clinical Endocrinologists http://www.aace.com/clin/guidelines/diabetes_2002.pdf

REFERENCES

- Chan NN et al: Metformin-associated lactic acidosis: a rare or very rare clinical entity? Diabet Med 1999; 16:273. [PMID: 10220200]
- Forsythe SM et al: Sodium bicarbonate for the treatment of lactic acidosis. Chest 2000;117:260. [PMID: 10631227]

Umesh Masharani, MB, BS; MRCP (UK)

Acidosis, Metabolic, Decreased or Normal Anion Gap

 KEY FEATURES

ESSENTIALS OF DIAGNOSIS

- The hallmark of this disorder is that the low HCO_3^- of metabolic acidosis is associated with hyperchloremia, so that the anion gap remains normal
- The anion gap helps determine the cause of the metabolic acidosis
- Decreased HCO_3^-, seen also in respiratory alkalosis, but the pH distinguishes between the two disorders

GENERAL CONSIDERATIONS

- The most common causes are gastrointestinal HCO_3^- loss and defects in renal acidification (renal tubular acidoses). The urinary anion gap can differentiate between these two common causes

HCO_3^- loss

- **Normal anion gap (6–12 mEq)**
- Gastrointestinal loss of HCO_3^-, eg, diarrhea, pancreatic ileostomy, or ileal loop bladder
- Renal tubular acidosis
- Recovery from diabetic ketoacidosis
- Dilutional acidosis from rapid administration of 0.9% NaCl
- Carbonic anhydrase inhibitors
- Chloride retention or administration of HCl equivalent or NH_4Cl
- **Decreased anion gap (<6 mEq)**
- Plasma cell dyscrasias, eg, multiple myeloma (cationic paraproteins accompanied by chloride and bicarbonate)
- Bromide or lithium intoxication
- **Decreased anion gap without acidosis**
- Hypoalbuminemia (decreased unmeasured anion)
- Severe hyperlipidemia

Renal tubular acidoses

- **Type I (distal H⁺ secretion defect)**
- Due to selective deficiency in H^+ secretion in the distal nephron
- Low serum K^+
- Despite acidosis, urinary pH cannot be acidified (urine pH >5.5)
- Associated with autoimmune disease, hypercalcemia
- **Type II (proximal HCO_3^- reabsorption defect)**
- Due to a selective defect in the proximal tubule's ability to adequately reabsorb filtered HCO_3^-
- Low serum K^+

- Urine pH <5.5
- Associated with multiple myeloma, drugs, eg, sulfa, carbonic anhydrase inhibitors (acetazolamide)
- **Type III (rare)**
- Associated with glomerular insufficiency [glomerular filtration rate (GFR) 20–30 mL/min]
- Ability to generate adequate NH_3 is impaired, with subsequent decreased $NH_4^+Cl^-$ excretion
- Normal serum K^+
- Urine pH <5.5
  – Further reduction in GFR results in increased anion gap acidosis of uremia
- **Type IV (hyporeninemic hypoaldosteronism)**
- The only renal tubular acidosis characterized by hyperkalemic, hyperchloremic acidosis
- The defect is aldosterone deficiency or antagonism, which impairs distal nephron Na^+ reabsorption and K^+ and H^+ excretion
- Urine pH <5.5
- Renal salt wasting is frequently present
- Most common in diabetic nephropathy, tubulointerstitial renal diseases, AIDS, and hypertensive nephrosclerosis

 CLINICAL FINDINGS

SYMPTOMS AND SIGNS

- Symptoms are mainly those of the underlying disorder
- Compensatory hyperventilation may be misinterpreted as a primary respiratory disorder
- When severe, Kussmaul respirations (deep, regular, sighing respirations) are seen

 DIAGNOSIS

LABORATORY TESTS

- See Table 83 (page 1270)
- Blood pH, serum HCO_3^-, and PCO_2 are decreased
- Anion gap is normal (hyperchloremic) or decreased
- Hyperkalemia may be seen
- Urinary anion gap from a random urine sample $[(Na^+ + K^+) - Cl^-]$ reflects the ability of the kidney to excrete NH_4Cl as in the following equation:

$$Na^+ + K^+ + NH_3^+ = Cl^- + 80$$

where 80 is the average value for the difference in the urinary anions and cations other than Na^+, K^+, NH_3^+, and Cl^-
- Therefore, urinary anion gap is equal to $(80 - NH_3^+)$, and thus aids in the distinction between gastrointestinal and renal causes of hyperchloremic acidosis
- If the cause of the metabolic acidosis is gastrointestinal HCO_3^- loss (diarrhea), renal acidification ability remains normal and NH_4Cl excretion increases in response to the acidosis. The urinary anion gap is negative (eg, −30 mEq/L)
- If the cause is distal renal tubular acidosis, the urinary anion gap is positive (eg, +25 mEq/L), since the basic lesion in the disorder is the inability of the kidney to excrete H^+ and thus the inability to increase NH_4Cl excretion
- Urinary pH may not as readily differentiate between the two causes

Acidosis, Metabolic, Decreased or Normal Anion Gap

 TREATMENT

MEDICATIONS

- See Table 83 (page 1270)
- In distal renal tubular acidosis, supplementation of bicarbonate is necessary since acid accumulates systemically
- In proximal renal tubular acidosis, correction of low serum bicarbonate is not indicated except in severe cases
- Potassium should be given when bicarbonate therapy is indicated in proximal renal tubular acidosis

 OUTCOME

COMPLICATIONS

- Drugs that can exacerbate the hyperkalemia include angiotensin-converting enzyme inhibitors, aldosterone receptor blockers such as spironolactone, and nonsteroidal antiinflammatory drugs

WHEN TO REFER

- If expertise is needed in determining the etiology of the metabolic acidosis
- If consultation is needed on whether bicarbonate should be administered

WHEN TO ADMIT

- Respiratory muscle weakness from severe hypokelemia

 EVIDENCE

PRACTICE GUIDELINES

- National Guideline Clearinghouse
  http://www.guideline.gov/summary/
  summary.aspx?doc_id=3099&nbr=2325
  &string=renal+tubular+acidosis

WEB SITES

- Dr. Rose's Peripheral Brain—Fluids and Electrolytes
  http://faculty.washington.edu/momus/
  PB/fluidand.htm
- Fluid and Electrolyte Disorders:
  MDAdvice.com
  http://www.mdadvice.com/library/ped/
  pedillsymp160.html

INFORMATION FOR PATIENTS

- National Kidney and Urologic Diseases Information Clearinghouse
  http://kidney.niddk.nih.gov/kudiseases/
  pubs/tubularacidosis/index.htm
- National Institutes of Health
  http://www.nlm.nih.gov/medlineplus/
  ency/article/000493.htm
  http://www.nlm.nih.gov/medlineplus/
  ency/article/000497.htmWEB SITES

REFERENCES

- Fall PJ: A stepwise approach to acid-base disorders. Practical patient evaluation for metabolic acidosis and other conditions. Postgrad Med 2000;107:249. [PMID: 10728149]
- Smulders YM et al: Renal tubular acidosis: pathophysiology and diagnosis. Arch Intern Med 1996;156:1629. [PMID: 8694660]

Masafumi Fukagawa, MD, PhD
Kiyoshi Kurokawa, MD, MACP
Maxine A. Papadakis, MD

Acidosis, Metabolic, Increased Anion Gap

 KEY FEATURES

ESSENTIALS OF DIAGNOSIS

- Decreased HCO_3^-, seen also in respiratory alkalosis, but the pH distinguishes between the two disorders
- Calculation of the anion gap is useful in determining the cause of the metabolic acidosis
- The hallmark of this disorder is that metabolic acidosis (thus low HCO_3^-) is associated with normal serum Cl^-, so that the anion gap increases

GENERAL CONSIDERATIONS

- Normochloremic (increased anion gap) metabolic acidosis generally results from addition to the blood of nonchloride acids such as lactate, acetoacetate, β-hydroxybutyrate, and exogenous toxins. An exception is uremia, with underexcretion of organic acids and anions

Etiology

- Lactic acidosis
  - Type A (tissue hypoxia): cardiogenic, septic, or hemorrhagic shock; seizure; carbon monoxide or cyanide poisoning
  - Type B (nonhypoxic): hepatic or renal failure, ischemic bowel, diabetes especially with metformin use, ketoacidosis, infection, leukemia or lymphoma, drugs (ethanol, methanol, salicylates, isoniazid), AIDS, idiopathic (usually in debilitated patients)
- Diabetic ketoacidosis
- Starvation ketoacidosis
- Alcoholic ketoacidosis
  - Frequently with mixed disorders (10% have triple acid-base disorder)
  - Acid-base disorders in alcoholism include three types of metabolic acidosis (ketoacidosis, lactic acidosis, or hyperchloremic acidosis from bicarbonate loss in urine from ketonuria); metabolic alkalosis from volume contraction and vomiting; respiratory alkalosis from alcohol withdrawal, pain, sepsis, or liver disease
- Uremic acidosis (usually at glomerular filtration rate <20 mL/min)
- Ethylene glycol toxicity
- Methanol toxicity
- Salicylate toxicity (mixed metabolic acidosis with respiratory alkalosis)
- Other: paraldehyde, isoniazid, iron, rhabdomyolysis

 CLINICAL FINDINGS

SYMPTOMS AND SIGNS

- Symptoms are mainly those of the underlying disorder
- Compensatory hyperventilation may be misinterpreted as a primary respiratory disorder
- When severe, Kussmaul respirations (deep, regular, sighing respirations) are seen

 DIAGNOSIS

LABORATORY TESTS

- See Table 82 (page 1269)
- Blood pH, serum HCO_3^-, and P_{CO_2} are decreased
- Anion gap is increased (normochloremic)
- Hyperkalemia may be seen
- In lactic acidosis, lactate levels are at least 4–5 mEq/L but commonly 10–30 mEq/L
- The diagnosis of alcoholic ketoacidosis is supported by the absence of a diabetic history and by no evidence of glucose intolerance after initial therapy

TREATMENT

MEDICATIONS

- Supplemental HCO_3^- is indicated for treatment of hyperkalemia but is controversial for treatment of increased anion gap metabolic acidosis
- Administration of large amounts of HCO_3^- may have deleterious effects, including hypernatremia, hyperosmolality, and worsening of intracellular acidosis
- In salicylate intoxication, alkali therapy must be started unless blood pH is already alkalinized by respiratory alkalosis, since the increment in pH converts salicylate to more impermeable salicylic acid and thus prevents central nervous system damage
- The amount of HCO_3^- deficit can be calculated as follows

$$\text{Amount of } HCO_3^- \text{ deficit} = 0.5 \times \text{body weight} \times (24 - HCO_3^-)$$

- Half of the calculated deficit should be administered within the first 3–4 h to avoid overcorrection and volume overload
- In methanol intoxication, ethanol administration works as a competitive substrate for alcohol dehydrogenase, which metabolizes methanol to formaldehyde

THERAPEUTIC PROCEDURES

- Treatment is aimed at the underlying disorder, such as insulin and volume resuscitation to restore tissue perfusion
- Lactate will later be metabolized to produce HCO_3^- and increase pH

 OUTCOME

PROGNOSIS

- The mortality rate of lactic acidosis exceeds 50%

WHEN TO ADMIT

- Because of the high mortality rate, all patients with lactic acidosis should be admitted and most others, as well

 EVIDENCE

PRACTICE GUIDELINES

- National Guideline Clearinghouse http://www.guideline.gov/summary/summary.aspx?doc_id=3582&nbr=2808&string=DKA

WEB SITES

- Dr. Rose's Peripheral Brain—Fluids and electrolytes http://faculty.washington.edu/momus/PB/fluidand.htm
- Fluid and Electrolyte Disorders: MDAdvice.com http://www.mdadvice.com/library/ped/pedillsymp160.html

INFORMATION FOR PATIENTS

- National Institutes of Health http://www.nlm.nih.gov/medlineplus/ency/article/000335.htm http://www.nlm.nih.gov/medlineplus/ency/article/001181.htm

REFERENCES

- Adrogue HJ et al: Management of life threatening acid base disorders. (Part 1.) N Engl J Med 1998;338:26. [PMID: 9414329]
- Adrogue HJ et al: Management of life-threatening acid-base disorders. Second of two parts. N Engl J Med 1998;338:107. [PMID: 9420343]
- John M et al: Hyperlactatemia syndromes in people with HIV infection. Curr Opin Infect Dis 2002;15:23. [PMID: 119649]
- Kraut JA et al: Use of base in the treatment of severe acidemic states. Am J Kidney Dis 2001;38:703. [PMID: 11576874]

Masafumi Fukagawa, MD, PhD
Kiyoshi Kurokawa, MD, MACP
Maxine A. Papadakis, MD

Acne Vulgaris

KEY FEATURES

ESSENTIALS OF DIAGNOSIS

- Occurs at puberty, though onset may be delayed into the third or fourth decade
- Open and closed comedones are the hallmark of acne vulgaris
- The most common of all skin conditions
- Severity varies from purely comedonal to papular or pustular inflammatory acne to cysts or nodules
- Face and trunk may be affected
- Scarring may be a sequela of the disease or picking and manipulating by the patient

GENERAL CONSIDERATIONS

- The disease is activated by androgens in those who are genetically predisposed
- The skin lesions parallel sebaceous activity
- Pathogenic events include plugging of the infundibulum of the follicles, retention of sebum, overgrowth of the acne bacillus *(Propionibacterium acnes)* with resultant release of and irritation by accumulated fatty acids, and foreign body reaction to extrafollicular sebum
- When a resistant case of acne is encountered in a woman hyperandrogenism may be suspected

DEMOGRAPHICS

- Acne vulgaris is more common and more severe in males
- 12% of women and 3% of men over age 25 have acne vulgaris

CLINICAL FINDINGS

SYMPTOMS AND SIGNS

- See Table 7 (page 1202)
- Mild soreness, pain, or itching
- Lesions occur mainly over the face, neck, upper chest, back, and shoulders
- Comedones are the hallmark
- Closed comedones are tiny, flesh-colored, noninflamed bumps that give the skin a rough texture or appearance
- Open comedones typically are a bit larger and have black material in them
- Inflammatory papules, pustules, ectatic pores, acne cysts, and scarring are also seen
- Acne may have different presentations at different ages

DIFFERENTIAL DIAGNOSIS

- Acne rosacea (face)
- Bacterial folliculitis (face or trunk)
- Tinea (face or trunk)
- Topical steroid use (face)
- Perioral dermatitis (face)
- Pseudofolliculitis barbae (ingrown beard hairs)
- Miliaria (heat rash) (trunk)
- Eosinophilic folliculitis (trunk)
- Hyperandrogenic states in women
- Pustules on the face can also be caused by tinea infections

DIAGNOSIS

LABORATORY TESTS

- Culture in refractory cases

TREATMENT

MEDICATIONS

- See Table 6 (page 1202)

Comedonal acne

- Soaps play little part and, if any are used, they should be mild
- Topical retinoids
  - Tretinoin is very effective: start with 0.025% cream (not gel) twice weekly at night, then build up to as often as nightly; a pea-sized amount is sufficient to cover half the entire face; wait 20 min after washing to apply
  - Adapalene gel 0.1% and reformulated tretinoin (Renova, Retin A Micro, Avita) are other options if standard tretinoin preparations cause irritation
  - Lesions may flare in the first 4 weeks of treatment; the drug is contraindicated in pregnancy
- Benzoyl peroxide is available in many concentrations but 2.5% is as effective as 10% and less irritating; topical antibiotics decrease comedonal lesions (see below)

Papular inflammatory acne

- Antibiotics are the mainstay, used topically or orally
- Mild acne
  - The first choice of topical antibiotics is the combination of erythromycin or clindamycin with benzoyl peroxide topical gel; clindamycin (Cleocin T) lotion (least irritating), gel, or solution, or topical erythromycin gel or solution may be used twice daily and benzoyl peroxide in the morning (a combination of erythromycin or clindamycin with benzoyl peroxide is available as a prescription item)
  - The addition of tretinoin 0.025% cream or 0.01% gel at night enhances efficacy
- Moderate acne
  - Tetracycline, 500 mg twice daily, erythromycin, 500 mg twice daily, doxycycline, 100 mg twice daily, and minocycline, 50–100 mg twice daily, are all effective; tetracycline, minocycline, and doxycycline are contraindicated in pregnancy

Acne Vulgaris

– If the skin is clear, taper the dose by 250 mg for tetracycline and erythromycin, by 100 mg for doxycycline, every 6–8 weeks—while treating with topicals—to arrive at the lowest systemic dose needed; lowering the dose to zero without other therapy usually results in recurrence of the acne

– Oral contraceptives or spironolactone (50–100 mg daily) may be added as an antiandrogen in women with antibiotic-resistant acne or in women in whom relapse occurs after isotretinoin therapy

• Severe cystic acne

– Isotretinoin (Accutane) should be used before significant scarring occurs or if symptoms are not promptly controlled by antibiotics

– Informed consent must be obtained before its use in all patients

– Dosage of 0.5–1 mg/kg/day for 20 weeks for a cumulative dose of at least 120 mg/kg is usually adequate

– The drug is teratogenic and must not be used in pregnancy; obtain two serum pregnancy tests before starting the drug in a female and every month thereafter; sufficient medication for only 1 month should be dispensed; two forms of effective contraception must be used

– Side effects of dry skin and mucous membranes occur in most patients; if headache occurs, consider pseudotumor cerebri; at higher dosages, elevation of cholesterol and triglycerides and a lowering of high-density lipoproteins can occur; minor elevations of liver function tests and fasting blood sugar can occur; moderate to severe myalgias necessitate decreasing the dosage or stopping the drug

• Monitor baseline and Q week cholesterol, triglycerides, and liver function studies when using isotretinoin

THERAPEUTIC PROCEDURES

• Comedones may be removed with a comedo extractor but will recur if not prevented by treatment

• In otherwise moderate acne, injection of triamcinolone acetonide (2.5 mg/mL, 0.05 mL per lesion) may hasten resolution of deeper papules and cysts

• Cosmetic improvement may be achieved by excision and punch-grafting of deep scars and by dermabrasion of inactive acne lesions, particularly flat, superficial scars

OUTCOME

COMPLICATIONS

• Cyst formation, pigmentary changes in pigmented patients, severe scarring, and psychological problems may result

PROGNOSIS

• The disease flares intermittently in spite of treatment

• The condition may persist through adulthood and may lead to severe scarring if left untreated

• Antibiotics continue to improve skin for the first 3–6 months of use

• Relapse during treatment may suggest the emergence of resistant *P acnes*

• Remissions following systemic treatment with isotretinoin may be lasting in up to 60% of cases

• Relapses after isotretinoin usually occur within 3 years and require a second course in up to 20% of patients

WHEN TO REFER

• Failure to respond to standard regimens

• When the diagnosis is in question

• Fulminant scarring disease (acne fulminans)

PREVENTION

• Foods do not cause or exacerbate acne

• Educate patients not to manipulate lesions

• Avoid topical exposure to oils, cocoa butter, and greases

EVIDENCE

PRACTICE GUIDELINES

• National Guideline Clearinghouse http://www.guideline.gov/summary/summary.aspx?doc_id=3389&nbr=2615&string=dermatologic

• American Academy of Dermatology http://www.aadassociation.org/Guidelines/vulgaris.html

WEB SITES

• American Academy of Dermatology http://www.aad.org

• Dermatology Handbook for Family Practice from the University of Iowa http://www.vh.org/Providers/ClinRef/FPHandbook/17.html

INFORMATION FOR PATIENTS

• American Academy of Dermatology http://www.aad.org/pamphlets/

• National Institute of Arthritis, and Musculoskeletal and Skin Diseases http://www.niams.nih.gov/hi/topics/acne/acne.htm

REFERENCES

• Johnson BA: Use of systemic agents in the treatment of acne vulgaris. Am Fam Physician 2000;62:1823. [PMID: 11057839]

• Thiboutot D: New treatments and therapeutic strategies for acne. Arch Fam Med 2000;9:179. [PMID: 10693736]

Timothy G. Berger, MD

Acromegaly & Gigantism

 KEY FEATURES

ESSENTIALS OF DIAGNOSIS

- Excessive growth of hands (increased glove and ring size), feet (increased shoe width), jaw (protrusion of lower jaw), and internal organs
- Gigantism if growth hormone (GH) excess before closure of epiphyses; acromegaly if after closure
- Coarsening of facial features; deeper voice
- Amenorrhea, headaches, visual field loss, sweating, weakness
- Soft, doughy, sweaty handshake
- Serum GH not suppressed following oral glucose
- Elevated insulin-like growth factor 1 (IGF-1)
- Radiographs: terminal phalangeal "tufting." CT or MRI: pituitary tumor in 90%

GENERAL CONSIDERATIONS

- GH exerts much of its effects through release of IGF-1 from liver and other tissues
- Nearly always caused by pituitary adenoma, usually macroadenomas (>1 cm). May be locally invasive but <1% are malignant
- GH-secreting pituitary tumors usually cause hypogonadism by cosecretion of prolactin or direct pressure on pituitary
- Usually sporadic, rarely familial
- May be associated with endocrine tumors of parathyroids or pancreas [multiple endocrine neoplasia type 1 (MEN-1)]
- Acromegaly may be seen in McCune-Albright syndrome and as part of Carney's complex (atrial myxoma, acoustic neuroma, and spotty skin pigmentation)
- Rarely caused by ectopic growth hormone-releasing hormone or GH secreted by lymphoma, hypothalamic tumor, bronchial carcinoid, or pancreatic tumor

 CLINICAL FINDINGS

SYMPTOMS AND SIGNS

- Tall stature
- Enlarged hands and soft, doughy, sweaty handshake
- Fingers widen and rings no longer fit
- Carpal tunnel syndrome is common
- Feet grow, particularly in width
- Facial features coarsen
- Hat size increases, tooth spacing widens
- Mandible becomes more prominent
- Macroglossia and hypertrophy of pharyngeal and laryngeal tissue cause deep, coarse voice and may cause obstructive sleep apnea
- Goiter may be noted
- Hypertension (50%) and cardiomegaly
- Weight gain
- Arthralgias, degenerative arthritis, and spinal stenosis may occur
- Colon polyps common
- Skin: hyperhidrosis, thickening, cystic acne, and acanthosis nigricans
- Symptoms of hypopituitarism
  - Hypogonadism: decreased libido, impotence, irregular menses or amenorrhea common
  - Secondary hypothyroidism sometimes occurs, hypoadrenalism is unusual
  - Headaches and temporal hemianopia

DIFFERENTIAL DIAGNOSIS

- Familial tall stature, coarse features, or large hands and feet
- Physiological growth spurt
- Pseudoacromegaly (acromegaly features, insulin resistance)
- Inactive ("burned-out") acromegaly (spontaneous remission due to pituitary adenoma infarction)
- Myxedema
- Isolated prognathism (jaw protrusion)
- Aromatase deficiency or estrogen receptor deficiency
- Other causes of increased growth hormone level: exercise or eating prior to test, acute illness or agitation, hepatic or renal failure, malnourishment, diabetes mellitus, drugs: estrogens, β-blockers, clonidine

 DIAGNOSIS

LABORATORY TESTS

- IGF-1 levels >5 times normal in most acromegalics
- Glucose tolerance test: glucose syrup 75 g PO, GH measured 60 min later; acromegaly excluded if GH <1 μg/L (IRMA or chemiluminescent assays) or <2 μg/L (older radioimmunoassays) and if IGF-1 is normal
- Prolactin may be elevated (cosecreted by many GH-secreting tumors)
- Insulin resistance usually present, often causing hyperglycemia (common) and diabetes mellitus (30%)
- Thyroid-stimulating hormone and free thyroxine may show secondary hypothyroidism
- Serum phosphorus frequently elevated
- Serum calcium elevated if hyperparathyroidism as in MEN-1

IMAGING STUDIES

- MRI shows pituitary tumor in 90%
- MRI superior to CT, especially postoperatively
- Skull x-rays may show enlarged sella and thickened skull
- Radiographs may show tufting of terminal phalanges of fingers and toes
- Lateral view of foot shows increased thickness of heel pad

Acromegaly & Gigantism

 TREATMENT

MEDICATIONS

- Dopamine agonists are used if surgery does not produce clinical remission or normalization of GH. Most successful if tumor secretes both prolactin and GH—with cabergoline 1–1.75 mg PO Q week, one-third of such tumors shrink by >50%
- Octreotide or lanreotide (somatostatin analogs) used if acromegaly persists despite pituitary surgery and suppress GH to <5 ng/mL in 60% of patients within 3–6 months
- Responders who tolerate short-acting octreotide 50 μg SQ TID are switched to long-acting octreotide 20 mg IM Q month
- Octreotide dose adjusted up to 40 mg IM Q month to maintain serum GH between 1 ng and 2.5 ng/mL, keeping IGF-1 levels normal
- Lanreotide SR 30 mg SQ Q 7–14 days (not available in the United States)
- Lanreotide Autogel 60–120 mg SQ Q 28 days, better tolerated than lanreotide SR (not available in the United States)
- Pegvisomant, a GH receptor antagonist, 10–30 mg/day SQ, following IGF-1 levels; restricted access in the United States

SURGERY

- Endoscopic transnsasal, transsphenoidal resection is treatment of choice for acromegaly caused by pituitary adenoma
- GH levels fall immediately
- About 10% get infection, cerebrospinal fluid leak, or hypopituitarism
- Hyponatremia can occur 4–13 days postoperatively, may be prevented by salt supplements

THERAPEUTIC PROCEDURES

- Pituitary irradiation suggested if not cured by surgical and medical therapy. Stereotactic radiosurgery (gamma knife) preferred

OUTCOME

FOLLOW-UP

- Postoperatively, normal pituitary function usually preserved
- Postoperative GH levels >5 ng/mL and rising IGF-1 levels usually indicate recurrent tumor
- Soft tissue swelling regresses but bone enlargement is permanent
- Hypertension frequently persists
- Carpal tunnel syndrome and diaphoresis often improve within a day of surgery

COMPLICATIONS

- Hypopituitarism
- Hypertension
- Glucose intolerance or frank diabetes mellitus
- Cardiac enlargement and cardiac failure
- Carpal tunnel syndrome
- Arthritis of hips, knees, and spine
- Spinal cord compression may be seen
- Visual field defects may be severe and progressive
- Tumor may be locally invasive, particularly into the cavernous sinus
- Acute loss of vision or cranial nerve palsy if tumor undergoes spontaneous hemorrhage and necrosis (pituitary apoplexy)
- Intubation may be difficult due to macroglossia and hypertrophy of pharyngeal and laryngeal tissue

PROGNOSIS

- Untreated or persistent acromegaly usually causes premature cardiovascular disease and progressive acromegalic symptoms
- Transsphenoidal pituitary surgery successful in 80–90% if tumor <2 cm and GH <50 ng/mL
- Conventional radiation therapy (alone) produces remission in 40% by 2 years and 75% by 5 years
- Gamma knife radiation reduces GH levels an average of 77%, with 20% in remission at 12 months
- Heavy particle pituitary radiation produces remission in 70% by 2 years and 80% by 5 years
- Radiation therapy usually produces some degree of hypopituitarism
- Conventional radiation therapy may cause some degree of organic brain syndrome and predisposes to small strokes

EVIDENCE

PRACTICE GUIDELINES

- Melmed S et al: Guidelines for acromegaly management. J Clin Endocrinol Metab 2002;87:4054. [PMID: 12213843]
- Scandinavian Workshop on the Treatment of Acromegaly. Treatment guidelines for acromegaly. Report from a Scandinavian workshop: first Scandinavian Workshop on the Treatment of Acromegaly. Growth Horm IGF Res 2001;11:72. [PMID: 11472072]

WEB SITE

- National Institute of Diabetes and Digestive and Kidney Diseases (NIDDK)—Endocrine and metabolic diseases http://www.niddk.nih.gov/health/endo/endo.htm

INFORMATION FOR PATIENTS

- Mayo Clinic—Acromegaly http://www.mayoclinic.com/invoke.cfm?id=DS00478

REFERENCES

- Bevan JS et al. Primary medical therapy for acromegaly: an open, prospective, multicenter study of the effects of subcutaneous and intramuscular slow-release octreotide on growth hormone, insulin-like growth factor-I, and tumor size. J Clin Endocrinol Metab 2002;87:4554. [PMID: 12364434]
- Costa AC et al: Assessment of disease activity in treated acromegalic patients using a sensitive GH assay: should we achieve strict normal GH levels for a biochemical cure? J Clin Endocrinol Metab 2002;87:3142. [PMID: 12107214]

Paul A. Fitzgerald, MD

Actinomycosis

 KEY FEATURES

ESSENTIALS OF DIAGNOSIS

- History of recent dental infection or abdominal trauma
- Chronic pneumonia or indolent intraabdominal or cervicofacial abscess
- Sinus tract formation

GENERAL CONSIDERATIONS

- Organisms are anaerobic, gram-positive, branching filamentous bacteria (1 μm in diameter) that may fragment into bacillary forms
- Occur in the normal flora of the mouth and tonsillar crypts
- When introduced into traumatized tissue and associated with other anaerobic bacteria, actinomycetes become pathogens
- The most common site of infection is the cervicofacial area (about 60% of cases)
- Infection typically follows extraction of a tooth or other trauma
- Lesions may develop in the gastrointestinal tract or lungs following ingestion or aspiration of the organism from its endogenous source in the mouth

 CLINICAL FINDINGS

SYMPTOMS AND SIGNS

Cervicofacial actinomycosis

- Develops slowly, becomes markedly indurated, and the overlying skin becomes reddish or cyanotic
- Abscesses eventually drain to the surface
- Persist for long periods
- Sulfur granules—masses of filamentous organisms—may be found in the pus
- There is usually little pain unless there is secondary infection

Thoracic actinomycosis

- Fever, cough, sputum production
- Night sweats, weight loss
- Pleuritic pain
- Multiple sinuses may extend through the chest wall to the heart or abdomen

Abdominal actinomycosis

- Pain in the ileocecal region
- Spiking fever and chills
- Vomiting
- Weight loss
- Irregular abdominal masses may be palpated
- Pelvic inflammatory disease caused by actinomycetes has been associated with prolonged use of an intrauterine contraceptive device
- Sinuses draining to the exterior may develop

DIFFERENTIAL DIAGNOSIS

- Lung cancer
- Tuberculous lymphadenitis (scrofula)
- Other cause of cervical lymphadenopathy
- Nocardiosis
- Crohn's disease
- Pelvic inflammatory disease due to another cause

 DIAGNOSIS

LABORATORY TESTS

- Organisms may be demonstrated as a granule or as scattered branching gram-positive filaments in the pus
- Anaerobic culture is necessary to distinguish from *Nocardia*

IMAGING STUDIES

- Chest x-ray shows areas of consolidation and, in many cases, pleural effusion
- Abdominal pelvic CT scanning reveals an inflammatory mass that may extend to involve bone

Actinomycosis

 TREATMENT

MEDICATIONS

- Penicillin G is the drug of choice, 10 to 20 million units IV for 2–4 weeks, followed by oral penicillin V, 500 mg four times daily
- Sulfonamides such as sulfamethoxazole may be an alternative regimen at a total daily dosage of 2–4 g

SURGERY

- Drainage and resection may be beneficial

THERAPEUTIC PROCEDURES

- Therapy should be continued for weeks to months after clinical manifestations have disappeared in order to ensure cure
- Response to therapy is slow

 OUTCOME

PROGNOSIS

- With penicillin and surgery, the prognosis is good
- The difficulties of diagnosis may result in extensive destruction of tissue before therapy is started

WHEN TO REFER

- Refer early to an infectious disease specialist for diagnosis and management

WHEN TO ADMIT

- All patients with thoracic or abdominal actinomycosis
- Patients with cervicofacial actinomycosis if the diagnosis is in question, to control symptoms, or initiate intravenous antibiotics

 EVIDENCE

PRACTICE GUIDELINES

- Cayley J et al: Recommendations for clinical practice: actinomyces-like organisms and intrauterine contraceptives. The Clinical and Scientific Committee. Br J Fam Plann 1998;23:137.

WEB SITE

- Karolinska Institute—Directory of bacterial infections and mycoses http://www.mic.ki.se/Diseases/c1.html

INFORMATION FOR PATIENTS

- National Institutes of Health http://www.nlm.nih.gov/medlineplus/ency/article/000599.htm http://www.nlm.nih.gov/medlineplus/ency/article/000074.htm

REFERENCES

- Lippes J: Pelvic actinomycosis: a review and preliminary look at prevalence. Am J Obstet Gynecol 1999;180(2 Part 1):265. [PMID: 9988785]
- Zitsch RP 3rd et al: Actinomycosis: a potential complication of head and neck surgery. Am J Otolaryngol 1999;20:260. [PMID: 10442782]

Henry F. Chambers, MD

Acute Respiratory Distress Syndrome (ARDS)

 KEY FEATURES

ESSENTIALS OF DIAGNOSIS

- Acute onset of respiratory failure
- Bilateral radiographic pulmonary infiltrates
- Absence of elevated left atrial pressure
- Ratio of $PaO_2/FIO_2 <200$, regardless of the level of peak end-expiratory pressure (PEEP)

GENERAL CONSIDERATIONS

- Acute hypoxemic respiratory failure following a sytsemic or pulmonary insult without evidence of heart failure
- Common risk factors include sepsis, aspiration of gastric contents, shock, infection, lung contusion, trauma, toxic inhalation, near drowning, and multiple blood transfusion (see Table 38, page 1231)
- Damage to capillary endothelial and alveolar epithelial cells is found, regardless of the cause of ARDS

Systemic causes

- Trauma, sepsis, shock, burns
- Pancreatitis
- Multiple transfusions
- Disseminated intravascular coagulation (DIC) and thrombotic thrombocytopenia purpura (TTP)
- Drugs: opioids, aspirin, phenothiazines, tricyclic antidepressants, amiodarone, chemotherapeutics, nitrofurantoin, protamine
- Cardiopulmonary bypass
- Head injury
- Paraquat

Pulmonary causes

- Aspiration of gastric contents
- Embolism of thrombus, fat, air, or amniotic fluid
- Miliary tuberculosis
- Diffuse pneumonia
- Acute eosinophilic pneumonia
- Bronchiolitis obliterans with organizing pneumonia (BOOP)
- Upper airway obstruction
- Free-base cocaine smoking
- Near drowning
- Toxic gas inhalation: nitrogen dioxide, chlorine, sulfur dioxide, ammonia, smoke inhalation
- Oxygen toxicity
- Lung contusion
- Radiation
- High-altitude exposure
- Lung reexpansion or reperfusion

 CLINICAL FINDINGS

SYMPTOMS AND SIGNS

- Rapid onset of profound dyspnea, usually 12–48 h after the initiating event
- Labored breathing and tachypnea, with crackles on examination
- Chest x-ray shows diffuse or patchy bilateral infiltrates that rapidly become confluent
- Air bronchograms are seen in 80% of cases
- Marked hypoxemia refractory to supplemental oxygen
- Multiple organ failure is seen in many patients

DIFFERENTIAL DIAGNOSIS

- Since ARDS is a syndrome, the concept of differential diagnosis applies only in considering the precipitating illness or injury
- Cardiogenic (hydrostatic) pulmonary edema
- Pneumonia
- Diffuse alveolar hemorrhage
- BOOP

 DIAGNOSIS

LABORATORY TESTS

- Tests to identify the systemic pulmonary causes of ARDS are indicated

IMAGING STUDIES

- Chest x-ray: features of congestive heart failure (pleural effusions, cardiomegaly, venous engorgement in upper lung zones) are absent

DIAGNOSTIC PROCEDURES

- When indicated to rule out cardiogenic pulmonary edema, Swan-Ganz catheterization will demonstrate pulmonary capillary wedge pressures <18 mm Hg

TREATMENT

MEDICATIONS

- Medications directed at the underlying cause of ARDS are indicated
- Intravascular volume should be maintained at the lowest level required to maintain adequate cardiac output
- Diuretics may be needed to reduce pulmonary capillary wedge pressure and improve oxygenation
- Judicious use of inotropes to maintain cardiac output at higher levels of PEEP may be necessary
- Achieving supranormal oxygen delivery through the use of inotropes and blood transfusion is not clinically useful and may be harmful
- Sedatives, analgesics, and antipyretics may be used to decrease oxygen consumption
- Systemic corticosteroids have not been shown to reliably improve outcomes

THERAPEUTIC PROCEDURES

- Intubation and mechanical ventilation are usually required to treat hypoxemia
- The lowest levels of PEEP and F_{IO_2} needed to maintain a PaO_2 >60 mm Hg
- The use of small tidal volume ventilation (6 mL/kg of ideal body weight) has been shown to reduce mortality by 10% in a large multicenter trial
- PEEP may be increased as long as cardiac output and O_2 delivery are not impaired and pulmonary pressures are not excessive
- Prone positioning may improve oxygenation in selected patients

 OUTCOME

FOLLOW-UP

- Efforts should be made to decrease F_{IO_2} below 60% as early as possible
- For patients who recover, no specific follow-up is required

COMPLICATIONS

- Complications are those associated with ICU level care and mechanical ventilation

PROGNOSIS

- Mortality is 30–40% in ARDS, 90% when associated with sepsis
- Median survival is 2 weeks
- Many patients with ARDS die when support is withdrawn
- Survivors of ARDS are left with some pulmonary symptoms, which tend to improve over time
- Mild abnormalities of oxygenation, diffusion capacity, and lung mechanics may persist in some survivors

WHEN TO REFER

- Care of patients with ARDS should involve a clinician who is familiar with the syndrome, typically an intensivist or pulmonologist

WHEN TO ADMIT

- Due to the profound hypoxemia that defines ARDS, all patients will need admission and intensive care

PREVENTION

- No measures have been identified to effectively prevent ARDS
- Prophylactic PEEP and methylprednisolone are not helpful in patients at risk

 EVIDENCE

INFORMATION FOR PATIENTS

- American Lung Association http://www.lungusa.org/diseases/ards_factsheet.html
- National Institutes of Health http://www.nlm.nih.gov/medlineplus/ency/article/000103.htm

REFERENCES

- Acute Respiratory Distress Syndrome Network: Ventilation with lower tidal volumes as compared with traditional tidal volumes for acute lung injury and the acute respiratory distress syndrome. N Engl J Med 2000;342:1301. [PMID: 10793162]
- Anonymous: International Consensus Conferences in Intensive Care Medicine: noninvasive positive pressure ventilation in acute respiratory failure. Am J Respir Crit Care Med 2001;163:283. [PMID: 11208659]
- Valta P et al: Acute respiratory distress syndrome: frequency, clinical course, and costs of care. Crit Care Med 1999;27:2367. [PMID: 10579250]
- Ware LB et al: The acute respiratory distress syndrome. N Engl J Med 2000;342:1334. [PMID: 10793167]

Mark S. Chesnutt, MD
Thomas J. Prenderast, MD

Adrenocortical Insufficiency, Acute (Adrenal Crisis)

 KEY FEATURES

ESSENTIALS OF DIAGNOSIS

- Weakness, abdominal pain, fever, confusion, nausea, vomiting, and diarrhea
- Low blood pressure, dehydration; skin pigmentation may be increased
- Serum potassium high, sodium low, blood urea nitrogen high
- Cosyntropin (ACTH$_{1-24}$) unable to stimulate a normal increase in serum cortisol

GENERAL CONSIDERATIONS

- Acute adrenal insufficiency is an emergency caused by insufficient cortisol
- May occur in course of chronic, treated adrenal insufficiency, or as its presenting manifestation
- Acute adrenal crisis is more common in primary adrenal insufficiency (adrenal gland disorder; Addison's disease) than secondary adrenocortical hypofunction (pituitary gland disorder)
- May occur following stress, eg, trauma, surgery, infection, or prolonged fasting in patient with latent insufficiency
- May result from withdrawal of adrenocortical hormone replacement in patient with chronic adrenal insufficiency or temporary insufficiency related to withdrawal of exogenous glucocorticoids
- May occur following bilateral adrenalectomy or removal of a functioning adrenal tumor that had suppressed the other adrenal
- May result from injury to both adrenals by trauma, hemorrhage, anticoagulant therapy, thrombosis, infection, or, rarely, metastatic carcinoma
- May occur after pituitary necrosis, or when thyroid hormone replacement is given to a patient with adrenal insufficiency
- Adrenal crisis may occur in infancy or childhood in congenital adrenal hyperplasia, congenital adrenal hypoplasia, Allgrove syndrome

 CLINICAL FINDINGS

SYMPTOMS AND SIGNS

- Headache, lassitude, nausea and vomiting, abdominal pain, and diarrhea
- Confusion or coma
- Fever, as high as 40.6°C or more
- Low blood pressure
- Recurrent hypoglycemia and reduced insulin requirements in patients with preexisting type 1 diabetes mellitus
- Cyanosis, dehydration, skin hyperpigmentation, and sparse axillary hair (if hypogonadism also present)
- Meningococcemia may cause purpura and adrenal insufficiency secondary to adrenal infarction (Waterhouse-Friderichsen syndrome)

DIFFERENTIAL DIAGNOSIS

- Other cause of shock, eg, sepsis, cardiogenic, hypovolemic, anaphylaxis
- Hyperkalemia due to other cause, eg, renal failure, rhabdomyolysis, angiotensin-converting enzyme inhibitors, angiotensin receptor blockers, spironolactone
- Hyponatremia due to other cause, eg, syndrome of inappropriate antidiuretic hormone, cirrhosis, vomiting
- Abdominal pain due to other cause

 DIAGNOSIS

LABORATORY TESTS

- Eosinophil count may be high
- Hyponatremia or hyperkalemia (or both) usually present
- Hypoglycemia common
- Hypercalcemia may be present
- Blood, sputum, or urine culture may be positive if bacterial infection is precipitating cause
- Cosyntropin stimulation test: synthetic ACTH$_{1-24}$ (cosyntropin), 0.25 mg, given SQ, IM, or IV, and serum cortisol obtained 45 min later. Normally, cortisol rises to ≥20 μg/dL. For patients on glucocorticoids, hydrocortisone must not be given for at least 8 h before test. Other glucocorticoids (eg, prednisone, dexamethasone) do not interfere with specific assays for cortisol
- Plasma ACTH markedly elevated if patient has primary adrenal disease (generally >200 pg/mL)

Adrenocortical Insufficiency, Acute (Adrenal Crisis)

 TREATMENT

MEDICATIONS

- If diagnosis is suspected, draw blood sample for cortisol determination and treat with hydrocortisone 100–300 mg IV and saline *immediately*, without waiting for results
- Then continue hydrocortisone 50–100 mg IV Q 6 h for first day, Q 8 h the second day, and taper as clinically appropriate
- Broad-spectrum antibiotics given empirically while waiting for initial culture results
- $D_{50}W$ to treat hypoglycemia with careful monitoring of serum electrolytes, blood urea nitrogen, and creatinine
- When patient is able to take oral medication, give hydrocortisone 10–20 mg PO Q 6 h, and taper to maintenance levels. Most require hydrocortisone twice daily: 10–20 mg QAM, 5–10 mg QPM
- Mineralocorticoid therapy is not needed when large amounts of hydrocortisone are being given, but as the dose is reduced, may need to add fludrocortisone 0.05–0.2 mg PO QD. Some never require fludrocortisone or become edematous at doses >0.05 mg once or twice weekly

THERAPEUTIC PROCEDURES

- Once the crisis is over, must assess degree of permanent adrenal insufficiency and establish cause if possible

 OUTCOME

FOLLOW-UP

- Repeat cosyntropin stimulation test

COMPLICATIONS

- Shock and death if untreated
- Sequelae of infection that commonly precipitate adrenal crisis

PROGNOSIS

- Rapid treatment usually life-saving
- Frequently unrecognized and untreated since manifestations mimic more common conditions; lack of treatment leads to shock that is unresponsive to volume replacement and vasopressors, resulting in death

 EVIDENCE

PRACTICE GUIDELINES

- Arlt W et al: Adrenal insufficiency. Lancet 2003;361:1881. [PMID: 12788587]
- Clinical practice parameters for hemodynamic support of pediatric and neonatal patients in septic shock. American College of Critical Care Medicine, 2002 http://www.sccm.org/pdf/hemodynamic%20peds%20guidelines.pdf
- Cooper MS et al: Corticosteroid insufficiency in acutely ill patients. N Engl J Med 2003;348:727. [PMID: 12594318]
- Oelkers W et al: Therapeutic strategies in adrenal insufficiency. Ann Endocrinol (Paris) 2001;62:212. [PMID: 11353897]

WEB SITE

- National Adrenal Disease Foundation http://medhelp.org/www/nadf.htm

INFORMATION FOR PATIENTS

- MEDLINEplus—Acute adrenal crisis http://www.nlm.nih.gov/medlineplus/ency/article/000357.htm
- Merck Source—Acute adrenal crisis http://www.mercksource.com/pp/us/cns/cns_hl_adam.jspzQzpgzEzzSzppdocszSzuszSzcnszSzcontentzSzadamzSzencyzSzarticlezSz000357zPzhtm

REFERENCES

- Marik PE et al: Adrenal insufficiency in the critically ill: a new look at an old problem. Chest 2002;122:1784. [PMID: 12426284]
- Vella A et al: Adrenal hemorrhage: a 25-year experience at the Mayo Clinic. Mayo Clin Proc 2001;76:161. [PMID: 11213304]

Paul A. Fitzgerald, MD

Adrenocortical Insufficiency, Chronic (Addison's Disease)

 ## KEY FEATURES

ESSENTIALS OF DIAGNOSIS

- Weakness, easy fatigability, anorexia, weight loss; nausea and vomiting, diarrhea; abdominal pain, muscle and joint pains; amenorrhea
- Sparse axillary hair; increased skin pigmentation, especially of creases, pressure areas, and nipples
- Hypotension, small heart
- Serum sodium may be low; potassium, calcium, and urea nitrogen may be elevated; neutropenia, mild anemia, eosinophilia, and relative lymphocytosis may be present
- Plasma cortisol levels low or fail to rise after administration of cosyntropin
- Plasma ACTH level elevated

GENERAL CONSIDERATIONS

- Autoimmune destruction of adrenals is most common cause in the United States. May occur alone or as part of an autoimmune polyglandular failure syndrome
- May be associated with autoimmune thyroid disease, hypoparathyroidism, type 1 diabetes mellitus, vitiligo, alopecia areata, celiac sprue, primary ovarian failure, testicular failure, and pernicious anemia
- Combination of Addison's disease and hypothyroidism is Schmidt's syndrome
- Tuberculosis is common cause in areas of high prevalence; now rare
- Bilateral adrenal hemorrhage may occur with sepsis, heparin-associated thrombocytopenia or anticoagulation, antiphospholipid antibody syndrome, surgery (postoperatively) or trauma, or spontaneously
- Adrenoleukodystrophy is an X-linked disorder accounting for one-third of Addison's disease in boys. May cause hypogonadism, psychiatric symptoms, and neurological deterioration
- Rare causes of adrenal insufficiency: lymphoma, metastatic carcinoma, coccidioidomycosis, histoplasmosis, cytomegalovirus (more frequent in AIDS), syphilitic gummas, scleroderma, amyloid disease, hemochromatosis, familial glucocorticoid deficiency, Allgrove syndrome, X-linked adrenal leukodystrophy, and congenital adrenal hypoplasia
- Congenital adrenal hyperplasia results from hereditary defects in adrenal enzymes for cortisol synthesis, eg, P-450c21 (21-hydroxylase). Severe cases manifest mineralocorticoid deficiency (salt wasting) in addition to deficient cortisol and excessive androgens

 ## CLINICAL FINDINGS

SYMPTOMS AND SIGNS

- Weakness and fatigability, weight loss, myalgias, arthralgias, fever
- Anorexia, nausea and vomiting
- Anxiety, mental irritability, and emotional changes common
- Diffuse tanning over nonexposed and exposed skin or multiple freckles; hyperpigmentation, especially knuckles, elbows, knees, posterior neck, palmar creases, nail beds, pressure areas, and new scars
- Vitiligo (10%)
- Hypoglycemia, when present, may worsen weakness and mental functioning, rarely leading to coma
- Other autoimmune disease manifestations
- Patients with established diabetes develop increased insulin sensitivity and hypoglycemic reactions
- Hypotension and orthostasis usual; 90% have SBP <110 mm Hg; SBP >130 mm Hg is rare
- Small heart
- Scant axillary and pubic hair (especially in women)
- Neuropsychiatric symptoms, sometimes without adrenal insufficiency, in adult-onset adrenoleukodystrophy

DIFFERENTIAL DIAGNOSIS

- Hypotension due to other cause, eg, medications
- Hyperkalemia due to other cause, eg, renal failure
- Gastroenteritis
- Occult cancer
- Anorexia nervosa
- Hyperpigmentation due to other cause, eg, hemochromatosis
- Isolated hypoaldosteronism

 ## DIAGNOSIS

LABORATORY TESTS

- WBC usually shows moderate neutropenia, lymphocytosis, and total eosinophil count >300/μL
- In *chronic* Addison's disease, serum sodium is usually low (90%) while potassium is elevated (65%). Patients with diarrhea may not be hyperkalemic
- Fasting blood glucose may be low
- Hypercalcemia may be present
- Plasma very-long-chain fatty acid levels to screen for adrenoleukodystrophy in young men with idiopathic Addison's disease
- Plasma cortisol level low (<5 mg/dL) at 8 AM is diagnostic, especially if accompanied by simultaneous elevated ACTH (usually >200 pg/mL)
- Cosyntropin stimulation test: synthetic $ACTH_{1-24}$ (cosyntropin), 0.25 mg, given parenterally, and serum cortisol obtained 45 min later. Normally, cortisol rises to ≥20 μg/dL. For patients on glucocorticoids, hydrocortisone must not be given for at least 8 h before test. Other glucocorticoids do not interfere with specific assays for cortisol
- Plasma ACTH markedly elevated if patient has primary adrenal disease (generally >200 pg/mL)
- Antiadrenal antibodies detected in 50% of autoimmune Addison's disease
- Antithyroid antibodies (45%) and other autoantibodies may be present
- Elevated plasma renin activity indicates depleted intravascular volume and need for higher doses of fludrocortisone replacement
- Plasma epinephrine levels low

IMAGING STUDIES

- Chest x-ray for tuberculosis, fungal infection, or cancer when Addison's disease not clearly autoimmune
- Abdominal CT shows small noncalcified adrenals in autoimmune Addison's disease. Adrenals enlarged in about 85% of cases of metastatic or granulomatous disease. Calcification noted in cases of tuberculosis (~50%), hemorrhage, fungal infection, and melanoma

Adrenocortical Insufficiency, Chronic (Addison's Disease)

 TREATMENT

MEDICATIONS

- Glucocorticoid and mineralocorticoid replacement required in most cases; hydrocortisone alone may be adequate in mild cases
- Hydrocortisone is drug of choice, usually 15–25 mg in two divided doses, two-thirds in AM and one-third in late PM or early evening
- Prednisone 2–3 mg PO QAM and 1–2 mg PO QPM or evening is an alternative
- Dose adjusted according to clinical response; proper dose usually results in normal WBC differential
- Glucocorticoid dose raised in case of infection, trauma, surgery, diagnostic procedures, or other stress. Maximum hydrocortisone dose for severe stress is 50 mg IV or IM Q 6 h. Lower doses, oral or parenteral, used for lesser stress. Dose tapered to normal as stress subsides
- Fludrocortisone, 0.05–0.3 mg PO QD or QOD required by many patients. Dose increased for postural hypotension, hyponatremia, hyperkalemia, fatigue, or elevated plasma renin activity. Dosage decreased for edema, hypokalemia, or hypertension
- Treat all infections immediately
- In some women with adrenal insufficiency, dehydroepiandrosterone (DHEA), 50 mg PO QAM improves sense of well-being, mood, and sexual performance

THERAPEUTIC PROCEDURES

- "Lorenzo's oil" for adrenoleukodystrophy normalizes serum very-long-chain fatty acid concentrations but is ineffective clinically. Hematopoietic stem cell transplantation from normal donors may improve neurological manifestations

 OUTCOME

FOLLOW-UP

- Follow clinically and adjust glucocorticoid and (if required) mineralocorticoid doses as needed
- Fatigue in treated patients may indicate suboptimal dosing of medication, electrolyte imbalance, or concurrent problems such as hypothyroidism or diabetes mellitus
- Glucocorticoid dose must be increased in case of physiological stress (see above)

COMPLICATIONS

- Complications of underlying disease (eg, tuberculosis) are more likely in chronic adrenal insufficiency
- Adrenal crisis may be precipitated by intercurrent infections
- Associated autoimmune diseases are common (see above)
- Fatigue often persists despite treatment of Addison's disease
- Excessive glucocorticoid replacement can cause Cushing's syndrome

PROGNOSIS

- Normal life expectancy if adrenal insufficiency is diagnosed and treated with appropriate doses of glucocorticoids and (if required) mineralocorticoids. Most able to live fully active lives
- However, associated conditions can pose additional health risks, eg, adrenoleukodystrophy or Allgrove syndrome may result in neurological disease; patients with adrenal tuberculosis may have serious systemic infection

PREVENTION

- Glucocorticoid and mineralocorticoid replacement must not be stopped
- Patients should wear medical alert bracelet or medal reading "Adrenal insufficiency—takes hydrocortisone"
- Higher doses of glucocorticoids must be administered to patients with infection, trauma, or surgery to prevent adrenal crisis

 EVIDENCE

PRACTICE GUIDELINES

- Arlt W et al: Adrenal insufficiency. Lancet 2003;361:1881. [PMID: 12788587]
- Don-Wauchope AC et al: Diagnosis and management of Addison's disease. Practitioner 2000;244:794. [PMID: 11048377]

WEB SITES

- Australian Addison's Disease Association http://www.addisons.org.au/
- National Adrenal Disease Foundation http://medhelp.org/www/nadf.htm

INFORMATION FOR PATIENTS

- Cleveland Clinic—Addison's Disease http://www.clevelandclinic.org/health/health-info/docs/0800/0853.asp?index=5484

REFERENCES

- Betterle C et al: Autoimmune adrenal insufficiency and autoimmune polyendocrine syndromes: autoantibodies, autoantigens, and their applicability in diagnosis and disease prediction. Endocr Rev 2002;23:327. [PMID: 12050123]
- Huebner A et al: ACTH resistance syndromes. J Pediatr Endocrinol Metab 1999;12(Suppl 1):277. [PMID: 10698592]
- Marik PE et al: Adrenal insufficiency in the critically ill: a new look at an old problem. Chest 2002;122:1784. [PMID: 12426284]
- Ten S et al: Clinical review 130: Addison's disease 2001. J Clin Endocrinol Metab 2001;86:2909. [PMID: 11443143]

Paul A. Fitzgerald, MD

Alcoholism

 ## KEY FEATURES

ESSENTIALS OF DIAGNOSIS

Major criteria

- Physiological dependence as evidenced by withdrawal when intake is interrupted
- Tolerance to the effects of alcohol
- Evidence of alcohol-associated illnesses, such as alcoholic liver disease
- Continued drinking despite strong medical and social contraindications
- Impairment in social and occupational functioning
- Depression
- Blackouts

Other signs

- Alcohol stigmas: alcohol odor on breath, alcoholic facies, flushed face, scleral injection, tremor, ecchymoses, peripheral neuropathy
- Surreptitious drinking
- Unexplained work absences
- Frequent accidents, falls, or injuries
- In smokers, cigarette burns on hands or chest

GENERAL CONSIDERATIONS

- The two-phase syndrome includes problem drinking and alcohol addiction
- Problem drinking is the repetitive use of alcohol, often to alleviate anxiety or solve other emotional problems
- Alcohol addiction is a true addiction
- Alcoholism is associated with a high prevalence of lifetime psychiatric disorders, especially depression

DEMOGRAPHICS

- The majority of suicides and intrafamily homicides involve alcohol
- Major factor in rapes and other assaults
- Male-to-female ratios of 4:1 are converging
- Adoption and twin studies indicate some genetic influence
- 40% of Japanese have aldehyde dehydrogenase deficiency, which increases susceptibility to the effects of alcohol

 ## CLINICAL FINDINGS

SYMPTOMS AND SIGNS

Acute intoxication

- Drowsiness, errors of commission, psychomotor dysfunction, disinhibition, dysarthria, ataxia, and nystagmus
- Presence of ataxia, dysarthria, and nausea and vomiting indicates a blood level above 150 mg/dL
- Lethal blood levels: 350–900 mg/dL
- Severe cases are marked by respiratory depression, stupor, seizures, shock syndrome, coma, and death
- Serious overdoses often include other sedatives combined with alcohol

Withdrawal

- Onset of withdrawal symptoms is usually 8–12 h, with peak intensity of symptoms 48–72 h after alcohol consumption is stopped
- Symptoms range from anxiety, decreased cognition, tremulousness, increasing irritability, and hyperreactivity to full-blown delirium tremens
- Symptoms of mild withdrawal, including tremor, elevated vital signs, and anxiety, begin about 8 h after the last drink and end by Day 3
- Generalized seizures occur within the first 24–38 h and are more prevalent in patients with previous withdrawal syndromes
- Delirium tremens is an acute organic psychosis
  - Usually manifest within 24–72 h after the last drink but may occur up to 7–10 days later
  - Characterized by mental confusion, tremor, sensory hyperacuity, visual hallucinations, autonomic hyperactivity, cardiac abnormalities, diaphoresis, dehydration, electrolyte disturbances (hypokalemia, hypomagnesemia), and seizures
- The acute withdrawal syndrome often unexpectedly occurs in patients hospitalized for some unrelated reason and presents as a diagnostic problem
- Possible persistence of sleep disturbances, anxiety, depression, excitability, fatigue, and emotional volatility for 3–12 months, becoming chronic in some cases

Alcoholic hallucinosis

- Paranoid psychosis without the tremulousness, confusion, and clouded sensorium seen in withdrawal syndromes

- Occurs either during heavy drinking or withdrawal
- The patient appears normal except for the auditory hallucinations, which are frequently persecutory and may cause the patient to behave aggressively and in a paranoid fashion

Chronic alcoholic brain syndromes

- Encephalopathies characterized by increasing erratic behavior, memory and recall problems, and emotional lability
- Wernicke's encephalopathy consists of the triad of confusion, ataxia, and ophthalmoplegia (typically sixth nerve)
- Korsakoff's psychosis is a sequelae characterized by both anterograde and retrograde amnesia, with confabulation early in the course

DIFFERENTIAL DIAGNOSIS

Alcohol dependence

- Primary alcoholism
- Alcoholism secondary to psychiatric disease, eg, depression, bipolar disorder, schizophrenia, borderline personality disorder
- Other sedative dependence, eg, benzodiazepines
- Other drug abuse, eg, opioids

Alcohol withdrawal

- Withdrawal from other sedatives, eg, benzodiazepines or opioids
- Drug intoxication, eg, cocaine
- Delirium due to medical illness, eg, hypoxia, hepatic encephalopathy, thiamine deficiency, bacteremia
- Anxiety disorder
- Hallucinosis due to other cause, eg, schizophrenia, amphetamine psychosis
- Seizure due to other cause, eg, hypoglycemia, epilepsy

 ## DIAGNOSIS

LABORATORY TESTS

- Blood alcohol levels below 50 mg/dL rarely cause much motor dysfunction
- Elevations of both γ-glutamyl transpeptidase (levels above 30 units/L are suggestive of heavy drinking) and mean corpuscular volume (>95 fL in men and >100 fL in women) make a serious drinking problem likely

DIAGNOSTIC PROCEDURES

- Suspect the problem early
- CAGE questionnaire (Table 99, page 1283)
- Before treating for withdrawal or hallucinosis, meticulous examination for other medical problems is necessary

TREATMENT

MEDICATIONS

Alcoholic addiction

- Disulfiram (250–500 mg/day orally); compliance depends on motivation
- Naltrexone (50 mg/day) lowers relapse rates over the 3–6 months after drinking cessation, apparently by lessening the pleasurable effects of alcohol

Alcoholic hallucinosis

- Haloperidol, 5 mg PO BID for the first day or so; taper drug over several days as the patient improves

Withdrawal symptoms

- Use adequate doses of sedative to cause moderate sedation
- Antipsychotic drugs should not be used
- For some outpatients, a short course of tapering benzodiazepines, eg, 20 mg of diazepam initially, decreasing by 5 mg daily, may be a useful adjunct
- In moderate to severe withdrawal, use diazepam (5–10 mg PO hourly depending on severity of withdrawal symptoms)
- In very severe withdrawal, IV diazepam
- After stabilization, diazepam (enough to maintain a sedated state) may be given orally every 8–12 h
- If withdrawal signs persist (eg, tremulousness), the dosage is increased until moderate sedation occurs
- The dosage is then gradually reduced by 20% every 24 h until withdrawal is complete, which usually requires a week or more of treatment
- Clonidine, 5μg/kg PO Q 2 h, or the patch formulation, suppresses cardiovascular signs of withdrawal
- Carbamazepine, 400–800 mg/day PO, compares favorably with benzodiazepines for alcohol withdrawal
- Atenolol, as an adjunct to benzodiazepines, can reduce symptoms of alcohol withdrawal but should not be used when bradycardia is present

- Atenolol dose is 100 mg/day PO when the heart rate is above 80 beats per minute and 50 mg/day for a heart rate between 50 and 80 beats per minute
- Phenytoin is not useful for alcohol withdrawal seizures unless there is a preexisting seizure disorder
- A general diet should be accompanied by vitamins in high doses: thiamine, 50 mg IV initially, then IM (IV glucose given prior to thiamine may precipitate Wernicke's syndrome; concurrent administration is satisfactory); pyridoxine, 100 mg/day; folic acid, 1 mg/day; and ascorbic acid, 100 mg BID

THERAPEUTIC PROCEDURES

- Maintain a nonjudgmental attitude
- Denial is best faced at the first meeting, preferably with family members
- Aversion behavioral therapy has been successful in some patients

OUTCOME

FOLLOW-UP

- Monitoring of vital signs and fluid and electrolyte levels is essential for the severely ill patient with withdrawal
- Alcoholic chronic brain syndrome patients require careful attention to their social and environmental care

COMPLICATIONS

- Nervous system complications include chronic brain syndromes, cerebellar degeneration, cardiomyopathy, and peripheral neuropathies
- Direct liver effects include cirrhosis and eventual hepatic failure
- Indirect effects include protein abnormalities, coagulation defects, hormone deficiencies, and an increased incidence of liver neoplasms
- Alcoholic hypoglycemia can occur even with low blood alcohol levels
- Traumatic subdural hematoma with liver-induced hypocoagulability
- Fetal alcohol syndrome

PROGNOSIS

- The mortality rate from delirium tremens has steadily decreased with early diagnosis and improved treatment

WHEN TO REFER

- Alcoholics Anonymous (AA)
- Al-Anon for the spouse

WHEN TO ADMIT

- Hallucinosis or severe withdrawal symptoms
- Comorbid conditions (eg, advanced liver disease) that may decompensate during alcohol withdrawal
- Hospitalization is usually not necessary

EVIDENCE

PRACTICE GUIDELINES

- National Guideline Clearinghouse http://www.guideline.gov/summary/summary.aspx?doc_id=1565&nbr=791&string=alcoholism

INFORMATION FOR PATIENTS

- JAMA patient page: Alcohol. JAMA 1999;281:1352. [PMID: 10208153]

REFERENCES

- Adams WL et al: Screening for problem drinking in older primary care patients. JAMA 1996;276:1964. [PMID: 897110650]
- Helping patients with alcohol problems. A health practitioner's guide. NIH Publication No. 03-3769, 2003.

Stuart J. Eisendrath, MD
Jonathan E. Lichtmacher, MD

Alkalosis, Metabolic

KEY FEATURES

ESSENTIALS OF DIAGNOSIS

- Characterized by high HCO_3^-, which is also seen in chronic respiratory acidosis but pH differentiates the two disorders
- Compensatory increase in P_{CO_2} rarely 55 mm Hg. A higher value implies a superimposed respiratory acidosis
- Effective circulating volume status and urinary chloride concentration help distinguish between saline-responsive and saline-unresponsive metabolic alkalosis

GENERAL CONSIDERATIONS

- Useful to classify the etiology into two groups—saline responsive or saline unresponsive (Table 84, page 1270)
- **Saline responsive**
- By far the more common disorder
- Characterized by normotensive extracellular volume contraction
- Less frequently, hypotension or orthostatic hypotension may be seen
- It is also generally associated with hypokalemia, due partly to the direct effect of alkalosis per se on renal potassium excretion and partly to secondary hyperaldosteronism from volume contraction
- **Saline unresponsive**
- Implies a volume-expanded state as from hyperaldosteronism with accompanying hypokalemia from the renal mineralocorticoid effect

Etiology

- **Saline responsive (U_{Cl} <10 mEq/day)**
- *Excessive body bicarbonate content*
- *Renal alkalosis*
- Diuretic therapy
- Poorly reabsorbable anion therapy: carbenicillin, penicillin, sulfate, phosphate
- Posthypercapnia
- Gastrointestinal alkalosis
- Loss of HCl from vomiting or nasogastric suction
- Intestinal alkalosis: chloride diarrhea
- Exogenous alkali
- $NaHCO_3$ (baking soda)
- Sodium citrate, lactate, gluconate, acetate
- Transfusions
- Antacids
- *Normal body bicarbonate content*
- Contraction alkalosis
- **Saline unresponsive (U_{Cl} >10 mEq/day)**
- *Excessive body bicarbonate content*

- *Renal alkalosis, normotensive*
- Bartter's syndrome (renal salt wasting and secondary hyperaldosteronism)
- Severe potassium depletion
- Refeeding alkalosis
- Hypercalcemia and hypoparathyroidism
- *Renal alkalosis, hypertensive*
- Endogenous mineralocorticoids
  - Primary aldosteronism
  - Hyperreninism
  - Adrenal enzyme deficiency: 11- and 17-hydroxylase
  - Liddle's syndrome
- Exogenous mineralocorticoids
  - Licorice

CLINICAL FINDINGS

SYMPTOMS AND SIGNS

- There are no characteristic symptoms or signs
- Orthostatic hypotension may be encountered
- Weakness and hyporeflexia occur if serum K^+ is markedly low
- Tetany and neuromuscular irritability occur rarely

DIAGNOSIS

LABORATORY TESTS

- Elevated arterial blood pH and bicarbonate
- The arterial P_{CO_2} is increased
- Serum potassium and chloride are decreased
- There may be an increased anion gap
- Urinary chloride is low (<10 mEq/day) in saline-responsive disorders, and urinary chloride is higher (>10 mEq/day) in saline-unresponsive disorders

TREATMENT

MEDICATIONS

Saline-responsive metabolic alkalosis

- Correct the extracellular volume deficit with adequate amounts of 0.9% NaCl and KCl
- For alkalosis due to nasogastric suction, discontinuation of diuretics and administration of H_2-blockers can be useful
- Acetazolamide, 250–500 mg intravenously every 4–6 h, can be used if cardiovascular status prohibits adequate volume repletion. Watch for the development of hypokalemia
- Administration of acid can be used as emergency therapy. HCl, 0.1 mol/L, is infused via a central vein (the solution is sclerosing). Dosage is calculated to decrease the HCO_3^- level by one-half over 2–4 h, assuming a HCO_3^- volume of distribution (L) of 0.5 × body weight (kg)

Saline-unresponsive metabolic alkalosis

- Blockage of aldosterone effect with an angiotensin-converting enzyme inhibitor or with spironolactone
- Metabolic alkalosis in primary aldosteronism can be treated only with potassium repletion

THERAPEUTIC PROCEDURES

- Mild alkalosis is generally well tolerated
- Severe or symptomatic alkalosis (pH >7.60) requires urgent treatment
- Patients with marked renal insufficiency may require dialysis

SURGERY

- Therapy for saline-unresponsive metabolic alkalosis includes surgical removal of a mineralocorticoid-producing tumor

 OUTCOME

WHEN TO ADMIT

- Persistent metabolic alkalosis in the absence of hypovelemia or associated with severe hypokalemia
- If administration of acid is needed for emergency therapy

EVIDENCE

PRACTICE GUIDELINE

- National Guideline Clearinghouse http://www.guideline.gov/summary/ summary.aspx?doc_id=3305&nbr=2531 &string=bicarbonate http://www.guideline.gov/summary/ summary.aspx?doc_id=3099&nbr= 2325&string=acid+base

WEB SITES

- Dr. Rose's Peripheral Brain—Fluids and electrolytes http://faculty.washington.edu/momus/ PB/fluidand.htm
- Fluid and Electrolyte Disorders: MDAdvice.com http://www.mdadvice. com/library/ped/pedillsymp160.html

INFORMATION FOR PATIENTS

- National Institutes of Health http://www.nlm.nih.gov/medlineplus/ ency/article/001183.htm
- American Association for Clinical Chemistry http://www.labtestsonline.org/ understanding/analytes/co2/test.html

REFERENCES

- Adrogue HJ et al: Management of life threatening acid base disorders. (Part 2.) N Engl J Med 1998;338:107. [PMID: 98069970]
- Galla JH: Metabolic alkalosis. J Am Soc Nephrol 2000;11:369. [PMID: 10665945]
- Khanna A: Metabolic alkalosis. Respir Care 2001;46:354. [PMID: 11262555]

Masafumi Fukagawa, MD, PhD
Kiyoshi Kurokawa, MD, MACP
Maxine A. Papadakis, MD

Allergy, Drug

KEY FEATURES

ESSENTIALS OF DIAGNOSIS

- An IgE-mediated reaction to a drug
- Many drugs have toxicities or idiosyncratic reactions that are not immune mediated and therefore are not drug allergies

GENERAL CONSIDERATIONS

- In previously sensitized individuals, immediate hypersensitivity is manifested by rapid development of urticaria, angioedema, or anaphylaxis
- Delayed onset of urticaria accompanied by fever, arthralgias, and nephritis may indicate the development of an immune complex–mediated disorder
- Drug fever and Stevens-Johnson syndrome are reactions that probably act by immune hypersensitivity mechanisms
- Some drugs are clearly more immunogenic than others, and this can be reflected in the incidence of drug hypersensitivity
- A partial list of drugs frequently implicated in drug reactions includes β-lactam antibiotics, sulfonamides, phenytoin, carbamazepine, allopurinol, muscle relaxants used for general anesthesia, nonsteroidal antiinflammatory drugs, antisera, and antiarrhythmic agents
- Drug toxicities, drug interactions, or idiosyncratic reactions must be distinguished from true hypersensitivity reactions because the prognosis and management differ

DEMOGRAPHICS

- Some estimate that 10% or less of adverse reactions to drugs are true hypersensitivity reactions

CLINICAL FINDINGS

SYMPTOMS AND SIGNS

- Urticaria
- Angioedema
- Anaphylaxis

DIFFERENTIAL DIAGNOSIS

- Vasculitis
- Erythema multiforme
- Contact dermatitis (eg, poison oak or ivy)
- Erythema migrans (Lyme disease)
- Arthropod bites (insect bites)
- Physical factors: heat, cold, solar, pressure, water, vibratory
- Cholinergic urticaria: exercise, excitement, hot showers
- Other allergic causes: feathers, dander, shellfish, tomatoes, strawberries, vaccines, chemicals, cosmetics
- Infection (eg, otitis media, sinusitis, hepatitis)
- Serum sickness
- Angioedema: hereditary or acquired complement mediated, angiotensin-converting enzyme inhibitors

DIAGNOSIS

LABORATORY TESTS

Allergy testing

- Observed allergic reaction in the setting of a new or old drug
- Skin testing (available for very few drugs, eg, penicillin)
- A negative penicillin skin test makes penicillin allergy unlikely
- If the likelihood of immunological reaction is low—based on the history and the assessment of likely offending agents—and if no allergy testing is available, judicious test dose challenges may be considered in a monitored setting (performed only by a practitioner skilled and experienced with these procedures)
- If the likelihood of IgE-mediated reaction is significant, these challenges are risky and rapid drug desensitization is indicated

Provocation tests

- Bronchoprovocation testing
  - Obtain serial determinations of peak expiratory flow rate (PEFR) using a portable peak flowmeter during periods of natural exposure to a suspected airborne allergen
  - May be helpful in some cases of occupational asthma
- Oral provocation
  - In most cases of suspected allergy to a food or drug, placebo-controlled oral challenge is the definitive test
  - Freeze-dried foods in large opaque capsules provide a sufficient dose of allergen for testing
  - This test should be conducted in a monitored setting and should not be administered to patients with suspected food-induced anaphylaxis

Alkalosis, Respiratory p. 1050. Alkaptonuria p. 1050. Allergic Bronchopulmonary Aspergillosis p. 1250.

Allergy, Drug

 TREATMENT

MEDICATIONS

- Same as other allergic reactions (antihistamines, steroids, or subcutaneous epinephrine)
- Acute rapid desensitization can be done if the drug (eg, penicillin or insulin) must be administered
- Rapid escalation of miniscule doses of the drug is followed by full-dose administration
- This is accomplished by a course of oral or parenteral doses starting with extremely low doses (dilutions of 1×10^{-6} or 1×10^{-5} units) and increasing to the full dose over a period of hours

 OUTCOME

WHEN TO REFER

- Refer to an allergist for specialized diagnostic or therapeutic interventions, such as oral provocation or rapid desensitization

WHEN TO ADMIT

- For rapid desensitization procedures, especially when there is a history of possible or probable anaphylaxis

PREVENTION

- The drug and all chemically related compounds should be avoided in the future.

 EVIDENCE

PRACTICE GUIDELINES

- National Guideline Clearinghouse http://www.guideline.gov/summary/summary.aspx?doc_id=1433&nbr=673&string=hypersensitivity
- Joint Task Force on Practice Parameters, the American Academy of Allergy, Asthma and Immunology, and the Joint Council of Allergy, Asthma and Immunology. Executive summary of disease management of drug hypersensitivity: a practice parameter. Ann Allergy Asthma Immunol 1999;83(6 Pt 3):665.

WEB SITES

- National Institutes of Health www.nih.gov/niams/healthinfo
- American Academy of Allergy, Asthma, and Immunology http://www.aaaai.org

INFORMATION FOR PATIENTS

- JAMA patient page: Allergies. JAMA. 2000;283:424. [PMID: 10647806]
- American College of Allergy, Asthma and Immunology http://www.medem.com/search/article_display.cfm?path=\\TANQUERAY\M_ContentItem&mstr=/M_Content Item/ZZZEA5MS2BC.html&soc=Medem_ACAAI&srch_typ=NAV_SERCH

REFERENCES

- Drain KL: Preventing and managing drug-induced anaphylaxis. Drug Safety 2001;24:843. [PMID: 11665871]
- Marshall GD: Determining allergic versus nonallergic drug reactions. Clin Allergy Immunol 2000;15:217. [PMID: 10943295]

Jeffrey L. Kishiyama, MD
Daniel C. Adelman, MD

Alzheimer's Disease

KEY FEATURES

ESSENTIALS OF DIAGNOSIS

- Persistent and progressive impairment in intellectual function
- Not due to delirium—diagnosis should not be made during an acute illness
- Primary deficit of short-term memory
- Must have other deficits (executive function, visuospatial function, language) as well

GENERAL CONSIDERATIONS

- A progressive, acquired impairment in multiple cognitive domains, at least one of which is memory
- The deficits must represent a decline in function significant enough to interfere with work or social life
- Frequently coexists with depression and delirium
- Patients have little cognitive reserve and can have acute cognitive or functional decline with a new medical illness

DEMOGRAPHICS

- Dementia is the fourth leading cause of death in the United States with a prevalence that doubles every 5 years in the older population, reaching 30–50% at age 85
- Women suffer disproportionately, as patients (even after age adjustment) and as caregivers
- Alzheimer's disease accounts for two-thirds of cases of dementia in the United States, with vascular dementia (either alone or combined with Alzheimer's disease) accounting for much of the rest
- Risk factors are older age, family history, lower education level, and female gender

CLINICAL FINDINGS

SYMPTOMS AND SIGNS

- Memory impairment with at least one or more of the following:
  - Language impairment (initially just word finding; later, difficulty following a conversation)
  - Apraxia (inability to perform previously learned tasks)
  - Agnosia (inability to recognize objects)
  - Impaired executive function (poor abstraction and judgment)
- Typical earliest deficits are in memory and visuospatial abilities
- Social graces may be retained despite advanced cognitive decline
- Personality changes and behavioral difficulties (wandering, inappropriate sexual behavior, agitation) may develop as the disease progresses
- Hallucinations typically observed only in moderate-to-severe dementia
- End-stage disease characterized by near-mutism, inability to sit up, hold up the head, or track objects with the eyes, difficulty with eating and swallowing, weight loss, bowel or bladder incontinence, and recurrent respiratory or urinary infections

DIFFERENTIAL DIAGNOSIS

- Dementia from other etiologies: eg, subcortical dementia, dementia with Lewy bodies [See *Dementia in elderly, non-Alzheimer's*]
- Depression
- Delirium
- Medication effect
- Potentially reversible cognitive decline: drug effect, depression, thyroid disease, vitamin B_{12} deficiency, hypercalcemia, subdural hematoma, HIV infection, and normal pressure hydrocephalus

DIAGNOSIS

LABORATORY TESTS

- Obtain tests for potentially reversible causes of dementia: complete blood count, electrolytes, calcium, creatinine, glucose, thyroid-stimulating hormone, vitamin B_{12}, HIV testing, rapid plasma reagin (RPR), heavy metal screen, and liver function tests

IMAGING STUDIES

- Obtain a head CT or MRI if other etiologies of dementia need to be excluded; those who are younger and those who have symptoms suggestive of other etiologies for dementia (focal neurological signs or symptoms, seizures, gait abnormalities, and an acute or subacute onset) are most likely to yield positive findings

DIAGNOSTIC PROCEDURES

- Assess mental status (Figure 1, page 1197)
- Evaluate for deficits related to cardiovascular accidents, Parkinsonism, or peripheral neuropathy
- The combination of the "clock draw" (in which the patient is asked to sketch a clock face, with all the numerals placed properly, the two clock hands positioned at a specified time) and the "three-item recall" is a fairly quick and good test; an abnormally drawn clock markedly increases the probability of dementia
- When patients fail either of these screening tests, further testing with the Mini-Mental State questionnaire (Figure 1, page 1197), neuropsychological testing, or other instruments is warranted
- Examine for comorbid conditions that may aggravate the disability

TREATMENT

MEDICATIONS

- Acetylcholinesterase inhibitors (donepezil, galantamine, rivastigmine)
  - Modest improvements in cognitive function in mild to moderate dementia
  - Modest benefit on functional outcomes in advanced disease
  - Starting doses: donepezil, 5 mg orally daily (maximum 10 mg daily); galantamine, 4 mg orally twice daily (maximum 12 mg twice daily); rivastigmine, 1.5 mg orally twice daily (maximum 6 mg twice daily)
  - Increase doses gradually as tolerated
  - Side effects include nausea, diarrhea, anorexia, and weight loss
- Choose medications based on symptoms—depression, anxiety, psychosis
- Anxiety may respond to buspirone, starting at 5–7.5 mg twice daily and advancing to 30 mg daily if necessary; takes weeks to show efficacy
- Acetylcholinesterase inhibitors may be modestly beneficial
- Haloperidol may modestly reduce aggression, but not agitation, but is associated with significant adverse effects
- Risperidone, olanzapine, and quetiapine are usually better tolerated than older agents, but are more expensive
- Starting and target neuroleptic dosages are low (eg, haloperidol 0.5–2.0 mg; risperidone 0.25–2 mg)
- Risperidone may be associated with increased strokes

THERAPEUTIC PROCEDURES

- Discontinue all nonessential drugs and correct, if possible, sensory deficits
- Exclude unrecognized delirium, pain, urinary obstruction, or fecal impaction
- Caregivers should speak simply to the patient, break down activities into simple component tasks, and employ a "distract, not confront" approach

OUTCOME

FOLLOW-UP

- Federal regulations require drug reduction efforts at least every 6 months if antipsychotic agents are used in a nursing home patient

COMPLICATIONS

- Clinicians should be alert for signs of elder abuse when working with stressed caregivers

PROGNOSIS

- The prevalence of fully reversible dementias is under 5%
- Life expectancy with Alzheimer's disease is typically 3–15 years
- Caregiver support, counseling, and respite care can prevent or delay nursing home placement

WHEN TO REFER

- Referral for neuropsychological testing may be helpful to distinguish dementia from depression, to diagnose dementia in persons of poor education or very high premorbid intellect, and to aid diagnosis when impairment is mild
- Referral to a geriatrician or neurologist is useful if the dementia does not have the classic features of Alzheimer's disease

WHEN TO ADMIT

- Dementia complicates other medical problems, and the threshold for admission should be lower

PREVENTION

- Nonsteroidal antiinflammatory drug use, HMG-CoA reductase inhibitor use, moderate alcohol intake, and strong social supports may decrease the risk of dementia

EVIDENCE

PRACTICE GUIDELINES

- American Geriatrics Society http://www.americangeriatrics.org/products/positionpapers/aan_dementia.shtml
- National Guideline Clearinghouse http://www.guideline.gov/summary/summary.aspx?doc_id=3157&nbr=2383&string=Alzheimers
- Agency for Healthcare Research and Quality http://hstat.nlm.nih.gov/hq/Hquest/fws/S/db/local.arahcpr.arclin.alzc/lhit/238/screen/Browse/s/60901/action/GetText/hitno/2/msr/1

WEB SITES

- AARP Guide to Internet Resources on Aging http://www.aarp.org/cyber/sd1_3.htm
- American Geriatrics Society http://www.americangeriatrics.org/
- Medicare Publications http://www.medicare.gov/NHCompare/home.asp
- Time-to-Death Prediction Calculator for Alzheimer's Disease http://cpmcnet.columbia.edu/dept/sergievsky/predictor.html

INFORMATION FOR PATIENTS

- Alzheimer's Association http://www.alz.org
- Alzheimer's Disease Education and Referral Center http://www.alzheimers.org/about.htm
- Alzheimer's Family Relief Program http://www.ahaf.org
- JAMA patient page: Alzheimer disease. JAMA 2001; 286:2194 [PMID: 1175749]

REFERENCE

- Trinh NH: Efficacy of cholinesterase inhibitors in the treatment of neuropsychiatric symptoms and functional impairment in Alzheimer disease: a meta-analysis. JAMA 2003;289:210. [PMID: 12517232]

C. Bree Johnston, MD
Kenneth E. Covinsky, MD

Amebiasis

KEY FEATURES

ESSENTIALS OF DIAGNOSIS

- Mild to severe colitis
- Amebas in stools; serological tests positive with severe colitis

GENERAL CONSIDERATIONS

- The *Entamoeba* complex contains two morphologically identical species: *E dispar* (about 90% of the complex), which remains in the colon in a stable asymptomatic carrier state, and *E histolytica*, whose virulence can range from asymptomatic to fulminant colitis and to extraintestinal infections
- Humans are the only established host
- The organisms exist in two forms: only cysts are infectious, since after ingestion they survive gastric acidity, which destroys trophozoites
- Transmission occurs through ingestion of cysts from fecally contaminated food or water. Flies and other arthropods also serve as mechanical vectors; transmission can result from contamination of food by the hands of food handlers
- Person-to-person contact is important in transmission; therefore, all household members and sexual partners should have their stools examined
- Corticosteroids and other immunosuppressive drugs may convert a commensal infection into an invasive one

DEMOGRAPHICS

- The infections are worldwide but are most prevalent in tropical areas with crowded conditions
- Urban outbreaks have occurred because of common-source water contamination
- Of 500 million persons worldwide infected with *Entamoeba*, an estimated 10% (50 million) are infected with *E histolytica*. Mortality is about 100,000 per year

CLINICAL FINDINGS

SYMPTOMS AND SIGNS

- Acute onset of severe diarrhea can occur as early as 8 days after infection
- Some patients may be asymptomatic or have mild recurrent symptoms for months to years before severe colitis or liver abscess appears
- Transition may occur from one type of intestinal infection to another, and each may give rise to hepatic abscess

Asymptomatic infection

- Mild to moderate colitis (nondysenteric colitis)
- Few semiformed stools a day; no blood
- Abdominal cramps, flatulence, fatigue, weight loss, abdominal distention and tenderness; fever is uncommon
- Periods of remission and recurrence may last days to weeks; during remissions, there may be constipation
- In some with chronic infection, the colon is thick and palpable, particularly over the cecum and descending colon
- Mild hepatomegaly and tenderness
- Severe colitis (dysenteric colitis)
- Several liquid stools with blood streaking
- With larger numbers of stools, 10–20 or more, little fecal material is present, but blood (fresh or dark) and bits of necrotic tissue may be evident
- The patient may become prostrate and toxic, with fever up to 40.5°C, colic, vomiting, diffuse abdominal tenderness, hepatic tenderness
- Localized ulcerative lesions of the colon
- Rectal ulcerations may result in passage of formed stools with bloody exudate
- Cecal ulcerations may induce mild diarrhea and simulate appendicitis
- Amebic appendicitis is rare
- Localized granulomatous lesions of the colon (ameboma)
- The masses may present as an irregular tumor(s) projecting into the bowel or as an annular constricting mass up to several centimeters in length
- May mimic colonic carcinoma, tuberculosis, or lymphogranuloma venereum
- Extraintestinal amebiasis
- See *Amebic liver disaese*
- Perianal skin infections
- Lungs, brain, genitalia, and elsewhere

DIFFERENTIAL DIAGNOSIS

- Inflammatory bowel disease
- Giardiasis
- *Shigella*, *Salmonella*, *Campylobacter*
- Irritable bowel syndrome
- Lactase deficiency
- Cryptosporidiosis, cyclosporiasis
- Annular carcinoma of the bowel

DIAGNOSIS

LABORATORY TESTS

Intestinal amebiasis

- Diagnosis is made by finding the organism or antigen in stool (antigen detection is more sensitive)
- Microscopic stool examination
- Testing three specimens obtained under optimal conditions will generally detect 80% of *Entamoeba* complex infections (but does not distinguish between *E histolytica* and *E dispar*); three additional tests will raise the diagnostic rate to 90%
- Collect three specimens at 2-day intervals or longer, with one of the three obtained after a laxative such as sodium sulfate or phosphate (Fleet's Phospho-Soda), 30–60 g in a glass of water; or bisacodyl 5–15 mL
- If the patient has received specific therapy, antibiotics, barium, antimalarials, antidiarrheal agents (containing bismuth, kaolin, or magnesium hydroxide), or mineral oil, specimen collection should be delayed
- The coproantigen TechLab *Entamoeba* test can differentiate between *E histolytica* and *E dispar* with a sensitivity of 93% and a specificity of 97%; however, fresh or frozen, but not preserved, stool specimens must be used
- Serology
- The ELISA and enzyme immunoassays are positive only in the case of *E histolytica* infection; about 70% of patients with active intestinal disease (the frequency is lower in mild colitis, higher in dysentery) and about 10% of asymptomatic *E histolytica* cyst passers will have postive serology; false-positive results are rare. The tests remain positive up to 10 years after successful treatment
- The agar gel immunodiffusion test becomes negative 3–6 months after eradication of the organism
- Other tests

- Detection of trophozoites that contain ingested red blood cells is nearly diagnostic for invasive *E histolytica*
- Fecal occult blood is frequently positive in amebic colitis, whereas findings for fecal leukocytes are noncontributory
- The white blood cell count can reach 20,000/μL or higher in amebic dysentery but is not elevated in mild colitis
- A low-grade eosinophilia is occasionally present

DIAGNOSTIC PROCEDURES

- Colonoscopy is preferred over sigmoidoscopy. The bowel should not be cleansed by laxative or enema as this washes exudate from the ulcers and destroys trophozoites
- Rectal biopsy (from the edge of the ulcer) may enhance diagnosis

TREATMENT

MEDICATIONS

- See Table 138 (page 1319)
- The decision to treat is based on finding *Entamoeba* cysts or trophozoites and, when feasible (rarely), differentiating *E histolytica* from *E dispar*; testing for *E histolytica* antigen in stool; and testing for serum antibody
- The **tissue amebicides** dehydroemetine and emetine act on organisms in the bowel wall but not on amebas in the bowel lumen; dehydroemetine may be the safer drug
- Chloroquine is principally active against amebas in the liver
- The **luminal amebicides** diloxanide furoate (not available in the United States), iodoquinol, and paromomycin act on organisms in the bowel lumen but are ineffective against amebas in the bowel wall or other tissues
- Metronidazole is effective both in the bowel lumen and bowel and in extraintestinal tissues

Mild to moderate intestinal disease

- In patients with intestinal symptoms with *Entamoeba* in the stool in whom *E dispar* and *E histolytica* cannot be differentiated, if both stool antigen and serum antibody tests are negative, the latter tests may be false negatives and *E histolytica* infection may be present. In such cases, proceed with anti–*E histolytica* treatment
- Metronidazole plus a luminal amebicide is the treatment of choice

Severe intestinal disease

- Fluid and electrolyte therapy and opioids to control bowel motility are necessary adjuncts. Use opioids cautiously because of the risk of toxic megacolon

THERAPEUTIC PROCEDURES

Asymptomatic intestinal infection

- In asymptomatic cyst-passers, if stool antigen and serum antibody tests are negative, the infection is presumed to be *E dispar*, and should not be treated
- Within endemic areas, asymptomatic carriers generally are not treated because of the frequency of reinfection

OUTCOME

FOLLOW-UP

- Examine at least three stools at 2- to 3-day intervals, starting 2–4 weeks after the end of treatment
- Colonoscopy and reexamination of stools within 3 months may be indicated

COMPLICATIONS

- See *Amebic liver disease*
- Rare complications include appendicitis, bowel perforation, massive mucosal sloughing, and hemorrhage. Death may follow

PROGNOSIS

- The mortality rate from untreated amebic dysentery or ameboma may be high. With chemotherapy instituted early in the course of the disease, the prognosis is good

WHEN TO REFER

- Progressive colitis despite therapy

WHEN TO ADMIT

- Severe colitis or hepatic abscess

PREVENTION

- Hand washing
- Water supplies can be boiled (briefly) or treated with iodine (0.5 mL tincture of iodine per liter for 20 min, or longer if the water is cold); cysts are resistant to standard concentrations of chlorine. Filters are also available to purify drinking water. Disinfection dips for fruits and vegetables are not advised, and no drug is effective in prophylaxis

EVIDENCE

PRACTICE GUIDELINES

- National Guideline Clearinghouse http://www.guideline.gov/summary/ summary.aspx?doc_id=2707&nbr=1933 &string=colitis http://www.guideline.gov/summary/ summary.aspx?doc_id=2791&nbr= 2017&string=colitis

INFORMATION FOR PATIENTS

- Centers for Disease Control http://www.cdc.gov/ncidod/dpd/ parasites/amebiasis/factsht_amebiasis. htm
- Nemours Foundation http://kidshealth.org/parent/infections/ parasitic/amebiasis.html

REFERENCES

- Blessmann J et al: Treatment of asymptomatic intestinal *Entamoeba histolytica* infection. N Engl J Med. 2002;347:1384. [PMID: 12397207]
- Petri WA: *Entamoeba histolytica:* clinical update and vaccine prospects. Curr Infect Dis Rep 2002;4:124. [PMID: 11927043]

Amebic Liver Disease

KEY FEATURES

ESSENTIALS OF DIAGNOSIS

- Fever, hepatomegaly, pain, localized tenderness
- Amebas in stool or abscess aspirate; positive serological tests
- Abscess by ultrasound or CT scan

GENERAL CONSIDERATIONS

- *Entamoeba histolytica* is hematogenously spread from the colon to the liver
- Hepatic abscesses range from a few millimeters to 15 cm or larger, usually are single, occur more often in the right lobe (particularly the upper portion), and are more common in men

DEMOGRAPHICS

- Of 500 million persons worldwide infected with *Entamoeba*, most are infected with nonpathogenic *E dispar* and an estimated 10% (50 million) with potentially pathogenic *E histolytica*. Invasive *E histolytica* may constitute 5 million cases, with mortality in the range of 100,000 per year
- Amebic liver abscess, although a relatively infrequent (3–9%) consequence of *E histolytica* intestinal amebiasis, is not uncommon given the large number of intestinal infections

CLINICAL FINDINGS

SYMPTOMS AND SIGNS

- Many patients do not have current or a past history of intestinal symptoms
- The onset of symptoms can be sudden or gradual, ranging from a few days to many months
- Cardinal manifestations are fever (often high), pain (continuous, stabbing, or pleuritic, and sometimes severe), and an enlarged and tender liver
- There may be malaise or prostration, sweating, chills, anorexia, and weight loss
- The liver enlargement may present subcostally, in the epigastrium, as a localized bulging of the rib cage, or, as a result of enlargement against the dome of the diaphragm, it may produce coughing and findings of consolidation at the right lung base
- Intercostal tenderness is common
- Localizing signs on the skin over the liver may be an area of edema or a point of maximum tenderness

DIFFERENTIAL DIAGNOSIS

- Pyogenic liver abscess
- Echinococcosis (hydatid disease)
- Cholecystitis or cholangitis
- Right lower lobe pneumonia
- Pancreatitis
- Hepatocellular carcinoma

DIAGNOSIS

LABORATORY TESTS

- The white blood cell count ranges from 15,000 to 25,000/μL without eosinophilia
- Liver function test abnormalities, when present, are usually minimal
- Examination of stools for antigen and the organism is frequently negative
- Serological tests (ELISA and enzyme immunoassay) are almost always positive by 1 week after onset of hepatic symptoms or earlier as a result of chronic intestinal infection
- The indirect hemagglutination test (a positive titer is 1:128 or a higher dilution) stays positive for as long as 10 years after successful treatment and does not distinguish between past and new infections
- The agar gel test, though less sensitive, is rapidly conducted and may detect current infection because it becomes negative 3–6 months after eradication of the organism
- Detection of trophozoites in stool that contains ingested red blood cells is nearly diagnostic for invasive *E histolytica* but may be confused with the occasional *E dispar* or macrophage that also contains the red blood cells

IMAGING STUDIES

- Elevation of the right dome of the diaphragm and the size and location of the abscess can be determined by ultrasonography (usually round or oval nonhomogeneous lesions, abrupt transition from normal liver to the lesion, hypoechoic center with diffuse echoes throughout the abscess), CT (well-defined, round, low-density lesions with an internal, nonhomogeneous structure), MRI, and radioisotope scanning
- After intravenous injection of contrast material, CT may show a hyperdense halo around the periphery of the abscess
- Gallium scans, infrequently useful, show a cold spot as opposed to the increased gallium uptake in the center of pyogenic abscesses

DIAGNOSTIC PROCEDURES

- As CT, MRI, and sonography do not distinguish amebic and pyogenic abscesses, percutaneous aspiration may be indicated; this is best done by an image-guided needle (risks described below)

- The aspirate is divided into serial 30- to 50-mL aliquots, but only the last sample is examined for amebas, since the organisms are found at the edge of the cyst
- Detection of amebic antigen in aspirate appears to be very sensitive

 ## TREATMENT

MEDICATIONS
- See Table 138 (page 1319)
- Treatment is metronidazole or tinidazole plus diloxanide furoate or iodoquinol followed by chloroquine
- There is no clinical evidence of metronidazole-resistant *E histolytica*
- Chloroquine has been included in treatment to avoid rare long-term failures
- Treatment also requires a luminal amebicide (diloxanide furoate or iodoquinol), whether or not the organism is found in the stool
- If a satisfactory clinical response does not occur in 3 days, the abscess should be drained for therapeutic purposes and to exclude pyogenic abscess. Continued failure to achieve an adequate clinical response requires changing to the potentially toxic alternative drug dehydroemetine (or emetine) plus chloroquine
- Antibiotics are added for concomitant bacterial liver abscess, although metronidazole itself is highly effective against anaerobic bacteria
- Adverse drug reactions (see *Amebiasis*)

THERAPEUTIC PROCEDURES
- Most treatments with metronidazole do not require therapeutic percutaneous drainage; when needed, the catheter method is preferred. Indications are a large abscess, threatening rupture; the presence of a left lobe abscess (which is associated with a higher rate of severe complications); and the absence of medical response after 3 days of metronidazole therapy to exclude pyogenic abscess
- The risks of aspiration or catheter drainage are bacterial superinfection, bleeding, peritoneal spillage, and inadvertent puncture of an infected hydatid cyst

 ## OUTCOME

FOLLOW-UP
- Imaging defects in the liver disappear slowly (range: 3–13 months) after treatment; some calcify

COMPLICATIONS
- Without prompt treatment, the abscess may rupture into the pleural, peritoneal, or pericardial space or other contiguous organs, and death may follow

PROGNOSIS
- With chemotherapy instituted early in the course of the disease, most patients are successfully treated

WHEN TO ADMIT
- All patients should be admitted

PREVENTION
- Hand washing
- Water supplies can be boiled (briefly) or treated with iodine (0.5 mL tincture of iodine per liter for 20 min, or longer if the water is cold); cysts are resistant to standard concentrations of chlorine
- Filters are available to purify drinking water
- Disinfection dips for fruits and vegetables are not advised, and no drug is effective in prophylaxis

 ## EVIDENCE

INFORMATION FOR PATIENTS
- National Institutes of Health http://www.nlm.nih.gov/medlineplus/ency/article/000211.htm
- Centers for Disease Control http://www.cdc.gov/ncidod/dpd/parasites/amebiasis/factsht_amebiasis.htm

REFERENCE
- Weinke T et al: Amebic liver abscess—rare need for percutaneous treatment modalities. Eur J Med Res 2002;7:25. [PMID: 11827837]

Amebic Meningoencephalitis, Primary

 ## KEY FEATURES

ESSENTIALS OF DIAGNOSIS

- A fulminating, hemorrhagic, necrotizing meningoencephalitis with a limited purulent exudate
- It occurs in healthy children and young adults and is rapidly fatal

GENERAL CONSIDERATIONS

- It is caused by free-living amebas, most commonly by the ameboflagellate *Naegleria fowleri*. Other causes are *Balamuthia mandrillaris* and the *Acanthamoeba* species, both of which may have a predilection for immunocompromised patients
- Nasal and throat swabs have shown a carrier state, and serological surveys suggest that inapparent infections occur
- The organism apparently invades the central nervous system through the cribriform plate
- The incubation period varies from 2 to 15 days

DEMOGRAPHICS

- *N fowleri* is a thermophilic organism found in fresh and polluted warm lake water, domestic water supplies, swimming pools, thermal water, and sewers
- Most patients give a history of exposure to fresh water; dust is also a possible source

 ## CLINICAL FINDINGS

SYMPTOMS AND SIGNS

- Early symptoms include headache, fever, and lethargy, often associated with rhinitis and pharyngitis
- Vomiting, disorientation, and other signs of meningoencephalitis develop within 1 or 2 days, followed by coma and then death on the fifth or sixth day
- There may also be nonspecific myocarditis

DIFFERENTIAL DIAGNOSIS

- No distinctive clinical features distinguish the infection from acute bacterial meningoencephalitis

 ## DIAGNOSIS

LABORATORY TESTS

Cerebrospinal fluid

- Lumbar or ventricular cerebrospinal fluid contains several hundred to 25,000 leukocytes/μL (50–100% neutrophils) and erythrocytes (up to several thousand/μL)
- Protein is usually somewhat elevated, and glucose is normal or moderately reduced
- If conventional examinations for bacteria and fungi are negative, the fluid is examined for free-living amebas. Phase contrast is preferred. A wet mount examined by an ordinary optical microscope with the aperture restricted or condenser down will enhance contrast and refractility; a warm stage is not needed. The fluid should not be centrifuged at speeds over $150 \times g$ or refrigerated, as this tends to immobilize the amebas (7–14 μm). Their brisk motility distinguishes them from leukocytes of various types, which they closely resemble. Staining, culture, and mouse inoculation should be performed
- Precise species identification is based on morphology, demonstration of flagellate transformation (*Naegleria* only), and various immunological methods
- Serological testing is only useful epidemiologically; patients die before antibodies are detectable

TREATMENT

MEDICATIONS

- A few well-documented survivors of *N fowleri* infection have been reported. One was treated with intravenous and intrathecal amphotericin B and another with a combination of amphotericin B, miconazole, and oral rifampin

OUTCOME

PROGNOSIS

- In *B mandrillaris* infections, the usual course is subacute, with death occurring within 1 week to several months. No treatment is available

WHEN TO ADMIT

- All patients with confirmed or suspected disease

EVIDENCE

PRACTICE GUIDELINES

- National Guideline Clearinghouse http://www.guideline.gov/summary/summary.aspx?doc_id=2446&nbr=1672&string=meningoencephalitis

INFORMATION FOR PATIENTS

- Centers for Disease Control http://www.cdc.gov/ncidod/dpd/parasites/naegleria/factsht_naegleria.htm
- National Institute of Allergy and Infectious Disease http://www.niaid.nih.gov/publications/microbes.htm

REFERENCE

- Doel I et al: Encephalitis due to a free-living amoeba (*Balamuthia mandrillaris*): case report with literature review. Surg Neurol 2000;53:611. [PMID: 10940434]

Amenorrhea, Secondary & Menopause

 ## KEY FEATURES

ESSENTIALS OF DIAGNOSIS

- Secondary amenorrhea: absence of menses for 3 consecutive months in women who have passed menarche
- Menopause: termination of naturally occurring menses; usually diagnosed after 6 months of amenorrhea

GENERAL CONSIDERATIONS

- **Causes of secondary amenorrhea**
- Pregnancy [high human chorionic gonadotropin (hCG)]: most common cause. Rare: ectopic secretion of hCG by choriocarcinoma or bronchogenic carcinoma
- Hypothalamic-pituitary causes [low-normal follicle-stimulating hormone (FSH)]
  - "Hypothalamic amenorrhea": idiopathic, stress, strict dieting, vigorous exercise, organic illness, or anorexia nervosa
  - Hyperprolactinemia, pituitary tumors, and glucocorticoid excess can suppress gonadotropins
- Hyperandrogenism (low-normal FSH): polycystic ovarian syndrome; anabolic steroids. Rare: adrenal P-450c21 deficiency, ovarian or adrenal malignancy, ectopic ACTH from malignancy, Cushing's disease
- Endometritis (normal FSH): scarring (Asherman's syndrome) occurring spontaneously, following delivery or D&C, or with tuberculosis or schistosomiasis in endemic areas
- Premature ovarian failure (high FSH) (primary hypogonadism before age 40): autoimmune, XO/XX chromosome mosaicism, bilateral oophorectomy, pelvic radiation therapy, and chemotherapy. Rare: myotonic dystrophy, galactosemia, mumps oophoritis, familial or idiopathic
- Menopause (high FSH)

DEMOGRAPHICS

- Normal age of menopause in the United States is 48–55 years (average 51.5 years)

 ## CLINICAL FINDINGS

SYMPTOMS AND SIGNS

- Nausea and breast engorgement suggest pregnancy
- Hot flushes suggest ovarian failure
- Headache or visual field abnormalities with pituitary tumor. Thirst and polyuria with diabetes insipidus due to hypothalamic or pituitary lesion. Acromegaly or gigantism indicate pituitary tumor
- Goiter suggests hyperthyroidism
- Weight loss, diarrhea, or skin darkening suggests adrenal insufficiency
- Weight loss with distorted body image suggests anorexia nervosa
- Galactorrhea suggests hyperprolactinemia due to pituitary tumor or various drugs
- Hirsutism or virilization occurs with hyperandrogenism
- Weakness, psychiatric changes, hypertension, central obesity, hirsutism, thin skin, ecchymoses suggest Cushing's syndrome or alcoholism
- Perform pelvic examination to check for uterine or adnexal enlargement
- Vasomotor instability (hot flushes), depression, irritability, fatigue, insomnia, headache, diminished libido, or rheumatological symptoms suggest menopause. Vasomotor instability in 80%, lasts seconds to many minutes; may be most severe at night or triggered by emotional stress, may persist for >5 years in 35%
- Urogenital atrophy, vaginal dryness, and dyspareunia; dysuria, frequency, and incontinence; osteoporotic fractures are late manifestations of estrogen deficiency

DIFFERENTIAL DIAGNOSIS

- Pregnancy
- Menopause or perimenopause
- Polycystic ovary syndrome
- Hypothalamic amenorrhea, eg, stress, weight change, exercise
- Hyperprolactinemia
- Hypothyroidism or hyperthyroidism
- Diabetes mellitus
- Premature ovarian failure
- Anorexia nervosa

 ## DIAGNOSIS

LABORATORY TESTS

- Serum pregnancy test for all women of childbearing age. False-positive tests may occur rarely with ectopic hCG secretion (eg, choriocarcinoma or bronchogenic carcinoma)
- Check serum prolactin, FSH, luteinizing hormone, thyroid-stimulating hormone, potassium, creatinine, and liver enzymes if not pregnant
- Check serum testosterone in hirsute or virilized women
- Perform 1-mg overnight dexamethasone suppression test (see *Cushing's syndrome*) if signs of hypercortisolism
- Perform Pap smear and vaginal smear to assess estrogen effect

IMAGING STUDIES

- Hyperprolactinemia or hypopituitarism without obvious cause should prompt pituitary MRI (see *Hypopituitarism*)

DIAGNOSTIC PROCEDURES

- Progestin withdrawal test: nonpregnant women with normal pelvic examination and laboratory tests are given a 10-day course of progestin (eg, medroxyprogesterone acetate 10 mg PO QD)
- Absence of withdrawal menses indicates possible pregnancy, uterine abnormality, or estrogen deficiency
- Occurrence of withdrawal bleeding indicates anovulation likely due to noncyclic gonadotropin secretion (eg, polycystic ovaries, idiopathic anovulation)

Amenorrhea, Secondary & Menopause

 TREATMENT

MEDICATIONS

- Hormone replacement for women with premature ovarian failure (<40 years of age)
  - **Uterus present:** conjugated estrogens 0.625 mg daily or estradiol 1 mg daily, with progestin 2.5 mg daily or progesterone 100–200 mg daily; cycled estrogen days 1–25 with progestin added days 16–25; oral combined contraceptive daily or cycled, transdermal ethinyl estradiol 0.05 mg/day with oral progestin daily or cycled
  - **Uterus absent:** daily estrogen alone
- Hormone replacement for women in menopause: doses of estrogen are kept low for short duration if possible (see *Menopausal syndrome*)
- Estrogen doses required for relief of vasomotor symptoms are sometimes higher than standard physiological replacement doses
- Progestins or phytoestrogens, and slow, deep breathing, can sometimes ameliorate hot flushes
- Postmenopausal women should be evaluated for osteoporosis and treated if appropriate (see *Osteoporosis*)
- Estrogen replacement (plus progestin if uterus is present) for premature ovarian failure

THERAPEUTIC PROCEDURES

- Treatment directed at underlying cause

 OUTCOME

FOLLOW-UP

- Hypothalamic amenorrhea: patients typically recover spontaneously but should have regular evaluations and a progestin withdrawal test about every 3 months to detect loss of estrogen effect

PROGNOSIS

- Ovarian failure (premature or menopausal): usually irreversible
- Menopause: increased bone osteoclastic activity increases risk for osteoporosis and fractures
- Menopause: increased LDL/HDL cholesterol ratio causes increased risk for atherosclerosis

PREVENTION

- Diet adequate in protein, calories, calcium, and vitamin D
- Calcium and vitamin D supplements and exercise for those at risk for osteoporosis
- Consider bisphosphonate if osteoporosis on bone densitometry
- Mammography recommended yearly for menopausal women receiving hormone replacement therapy
- Tamoxifen and raloxifene offer protection against osteoporosis but aggravate hot flushes

 EVIDENCE

PRACTICE GUIDELINES

- Hormone replacement therapy: collaborative decision making and management. Institute for Clinical Systems Improvement, 2002 http://www.icsi.org/knowledge/detail. asp?catID=29&itemID=172

WEB SITE

- American Academy of Family Physicians—Menopause http://familydoctor.org/healthfacts/125/ index.html

INFORMATION FOR PATIENTS

- Mayo Clinic—Menopause http://www.mayoclinic.com/invoke. cfm?id=DS00119

REFERENCES

- Falsetti L et al: Long-term follow-up of functional hypothalamic amenorrhea and prognostic factors. J Clin Endocrinol Metab 2002;87:500. [PMID: 11836275]
- Grady D et al: Cardiovascular disease outcomes during 6.8 years of hormone therapy: Heart and Estrogen/Progestin Replacement Study follow-up (HERS II). JAMA 2002;288:49. [PMID: 12090862]
- Grady D et al: Effect of postmenopausal hormone therapy on cognitive function: the Heart and Estrogen/Progestin Replacement Study. Am J Med 2002;113:543. [PMID: 12459399]
- Hulley S et al: Noncardiovascular disease outcomes during 6.8 years of hormone therapy: Heart and Estrogen/Progestin Replacement Study follow-up (HERS II). JAMA 2002;288:58. [PMID: 12090863]
- Rossouw JE et al: Risks and benefits of estrogen plus progestin in healthy postmenopausal women: principal results from the Women's Health Initiative randomized controlled study. JAMA 2002;288:321. [PMID: 12117397]

Paul A. Fitzgerald, MD

Amphetamine & Cocaine Overdose

 ## KEY FEATURES

ESSENTIALS OF DIAGNOSIS

- Agitation, paranoia, psychosis
- Seizures, hyperthermia
- Hypertension, tachycardia
- Hyponatremia may occur with methyl-enedioxymethamphetamine (MDMA, "ecstasy")

GENERAL CONSIDERATIONS

- Amphetamines and cocaine are widely abused for their euphorigenic and stimulant properties. Both drugs may be smoked, snorted, ingested, or injected
- The toxic dose of each drug is highly variable and depends on the route of administration and individual tolerance
- Amphetamine derivatives and related drugs include methamphetamine ("crystal meth," "crank"), MDMA, ephedrine ("herbal ecstasy"), and methcathinone ("cat")
- Nonprescription medications and nutritional supplements may contain stimulant or sympathomimetic drugs such as ephedrine or caffeine

 ## CLINICAL FINDINGS

SYMPTOMS AND SIGNS

- Amphetamines and cocaine produce central nervous system stimulation and a generalized increase in central and peripheral sympathetic activity
- The onset of effects is most rapid after intravenous injection or smoking
- There may be anxiety, tremulousness, tachycardia, hypertension, diaphoresis, dilated pupils, agitation, muscular hyperactivity, and psychosis
- In severe intoxication, seizures and hyperthermia may occur

DIFFERENTIAL DIAGNOSIS

- Ephedrine
- Pseudoephedrine
- Anticholinergic poisoning
- Psychosis
- Heat stroke

 ## DIAGNOSIS

LABORATORY TESTS

- Amphetamines, cocaine, or the cocaine metabolite benzoylecgonine is found in the urine
- Blood screening is not sensitive enough to detect these drugs
- Metabolic acidosis may occur
- Hyponatremia has been reported after MDMA use
- Masssive cocaine intoxication can cause QRS interval prolongation similar to tricyclic antidepressant overdose

TREATMENT

MEDICATIONS

Emergency and supportive measures

- Rapidly lower the body temperature (see *Hyperthermia*) in patients who are hyperthermic (40°C)
- Treat agitation or psychosis with a benzodiazepine—lorazepam, 2–3 mg intravenously (repeated as needed up to 8–10 mg) or midazolam, 0.1–0.2 mg/kg intramuscularly
- For poisoning by ingestion, administer activated charcoal
- Do *not* induce emesis, because of the risk of seizures

Specific treatment

- Treat agitation with a sedative such as lorazepam, 2–3 mg intravenously
- Treat seizures with lorazepam or phenobarbital
- Treat hypertension with a vasodilator drug such as phentolamine (1–5 mg intravenously) or nifedipine (10–20 mg orally) or a combined α- and β-adrenergic blocker such as labetalol (10–20 mg intravenously). Do *not* administer a pure β-blocker such as propranolol alone, as this may result in paradoxic worsening of the hypertension as a result of unopposed α-adrenergic effects
- Treat tachycardia or tachyarrhythmias with a short-acting β-blocker such as esmolol (25–100 μg/kg/min by intravenous infusion)
- Treat hyponatremia (see *Hyponatremia*)

OUTCOME

COMPLICATIONS

- Sustained or severe hypertension may result in intracranial hemorrhage, aortic dissection, or myocardial infarction
- Hyperthermia may cause multiorgan failure or permanent brain damage

PROGNOSIS

- Good if only a single brief seizure or mild-moderate agitation or cardiovascular effects
- Poor after severe hyperthermia (eg, T >104°C) or intracranial hemorrhage

WHEN TO ADMIT

- Persistent hypertension, tachycardia
- Hyperthermia
- Multiple or prolonged seizures

EVIDENCE

PRACTICE GUIDELINES

- National Guideline Clearinghouse http://www.guideline.gov/summary/summary.aspx?doc_id=2540&nbr=1766&string=cocaine http://www.guideline.gov/summary/summary.aspx?doc_id=3169&nbr=2395&string=cocaine

WEB SITES

- Agency for Toxic Substances and Disease Registry (ATSDR) http://www.cdc.gov/niosh/nasd/srd/og56400.html
- Carbon monoxide poisonings http://www.cdc.gov/mmwr/preview/mmwrhtml/00039315.htm
- Pesticide poisonings: National Pesticide Information Center http://ace.orst.edu/info/npic/rmpp.htm
- Toxicology—eMedicine http://www.emedicine.com/cgi-bin/foxweb.exe/showsection@d:/em/ga?book=emerg&sct=TOXICOLOGY

INFORMATION FOR PATIENTS

- JAMA patient page: Cocaine addiction. JAMA 2002;287:146.
- JAMA patient page: Drug abuse. JAMA 2000;283:1378.

REFERENCES

- Albertson TE et al: Methamphetamine and the expanding complications of amphetamines. West J Med 1999;170: 214. [PMID: 10344175]
- Haller CA et al: Adverse cardiovascular and central nervous system events associated with dietary supplements containing ephedra alkaloids. N Engl J Med 2000;343:1833. [PMID: 11117974]
- Parrott AC: Recreational ecstasy/MDMA, the serotonin syndrome, and serotonergic neurotoxicity. Pharmacol Biochem Behav 2002;71:837. [PMID: 11888574]

Kent R. Olson, MD

Amyloidosis

 ## KEY FEATURES

ESSENTIALS OF DIAGNOSIS

- The diagnosis is based on clinical suspicion, family history, and preexisting long-standing infection or debilitating illness
- Microscopic examination of biopsy (eg, gingival, renal, rectal) or surgical specimens is diagnostic
- Fine-needle biopsy of subcutaneous abdominal fat is a simple and reliable method for diagnosing secondary systemic amyloidosis

GENERAL CONSIDERATIONS

- A group of disorders characterized by impaired organ function due to infiltration with insoluble protein fibrils
- Different fibrils are correlated with the clinical syndromes
- In primary amyloidosis (AL), the protein fibrils are monoclonal immunoglobulin light chains
- Secondary amyloid (AA) proteins are derived from acute-phase reactant apolipoprotein precursors
- Familial syndromes commonly cause infiltrative neuropathies
- Other types of amyloidosis may also be hereditary
- Over 20 types of fibrils have been identified in amyloid deposits
- Amyloidosis due to deposition of β_2-microglobulin in carpal ligaments occurs in chronic hemodialysis patients

 ## CLINICAL FINDINGS

SYMPTOMS AND SIGNS

- Related to malfunction of the infiltrated organ
- The hereditary amyloidoses usually cause neuropathies

Primary amyloidosis

- Causes widespread disease
- Nephrotic syndrome and renal failure
- Cardiomyopathy and cardiac conduction defects
- Intestinal malabsorption and pseudo-obstruction
- Carpal tunnel syndrome
- Macroglossia
- Peripheral neuropathy
- End-organ insufficiency of endocrine glands
- Respiratory failure
- Capillary damage with ecchymosis

Secondary amyloidosis

- Usually limited to the liver, spleen, and adrenals

DIFFERENTIAL DIAGNOSIS

- Multiple myeloma
- Hemochromatosis
- Sarcoidosis
- Waldenström's macroglobulinemia
- Metastatic cancer
- Other cause of nephrotic syndrome, eg, lupus nephritis

 ## DIAGNOSIS

LABORATORY TESTS

- Monoclonal gammopathy on serum protein electrophoresis (in primary amyloidosis)

DIAGNOSTIC PROCEDURES

- Abdominal fat pad, rectal, or gingival biopsy with microscopic examination revealing amyloid protein (green birefringence under polarizing microscope after Congo red staining)
- In systemic disease, rectal or gingival biopsies show a sensitivity of about 80%, bone marrow biopsy about 50%, and abdominal fat aspiration between 70% and 80%

Amyloidosis

 TREATMENT

MEDICATIONS

- Myeloma- or AL-associated amyloid can be treated with melphalan and prednisone

SURGERY

- Treatment of localized amyloid tumors is by surgical excision
- Some hereditary forms of amyloid are being treated with liver transplantation

THERAPEUTIC PROCEDURES

Systemic amyloidosis

- There is no effective treatment
- Supportive care/specific care pertinent to involved organs
- Hemodialysis and immunosuppressive therapy may be useful

Secondary disease

- Usually approached by aggressively treating the predisposing disease, but remission of fibril deposition does not occur
- Bone marrow transplant after chemotherapy has been employed in selected patients

 OUTCOME

PROGNOSIS

- Death usually occurs within 1–3 years of diagnosis with systemic amyloidosis

WHEN TO REFER

- Refer to a hematologist to confirm the diagnosis and for management
- Refer to specialist of the organ(s) involved (eg, cardiologist, nephrologist)

 EVIDENCE

PRACTICE GUIDELINES

- National Clearinghouse Guidelines
  http://www.guideline.gov/search/
  searchresults.aspx?Type=3&txtSearch=
  amyloidosis&num=20
- National Comprehensive Cancer Network
  http://www.nccn.org/physician_gls/
  PDF/myeloma.pdf

WEB SITE

- National Institutes of Health
  www.nih.gov/niams/healthinfo

INFORMATION FOR PATIENTS

- Mayo Clinic
  http://www.mayoclinic.org/
  amyloidosis-rst/
- U.S. National Institute of Diabetes & Digestive & Kidney Diseases
  http://www.niddk.nih.gov/health/
  kidney/pubs/kidney-failure/amyloidosis/
  amyloidosis.htm
- National Institute of Arthritis and Musculoskeletal and Skin Diseases
  http://www.niams.nih.gov/hi/index.
  htm#ip

REFERENCE

- Kyle RA: Clinical aspects of multiple myeloma and related disorders including amyloidosis. Pathol Biol (Paris) 1999;47:148. [PMID: 10192881]

Jeffrey L. Kishiyama, MD
Daniel C. Adelman, MD

Anaphylaxis

KEY FEATURES

ESSENTIALS OF DIAGNOSIS

- Anaphylaxis is a systemic reaction with cutaneous symptoms, associated with dyspnea, visceral edema, and hypotension
- Urticaria is characterized by large, irregularly shaped, pruritic, erythematous wheals
- Angioedema is painless, deep, subcutaneous swelling, often involving periorbital, circumoral, and facial regions
- These disorders may be diagnosed clinically, especially in the context of allergen exposure; detection of specific IgE or elevated serum tryptase can confirm diagnosis

GENERAL CONSIDERATIONS

- The most common allergens that induce this IgE antibody–mediated response are drugs, insect venoms, and foods
- A generalized release of mediators from mast cells can result in systemic anaphylaxis
- Can affect both nonatopic and atopic persons
- Isolated urticaria and angioedema are more common cutaneous forms of anaphylaxis with a better prognosis
- In about 10% of cases, chronic relapsing urticaria, angioedema, and anaphylaxis are not due to IgE-mediated hypersensitivity; consider underlying systemic disorders such as systemic mastocytosis or subclinical infection or inflammatory disorders
- Idiopathic autoimmune processes include the production of histamine-liberating autoantibodies directed against Fcε mast cell membrane receptors
- Twenty percent of the population will experience urticaria or angioedema during their lifetime

DEMOGRAPHICS

In the United States

- The estimated prevalence of idiopathic anaphylaxis is 34,000 patients
- Food allergies cause an estimated 150 fatalities per year
- Most food allergy fatalities are due to peanuts, tree nuts, shellfish, and fish
- β-Lactam antibiotics may be involved in 400–800 fatalities per year
- Stinging insect venom causes about 50 fatalities per year

CLINICAL FINDINGS

SYMPTOMS AND SIGNS

- Hypotension/shock from widespread vasodilatation
- Respiratory distress from bronchospasm or laryngeal edema
- Gastrointestinal or uterine smooth muscle contraction
- Flushing, pruritus, urticaria, and angioedema

DIFFERENTIAL DIAGNOSIS

- Other causes of shock
  - Sepsis
  - Cardiogenic
  - Hypovolemic
  - Neurogenic
- Asthma
- Adrenal insufficiency
- Vasovagal reaction

DIAGNOSIS

LABORATORY TESTS

- Based on the clinical presentation and a history of allergen exposure
- An elevated serum tryptase (a mast cell protease) measured during the episode can confirm the diagnosis
- Detection of a specific IgE, skin testing, or radioallergosorbent test (RAST) against the suspected antigen can confirm the allergic diathesis

Anaphylaxis

 ## TREATMENT

MEDICATIONS

Anaphylaxis

- Epinephrine 1:1000 in a dose of 0.2–0.5 mL (0.2–0.5 mg) injected IM in the anterolateral thigh (more predictable and rapidly absorbed than injecting in the arm); repeated injections can be given every 5–15 min if necessary
- Rapid infusions of normal saline
- SQ epinephrine, inhaled β_2-adrenergic agonists, or IV aminophylline for bronchospasm
- Antihistamines (H_1 and H_2 receptor antagonists)
- Intravenous corticosteroids (which may mitigate the late-phase response that occurs 24 h after onset)
- 12–24 h of observation
- See *Urticaria & angioedema*

THERAPEUTIC PROCEDURES

- Endotracheal intubation for laryngeal edema or severe bronchospasm

 ## OUTCOME

FOLLOW-UP

- Follow up with an allergist and receive a subcutaneous epinephrine self-injection kit; further management may involve antihistamines or immunotherapy

WHEN TO REFER

- Early referral to an allergist may help with management
- Refer for desensitization and immunotherapy

WHEN TO ADMIT

- Patients with anaphylaxis should be admitted for 12–24 h of observation for recurrence of symptoms

PREVENTION

- Long-term combined oral antihistamine and prednisone therapy reduces the number and severity of attacks of life-threatening idiopathic anaphylaxis
- Medical therapy does not reliably prevent true IgE-mediated hypersensitivity reactions

Venom immunotherapy

- Patients with immediate hypersensitivity reactions to stinging insects and documented venom-specific IgE on allergy testing should receive venom immunotherapy for prevention of anaphylaxis
- Untreated individuals have a 50–60% risk of anaphylactic response to subsequent stings
- Venom immunotherapy provides 98% protection from life-threatening reactions on rechallenge

 ## EVIDENCE

PRACTICE GUIDELINES

- The diagnosis and management of anaphylaxis. Joint Task Force on Practice Parameters, Work Group on Diagnosis and Management of Anaphylaxis. J Allergy Clin Immunol 1998;101:S465.
- Joint Council of Allergy, Asthma and Immunology http://www.guideline.gov/summary/summary.aspx?doc_id=1433&nbr=673&string=anaphylaxis

WEB SITES

- National Institutes of Health www.nih.gov/niams/healthinfo
- American Academy of Allergy, Asthma, and Immunology http://www.aaaai.org

INFORMATION FOR PATIENTS

- JAMA patient page: Allergies. JAMA 2000;283:424. [PMID: 10647806]
- American College of Allergy, Asthma and Immunology http://www.medem.com/search/article_display.cfm?path=\\TANQUERAY\M_ContentItem&mstr=/M_ContentItem/ZZZFNLSBZ6C.html&soc=ACAAI&srch_typ=NAV_SERCH
- American Academy of Family Physicians http://familydoctor.org/handouts/340.html

REFERENCES

- Charous BL: Natural rubber latex allergy after 12 years: recommendations and perspectives. J Allergy Clin Immunol 2002;109:31. [PMID: 11799362]
- Kaplan AP: Diagnostic tests for urticaria and angioedema. Clin Allergy Immunol 2000;15:111. [PMID: 10943290]
- Kemp SF: Anaphylaxis: a review of causes and mechanisms. J Allergy Clin Immunol 2002:110:341. [PMID: 12209078]

Jeffrey L. Kishiyama, MD
Daniel C. Adelman, MD

Anemia, Aplastic

KEY FEATURES

ESSENTIALS OF DIAGNOSIS

- Pancytopenia
- No abnormal cells seen
- Hypocellular bone marrow

GENERAL CONSIDERATIONS

- In aplastic anemia, bone marrow failure and pancytopenia arise from injury to or abnormal expression of the hematopoietic stem cell

Causes of aplastic anemia

- "Idiopathic" (probably autoimmune)
- Drugs: chloramphenicol, phenylbutazone, gold salts, sulfonamides, phenytoin, carbamazepine, quinacrine, tolbutamide
- Viruses: hepatitis, Epstein-Barr virus, HIV, parvovirus B19
- Systemic lupus erythematosus
- Chemotherapy
- Radiation therapy
- Toxins: benzene, toluene, insecticides
- Posthepatitis
- Pregnancy
- Paroxysmal nocturnal hemoglobinuria
- Congenital (rare)

CLINICAL FINDINGS

SYMPTOMS AND SIGNS

- Weakness and fatigue from anemia
- Vulnerability to bacterial infections from neutropenia
- Mucosal and skin bleeding from thrombocytopenia
- Pallor, purpura, and petechiae
- Hepatosplenomegaly, lymphadenopathy, or bone tenderness should *not* be present

DIFFERENTIAL DIAGNOSIS

- Acute leukemia
- Myelodysplastic syndrome
- Bone marrow infiltrative process, eg, tumor, infection, granulomatous disease
- Hypersplenism
- Viral infection, eg, parvovirus B19, hepatitis, HIV
- Systemic lupus erythematosus

DIAGNOSIS

LABORATORY TESTS

- Pancytopenia, though in early disease, only one or two cell lines may be reduced
- Anemia may be severe
- Reticulocytes always decreased
- Red blood cell morphology unremarkable
- Neutrophils and platelets reduced in number, no immature or abnormal forms seen
- Severe aplastic anemia defined by neutrophils <500/μL, platelets <20,000/μL, reticulocytes <1%, and bone marrow cellularity <20%

DIAGNOSTIC PROCEDURES

- Bone marrow aspirate and bone marrow biopsy appear hypocellular, with scant amounts of normal hematopoietic progenitors; no abnormal cells are seen

Anemia, Aplastic

TREATMENT

MEDICATIONS

- Antibiotics to treat infections
- Immunosuppression with antithymocyte globulin (ATG) plus cyclosporine for severe aplastic anemia in adults aged >50 or those without HLA-matched siblings
- Useful regimen is ATG 40 mg/kg/day IV for 4 days, in combination with cyclosporine, 6 mg/kg PO BID, given in hospital in conjunction with corticosteroids, and transfusion and antibiotic support
- Corticosteroids are given with ATG (prednisone 1–2 mg/kg/day initially, followed by rapid taper) to avoid complications of serum sickness
- High-dose cyclophosphamide (200 mg/kg) immunosuppression for refractory cases and in patients without suitable bone marrow donors
- Antibiotics and transfusion often required for prolonged pancytopenia (median 7 weeks of neutropenia)
- Androgens, eg, oxymetholone 2–3 mg/kg PO QD, used commonly in past
- Despite low response rate, some patients can be maintained successfully with androgens

THERAPEUTIC PROCEDURES

- Supportive measures only for mild cases
- Allogeneic bone marrow transplantation for severe aplastic anemia in adults aged <50 with HLA-matched siblings
- Allogeneic transplantation using unrelated donor for severe aplastic anemia in children or adults aged <30
- Red blood cell and platelet transfusions as necessary

OUTCOME

COMPLICATIONS

- Infections
- Bleeding

PROGNOSIS

- Median survival in severe aplastic anemia without treatment is ~3 months, and 1-year survival is only 20%
- Allogeneic bone marrow transplantation is highly successful in children and young adults with HLA-matched siblings, with durable complete response rate >80%
- ATG treatment produces partial response in ~ 60% of adults, usually in 4–12 weeks; long-term prognosis of responders is good
- Paroxysmal nocturnal hemoglobinuria or myelodysplasia or other clonal hematological disorders develop in <25% of nontransplanted patients after many years of follow-up

EVIDENCE

PRACTICE GUIDELINES

- Ball SE: The modern management of severe aplastic anaemia. Br J Haematol 2000;110:41. [PMID: 10930978]
- Paquette RL: Diagnosis and management of aplastic anemia and myelodysplastic syndrome. Oncology (Huntingt) 2002;16(9 Suppl 10):153. [PMID: 12380966]

WEB SITE

- American Cancer Society—Aplastic anemia
  http://www.cancer.org/docroot/CRI/CRI_2_3x.asp?dt=77

INFORMATION FOR PATIENTS

- Aplastic Anemia & MDS International Foundation—Aplastic anemia
  http://www.aplastic.org/cgi-bin/byteserver.pl/pdfs/Acquired-aplastic-anemia-basic-explanations.pdf
- Mayo Clinic—Aplastic anemia
  http://www.mayoclinic.com/invoke.cfm?objectid=BBF63113-1AC6-4EAB-B10232C099C4C55E

REFERENCES

- Brodsky RA et al: Durable treatment-free remission after high-dose cyclophosphamide therapy for previously untreated severe aplastic anemia. Ann Intern Med 2001;135:477. [PMID: 11578150]
- Storb R et al: Cyclophosphamide and antithymocyte globulin to condition patients with aplastic anemia for allogeneic marrow transplantation: the experience in four centers. Biol Blood Marrow Transplant 2001;7:39. [PMID: 11215697]
- Young NS: Acquired aplastic anemia. Ann Intern Med 2002;136:534. [PMID: 11926789]

Charles A. Linker, MD

Anemia, Autoimmune Hemolytic

 ## KEY FEATURES

ESSENTIALS OF DIAGNOSIS

- Acquired anemia caused by immunoglobulin G (IgG) autoantibody
- Spherocytes and reticulocytosis on peripheral blood smear
- Positive Coombs test

GENERAL CONSIDERATIONS

- Acquired disorder in which IgG autoantibody binds to red blood cell (RBC) membrane.
  - Macrophages in spleen and other portions of reticuloendothelial system then remove portion of RBC membrane, forming a spherocyte because of decreased surface-to-volume ratio of RBC
  - Spherocytes less deformable and become trapped in spleen
- Causes include idiopathic (~50% of cases), systemic lupus erythematosus, chronic lymphocytic leukemia, or lymphomas
- Must be distinguished from drug-induced hemolytic anemia, eg, penicillin (and other drugs) coat RBC membrane, and antibody is directed against membrane–drug complex
- Typically produces anemia of rapid onset that may be life-threatening

 ## CLINICAL FINDINGS

SYMPTOMS AND SIGNS

- Fatigue, angina pectoris, or symptoms of congestive heart failure
- Jaundice and splenomegaly may be present

DIFFERENTIAL DIAGNOSIS

- Coombs positive (immune) hemolytic anemia: autoimmune, drugs, infection, lymphoproliferative disease, Rh or ABO incompatibility
- Coombs negative hemolytic anemia
- Hereditary spherocytosis
- Glucose-6-phosphate dehydrogenase deficiency, pyruvate kinase deficiency
- Microangiopathic hemolytic anemia: thrombotic thrombocytopenic purpura, hemolytic uremic syndrome, disseminated intravascular coagulation
- Splenic sequestration

 ## DIAGNOSIS

LABORATORY TESTS

- Anemia of variable severity, though hematocrit may be <10%
- Reticulocytosis usually present
- Spherocytes on peripheral blood smear
- Indirect bilirubin increased
- Coincident immune thrombocytopenia (Evans syndrome) in ~10%
- Coombs antiglobulin test is basis for diagnosis; reagent is rabbit IgM antibody against human IgG or human complement
- Direct Coombs test positive: patient's RBCs mixed with Coombs reagent; agglutination indicates antibody on RBC surface
- Indirect Coombs test may or may not be positive: patient's serum mixed with panel of type O RBCs, then Coombs reagent added; agglutination indicates presence of large amount of autoantibody that has saturated binding sites on RBC and consequently appears in serum
- Micro-Coombs test is more sensitive and is necessary to make diagnosis in approximately 10% of cases; test indicated in patient with acquired spherocytic hemolytic anemia that may be autoimmune who has a negative direct Coombs test

TREATMENT

MEDICATIONS

- Prednisone, 1–2 mg/kg/day in divided doses is initial therapy
- Splenectomy if prednisone ineffective or if disease recurs on tapering dose
- Immunosuppressive agents, eg, cyclophosphamide, azathioprine, or cyclosporine in refractory cases
- Danazol, 600–800 mg/day is less effective than in immune thrombocytopenia
- High-dose IVIG (1 g daily for 1 or 2 days) may be highly effective in controlling hemolysis; benefit is short lived (1–3 weeks) and it is expensive
- Rituximab, 375 mg/m² IV Q weeks for 4 weeks is effective in some cases

SURGERY

- Splenectomy is often successful

THERAPEUTIC PROCEDURES

- Transfusion may be difficult because of difficulty in performing cross-match, thus incompatible blood may be given
- If compatible, most transfused blood survives similarly to patient's own RBCs

 ## OUTCOME

COMPLICATIONS

- Possible transfusion reactions

PROGNOSIS

- Long-term prognosis is good, especially if there is no underlying autoimmune disorder or lymphoma

WHEN TO REFER

- Decisions regarding transfusions should be made in consultation with a hematologist

 ## EVIDENCE

PRACTICE GUIDELINES

- Gehrs BC et al: Autoimmune hemolytic anemia. Am J Hematol 2002;69:258. [PMID: 11921020]
- Hashimoto C: Autoimmune hemolytic anemia. Clin Rev Allergy Immunol 1998;16:285. [PMID: 9773255]
- Petz LD: Treatment of autoimmune hemolytic anemias. Curr Opin Hematol 2001;8:411. [PMID: 11604584]

WEB SITES

- MEDLINEplus—Idiopathic autoimmune hemolytic anemia http://www.nlm.nih.gov/medlineplus/ency/article/000579.htm
- American Autoimmune Related Disease Association—Autoimmune hemolytic anemia http://www.aarda.org/patient_information.php

INFORMATION FOR PATIENTS

- The Regional Cancer Center http://www.trcc.org/blood/10b_autoimmune.pdf
- UCSF Childrenís Hospital—Hemolytic anemia http://www.ucsfhealth.org/childrens/medical_services/cancer/blood/conditions/h_anemia/signs.html
- University of Maryland—Hemolytic anemia http://www.umm.edu/blood/anehemol.htm

REFERENCES

- Kokori SI et al: Autoimmune hemolytic anemia in patients with systemic lupus erythematosus. Am J Med 2000;108:198. [PMID: 10723973]
- Mauro FR et al: Autoimmune hemolytic anemia in chronic lymphocytic leukemia: clinical, therapeutic, and prognostic features. Blood 2000;95:2786. [PMID: 10779422]

Charles A. Linker, MD

Anemia, Iron Deficiency

 KEY FEATURES

ESSENTIALS OF DIAGNOSIS

- Absent bone marrow iron stores or serum ferritin <12 μg/L are both pathognomonic
- Caused by bleeding in adults unless proved otherwise
- Response to iron therapy

GENERAL CONSIDERATIONS

- Most common cause of anemia worldwide
- Causes: blood loss [gastrointestinal (GI), menstrual, repeated blood donation]; deficient diet; increased requirements (pregnancy, lactation); hemoglobinuria, eg, paroxysmal nocturnal hemoglobinuria; malabsorption, eg, gastric surgery, celiac disease; hemolysis; pulmonary hemosiderosis (iron sequestration)
- Women with heavy menstrual losses may require more iron than can reasonably be absorbed, thus they often become iron deficient
- Pregnancy and lactation also increase requirement for iron, necessitating medicinal iron supplementation
- Blood loss, especially GI bleeding, is by far the most important cause of iron deficiency anemia
- Chronic aspirin use may cause blood loss even without documented structural lesion
- In iron deficiency, search for source of GI bleeding if other sites of blood loss (menorrhagia, other uterine bleeding, and repeated blood donations) are excluded
- Diagnosis of iron deficiency anemia can involve demonstrating iron-deficient state or evaluating response to a therapeutic trial of iron replacement

DEMOGRAPHICS

- More common in women due to menstrual losses

 CLINICAL FINDINGS

SYMPTOMS AND SIGNS

- Symptoms of anemia, eg, easy fatigability, tachycardia, palpitations and tachypnea on exertion
- Skin and mucosal changes, eg, smooth tongue, brittle nails, and cheilosis, in severe deficiency
- Dysphagia due to esophageal webs (Plummer-Vinson syndrome)
- Pica, ie, craving for specific foods (ice chips, lettuce, etc) often not rich in iron, in many

DIFFERENTIAL DIAGNOSIS

- Microcytic anemia due to other causes: thalassemia, anemia of chronic disease, sideroblastic anemia, or lead poisoning

 DIAGNOSIS

LABORATORY TESTS

- Hematocrit low, but initially mean corpuscular hemoglobin (MCV) normal, later MCV low
- Platelet count often increased
- Serum ferritin low; value <30 μg/L highly reliable indicator of iron deficiency
- Serum total iron-binding capacity (TIBC) rises
- Serum iron <30 μg/dL and transferrin saturation <15% after iron stores depleted
- Blood smear shows hypochromic microcytic cells, anisocytosis [variations in red blood cell (RBC) size], and poikilocytosis (variation in RBC shape)
- Severely hypochromic cells, target cells, hypochromic pencil-shaped cells, and occasionally small numbers of nucleated RBCs in severe iron deficiency
- Fecal occult blood testing often positive with GI bleeding

DIAGNOSTIC PROCEDURES

- Colonoscopy or flexible sigmoidoscopy may be required in evaluation of suspected GI bleeding

TREATMENT

MEDICATIONS

- Ferrous sulfate, 325 mg PO TID, is treatment of choice; may cause GI side effects
- Compliance improved by starting 325 mg PO QD with food, then gradually escalating dose
- Continue iron therapy for 3–6 months after restoration of normal hematological values to replenish iron stores
- Failure of response to iron therapy usually due to noncompliance; occasional patients absorb iron poorly; other reasons include incorrect diagnosis (anemia of chronic disease, thalassemia) and ongoing GI blood loss
- Parenteral iron indicated in intolerance of oral iron, refractoriness to oral iron, GI disease (usually inflammatory bowel disease) precluding use of oral iron, and continued blood loss that cannot be corrected
- Parenteral iron used only for persistent anemia after reasonable trial of oral therapy due to risk of anaphylaxis
- Dose of IV iron (total 1.5–2 g) is calculated by estimating decrease in volume of RBC mass and supplying 1 mg of iron for each milliliter of volume below normal
  - Then add approximately 1 g for storage iron
  - Entire dose may be given as IV infusion over 4–6 h
  - Test dose of dilute solution given first; observe patient during entire infusion for anaphylaxis

THERAPEUTIC PROCEDURES

- Treat underlying cause such as source of GI bleeding

 OUTCOME

FOLLOW-UP

- Recheck complete blood cell count to observe for response to iron replacement by return of hematocrit to halfway toward normal within 3 weeks and fully to baseline after 2 months

PREVENTION

- Iron supplementation during pregnancy and lactation—included in prenatal vitamin

 EVIDENCE

PRACTICE GUIDELINES

- American Gastroenterological Association medical position statement: evaluation and management of occult and obscure gastrointestinal bleeding. Gastroenterology 2000;118:197. [PMID: 10611169]
- CDC Recommendations to prevent and control iron deficiency in the United States ftp://ftp.cdc.gov/pub/Publications/mmwr/rr/rr4703.pdf
- Goddard AF et al: Guidelines for the management of iron deficiency anaemia. British Society of Gastroenterology. Gut 2000;46(Suppl 3–4):IV1. [PMID: 10862605]

WEB SITES

- MEDLINEplus—Iron deficiency anemia http://www.nlm.nih.gov/medlineplus/ency/article/000584.htm
- National Heart, Lung, and Blood Institute http://hin.nhlbi.nih.gov/2010Objs/19Nutrition.pdf

INFORMATION FOR PATIENTS

- American Academy of Family Physicians—Anemia: when low iron is the cause http://familydoctor.org/healthfacts/009/index.html
- Mayo Clinic—Iron deficiency anemia http://www.mayoclinic.com/invoke.cfm?objectid=072ADD99-C40D-4E6A-82DAA8347C662BDD

REFERENCES

- Goddard AF et al: Guidelines for the management of iron deficiency anaemia. British Society of Gastroenterology. Gut 2000;46(Suppl 3–4):IV1. [PMID: 10862605]
- Goodnough LT et al: Erythropoietin, iron, and erythropoiesis. Blood 2000;96:823. [PMID: 10910892]

Charles A. Linker, MD

Aneurysm, Intracranial

 ## KEY FEATURES

ESSENTIALS OF DIAGNOSIS

- Subarachnoid hemorrhage or focal deficit
- Abnormal imaging studies

GENERAL CONSIDERATIONS

- Most aneurysms are located on the anterior part of the circle of Willis—particularly on the anterior or posterior communicating arteries, at the bifurcation of the middle cerebral artery, and at the bifurcation of the internal carotid artery
- Saccular aneurysms ("berry" aneurysms) occur at arterial bifurcations, are more common in adults than in children, are frequently multiple (20% of cases), and are usually asymptomatic
- May be associated with polycystic kidney disease and coarctation of the aorta

DEMOGRAPHICS

- Risk factors for aneurysm formation include smoking, hypertension, and hypercholesterolemia

 ## CLINICAL FINDINGS

SYMPTOMS AND SIGNS

- May cause a focal neurological deficit by compressing adjacent structures
- Most are asymptomatic or produce only nonspecific symptoms until they rupture, causing a subarachnoid hemorrhage
- Focal neurological signs may be absent in subarachnoid hemorrhage and secondary to a focal hematoma or ischemia in the territory of the vessel with the ruptured aneurysm
- Focal arterial spasm in the area of the ruptured aneurysm may occur after 1–14 days, causing hemiplegia or other focal deficits
- Cause of vasospasm is unknown and likely multifactorial
- Vasospasm may lead to significant cerebral ischemia or infarction and increase in intracranial pressure
- Subacute hydrocephalus due to interference with the flow of cerebrospinal fluid may occur after 2 or more weeks; leads to delayed clinical deterioration and is relieved by shunting
- "Warning leaks" of a small amount of blood from the aneurysm sometimes precede the major hemorrhage by a few hours or days, leading to headaches, nausea, and neck stiffness

DIFFERENTIAL DIAGNOSIS

- Meningitis or meningoencephalitis
- Ischemic stroke
- Space-occupying lesion, eg, brain tumor
- Subdural hemorrhage
- Epidural hemorrhage
- Migraine

 ## DIAGNOSIS

LABORATORY TESTS

- Cerebrospinal fluid is bloodstained if subarachnoid hemorrhage has occurred
- Electrocardiographic evidence of arrhythmias or myocardial ischemia may occur and probably relates to excessive sympathetic activity
- Peripheral leukocytosis and transient glycosuria also common

IMAGING STUDIES

- CT scan generally confirms that subarachnoid hemorrhage has occurred, but may be normal
- Angiography (bilateral carotid and vertebral studies) indicates the size and site of the lesion, sometimes reveals multiple aneurysms, and may show arterial spasm
- If subarachnoid hemorrhage is confirmed by lumbar puncture or CT scanning but arteriogram is normal, the examination should be repeated after 2 weeks, because vasospasm may prevent detection of an aneurysm during the initial study

Aneurysm, Intracranial

 TREATMENT

MEDICATIONS

- Phenytoin to prevent seizures
- Calcium channel-blocking agents reduce or reverse experimental vasospasm, and nimodipine reduces ischemic deficits from arterial spasm without any side effects (60 mg every 4 h for 21 days)

SURGERY

- Definitive treatment requires surgery and clipping of the aneurysm base, or endovascular treatment by interventional radiology

THERAPEUTIC PROCEDURES

- Major aim is to prevent further hemorrhages
- Conscious patients are confined to bed, advised against exertion or straining, treated symptomatically for headache and anxiety, and given laxatives or stool softeners
- Lower blood pressure gradually for severe hypertension, but not below a diastolic level of 90 mm Hg
- Medical management as outlined for subarachnoid hemorrhage is continued for about 6 weeks and followed by gradual mobilization

 OUTCOME

FOLLOW-UP

- After surgical obliteration of aneurysms, symptomatic vasospasm may be treated by intravascular volume expansion, induced hypertension, or transluminal balloon angioplasty of involved intracranial vessels

PROGNOSIS

- Unruptured aneurysms that are symptomatic merit prompt treatment, whereas small asymptomatic ones discovered incidentally are often followed arteriographically and corrected surgically only if greater than 10 mm
- Greatest risk of further hemorrhage is within a few days of initial bleed; thus, early obliteration (within 2 days) is preferred
- Approximately 20% of patients will have further bleeding within 2 weeks and 40% within 6 months

WHEN TO ADMIT

- All patients need admission and referral to specialized care

 EVIDENCE

PRACTICE GUIDELINES

- National Guideline Clearinghouse http://www.guideline.gov/summary/summary.aspx?doc_id=2437&nbr=1663&string=intracranial+aneurysm
- Bederson JB et al: Recommendations for the management of patients with unruptured intracranial aneurysms: a statement for healthcare professionals from the Stroke Council of the American Heart Association. Stroke 2000;31:2742.
- Johnston SC et al: Recommendations for the endovascular treatment of intracranial aneurysms: a statement for healthcare professionals from the Committee on Cerebrovascular Imaging of the American Heart Association Council on Cardiovascular Radiology. Stroke 2002;33:2536.

WEB SITE

- 3-D Visualization of brain aneurysms http://everest.radiology.uiowa.edu/nlm/app/aneur/brain/aneur.html

INFORMATION FOR PATIENTS

- Brain Aneurysm Foundation http://www.bafound.org/faq.htm
- National Institute of Neurological Disorders and Stroke http://www.ninds.nih.gov/health_and_medical/disorders/ceraneur_doc.htm

REFERENCES

- International Study of Unruptured Intracranial Aneurysms Investigators: Unruptured intracranial aneurysms: risks of rupture and risks of surgical intervention. N Engl J Med 1998;339:1725. [PMID: 9867550]
- Johnston SC et al: Which unruptured cerebral aneurysms should be treated? A cost-utility analysis. Neurology 1999;52:1806. [PMID: 10371527]
- Wardlaw JM et al: The detection and management of unruptured intracranial aneurysms. Brain 2000;123:205. [PMID: 10648430]

Michael J. Aminoff, DSc, MD, FRCP

Angina Pectoris

KEY FEATURES

ESSENTIALS OF DIAGNOSIS

- Precordial chest pain, usually precipitated by stress or exertion, and rapidly relieved by resting or nitrates
- Electrocardiographic, echocardiographic, or scintigraphic evidence of ischemia during pain or stress testing
- Angiographic evidence of significant obstruction of major coronary arteries

GENERAL CONSIDERATIONS

- Usually due to atherosclerotic coronary artery disease
- Less common causes: coronary vasospasm, congenital anomalies, emboli, arteritis, dissection, severe hypertrophy, severe aortic stenosis or regurgitation
- Commonly exacerbated by increased metabolic demands (eg, hyperthyroidism, anemia, tachycardias)
- Coronary vasospasm may occur spontaneously, or by exposure to cold, emotional stress, vasoconstricting medications, or cocaine

DEMOGRAPHICS

- Underdiagnosed in postmenopausal women

CLINICAL FINDINGS

SYMPTOMS AND SIGNS

- Diagnosis depends primarily on the history
- Angina most commonly arises during activity and is relieved by rest
- Patient often prefers to remain upright rather than lie down
- Rather than "pain," patient may describe tightness, squeezing, burning, pressure, choking, aching
- Discomfort behind or slightly to the left of the mid-sternum (in 80–90%)
- May radiate to the left shoulder and upper arm; the medial aspect of the arm, elbow, forearm, wrist, and fourth and fifth fingers; or to the lower jaw, nape of the neck, and interscapular area
- Diagnosis strongly supported if sublingual nitroglycerin aborts or attenuates length of attack
- Physical examination during an attack often reveals a significant elevation in systolic and diastolic blood pressure
- Hypotension is a more ominous sign
- An S_3 or arrhythmia may occur (bradycardia more common with involvement of the right coronary artery)

DIFFERENTIAL DIAGNOSIS

- Myocardial infarction, pericarditis, aortic dissection, pulmonary embolism, tension pneumothorax, esophageal rupture
- *Cardiovascular:* myocardial infarction, pericarditis, aortic stenosis, aortic dissection, pulmonary embolism, cardiomyopathy, myocarditis, mitral valve prolapse, pulmonary hypertension, hypertrophic cardiomyopathy, carditis in acute rheumatic fever, aortic insufficiency, right ventricular hypertrophy
- *Pulmonary:* pneumonia, pleuritis, bronchitis, pneumothorax, tumor, mediastinitis
- *Gastrointestinal:* esophageal rupture, gastroesophageal reflux disease, esophageal spasm, Mallory-Weiss tear, peptic ulcer disease, biliary disease, pancreatitis, functional gastrointestinal pain
- *Musculoskeletal:* cervical or thoracic disk disease or arthritis, shoulder arthritis, costochondritis or Tietze's syndrome, subacromial bursitis
- *Other:* anxiety, herpes zoster, breast disorders, chest wall tumors, thoracic outlet syndrome

DIAGNOSIS

LABORATORY TESTS

- Obtain a fasting lipid profile
- Rule out diabetes mellitus and anemia
- Exercise testing (treadmill or bicycle) is the least expensive and most useful non-invasive procedure to confirm the diagnosis of angina, determine the severity of limitation of angina, assess prognosis, and evaluate responses to therapy

IMAGING STUDIES

- Stress scintigraphy (thallium or technetium) is indicated when patients are physically unable to exercise, the ECG is difficult to interpret (eg, LBBB), results of exercise testing contradict the clinical impression, the ischemia needs to be more precisely localized, to assess the completeness of revascularization, or as a prognostic indicator
- Scintigraphy can provide more information about the presence, location, and extent of coronary artery disease than exercise testing
- Scintigraphy is performed both at rest and during stressing (exercise or pharmacological stimulation)

DIAGNOSTIC PROCEDURES

- Obtain an electrocardiogram (ECG) in all patients and, if possible, compare ECGs when pain is and is not present
- During anginal episodes, the ECG may reveal horizontal or downsloping ST-segment depression, or T wave flattening or inversion, that reverses after ischemia disappears, or, less commonly, ST-segment elevation
- The ECG is normal in about 25% of patients with angina
- Coronary arteriography is the definitive diagnostic procedure
- Arteriography has a mortality rate of ~0.1% and morbidity of ~1–5%, but it is expensive
- Left ventricular angiography performed at the same time assesses left ventricular function and mitral regurgitation

Angina Pectoris

 # TREATMENT

MEDICATIONS

- Nitroglycerin, 0.3–0.6 mg sublingual or 0.4–0.8 mg by spray, with onset of symptoms or prophylactically 5 min before activity
- Long-acting nitrates (isosorbide dinitrate or mononitrate) for symptom management: avoid use for 8–10 h each day to avoid tolerance
- Nitrates relieve symptoms but do not benefit mortality
- β-Blockers reduce myocardial oxygen demand and benefit mortality
- Calcium channel blockers are generally not indicated except to treat coronary vasospasm
- Platelet inhibitors reduce the risk of coronary thromboembolism: aspirin (81 to 325 mg QD), or clopidogrel in aspirin-intolerant patients, benefits mortality

SURGERY

- Revascularization (coronary bypass or angioplasty) is indicated when symptoms are unacceptable despite maximal medical therapy, there is greater than 50% stenosis of the left main coronary artery with or without symptoms, triple-vessel disease coexists with either an ejection fraction <50% or a prior myocardial infarction (MI), unstable angina is present, and angina or severe ischemia persists on noninvasive testing after MI
- Coronary bypass is generally reserved for left main and triple-vessel disease

THERAPEUTIC PROCEDURES

- Angioplasty or stenting performed during angiography
  - The procedure of choice for single-vessel disease in the setting of refractory symptoms
  - Superior to medical therapy for symptom relief, but not in preventing infarction or death
  - A high rate (~40%) of restenosis may be reduced with newer stents

 # OUTCOME

WHEN TO ADMIT

- Admit patients with unremitting or unstable angina (see *Angina, unstable*) for cardiology evaluation, to rule out MI, and to maximize therapy, including possible emergent revascularization

PREVENTION

- Smoking cessation
- β-Blockers, nitrates, and aspirin
- Vigorous treatment of hyperlipidemia (goal LDL <100, HDL >45)
- Tight control of diabetes mellitus
- Goal blood pressure (<140/90)
- Avoiding aggravating factors: strenuous activity, cold temperatures, strong emotion

EVIDENCE

PRACTICE GUIDELINES

- Diagnosis of chest pain. Institute for Clinical Systems Improvement, 2001 http://www.icsi.org/knowledge/detail. asp?catID=29&itemID=169
- ACC/AHA 2002 guideline update for the management of patients with unstable angina and non-ST-segment elevation myocardial infarction. A report of the American College of Cardiology/ American Heart Association Task Force on Practice Guidelines (Committee on the Management of Patients With Unstable Angina). American College of Cardiology Foundation, American Heart Association, 2002 http://www.acc.org/clinical/guidelines/ unstable/unstable.pdf

WEB SITES

- American Heart Association http://www.americanheart.org/ presenter.jhtml?identifier=4472
- National Heart, Lung, & Blood Institute http://www.nhlbi.nih.gov/ health/ public/heart/other/angina.htm
- National Institutes of Health Patient Education Institute: Angina http://www.nlm.nih.gov/medlineplus/ tutorials/angina.html

INFORMATION FOR PATIENTS

- JAMA patient page: Heart attack. JAMA 1999;282(4):402. [PMID: 10432039]
- National Women's Health Information Center—Angina http://www.4woman.gov/faq/angina. htm?src=ng
- American Academy of Family Physicians—Angina and Heart Disease http://familydoctor.org/handouts/ 233.html
- MEDLINEplus—Angina http://www.nlm.nih.gov/medlineplus/ ency/article/001107.htm

Barry Massie, MD
Thomas Amidon, MD

Angiostrongyliasis Cantonensis

 KEY FEATURES

ESSENTIALS OF DIAGNOSIS

- Meningoencephalitis
- Transient cranial neuropathies

GENERAL CONSIDERATIONS

- A nematode of rats, *Angiostrongylus cantonensis*, is the causative agent of a form of eosinophilic meningoencephalitis
- Human infection results from the ingestion of infective larvae contained in uncooked food—either the intermediate mollusk hosts (snails, slugs, planarians) or transport hosts that have ingested mollusks (crabs, shrimp, fish)
- Leafy vegetables contaminated by small mollusks or by mollusk slime may also be the source of infection, as can fingers during collection and preparation of snails for cooking
- The mollusks become infected by ingesting larvae excreted in feces of infected rodents, the definitive host
- The incubation period in humans is 1–3 weeks. Ingested larvae (0.5 × 0.025 mm) invade the central nervous system, where, during migration, they may cause extensive tissue damage; at their death, a local inflammatory reaction ensues

DEMOGRAPHICS

- The disease has been reported from Hawaii and other Pacific islands, Southeast Asia, Japan, China, Taiwan, Hong Kong, Australia, Egypt, Madagascar, Nigeria, Bombay, Cuba, Puerto Rico, Bahamas, Brazil, and New Orleans

 CLINICAL FINDINGS

SYMPTOMS AND SIGNS

- Meningoencephalitis, including severe headache, fever, neck stiffness, nausea and vomiting
- Multiple neurological findings, particularly asymmetric transient cranial neuropathies
- Worms in the spinal cord may result in sensory abnormalities in the trunk or extremities
- Worms can occur in the eye

DIFFERENTIAL DIAGNOSIS

- Tuberculous, coccidioidal, or aseptic meningitis
- Neurocysticercosis
- Neurosyphilis
- Lymphoma
- Paragonimiasis
- Echinococcosis
- Gnathostomiasis

 DIAGNOSIS

LABORATORY TESTS

- The spinal fluid characteristically shows elevated protein, eosinophilic pleocytosis, and normal glucose. Occasionally, the parasite can be recovered from spinal fluid
- Peripheral eosinophilia with a low-grade leukocytosis is common
- A serological test is available from the Centers for Disease Control and Prevention

IMAGING STUDIES

- CT and MRI may show a central nervous system lesion

Angiostrongyliasis Cantonensis

 ## TREATMENT

MEDICATIONS

- No specific treatment is available; however, albendazole (400 mg twice daily for 7 days), thiabendazole (25 mg/kg three times daily for 3 days; this dose may be toxic and need to be reduced), mebendazole (100 mg twice daily for 5 days), or ivermectin can be tried

 ## OUTCOME

COMPLICATIONS

- Parasite deaths may exacerbate central nervous system inflammatory lesions. Symptomatic treatment with analgesics or corticosteroids may be necessary

PROGNOSIS

- The illness usually persists for weeks to months, the parasite dies, and the patient then recovers spontaneously, usually without sequelae. However, fatalities have been recorded

WHEN TO ADMIT

- All patients

PREVENTION

- Prevention is by rat control; by cooking of snails, prawns, fish, and crabs for 3–5 min or by freezing them (−15°C for 24 h); and by examining vegetables for mollusks before eating
- Washing contaminated vegetables to eliminate larvae contained in mollusk mucus is not always successful

 ## EVIDENCE

PRACTICE GUIDELINES

- National Guideline Clearinghouse http://www.guideline.gov/summary/summary.aspx?doc_id=2446&nbr=1672&string=meningoencephalitis

INFORMATION FOR PATIENTS

- National Institute of Allergy and Infectious Disease http://www.niaid.nih.gov/publications/microbes.htm
- Centers for Disease Control http://www.dpd.cdc.gov/dpdx/HTML/Angiostrongyliasis.htm

REFERENCE

- Wang X et al: A clinical study of eosinophilic meningoencephalitis caused by angiostrongyliasis. Chin Med J (Engl) 2002;115:1312. [PMID: 12411101]

Anisakiasis

 KEY FEATURES

ESSENTIALS OF DIAGNOSIS

- The majority of acute cases present as gastric anisakiasis with symptoms of nausea, vomiting, and progressive epigastric pain
- Occasionally, acute infection is followed by a chronic course
- Infection is by larval invasion of the stomach or intestinal wall by anisakid nematodes

GENERAL CONSIDERATIONS

- Humans are infected when they ingest larvae in marine fish or squid eaten raw, undercooked, salted, or lightly pickled
- Larvae liberated in the stomach attach to or partially penetrate the gastric or intestinal mucosa (small bowel is more common; colon is rare), resulting in localized ulceration, edema, and eosinophilic granuloma formation; eventually, the parasite dies
- In the **acute form**, the infection may mimic surgical abdomen; in the **chronic form**, mild symptoms may persist for weeks to years
- Rarely, worms are coughed up and expectorated or penetrate the gut wall, enter the peritoneal cavity, and migrate. Most larvae, however, probably fail to cause infection and are passed in feces

DEMOGRAPHICS

- The infection occurs worldwide, but most cases have been reported in Japan and The Netherlands, with a few in the United States, Scandinavia, Chile, and other countries with high fish consumption
- Raw sashimi in Japan, pickled herring in the Netherlands, and ceviche (seviche) in Latin America are sources of infection

 CLINICAL FINDINGS

SYMPTOMS AND SIGNS

Acute gastric anisakiasis

- Within hours after larval ingestion, there is nausea, vomiting, and epigastric pain that progressively becomes more severe
- Allergic reactions, including rare anaphylaxis, can occur
- Chest pain and hematemesis are rare

Intestinal anisakiasis

- Acute disease: within 1–7 days, colicky pain appears in the lower abdomen, often localized at the ileocecal region, accompanied by diarrhea, nausea, vomiting, diffuse abdominal tenderness, and mild fever
- Chronic disease: for weeks to several years, symptoms may continue that mimic gastric ulcer, gastritis, gastric tumor, bowel obstruction, or inflammatory bowel disease

DIFFERENTIAL DIAGNOSIS

- Norwalk or rotavirus
- "Food poisoning" by toxins from *Bacillus cereus, Staphylococcus aureus, Clostridium perfringens*
- Appendicitis
- Peptic ulcer disease or gastritis
- Inflammatory bowel disease

 DIAGNOSIS

LABORATORY TESTS

- Stools may show occult blood, but eggs are not produced
- Mild leukocytosis and eosinophilia may be present
- ELISA and RAST serological tests may be helpful but are not reliable in chronic disease

IMAGING STUDIES

- In acute infections, x-rays of the stomach may show a localized edematous, ulcerated area with an irregularly thickened wall, decreased peristalsis, and rigidity. Double-contrast technique may show the threadlike larvae. Small bowel x-rays may show thickened mucosa and segments of stenosis with proximal dilation
- Ultrasound examination of gastric and intestinal lesions may also be useful
- In the chronic stage, x-rays of the stomach—but not of the bowel—may be helpful

DIAGNOSTIC PROCEDURES

- In acute infection, gastroscopy is preferred because the larvae sometimes can be seen and removed from the stomach
- In the chronic stage, stomach endoscopy—but not of the bowel—may be helpful
- The diagnosis is often made only at laparotomy with surgical removal of the parasite

TREATMENT

MEDICATIONS

- There is no drug treatment, although one report suggests efficacy for albendazole

SURGERY

- Surgical excision of the worm may be necessary in severe cases

THERAPEUTIC PROCEDURES

- Treatment of acute and chronic lesions is limited to symptomatic measures; symptoms generally improve in 1–2 weeks
- At times, larvae can be removed by fiberoptic gastroscopy or colonoscopy

 OUTCOME

COMPLICATIONS

- Chronic intestinal anisakiasis

WHEN TO REFER

- Refer for consideration of mechanical removal of the worm

PREVENTION

- Prevention is by avoidance of ingestion of raw or incompletely cooked squid or marine fish, especially salmon, rockfish, herring, and mackerel; early evisceration of fish is recommended
- Larvae within fish may with difficulty be seen as colorless, tightly coiled or spiraled worms in 3-mm whorls or as reddish or pigmented larvae lying open in muscles or viscera
- The larvae are killed by temperatures above 60°C or by freezing at −20°C for 24 h (7 days is advised by some workers)
- Smoking procedures that do not bring the temperature to 60°C, marinating in vinegar, and salt-curing are not reliable

 EVIDENCE

PRACTICE GUIDELINES

- National Guideline Clearinghouse http://www.guideline.gov/summary/ summary.aspx?doc_id=2707&nbr=1933 &string=foodborne http://www.guideline.gov/summary/ summary.aspx?doc_id=2791&nbr= 2017&string=foodborne

INFORMATION FOR PATIENTS

- National Institute of Allergy and Infectious Disease http://www.niaid.nih.gov/publications/ microbes.htm
- Centers for Disease Control http://www.dpd.cdc.gov/dpdx/HTML/ Anisakiasis.htm

REFERENCES

- Audicana MT et al: Anisakis simplex: dangerous—dead and alive? Trends Parasitol 2002;18:20. [PMID: 11850010]
- Moore DA et al: Treatment of anisakiasis with albendazole. Lancet 2002;360:54. [PMID: 12114042]

Ankylosing Spondylitis

 ## KEY FEATURES

ESSENTIALS OF DIAGNOSIS

- Chronic low backache in young adults
- Progressive limitation of back motion and chest expansion
- Transient (50%) or permanent (25%) peripheral arthritis
- Anterior uveitis in 20–25%
- Diagnostic x-ray changes in sacroiliac joints
- Accelerated erythrocyte sedimentation rate and negative serological tests for rheumatoid factor
- HLA-B27 usually positive

GENERAL CONSIDERATIONS

- Chronic inflammatory disease of the joints of the axial skeleton, manifested clinically by pain and progressive stiffening of the spine
- Hallmark of the disease is enthesopathy, inflammation of tendons and ligaments

DEMOGRAPHICS

- The age at onset is usually in the late teens or early 20s
- The incidence is greater in males than in females

 ## CLINICAL FINDINGS

SYMPTOMS AND SIGNS

- Gradual onset, with intermittent bouts of back pain that may radiate down the thighs
- Symptoms progress in a cephalad direction
- Motion becomes limited, with the normal lumbar curve flattened and the thoracic curvature exaggerated
- Chest expansion is often limited as a consequence of costovertebral joint involvement
- In advanced cases, the entire spine becomes fused, allowing no motion in any direction
- Transient acute arthritis of the peripheral joints occurs in about 50% of cases, and permanent changes—most commonly the hips, shoulders, and knees—are seen in about 25%
- Anterior uveitis in up to 25% of cases
- Constitutional symptoms similar to those of rheumatoid arthritis are absent in most patients

DIFFERENTIAL DIAGNOSIS

- Rheumatoid arthritis predominantly affects multiple, small, peripheral joints of the hands and feet and usually spares the sacroiliac joints with little effect on the rest of the spine except for C1–C2
- In ankylosing hyperostosis [diffuse idiopathic skeletal hyperostosis (DISH), Forestier's disease], there is exuberant osteophyte formation. The osteophytes are thicker and more anterior than the syndesmophytes of ankylosing spondylitis, and the sacroiliac joints are not affected
- Other causes or mimics of sacroiliitis: reactive arthritis (Reiter's syndrome), psoriatic arthritis, inflammatory bowel disease, osteitis condensans ilii, hyperparathyroidism, Whipple's disease
- DISH; in elderly
- Synovitis-acne-pustulosis-hyperostosis-osteitis (SAPHO) syndrome
- Sciatica
- Lumbar disk herniation, spinal stenosis, or facet joint degenerative arthritis

 ## DIAGNOSIS

LABORATORY TESTS

- The erythrocyte sedimentation rate is elevated in 85% of cases
- Serological tests for rheumatoid factor are characteristically negative
- HLA-B27 is found in 90% of patients with ankylosing spondylitis (occurs in 8% of the normal population)

IMAGING STUDIES

- The earliest radiographic changes of sclerosis and erosion are usually in the sacroiliac joints (early on may be detectable only by CT)
- Involvement of the apophysial joints of the spine, ossification of the annulus fibrosus, calcification of the anterior and lateral spinal ligaments, and squaring and generalized demineralization of the vertebral bodies may occur in more advanced stages
- "Bamboo spine"describes the late radiographic appearance of the spinal column

Ankylosing Spondylitis

TREATMENT

MEDICATIONS

- Postural and breathing exercises
- Nonsteroidal antiinflammatory drugs (NSAIDs)
- Sulfasalazine (1000 mg twice daily) is sometimes useful for the peripheral arthritis but has little symptomatic effect on spinal and sacroiliac joint disease
- Tumor necrosis factor inhibitors are highly effective in both the spinal and peripheral arthritis. Either etanercept (25 mg subcutaneously twice a week) or infliximab (5 mg/kg every other month) is reasonable for patients whose symptoms are refractory to physical therapy and other interventions

SURGERY

- Total hip replacement benefits those with severe hip involvement

OUTCOME

COMPLICATIONS

- Spondylitic heart disease, characterized chiefly by atrioventricular conduction defects and aortic insufficiency, occurs in 3–5% of patients with long-standing severe disease
- Pulmonary fibrosis of the upper lobes, with progression to cavitation and bronchiectasis mimicking tuberculosis, may occur

PROGNOSIS

- Almost all patients have persistent symptoms over decades
- The severity of disease varies greatly, with about 10% of patients having work disability after 10 years
- Absence of severe hip disease after the first 5 years is an excellent prognostic sign

WHEN TO REFER

- Refer to a rheumatologist when diagnosis is in doubt or when the patient fails to improve on NSAIDs
- Refer to an ophthalmologist for symptoms of uveitis
- Refer for hip replacement

PREVENTION

- Avoid cigarette smoking, since patients are already at risk for restrictive lung disease
- Use a small pillow at night to avoid accelerating flexion deformities of the spine

EVIDENCE

PRACTICE GUIDELINES

- National Guideline Clearinghouse http://www.guideline.gov/summary/summary.aspx?doc_id=3498&nbr=2724&string=ankylosing+spondylitis

INFORMATION FOR PATIENTS

- Arthritis Foundation http://www.arthritis.org/conditions/DiseaseCenter/ankylosing_spondylitis.asp
- Mayo Clinic http://www.mayoclinic.com/invoke.cfm?id=DS00483

REFERENCES

- Braun J et al: Anti-tumour necrosis factor-alpha therapy for ankylosing spondylitis: international experience. Ann Rheum Dis 2002;61(Suppl 3):iii51. [PMID: 12381511]
- Khan MA: Update on spondyloarthropathies. Ann Intern Med 2002;136:896.
- Reveille JD et al: HLA-B27 and genetic predisposing factors in spondyloarthropathies. Curr Opin Rheumatol 2001;13:265. [PMID: 11555726]

David B. Hellmann, MD, FACP
John H. Stone, MD, MPH

Anorexia Nervosa

 ## KEY FEATURES

ESSENTIALS OF DIAGNOSIS

- Disturbance of body image and intense fear of becoming fat
- Weight loss, leading to body weight 15% below expected
- In females, absence of three consecutive menstrual cycles
- Fear of weight gain and of loss of control over food intake

GENERAL CONSIDERATIONS

- Begins in the years between adolescence and young adulthood
- Occurs most commonly in females (90%), predominantly middle and upper income
- Estimated prevalence: 270 cases per 100,000 population for females and 22 per 100,000 for males
- Cause not known, probably of primary psychiatric origin
- Medical or psychiatric illnesses that can account for anorexia and weight loss must be excluded

 ## CLINICAL FINDINGS

SYMPTOMS AND SIGNS

- Loss of body fat with severe emaciation
- Dry and scaly skin
- Increased lanugo body hair
- Parotid enlargement and edema
- In severe cases, bradycardia, hypotension, and hypothermia
- Cold intolerance
- Constipation
- Amenorrhea

DIFFERENTIAL DIAGNOSIS

- Endocrine and metabolic disorders such as panhypopituitarism, Addison's disease, hyperthyroidism, and diabetes mellitus
- Gastrointestinal disorders, eg, malabsorption, pancreatic insufficiency, Crohn's disease, and celiac sprue
- Chronic infections, eg, tuberculosis
- Cancer, eg, lymphoma
- Rare central nervous system disorders such as hypothalamic tumors
- Severe malnutrition
- Depression
- Obsessive-compulsive disorder
- Body dysmorphic disorder
- Malignancy
- AIDS
- Substance abuse

 ## DIAGNOSIS

LABORATORY TESTS

- Check for anemia, leukopenia, electrolyte abnormalities, and elevations of BUN and serum creatinine
- Serum cholesterol—level often increased
- Luteinizing hormone—depressed level and impaired response to luteinizing hormone-releasing hormone

TREATMENT

MEDICATIONS

- Tricyclic antidepressants, selective serotonin reuptake inhibitors, and lithium carbonate are effective in some cases

THERAPEUTIC PROCEDURES

- Treatment goal: restoration of normal body weight and resolution of psychological difficulties
- Supportive care
- Structured behavioral therapy
- Intensive psychotherapy
- Family therapy
- Hospitalization may be necessary
- Treatment by experienced teams successful in about two-thirds of cases

 OUTCOME

COMPLICATIONS

- Poor dentition
- Pharyngitis
- Esophagitis
- Aspiration
- Gastric dilatation
- Pancreatitis
- Constipation
- Hemorrhoids
- Dehydration
- Electrolyte abnormalities

PROGNOSIS

- 50% of patients continue to experience difficulties with eating behavior and psychiatric problems
- 2% to 6% of patients die from the complications of the disorder or from suicide

EVIDENCE

PRACTICE GUIDELINES

- Position of the American Dietetic Association: Nutrition intervention in the treatment of anorexia nervosa, bulimia nervosa, and binge eating. J Am Diet Assoc 2001;101:810. [PMID: 11478482]
- American Dietetic Association http://www.eatright.org/aanorexiainter.html.

WEB SITES

- National Association of Anorexia Nervosa and Associated Disorders (ANAD) http://www.altrue.net/site/anadweb/content.php?type=1&id=6982
- National Eating Disorders Association http://www.nationaleatingdisorders.org/p.asp?WebPage_ID=286&Profile_ID=41142

INFORMATION FOR PATIENTS

- American Academy of Family Physicians—Anorexia nervosa http://familydoctor.org/handouts/063.|html
- MEDLINEplus—Anorexia nervosa http://www.nlm.nih.gov/medlineplus/ency/article/000362.htm

REFERENCES

- Brown JM et al: Medical complications occurring in adolescents with anorexia nervosa. West J Med 2000;172:189. [PMID: 10734811]
- Hetherington MM: Eating disorders: diagnosis, etiology and prevention. Nutrition 2000;16:547. [PMID: 10906551]
- Kaplan AS: Psychological treatments for anorexia nervosa: a review of published studies and promising new directions.Can J Psychiatry 2002; 47:235. [PMID: 11987474]
- Steinhausen HC: The outcome of anorexia nervosa in the 20th century. Am J Psychiatry 2002;159:1284.
- Zhu AJ et al: Pharmacologic treatment of eating disorders. Can J Psychiatry 2002; 47:227. [PMID: 11987473]

Robert B. Baron, MD, MS

Anthrax

KEY FEATURES

ESSENTIALS OF DIAGNOSIS

- Appropriate epidemiological setting, eg, exposure to animals or animal hides, or potential exposure resulting from an act of bioterrorism
- A cutaneous black eschar, typically painless and on exposed areas of the skin, with marked surrounding edema and vesicles
- Nonspecific flu-like symptoms that rapidly progress to extreme dyspnea and shock in association with mediastinal widening and pleural effusions on chest x-ray

GENERAL CONSIDERATIONS

- Naturally occurring anthrax is a disease of sheep, cattle, horses, goats, and swine
- *Bacillus anthracis* is a gram-positive spore-forming aerobic rod. Spores—not vegetative bacteria—are the infectious form of the organism
- Transmitted to humans from contaminated animals, animal products, or soil by inoculation of broken skin or mucous membranes; by inhalation of aerosolized spores; or, rarely, by ingestion resulting in cutaneous, inhalational, or gastrointestinal forms of anthrax, respectively
- Spores entering the lungs are ingested by macrophages and carried via lymphatics to regional lymph nodes, where they germinate. The bacteria rapidly multiply within the lymphatics, causing a hemorrhagic lymphadenitis. Invasion of the bloodstream leads to overwhelming sepsis, killing the host

CLINICAL FINDINGS

SYMPTOMS AND SIGNS

Cutaneous anthrax

- Onset occurs within 2 weeks after exposure to spores
- The initial lesion is an erythematous papule, often on an exposed area of skin, that vesiculates and then ulcerates and undergoes necrosis, ultimately progressing to a purple to black eschar
- The surrounding area is edematous and vesicular but not purulent
- The infection is usually self-limited

Inhalational anthrax

- Nonspecific viral-like symptoms
- Anterior chest pain is an early symptom of mediastinitis
- Within hours to a few days, the patient progresses to the fulminant stage of infection in which signs and symptoms of overwhelming sepsis predominate
- Dissemination may occur, resulting in meningitis

Gastrointestinal anthrax

- Symptoms begin 2–5 days after ingestion of meat contaminated with anthrax spores
- Fever, diffuse abdominal pain, rebound abdominal tenderness, vomiting, constipation, and diarrhea occur
- Because the primary lesion is ulcerative, emesis is blood-tinged or coffee-grounds and stool may be blood-tinged or melenic
- Bowel perforation can occur

DIFFERENTIAL DIAGNOSIS

- *Cutaneous anthrax*
  - Ecthyma gangrenosum (neutropenic, *Pseudomonas*)
  - Tularemia
  - Plague
  - Brown recluse spider bite
  - Aspergillosis or mucormycosis
  - Antiphospholipid antibody syndrome
  - Warfarin necrosis
  - Rat-bite fever
  - Rickettsialpox
  - Orf (parapoxvirus infection)
  - Cutaneous mycobacterial infection
  - Cutaneous leishmaniasis
- *Inhalational anthrax*
  - Influenza

- Bacterial mediastinitis
- Fibrous mediastinitis due to histoplasmosis, coccidioidomycosis, atypical or viral pneumonia, silicosis, sarcoidosis
- Other causes of mediastinal widening, eg, ruptured aortic aneurysm, lymphoma, superior vena cava syndrome
- Tuberculosis
- *Gastrointestinal anthrax*
  - Bowel obstruction
  - Perforated viscus
  - Peritonitis
  - Gastroenteritis
  - Peptic ulcer disease

DIAGNOSIS

LABORATORY TESTS

- Pleural fluid in inhalational anthrax is hemorrhagic with few white blood cells; cerebrospinal fluid from meningitis cases is hemorrhagic
- Gram stain of fluid from a cutaneous lesion, pleural fluid, cerebrospinal fluid, unspun blood, or blood culture may show the characteristic boxcar-shaped encapsulated rods in chains
- The diagnosis is established by isolation of the organism from culture of the skin lesion (or fluid expressed from it), blood, or pleural fluid—or cerebrospinal fluid in cases of meningitis
- In the absence of prior antimicrobial therapy, cultures are invariably positive

IMAGING STUDIES

- The chest x-ray is the most sensitive test for inhalational disease, being abnormal initially in every case of bioterrorism-associated disease
- Mediastinal widening due to hemorrhagic lymphadenitis in 70% of the bioterrorism-related cases
- Pleural effusions were present initially or occurred over the course of illness in all cases, and approximately three-fourths had pulmonary infiltrates or signs of consolidation

TREATMENT

MEDICATIONS

- *B anthracis* may express β-lactamases that confer resistance to cephalosporins and penicillins. For this reason, penicillin or amoxicillin is no longer recommended for use as a single agent in treatment of disseminated disease
- Ciprofloxacin is considered the drug of choice (Table 130, page 1313); other fluoroquinolones are probably as effective
- Doxycycline is an alternative first-line agent

 OUTCOME

PROGNOSIS

- The prognosis in cutaneous infection is excellent. Death is unlikely if the infection has remained localized, and lesions heal without complications in most cases
- The reported mortality rate for gastrointestinal and inhalational infections is up to 85%

WHEN TO REFER

- Any suspected case of anthrax should be immediately reported to the Centers for Disease Control and Prevention so that a complete investigation can be conducted

PREVENTION

- Ciprofloxacin is considered the drug of choice (Table 130, page 1313) for treatment and for prophylaxis following exposure to anthrax spores
- There is an FDA-approved vaccine for persons at high risk of exposure to anthrax spores

 EVIDENCE

PRACTICE GUIDELINES

- National Guideline Clearinghouse http://www.guideline.gov/summary/summary.aspx?doc_id=3220&nbr=2446&string=anthrax http://www.guideline.gov/summary/summary.aspx?doc_id=2652&nbr=1878&string=anthrax

WEB SITES

- CDC web site: Anthrax and other bioterrorism-related issues http://www.bt.cdc.gov/
- Karolinska Institute—Directory of bacterial infections and mycoses http://www.mic.ki.se/Diseases/c1.html

INFORMATION FOR PATIENTS

- JAMA patient page: Anthrax. JAMA 2001;286:2626.
- Centers for Disease Control http://www.cdc.gov/ncidod/dbmd/diseaseinfo/anthrax_g.htm

REFERENCES

- Borio L et al: Death due to bioterrorism-related inhalational anthrax: report of 2 patients. JAMA 2001;286:2554. [PMID: 11722269]
- Dixon TC et al: Anthrax. N Engl J Med 1999;341:815. [PMID: 10477781]
- Inglesby TV et al: Anthrax as a biological weapon: medical and public health management. Working Group on Civilian Biodefense. JAMA 1999;281:1735. [PMID: 10328075]
- Jernigan JA et al: Bioterrorism-related inhalational anthrax: the first 10 cases reported in the United States. Emerg Infect Dis 2001;7:933. [PMID: 11747719]
- Kuehnert MJ et al: Clinical features that discriminate inhalational anthrax from other acute respiratory illnesses. Clin Infect Dis 2003;36:328. [PMID: 12539075]
- Roche KJ et al: Images in clinical medicine. Cutaneous anthrax infection. N Engl J Med 2001;345:1611. [PMID: 11704684]

Henry F. Chambers, MD

Anticoagulant Overdose

 ## KEY FEATURES

ESSENTIALS OF DIAGNOSIS

- Prolonged prothrombin time (PT)

GENERAL CONSIDERATIONS

- Warfarin and related compounds (including ingredients of many commercial rodenticides) inhibit the clotting mechanism by blocking hepatic synthesis of vitamin K–dependent clotting factors
- Half-life of the "super warfarins" used as rodenticides can be weeks or longer

 ## CLINICAL FINDINGS

SYMPTOMS AND SIGNS

- Initially asymptomatic, as evidence of anticoagulant effect usually delayed for 12–24 h
- Hemoptysis
- Gross hematuria
- Bloody stools
- Hemorrhages into organs
- Widespread bruising
- Bleeding into joint spaces

DIFFERENTIAL DIAGNOSIS

- Liver disease
- Hemophilia
- Aspirin overdose

 ## DIAGNOSIS

LABORATORY TESTS

- The PT is increased within 12–24 h (peak 36–48 h) after a single overdose
- After ingestion of brodifacoum and indanedione rodenticides (so-called super-warfarins), inhibition of clotting factor synthesis may persist for several weeks or even months after a single dose

DIAGNOSTIC PROCEDURES

- Obtain daily PT/INR for 2 days

Anticoagulant Overdose

 ## TREATMENT

 ## OUTCOME

 ## EVIDENCE

MEDICATIONS

Emergency and supportive measures

- Discontinue the drug at the first sign of gross bleeding, and determine the PT
- If the patient has ingested an acute overdose, administer activated charcoal

Activated charcoal

- Administer activated charcoal, 60–100 g orally or via gastric tube, mixed in aqueous slurry

Specific treatment

- Do not treat prophylactically—wait for the evidence of anticoagulation (elevated PT)
- If the PT is elevated, give phytonadione (vitamin K_1), 10–25 mg orally, and additional doses as needed to restore the PT to normal
- Give fresh-frozen plasma as needed to rapidly correct the coagulation factor deficit if there is serious bleeding
- If the patient is chronically anticoagulated and has strong medical indications for being maintained in that status (eg, prosthetic heart valve), give much smaller doses of vitamin K (1 mg) and fresh-frozen plasma (or both) to titrate to the desired PT
- If the patient has ingested brodifacoum or a related superwarfarin, prolonged observation (over weeks) and repeated administration of large doses of vitamin K may be required

FOLLOW-UP

- Serial evaluation of PT

COMPLICATIONS

- Bleeding

WHEN TO ADMIT

- Admit all patients with a history of superwarfarin ingestion for 2-day observation of the PT
- Admit all patients with active bleeding

PROGNOSIS

- Very good if no active bleeding and if close outpatient follow-up is maintained (for several weeks or longer after brodifacoum overdose)

PRACTICE GUIDELINES

- National Guideline Clearinghouse http://www.guideline.gov/summary/ summary.aspx?doc_id=2907&nbr=2133 &string=anticoagulant+overdose

WEB SITES

- Agency for Toxic Substances and Disease Registry (ATSDR) http://www.cdc.gov/niosh/nasd/srd/ og56400.html
- Carbon monoxide poisonings http://www.cdc.gov/mmwr/preview/ mmwrhtml/00039315.htm
- Pesticide Poisonings: National Pesticide Information Center http://ace.orst.edu/ info/npic/rmpp.htm
- Toxicology—eMedicine http://www.emedicine.com/cgi-bin/ foxweb.exe/showsection@d:/em/ ga?book=emerg&sct=TOXICOLOGY

INFORMATION FOR PATIENTS

- National Institutes of Health http://www.nlm.nih.gov/medlineplus/ druginfo/uspdi/202050.html

REFERENCES

- Chua JD et al: Superwarfarin poisoning. Arch Intern Med 1998;158:1929. [PMID: 9759690]
- Ingels M et al: A prospective study of acute, unintentional, pediatric superwarfarin ingestions managed without decontamination. Ann Emerg Med 2002;40:73. [PMID: 12085076]

Kent R. Olson, MD

Anticonvulsant Overdose

 KEY FEATURES

ESSENTIALS OF DIAGNOSIS

- Ataxia, slurred speech, somnolence
- Valproic acid can cause hypernatremia, metabolic acidosis, hyperammonemia

GENERAL CONSIDERATIONS

- Rapid intravenous injection of phenytoin can cause acute myocardial depression and cardiac arrest owing to the solvent propylene glycol. (Does not occur with fosphenytoin injection)
- Phenytoin intoxication can occur with only slightly increased doses because of the small toxic-therapeutic window

 CLINICAL FINDINGS

SYMPTOMS AND SIGNS

Phenytoin

- The overdose syndrome is usually mild even with high serum levels
- The most common manifestations are ataxia, nystagmus, and drowsiness
- Choreoathetoid movements have been described

Carbamazepine

- Drowsiness, stupor, and, with high levels, coma and seizures
- Dilated pupils and tachycardia are common

Valproic acid

- Encephalopathy, which may be associated with hyperammonemia, metabolic acidosis, cerebral edema
- Valproic acid intoxication produces a unique syndrome consisting of hypernatremia (from the sodium component of the salt), metabolic acidosis, hypocalcemia, elevated serum ammonia, and mild liver aminotransferase elevation Hypoglycemia may occur as a result of hepatic metabolic dysfunction
- Coma with small pupils, which can mimic opioid poisoning

DIFFERENTIAL DIAGNOSIS

- Opioid intoxication

 DIAGNOSIS

LABORATORY TESTS

- Carbamazepine toxicity may be seen with serum levels greater than 20 mg/L, though severe poisoning is usually associated with concentrations greater than 30–40 mg/L. Because of erratic and slow absorption, intoxication may progress over several hours to days
- Phenytoin levels >20 mg/L associated with ataxia, nystagmus, drowsiness
- Valproic acid: obtain frequent repeated levels to rule out delayed absorption from sustained-release formulations (eg, Depakote, Depakote ER)

TREATMENT

MEDICATIONS

Repeat-dose charcoal

- Repeated doses of activated charcoal, 20–30 g every 3–4 h, are indicated for massiove ingestions of valproic acid or carbamazepine
- Sorbitol or other cathartics should *not* be used with each dose, or resulting large stool volumes may lead to dehydration or hypernatremia

Whole bowel irrigation

- For large ingestions of carbamazepine or valproic acid—especially of sustained-release formulations—consider whole bowel irrigation
- Administer the balanced polyethylene glycol-electrolyte solution (CoLyte, GoLYTELY) into the stomach via gastric tube at a rate of 1–2 L/h until the rectal effluent is clear

Specific treatment

- There are no antidotes
- Naloxone has been reported to reverse valproic acid overdose in a few anecdotal case reports.

THERAPEUTIC PROCEDURES

- Consider hemodialysis for massive intoxication of valproic acid with levels >1000 mg/L
- Consider hemoperfusion for massive intoxication (eg, carbamazepine levels >100 mg/L or valproic acid levels >1000 mg/L)

 OUTCOME

WHEN TO ADMIT

- For phenytoin-induced ataxia if adequate home care is not available
- After overdose of any drug with symptoms

 EVIDENCE

PRACTICE GUIDELINES

- National Guideline Clearinghouse http://www.guideline.gov/summary/summary.aspx?doc_id=3169&nbr=2395&string=anticonvulsant

WEB SITES

- Agency for Toxic Substances and Disease Registry (ATSDR) http://www.cdc.gov/niosh/nasd/srd/og56400.html
- Toxicology—eMedicine http://www.emedicine.com/cgi-bin/foxweb.exe/showsection@d:/em/ga?book=emerg&sct=TOXICOLOGY

INFORMATION FOR PATIENTS

- Epilepsy Foundation http://www.epilepsyfoundation.org/answerplace/Life/adults/women/weimeds.cfm
- National Institutes of Health http://www.nlm.nih.gov/medlineplus/druginfo/uspdi/202052.html http://www.nlm.nih.gov/medlineplus/druginfo/uspdi/202053.html http://www.nlm.nih.gov/medlineplus/druginfo/uspdi/202051.html

REFERENCES

- Cameron RJ et al: Efficacy of charcoal hemoperfusion in massive carbamazepine poisoning. J Toxicol Clin Toxicol 2002;40:507. [PMID: 12217004]
- Chua HC et al: Elimination of phenytoin in toxic overdose. Clin Neurol Neurosurg 2000;102:6. [PMID: 10717394]
- Franssen EJ et al: Valproic acid toxicokinetics: serial hemodialysis and hemoperfusion. Ther Drug Monit 1999;21:289. [PMID: 10365638]

Kent R. Olson, MD

Anxiety & Dissociative Disorders

 KEY FEATURES

ESSENTIALS OF DIAGNOSIS

- Overt anxiety or an overt manifestation of a defense mechanism (such as a phobia), or both
- Not limited to an adjustment disorder
- Somatic symptoms referable to the autonomic nervous system or to a specific organ system (eg, dyspnea, palpitations, paresthesias)
- Not a result of physical disorders, psychiatric conditions (eg, schizophrenia), or drug abuse

GENERAL CONSIDERATIONS

- Group of disorders
  - Generalized anxiety disorder (GAD 300.02)
  - Panic disorder (300.01)
  - Obsessive-compulsive disorder (OCD 300.3)
  - Phobic disorder (300.2)
  - Dissociative disorder
- In *GAD*, symptoms are brought on by everyday activities and are present on most days for at least 6 months
- In *panic disorder*, symptoms occur in recurrent, short-lived episodes with unpredictable triggers. Somatic symptoms are often marked
- In *OCD*, patients experience recurrent intrusive thoughts or obsessions. They engage in compulsive actions or rituals to maintain control
- In *phobic disorder*, symptoms occur predictably, following exposure to certain objects or situations
- In *dissociative disorder*, the reaction is precipitated by emotional crisis. The symptom produces anxiety reduction and a temporary solution of the crisis. Mechanisms include repression and isolation, as well as particularly limited concentration, as seen in hypnotic states

DEMOGRAPHICS

- Incidence: *OCD*: 2–5%
- Prevalence: *Panic disorder*: 3–5%, 25% with coincident *OCD*
- Age: *Panic disorder*: onset <25; *OCD*: onset 20–35
- Risk factors: *OCD*: divorce or separation, unemployment

 CLINICAL FINDINGS

SYMPTOMS AND SIGNS

- Anxiety or fear
- Apprehension or worry
- Difficulty concentrating
- Insomnia and fatigue
- Irritability
- Feelings of impending doom
- Recurrent thoughts or fears
- Repetitive actions and rituals
- Avoidant behaviors
- Sympathomimetic symptoms: tachycardia, hyperventilation, tremor, sweating
- Somatic symptoms: headache, paresthesias, dizziness, nausea, bloating, chest pain, palpitations
- Fugue (the sudden, unexpected travel away from one's home with inability to recall one's past), amnesia, somnambulism, dissociative identity disorder (multiple personality disorder), and depersonalization are all dissociative states

DIFFERENTIAL DIAGNOSIS

- Hyperthyroidism
- Pheochromocytoma
- Sympathomimetic drug use
- Myocardial infarction
- Hypoglycemia
- Adjustment disorders
- Dissociative symptoms are similar to symptoms of temporal lobe dysfunction

 DIAGNOSIS

LABORATORY TESTS TO CONSIDER

- Thyroid-stimulating hormone
- Complete blood cell count
- Toxicology screen (if suspected)
- Glucose (as appropriate to rule out medical disorders)

IMAGING STUDIES

- Chest x-ray may be indicated
- Head CT may be useful in dissociative symptoms to rule out temporal lobe dysfunction

DIAGNOSTIC PROCEDURES

- EKG
- EEG may be useful in dissociative symptoms to rule out temporal lobe dysfunction

Anxiety & Dissociative Disorders

 TREATMENT

MEDICATIONS

- See Table 101 (page 1285)
- *GAD*: benzodiazepines initially [diazepam 5–10 mg PO TID (or equivalent)], buspirone (start 15–60 mg divided TID), venlafaxine (start 37.5–75 mg QD), possibly selective serotonin reuptake inhibitors (SSRIs)
- *Panic disorder*: lorazepam (0.5–2 mg) or alprazolam (0.5–1 mg) SL as acute treatment, SSRIs (eg, sertraline 25 mg QD, titrate upward after 1 week) for ongoing treatment
- *OCD*: SSRIs, usually in doses higher than for depression (eg, fluoxetine, up to 60–80 mg QD); clomipramine
- *Phobic disorder*: SSRIs (paroxetine, sertraline, fluvoxamine); monoamine oxidase inhibitors; gabapentin (900–3600 mg divided TID) for global social phobia. Propranolol 20–40 mg 1 h prior to exposure for specific phobias (eg, performance)

SURGERY

- Stereotactic modified cingulotomy of limited use in severe, unremitting OCD

THERAPEUTIC PROCEDURES

Behavioral/cognitive

- Frequently used in conjunction with medical therapies
- Relaxation techniques (particularly effective for physiological symptoms in *Panic disorder*)
- Desensitization, via graded exposure to a phobic object
- Emotive imagery (imagining anxiety-provoking situation while employing relaxation techniques)
- Cognitive therapy

Social

- Support groups
- Family counseling
- School, vocational counseling

 OUTCOME

FOLLOW-UP

- Every 1–2 weeks until stabilized, then as agreed upon with patient

COMPLICATIONS

- Alcohol and substance abuse

WHEN TO REFER

- Refer to a psychiatrist if the diagnosis is in question, to receive recommendations on therapy or if first-line therapy has failed, or in patients who present with management problems

PROGNOSIS

- Usually long-standing and difficult to treat
- All disorders relieved to varying degrees by medication and behavioral techniques (eg, 60% response rate to SSRIs for *OCD*)

 EVIDENCE

PRACTICE GUIDELINES

- National Guideline Clearinghouse http://www.guideline.gov/summary/summary.aspx?doc_id=3350&nbr=2576&string=alcoholism
- Bandelow B et al: World Federation of Societies of Biological Psychiatry (WFSBP) guidelines for the pharmacological treatment of anxiety, obsessive-compulsive and posttraumatic stress disorders. World J Biol Psychiatry 2002;3:171. [PMID: 12516310]

WEB SITES

- American Psychiatric Association http://www.psych.org/
- Internet Mental Health http://www.mentalhealth.com/t30.html

INFORMATION FOR PATIENTS

- JAMA patient page: Obsessive-compulsive disorder. JAMA 1998;280:1806. [PMID: 9842960]
- National Institutes of Health http://www.nimh.nih.gov/anxiety/anxiety.cfm

REFERENCES

- McDonough M, Kennedy N: Pharmacological management of obsessive-compulsive disorders: a review for clinicians. Harvard Rev Psychiatry 2002;10:127.
- Pohl RB et al: Sertraline in the treatment of panic disorder: a double-blind multicenter trial. Am J Psychiatry 1998;155:1189.
- Stein DJ et al: Efficacy of paroxetine for relapse prevention in social anxiety disorder: a 24-week study. Arch Gen Psychiatry 2002;59:1111.

Stuart J. Eisendrath, MD
Jonathan E. Lichtmacher, MD

Aortic Dissection

 KEY FEATURES

ESSENTIALS OF DIAGNOSIS

- A history of hypertension or Marfan's syndrome is often present
- Sudden severe chest pain with radiation to the back, occasionally migrating to the abdomen and hips or groin
- Patient appears to be in shock, but blood pressure is normal or elevated; pulse discrepancy in many patients
- Acute aortic regurgitation

GENERAL CONSIDERATIONS

- Aortic dissection caused by an intimal tear allows creation of a false lumen between the media and adventitia
- Over 95% of intimal tears occur either in the ascending aorta just distal to the aortic valve (Stanford type A) or just distal to the left subclavian artery (Stanford type B)
- A false lumen can rupture into the left pleural space, retroperitoneum, pericardium, or abdominal cavity, but more commonly propagates distally to involve aortic branch vessels, producing acute ischemia of the spinal cord (3%), viscera (9%), kidney (12%), or lower extremity (9%)
- Antegrade extension can produce acute aortic regurgitation, myocardial infarction, and intrapericardial rupture with tamponade
- Risk factors include hypertension (80% of patients), Marfan's syndrome, pregnancy, bicuspid aortic valve, and coarctation of the aorta

 CLINICAL FINDINGS

SYMPTOMS AND SIGNS

- Sudden excruciating ("ripping") pain in the chest or upper back, radiating into the abdomen, neck, or groin in 85%
- Hypertension in most patients
- Syncope, hemiplegia, lower extremity paralysis, or abdominal pain
- Physical examination: diminished or unequal peripheral pulses and blood pressures
- Diastolic murmur of aortic regurgitation

DIFFERENTIAL DIAGNOSIS

- Acute myocardial infarction
- Pulmonary embolus
- Esophageal rupture
- Strangulated paraesophageal hernia
- Mesenteric ischemia
- Symptomatic aortic aneurysm
- Pneumothorax/pneumonia

 DIAGNOSIS

LABORATORY TESTS

- Electrocardiogram may be normal but often reveals left ventricular hypertrophy
- Acute ischemia suggests coronary artery involvement
- Because dissections preferentially extend into the right coronary ostium, inferior wall ischemic changes predominate

IMAGING STUDIES

- Chest x-ray: abnormal aortic contour or a widened superior mediastinum, pleural or pericardial effusion
- Dynamic CT scanning, angiography, MRI, and transesophageal echocardiography (TEE) are all useful in diagnosis
- TEE has high sensitivity (98%) and specificity (99%)
- CT or MRI useful for serial follow-up

TREATMENT

MEDICATIONS

Acute management

- Vasodilator: nitroprusside (0.3–10 µg/kg/min) or fenoldopam (0.1–1.6 µg/kg/min) by continuous IV infusion to maintain a systolic blood pressure of 100–120 mm Hg (see Table 50, page 1248)
- β-Blocker: esmolol (50–300 µg/kg/min IV), metoprolol (5–10 mg IV Q 15 min), or labetalol (20–80 mg IV Q 10 min or 1–2 mg/min) to decrease heart rate (see Table 50, page 1248)

Chronic management

- β-Blocker (eg, metoprolol 25–100 mg PO BID, atenolol 50–100 mg PO QD), often in combination with
  – Clonidine, 0.1–0.3 mg PO BID (0.1–0.3 mg TTS patch topically Q 24 h), or
  – Hydralazine, 10–50 mg PO QID, or
  – Amlodipine, 2.5–10 mg PO QD, or
  – Enalapril, 2.5–20 mg PO QD

SURGERY

- Type A dissection: warrants emergent surgical repair
- Replace ascending aorta and, if necessary, the aortic valve and arch with reimplantation of the coronary and brachiocephalic vessels
- Type B dissection: manage aggressively with medications initially
- Indications for surgical treatment of type B dissections: aortic rupture; severe intractable pain; mesenteric, renal, or limb ischemia; and progression of the dissection
- Surgery involves obliteration of the false lumen and secondary arterial bypass if this fails to restore blood flow
- Obliteration of the false lumen involves resection of the entry point of the dissection and prosthetic tube graft interposition, open or endovascular fenestration of the dissection flap, or stent graft deployment to cover the entry point
- Chronic type B dissections: repair if patients are symptomatic or aneurysm diameter is >6 cm

THERAPEUTIC PROCEDURES

- Bedrest
- Opioids for pain relief
- Arterial line for continuous blood pressure monitoring
- Reduce aortic pressure and pulsatile flow (dP/dt) by lowering systemic vascular resistance and cardiac output (heart rate)

 OUTCOME

FOLLOW-UP

- Acute: if nitroprusside is administered for ≥48 h, check serum thiocyanate level and stop the infusion if level is >10 mg/dL to avoid toxicity
- Chronic: follow unoperated patients with annual CT scan or MRI

PROGNOSIS

- Mortality in untreated type A dissection is 50% at 48 h and 90% at 1 month
- Mortality in untreated type B dissection is 10–20%
- Operative mortality of type A dissection approaches 20%
- Operative mortality of type B dissection is twice that of type A dissection
- 5-year survival is 70–80% for repaired type A dissections and 50–70% for repaired type B dissections

WHEN TO REFER

- Any acute aortic dissection
- Chronic dissection with diameter >4 cm or evidence of progression

WHEN TO ADMIT

- Any acute aortic dissection
- Any symptomatic dissection

PREVENTION

- Control of hypertension
- Control of hyperlipidemia

EVIDENCE

PRACTICE GUIDELINES

- ACR Appropriateness Criteria for acute chest pain—suspected aortic dissection. American College of Radiology, 1999 http://www.acr.org/dyna/?id=appcrit& pdf=0001-6_acute_chest_pain_susp_ aortic_diss-ac
- Erbel R et al: Diagnosis and management of aortic dissection. Eur Heart J 2001;22:1642. [PMID: 11511117]

WEB SITE

- American Heart Association http://www.americanheart.org/ presenter.jhtml?identifier=8458

INFORMATION FOR PATIENTS

- MEDLINEplus—Aortic dissection http://www.nlm.nih.gov/medlineplus/ ency/article/000181.htm

REFERENCES

- Beregi J-P et al: Endovascular treatment for dissection of the descending aorta. Lancet 2000;356:482. [PMID: 10981895]
- Buffolo E et al: Revolutionary treatment of aneurysms and dissections of descending aorta: the endovascular approach. Ann Thorac Surg 2002;74:S1815. [PMID: 12440672]
- Genoni M et al: Chronic β–blocker therapy improves outcome and reduces treatment costs in chronic type B aortic dissection. Eur J Cardiothorac Surg 2001;19:606. [PMID: 11343940]
- Hagan P et al: The international registry of acute aortic dissection (IRAD): new insights into an old disease. JAMA 2000;283:897. [PMID: 10685714]

Louis M. Messina, MD
Laura K. Pak, MD
Lawrence M. Tierney, Jr., MD

Appendicitis

 KEY FEATURES

ESSENTIALS OF DIAGNOSIS

- Early: periumbilical pain; later: right lower quadrant pain and tenderness
- Anorexia, nausea and vomiting, obstipation
- Tenderness or localized rigidity at McBurney's point
- Low-grade fever and leukocytosis

GENERAL CONSIDERATIONS

- The most common abdominal surgical emergency, affecting ~ 10% of the population
- Occurs most commonly between the ages of 10 and 30 years
- Caused by obstruction of the appendix by a fecalith, inflammation, foreign body, or neoplasm
- If untreated, gangrene and perforation develop within 36 h

 CLINICAL FINDINGS

SYMPTOMS AND SIGNS

- Vague, often colicky, periumbilical or epigastric pain
- Within 12 h, pain shifts to right lower quadrant, steady ache worsened by walking or coughing
- Nausea and one or two episodes of vomiting in almost all
- Constipation
- Low-grade fever (<38°C)
- Localized tenderness with guarding in the right lower quadrant
- Rebound tenderness
- Psoas sign (pain on passive extension of the right hip)
- Obturator sign (pain with passive flexion and internal rotation of the right hip)
- "Atypical" presentations include
  - Pain less intense and poorly localized; tenderness minimal in the right flank
  - Pain in the lower abdomen, often on the left; urge to urinate or defecate
  - Abdominal tenderness absent, but tenderness on pelvic or rectal examination

DIFFERENTIAL DIAGNOSIS

- Gastroenteritis or colitis
- Gynecologic: pelvic inflammatory disease, tuboovarian abscess, ovarian torsion, ruptured ectopic pregnancy or ovarian cyst, mittelschmerz, endometriosis
- Urologic: testicular torsion, acute epididymitis
- Urinary calculus
- Pyelonephritis
- Diverticulitis
- Meckel's diverticulitis
- Carcinoid of the appendix
- Perforated colon cancer
- Crohn's ileitis
- Perforated peptic ulcer
- Cholecystitis
- Mesenteric adenitis
- Typhlitis (neutropenic colitis)
- Parasites, eg, ascariasis

 DIAGNOSIS

LABORATORY TESTS

- Moderate leukocytosis (10,000–20,000/μL) with neutrophilia
- Microscopic hematuria and pyuria in 25%

IMAGING STUDIES

- No imaging necessary in typical appendicitis; imaging may be useful in patients in whom the diagnosis is uncertain
- Abdominal or transvaginal ultrasound: diagnostic accuracy of >85%, useful in the exclusion of adnexal disease in younger women
- Abdominal CT: useful in suspected appendiceal perforation to diagnose a peri-appendiceal abscess

Aortic Regurgitation p. 1058. Aortic Stenosis p. 1059. Aphthous Ulcer p. 1060.

Appendicitis

 TREATMENT

MEDICATIONS

- Systemic antibiotics reduce the incidence of postoperative wound infections

SURGERY

- Surgical appendectomy by laparotomy or by laparoscopy in patients with uncomplicated appendicitis
- Emergency appendectomy in patients with perforated appendicitis with generalized peritonitis

THERAPEUTIC PROCEDURES

- Percutaneous CT-guided drainage of periappendiceal abscess, intravenous fluids and antibiotics, and interval appendectomy after 6 weeks in stable patients with perforated appendicitis

 OUTCOME

COMPLICATIONS

- Perforation in 20%
- Periappendiceal abscess
- Suppurative peritonitis
- Septic thrombophlebitis (pylephlebitis) of the portal venous system

PROGNOSIS

- Mortality of uncomplicated appendicitis is extremely low
- Mortality of perforated appendicitis is 0.2%, but 15% in the elderly

 EVIDENCE

PRACTICE GUIDELINES

- American College of Emergency Physicians (ACEP). Clinical policy: critical issues for the initial evaluation and management of patients presenting with a chief complaint of nontraumatic acute abdominal pain, 2000 http://www.acep.org/library/pdf/cp402130.pdf
- Eypasch E et al: Laparoscopic versus open appendectomy: between evidence and common sense. Dig Surg 2002; 19:518. [PMID: 12499748]

WEB SITES

- American Academy of Family Physicians http://familydoctor.org/
- National Institute of Diabetes and Digestive and Kidney Diseases (NIDDK) NIH http://www.niddk.nih.gov

INFORMATION FOR PATIENTS

- JAMA patient page: Detecting appendicitis in your children http://www.ama-assn.org/insight/spec_con/patient/pat068.pdf
- Mayo Clinic http://www.mayoclinic.com/invoke.cfm?id=DS00274
- NDDIC–NIH http://digestive.niddk.nih.gov/ddiseases/pubs/appendicitis/index.htm

REFERENCES

- Jones PF: Suspected acute appendicitis: trends in management over 30 years. Br J Surg 2001;88:1570. [PMID: 11736966]
- Kraemer M et al: Acute appendicitis in late adulthood: incidence, presentation, and outcome. Results of a prospective multicenter acute abdominal pain study and review of the literature. Langenbecks Arch Surg 2000;385:470. [PMID: 11131250]

Kenneth R. McQuaid, MD

Arteriovenous Malformations, Intracranial

 ## KEY FEATURES

ESSENTIALS OF DIAGNOSIS

- Sudden onsest of subarachnoid or intracerebral hemorrage
- Distinctive neurological signs reflect the region of the brain involved
- Signs of meningeal irritation in patients presenting with subarachnoid hemorrhage
- Seizures or focal deficits may occur

GENERAL CONSIDERATIONS

- See Table 92 (page 1276)
- Congenital vascular malformations that result from a localized maldevelopment of part of the primitive vascular plexus
- Vary in size, ranging from massive lesions fed by multiple vessels to small lesions that are hard to identify at arteriography, surgery, or autopsy
- Approximately 10% of cases are associated with arterial aneurysm, while 1–2% of patients with aneurysms have arteriovenous malformations
- Symptoms may relate to hemorrhage or to cerebral ischemia due to diversion of blood by the anomalous arteriovenous shunt or venous stagnation

Supratentorial lesions

- Most cerebral arteriovenous malformations are supratentorial and in the middle cerebral artery territory
- Small arteriovenous malformations are more likely to bleed than large ones
- Arteriovenous malformations that have bled once are more likely to bleed again
- Bleeding unrelated to sex or lesion site
- Hemorrhage is intracerebral and subarachnoid (with 10% of cases fatal)

DEMOGRAPHICS

- Up to 70% of arteriovenous malformations bleed, most commonly before the age of 40

 ## CLINICAL FINDINGS

SYMPTOMS AND SIGNS

Supratentorial lesions

- Initial symptoms consist of hemorrhage in 30–60% of cases, recurrent seizures in 20–40%, headache in 5–25%, and miscellaneous complaints (including focal deficits) in 10–15%
- Focal or generalized seizures may accompany or follow hemorrhage, or may be the initial presentation, especially with frontal or parietal arteriovenous malformations
- Headaches, especially when the external carotid arteries are involved (sometimes simulate migraine but usually are nonspecific in character)
- In patients with subarachnoid hemorrhage, examination may reveal an abnormal mental status and signs of meningeal irritation
- Symptoms of increased intracranial pressure may be present—headache, visual obscurations, obtundation
- A cranial bruit may be present, but may also be found with aneurysms, meningiomas, acquired arteriovenous fistulas, and arteriovenous malformations involving the scalp, calvarium, or orbit
- Bruits are best heard over the ipsilateral eye or mastoid region and help in lateralization but not localization
- Absence of a bruit does not exclude an arteriovenous malformation

Infratentorial lesions

- Brainstem arteriovenous malformations are often clinically silent, but may hemorrhage, cause obstructive hydrocephalus, or lead to progressive or relapsing brainstem deficits
- Cerebellar arteriovenous malformations may also be clinically inconspicuous but sometimes lead to cerebellar hemorrhage

DIFFERENTIAL DIAGNOSIS

- Aneurysmal hemorrhage
- Intracerebral hemorrhage from other causes
- Space-occupying lesion, eg, brain tumor

DIAGNOSIS

IMAGING STUDIES

- CT scanning indicates whether subarachnoid or intracerebral bleeding has recently occurred, helps to localize its source, and may reveal the arteriovenous malformation
- If the source of hemorrhage is not evident on the CT scan, arteriography is necessary to exclude aneurysm or arteriovenous malformation. MR angiography is not always sensitive enough for this purpose
- Even if the findings on CT scan suggest arteriovenous malformation, bilateral arteriography of the internal and external carotid and vertebral arteries is required to establish the nature of the lesion
- Arteriovenous malformations typically appear as a tangled vascular mass with distended tortuous afferent and efferent vessels, a rapid circulation time, and arteriovenous shunting
- MRI typically reveals the lesion but does not define its blood supply
- Plain radiographs of the skull are often normal unless an intracerebral hematoma is present, in which case there may be changes suggestive of raised intracranial pressure and displacement of a calcified pineal gland

DIAGNOSTIC PROCEDURES

- If the CT scan shows no evidence of bleeding but subarachnoid hemorrhage is diagnosed clinically, the cerebrospinal fluid should be examined
- Electroencephalography is usually indicated in patients presenting with seizures and may show consistently focal or lateralized abnormalities resulting from the underlying cerebral arteriovenous malformation

Arteriovenous Malformations, Intracranial

 TREATMENT

MEDICATIONS

- In patients presenting solely with seizures, anticonvulsant drug treatment is usually sufficient, and surgery is unnecessary

SURGERY

- Surgical treatment to prevent further hemorrhage is justified with arteriovenous malformations that have bled, provided that the lesion is accessible and the patient has a reasonable life expectancy
- Surgical treatment is appropriate if intracranial pressure is increased and to prevent further progression of a focal neurological deficit
- Definitive operative treatment consists of excision of the arteriovenous malformation if it is surgically accessible

THERAPEUTIC PROCEDURES

- Inoperable arteriovenous malformations are sometimes treated solely by embolization; although the risk of hemorrhage is not reduced, neurological deficits may be stabilized or even reversed by this procedure
- Other techniques are injection of a vascular occlusive polymer through a flow-guided microcatheter and permanent occlusion of feeding vessels by positioning detachable balloon catheters in the desired sites and then inflating them with quickly solidifying contrast material
- Stereotactic radiosurgery with the gamma knife is also useful in the management of inoperable cerebral arteriovenous malformations

 OUTCOME

FOLLOW-UP

- Serial MRIs help to monitor malformations that are not treated surgically

COMPLICATIONS

- Communicating or obstructive hydrocephalus may occur and lead to symptoms

PROGNOSIS

- Depends on site of malformation and whether it has bled

WHEN TO REFER

- All patients

 EVIDENCE

PRACTICE GUIDELINES

- Ogilvy CS et al: AHA Scientific Statement: recommendations for the management of intracranial arteriovenous malformations. Stroke 2001;32:1458. [PMID: 11387517]
- National Guideline Clearinghouse http://www.guideline.gov/summary/summary.aspx?doc_id=2437&nbr=1663&string=arteriovenous+malformations

INFORMATION FOR PATIENTS

- National Institute of Neurological Disorders and Stroke http://www.ninds.nih.gov/health_and_medical/disorders/avms_html.htm http://www.ninds.nih.gov/health_and_medical/pubs/arteriovenous.htm

REFERENCE

- Al-Shahi R et al: A systematic review of the frequency and prognosis of arteriovenous malformations of the brain in adults. Brain 2001;124:1900. [PMID: 11571210]

Michael J. Aminoff, MD, DSc, FRCP

Arthritis, Gonococcal

 KEY FEATURES

ESSENTIALS OF DIAGNOSIS

- Prodromal migratory polyarthralgias
- Tenosynovitis most common sign
- Purulent monarthritis in 50%
- Characteristic skin rash
- Most common in young women during menses or pregnancy
- Symptoms of urethritis frequently absent
- Dramatic response to antibiotics

GENERAL CONSIDERATIONS

- Usually occurs in otherwise healthy individuals
- Most common cause of infectious arthritis in large urban areas

Associated conditions

- Menses or pregnancy
- Complement deficiency
- Reiter's syndrome can produce acute monarthritis in a young person but is distinguished by negative cultures, sacroiliitis, and failure to respond to antibiotics
- Lyme disease involving the knee is less acute, does not show positive cultures, and may be preceded by known tick exposure and characteristic rash
- Infective endocarditis with septic arthritis can mimic disseminated gonococcal infection

DEMOGRAPHICS

- Two to three times more common in women than in men, and is especially common during menses and pregnancy
- Gonococcal arthritis is also common in male homosexuals
- Rare after age 40

 CLINICAL FINDINGS

SYMPTOMS AND SIGNS

- One to 4 days of migratory polyarthralgias involving the wrist, knee, ankle, or elbow
- Thereafter, two patterns emerge, one (60%) characterized by tenosynovitis and the other (40%) by purulent monarthritis, most frequently involving the knee
- Less than half of patients have fever
- Less than one-fourth have genitourinary symptoms
- Most patients will have asymptomatic but highly characteristic skin lesions: two to ten small necrotic pustules distributed over the extremities, especially the palms and soles

DIFFERENTIAL DIAGNOSIS

- Reactive arthritis (Reiter's syndrome)
- Nongonococcal septic arthritis
- Gout or pseudogout
- Rheumatic fever
- Endocarditis
- Lyme disease
- Sarcoidosis
- Meningococcemia

 DIAGNOSIS

LABORATORY TESTS

- The synovial fluid white blood cell count is typically over 50,000 cells/mL
- The synovial fluid Gram stain is positive in one-fourth of cases and culture in less than half
- Positive blood cultures are seen in 40% of patients with tenosynovitis and virtually never in patients with suppurative arthritis
- Urethral, throat, and rectal cultures should be done in all patients, since they are often positive in the absence of local symptoms
- The peripheral blood is elevated in less than one-third of patients

IMAGING STUDIES

- Radiographs are usually normal or show only soft tissue swelling

Arthritis, Gonococcal

 TREATMENT

MEDICATIONS

- Approximately 25% of patients have absolute or relative resistance to penicillin. Therefore, give ceftriaxone, 1 g intravenously daily (or cefotaxime, 1 g intravenously every 8 h; or ceftizoxime, 1 g intravenously every 8 h; or spectinomycin, 2 g intramuscularly every 12 h, for patients with β-lactam allergy)
- Once improvement from parenteral antibiotics has been achieved for 24–48 h, patients can be switched to oral cefixime, 400 mg orally twice daily, or ciprofloxacin, 500 mg orally twice daily, to complete a 7- to 10-day course

THERAPEUTIC PROCEDURES

- Generally responds dramatically in 24–48 h after initiation of antibiotics so that daily joint aspirations are rarely needed

 OUTCOME

PROGNOSIS

- Complete recovery is the rule

WHEN TO REFER

- When diagnosis is in doubt
- Report to the public health department for tracing contacts

WHEN TO ADMIT

- While outpatient treatment has been recommended in the past, the rapid rise in gonococci resistant to penicillin makes initial inpatient treatment advisable
- Patients suspected of having gonococcal arthritis should be admitted to the hospital to confirm the diagnosis, to exclude endocarditis, and to start treatment

EVIDENCE

PRACTICE GUIDELINES

- National Guideline Clearinghouse http://www.guideline.gov/summary/summary.aspx?doc_id=3045&nbr=2271&string=reactive+arthritis

INFORMATION FOR PATIENTS

- National Institutes of Health http://www.nlm.nih.gov/medlineplus/ency/article/000453.htm
- National Institute of Arthritis and Musculoskeletal and Skin Diseases http://www.niams.nih.gov/hi/topics/reactive/reactive.htm#rea_a

REFERENCE

- Sieper J et al: Diagnosing reactive arthritis: role of clinical setting in the value of serologic and microbiologic assays. Arthritis Rheum 2002;46:319.

David B. Hellmann, MD, FACP
John H. Stone, MD, MPH

Arthritis, Nongonococcal Acute Bacterial (Septic)

 ## KEY FEATURES

ESSENTIALS OF DIAGNOSIS

- Sudden onset of acute arthritis, usually monarticular, most often in large weight-bearing joints and wrists
- Previous joint damage or intravenous drug abuse are common risk factors
- Infection with causative organisms commonly found elsewhere in body
- Joint effusions are usually large, with white blood cell counts commonly >50,000/mL

GENERAL CONSIDERATIONS

- A disease of an abnormal host
- Key risk factors are persistent bacteremia (eg, intravenous drug use, endocarditis) and damaged joints (eg, rheumatoid arthritis)
- *Staphylococcus aureus* is the most common cause of nongonococcal septic arthritis, followed by group A and group B streptococci
- Gram-negative septic arthritis is seen in intravenous drug abusers and in other immunocompromised hosts
- *Staphylococcus epidermidis* is the usual organism in prosthetic joint arthritis

 ## CLINICAL FINDINGS

SYMPTOMS AND SIGNS

- Sudden onset, with pain, swelling, and heat of one joint—most frequently the knee
- Unusual sites, such as the sternoclavicular or sacroiliac joint, can be involved in intravenous drug abusers
- Chills and fever are common but are absent in up to 20% of patients
- Infection of the hip usually does not produce apparent swelling but results in groin pain greatly aggravated by walking

DIFFERENTIAL DIAGNOSIS

- Gout and pseudogout are excluded by the failure to find crystals on synovial fluid analysis
- Acute rheumatic fever and rheumatoid arthritis commonly involve many joints
- Still's disease may mimic septic arthritis, but laboratory evidence of infection is absent

 ## DIAGNOSIS

LABORATORY TESTS

- Blood cultures are positive in approximately 50% of patients
- The leukocyte count of the synovial fluid exceeds 50,000 and often 100,000/mL, with 90% or more polymorphonuclear cells
- Gram stain of the synovial fluid is positive in 75% of staphylococcal infections and in 50% of gram-negative infections

IMAGING STUDIES

- Radiographs are usually normal early in the disease, but evidence of demineralization may be present within days of onset
- Bony erosions and narrowing of the joint space followed by osteomyelitis and periostitis may be seen within 2 weeks

DIAGNOSITIC PROCEDURES

- Joint aspiration is required to establish the diagnosis

TREATMENT

MEDICATIONS

- Prompt systemic antibiotic therapy of any septic arthritis should be based on the best clinical judgment of the causative organism
- If the organism cannot be determined clinically, treatment should be started with bactericidal antibiotics effective against staphylococci, pneumococci, and gram-negative organisms

SURGERY

- Immediate surgical drainage is reserved for septic arthritis of the hip, because that site is inaccessible to repeated aspiration
- For most other joints, surgical drainage is used only if medical therapy fails over 2–4 days to improve the fever and the synovial fluid volume, white blood cell count, and culture results

THERAPEUTIC PROCEDURES

- Rest, immobilization, and elevation are used at the onset of treatment. Early active motion exercises within the limits of tolerance will hasten recovery
- Frequent (even daily) local aspiration is indicated to complement antibiotic therapy when synovial fluid rapidly reaccumulates and causes symptoms

OUTCOME

COMPLICATIONS

- Bony ankylosis and articular destruction occur if treatment is delayed or inadequate

PROGNOSIS

- With prompt antibiotic therapy and no serious underlying disease, functional recovery is usually good
- Five to 10% of patients with an infected joint die, chiefly from respiratory complications of sepsis
- The mortality rate is 30% for patients with polyarticular sepsis

WHEN TO REFER

- Refer to an orthopedist if the infected joint is not easy to aspirate repeatedly (eg, hip)

WHEN TO ADMIT

- Admit for presumed or confirmed septic arthritis

EVIDENCE

PRACTICE GUIDELINES

- American College of Rheumatology http://www.rheumatology.org/research/ guidelines/musc/musc-dis.html

INFORMATION FOR PATIENTS

- American Association for Clinical Chemistry http://www.labtestsonline.org/ understanding/conditions/septic.html
- National Institues of Health http://www.nlm.nih.gov/medlineplus/ ency/article/000430.htm

REFERENCES

- Ho G Jr: Bacterial arthritis. Curr Opin Rheumatol 2001;13:310. [PMID: 11555734]
- Ross JJ: Pneumococcal septic arthritis. Clin Infect Dis 2003;36:319. [PMID: 12539074]
- Shirtliff ME, Mader JT: Acute septic arthritis. Clin Microbiol Rev 2002; 15:527. [PMID: 12364368]

David B. Hellmann, MD, FACP
John H. Stone, MD, MPH

Arthritis, Reactive (Reiter's Syndrome)

 KEY FEATURES

ESSENTIALS OF DIAGNOSIS

- Fifty to 80% of patients are HLA-B27 positive
- Oligoarthritis, conjunctivitis, urethritis, and mouth ulcers most common features
- Usually follows dysentery or a sexually transmitted infection

GENERAL CONSIDERATIONS

- Also called "reactive arthritis"
- Reiter's syndrome is a clinical tetrad of urethritis, conjunctivitis (or, less commonly, uveitis), mucocutaneous lesions, and aseptic arthritis
- Most cases develop within days or weeks after definite or implicated triggers
  - Dysentery: *Shigella, Salmonella, Yersinia, Campylobacter*
  - Sexually transmitted disease: *Chlamydia trachomatis, Ureaplasma urealyticum,* gonorrhea
  - Other: *Chlamydia pneumoniae, Clostridium difficile*
- Gonococcal arthritis can initially mimic Reiter's syndrome, but the marked improvement after 24–48 h of antibiotic administration and the culture results distinguish the two disorders

DEMOGRAPHICS

- Most commonly in young men
- The gender ratio: 1:1 after enteric infections but 9:1 with male predominance after sexually transmitted infections
- Associated with HLA-B27 in 80% of white patients and 50–60% of blacks

 CLINICAL FINDINGS

SYMPTOMS AND SIGNS

- The arthritis is most commonly asymmetric and frequently involves the large weight-bearing joints (chiefly the knee and ankle)
- Sacroiliitis or ankylosing spondylitis is observed in at least 20% of patients
- Systemic symptoms including fever and weight loss are common at the onset of disease
- The mucocutaneous lesions may include circinate balanitis, stomatitis, and keratoderma blenorrhagicum, indistinguishable from pustular psoriasis
- Carditis and aortic regurgitation may occur

DIFFERENTIAL DIAGNOSIS

- Gonococcal arthritis
- Psoriatic arthritis
- Ankylosing spondylitis
- Rheumatoid arthritis
- Arthritis associated with inflammatory bowel disease

 DIAGNOSIS

LABORATORY TESTS

- HLA-B27 test is useful in the diagnosis

IMAGING STUDIES

- X-ray signs of permanent or progressive joint disease may be seen in the sacroiliac as well as the peripheral joints

Arthritis, Reactive (Reiter's Syndrome)

TREATMENT

MEDICATIONS

- Nonsteroidal antiinflammatory drugs (NSAIDs) have been the mainstay of therapy
- Glucocorticoids are typically not helpful
- Tetracycline (250 mg four times daily) given for 3 months to patients with Reiter's syndrome associated with *C trachomatis* reduces the duration of symptoms
- Patients who fail NSAIDs and tetracycline may respond to sulfasalazine, 1000 mg twice daily
- Anti-tumor necrosing factor agents (etanercept, infliximab) are reasonable therapies for patients with refractory disease

OUTCOME

PROGNOSIS

- While most signs of the disease disappear within days or weeks, the arthritis may persist for several months or even years
- Recurrences involving any combination of the clinical manifestations are common and are sometimes followed by permanent sequelae, especially in the joints

WHEN TO REFER

- Refer to a rheumatologist for progressive symptoms despite therapy

PREVENTION

- Antibiotics given at the time of a nongonococcal sexually transmitted infection reduce the chance that the individual will develop Reiter's syndrome

EVIDENCE

PRACTICE GUIDELINES

- National Guideline Clearinghouse http://www.guideline.gov/summary/summary.aspx?doc_id=3045&nbr=2271&string=reactive+arthritis

INFORMATION FOR PATIENTS

- American Academy of Family Physicians http://familydoctor.org/handouts/448.html
- National Institute of Arthritis and Musculoskeletal and Skin Diseases http://www.niams.nih.gov/hi/topics/reactive/reactive.htm

REFERENCES

- Sieper J et al: Diagnosing reactive arthritis: role of clinical setting in the value of serologic and microbiologic assays. Arthritis Rheum 2002;46:319.
- Toivanen A et al: Reactive arthritis. Isr Med Assoc J 2001;3:681. [PMID: 11574987]

David B. Hellmann, MD, FACP
John H. Stone, MD, MPH

Ascariasis

 ## KEY FEATURES

ESSENTIALS OF DIAGNOSIS

- Pulmonary phase: transient cough, dyspnea, wheezing, urticaria, with eosinophilia and transient pulmonary infiltrates
- Intestinal phase: vague upper abdominal discomfort; occasional vomiting, abdominal distension
- Eggs in stools; worms passed per rectum, nose, or mouth

GENERAL CONSIDERATIONS

- *Ascaris lumbricoides* is the most common intestinal helminth
- Adult worms live in the upper small intestine. After fertilization, the female produces enormous numbers of eggs that pass in feces
- Direct transmission between humans does not occur, as the eggs must remain on the soil for 2–3 weeks before they become infective. Thereafter, they can survive for years
- Infection occurs through ingestion of mature eggs in fecally contaminated food and drink
- Egg production begins 60–75 days after ingestion of infective eggs. Adult worms (20–40 cm × 3–6 mm) live for 1 year or more
- As a result of their migration and induction of hypersensitivity, larvae in the lung cause capillary and alveolar damage and symptoms of the pulmonary phase

DEMOGRAPHICS

- An estimated 1 billion people are infected worldwide
- It is cosmopolitan in distribution and is found in high prevalence wherever there are low standards of hygiene and sanitation (including focally in the southeastern United States) or where human feces are used as fertilizer

 ## CLINICAL FINDINGS

SYMPTOMS AND SIGNS

- Pulmonary phase: low-grade fever, nonproductive cough, blood-tinged sputum, wheezing, dyspnea, and substernal pain
- There may be urticaria and localized rales
- Rarely, larvae lodge ectopically in the brain, kidney, eye, spinal cord, etc, and may be symptomatic
- Small numbers of adult worms in the intestine usually produce no symptoms With heavy infection, peptic ulcer–like symptoms or vague pre- or postprandial abdominal discomfort may be seen
- Adult worms may be coughed up, vomited, or emerge through the nose or anus
- Adult worms may migrate into the common bile duct, pancreatic duct, appendix, diverticula, and other sites, which may lead to cholangitis, cholecystitis, pyogenic liver abscess, pancreatitis, or obstructive jaundice
- With very heavy infestations, masses of worms may cause intestinal obstruction, volvulus, intussusception, or death

DIFFERENTIAL DIAGNOSIS

- Asthma
- Allergic bronchopulmonary aspergillosis (ABPA)
- Acute eosinophilic pneumonia (Löffler's syndrome)
- Paragonimiasis
- Tropical pulmonary eosinophilia (*Wuchereria bancrofti, Brugia malayi*)
- Hookworm disease
- Strongyloidiasis
- Toxocariasis (visceral larva migrans)
- Peptic ulcer disease
- Other causes of cholangitis, cholecystitis, pancreatitis, appendicitis, diverticulitis

DIAGNOSIS

LABORATORY TESTS

- During the pulmonary phase, eosinophils may reach 30–50% and remain high for about a month; larvae are occasionally found in sputum
- During the intestinal phase, diagnosis usually depends on finding the characteristic eggs in feces
- Occasionally, an adult worm spontaneously passed per rectum or orally reveals an unsuspected infection
- Serological tests are not useful, and there is no eosinophilia in the intestinal phase

IMAGING STUDIES

- During the larval migratory phase, chest radiographs may show transitory, patchy, ill-defined asymmetric infiltrations (Löffler's syndrome)
- Radiological examination of the abdomen (with or without barium) may show the presence of worms
- In intestinal obstruction, plain abdominal films show air-filled levels and multiple linear images of ascarides in dilated bowel loops; ultrasonography can also demonstrate the dilated bowel and worm mass

DIAGONISTIC PROCEDURES

- The diagnosis of biliary ascariasis can be made by endoscopic retrograde cholangiopancreatography, which has the therapeutic potential of removing the worms

Ascariasis

TREATMENT

MEDICATIONS

- Albendazole and pyrantel pamoate are the treatments of choice
- Ascariasis, hookworm, and trichuriasis infections, which often occur together, may be treated simultaneously by albendazole, mebendazole, or oxantel–pyrantel pamoate
- In pregnancy, ascariasis should be treated after the first trimester
- Drug treatment should not be used in the migratory phase

Albendazole

- In light infections, a single dose of albendazole (400 mg) results in cure rates over 95%; in heavy infections, a 2- to 3-day course is indicated
- Side effects, including migration of ascaris through the nose or mouth, are rare
- The drug is contraindicated in pregnancy

Pyrantel pamoate

- Pyrantel pamoate as a single oral dose of 10 mg base/kg (maximum, 1 g) results in 85–100% cure rates. It may be given before or after meals
- Infrequent and mild side effects include vomiting, diarrhea, headache, dizziness, and drowsiness

Mebendazole

- Although mebendazole is highly effective when given in a dosage of 100 mg twice daily before or after meals for 3 days, a single 500-mg dose is often sufficient
- Gastrointestinal side effects are infrequent
- The drug is contraindicated in pregnancy

Piperazine

- The dosage for piperazine (as the hexahydrate) is 75 mg/kg body weight (maximum, 3.5 g) for 2 days in succession, giving the drug orally before or after breakfast
- For heavy infestations, treatment should be continued for 4 days in succession or the 2-day course should be repeated after 1 week
- Gastrointestinal symptoms and headache occur occasionally; central nervous system symptoms (temporary ataxia and exacerbation of seizures) are rare

- Allergic symptoms have been attributed to piperazine
- The drug should not be used for patients with hepatic or renal insufficiency or in those with a history of seizures or chronic neurological disease

Levamisole

- Levamisole is highly effective as a single oral dose of 150 mg
- Occasional mild and transient side effects are nausea, vomiting, abdominal pain, headache, and dizziness

THERAPEUTIC PROCEDURES

- In intestinal obstruction or biliary ascariasis, surgery may be avoided by nasogastric suction followed by a standard dose of an anthelmintic given via the tube
- In biliary ascariasis, endoscopic removal of the worm under ultrasonographic guidance is often successful; treatment by injection of a solution of albendazole or piperazine into the common duct followed by systemic treatment has also been effective

OUTCOME

FOLLOW-UP

- Stools should be rechecked at 2 weeks after treatment and patients retreated until all ascarids are removed
- Because anesthesia stimulates worms to hypermotility, they should be removed in advance in infected patients undergoing elective surgery
- The complications caused by wandering adult worms require that all *Ascaris* infections be treated and eradicated

WHEN TO REFER

- If there is difficulty in making the diagnosis or progressive symptoms despite therapy

WHEN TO ADMIT

- Intestinal obstruction or biliary ascariasis

EVIDENCE

PRACTICE GUIDELINES

- National Guideline Clearinghouse
http://www.guideline.gov/summary/summary.aspx?doc_id=2707&nbr=1933&string=abdominal+pain

INFORMATION FOR PATIENTS

- National Institute of Allergy and Infectious Disease
http://www.niaid.nih.gov/factsheets/roundwor.htm
- Nemours Foundation
http://kidshealth.org/parent/infections/stomach/ascariasis.html

REFERENCES

- Crompton DW: Ascaris and ascariasis. Adv Parasitol 2001;48:285. [PMID: 11013758]
- Dib J et al: Hepato-biliary ascariasis. Gastrointest Endosc 2000;51:594. [PMID: 10805849]
- Misra SP et al: Clinical features and management of biliary ascariasis in non-endemic areas. Postgrad Med J 2000;76:29. [PMID: 10622777]
- Ogata H et al: Multilocular pyogenic hepatic abscess complicating *Ascaris lumbricoides* infestation. Intern Med 2000;39:228. [PMID: 10772125]

Ascites

 KEY FEATURES

ESSENTIALS OF DIAGNOSIS

- Pathological accumulation of fluid in the peritoneal cavity

GENERAL CONSIDERATIONS

- Two broad categories of ascites: one associated with a normal peritoneum and the other due to a diseased peritoneum (Table 53, page 1250)
- Most common cause is portal hypertension secondary to chronic liver disease (>80% of cases)
- Other causes include infections (tuberculous peritonitis), intraabdominal malignancy, inflammatory disorders of the peritoneum, and ductal disruptions (chylous, pancreatic, biliary)
- Risk factors for ascites include causes of liver disease: ethanol consumption, transfusions, tattoos, intravenous drug use, a history of viral hepatitis or jaundice, and birth in an area endemic for hepatitis
- History of cancer or marked weight loss suggests malignancy
- Fevers suggest infected peritoneal fluid, including bacterial peritonitis (spontaneous or secondary)

DEMOGRAPHICS

- Tuberculous peritonitis occurs in immigrants, immunocompromised hosts, or severely malnourished alcoholics
- Cirrhosis with portal hypertensive ascites most commonly caused by chronic alcoholism or chronic viral infection (hepatitis B or C)

 CLINICAL FINDINGS

SYMPTOMS AND SIGNS

- Increasing abdominal girth
- Abdominal pain
- Large abdominal wall veins with cephalad flow in portal hypertension; inferiorly directed flow implies hepatic vein obstruction
- Palmar erythema, cutaneous spider angiomas, gynecomastia, Dupuytren's contracture, and asterixis in portal hypertension and chronic liver disease
- Elevated jugular venous pressure in right-sided congestive heart failure or constrictive pericarditis
- Large tender liver in acute alcoholic hepatitis or Budd-Chiari syndrome
- Anasarca in congestive heart failure or nephrotic syndrome
- Firm lymph nodes in the left supraclavicular region or umbilicus in malignancy

DIFFERENTIAL DIAGNOSIS

- See Table 53 (page 1250)
- Cirrhosis (80–85%)
- Malignancy (10%)
- Congestive heart failure (3%)
- Tuberculous peritonitis
- Dialysis-related
- Bile or pancreatic ascites
- Lymphatic tear (chylous ascites)
- Nephrotic syndrome

 DIAGNOSIS

LABORATORY TESTS

- Ascitic fluid cell count: normal cell count is <500 leukocytes/μL and <250 polymorphonuclear neutrophils (PMNs)/μL
- PMN count of >250/μL (neutrocytic ascites), with >75% of all white blood cells (WBCs) being PMNs in bacterial peritonitis
- Elevated WBCs with a predominance of lymphocytes occur in tuberculosis or peritoneal carcinomatosis
- Cloudy ascitic fluid suggests infection
- Milky fluid occurs in chylous ascites
- Bloody fluid suggests traumatic paracentesis, malignant ascites
- Serum-ascites albumin gradient (SAAG) classifies ascites into portal hypertensive and nonportal hypertensive causes (Table 53, page 1250)
- SAAG is calculated by subtracting the ascitic fluid albumin from the serum albumin
- SAAG >1.1 g/dL suggests underlying portal hypertension, while SAAG <1.1 g/dL implicates nonportal hypertensive causes
- ~ 4% of patients have "mixed ascites," due to underlying cirrhosis with portal hypertension complicated by a second cause for ascites (such as malignancy or tuberculosis)
- An elevated SAAG and a high ascitic fluid total protein level (>2.5 g/dL) occurs in hepatic congestion secondary to cardiac disease or Budd-Chiari syndrome, and in up to 20% of cases of uncomplicated cirrhosis
- Ascitic fluid glucose is low in tuberculous peritonitis
- Ascitic fluid amylase is elevated in pancreatic ascites or a perforation of the gastrointestinal tract
- Ascitic fluid bilirubin concentration is greater than the serum bilirubin in perforation of the biliary tree
- Ascitic fluid creatinine is elevated in leakage of urine from the bladder or ureters
- Ascitic fluid culture and Gram stain in suspected peritonitis

IMAGING STUDIES

- Ultrasound and CT imaging useful in distinguishing between causes of portal and nonportal hypertensive ascites, thrombosis of the hepatic veins (Budd-Chiari syndrome) or portal veins, detecting lymphadenopathy and masses, permiting directed percutaneous needle biopsies

DIAGNOSTIC PROCEDURES

- Physical examination is insensitive for detecting ascitic fluid until >1500 mL of fluid
- Abdominal ultrasound confirms presence of ascites and facilitates paracentesis
- Cytological examination if peritoneal carcinomatosis is suspected
- Laparoscopy permits direct visualization and biopsy of the peritoneum, liver, and some intraabdominal lymph nodes in suspected peritoneal tuberculosis or malignancy
- Abdominal paracentesis indicated in all patients with new onset of ascites to diagnose bacterial peritonitis, in all patients admitted to the hospital with cirrhosis and ascites, and when patients with known ascites develop clinical deterioration (fever, abdominal pain, rapid worsening of renal function, or worsened hepatic encephalopathy)

 TREATMENT

MEDICATIONS

- Portal hypertensive ascites: diuretics: spironolactone, 100 mg/day, and furosemide, 40 mg/day
- Dose increased every 5–7 days until diuresis achieved to maximum of 400 mg/day aldactone and 160 mg/day furosemide
- Goal is to lose 0.5 kg/day
- Careful monitoring of serum sodium, potassium, and creatinine required

SURGERY

- Peritovenous shunt in patients with refractory ascites due to portal hypertension

THERAPEUTIC PROCEDURES

- In ascites caused by portal hypertension, dietary sodium restriction to 1–2 g/day; fluid intake restriction if serum Na <125 mEq/L
- TIPS (transjugular intrahepatic portosystemic shunt) effectively controls 75% of patients with portal hypertension and refractory ascites
- Large-volume paracentesis (4–6 L) is indicated for patients with massive ascites or ascites refractory to diuretics
- Intravenous albumin should be administered to reduce acute and long-term complication: 10 g albumin/L of ascites removed

 OUTCOME

COMPLICATIONS

- Portal hypertensive ascites: spontaneous bacterial peritonitis occurs in 20–30%; patients with ascites total protein <1 g/dL are at higher risk (40%)
- Massive ascites: ruptured umbilical hernia, hepatic hydrothorax, respiratory compromise, poor nutritional intake
- Peritoneovenous shunts: shunt occlusion, disseminated intravascular coagulation, bacterial infection, variceal hemorrhage
- TIPS: encephalopathy 30% and shunt stenosis or occlusion in 30–60% within 1 year, requiring periodic revisions

PROGNOSIS

- In patients with cirrhosis, ascites is a poor prognostic indicator, with 50% survival at 2 years

WHEN TO ADMIT

- Suspected peritonitis

 EVIDENCE

PRACTICE GUIDELINES

- Salerno F et al: Clinical practice guidelines for the management of cirrhotic patients with ascites. Committee on Ascites of the Italian Association for the Study of the Liver. Ital J Gastroenterol Hepatol 1999;31:626. [PMID: 10604107]
- Stephenson J et al: The development of clinical guidelines on paracentesis for ascites related to malignancy. Palliat Med 2002;16:213. [PMID: 12046997]

WEB SITES

- National Institute of Diabetes and Digestive and Kidney Diseases (NIDDK), NIH http://www.niddk .nih.gov

INFORMATION FOR PATIENTS

- Cancerbacup http://www.cancerbacup.org.uk/info/ascites.htm
- MEDLINEplus http://www.nlm.nih.gov/medlineplus/ency/article/000286.htm
- Merck Manual http://www.merck.com/pubs/mmanual/section4/chapter38/38e.htm

REFERENCES

- Jeffrey J et al: Ascitic fluid analysis: the role of biochemistry and haematology. Hosp Med 2001;62:282. [PMID: 11885888]
- Krige JE et al: ABC of diseases of the liver, pancreas, and biliary system: portal hypertension 2. Ascites, encephalopathy, and other conditions. BMJ 2001;322:416. [PMID: 11179165]
- Runyon BA: Ascites. Clin Liver Dis 2000;4:151. [PMID: 11232182]

Kenneth R. McQuaid, MD

Asthma

KEY FEATURES

ESSENTIALS OF DIAGNOSIS

- Episodic or chronic symptoms of airflow obstruction: breathlessness, cough, wheezing, and chest tightness
- Symptoms frequently worse at night or in the early morning
- Prolonged expiration and diffuse wheezes on physical examination
- Limitation of airflow on pulmonary function testing or positive bronchoprovocation challenge
- Complete or partial reversibility of airflow obstruction, either spontaneously or following bronchodilator therapy

GENERAL CONSIDERATIONS

- Affects 5% of the population
- Accounts for 470,000 hospital admissions and 5000 deaths annually in the United States
- Prevalence, hospitalizations, and fatal asthma have all increased in the United States over the past 20 years

DEMOGRAPHICS

- Men and women are affected equally
- Hospitalization rates have been highest among blacks and children
- Death rates for asthma are consistently highest among blacks aged 15–24 years

CLINICAL FINDINGS

SYMPTOMS AND SIGNS

- See Tables 12 and 13 (pages 1210 and 1211)
- Episodic wheezing and difficulty breathing, chest tightness, and cough
- Symptoms are frequently worse at night
- Common aeroallergens include dust mites, cockroaches, cats, and pollen
- Nonspecific precipitants include exercise, respiratory tract infections, postnasal drip, aspiration, gastroesophageal reflux, changes in weather, and stress
- Tobacco smoke increases symptoms and decreases lung function
- Certain medications (including aspirin and nonsteroidal antiinflammatory drugs) may be triggers
- Nasal findings consistent with allergy and evidence of allergic skin disorders
- Wheezing with normal breathing or a prolonged forced expiratory phase

DIFFERENTIAL DIAGNOSIS

Upper airway disorders

- Vocal cord paralysis
- Vocal cord dysfunction syndrome
- Foreign body aspiration
- Laryngotracheal mass
- Tracheal stenosis
- Tracheomalacia
- Angioedema
- Airway edema from inhalation injury

Lower airway disorders

- Chronic obstructive pulmonary disease
- Bronchiectasis
- Allergic bronchopulmonary aspergillosis
- Cystic fibrosis
- Eosinophilic pneumonia
- Bronchiolitis obliterans

Other

- Congestive heart failure (cardiac asthma)
- Gastroesophageal reflux disease
- Pulmonary embolism
- Churg-Strauss

Psychiatric

- Conversion disorder

DIAGNOSIS

LABORATORY TESTS

- See Tables 12 and 13 (pages 1210 and 1211)
- Spirometry (FEV_1, FVC, FEV_1/FVC) before and after the administration of a short-acting bronchodilator
- Significant reversibility of obstruction is demonstrated by an increase of >12% and 200 mL in FEV_1 or >15% and 200 mL in FVC after inhaling a bronchodilator
- Arterial blood gases may show a respiratory alkalosis and an increase in the alveolar–arterial oxygen difference; in severe exacerbations, hypoxemia develops and the $PaCO_2$ normalizes
- An increased $PaCO_2$ and respiratory acidosis may portend respiratory failure

IMAGING STUDIES

- Chest x-rays show only hyperinflation, but may include bronchial wall thickening and diminished peripheral lung vascular shadows
- Chest x-rays if pneumonia or complications of asthma are suspected

DIAGNOSTIC PROCEDURES

- Bronchial provocation testing with histamine, methacholine, or exercise is useful when asthma is expected and spirometry is nondiagnostic
- Skin testing for sensitivity to environmental allergens may be useful in persistent asthma

TREATMENT

MEDICATIONS

- See Tables 14 and 15 (pages 1212 and 1213)

Long-term control therapy

- Inhaled corticosteroids
- Systemic corticosteroids
- Long-acting β_2-agonists
- Combination inhaled corticosteroid and long-acting β_2-agonist
- Leukotriene modifiers
- Mediator inhibitors
- Phosphodiesterase inhibitors

Ascites, Malignant p. 1062. Aspergillosis p. 1062. Aspiration of Gastric Contents, Acute, p. 1063. Aspiration of Gastric Contents, Chronic p. 1064.

Asthma

Quick-relief therapy

- See Table 16 (page 1215)
- Short-acting inhaled β_2-agonists
- Anticholinergics
- Glucocorticoids
- Antimicrobials
  - No role in routine asthma exacerbations
  - Fever and purulent sputum and evidence of pneumonia or bacterial sinusitis may suggest a benefit
- Acute exacerbations
  - Repetitive or continuous use of inhaled short-acting β_2-agonist
  - Early administration of systemic corticosteroids
  - Treatment or removal of any identified trigger to the exacerbation
  - Mild exacerbations [peak expiratory flow (PEF) >80%]: double the usual dose of inhaled steroids after acute treatment
- Moderate exacerbations (PEF 50–80%): a course of oral corticosteroids
- Severe exacerbations (PEF <50%): rapid inititiation of high-dose bronchodilators and systemic corticosteroids, and careful observation
- Chronic asthma
  - Treatment is guided by an assessment of asthma severity (see Table 12, page 1210)
- Mild intermittent asthma
  - Short-acting β_2-agonists
  - Control therapy added if >2 uses/week
- Mild persistent asthma
  - Daily use of either low-dose inhaled steroid OR cromolyn or neodocromil
  - Sustained-release theophylline or leukotriene modifier is less desirable
  - Short-acting β_2-agonists
- Moderate persistent asthma
  - Daily use of medium-dose OR low–medium-dose inhaled steroid with long-acting inhaled β_2-agonist
  - Daily use of long-acting inhaled β_2-agonist OR sustained-release theophylline or long-acting β_2-agonist tablets
  - Short-acting β_2-agonists
- Severe persistent asthma
  - Daily use of high-dose inhaled corticosteroid AND long-acting bronchodilator or sustained-release theophylline or long-acting β_2-agonist tablets
  - Daily use of systemic corticosteroids
  - Short-acting β_2-agonists

THERAPEUTIC PROCEDURES

- Desensitization to specific allergens
- Intubation and mechanical ventilation for patients with impending respiratory failure; permissive hypercapnia to limit airway pressures

OUTCOME

FOLLOW-UP

- Patient self-assesment is a primary method of monitoring
- PEF monitoring can provide objective measurement to guide treatment
  - A 20% change in PEF from day to day or AM to PM suggests inadequate control
  - PEF <200 L/min indicates severe obstruction
- Follow-up visits should be at least biannual to maintain control and evaluate medication adjustments
- Repeat spirometry at least every 1–2 years after symptoms have stabilized

COMPLICATIONS

- Exhaustion, dehydration, and tussive syncope
- Cor pulmonale
- Airway infection
- Acute hypercapnic and hypoxic respiratory failure in severe disease

PROGNOSIS

- Good with regular follow-up and care

WHEN TO REFER

- Lack of response to therapy or progressive disease

WHEN TO ADMIT

- Patients with acute exacerbations who have an inadequate response to initial therapy
- Admission should be considered for patients with a PEF or FEV_1 <70% of predicted; admission is likely for PEF <50%
- The duration and severity of symptoms, as well as severity of prior exacerbations and psychosocial issues, should be taken into account

PREVENTION

- Patients should be taught to recognize early symptoms of an exacerbation and initiate a predetermined action plan
- Pneumococcal and annual influenza vaccination
- Environmental measures to reduce exposure to allergens should occur

 EVIDENCE

PRACTICE GUIDELINES

- National Asthma Education and Prevention Program: Expert Panel Report 2: Guidelines for the diagnosis and management of asthma. National Institutes of Health, Pub No. 97-4051, Bethesda, MD, 1997
- National Guideline Clearinghouse http://www.guideline.gov/summary/summary.aspx?doc_id=3734&nbr=2960&string=asthma
- National Intitutes of Health http://www.nhlbi.nih.gov/guidelines/asthma/asthgdln.htm http://www.nhlbi.nih.gov/guidelines/asthma/index.htm

WEB SITES

- National Institute of Allergy and Infectious Disease http://www.niaid.nih.gov/newsroom/focuson/asthma01/basics.htm
- National Heart, Lung and Blood Institute http://www.nhlbi.nih.gov/health/public/lung/asthma/asth_fs.pdf

INFORMATION FOR PATIENTS

- JAMA patient page: Asthma.JAMA 1999;281:2160. [PMID: 10367828]

REFERENCES

- Busse WW et al: Asthma. N Engl J Med 2001;344:350. [PMID: 11172168]
- Naureckas ET et al: Clinical practice. Mild asthma. N Engl J Med 2001; 345:1257. [PMID: 11680447]
- Suissa S et al: Low-dose inhaled corticosteroids and the prevention of death from asthma. N Engl J Med 2000;343:332. [PMID: 10922423]
- Woodruff PG et al: Asthma: prevalence, pathogenesis, and prospects for novel therapies. JAMA 2001;286:395. [PMID: 11466111]

Mark S. Chesnutt, MD
Thomas J. Prenderast, MD

Auditory Tube Dysfunction

 ## KEY FEATURES

ESSENTIALS OF DIAGNOSIS

- Aural fullness
- Fluctuating hearing
- Discomfort with barometric pressure change

GENERAL CONSIDERATIONS

- The tube that connects the middle ear to the nasopharynx—the auditory tube, or eustachian tube—provides ventilation and drainage for the middle ear cleft
- The auditory tube is normally closed, opening only during the act of swallowing or yawning

Hypofunctioning (narrowed) auditory tube

- When auditory tube function is compromised, air trapped within the middle ear becomes absorbed and negative pressure results
- The most common causes are diseases associated with edema of the tubal lining, such as viral upper respiratory tract infections and allergy

Overly patent auditory tube

- A relatively uncommon problem that may be quite distressing
- May develop during rapid weight loss, or may be idiopathic

 ## CLINICAL FINDINGS

SYMPTOMS AND SIGNS

Hypofunctioning auditory tube

- Usually there is a sense of fullness in the ear and mild to moderate impairment of hearing
- When the tube is only partially blocked, swallowing or yawning may elicit a popping or crackling sound
- Examination reveals retraction of the tympanic membrane and decreased mobility on pneumatic otoscopy

Overly patent auditory tube

- Fullness in the ear
- Autophony, an exaggerated ability to hear oneself breathe and speak
- In contrast to a hypofunctioning auditory tube, the aural pressure is often made worse by exertion and may diminish during an upper respiratory tract infection.
- Although physical examination is usually normal, respiratory excursions of the tympanic membrane may occasionally be detected during vigorous breathing

DIFFERENTIAL DIAGNOSIS

- Cerumen impaction (ear wax)
- Acute or chronic otitis media
- Temporomandibular joint disfunction
- Paget's disease
- Head trauma

 ## DIAGNOSIS

DIAGNOSTIC PROCEDURES

- Clinical diagnosis

TREATMENT

MEDICATIONS

Hypofunctioning auditory tube

- Systemic and intranasal decongestants (eg, pseudoephedrine, 60 mg orally every 4 h; oxymetazoline, 0.05% spray every 8–12 h) combined with autoinflation by forced exhalation against closed nostrils may hasten relief
- Allergic patients may also benefit from desensitization or intranasal corticosteroids (eg, beclomethasone dipropionate, two sprays in each nostril twice daily for 2–6 weeks)

Overly patent auditory tube

- Avoidance of decongestant products

SURGERY

Hypofunctioning auditory tube

- In medically refractory tube hypofunction, insertion of a tympanostomy tube is often helpful

Overly patent auditory tube

- Rarely, surgical narrowing of the auditory tube is indicated, and the same is true of insertion of a ventilating tube to reduce the outward stretch of the ear drum during phonation

THERAPEUTIC PROCEDURES

- Autoinflation should not be recommended to patients with active intranasal infection, since this maneuver may precipitate middle ear infection

 OUTCOME

PROGNOSIS

- Following a viral illness, this disorder is usually transient, lasting days to weeks

WHEN TO REFER

- Refer to an otolaryngologist if symptoms persist despite medical therapy or if there is persistent hearing loss

PREVENTION

- Avoid chronic decongestant use
- Avoid exacerbants of air travel, rapid altitudinal change, and underwater diving
- Control associated sinonasal disease

 EVIDENCE

PRACTICE GUIDELINES

National Guideline Clearinghouse
http://www.guideline.gov/summary/
summary.aspx?doc_id=2622&nbr=1848
&string=auditory+tube+dysfunction

WEB SITES

- Ear, Nose, and Throat Information Center
  http://www.netdoor.com/entinfo/
- Otolaryngology Resources on the Internet
  http://www.bcm.tmc.edu/oto/
  othersa.html

INFORMATION FOR PATIENTS

- American Academy of Otolaryngology-Head and Neck Surgery. Ears and Altitude
  http://www.entnet.org/healthinfo/ears/
  altitude.cfm
- National Institutes of Health
  http://www.nlm.nih.gov/medlineplus/
  hearingdisordersdeafness.html

REFERENCES

- Derebery MJ et al: Allergic eustachian tube dysfunction: diagnosis and treatment. Am J Otolaryngol 1997;18:160. [PMID: 9093670]
- Monsell EM et al: Eustachian tube dysfunction. Otolaryngol Clin North Am 1996;29:437. [PMID: 8743342]

Robert K. Jackler, MD
Michael J. Kaplan, MD

Babesiosis

 ## KEY FEATURES

ESSENTIALS OF DIAGNOSIS

- Fever, chills, headache, myalgia, fatigue
- Nausea, vomiting
- Hemolytic anemia, moderate
- Intraerythrocytic parasites on staining of thick and thin blood smears; no gametocytes
- Specific IgM antibody in 1–4 weeks

GENERAL CONSIDERATIONS

- Babesiae are tick-borne protozoal parasites of wild and domestic animals
- In Europe, the infection is caused by *Babesia divergens*; in the United States, Taiwan, China, Egypt, South Africa, Mexico, and South America, the infection is caused by *B microti*
- New *Babesia* species or strains (WA1 and others) have been described in California, Washington, and Georgia
- Natural hosts for *B microti* are wild and domestic animals, particularly the white-footed mouse and white-tailed deer. The extension of the deer's habitat is increasing human infection
- Humans are infected as a result of *Ixodes scapularis* (*I dammini*) tick bites (mainly nymphal) but also by blood transfusion and perinatally
- Coinfections with Lyme disease and ehrlichiosis occur
- Without passing through an exoerythrocytic stage, *B microti* enters the red blood cell and multiplies, resulting in cell rupture followed by infection of other cells
- The incubation period is 1 week to several months; parasitemia is evident in 2–4 weeks
- All *B divergens* infections (transmitted by *I ricinus*) have been in splenectomized patients

DEMOGRAPHICS

- In the United States, *B microti* infections have occurred in the coastal and island areas of northeastern and mid-Atlantic states as well as Wisconsin, Minnesota, Missouri, Washington, and California

 ## CLINICAL FINDINGS

SYMPTOMS AND SIGNS

- Irregular fever, chills, headache, diaphoresis, myalgia, and fatigue but without malaria-like periodicity of symptoms
- Nausea, vomiting, jaundice, arthralgia, and emotional lability
- Some patients have hemoglobinuria, hepatosplenomegaly, or thrombocytopenia
- *B divergens* infections in splenectomized patients present with rapidly progressive high fever, severe hemolytic anemia, jaundice, hemoglobinuria, and renal failure

DIFFERENTIAL DIAGNOSIS

- Malaria
- Infectious mononucleosis
- Viral hepatitis
- Ehrlichiosis
- Lyme disease

 ## DIAGNOSIS

LABORATORY TESTS

- The intraerythrocytic parasite (2–3 μm) can be identified on Wright- or Giemsa-stained thick and thin blood smears; no gametocytes and no intracellular pigment are seen
- A single red cell may contain different stages of the parasite, and parasitemia can exceed 10%. Repeated smears may be necessary
- The organism must be differentiated from malarial parasites, particularly *Plasmodium falciparum*
- Isolation can be attempted by inoculating patient blood into hamsters or gerbils
- Antibody is detectable within 1–4 weeks after onset of symptoms and persists for 6–12 months
- Testing with specific antigens in the immunofluorescent test is relatively species specific, with a titer of 1:1024 or greater considered diagnostic; antibody titers against *Plasmodium* are generally low or absent
- Detection of specific IgM antibody confirms the diagnosis
- The polymerase chain reaction method, where available, is more sensitive for low parasitemias but of equal specificity
- Other findings include hemolytic anemia, thrombocytopenia, low-grade leukocytosis or leukopenia, and abnormal liver and renal function tests

IMAGING STUDIES

- Imaging studies may detect morphological changes in the spleen

Babesiosis

 ## TREATMENT

MEDICATIONS

- No drug treatment is fully satisfactory
- Everyone, even those mildly ill, should be treated with a 7–10 day course of quinine (650 mg three times a day) plus clindamycin (1.2 g twice daily intravenously or 650 mg orally three times a day)
- A secondary mode of treatment is with azithromycin (500 mg twice daily for 3 days followed by 500 mg daily for 7 days) plus atovaquone (750 mg twice daily for 7–10 days)
- Exchange transfusion with antibiotics has been successful in several severely ill asplenic patients with parasitemia greater than 10%
- Management of *B divergens* infection can be attempted with exchange transfusion and clindamycin-quinine therapy

 ## OUTCOME

COMPLICATIONS

- Severe complications include acute respiratory, cardiac, and renal failure

PROGNOSIS

- Although parasitemia may continue for months, with or without symptoms, the disease is self-limited and, after several weeks or months, most patients recover without sequelae
- Splenectomized, older, or immunosuppressed persons are most likely to have severe manifestations; case fatality rates in the United States may reach 5%
- Splenectomized patients with *B divergens* infections have a death rate of over 40%

WHEN TO REFER

- Patients not responding to therapy

WHEN TO ADMIT

- All splenectomized, older, or immunosuppressed patients

 ## EVIDENCE

PRACTICE GUIDELINES

- National Guideline Clearinghouse http://www.guideline.gov/summary/summary.aspx?doc_id=2767&nbr=1993&string=tick+bites http://www.guideline.gov/summary/summary.aspx?doc_id=2672&nbr=1898&string=tick+bites

INFORMATION FOR PATIENTS

- American Academy of Family Physicians http://familydoctor.org/handouts/689.html
- American College of Emergency Physicians http://www.acep.org/1,2737,0.html

REFERENCES

- Krause PJ: Babesiosis. Med Clin North Am 2002;86:361. [PMID: 11982307]
- Krause PJ et al: Disease-specific diagnosis of coinfecting tickborne zoonoses: babesiosis, human granulocytic ehrlichiosis, and Lyme disease. Clin Infect Dis 2002;34:1184. [PMID: 11941544]
- Ranque S: The treatment of babesiosis. N Engl J Med 2000;343:1454. [PMID 11236790]

Baldness

KEY FEATURES

ESSENTIALS OF DIAGNOSIS

Forms of hair loss

- Baldness due to scarring (cicatricial baldness)
- Baldness not due to scarring
- Androgenetic (male pattern) baldness
- Telogen effluvium
- Alopecia areata
- Drug-induced alopecia
- Trichotillomania (the pulling out of one's own hair)

GENERAL CONSIDERATIONS

Baldness due to scarring

- Irreversible and permanent, thus it is important to treat the scarring process as early as possible
- May occur following chemical or physical trauma, lichen planopilaris, severe bacterial or fungal infections, severe herpes zoster, chronic discoid lupus erythematosus, scleroderma, and excessive ionizing radiation
- The specific cause is often suggested by the history, the distribution of hair loss, and the appearance of the skin, as in lupus erythematosus

Baldness not due to scarring

- Nonscarring alopecia may occur in association with various systemic diseases such as systemic lupus erythematosus, secondary syphilis, hyper- or hypothyroidism, iron deficiency anemia, and pituitary insufficiency

Androgenetic baldness

- The most common form of alopecia is of genetic predetermination

Telogen effluvium

- A transitory increase in the number of hairs in the telogen (resting) phase of the hair growth cycle
- May occur spontaneously, may appear at the termination of pregnancy, may be precipitated by "crash dieting," high fever, stress from surgery or shock, or malnutrition, or may be provoked by hormonal contraceptives
- Latent period of 2–4 months
- The prognosis is generally good
- A major important cause is iron deficiency

Alopecia areata

- Unknown cause but is believed to be an immunological process
- Occasionally associated with Hashimoto's thyroiditis, pernicious anemia, Addison's disease, and vitiligo

Drug-induced alopecia

- Becoming increasingly important
- Incriminated drugs include thallium, excessive and prolonged use of vitamin A, retinoids, antimitotic agents, anticoagulants, antithyroid drugs, oral contraceptives, trimethadione, allopurinol, propranolol, indomethacin, amphetamines, salicylates, gentamicin, and levodopa
- While chemotherapy-induced alopecia is very distressing, it must be emphasized to the patient before treatment that it is invariably reversible

CLINICAL FINDINGS

SYMPTOMS AND SIGNS

Androgenetic baldness

- The earliest changes occur at the anterior portions of the calvarium on either side of the "widow's peak" and on the crown (vertex) of the skull
- The extent of hair loss is variable and unpredictable
- Occurs in both women and men

Alopecia areata

- Typically, there are patches that are perfectly smooth and without scarring
- Tiny hairs 2–3 mm in length, called "exclamation hairs," may be seen
- Telogen hairs are easily dislodged from the periphery of active lesions
- The beard, brows, and lashes may be involved
- Involvement may extend to all of the scalp hair (alopecia totalis) or to all scalp and body hair (alopecia universalis)

Trichotillomania

- The patches of hair loss are irregular and growing hairs are always present, since they cannot be pulled out until they are long enough

DIFFERENTIAL DIAGNOSIS

- Scarring (cicatricial)
  - Chemical or physical trauma
  - Lichen planopilaris

  - Bacterial or fungal infection (severe)
  - Herpes zoster (shingles) (severe)
  - Discoid lupus erythematosus
  - Scleroderma
  - Excessive ionizing radiation
- Nonscarring
  - Androgenic (male pattern) baldness
  - Telogen effluvium
  - Alopecia areata
  - Trichotillomania
  - Drug-induced alopecia (eg, thallium, excessive vitamin A, retinoids, chemotherapy, anticoagulants, antithyroid drugs, oral contraceptives, trimethadione, allopurinol, propranolol, indomethacin, amphetamines, salicylates, gentamicin, levodopa)
  - Systemic lupus erythematosus
  - Secondary syphilis
  - Hyperthyroidism
  - Hypothyroidism
  - Iron deficiency anemia
  - Pituitary insufficiency

DIAGNOSIS

LABORATORY TESTS

- Hair loss in women
- Serum testosterone, DHEAS, iron, total iron-binding capacity, and thyroid function tests and a complete blood cell count will identify most other causes of hair thinning in premenopausal women

Telogen effluvium

- Diagnosed by the presence of large numbers of hairs with white bulbs coming out upon gentle tugging
- Counts of hairs lost on combing or shampooing often exceed 150 per day, compared to an average of 70–100

DIAGNOSTIC PROCEDURES

- Biopsy is useful in the diagnosis of scarring alopecia, but specimens must be taken from the active border and not from the scarred central zone

Bacteremia, *Salmonella* p. 1067. Bacteremia, Staphylococcal p. 1068. Bacterial Overgrowth, Small Intestine p. 1068. Balantidiasis p. 1069.

 Baldness

 # TREATMENT

MEDICATIONS

Androgenetic baldness

- Rogaine extra strength
  - Solution containing 50 mg/mL of minoxidil; available over the counter; best results achieved in persons with recent onset (<5 years) and smaller areas of alopecia
  - Approximately 40% of patients treated twice daily for a year will have moderate to dense growth
- Finasteride (Propecia): 1 mg orally daily, has similar efficacy to Rogaine and may be additive to minoxidil; used only in males

Hair loss or thinning in women

- May be treated with minoxidil

Alopecia areata

- Intralesional corticosteroids are frequently effective
- Triamcinolone acetonide in a concentration of 2.5–10 mg/mL is injected in aliquots of 0.1 mL at approximately 1- to 2-cm intervals, not exceeding a total dose of 30 mg per month for adults
- Alternatively, anthralin 0.5% ointment used daily, may help some patients

THERAPEUTIC PROCEDURES

Baldness not due to scarring

- The only treatment necessary is prompt and adequate control of the underlying disorder, in which case hair loss may be reversible

Alopecia areata

- Alopecia areata is usually self-limiting, with complete regrowth of hair in 80% of patients, but some mild cases are resistant
- Support groups for patients with extensive alopecia areata are very beneficial

 # OUTCOME

FOLLOW-UP

- Women who complain of thin hair but show little evidence of alopecia need follow-up, because more than 50% of the scalp hair can be lost before the clinician can perceive it

COMPLICATIONS

- Scarring alopecia can be very disfiguring

WHEN TO REFER

- All scarring alopecias except clearly diagnosed discoid lupus erythematosis and posttraumatic
- Diagnosis and management questions

 # EVIDENCE

PRACTICE GUIDELINES

- Drake LA et al: Guidelines of care for androgenetic alopecia. J Am Acad Dermatol 1996;35(3 Pt 1):465.
- American Academy of Dermatology http://www.aadassociation.org/Guidelines/areata.html

WEB SITES

- American Academy of Dermatology http://www.aad.org
- An Introduction to Basic Dermatology http://www.vh.org/Providers/Lectures/PietteDermatology/BasicDermatology.html
- Dermatology Handbook for Family Practice from the University of Iowa http://www.vh.org/Providers/ClinRef/FPHandbook/17.html

INFORMATION FOR PATIENTS

- American Academy of Dermatology http://www.aad.org/pamphlets/
- Mayo Clinic http://www.mayoclinic.com/invoke.cfm?id=DS00278

REFERENCES

- Bertolino AP: Alopecia areata. A clinical overview. Postgrad Med 2000;107:81. [PMID: 10887448]
- Madani S et al: Alopecia areata update. J Am Acad Dermatol 2000;42:549. [PMID: 10727299]
- Price VH: Treatment of hair loss. N Engl J Med 1999;341:964. [PMID: 10498493]

Timothy G. Berger, MD

Basal Cell Carcinoma

 KEY FEATURES

ESSENTIALS OF DIAGNOSIS

- Slow-growing lesions
- Pearly or translucent appearance
- Telangiectatic vessels easily visible

GENERAL CONSIDERATIONS

- Most common form of cancer
- They occur on sun-exposed skin in otherwise normal fair-skinned individuals
- Clinicians should examine the skin routinely, looking for bumps, patches, and scabbed lesions

 CLINICAL FINDINGS

SYMPTOMS AND SIGNS

- The most common presentation is a papule or nodule that may have a scab or erosion
- Occasionally the nodules have a brown-gray color or have stippled pigment (pigmented basal cell carcinoma)
- Grow slowly, attaining a size of 1–2 cm or more in diameter, often after years of growth
- There is a waxy, "pearly" appearance, with telangiectatic vessels easily visible
- Pearly or translucent quality of the lesions is most diagnostic, a feature best appreciated if the skin is stretched
- Less common types include morpheaform or scar-like lesions; these are hypopigmented, somewhat thickened plaques
- On the back and chest, basal cell carcinomas appear as reddish, somewhat shiny, scaly plaques
- When examining the face, look at the eyelid margins and medial canthi, the nose and alar folds, the lips, and then around and behind the ears
- Basal cell carcinomas of the medial canthi are particularly dangerous

DIFFERENTIAL DIAGNOSIS

- Squamous cell carcinoma
- Actinic keratosis
- Intradermal nevi
- Fibrous papule of the nose
- Seborrheic keratosis (unpigmented type)
- Sebaceous (epidermal inclusion) cyst
- Sebaceous hyperplasia
- Keratoacanthoma
- Molluscum contagiosum
- Melanoma
- Paget's disease

 DIAGNOSIS

DIAGNOSTIC PROCEDURES

- Lesions suspected to be basal cell carcinomas should be biopsied, by shave or punch biopsy
- Biopsy confirms the diagnosis

Basal Cell Carcinoma

 ## TREATMENT

MEDICATIONS

- Imiquimod cream 5% three times a week for 10 weeks may be effective for nonfacial, superficial (by biopsy) basal cell cancers

SURGERY

- Therapy is aimed at eradication with minimal cosmetic deformity, often by excision and suturing with recurrence rates of 5% or less
- The technique of three cycles of curettage and electrodesiccation depends on the skill of the operator and is not recommended for head and neck lesions
- After 4–6 weeks of healing, it leaves a broad, hypopigmented, at times hypertrophic scar
- Mohs surgery—removal of the tumor followed by immediate frozen section histopathological examination of margins with subsequent reexcision of tumor-positive areas and final closure of the defect—gives the highest cure rates (98%) and results in least tissue loss

THERAPEUTIC PROCEDURES

- Radiotherapy is effective and sometimes appropriate for older individuals (over 65), but recurrent tumors after radiation therapy are more difficult to treat and may be more aggressive

 ## OUTCOME

FOLLOW-UP

- Patients must be followed for the first 1 to 2 years to detect new or recurrent lesions

COMPLICATIONS

- Neglected lesions may ulcerate and produce great destruction

PROGNOSIS

- Metastases almost never occur
- Most recurrences appear in the first 1 to 2 years
- Recurrent lesions around the nose and ears may track along cartilage underneath the skin, requiring treatment of much more extensive areas than are apparent from inspection

WHEN TO REFER

- If confirmation of the need for biopsy is required or to perform biopsy

PREVENTION

- Sun avoidance, particularly in children, is essential to lower the incidence of new basal cell cancers

EVIDENCE

PRACTICE GUIDELINES

- National Guideline Clearinghouse http://www.guideline.gov/summary/summary.aspx?doc_id=2662&nbr=1888&string=basal+cell+carcinoma
- The National Comprehensive Cancer Network (NCCN). Miller SJ: Guidelines of care for nonmelanoma skin cancers. Dermatol Surg 2000; 26(3):289.

WEB SITES

- American Academy of Dermatology http://www.aad.org
- An Introduction to Basic Dermatology http://www.vh.org/Providers/Lectures/PietteDermatology/BasicDermatology.html
- Dermatology Handbook for Family Practice from the University of Iowa http://www.vh.org/Providers/ClinRef/FPHandbook/17.html

INFORMATION FOR PATIENTS

- American Academy of Dermatology http://www.aad.org/pamphlets/
- JAMA patient page: Skin cancer. JAMA 1999;281(7):676.

REFERENCES

- Garner KL et al: Basal and squamous cell carcinoma. Prim Care 2000;27:447. [PMID: 10815054]
- Jerant AF et al: Early detection and treatment of skin cancer. Am Fam Physician 2000;62:357. [PMID: 10929700]

Timothy G. Berger, MD

Bell's Palsy

 ## KEY FEATURES

ESSENTIALS OF DIAGNOSIS

- Sudden onset of lower motor neuron facial palsy
- May have hyperacusis or impaired taste
- No other neurological abnormalities

GENERAL CONSIDERATIONS

- Idiopathic lower motor neuron facial paresis
- Attributed to an inflammatory reaction of the facial nerve near the stylomastoid foramen or in the bony facial canal
- Reactivation of herpes simplex virus has been postulated

 ## CLINICAL FINDINGS

SYMPTOMS AND SIGNS

- Generally comes on abruptly, but it may worsen over one or two days
- Pain about the ear often precedes or accompanies the weakness but usually lasts for only a few days
- There may be ipsilateral restriction of eye closure and difficulty with eating and fine facial movements
- A disturbance of taste is common, owing to involvement of chorda tympani fibers, and hyperacusis due to involvement of fibers to the stapedius occurs occasionally

DIFFERENTIAL DIAGNOSIS

- HIV-related facial neuropathies
- Lyme disease
- Sarcoidosis
- Ramsay Hunt syndrome (herpes zoster of geniculate ganglion)
- Acoustic neuroma
- Acute or chronic otitis media
- Malignant otitis externa
- Guillain-Barré syndrome
- Tumor, eg, parotid, temporal bone tumor
- Brainstem infarct

 ## DIAGNOSIS

- The clinical features are characteristic
- Electromyography and nerve excitability or conduction studies provide a guide to prognosis

LABORATORY TESTS

- To exclude other causes of facial neuropathy (see Differential Diagnosis)

TREATMENT

MEDICATIONS

- The only medical treatment that may influence the outcome is administration of corticosteroids with or without acyclovir, but studies supporting this approach have been criticized
- Many clinicians nevertheless routinely prescribe corticosteroids for patients seen within 5 days of onset. Others prescribe them only when the palsy is clinically complete or there is severe pain
- Treatment with prednisone, 60 or 80 mg daily in divided doses for 4 or 5 days, followed by tapering of the dose over the next 7–10 days, is a satisfactory regimen
- It is helpful to protect the eye with lubricating drops (or lubricating ointment at night) and a patch if eye closure is not possible

SURGERY

- There is no evidence that surgical procedures to decompress the facial nerve are of benefit

THERAPEUTIC PROCEDURES

- The management is controversial
- Approximately 60% recover completely without treatment. Considerable improvement occurs in most other cases, and only about 10% of all patients have permanent disfigurement or other long-term sequelae
- Treatment is unnecessary in most cases but is indicated when an unsatisfactory outcome can be predicted. The best clinical guide to progress is the severity of the palsy during the first few days after presentation

 OUTCOME

PROGNOSIS

- Patients with clinically complete palsy when first seen are less likely to make a full recovery than those with an incomplete one
- A poor prognosis for recovery is also associated with advanced age, hyperacusis, and severe initial pain

 EVIDENCE

PRACTICE GUIDELINES

- Grogan PM et al: Practice parameter: steroids, acyclovir, and surgery for Bell's palsy (an evidenced-based review): report of the Quality Standards Subcommittee of the American Academy of Neurology. Neurology 2001;56:830. [PMID: 11294918]

INFORMATION FOR PATIENTS

- National Institute of Neurological Disorders and Stroke http://www.ninds.nih.gov/health_and_medical/disorders/ bells_doc.htm
- American Academy of Otolaryngology —Head and Neck Surgery http://www.entnet.org/healthinfo/ topics/bells.cfm

REFERENCE

- Ramsey MJ et al: Corticosteroid treatment for idiopathic facial nerve paralysis: a meta-analysis. Laryngoscope 2000;110:335. [PMID: 10718415]

Michael J. Aminoff, DSc, MD, FRCP

Benign Prostatic Hyperplasia

 KEY FEATURES

ESSENTIALS OF DIAGNOSIS

- Obstructive or irritative voiding symptoms
- May have enlarged prostate on rectal examination
- Absence of urinary tract infection, neurological disorder, stricture disease, prostatic or bladder malignancy

GENERAL CONSIDERATIONS

- Smooth, firm, elastic enlargement of the prostate

Etiology

- Multifactorial
- Endocrine: dihydrotestosterone (DHT)
- Aging

DEMOGRAPHICS

- The most common benign tumor in men
- Incidence is age related
- Prevalence: ~20% in men aged 41–50; ~50% in men aged 51–60; >90% in men aged 80 and older
- Symptoms are also age related: at age 55, ~25% of men report obstructive voiding symptoms

 CLINICAL FINDINGS

SYMPTOMS AND SIGNS

- Can be divided into obstructive and irritative complaints
- Obstructive symptoms: hesitancy, decreased force and caliber of stream, sensation of incomplete bladder emptying, double voiding (urinating a second time within 2 h), straining to urinate, and postvoid dribbling
- Irritative symptoms: urgency, frequency, and nocturia
- American Urological Association (AUA) Symptom Index (Table 86A, page 1271) should be calculated for all patients starting therapy
- Seven questions quantitate the severity of obstructive or irritative complaints on a scale of 0–5. Thus, the score can range from 0 to 35

DIFFERENTIAL DIAGNOSIS

- Prostate cancer, urinary tract infection, neurogenic bladder, or urethral stricture

 DIAGNOSIS

DIAGNOSTIC PROCEDURES

- History to exclude other possible causes of symptoms
- Physical examination, digital rectal examination (DRE), and a focused neurological examination
- DRE: note size and consistency of the prostate
- Examine lower abdomen for a distended bladder
- If possibility of cancer, further evaluation is needed by serum prostate-specific antigen (PSA), transrectal ultrasound, and biopsy

TREATMENT

MEDICATIONS

- α-Blockers
  - Prazosin 1 mg PO QHS for 3 nights, increasing to 1 mg PO BID and then titrating up to 2 mg PO BID if necessary
  - Terazosin 1 mg PO QD for 3 days, increasing to 2 mg PO QD for 11 days, then 5–10 mg PO QD if necessary
  - Doxazosin 1 mg PO QD for 7 days, increasing to 2 mg PO QD for 7 days, then 4–8 mg PO QD if necessary
  - Tamsulosin 0.4 mg PO QD, increased to 0.8 mg PO QD if necessary
- 5α-Reductase inhibitors
  - Finasteride 5 mg PO QD—6 months of therapy required for maximum effects on prostate size (20% reduction) and symptomatic improvement
- Combination therapy
  - α-Blocker and 5α-reductase inhibitor

SURGERY

- Indicated for refractory urinary retention (failing at least one attempt at catheter removal), large bladder diverticula, recurrent urinary tract infection, recurrent gross hematuria, bladder stones, or renal insufficiency
- Transurethral resection of the prostate (TURP): operative complications include bleeding, urethral stricture or bladder neck contracture, perforation of the prostate capsule with extravasation, and transurethral resection syndrome, a hypervolemic, hyponatremic state resulting from the absorption of the hypotonic irrigating solution. Postoperative complications include retrograde ejaculation (75%), impotence (5–10%), and urinary incontinence (<1%)
- Transurethral incision of the prostate (TUIP)—lower rate of retrograde ejaculation reported (25%)
- Open simple prostatectomy—when prostate is too large to remove endoscopically (>100 g), concomitant bladder diverticulum, bladder stone, when dorsal lithotomy positioning is not possible

Minimally invasive

- Laser therapy—(Nd:YAG) and holmium-YAG lasers used
- TULIP (transurethral laser-induced prostatectomy) under transrectal ultrasound guidance
- Visually directed laser techniques under cystoscopic control
- Interstitial laser therapy usually under cystoscopic control
- Advantages to laser surgery include outpatient surgery, minimal blood loss, rare occurrence of transurethral resection syndrome, and ability to treat patients while on anticoagulation therapy. Disadvantages include lack of tissue for pathological examination, longer postoperative catheterization time, more frequent irritative voiding complaints, and expense of laser fibers and generators
- Transurethral needle ablation of the prostate (TUNA)
- Transurethral electrovaporization of the prostate
- Hyperthermia—microwave thermotherapy
- High-intensity focused ultrasound (HIFU)
- Intraurethral stents

THERAPEUTIC PROCEDURES

- Watchful waiting: only for patients with mild symptoms (AUA scores 0–7)
- With watchful waiting, ~10% progress to urinary retention, and half demonstrate marked improvement or resolution of symptoms

OUTCOME

FOLLOW-UP

- Follow American Urological Association Symptom Index for benign prostatic hyperplasia (Table 86A, page 1271)

EVIDENCE

PRACTICE GUIDELINES

- AUA Practice Guidelines Committee. AUA guideline on management of benign prostatic hyperplasia (2003). Chapter 1: Diagnosis and treatment recommendations. J Urol 2003;170(2 Pt 1):530. [PMID: 12853821]

WEB SITE

- National Cancer Institute—Understanding prostate changes: a health guide for all men http://www.cancer.gov/cancerinfo/understanding-prostate-changes/page3

INFORMATION FOR PATIENTS

- MEDLINEplus—Benign prostatic hyperplasia http://www.nlm.nih.gov/medlineplus/ency/article/000381.htm

REFERENCES

- Arai Y et al: Impact of interventional therapy for benign prostatic hyperplasia on quality of life and sexual function: a prospective study. J Urol 2000;164:1206. [PMID: 10992367]
- Djavan B et al: Prospective randomized comparison of high energy transurethral microwave thermotherapy versus alpha-blocker treatment of patients with benign prostatic hyperplasia. J Urol 1999;161:139. [PMID: 10037386]
- Medina JJ et al: Benign prostatic hyperplasia (the aging prostate). Med Clin North Am 1999;83:1213. [PMID: 10503061]
- Wilde MI et al: Finasteride: an update of its use in the management of symptomatic benign prostatic hyperplasia. Drugs 1999;57:557. [PMID: 10235693]

Marshall L. Stoller, MD
Peter R. Carroll, MD

Biliary Tract Carcinoma

 ## KEY FEATURES

ESSENTIALS OF DIAGNOSIS

- Presents with obstructive jaundice, usually painless, often with dilated biliary tree
- Pain is more common in gallbladder carcinoma than cholangiocarcinoma
- A Courvoisier (dilated) gallbladder may be detected
- In general, the prognosis is poor, with few patients surviving for more than 12 months after surgery

GENERAL CONSIDERATIONS

Gallbladder carcinoma

- The diagnosis is often made unexpectedly at surgery
- Spread of the cancer—by direct extension into the liver or to the peritoneal surface—may be the initial manifestation
- Cholelithiasis (often large, symptomatic stones) is usually present
- **Risk factors**
- Chronic infection of the gallbladder with *Salmonella typhi*
- Gallbladder polyps over 1 cm in diameter
- Mucosal calcification of the gallbladder (porcelain gallbladder)
- Anomalous pancreaticobiliary ductal junction
- **TNM classification**
- Tis, carcinoma in situ
- T1, invasion of the subepithelial fibro-(muscular) connective tissue
- T2, invasion beyond the wall of the bile duct
- T3, invasion of branches of the portal vein (right or left), hepatic artery, or liver
- T4, invasion of the main portal vein, common hepatic artery, and/or regional organs

Carcinoma of the bile ducts (cholangiocarcinoma)

- Two-thirds arise at the confluence of the hepatic ducts (Klatskin tumors), and one-fourth arise in the distal extrahepatic bile duct; the remainder are intrahepatic
- Staging is similar to that for carcinoma of the gallbladder
- There is an increased incidence with ulcerative colitis, especially with primary sclerosing cholangitis

- In southeast Asia, infection of the bile ducts with helminths (*Clonorchis sinensis, Opisthorchis viverrini, Fasciola hepatica*) is associated with chronic cholangitis and an increased risk of cholangiocarcinoma

DEMOGRAPHICS

Carcinoma of the bile ducts

- Accounts for 3% of all cancer deaths in the United States, and the incidence and mortality rates have increased dramatically in the past 2 decades
- Affects both sexes equally but is more prevalent in individuals aged 50–70
- Found in approximately 2% of people operated on for biliary tract disease

 ## CLINICAL FINDINGS

SYMPTOMS AND SIGNS

- Progressive jaundice is the most common symptom
- Pain in the right upper abdomen with radiation into the back is usually present early in the course of gallbladder carcinoma, but this occurs later in the course of bile duct carcinoma
- Anorexia and weight loss are common and often associated with fever and chills due to cholangitis
- Rarely, hematemesis or melena results from erosion of tumor into a blood vessel (hemobilia). Fistula formation between the biliary system and adjacent organs may also occur
- The course is usually one of rapid deterioration, with death occurring within a few months
- A palpable gallbladder with obstructive jaundice usually is said to signify malignant disease (Courvoisier's law); however, this clinical generalization has proved to be only 50% accurate
- Hepatomegaly is usually present and is associated with liver tenderness
- Ascites may occur with peritoneal implants
- Pruritus and skin excoriations

DIFFERENTIAL DIAGNOSIS

- Biliary stricture
- Hepatocellular or pancreatic carcinoma
- Primary sclerosing cholangitis
- Primary biliary cirrhosis
- Choledocholithiasis

 ## DIAGNOSIS

LABORATORY TESTS

- Predominantly conjugated hyperbilirubinemia, with total serum bilirubin values ranging from 5 to 30 mg/dL
- There is usually concomitant elevation of the alkaline phosphatase and serum cholesterol. Aspartate aminotransferase is normal or minimally elevated
- An elevated CA 19-9 level may help distinguish cholangiocarcinoma from a benign biliary stricture (in the absence of cholangitis)

IMAGING STUDIES

- Ultrasonography and CT may show a gallbladder mass in gallbladder carcinoma and intrahepatic mass or biliary dilation in carcinoma of the bile ducts CT may also show involved regional lymph nodes
- MRI with magnetic resonance cholangiopancreatography permits visualization of the biliary tree and detection of vascular invasion and obviates the need for angiography
- Positron emission tomography (PET) may detect cholangiocarcinomas as small as 1 cm

DIAGNOSTIC PROCEDURES

- The most helpful diagnostic studies before surgery are either percutaneous transhepatic or endoscopic retrograde cholangiography with biopsy and cytological specimens, though false-negative biopsy and cytology results are common
- Fine-needle aspiration of tumors under endoscopic ultrasonographic guidance, choledochoscopy, and intraductal ultrasonography has a potential role in the diagnosis of cholangiocarcinoma

Biliary Tract Carcinoma

TREATMENT

MEDICATIONS

- There is limited response to chemotherapy such as with gemcitabine

SURGERY

- In young and fit patients, curative surgery may be attempted if the tumor is well localized
- If the tumor is unresectable at laparotomy, cholecystoduodenostomy or T-tube drainage of the common duct can be performed
- Although cholangiocarcinoma is generally considered a contraindication to liver transplantation because of rapid tumor recurrence, a 60% 5-year survival rate has been reported in patients with a single peripheral cholangiocarcinoma undergoing either transplantation or resection, with clear resection margins and no lymph node involvement

THERAPEUTIC PROCEDURES

- When disease progresses despite treatment, meticulous efforts at palliative care are essential
- Palliation can be achieved by placement of a self-expandable metal stent via the endoscopic or percutaneous transhepatic route. Plastic stents are less expensive but more prone to occlude than metal ones; they are suitable for patients expected to survive only a few months
- There may be a role for palliative photodynamic therapy. Radiotherapy may relieve pain and contribute to biliary decompression

OUTCOME

PROGNOSIS

- The 5-year survival rate for localized carcinoma of the gallbladder (stage 1, T1a, N0, M0) is as high as 80% with laparoscopic cholecystectomy but drops to 15%, even with a more extended open resection, if there is muscular invasion (T1b)
- Carcinoma of the bile ducts is curable by surgery in less than 10% of cases

PREVENTION

- The frequency of carcinoma with choledochal cysts is over 14% at 20 years, and surgical excision is recommended

EVIDENCE

PRACTICE GUIDELINES

- Khan SA et al: British Society of Gastroenterology. Guidelines for the diagnosis and treatment of cholangiocarcinoma: consensus document. Gut 2002;51(Suppl 6):VI1.

WEB SITE

- Carcinoma of the Ampulla of Vater Demonstration Case http://www.brighamrad.harvard.edu/ Cases/bwh/hcache/43/full.html

INFORMATION FOR PATIENTS

- National Institutes of Health http://www.nlm.nih.gov/medlineplus/ ency/article/000291.htm http://www.cancer.gov/cancerinfo/pdq/ treatment/gallbladder/patient

REFERENCES

- Abraham NS et al: Palliation of malignant biliary obstruction: a prospective trial examining impact on quality of life. Gastrointest Endosc 2002;56:835.
- Jarnagin WR et al: Staging, resectability, and outcome in 225 patients with hilar cholangiocarcinoma. Ann Surg 2001;234:507. [PMID: 11573044]
- Watanapa P et al: Liver-fluke-associated cholangiocarcinoma. Br J Surg 2002;89:962.

Lawrence S. Friedman, MD

Bipolar Disorder

 ## KEY FEATURES

ESSENTIALS OF DIAGNOSIS

- Episodic mood shifts into mania, major depression, hypomania, and mixed states

For manic episodes

- Mood ranging from euphoria to irritability
- Sleep disruption
- Hyperactivity
- Racing thoughts
- Grandiosity
- Variable psychotic symptoms

Present in most depressions

- Lowered mood, varying from mild sadness to intense feelings of guilt, worthlessness, and hopelessness
- Difficulty in thinking, including inability to concentrate, ruminations, and lack of decisiveness
- Loss of interest, with diminished involvement in work and recreation
- Somatic complaints such as headache; disrupted, lessened, or excessive sleep; loss of energy; change in appetite; decreased sexual drive
- Anxiety

Present in some severe depressions

- Psychomotor retardation or agitation
- Delusions of a hypochondriacal or persecutory nature
- Withdrawal from activities
- Physical symptoms of major severity, eg, anorexia, insomnia, reduced sexual drive, weight loss, and various somatic complaints
- Suicidal ideation

GENERAL CONSIDERATIONS

- Manic episodes begin abruptly and may be triggered by life stresses
- Manic episodes last days to months—generally shorter than depressive episodes
- Manic episodes are most common in spring and summer months

Cyclothymia

- Chronic mood disturbances with episodes of depression and hypomania
- Symptoms are milder than those in a manic or depressive episode, but have at least a 2-year duration
- Symptoms will occasionally escalate to a full-blown manic or depressive episode, warranting a diagnosis of bipolar I or bipolar II disorder

 ## CLINICAL FINDINGS

SYMPTOMS AND SIGNS

Manic episodes

- Overinvolvement in life activities
- Flight of ideas with distractibility
- Little need for sleep
- Behaviors may initially attract others
- Irritability, mood lability, aggression, and grandiosity usually lead to problems in relationships
- Excessive spending, resignation from a job, a hasty marriage or divorce, sexual acting out, or exhibitionism may occur
- Atypical episodes involve gross delusions, paranoid ideations, and auditory hallucinations
- "Rapid cyclers" experience four or more discrete episodes of mood disturbance per year

DIFFERENTIAL DIAGNOSIS

- Schizophrenia and other psychotic disorders
- Intoxication with stimulants
- Major depressive episode
- Hypothryoidism
- Dysthymia

 ## DIAGNOSIS

LABORATORY TESTS

- Consider thyroid-stimulating hormone
- Consider toxicology screen

TREATMENT

MEDICATIONS

For mania

- Haloperidol (5–10 mg PO or IM Q 2–3 h)
- Alternatively, atypical neuroleptics (olanzapine 5–20 mg QD) may be used initially to treat agitation and psychosis
- Clonazepam (1–2 mg PO Q 4–6 h) may be used in lieu of or in conjunction with a neuroleptic to control acute behavioral symptoms
- Lithium (1200–1800 mg/day targeted to therapeutic serum level) is effective in acute mania or hypomania, but takes several days to take effect. As prophylaxis, it can limit the frequency and severity of mood swings in 70% of patients
- Valproic acid (750 mg/day divided and titrated to therapeutic levels) can be loaded to therapeutic levels in 2–3 days
- Carbamazepine (800–1600 mg/day) is used in patients intolerant or unresponsive to lithium. It is also more effective than lithium in rapid cyclers
- Calcium channel blockers (verapamil) have been used in refractory patients
- Anticonvulsants such as lamotrigine (25–50 mg/day titrated slowly upward) and topiramate are beginning to be used

For depression

- See *Depression*

THERAPEUTIC PROCEDURES

- Electroconvulsive therapy is effective in treatment of manic disorders in pregnant women, where medications are contraindicated

OUTCOME

FOLLOW-UP

- Lithium levels should be measured 5–7 days after initiation and dose changes, monthly to bimonthly early in treatment, and Q 6–12 months in stable patients
- Thyroid and kidney function should be monitored Q 3–4 months in patients on lithium
- Liver function and blood counts must be monitored in patients taking valproic acid or carbamazepine

COMPLICATIONS

- Suicide (see *Depression*)
- Drug-drug interactions complicate therapy with all agents—careful review of concomitant medications is needed
- Lithium toxicity occurs at serum levels >2 mEq/L (see *Lithium toxicity*)
- Long-term lithium use can cause cogwheel rigidity and other extrapyramidal signs

PROGNOSIS

- Good prognosis with adequate treatment
- Compliance with lithium is adversely affected by the loss of some hypomanic experiences valued by the patient

WHEN TO REFER

- When diagnosis is in question or when standard management strategies are inefffective
- Any question of suicidiality or irrational behavior

WHEN TO ADMIT

- In a depressive episode, patients must be admitted when there is risk of suicide or self-harm
- Manic patients should be admitted when their judgment is sufficiently impaired to make them a risk to themselves or others

EVIDENCE

PRACTICE GUIDELINES

- National Guideline Clearinghouse http://www.guideline.gov/summary/summary.aspx?doc_id=3302&nbr=2528&string=bipolar+disorder

WEB SITES

- American Psychiatric Association http://www.psych.org/
- Internet Mental Health http://www.mentalhealth.com/t30.html
- Psychopharmacology Tips http://www.dr-bob.org/tips/
- Psychiatry On Line http://www.priory.com/psych.htm

INFORMATION FOR PATIENTS

- JAMA patient page: Depression. JAMA 2000;284:1606.
- National Institute of Mental Health http://www.nimh.nih.gov/publicat/bipolar.cfm

REFERENCES

- Viguera AC et al: Reproductive decisions by women with bipolar disorder after prepregnancy psychiatric consultation. Am J Psychiatry 2002;159:2102.
- Young LT et al: Double-blind comparison of addition of second mood stabilizer versus an anti-depressant to an initial mood stabilizer for treatment of patients with bipolar depression. Am J Psychiatry 2000;157:124. [PMID: 10618026]

Stuart J. Eisendrath, MD
Jonathan E. Lichtmacher, MD

Bites, Animal & Human

 KEY FEATURES

ESSENTIALS OF DIAGNOSIS

- Cat and human bites are more likely to become infected than dog bites
- Bites to the hand are of special concern because of the possiblity of closed-space infection
- Antibiotic prophylaxis indicated for noninfected bites of the hand and hospitalization required for infected hand bites
- All infected wounds need to be cultured to direct therapy

GENERAL CONSIDERATIONS

- Biting animals are usually known by their victims, and most biting incidents are provoked (ie, bites occur while playing with the animal or after surprising the animal or waking it abruptly from sleep)
- Failure to elicit a history of provocation is important, because an unprovoked attack raises the possibility of rabies
- **Human bites** are usually inflicted by children while playing or fighting; in adults, bites are associated with alcohol use and closed-fist injuries that occur during fights
- The animal inflicting the bite, the location of the bite, and the type of injury inflicted are all important determinants of whether they become infected
- **Cat bites** are more likely to become infected than human bites—between 30% and 50% of all cat bites become infected
- Infections following human bites are variable. Those inflicted by children rarely become infected, because they are superficial; and bites by adults become infected in 15–30% of cases, with a particularly high rate of infection in closed-fist injuries
- **Dog bites,** for unclear reasons, become infected only 5% of the time
- Bites of the head, face, and neck are less likely to become infected than bites on the extremities
- **Puncture wounds** become infected more frequently than lacerations, probably because the latter are easier to irrigate and debride
- The bacteriology of bite infections depends on the biting animal and when the infection occurs after the biting incident
- Early infections (within 24 h after the bite) following dog and cat bites are most frequently caused by *Pasteurella multocida*
- Early infections following human bites are usually caused by mixed aerobic and anaerobic mouth flora. Late infections (longer than 24 h after the bite) are caused mainly by staphylococci, streptococci, and anaerobes (*Fusobacterium, Bacteroides, Prevotella*), but innumerable organisms have been implicated. *Capnocytophaga canimorsus* (formerly called a DF2 organism), a gram-negative organism that is part of canine oral flora; *Eikenella corrodens*, another gram-negative organism that can be part of human mouth flora and has been recovered in up to 25% of infections following human bites; *Haemophilus* species, *Pseudomonas* species, and other gram-negative organisms—all have been implicated in bite infections
- There have been no documented cases of HIV transmission by human bites

DEMOGRAPHICS

- About 900 dog bite injuries require emergency department attention each day, most often in urban areas
- Dog bites occur most commonly in the summer months

 CLINICAL FINDINGS

SYMPTOMS AND SIGNS

Dog and cat bites

- Early infections (within 24 h after the bite) are characterized by rapid onset and progression, fever, chills, cellulitis, and local adenopathy

Human bites

- **Early infections** can produce a rapidly progressive necrotizing infection
- **Late infections** (longer than 24 h after the bite) present with local swelling and erythema. Drainage and systemic symptoms may or may not be present

 DIAGNOSIS

LABORATORY TESTS

- Because the bacteriology of the infections is so variable, always culture infected wounds and adjust therapy appropriately, especially if the patient is not responding to initial empirical treatment

IMAGING STUDIES

- X-rays should be obtained to look for fractures and the presence of foreign bodies

TREATMENT

MEDICATIONS

Prophylactic antibiotics

- Prophylaxis is indicated in high-risk bites, eg, cat bites in any location (dicloxacillin, 0.5 g orally four times a day for 3–5 days) and hand bites by any animal or by humans (penicillin V, 0.5 g orally four times a day for 3–5 days)
- Broader-spectrum agents include cefuroxime, amoxicillin-clavulanic acid, and, in the penicillin-allergic patient, clindamycin plus a fluoroquinolone
- Immunocompromised and asplenic patients are at risk for developing overwhelming bacteremia and sepsis following animal bites and should also receive prophylaxis, even for low-risk bites

Antibiotics

- Infected wounds require antibiotics, administered either orally or intravenously), depending on individualized clinical decisions
- *Pasteurella multocida* is best treated with penicillin or a tetracycline. Other active agents include second- and third-generation cephalosporins, fluoroquinolones, or azithromycin and clarithromycin. Response to therapy is slow, and therapy should be continued for at least 2–3 weeks
- Human bites frequently require intravenous therapy with a β-lactam plus a β-lactamase inhibitor combination (Unasyn, Timentin, Zosyn), a second-generation cephalosporin with anaerobic activity (cefoxitin, cefotetan, cefmetazole), or, in the penicillin-allergic patient, clindamycin plus a fluoroquinolone

THERAPEUTIC PROCEDURES

Local care

- Careful examination to assess the extent of the injury (tendon laceration, joint space penetration) is critical to appropriate care
- Vigorous cleansing and irrigation of the wound as well as debridement of necrotic material are the most important factors in decreasing the incidence of infections

Suturing

- If wounds require closure for cosmetic or mechanical reasons, suturing can be done
- Never suture an infected wound, and wounds of the hand should generally not be sutured since a closed-space infection of the hand can result in loss of function

OUTCOME

FOLLOW-UP

- Careful follow-up is requred every 1–2 days to assess improvement

COMPLICATIONS

- Osteomyelitis
- Tendon rupture
- Abscess

PROGNOSIS

- Generally good, but resolution may be slow, especially with *Pasteurella* infections

WHEN TO REFER

- Bites to the hand
- Failure to improve within 2–3 days

WHEN TO ADMIT

- Human bites to the hand are usually admitted to the hospital

PREVENTION

- All patients must be evaluated for the need for tetanus (Tables 127 and 128, pages 1310 and 1311) and rabies prophylaxis (see *Rabies*)

EVIDENCE

PRACTICE GUIDELINES

- Update on emerging infections from the Centers for Disease Control and Prevention. Update rabies postexposure prophylaxis guidelines. Ann Emerg Med 1999;33:590. [PMID: 10216339]

INFORMATION FOR PATIENTS

- The Mayo Clinic http://www.mayoclinic.com/invoke. cfm?id=FA00044 http://www.mayoclinic.com/invoke.cfm? id=FA00057

REFERENCES

- Medeiros I et al: Antibiotic prophylaxis for mammalian bites. Cochrane Database Syst Rev 2001;(2)CD001738. [PMID: 11406003]
- Smith PF et al: Treating mammalian bite wounds. J Clin Pharm Ther 2000;25:85. [PMID: 10849186]
- Talan DA et al: Bacteriologic analysis of infected dog and cat bites. N Engl J Med 1999;340:85. [PMID: 9887159]

Richard A. Jacobs, MD, PhD

Bites, Insect

KEY FEATURES

ESSENTIALS OF DIAGNOSIS

- Localized rash with pruritus
- Furuncle-like lesions containing live arthropods
- Tender erythematous patches that migrate ("larva migrans")
- Generalized urticaria or erythema multiforme in some patients

GENERAL CONSIDERATIONS

- Some arthropods (eg, most pest mosquitoes and biting flies) are readily detected as they bite, whereas in others reactions may be delayed for many hours; many are allergic
- Patients are most apt to consult a clinician when the lesions are multiple and pruritus is intense
- Body lice, fleas, bedbugs, and mosquitoes should be considered
- Spiders are often incorrectly believed to be the source of bites; they rarely attack humans, though the brown spider (*Loxosceles laeta*, *Loxosceles reclusa*) may cause severe necrotic reactions and death due to intravascular hemolysis, and the black widow spider (*Latrodectus mactans*) may cause severe systemic symptoms and death
- In addition to arthropod bites, the most common lesions are venomous stings (wasps, hornets, bees, ants, scorpions) or bites (centipedes), furuncle-like lesions due to fly maggots or sand fleas in the skin, and a linear creeping eruption due to a migrating larva
- Fleas: *Ctenocephalides felis* and *Ctenocephalides canis* are the most common species found on cats and dogs, and both species attack humans; the human flea is *Pulex irritans*
- Bedbugs: found in crevices of beds or furniture
- Ticks: usually picked up by brushing against low vegetation; ticks may transmit Rocky Mountain spotted fever, Lyme disease, relapsing fever, and ehrlichiosis (see separate diagnoses)
- Chiggers or red bugs are larvae of trombiculid mites
- Bird and rodent mites: larger than chiggers, bird mites infest pigeon lofts or nests of birds in eaves; bites are multiple anywhere on the body
- Mites in stored products
  - White and almost invisible; infest products such as vanilla pods, sugar, straw, cottonseeds, cereals
  - Persons who handle these products may be attacked, on the hands and forearms and sometimes on the feet
- Caterpillars of moths with urticating hairs: hairs are blown from cocoons or carried by emergent moths, causing severe and often seasonally recurrent outbreaks after mass emergence; the gypsy moth is a cause in eastern United States
- Tungiasis
  - Due to the burrowing flea known as *Tunga penetrans* and found in Africa, the West Indies, and South and Central America
  - The female burrows under the skin, sucks blood, swells to 0.5 cm, and then ejects her eggs onto the ground

CLINICAL FINDINGS

SYMPTOMS AND SIGNS

- Individual bites are often in clusters and tend to occur either on exposed parts (eg, midges and gnats) or under clothing, especially around the waist or at flexures (eg, small mites or insects in bedding or clothing)
- The reaction is often delayed for 1–24 h or more
- Pruritus is almost always present and may be all but intolerable once the patient starts to scratch
- Secondary infection may follow scratching
- Urticarial wheals are common; papules may become vesicular
- Flea saliva and bedbugs produce papular urticaria in sensitized individuals
- Chiggers or red bugs
  - A few species attack humans, often around the waist, on the ankles, or in flexures, raising intensely itching erythematous papules after a delay of many hours
  - The red chiggers may sometimes be seen in the center of papules that have not yet been scratched
- Tungiasis: ulceration, lymphangitis, gangrene, and septicemia may result, in some cases with lethal effect

DIFFERENTIAL DIAGNOSIS

- Scabies
- Lice
- Fleas
- Bedbugs
- Ticks
- Chiggers or red bugs
- Bird or rodent mites
- Tungiasis (burrowing flea)

DIAGNOSIS

- Diagnosis is based on the clinical features, but may be aided by searching for exposure to arthropods and by considering the patient's occupation and recent activities

TREATMENT

MEDICATIONS

- Corticosteroid lotions or creams are helpful
- Calamine lotion or a cool wet dressing is always appropriate
- Topical antibiotics may be applied if secondary infection is suspected
- Localized persistent lesions may be treated with intralesional corticosteroids
- Stings produced by many arthropods may be alleviated by applying papain powder (Adolph's Meat Tenderizer) mixed with water, or aluminum chloride hexahydrate (Xerac AC)
- To break the life cycle of the flea, one must repeatedly treat the home and pets, using quick-kill insecticides, residual insecticides, and a growth regulator
- Tungiasis: ethyl chloride spray will kill the insect when applied to the lesion, and disinfestation may be accomplished with insecticide applied to the terrain; simple surgical excision is usually performed

THERAPEUTIC PROCEDURES

- Living arthropods should be removed carefully with tweezers after application of alcohol and preserved in alcohol for identification

 OUTCOME

WHEN TO REFER

- If there is a question about the diagnosis, if recommended therapy is ineffective, or specialized treatment is necessary

PREVENTION

- Arthropod infestations are best prevented by avoidance of contaminated areas, personal cleanliness, and disinfection of clothing, bedclothes, and furniture as indicated; benzyl benzoate and dimethylphthalate are excellent acaricides; clothing should be impregnated by spray or by dipping in a soapy emulsion

 EVIDENCE

PRACTICE GUIDELINES

- National Guideline Clearinghouse
  http://www.guideline.gov/summary/
  summary.aspx?doc_id=2672&nbr=1898
  &string=lyme+disease
  http://www.guideline.gov/summary/
  summary.aspx?doc_id=3047&nbr=2273
  &string=lice_
  http://www.guideline.gov/summary/
  summary.aspx?doc_id=3225&nbr=
  2451&string=lice

WEB SITES

- American Academy of Dermatology
  http://www.aad.org
- Dermatology Handbook for Family Practice from the University of Iowa
  http://www.vh.org/Providers/ClinRef/
  FPHandbook/17.html

INFORMATION FOR PATIENTS

- Centers for Disease Control and Prevention
  http://www.cdc.gov/travel/bugs.htm
- Mayo Clinic
  http://www.mayoclinic.com/invoke.cfm?
  id=fa00046

REFERENCE

- Elston DM et al: What's eating you? Bedbugs. Cutis 2000;65:262. [PMID: 10826083]

Timothy G. Berger, MD

Bladder Cancer

 ## KEY FEATURES

ESSENTIALS OF DIAGNOSIS

- Irritative voiding symptoms
- Gross or microscopic hematuria
- Positive urinary cytology in most patients
- Filling defect within bladder noted on imaging

GENERAL CONSIDERATIONS

- Second most common urological cancer
- More common in men than women (2.7:1)
- Mean age at diagnosis is 65 years
- Risk factors: cigarette smoking, exposure to industrial dyes and solvents

 ## CLINICAL FINDINGS

SYMPTOMS AND SIGNS

- Hematuria is the presenting symptom in 85–90%
- Irritative voiding symptoms in a small percent
- Masses detected on bimanual examination with large-volume or deeply infiltrating cancers
- Lymphedema of the lower extremities with locally advanced cancers or metastases to pelvic lymph nodes
- Hepatomegaly or supraclavicular lymphadenopathy with metastatic disease

 ## DIAGNOSIS

LABORATORY TESTS

- Urinalysis—hematuria; on occasion, pyuria
- Azotemia
- Anemia

IMAGING STUDIES

- Intravenous urography, ultrasound, CT, MRI show filling defects within the bladder

Pathology

- Transitional cell carcinomas (~90%)
- Squamous cell cancers ~7%
- Adenocarcinomas ~2%
- Bladder cancer staging is based on the extent of bladder wall penetration and the presence of either regional or distant metastases
- Natural history is based on tumor recurrence and progression to higher stage disease. Both are related to tumor grade and stage

DIAGNOSTIC PROCEDURES

- Cytology useful in detecting disease at initial presentation or recurrence
- Cytology very sensitive (80–90%) in detecting cancers of higher grade and stage. Sensitivity enhanced by flow cytometry
- Imaging done primarily for evaluating the upper urinary tract and staging
- Cystourethroscopy and biopsy
- Diagnosis and staging are by cystoscopy and transurethral resection of bladder (TURB)
- TURB under general or regional anesthesia
- Resection down to muscular elements of the bladder
- Random bladder and, on occasion, prostatic urethral biopsies

Bladder Cancer

 TREATMENT

MEDICATIONS

- Patients with superficial cancers (Ta, T1) are treated with complete TURB and the selective use of intravesical chemotherapy
- Patients with large, high-grade, recurrent Ta lesions, T1 cancers, and carcinoma in situ are treated with intravesical chemotherapy
- Patients with more invasive (T2, T3) but still localized cancers require more aggressive surgery, irradiation, or the combination of chemotherapy and selective surgery or irradiation
- Patients with evidence of lymph node or distant metastases should undergo systemic chemotherapy

Intravesical chemotherapy

- Immuno- or chemotherapeutic agents administered weekly for 6–12 weeks
- Maintenance therapy after the initial induction regimen includes thiotepa, mitomycin, doxorubicin, and BCG

SURGERY

- Transurethral resection is diagnostic, allows for proper staging, and controls superficial cancers
- Partial cystectomy indicated in patients with solitary lesions and cancers in a bladder diverticulum
- Radical cystectomy
- Urinary diversion—a conduit of small or large bowel
- Continent forms of diversion available

THERAPEUTIC PROCEDURES

- Radiotherapy: external beam therapy over a 6- to 8-week period

Chemotherapy (systemic)

- Cisplatin-based combination chemotherapy
- Adjuvant chemotherapy when the primary tumor invades perivesical fat or adjacent organs or when lymph nodes are found to have metastatic disease—used for patients being treated with radical cystectomy
- Combination radiotherapy and systemic chemotherapy or surgery, radiotherapy, and systemic chemotherapy

 OUTCOME

COMPLICATIONS

- Intravesical chemotherapy: side effects include irritative voiding symptoms and hemorrhagic cystitis
- Radiotherapy: approximately 10–15% of patients develop bladder, bowel, or rectal complications; local recurrence is common (30–70%)

PROGNOSIS

- Chemotherapy (systemic): partial response in 15–35%; complete response in 15–45%

 EVIDENCE

PRACTICE GUIDELINES

- Oosterlinck W et al: Guidelines on bladder cancer. Eur Urol 2002;41:105. [PMID: 12074395]
- Scher H et al: NCCN urothelial cancer practice guidelines. National Comprehensive Cancer Network. Oncology (Huntingt) 1998;12:225. [PMID: 9699218]

WEB SITES

- American Cancer Society—What is bladder cancer? http://www.cancer.org/docroot/cri/content/cri_2_4_1x_what_is_bladder_cancer_44.asp?sitearea=cri
- American Urological Association — Bladder cancer http://www.urologyhealth.org/adult/index.cfm?cat=03&topic=37

INFORMATION FOR PATIENTS

- Cleveland Clinic — Bladder cancer http://www.clevelandclinic.org/health/health-info/docs/1300/1379.asp?index=6150

REFERENCES

- Kim HL et al: The current status of bladder preservation in the treatment of muscle invasive bladder cancer. J Urol 2000;164(3 Part 1):627. [PMID: 10953112]
- Smith JA Jr et al: Bladder cancer clinical guidelines panel summary report on the management of nonmuscle invasive bladder cancer (stages Ta, T1 and Tis). The American Urological Association. J Urol 1999;162:1697. [PMID: 10524909]

Marshall L. Stoller, MD
Peter R. Carroll, MD

Bone Tumors & Tumor-Like Lesions

 KEY FEATURES

ESSENTIALS OF DIAGNOSIS

- Persistent pain, swelling, or tenderness of a skeletal part
- Pathological ("spontaneous") fractures
- Suspicious areas of bony enlargement, deformity, radiodensity, or radiolucency on x-ray
- Histological evidence of bone neoplasm on biopsy specimen

GENERAL CONSIDERATIONS

- Primary tumors of bone are relatively uncommon in comparison with secondary or metastatic neoplasms

DEMOGRAPHICS

- Osteosarcoma, the most common malignancy of bone, typically occurs in adolescents

 CLINICAL FINDINGS

SYMPTOMS AND SIGNS

- Persistent skeletal pain and swelling, with or without limitation of motion of adjacent joints
- Spontaneous fracture
- Osteosarcoma may present as pain or swelling in a bone or joint (especially in or around the knee). When the symptoms often appear to begin following a sports-related injury, accurate diagnosis may be delayed

DIFFERENTIAL DIAGNOSIS

- Benign developmental skeletal abnormalities
- Metastatic neoplastic disease
- Infections (eg, osteomyelitis)
- Posttraumatic bone lesions
- Metabolic disease of bone
- Osteoid osteomas
- Osteosarcoma
- Fibrosarcomas
- Enchondromas
- Chondromyxoid fibromas
- Chondrosarcomas
- Giant cell tumors (osteoclastomas)
- Chondroblastomas
- Ewing's sarcoma

 DIAGNOSIS

DIAGNOSTIC PROCEDURES

- Biopsy (which is not always definitive)

TREATMENT

MEDICATIONS

- Chemotherapy for some

SURGERY

- Osteosarcomas are treated by resection and chemotherapy
- Osteoid osteomas are benign tumors of children and adolescents that should be surgically removed

 OUTCOME

PROGNOSIS

- Patients with osteosarcomas treated by resection and chemotherapy have a 5-year survival rate of 60%
- Tumors derived from cartilage treated with appropriate curettement or surgery have a good prognosis
- Ewing's sarcoma, which affects children, adolescents, and young adults, has a 50% mortality rate in spite of chemotherapy, irradiation, and surgery

 EVIDENCE

INFORMATION FOR PATIENTS

- National Cancer Institute
  http://www.nci.nih.gov/cancerinfo/types/bone/
- American Cancer Society
  http://www.cancer.org/docroot/cri/content/cri_2_4_1x_what_is_bone_cancer_2.asp?

REFERENCE

- Arndt C et al: Common musculoskeletal tumors of childhood and adolescence. N Engl J Med 1999;341:342. [PMID: 10423470]

David B. Hellmann, MD, FACP
John H. Stone, MD, MPH

Botulism

 ## KEY FEATURES

ESSENTIALS OF DIAGNOSIS

- History of recent ingestion of home-canned or smoked foods or of injection drug use and demonstration of toxin in serum or food
- Sudden onset of diplopia, dry mouth, dysphagia, dysphonia, and muscle weakness progressing to respiratory paralysis
- Pupils are usually fixed and dilated

GENERAL CONSIDERATIONS

- A paralytic disease caused by botulinum neurotoxin, which is produced by *Clostridium botulinum*, a ubiquitous, strictly anaerobic, spore-forming bacillus found in soil
- Four toxin types—A, B, E, and F—cause human disease
- Botulinum toxin inhibits release of acetylcholine at the neuromuscular junction
- Naturally occurring botulism occurs in one of three forms: food-borne botulism, infant botulism, or wound botulism
- Food-borne botulism is caused by ingestion of preformed toxin present in canned, smoked, or vacuum-packed foods such as home-canned vegetables, smoked meats, and vacuum-packed fish
- Infant botulism is associated with ingestion of honey. Honey consumption is safe for children 1 year of age or older
- Wound botulism typically occurs in association with injection drug use. It result from organisms present in the gut or wound that elaborate toxin in vivo
- Botulinum toxin is extremely potent and is classified by the Centers for Disease Control and Prevention (CDC) as a high-priority agent because of its potential for use as an agent of bioterrorism

DEMOGRAPHICS

- Approximately 170 cases of botulism have been reported to the CDC over a year's time. Of these, food-borne and wound botulism were each one-fifth of cases, and the remainder were infant botulism

 ## CLINICAL FINDINGS

SYMPTOMS AND SIGNS

- Twelve to 36 h after ingestion of the toxin, visual disturbances appear, particularly diplopia and loss of accommodation
- Ptosis, cranial nerve palsies with impairment of extraocular muscles, and fixed dilated pupils are characteristic signs
- Other symptoms are dry mouth, dysphagia, and dysphonia
- The sensory examination is normal
- The sensorium remains clear and the temperature normal
- Respiratory paralysis may lead to death unless mechanical assistance is provided

DIFFERENTIAL DIAGNOSIS

- Poliomyelitis
- Guillain-Barré syndrome
- Myasthenia gravis
- Brainstem infarct or vertebrobasilar insufficiency
- Tick paralysis
- Organophosphate poisoning

 ## DIAGNOSIS

LABORATORY TESTS

- Toxin in patients' serum and in suspected foods may be shown by mouse inoculation and identified with specific antiserum

TREATMENT

MEDICATIONS

- If botulism is suspected, the CDC should be contacted for advice and help with procurement of botulinus antitoxin and for assistance in obtaining assays for toxin. During off hours, the CDC provides assistance via a recorded message at 404-639-2206

THERAPEUTIC PROCEDURES

- Respiratory failure is managed with intubation and mechanical ventilation

OUTCOME

PROGNOSIS

- Early nervous system involvement leads to respiratory paralysis and death in untreated cases

WHEN TO REFER

- All cases should be reported to the public health authorities
- Obtain immediate expert infectious and neurologist consultation

WHEN TO ADMIT

- All suspected and proven cases because of the high fatality rate

PREVENTION

- Botulism toxin is destroyed by high temperatures; persons who eat home-canned foods should consider boiling the food for 10 min before eating it

EVIDENCE

PRACTICE GUIDELINES

- National Guideline Clearinghouse
  http://www.guideline.gov/summary/summary.aspx?doc_id=3619&nbr=2845&string=botulism
  http://www.guideline.gov/summary/summary.aspx?doc_id=2707&nbr=1933&string=botulism

WEB SITES

- CDC—Division of Bacterial and Mycotic Diseases
  http://www.cdc.gov/ncidod/dbmd/
- Karolinska Institute—Directory of bacterial infections and mycoses
  http://www.mic.ki.se/Diseases/c1.html

INFORMATION FOR PATIENTS

- Centers for Disease Control—Bioterrorism
  http://www.bt.cdc.gov/
- JAMA patient page: Food-borne illnesses. JAMA 1999;281:1866. [PMID: 10340376]

REFERENCES

- Merrison AF et al: Wound botulism associated with subcutaneous drug use. BMJ 2002;326:1020. [PMID: 12411365]
- Shapiro RL et al: Botulism in the United States: A clinical and epidemiologic review. Ann Intern Med 1998;129:221. [PMID: 9696731]

Henry F. Chambers, MD

Brain Abscess

 ## KEY FEATURES

ESSENTIALS OF DIAGNOSIS

- Symptoms and signs of expanding intracranial mass
- May be signs of primary infection or congenital heart disease
- Fever may be absent

GENERAL CONSIDERATIONS

- Presents as an intracranial space-occupying lesion
- May be a sequela of ear or nose disease, a complication of infection elsewhere in the body, or an infection introduced intracranially by trauma or surgical procedures
- Most common infective organisms are streptococci, staphylococci, and anaerobes; mixed infections are not uncommon

 ## CLINICAL FINDINGS

SYMPTOMS AND SIGNS

- Headache, drowsiness, inattention, confusion, and seizures are early symptoms
- Increasing intracranial pressure and focal neurological deficits are later signs
- There may be little or no systemic evidence of infection

DIFFERENTIAL DIAGNOSIS

- Other rapidly expanding intracranial space-occupying lesions

 ## DIAGNOSIS

LABORATORY TESTS

- Examination of the cerebrospinal fluid does not help in diagnosis and may precipitate a herniation syndrome

IMAGING STUDIES

- CT scan of the head characteristically shows an area of contrast enhancement surrounding a low-density core (similar to metastatic neoplasms)
- MRI permits earlier recognition of focal cerebritis or an abscess
- Arteriography indicates the presence of a space-occupying lesion (avascular mass with displacement of normal cerebral vessels) but provides no clue to the nature of the lesion

Brain Abscess

 ## TREATMENT

MEDICATIONS

- Intravenous antibiotics, combined with surgical drainage (aspiration or excision) if necessary to reduce the mass effect, or to establish the diagnosis
- Broad-spectrum antibiotics are used if the infecting organism is unknown (Table 123, page 1306); a common regimen is penicillin G (2 million units every 2 h intravenously) plus either chloramphenicol (1–2 g intravenously every 6 h), metronidazole (750 mg intravenously every 6 h), or both; nafcillin is added if *Staphylococcus aureus* is suspected
- Antimicrobial treatment is usually continued parenterally for 6–8 weeks, then orally for another 2–3 weeks
- Dexamethasone (4–25 mg four times daily, depending on severity, followed by tapering of dose, depending on response) may reduce any associated edema; intravenous mannitol is sometimes required

THERAPEUTIC PROCEDURES

- Aspiration or excision if necessary to reduce mass effect or to establish the diagnosis

 ## OUTCOME

FOLLOW-UP

- Monitor patient by serial CT scans or MRI every 2 weeks and at deterioration

COMPLICATIONS

- Seizures
- Focal neurological deficits

PROGNOSIS

- Abscesses smaller than 2 cm can often be cured medically

WHEN TO ADMIT

- When the diagnosis is suspected

 ## EVIDENCE

PRACTICE GUIDELINES

- Evaluation and management of intracranial mass lesions in AIDS. Report of the Quality Standards Subcommittee of the American Academy of Neurology. Neurology 1998;50:21.
- National Guideline Clearinghouse http://www.guideline.gov/summary/summary.aspx?doc_id=2446&nbr=1672&string=brain+abscess

WEB SITES

- The Whole Brain Atlas http://www.med.harvard.edu:80/AANLIB/home.html
- CNS Pathology Index http://medstat.med.utah.edu/WebPath/CNSHTML/CNSIDX.html

INFORMATION FOR PATIENTS

- National Institutes of Health http://www.nlm.nih.gov/medlineplus/ency/article/000783.htm

REFERENCE

- Roos KL: Acute bacterial infections of the central nervous system. In: *Neurology and General Medicine*, ed 3. Aminoff MJ (editor). Churchill Livingstone, 2001.

Michael J. Aminoff, DSc, MD, FRCP

Brain Death

 KEY FEATURES

ESSENTIALS OF DIAGNOSIS

- The definition of brain death is controversial
- Irreversible coma without any brainstem reflexes for at least 6 h

GENERAL CONSIDERATIONS

- To establish brain death, the irreversibly comatose patient must be shown to have lost all brainstem reflex responses, including the pupillary, corneal, oculovestibular, oculocephalic, oropharyngeal, and respiratory reflexes, and should have been in this condition for at least 6 h
- Spinal reflex movements do not exclude the diagnosis, but ongoing seizure activity or decerebrate or decorticate posturing is not consistent with brain death

 CLINICAL FINDINGS

SYMPTOMS AND SIGNS

- Coma (irreversible)
- No response to external stimulation
- No brainstem reflexes
- No spontaneous respirations and no respirations during apnea test

DIFFERENTIAL DIAGNOSIS

- Reversible coma simulating brain death may be seen with hypothermia (temperature <32°C) and overdosage with central nervous system depressant drugs
- Persistent vegetative state
- Locked-in syndrome (deefferented state)

 DIAGNOSIS

LABORATORY TESTS

- The apnea test (presence or absence of spontaneous respiratory activity at a $PaCO_2$ of at least 60 mm Hg) serves to determine whether the patient is capable of respiratory activity
- Certain ancillary tests may assist the determination of brain death but are not essential. An isoelectric electroencephalogram recorded according to the recommendations of the American Electroencephalographic Society is especially helpful in confirming the diagnosis

IMAGING STUDIES

- Alternatively, the demonstration of an absent cerebral circulation by intravenous radioisotope cerebral angiography or four-vessel contrast cerebral angiography can be confirmatory

TREATMENT

THERAPEUTIC PROCEDURES

• Palliative care

 OUTCOME

PROGNOSIS

• Will not recover

EVIDENCE

PRACTICE GUIDELINES

• National Guideline Clearinghouse
http://www.guideline.gov/summary/
summary.aspx?doc_id=3121&nbr=2347
&string=brain+death
• American Academy of Neurology
http://www.aan.com/professionals/
practice/pdfs/gl0065.pdf

WEB SITE

• Brain Death Demonstration Case
http://www.brighamrad.harvard.edu/
Cases/bwh/hcache/20/full.html

INFORMATION FOR PATIENTS

• National Institute of Neurological
Disorders and Stroke
http://www.ninds.nih.gov/health_and_
medical/disorders/ coma_doc.htm
• University of Michigan
http://www.transweb.org/qa/qa_don/
br_death.htm

REFERENCE

• Wijdicks EFM: Brain death worldwide.
Neurology 2002;58:20. [PMID:
11781400]

Michael J. Aminoff, DSc, MD, FRCP

Brain Tumor, Primary

 KEY FEATURES

ESSENTIALS OF DIAGNOSIS

- Generalized or focal disturbance of cerebral function, or both
- Increased intracranial pressure in some patients
- Neuroradiological evidence of space-occupying lesion

GENERAL CONSIDERATIONS

- Half of all primary intracranial neoplasms (Table 95, page 1279) are gliomas and the remainder meningiomas, pituitary adenomas, neurofibromas, and other tumors
- Certain tumors (eg, neurofibromas, hemangioblastomas, and retinoblastomas) have a familial basis
- May lead to a generalized disturbance of cerebral function and symptoms of increased intracranial pressure

DEMOGRAPHICS

- Tumors may occur at any age, but some gliomas are age-specific (Table 95, page 1279)

 CLINICAL FINDINGS

SYMPTOMS AND SIGNS

- Personality changes, intellectual decline, emotional lability, seizures, headaches, nausea, and malaise
- Increased pressure may cause herniation of brain tissue into a compartment with lower pressure
- Intracranial tumors may lead to focal deficits depending on the location

Herniation symptoms

- Temporal lobe uncus herniation with compression of the third cranial nerve, midbrain, and posterior cerebral artery
  - Ipsilateral pupillary dilation
  - Followed by stupor, coma, decerebrate posturing, and respiratory arrest
- Cerebellar tonsillar displacement causing medullary compression; apnea, circulatory collapse, and death

Focal deficits

- **Frontal lobe lesions**
- Progressive intellectual decline, slowing of mental activity, personality changes, and contralateral grasp reflexes
- Expressive aphasia if the posterior part of the left inferior frontal gyrus is involved

- Anosmia secondary to pressure on the olfactory nerve
- Precentral lesions may cause focal motor seizures or contralateral pyramidal deficits
- **Temporal lobe lesions**
- Seizures with olfactory or gustatory hallucinations, motor automatisms, and impairment of external awareness without actual loss of consciousness
- Depersonalization, emotional changes, behavioral disturbances, sensations of déjà vu or jamais vu
- Micropsia or macropsia (objects appear smaller or larger than they are), visual field defects (crossed upper quadrantanopia), and auditory illusions or hallucinations
- Left-sided lesions may lead to dysnomia and receptive aphasia, while right-sided involvement may disturb the perception of musical notes and melodies
- **Parietal lobe lesions**
- May cause sensory seizures
- Contralateral disturbances of sensation, sensory loss or inattention (cortical in type and involves postural sensibility and tactile discrimination, so that the appreciation of shape, size, weight, and texture is impaired)
- Objects placed in the hand may not be recognized (astereognosis)
- Extensive lesions may produce contralateral hyperpathia and spontaneous pain (thalamic syndrome)
- Optic radiation involvement leads to a contralateral homonymous field defect that sometimes consists solely of lower quadrantanopia
- Left angular gyrus lesions cause Gerstmann's syndrome (alexia, agraphia, acalculia, right-left confusion, and finger agnosia), whereas involvement of the left submarginal gyrus causes ideational apraxia
- Anosognosia (denial, neglect, or rejection of a paralyzed limb) is seen in patients with lesions of the nondominant (right) hemisphere
- Constructional apraxia and dressing apraxia may also occur with right-sided lesions
- **Occipital lobe lesions**
- Crossed homonymous hemianopia or a partial field defect
- Left-sided or bilateral lesions may cause visual agnosia; irritative lesions on either side can cause unformed visual hallucinations
- Bilateral occipital lobe involvement causes cortical blindness with preserva-

tion of pupillary responses to light and lack of awareness of the defect by the patient
- Loss of color perception, prosopagnosia (inability to identify a familiar face), simultagnosia (inability to integrate and interpret a composite scene as opposed to its individual elements), and Balint's syndrome (failure to turn the eyes to a particular point in space, despite preservation of spontaneous and reflex eye movements), denial of blindness or a field defect (Anton's syndrome)
- **Brainstem and cerebellar lesions**
- Brainstem lesions lead to cranial nerve palsies, ataxia, incoordination, nystagmus, and pyramidal and sensory deficits in the limbs
- Intrinsic brainstem tumors, such as gliomas, cause an increase in intracranial pressure, usually late
- Marked ataxia of the trunk if the vermis cerebelli is involved
- Ipsilateral appendicular deficits (ataxia, incoordination and hypotonia of the limbs) if the cerebellar hemispheres are affected
- **False localizing signs**
- Neurological signs other than by direct compression or infiltration, leading to errors of clinical localization
- Include third or sixth nerve palsy and bilateral extensor plantar responses produced by herniation syndromes, and an extensor plantar response occurring ipsilateral to a hemispheric tumor because the opposite cerebral peduncle is compressed against the tentorium

DIFFERENTIAL DIAGNOSIS

- Metastatic intracranial tumors
  - Cerebral metastases
  - Leptomeningeal metastases (carcinomatous meningitis)
- Intracranial mass lesions in AIDS patients

Brain Tumor, Primary

 DIAGNOSIS

IMAGING STUDIES

- MRI with gadolinium or CT scanning
- MRI is best for tumors in the posterior fossa
- The characteristic appearance of meningiomas on CT scanning is virtually diagnostic: noncontrast CT shows a lesion in the parasagittal and sylvian regions, olfactory groove, sphenoidal ridge, or tuberculum sellae with a homogeneous area of increased density, which enhances uniformly with contrast
- Arteriography may show stretching or displacement of normal cerebral vessels by the tumor and tumor vascularity. An avascular mass may be due to tumor, hematoma, abscess, or any space-occupying lesion; in patients with normal hormone levels and an intrasellar mass, angiography used to distinguish between a pituitary adenoma and an arterial aneurysm

DIAGNOSTIC PROCEDURES

- Lumbar puncture is rarely necessary; the findings are seldom diagnostic, herniation syndrome is a risk

 TREATMENT

MEDICATIONS

- Corticosteroids help reduce cerebral edema and are usually started before surgery
- Herniation is treated with intravenous dexamethasone (10–20 mg as a bolus, followed by 4 mg every 6 h) and intravenous mannitol (20% solution given in a dose of 1.5 g/kg over about 30 min)
- Anticonvulsants in standard doses (Table 94, page 1278): controversial whether to start these prophylactically or only after a first seizure

SURGERY

- Complete surgical removal if the tumor is extraaxial (eg, meningioma, acoustic neuroma) or is not in a critical or inaccessible region of the brain (eg, cerebellar hemangioblastoma)
- Surgery may be diagnostic and may relieve intracranial pressure symptoms even if the neoplasm cannot be completely removed
- Simple surgical shunting procedures help in cases with obstructive hydrocephalus

THERAPEUTIC PROCEDURES

- Treatment depends on the type and site of the tumor (Table 95, page 1279) and the condition of the patient
- For those patients whose disease deteriorates despite treatment, palliative care is important
- With malignant gliomas, radiation therapy increases median survival rates regardless of preceding surgery; chemotherapy provides additional benefit
- Indications for irradiation for other primary intracranial neoplasms depend on tumor type and accessibility and the feasibility of complete surgical removal

 OUTCOME

WHEN TO REFER

- All patients should be referred to specialized care

WHEN TO ADMIT

- Altered sensorium
- Specialized treatment or surgery

 EVIDENCE

PRACTICE GUIDELINES

- National Guideline Clearinghouse http://www.guideline.gov/summary/ summary.aspx?doc_id=2438&nbr=1664 &string=primary+intracerebral+ neoplasm

WEB SITES

- Anaplastic Astrocytoma Demonstration Case http://www.brighamrad.harvard.edu/ Cases/bwh/hcache/49/full.html
- List of Clinical Trials for Brain Tumors http://www.virtualtrials.com

INFORMATION FOR PATIENTS

- Patient Education Institute http://www.nlm.nih.gov/medlineplus/ tutorials/braincancer.html
- National Cancer Institute http://www.cancer.gov/cancerinfo/ wyntk/brain

REFERENCES

- Whittle IR: Surgery for gliomas. Curr Opin Neurol 2002;15:663. [PMID: 12447103]
- Wrensch M et al: Epidemiology of primary brain tumors: current concepts and review of the literature. Neuro-oncology 2002;4:278. [PMID: 12356358]

Michael J. Aminoff, MD, DSc, FRCP

Breast Cancer, Female

 ## KEY FEATURES

ESSENTIALS OF DIAGNOSIS

- Early findings: single, nontender, firm to hard mass with ill-defined margins; mammographic abnormalities and no palpable mass
- Later findings: skin or nipple retraction; axillary lymphadenopathy; breast enlargement, redness, edema, pain; fixation of mass to skin or chest wall

GENERAL CONSIDERATIONS

- Second most common cancer in women
- Second most common cause of cancer death in women
- 1 out of every 8–9 American women will develop breast cancer in her lifetime
- ~203,500 new cases of breast cancer and ~40,000 deaths from this disease in U.S. women in 2002

DEMOGRAPHICS

- Mean and median age: 60–61 years
- More common in whites
- 3–4 times increased risk in those whose mother or sister had breast cancer, risk further increased if family member had premenopausal or bilateral disease
- 1.5 times increased incidence if nulliparous or first full-term pregnancy at age >35
- Slight increased risk if menarche at age <12 or natural menopause at age >50
- Increased incidence in fibrocystic disease with proliferative changes, papillomatosis, or atypical ductal epithelial hyperplasia
- Women with prior breast cancer develop contralateral cancer at a rate of 1–2% per year
- Increased risk with long-term use of hormone replacement therapy
- Increased risk if history of uterine cancer
- 85% lifetime risk in women with *BRCA1* gene mutations
- Increased risk with *BRCA2*, ataxia-telangiectasia, and *P53* gene mutations

 ## CLINICAL FINDINGS

SYMPTOMS AND SIGNS

- Presenting complaint in 70% is a lump (usually painless)
- Less frequently
  - Breast pain
  - Nipple discharge
  - Erosion, retraction, enlargement, or itching of the nipple
  - Redness, generalized hardness, enlargement, or shrinking of the breast
  - Axillary mass or swelling of the arm (rare)
- With metastatic disease, back or bone pain, jaundice, or weight loss
- Physical examination is done with patient sitting arms at sides and then overhead, and supine with arm abducted
- Findings include
- Nontender, firm or hard mass with poorly delineated margins
  - Skin or nipple retraction
  - Breast asymmetry
  - Erosions of nipple epithelium
  - Watery, serous or bloody discharge
- Metastatic disease suggested by
  - Firm or hard axillary nodes >1 cm
  - Axillary nodes that are matted or fixed to skin or deep structures indicate advanced disease (at least stage III)
- Advanced stage (stage IV) cancer suggested by ipsilateral supraclavicular or infraclavicular nodes

DIFFERENTIAL DIAGNOSIS

- Fibrocystic disease or cyst
- Fibroadenoma
- Intraductal papilloma
- Lipoma
- Fat necrosis
- Breast abscess
- Phyllodes tumor

 ## DIAGNOSIS

LABORATORY TESTS

- Increased erythrocyte sedimentation rate with metastatic disease
- Increased alkaline phosphatase with liver or bone metastases
- Increased calcium with advanced disease
- Carcinoembryonic antigen (CEA) and CA 15-3 or CA 27-29 are tumor markers for recurrent breast cancer
- Cytological examination of breast nipple discharge occasionally helpful

IMAGING STUDIES

- Mammography
- Breast ultrasound may differentiate cystic from solid masses
- MRI and PET may play a role in imaging atypical lesions but only after diagnostic mammography
- CT scan of chest, abdomen, pelvis, and brain may demonstrate metastases
- Bone scan may show bony metastases in symptomatic patients
- PET scan is under investigation as single test for evaluation of breast, lymphatics, and metastases

DIAGNOSTIC PROCEDURES

- Fine needle aspiration (FNA) or core biopsy
- Open biopsy under local anesthesia if needle biopsy inconclusive
- Computerized stereotactic guided core needle biopsies for nonpalpable lesions found on mammogram
- TNM staging (I–IV)

Breast Cancer, Female

TREATMENT

MEDICATIONS

Potentially curable disease

- Adjuvant chemotherapy improves survival
- Tamoxifen in all hormone receptor–positive patients
- CMF (cyclophosphamide, methotrexate, fluorouracil)
- AC [Adriamycin (doxorubicin), cyclophosphamide] with taxanes (docetaxel or paclitaxel)
- Tamoxifen plus chemotherapy with AC or PAF (prednisone, adriamycin, fluorouracil) lowers recurrence rates more than tamoxifen alone in postmenopausal women with estrogen receptor (ER)–positive tumors

Metastatic disease

- For hormone receptor–positive patients, palliative tamoxifen 20 mg PO QD can be effective
- For patients who initially respond to tamoxifen, but then relapse, consider diethylstilbestrol, megestrol acetate, or aromatase inhibitors
- For metastatic disease, chemotherapy should be considered if visceral metastases (especially brain or lung lymphangitic); hormonal treatment is unsuccessful or the disease has progressed after an initial response to hormonal manipulation; or the tumor is ER-negative
- AC achieves response rate of ~85%
- Combinations of cyclophosphamide, vincristine, methotrexate, fluorouracil, and taxanes achieve response rates of up to 60–70%
- Paclitaxel achieves response rate of 30–40%
- Trastuzumab, a monoclonal antibody that binds to HER-2/*neu* receptors on the cancer cell, is highly effective in HER-2/*neu*–expressive cancers
- High-dose chemotherapy and autologous bone marrow or stem cell transplantation produce no improvement in survival over conventional chemotherapy

SURGERY

- Indicated for stage I and stage II cancers
- Disease-free survival rates are similar with partial mastectomy plus axillary dissection followed by radiation therapy and with modified radical mastectomy (total mastectomy plus axillary dissection)
- Large size, subareolar, and multifocal tumors, fixation to the chest wall, or involvement of the nipple or overlying skin are relative contraindications to breast-conserving therapy
- Axillary dissection generally indicated in all women with invasive cancer
- Sentinel node biopsy is an alternative to axillary dissection in selected patients

THERAPEUTIC PROCEDURES

- Radiotherapy after partial mastectomy improves survival: 5–6 weeks of 5 daily fractions to a total dose of 5000–6000 cGy; may also improve survival after total mastectomy

OUTCOME

FOLLOW-UP

- For the first 3 years after diagnosis, examine the patient every 6 months; thereafter, annually

COMPLICATIONS

- Pleural effusion occurs in almost half of patients with metastatic breast cancer
- Local recurrence occurs in 8%
- Significant edema of the arm occurs in about 10–30%; more commonly if radiotherapy to axilla

PROGNOSIS

- Stage of breast cancer is the most reliable indicator of prognosis
- Increasing number of involved axillary nodes correlates directly with lower survival rates
- Estrogen and progesterone receptor–positive primary tumors have a more favorable course
- Tumors with marked aneuploidy have a poor prognosis
- HER-2/*neu* oncogene amplification, epidermal growth factor receptors, and cathepsin D have some prognostic value
- Clinical cure rate of localized breast cancer treated with most accepted methods of therapy is 75–90%
- When axillary lymph nodes are involved, the survival rate drops to 40–50% at 5 years and 25% at 10 years

WHEN TO REFER

- Women with exceptional family histories should be referred for genetic counseling and testing

WHEN TO ADMIT

- For definitive therapy by lumpectomy, axillary node dissection or sentinel node biopsy, or mastectomy after diagnosis by FNA or core needle biopsy

PREVENTION

- Screening requires combination of clinical examination and mammography: 35–50% detectable only by mammogram; 40% detectable only by examination
- Monthly breast self-examination
- Clinical examination every 2–3 years in women age 20–40, annually in women age >40
- Mammography every 1–2 years in women 50–79
- For women at high risk of developing breast cancer tamoxifen yields a 50% reduction in breast cancer if taken for 5 years; raloxifene studies are ongoing

EVIDENCE

WEB SITE

- NIH—Patient Education Institute: Breast cancer
  http://www.nlm.nih.gov/medlineplus/tutorials/breastcancernew.html

INFORMATION FOR PATIENTS

- Mayo Clinic Breast cancer
  http://www.mayoclinic.com/invoke.cfm?objectid=B105D3F6-BFE9-4D89-A5E53914589F7E86

REFERENCES

- Abrams JS: Adjuvant therapy for breast cancer—results from the USA Consensus Conference. Breast Cancer 2001;8:298. [PMID: 11791121]
- Hartmann LC et al: Efficacy of bilateral prophylactic mastectomy in women with a family history of breast cancer. N Engl J Med 1999;340:77. [PMID: 9887158]
- Rossouw JE et al: Risks and benefits of estrogen plus progestin in healthy postmenopausal women: principal results from the Women's Health Initiative randomized controlled trial. JAMA 2002;288:321. [PMID: 12117397]

Armando E. Giuliano, MD

Bronchiectasis

 KEY FEATURES

ESSENTIALS OF DIAGNOSIS

- Chronic cough with copious purulent sputum production
- Recurrent pulmonary infections
- A preceding history of recurrent pulmonary infection or inflammation or a condition predisposing to this
- Radiographic findings of dilated airways

GENERAL CONSIDERATIONS

- A congenital or acquired disorder of large bronchi characterized by abnormal dilation and destruction of bronchial walls
- Abnormal bronchi may be localized or diffuse
- May be caused by recurrent inflammation or infection
- Cystic fibrosis causes 50% of all cases
- Can result from abnormal lung defenses (immunodeficiency states, α_1-antiprotease deficiency, mucociliary clearance disorders, rheumatic disease)
- Localized airway obstruction
- Airways are often colonized with gram-negative bacilli (especially *Pseudomonas*), *Staphylococcus aureus*, and *Aspergillus* species

Etiology

- Cystic fibrosis
- Infection: tuberculosis, fungal, abscess, pneumonia
- Abnormal lung defense mechanisms
  - Hypogammaglobulinemia
  - Common variable immunodeficiency
  - Selective IgA, IgM, and IgG subclass deficiency
  - Acquired immunodeficiency from cytotoxic drugs, AIDS, lymphoma, leukemia, multiple myeloma, chronic renal disease, chronic liver disease
  - α_1-Antiprotease deficiency with cigarette smoking
  - Mucociliary clearance disorders (immotile cilia syndrome)
  - Rheumatic disease, eg, rheumatoid arthritis
- Localized airway obstruction

 CLINICAL FINDINGS

SYMPTOMS AND SIGNS

- Chronic cough with production of copious, purulent sputum
- Recurrent pneumonia
- Hemoptysis
- Weight loss and anemia are common
- Persistent basilar crackles are commonly found on examination
- Clubbing is infrequent in mild cases, but present in severe disease
- Obstructive pulmonary dysfunction with hypoxemia is seen in moderate or severe disease

DIFFERENTIAL DIAGNOSIS

- Chronic obstructive pulmonary disease
- Asthma
- Bronchiolitis
- Allergic bronchopulmonary aspergillosis

 DIAGNOSIS

LABORATORY TESTS

- Sputum smear and culture for bacterial, mycobacterial and fungal organisms
- Sweat chloride testing
- Quantitative immunoglobulins
- α_1-Antitrypsin level
- Excluding patients with humoral immunodeficiencies, most patients have panhypergammaglobulinemia, reflecting an immune response to chronic airway infection

IMAGING STUDIES

- Chest x-ray shows crowded bronchial markings related to peribronchial fibrosis and small cystic spaces at lung bases
- High-resolution CT scanning is the diagnostic test of choice

Bronchiectasis

 ## TREATMENT

MEDICATIONS

- Antibiotics should be used in acute exacerbations
- Empiric therapy for 10–14 days with amoxicillin or amoxicillin clavulanate, ampicillin or tetracycline, or trimethoprim-sulfamethoxazole
- Sputum smears and cultures should guide therapy where possible
- Preventive or suppressive antibiotics are frequently given to patients with increased purulent sputum, though this practice is not guided by clinical trial data
- Inhaled aerosolized aminoglycosides reduce *Pseudomonas* colonization, but improve FEV_1 and reduce hospitalizations only in cystic fibrosis patients
- Inhaled bronchodilators are commonly used as maintenance therapy and in acute exacerbations

SURGERY

- Resection is reserved for the few patients with localized bronchiectasis and adequate pulmonary function who fail to respond to conservative treatment
- Surgical treatment may be necessary to stop bleeding in some cases of massive hemoptysis

THEREAPEUTIC PROCEDURES

- Daily chest physiotherapy with postural drainage and chest percussion
- Bronchoscopy may be needed to evaluate hemoptysis, remove retained secretions, and rule out obstructing lesions
- Pulmonary angiography with embolization may be required to control massive hemoptysis

 ## OUTCOME

FOLLOW-UP

- Monitor serial pulmonary function tests and sputum cultures

COMPLICATIONS

- Hemoptysis
- Hypoxemia
- Cor pulmonale
- Amyloidosis
- Secondary visceral abscesses at distal sites

PROGNOSIS

- Depends on etiology and severity

WHEN TO REFER

- Most cases should be referred to a pulmonary, allergy, clinical immunology, or infectious disease specialist to assist in the evaluation and treatment

WHEN TO ADMIT

- Hypoxia
- Moderate to severe acute airflow obstruction
- Severe infection

PREVENTION

- Influenza vaccine
- Pneumococcal vaccine
- Regular chest physiotherapy

 ## EVIDENCE

INFORMATION FOR PATIENTS

- American Lung Association
  http://www.lungusa.org/diseases/bronchiectasis.html
- National Institutes of Health
  http://www.nlm.nih.gov/medlineplus/ency/article/000144.htm

REFERENCES

- Barker AF et al: Tobramycin solution for inhalation reduces sputum *Pseudomonas aeruginosa* density in bronchiectasis. Am J Respir Crit Care Med 2000;162:481. [PMID: 10934074]
- Barker AF: Medical progress: bronchiectasis. N Engl J Med 2002;346;1383.

Mark S. Chesnutt, MD
Thomas J. Prendergast, MD

Bronchiolitis Obliterans & Organizing Pneumonia

 ## KEY FEATURES

ESSENTIALS OF DIAGNOSIS

- Dry cough, dyspnea, and a flu-like illness of abrupt onset, but lasting from days to several months
- Patchy, bilateral ground glass or alveolar infiltrates on chest x-ray.
- Pulmonary function tests (PFTs) demonstrate restrictive pattern and hypoxemia
- Lung biopsy may be necessary to confirm diagnosis

GENERAL CONSIDERATIONS

- Diagnosis is difficult on clinical grounds alone

DEMOGRAPHICS

- Affects men and women equally
- Most patients between ages 50 and 70

 ## CLINICAL FINDINGS

SYMPTOMS AND SIGNS

- Onset is abrupt, frequently weeks to a few months after a flu-like illness
- Dyspnea and dry cough are common
- Constitutional symptoms such as fatigue, fever, and weight loss are common
- Crackles are heard in most patients and wheezing in approximately one-third
- Clubbing is uncommon

DIFFERENTIAL DIAGNOSIS

- Idiopathic interstitial pneumonias
- Idiopathic pulmonary fibrosis
- Interstitial lung disease due to infection (eg, fungal, tuberculosis, *Pneumocystis jiroveci* pneumonia, viral)
- Drug-induced fibrosis, eg, amiodarone, bleomycin
- Sarcoidosis
- Pneumoconiosis
- Hypersensitivity pneumonitis
- Asbestosis

 ## DIAGNOSIS

LABORATORY TESTS

- PFTs typically show a restrictive pattern with hypoxemia, but obstruction is seen in 25%
- High-resolution CT scan shows subpleural consolidation and bronchial wall thickening and dilation

IMAGING STUDIES

- Chest x-ray typically shows bilateral ground glass or alveolar infiltrates
- Solitary pneumonia-like infiltrates or a diffuse interstitial pattern may be seen

DIAGNOSTIC PROCEDURES

- Lung biopsy shows buds of loose connective tissue and inflammatory cells filling alveoli and distal bronchioles

TREATMENT

MEDICATIONS

- Prednisone, 1 mg/kg/day for 2–3 months, tapered slowly to 20–40 mg/day and usually continued for at least 6 months

 OUTCOME

FOLLOW-UP

- Monitor serial chest x-rays and PFTs

COMPLICATIONS

- Irreversible scarring or fibrosis of the lung
- Respiratory failure
- Complications of chronic steroid use

PROGNOSIS

- Two-thirds of patients respond rapidly to corticosteroids
- Long-term prognosis is generally good for steroid-responsive patients
- Relapses are common

WHEN TO REFER

- The majority of patients with suspected or confirmed disease should be seen by a pulmonologist

WHEN TO ADMIT

- Respiratory failure
- Signs of acute infection

PREVENTION

- Measures to prevent steroid-induced bone mineral loss

 EVIDENCE

PRACTICE GUIDELINES

- National Guideline Clearinghouse http://www.guideline.gov/summary/summary.aspx?doc_id=2665&nbr=1891&string=pneumonia

INFORMATION FOR PATIENTS

- American Lung Association http://www.lungusa.org/diseases/lungpneumoni.html
- JAMA patient page: Pneumonia. JAMA 2000;283:832.

REFERENCES

- Epler GR: Bronchiolitis obliterans organizing pneumonia. Arch Intern Med 2001;161:158. [PMID: 11176728]
- Schlesinger C et al: Bronchiolitis: update 2001. Curr Opin Pulmon Med 2002;8:112. [PMID: 11845006]
- Wright JL: Diseases of the small airways. Lung 2001;179:375. [PMID: 12040427]

Mark S. Chesnutt, MD
Thomas J. Prendergast, MD

Bronchogenic Carcinoma

 ## KEY FEATURES

ESSENTIALS OF DIAGNOSIS

- New cough or change in chronic cough
- Dyspnea, hemoptysis, anorexia
- New or enlarging mass; persistent infiltrate, atelectasis, or pleural effusion on chest radiograph or CT scan
- Cytological or histological findings of lung cancer in sputum, pleural fluid, or biopsy specimen

GENERAL CONSIDERATIONS

- Leading cause of cancer deaths
- 90% of lung cancer in men and 79% in women are attributable to smoking
- **Small cell lung cancer** (SCLC) is prone to early hematogenous spread, is rarely amenable to resection, and has a very aggressive course
- **Non–small cell lung cancer** (NSCLC) spreads more slowly and early disease may be cured with resection
- Histological types
  - Squamous cell carcinoma (25–35%) arises from bronchial epithelium; it is usually centrally located and intraluminal
  - Adenocarcinoma (35–40%) arises from mucous glands as a peripheral nodule or mass
  - Small cell carcinoma (15–20%) is of bronchial origin, begins centrally, and infiltrates submucosally
  - Large cell carcinoma (5–10%) is a heterogeneous group and presents as a central or peripheral mass
  - Bronchioloalveolar cell carcinoma (2%) arises from epithelial cells distal to the terminal bronchiole and spreads intraalveolarly

DEMOGRAPHICS

- Mean age at diagnosis is 60
- Environmental risk factors include tobacco smoke, radon gas, asbestos, metals, and industrial carcinogens
- A familial predisposition is recognized
- Chronic obstructive pulmonary disease, pulmonary fibrosis, and sarcoidosis are associated with an increased risk of lung cancer

 ## CLINICAL FINDINGS

SYMPTOMS AND SIGNS

- 75–90% are symptomatic at diagnosis; the presentation depends on type and location of tumor, extent of spread, and presence of paraneoplastic syndromes
- Anorexia, weight loss, and asthenia in 55–90%
- New or changed cough in up to 60%
- Hemoptysis in 5–30%
- Pain, often from bony metastases, is present in 25–40%
- Local spread may result in endobronchial obstruction and postobstructive pneumonia, effusions, or a change in voice due to recurrent laryngeal nerve involvement
- Superior vena cava (SVC) syndrome and Horner's syndrome
- Liver metastases are associated with asthenia and weight loss
- Brain metastases may present with headache, nausea and vomiting, seizures, or altered mental status
- **Paraneoplastic syndromes** (Table 151, page 1339) are not necessarily indicative of metastasis: syndrome of inappropriate antidiuretic hormone secretion occurs in 15% of SCLC patients and hypercalcemia in 10% of squamous cell cases

DIFFERENTIAL DIAGNOSIS

- Pneumonia
- Tuberculosis
- Metastatic cancer to lung
- Benign pulmonary nodule or nodules
- Lymphoma
- *Mycobacterium avium* complex
- Sarcoidosis
- Fungal pneumonia
- Bronchial carcinoid tumor
- Foreign body aspiration (retained)

DIAGNOSIS

LABORATORY TESTS

- See Tables 25 and 26 (pages 1222 and 1223)
- Tissue or cytology specimen is needed for diagnosis
- Sputum cytology is highly specific, but insensitive; yield is best with lesions in central airways
- Serum tumor markers are neither sensitive nor specific

- Complete blood cell count, renal panel, calcium, liver function tests, and lactate dehydrogenase are a routine part of staging
- Pulmonary function tests are required in all NSLC patients prior to surgery:
  - Preop FEV_1 >2 L is adequate to undergo surgery
  - Estimate of postresection FEV_1 is needed if <2 L preresection
  - Postresection FEV_1 >800 mL or >40% predicted is associated with a low incidence of perioperative complications

IMAGING STUDIES

- Nearly all patients have abnormal findings on chest x-ray or CT
  - Hilar adenopathy and mediastinal thickening (squamous cell)
  - Infiltrates, single or multiple nodules (bronchioloalveolar cell)
  - Central or peripheral masses (large cell)
  - Hilar and mediastinal abnormalities (small cell)
- Chest CT is the most important modality in staging to determine resectability
- For staging, brain MRI, abdominal CT, or radionuclide bone scanning should be targeted to symptoms or signs
- PET imaging can help confirm no metastates in NSCLC patients who are candidates for surgical resection

DIAGNOSISTIC PROCEDURES

- Thoracentesis can be diagnostic in the setting of malignant effusions (50–65%)
- If pleural fluid cytology is nondiagnostic after two thoracenteses, thoracoscopy is preferred to blind pleural biopsy
- Fine needle aspiration of palpable supraclavicular or cervical lymph nodes is frequently diagnostic
- Tissue diagnostic yield from bronchoscopy is 10–90%
- Transthoracic needle biopsy has a sensitivity of 50–90%
- Mediastinoscopy, VATS, or thoracotomy is necessary where less invasive techniques are not diagnostic

Staging

- See Table 25 (page 1222)
- NSCLC is staged with the TNM international staging system:
  - Stage I and II disease may be cured surgically
  - Stage IIIA disease may benefit from surgery
  - Stage IIIB and IV disease does not benefit from surgery

TREATMENT

MEDICATIONS

- See Table 149 (page 1337)

Neoadjuvant chemotherapy in NSCLC

- Administration in advance of surgery or radiation therapy
- There is no consensus on the survival impact in stage I and II disease but it is widely used in stage IIIA and IIIB disease

Adjuvant chemotherapy in NSCLC

- Administration of drugs following surgery or radiation therapy
- Multidrug platinum-based therapy shows a trend toward improved survival in stage I and N0 stage II disease (on the order of 3 months at 5 years)
- Data are conflicting for stage IIIA or node-positive stage II disease
- Stage IIIA and IIIB disease, which cannot be treated surgically, has improved survival when treated with combination chemo- and radiation therapy
- Performance status and symptom control in stage IIIB and stage IV disease may be improved by chemotherapy

Chemotherapy in SCLC

- 80–100% response to cisplatin/etoposide in limited stage disease (50–70% complete response)
- 60–80% response to cisplatin/etoposide in extensive disease (15–40% complete response)
- Remissions last a median of 6–8 months
- Median survival is 3–4 months after recurrence

SURGERY

- Resection of solitary brain metastases does not improve survival, but may improve quality of life in combination with radiation therapy

NSCLC

- Stages I and II are treated with surgical resection where possible
- Stage IIIA disease should be treated with multimodal protocols
- Selected stage IIIB patients who undergo resection after multimodal therapy have shown long-term survival
- Stage IV patients are treated palliatively

THERAPEUTIC PROCEDURES

- Radiation therapy is used as part of multimodal regimens in NSCLC
- Intraluminal radiation is an alternative palliative approach to intraluminal disease

Palliative care

- Pain control at the end of life is essential
- External beam radiation therapy is used to control dyspnea, hemoptysis, pain from bony metastases, obstruction from SVC syndrome, and solitary brain metastases

 OUTCOME

FOLLOW-UP

- Depends on type and stage of cancer as well as the patient's functional status and comorbid conditions

COMPLICATIONS

- SVC syndrome
- Paraneoplastic syndromes
- Venous thrombosis
- Postobstructive pneumonia

PROGNOSIS

- See Table 27 (page 1223)
- The overall 5-year survival is 15%
- Squamous cell carcinoma may have a better prognosis than adenocarcinoma or large cell carcinoma

WHEN TO REFER

- All patients deserve an evaluation by a multidisciplinary lung cancer evaluation and treatment program
- A palliative care specialist should be involved in advanced disease care

WHEN TO ADMIT

- Respiratory distress, altered mental status, pain control

PREVENTION

- Smoking cessation
- Screening in high-risk, asymptomatic patients has no proven benefit

 EVIDENCE

PRACTICE GUIDELINES

- Back PB: Screening for lung cancer. The guidelines. Chest 2003;123:83S.
- Rivera MP et al: Diagnosis of lung cancer: the guidelines. Chest 2003;123 (1 Suppl):129S.

INFORMATION FOR PATIENTS

- American Lung Association http://www.lungusa.org/diseases/lungcanc.html
- JAMA patient page: Lung cancer. JAMA 2003;289:380. [PMID: 12532974]

REFERENCES

- Detterbeck FC: Lung cancer. Special treatment issues. Chest 2003;123:244S. [PMID: 12527583]
- Griffin JP et al: End-of-life care in patients with lung cancer. Chest 2003;123(1 Suppl):312S. [PMID: 12527587]

Mark S. Chesnutt, MD
Thomas J. Prendergast, MD

Brucellosis

 KEY FEATURES

ESSENTIALS OF DIAGNOSIS

- History of animal exposure, ingestion of unpasteurized milk or cheese
- Insidious onset: easy fatigability, headache, arthralgia, anorexia, sweating, irritability
- Intermittent fever, especially at night, which may become chronic and undulant
- Cervical and axillary lymphadenopathy; hepatosplenomegaly
- Lymphocytosis, positive blood culture, elevated agglutination titer

GENERAL CONSIDERATIONS

- The infection is transmitted from animals to humans. *Brucella abortus* (cattle), *Brucella suis* (hogs), and *Brucella melitensis* (goats) are the main agents
- Transmission to humans occurs by contact with infected meat (slaughterhouse workers), placentae of infected animals (farmers, veterinarians), or ingestion of infected unpasteurized milk or cheese
- The incubation period varies from a few days to several weeks
- The disorder may become chronic

DEMOGRAPHICS

- In the United States, brucellosis is very rare except in the midwestern states (*B suis*) and in visitors or immigrants from countries where brucellosis is endemic (eg, Mexico, Spain, South American countries)

 CLINICAL FINDINGS

SYMPTOMS AND SIGNS

- Insidious onset of weakness, weight loss, low-grade fevers, sweats, and exhaustion with minimal activity
- Headache, abdominal or back pains with anorexia and constipation, and arthralgia
- Epididymitis occurs in 10% of cases in men
- 50% of cases have peripheral lymph node enlargement and splenomegaly; hepatomegaly is less common
- The chronic form may assume an undulant nature, with periods of normal temperature between acute attacks; symptoms may persist for years, either continuously or intermittently

DIFFERENTIAL DIAGNOSIS

- Lymphoma
- Tuberculosis
- Infective endocarditis
- Q fever
- Typhoid fever
- Tularemia
- Malaria
- Infectious mononucleosis
- Influenza
- HIV infection
- Disseminated fungal infection, eg, histoplasmosis, coccidioidomycosis

 DIAGNOSIS

LABORATORY TESTS

- Early in the course of infection, the organism can be recovered from the blood, cerebrospinal fluid, urine, and bone marrow
- Most modern culture systems can detect growth of the organism in blood by 7 days; cultures are more likely to be negative in chronic cases
- The diagnosis often is made by serological testing
- Rising serological titers or an absolute agglutination titer of greater than 1:100 supports the diagnosis

TREATMENT

MEDICATIONS

- Combination regimens of two or three drugs are more effective. Either doxycycline plus rifampin or streptomycin (or both) *or* trimethoprim-sulfamethoxazole plus rifampin or streptomycin (or both) is effective in doses as follows for 21 days: doxycycline, 100–200 mg/day in divided doses; trimethoprim 320 mg/day plus sulfamethoxazole 1600 mg/day in divided doses; rifampin, 600–1200 mg/day; and streptomycin, 500 mg intramuscularly twice a day
- Longer courses of therapy (eg, several months) may be required to cure relapses, osteomyelitis, or meningitis

OUTCOME

COMPLICATIONS

Most frequent

- Bone and joint lesions such as spondylitis and suppurative arthritis (usually of a single joint)
- Endocarditis
- Meningoencephalitis

Less common

- Pneumonitis with pleural effusion
- Hepatitis
- Cholecystitis

WHEN TO REFER

- Refer to an infectious disease specialist to confirm the diagnosis or for management of proven cases

WHEN TO ADMIT

- Suspected or known complications such as endocarditis or meningoencephalitis

EVIDENCE

WEB SITES

- CDC—Division of Bacterial and Mycotic Diseases
  http://www.cdc.gov/ncidod/dbmd/
- Karolinska Institute—Directory of bacterial infections and mycoses
  http://www.mic.ki.se/Diseases/c1.html

INFORMATION FOR PATIENTS

- Centers for Disease Control
  http://www.cdc.gov/ncidod/dbmd/diseaseinfo/brucellosis_g.htm
- National Institutes of Health
  http://www.nlm.nih.gov/medlineplus/ency/article/000597.htm

REFERENCE

- Yagupsky P: Detection of brucellae in blood cultures. J Clin Microbiol 1999;37:3437. [PMID: 10523530]

Henry F. Chambers, MD

Bulimia Nervosa

 KEY FEATURES

ESSENTIALS OF DIAGNOSIS

- Uncontrolled episodes of binge eating at least twice weekly for 3 months
- Recurrent inappropriate compensation to prevent weight gain, such as self-induced vomiting, laxatives, diuretics, fasting, or excessive exercise
- Overconcern with weight and body shape

GENERAL CONSIDERATIONS

- Occurs predominantly in young, white, middle- and upper-class women
- Prevalence may be as high as 19% in college-age women

 CLINICAL FINDINGS

SYMPTOMS AND SIGNS

- Consuming large quantities of easily ingested high-calorie foods, usually in secrecy, followed by vomiting, cathartics, or diuretics accompanied by feelings of guilt or depression; several episodes a day for a few days or regular and persistent patterns of binge eating may occur
- Body weight fluctuates but generally within 20% of desirable weight
- Menstruation is usually preserved

DIFFERENTIAL DIAGNOSIS

- Anorexia nervosa
- Depression
- Obsessive-compulsive disorder
- Personality disorder
- Substance abuse

 DIAGNOSIS

DIAGNOSTIC PROCEDURES

- History
- Identification of behavioral features

TREATMENT

MEDICATIONS

- Antidepressant medications such as flu-oxetine hydrochloride and other selective serotonin reuptake inhibitors

THERAPEUTIC PROCEDURES

- Supportive care
- Psychotherapy (individual, group, family)
- Behavioral therapy

 OUTCOME

COMPLICATIONS

- Poor dentition
- Pharyngitis
- Esophagitis
- Aspiration
- Gastric dilatation
- Pancreatitis
- Constipation
- Hemorrhoids
- Dehydration
- Electrolyte abnormalities

PROGNOSIS

- Death is rare
- Long-term psychiatric prognosis in severe bulimia is worse than in anorexia nervosa

EVIDENCE

PRACTICE GUIDELINES

- Position of the American Dietetic Association: nutrition intervention in the treatment of anorexia nervosa, bulimia nervosa, and eating disorders not otherwise specified (EDNOS). J Am Diet Assoc 2001;101:810. [PMID: 11478482]

INFORMATION FOR PATIENTS

- MEDLINEplus—Bulimia http://www.nlm.nih.gov/medlineplus/ency/article/000341.htm

WEB SITES

- National Association of Anorexia Nervosa and Associated Disorders (ANAD) http://www.altrue.net/site/anadweb/content.php?type=1&id=6982
- National Eating Disorders Association http://www.nationaleatingdisorders.org/p.asp?WebPage_ID=286&Profile_ID=41141

REFERENCES

- Arnold LM et al: A placebo-controlled, randomized trial of fluoxetine in the treatment of binge-eating disorder. J Clin Psychiatry 2002;63:1028. [PMID: 12444817]
- Dingemans AE et al: Binge eating disorder: a review. Int J Obes Relat Metab Disord 2002;26:299. [PMID: 11896484]
- Fitzgibbon ML et al: Binge eating disorder and bulimia nervosa: differences in the quality and quantity of binge eating episodes. Int J Eat Disord 2000;27:238. [PMID: 2012578]
- Wells LA et al: Bulimia nervosa: an update and treatment recommendations. Curr Opin Pediatr 2001;13:591. [PMID: 11753113]

Robert B. Baron, MD, MS

Bullous Pemphigoid

 KEY FEATURES

ESSENTIALS OF DIAGNOSIS

- Large, tense blisters that rupture, leaving denuded areas that heal without scarring
- Predilection for groin, axillae, flexor forearms, thighs and shins; may occur anywhere; some have oral involvement
- Caused by autoantibodies to two specific components of the hemidesmosome

GENERAL CONSIDERATIONS

- Relatively benign pruritic disease characterized by tense blisters in flexural areas, usually remitting in 5 or 6 years, with a course characterized by exacerbations and remissions
- Oral lesions are present in about one-third of affected persons
- The disease may occur in various forms, including localized and urticarial
- There is no statistical association with internal malignant disease

DEMOGRAPHICS

- Most patients are over the age of 60 (often in their 70s and 80s)
- Men are affected twice as frequently as women

 CLINICAL FINDINGS

SYMPTOMS AND SIGNS

- See Table 7 (page 1202)
- Characterized by tense blisters in flexural areas
- Appearance of blisters may be preceded by urticarial or edematous lesions for months
- May occur in various forms, including localized, vesicular, vegetating, erythematous, erythrodermic, and nodular
- Course characterized by exacerbations and remissions

DIFFERENTIAL DIAGNOSIS

- Pemphigus
- Drug eruptions
- Erythema multiforme major or toxic epidermal necrolysis
- Bullous impetigo
- Contact dermatitis
- Dermatitis herpetiformis
- Cicatricial pemphigoid
- Paraneoplastic pemphigus
- Linear IgA dermatosis
- Pemphigus foliaceus
- Porphyria cutanea tarda
- Epidermolysis bullosa
- Staphylococcal scalded skin syndrome
- Herpes gestationis
- Graft-versus-host disease

 DIAGNOSIS

LABORATORY TESTS

- Circulating anti-basement membrane antibodies can be found in the sera of patients in about 70% of cases

DIAGNOSTIC PROCEDURES

- The diagnosis is made by biopsy and direct immunofluorescence examination
- Light microscopy shows a subepidermal blister
- With direct immunofluorescence, IgG and C3 are found at the dermal–epidermal junction

TREATMENT

MEDICATIONS

- If the patient has only a few blisters, ultrapotent topical steroids may be adequate (Table 6, page 1199)
- Prednisone at dosages of 60–80 mg/day is often used to achieve rapid control of more widespread disease
- Although slower in onset of action, tetracycline or erythromycin, 1–1.5 g/day, alone or combined with nicotinamide—not nicotinic acid or niacin!—(up to 1.5 g/day), if tolerated, may control the disease in patients who cannot use corticosteroids or may allow decreasing or eliminating steroids after control is achieved
- Dapsone is particularly effective in mucous membrane pemphigoid
- If these drugs are not effective, methotrexate, 5–25 mg weekly, or azathioprine, 50 mg one to three times daily, may be used as steroid-sparing agents
- Mycophenolate mofetil (1 g twice daily) or intravenous immunoglobulin as used for pemphigus vulgaris may be used in refractory cases

 ## OUTCOME

PROGNOSIS

- Usually remitting in 5–6 years

WHEN TO REFER

- If there is a question about the diagnosis, if recommended therapy is ineffective, or specialized treatment is necessary

 ## EVIDENCE

PRACTICE GUIDELINES

- British Association of Dermatologists. Wojnarowska F et al: Guidelines for the management of bullous pemphigoid. Br J Dermatol 2002;147:214.

WEB SITES

- American Academy of Dermatology http://www.aad.org
- An Introduction to Basic Dermatology http://www.vh.org/Providers/Lectures/PietteDermatology/BasicDermatology.html
- Dermatology Handbook for Family Practice from the University of Iowa http://www.vh.org/Providers/ClinRef/FPHandbook/17.html

INFORMATION FOR PATIENTS

- American Academy of Dermatology http://www.aad.org/pamphlets/
- National Institutes of Health http://www.nlm.nih.gov/medlineplus/ency/article/000883.htm

REFERENCES

- Ahmed AR: Intravenous immunoglobulin therapy for patients with bullous pemphigoid unresponsive to conventional immunosuppressive treatment. J Am Acad Dermatol 2001;45:825. [PMID: 11756944]
- Heilborn JD et al: Low-dose oral pulse methotrexate as monotherapy in elderly patients with bullous pemphigoid. J Am Acad Dermatol 1999;40(5 Part 1):741. [PMID: 10321603]
- Nousari HC et al: Pemphigus and bullous pemphigoid. Lancet 1999;354:667. [PMID: 10466686]

Timothy G. Berger, MD

Burns

KEY FEATURES

ESSENTIALS OF DIAGNOSIS

- Assess body surface area affected by burns
- Evaluate depth of burn to categorize as first- or second-degree burn
- Consider patient age and associated illness or injury

GENERAL CONSIDERATIONS

- Only second- and third-degree burns are included in calculating the total burn surface area (TBSA)
- Distinguishing between second- and third-degree burns is not necessary because both are generally treated as full-thickness (third-degree) burns with early excision and grafting

DEMOGRAHICS

- About 1.25 million burn injuries occur yearly in the United States
- About 51,000 victims of acute burns are hospitalized each year in the United States

CLINICAL FINDINGS

SYMPTOMS AND SIGNS

- First-degree burns do not blister initially
- Second-degree burns blister. Hairs are absent or easily extracted, sweat glands become less visible, and the skin appears smoother

DIAGNOSIS

IMAGING STUDIES

- Chest radiographs, usually normal initially, may show acute respiratory distress syndrome in 24–48 h with severe inhalation injury

TREATMENT

MEDICATIONS

- **Crystalloids:** fluid resuscitation may be instituted simultaneously with initial resuscitation
  - The Parkland formula for fluid requirement in the first 24 h is lactated Ringer's injection, estimated as 4 mL/kg body weight per percent of body surface area burned
  - Deep electrical burns and inhalation injury increase the fluid requirement
  - Adequacy of resuscitation is determined by clinical parameters, including urine output and specific gravity, blood pressure, and central venous catheter or, if necessary, Swan-Ganz catheter readings
  - Half the calculated fluid is given in the first 8-h period (measured from the hour of injury). The remaining fluid, divided into two equal parts, is delivered over the next 16 h
  - An extremely large volume of fluid may be required
- **β-Blockade:** routine β-blockade (propranolol, adjusting dose to decrease resting heart rate by 20%, for up to 4 weeks) may reverse some of the catecholamine-mediated hypermetabolic response after severe burns
- **Colloids:** avoid colloids in routine burn resuscitation because of potential decline in glomerular filtration and its association with pulmonary edema

SURGERY

- Because a full-thickness circumferential burn may develop ischemia under a constricting eschar, escharotomy incisions through the anesthetic eschar can save life and limb
- Early excision and grafting of burned areas, as soon as 24 h after injury or when the patient will hemodynamically tolerate the excision and grafting procedure, are critical
- Wounds that will not heal in 7–10 days (ie, deep second-degree or third-degree burns) are best treated by excision and autograft

THERAPEUTIC PROCEDURES

- Establish an airway, evaluate the cervical spine and head injuries, and stabilize fractures
- Give supplemental oxygen

- **Vascular access:** remove all clothing and establish a venous access, preferably with a percutaneous large-bore (14- or 16-gauge) intravenous line through non-burned skin (eg, femoral lines), since hypovolemic shock may develop with major burns
  - Avoid emergent subclavian lines in a volume-depleted patient because of the risk of pneumothorax and subclavian vein laceration
  - *All lines—without exception—placed in the emergency department should be changed within 24 h because of the high risk of nonsterile placement*
- Protect the wound by application of topical antibiotic, such as silver sulfadiazine or mafenide acetate
- Clean burned areas thoroughly

OUTCOME

FOLLOW-UP

- A Foley catheter is essential for monitoring urinary output
- Follow inhalation injuries with serial blood gas determination and bronchoscopy

COMPLICATIONS

- Suspect smoke inhalation injury when the nasal hairs are singed, the mechanism of burn involves closed spaces, the sputum is carbonaceous, or the carboxyhemoglobin level exceeds 5% in nonsmokers
- Electrical injury that causes burns may also produce cardiac arrhythmias that require immediate attention
- Pancreatitis occurs in severe burns
- Prior alcohol exposure may exacerbate the pulmonary components of burn injury
- Nearly all burn patients have one or more septicemic episodes during their hospital course

PROGNOSIS

- The Baux Score (age + percent burn) predicts mortality after major burn
- A base deficit during resuscitation of greater than −6 mmol/L predicts a far higher incidence of multiple organ dysfunction and death

WHEN TO REFER

- Burn units offer the extensive support needed for patients with burns

PREVENTION

- Prophylactic antibiotics in burn patients are increasingly being used
- Prophylactic administration of trimethoprim-sulfamethoxazole may prevent methicillin-resistant *S aureus* (MRSA) infection in ventilator-dependent burn patients
- Maintain normal core body temperature with burns >20% of TBSA
- If tube feedings are not tolerated, begin total parenteral nutrition because of markedly increased metabolic rate. As much as 4000–6000 kcal/day may be required in the postburn period

EVIDENCE

WEB SITE

- Merck Manual—Disorder due to physical agents
  http://www.merck.com/pubs/mmanual/section20/sec20.htm

INFORMATION FOR PATIENTS

- JAMA patient page: Burn injuries. JAMA 2003;290:844.
- The Mayo Clinic
  http://www.mayoclinic.com/invoke.cfm?id=FA00022

REFERENCES

- Cumming J et al: Objective estimates of the incidence and consequences of multiple organ dysfunction and sepsis after burn trauma. J Trauma 2001;50:510. [PMID: 11265031]
- Marik PE et al: Early enteral nutrition in acutely ill patients: a systematic review. Crit Care Med 2001;29:2264. [PMID: 11801821]

Richard Cohen, MD, MPH
Brent R.W. Moelleken, MD, FACS

Cancer, Overview

 KEY FEATURES

ESSENTIALS OF DIAGNOSIS

- In the United States, second most common cause of death after cardiovascular disease
- In 2002, >1.3 million new cases of invasive cancer and >550,000 cancer deaths
- One of every 2 men and 1 of every 3 women will develop invasive cancer

GENERAL CONSIDERATIONS

- Cause of most cancers unknown
- DNA mutations in protooncogenes or deletion of tumor suppressor genes (eg, *P53*), or both, cause abnormal cellular proliferation
- Overexpression of *Bcl-2* in breast, colon, prostate, head and neck, and ovarian cancer confers resistance to chemotherapy and radiation therapy
- Certain chromosomal abnormalities are associated with specific malignancies and can be used to assess prognosis
- Autoimmune suppression may contribute to development of cancer
- Hereditary predisposition to some cancers is linked to gene mutations
- Somatic genetic mutations can be caused by environmental exposure, genetic susceptibility to environmental toxins, infectious agents, physical agents, and drugs, including chemotherapeutic agents such as alkylating agents and topoisomerase II inhibitors

DEMOGRAPHICS

- U.S. incidence and mortality data for common cancers in Table 146 (page 1328)
- Lifetime risk of diagnosis or death for 5 leading cancers in the United States is listed in Table 147 (page 1328)
- Median age at diagnosis of cancer is 68
- Risk factors for cancer: tobacco use, diet, alcohol consumption, obesity, parity, length of lactation, and occupation

 CLINICAL FINDINGS

SYMPTOMS AND SIGNS

- Anorexia
- Malaise
- Weight loss
- Fever
- Local effects of tumor growth
- Paraneoplastic syndromes (Table 151, page 1339)

DIFFERENTIAL DIAGNOSIS

- Depression
- Thyroid disease
- Metabolic disorders (renal, liver disease)
- Chronic infection
- Rheumatologic disease

 DIAGNOSIS

LABORATORY TESTS

- Tumor markers primarily used for assessing response to therapy in advanced disease

IMAGING STUDIES

- Plain x-rays occasionally helpful
- CT, MRI
- PET scan may be more sensitive for certain cancers
- Bone scan to assess for skeletal metastases

DIAGNOSTIC PROCEDURES

- Surgical staging
- Sentinel lymph node biopsy under investigation

Staging

- TNM system: used clinically to indicate the extension of cancer before definitive therapy begins: extent of untreated primary tumor (T); regional lymph node involvement (N); distant metastases (M)
- Staging of certain tumors (lymphomas, Hodgkin's disease) differs to reflect their natural history and to better direct treatment decisions
- Pathological characteristics of certain tumors add prognostic information
- Overexpression or underproduction of oncogene products (Her-2/*neu* in breast cancer), infection of cancer cells with specific viral genomes (HPV18 in cervical cancer), and certain chromosomal

translocations or deletions (alteration of the retinoic acid receptor gene in acute promyelocytic leukemia) have prognostic significance and may direct therapy

TREATMENT

MEDICATIONS

- Systemic chemotherapy can be used
  - As curative therapy for certain malignancies
  - Preoperatively, as "neoadjuvant" therapy to reduce the size and extent of the primary tumor, allowing complete excision at surgery
  - As adjuvant therapy to decrease the rate of relapse, improve the disease-free interval, and improve cure rate
  - As palliative therapy for symptoms and to prolong survival in some patients with incurable malignancies
  - As intensive therapy, in combination with bone marrow transplant to improve cure rate in certain cancers
- Regional administration of active chemotherapeutic agents into the tumor site can result in palliation and prolonged survival
- Types of cancer responsive to chemotherapy and current treatments of choice in Table 148 (page 1329)
- Dosage schedules and toxicities of most commonly used chemotherapeutic agents in Table 149 (page 1332)
- Hormonal therapy (or ablation) used in treatment and palliation of breast, prostate, endometrial cancers
- Bisphosphonates used to reduce bone pain and fractures in bone metastases

SURGERY

- Resection is treatment of choice for gastrointestinal, genitourinary, central nervous system, breast, thyroid, or skin cancers and sarcomas
- Cryosurgical ablation being evaluated for localized breast and prostate cancer
- Resection of isolated metastases and limited recurrences may result in long-term disease-free survival

THERAPEUTIC PROCEDURES

- Radiation therapy may be used primarily or in combination with surgery and/or chemotherapy for cancers of the larynx, oral cavity, pharynx, esophagus, uterine

Cancer, Overview

cervix, vagina, prostate, skin, Hodgkin's lymphoma and non-Hodgkin's lymphoma, brain and spinal cord

 OUTCOME

FOLLOW-UP

- Monitor for toxicities and need for dosage modification (Table 150, page 1338)
- Evaluate tumor response by examination and radiographic imaging
  - Partial response (PR) = 50% or greater reduction in the original tumor mass
  - Complete response (CR) = complete disappearance of detectable tumor
  - Progression = increase in size of tumor by 25% or more or any new lesions
- Tumor markers used to monitor response

COMPLICATIONS

Of cancer

- Spinal cord compression
- Hypercalcemia
- Hyperuricemia and acute urate nephropahty
- Malignant carcinoid syndrome
- Malignant effusions
- Infection
- Paraneoplastic syndromes (Table 151, page 1339)

Of therapy

- Toxicities of most commonly used chemotherapeutic agents in Table 149 (page 1337)
- Acute radiation toxicity: fatigue, malaise, anorexia, nausea, vomiting, local skin changes, diarrhea, mucosal ulceration of irradiated area, bone marrow suppression, pneumonitis, congestive heart failure, gastroenteritis
- Long-term radiation toxicity: increased cardiac mortality with chest radiation, secondary leukemias and solid tumors, decreased function of the radiated organ, myelopathy, osteonecrosis, and hyperpigmentation of the involved skin

PROGNOSIS

- Functional status at diagnosis (or at start of treatment) is a major prognostic factor and determinant of outcome with or without tumor-directed therapy
- Depends on stage

WHEN TO REFER

- Patients with strong family histories of cancer should be referred for genetic screening and counseling

WHEN TO ADMIT

- Oncological emergencies
- Fever and neutropenia after chemotherapy
- Intractable pain

PREVENTION

Primary prevention

- Smoking cessation
- Diets rich in vegetables and fruit and low in saturated fats
- Reduced exposure to UV light and regular use of sunscreen
- Aspirin and nonsteroidal antiinflammatory drugs for colon cancer, polyps
- Vitamin E for prostate cancer
- Calcium for colon polyps and selenium for prostate cancer
- Tamoxifen for breast cancer
- Oral contraceptives for ovarian cancer
- Bilateral prophylactic oophorectomy or mastectomy

Secondary prevention

- Mammography
- Pap smear and human papillomavirus testing
- Fecal occult blood testing (FOBT), sigmoidoscopy, and colonoscopy
- Prostate-specific antigen in combination with digital rectal examination controversial for prostate cancer screening

 EVIDENCE

PRACTICE GUIDELINES

- www.nccn.org (cancer diagnosis and treatment guidelines)
- www.cancer.org (cancer screening guidelines)

WEB SITES

- www.cancernet.nci.nih.gov
- www.cancertrials.nci.gov (cancer trial information)
- www.cancer.org (cancer screening guidelines)

INFORMATION FOR PATIENTS

- www.PeopleLivingWithCancer.org

REFERENCES

- *AJCC Cancer Staging Manual/American Joint Committee on Cancer*, ed 6. Springer, 2002. (The newly revised bible of TNM staging.)
- Chlebowski RT et al: Reducing the risk of breast cancer. N Engl J Med 2000;343:191. [PMID: 10900280]
- Janne PA et al: Chemoprevention of colorectal cancer. N Engl J Med 2000;342:1960. [PMID: 10874065]
- Lieberman DA et al: Use of colonoscopy to screen asymptomatic adults for colorectal cancer. N Engl J Med 2000;343:162. [PMID: 10900274]
- Mandel JS et al: The effect of fecal occult-blood screening on the incidence of colorectal cancer. N Engl J Med 2000;343:1603. [PMID: 11096167]
- Sawaya GF et al: Current approaches to cervical cancer screening. N Engl J Med 2001;344:1603. [PMID: 11372013]
- Smith TJ et al: American Society of Clinical Oncology 1998 Update of Recommended Breast Cancer Surveillance Guidelines. J Clin Oncol 1999;17:1080. [PMID: 10071303]

Hope Rugo, MD

Candidiasis

 KEY FEATURES

ESSENTIALS OF DIAGNOSIS

- Common normal flora and opportunistic pathogen
- Gastrointestinal mucosal disease most common, particularly esophagitis
- Catheter-associated fungemia in hospitalized patients
- Diagnosis of invasive systemic disease requires biopsy or evidence of retinal disease

GENERAL CONSIDERATIONS

- Cutaneous and oral lesions
- Persistent oral or vaginal candidiasis should arouse suspicion of HIV infection
- Fungemia in immunocompromised patients on fluconazole prophylaxis is increasingly due to imidazole-resistant *Candida albicans* or non-*albicans* species

DEMOGRAPHICS

- Mucocutaneous disease occurs with cellular immunodeficiency
- Vulvovaginal candidiasis occurs with pregnancy, uncontrolled diabetes mellitus, broad-spectrum antibiotics, corticosteroids, HIV
- Invasive candidiasis occurs with prolonged neutropenia, recent surgery, broad-spectrum antibiotics, IV catheters (especially for total parenteral nutrition), IV drug use
- Candidal endocarditis occurs with repeated inoculation with IV drug use and direct inoculation during valvular heart surgery causing infection of prosthetic valves in first few months following surgery

 CLINICAL FINDINGS

SYMPTOMS AND SIGNS

- Esophageal candidiasis
  - Substernal odynophagia, gastroesophageal reflux, or nausea without substernal pain
  - Oral candidiasis may not be present
- Vulvovaginal candidiasis: acute vulvar pruritus, burning vaginal discharge, and dyspareunia
- Disseminated candidiasis
  - Fluffy white retinal infiltrates (in <50%)
  - Raised, erythematous skin lesions that may be painful (in <50%)
  - Brain, meninges, and myocardial involvement
- Hepatosplenic candidiasis: fever and variable abdominal pain weeks after chemotherapy for hematological cancers, when neutrophil counts have recovered
- Candidal endocarditis: splenomegaly, petechiae, large-vessel embolization

DIFFERENTIAL DIAGNOSIS

- Esophageal
  - Herpes simplex virus (HSV) esophagitis
  - Cytomegalovirus (CMV) esophagitis
  - Varicella-zoster virus esophagitis
  - Pill esophagitis, eg, nonsteroidal anti-inflammatory drugs, bisphosphonates, KCl
  - Gastroesophageal reflux disease
- Vulvovaginal
  - Bacterial vaginosis
  - *Trichomonas* vaginitis
  - Normal vaginal discharge
- Disseminated
  - Histoplasmosis
  - Coccidioidomycosis
  - Tuberculosis
  - Bacterial endocarditis
  - Aspergillosis

DIAGNOSIS

LABORATORY TESTS

- Disseminated candidiasis: blood cultures positive in only 50%
- Hepatosplenic candidiasis: blood cultures generally negative, alkaline phosphatase elevated, diagnosis established by liver biopsy and culture
- Candidal endocarditis: positive culture from emboli or from vegetations found during valve replacement

IMAGING STUDIES

- Esophageal candidiasis: difficult to distinguish from CMV or HSV esophagitis on barium swallow
- Hepatosplenic candidiasis: abdominal CT shows hepatosplenomegaly with multiple low-density defects in the liver

DIAGNOSTIC PROCEDURES

- Esophageal candidiasis best confirmed by endoscopy with biopsy and culture
- Fundoscopic examination helpful in suspected fungemia

TREATMENT

MEDICATIONS

- Esophageal candidiasis
  - Fluconazole, 100 mg PO QD, or itraconazole solution, 100 mg PO QD for 10–14 days
  - Amphotericin, B 0.3 mg/kg/day IV for 10–14 days if ill, cannot take PO, or developed esophagitis while on fluconazole
  - Caspofungin acetate, 50 mg/day IV, has equivalent efficacy to amphotericin B without significant toxicity
- Vulvovaginal candidiasis
  - Topical azole, eg, clotrimazole, 100 mg vaginally QD for 7 days, or miconazole, 200 mg vaginally QD for 3 days
  - Fluconazole, 150 mg PO once, has equivalent efficacy with better patient acceptance
- Candidal funguria
  - Benefit from treatment of asymptomatic candiduria not demonstrated
  - Frequently resolves with discontinuance of antibiotics or removal of bladder catheter
  - Fluconazole, 200 mg PO QD for 7–14 days if symptoms persist
- Candidal fungemia
  - Amphotericin, B 0.3–0.5 mg/kg/day
  - Flucytosine, 150 mg/kg/day PO divided QID, is added if CNS involvement
  - Fluconazole 200–800 mg/day IV, if amphotericin B not tolerated
  - Lipid formulations of amphotericin B reduce nephrotoxicity, allowing administration of higher doses, but are more costly
- Hepatosplenic candidiasis: fluconazole, 400 mg daily, or a lipid formulation of amphotericin B until clinical and radiographic improvement
- Candidal endocarditis: amphotericin B usually to total dose of 1–1.5 g IV

SURGERY

- Removal or exchange of IV catheters decreases duration of candidemia
- Candidal endocarditis: surgical valve replacement needed in addition to amphotericin

 OUTCOME

COMPLICATIONS

- Candidal funguria: rare ureteral obstruction and dissemination
- Candidal fungemia: endophthalmitis; often no complications if fungemia resolves with removal of IV catheters
- Candidal endocarditis: valve destruction (usually aortic or mitral) is common

PROGNOSIS

- Esophageal candidiasis: relapse common in HIV infection

PREVENTION

- Fluconazole prophylaxis for high-risk patients undergoing induction chemotherapy
- Minimize unnecessary broad-spectrum antibiotics and IV catheters

 EVIDENCE

PRACTICE GUIDELINES

- Infectious Diseases Society of America—Practice guidelines for the treatment of candidiasis.
  http://www.journals.uchicago.edu/CID/journal/issues/v30n4/990667/990667.web.pdf

WEB SITE

- Project Inform
  http://www.ProjectInform.org

INFORMATION FOR PATIENTS

- CDC Disease Information
  http://www.cdc.gov/ncidod/dbmd/diseaseinfo/candidiasis_g.htm
- JAMA patient page: HIV infection: the basics. JAMA 2002;288:268. [PMID: 12123237]
- Mayo Clinic
  http://www.mayoclinic.com/invoke.cfm?id=DS00408
- MEDLINEplus
  http://www.nlm.nih.gov/medlineplus/ency/article/000626.htm

REFERENCES

- Kontoyiannis DP et al: Fluconazole vs. amphotericin B for the management of candidaemia in adults: a meta-analysis. Mycoses 2001;44:125. [PMID: 11486448]
- Mora-Duarte J et al: Comparison of caspofungin and amphotericin B for invasive candidiasis. N Engl J Med 2002;347:2020. [PMID: 12490683]
- Rex JH et al: Practice guidelines for the treatment of candidiasis. Clin Infect Dis 2000;30:662. [PMID: 10770728]

Richard J. Hamill, MD

Candidiasis, Mucocutaneous

Candidiasis, Oral p. 1078. Carbon Monoxide Poisoning p. 1078. Carcinoid Syndrome, Malignant p. 1079.

 ## KEY FEATURES

ESSENTIALS OF DIAGNOSIS

- Candidal intertrigo
- Oral candidiasis
- Angular cheilitis
- Perianal candidiasis
- Candidal paranonychia
- Severe pruritus of vulva, anus, or body folds
- Superficial denuded, beefy-red areas with or without satellite vesicopustules
- Whitish curd-like concretions on the oral and vaginal mucous membranes
- Yeast on microscopic examination of scales or curd

GENERAL CONSIDERATIONS

- Superficial fungal infection that may involve almost any cutaneous or mucous surface of the body
- Particularly likely to occur in diabetics, during pregnancy, and in obese persons who perspire freely
- Antibiotics and oral contraceptive agents may be contributory

DEMOGRAPHICS

- Oral candidiasis more common in elderly, debilitated, malnourished, diabetic, or HIV-infected patients as well as those taking antibiotics, systemic steroids, or chemotherapy

 ## CLINICAL FINDINGS

SYMPTOMS AND SIGNS

- See Table 7 (page 1202)
- Itching may be intense
- Burning is reported, particularly around the vulva and anus
- Lesions consist of superficially denuded, beefy-red areas in the depths of the body folds such as in the groin and the intergluteal cleft, beneath the breasts, at the angles of the mouth, and in the umbilicus; the peripheries of these denuded lesions are superficially undermined, and there may be satellite vesicopustules
- Whitish, curd-like concretions may be present on the surface of the mucosal lesions
- Paronychia and interdigital erosions may occur

DIFFERENTIAL DIAGNOSIS

Cutaneous candidiasis

- Intertrigo
- Seborrheic dermatitis
- Tinea cruris (jock itch)
- Psoriasis of body folds ("inverse psoriasis")
- Erythrasma
- Contact dermatitis
- Tinea versicolor (pityriasis versicolor) (rarely)

Oral candidiasis

- Leukoplakia
- Lichen planus
- Dysplasia or carcinoma
- Geographic tongue
- Herpes simplex
- Erythema multiforme
- Pemphigus
- Oral hairy leukoplakia

DIAGNOSIS

LABORATORY TESTS

- Clusters of budding cells and hyphae can be seen under high power when skin scales or curd-like lesions have been cleared in 10% KOH

Candidiasis, Mucocutaneous

 ## TREATMENT

MEDICATIONS

- See Table 6 (page 1202)

Nails and skin

- Apply ciclopirox cream, nystatin cream, 100,000 units/g, or miconazole, econazole, ketoconazole, or clotrimazole cream three or four times daily
- Gentian violet, 1%, or carbolfuchsin paint (Castellani's paint) may be applied once or twice weekly as an alternative, but these preparations are messy

Vaginal candidiasis

- Single-dose fluconazole (150 mg) is effective; intravaginal clotrimazole, miconazole, terconazole, or nystatin may also be used
- Chronic suppressive therapy may be required for recurrent or "intractable" cases
- Non-*albicans* candidal species may be identified by culture in some refractory cases and may respond to oral itraconazole, 200 mg twice daily for 2–4 weeks

Balanitis

- Most frequent in uncircumcised men
- Topical imidazole cream or nystatin ointment is the initial treatment if the lesions are mildly erythematous or superficially erosive
- Soaking with dilute aluminum acetate for 15 min twice daily may quickly relieve burning or itching
- Chronicity and relapses, especially after sexual contact, suggest reinfection from a sexual partner who should be treated
- Severe purulent balanitis is usually due to bacteria; if it is so severe that phimosis occurs, oral antibiotics—some with activity against anaerobes—are required; if rapid improvement does not occur, urological consultation is indicated

THERAPEUTIC PROCEDURES

- Affected parts should be kept dry and exposed to air as much as possible
- If possible, discontinue systemic antibiotics

 ## OUTCOME

PROGNOSIS

- Cases of cutaneous candidiasis range from the easily cured to the intractable and prolonged

WHEN TO REFER

- If there is a question about the diagnosis, if recommended therapy is ineffective, or if specialized treatment is necessary

PREVENTION

- Keep skin dry and cool
- Keep good glucose control in diabetics

EVIDENCE

PRACTICE GUIDELINES

- National Guideline Clearinghouse http://www.guideline.gov/summary/summary.aspx?doc_id=2670&nbr=1896&string=candidiasis
- American Academy of Dermatology http://www.aadassociation.org/Guidelines/mucocand.html

WEB SITES

- American Academy of Dermatology http://www.aad.org
- Dermatology Handbook for Family Practice from the University of Iowa http://www.vh.org/Providers/ClinRef/FPHandbook/17.html

INFORMATION FOR PATIENTS

- National Institutes of Health Medical Encyclopedia http://www.nlm.nih.gov/medlineplus/ency/article/000880.htm
- The Nemours Foundation http://kidshealth.org/parent/infections/common/candidiasis.html

REFERENCE

- Ringdahl EN: Treatment of recurrent vulvovaginal candidiasis. Am Fam Physician 2000;61:3306. [PMID: 10865926]

Timothy G. Berger, MD

Celiac Disease

Cardiomyopathy, Hypertrophic p. 1080. Cardiomyopathy, Peripartum p. 1080. Cardiomyopathy, Primary Dilated p. 1081. Carotid Artery Aneurysm p. 1081.

 ## KEY FEATURES

ESSENTIALS OF DIAGNOSIS

- Typical symptoms: weight loss, chronic diarrhea, abdominal distension, growth retardation
- Atypical symptoms: dermatitis herpetiformis, iron deficiency anemia, osteoporosis
- Abnormal serological test results
- Abnormal small bowel biopsy
- Clinical improvement on gluten-free diet

GENERAL CONSIDERATIONS

- Also known as gluten enteropathy or celiac sprue
- Diffuse damage to the proximal small intestinal mucosa results in malabsorption of most nutrients
- Typical symptoms commonly manifest between 6 months and 24 months of age
- Up to 50% of cases present with atypical symptoms in childhood or adulthood
- More than 10% of adults with iron deficiency have undiagnosed celiac disease
- Removal of gluten from the diet results in resolution of symptoms and intestinal healing in most patients
- Celiac disease may be associated with other autoimmune disorders

DEMOGRAPHICS

- Occurs in 1:250 whites of Northern European ancestry but is rare in Africans and Asians
- Clinical diagnosis made in only 1:5000 persons in the United States, so most cases are undiagnosed

 ## CLINICAL FINDINGS

SYMPTOMS AND SIGNS

- Infants (<2 years): diarrhea, weight loss, abdominal distension, weakness, muscle wasting, or growth retardation; stools characteristically loose to soft, large, floating, oily or greasy, and foul-smelling, may also be watery and frequent in number (up to 10–12 daily)
- Children and adults: chronic diarrhea or flatulence, weight loss (variable), fatigue, short stature, osteoporosis, dental enamel hypoplasia, and anemia
- Physical examination may be normal in mild cases; may reveal signs of malabsorption, loss of muscle mass or subcutaneous fat, pallor, easy bruising, hyperkeratosis, or bone pain in more severe cases
- Abdominal examination may reveal distension with hyperactive bowel sounds
- Dermatitis herpetiformis in <10%

DIFFERENTIAL DIAGNOSIS

- Irritable bowel syndrome
- Malabsorption due to other cause, eg, pancreatic insufficiency, reduced bile salts, lymphatic obstruction, bacterial overgrowth, tropical sprue
- Lactase deficiency
- Viral gastroenteritis, eosinophilic gastroenteritis
- Whipple's disease
- Giardiasis
- Mucosal damage caused by acid hypersecretion associated with gastrinoma

 ## DIAGNOSIS

LABORATORY TESTS

- Obtain complete blood cell count, prothrombin time, and serum iron or ferritin, red cell folate, vitamin B_{12} level, serum calcium, alkaline phosphatase, albumin, and β-carotene
- Iron deficiency or megaloblastic anemia occurs due to iron or folate or vitamin B_{12} malabsorption
- Dual-energy x-ray densitometry scanning for osteoporosis
- Elevations of prothrombin time
- Nonanion gap acidosis and hypokalemia in severe diarrhea
- Steatorrhea detected by a qualitative (Sudan stain) or quantitative 72-h stool assessment for fecal fat while patients are consuming a 100-g fat diet; excretion of more than 10 g/day of fat is abnormal
- D-Xylose test for malabsorption

Serological tests

- IgG and IgA antigliadin antibodies present in >90%, IgG antibody is more sensitive, IgA antibody is more specific, a combination of the two tests provides sensitivity and specificity of >95%
- The IgA endomysial antibody test has >90% sensitivity and specificity
- Tissue transglutaminase antibody has >95% sensitivity and specificity; may be preferred serological test
- Serological tests become negative 6–12 months after dietary gluten withdrawal

DIAGNOSTIC PROCEDURES

- Mucosal biopsy: endoscopic mucosal biopsy of the distal duodenum or proximal jejunum confirms diagnosis

Celiac Disease

 ## TREATMENT

- Removal of all gluten from the diet
- Most patients with celiac disease also have lactose intolerance either temporarily or permanently and should avoid dairy products until the intestinal symptoms have improved on the gluten-free diet

MEDICATIONS

- Nutrient supplements (folate, iron, vitamin B_{12}, calcium, vitamins A and D) in initial stages of therapy, as necessary
- Calcium, vitamin D, and bisphosphonate therapy for osteoporosis

 ## OUTCOME

FOLLOW-UP

- Improvement in symptoms within a few weeks on the gluten-free diet

PROGNOSIS

- If appropriately diagnosed and treated, excellent prognosis
- Celiac disease that is truly refractory to gluten withdrawal carries a poor prognosis; may be caused by ulcerative jejunitis or enteropathy or by associated T cell lymphoma, which occurs in up to 10% of patients

 ## EVIDENCE

PRACTICE GUIDELINES

- American Gastroenterological Association medical position statement: celiac sprue. Reviewed 2001 http://www2.gastrojournal.org/scripts/om.dll/serve?action=get-media&id=a0060101522&trueID=pdf_0060101522&location=jgast0112006&type=pdf&name=x.pdf
- Ciclitira PJ et al: AGA technical review on celiac sprue. American Gastroenterological Association. Gastroenterology. 2001;120:1526. [PMID: 11313324]

WEB SITES

- Celiac Sprue Association http://www.csaceliacs.org/
- National Institute of Diabetes and Digestive and Kidney Diseases (NIDDK), NIH http://www.niddk.nih.gov/

INFORMATION FOR PATIENTS

- Celiac Disease Foundation http://www.celiac.org
- Celiac Disease http://www.ama-assn.org/public/journals/patient/archive/jpg032002.htm
- National Institute of Diabetes and Digestive and Kidney Diseases (NIDDK), NIH http://digestive.niddk.nih.gov/ddiseases/pubs/celiac/index.htm

REFERENCES

- American Gastroenterological Association medical position statement: Celiac sprue. Gastroenterology 2001;120:1522. [PMID: 11313323]
- Farrell RJ et al: Celiac sprue. N Engl J Med 2002;346:180. [PMID: 11796853]
- Shan L et al: Structural basis for gluten intolerance in celiac sprue. Science 2002;297:2275. [PMID: 12351792]

Kenneth R. McQuaid, MD

Cerebrovascular Disease, Occlusive

 KEY FEATURES

ESSENTIALS OF DIAGNOSIS

- A stroke is defined as a sudden onset of a neurological deficit that persists beyond 24 h
- A transient ischemic attack (TIA) is defined as the sudden onset of a neurological deficit that resolves completely within 24 h

GENERAL CONSIDERATIONS

- Most strokes are caused by emboli occluding small cerebral arteries
- Emboli consist of platelet aggregates that form on irregular or ulcerated surfaces, or plaque debris liberated by turbulent flow and intraplaque hemorrhage from the carotid bifurcation, from the heart (eg, mural thrombus or atrial myxoma), or from the aortic arch
- Stroke is also caused by intracerebral hemorrhage (from trauma, hypertension, or a ruptured cerebral aneurysm) or by small vessel occlusive disease in the pons, basal ganglia, and internal capsule (lacunar infarcts)
- Risk of stroke for carotid artery stenosis <60% is 1.6% per year; >60% is 3.2% per year; >80% is 5–10% per year
- Increased stroke risk is also associated with rapid progression of carotid disease and with plaque heterogeneity or ulceration
- Risk factors for carotid disease include hypertension, diabetes mellitus, hypercholesterolemia, advanced age, smoking, and coronary artery disease
- A single TIA is associated with a 30% risk of subsequent stroke

DEMOGRAPHICS

- Every year, half a million people in the United States suffer a stroke
- 15–30% of strokes are fatal

 CLINICAL FINDINGS

SYMPTOMS AND SIGNS

- Carotid artery occlusive disease: contralateral weakness or sensory loss, expressive aphasia, and amaurosis fugax (transient partial or complete loss of vision in the ipsilateral eye)
- Vertebrobasilar occlusive disease: brainstem and cerebellar symptoms, including dysarthria, diplopia, vertigo, ataxia, and hemiparesis or quadriparesis
- Cervical bruits
- Diminished or absent pulses in the neck or arms
- Hollenhorst plaques (bright, refractile cholesterol emboli) in the retinal arteries
- Blood pressure difference between the two arms of >10 mm Hg

DIFFERENTIAL DIAGNOSIS

- Acute myocardial infarction
- Carotid dissection
- Syncope
- Intracranial hemorrhage

 DIAGNOSIS

IMAGING STUDIES

- Duplex carotid ultrasonography provides both physiological (flow) and anatomic (plaque characterization) information; percent stenosis is derived from measurement of blood flow velocities, with sensitivity and specificity >90%
- Gadolinium-enhanced magnetic resonance angiography (MRA) or CT angiography (CTA) provides anatomic information, cross-sectional imaging for measurement of degree of stenosis, and characterizes the arch intracranial circulation and vertebral arteries
  - MRA can provide more detailed information about plaque composition, but is time-consuming and can overestimate degree of stenosis
  - CTA is fast but requires contrast and can be limited in cases with severe arterial calcification
- Ultrasound plus MRA or CTA estimates percent stenosis better than conventional angiography
- Conventional or CT angiography is used in cases of suspected carotid occlusion before nonoperative management is elected because a small percentage will have internal carotid artery "string sign" lesions that require urgent revascularization
- Because catheter angiography has a 1% risk of procedure-related stroke, it is reserved for patients with greatly disparate ultrasound and CTA or MRA findings, those suspected of vertebrobasilar insufficiency or intracranial lesions, those unable to undergo MRA or CTA, and those potentially requiring endovascular intervention
- Noncontrast CT head for any patients with TIA/CVA

Cerebrovascular Disease, Occlusive

 ## TREATMENT

MEDICATIONS

- Asymptomatic diagnosis: antiplatelet medication, eg, aspirin, 325 mg PO QD; ticlopidine, 250 mg PO BID; or clopidogrel, 75 mg PO BID, to reduce the likelihood of thrombosis and microemboli
- Acute TIA: heparin by continuous infusion for urgent surgery
- Acute stroke: heparin then coumadin in preparation for surgery in 5—8 weeks
- Warfarin or clopidogrel for patients with neurological symptoms secondary to intracerebral disease not amenable to surgical reconstruction

SURGERY

Acute stroke

- Delay surgery until neurological examination stabilizes (5–8 weeks)
- Carotid endarterectomy, antiplatelet therapy, and risk factor modification

Transient ischemic attacks

- Carotid endarterectomy plus antiplatelet or anticoagulant therapy, and risk factor modification
  - Highly effective in preventing stroke and death in symptomatic patients with >70% carotid stenosis
  - More modest benefit/risk ratio in symptomatic patients with 50–69% carotid stenosis

Asymptomatic carotid stenosis

- Risk of stroke is ~5% per year in asymptomatic patients with >80% carotid stenosis
- Carotid endarterectomy in good-risk asymptomatic patients with >60% stenosis affords an overall risk reduction of 53% compared to aspirin alone

THERAPEUTIC PROCEDURES

- Percutaneous techniques: carotid angioplasty and stenting indicated in patients who are not good candidates for surgery

 ## OUTCOME

COMPLICATIONS

- Carotid endarterectomy morbidity–mortality rate is <5%; endarterectomy has a ~1–2% mortality rate and ~1–4% risk of neurological complications
- Carotid stenting has a 5–18% risk of periprocedural stroke or TIA and 8–14% per year incidence of recurrent stenosis (compared with <4% per year with surgery)

PROGNOSIS

- In symptomatic patients, endarterectomy reduces stroke risk 5- to 10-fold at 5 years; there is a 5–15% incidence of late stroke after uncomplicated endarterectomy often related to contralateral carotid or intracranial disease
- Restenosis occurring <2 years after endarterectomy is due to intimal hyperplasia, which responds well to angioplasty and stenting
- Restenosis >2 years after endarterectomy is more often related to progression of atherosclerotic disease
- Repeat surgery or stenting is advised for symptomatic restenoses or >80% stenoses

WHEN TO REFER

- Asymptomatic carotid stenosis >60%
- Symptomatic carotid disease

WHEN TO ADMIT

- Patients with acute or crescendo TIAs for heparin anticoagulation and evaluation for surgery.

PREVENTION

- Risk factor modification: control of hypertension, hyperlipidemia, and diabetes

 ## EVIDENCE

PRACTICE GUIDELINES

- Moore WS et al: Guidelines for carotid endarterectomy. A multidisciplinary consensus statement from the Ad Hoc Committee, American Heart Association. Circulation 1995;91:566. [PMID: 7805271]
- Streefkerk HJ et al: Cerebral revascularization. Adv Tech Stand Neurosurg 2003;28:145. [PMID: 12627810]

WEB SITES

- American Stroke Association—What is stroke? http://www.strokeassociation.org/presenter.jhtml?identifier=2528
- MEDLINEplus—Stroke secondary to atherosclerosis http://www.nlm.nih.gov/medlineplus/ency/article/000738.htm
- National Institute of Neurological Disorders and Stroke http://www.ninds.nih.gov/

INFORMATION FOR PATIENTS

- Cleveland Clinic—Understanding stroke http://www.clevelandclinic.org/health/health-info/docs/2100/2179.asp?index=9074
- JAMA patient page: Stroke prevention http://www.ama-assn.org/insight/spec_con/patient/pat045.pdf
- Mayo Clinic—Stroke http://www.mayoclinic.com/invoke.cfm?objectid=487C37FA-C927-45BF-84821670F1635148

REFERENCES

- Barnett HJM et al: Causes and severity of ischemic stroke in patients with internal carotid artery stenosis. JAMA 2000;283:1429. [PMID: 10732932]
- Endovascular versus surgical treatment in patients with carotid stenosis in the Carotid and Vertebral Artery Transluminal Angioplasty Study (CAVATAS): a randomised trial. Lancet 2001;357:1729. [PMID: 11403808]

Louis M. Messina, MD
Laura K. Pak, MD
Lawrence M. Tierney, Jr., MD

Cervical Cancer

 KEY FEATURES

ESSENTIALS OF DIAGNOSIS

- Abnormal uterine bleeding and vaginal discharge
- Cervical lesion may be visible on inspection as a tumor or ulceration
- Vaginal cytology usually positive; must be confirmed by biopsy

GENERAL CONSIDERATIONS

- Cancer appears first in the intraepithelial layers (the preinvasive stage, or carcinoma in situ)
- Preinvasive cancer (CIN III) is a common diagnosis in women 25–40 years of age and is etiologically related to infection with the human papillomavirus

DEMOGRAPHICS

- Multiparity
- Smoker
- Early initiation of intercourse
- Multiple sex partners

 CLINICAL FINDINGS

SYMPTOMS AND SIGNS

- The most common signs are metrorrhagia, postcoital spotting, and cervical ulceration
- Bloody or purulent, odorous, nonpruritic discharge may appear after invasion
- Bladder and rectal dysfunction or fistulas and pain are late symptoms

DIFFERENTIAL DIAGNOSIS

- Cervical intraepithelial neoplasia
- Cervical ectropion
- Cervical ectopy (columnar epithelium on face of os, common in adolescence)
- Genital warts (condyloma acuminata)
- Cervical polyp
- Cervicitis
- Nabothian cyst
- Granuloma inguinale

DIAGNOSIS

LABORATORY TESTS

- Positive Papanicolaou smear

IMAGING STUDIES

- Further staging assessment beyond biopsy may be carried out by abdominal and pelvic CT scanning or MRI

DIAGNOSTIC PROCEDURES

Cervical biopsy and endocervical curettage, or conization

- These procedures are necessary steps after a positive Papanicolaou smear to determine the extent and depth of invasion of the cancer
- Even if the smear is positive, treatment is never justified until definitive diagnosis has been established through biopsy

"Staging," or estimate of gross spread of cancer of the cervix

- The depth of penetration of the malignant cells beyond the basement membrane is a reliable clinical guide to the extent of primary cancer within the cervix and the likelihood of metastases
- It is customary to stage cancers of the cervix under anesthesia as shown in Table 63 (page 1257)

Cervical Cancer

TREATMENT

SURGERY

Carcinoma in situ (stage 0)

- In women who have completed child-bearing, total hysterectomy is the treatment of choice
- In women who wish to retain the uterus, acceptable alternatives include cervical conization or ablation of the lesion with cryotherapy or laser

Invasive carcinoma

- Microinvasive carcinoma (stage IA) is treated with simple, extrafascial hysterectomy
- Stage IB and stage IIA cancers may be treated with either radical hysterectomy or radiation therapy
- Stage IIB and stage III and IV cancers must be treated with radiation therapy
- Because radical surgery results in fewer long-term complications than irradiation and may allow preservation of ovarian function, it may be the preferred mode of therapy in younger women without contraindications to major surgery

Emergency measures

- Vaginal hemorrhage originates from gross ulceration and cavitation in stage II–IV cervical carcinoma
- Ligation and suturing of the cervix are usually not feasible, but ligation of the uterine or hypogastric arteries may be lifesaving when other measures fail
- Styptics such as Monsel's solution or acetone are effective, although delayed sloughing may result in further bleeding
- Wet vaginal packing is helpful
- Emergency irradiation usually controls bleeding

OUTCOME

FOLLOW-UP

- Carcinoma in situ
- Close follow-up with Papanicolaou smears every 3 months for 1 year and every 6 months for another year is necessary after cryotherapy or laser

COMPLICATIONS

- Metastases to regional lymph nodes occur with increasing frequency from stage I to stage IV
- The ureters are often obstructed lateral to the cervix, causing hydroureter, hydronephrosis, and renal insufficiency
- Almost two-thirds of untreated patients die of uremia when ureteral obstruction is bilateral
- Pain in the back, in the distribution of the lumbosacral plexus, is often indicative of neurological involvement
- Gross edema of the legs may be indicative of vascular and lymphatic stasis due to tumor
- Vaginal fistulas to the rectum and urinary tract
- 10–20% of patients with extensive invasive carcinoma die of hemorrhage

PROGNOSIS

- Two to 10 years are required for carcinoma to penetrate the basement membrane and invade the tissues; death usually occurs in 3–5 years in untreated or unresponsive patients
- The overall 5-year relative survival rate is 68% in white women and 55% in black women in the United States
- Survival rates are inversely proportional to the stage of cancer: stage 0, 99–100%; stage IA, >95%; stage IB–IIA, 80–90%; stage IIB, 65%; stage III, 40%; stage IV, <20%

WHEN TO REFER

- All patients with invasive cervical cancer should be referred to a gynecological oncologist

PREVENTION

- Regular Papanicolaou smears (Table 145, page 1327)
- Smoking cessation

EVIDENCE

PRACTICE GUIDELINES

- National Guideline Clearinghouse
  http://www.guideline.gov/summary/summary.aspx?doc_id=3286&nbr=2512&string=cervical+cancer
  http://www.guideline.gov/summary/summary.aspx?doc_id=3533&nbr=2759&string=cervical+cancer

WEB SITES

- Cervical Cancer
  http://www.cancer.gov/cancer_information/cancer_type/cervical/
- Cervical Cancer—National Cancer Institute—CancerNet
  http://cancernet.nci.nih.gov/cgi-bin/srchcgi.exe?DBID=pdq&TYPE=search&UID=208+00103&ZFILE=professional&SFMT=pdq_treatment/1/0/0
- Cervical Cancer Screening: Collection of articles
  http://bmj.com/cgi/collection/cervical_screening
- Pap Smear Cytopathology Tutorial
  http://medlib.med.utah.edu/WebPath/TUTORIAL/CYTOPATH/CYTOPATH.html

INFORMATION FOR PATIENTS

- National Cancer Institute
  http://www.cancer.gov/cancerinfo/wyntk/cervix
- JAMA patient page: Cervical cancer. JAMA 2000;283:1094.
- JAMA patient page: Pap test. JAMA 1999;28:1666.

REFERENCES

- Canavan TP et al: Cervical cancer. Am Family Physician 2000;61:1369. [PMID: 10735343]
- Ferrante JM et al: Clinical and demographic predictors of late-stage cervical cancer. Arch Fam Med 2000;9:439. [PMID: 10810949]

H. Trent MacKay, MD, MPH

Cervical Intraepithelial Neoplasia

 ## KEY FEATURES

ESSENTIALS OF DIAGNOSIS

- The presumptive diagnosis is made by an abnormal Pap smear of an asymptomatic woman with no grossly visible cervical changes
- Diagnose by colposcopically directed biopsy
- Increased in women with HIV

GENERAL CONSIDERATIONS

- Cervical infection with the human papillomavirus (HPV) is associated with a high percentage of all cervical dysplasias and cancers
- There are over 60 recognized HPV subtypes, of which types 6 and 11 tend to cause mild dysplasia, while types 16, 18, 31, and others cause higher-grade cellular changes
- The varying degrees of dysplasia are defined by the degree of cellular atypia (Table 62, page 1257)
- The cervical intraepithelial neoplasia (CIN) classification is used along with a description of abnormal cells, including evidence of HPV. The term "squamous intraepithelial lesions (SIL)," low-grade or high-grade, is increasingly used
- HPV testing of cytological smears may be useful for triage of atypia (atypical squamous cells of unknown significance; ASCUS)

DEMOGRAPHICS

- Cervical cancer almost never occurs in virginal women; it is epidemiologically related to the number of sexual partners a woman has had and the number of other female partners a male partner has had
- Women with HIV infection appear to be at increased risk of the disease and of recurrent disease after treatment

 ## CLINICAL FINDINGS

SYMPTOMS AND SIGNS

- There are no specific symptoms or signs of cervical intraepithelial neoplasia

DIFFERENTIAL DIAGNOSIS

- Cervical cancer
- Cervical ectropion
- Cervical ectopy (columnar epithelium on face of os, common in adolescence)
- Genital warts (condyloma acuminata)
- Cervical polyp
- Cervicitis
- Nabothian cyst
- Granuloma inguinale

 ## DIAGNOSIS

LABORATORY TESTS

Cytological examination (Papanicolaou smear)

- Specimens should be taken from a non-menstruating patient, spread on a single slide, and fixed or rinsed directly into preservative solution if a thin-layer slide system (ThinPrep) is to be used
- A specimen should be obtained from the squamocolumnar junction with a wooden or plastic spatula and from the endocervix with a cotton swab or nylon brush

DIAGNOSTIC PROCEDURES

Colposcopy

- Viewing the cervix with 10–20 × magnification allows for assessment of the size and margins of an abnormal transformation zone and determination of extension into the endocervical canal
- The application of 3–5% acetic acid (vinegar) dissolves mucus, and the acid's desiccating action sharpens the contrast between normal and actively proliferating squamous epithelium
- Abnormal changes include white patches and vascular atypia, which indicate areas of greatest cellular activity
- Paint the cervix with Lugol's solution [strong iodine solution (Schiller's test)]. Normal squamous epithelium will take the stain; nonstaining squamous epithelium should be biopsied. (The single-layered, mucus-secreting endocervical tissue will not stain either but can readily be distinguished by its darker pink, shinier appearance.)

Biopsy

- Colposcopically directed punch biopsy and endocervical curettage are office procedures
- If colposcopic examination is not available, the normal-appearing cervix shedding atypical cells can be evaluated by endocervical curettage and multiple punch biopsies of nonstaining squamous epithelium or biopsies from each quadrant of the cervix
- All visibly abnormal cervical lesions should be biopsied

TREATMENT

SURGERY

Conization of the cervix

- Conization is surgical removal of the entire transformation zone and endocervical canal
- It should be reserved for cases of severe dysplasia or cancer in situ (CIN III), particularly those with endocervical extension
- The procedure can be performed with the scalpel, the CO_2 laser, the needle electrode, or by large-loop excision

THERAPEUTIC PROCEDURES

- Treatment varies depending on the degree and extent of cervical intraepithelial neoplasia
- Biopsies should always precede treatment

Cauterization or cryosurgery

- The use of either hot cauterization or freezing (cryosurgery) is effective for noninvasive small lesions visible on the cervix without endocervical extension

CO_2 laser

- This well-controlled method minimizes tissue destruction
- It is colposcopically directed and requires special training
- May be used with large visible lesions
- Involves the vaporization of the transformation zone on the cervix and the distal 5–7 mm of the endocervical canal

Loop resection

- When the CIN is clearly visible in its entirety, a wire loop can be used for excisional biopsy
- Cutting and hemostasis are effected with a low-voltage electrosurgical machine (Bovie)
- This office procedure with local anesthesia is quick and uncomplicated

 OUTCOME

FOLLOW-UP

- All types of dysplasia must be observed and treated if they persist or become more severe
- Because recurrence is possible—especially in the first 2 years after treatment—and because the false-negative rate of a single cervical cytological test is 20%, close follow-up is imperative
- Vaginal cytological examination should be repeated at 3-month intervals for at least 1 year

PROGNOSIS

- At present, the malignant potential of a specific lesion cannot be predicted. Some lesions remain stable for long periods of time; some regress; and others advance
- Adequately treated CIN very rarely progresses to invasive disease

WHEN TO REFER

- Patients with abnormal Papanicolaou smears or visible cervical lesions should be referred for colposcopy

PREVENTION

- Preventive measures include the following
  - Regular cytological screening to detect abnormalities
  - Limiting the number of sexual partners
  - Using a diaphragm or condom for coitus
  - Stopping smoking
- Women with HIV infection should receive regular cytological screening and should be followed closely after treatment for cervical intraepithelial neoplasia
- Because of the very low rate of abnormal Papanicolaou smears in women who have undergone hysterectomy for benign disease, routine screening is not justified in this population

 EVIDENCE

PRACTICE GUIDELINES

- National Guideline Clearinghouse
  http://www.guideline.gov/summary/summary.aspx?doc_id=3286&nbr=2512&string=cervical+intraepithelial+neoplasia
  http://www.guideline.gov/summary/summary.aspx?doc_id=3240&nbr=2466&string=cervical+intraepithelial+neoplasia

WEB SITE

- Colposcopy Atlas
  http://lib-sh.lsumc.edu/fammed/atlases/colpo.html

INFORMATION FOR PATIENTS

- National Cancer Institute
  http://www.cancer.gov/cancerinfo/wyntk/cervix
- JAMA patient page: Papillomavirus JAMA 2002 287(18):2452. [PMID: 12004891]
- JAMA patient page: Pap test. JAMA 1999;28:1666.

REFERENCES

- Sawaya GF et al: Current practice. Current approaches to cervical-cancer screening. N Engl J Med 2001;344:1603. [PMID: 11372013]
- Sherman ME et al: Effects of age and human papilloma viral load on colposcopy triage: data from the Randomized Atypical Squamous Cells of Undetermined Significance/Low-grade Squamous Intraepithelial Lesion Triage Study (ALTS). J Natl Cancer Inst 2002;94:102. [PMID: 11792748]

H. Trent MacKay, MD, MPH

Cholangitis & Choledocholithiasis

 KEY FEATURES

ESSENTIALS OF DIAGNOSIS

- Often a history of biliary colic or jaundice
- Sudden onset of severe right upper quadrant or epigastric pain, which may radiate to the right scapula or shoulder
- Occasional patients present with painless jaundice
- Nausea and vomiting
- Fever, which may be followed by hypothermia and gram-negative shock, jaundice, and leukocytosis
- Abdominal films may reveal gallstones

GENERAL CONSIDERATIONS

- Common duct stones usually originate in the gallbladder but may also form spontaneously in the common duct after cholecystectomy
- The stones are frequently "silent" unless there is obstruction
- Biliary colic results from rapid increases in common bile duct pressure due to obstructed bile flow

DEMOGRAPHICS

- About 15% of patients with gallstones have choledocholithiasis (common bile duct stones). The percentage rises with age, and the frequency in elderly people with gallstones may be as high as 50%

 CLINICAL FINDINGS

SYMPTOMS AND SIGNS

- See Table 60 (page 1256)
- Biliary colic with jaundice
- Frequently recurring attacks of right upper abdominal pain that is severe and persists for hours
- Chills and fever associated with severe colic
- **Charcot's triad** [pain, fever (and chills), and jaundice] is characteristic of cholangitis
- Altered sensorium, lethargy, and septic shock connote acute suppurative cholangitis and constitute an endoscopic or surgical emergency
- Hepatomegaly may be present in calculous biliary obstruction, and tenderness is usually present in the right upper quadrant and epigastrium

DIFFERENTIAL DIAGNOSIS

- Cancer of the pancreas, ampulla of Vater, or common duct
- Acute hepatitis
- Biliary stricture
- Chronic cholestatic liver disease, eg, primary biliary cirrhosis, primary sclerosing cholangitis, drug toxicity
- Pancreatitis
- Sepsis due to other cause
- Underlying ascaris or clonorchis, or hydatid disease

 DIAGNOSIS

LABORATORY TESTS

- Bilirubinuria and elevation of serum bilirubin are present if the common duct is obstructed; levels commonly fluctuate
- Serum alkaline phosphatase elevation is suggestive of obstructive jaundice
- Serum amylase elevations may be present in secondary pancreatitis
- Acute obstruction of the bile duct rarely produces a transient striking increase in serum aminotransferase levels (>1000 units/L)
- Hypoprothrombinemia can result from obstructed flow of bile to the intestine
- When extrahepatic obstruction persists for more than a few weeks, differentiation of obstruction from chronic cholestatic liver disease becomes progressively more difficult

IMAGING STUDIES

- Ultrasonography, CT scan, and radionuclide imaging may demonstrate dilated bile ducts and impaired bile flow
- Endoscopic ultrasonography, helical CT, and MR cholangiography can accurately demonstrate common duct stones and, if available, may be used when there is low or intermediate risk for choledocholithiasis

DIAGNOSTIC PROCEDURES

- Endoscopic retrograde cholangiopancreatography (ERCP) or percutaneous transhepatic cholangiography is the best means to determine the cause, location, and extent of obstruction
- If the likelihood that obstruction is caused by a stone is high, ERCP is the procedure of choice because it permits papillotomy or balloon dilation of the papilla with stone extraction or stent placement

Cholangitis & Choledocholithiasis

TREATMENT

MEDICATIONS

Hypoprothrombinemia

- Treat with 10 mg of parenteral vitamin K or water-soluble oral vitamin K (phytonadione, 5 mg) in 24–36 h

Cholangitis

- Ciprofloxacin, 250 mg intravenously every 12 h
- Alternatively, in severely ill patients, give mezlocillin, 3 g intravenously every 4 h, plus either metronidazole, 500 mg intravenously every 6 h (if there has been no prior manipulation of the duct) or gentamicin (2 mg/kg intravenously as loading dose, plus 1.5 mg/kg every 8 h adjusted for renal function) (or both)
- Aminoglycosides should not be given for more than a few days because the risk of aminoglycoside nephrotoxicity is increased in patients with cholestasis

SURGERY

- At cholecystectomy, operative cholangiography via the cystic duct should be considered. If stones in the common duct are found, common duct exploration can be performed or a postoperative ERCP and sphincterotomy can be planned
- Following operative choledochostomy, a simple catheter or T tube is placed in the common duct for decompression. A properly placed tube should drain bile at the operating table and continuously thereafter; otherwise, it should be considered blocked or dislocated. The volume of bile drainage varies from 100 to 1000 mL daily (average, 200–400 mL). Above-average drainage may be due to obstruction at the ampulla (usually by edema)
- Choledocholithiasis discovered at laparoscopic cholecystectomy may be managed via laparoscopic removal or, if necessary, conversion to open surgery or by postoperative endoscopic sphincterotomy

THERAPEUTIC PROCEDURES

- Nutrition should be restored by a high-carbohydrate, high-protein diet and vitamin supplementation
- Common duct stone with cholelithiasis and cholecystitis is usually treated by endoscopic papillotomy and stone extraction followed by laparoscopic

cholecystectomy. For the poor-risk patient, cholecystectomy may be deferred because the risk of subsequent cholecystitis is low

- ERCP should be performed before cholecystectomy in patients with gallstones and jaundice (serum total bilirubin >2 mg/dL), a dilated common bile duct (>7 mm), or stones in the bile duct seen on ultrasound or CT
- When biliary pancreatitis resolves rapidly, the stone usually passes into the intestine, and ERCP prior to cholecystectomy is not necessary if an intraoperative cholangiogram is done
- In the postcholecystectomy patient with choledocholithiasis, endoscopic papillotomy with stone extraction is preferable to transabdominal surgery
- Lithotripsy (endoscopic or external), direct cholangioscopy, or biliary stenting may be therapeutic for large stones. For the patient with a T tube and common duct stone, the stone may be extracted via the T tube
- Urgent ERCP, sphincterotomy, and stone extraction are generally indicated for choledocholithiasis complicated by ascending cholangitis
- Emergent decompression of the bile duct, generally by ERCP, for patients who are septic or fail to improve on antibiotics within 12–24 h
- If sphincterotomy cannot be performed, decompression by a biliary stent or nasobiliary catheter can be done. Once decompressed, antibiotics are generally continued for another 3 days

OUTCOME

FOLLOW-UP

- Postoperative antibiotics are not given routinely after biliary tract surgery; intraoperative bile cultures are taken
- If biliary tract infection was present preoperatively or is apparent at operation, ampicillin (500 mg every 6 h intravenously) with gentamicin (1.5 mg/kg every 8 h) and metronidazole (500 mg every 6 h) or ciprofloxacin (250 mg intravenously every 12 h) or a third-generation cephalosporin (eg, cefoperazone, 1–2 g intravenously every 12 h) is administered postoperatively until the sensitivity tests on culture specimens are available
- A T-tube cholangiogram should be done before the tube is removed, usually

about 3 weeks after surgery. A small amount of bile frequently leaks from the tube site for a few days

COMPLICATIONS

- Common duct obstruction lasting longer than 30 days results in liver damage leading to cirrhosis
- Hepatic failure with portal hypertension occurs in untreated cases

PROGNOSIS

- Medical therapy alone is most likely to fail in patients with tachycardia, serum albumin <3 g/dL, serum bilirubin >50 μmol/L, and prothombin time >14 s on admission

EVIDENCE

PRACTICE GUIDELINES

- National Guideline Clearinghouse http://www.guideline.gov/summary/ summary.aspx?doc_id=1704&nbr=930 &string=choledocholithiasis

WEB SITE

- Choledocholithiasis Demonstration Case http://www.brighamrad.harvard.edu/ Cases/bwh/hcache/99/full.html

INFORMATION FOR PATIENTS

- National Institutues of Health http://www.nlm.nih.gov/medlineplus/ ency/article/000290.htm http://www.nlm.nih.gov/medlineplus/ ency/article/000274.htm

REFERENCE

- Boerma D et al: Wait-and-see policy or laparoscopic cholecystectomy after endoscopic sphincterotomy for bile-duct stones: a randomized trial. Lancet 2002;360:761.

Lawrence S. Friedman, MD

Cholecystitis, Acute

 ## KEY FEATURES

ESSENTIALS OF DIAGNOSIS

- Steady, severe pain and tenderness in the right hypochondrium or epigastrium
- Nausea and vomiting
- Fever and leukocytosis

GENERAL CONSIDERATIONS

- Associated with gallstones in over 90% of cases
- Occurs when a stone becomes impacted in the cystic duct and inflammation develops behind the obstruction
- Acalculous cholecystitis should be considered when unexplained fever or right upper quadrant pain occurs within 2–4 weeks of major surgery or in a critically ill patient who has had no oral intake for a prolonged period
- Primarily as a result of ischemic changes secondary to distension, gangrene may develop, resulting in perforation. Although generalized peritonitis is possible, the leak usually remains localized and forms a chronic, well-circumscribed abscess cavity
- Acute cholecystitis caused by infectious agents (eg, cytomegalovirus, cryptosporidiosis, or microsporidiosis) may occur in patients with AIDS

 ## CLINICAL FINDINGS

SYMPTOMS AND SIGNS

- The acute attack is often precipitated by a large or fatty meal
- The attack is characterized by relatively sudden, severe, steady pain that is localized to the epigastrium or right hypochondrium and may gradually subside over a period of 12–18 h
- Vomiting occurs in about 75% of patients and in half of instances affords variable relief
- Right upper quadrant abdominal tenderness is almost always present and is usually associated with muscle guarding and rebound pain
- A palpable gallbladder is present in about 15% of cases
- Jaundice is present in about 25% of cases and, when persistent or severe, suggests the possibility of choledocholithiasis. Jaundice also may result from compression of the common bile or hepatic duct by a cystic duct that is inflamed because of an impacted stone (Mirizzi's syndrome)
- Fever is usually present

DIFFERENTIAL DIAGNOSIS

- Perforated viscus, eg, peptic ulcer, diverticulitis
- Acute pancreatitis
- Appendicitis
- Acute hepatitis or liver abscess
- Right lower lobe pneumonia
- Myocardial infarction
- Radicular pain in T6–T10 dermatome, eg, preeruptive zoster

 ## DIAGNOSIS

LABORATORY TESTS

- The white blood cell count is usually high (12,000–15,000/μL)
- Total serum bilirubin values of 1–4 mg/dL may be seen even in the absence of common duct obstruction
- Serum aminotransferase and alkaline phosphatase are often elevated—the former as high as 300 units/mL, or even higher when associated with ascending cholangitis
- Serum amylase may also be moderately elevated

IMAGING STUDIES

- Plain films of the abdomen may show radiopaque gallstones in 15% of cases
- ^{99m}Tc hepatobiliary imaging (using iminodiacetic acid compounds) (HIDA scan) is useful in demonstrating an obstructed cystic duct, which is the cause of acute cholecystitis in most patients. This test is reliable if the bilirubin is under 5 mg/dL (98% sensitivity and 81% specificity for acute cholecystitis)
- Right upper quadrant abdominal ultrasound may show the presence of gallstones but is not sensitive for acute cholecystitis (67% sensitivity, 82% specificity)

Cholecystitis, Acute

 TREATMENT

MEDICATIONS

- Will usually subside on a conservative regimen (withholding of oral feedings, intravenous alimentation, analgesics, and antibiotics)
- Meperidine may be preferable to morphine for pain because of less spasm of the sphincter of Oddi

SURGERY

- Because of the high risk of recurrent attacks (up to 10% by 1 month and over 30% by 1 year), cholecystectomy—generally laparoscopically—should generally be performed within 2–3 days after hospitalization
- Surgical treatment of chronic cholecystitis is the same as for acute cholecystitis. If indicated, cholangiography can be performed during laparoscopic cholecystectomy. Choledocholithiasis can also be excluded by either pre- or postoperative endoscopic retrograde or magnetic resonance cholangiopancreatography

THERAPEUTIC PROCEDURES

- In high-risk patients, ultrasound-guided aspiration of the gallbladder or percutaneous cholecystostomy may postpone or even avoid the need for surgery. Cholecystectomy is mandatory when there is evidence of gangrene or perforation

 OUTCOME

FOLLOW-UP

- If nonsurgical treatment has been elected, watch the patient (especially if diabetic or elderly) for recurrent symptoms, evidence of gangrene of the gallbladder, or cholangitis

COMPLICATIONS

Gangrene of the gallbladder

- Continuation or progression of right upper quadrant abdominal pain, tenderness, muscle guarding, fever, and leukocytosis after 24–48 h suggests severe inflammation and possible gangrene of the gallbladder
- Necrosis may develop without definite signs in the obese, diabetic, elderly, or immunosuppressed patient
- See *Cholangitis & choledocholithiasis*

Chronic cholecystitis

- Results from repeated episodes of acute cholecystitis or chronic irritation of the gallbladder wall by stones
- Calculi are usually present
- In about 5% of cases, the villi of the gallbladder undergo polypoid enlargement due to deposition of cholesterol ("strawberry gallbladder," cholesterolosis). In other instances, adenomatous hyperplasia of the gallbladder wall may be so marked as to give the appearance of a myoma (pseudotumor)
- Hydrops of the gallbladder results when acute cholecystitis subsides but cystic duct obstruction persists, producing distension of the gallbladder with a clear mucoid fluid
- A stone in the neck of the gallbladder may compress the bile duct and cause jaundice (Mirizzi's syndrome)
- Cholelithiasis with chronic cholecystitis may be associated with acute exacerbations of gallbladder inflammation, common duct stone, fistulization to the bowel, pancreatitis, and, rarely, carcinoma of the gallbladder
- Calcified (porcelain) gallbladder may have a high association with gallbladder carcinoma (particularly when the calcification is mucosal rather than intramural) and appears to be an indication for cholecystectomy

PROGNOSIS

- The mortality rate of cholecystectomy is less than 1%, but hepatobiliary tract surgery in the elderly has a mortality rate of 5–10%
- A successful surgical procedure is generally followed by complete resolution of symptoms

 EVIDENCE

PRACTICE GUIDELINES

- National Guideline Clearinghouse http://www.guideline.gov/summary/summary.aspx?doc_id=1704&nbr=930&string=acute+cholecystitis http://www.guideline.gov/summary/summary.aspx?doc_id=2402&nbr=1628&string=acute+cholecystitis

WEB SITES

- Acute Acalculous Cholecystitis Demonstration Case http://www.brighamrad.harvard.edu/Cases/bwh/hcache/55/full.html
- Acute Cholecystitis Demonstration Case http://www.brighamrad.harvard.edu/Cases/bwh/hcache/96/full.html

INFORMATION FOR PATIENTS

- JAMA patient page: Acute cholecystitis. JAMA 2003;289:124.
- National Institutes of Health http://www.nlm.nih.gov/medlineplus/ency/article/000264.htm

REFERENCES

- Spira RM et al: Percutaneous transhepatic cholecystostomy and delayed laparoscopic cholecystectomy in critically ill patients with acute calculus cholecystitis. Am J Surg 2002;183:62.
- Trowbridge RL et al: Does this patient have acute cholecystitis? JAMA 2003;289:80.

Lawrence S. Friedman, MD

Cholelithiasis (Gallstones)

 KEY FEATURES

ESSENTIALS OF DIAGNOSIS

- Biliary colic
- Gallstones in gallbladder on ultrasound
- Patients may be asymptomatic

GENERAL CONSIDERATIONS

- Gallstones are classified according to their predominant chemical composition as cholesterol or calcium bilirubinate stones. The latter comprise less than 20% of the stones found in Europe or the United States but 30–40% of stones found in Japan
- Three compounds comprise 80–95% of the total solids dissolved in bile: conjugated bile salts, lecithin, and cholesterol. Cholesterol is a neutral sterol, and lecithin is a phospholipid; both are almost completely insoluble in water. However, bile salts in combination with lecithin are able to form multimolecular aggregates (and micelles) or vesicles that solubilize cholesterol in an aqueous solution. Precipitation of cholesterol microcrystals may come about because of increased biliary secretion of cholesterol, defective formation of vesicles, an excess of factors promoting the nucleation of cholesterol crystals (or deficiency of antinucleating factors), or delayed emptying of the gallbladder

DEMOGRAPHICS

- Gallstones are more common in women than in men and increase in incidence in both sexes and all races with aging
- In the United States, over 10% of men and 20% of women have gallstones by age 65; the total exceeds 20 million people. Although cholesterol gallstones are less common in black people, cholelithiasis attributable to hemolysis occurs in over a third of individuals with sickle cell anemia
- Native Americans of both the Northern and Southern Hemispheres have a high rate of cholesterol cholelithiasis, probably because of a predisposition resulting from "thrifty" (*LITH*) genes that promote efficient calorie utilization and fat storage
- As many as 75% of Pima and other American Indian women over the age of 25 years have cholelithiasis
- Obesity is a risk factor for gallstones, especially in women, while rapid weight loss increases the risk of symptomatic gallstone formation

- Diabetes and elevated serum insulin levels (insulin resistance syndrome) are risk factors for gallstones
- Prolonged fasting (over 5–10 days) can lead to formation of biliary "sludge" (microlithiasis), which usually resolves with refeeding but can lead to gallstones or biliary symptoms
- Pregnancy is associated with an increased risk of gallstones and of symptomatic gallbladder disease
- Hormone replacement therapy conveys a slight risk for biliary tract surgery

 CLINICAL FINDINGS

SYMPTOMS AND SIGNS

- See Table 60 (page1256)
- Cholelithiasis is frequently asymptomatic and is discovered incidentally
- "Symptomatic" cholelithiasis usually means characteristic right upper quadrant or epigastric discomfort or pain (biliary colic)
- Occasional patients present with small intestinal obstruction due to "gallstone ileus" as the initial manifestation of cholelithiasis

DIFFERENTIAL DIAGNOSIS

- Acute cholecystitis
- Acute pancreatitis
- Peptic ulcer disease
- Appendicitis
- Acute hepatitis
- Myocardial infarction
- Radicular pain in T6–T10 dermatome, eg, preeruptive zoster

 DIAGNOSIS

LABORATORY TESTS

- Table 60 (page 1256)
- Laboratory tests are normal in asymptomatic gallstones

IMAGING STUDIES

- Ultrasound is the most sensitive imaging modality
- CT is an alternative but usually not necessary

DIAGNOSTIC PROCEDURES

- See *Cholecystitis, acute* or *Cholangitis & choledocholithiasis*

TREATMENT

MEDICATIONS

- Cheno- and ursodeoxycholic acids are bile salts that when given orally for up to 2 years dissolve some cholesterol stones and may be considered in selected patients who refuse cholecystectomy. The dose is 7 mg/kg/day of each or 8–13 mg/kg of ursodeoxycholic acid in divided doses daily. They are most effective in patients with a functioning gallbladder, as determined by gallbladder visualization on oral cholecystography, and multiple small "floating" gallstones (representing not more than 15% of patients with gallstones). In half of patients, gallstones recur within 5 years after treatment is stopped

SURGERY

- There is generally no need for prophylactic cholecystectomy in an asymptomatic person unless the gallbladder is calcified or gallstones are over 3 cm in diameter
- Laparoscopic cholecystectomy is the treatment of choice for symptomatic gallbladder disease. The minimal trauma to the abdominal wall makes it possible for patients to go home within 2 days after the procedure and to return to work within 7 days (instead of weeks for those undergoing standard open cholecystectomy). If problems are encountered, the surgery can be converted to a conventional open cholecystectomy. See *Cholangitis & choledocholithiasis*
- A conservative approach to biliary colic is advised in pregnant patients, but for patients with repeated attacks of biliary colic or acute cholecystitis, cholecystectomy can be performed—even by the laparoscopic route—preferably in the second trimester

THERAPEUTIC PROCEDURES

- Enterolithotomy alone is considered adequate treatment in most patients with gallstone ileus.
- Lithotripsy in combination with bile salt therapy for single radiolucent stones less than 20 mm in diameter is no longer generally employed in the United States

 ## OUTCOME

COMPLICATIONS

- Cholecystectomy may increase the risk of esophageal and proximal small intestinal adenocarcinoma because of increased duodenogastric reflux and changes in intestinal exposure to bile, respectively
- There may be persistence of symptoms after removal of the gallbladder (see *Cholecystectomy, pre- and post-syndrome*)

PROGNOSIS

- Symptoms (biliary colic) develop in 10–25% of patients with gallstones by 10 years

PREVENTION

- Low-carbohydrate diet and physical activity may help prevent gallstones, and consumption of caffeinated coffee appears to protect against gallstones in women

 ## EVIDENCE

PRACTICE GUIDELINES

- National Guideline Clearinghouse http://www.guideline.gov/summary/ summary.aspx?doc_id=2263&nbr=1489 &string=gallstones http://www.guideline.gov/summary/ summary.aspx?doc_id=1704&nbr= 930&string=gallstones

WEB SITE

- Choledocholithiasis Demonstration Case http://www.brighamrad.harvard.edu/ Cases/bwh/hcache/99/full.html

INFORMATION FOR PATIENTS

- National Institutes of Health http://www.nlm.nih.gov/medlineplus/ ency/article/000273.htm
- National Digestive Diseases Information Clearinghouse http://www.niddk.nih.gov/health/ nutrit/pubs/dietgall.htm

REFERENCES

- Johnson CD: ABC of the upper gastrointestinal tract. Upper abdominal pain: Gall bladder. BMJ 2001;323:1170. [PMID: 11711412]
- Simon JA et al: Effect of estrogen plus progestin on risk for biliary tract surgery in postmenopausal women with coronary artery disease: The Heart and Estrogen/Progestin Replacement Study. Ann Intern Med 2001;135:493. [PMID: 11578152]
- Zacks SL et al: A population-based cohort study comparing laparoscopic cholecystectomy and open cholecystectomy. Am J Gastroenterol 2002;97:334.

Lawrence S. Friedman, MD

Cholera

 KEY FEATURES

ESSENTIALS OF DIAGNOSIS

- History of travel in endemic area or contact with infected person
- Voluminous diarrhea
- Stool is liquid, gray, turbid, and without fecal odor, blood, or pus ("rice water stool")
- Rapid development of marked dehydration
- Positive stool cultures and agglutination of vibrios with specific contaminated food or water

GENERAL CONSIDERATIONS

- An acute diarrheal illness caused by certain serotypes of *Vibrio cholerae*
- The toxin activates adenylyl cyclase in intestinal epithelial cells of the small intestines, producing hypersecretion of water and chloride ion and a massive diarrhea of up to 15 L/day
- Occurs in epidemics under conditions of crowding, war, and famine (eg, in refugee camps) and where sanitation is inadequate
- Infection is acquired by ingestion of contaminated food or water

DEMOGRAPHICS

- Rarely seen in the United States until 1991, when epidemic cholera returned to the Western Hemisphere, originating as an outbreak in coastal cities of Peru. The epidemic spread to involve several countries in South and Central America as well as Mexico, and cases have been imported into the United States
- A major cause of epidemic diarrhea throughout the developing world

 CLINICAL FINDINGS

SYMPTOMS AND SIGNS

- See Table 126 (page 1309)
- A sudden onset of severe, frequent watery diarrhea (up to 1 L/h)
- The liquid stool is gray, turbid, and without fecal odor, blood, or pus ("rice water stool")
- Dehydration and hypotension develop rapidly
- The disease is toxin mediated, and fever is unusual

DIFFERENTIAL DIAGNOSIS

- Viral gastroenteritis
- Other small intestinal diarrhea, eg, salmonellosis, enterotoxigenic *Escherichia coli*
- Vasoactive intestinal polypeptide-producing pancreatic tumor (pancreatic cholera)
- Food poisoning, eg, *Staphylococcus aureus*

 DIAGNOSIS

LABORATORY TESTS

- Stool culture

TREATMENT

MEDICATIONS

- Antimicrobial therapy will shorten the course of illness
- Several antimicrobials are active against *V cholerae*, including tetracycline, ampicillin, chloramphenicol, trimethoprim-sulfamethoxazole, and fluoroquinolones

THERAPEUTIC PROCEDURES

- Fluid replacement
- In mild or moderate illness, oral rehydration usually is adequate

 OUTCOME

COMPLICATIONS

- Death results from profound hypovolemia

PROGNOSIS

- 25–50% fatality if untreated

WHEN TO ADMIT

- Severe diarrhea
- Moderate to severe dehydration in need of parenteral fluid replacement
- Inability to maintain fluid replacement because there can be rapid development of dehydration

PREVENTION

- A vaccine is available that confers short-lived, limited protection
- Vaccine may be required for entry into or reentry after travel to some countries
- Vaccine is administered in two doses 1–4 weeks apart. A booster dose every 6 months is recommended for persons remaining in areas where cholera is a hazard
- Vaccination programs are expensive and not particularly effective in managing outbreaks of cholera. When outbreaks occur, efforts should be directed toward establishing clean water and food sources and proper waste disposal

 EVIDENCE

PRACTICE GUIDELINES

- National Guideline Clearinghouse http://www.guideline.gov/summary/summary.aspx?doc_id=2791&nbr=2017&string=cholera

WEB SITES

- CDC—Division of Bacterial and Mycotic Diseases http://www.cdc.gov/ncidod/dbmd/
- Karolinska Institute—Directory of bacterial infections and mycoses http://www.mic.ki.se/Diseases/c1.html

INFORMATION FOR PATIENTS

- JAMA patient page: Preventing dehydration from diarrhea. JAMA 2001; 185:362.
- Centers for Disease Control http://www.cdc.gov/ncidod/dbmd/diseaseinfo/cholera_g.htm

REFERENCE

- Guerrant RL et al: How intestinal bacteria cause disease. J Infect Dis 1999; 179(Suppl 2):S331. [PMID: 10081504]

Henry F. Chambers, MD

Chronic Fatigue Syndrome

 KEY FEATURES

ESSENTIALS OF DIAGNOSIS

- Weight loss
- Fever
- Sleep-disordered breathing
- Substance use
- Depression

GENERAL CONSIDERATIONS

- Fatigue often attributable to overexertion, poor physical conditioning, sleep disturbance, obesity, undernutrition, and emotional problems
- The lifetime prevalence of significant fatigue (present for at least 2 weeks) is about 25%

 CLINICAL FINDINGS

SYMPTOMS AND SIGNS

- Screen for psychiatric disorders
- Evaluation and classification of unexplained chronic fatigue involves history and physical examination, mental status examination (abnormalities require appropriate psychiatric, psychological, or neurological examination), and screening laboratory tests
- Fatigue is classified as chronic fatigue syndrome if criteria for severity of fatigue are met and four or more of the following symptoms are concurrently present for 6 or more months
  - Impaired memory or concentration
  - Sore throat
  - Tender cervical or axillary lymph nodes
  - Muscle pain
  - Multijoint pain
  - New headaches
  - Unrefreshing sleep
  - Postexertion malaise
- Fatigue is classified as idiopathic chronic fatigue if criteria for fatigue severity or the symptoms are not met

DIFFERENTIAL DIAGNOSIS

- Hypothyroidism
- Anemia
- Depression
- Obstructive sleep apnea or insufficient sleep
- Infection, eg, tuberculosis, hepatitis, endocarditis, HIV, Lyme disease
- Diabetes mellitus
- Congestive heart failure, chronic obstructive pulmonary disease, or chronic renal failure
- Cancer
- Alcoholism
- Hypercalcemia
- Drugs, eg, sedatives, β-blockers
- Chronic fatigue syndrome
- Somatoform disorder (somatization)
- Fibromyalgia
- Mononucleosis
- Autoimmune disease

 DIAGNOSIS

LABORATORY TESTS

- Obtain complete blood count, erythrocyte sedimentation rate, serum electrolytes, glucose, blood urea nitrogen, creatinine, calcium, liver and thyroid function tests, antinuclear antibody, urinalysis, and tuberculin skin test
- Consider, as indicated, serum cortisol, rheumatoid factor, immunoglobulin levels, Lyme serology in endemic areas, and HIV antibody test

TREATMENT

MEDICATIONS

- Treat affective or anxiety disorder
- Treat postural hypotension with fludro-cortisone, 0.1 mg/day, and increased dietary sodium

THERAPEUTIC PROCEDURES

- For chronic fatigue syndrome, treatment involves a comprehensive multidisciplinary intervention
  - Optimal medical management of co-existing disorders, eg, depression
  - Cognitive-behavioral therapy
  - Graded exercise program

 OUTCOME

PROGNOSIS

- Although few patients are cured, the treatment effect is substantial
- Full recovery is eventually possible in most cases

 EVIDENCE

PRACTICE GUIDELINES

- Chronic fatigue syndrome. Clinical practice guidelines—2002. Med J Aust 2002;176 suppl:S23. [PMID: 12056987]
- AHRQ—Defining and managing chronic fatigue syndrome http://www.ahrq.gov/clinic/epcsums/cfssum.htm

WEB SITES

- Centers for Disease Control and Prevention—Chronic fatigue syndrome (CFS) home page http://www.cdc.gov/ncidod/diseases/cfs/

INFORMATION FOR PATIENTS

- Cleveland Clinic—Cancer related fatigue http://www.clevelandclinic.org/health/health-info/docs/0300/0305.asp?index=5230
- Chronic Fatigue and Immune Dysfunction Syndrome Association of America http://www.cfids.org
- National Chronic Fatigue Syndrome & Fibromyalgia Association http://www.ncfsfa.org/
- The American Association for Chronic Fatigue Syndrome www.aacfs.org

REFERENCES

- Powell P et al: Randomised controlled trial of patient education to encourage graded exercise in chronic fatigue syndrome. BMJ 2001;322:1. [PMID: 11179154]
- Whiting P et al: Interventions for the treatment and management of chronic fatigue syndrome: a systematic review. JAMA 2001;286:1360. [PMID: 11560542]

Ralph Gonzales, MD

Chronic Obstructive Pulmonary Disease (COPD)

 KEY FEATURES

ESSENTIALS OF DIAGNOSIS

- History of cigarette smoking
- Chronic cough and sputum production (bronchitis) and dyspnea (emphysema)
- Rhonchi, decreased intensity of breath sounds, and prolonged expiration on physical examination
- Airflow limitation on pulmonary function testing

GENERAL CONSIDERATIONS

- Airflow obstruction due to chronic bronchitis or emphysema; most patients have features of both
- Obstruction is progressive, may be accompanied by airway hyperreactivity, and may be partially reversible
- Chronic bronchitis is characterized by excessive mucous secretions with productive cough for 3 months or more in at least 2 consecutive years
- Emphysema is abnormal enlargement of distal air spaces and destruction of bronchial walls without fibrosis
- Cigarette smoking is the most important cause; about 80% of patients have had a significant exposure to tobacco smoke
- Air pollution, airway infection, familial factors, and allergy have been implicated in chronic bronchitis
- α_1-Antitrypsin deficiency has been implicated in emphysema

 CLINICAL FINDINGS

SYMPTOMS AND SIGNS

- Presentation is usually at 40–50 years of age with cough, sputum production, and shortness of breath
- Dyspnea initially occurs only with heavy exertion, progressing to symptoms at rest in severe disease
- Frequent exacerbations leading to eventual disability
- Viral infections precede exacerbations in the majority of patients
- Pneumonia, pulmonary hypertension, cor pulmonale, and respiratory failure characterize late-stage COPD
- Death usually occurs during an exacerbation of COPD in association with respiratory failure
- Clinical findings may be absent early
- Often dichotomized as "pink puffers" or "blue bloaters" depending on whether emphysema or bronchitis predominates (Table 17, page 1216)

DIFFERENTIAL DIAGNOSIS

- Bronchial asthma
- Bronchiectasis, which features recurrent pneumonia and hemoptysis, with distinct radiographic findings
- Severe α_1-antiprotease deficiency
- Cystic fibrosis, which is seen in children and young adults

 DIAGNOSIS

LABORATORY TESTS

- Sputum examination may reveal *Streptococcus pneumoniae*, *Haemophilus influenzae*, or *Moraxella catarrhalis*, though cultures correlate poorly with exacerbations
- ECG shows sinus tachycardia, abnormalities consistent with cor pulmonale in severe disease, and/or supraventricular tachycardias and ventricular irritability
- Arterial blood gas
  - May show only an increased A–a DO_2 in early disease
  - Is unnecessary unless hypoxemia or hypercapnia is suspected
  - Hypoxemia in advanced disease
  - Compensated respiratory acidosis with worsening acidemia during exacerbations
- Spirometry
  - Objectively measures pulmonary function and assesses severity
  - Early changes are reductions in midexpiratory flow and abnormal closing volumes
  - FEV_1 and FEV_1/FVC are reduced later in disease
  - FVC is reduced in severe disease
  - Lung volume measurements show an increase in total lung capacity (TLC), residual volume (RV), and an elevation of RV/TLC indicating air trapping
- α_1-Antitrypsin level in young patients with emphysema

IMAGING STUDIES

- Chest x-ray may show hyperinflation, especially when emphysema predominates
  - Parenchymal bullae or subpleural blebs are pathognomonic of emphysema
  - Nonspecific peribronchial and perivascular markings with chronic bronchitis
  - Enlargement of central pulmonary arteries in advanced disease

TREATMENT

MEDICATIONS

- Supplemental oxygen
  - In hospitalized patients, O_2 should not be withheld for fear of worsening acidemia
  - Longer survival, reduced hospitalizations, and better quality of life in advanced disease
  - Unless therapy is intended only for nighttime or exercise use, 15 h of nasal oxygen per day is required
  - For most patients, a flow rate of 1–3 L achieves a PaO_2 >55%
  - Medicare covers 80% of costs for patients who meet requirements (Table 18, page 1217)
- Bronchodilators are the most important pharmacological agents (Tables 15 and 16, pages 1214 and 1216)
  - **Ipratropium bromide** (2–4 puffs via MDI Q 6 h) is first-line therapy, as it is longer-acting and without sympathomimetic side effects
  - Short-acting β-agonists (**albuterol, metaproterenol**) have a shorter onset of action and are cheaper
  - At maximal doses, bronchodilation of β-agonists is equivalent to ipratropium, but with side effects of tremor, tachycardia, and hypokalemia
  - Ipratropium and β-agonists together are more effective than either alone
  - Oral **theophylline** is a third-line agent for patients who fail ipratropium or β-agonists
- Corticosteroids
  - COPD is generally not steroid responsive; 10% of stable outpatients will have more than a 20% increase in FEV_1 compared with placebo
- Antibiotics improve outcomes slightly when used to treat acute exacerbations
  - Regimens include tremethoprim-sulfamethoxaxole, 160/800 mg BID, amoxicillin or amoxicillin-clavulanate, 500 mg TID, or doxycycline, 100 mg BID
- Opioids: severe dyspnea in spite of optimal management may warrant a trial of an opioid
- Sedative-hypnotic drugs (diazepam 5 mg TID) may benefit very anxious patients with intractable dyspnea

SURGERY

- The 2-year survival with lung transplantation is 75%, which offers substantial improvement in pulmonary function and exercise performance
- 20–30% lung volume reduction surgery results in modest improvements in pulmonary function, exercise performance, and dyspnea; surgical mortality rates at experienced centers are 4–10%

THERAPEUTIC PROCEDURES

- Noninvasive positive-pressure ventilation reduces the need for intubation, shortens ICU lengths of stay, and may reduce the risk of nosocomial infection and antibiotic use
- Smoking cessation is the single most important goal
- Cough suppressants and sedatives should be avoided as routine measures
- Graded physical exercise programs
- Measure theophylline levels in hospitalized patients

OUTCOME

COMPLICATIONS

- Pulmonary hypertension, cor pulmonale, and chronic respiratory failure are common in advanced disease
- Spontaneous pneumothorax occurs in a small fraction of emphysematous patients
- Hemoptysis may result from chronic bronchitis or bronchogenic carcinoma

PROGNOSIS

- Median survival for severe disease (FEV_1 <1 L) is 4 years
- Degree of dysfunction at presentation is the most important predictor of survival

WHEN TO REFER

- Progressive and/or severe airflow obstruction and/or symptoms
- α_1-Antitrypsin deficiency
- Large bullae

WHEN TO ADMIT

- Acute exacerbations that fail to respond to measures for ambulatory patients
- Acute respiratory failure
- Cor pulmonale or pneumothorax

PREVENTION

- Largely preventable by eliminating chronic exposure to tobacco smoke
- Smoking cessation slows the decline in FEV_1 in middle-aged smokers with mild obstructive disease
- Vaccination against influenza and pneumococcal infection

EVIDENCE

PRACTICE GUIDELINES

- National Guideline Clearinghouse
  http://www.guideline.gov/summary/summary.aspx?doc_id=3145&nbr=2371&string=COPD
  http://www.guideline.gov/summary/summary.aspx?doc_id=2779&nbr=2005&string=COPD

INFORMATION FOR PATIENTS

- JAMA patient page: Chronic obstructive pulmonary disease. JAMA 2003;290:2362. [PMID: 14600198]

REFERENCES

- Bach PB et al: Management of acute exacerbations of chronic obstructive pulmonary disease: a summary and appraisal of published evidence. Ann Intern Med 2001;134:600. [PMID: 11296189]
- Crockett AJ et al: Domiciliary oxygen for chronic obstructive pulmonary disease. Cochrane Database of Systematic Reviews 2000;(2):CD001744. [PMID: 10796666]

Mark S. Chesnutt, MD
Thomas J. Prendergast, MD

Cirrhosis

 KEY FEATURES

ESSENTIALS OF DIAGNOSIS

- End result of injury that leads to both fibrosis and nodular regeneration
- Generally irreversible
- The clinical features result from hepatic cell dysfunction, portosystemic shunting, and portal hypertension

GENERAL CONSIDERATIONS

- The most common histological classification is micronodular, macronodular, and mixed forms cirrhosis. Each form may be seen at different stages of the disease

Micronodular cirrhosis

- Regenerating nodules are ≤1 mm
- Typical of alcoholic liver disease (Laennec's cirrhosis)

Macronodular cirrhosis

- Characterized by larger nodules, up to several centimeters in diameter, and may contain central veins
- Corresonds to postnecrotic (posthepatic) cirrhosis; but may not follow episodes of massive necrosis

Etiology of cirrhosis

- Chronic hepatitis C or B
- Alcoholism
- Nonalcoholic fatty liver disease
- Cryptogenic
- Metabolic, eg, hemochromatosis, Wilson's disease, α_1-antiprotease deficiency
- Primary biliary cirrhosis
- Secondary biliary cirrhosis (chronic obstruction due to stone, stricture, neoplasm)
- Congestive heart failure or constrictive pericarditis
- Other: Budd-Chiari syndrome, cystic fibrosis, autoimmune hepatitis, *Clonorchis sinensis* infection, glycogen storage disease

DEMOGRAPHICS

- Eighth leading cause of death in the United States

 CLINICAL FINDINGS

SYMPTOMS AND SIGNS

- Can be asymptomatic for long periods
- Symptoms may be insidious or, less often, abrupt
- Weakness, fatigability, disturbed sleep, muscle cramps, anorexia, and weight loss are common
- Nausea and occasional vomiting
- Jaundice—usually not an initial sign—is mild at first, increasing in severity
- Abdominal pain from hepatic enlargement and stretching of Glisson's capsule or from ascites
- Hematemesis is the presenting symptom in 15–25%
- Amenorrhea, impotence, loss of libido, sterility, and gynecomastia in men
- In 70% of cases, the liver is enlarged and firm with a sharp or nodular edge; the left lobe may predominate
- Splenomegaly occurs in 35–50%
- Ascites, pleural effusions, peripheral edema, and ecchymoses are late findings
- Fever may be a presenting symptom in up to 35% and usually reflects associated alcoholic hepatitis, spontaneous bacterial peritonitis, or intercurrent infection

Encephalopathy

- Day-night reversal, asterixis, tremor, dysarthria, delirium, drowsiness
- Coma occurs late except when precipitated by an acute hepatocellular insult or gastrointestinal bleeding

Skin

- Spider nevi on the upper half of the body
- Palmar erythema, Dupuytren's contractures
- Glossitis and cheilosis from vitamin deficiencies are common
- Dilated superficial veins of the abdomen and thorax that fill from below when compressed

 DIAGNOSIS

LABORATORY TESTS

- Laboratory abnormalities are either absent or minimal in quiescent cirrhosis
- Anemia, usually macrocytic, from suppression of erythropoiesis by alcohol, folate deficiency, hypersplenism, hemolysis, and blood loss from the gastrointestinal tract
- The white blood cell count may be low, reflecting hypersplenism, or high, suggesting infection; thrombocytopenia is secondary to alcoholic marrow suppression, sepsis, folate deficiency, or splenic sequestration
- Prolongation of the prothrombin time from failure of hepatic synthesis of clotting factors
- Modest elevations of aspartate aminotransferase and alkaline phosphatase and progressive elevation of the bilirubin. Serum albumin is low; γ-globulin is increased and may be as high as in autoimmune hepatitis
- Patients with alcoholic cirrhosis may have elevated serum cardiac troponin I levels of uncertain significance
- See *Ascites* or *Peritonitis, spontaneous bacterial*

IMAGING STUDIES

- Upper gastrointestinal barium studies may show esophageal or gastric varices
- Ultrasound can assess liver size and detect ascites or hepatic nodules, including small hepatocellular carcinomas. Together with Doppler studies, it may establish patency of the splenic, portal, and hepatic veins
- Hepatic nodules can be characterized by contrast-enhanced CT scan or MRI. Nodules suspicious for malignancy may be biopsied under ultrasound or CT guidance

DIAGNOSTIC PROCEDURES

- Perform diagnostic paracentesis for new ascites
- Esophagogastroduodenoscopy confirms the presence of varices and detects specific causes of bleeding
- Liver biopsy

TREATMENT

MEDICATIONS

Ascites and edema

- Restrict sodium intake to 400–800 mg/day
- Restrict fluid intake (800–1000 mL/day) for hyponatremia (sodium <125 mEq/L)
- Ascites may rapidly decrease on bed rest and dietary sodium restriction alone
- **Diuretics**
- Use spironolactone if there is no response to salt restriction. The initial dose is 100 mg daily and may be increased by 100 mg every 3–5 days (up to a maximal conventional daily dose of 400 mg/day, though higher doses have been used) until diuresis is achieved, typically preceded by a rise in the urinary sodium concentration. Monitor for hyperkalemia
- Substitute amiloride, 5–10 mg orally daily if painful gynecomastia develops from spironolactone
- Diuresis can be augmented with the addition of furosemide, 40–160 mg/day Monitor for prerenal azotemia, blood pressure, urine output, mental status, and serum electrolytes, especially potassium

Anemia

- For iron deficiency anemia, give ferrous sulfate, 0.3 g enteric-coated tablets, one tablet three times daily after meals
- Treat macrocytic anemia associated with alcoholism with folic acid, 1 mg/day orally
- Packed red blood cell transfusions may be necessary to replace blood loss

Hemorrhagic tendency

- Treat severe hypoprothrombinemia with vitamin K (eg, phytonadione, 5 mg orally or subcutaneously daily)
- When this treatment is ineffective, use large volumes of fresh frozen plasma. Because the effect is transient, plasma infusions are indicated only for active bleeding or before an invasive procedure
- Use of recombinant factor VII may be an alternative

SURGERY

- Liver transplantation is indicated in selected cases of irreversible, progressive liver disease

- Absolute contraindications include malignancy (except small hepatocellular carcinomas in a cirrhotic liver), sepsis, and advanced cardiopulmonary disease (except pulmonary arteriovenous shunting due to portal hypertension and cirrhosis)

THERAPEUTIC PROCEDURES

- The most important principle is abstinence from alcohol
- The diet should have adequate calories (25–35 kcal/kg/day) in compensated cirrhosis and 35–40 kcal/kg/day in those with malnutrition. Protein should include 1.0–1.2 g/kg/day in compensated cirrhosis and 1.5 g/kg/day in those with malnutrition
- For hepatic encephalopathy, protein intake should be reduced to 60–80 g/day
- Vitamin supplementation is desirable
- The goal of weight loss with ascites without associated peripheral edema should not exceed 0.5–0.7 kg/day
- In refractory ascites, transjugular intrahepatic portosystemic shunt (TIPS) reduces ascites recurrence and the risk of hepatorenal syndrome but increases the rate of hepatic encephalopathy compared with repeated large-volume paracentesis, but a survival benefit has not been shown
- TIPS is now preferred for refractory ascites because of the high rate of complications from peritoneovenous shunts

 OUTCOME

COMPLICATIONS

- Upper gastrointestinal tract bleeding from varices, portal hypertensive gastropathy, or gastroduodenal ulcer
- Hepataocellular carcinoma
- Spontaneous bacterial peritonitis
- Hepatorenal or hepatopulmonary syndrome
- Increased risk of systemic infection
- Increased risk of diabetes mellitus

PROGNOSIS

- Factors determining survival include ability to stop alcohol intake and the Child-Turcotte-Pugh class (Table 59, page 1254)
- The Model for End-Stage Liver Disease (MELD) is used to determine priorities

for donor livers. Hematemesis, jaundice, and ascites are unfavorable signs
- In established cases with severe hepatic dysfunction (serum albumin <3 g/dL, bilirubin >3 mg/dL, ascites, encephalopathy, cachexia, and upper gastrointestinal bleeding), only 50% survive 6 months. The risk of death is associated with renal insufficiency, cognitive dysfunction, ventilatory insufficiency, age ≥65 years, and prothrombin time ≥16 s
- Liver transplantation has markedly improved survival, particularly for patients referred for evaluation early

EVIDENCE

PRACTICE GUIDELINES

- National Guideline Clearinghouse http://www.guideline.gov/summary/ summary.aspx?doc_id=3520&nbr=2746 &string=cirrhosis http://www.guideline.gov/summary/ summary.aspx?doc_id=3450&nbr= 2676&string=cirrhosis

WEB SITE

- Diseases of the Liver http://cpmcnet.columbia.edu/dept/gi/ disliv.html

INFORMATION FOR PATIENTS

- American Gastroenterological Association http://www.gastro.org/ public/brochures/cirrhosis.html

REFERENCES

- Blei AT et al: Hepatic encephalopathy. Am J Gastroenterol 2001;96:1968.
- Kim WR et al: Burden of liver disease in the United States: summary of a workshop. Hepatology 2002;36:227.

Lawrence S. Friedman, MD

Cirrhosis, Primary Biliary

 ## KEY FEATURES

ESSENTIALS OF DIAGNOSIS

- Middle-aged women
- Often asymptomatic
- Elevation of alkaline phosphatase, antimitochondrial antibodies (+AMA), elevated IgM, increased cholesterol
- Characteristic liver biopsy
- In later stages, can present with fatigue, jaundice, features of cirrhosis, xanthelasma, xanthomata, steatorrhea

GENERAL CONSIDERATIONS

- Chronic disease of the liver characterized by autoimmune destruction of intrahepatic bile ducts and cholestasis
- Insidious in onset, occurs usually in women aged 40–60, and is often detected by the chance finding of elevated alkaline phosphatase levels
- Infection with *Chlamydia pneumoniae* may be a triggering or causative agent; viral triggers are also suspected
- Patients with a clinical and histological picture of primary biliary cirrhosis but no AMAs are said to have "autoimmune cholangitis," which has been associated with lower serum IgM levels and a greater frequency of smooth muscle and antinuclear antibodies

DEMOGRAPHICS

- Estimated incidence and prevalence rates in the United States are 4.5 and 65.4 per 100,000, respectively, in women, and 0.7 and 12.1 per 100,000, respectively, in men

 ## CLINICAL FINDINGS

SYMPTOMS AND SIGNS

- Many are asymptomatic for years
- The onset of clinical illness is insidious and is heralded by fatigue and pruritus. With progression, physical examination reveals hepatosplenomegaly
- Xanthomatous lesions may occur in the skin and tendons and around the eyelids
- Jaundice and signs of portal hypertension are late findings
- The risk of osteoporosis is increased, as in patients with other forms of chronic liver disease

DIFFERENTIAL DIAGNOSIS

- Chronic biliary tract obstruction (stone or stricture)
- Carcinoma of the bile ducts
- Primary sclerosing cholangitis
- Sarcoidosis
- Cholestatic drug toxicity (eg, chlorpromazine)
- Chronic hepatitis
- Fascioliasis (sheep liver fluke)
- Some patients have overlapping features of primary biliary cirrhosis and autoimmune hepatitis

 ## DIAGNOSIS

LABORATORY TESTS

- Blood cell counts are normal early in the disease
- Liver biochemical tests reflect cholestasis with elevation of alkaline phosphatase, cholesterol (especially high-density lipoproteins), and, in later stages, bilirubin
- AMAs (directed against pyruvate dehydrogenase or other 2-oxo-acid enzymes in mitochondria) are present in 95% of patients, and serum IgM levels are elevated

DIAGNOSTIC PROCEDURES

- Liver biopsy permits histological staging: I, portal inflammation with granulomas; II, bile duct proliferation, periportal inflammation; III, interlobular fibrous septa; and IV, cirrhosis

TREATMENT

MEDICATIONS

- Treatment is primarily symptomatic
- Cholestyramine (4 g) or colestipol (5 g) in water or juice three times daily may be beneficial for the pruritus
- Rifampin, 150–300 mg orally twice daily, is inconsistently beneficial
- Opioid antagonists (eg, naloxone, 0.2 µg/kg/min by intravenous infusion, or naltrexone, 50 mg/day by mouth) may help the pruritus. The 5-HT$_3$ serotonin receptor antagonist ondansetron may also provide some benefit
- Deficiencies of vitamins A, K, and D may occur if steatorrhea is present and is aggravated when cholestyramine or colestipol is administered
- Calcium supplementation (500 mg three times daily) may help prevent osteomalacia but is of uncertain benefit in osteoporosis
- Because of its lack of toxicity, ursodeoxycholic acid (10–15 mg/kg/day in one or two doses) is the preferred medical treatment and slows the progression of disease, improves long-term survival, reduces the risk of developing esophageal varices, and delays the need for liver transplantation
- Colchicine (0.6 mg twice daily) and methotrexate (15 mg/week) may improve symptoms and serum levels of alkaline phosphatase and bilirubin
- Methotrexate may also improve liver histology
- Penicillamine, corticosteroids, and azathioprine are not beneficial
- Mycophenolate mofetil is under study

SURGERY

- For patients with advanced disease, liver transplantation is the treatment of choice

 ## OUTCOME

COMPLICATIONS

- Steatorrhea, xanthomas, xanthelasma, osteoporosis, osteomalacia, and portal hypertension
- It may be associated with Sjögren's syndrome, autoimmune thyroid disease, Raynaud's syndrome, scleroderma, hypothyroidism, and celiac disease

PROGNOSIS

- The disease is progressive. Without liver transplantation, survival averages 7–10 years once symptoms develop
- In advanced disease, adverse prognostic markers are older age, high serum bilirubin, edema, low albumin, prolonged prothrombin time, and variceal hemorrhage
- Among asymptomatic patients, at least one-third will become symptomatic within 15 years
- The risk of hepatobiliary malignancies appears to be increased
- Liver transplantation is associated with a 1-year survival rate of 85–90%. The disease recurs in the graft in 20% of patients by 3 years, but this does not seem to affect survival

 ## EVIDENCE

PRACTICE GUIDELINES

- National Guideline Clearinghouse http://www.guideline.gov/summary/summary.aspx?doc_id=3445&nbr=2671&string=primary+biliary+cirrhosis http://www.guideline.gov/summary/summary.aspx?doc_id=3449&nbr=2675&string=primary+biliary+cirrhosis

WEB SITES

- Diseases of the Liver http://cpmcnet.columbia.edu/dept/gi/disliv.html
- Pathology Index http://www-medlib.med.utah.edu/WebPath/LIVEHTML/LIVERIDX.html

INFORMATION FOR PATIENTS

- National Digestive Diseases Information Clearinghouse http://digestive.niddk.nih.gov/ddiseases/pubs/primarybiliarycirrhosis/index.htm
- National Institutes of Health http://www.nlm.nih.gov/medlineplus/ency/article/000282.htm

REFERENCES

- Collier JD et al: Guidelines on the management of osteoporosis associated with chronic liver disease. Gut 2002; 50(Suppl 1):i1. [PMID: 11788576]
- Corpechot C et al: Primary biliary cirrhosis: incidence and predictive factors of cirrhosis development in ursodiol-treated patients. Gastroenterology 2002;122:652.

Lawrence S. Friedman, MD

Clonorchiasis & Opisthorchiasis

 KEY FEATURES

ESSENTIALS OF DIAGNOSIS

- Clinically and epidemiologically, opisthorchiasis and clonorchiasis are identical
- Acute symptoms are fever, tender liver, urticaria, and arthralgias
- Cholangiocarcinoma has been causally linked with prolonged *Clonorchis* and *Opisthorchis* infection

GENERAL CONSIDERATIONS

- Snails become infected when they ingest opisthorchiasis and clonorchiasis eggs shed into water in human or animal feces. Larval forms escape from the snails, penetrate the flesh of various freshwater fish, and encyst as metacercariae. Fish-eating mammals—including dogs, cats, and pigs—and humans maintain the life cycle
- Human infection results from eating either raw or undercooked fish
- In humans, the ingested parasites excyst in the duodenum and ascend the bile ducts, where they mature and remain throughout their lives (15–25 years), shedding eggs in the bile
- In size, the worms are 7–20 × 1.5–3 mm
- In chronic infection, bile duct thickening, periductal fibrosis, dilation, biliary stasis, and secondary infection occcur. Little fibrosis occurs in the portal tracts

DEMOGRAPHICS

- Infection by *Clonorchis sinensis*, the Chinese liver fluke, is endemic in areas of Japan, Korea, China, Taiwan, Southeast Asia, and the far eastern part of Russia. Over 20 million people are affected
- Opisthorchiasis is caused by worms of the genus *Opisthorchis*, generally either *O felineus* (central, eastern, and southern Europe, eastern Asia, Southeast Asia, India) or *O viverrini* (Thailand, Laos, Vietnam)

 CLINICAL FINDINGS

SYMPTOMS AND SIGNS

- Most patients are asymptomatic
- Acute symptoms follow entry of immature worms into the biliary ducts and may persist for several weeks. Findings include malaise, low-grade fever, an enlarged, tender liver, pain in the hepatic area or epigastrium, urticaria, arthralgia, and jaundice
- In chronic infections, findings include weakness, anorexia, epigastric pain, diarrhea, prolonged low-grade fever, intermittent episodes of right upper quadrant pain, localized hepatic area tenderness, and progressive hepatomegaly

DIFFERENTIAL DIAGNOSIS

- Opisthorchiasis (clinically identical)
- Fascioliasis (sheep liver fluke)
- Ascariasis
- Toxocariasis (visceral larva migrans)
- Echinococcosis (hydatid disease)
- Whipple's disease
- Celiac sprue or tropical sprue

 DIAGNOSIS

LABORATORY TESTS

Acute Infection

- Difficult to diagnose, since ova may not appear in the feces until 3–4 weeks after onset of symptoms
- There may be leukocytosis, eosinophilia, elevated serum alanine aminotransferase, and elevated bilirubin
- Diagnosis is made by finding characteristic eggs in stools (repeated tests may be necessary) or duodenal aspirate (sensitivity approaches 100%)
- In severe infection, the number of eggs per gram of feces may not reflect the heavy worm burden; and in complete biliary obstruction, eggs can be detected in bile only by needle aspiration or at surgery

Chronic infection

- Liver function tests are normal except in severe cases
- Leukocytosis varies according to the intensity of infection; eosinophilia may be present
- In advanced chronic disease, liver function tests will indicate parenchymal damage
- The ELISA is the preferred serological test (sensitivity, 77%); however, unless a specific monoclonal antibody is used, cross-reactions are common with other trematode and cestode infections, tuberculosis, and liver cancer

IMAGING STUDIES

- In advanced chronic disease, CT and sonography may show diffuse dilation of small intrahepatic bile ducts with no or minimal dilation of the large intra- and extrahepatic ducts

DIAGNOSTIC PROCEDURES

- In advanced chronic disease, transhepatic cholangiograms may show alternating stricture and dilation of the biliary tree, with worms visualized as filling defects

Clonorchiasis & Opisthorchiasis

TREATMENT

MEDICATIONS

- The drug of choice is praziquantel. The dosage is 25 mg/kg three times daily for 2 days (with a 4- to 6-h interval between doses) for *Clonorchis* infections and 1 day of treatment may be sufficient for *Opisthorchis* infections
- Albendazole, at a dosage of 400 mg twice daily for 7 days, appears to be less effective (cures, 40–65%)
- In relapsing cholangitis, antibiotics are indicated to cover biliary pathogens

OUTCOME

COMPLICATIONS

- Intrahepatic bile duct calculi may occur that may lead to recurrent pyogenic cholangitis, biliary abscess, or endophlebitis of the portal-venous branches. This may gradually result in destruction of the liver parenchyma, fibrosis, and, rarely, cirrhosis with jaundice and ascites
- Chronic cholecystitis, cholelithiasis, and a nonfunctional, enlarged gallbladder may occur
- Flukes may enter the pancreatic duct, causing acute pancreatitis or cholelithiasis
- Cholangiocarcinoma has been causally linked with prolonged *Clonorchis* and *Opisthorchis* infection

PROGNOSIS

- Treatment cure rates over 95% can be anticipated for *Clonorchis* infections treated with praziquantel
- The disease is rarely fatal, but patients with advanced infections and impaired liver function may succumb more readily to other diseases

PREVENTION

- Pickling, smoking, or drying may not suffice to kill the metacercariae

EVIDENCE

PRACTICE GUIDELINES

- National Guideline Clearinghouse http://www.guideline.gov/summary/ summary.aspx?doc_id=2707&nbr=1933 &string=foodborne

INFORMATION FOR PATIENTS

- National Institute of Allergy and Infectious Disease http://www.niaid.nih.gov/publications/ microbes.htm
- Centers for Disease Control http://www.dpd.cdc.gov/dpdx/HTML/ Clonorchiasis.htm http://www.dpd.cdc.gov/dpdx/HTML/ opisthorchiasis.htm

REFERENCES

- Chan HH et al: The clinical and cholangiographic picture of hepatic clonorchiasis. J Clin Gastroenterol 2002;34:183. [PMID: 11782616]
- Watanapa P et al: Liver fluke-associated cholangiocarcinoma. Br J Surg 2002;89:962. [PMID: 12153620]

Clostridial Myonecrosis

 KEY FEATURES

ESSENTIALS OF DIAGNOSIS

- Sudden onset of pain and edema in an area of wound contamination
- Prostration and systemic toxicity
- Brown to blood-tinged watery exudate, with skin discoloration of surrounding area
- Gas in the tissue by palpation or x-ray
- Gram-positive rods in culture or smear of exudate

GENERAL CONSIDERATIONS

- Gas gangrene or clostridial myonecrosis is produced by entry of one of several clostridia (*Clostridium perfringens, Clostridium ramosum, Clostridium bifermentans, Clostridium histolyticum, Clostridium novyi,* etc) into devitalized tissues
- Toxins produced under anaerobic conditions result in shock, hemolysis, and myonecrosis

 CLINICAL FINDINGS

SYMPTOMS AND SIGNS

- The onset is usually sudden
- Rapidly increasing pain in the affected area
- Hypotension and tachycardia
- Fever is present but is not proportionate to the severity of the infection
- In the last stages of the disease, severe prostration, stupor, delirium, and coma occur
- The wound becomes swollen, and the surrounding skin is pale
- There is a foul-smelling brown, blood-tinged serous discharge
- As the disease advances, the surrounding tissue changes from pale to dusky and finally becomes deeply discolored, with coalescent, red, fluid-filled vesicles
- Gas may be palpable in the tissues

DIFFERENTIAL DIAGNOSIS

- Other gas-forming infections (mixed aerobic and anaerobic enteric organisms)
- Cellulitis due to staphylococcal or streptococcal infection
- Necrotizing fasciitis
- Shock due to other causes

 DIAGNOSIS

LABORATORY TESTS

- The smear shows a remarkable absence of neutrophils and the presence of gram-positive rods
- Anaerobic culture confirms the diagnosis

IMAGING STUDIES

- Radiographic studies may show gas within the soft tissues, but this finding is not specific

DIAGNOSTIC PROCEDURES

- Gas gangrene is a clinical diagnosis, and empirical therapy is indicated if the diagnosis is suspected

TREATMENT

MEDICATIONS

- Penicillin, 2 million units every 3 h intravenously
- Other agents (eg, tetracycline, clindamycin, metronidazole, chloramphenicol, cefoxitin) are probably effective

SURGERY

- Adequate surgical debridment and exposure of infected areas is essential, with radical surgical excision often necessary

THERAPEUTIC PROCEDURES

- Hyperbaric oxygen therapy has been used empirically but must be used in conjunction with administration of an appropriate antibiotic and surgical debridement

 ## OUTCOME

COMPLICATIONS

- Serious puerperal infection with hemolysis due to a lecithinase elaborated by the organism

 ## EVIDENCE

WEB SITES

- Baron's Medical Microbiology Textbook http://www.md.huji.ac.il/microbiology/book/toc.htm
- CDC—Division of Bacterial and Mycotic Diseases http://www.cdc.gov/ncidod/dbmd/
- CliniWeb International—Directory of Bacterial Infections and Mycoses http://www.ohsu.edu/cliniweb/C1/C1.html
- Karolinska Institute—Directory of Bacterial Infections and Mycoses http://www.mic.ki.se/Diseases/c1.html

INFORMATION FOR PATIENTS

- Nemours Foundation http://kidshealth.org/parent/infections/bacterial_viral/clostridium.html
- National Institutes of Health http://www.nlm.nih.gov/medlineplus/ency/article/000620.htm

REFERENCE

- Petit L et al: *Clostridium perfringens:* toxinotype and genotype. Trends Microbiol 1999;7:104. [PMID: 10203838]

Henry F. Chambers, MD

Coccidioidomycosis

 KEY FEATURES

ESSENTIALS OF DIAGNOSIS

- Influenza-like illness with malaise, fever, backache, headache, and cough
- Arthralgia and periarticular swelling of knees and ankles
- Erythema nodosum common
- Dissemination may result in meningitis, bone lesions, or skin and soft tissue abscesses
- Chest x-ray (CXR) varies widely from pneumonitis to cavitation
- Serological tests useful
- Spherules containing endospores demonstrable in sputum or tissues

GENERAL CONSIDERATIONS

- Consider this diagnosis in any obscure illness in a patient who has been in an endemic area
- Infection results from inhalation of *Coccidioides immitis*, a mold that grows in soil of southwestern United States, Mexico, and Central and South America
- Dissemination occurs in <1% of immunocompetent hosts, but mortality of disseminated disease is high

DEMOGRAPHICS

- Disseminated coccidioidomycosis occurs in about 0.1% of white and 1% of nonwhite patients. Filipinos and blacks and pregnant women of all races especially susceptible
- In HIV-infected people in endemic areas, coccidioidomycosis is a common opportunistic infection

 CLINICAL FINDINGS

SYMPTOMS AND SIGNS

Primary coccidioidomycosis

- Incubation period is 10–30 days
- Symptoms, usually respiratory, in 40%
- Nasopharyngitis with fever and chills; bronchitis with dry or slightly productive cough; pleuritic chest pain
- Arthralgias with periarticular swelling of knees and ankles
- Erythema nodosum 2–20 days after symptom onset
- Persistent pulmonary lesions in ~5%

Disseminated coccidioidomycosis

- Can involve any organ
- Productive cough
- Enlarged mediastinal lymph nodes
- Lung abscesses, empyema
- Fungemia, with diffuse miliary infiltrates on CXR and early death, in immunocompromised patients
- Meningitis in 30–50%
- Bone lesions at bony prominences
- Subcutaneous abscesses and verrucous skin lesions
- Lymphadenitis may progress to suppuration
- Mediastinal and retroperitoneal abscesses
- Disseminated in HIV-infected patients more often shows miliary infiltrates, lymphadenopathy, multiple organ involvement and meningitis, but skin lesions are uncommon

DIFFERENTIAL DIAGNOSIS

- Histoplasmosis, cryptococcosis, nocardiosis, blastomycosis
- Sarcoidosis
- Pneumoconiosis, eg, silicosis
- Tuberculosis
- Upper respiratory tract infection
- Atypical pneumonia
- Lymphoma (including lymphocytic interstitial pneumonitis)

 DIAGNOSIS

LABORATORY TESTS

- In primary coccidioidomycosis, moderate leukocytosis and eosinophilia
- IgM antibodies are positive in early disease
- In disseminated coccidioidomycosis, persistent or rising serum complement fixation titer (≥1:16); titers can be used to assess treatment adequacy. Complement fixation titer may be low in meningitis without other disseminated disease. In HIV-infected patients, complement fixation false-negative rate is as high as 30%
- In coccidioidal meningitis, cerebrospinal fluid (CSF) complement-fixing antibodies in >90%. CSF shows increased cell count, lymphocytosis, and reduced glucose; positive culture in 30%
- Spherules filled with endospores in biopsy specimens, can be cultured
- Blood cultures rarely positive in disseminated disease

IMAGING STUDIES

- CXR findings vary: nodular infiltrates and thin-walled cavities most common; hilar lymphadenopathy suggests localized disease, mediastinal adenopathy suggests dissemination; pleural effusions, abscesses, bronchiectasis, and lytic bone lesions

Coccidioidomycosis

 ## TREATMENT

MEDICATIONS

- For disease limited to the chest with no evidence of progression, symptomatic therapy
- For progressive pulmonary or extrapulmonary disease, IV amphotericin B until favorable clinical response and declining complement fixation titer
- For severe meningitis, lumbar intrathecal amphotericin B daily in increasing doses up to 1–5 mg/day, usually given with IV amphotericin B 0.6 mg/kg/day, until clinically stable. Then, taper intrathecal amphotericin to once every 6 weeks, or give oral azole therapy for several years
- For mild meningitis, fluconazole, 400 mg PO QD suppresses manifestations in about 75% of patients, but must be continued indefinitely, probably lifelong
- For chest, bone, and soft tissue disease, fluconazole, 200–400 mg PO QD, or itraconazole, 400 mg PO QD, continued for ≥6 months after disease inactive to prevent relapse

SURGERY

- Thoracic surgery is occasionally indicated for giant, infected, or ruptured cavities
- Surgical drainage useful for soft tissue abscesses and bone disease
- Following extensive surgical manipulation of infected tissue, give amphotericin B, 1 mg/kg/day IV, until disease is inactive, then change to oral azole therapy

 ## OUTCOME

FOLLOW-UP

- Follow the decrease in serum complement fixation titers
- Perform serial complement fixation titers after therapy; rising titers indicate relapse and warrant reinstitution of therapy

COMPLICATIONS

- Lung abscesses may rupture into pleural space, producing empyema, and may extend to bones, skin, and occasionally pericardium and myocardium

PROGNOSIS

- Good for patients with limited disease
- Nodules, cavities, and fibrosis may rarely progress after long periods of stability or regression
- Disseminated and meningeal forms have mortality rates exceeding 50% in the absence of therapy

 ## EVIDENCE

PRACTICE GUIDELINES

- 2001 USPHS/IDSA guidelines for the prevention of opportunistic infections in persons infected with human immunodeficiency virus. U.S. Department of Health and Human Services, Public Health Service
http://aidsinfo.nih.gov/guidelines/op_infections\OI_112801.pdf
- Infectious Diseases Society of America— Practice guidelines for the treatment of coccidioidomycosis
http://www.journals.uchicago.edu/CID/journal/issues/v30n4/990665/990665.web.pdf

WEB SITE

- AIDS Info by the USDHHS
http://aidsinfo.nih.gov/

INFORMATION FOR PATIENTS

- CDC—Coccidioidomycosis
http://www.cdc.gov/ncidod/dbmd/diseaseinfo/coccidioidomycosis_t.htm
- MEDLINEplus
http://www.nlm.nih.gov/medlineplus/ency/article/001322.htm

REFERENCES

- Galgiani JN et al: Practice guidelines for the treatment of coccidioidomycosis. Clin Infect Dis 2000;30:658. [PMID: 10770727]
- Stevens DA et al: Intrathecal amphotericin in the management of coccidioidal meningitis. Semin Respir Infect 2001;16:263. [PMID: 11739548]

Richard J. Hamill, MD

Colitis, Antibiotic-Associated

KEY FEATURES

ESSENTIALS OF DIAGNOSIS

- Most cases of antibiotic-associated diarrhea are not attributable to *Clostridium difficile* and are usually mild and self-limited
- Symptoms of antibiotic-associated colitis vary from mild to fulminant; almost all colitis is attributable to *C difficile*
- Diagnosis in mild to moderate colitis is established by stool toxin assay
- Flexible sigmoidoscopy provides most rapid diagnosis in severe colitis

GENERAL CONSIDERATIONS

- Antibiotic-associated diarrhea is common
- Characteristically occurs during antibiotic exposure, is dose related, and resolves spontaneously after discontinuation
- Most cases of diarrhea are mild, self-limited, and do not require evaluation or treatment
- Antibiotic-associated colitis is almost always caused by *C difficile*, which colonizes 5% of healthy adults, >20% of hospitalized patients
- *C difficile*–induced colitis most often occurs in hospitalized patients who are severely ill or malnourished or receiving chemotherapy or enteral tube feedings
- *C difficile* is the major cause of diarrhea in patients hospitalized for >3 days, affecting 7:1000 patients
- *C difficile*–induced colitis most commonly develops after use of ampicillin, clindamycin, and third-generation cephalosporins
- Symptoms begin during or shortly after antibiotic therapy but may be delayed for up to 8 weeks

DEMOGRAPHICS

- Hospitalized or recently hospitalized patients
- Elderly or debilitated patients
- Recent antibiotic exposure
- External tube feeding
- Recent abdominal surgery

CLINICAL FINDINGS

SYMPTOMS AND SIGNS

- Mild to moderate greenish, foul-smelling watery diarrhea with lower abdominal cramps in most patients
- Physical examination normal, or mild left lower quadrant tenderness
- With more serious illness, abdominal pain, profuse watery diarrhea with up to 30 stools per day
- Usually low-grade fever
- Abdominal tenderness mild unless severe disease

DIFFERENTIAL DIAGNOSIS

- Antibiotic-associated diarrhea (not related to *C difficile*)
- Other drug reaction
- Diarrhea due to enteral feedings
- Ischemic colitis
- Other bacterial diarrhea
- Inflammatory bowel disease
- Rarely, other organisms (staphylococci, *Clostridium perfringens*) are associated with pseudomembranous colitis

DIAGNOSIS

LABORATORY TESTS

- No or minimal leukocytosis with mild disease; in severe disease, leukocytosis as high as 50,000/µL
- Fecal leukocytes present in only 50%
- Stool toxin cytotoxicity assay (toxin B) has sensitivity of 95% and specificity of 90%
- Rapid enzyme immunoassays (EIA) (2–4 h) for toxins A and B have a 70–85% sensitivity with 1 stool specimen, 90% sensitivity with 2 specimens
- Culture for *C difficile* is the most sensitive test, but it is slower (2–3 days), more costly, and less specific, so is not used in most clinical settings

IMAGING STUDIES

- Abdominal radiographs: useful in detecting toxic dilation or megacolon, mucosal edema, or "thumbprinting"
- Abdominal CT: useful in detecting colonic edema

DIAGNOSTIC PROCEDURES

- Flexible sigmoidoscopy: no abnormalities or only patchy or diffuse, nonspecific colitis in mild to moderate symptoms, but true pseudomembranous colitis, most severe in the distal colon and rectum, in severe illness

Colitis, Antibiotic-Associated

 TREATMENT

 OUTCOME

 EVIDENCE

MEDICATIONS

Acute therapy

- Metronidazole, 500 mg PO TID for 10–14 days
- Vancomycin, 125 mg PO QID is equally effective, but more expensive, so reserved for patients who are intolerant of metronidazole, for pregnant women and children, for patients with severe disease who do not respond rapidly to metronidazole, and for patients who fail to respond to metronidazole

Relapse therapy

- Vancomycin, 125 mg PO QID for 7 days; BID for 7 days; QD for 7 days; QOD for 7 days; and Q3D for 2 weeks
- *Saccharomyces boulardii* (nonpathogenic yeast) 1 g/day for 4 weeks in combination with antibiotic reduces recurrences

SURGERY

- Total abdominal colectomy may be required in patients with toxic megacolon, perforation, sepsis, or hemorrhage

THERAPEUTIC PROCEDURES

- Discontinue offending antibiotic, if possible

COMPLICATIONS

- Weight loss and protein-losing enteropathy in chronic untreated colitis
- Dehydration, electrolyte imbalance, toxic megacolon, perforation, and death in fulminant disease

PROGNOSIS

- Relapse occurs in 10–25%
- Fulminant colitis with progression to toxic megacolon: high fever, profound leukocytosis (>20,000/μL), diarrhea, or paradoxical ileus with decreased bowel movement, dilation, and thickening of colon on CT

WHEN TO REFER

- Lack of improvement after 3–5 days of therapy
- Fulminant colitis or toxic megacolon
- Multiple relapses

WHEN TO ADMIT

- Severe colitis: pain, diarrhea, dehydration, temperature >38.5°C, abdominal tenderness, leukocytosis

PREVENTION

- Fastidious hand washing and use of disposable gloves minimize transmission of *C difficile*

PRACTICE GUIDELINES

- Fekety R: Guidelines for the diagnosis and management of *Clostridium difficile*-associated diarrhea and colitis. American College of Gastroenterology, Practice Parameters Committee. Am J Gastroenterol 1997;92:739. [PMID: 9149180]
- Fekety R et al: Evaluation of new anti-infective drugs for the treatment of antibiotic-associated colitis. Infectious Diseases Society of America and the Food and Drug Administration. Clin Infect Dis 1992;15(Suppl 1):S263. [PMID: 1477241]
- Jabbar A et al: Gastroenteritis and antibiotic-associated diarrhea. Prim Care 2003;30:63. [PMID: 12825250]

WEB SITES

- MEDLINEplus—Pseudomembranous colitis
  http://www.nlm.nih.gov/medlineplus/ency/article/000259.htm
- Merck Manual—Antibiotic associated colitis
  http://www.merck.com/mrkshared/mmanual_home/sec9/109.jsp

INFORMATION FOR PATIENTS

- Mayo Clinic—Antibiotic associated colitis
  http://www.mayoclinic.com/invoke.cfm?objectid=1CA38BA4-1AD5- 47B4-BFFE6A66CF08493C
- MD consult—Antibiotic associated diarrhea
  http://home.mdconsult.com/das/patient/view/30835332/10002/11145.html/top?sid=202796124

REFERENCES

- Buchner A et al: Medical diagnoses and procedures associated with *Clostridium difficile* colitis. Am J Gastroenterol 2001;96:766. [PMID: 11280548]
- Yassin S et al: *Clostridium difficile* colitis-associated diarrhea and colitis. Mayo Clin Proc 2001;76:725. [PMID: 11444405]

Kenneth R. McQuaid, MD

Colonic Pseudoobstruction, Acute (Ogilvie's Syndrome)

 KEY FEATURES

ESSENTIALS OF DIAGNOSIS

- Severe abdominal distension
- Massive dilation of cecum or right colon
- Arises in postoperative state or with severe medical illness
- May be precipitated by electrolyte imbalances, medications
- Absent to mild abdominal pain; minimal tenderness

GENERAL CONSIDERATIONS

- Spontaneous massive dilation of the cecum and proximal colon in hospitalized patients
- Progressive cecal dilation may lead to spontaneous perforation
- Etiology unknown

Associated conditions

- Trauma, burns
- Respiratory failure
- Malignancy
- Myocardial infarction or CHF
- Pancreatitis
- Stroke or subarachnoid hemorrhage
- Ischemic colitis
- Use of drugs, eg, opioids, anticholinergics

DEMOGRAPHICS

- Occurs mainly in hospitalized patients with recent trauma, surgery (especially cardiothoracic), or severe medical illness
- May be precipitated by electrolyte imbalance or narcotics

 CLINICAL FINDINGS

SYMPTOMS AND SIGNS

- Sometimes asymptomatic
- Constant but mild abdominal pain
- Nausea and vomiting
- Abdominal distension
- Bowel movements absent
- Abdominal tenderness with some degree of guarding or rebound tenderness
- Fever suggests colonic perforation

DIFFERENTIAL DIAGNOSIS

- Mechanical colonic obstruction, eg, malignancy, diverticulitis, volvulus, fecal impaction
- Toxic megacolon due to inflammatory bowel disease or *Clostridium difficile* colitis, cytomegalovirus

 DIAGNOSIS

LABORATORY TESTS

- Obtain complete blood cell count, serum sodium, potassium, magnesium, phosphorus, and calcium
- Leukocytosis suggests colonic perforation

IMAGING STUDIES

- Plain film radiographs demonstrate colonic dilation, usually cecum and proximal colon
- Varying amounts of small intestinal dilation and air-fluid levels
- Cecal diameter >10–12 cm associated with increased risk of colonic perforation

DIAGNOSTIC PROCEDURES

- Hypaque (diatrizoate meglumine) enema to exclude colonic obstruction and to decompress the colon and evacuate distal fecal material

Colonic Pseudoobstruction, Acute (Ogilvie's Syndrome)

TREATMENT

MEDICATIONS

- Discontinue opioids, anticholinergics, and calcium channel blockers, if possible
- Correct electrolyte abnormalities
- Oral laxatives are not helpful and may cause perforation
- In patients with sustained or progressive cecal dilation to ≥10–12 cm and in those with signs of clinical deterioration, administering neostigmine, 2 mg IV as a single dose, results in rapid (within 30 min) colonic decompression in 75–90%

SURGERY

- In patients in whom colonoscopy is unsuccessful, a tube cecostomy placed through a small laparotomy or percutaneously with radiological guidance can decompress the colon

THERAPEUTIC PROCEDURES

- Treat underlying illness
- Conservative treatment is recommended if no or minimal abdominal tenderness, no fever, no leukocytosis, and a cecal diameter <12 cm
- Place a nasogastric tube and a rectal tube
- Patients periodically rolled from side to side
- Enemas if large amounts of stool on radiography
- Conservative treatment successful in >80%
- Colonoscopic decompression in patients who fail to respond to neostigmine, successful in up to 90%; dilation recurs in up to 50%

OUTCOME

FOLLOW-UP

- Watch for signs of worsening distension or abdominal tenderness
- Assess cecal size by abdominal radiographs Q 12 h
- Cardiac monitoring following neostigmine for possible bradycardia that may require atropine administration

COMPLICATIONS

- Colonic perforation

PROGNOSIS

- Prognosis related to the underlying illness
- With aggressive therapy, perforation unusual

WHEN TO REFER

- Failure to improve within 24 h of conservative therapy
- Signs of perforation

WHEN TO ADMIT

- Usually occurs in hospitalized patients

EVIDENCE

PRACTICE GUIDELINES

- Cappell MS et al: The role of sigmoidoscopy and colonoscopy in the diagnosis and management of lower gastrointestinal disorders: endoscopic findings, therapy, and complications. Med Clin North Am 2002;86:1253. [PMID: 12510454]
- Dorudi S et al: Acute colonic pseudoobstruction. Br J Surg 1992;79:99. [PMID: 1555081]
- Eisen GM et al: Standards of Practice Committee of the American Society for Gastrointestinal Endoscopy. Acute colonic pseudo-obstruction. Gastrointest Endosc 2002;56:789. [PMID: 12447286]

WEB SITE

- International Foundation for Functional Gastrointestinal Disorders (IFFGD) Inc. Motility disorders http://www.iffgd.org/GIDisorders/GIAdults.html#GIMot

INFORMATION FOR PATIENTS

- MEDLINEplus—Primary or idiopathic intestinal pseudo-obstruction http://www.nlm.nih.gov/medlineplus/ency/article/000253.htm
- NIDDK/NIH—Intestinal pseudo-obstruction http://digestive.niddk.nih.gov/ddiseases/pubs/intestinalpo/index.htm

REFERENCES

- De Giorgio R et al: Review article: the pharmacologic treatment of acute colonic pseudo-obstruction. Aliment Pharmacol Ther 2001;15:1717. [PMID: 11683685]
- Eisen GM et al: Acute colonic pseudo-obstruction. Gastrointest Endosc 2002;56:789. [PMID: 12447286]
- Loftus C et al: Assessment of predictors of response to neostigmine for acute colonic pseudo-obstruction. Am J Gastroenterol 2002;97:3118. [PMID: 12492198]

Kenneth R. McQuaid, MD

Colorectal Cancer

 KEY FEATURES

ESSENTIALS OF DIAGNOSIS

- Symptoms or signs dependent on tumor location
- Proximal colon: fecal occult blood, anemia
- Distal colon: change in bowel habits, hematochezia
- Characteristic findings on barium enema
- Diagnosis established with colonoscopy and biopsy

GENERAL CONSIDERATIONS

- Almost all colon cancers are adenocarcinomas
- ~50% occur in the rectosigmoid; ~25% in the cecum and ascending colon
- The majority of colorectal cancers arise from malignant transformation of an adenomatous polyp
- Approximately 3% of colorectal cancers are caused by inherited autosomal dominant germline mutations resulting in polyposis syndromes or hereditary non-polyposis colorectal cancer
- Risk factors: age; history of colorectal cancer or adenomatous polyps, breast, uterine, or ovarian cancer; family history of colorectal cancer; inflammatory bowel disease (ulcerative colitis and Crohn's colitis); diets rich in fats and red meat; race (higher in blacks than in whites)

DEMOGRAPHICS

- Second leading cause of death due to malignancy in the United States
- ~6% of Americans will develop colorectal cancer and 40% of those will die of the disease
- ~134,000 new cases and 55,000 deaths occur annually in the United States

 CLINICAL FINDINGS

SYMPTOMS AND SIGNS

- Adenocarcinomas grow slowly and may be asymptomatic
- Symptoms depend on the location of the cancer
- Right-sided colon cancers cause iron deficiency anemia, fatigue, and weakness from chronic blood loss
- Left-sided colon cancers cause obstructive symptoms, colicky abdominal pain, change in bowel habits, constipation alternating with loose stools, and stool streaked with blood
- Rectal cancers cause rectal tenesmus, urgency, and recurrent hematochezia
- Physical examination usually normal, except in advanced disease: mass may be palpable in the abdomen
- Hepatomegaly suggests metastatic spread

DIFFERENTIAL DIAGNOSIS

- Diverticulosis or diverticulitis
- Hemorrhoids
- Adenomatous polyps
- Ischemic colitis
- Inflammatory bowel disease
- Irritable bowel syndrome
- Infectious colitis
- Iron deficiency due to other cause

 DIAGNOSIS

LABORATORY TESTS

- Complete blood cell count reveals iron deficiency anemia
- Liver function tests elevated in metastatic disease
- Fecal occult blood tests positive
- Carcinoembryonic antigen (CEA) level elevated in 70%, should normalize after complete surgical resection

IMAGING STUDIES

- Barium enema or CT colonography ("virtual colonoscopy") for initial diagnosis, if colonoscopy not available
- Abdominal and chest CT scan for preoperative staging
- Pelvic MRI and endorectal ultrasonography may guide operative management of rectal cancer

DIAGNOSTIC PROCEDURES

- Colonoscopy is the diagnostic procedure of choice because it visualizes the whole colon and permits biopsy of lesions
- Staging by TNM system correlates with the patient's long-term survival, used to determine which patients should receive adjuvant therapy (Table 55A, page 1252)

TREATMENT

MEDICATIONS

- Postoperative adjuvant chemotherapy with fluorouracil and leucovorin for 6 months for stage III disease improves 5-year disease-free survival to 64%; alternatively, chemotherapy with a combination of fluorouracil and levamisole for 1 year
- Combination therapy with fluorouracil, leucovorin, and irinotecan for stage IV disease yields tumor response rate of 40% and increases overall survival (mean 15 months)

SURGERY

- Resection of the primary colonic or rectal cancer
- Regional lymph node removal to determine staging
- For rectal carcinoma, in selected patients, transanal excision
- For all other patients with rectal cancer, low anterior resection with a colorectal anastomosis or an abdominoperineal resection with a colostomy
- For unresectable rectal cancer, diverting colostomy, laser fulguration, or placement of an expandable wire stent
- For metastatic disease, resection of isolated (1 to 3) liver or lung metastases

THERAPEUTIC PROCEDURES

- Radiation therapy used for selected patients with locally advanced (T3 or T4) colon cancer
- Combined postoperative adjuvant pelvic radiation and chemotherapy with fluorouracil for both stage II and stage III rectal cancers
- Local ablative techniques (cryosurgery, embolization) for unresectable hepatic metastases

 OUTCOME

FOLLOW-UP

- After resection surgery, patients should be evaluated every 3–6 months for 3–5 years with history, physical examination, fecal occult blood testing, liver function tests, and CEA determinations
- A rise in CEA levels that had normalized initially after surgery is suggestive of cancer recurrence
- Colonoscopy within 6–12 months and then every 3–5 years
- Change in the patient's clinical picture, abnormal liver function tests, or a rising CEA level warrant chest radiography and abdominal CT

PROGNOSIS

- 5-year survival rates: stage I: 80–100%, even with no adjuvant therapy; stage II (node-negative disease), 50–75%, with no adjuvant therapy, though patients with advanced local stage II disease (T3–T4) should be considered for study protocols of adjuvant chemotherapy or radiotherapy; stage III (node-positive) disease, 30–50%, improved by postoperative adjuvant chemotherapy
- Long-term survival rates: stage I, >90%; stage II, >70%; stage III with fewer than four positive lymph nodes, 67%; stage III with more than four positive lymph nodes, 33%; and stage IV, <5%
- For each stage, rectal cancers have a worse prognosis
- Tumors that have microsatellite instability have a more favorable prognosis

PREVENTION

- Screening for colorectal neoplasms should be offered to every patient age >50 (Table 55B, page 1252)
- Chemoprevention: prolonged regular use of aspirin and other nonsteroidal antiinflammatory drugs may decrease the risk of colorectal neoplasia, however, routine use as chemotherapeutic agent not recommended currently

 EVIDENCE

PRACTICE GUIDELINES

- Practice parameters for the detection of colorectal neoplasms. American Society of Colon and Rectal Surgeons, 1999 http://www.fascrs.org/ascrspp-docn-r.html
- Screening for colorectal cancer: recommendations and rationale. United States Preventive Services Task Force, 2002 http://www.ahrq.gov/clinic/3rduspstf/colorectal/

WEB SITES

- American Cancer Society—What is colorectal cancer? http://www.cancer.org/docroot/CRI/content/CRI_2_2_1X_What_is_colon_and_rectum_cancer_10.asp?sitearea=CRI
- MEDLINEplus—Colorectal cancer http://www.nlm.nih.gov/medlineplus/colorectalcancer.html
- Rectal cancer—National Cancer Institute—Cancer Net http://cancernet.nci.nih.gov

INFORMATION FOR PATIENTS

- JAMA patient page: Colon cancer screening http://www.ama-assn.org/public/journals/patient/archive/jpg031203.htm

REFERENCES

- Blumberg D et al: Treatment of colon and rectal cancer. J Clin Gastroenterol 2002;34:15. [PMID: 11743241]
- Ransohoff D et al: Clinical practice. Screening for colorectal cancer. N Engl J Med 2002;346:40. [PMID: 11778002]
- Screening for colorectal cancer: recommendations and rationale. Ann Intern Med 2002;137:129. [PMID: 11821507]
- Yee J et al: Colorectal neoplasia: performance characteristics of CT colonography for detection in 300 patients. Radiology 2001;219:685. [PMID: 11376255]

Kenneth R. McQuaid, MD

Common Variable Immunodeficiency

 KEY FEATURES

ESSENTIALS OF DIAGNOSIS

- Defect in terminal differentiation of B cells, with absent plasma cells and deficient synthesis of secreted antibody
- Increased susceptibility to pyogenic infections–frequent sinopulmonary infections
- Confirmation by evaluation of serum immunoglobulin levels and deficient functional antibody responses

GENERAL CONSIDERATIONS

- A heterogeneous immunodeficiency disorder clinically characterized by an increased incidence of recurrent infections, autoimmune phenomena, and neoplastic diseases
- The most common cause of panhypogammaglobulinemia in adults
- The onset is usually during adolescence or early adulthood but can occur at any age
- Paradoxically, there is an increased incidence of autoimmune disease (20%), though patients may not display the usual serological markers
- Gastrointestinal disorders are commonly associated

DEMOGRAPHICS

- The prevalence is about 1:80,000 in the United States

 CLINICAL FINDINGS

SYMPTOMS AND SIGNS

- Increased susceptibility to pyogenic infections
- Virtually all patients suffer from recurrent sinusitis
- Bronchitis, otitis, pharyngitis, and pneumonia are also common
- Autoimmune disease
- Sprue-like syndrome, with diarrhea, steatorrhea, malabsorption, protein-losing enteropathy, and hepatosplenomegaly
- Lymphadenopathy
- Increased incidence of cancers—lymphoma, gastric, and skin

DIFFERENTIAL DIAGNOSIS

- Secondary immunodeficiency, eg, AIDS, corticosteroid use, leukemia
- Selective IgA deficiency
- Multiple myeloma
- Cystic fibrosis
- Asplenism
- Celiac sprue
- Systemic lupus erythematosus
- X-linked agammaglobulinemia
- Immunodeficiency with thymoma
- Wegener's granulomatosis

 DIAGNOSIS

LABORATORY TESTS

- The pattern of immunoglobulin isotype deficiency is variable
- Typically present with significantly depressed IgG levels (usually less than 250 mg/dL), but over time all antibody classes (IgG, IgA, and IgM) may decrease
- Decreased to absent functional antibody responses to protein antigen immunizations establish the diagnosis
- Autoimmune cytopenias are common

DIAGNOSTIC PROCEDURES

- Biopsies of enlarged lymph nodes show marked reduction in plasma cells
- Noncaseating granulomas are frequently found in the spleen, liver, lungs, or skin

TREATMENT

MEDICATIONS

- Systolic dysfunction: a diuretic and an angiotensin-converting enzyme (ACE) inhibitor (or angiotensin receptor blocker in ACE-intolerant patients) with subsequent addition of a β-blocker
- Diuretics (Table 44, page 1237): thiazide, loop, thiazide and loop, or thiazide and spironolactone
- Aldosterone blockers: spironolactone 25 mg QD; may decrease to 12.5 mg or increase to 50 mg depending on renal function, K^+, and symptoms
- ACE inhibitors (Table 46, page 1241), started at low doses and titrated to dosages proved effective in clinical trials (eg, captopril 50 mg PO TID, enalapril 10 mg PO BID, lisinopril 10 mg PO QD) over 1–3 months
- Angiotensin receptor blockers (Table 46, page 1241) for ACE-intolerant patients
- β-Blockers (Table 45, page 1239): in stable patients, started at low doses and titrated gradually and with great care, eg, carvedilol started at 3.125 mg PO BID, increased to 6.25, 12.5, and 25 mg BID at intervals of ~2 weeks, or extended-release metoprolol, starting at 12.5 or 25 mg once daily and increasing to 50, 75, 100, 150, and 200 mg at 2-week or longer intervals
- Digoxin
- Positive inotropic agents (eg, dobutamine and milrinone): use limited to patients with hypoperfusion, rapidly deteriorating renal function, failed response to intravenous diuretics, and awaiting cardiac transplantation
- Anticoagulation: for patients with LV CHF associated with atrial fibrillation or large recent (within 3–6 months) MI
- Diastolic dysfunction: diuretics, rigorous blood pressure control

SURGERY

- Coronary revascularization may improve symptoms and prevent progression
- Bypass surgery provides more complete revascularization than angioplasty
- Cardiac transplantation for advanced heart failure
- Implantable defibrillators for sudden death and unexplained syncope

THERAPEUTIC PROCEDURES

- Moderate salt restriction (2–2.5 g sodium or 5–6 g salt per day)
- Temporary restriction of activity

 ## OUTCOME

FOLLOW-UP

- Monitor patients on diuretics and ACE inhibitors for hypokalemia, renal failure
- Case management, home monitoring of weight and clinical status, and patient adjustment of diuretics can prevent rehospitalizations

COMPLICATIONS

- Myocardial ischemia in patients with underlying coronary artery disease
- Asymptomatic and symptomatic arrhythmias, especially nonsustained ventricular tachycardia
- Sudden death and unexplained syncope

PROGNOSIS

- Poor prognosis, with annual mortality rates ~5% in stable patients with mild symptoms to ~30–50% in patients with advanced, progressive symptoms
- Poorer prognosis with severe LV dysfunction (ejection fractions <20%), nonsustained ventricular tachycardia, major limitation of exercise capacity, secondary renal insufficiency, hyponatremia, and elevated plasma catecholamine levels
- 30–50% of hospitalized patients will be readmitted within 3–6 months
- Posttransplant 1-year survival rate ≥80-90%, and 5-year survival rate ≥70%

PREVENTION

- Antihypertensive therapy
- Antihyperlipidemic therapy
- Treat valvular lesions early (aortic stenosis and mitral and aortic regurgitation)

EVIDENCE

PRACTICE GUIDELINES

- ACC/AHA Guidelines for the evaluation and management of chronic heart failure in the adult: executive summary. J Am Coll Cardiol 2001;38:2101

WEB SITES

- Heart Failure Society of America http://www.abouthf.org/
- American Heart Association Learning about heart failure http://www.americanheart.org/presenter.jhtml?identifier=337

INFORMATION FOR PATIENTS

- JAMA patient page: Heart failure. JAMA 2002;287:676. [PMID: 11842812] http://www.ama-assn.org/public/journals/patient/archive/pat0206.htm

REFERENCES

- Angeja BG et al: Evaluation and management of diastolic heart failure. Circulation 2003;107:659. [PMID: 12578862]
- Coats AJ : Angiotensin type-1 receptor blockers in heart failure. Prog Cardiovasc Dis 2002;44:231. [PMID: 12007079]
- Foody JM et al: Beta-blocker therapy in heart failure: scientific review. JAMA 2002;287:883. [PMID: 11851582]
- Maisel AS et al: Rapid measurement of B-type natriuretic peptide in the emergency diagnosis of heart failure. N Engl J Med 2002;347:161. [PMID: 12124404]

Barry M. Massie, MD
Thomas M. Amidon, MD

Conjunctivitis

 KEY FEATURES

ESSENTIALS OF DIAGNOSIS

- The most common eye disease, also known as "pink eye"
- Diffuse redness of the bulbar and tarsal conjunctiva
- Usually mild to moderate ocular irritation and discharge, clear cornea, and normal visual acuity

GENERAL CONSIDERATIONS

- Usually due to bacterial (including gonococcal or chlamydial) or viral infections
- Other common causes include atopy, chemical irritants, and keratoconjunctivitis sicca (dry eyes)
- Mode of transmission of infectious conjunctivitis is usually direct contact via fingers, towels, etc to the other eye, or to other persons
- Clinically important to differentiate conjunctivitis from acute uveitis, acute glaucoma, and corneal disorders

DEMOGRAPHICS

- Precise incidence is unknown, but very common
- Men and women affected equally
- Age group affected depends on the underlying cause
- Trachoma (*Chlamydia trachomatis*) is a major cause of blindness worldwide
- Gonococcal conjunctivitis and inclusion conjunctivitis (*C trachomatis*) are caused by the agents involved in the respective genital tract diseases and typically occur in sexually active adults
- Viral conjunctivitis is more common in children than adults, with contaminated swimming pools or ophthalmologists' offices often being the source of epidemics
- Keratoconjunctivitis sicca is common in elderly women and sometimes associated with systemic diseases (Sjögren's syndrome)
- Allergic eye disease typically begins in late childhood or young adulthood and usually in people with atopy

 CLINICAL FINDINGS

SYMPTOMS AND SIGNS

Bacterial conjunctivitis

- Staphylococci, streptococci, *Haemophilus, Pseudomonas,* and *Moraxella* are the most common organisms isolated
- Purulent discharge
- Usually self-limited, lasting 10–14 days if untreated

Gonococcal conjunctivitis

- Exposure to infected genital secretions is the usual mode of transmission
- Copious purulent discharge
- An ophthalmological emergency because corneal involvement may rapidly lead to perforation and blindness.

Chlamydial conjunctivitis

- Trachoma usually causes recurrent conjunctivitis and epithelial keratitis during childhood leading to corneal scarring in adulthood
- Inclusion conjunctivitis produces follicular conjunctivitis with redness, discharge, and irritation, and nontender preauricular lymphadenopathy

Viral conjunctivitis

- The most common causative agents are adenoviruses
- Copious watery discharge with severe ocular irritation and possibly visual loss due to keratitis
- Subconjunctival hemorrhages occasionally occur
- There may be pharyngitis, fever, malaise, and preauricular lymphadenopathy

Keratoconjunctivitis sicca

- Due to hypofunction of the lacrimal glands, excessive evaporation of tears, abnormalities of the lipid component of tears, or mucin deficiency
- Ocular dryness, redness, or foreign body sensation
- Marked discomfort, photophobia, and excessive mucus in severe cases
- Corneal ulceration may develop

Allergic eye disease

- Itching is strongly suggestive of allergic eye disease
- Allergic conjunctivitis is a benign disease characterized by conjunctival hyperemia and edema, often of sudden onset, that

may be seasonal (hay fever conjunctivitis) or perennial
- Vernal keratoconjunctivitis, characterized by large "cobblestone" papillae on the upper tarsal conjunctiva, and atopic keratoconjunctivitis, characterized by chronic papillary conjunctivitis with fibrosis, are potentially blinding diseases

DIFFERENTIAL DIAGNOSIS

- See Table 9 (page 1205)
- Acute anterior uveitis (iritis)
- Acute (angle-closure) glaucoma
- Corneal trauma (eg, foreign body or abrasion)
- Corneal infection or inflammation (eg, corneal ulcer or herpes simplex keratitis)
- Scleritis or episcleritis

DIAGNOSIS

- Diagnosis is usually clinical
- If there is copious purulent discharge, conjunctival swab for gram stain and bacterial culture to identify gonococcal infection
- For suspected inclusion conjunctivitis or trachoma, chlamydial culture and examination of Giemsa-stained conjunctival scrapings
- For suspected keratoconjunctivitis sicca, Schirmer's test to measure tear production may be helpful

TREATMENT

MEDICATIONS

- See Table 10 (page 1206)
- Choice of therapeutic agent should be dictated by underlying cause
- Mild bacterial conjunctivitis: sulfonamide or erythromycin ophthalmic solution or ointment
- Gonococcal conjunctivitis: ceftriaxone 1 g IM but admit if corneal involvement
- Chlamydial conjunctivitis: oral tetracycline, erythromycin, doxycyline for 2–5 weeks or single-dose therapy with azithromycin
- Viral conjunctivitis: weak topical steroids under the supervision of an ophthalmologist for corneal involvement
- Keratoconjunctivitis sicca: artificial tears (preparations with methylcellulose or polyvinyl alcohol are longer lasting)
- Allergic keratoconjunctivitis: topical antihistamine, nonsteroidal antiinflammatory or mast cell stabilizing agents, or if severe, topical corticosteroids under the supervision of an ophthalmologist

SURGERY

- Correction of eyelid deformities and corneal transplantation in the later stages of trachoma

THERAPEUTIC PROCEDURES

- Warm compresses and rest can be helpful and are often the only therapy necessary for mild bacterial or viral conjunctivitis

 OUTCOME

FOLLOW-UP

- Most cases of bacterial or viral conjunctivitis do not require follow-up
- Recurrent bacterial conjunctivitis requires ophthalmological assessment for predisposing factors such as blepharitis
- Gonococcal and inclusion conjunctivitis require follow-up for other sexually transmitted diseases
- Chronic moderate or severe allergic eye disease or keratoconjunctivitis sicca should be managed by an ophthalmologist

COMPLICATIONS

- Corneal ulceration, perforation or scarring, resulting in visual loss, may complicate gonococcal conjunctivitis, trachoma, keratoconjunctivitis sicca, or severe allergic eye disease

PROGNOSIS

- Most cases of conjunctivitis have an excellent prognosis, although long-term treatment may be required in keratoconjunctivitis sicaa and chronic allergic eye disease

WHEN TO REFER

- Refer patients with copious purulent disharge, corneal involvement, loss of visual acuity, severe pain, or lack of response to treatment to an ophthalmologist
- Refer patients (or their mothers in the case of neonates) with inclusion conjunctivitis or gonococcal conjunctivitis for identification of genital tract infection and other sexually transmitted diseases to an internist or gynecologist

WHEN TO ADMIT

- Admit patients with gonococcal conjunctivitis involving the cornea

 EVIDENCE

PRACTICE GUIDELINES

- American Academy of Opthalmology http://www.aao.org/aao/education/library/ppp/loader.cfm?url=/commonspot/security/getfile.cfm&PageID=23346
- American Family Physician (Cochrane Interpretation) http://www.aafp.org/afp/20021101/cochrane.html

WEB SITES

- Allergic eye disease http://www.medem.com/MedLB/articledetaillb.cfm?article_ID=ZZZL7E331CC&sub_cat=37
- American Academy of Opthalmology http://www.aao.org
- Keratoconjunctivitis sicca http://www.medem.com/MedLB/article_detaillb.cfm?article_ID=ZZZXQXXV1ED&sub_cat=37
- National Eye Institute http://www.nei.nih.gov

INFORMATION FOR PATIENTS

- MD Consult http://home.mdconsult.com/das/patient/view/29760586/10055/6553.html/top?sid=192484919
- MEDLINE plus http://www.nlm.nih.gov/medlineplus/ency/article/001010.htm

REFERENCES

- Kalayoglu MV: Ocular chlamydial infections: pathogenesis and emerging treatment strategies. Curr Drug Targets Infect Disord 2002;2:85. [PMID: 12462156]
- Lee JS et al: Gonococcal keratoconjunctivitis in adults. Eye 2002;16:646. [PMID: 12194086]
- Robert PY et al: Comparative review of topical ophthalmic antibacterial preparations. Drugs 2001;61:175. [PMID: 11270936]

Paul Riordan-Eva, FRCOphth
Richard A. Jacobs, MD, PhD

Constipation

 KEY FEATURES

ESSENTIALS OF DIAGNOSIS

- Defined as two or fewer bowel movements per week or excessive difficulty and straining at defecation

GENERAL CONSIDERATIONS

- Common complaint
- May be intermittent or chronic
- Most commonly caused by diet, medications, or immobility
- May be caused by systemic diseases, structural abnormalities, or abnormal motility
- Fecal impaction: predisposing factors: severe psychiatric disease, prolonged bed rest and debility, neurogenic disorders of the colon, and spinal cord disorders

DEMOGRAPHICS

- Increased incidence with advancing age

 CLINICAL FINDINGS

SYMPTOMS AND SIGNS

- Decreased appetite
- Nausea and vomiting
- Abdominal pain and distention
- Paradoxical "diarrhea"
- Firm feces palpable on digital rectal examination

DIFFERENTIAL DIAGNOSIS

- Inadequate fiber or fluid intake
- Poor bowel habits
- Irritable bowel syndrome

Systemic disease

- Endocrine: hypothyroidism, hyperparathyroidism, diabetes mellitus
- Metabolic: hypercalcemia, hypokalemia, uremia, porphyria
- Neurological: Parkinson's disease, multiple sclerosis, sacral nerve damage (pelvic surgery, tumor), paraplegia, autonomic neuropathy
- Rheumatological: scleroderma, amyloidosis
- Medications: narcotics, diuretics, calcium channel blockers, anticholinergics, psychotropic, calcium, iron, nonsteroidal antiinflammatory drugs, clonidine, sucralfate, cholestyramine
- Infectious: typhoid fever

Structural abnormalities

- Anorectal: rectal prolapse, rectocele, rectal intussusception, anorectal stricture, anal fissure, solitary rectal ulcer syndrome
- Pelvic floor dysfunction (hysterectomy)
- Obstructing colonic mass (cancer)
- Colonic stricture: radiation, ischemia, diverticulosis
- Hirschsprung's disease
- Chagas disease

Slow colonic transit

- Idiopathic: isolated to colon
- Psychogenic
- Eating disorders
- Chronic intestinal pseudoobstruction

 DIAGNOSIS

LABORATORY TESTS

- Complete blood cell count
- Serum electrolytes
- Serum calcium
- Serum thyroid-stimulating hormone
- Fecal occult blood test

IMAGING STUDIES

- Colonoscopy or flexible sigmoidoscopy and barium enema

DIAGNOSTIC PROCEDURES

- Diet, fluid, and medication history
- Physical examination
- Colonic transit and pelvic floor function studies for severe constipation unresponsive to life-style changes and laxatives

Constipation

 ## TREATMENT

MEDICATIONS

- Stool surfactant agents: docusate sodium, 50–200 mg/day, or mineral oil, 14–45 mL/day, orally or rectally
- Saline laxatives: magnesium-containing saline laxatives (milk of magnesia, magnesium sulfate); sodium phosphate or magnesium citrate
- Nonabsorbable carbohydrate laxatives: sorbitol (70%) or lactulose, 15–30 mL PO QD or BID
- Polyethylene glycol 3350 powder (Miralax), 17 g once or twice daily
- Stimulant agents: bisacodyl, senna, cascara, and castor oil
- Fecal impaction: Initial treatment: enemas (saline, mineral oil, or diatrizoate) or digital disruption; long-term treatment: maintaining soft stools and regular bowel movements

SURGERY

- Subtotal colectomy with ileorectal anastomosis rarely required for severe intractable colonic inertia
- Disimpaction under anesthesia sometimes required for severe impaction

THERAPEUTIC PROCEDURES

- Biofeedback therapy for pelvic floor dysfunction

 ## OUTCOME

COMPLICATIONS

- Fecal impaction
- Large bowel obstruction with pain, distension, nausea and vomiting

PROGNOSIS

- Most patients successfully treated with life-style changes and intermittent or chronic laxatives

WHEN TO REFER

- Severe constipation unresponsive to laxatives
- Suspected pelvic floor dysfunction (prolonged straining, difficulty with evacuation)

WHEN TO ADMIT

- Severe fecal impaction

 ## EVIDENCE

PRACTICE GUIDELINES

- American Gastroenterological Association medical position statement: guidelines on constipation. American Gastroenterological Association, 2001 http://www2.gastrojournal.org/scripts/om.dll/serve?action=get-media&id=a0060001761&trueID=pdf_0060001761&location=jgast0011906&type=pdf&name=x.pdf
- Jones MP et al: Lack of objective evidence of efficacy of laxatives in chronic constipation. Dig Dis Sci 2002;47:2222. [PMID: 12395895]
- Petticrew M et al: Effectiveness of laxatives in adults. Qual Health Care 2001;10:268. [PMID: 11743157]

WEB SITES

- Cleveland Clinic—Constipation http://www.clevelandclinic.org/health/health-info/docs/0000/0062.asp?index=4059
- Mayo Clinic—Constipation http://www.mayoclinic.com/invoke.cfm?objectid=2D434692-F005-495C-A5EB2AFBD98CA2A5

INFORMATION FOR PATIENTS

- American Academy of Family Physicians—Constipation http://familydoctor.org/healthfacts/037/
- National Digestive Diseases Information Clearinghouse—Constipation http://digestive.niddk.nih.gov/ddiseases/pubs/constipation/index.htm

REFERENCES

- American Gastroenterological Association Medical position statement: guidelines on constipation. Gastroenterology 2000;119:1761. [PMID: 11113098]
- Schiller LR: Review article: the therapy of constipation. Aliment Pharmacol Ther 2001;15:749. [PMID: 11380313]

Kenneth R. McQuaid, MD

Contraception, IUD & Barrier Methods

 KEY FEATURES

GENERAL CONSIDERATIONS

- Contraception should be available to all women and men of reproductive ages
- Education about and access to contraception are especially important for sexually active teenagers and for women following childbirth or abortion
- IUDs are not abortifacients

Intrauterine devices

- IUDs include the Mirena (which releases levonorgestrel) and the copper-bearing TCu380A
- The hormone-containing IUDs have the advantage of reducing cramping and menstrual flow
- Nulliparity is not a contraindication to IUD use
- The Mirena may have a protective effect against upper tract infection similar to that of oral contraceptives
- Contraindications to use of IUDs are outlined in Table 67 (page 1261)
- A copper-containing IUD can be inserted within 5 days following a single episode of unprotected mid-cycle coitus as a postcoital contraceptive
- An IUD should not be inserted into a pregnant uterus
- If pregnancy occurs as an IUD failure, there is a greater chance of spontaneous abortion if the IUD is left in situ (50%) than if it is removed (25%)
- Spontaneous abortion with an IUD in place is associated with a high risk of severe sepsis, and death can occur rapidly
- Women using an IUD who become pregnant should have the IUD removed if the string is visible
- It can be removed at the time of abortion if this is desired
- If the string is not visible and the patient wants to continue the pregnancy, she should be informed of the serious risk of sepsis and, occasionally, death with such pregnancies
- She should be informed that any flu-like symptoms such as fever, myalgia, headache, or nausea warrant immediate medical attention for possible septic abortion
- Since the ratio of ectopic to intrauterine pregnancies is increased among IUD wearers, clinicians should search for adnexal masses in early pregnancy and should always check the products of

conception for placental tissue following abortion

Diaphragm & cervical cap

- The diaphragm (with contraceptive jelly) is a safe and effective contraceptive method with features that make it acceptable to some women and not others
- Failure rates range from 2% to 20%, depending on the motivation of the woman and the care with which the diaphragm is used
- The advantages of this method are that it has no systemic side effects and gives significant protection against pelvic infection and cervical dysplasia as well as pregnancy
- The disadvantages are that it must be inserted near the time of coitus and that pressure from the rim predisposes some women to cystitis after intercourse
- The cervical cap (with contraceptive jelly) is similar to the diaphragm but fits snugly over the cervix only (the diaphragm stretches from behind the cervix to behind the pubic symphysis)
- The cervical cap is more difficult to insert and remove than the diaphragm
- The main advantages are that it can be used by women who cannot be fitted for a diaphragm because of a relaxed anterior vaginal wall or by women who have discomfort or develop repeated bladder infections with the diaphragm
- Because of the small risk of toxic shock syndrome, a cervical cap or diaphragm should not be left in the vagina for over 12–18 h, nor should these devices be used during the menstrual period (see above)

Contraceptive foam, cream, film, sponge, jelly, & suppository

- These products are available without prescription, are easy to use, and are fairly effective, with reported failure rates of 2–30%. All contain the spermicide nonoxynol-9, which also has some virucidal and bactericidal activity. Nonoxynol-9 does not appear to adversely affect the vaginal colonization of hydrogen peroxide–producing lactobacilli. Recent unpublished data suggest that nonoxynol-9 may not be protective against HIV infection, particularly in women who have frequent intercourse. The products have the advantages of being simple to use and easily available. Their disadvantage is a slightly higher failure rate than the diaphragm or condom

Condom

- The male sheath of latex or animal membrane affords good protection against pregnancy—equivalent to that of a diaphragm and spermicidal jelly; latex (but not animal membrane) condoms also offer protection against sexually transmitted disease and cervical dysplasia. Men and women seeking protection against HIV transmission are advised to use a latex condom along with spermicide during vaginal or rectal intercourse. When a spermicide such as vaginal foam is used with the condom, the failure rate approaches that of oral contraceptives. Condoms coated with spermicide are available in the United States. The disadvantages of condoms are dulling of sensation and spillage of semen due to tearing, slipping, or leakage with detumescence of the penis
- The polyurethane female condom has failure rates from 5% to 21%; the efficacy is comparable to that of the diaphragm. This is the only female-controlled method that offers significant protection from both pregnancy and sexually transmitted diseases

Contraception, IUD & Barrier Methods

TREATMENT

THERAPEUTIC PROCEDURES

IUDS

- IUD insertion can be performed during or after the menses, at midcycle to prevent implantation, or later in the cycle if the patient is not pregnant
- Wait for 6–8 weeks postpartum before inserting an IUD
- When insertion is performed during lactation, there is greater risk of uterine perforation or embedding of the IUD
- Insertion immediately following abortion is acceptable if there is no sepsis and if follow-up insertion a month later will not be possible; otherwise, it is wise to wait until 4 weeks postabortion
- IUDs can be tried in these cases, as they often cause decreased bleeding and cramping with menses. Nonsteroidal antiinflammatory drugs are also helpful in decreasing bleeding and pain

OUTCOME

COMPLICATIONS

Pelvic infection

- There is an increased risk of pelvic infection during the first month following insertion. The subsequent risk of pelvic infection appears to be primarily related to the risk of acquiring STDs. Infertility rates do not appear to be increased among women who have previously used the currently available IUDs. At the time of insertion, women with an increased risk of STDs should be screened for gonorrhea and chlamydiosis. Women with a history of recent or recurrent pelvic infection are not good candidates for IUD use

Menorrhagia or severe dysmenorrhea

- The copper IUD can cause heavier menstrual periods, bleeding between periods, and more cramping, so it is generally not suitable for women who already suffer from these problems. However, hormone-releasing IUDs can be tried in these cases, as they often cause decreased bleeding and cramping with menses. Nonsteroidal anti-inflammatory drugs are also helpful in decreasing bleeding and pain

Complete or partial expulsion

- Spontaneous expulsion of the IUD occurs in 10–20% of cases during the first year of use. Any IUD should be removed if the body of the device can be seen or felt in the cervical os

Missing IUD strings

- If the transcervical tail cannot be seen, this may signify unnoticed expulsion, perforation of the uterus with abdominal migration of the IUD, or simply retraction of the string into the cervical canal or uterus owing to movement of the IUD or uterine growth with pregnancy. Once pregnancy is ruled out, probe for the IUD with a sterile sound or forceps designed for IUD removal, after administering a paracervical block. If the IUD cannot be detected, pelvic ultrasound will demonstrate the IUD if it is in the uterus. Or obtain anteroposterior and lateral x-rays of the pelvis with another IUD or a sound in the uterus as a marker, to confirm an extrauterine IUD. If the IUD is in the abdominal cavity, it should be removed by laparoscopy or laparotomy. Open-looped all-plastic IUDs such as the Lippes Loop can be left in the pelvis without danger, but ring-shaped IUDs may strangulate a loop of bowel and copper-bearing IUDs may cause tissue reaction and adhesions

PROGNOSIS

- The IUD is highly effective, with failure rates similar to those achieved with surgical sterilization
- Women who are not in mutually monogamous relationships should use condoms for protection from STDs
- The Mirena is approved for 5 years use and the Tcu380A for 10 years

PREVENTION

- Perforations of the uterus are less likely if insertion is performed slowly, with care taken to follow directions applicable to each type of IUD

EVIDENCE

PRACTICE GUIDELINES

- National Guideline Clearinghouse
  http://www.guideline.gov/summary/
  summary.aspx?doc_id=3230&nbr=2456
  &string=barrier+methods

WEB SITES

- Gynecology Handbook for Family Practitioners
  http://www.vh.org/Providers/ClinRef/
  FPHandbook/13.html

INFORMATION FOR PATIENTS

- American College of Obstetricians and Gynecologists
  http://www.medem.com/MedLB/
  article_detaillb.cfm?article_ID=
  |ZZZ48OI527C&sub_cat=5
- Food and Drug Administration
  http://www.fda.gov/fdac/features/1997/
  babytabl.html

REFERENCES

- Grimes DA: Intrauterine device and upper-genital-tract infection. Lancet 2000;356:1013. [PMID: 11041414]
- Richardson BA et al: Use of nonoxynol-9 and changes in vaginal lactobacilli. J Infect Dis 1998;178:441. [PMID: 9697724]
- Rosen AD et al: Study of condom integrity after brief exposure to over-the-counter vaginal preparations. South Med J 1999;92:305. [PMID: 10094272]

H. Trent MacKay, MD, MPH

Contraception, Oral, Injections, & Implants

 KEY FEATURES

GENERAL CONSIDERATIONS

- Contraception should be available to all women and men of reproductive ages
- Education about contraception and access to contraceptive pills or devices are especially important for sexually active teenagers and for women following childbirth or abortion

 TREATMENT

MEDICATIONS

Oral contraceptives

- **Combined Oral Contraceptives**
- Oral contraceptives have a theoretical failure rate of less than 0.5% if taken absolutely on schedule and a typical failure rate of 3%
- The primary mode of action is suppression of ovulation
- The pills are initially started on the first or fifth day of the ovarian cycle and taken daily for 21 days, followed by 7 days of placebos or no medication, and this schedule is then continued for each cycle. If a pill is missed at any time, two pills should be taken the next day, and another method of contraception should be used for the rest of the cycle (eg, condoms or foam)
- A backup method should also be used during the first cycle if the pills are started later than the fifth day
- Low-dose oral contraceptives are no longer contraindicated in women aged 35–50 who are nonsmokers and have no risk factors for cardiovascular disease
- **Benefits of Oral Contraceptives**
- There are many noncontraceptive advantages to oral contraceptives. Menstrual flow is lighter, resultant anemia is less common, and dysmenorrhea is relieved for most women
- Functional ovarian cysts generally disappear with oral contraceptive use, and new cysts do not occur
- Pain with ovulation and postovulatory aching are relieved
- The risk of ovarian and endometrial cancer is decreased, and the risks of salpingitis and ectopic pregnancy may be diminished
- Acne is usually improved
- The frequency of developing myomas is lower in long-term users (>4 years). There is a beneficial effect on bone mass
- **Selection of an Oral Contraceptive**
- Any of the combination oral contraceptives containing less than 50 μg of estrogen are suitable for most women
- There is some variation in potency of the various progestins in the pills, but there are essentially no clinically significant differences for most women among the progestins in the low-dose pills
- Women who have acne or hirsutism may benefit from use of one of the pills containing the third-generation progestins, desogestrel or norgestimate, as they are the least androgenic
- The low-dose oral contraceptives commonly used in the United States are listed in Table 65 (page 1260)
- **Drug Interactions**
- Drugs that interact with oral contraceptives to decrease their efficacy include phenytoin, phenobarbital (and other barbiturates), primidone, carbamazepine, and rifampin. Women taking these drugs should use another means of contraception for maximum safety
- **Contraindications and Adverse Effects**
- Oral contraceptives have been associated with many adverse effects (Table 66, page 1261)
- **Minor Side Effects**
- Nausea and dizziness may occur in the first few months of pill use
- A weight gain of 2–5 lb commonly occurs
- Spotting or breakthrough bleeding between menstrual periods may occur, especially if a pill is skipped or taken late; this may be helped by switching to a pill of slightly greater potency
- Missed menstrual periods may occur, especially with low-dose pills. A pregnancy test should be performed if pills have been skipped or if two or more menstrual periods are missed
- Depression, fatigue, and decreased libido can occur
- Chloasma may occur, as in pregnancy, and is increased by exposure to sunlight

Progestin minipill

- **Efficacy and Methods of Use**
- Formulations containing 0.35 mg of norethindrone or 0.075 mg of norgestrel are available in the United States
- Efficacy is slightly lower than that of combined oral contraceptives, with failure rates of 1–4% being reported
- The minipill is begun on the first day of a menstrual cycle and then taken continuously for as long as contraception is desired
- **Advantages**
- The low dose and absence of estrogen make the minipill safe during lactation; it may increase the flow of milk
- It is often tried by women who want minimal doses of hormones and by patients who are over age 35
- It can be used by women with uterine myomas or sickle cell disease (S/S or S/C)

- Like the combined pill, the minipill decreases the likelihood of pelvic inflammatory disease by its effect on cervical mucus

- **Complications and Contraindications**

- Minipill users often have bleeding irregularities (eg, prolonged flow, spotting, or amenorrhea); such patients may need monthly pregnancy tests

- Ectopic pregnancies are more frequent, and complaints of abdominal pain should be investigated with this in mind

- The contraindications listed in Table 66 (page 1261) apply to the minipill

- Minor side effects of combination oral contraceptives such as weight gain and mild headache may also occur with the minipill

Contraceptive injections and implants

- **Long-Acting Progestins**

- Progestin medroxyprogesterone acetate IM, 150 mg every 3 months

- It has a contraceptive efficacy of 99.7%

- Common side effects include irregular bleeding, amenorrhea, weight gain, and headache. Bone mineral loss may occur

- Users commonly have irregular bleeding initially and subsequently develop amenorrhea

- Ovulation may be delayed after the last injection

- Contraindications are similar to those for the minipill

- A monthly injectable containing both depot medroxyprogesterone acetate and an estrogen, estradiol cypionate (Lunelle), is highly effective, with a first-year pregnancy rate of 0.2% and a side effect profile similar to that of oral contraceptives

- The other long-acting progestin is the Norplant system, a contraceptive implant containing levonorgestrel, which is no longer marketed in the United States

Other hormonal methods

- A transdermal contraceptive patch containing 150 μg norelgestromin and 20 μg ethinyl estradiol and measuring 20 cm² is available. The patch is applied to the lower abdomen, upper torso, or buttock once a week for 3 consecutive weeks, followed by 1 week without the patch. The mechanism of action, side effects, and efficacy are similar to those associated with oral contraceptives, though compliance may be better

- A contraceptive vaginal ring that releases 120 μg of etonogestrel and 15 μg of

ethinyl estradiol daily is available. The ring is soft and flexible and is placed in the upper vagina for 3 weeks, removed, and replaced 1 week later. The efficacy, mechanism of action, and systemic side effects are similar to those associated with oral contraceptives. In addition, users may experience an increased incidence of vaginal discharge

OUTCOME

FOLLOW-UP

- Patients using hormonal contraception are usually seen annually for a review of pertinent history, breast and pelvic examination with Pap smear

COMPLICATIONS

- Serious complications of combined hormonal contraception include
  - Venous thromboembolism: 10–30/100,000 annually
  - Myocardial infarction: 40/100,000 annually in smokers over age 35
  - Hypertension: 1% incidence

EVIDENCE

PRACTICE GUIDELINES

- FFPRHC Guidance: emergency contraception (April 2003). J Fam Plan Reprod Health Care. 2003;29:9.

- Mishell Dr Jr et al: Practice guidelines for OC selection. Dialogues Contracept 1996;4:1.

WEB SITE

- Gynecology Handbook for Family Practitioners http://www.vh.org/Providers/ClinRef/FPHandbook/13.html

INFORMATION FOR PATIENTS

- American College of Obstetricians and Gynecologists http://www.medem.com/MedLB/article_detaillb.cfm?article_ID=ZZZ48OI527C&sub_cat=5

- The Nemours Foundation http://kidshealth.org/teen/sexual_health/contraception/contraception_birth.html

- National Women's Health Information http://www.4woman.gov/faq/econtracep.htm

REFERENCES

- Beral V et al: Mortality associated with oral contraceptive use: 25 year follow up of cohort of 46,000 women from Royal College of General Practitioners' oral contraceptive study. BMJ 1999;318:96. [PMID: 9880284]

- Grabrick DM et al: Risk of breast cancer with oral contraceptive use in women with a family history of breast cancer. JAMA 2000;284:1791. [PMID: 11025831]

- Kaunitz AM: Injectable long-acting contraceptives. Clin Obstet Gynecol 2001;44:73. [PMID: 11219248]

H. Trent MacKay, MD, MPH

Cough

KEY FEATURES

ESSENTIALS OF DIAGNOSIS

- Duration of cough
- Dyspnea (at rest or with exertion)
- Constitutional symptoms
- Tobacco use history
- Vital signs (temperature, respiratory rate, heart rate)
- Chest examination

GENERAL CONSIDERATIONS

- Cough results from stimulation of mechanical or chemical afferent nerve receptors in the bronchial tree
- Cough illness syndromes are defined as acute (<3 weeks) or persistent (>3 weeks)
- In about 25% of cases, persistent cough has multiple contributors

CLINICAL FINDINGS

SYMPTOMS AND SIGNS

- The timing and character of cough usually not useful in establishing cause
- Acute cough syndromes: most due to viral respiratory tract infections; less common causes include congestive heart failure (CHF), hay fever (allergic rhinitis), and environmental factors
- Search for additional features of infection such as fever, nasal congestion, and sore throat
- Dyspnea (at rest or with exertion) may reflect a more serious condition
- Persistent cough: usually due to angiotensin-converting enzyme (ACE) inhibitor therapy, postnasal drip, asthma, or gastroesophageal reflux disease (GERD); less common causes include bronchogenic carcinoma, chronic bronchitis, bronchiectasis, other chronic lung disease, and CHF
- Signs of pneumonia: tachycardia, tachypnea, fever, rales, decreased breath sounds, fremitus, egophony
- Signs of acute bronchitis: wheezing and rhonchi
- Signs of chronic sinusitis: postnasal drip
- Signs of chronic obstructive pulmonary disease (COPD): abnormal match test (inability to blow out a match from 10 inches away) and maximum laryngeal height <4 cm (measured from the sternal notch to the cricoid cartilage at end expiration)
- Signs of CHF: abnormal jugular venous pressure and positive hepatojugular reflux

DIFFERENTIAL DIAGNOSIS

Acute cough

- Viral upper respiratory infection or postviral cough (most common)
- Postnasal drip (allergic rhinitis)
- Pneumonia
- Pulmonary edema
- Pulmonary embolism
- Aspiration pneumonia

Persistent cough

- Top three causes: postnasal drip, asthma, GERD
- *Pulmonary infection:* postviral, chronic bronchitis especially in smokers, bronchiectasis, tuberculosis, cystic fibrosis, *Mycobacterium avium* complex, pertussis, *Mycoplasma, Chlamydia,*

respiratory syncytial virus (underrecognized in adults)
- *Pulmonary noninfectious:* asthma (cough-variant asthma), β-blockers causing asthma, COPD, ACE inhibitors, irritant inhalation, eg, smoking, endobronchial lesion, eg, tumor, interstitial lung disease, sarcoidosis, chronic microaspiration
- *Nonpulmonary:* GERD, postnasal drip (allergic rhinitis), sinusitis, CHF, laryngitis, ear canal or tympanic membrane irritation, psychogenic or habit cough

DIAGNOSIS

LABORATORY TESTS

- Pulse oximetry or arterial blood gas measurement to assess hypoxemia
- Peak expiratory flow rate or spirometry to assess airflow obstruction

IMAGING STUDIES

- Chest radiography to evaluate for parenchymal disease
- Acute cough: obtain chest radiograph if abnormal vital signs or chest examination; higher index of suspicion in elderly and/or immunocompromised
- Persistent cough: obtain chest radiograph if unexplained cough lasts more than 3–6 weeks

DIAGNOSTIC PROCEDURES

- Reserve procedures for patients who do not respond to therapuetic trials
- Sinus CT scan for cough with postnasal drip
- Spirometry (if normal, possible methacholine challenge) for cough with wheezing or possible asthma, though pulmonary function tests are often normal in cough variant asthma
- Esophageal pH monitoring for cough with GERD symptoms

Cough

TREATMENT

MEDICATIONS

- If symptoms of postnasal drip, asthma, or GERD, begin with treatment for that condition, otherwise, undertake empiric trials with a maximum strength regimen for one condition for 2–4 weeks, followed by the next if no response
- For postnasal drip: decongestants, nasal steroids, with or without antibiotics
- For asthma: inhaled albuterol
- For GERD: proton pump inhibitors

OUTCOME

WHEN TO REFER

- Refer patients with cough due to chronic sinusitis unresponsive to medications to ENT surgeon
- Refer patients with cough due to GERD unresponsive to medications to gastroenterologist or surgeon

WHEN TO ADMIT

- Pneumonia
- Bronchiectasis exacerbation
- COPD exacerbation

EVIDENCE

PRACTICE GUIDELINES

- Irwin RS et al: Managing cough as a defense mechanism and symptom. A consensus panel report of the American College of Chest Physicians. Chest 1998;114(2 Suppl):133S. [PMID: 9725800]
- Institute for Clinical Systems Improvement (ICSI): Chronic obstructive pulmonary disease, 2001. http://www.icsi.org/knowledge/detail.asp?catID=29&itemID=157
- Institute for Clinical Systems Improvement (ICSI): Viral upper respiratory infection (VURI) in adults and children, 2002 http://www.icsi.org/knowledge/detail.asp?catID=29&itemID=203

WEB SITES

- American Academy of Family Physicians http://www.familydoctor.org/
- National Heart, Lung, and Blood Institute http://www.nhlbi.nih.gov/

INFORMATION FOR PATIENTS

- JAMA patient page: Asthma. JAMA 1999;281:2160. [PMID: 10367828]
- American Academy of Family Physicians: Chronic cough http://familydoctor.org/handouts/237.html
- MEDLINEplus http://www.nlm.nih.gov/medlineplus/ency/article/003072.htm

REFERENCES

- Gonzales R et al: Principles of appropriate antibiotic use for treatment of acute respiratory tract infections in adults: background, specific aims, and methods. Ann Intern Med 2001;134:479. [PMID: 11255524]
- Metlay JP, Fine JM: Testing strategies in the initial management of patients with community-acquired pneumonia. Ann Intern Med 2003;138:109. [PMID: 12529093]

Ralph Gonzales, MD

Crohn's Disease

 KEY FEATURES

ESSENTIALS OF DIAGNOSIS

- Insidious onset
- Intermittent bouts of low-grade fever, diarrhea, and right lower quadrant pain
- Right lower quadrant mass and tenderness
- Perianal disease with abscess, fistulas
- Radiographic evidence of ulceration, stricturing, or fistulas of the small intestine or colon

GENERAL CONSIDERATIONS

- Crohn's disease is a transmural process
- Crohn's may involve the small bowel only, most commonly the terminal ileum (ileitis) in ~33% of cases, the small bowel and colon, most often the terminal ileum and adjacent proximal ascending colon (ileocolitis) in ~50%; or the colon alone in 20%
- Chronic illness with exacerbations and remissions
- Treatment is directed both toward symptomatic improvement and controlling the disease process

DEMOGRAPHICS

- Increased in Europeans, North Americans, and Ashkenazi Jews
- Increased risk among first-degree relatives
- Increased risk in smokers

 CLINICAL FINDINGS

SYMPTOMS AND SIGNS

- Fevers
- Abdominal pain
- Liquid bowel movements
- Abdominal tenderness or abdominal mass

Chronic inflammatory disease

- Malaise, loss of energy
- Diarrhea, nonbloody, intermittent
- Cramping or steady right lower quadrant or periumbilical pain
- Focal tenderness, right lower quadrant
- Palpable, tender mass in the lower abdomen

Intestinal obstruction

- Postprandial bloating, cramping pains, and loud borborygmi

Fistulization with or without infection

- Sinus tracts and fistulas can result in intraabdominal or retroperitoneal abscesses manifested by fevers, chills, a tender abdominal mass
- Bacterial overgrowth with diarrhea, weight loss, and malnutrition
- Bladder or vagina recurrent infections
- Cutaneous fistulas
- Perianal disease: anal fissures, perianal abscesses, and fistulas

Extraintestinal manifestations

- Oral aphthous lesions
- Gallstones
- Nephrolithiasis with stones

DIFFERENTIAL DIAGNOSIS

- Ulcerative colitis
- Irritable bowel syndrome
- Appendicitis
- *Yersinia enterocolitica* enteritis
- Mesenteric adenitis
- Intestinal lymphoma
- Segmental colitis due to ischemic colitis, tuberculosis, amebiasis, chlamydia
- Diverticulitis with abscess
- Nonsteroidal antiinflammatory drug–induced colitis
- Perianal fistula due to other cause

 DIAGNOSIS

LABORATORY TESTS

- Obtain complete blood cell count, erythrocyte sedimentation rate or C-reactive protein, serum albumin
- Anemia of chronic inflammation, blood loss, iron deficiency, or vitamin B_{12} malabsorption
- Leukocytosis with abscesses
- Sedimentation rate or C-reactive protein elevated
- Stool for routine pathogens, ova and parasites, and *Clostridium difficile* toxin
- Antibodies to the yeast *Saccharomyces cerevisiae* (ASCA) are found in 60–70%

IMAGING STUDIES

- Upper gastrointestinal series with small bowel follow-through
- Barium enema

DIAGNOSTIC PROCEDURES

- Colonoscopy
- Biopsy of intestine reveals granulomas in 25%

Crohn's Disease

TREATMENT

MEDICATIONS

Treatment of diarrhea

- Cholestyramine (2–4 g) or colestipol (5 g) PO BID–TID before meals in terminal ileal Crohn's
- Broad-spectrum antibiotics if bacterial overgrowth
- Antidiarrheal agents: loperamide (2–4 mg), diphenoxylate with atropine (one tablet), or tincture of opium (5–15 drops) QID PRN; not used in patients with active severe colitis

Treatment of exacerbations

- 5-Aminosalicylic acid agents: sulfasalazine, 1.5–2 g PO BID; mesalamine (Asacol), 0.8–1.2 g PO QID, or its slow-release form (Pentasa), 1 g PO QID, for mild to moderate small bowel and ileocecal disease
- Antibiotics: metronidazole, 10 mg/kg/day for ileocolitis, colitis, or perianal disease, ciprofloxacin, 500 mg PO BID for ileitis or perianal disease
- Broad-spectrum antibiotics, and if malnourished TPN, for abscess
- Corticosteroids: prednisone, 40–60 mg/day for 2–3 weeks, tapering by 5 mg/week until dosage is 20 mg/day, then by 2.5 mg/week or every other week
- Ileal-release preparation of topically active compound budesonide, 9 mg PO QD for 8 weeks for terminal ileal disease
- Immunomodulatory drugs
  - Azathioprine (2–2.5 mg/kg) and mercaptopurine (1–1.5 mg/kg) useful for fistulas and in long-term treatment
  - Methotrexate (25 mg IM weekly for 12 weeks, followed by 12.5–15 mg IM once weekly) for patients who fail to respond to azathioprine
  - Infliximab, 5 mg/kg single dose, may repeat every 8 weeks, is useful in moderate to severe Crohn's disease; infliximab, 5 mg/kg given at 0, 2, and 6 weeks results in closure of fistulas in ~50% and improvement in ~75%

Maintenance of remission

- Mesalamine (Asacol), 800 mg PO TID or Pentasa, 500–750 mg PO QID
- Corticosteroids should not be used
- Azathioprine, mercaptopurine, and methotrexate help maintain remission
- Chronic infliximab (every 8 weeks) appropriate for some patients with moderate to severe disease

SURGERY

- At least one surgical procedure required by >50% of patients
- Indications for surgery are intractability to medical therapy, intraabdominal abscess, massive bleeding, and obstruction with fibrous stricture
- Incision and drainage for abscess
- Surgical resection of the stenotic area or stricturoplasty in small bowel obstruction
- Surgical fistulotomy; avoid in active Crohn's disease

THERAPEUTIC PROCEDURES

- Percutaneous drainage for abscess
- Nasogastric suction and intravenous fluids for small bowel obstruction
- Well-balanced diet
- Avoid lactose-containing foods since lactose intolerance is common
- Fiber supplementation for patients with colonic involvement
- Low-roughage diet for patients with obstructive symptoms
- Low-fat diet for patients with fat malabsorption
- Iron supplement if documented deficiency
- Vitamin B_{12} 100 µg IM every month if prior terminal ileal resection
- Total parenteral nutrition (TPN) used short term in patients with active disease and progressive weight loss or in malnourished patients awaiting surgery
- TPN used long term in subset of patients with extensive intestinal resections resulting in short bowel syndrome with malnutrition

OUTCOME

COMPLICATIONS

- Abscess
- Small bowel obstruction
- Fistulas
- Perianal disease
- Hemorrhage (unusual)
- Malabsorption

PROGNOSIS

- With proper medical and surgical treatment, the majority of patients are able to cope with this chronic disease and its complications
- Few patients die of Crohn's disease

WHEN TO ADMIT

- Hospitalize patients with persisting symptoms despite oral steroids or those with high fever, persistent vomiting, evidence of intestinal obstruction, severe weight loss, severe abdominal tenderness, or suspicion of an abscess

PREVENTION

- Colonoscopy screening to detect dysplasia or cancer recommended for patients with a history of 8 or more years of Crohn's colitis

EVIDENCE

PRACTICE GUIDELINES

- ACR Appropriateness criteria for imaging recommendations for patients with Crohn's disease. American College of Radiology, 2001 http://www.acr.org/cgi-bin/fr?tmpl: appcrit,pdf:0181-192_crohns_disease_ac.pdf
- Management of Crohn's disease in adults. American College of Gastroenterology, 2001 http://www-east.elsevier.com/ajg/issues/9603/ajg3671fla.htm

WEB SITES

- Crohn's & Colitis Foundation of America http://www.ccfa.org/medinfo/medinfo/aboutcd.html
- NIH—Crohn's disease http://www.nih.gov/news/WordonHealth/dec2001/story02.htm

INFORMATION FOR PATIENTS

- Cleveland Clinic—Crohn's disease http://www.clevelandclinic.org/health/health-info/docs/2300/2371.asp?index=9357
- NIH—Patient Education Institute—Crohn's http://www.nlm.nih.gov/medlineplus/tutorials/crohnsdiseas.html

REFERENCES

- Regueiro M: Update in medical treatment of Crohn's disease. J Clin Gastroenterol 2000;31:282. [PMID: 11129268]
- Ricart E et al: Infliximab in Crohn's disease in clinical practice at the Mayo Clinic: the first 100 patients. Am J Gastroenterol 2001;96:722. [PMID: 11280541]

Kenneth R. McQuaid, MD

Cryptococcosis

 KEY FEATURES

ESSENTIALS OF DIAGNOSIS

- Infection caused by *Cryptococcus neoformans*, an encapsulated budding yeast found worldwide in soil and on dried pigeon dung
- Most common cause of fungal meningitis

GENERAL CONSIDERATIONS

- Infection acquired by inhalation. In the lung, infection may remain localized, heal, or disseminate
- Predisposing factors: Hodgkin's disease, corticosteroid therapy, HIV infection

DEMOGRAPHICS

- Symptomatic cryptococcal pneumonia rarely develops in immunocompetent hosts
- Progressive lung disease and dissemination usually occur in immunocompromised patients, eg, those with HIV infection, corticosteroid therapy, Hodgkin's disease, or hematological malignancy

 CLINICAL FINDINGS

SYMPTOMS AND SIGNS

- Disseminated cryptococcosis most commonly manifests as meningitis, which usually begins with headache, then confusion; cranial nerve abnormalities, nausea, and vomiting may occur
- Nuchal rigidity and meningeal signs in about 50%, but uncommon in HIV-infected patients
- Intracerebral mass lesions (cryptococcomas) are rare
- Obstructive hydrocephalus may occur
- In AIDS, extrameningeal disease (lungs, blood, urinary tract) is common

DIFFERENTIAL DIAGNOSIS

- Histoplasmosis
- Coccidioidomycosis
- Tuberculous meningitis
- Neurosyphilis
- *Acanthamoeba* (amebic encephalitis)
- Toxoplasmosis
- Lyme meningitis

 DIAGNOSIS

LABORATORY TESTS

- In HIV-infected patients with cryptococcosis, serum cryptococcal antigen positive in 95%
- In patients with cryptococcal meningitis, cerebrospinal fluid (CSF) shows increased opening pressure, variable pleocytosis, increased protein, decreased glucose, and budding encapsulated fungus cells
- Up to 50% of AIDS patients have no CSF pleocytosis
- CSF positive for cryptococcal capsular antigen in >90%
- CSF positive culture in >90%

TREATMENT

MEDICATIONS

Acute therapy

- Mild AIDS-related cryptococcal meningitis: fluconazole, 400 mg PO QD, for minimum of 10 weeks for patients with intact level of consciousness and CSF cryptococcal antigen titer <1:128. Fluconazole plus flucytosine may also be efficacious
- Higher-risk patients: amphotericin B, 0.7–1 mg/kg/day IV for 14 days, followed by 8 weeks of fluconazole, 400 mg PO QD, achieves clinical response and CSF sterilization in about 70%. The switch from amphotericin B to fluconazole should be guided by clinical improvement and conversion of CSF culture to negative
- Early addition of flucytosine, 100 mg/kg/day PO divided QID, prevents late relapses but does not substantially improve cure rates
- For non–AIDS-related cryptococcal meningitis, similar treatment, though mortality is higher. Because of underlying illnesses and older age, this group does not tolerate higher doses of amphotericin B. Lipid formulations of amphotericin B have equivalent efficacy with reduced nephrotoxicity. Therapy is continued until CSF culture is negative and CSF antigen titers are <1:8

Maintenance therapy

- AIDS-related cryptococcal meningitis: fluconazole, 200 mg PO QD chronically, is needed after acute therapy, otherwise >50% relapse rate
- Non–AIDS-related cryptococcal meningitis: fluconazole, 200 mg PO QD for 3 months, is recommended by some experts

THERAPEUTIC PROCEDURES

- Repeated lumbar punctures or ventricular shunting is done to relieve high CSF pressures or hydrocephalus

OUTCOME

COMPLICATIONS

- Obstructive hydrocephalus

PROGNOSIS

- Poor prognosis indicated by activity of predisposing conditions, older age, organ failure, lack of CSF pleocytosis, high initial antigen titer in serum or CSF, decreased mental status, and disease outside CNS
- Fluconazole maintenance therapy after HIV-related meningitis decreases relapse rate 10-fold compared with placebo and 3-fold compared with weekly amphotericin B in patients whose CSF has been sterilized by induction therapy

EVIDENCE

PRACTICE GUIDELINES

- Practice Guidelines from the Infectious Diseases Society of America http://www.journals.uchicago.edu/CID/journal/issues/v30n4/991230/991230.web.pdf 2001
- USPHS/IDSA guidelines for the prevention of opportunistic infections in persons infected with human immunodeficiency virus. U.S. Department of Health and Human Services, Public Health Service http://aidsinfo.nih.gov/guidelines/op_infections\OI_112801. pdf

WEB SITE

- CDC http://www.cdc.gov/ncidod/dbmd/diseaseinfo/cryptococcosis_t.htm

INFORMATION FOR PATIENTS

- CDC—Cryptococcosis http://www.cdc.gov/ncidod/dbmd/diseaseinfo/cryptococcosis_t.htm
- JAMA patient page: HIV infection: the basics. JAMA 2002;288:268. [PMID: 12123237]
- MEDLINEplus—cryptococcosis http://www.nlm.nih.gov/medlineplus/ency/article/001328.htm

REFERENCES

- Kirk O et al: Safe interruption of maintenance therapy against previous infection with four common HIV-associated opportunistic pathogens during potent antiretroviral therapy. Ann Intern Med 2002;137:239. [PMID: 12186514]
- Pappas PG et al: Cryptococcosis in human immunodeficiency virus-negative patients in the era of effective azole therapy. Clin Infect Dis 2001;33:690. [PMID: 11477526]
- Saag MS et al: Practice guidelines for the management of cryptococcal disease. Clin Infect Dis 2000;30:710. [PMID: 10770733]

Richard J. Hamill, MD

Cryptosporidiosis

 ## KEY FEATURES

ESSENTIALS OF DIAGNOSIS

In immunocompetent patients

- Diarrhea, mild to severe with flatulence and bloating. Mucus but no blood
- Low-grade fever, malaise, weight loss
- Generally self-limited in days to weeks

In immunocompromised patients

- Severe watery diarrhea
- Malabsorption, weight loss
- Blood and leukocytes seldom present

GENERAL CONSIDERATIONS

- Coccidiosis is an intracellular infection of intestinal epithelial cells by spore-forming protozoa
- The causes of coccidiosis are *Cryptosporidium parvum, Isospora belli, Cyclospora cayetanensis, Sarcocystis bovihominis,* and *S suihominis*; all but the *Sarcocystis* species complete their life cycle in a single host
- Cryptosporidiosis is a zoonosis in which infections in farm animals (cattle, goats, turkeys, and others) can be transmitted to humans; however, most human infections are acquired from humans
- The organism is highly infectious (few parasites can induce infection) and readily transmitted in health and day care settings and in households
- The incubation period is about 5–21 days
- Humans may be infected by species of *Cryptosporidium* other than *parvum*

DEMOGRAPHICS

- These infections occur worldwide, particularly in the tropics and in regions where hygiene is poor
- Clustering occurs in households, day care centers, and among sexual partners
- The prevalence of asymptomatic human carriers in the United States is estimated to be about 1.5%
- Outbreaks are of particular concern, as exemplified by the 1993 epidemic in Milwaukee in which 400,000 persons became ill

 ## CLINICAL FINDINGS

SYMPTOMS AND SIGNS

In immunocompetent patients

- Infection varies from no symptoms, to a mild diarrhea with flatulence and bloating, to severe and frequent watery diarrhea in which the onset may be explosive
- Mucus may be present in stools, but no microscopic or gross blood
- May also have low-grade fever, malaise, anorexia, abdominal cramps, vomiting, and myalgia
- Symptoms are generally self-limited, lasting a few days to several weeks
- Weight loss can be marked

In immunodeficient patients

- The diarrhea can be profuse (up to 15 L daily has been reported), with cholera-like watery movements, accompanied by severe malabsorption, electrolyte imbalance, and marked weight loss
- Mucus is seen in the stools, but blood and leukocytes are seldom present
- The diarrhea may recur or persist
- Fever is uncommon
- In AIDS, infection may involve any part of the gastrointestinal tract, including the biliary tract (sclerosing cholangitis); respiratory tract infection, hepatitis, pancreatitis, lymphadenopathy, and hepatosplenomegaly may occur, as well as multisystem involvement

DIFFERENTIAL DIAGNOSIS

- *Isospora belli, Cyclospora cayetanensis*, and *Sarcocystis bovihominis*
- Giardiasis
- Viral gastroenteritis, eg, rotavirus
- Other traveler's diarrhea, eg, *Escherichia coli*
- Cholera
- Other cause of diarrhea in AIDS, eg, cytomegalovirus colitis

 ## DIAGNOSIS

LABORATORY TESTS

- Three stool specimens should be obtained fresh and in preservative over 5–7 days
- Diagnosis is by detecting the organism by the modified acid-fast staining method; a minimum of two concentrated specimens should be tested
- Commercially available antigen detection kits improve on the diagnosis: direct fluorescent antibody methods have sensitivities and specificities of 99–100%; enzyme immunoassays have sensitivities and specificities of 93–100%. Some of the kits can be used with both fresh and frozen specimens; others, however, can be used only if the specimen is fresh
- The polymerase chain reaction offers an alternative mode of diagnosis
- Tests for serum antibody are useful epidemiologically but not for patient diagnosis
- Stools rarely show white or red blood cells
- Blood leukocytosis and eosinophilia are uncommon

IMAGING STUDIES

- Radiological changes have been reported in the stomach, intestines, and bile ducts in severe disease

DIAGNOSTIC PROCEDURES

- The organisms can also be detected by duodenal aspiration or biopsy
- In AIDS patients with unexplained diarrhea, the organism should also be looked for in sputum and bronchoalveolar lavage fluid; specimens obtained from lung tissue have sometimes been positive in patients with negative stool specimens

TREATMENT

MEDICATIONS

- No treatment has been successful. The following have been attempted
  - Roxithromycin (300 mg twice daily for 4 weeks)
  - Spiramycin (1 g three times daily for 2 weeks or longer)
  - Paromomycin (25–35 mg/kg/day in three or four divided doses; duration uncertain)
  - Zidovudine (AZT), azithromycin (600 mg daily), octreotide, eflornithine, letrazuril, nitazoxanide, and hyperimmune bovine colostrum

THERAPEUTIC PROCEDURES

- Most acute infections in immunocompetent persons are self-limited and do not require treatment
- Supportive treatment for severe or chronic diarrhea includes fluid and electrolyte replacement and, in chronic cases, parenteral nutrition

OUTCOME

FOLLOW-UP

- Symptoms are generally self-limited in **immunocompetent patients**
- Parasitological clearance, however, may take several months
- The diarrhea may recur or persist in **immunodeficient patients,** and passage of organisms continues for months to indefinitely
- Oocysts passed in stools are fully sporulated and infectious; therefore, hospitalized patients should be isolated and stool precautions strictly observed

WHEN TO REFER

- Persistent diarrhea, particularly in the immunocompromised patient
- Malabsoption, progressive weight loss

WHEN TO ADMIT

- Profuse diarrhea causing hypotension or electrolyte imbalance

PREVENTION

- Measures to reduce exposure to the organisms are recommended for immunodeficient patients. These include reduced exposure to swimming in fresh water
- Since chlorine disinfection of water is not effective, adequate filtration is required. However, because of the oocysts' small size (2–5 μm), filtration is difficult and unreliable (the <1-μm filters used frequently become obstructed)

EVIDENCE

PRACTICE GUIDELINES

- National Guideline Clearinghouse
  http://www.guideline.gov/summary/
  summary.aspx?doc_id=3080&nbr=2306
  &string=cryptosporidiosis
  http://www.guideline.gov/summary/
  summary.aspx?doc_id=2573&nbr=
  1799&string=cryptosporidiosis

INFORMATION FOR PATIENTS

- Centers for Disease Control
  http://www.cdc.gov/ncidod/dpd/
  parasites/cryptosporidiosis/factsht_
  cryptosporidiosis.htm
  http://www.cdc.gov/ncidod/dpd/
  parasites/cryptosporidiosis/factsht_
  crypto_prevent_water.htm

REFERENCES

- Chappell CL et al: Cryptosporidiosis. Curr Opin Infect Dis 2002;15:523. [PMID: 12686887]
- Chen XM et al: Cryptosporidiosis. N Engl J Med 2002;346:1723. [PMID: 12037153]

Cushing's Syndrome (Hypercortisolism)

 KEY FEATURES

ESSENTIALS OF DIAGNOSIS

- Central obesity, muscle wasting, thin skin, easy bruisability, psychological changes, hirsutism, purple striae
- Osteoporosis, hypertension, poor wound healing
- Hyperglycemia, glycosuria, leukocytosis, lymphocytopenia, hypokalemia
- Elevated serum cortisol and urinary free cortisol. Lack of normal suppression by dexamethasone

GENERAL CONSIDERATIONS

- Cushing's "syndrome" refers to manifestations of excessive corticosteroids
- Commonly due to supraphysiological doses of glucocorticoid drugs; rarely due to excessive corticosteroid production
- Excessive corticosteroid production is often due to Cushing's "disease" (~43% of cases), ie, hypercortisolism due to ACTH hypersecretion by the pituitary. Usually caused by benign pituitary adenoma
- ~10% due to nonpituitary neoplasms (eg, small-cell lung carcinoma) that produce excessive ectopic ACTH
- ~15% due to ACTH from a source that cannot be initially located
- ~32% due to excessive autonomous secretion of cortisol by the adrenals independent of ACTH (serum ACTH usually low). Usually due to unilateral adrenal tumor of three types. Benign adrenal adenomas are generally small tumors that produce mostly cortisol. Adrenal carcinomas usually large and can produce excessive androgens as well as cortisol. ACTH-independent bilateral adrenal hyperplasia can also produce hypercortisolism

DEMOGRAPHICS

- Spontaneous Cushing's syndrome is rare: 2.6 new cases yearly per million population
- ACTH-secreting pituitary adenoma (Cushing's "disease") >3 times more frequent in women than men

 CLINICAL FINDINGS

SYMPTOMS AND SIGNS

- Central obesity with plethoric "moon face," "buffalo hump," supraclavicular fat pads, protuberant abdomen, and thin extremities
- Oligomenorrhea or amenorrhea (or impotence in males)
- Weakness, backache, headache
- Hypertension
- Osteoporosis or avascular bone necrosis
- Acne, superficial skin infections, purple striae (especially around the thighs, breasts, and abdomen), easy bruising, and impaired wound healing
- Thirst and polyuria (with or without glycosuria); renal calculi
- Glaucoma
- Mental symptoms range from diminished concentration to increased mood lability to psychosis
- Increased susceptibility to opportunistic infections
- Hirsutism and virilization may occur with adrenal carcinomas

DIFFERENTIAL DIAGNOSIS

- Chronic alcoholism (alcoholic pseudo-Cushing's syndrome)
- Diabetes mellitus
- Depression (may have hypercortisolism)
- Osteoporosis due to other cause
- Obesity due to other cause
- Primary hyperaldosteronism
- Anorexia nervosa (high urine free cortisol)
- Striae distensae ("stress marks") seen in adolescence and in pregnancy
- Lipodystrophy from antiretroviral agents

 DIAGNOSIS

LABORATORY TESTS

- Glucose tolerance impaired due to insulin resistance
- Polyuria and glycosuria
- Leukocytosis with relative granulocytosis and lymphopenia
- Hypokalemia (but not hypernatremia) may be present, particularly with ectopic ACTH secretion
- Dexamethasone suppression test is the easiest screening test for hypercortisolism. Give dexamethasone, 1 mg PO, at 11 PM and measure serum cortisol at about 8 AM next morning. Plasma cortisol <5 µg/dL (fluorometric assay) or <2 µg/dL (HPLC assay) excludes Cushing's syndrome with 98% certainty
- If not excluded, measure 24-h urine for free cortisol and creatinine. High 24-h urine free cortisol (or free cortisol to creatinine ratio of >95 µg cortisol/g creatinine) helps confirm hypercortisolism. Misleadingly high urine free cortisol occurs with high fluid intake
- In uncertain cases, dexamethasone suppression test can be done by giving dexamethasone, 0.5 mg PO Q 6 h for 48 h, with 24-h urine collected on second day. Urine free cortisol >20 µg/day or urine 17-hydroxycorticosteroid >4.5 mg/day helps confirm hypercortisolism
- Midnight serum cortisol level >7.5 µg/dL is indicative of Cushing's syndrome and distinguishes it from other conditions associated with high urine free cortisol (pseudo-Cushing states, depression, anorexia nervosa). Must be NPO for 3 h and have IV established in advance for blood draw
- Drugs (eg, estrogens, phenytoin, phenobarbital, primidone) may cause false-positive dexamethasone suppression test
- If hypercortisolism is confirmed, plasma ACTH below normal indicates probable adrenal tumor; high or normal ACTH indicates pituitary or ectopic tumors

IMAGING STUDIES

- Pituitary MRI shows adenoma in ~50% of cases of ACTH-dependent Cushing's syndrome
- CT of chest and abdomen can help locate source of ectopic ACTH, in lungs (carcinoid or small-cell carcinomas), thymus, pancreas, or adrenals. Chest masses are frequently due to opportunistic infections, so biopsy is required prior to resection
- CT of adrenals can localize adrenal tumor in most cases of non–ACTH-dependent Cushing's syndrome

DIAGNOSTIC PROCEDURES

- If pituitary MRI normal or shows irregularity that may be incidental, selective inferior petrosal venous sampling for ACTH is performed (with corticotropin-releasing hormone stimulation) where available to confirm pituitary ACTH source, distinguishing it from an occult nonpituitary tumor secreting ACTH

TREATMENT

MEDICATIONS

- Hydrocortisone replacement required temporarily after resection of pituitary adenoma or adrenal adenoma (see above)
- Ketoconazole, 200 mg PO Q 6 h, for patients with Cushing's disease who are not surgical candidates; must monitor liver enzymes
- Mitotane for metastatic adrenal carcinomas; ketoconazole or metyrapone may suppress hypercortisolism in unresectable adrenal carcinoma; however, metyrapone may exacerbate female virilization
- Bisphosphonates for patients with osteoporosis

SURGERY

- Selective transsphenoidal resection of pituitary adenoma indicated in Cushing's disease, after which remainder of pituitary usually returns to normal function. However, corticotrophs require 6–36 months to recover normal function; thus, hydrocortisone replacement is required temporarily
- Bilateral laparoscopic adrenalectomy if no remission (or recurrence) after pituitary surgery
- Laparoscopic resection for adrenal neoplasms secreting cortisol. Because contralateral adrenal is suppressed, postoperative hydrocortisone replacement is required until recovery
- Surgical resection of ectopic ACTH-secreting tumors

THERAPEUTIC PROCEDURES

- Stereotactic pituitary radiosurgery (gamma knife) normalizes urine free cortisol in two-thirds of patients within 12 months
- Conventional radiation therapy cures 23%

OUTCOME

COMPLICATIONS

- If untreated, produces serious morbidity and even death
- Complications of hypertension or diabetes
- Increased susceptibility to infections
- Compression fractures of osteoporotic spine, aseptic necrosis of femoral head
- Nephrolithiasis
- Depression, dementia, psychosis
- Following bilateral adrenalectomy for Cushing's disease, progressive enlargement of pituitary adenoma may cause local effects (eg, visual field impairment) and hyperpigmentation (Nelson's syndrome)

PROGNOSIS

- Cushing's syndrome due to benign adrenal adenoma has 5-year survival of 95% and 10-year survival of 90% following successful adrenalectomy
- Patients with Cushing's disease from pituitary adenoma have similar survival if pituitary surgery is successful
- Transsphenoidal surgery fails in ~10–20%
- Despite complete remission after transsphenoidal surgery, ~15–20% recur over 10 years
- Bilateral laparoscopic adrenalectomy may be required, but is often complicated by infection; recurrence of hypercortisolism may occur due to growth of adrenal remnant stimulated by high ACTH levels
- Prognosis with ectopic ACTH-producing tumors dependent on aggressiveness and stage of tumor
- Patients with ACTH of unknown source have 5-year survival rate of 65% and 10-year survival rate of 55%
- Patients with adrenal carcinoma have median survival of 7 months

WHEN TO REFER

- If abnormal dexamethasone suppression test

WHEN TO ADMIT

- Transsphenoidal hypophysectomy

EVIDENCE

PRACTICE GUIDELINES

- Morris D et al: The medical management of Cushing's syndrome. Ann NY Acad Sci 2002;970:119. [PMID: 12381547]
- Nieman LK: Diagnostic tests for Cushing's syndrome. Ann NY Acad Sci 2002;970:112. [PMID: 12381546]

WEB SITE

- American Academy of Family Physicians—Cushing's syndrome and cushing's disease http://familydoctor.org/handouts/623.html

INFORMATION FOR PATIENTS

- NIDDK/NIH—Cushing's syndrome http://www.niddk.nih.gov/health/endo/pubs/cushings/cushings.htm

REFERENCES

- Boscaro M et al: The diagnosis of Cushing's syndrome: atypical presentations and laboratory shortcomings. Arch Intern Med 2001;161:1780. [PMID: 11074733]
- Kirk LF et al: Cushing's disease: clinical manifestations and diagnostic evaluation. Am Fam Physician 2000;62:1119:1133. [PMID: 10997535]
- Ng L et al: Adrenocortical carcinoma: diagnosis, evaluation and treatment. J Urol 2003;169:5. [PMID: 12478091]

Paul A. Fitzgerald, MD

Cyclosporiasis

 KEY FEATURES

ESSENTIALS OF DIAGNOSIS

In immunocompetent patients

- Mild to severe diarrhea. Mucus may be present in the stool but blood is absent
- Low-grade fever, vomiting, malaise

In immunodeficient patients

- Diarrhea may be profuse
- Occasionally, severe malabsorption and weight loss
- Blood and leukocytes are seldom present

GENERAL CONSIDERATIONS

- The causes of coccidiosis are *Cryptosporidium parvum*, *Isospora belli*, *Cyclospora cayetanensis*, *Sarcocystis bovihominis*, and *S suihominis*; all but the *Sarcocystis* species complete their life cycle in a single host. Diarrhea caused by any of these organisms is usually clinically similar
- The *Cyclospora* species in humans appear to be distinct to humans only
- The infectious agents are oocysts (spores) transmitted directly from person to person or by contaminated water or food
- *Cyclospora* require time outside the host to sporulate and become infectious
- Outbreaks in the United States have been attributed to imported fresh fruit and vegetables
- Is a cause of traveler's diarrhea; institutional and community outbreaks of diarrhea; and acute and chronic diarrhea in immunodeficient patients, including those with AIDS, in whom the infection can be life-threatening
- The pathogenesis of the diarrhea is not well understood. No enterotoxin has been identified

DEMOGRAPHICS

- Occurs worldwide, particularly in the tropics and in regions where hygiene is poor

 CLINICAL FINDINGS

SYMPTOMS AND SIGNS

- The diarrhea caused by the coccidial and microsporidial agents is clinically indistinguishable
- The incubation period is 2–11 days
- Rarely, the organisms invade the biliary tree. Voluminous secretory or malabsorption diarrhea (including vitamin B_{12}, D-xylose, and fat absorption dysfunction) can result

In immunocompetent patients

- Infection varies from no symptoms, to a mild diarrhea with flatulence and bloating, to severe and frequent watery diarrhea in which the onset may be explosive
- Mucus may be present in stools, but no microscopic or gross blood is found
- There may be low-grade fever, malaise, anorexia, abdominal cramps, vomiting, and myalgia. These symptoms are generally self-limited, lasting a few days to several weeks
- Weight loss can be marked

In immunodeficient patients

- The diarrhea can be profuse (up to 15 L daily has been reported), with cholera-like watery movements, accompanied by severe malabsorption, electrolyte imbalance, and marked weight loss
- Fever is uncommon
- Mucus is seen in the stools, but blood and leukocytes are seldom present
- The diarrhea may recur or persist

DIFFERENTIAL DIAGNOSIS

- *Cryptosporidium parvum*, *Isospora belli*, *Sarcocystis bovihominis*, and *S suihominis*
- Giardiasis
- Viral gastroenteritis, eg, rotavirus
- Other traveler's diarrhea, eg, *Escherichia coli*
- Cholera
- Other causes of diarrhea in AIDS, eg, cytomegalovirus colitis

 DIAGNOSIS

LABORATORY TESTS

- Three stool specimens collected over 5–7 days should be stored both as fresh specimens and in preservative and processed by flotation or concentration methods to detect the distinctive oocysts (8–10 μm)
- The laboratory should be notified that *Cyclospora* are being investigated because specific fecal examinations are needed
- Antibodies have been detected and titers increase during convalescence

Cyclosporiasis

 TREATMENT

MEDICATIONS

- Trimethoprim (TMP, 160 mg)-sulfamethoxazole (SMZ, 800 mg) twice daily for 7 days is effective; in HIV infections, higher doses (four times daily for 10 days) and long-term maintenance (three times weekly) are needed
- For patients intolerant of TMP-SMZ, ciprofloxacin can be tried

THERAPEUTIC PROCEDURES

- Most acute infections in immunocompetent persons are self-limited and do not require treatment
- Supportive treatment for severe or chronic diarrhea includes fluid and electrolyte replacement and, in chronic cases, parenteral nutrition

 OUTCOME

FOLLOW-UP

- Parasitological clearance may take several months even in immunocompetent patients
- Passage of organisms continues for months to indefinitely in immunoimpaired persons

WHEN TO REFER

- Refer to an infectious disease specialist or gastroenterologist if diarrhea persists despite antibiotic therapy, particularly in immunocompromised patients
- Refer for secretory or malabsorption diarrhea
- Refer for progressive weight loss

WHEN TO ADMIT

- Profuse diarrhea causing hypotension or electrolyte imbalance

PREVENTION

- Measures to reduce exposure to the organism is recommended for immunocompromised patients. These include reduced exposure to swimming in fresh water and boiling of drinking water (1 min) or use of a filter that removes particles over 1 μm in size

 EVIDENCE

PRACTICE GUIDELINES

- National Guideline Clearinghouse
  http://www.guideline.gov/summary/
  summary.aspx?doc_id=3080&nbr=2306
  &string=cryptosporidiosis
  http://www.guideline.gov/summary/
  summary.aspx?doc_id=2573&nbr=
  1799&string=cryptosporidiosis

INFORMATION FOR PATIENTS

- Centers for Disease Control
  http://www.cdc.gov/ncidod/dpd/
  parasites/cyclospora/factsht_cyclospora.
  htm
  http://www.cdc.gov/ncidod/dbmd/
  diseaseinfo/travelersdiarrhea_g.htm

REFERENCES

- Eberhand ML et al: *Cyclospora* spp. Curr Opin Infect Dis 2002;15:519. [PMID: 12686886]
- Herwaldt BL: *Cyclospora cayetanensis*: a review, focusing on the outbreaks of cyclosporiasis in the 1990s. Clin Infect Dis 2000;31:1040. [PMID: 11049789]

Cystic Fibrosis

 ## KEY FEATURES

ESSENTIALS OF DIAGNOSIS

- Chronic or recurrent cough, sputum production, dyspnea, and wheezing
- Recurrent infections or chronic colonization of the airways with *Haemophilus influenzae, Pseudomonas aeruginosa, Staphylococcus aureus*, or *Burkholderia cepacia*
- Pancreatic insufficiency, recurrent pancreatitis, distal intestinal obstruction syndrome, chronic hepatic disease, nutritional deficiencies, or male urogenital abnormalities
- Bronchiectasis and scarring on chest radiographs
- Airflow obstruction on spirometry
- Sweat chloride concentration above 60 mEq/L on two occasions or mutations in genes known to cause cystic fibrosis

GENERAL CONSIDERATIONS

- Most common fatal hereditary disorder of whites in the United States
- Autosomal recessive disorder due to mutations affecting a membrane chloride channel (the cystic fibrosis transmembrane conductance regulator, or CFTR)
- At least 1000 mutations to the CFTR gene are described, with "DeltaF508" accounting for 60% of cases
- Pathophysiology results from production of an abnormal mucous in exocrine glands, which leads to tissue distruction and, in the respiratory tract, impairs mucociliary clearance
- Variety of mutations is reflected in wide range of pulmonary and nonpulmonary manifestations

DEMOGRAPHICS

- Affects 1 in 3200 whites; 1 in 25 is a carrier

 ## CLINICAL FINDINGS

SYMPTOMS AND SIGNS

- Disease should be suspected in young adults with a history of chronic lung disease, pancreatitis, or infertility
- Productive cough, decreased exercise tolerance, and recurrent hemoptysis are typical
- Sinus pain or pressure with purulent nasal discharge is frequent
- Pulmonary manifestations include bronchitis, bronchiectasis, pneumonia, atelectasis, and peribronchial and parenchymal scarring
- Steatorrhea, diarrhea, and abdominal pain are common extrapulmonary manifestations
- Hypoxemia, hypercapnia, and cor pulmonale occur in advanced disease
- Nearly all male patients have congenital absence of the vas deferens with azoospermia
- Findings include digital clubbing, increased anterioposterior chest diameter, and apical crackles

DIFFERENTIAL DIAGNOSIS

- Chronic obstructive pulmonary disease
- Asthma
- α_1-Antiprotease deficiency
- Bronchiolitis
- Celiac disease (celiac sprue)
- Chronic sinusitis

 ## DIAGNOSIS

LABORATORY TESTS

- Arterial blood gases reveal hypoxemia, with compensated respiratory acidosis in advanced disease
- Pulmonary function tests
  - A mixed obstructive and restrictive pattern
  - Reduced FVC, airflow rates, and total lung capacity
  - Air trapping and reduced diffusion capacity are common
- Genotyping, measurement of nasal membrane potential difference, semen analysis, or assessment of pancreatic function can play a role in diagnosis
- Sputum cultures frequently show *S aureus* and *P aeruginosa*; *H influenzae, Stenotrophomonas maltophilia,* and *B cepacia* are occasionally isolated

IMAGING STUDIES

- Hyperinflation is seen early in chest x-rays
- Peribronchial cuffing, mucus plugging, bronchiectasis, atelectasis, and increased interstitial markings are sometimes seen
- High-resolution CT is the test of choice to confirm bronchiectasis

DIAGNOSTIC PROCEDURES

- Chloride sweat test reveals elevated sodium and chloride levels; two tests on different days are required for accurate diagnosis
- A normal sweat chloride test does not exclude the diagnosis

TREATMENT

MEDICATIONS

- Inhaled bronchodilators should be considered in patients who demonstrate an increase in FEV_1 of 12% in response to treatment
- rhDNase, 2.5 mg nebulized daily, thins sputum by cleaving extracellular DNA from neutrophils that accumulate in sputum and increase viscosity
- Antibiotics are used to treat airway infection based on results of sputum culture and sensitivity testing
- Aerosolized antibiotics (tobramycin and others) are sometimes helpful, but there is concern regarding development of resistant *B cepacia* and side effects such as bronchospasm

SURGERY

- Lung transplantation is the only definitive therapy for advanced disease; double lung or heart-lung transplantation is required
- 3-year survival rates following transplantation are about 55%

THERAPEUTIC PROCEDURES

- Mechanical interventions to clear lower airway secretions: postural drainage, chest percussion or vibration, positive expiratory pressure, flutter valve breathing devices, and directed cough

OUTCOME

FOLLOW-UP

- Regular assessment of FEV_1
- Nutritional status

COMPLICATIONS

- Pneumothorax and hemoptysis are common
- Cor pulmonale is seen in late disease
- Patients have increased risk of gastrointestinal malignancies, osteopenia, and arthropathies
- Biliary cirrhosis, gallstones, and pancreatitis are seen
- Resistant infections, including methicillin-resistant *Staphylococcus aureus* and *B cepacia*

PROGNOSIS

- Median survival is at 31 years, but is increasing
- Death results from pulmonary infections or as a result of chronic respiratory failure and cor pulmonale

WHEN TO REFER

- All patients with suspected or confirmed cystic fibrosis should be referred to a Cystic Fibrosis Center of Excellence for evaluation and treatment recommendations

WHEN TO ADMIT

- Increased cough, sputum production, shortness of breath, decline in FEV_1, weight loss, constitutional symptoms, hemoptysis

PREVENTION

- Vaccination against pneumococcal infection and annual influenza vaccination are recommended
- Screening of family members and genetic counseling are suggested

EVIDENCE

PRACTICE GUIDELINES

- National Guideline Clearinghouse http://www.guideline.gov/summary/ summary.aspx?doc_id=3273&nbr=2499 &string=cystic+fibrosis

INFORMATION FOR PATIENTS

- Cystic Fibrosis Foundation website www.cff.org
- National Heart, Lung and Blood Institute http://www.nhlbi.nih.gov/health/ public/lung/other/cf.htm
- Mayo Clinic http://www.mayoclinic.com/invoke. cfm?id=DS00287

REFERENCES

- Liou TG et al: Survival effect of lung transplantation among patients with cystic fibrosis. JAMA 2001;286:2683. [PMID: 11730443]
- Rosenstein BJ et al: The diagnosis of cystic fibrosis: a consensus statement. J Pediatr 1998;132:589. [PMID: 9580754]
- Rubin BK: Emerging therapies for cystic fibrosis lung disease. Chest 1999;115: 1120. [PMID: 10208218]
- Ryan G et al: Nebulised antipseudomonal antibiotics for cystic fibrosis. Cochrane Database Syst Rev 2000(2):CD001021. [PMID: 10796732]

Mark S. Chesnutt, MD
Thomas J. Prendergast, MD

Cysticercosis

 KEY FEATURES

ESSENTIALS OF DIAGNOSIS

- History of exposure to *Taenia solium* in an endemic region; concomitant or past intestinal tapeworm infection
- Seizures, headache, and other findings of a focal space-occupying central nervous system (CNS) lesion
- Subcutaneous or muscular nodules (5–10 mm); calcified lesions on x-rays of soft tissues
- Calcified or uncalcified cysts by CT scan or MRI; positive serological tests

GENERAL CONSIDERATIONS

- Human cysticercosis is infection by the larval (cysticercus) stage of the tapeworm *T solium*
- Cysticerci complete their development within 2–4 months after larval entry and live for months to years
- Initially, the live larva within a thin-walled cyst (vesicular cyst) is minimally antigenic. When the host immune response or chemotherapy results in gradual death of the cyst, there may be cyst enlargement (colloidal cyst) with mechanical compression, inflammation with pericyst edema, and (sometimes) vasculitis that can result in small cerebral infarcts; increased intracranial pressure and cerebrospinal fluid changes may follow. As the cyst degenerates over 2–7 years, it may disappear or be replaced by a granuloma, calcification, or residual fibrosis. Cysts at different life cycle stages—active (live), transitional, and inactive (dead)—may be in the same organ
- Locations of cysts in order of frequency are the CNS, subcutaneous tissues and striated muscle, globe of the eye, and, rarely, other tissues. Cysts reach 5–10 mm in soft tissues but may be larger (up to 5 cm) in the CNS

DEMOGRAPHICS

- Worldwide, an estimated 20 million persons are infected and 50,000 deaths occur yearly. Antibody prevalence rates to 10% are recognized in some endemic areas

 CLINICAL FINDINGS

SYMPTOMS AND SIGNS

Neurocysticercosis

- May be asymptomatic

- When symptomatic, the incubation period is highly variable (usually from 1 to 5 years but sometimes shorter)
- Acute invasive stage results from extensive acute spread of cysticerci to the brain parenchyma. Rarely, fever, headache, myalgia, marked eosinophilia, and coma may occur
- Parenchymal cysts can present singly or multiply and may be scattered or in clumps. Findings include epilepsy (focal or generalized), focal neurological deficits, intracranial hypertension, and altered mental status
- Subarachnoid space and meningeal cysts may result in obstructive hydrocephalus, intracranial hypertension, arterial thrombosis, and cranial nerve palsy (most often of the optic nerve)
- Ventricular cysts may float freely (usually singly) or may be attached to the ventricular wall. They are usually asymptomatic but can cause increased intracranial pressure
- Racemose cysts are rare grape-like irregular clusters and may reach over 10 cm in diameter. They can cause marked adhesive arachnoiditis and obstructive hydrocephalus
- Spinal cord cysts can cause arachnoiditis (meningitis, radiculopathy) or pressure symptoms

Ophthalmocysticercosis

- Usually there is a single cyst, free-floating in the vitreous or under the retina
- Presenting symptoms include periorbital pain, scotomas, and progressive deterioration of visual acuity
- Findings may include disk hemorrhage, retinal detachment, iridocyclitis, and chorioretinitis

Subcutaneous and striated muscle cysticercosis

- Usually asymptomatic
- May present as nodules that tend to appear and disappear, or they may die and calcify and be detected on radiographs

DIFFERENTIAL DIAGNOSIS

- Seizure due to other cause, eg, epilepsy, bacterial meningitis
- Primary or metastatic cancer
- Tuberculoma
- Echinococcosis (hydatid disease)
- Bacterial or fungal brain abscess
- Toxoplasmosis
- Neurosyphilis

 DIAGNOSIS

LABORATORY TESTS

- With serum, the enzyme-linked immunoelectrotransfer blot (EITB) assay has nearly 100% specificity and 94–98% sensitivity; when used with cerebrospinal fluid, however, both parameters are lower. The EITB sensitivity drops about 50% if only one or two cysts are present and is also low in patients with only calcified cysts
- The older ELISA has a 63% specificity and 65% sensitivity with serum; paradoxically, the ELISA with cerebrospinal fluid has a high specificity (95%) and sensitivity (87%) for both IgM and IgG antibody. False-positives can occur with previous exposure
- Cerebrospinal fluid typically shows increased protein, decreased glucose, and a cellular reaction of mainly lymphocytes and eosinophils; eosinophilia may be over 20% and is diagnostically important. Lumbar puncture is contraindicated in case of increased intracerebral pressure

IMAGING STUDIES

- Initially, use nonenhanced CT and then MRI and enhanced CT. Brain or spinal cord cystic lesions can show the scolex ("hole-with-dot")
- Spinal cysticercosis is evaluated by CT myelography or MRI
- Plain radiographs of muscle may detect oval or linear calcified lesions (4–10 × 2–5 mm). Plain skull films may demonstrate one or more cerebral calcifications (generally 5–10 mm; sometimes 1–2 mm when only the scolex is calcified)

DIAGNOSTIC PROCEDURES

- The diagnosis of neurocysticercosis is by demonstration of characteristic lesions on CT or MRI scan; by visualization of the parasite by ophthalmoscopic examination (subretinal or in the anterior chamber); or by finding the parasite in histological sections of brain or spinal cord tissue (not usually recommended)
- A probable diagnosis is based on the presence of various combinations of other major and minor criteria
- Highly suggestive of the diagnosis is finding the organism in excisional biopsies of skin or subcutaneous pea-sized nodules or a varied radiological appearance on brain scans

TREATMENT

MEDICATIONS

- Single enhancing lesions may be treated only with anticonvulsants; some experts do add albendazole or praziquantel treatment; however, patients with only calcified cysts do not need these drugs
- During the acute phase of encephalitis, if intracranial hypertension is present, mannitol (2 g/kg/day) and corticosteroids are used but drug treatment is withheld

Albendazole

- The dosage is 400 mg twice daily with a fatty meal
- Seven to 14 days of treatment may be sufficient, but a longer course (up to 28 days) is advisable; it can be repeated as necessary
- Up to 3 months of treatment may be needed for ventricular and subarachnoid cysts

Praziquantel

- Give 50–100 mg/kg/day in three divided doses for 15–30 days
- For both drugs, ingestion with a fatty meal enhances absorption

Other measures

- Phenytoin, phenobarbital, carbamazepine, cimetidine, and corticosteroids, when administered with praziquantel, reduce serum levels of the latter
- For patients with seizures, anticonvulsants should be given during drug treatment and probably for an indefinite time afterward
- Give corticosteroids at time of treatment to prevent the marked inflammatory reactions around dying parasites. Prednisone, 1 mg/kg/day in two or three divided doses, starting 1–2 days before use of the drug and continuing at diminishing doses for about 14 days afterward, is used. The reaction usually subsides in 48–72 h, but continuing severity may require steroids in higher dosage and mannitol
- Subarachnoiditis and vasculitis are treated with albendazole or praziquantel plus a corticosteroid
- An ophthalmological examination should be done; if cysticercocidal drugs are given in the presence of ocular or spinal cysts, irreparable damage can occur

SURGERY

- Surgery can remove accessible orbital, cisternal, ventricular, cerebral, meningeal, and spinal cord cysts. Obstructive hydrocephalus requires cerebrospinal fluid diversion plus a corticosteroid

THERAPEUTIC PROCEDURES

- Medical treatment, which is usually preferable to surgery, is most effective for parenchymal cysts; less effective for intraventricular, subarachnoid, or racemose cysts
- When only one or a few live parenchymal cysts are present, it is unclear whether medical treatment is preferable to symptomatic management followed by normal death of the parasites. Some clinicians wait 3 months with selected patients to see if cysts will spontaneously disappear

 ## OUTCOME

PROGNOSIS

- The fatality rate for untreated neurocysticercosis is about 50%. Drug treatment has reduced the mortality rate to about 5–15%
- Surgical procedures to relieve intracranial hypertension along with use of steroids to reduce edema improve the prognosis for those not effectively treated with the drugs

WHEN TO REFER

- All patients should be referred to a clinician with expertise in these disorders

WHEN TO ADMIT

- Treatment should be conducted in a hospital

PREVENTION

- All family members should examine their stools over several days for passage of proglottids, and stool specimens should be sent to the laboratory to be examined for proglottids and eggs

 ## EVIDENCE

PRACTICE GUIDELINES

- Garcia HH et al: Current consensus guidelines for treatment of neurocysticercosis. Clin Microbiol Rev 2002;15:747. [PMID: 12364377]

INFORMATION FOR PATIENTS

- Centers for Disease Control http://www.cdc.gov/ncidod/dpd/parasites/cysticercosis/factsht_cysticercosis.htm
- National Institute of Allergy and Infectious Diseases http://www.niaid.nih.gov/publications/microbes.htm

REFERENCES

- Katti MK: Proposed diagnostic criteria for neurocysticercosis. Neurology 2002;58(8):1315. [PMID: 11973827]
- Thaler DE, Frosch MP: Case records of the Massachusetts General Hospital. Weekly clinicopathological exercises. Case 16-2002. A 41-year-old woman with global headache and an intracranial mass. N Engl J Med 2002;346(21):1651. [PMID: 12023999]
- Verma L et al: Optic nerve cysticercosis. Arch Ophthalmol 2002;120(10):1408. [PMID: 12365933]

Cystitis, Acute

 KEY FEATURES

ESSENTIALS OF DIAGNOSIS

- Irritative voiding symptoms
- Patient usually afebrile
- Positive urine culture; blood cultures may also be positive

 CLINICAL FINDINGS

SYMPTOMS AND SIGNS

- Frequency, urgency, dysuria, suprapubic discomfort, gross hematuria
- Suprapubic tenderness, no systemic toxicity

DIFFERENTIAL DIAGNOSIS

- In women: vulvovaginitis, pelvic inflammatory disease
- In men: urethritis, prostatitis, cystitis (rare)
- In both: pelvic irradiation, chemotherapy (cyclophosphamide), bladder carcinoma, interstitial cystitis, voiding dysfunction disorders, and psychosomatic disorders

 DIAGNOSIS

LABORATORY TESTS

- Urinalysis: pyuria, hematuria, bacteriuria
- Urine culture: positive, but colony counts >10^5/mL not essential
- Urine culture and sensitivity

IMAGING STUDIES

- Imaging warranted only if pyelonephritis, recurrent infections, or anatomic abnormalities are suspected

TREATMENT

MEDICATIONS

- Uncomplicated cystitis: cephalexin, nitrofurantoin, or fluoroquinolone single-dose or 1–3 days of therapy (see regimens below)
- Avoid trimethoprim-sulfamethoxazole due to resistant organisms.
- Cephalexin, 250–500 mg PO q6h for 1–3 days
- Ciprofloxacin, 250–500 mg PO q12h for 1–3 days
- Nitrofurantoin (macrocrystals), 100 mg PO q12h for 7 days
- Norfloxacin, 400 mg PO q12h for 1–3 days
- Ofloxacin, 200 mg PO q12h for 1–3 days
- Trimethoprim-sulfamethoxazole, 160/800 mg, 2 tablets PO once; increasing resistance noted (up to 20%)

THERAPEUTIC PROCEDURES

- Symptomatic relief: hot sitz baths or urinary analgesics (phenazopyridine, 200 mg PO TID)
- Uncomplicated cystitis in men warrants elucidation of underlying problem

OUTCOME

PROGNOSIS

- Infections typically respond rapidly to treatment
- Failure to respond suggests resistance to the selected drug or anatomic abnormalities requiring further investigation

EVIDENCE

PRACTICE GUIDELINES

- Rubin RH et al: Evaluation of new anti-infective drugs for the treatment of urinary tract infection. Infectious Diseases Society of America and the Food and Drug Administration. Clin Infect Dis 1992;15(Suppl 1):S216. [PMID: 1477233]
- Warren JW et al: Guidelines for antimicrobial treatment of uncomplicated acute bacterial cystitis and acute pyelonephritis in women. Infectious Diseases Society of America (IDSA). Clin Infect Dis 1999;29:745. [PMID: 10589881] http://www.journals.uchicago.edu/IDSA/guidelines/p745.pdf

WEB SITE

- American College of Obstetricians and Gynecologists—Urinary tract infections http://www.medem.com/MedLB/article_detaillb.cfm?article_ID=ZZZ1LJ5770D&sub_cat=2008

INFORMATION FOR PATIENTS

- JAMA patient page: Urinary tract infections http://www.ama-assn.org/insight/spec_con/patient/pat093.pdf

REFERENCES

- Gupta K et al: Increasing prevalence of antimicrobial resistance among uropathogens causing acute uncomplicated cystitis in women. JAMA 1999;281:736. [PMID: 10052444]
- Proceedings of the 5th International Symposium on Clinical Evaluation of Drug Efficacy in Urinary Tract Infection and of the Urinary Tract Infections Symposia of the Commission for Treatment of Urinary Tract Infection of the International Society of Chemotherapy, 29 June–3 July 1997, Sydney, Australia. Int J Antimicrob Agents 1999;11:183. [PMID: 10465618]

Marshall L. Stoller, MD
Peter R. Carroll, MD

Cystitis, Interstitial

 KEY FEATURES

ESSENTIALS OF DIAGNOSIS

- Pain with bladder filling that is relieved by emptying
- Often associated with urgency and frequency
- Submucosal petechiae on cystoscopic examination
- Diagnosis of exclusion

GENERAL CONSIDERATIONS

- Etiology unknown
- Most likely several diseases with similar symptomatology
- Associated diseases include severe allergies, irritable bowel syndrome, or inflammatory bowel disease

DEMOGRAPHICS

- Prevalence of between 18 and 40 per 100,000 people
- Both sexes
- Majority of patients are women
- Mean age at onset of 40 years

 CLINICAL FINDINGS

SYMPTOMS AND SIGNS

- History: pain with bladder filling that is relieved with urination, or urgency, frequency, and nocturia
- Physical examination: should exclude genital herpes, vaginitis, or a urethral diverticulum

DIFFERENTIAL DIAGNOSIS

- Exposure to radiation (radiation cystitis) or cyclophosphamide (chemical cystitis), bacterial vaginitis, genital herpes, urethral diverticulum, urethral carcinoma, bladder carcinoma, eosinophilic cystitis, and tuberculous cystitis

 DIAGNOSIS

LABORATORY TESTS

- Negative urine culture and cytology
- Urinalysis and urine culture to exclude infectious causes
- Urinary cytology to exclude bladder malignancy

DIAGNOSTIC PROCEDURES

- Urodynamic testing assesses bladder sensation and compliance and excludes detrusor instability
- The bladder is distended with fluid (hydrodistension) to detect glomerulations (submucosal hemorrhage), which must be present in at least three quadrants of the bladder
- Bladder biopsy to exclude other causes

TREATMENT

MEDICATIONS

- Amitriptyline
- Nifedipine and other calcium channel blockers
- Pentosan polysulfate sodium (Elmiron)—an oral synthetic sulfated polysaccharide helps restore integrity to the epithelium of the bladder
- Intravesical instillation of dimethyl sulfoxide (DMSO)
- Intravesical instillation of heparin and BCG

SURGERY

- Cystourethrectomy with urinary diversion

PROCEDURES

- Symptomatic relief from hydrodistension

 OUTCOME

PROGNOSIS

- No cure, but most patients achieve symptomatic relief

 EVIDENCE

PRACTICE GUIDELINES

- Lukban JC et al: Current management of interstitial cystitis. Urol Clin North Am 2002;29:649. [PMID: 12476528]
- MaLossi J et al: Interstitial cystitis: diagnosis and treatment options. Curr Womens Health Rep 2002;2:298. [PMID: 12150758]

WEB SITES

- Interstitial Cystitis Association—Most frequently asked questions about IC http://www.ichelp.org/WhatIsIC/TheMostFAQ.html
- National Kidney and Urologic Diseases Information Clearinghouse—Interstitial cystitis http://kidney.niddk.nih.gov/kudiseases/pubs/interstitialcystitis/index.htm

INFORMATION FOR PATIENTS

- Mayo Clinic—Interstitial cystitis http://www.mayoclinic.com/invoke.cfm?objectid=CBC4AE4E-273C-4A16-813E4F06BFB5F959

REFERENCES

- Hanno PM et al: The diagnosis of interstitial cystitis revisited: lessons learned from the National Institutes of Health Interstitial Cystitis Database Study. J Urol 1999;161:553. [PMID: 99112653]
- Jepsen JV et al: Long-term experience with pentosanpolysulfate in interstitial cystitis. Urology 1998;51:381. [PMID: 9510339]
- Propert KJ et al: A prospective study of interstitial cystitis: results of longitudinal followup of the interstitial cystitis data base cohort. The Interstitial Cystitis Data Base Study Group. J Urol 2000;163:1434. [PMID: 10751852]
- Sant GR et al: Interstitial cystitis. Curr Opin Urol 1999;9:297. [PMID: 10459464]

Marshall L. Stoller, MD
Peter R. Carroll, MD

Decompression Sickness

 KEY FEATURES

ESSENTIALS OF DIAGNOSIS

- Respiratory gases are compressed into the blood and other tissues by the greatly increased pressures at low depths
- Gases dissolved in the blood and other tissues escape as the external pressure decreases during ascent from depths greater than 9 m (30 ft)

GENERAL CONSIDERATIONS

- The appearance of symptoms depends on the depth and duration of submersion; the degree of physical exertion; the age, weight, and physical condition of the diver; and the rate of ascent
- The release of gas bubbles and (particularly) the location of their release determine the symptoms. The size and number of gas bubbles (notably nitrogen) escaping from the tissues depend on the difference between the atmospheric pressure and the partial pressure of the gas dissolved in the tissues
- Predisposing factors include exercise, injury, patent foramen ovale, obesity, dehydration, alcoholic excess, hypoxia, some medications (eg, narcotics, antihistamines), and cold
- Asthma, pneumothorax, reduced pulmonary function, lung cysts, or thoracic trauma may be contraindications to diving

 CLINICAL FINDINGS

SYMPTOMS AND SIGNS

- The onset of acute symptoms occurs within 30 min in 50% of cases and almost invariably within 6 h
- Symptoms, which are highly variable, include pain (largely in the joints) from gas bubble formation (bends), headache, fatigue, numbness, confusion, pruritic rash, visual disturbances, nausea, vomiting, loss of hearing, weakness, paralysis, dizziness, vertigo, dyspnea, paresthesias, aphasia, and coma
- Pulmonary decompression sickness (chokes) presents with burning, pleuritic substernal pain, cough, and dyspnea

 DIAGNOSIS

DIAGNOSTIC PROCEDURES

- Early recognition is very important

Decompression Sickness

 TREATMENT

MEDICATIONS
- Aspirin may be given for pain
- Narcotics should be used very cautiously to avoid obscuring the patient's response to recompression

THERAPEUTIC PROCEDURES
- Prompt treatment is extremely important
- Complete alleviation of decompression symptoms is possible, however, with treatment given up to 2 weeks postinjury
- Administer continuous oxygen as a first aid measure whether or not cyanosis is present

 OUTCOME

COMPLICATIONS
Sequelae
- Hemiparesis
- Neurological dysfunction
- Bone damage

WHEN TO REFER
- Rapid transportation to a treatment facility for recompression, hyperbaric oxygen, hydration treatment of plasma deficits, and supportive measures are necessary not only to relieve symptoms but also to prevent permanent impairment
- Call the local public health department or nearest naval facility for information on the nearest compression center
- The National Divers Alert Network at Duke University (919-684-8111) provides assistance in the management of underwater diving accidents

EVIDENCE

PRACTICE GUIDELINES
- British Thoracic Society Fitness to Dive Group, Subgroup of the British Thoracic Society Standards of Care Committee. British Thoracic Society guidelines on respiratory aspects of fitness for diving. Thorax 2003;58:3. [PMID: 12511710]
- Moon RE et al: Guidelines for treatment of decompression illness. Aviat Space Environ Med 1997;68:234. [PMID: 9056035]

WEB SITE
- Merck Manual—Disorder due to physical agents http://www.merck.com/pubs/mmanual/section20/sec20.htm

INFORMATION FOR PATIENTS
- American Academy of Family Physicians http://familydoctor.org/handouts/156.html
- American Red Cross http://www.redcross.org/services/hss/tips/healthtips/safetywater.html#scuba

REFERENCES
- Moon RE: Treatment of diving emergencies. Crit Care Clin 1999;15:429. [PMID: 10331136]
- Strauss MB et al: Diving medicine: contemporary topics and their controversies. Am J Emerg Med 2001;19:232. [PMID: 11326354]
- Van Meter K: Medical field management of the injured diver. Respir Care Clin North Am 1999;5:137. [PMID: 10205815].)

Richard Cohen, MD, MPH
Brent R.W. Moelleken, MD, FACS

Decubitus Ulcers

 KEY FEATURES

ESSENTIALS OF DIAGNOSIS

- A special type of ulcer caused by impaired blood supply and tissue nutrition
- Results from prolonged pressure over bony or cartilaginous prominences

GENERAL CONSIDERATIONS

- Occur most readily in the elderly, paralyzed, debilitated, and unconscious patients

 CLINICAL FINDINGS

SYMPTOMS AND SIGNS

- The skin overlying the sacrum and hips is most commonly involved, but bedsores may also be seen over the occiput, ears, elbows, heels, and ankles

DIFFERENTIAL DIAGNOSIS

- Herpes simplex virus: in immunocompromised patients, particularly if there is a scalloped border, representing the erosions of herpetic vesicles
- Skin cancer: in the perianal area, a non-healing ulcer may be cancer
- Pyoderma gangrenosum: rapidly expanding ulcers associated with inflammatory bowel disease
- Ecthyma gangrenosum: ulcerating lesion, commonly due to *Pseudomonas*, observed in neutropenic patients

 DIAGNOSIS

LABORATORY TESTS

- Based on clinical appearance
- Suspect an alternative diagnosis if ulcers not healing properly

TREATMENT

MEDICATIONS

- See Table 6 (page 1199)

Early lesions

- Treat with topical antibiotic powders and adhesive absorbent bandage (Gelfoam)
- Once clean, they may be treated with hydrocolloid dressings such as DuoDerm

Established lesions

- Topical antiseptics are not recommended
- Systemic antibiotics may be required for deep infections if the patient is systemically ill, but should otherwise be avoided because they will promote antibiotic resistance

SURGERY

- Established lesions require surgery for debridement, cleansing, and dressing

THERAPEUTIC PROCEDURES

- For established lesions a spongy foam pad placed under the patient may work best in some cases

 OUTCOME

COMPLICATIONS

- Low-grade infection may occur

WHEN TO REFER

- If there is a question about the diagnosis, if recommended therapy is ineffective, or if specialized treatment is necessary

PREVENTION

- Good nursing care, good nutrition, and maintenance of skin hygiene are important preventive measures
- The skin and the bed linens should be kept clean and dry
- Bedfast, paralyzed, moribund, listless, or incontinent patients who are candidates for the development of decubiti must be turned frequently (at least every hour) and must be examined at pressure points for the appearance of small areas of redness and tenderness
- Water-filled mattresses, rubber pillows, alternating-pressure mattresses, and thick papillated foam pads are useful in prevention and in the treatment of lesions
- "Donut" devices should not be used

EVIDENCE

PRACTICE GUIDELINES

- National Guideline Clearinghouse http://www.guideline.gov/summary/summary.aspx?doc_id=3457&nbr=2683&string=decubitus+ulcers

WEB SITES

- American Academy of Dermatology http://www.aad.org
- Dermatology Handbook for Family Practice from the University of Iowa http://www.vh.org/Providers/ClinRef/FPHandbook/17.html

INFORMATION FOR PATIENTS

- American Academy of Dermatology http://www.aad.org/pamphlets/
- American Academy of Family Practice http://familydoctor.org/handouts/039.html

REFERENCE

- Theaker C: Risk factors for pressure sores in the critically ill. Anaesthesia 2000;55:221. [PMID: 10671839]

Timothy G. Berger, MD

Deep Vein Thrombosis

KEY FEATURES

ESSENTIALS OF DIAGNOSIS

- Pain in the calf or thigh, new leg edema
- History of congestive heart failure, recent surgery, trauma, neoplasia, oral contraceptive use, or prolonged inactivity
- Physical signs unreliable
- Duplex ultrasound is diagnostic

GENERAL CONSIDERATIONS

- Cause often multifactorial
- Virchow's triad: stasis, vascular injury, and hypercoagulability
- Chronic venous insufficiency with venous stasis disease occurs in ~35% of patients
- In 80% of patients thrombosis begins in the deep veins of the calf
- Propagation into the popliteal and femoral veins then occurs in ~25% of patients
- About 3% of patients undergoing major general surgical procedures develop symptomatic deep vein thrombosis
- Major risk factors: certain operations, particularly total hip replacement; prolonged bed rest or immobility; hypercoagulable state; occult or known malignancy
- Other risk factors: advanced age, type A blood group, obesity, previous thrombosis, multiparity, use of oral contraceptives, inflammatory bowel disease, and systemic lupus erythematosus

DEMOGRAPHICS

- 800,000 new cases per year

CLINICAL FINDINGS

SYMPTOMS AND SIGNS

- Half of patients have no symptoms or signs
- Dull ache, tightness, or pain in the calf or leg, especially when walking
- Edema of the involved calf, distension of the superficial venous collaterals, low-grade fever, and tachycardia
- Homans' sign positive in 50% of patients
- Cyanosis of the skin (phlegmasia cerulea dolens) in iliofemoral venous thrombosis
- A pale, cool extremity (phlegmasia alba dolens) if reflex arterial spasm is superimposed

DIFFERENTIAL DIAGNOSIS

- Localized muscle strain or contusion
- Baker's cyst (rupture or obstruction of popliteal vein)
- Achilles tendon rupture
- Cellulitis
- Superficial thrombophlebitis
- Lymphedema from lymphatic obstruction, eg, by pelvic tumor
- Reflex sympathetic dystrophy
- Tumor or retroperitoneal fibrosis obstructing iliac vein or inferior vena cava
- May-Thurner syndrome (external compression of the left iliac vein by the right common iliac artery)
- Edema secondary to heart, liver, or kidney failure, or pregnancy

DIAGNOSIS

LABORATORY TESTS

- Obtain complete blood cell count, prothrombin time, partial thromboplastin time (PTT)
- Consider hypercoagulable workup in cases of recurrent or spontaneous deep vein thrombosis or with family history of hypercoagulable state

IMAGING STUDIES

- Duplex ultrasonography has high sensitivity and specificity
- Ascending contrast venography has 100% sensitivity and 96% specificity but is invasive and rarely indicated to make the diagnosis
- MRA is considered in cases in which there is high clinical suspicion of deep venous thrombosis but ultrasound is negative

TREATMENT

MEDICATIONS

- Patients with thrombus in the deep veins or with symptomatic calf vein thrombosis should be anticoagulated
- Unfractionated heparin (initial bolus 100 units/kg, followed by 10 units/kg/h, dosed to a goal PTT = 1.5–2 times normal) or therapeutic dose low-molecular-weight heparin, eg, enoxaparin, 1 mg/kg SQ BID
- Warfarin is started after therapeutic heparinization to maintain a goal INR = 2.0–3.0 for 3–6 months
- Lifelong anticoagulation is recommended after a second episode of deep venous thrombosis (DVT), and in factor V Leiden mutations, homozygous activated protein C resistance, antiphospholipid antibody, and deficiencies of antithrombin III and of protein C or protein S
- Fibrinolytic agents, eg, alteplase, indicated for acute iliofemoral venous thrombosis complicated by phlegmasia within 1 week after clot formation

OUTCOME

FOLLOW-UP

- Patients with asymptomatic calf vein thrombosis may be followed expectantly (without anticoagulation) with serial ultrasound examination

COMPLICATIONS

- Pulmonary embolism
- Varicose veins
- Chronic venous insufficiency
- Bleeding complications (more common with alteplase than anticoagulants)

PROGNOSIS

- Mortality is related to pulmonary embolism, which occurs in 60% of patients with inadequately treated proximal lower extremity DVT

PREVENTION

- Elevation of the foot of the bed
- Footboard
- Early ambulation
- Graduated compression stockings
- Sequential compression devices
- Unfractionated heparin, 5000 units SQ BID, or low-molecular-weight heparin (LMWH), eg, enoxaparin, 30 mg SQ BID
- LMWH is more effective and has lower risk of bleeding complications in orthopedic surgery patients
- Avoidance of dehydration and femoral catheters or blood draws

EVIDENCE

PRACTICE GUIDELINES

- American College of Emergency Physicians (ACEP) Clinical Policies Committee; ACEP Clinical Policies Subcommittee on Suspected Lower-Extremity Deep Venous Thrombosis. Clinical policy: critical issues in the evaluation and management of adult patients presenting with suspected lower-extremity deep venous thrombosis. Ann Emerg Med 2003;42:124. [PMID: 12827132]

WEB SITE

- American Academy of Orthopaedic Surgeons—Deep vein thrombosis http://orthoinfo.aaos.org/fact/thr_report.cfm?Thread_ID=264&topcategory=Hip&all=all

INFORMATION FOR PATIENTS

- Mayo Clinic—Thrombophlebitis http://www.mayoclinic.com/invoke.cfm?id=DS00223
- MEDLINEplus—Deep venous thrombosis http://www.nlm.nih.gov/medlineplus/ency/article/000156.htm

REFERENCES

- Breddin HK et al: Effects of a low-molecular weight heparin on thrombus regression and recurrent thromboembolism in patients with deep-vein thrombosis. N Engl J Med 2001;344:626. [PMID: 11228276]
- Forster A et al: Tissue plasminogen activator for the treatment of deep venous thrombosis of the lower extremity: a systematic review. Chest 2001;119:572. [PMID: 11171740]
- Lopez-Beret P et al: Systematic study of occult pulmonary thromboembolism in patients with deep venous thrombosis. J Vasc Surg 2001;33:515. [PMID: 11241121]

Louis M. Messina, MD
Laura K. Pak, MD
Lawrence M. Tierney, Jr., MD

Delirium

 KEY FEATURES

ESSENTIALS OF DIAGNOSIS

- Acute confusional state
- Transient global disorder of attention, with clouding of consciousness
- Uually a result of systemic problems (eg, drugs, hypoxemia)

GENERAL CONSIDERATIONS

- The organic problem may be a primary brain disease or a secondary manifestation of some general disorder
- The causes of cognitive disorders are listed in Table 105 (page 1289)
- Should be considered a syndrome of acute brain dysfunction analogous to acute renal failure
- Delirium can coexist with dementia

DEMOGRAPHICS

- Alcohol or substance withdrawal is the most common cause of delirium in the general hospital

 CLINICAL FINDINGS

SYMPTOMS AND SIGNS

- Onset is usually rapid
- The mental status fluctuates (impairment is usually least in the morning), with varying inability to concentrate, maintain attention, and sustain purposeful behavior
- "Sundowning"—mild to moderate delirium at night—is more common in patients with preexisting dementia and may be precipitated by hospitalization, drugs, and sensory deprivation
- There is a marked deficit of memory and recall
- Anxiety and irritability are common
- Amnesia is retrograde (impaired recall of past memories) and anterograde (inability to recall events after the onset of the delirium)
- Orientation problems follow the inability to retain information
- Perceptual disturbances (often visual hallucinations) and psychomotor restlessness with insomnia are common
- Autonomic changes include tachycardia, dilated pupils, and sweating
- Physical findings will naturally vary according to the cause

DIFFERENTIAL DIAGNOSIS

- *Drugs:* opioids, alcohol, sedatives, antipsychotics
- *Metabolic:* hypoxia, hypoglycemia, hyperglycemia, hypercalcemia, hypernatremia, hyponatremia, uremia, hepatic encephalopathy, hypothyroidism, hyperthyroidism, vitamin B_{12} or thiamine deficiency, carbon monoxide poisoning, Wilson's disease
- *Infectious:* meningitis, encephalitis, bacteremia, urinary tract infections, pneumonia, neurosyphilis
- *Structural:* space-occupying lesion, eg, brain tumor, subdural hematoma, hydrocephalus
- *Vascular:* stroke, subarachnoid hemorrhage, hypertensive encephalopathy, CNS vasculitis, thrombotic thrombocytopenic purpura, disseminated intravascular coagulation, hyperviscosity
- *Psychiatric:* schizophrenia, depression
- *Other:* seizure, hypothermia, heat stroke, ICU psychosis

 DIAGNOSIS

LABORATORY TESTS

- Comprehensive physical examination including a search for neurological abnormalities, infection, or hypoxia
- Routine laboratory tests may include serum electrolytes, serum glucose, blood urea nitrogen, serum creatinine, liver function tests, thyroid function tests, arterial blood gases, complete blood count, serum calcium, phosphorus, magnesium, vitamin B_{12}, folate, blood cultures, urinalysis, and cerebrospinal fluid analysis
- See Table 105 (page 1289)

IMAGING STUDIES

- Electroencephalography, CT, MRI, positron emission tomography, and single-photon emission computed tomography evaluations may be helpful in diagnosis

DIAGNOSTIC PROCEDURES

- The EEG usually shows generalized slowing

TREATMENT

MEDICATIONS

- The first aim of treatment is to identify and correct the etiological medical problem
- Discontinue drugs that may be contributing to the problem (eg, analgesics, corticosteroids, cimetidine, lidocaine, anticholinergic drugs, central nervous system depressants, mefloquine)
- Ideally, the patient should be monitored without further medications while the evaluation is carried out
- There are, however, two indications for medication in delirious states: behavioral control (eg, pulling out lines) and subjective distress (eg, pronounced fear due to hallucinations). If these indications are present, medications may be employed
- If there is any hint of alcohol or substance withdrawal, a benzodiazepine such as lorazepam (1–2 mg every hour) can be given parenterally
- If there is little likelihood of withdrawal syndrome, haloperidol is often used in doses of 1–10 mg every hour
- Once the underlying condition has been identified and treated, adjunctive medications can be tapered

THERAPEUTIC PROCEDURES

- In addition to the medication, a pleasant, comfortable, nonthreatening, and physically safe environment with adequate nursing or attendant services should be provided

OUTCOME

PROGNOSIS

- The prognosis is good for recovery of mental functioning in delirium when the underlying condition is reversible
- The average duration is about 1 week, with full recovery in most cases

EVIDENCE

PRACTICE GUIDELINES

- National Guideline Clearinghouse http://www.guideline.gov/summary/summary.aspx?doc_id=2180&nbr=1406&string=delirium http://www.guideline.gov/summary/summary.aspx?doc_id=1344&nbr=536&string=delirium

WEB SITES

- American Psychiatric Association http://www.psych.org/
- Internet Mental Health http://www.mentalhealth.com/t30.html
- Psychopharmacology Tips http://www.dr-bob.org/tips/
- Psychiatry On Line http://www.priory.com/psych.htm

INFORMATION FOR PATIENTS

- National Cancer Institute http://www.cancer.gov/cancerinfo/pdq/supportivecare/delirium/patient
- National Institutes of Health http://www.nlm.nih.gov/medlineplus/ency/article/000740.htm

REFERENCES

- Gleason OC: Delirium. Am Fam Physician 2003;67:1027.
- Sirois F: Steroid psychosis: a review. Gen Hosp Psychiatry 2003;25:27.

Stuart J. Eisendrath, MD
Jonathan E. Lichtmacher, MD

Delirium in Elderly

 KEY FEATURES

ESSENTIALS OF DIAGNOSIS

- Rapid onset of acute confusional state, usually lasting less than 1 week
- Fluctuates during the day
- Inability to concentrate, maintain attention, or sustain purposeful behavior
- Increased anxiety and irritability
- The vast majority of delirium is initiated by problems outside the central nervous system

GENERAL CONSIDERATIONS

- Delirium is the pathophysiological consequence of an underlying general medical condition such as infection, coronary ischemia, hypoxemia, or metabolic derangement
- Although the acutely agitated, "sundowning" elderly patient often comes to mind when considering delirium, many episodes are more subtle
- A key component is review of medications, as a large number of drugs, the addition of a new agent, or the discontinuation of an agent known to cause withdrawal symptoms is associated with the development of delirium

DEMOGRAPHICS

- Approximately 25% of delirious patients are demented, and 40% of demented hospitalized patients are delirious
- Cognitive impairment is an important risk factor
- Other risk factors are male sex, severe illness, hip fracture, fever or hypothermia, hypotension, malnutrition, polypharmacy and use of psychoactive medications, sensory impairment, use of restraints, use of intravenous lines or urinary catheters, metabolic disorders, depression, and alcoholism

 CLINICAL FINDINGS

SYMPTOMS AND SIGNS

- An acute, fluctuating disturbance of consciousness
- Change in cognition or the development of perceptual disturbances
- Inattention, inability to focus on tasks
- Disorientation, confusion
- Irritability
- Mental status may fluctuate throughout the day
- Agitation or may be subdued
- Mental slowing
- Hallucinations are common

DIFFERENTIAL DIAGNOSIS

- Almost any medical condition and many medications
- Depression
- Dementia, especially Lewy body dementia
- Psychosis
- Hypoxemia
- Hypercalcemia
- Hyponatremia
- Infection
- Thiamine deficiency
- Medication side effect
- Pain

DIAGNOSIS

LABORATORY TESTS

- Laboratory evaluation is aimed at finding an underlying medical condition
- Routine studies include complete blood cell count, electrolytes, blood urea nitrogen and serum creatinine, glucose, calcium, albumin, liver function studies, urinalysis, and electrocardiography
- In selected cases, serum magnesium, serum drug levels, arterial blood gas measurements, blood cultures, chest radiography, and urinary toxin screens may be helpful

IMAGING STUDIES

- CT may be indicated if there is a history of falls or if the patient does not respond to other measures

DIAGNOSTIC PROCEDURES

- Most cases of delirium do not require lumbar puncture. Consider lumbar puncture if sign of infection (fever, high white count), if no other obvious cause, or no clinical response to other measures
- EEG may sometimes be helpful if seizures are in the differential diagnosis

TREATMENT

MEDICATIONS

- Management entails treatment of the underlying cause, eliminating unnecessary medications, and avoidance of restraints
- For refractory cases in which the patient's or others' welfare is at risk, an antipsychotic such as risperidone 0.25–0.5 mg or haloperidol 0.5–1.0 mg at bedtime or twice a day may be necessary
- In emergency situations, starting haloperidol at 0.5 mg by mouth or intramuscularly and repeating every 30 min until the agitation is controlled may be necessary, but is often followed by prolonged sedation or other complications

 OUTCOME

FOLLOW-UP

- Patients who suffer prolonged episodes of delirium merit closer follow-up for the development of dementia if not already diagnosed

COMPLICATIONS

- May lead to increased number of iatrogenic events

PROGNOSIS

- Delirium is associated with worse clinical outcomes (higher in-hospital and postdischarge mortality, longer lengths of stay, greater probability of placement in a nursing facility), though it is unclear if delirium causes worse outcomes or is simply an ominous marker
- Most episodes clear in a matter of days after correction of the precipitant

WHEN TO REFER

- Patients in whom restraints are being considered should be referred to a geriatrician or geropsychiatrist
- Refer to a neurologist, geriatrician, or psychiatrist when the etiology is not clear or the patient is not responding to therapy

WHEN TO ADMIT

- Delirium generally signifies an underlying serious medical issue in need of treatment
- Most patients with delirium should be admitted, unless the cause is obvious, treatment is expected to result in rapid response, and they have good social support
- Uncontrollable patients should be admitted

PREVENTION

- Preventive measures include improving cognition (frequent reorientation, activities), sleep (massage, noise reduction), mobility, vision (visual aids and adaptive equipment), hearing (portable amplifiers, cerumen disimpaction), and hydration status (volume repletion)

 EVIDENCE

PRACTICE GUIDELINES

- National Guideline Clearinghouse http://www.guideline.gov/summary/summary.aspx?doc_id=1344&nbr=536&string=delirium+and+elderly
- American Psychiatric Association http://www.psych.org/clin_res/pg_delirium.cfm

WEB SITES

- Mayo Clinic—Topics in geriatrics http://www.mayo.edu/geriatrics-rst/GeriArtcls.html
- Administration on Aging http://www.aoa.dhhs.gov
- AARP Guide to Internet Resources on Aging http://www.aarp.org/cyber/sd1_3.htm

INFORMATION FOR PATIENTS

- JAMA patient page: Psychiatric illness in the older adults. JAMA 2000;283;2886. [PMID: 10896524]
- American Psychiatric Association http://www.psych.org/clin_res/Delirium.pdf

REFERENCES

- Elie M: Delirium risk factors in elderly hospitalized patients. J Gen Intern Med 1998;13:204. [PMID: 9541379]
- Inouye SK: A multicomponent intervention to prevent delirium in hospitalized older patients. N Engl J Med 1999;340:669. [PMID: 10053175]
- Marcantonio ER: Reducing delirium after hip fracture: a randomized trial. J Am Geriatr Soc 2001;49:516. [PMID: 11380742]

C. Bree Johnston, MD
William L. Lyons, MD
Kenneth E. Covinsky, MD

Dementia in Elderly, Non-Alzheimer's

 ## KEY FEATURES

ESSENTIALS OF DIAGNOSIS

- Persistent and progressive impairment in intellectual function
- Not due to delirum—diagnosis should not be made during an acute illness
- Primary deficit of short-term memory
- Must have other deficits (executive function, visuospatial function, language) as well

GENERAL CONSIDERATIONS

- A progressive, acquired impairment in multiple cognitive domains, at least one of which is memory
- The deficits must represent a decline in function significant enough to interfere with work or social life
- Frequently coexists with depression and delirium
- Patients are at high risk of acute cognitive or functional decline in the setting of new medical illness

Classification of dementia

- See *Alzheimer's disease*
- "Subcortical" dementias (Parkinson's disease, vascular dementia)
- Dementia with Lewy bodies
- Frontotemporal dementias (Pick's disease, dementia associated with amyotrophic lateral sclerosis)
- Dementia with motor findings (progressive supranuclear palsy, corticobasal ganglionic degeneration, olivopontocerebellar atrophy)

DEMOGRAPHICS

- Fourth leading cause of death in the United States with a prevalence that doubles every 5 years in the older population, reaching 30–50% at age 85
- Women suffer disproportionately, as patients (even after age adjustment) and as caregivers
- Alzheimer's disease accounts for two-thirds of cases in the United States, with vascular dementia (either alone or combined with Alzheimer's disease) accounting for much of the rest

 ## CLINICAL FINDINGS

SYMPTOMS AND SIGNS

- Memory impairment with at least one or more of the following
  - Language impairment (initially just word finding; later, difficulty following a conversation; finally, mutism)
  - Apraxia (inability to perform previously learned tasks, such as cutting a loaf of bread, despite intact sensory and motor function)
  - Agnosia (inability to recognize objects)
  - Impaired executive function (poor abstraction, mental flexibility, planning, and judgment)
- "Subcortical" dementias: psychomotor slowing, reduced attention, early loss of executive function, personality changes, and benefit from cuing in tests of memory
- Dementia with Lewy bodies
  - May be confused with delirium, as fluctuating cognitive impairment is frequently observed
  - Rigidity and bradykinesia are primarily noted; tremor is rare
  - Hallucinations—classically visual and bizarre—may occur
- Frontotemporal dementias
  - Personality change (euphoria, disinhibition, apathy) and compulsive behaviors
  - In contrast to Alzheimer's disease, visuospatial function is relatively preserved
- Dementia with motor findings: extrapyramidal features or ataxia

DIFFERENTIAL DIAGNOSIS

- Depression
- Delirium
- Medication effect
- Potentially reversible cognitive impairment: drug effect, depression, thyroid disease, vitamin B_{12} deficiency, hypercalcemia, subdural hematoma, HIV infection, and normal pressure hydrocephalus

 ## DIAGNOSIS

LABORATORY TESTS

- Obtain a complete blood cell count, electrolytes, calcium, creatinine, glucose, thyroid-stimulating hormone, and vitamin B_{12} levels
- HIV testing, rapid plasma reagin (RPR), heavy metal screen, and liver function tests in selected patients

IMAGING STUDIES

- Head CT or MRI is most likely to yield positive findings in those who are younger, have focal neurological signs or symptoms, seizures, gait abnormalities, and an acute or subacute onset

DIAGNOSTIC PROCEDURES

- Assess mental status (Figure 1, page 1197)
- Evaluate for deficits related to previous cardiovascular accidents, Parkinsonism, or peripheral neuropathy
- The combination of the "clock draw" (in which the patient is asked to sketch a clock face, with all the numerals placed properly, the two clock hands positioned at a specified time) and the "three-item recall" is a fairly quick and good test; an abnormally drawn clock markedly increases the probability of dementia
- When patients fail either of these screening tests, further testing with the Mini-Mental State questionnaire (Figure 1, page 1197), neuropsychological testing, or other instruments is warranted
- Examine for comorbid conditions that may aggravate the disability

TREATMENT

MEDICATIONS

- Acetylcholinesterase inhibitors (donepezil, galantamine, rivastigmine)
  - Modest improvements in cognitive function in mild to moderate dementia
  - Modest benefit on functional outcomes in advanced disease
  - Starting doses: donepezil, 5 mg orally daily (maximum 10 mg daily); galantamine, 4 mg orally twice daily (maximum 12 mg twice daily); rivastigmine 1.5 mg orally twice daily (maximum 6 mg twice daily)
  - Increase doses gradually as tolerated
  - Side effects include nausea, diarrhea, anorexia, and weight loss
- Choose medications based on symptoms—depression, anxiety, psychosis
- Anxiety may respond to buspirone, starting at 5–7.5 mg twice daily and advancing to 30 mg daily if necessary; takes weeks to show efficacy
- Acetylcholinesterase inhibitors may be modestly beneficial
- Haloperidol may modestly reduce aggression, but not agitation, but is associated with significant adverse effects
- Risperidone, olanzapine, and quetiapine are usually better tolerated than older agents, but are more expensive
- Starting and target neuroleptic dosages are low (eg, haloperidol 0.5–2.0 mg, risperidone 0.25–2 mg)
- Risperidone may be associated with increased strokes
- Behavioral symptoms in Lewy body dementia improve with rivastigmine

THERAPEUTIC PROCEDURES

- Discontinue all nonessential drugs and correct, if possible, sensory deficits
- Exclude unrecognized delirium, pain, urinary obstruction, or fecal impaction
- Caregivers should speak simply to the patient, break down activities into simple component tasks, and employ a "distract, not confront" approach

 OUTCOME

FOLLOW-UP

- Federal regulations require drug reduction efforts at least every 6 months if antipsychotic agents are used in a nursing home patient

PROGNOSIS

- The prevalence of fully reversible dementias is under 5%
- Life expectancy with neurodegenerative dementias, such as dementia with Lewy bodies, show a rapid decline (<3 years)

WHEN TO REFER

- Referral for neuropsychological testing may be helpful to distinguish dementia from depression, to diagnose dementia in persons of poor education or very high premorbid intellect, and to aid diagnosis when impairment is mild
- Referral to a geriatrician or neurologist is useful if the dementia does not have the classic features of Alzheimer's disease

WHEN TO ADMIT

- Dementia complicates other medical problems, and the threshold for admission should be lower

PREVENTION

- Use of nonsteroidal antiinflammatory drugs and HMG-CoA reductase inhibitors, moderate alcohol intake, and strong social supports may decrease the risk of dementia

 EVIDENCE

PRACTICE GUIDELINES

- National Guideline Clearinghouse http://www.guideline.gov/summary/summary.aspx?doc_id=1805&nbr=1031&string=dementia
- American Academy of Neurology http://www.aan.com/professionals/practice/pdfs/dementia_guideline.pdf
- American Geriatrics Society http://www.americangeriatrics.org/products/positionpapers/aan_dementia.shtml

WEB SITES

- AARP Guide to Internet Resources on Aging http://www.aarp.org/cyber/sd1_3.htm
- Administration on Aging http://www.aoa.dhhs.gov
- American Geriatrics Society http://www.americangeriatrics.org/
- Medicare Publications http://www.medicare.gov/nhcompare/home.asp

INFORMATION FOR PATIENTS

- American Academy of Family Phsysicians http://familydoctor.org/handouts/022.html http://familydoctor .org/handouts/662.html htp://familydoctor.org/handouts/662.html
- JAMA patient page: Psychiatric illness in older adults. JAMA 2000;283:1886. [PMID: 10896524]

REFERENCE

- Trinh NH: Efficacy of cholinesterase inhibitors in the treatment of neuropsychiatric symptoms and functional impairment in Alzheimer disease: a meta-analysis. JAMA 2003;289:210. [PMID: 12517232]

C. Bree Johnston, MD
Kenneth E. Covinsky, MD

Depression

KEY FEATURES

ESSENTIALS OF DIAGNOSIS

Present in most depressions

- Lowered mood, from mild sadness to intense guilt, worthlessness, and hopelessness
- Difficulty in thinking and concentration, with rumination and indecision
- Loss of interest, with diminished involvement in activities
- Somatic complaints
- Disrupted, reduced, or excessive sleep
- Loss of energy, appetite, and sex drive
- Anxiety

Present in some severe depressions

- Psychomotor disturbance: retardation or agitation
- Delusions of a hypochondriacal or persecutory nature
- Withdrawal from activities
- Suicidal ideation

GENERAL CONSIDERATIONS

- Sadness and grief are normal responses to loss; depression is not
- Unlike grief, depression is marked by a disturbance of self-esteem, with a sense of guilt and worthlessness
- Dysthymia is a chronic depressive disturbance with symptoms generally milder than in a major depressive episode

DEMOGRAPHICS

- Up to 30% of primary care patients have depressive symptoms

CLINICAL FINDINGS

SYMPTOMS AND SIGNS

- Anhedonia
- Withdrawal from activities
- Feelings of guilt
- Poor concentration and cognitive dysfunction
- Anxiety
- Chronic fatigue and somatic complaints
- Diurnal variation with improvement as the day progresses
- Vegetative signs: insomnia, anorexia, constipation
- Occasionally, severe agitation and psychotic ideation are present
- Atypical features are hypersomnia, overeating, lethargy, and rejection sensitivity
- Unlike normal sadness and grief, depression often produces frustration and irritation in the clinician

DIFFERENTIAL DIAGNOSIS

- Bipolar disorder or cyclothymia
- Adjustment disorder with depressed mood
- Dysthymia
- Premenstrual dysphoric disorder
- Major depression with postpartum onset: usually 2 weeks to 6 months postpartum
- Seasonal affective disorder: symptoms include carbohydrate craving, lethargy, hyperphagia, and hypersomnia

DIAGNOSIS

LABORATORY TESTS

- Complete blood cell count
- Thyroid-stimulating hormone
- Folate
- Toxicology screen may be indicated

TREATMENT

MEDICATIONS

- See Table 104 and Figure 9 (pages 1288 and 1282)
- Selective serotonin reuptake inhibitors (SSRIs) and atypical antidepressants
  - Generally lack anticholinergic or cardiovascular side effects
  - Most are activating and should be given in the morning. Some patients may experience sedation with paroxetine, fluvoxamine, and mirtazapine
  - Clinical response varies from 2 to 6 weeks
  - Common side effects are headache, nausea, tinnitus, insomnia, nervousness
  - Sexual side effects are very common and may respond to sildenafil
  - "Serotonin syndrome" may occur when taken in conjunction with monoamine oxidase inhibitors or selegeline
  - With the exception of paroxetine, this class should be tapered over weeks to months to avoid a withdrawal syndrome
  - Fluoxetine, fluvoxamine, paroxetine, sertraline, and venlafaxine appear to be safe in pregnancy. Use should be weighed against the risks of an untreated depression in the mother
- Tricyclic antidepressants (TCAs)
  - Mainstay of treatment prior to SSRIs
  - Clinical response lags several weeks
  - With all TCAs, start low dose and increase by 25 mg weekly to avoid sedation and anticholinergic side effects
  - Overdose can be serious
- Monoamine oxidase inhibitors (MAOIs)
  - Third-line agents due to dietary restrictions and drug-drug interactions
  - Commonly cause orthostatic hypotension and sympathomimetic effects
  - Potential for withdrawal syndromes requires gradual tapering

- Drug selection influenced by any history of prior responses
- If response is inadequate to first agent at 6 weeks, a second agent from a different group should be substituted
- Lithium should be added when a second drug fails to produce a response
- Thyroid drug (liothyronine 25 μg/day) may be added as augmentatinve therapy if a second agent fails
- Stimulants such as dextroamphetamine (5–30 mg/day) and methylphenidate (10–45 mg/day) can be used for short-term treatment of medically ill and geriatric patients or in refractory cases

THERAPEUTIC PROCEDURES

- Electroconvulsive therapy (ECT) is the most effective (70–85%) treatment for severe depression
  - Indications are contraindications to medications or depression refractory to medications
  - Most common side effects are headache and memory disturbances, which are usually short-lived

Psychological

- Medication and psychotherapy are more effective than either modality alone
- Psychotherapy is seldom possible in the acute phase of severe depression

Social

- In depressions involving alcohol abuse, early involvement in recovery programs is important to future success
- Family, employers, and friends can help to mobilize a recently depressed patient

⛰ OUTCOME

FOLLOW-UP

- Medication trials should be monitored Q 1–2 weeks until 6 weeks, when the effectiveness of the medication can be assessed
- If successful, medications should be continued for 6–12 months before tapering is considered
- Medications should be continued indefinitely in patients with their first episode prior to age 20, more than two episodes after age 40, or a single episode after age 50
- Tapering of medications should occur gradually over several months

COMPLICATIONS

- There is a lifetime risk of 10–15% of suicide among patients with depression
- Four major groups who attempt suicide
  - Those who are overwhelmed by problems in living
  - Those who are clearly attempting to control others
  - Those with severe depressions
  - Those with psychotic illness

PROGNOSIS

- Frequently responds well to a full trial of drug treatment

WHEN TO REFER

- When depression is refractory to antidepressant therapy
- When depression is moderate to severe
- When suicidality or significant loss of function is present
- Actively psychotic, or history of mania

WHEN TO ADMIT

- Patients at risk for suicide
- Complex treatment modalities are required

PREVENTION

- Patients at risk for suicide should receive medications in small amounts
- Guns and drugs should be removed from the patient's house
- High-risk patients should be asked not to drive

EVIDENCE

PRACTICE GUIDELINES

- National Guideline Clearinghouse
  http://www.guideline.gov/summary/
  summary.aspx?doc_id=3354&nbr=2580
  &string=depression
  http://www.guideline.gov/summary/
  summary.aspx?doc_id=3432&nbr=
  2658&string=depression

WEB SITES

- American Psychiatric Association
  http://www.psych.org/
- ECT On-Line
  http://www.priory.co.uk/psych/ectol.
  htm

INFORMATION FOR PATIENTS

- American Medical Association
  http://www.medem.com/medlb/
  article_detaillb.cfm?article_ID=
  ZZZZ9FG0VGD&sub_cat=128
- National Institute of Mental Health
  http://www.nimh.nih.gov/publicat/
  depression.cfm
- JAMA patient page: Depression. JAMA 1998;279:1760. [PMID: 9624033]

REFERENCES

- Glass RM: Treating depression as a recurrent or chronic disease. JAMA 1999;281:83. [PMID: 9892456]
- Glassman AH et al: Sertraline treatment of major depression in patients with acute MI or unstable angina. JAMA 2002;288:701. Erratum in JAMA 2002;288:1720. [PMID: 12169073]
- Nurnberg HG et al: Treatment of antidepressant-associated sexual dysfunction with sildenafil: a randomized controlled trial. JAMA 2003;289:56.
- Reynolds CF et al: Nortriptyline and interpersonal psychotherapy as maintenance therapies for recurrent major depression: a randomized controlled trial in patients older than 59 years. JAMA 1999;281:39. [PMID: 9892449]

Stuart J. Eisendrath, MD
Jonathan E. Lichtmacher, MD

Depression in Elderly

KEY FEATURES

ESSENTIALS OF DIAGNOSIS

- Older patients often present without complaining of depressed mood
- Somatization is a frequent presentation
- Older people not meeting diagnostic criteria for major depression may still have clinically significant depressive symptoms

GENERAL CONSIDERATIONS

- Compared to younger patients, geriatric patients with depression are more likely to have somatic complaints, less likely to report depressed mood or feelings of guilt, and are more likely to experience delusions
- Depression should be ruled out in any geriatric patient with unexplained functional decline
- Depression and dementia frequently co-exist, and should be considered as a potential exacerbating comorbidity

DEMOGRAPHICS

- Medical illness and disability—more common in older adults—are risk factors for depression
- Stroke and Parkinson's disease appear to predispose to depression
- Depression in older adults is associated with disability, increased rates of hospitalization and nursing home admission, and higher mortality
- Major depressive disorder has a slightly lower prevalence in older adults than in younger populations

CLINICAL FINDINGS

SYMPTOMS AND SIGNS

- *DSM-IV* diagnosis requires at least five of the following symptoms for a diagnosis of major depression
  - Low mood (must be one of the symptoms)
  - Diminished interest or pleasure in most activities (must be one of the symptoms)
  - Significant weight loss or weight gain
  - Insomnia or hypersomnia
  - Fatigue
  - Feelings of worthlessness or guilt
  - Diminished ability to think or concentrate
  - Recurrent thoughts of death

DIFFERENTIAL DIAGNOSIS

- Substance-induced mood disorder (alcoholism)
- Bipolar disorder
- Grief reaction

DIAGNOSIS

LABORATORY TESTS

- A simple two-question screen, "Over the last month, have you often been bothered by feeling sad, depressed or hopeless?" and "During the last month, have you often been bothered by little inteerst or pleasure in doing things? " is at least 96% sensitive for detecting major depression
- Positive responses can be followed up with more comprehensive interviews such as the Yesavage's Geriatric Depression Scale (Table 4, page 1198)
- Question patient and family about medication use (including steroids, benzodiazepines, cimetidine, β-blockers, and clonidine)
- Laboratory determination of complete blood cell count; liver, thyroid, and renal function; and calcium may be helpful to rule out medical problems presenting as or contributing to depression

TREATMENT

MEDICATIONS

- Longer trials of antidepressants (at least 9 weeks) may be needed in elderly patients than in younger ones
- Of antidepressant drugs sertraline, citalopram, venlafaxine, and mirtazapine are best tolerated in the elderly (Table 104, page 1288)
- See *Depression*

OUTCOME

FOLLOW-UP

- A significant number of older patients who develop depression may represent individuals with neurodegenerative disorders (eg, dementia)
- Close follow-up of a newly diagnosed patient, with frequent assessment of mental status and neurological examination, may disclose an additional or alternative diagnosis

COMPLICATIONS

- Risk for suicide, the most dreaded complication of depression, is highest in the geriatric age group

PROGNOSIS

- Chances for recovery are good, but it often takes over 4 weeks to respond to an antidepressant
- Patients not responding to one antidepressant will often respond to another agent

WHEN TO REFER

- Suicidal ideation
- Possibility of bipolar disorder
- Unresponsive to treatment
- Coexisting substance use disorder

WHEN TO ADMIT

- Suicidal ideation, especially if active plan and/or patient will not contract to seek assistance if thoughts worsen
- Patient unable to care for self
- Psychotic symptoms

PREVENTION

- Some evidence suggests increasing social activity may be helpful
- Rates of recurrence are high; a high index of suspicion is required in a patient with a previous episode

EVIDENCE

PRACTICE GUIDELINES

- American Psychiatric Association http://\www.psych.org/clin_res/Depression2e.book.cfm
- National Guideline Clearinghouse http://www.guideline.gov/summary/summary.aspx?doc_id=1503&nbr=729&string=depression+and+geriatric

WEB SITES

- American Psychiatric Association http://www.psych.org/
- ECT On-Line http://www.priory.co.uk/psych/ectol.htm
- Psychopharmacology Tips http://www.dr-bob.org/tips/
- Depression http://www.guideline.gov/FRAMESETS/guideline_fs.asp?guideline=001008&sSearch_string=depression

INFORMATION FOR PATIENTS

- JAMA patient page: Depression. JAMA 2000;284:1606.
- JAMA patient page: Psychiatric illness in older adults. JAMA 2000;283:2886. [PMID: 10896524]
- American Academy of Family Physicians http://familydoctor.org/handouts/588.html

REFERENCES

- Covinsky KE: Depressive symptoms and 3-year mortality in older hospitalized medical patients. Ann Intern Med 1999;130:563. [PMID: 10189325]
- Schulz R: Association between depression and mortality in older adults: the Cardiovascular Health Study. Arch Intern Med 2000;160:1761. [PMID: 10871968]

C. Bree Johnston, MD
Kenneth E. Covinsky, MD

Dermatitis, Atopic

 KEY FEATURES

ESSENTIALS OF DIAGNOSIS

- Pruritic, exudative, or lichenified eruption on face, neck, upper trunk, wrists, hands, antecubital and popliteal folds
- Personal or family history of allergies or asthma
- Peripheral eosinophilia, increased IgE — not needed for the diagnosis

GENERAL CONSIDERATIONS

- A chronic or intermittent pruritic, exudative, or lichenified eruption with typical distribution
- Poor prognostic factors for persistence: onset early in childhood, early generalized disease, asthma
- Personal or family history of allergic manifestations (eg, asthma, allergic rhinitis, atopic dermatitis)

 CLINICAL FINDINGS

SYMPTOMS AND SIGNS

- See Table 6 (page 1199)
- Distribution of lesions is characteristic: face, neck, and upper trunk ("monk's cowl"), bends of elbows and knee
- Looks different at different ages and in different races, but most patients have scaly dry skin at some point
- Acute flares may present with red patches that are weepy, shiny, or lichenified and plaques and papules
- Fissures, crusts, erosions, or pustules indicate staphylococcal infection so dicloxacillin or first-generation cephalosporins may help in flares
- Pigmented persons tend to present with a papular eruption, and hypopigmented patches (pityriasis alba) are commonly seen on the cheeks and extremities

DIFFERENTIAL DIAGNOSIS

- Seborrheic dermatitis
- Contact dermatitis
- Impetigo
- Psoriasis
- Lichen simplex chronicus (circumscribed neurodermatitis)

 DIAGNOSIS

LABORATORY TESTS

- Clinical diagnositic criteria: pruritus, typical morphology and distribution (flexural lichenification), and a tendency toward chronicity
- Also helpful: a personal or family history of atopic disease, xerosis-ichthyosis, facial pallor with infraorbital darkening, elevated serum IgE, fissures under the ear lobes, tendency toward hand dermatitis, tendency toward repeated skin infections, and nipple eczema

TREATMENT

MEDICATIONS

Local treatments

- Corticosteroids: apply sparingly 2–4 times daily; begin with hydrocortisone, Aclovate, or Desonide and use triamcinolone 0.1% for short periods
- Taper corticosteroids when the dermatitis clears to avoid both tachyphylaxis, steroid side effects, and to prevent rebounds
- Doxepin cream 5%: may use up to 4 times daily; is best applied simultaneously with the topical steroid; stinging and drowsiness occur in 25%
- Tacrolimus ointment (Protopic): effective as a first-line steroid-sparing agent, available in 0.03% and 0.1% and applied twice daily
- Burning on application occurs in about half but may resolve with continued treatment; does not appear to cause steroid side effects and is safe on the face and eyelids
- Pimecrolimus (Elidel) cream 1% is similar, but burns less

Systemic and adjuvant therapies

- Immunosuppressives, oral antipruritic agents, and phototherapy

Treatment by stage of dermatitis

- Acute weeping lesions: use saline or aluminum subacetate solution (Domeboro tablets) or colloidal oatmeal (Aveeno; dispense one box) as soothing or astringent soaks or wet dressings for 10–30 min 2–4 times a day
- Lesions on extremities may be bandaged for protection at night
- Steroid lotions or creams are preferred to ointments
- Tacrolimus may not be tolerated; systemic steroids are last resort

Subacute or scaly lesions (lesions are dry but still red and pruritic)

- Mid- to high-potency steroids in ointment form if tolerated—creams if not—should be continued until scaling and elevated skin lesions are cleared and itching is decreased; then begin a 2- to 4-week taper with topical steroids

THERAPEUTIC PROCEDURES

- Avoid things that dry or irritate the skin: low humidity and dry air
- Other triggers: sweating, overbathing, animal danders, scratchy fabrics
- Do not bathe more than once daily and use soap only on armpits, groin, and feet; preferred: Dove, Eucerin, Aveeno, Basis, Alpha Keri, Purpose
- After rinsing, pat the skin dry (not rub) and then, before it dries completely, cover with a thin film of emollient such as Aquaphor, Eucerin, Vaseline
- Triceram cream is a less greasy moisturizer and antiinflammatory, but is much more expensive

OUTCOME

COMPLICATIONS

- Treatment complications
  - Monitor for skin atrophy
  - Eczema herpeticum, a generalized herpes simplex infection manifested by monomorphic vesicles, crusts, or erosions superimposed on atopic dermatitis or other extensive eczematous processes
- Smallpox vaccination is absolutely contraindicated in patients with atopic dermatitis or a history thereof because of the risk of eczema vaccinatum
- Atopic dermatitis patients may develop generalized vaccinia by contact with recent vaccine recipients who still have pustular or crusted vaccination sites

PROGNOSIS

- Runs a chronic or intermittent course
- Affected adults may have only hand dermatitis
- Poor prognostic factors for persistence into adulthood: onset early in childhood, early generalized disease, and asthma; only 40–60% of these patients have lasting remissions

WHEN TO REFER

- If there is a question about the diagnosis, if recommended therapy is ineffective, or if specialized treatment is necessary

EVIDENCE

PRACTICE GUIDELINES

- American Academy of Dermatology http://www.aadassociation.org/Guidelines/atopic.html

WEB SITES

- American Academy of Dermatology http://www.aad.org
- Dermatology Handbook for Family Practice from the University of Iowa http://www.vh.org/Providers/ClinRef/FPHandbook/17.html

INFORMATION FOR PATIENTS

- American Academy of Dermatology http://www.aad.org/pamphlets/
- National Institute of Arthritis and Musculoskeletal and Skin Diseases http://www.niams.nih.gov/hi/topics/dermatitis/index.html

REFERENCES

- Jaffe R: Atopic dermatitis. Prim Care 2000;27:503. [PMID: 10815058]
- Leung DY et al: Atopic dermatitis. Lancet 2003:361:151. [PMID: 12531593]

Timothy G. Berger, MD

Dermatitis, Contact

 KEY FEATURES

ESSENTIALS OF DIAGNOSIS

- Erythema and edema, with pruritus, often followed by vesicles and bullae in an area of contact with a suspected agent
- Later, weeping, crusting, or secondary infection
- A history of previous reaction to suspected contactant
- Patch test with agent positive

GENERAL CONSIDERATIONS

- An acute or chronic dermatitis that results from direct skin contact with chemicals or allergens
- Eighty percent of cases are due to excessive exposure to or additive effects of primary or universal irritants (eg, soaps, detergents, organic solvents) and are called irritant contact dermatitis
- The minority are due to actual contact allergy such as poison ivy or poison oak
- The most common topicals causing allergic rashes include antimicrobials (especially neomycin), antihistamines, anesthetics (benzocaine), hair dyes, preservatives (eg, parabens), latex, and adhesive tape
- Occupational exposure is an important cause of allergic contact dermatitis
- Weeping and crusting are typically due to allergic and not irritant dermatitis, which often appears red and scaly
- Contact dermatitis due to latex rubber in gloves is of special concern in health care workers
- Etiology of allergic contact dermatitis
  - Antimicrobials (eg, neomycin)
  - Antihistamines
  - Anesthetics (eg, benzocaine)
  - Hair dyes
  - Preservatives (eg, parabens)
  - Latex
  - Adhesive tape
- Etiology of irritant contact dermatitis
  - Soaps
  - Detergents
  - Organic solvents

 CLINICAL FINDINGS

SYMPTOMS AND SIGNS

- See Table 7 (page 1202)
- The acute phase is characterized by tiny vesicles and weepy and crusted lesions
- Resolving or chronic contact dermatitis presents with scaling, erythema, and possibly thickened skin; itching, burning, and stinging may be severe
- The lesions, distributed on exposed parts or in bizarre asymmetric patterns, consist of erythematous macules, papules, and vesicles
- The affected area is often hot and swollen, with exudation and crusting, simulating and at times complicated by infection
- The pattern of the eruption may be diagnostic (eg, typical linear streaked vesicles on the extremities in poison oak or ivy dermatitis)
- The location will often suggest the cause: scalp involvement suggests hair tints, sprays, or tonics; face involvement, creams, cosmetics, soaps, shaving materials, nail polish; neck involvement, jewelry, hair dyes, etc

DIFFERENTIAL DIAGNOSIS

- Impetigo
- Scabies
- Dermatophytid reaction (allergy or sensitivity to fungi)
- Atopic dermatitis
- Pomphylox
- Asymmetric distribution, blotchy erythema around the face, linear lesions, and a history of exposure help distinguish contact dermatitis from other skin lesions
- The most commonly confused diagnosis is impetigo, in which case Gram stain and culture will rule out impetigo or secondary infection (impetiginization)

 DIAGNOSIS

LABORATORY TESTS

- During the acute episode, patch testing cannot be performed; after the episode has cleared, the patch test may be useful, but not all potential allergens are available for testing; in the event of a positive reaction, the clinical relevance of the chemical agent to the dermatitis must be determined

DIAGNOSTIC PROCEDURES

- If itching is generalized and impetiginized scabies is considered, a scraping for mites should be done

TREATMENT

MEDICATIONS

- See Table 6 (page 1199)
- Vesicular and weepy lesions often require systemic steroid therapy
- Localized involvement (except on the face) can often be managed solely with topical agents
- Irritant contact dermatitis is treated by protection from the irritant and use of topical steroids as for atopic dermatitis

Local measures

- Acute weeping dermatitis
  - Compresses are most often used
  - Calamine or starch shake lotions may sometimes be used in intervals between wet dressings, especially for involvement of intertriginous areas or when oozing is not marked
  - Lesions on the extremities may be bandaged with wet dressings for 30–60 min several times a day
  - Potent topical corticosteroids in gel or cream form may help suppress acute contact dermatitis and relieve itching
  - In cases where weeping is marked or in intertriginous areas, ointments will make the skin even more macerated and should be avoided
  - Suggested topical steroid preparations are fluocinonide gel, 0.05%, used two or three times daily with compresses, or clobetasol or halobetasol cream, used twice daily for a maximum of 2 weeks—not in body folds or on the face; this should be followed by tapering of the number of applications per day or use of a mid-potency steroid such as triamcinolone 0.1% cream to prevent rebound of the dermatitis
  - A soothing formulation is 0.1% triamcinolone acetonide in Sarna lotion (0.5% camphor, 0.5% menthol, 0.5% phenol)
- Subacute dermatitis (subsiding)
  - Mid-potency (triamcinolone 0.1%) to high-potency steroids (amcinonide, fluocinonide, desoximetasone) are the mainstays of therapy
- Chronic dermatitis (dry and lichenified)
  - High- to highest-potency steroids are used in ointment form

Systemic therapy

- For acute severe cases, give prednisone orally for 12–21 days

- Prednisone, 60 mg for 4–7 days, 40 mg for 4–7 days, and 20 mg for 4–7 days without a further taper is one useful regimen or dispense 78 5-mg pills to be taken 12 the first day, 11 the second day, and so on
- The key is to use enough corticosteroid (and as early as possible) to achieve a clinical effect and to taper slowly enough to avoid rebound
- A Medrol Dosepak (methylprednisolone) with 5 days of medication is inappropriate on both counts

OUTCOME

PROGNOSIS

- Self-limited if reexposure is prevented but often takes 2–3 weeks for full resolution

WHEN TO REFER

- Occupational allergic contact dermatitis should be referred to a dermatologist

PREVENTION

- Prompt and thorough removal of allergens by washing with water or solvents or other chemical agents may be effective if done very shortly after exposure to poison oak or ivy
- Several barrier creams (eg, Stokogard, Ivy Shield) offer some protection to patients at high risk for poison oak and ivy dermatitis if applied before exposure
- Iodoquinol cream (Vioform) may benefit nickel allergic patients
- Ingestion of rhus antigen is of limited clinical value for the induction of tolerance
- The mainstay of prevention is identification of agents causing the dermatitis and avoidance of exposure or use of protective clothing and gloves

EVIDENCE

PRACTICE GUIDELINES

- Bourke J et al: Guidelines for care of contact dermatitis. Br J Dermatol 2001;145(6):877.
- American Academy of Dermatology http://www.aadassociation.org/ Guidelines/contderm.html

WEB SITES

- American Academy of Dermatology http://www.aad.org
- Dermatology Handbook for Family Practice from the University of Iowa http://www.vh.org/Providers/ClinRef/ FPHandbook/17.html

INFORMATION FOR PATIENTS

- American Academy of Dermatology http://www.aad.org/pamphlets/
- American Academy of Pediatrics http://www.medem.com/search/article_ display.cfm?path=\\TANQUERAY\M_ ContentItem&mstr=/M_ContentItem/ ZZZO4AUVQ7C.html&soc=AAP& srch_typ=NAV_SERCH
- American Academy of Family Physicians http://familydoctor.org/handouts/176. html

REFERENCES

- Belsito DV: The diagnostic evaluation, treatment, and prevention of allergic contact dermatitis in the new millennium. J Allergy Clin Immunol 2000;105:409. [PMID: 10719287]
- Tanner TL: Rhus (Toxicodendron) dermatitis. Prim Care 2000;27:493. [PMID: 10815057]

Timothy G. Berger, MD

Dermatitis, Exfoliating

 KEY FEATURES

ESSENTIALS OF DIAGNOSIS

- Scaling and erythema over most of the body
- Itching, malaise, fever, chills, weight loss

GENERAL CONSIDERATIONS

- A preexisting dermatosis is the cause in up to 65% of cases, including psoriasis, atopic dermatitis, contact dermatitis, pityriasis rubra pilaris, and seborrheic dermatitis
- Reactions to topical or systemic drugs (eg, sulfonamides) account for perhaps 20–40% of cases and cancer (cutaneous T cell lymphoma, Sézary syndrome) for 10–20%
- Causation of the remainder is indeterminable
- At the time of acute presentation, without a clear-cut prior history of skin disease or drug exposure, it may be impossible to make a specific diagnosis of the underlying condition, and diagnosis may require observation
- Generalized lymphadenopathy may be due to lymphoma or leukemia or may be part of the clinical picture of the skin disease (dermatopathic lymphadenitis)

Etiology

- Idiopathic
- Drug eruption
- Seborrheic dermatitis
- Contact dermatitis
- Atopic dermatitis
- Psoriasis
- Cancer (Sézary syndrome of cutaneous T cell lymphoma, Hodgkin's disease)
- Pityriasis rubra pilaris

 CLINICAL FINDINGS

SYMPTOMS AND SIGNS

- See Table 7 (page 1202)
- Symptoms may include itching, weakness, malaise, fever, and weight loss
- Chills are prominent
- Redness and scaling may be generalized and sometimes includes loss of hair and nails
- Generalized lymphadenopathy
- The mucosa is spared

DIFFERENTIAL DIAGNOSIS

- Psoriasis
- Seborrheic dermatitis
- Drug eruption

 DIAGNOSIS

LABORATORY TESTS

- Peripheral leukocytes may show clonal rearrangements of the T cell receptor in Sézary syndrome

DIAGNOSTIC PROCEDURES

- A skin biopsy is required and may show changes of a specific inflammatory dermatitis or cutaneous T cell lymphoma or leukemia

TREATMENT

MEDICATIONS

- See Table 6 (page 1199)
- Stop all drugs, if possible
- Systemic corticosteroids may provide spectacular improvement in severe or fulminant exfoliative dermatitis, but long-term therapy should be avoided
- For cases of psoriatic erythroderma and pityriasis rubra pilaris, either acitretin or methotrexate may be indicated
- Erythroderma secondary to lymphoma or leukemia requires specific topical or systemic chemotherapy
- Suitable antibiotic drugs with coverage for *Staphylococcus* should be given when there is evidence of bacterial infection

THERAPEUTIC PROCEDURES

- Home treatment is with cool to tepid baths and application of mid-potency steroids under wet dressings or with the use of an occlusive plastic suit

 OUTCOME

FOLLOW-UP

- It may be impossible to identify the cause of exfoliative dermatitis early in the course of the disease, so careful follow-up is necessary
- Psoriasis, severe seborrheic dermatitis, and drug eruptions may have an erythrodermic phase

COMPLICATIONS

- Debility (protein loss) and dehydration may develop in patients with generalized inflammatory exfoliative erythroderma
- Sepsis
- Systemic corticosteroids must be used with caution because some patients with erythroderma have psoriasis and could develop pustular psoriasis

PROGNOSIS

- Most patients recover completely or improve greatly over time but may require chronic therapy
- Deaths are rare in the absence of cutaneous T cell lymphoma
- A minority of patients will suffer from undiminished erythroderma for indefinite periods

WHEN TO REFER

- Early referral is frequently helpful

WHEN TO ADMIT

- If the exfoliative erythroderma becomes chronic and is not manageable in an outpatient setting, hospitalize the patient
- Keep the room at a constant warm temperature and provide the same topical treatment as for an outpatient

EVIDENCE

WEB SITES

- American Academy of Dermatology
  http://www.aad.org
- Dermatology Handbook for Family Practice from the University of Iowa
  http://www.vh.org/Providers/ClinRef/FPHandbook/17.html

INFORMATION FOR PATIENTS

- American Academy of Dermatology
  http://www.aad.org/pamphlets/
- Mayo Clinic
  http://www.mayoclinic.com/invoke.cfm?id=DS00339
- National Institutes of Health Medical Encyclopedia
  http://www.nlm.nih.gov/medlineplus/ency/article/001610.htm

REFERENCES

- Karakayli G et al: Exfoliative dermatitis. Am Fam Physician 1999;59:625. [PMID: 10029788]
- Levine N: Exfoliative erythroderma. Skin biopsy is required to determine the cause of this pruritic eruption. Geriatrics 2000;55:25. [PMID: 10953683]

Timothy G. Berger, MD

Dermatitis, Seborrheic

 KEY FEATURES

 CLINICAL FINDINGS

 DIAGNOSIS

ESSENTIALS OF DIAGNOSIS

- Dry scales and underlying erythema
- Scalp, central face, presternal, interscapular areas, umbilicus, and body folds

GENERAL CONSIDERATIONS

- An acute or chronic papulosquamous dermatitis
- May represent an inflammatory reaction to *Malassezia furfur* yeasts

SYMPTOMS AND SIGNS

- See Table 7 (page 1202)
- Clinical spectrum ranges from simple dandruff to seborrheic dermatitis to scalp psoriasis
- The scalp, face, chest, back, umbilicus, eyelid margins, and body folds have dry scales or oily yellowish scurf
- Fissuring and secondary infection are occasionally present
- On the scalp, the presence of well-demarcated red plaques is termed psoriasis, and general erythema without tight, thick, silvery scale is called seborrheic dermatitis; the presence of mild scaling without any erythema is termed simple dandruff
- Scaling of the scalp due to tinea capitis may simulate dandruff or seborrheic dermatitis, but alopecia is usually present in tinea capitis; pruritus is an inconstant finding
- May be seen in Parkinson's disease or in patients with HIV infection

DIFFERENTIAL DIAGNOSIS

- Psoriasis
- Atopic dermatitis (eczema)
- Impetigo
- Tinea capitis
- Contact dermatitis
- Tinea versicolor
- Pityriasis rosea

LABORATORY TESTS

- Diagnosis made clinically

TREATMENT

MEDICATIONS

- See Table 8 (page 1203)

The scalp

- Shampoos that contain zinc pyrithione or selenium are used daily if possible
- These may be alternated with ketoconazole shampoo (1% or 2%) used twice weekly; a combination of shampoos is used in refractory cases
- Tar shampoos are also effective for milder cases and for scalp psoriasis
- Topical corticosteroid solutions or lotions are then added if necessary and are used twice daily

Facial

- A mild corticosteroid (hydrocortisone 1%, alclometasone, desonide) used intermittently and not near the eyes; these are rarely indicated for seborrheic dermatitis
- If this is not effective, ketoconazole (Nizoral) 2% cream is added twice daily
- Topical tacrolimus (Protopic) and pimecrolimus (Elidel) are steroid-sparing alternatives

Nonhairy areas

- Low-potency steroid creams—ie, 1% or 2.5% hydrocortisone, desonide, or alclometasone dipropionate—are highly effective

Intertriginous areas

- Avoid greasy ointments
- Apply low-potency steroid lotions or creams twice daily for 5–7 days and then once or twice weekly for maintenance as necessary
- Ketoconazole cream may be a useful adjunct
- Tacrolimus or pimecrolimus topically may avoid steroid atrophy in chronic cases

THERAPEUTIC PROCEDURES

- "Marginal blepharitis" usually responds to gentle cleaning of the lid margins nightly with undiluted Johnson and Johnson Baby Shampoo

 ## OUTCOME

COMPLICATIONS

- Potent fluorinated corticosteroids used on the face may produce steroid rosacea or atrophy and telangiectasia

PROGNOSIS

- The tendency is to lifelong recurrences, with outbreaks lasting weeks, months, or years

WHEN TO REFER

- If there is a question about the diagnosis, if recommended therapy is ineffective, or if specialized treatment is necessary

 ## EVIDENCE

PRACTICE GUIDELINES

- National Guideline Clearinghouse http://www.guideline.gov/summary/summary.aspx?doc_id=3392&nbr=2618&string=seborrheic+dermatitis

WEB SITES

- American Academy of Dermatology http://www.aad.org
- Dermatology Handbook for Family Practice from the University of Iowa http://www.vh.org/Providers/ClinRef/FPHandbook/17.html

INFORMATION FOR PATIENTS

- American Academy of Family Physicians http://familydoctor.org/handouts/157.html
- National Institutes of Health http://www.nlm.nih.gov/medlineplus/ency/article/000963.htm

REFERENCE

- Johnson BA et al: Treatment of seborrheic dermatitis. Am Fam Physician 2000;61:2703. [PMID: 10821151]

Timothy G. Berger, M.D

Dermatophytid

 KEY FEATURES

ESSENTIALS OF DIAGNOSIS

- Pruritic, grouped vesicular lesions involving the sides and flexor aspects of the fingers and the palms
- Fungal infection elsewhere on the body, usually the feet
- No fungus demonstrable in lesions

GENERAL CONSIDERATIONS

- Dermatophytid must be considered in the differential diagnosis of vesicles on the hands and feet
- It is a hypersensitivity reaction to an active focus of inflammatory dermatophytosis elsewhere on the body, usually the feet
- Fungi are present in the primary lesions but are not present in the lesions of dermatophytid
- The hands are most often affected, but dermatophytid may occur on other areas

 CLINICAL FINDINGS

SYMPTOMS AND SIGNS

- See Table 7 (page 1203)
- Itching is the only symptom
- Vesicular eruptions of the hands

DIFFERENTIAL DIAGNOSIS

- Contact dermatitis
- Pomphylox
- Photosensitive drug eruption
- Scabies
- Vesicular tinea
- "id" reaction to other infectious or inflammatory conditions

 DIAGNOSIS

LABORATORY TESTS

- This entity is best diagnosed morphologically and by response to treatment

TREATMENT

MEDICATIONS

- See Table 6 (page 1199)
- The primary focus of tinea should be treated with an oral antifungal or by local measures
- Topical steroids with occlusion may benefit

 OUTCOME

PROGNOSIS

- Clears with adequate treatment of the primary infection elsewhere on the body
- An initial flare can occur when oral therapy is started
- Recurrences are not uncommon

WHEN TO REFER

- If there is a question about the diagnosis, if recommended therapy is ineffective, or specialized treatment is necessary

EVIDENCE

PRACTICE GUIDELINES

- American Academy of Dermatology http://www.aadassociation.org/ Guidelines/tineacapitis.html
- Drake LA et al: Guidelines of care for superficial mycotic infections of the skin: pityriasis (tinea) versicolor. Guidelines/Outcomes Committee. American Academy of Dermatology. J Am Acad Dermatol 1996;34(2 Pt 1):287.

WEB SITES

- American Academy of Dermatology http://www.aad.org
- Dermatology Handbook for Family Practice from the University of Iowa http://www.vh.org/Providers/ClinRef/ FPHandbook/17.html

INFORMATION FOR PATIENTS

- American Academy of Dermatology http://www.aad.org/pamphlets/
- American Academy of Family Physicians http://familydoctor.org/handouts/316. html

REFERENCE

- Busch RF: Dermatophytid reaction and chronic otitis externa. Otolaryngol Head Neck Surg 1998;118(3 Part 1):420. [PMID: 9727132]

Timothy G. Berger, MD

Diabetes Insipidus

 ## KEY FEATURES

ESSENTIALS OF DIAGNOSIS

- Polyuria (2–20 L/day); polydipsia
- Urine specific gravity usually <1.006 during ad libitum fluid intake
- Urine is otherwise normal
- Vasopressin reduces urine output except in nephrogenic diabetes insipidus (DI)

GENERAL CONSIDERATIONS

- Uncommon disease caused by a deficiency of or resistance to vasopressin

Deficiency of vasopressin

- Primary DI (no lesion on MRI of pituitary and hypothalamus) may be familial or idiopathic
- Secondary DI is due to damage to hypothalamus or pituitary stalk by tumor, anoxic encephalopathy, surgical or accidental trauma, infection (eg, encephalitis, tuberculosis, syphilis), sarcoidosis, or multifocal Langerhans cell (eosinophilic) granulomatosis ("histiocytosis X")
- Metastases to pituitary cause DI more than pituitary adenomas (33% vs. 1%)
- Vasopressinase-induced DI may occur in last trimester of pregnancy and postpartum, often associated with oligohydramnios, preeclampsia, or hepatic dysfunction

"Nephrogenic" diabetes insipidus

- Due to defect in kidney tubules that interferes with water reabsorption
- Polyuria is unresponsive to vasopressin and patients have normal vasopressin secretion
- Congenital nephrogenic DI is X-linked, present from birth, and due to defective expression of renal vasopressin V2 receptors or vasopressin-sensitive water channels
- Acquired form less severe, seen in pyelonephritis, amyloidosis, multiple myeloma, hypokalemia, Sjögren's syndrome, sickle cell anemia, hypercalcemia, recovery from acute tubular necrosis
- May be caused by drugs, eg, glucocorticoids, diuretics, demeclocycline, tetracycline, lithium, foscarnet, methicillin

DEMOGRAPHICS

- In familial autosomal dominant central DI, symptoms begin at about age 2 years

 ## CLINICAL FINDINGS

SYMPTOMS AND SIGNS

- Intense thirst, especially for ice water
- Polyuria
- 2 L to 20 L of fluid ingested daily, with corresponding urine volumes
- Although most patients with DI maintain fluid balance, dehydration and hypernatremia occur if patients are unable to drink or if hypothalamic thirst center is damaged by shock, anoxia, or tumor
- Partial DI presents with less intense symptoms and should be suspected in unremitting enuresis

DIFFERENTIAL DIAGNOSIS

- Central DI
- Nephrogenic DI
- Osmotic diuresis, eg, diabetes mellitus
- Polyuria from Cushing's syndrome, glucocorticoids, or lithium
- Excessive fluid intake: psychogenic polydipsia, IV fluids, CNS sarcoidosis

 ## DIAGNOSIS

LABORATORY TESTS

- 24 h urine collection for volume (<2 L/day rules out DI in adults), glucose (to screen for diabetes mellitus), creatinine (to ensure accurate collection and assess creatinine clearance)
- Serum for osmolality, glucose (to screen for diabetes mellitus as cause for polyuria), potassium (hypokalemia causes polyuria), sodium, uric acid
- Urinalysis: low specific gravity but is otherwise normal, without glucosuria seen in diabetes mellitus
- Serum osmolality greater than urine osmolality
- Hypernatremia
- In nephrogenic DI, serum vasopressin is high during modest fluid restriction
- Hyperuricemia implicates central DI
- "Vasopressin challenge test" if suspect central DI
  - Desmopressin acetate, 0.05–0.1 mL (5–10 µg) intranasally or 1 µg SQ or IV, measuring urine volume for 12 h prior to and 12 h after administration
  - Obtain serum sodium immediately if symptoms of hyponatremia
  - Patients with central DI notice reduction in thirst and polyuria
  - Serum sodium remains normal except in some salt-losing conditions
  - If marginal response, desmopressin dosage is doubled

IMAGING STUDIES

- In nonfamilial central DI, MRI of pituitary and hypothalamus is done to look for mass lesions
- Absence of a posterior pituitary "bright spot" on T1-weighted MRI is suggestive of central DI

DIAGNOSTIC PROCEDURES

- Diagnosis of DI as cause of polyuria or hypernatremia mostly requires clinical judgment

Diabetes Insipidus

TREATMENT

MEDICATIONS

- Mild cases require only adequate fluid intake
- Reduction of aggravating factors (eg, glucocorticoids) improves polyuria
- Desmopressin is treatment of choice for central DI
- Desmopressin useful for DI in pregnancy or postpartum, since it is resistant to degradation by vasopressinase
- Intranasal: start at 0.05–0.1 mL (100 µg/mL solution) intranasally Q 12–24 h, then individualize according to thirst and polyuria. May cause sinusitis
- Parenteral: dose is 1–4 µg IV, IM, or subcutaneously Q 12–24 h PRN thirst or hypernatremia
- Oral: start at 0.05 mg PO BID, increase up to 0.4 mg Q 8 h; especially useful for patients with sinusitis from nasal preparation. May cause hepatic enzymes elevation; avoid use in liver disease
- Hyponatremia is uncommon if minimum effective doses are used and occasional thirst is allowed
- Central and nephrogenic DI respond partially to hydrochlorothiazide 50–100 mg/day (with potassium supplement or amiloride)
- Nephrogenic DI may respond to indomethacin, 50 mg PO Q 8 h, or to combined indomethacin-hydrochlorothiazide, indomethacin-desmopressin, or indomethacin-amiloride
- Psychotherapy for patients with compulsive water drinking. Thioridazine and lithium are best avoided if drug therapy needed, since they cause polyuria

OUTCOME

COMPLICATIONS

- Without water, excessive urine output leads to severe dehydration
- Patients with impaired thirst mechanism are prone to hypernatremia, particularly when impaired mentation causes them to forget to take desmopressin
- With desmopressin acetate therapy, there is risk of water intoxication
- Desmopressin may cause nasal irritation, sinusitis, agitation, erythromelalgia

PROGNOSIS

- Chronic central DI is more an inconvenience than a dire medical condition. Desmopressin treatment allows normal sleep and activity
- Central DI appearing after pituitary surgery usually remits after days to weeks but may be permanent if upper pituitary stalk is cut
- Central DI is made transiently worse by glucocorticoids in high doses frequently given perioperatively
- Hypernatremia can occur, especially when thirst center is damaged
- Central DI itself does not reduce life expectancy if hypothalamic thirst center is intact. Prognosis is that of underlying disorder

EVIDENCE

PRACTICE GUIDELINES

- Dehydration and fluid maintenance. American Medical Directors Association, 2001
  http://www.guidelines.gov/summary/summary.aspx?doc_id=3305&nbr=2531&string=Diabetes+Insipidus
- Singer PA et al: Postoperative endocrine management of pituitary tumors. Neurosurg Clin North Am 2003;14:123. [PMID: 12690984]

WEB SITES

- Diabetes Insipidus Foundation http://www.diabetesinsipidus.org/
- MEDLINEplus—Diabetes Insipidus http://www.nlm.nih.gov/medlineplus/diabetesinsipidus.html
- Nephrogenic Diabetes Insipidus Foundation http://www.ndif.org/

INFORMATION FOR PATIENTS

- Mayo Clinic—Diabetes insipidus http://www.mayoclinic.com/invoke.cfm?id=AN00126
- MEDLINEplus—Diabetes insipidus http://www.nlm.nih.gov/medlineplus/diabetesinsipidus.html
- NIDDK/NIH—Diabetes insipidus http://kidney.niddk.nih.gov/kudiseases/pubs/insipidus/index.htm

REFERENCES

- Maghnie M et al: Central diabetes insipidus in children and young adults. N Engl J Med 2000;343:998. [PMID: 11018166]
- Wong LL et al: Systemic diseases associated with disorders of water homeostasis. Endocrinol Metab Clin North Am 2002;231:121. [PMID: 12055984]

Paul A. Fitzgerald, MD

Diabetes Mellitus, Gestational

 KEY FEATURES

ESSENTIALS OF DIAGNOSIS

- Euglycemia should be established before pregnancy
- Fasting and preprandial glucose values are lower during pregnancy in both diabetic and nondiabetic women
- During pregnancy, euglycemia is 60–80 mg/dL while fasting and 30–45 min before meals and <120 mg/dL 2 h after meals
- At least two abnormal values on a 3-h glucose tolerance test (GTT)

GENERAL CONSIDERATIONS

- Pregnancy is a natural state of insulin resistance from placental lactogen and elevated circulating estrogens and progesterone
- Depending on the population screened, a significant proportion may evidence glucose intolerance, which can have implications for adverse fetal outcome
- Type I diabetics express particular HLA haplotypes with antiislet cell antibodies
- Type II diabetics have minimal risk of ketoacidosis

DEMOGRAPHICS

- Women at higher risk include those of Hispanic, African-American, Native American, Asian, Pacific Island, or Indigenous Australian ancestry
- Prior history of gestational diabetes
- Prior history of adverse pregnancy outcome
- First-degree relative with diabetes mellitus
- Body mass index ≥30

 CLINICAL FINDINGS

SYMPTOMS AND SIGNS

- Polyuria and thirst
- Weakness or fatigue
- Recurrent blurred vision
- Macrosomia
- Polyhydramnios
- Often asymptomatic

DIFFERENTIAL DIAGNOSIS

- Drugs: glucocorticoids, thiazides, tacrolimus
- Diabetes insipidus
- Psychogenic polydipsia
- Nondiabetic glycosuria (benign)

 DIAGNOSIS

LABORATORY TESTS

- See Table 70 (page 1262)
- The target for glycemic control during pregnancy is euglycemia of 60–80 mg/dL while fasting and 30–45 min before meals and <120 mg/dL 2 h after meals
- Glycated hemoglobin levels help determine the quality of glucose control both before and during pregnancy
- Glucose challenge test at 24–28 weeks with 50 g oral glucose load and venous sample 1 h later
- Cut-off value of 130 mg/dL or higher requires follow-up with 3-h GTT
- Normal values for glucose challenge test and fasting blood sugar are 95 mg/dL; 1 h 180 mg/dL; 2 h 155 mg/dL; 3 h 140 mg/dL
- Two or more abnormal values required for diagnosis of gestational diabetes

TREATMENT

MEDICATIONS

Before pregnancy

- Subcutaneous insulin in a split-dose regimen with frequent dosage adjustments
- Patients taking oral agents prior to pregnancy should be switched to insulin but glyburide may be safe and effective in pregnancy

During pregnancy

- 15% of patients with gestational diabetes require insulin during pregnancy
- Dietary therapy with 1800–2200 kcal/day
- Insulin therapy for persistent fasting blood sugar at ≥90 mg/dL or 2 h postprandial values of ≥120 mg/dL
- Glyburide may be safe and effective in pregnancy
- Continuous insulin pump therapy is very useful in type 1 diabetes mellitus

SURGERY

- Cesarean sections are performed for obstetric indications

THERAPEUTIC PROCEDURES

- The risk of fetal demise in the third trimester (stillbirth) and neonatal death increases with the level of hyperglycemia. Consequently, pregnant women with diabetes must receive regular antepartum fetal testing (nonstress testing, contraction stress testing, biophysical profile) during the third trimester

Timing of delivery

- Dictated by the quality of diabetic control, the presence or absence of medical complications, and fetal status
- The goal is to reach 39 weeks (38 completed weeks) and then proceed with delivery
- Confirmation of lung maturity is necessary only for delivery prior to 39 weeks

 OUTCOME

FOLLOW-UP

- Patients should be evaluated 6–8 weeks postpartum by a 2-h oral glucose tolerance test (75 g glucose load)
- Following delivery insulin dosage needs to be adjusted down to prepregnancy levels

COMPLICATIONS

- Infants of diabetic mothers are at risk for macrosomia
- Congenital anomalies result from hyperglycemia during the first 4–8 weeks of pregnancy. They occur in 4–10% of diabetic pregnancies (two to three times the rate in nondiabetic pregnancies)
- Euglycemia in the early weeks of pregnancy, when organogenesis is occurring, reduces the rate of anomalies to near-normal levels. Even so, because euglycemia is not consistently achieved, congenital anomalies are the principal cause of perinatal fetal deaths in diabetic pregnancies
- Hydramnios, preeclampsia-eclampsia, infections, and prematurity are increased even in carefully managed diabetic pregnancies

PROGNOSIS

- Pregnancy does not appear to alter the long-term consequences of diabetes, but retinopathy and nephropathy may first appear or become worse during pregnancy

WHEN TO REFER

- All women with diabetes should receive prepregnancy management by physicians experienced in diabetic pregnancies

WHEN TO ADMIT

- Failed intensive outpatient management of hypo- or hyperglycemia
- Diagnosis of ketoacidosis
- Major complication of pregnancy

PREVENTION

- Prepregnancy HbA_{1c} levels of less than 8% should be achieved to reduce the incidence of congenital anomalies

 EVIDENCE

PRACTICE GUIDELINES

- National Guideline Clearinghouse
  http://www.guideline.gov/summary/
  summary.aspx?doc_id=3580&nbr=2806
  &string=gestational+diabetes
  http://www.guideline.gov/summary/
  summary.aspx?doc_id=3493&nbr=
  2719&string=gestational+diabetes

WEB SITES

- Clinical Guidelines in Obstetrics and Gynecology
  http://www.rcog.org.uk/guidelines.asp?
  PageID=105
- Guidelines, Recommendations, and Evidence-Based Medicine in Obstetrics
  http://matweb.hcuge.ch/matweb/endo/
  cours_4e_MREG/obstetrics_
  gynecology_guidelines.htm

INFORMATION FOR PATIENTS

- Patient Information for Obstetrics and Gynecology
  http://www.vh.org/Patients/IHB/
  ObGyn.html
- National Institute of Child Health and Human Development
  http://www.nichd.nih.gov/about/
  womenhealth/disorders_of_pregnancy.
  cfm

REFERENCES

- Diabetes and Pregnancy. ACOG technical bulletin No. 200, 2001. Compendium of Selected Publications, American College of Obstetricians and Gynecologists. 2000:393. [PMID: 11547793]
- Gabbe SG et al: Benefits, risks, costs and patient satisfaction associated with insulin pump therapy for the pregnancy complicated by type 1 diabetes mellitus. Am J Obstet Gynecol 2000;182:1283. [PMID: 10871440]
- Temple R et al: Association between outcome of pregnancy and glyceamic control in early pregnancy in type I diabetics: population based study. BMJ 2002;325(7375):1275. [PMID: 12458245]

William R. Crombleholme, MD

Diabetes Mellitus, Type 1

 ## KEY FEATURES

ESSENTIALS OF DIAGNOSIS

- Polyuria, polydipsia, and weight loss associated with random plasma glucose ≥200 mg/dL
- Plasma glucose of 126 mg/dL or higher after an overnight fast, documented on more than one occasion
- Ketonemia, ketonuria, or both

GENERAL CONSIDERATIONS

- Due to pancreatic islet B cell destruction
- Destruction immune mediated in over 90% of cases and idiopathic in the remainder
- About 95% of type 1 patients possess either HLA-DR3 or HLA-DR4, compared with 50% of white controls. HLA-DQB1*0302 is an even more specific marker for susceptibility
- As many as 85% are positive for islet cell antibodies, anti-glutamic acid decarboxylase (GAD), antiinsulin, and anti-ICA 512 (tyrosine phosphatase) antibodies at diagnosis
- The rate of pancreatic B cell destruction ranges from rapid to slow
- Prone to ketoacidosis
- C-peptide negative 1 to 5 years after diagnosis; plasma glucagon is elevated

DEMOGRAPHICS

- Occurs mainly in 10- to 14-year olds, but may occur in adults, especially when hyperglycemia first appears in the nonobese or elderly
- The highest incidence is in Scandinavia; the yearly incidence per 100,000 10 to 14-year-olds is 37 in Finland. The United States averages 15 per 100,000, with higher incidences in states densely populated with persons of Scandinavian descent such as Minnesota. The lowest incidence is less than 1 per 100,000 per year in China and parts of South America
- An estimated 16 million Americans have diabetes, of whom 1.4 million have type 1 diabetes

 ## CLINICAL FINDINGS

SYMPTOMS AND SIGNS

- Increased thirst and urination
- Polyphagia with weight loss
- Ketoacidosis
- Paresthesias
- Recurrent blurred vision
- Vulvovaginitis or pruritus
- Nocturnal enuresis
- Postural hypotension from lowered plasma volume

DIFFERENTIAL DIAGNOSIS

- Type 2 diabetes
- Hyperglycemia due to other causes (glucocorticoids, Cushing's syndrome, glucagonoma, acromegaly, pheochromocytoma, pentamidine)
- Metabolic acidosis of other etiologies (alcoholic ketoacidosis)
- Nondiabetic glycosuria (renal glycosuria)

 ## DIAGNOSIS

LABORATORY TESTS

- Fasting plasma glucose >126 mg/dL or >200 mg/dL 2 h after glucose load (Table 107, page XX)
- Ketonemia, ketonuria, or both
- Glucosuria (Clinistix, Diastix)
- Ketonuria (Acetest, Ketostix)
- Glycosylated hemoglobin (hemoglobin A_{1c})—reflects glycemic control over preceding 8–12 weeks
- Serum fructosamine—reflects glycemic control over preceding 2 weeks. Helpful in presence of abnormal hemoglobins or ascertaining glycemic control at time of conception of diabetic woman
- Lipoprotein abnormalities. Unlike type 2 diabetes, moderately deficient control of hyperglycemia in type 1 diabetes is associated with only slight elevation of low-density lipoprotein (LDL) cholesterol and serum triglycerides and minimal change in high-density lipoprotein (HDL) cholesterol

TREATMENT

MEDICATIONS

Use of insulin

- See Tables 111 and 112 (page 1293 and Figure 10 (page 1291)
- Preprandial rapid-acting insulin, plus basal insulin replacement with intermediate- or long-acting insulin
- Ultra-short-acting insulin: insulin lispro, insulin aspart
- Short-acting insulins "Purified": regular, regular humulin, regular iletin II, velosulin
- Intermediate-acting insulins "Purified": lente humulin, lente iletin II, lente novalin, neutral protamine Hagedorn (NPH) humulin, NPH iletin II, NPH novalin
- Premixed insulins (% NPH/% regular): novalin 70/30, humulin 70/30 (% NPH, % insulin lispro: humulog mix 75/25)
- Long-acting insulins "Purified": ultralente humulin, insulin glargine

SURGERY

- Infuse intraoperatively and in the immediate postoperative period: D5 0.9% saline containing 20 mEq KCl IV at a rate of 100–200 mL/h. Infuse regular human insulin (25 units/250 mL 0.9% saline) into the IV tubing at a rate of 1–3 units/h
- Initially, monitor blood glucose hourly and adjust infusion for target glucose levels 100–190 mg/dL
- Patients undergoing simultaneous pancreas and kidney transplantation have an 85% chance of pancreatic graft survival and a 92% chance of renal graft survival after 1 year. Solitary pancreas transplant only for recurrent life-threatening metabolic instability
- Islet transplantation is minimally invasive. Application is limited by the need for multiple donors and potent long-term immunotherapy

THERAPEUTIC PROCEDURES

- Eucaloric healthy diet
- Limit cholesterol to 300 mg QD, protein intake to 10–20% of total calories, keep saturated fats <8–9% of total calories, remainder of diet to be made up of monounsaturated fats and carbohydrates with 20–35 g of dietary fiber

- Treat microalbuminuria with angiotensin-converting enzyme (ACE)-I inhibitor to retard diabetic nephropathy
- Treat hypertension and hyperlipidemia (reduce LDL <100 mg/dL)
- Attempts have been made to prolong the partial clinical remission ("honeymoon") using drugs that may induce immune tolerance

OUTCOME

FOLLOW-UP

- Glycemic control of HbA_{1c} no higher than 2% above upper limits of normal has 60% reduction in risk of diabetic retinopathy, nephropathy, and neuropathy

COMPLICATIONS

- Diabetic ketoacidosis
- Hypoglycemia and altered awareness of hypoglycemia
- Diabetic retinopathy, cataracts
- Nephropathy
- Neuropathy
- Diabetic atherothrombosis (coronary artery disease, peripheral vascular disease)
- Lipodystrophy at injection sites

PROGNOSIS

- The Diabetes Control and Complications Trial (DCCT) showed that the poor prognosis for 40% of patients with type 1 diabetes is markedly improved by optimal care
- Patients can have a full life
- Tight control (mean HbA_{1c} 7.2% (normal: <6%) in the DCCT was associated with a threefold greater risk of serious hypoglycemia as well as more weight gain. However, no deaths occurred because of hypoglycemia, and no evidence of posthypoglycemic cognitive damage was detected
- Subsequent renal failure predicted by microalbuminuria >30 μg/min. Risk decreased by treatment with ACE-I

WHEN TO REFER

- Team educational approach is critical. Enlist nutritionist
- Poorly controlled diabetes

WHEN TO ADMIT

- Altered mental status
- Diabetic ketoacidosis
- Marked volume disorders
- Marked electrolyte disorders
- Unstable comorbid conditions

PREVENTION

- Acetylsalicylic acid (aspirin) 81–325 mg (enteric-coated) a day to reduce risk of diabetic atherothrombosis without increasing risk of vitreous bleeding
- Instruction in personal hygiene, in particular, care of feet, skin, and teeth
- Yearly diabetic eye examination
- Patient self-management training
- Self-monitoring of blood glucose
- Exercise

EVIDENCE

PRACTICE GUIDELINES

- American Diabetes Association: Clinical practice recommendations. Diabetes Care 2002;25(Suppl 1):S1.

WEB SITES

- CDC Diabetes Web Site http://www.cdc.gov/diabetes/
- American Diabetes Association http://www.diabetesnet.com/ada.html

INFORMATION FOR PATIENTS

- JAMA patient page: Type 1 diabetes. JAMA 2003;290:2216. [PMID: 14570956]

REFERENCE

- Atkinson MA: Type 1 diabetes: new perspectives on disease pathogenesis and treatment. Lancet 2001;358:221. [PMID: 11476858]

Umesh Masharani, MB, BS; MRCH (UK)

Diabetes Mellitus, Type 2

 ## KEY FEATURES

ESSENTIALS OF DIAGNOSIS

- Typically over 40 years of age
- Obesity
- Polyuria and polydipsia
- Candidal vaginitis sometimes an initial manifestation
- Often few or no symptoms
- After an overnight fast, plasma glucose of 126 mg/dL or higher more than once
- After 75 g oral glucose, diagnostic values are 200 mg/dL or more 2 h after the oral glucose
- Often associated with hypertension, dyslipidemia, and atherosclerosis

GENERAL CONSIDERATIONS

- Circulating endogenous insulin is sufficient to prevent ketoacidosis but inadequate to prevent hyperglycemia from tissue insensitivity
- Strong genetic influences
- Prevalence of obesity in type 2 diabetes mellitus is 30% in Chinese and Japanese, 60–70% in North Americans, Europeans, and Africans, and nearly 100% in Pima Indians and Pacific Islanders from Nauru or Samoa
- Enhancers of insulin resistance are aging, sedentary life-style, and abdominal-visceral obesity
- Abdominal fat, with an abnormally high waist-to-hip ratio, is generally associated with obesity in type 2 diabetes. This visceral obesity correlates with insulin resistance, whereas subcutaneous fat seems to have less of an association
- Both the tissue resistance to insulin and the impaired B cell response to glucose are further aggravated by increased hyperglycemia, and both defects improve with decreased hyperglycemia

DEMOGRAPHICS

- 14.5 million Americans, or more than 90% of all diabetics in the United States, have type 2 diabetes
- Middle-aged adults but occasionally juveniles
- No sex predominance

 ## CLINICAL FINDINGS

SYMPTOMS AND SIGNS

- Polyuria and thirst
- Weakness or fatigue
- Recurrent blurred vision
- Vulvovaginitis or pruritis
- Peripheral neuropathy
- Often asymptomatic

DIFFERENTIAL DIAGNOSIS

Hyperglycemia

- Endocrinopathies: type 1 diabetes mellitus, Cushing's syndrome, acromegaly, pheochromocytoma, glucagonoma, somatostatinoma
- Drugs: glucocorticoids, thiazides, phenytoin, niacin, oral contraceptives, pentamidine
- Pancreatic insufficiency: subtotal pancreatectomy, chronic pancreatitis, hemochromatosis ("bronze diabetes"), cystic fibrosis, hemosiderosis
- Other: gestational diabetes, cirrhosis, Schmidt's syndrome (polyglandular failure: Addison's disease, autoimmune thyroiditis, diabetes)

Polyuria

- Diabetes insipidus

Hypercalcemia

- Psychogenic polydipsia

Nondiabetic glycosuria (benign)

- Genetic
- Fanconi's syndrome
- Chronic renal failure
- Pregnancy

 ## DIAGNOSIS

LABORATORY TESTS

- Fasting plasma glucose ≥126 mg/dL or ≥200 mg/dL 2 h after glucose load (Table 107, page 1290)
- Glucosuria (Clinistix, Diastix)
- Ketonuria on occasion without ketonemia (Acetest, Ketostix)
- Glycosylated hemoglobin (HbA_{1c}) reflects glycemic control over preceding 8–12 weeks
- Serum fructosamine reflects glycemic control over preceding 2 weeks. Helpful in the presence of abnormal hemoglobins or in ascertaining glycemic control at time of conception in diabetic women
- Lipoprotein abnormalities in obese type 2 diabetics include high serum triglyceride (300–400 mg/dL), low high-density lipoprotein (HDL) cholesterol (<30 mg/dL), and a qualitative change in low-density lipoprotein (LDL) particles, differing from type 1 diabetes, which is associated with only slight elevation of LDL cholesterol and serum triglycerides and minimal change in HDL cholesterol

TREATMENT

MEDICATIONS

- Oral agents that stimulate insulin secretion: sulfonylureas, meglitinide analogs, D-phenylalanine derivative (Table 108, page 1291)
- Insulin-sparing oral agents: buguanides, thiazolidinediones, α-glucosidase inhibitors (Table 109 and 110, pages 1291 and 1292)
- Combination oral agents: glyburide-metformin combination available but limits optimal dose adjustment of individual drugs
- Insulin: indicated for type 2 diabetics with insulinopenia and hyperglycemia unresponsive to diet and oral hypoglycemic agents
- Preprandial rapid-acting insulin plus basal insulin replacement with an intermediate-acting or long-acting insulin used to attain acceptable control of blood glucose (Tables 111 and 112, pages 1293 and Figure 10, page 1291)

SURGERY

Major surgery

- Insulin during major surgery necessary for most type 2 diabetics, even if not previously taking insulin
- Infuse IV intraoperatively and in the immediate postoperative period: 1 L D_5W with 20 mEq KCl and 10 U regular insulin at rate of about 100 mL/h
- Monitor blood glucose hourly and adjust infusion for target glucose levels 100–250 mg/dL. If blood glucose remains >250 mg/dL after 1–2 h, increase insulin infusion to 15 U/L

Minor surgery

- Regular human insulin or insulin lispro prn SQ to maintain glucose <250 mg/dL
- Avoid glucose-containing solutions

THERAPEUTIC PROCEDURES

- *Diet:* Limit cholesterol to 300 mg QD, protein intake 10–20% of total calories, saturated fats <8–9% of total calories, with remainder of diet monounsaturated fats and carbohydrates with 20–35 g of dietary fiber

OUTCOME

FOLLOW-UP

- Self-monitoring
- HbA_{1c} quarterly
- Annual screen for microalbuminuria
- Serum lipids
- Feet examination annually
- Yearly diabetic eye examination
- Treatment goals: self-monitored blood glucose, 80–120 mg/dL before meals; 100–140 mg/dL at bedtime; <180 mg/dL 1.5–2.0 h postprandially. HbA_{1c} <7.0%

COMPLICATIONS

- Hypoglycemia
- Ocular (diabetic cataracts and retinopathy)
- Diabetic nephropathy (microalbuminuria, progressive diabetic nephropathy)
- Gangrene of the feet
- Diabetic neuropathy (peripheral neuropathy, distal symmetric polyneuropathy, isolated peripheral neuropathy, painful diabetic neuropathy, autonomic neuropathy)
- Skin and mucous membranes (pyogenic infections, eruptive xanthomas from hypertriglyceridemia associated with poor glucose control, necrobiosis lipoidica diabeticorum, shin spots, intertriginous candida, vulvovaginitis)

WHEN TO REFER

- Team-oriented educational approach, including a nutritionist, is critical
- Poorly controlled diabetes

WHEN TO ADMIT

- Altered mental status
- Diabetic ketoacidosis
- Marked volume disorders
- Marked electrolyte disorders
- Unstable comorbid conditions

PROGNOSIS

- Antihypertensive control to a mean of 144/82 mm Hg had beneficial effects on all microvascular and all diabetes-related end points in the United Kingdom Prospective Diabetes Study

PREVENTION

- Goal of therapy is to prevent acute illness and reduce risk of long-term complications
- Life-style modifications can prevent or slow the development of diabetes
- Daily vigorous exercise prevents accumulation of visceral fat, which can prevent the development of diabetes
- Screen with fasting glucose at 3-year intervals beginning at age 45; screen earlier and more frequently if risk factors present

EVIDENCE

PRACTICE GUIDELINES

- National Guideline Clearinghouse http://www.guideline.gov/summary/summary.aspx?doc_id=3172&nbr=2398&string=diabetes+type+II http://www.guideline.gov/summary/summary.aspx?doc_id=3127&nbr=2353&string=diabetes+type+II
- American Association of Clinical Endocrinologists http://www.aace.com/clin/guidelines/diabetes_2002.pdf

WEB SITES

- http://www.cdc.gov/diabetes/
- http://www.joslin.harvard.edu/

INFORMATION FOR PATIENTS

- American Dietetic Association http://www.eatright.org/Public/
- JAMA patient page: The ABCs of diabetes. JAMA 2002;287(19):2608. [PMID: 12025825]

REFERENCES

- American Diabetes Association: Clinical practice recommendations. Diabetes Care 2002;25(Suppl 1):S1
- UK Prospective Diabetes Study (UKPDS) Group. Lancet 1998;352:854.

Umesh Masharani, MB, BS; MRCH (UK)

Diabetic Ketoacidosis

 KEY FEATURES

ESSENTIALS OF DIAGNOSIS

- Hyperglycemia >250 mg/dL
- Acidosis with blood pH <7.3
- Serum bicarbonate <15 mEq/L
- Serum positive for ketones

GENERAL CONSIDERATIONS

- May be the initial manifestation of type 1 diabetes
- Commonly occurs with poor compliance in type 1 diabetics, particularly when episodes are recurrent
- Develops in type 1 diabetics with increased insulin requirements during infection, trauma, myocardial infarction, or surgery
- May develop in type 2 diabetics under severe stress such as sepsis or trauma
- Common serious complication of insulin pump therapy

DEMOGRAPHICS

- Incidence is five to eight episodes per 1000 diabetic subjects annually
- Incidence in insulin pump therapy is one per 80 patient-months of treatment

 CLINICAL FINDINGS

SYMPTOMS AND SIGNS

- May begin with a day or more of polyuria, polydipsia, marked fatigue, nausea and vomiting, and, finally, mental stupor that can progress to coma
- Dehydration, possible stupor
- Rapid deep breathing and a "fruity" breath odor of acetone
- Hypotension with tachycardia indicates profound fluid and electrolyte depletion
- Mild hypothermia usually present; elevated or even a normal temperature may suggest infection
- Abdominal pain and tenderness in the absence of abdominal disease. Conversely, cholecystitis or pancreatitis may occur with minimal symptoms and signs

DIFFERENTIAL DIAGNOSIS

- Lactic acidosis in type 1 diabetics, including the use of metformin
- Alcoholic ketoacidosis
- Hypoglycemia
- Hyperglycemic hyperosmolar state
- Uremia
- Starvation ketoacidosis
- Salicylate poisoning

 DIAGNOSIS

LABORATORY TESTS

- 4+ glycosuria, hyperglycemia
- Strong ketonuria and ketonemia [acetoacetic acid measured by nitroprusside reagents (Acetest and Ketostix)]. The more prevalent β-hydroxybutyric acid has no ketone group and is therefore not detected by conventional nitroprusside tests
- Strong ketonuria, anion-gap ketoacidosis
- Serum potassium often elevated despite total body potassium depletion
- Elevated serum amylase from salivary as well as pancreatic amylase. An elevated serum amylase is not specific for acute pancreatitis
- Serum lipase may be useful if the diagnosis of pancreatitis is being seriously considered
- Leukocytosis up to 25,000/μL with a left shift may occur with or without associated infection
- Hyperchloremic metabolic acidosis can develop during initial therapy, as keto acids are lost in the urine and a portion of the bicarbonate deficit is replaced with chloride ions from the saline therapy. This relatively benign condition reverses over a day once intravenous saline is stopped

TREATMENT

MEDICATIONS

Regular insulin

- Initially in severe ketoacidosis, use only regular insulin. Begin with loading dose of 0.1 unit/kg as an intravenous bolus followed by 0.1 unit/kg/h, continuously infused or given hourly as an intramuscular injection. "Piggy-back" insulin into the fluid line so the rate of fluid replacement can be changed without altering the insulin delivery rate. If plasma glucose level fails to fall at least 10% in the first hour, give repeat loading dose

Fluids

- Fluid deficit is usually 4–5 L. In the first hour, give at least 1 L of 0.9% saline to reexpand contracted vascular volume
- One can then switch to 0.45% saline at a rate of 300–500 mL/h, depending on the severity of the dehydration and the cardiac and renal status
- Failure to give enough volume replacement (at least 3–4 L in 8 h) to restore normal perfusion affects satisfactory recovery
- Excessive fluid replacement (more than 5 L in 8 h) may contribute to acute respiratory distress syndrome or cerebral edema

Electrolytes

- Use sodium bicarbonate only for pH <7.1. For arterial pH 6.9–7.0, add one ampule of 7.5% sodium bicarbonate (44 mEq/L) to 200 mL of sterile water intravenously at a rate of 200 mL/h. If the pH is below 6.9, use two ampules of sodium bicarbonate (88 mEq) in 400 mL of sterile water at the same rate of 200 mL/h. For each ampule of sodium bicarbonate, add 15 mEq/L of potassium chloride as long as the serum potassium does not exceed 5.5 mEq/L. Stop bicarbonate when pH reaches 7.1
- When blood glucose falls to 250 mg/dL or less, use 5% glucose solutions to maintain blood glucose 200–300 mg/dL while continuing insulin to clear ketonemia
- Total body potassium loss from polyuria and vomiting may be several hundred milliequivalents. However, initial serum potassium is usually normal or high because of extracellular shifts from acidosis. Potassium infusion 20–30 mEq/h should begin 2–3 h after beginning therapy, or sooner if initial serum potassium is low. Defer potassium replacement if serum potassium remains above 5 mEq/L, as in renal insufficiency
- Phosphate replacement is seldom required. However, if severe hypophosphatemia of less than 0.35 mmol/L (<1 mg/dL) develops during insulin therapy, a small amount of phosphate can be replaced as the potassium salt. To minimize the risk of tetany from an overload of phosphate replacement, an average deficit of 40–50 mmol phosphate should be replaced by intravenous infusion at a rate not to exceed 3 mmol/h. A stock solution (Abbott Laboratories) provides a mixture of 1.12 g KH_2PO_4 and 1.18 g K_2HPO_4 in a 5-mL single-dose vial representing 22 mEq potassium and 15 mmol phosphate (27 mEq); 5 mL of this stock solution in 2 L of 0.45% saline or 5% dextrose in water, infused at 400 mL/h, will replace the phosphate at the optimal rate of 3 mmol/h and provide 4.4 mEq of potassium per hour. If serum phosphate remains below 0.35 mmol/L (1 mg/dL), repeat a 5-h infusion of potassium phosphate at a rate of 3 mmol/h

THERAPEUTIC PROCEDURES

- Use a flow sheet listing vital signs, time sequence of laboratory values (arterial pH, plasma glucose, acetone, bicarbonate, serum urea nitrogen, electrolytes, serum osmolality) in relation to therapy
- Careful monitoring of serum potassium during fluid replacement

 OUTCOME

COMPLICATIONS

- Acute myocardial infarction and infarction of the bowel following prolonged hypotension
- Renal failure, especially with prior kidney dysfunction
- Cerebral edema occurs rarely. This is best prevented by avoiding sudden reversal of marked hyperglycemia. Maintaining glycemic levels of 200–300 mg/dL for the initial 24 h after correction of severe hyperglycemia reduces this risk

PROGNOSIS

- Life-threatening medical emergency with a mortality rate just under 5% in individuals under 40 years of age, but with a more serious prognosis in the elderly, who have mortality rates over 20%

WHEN TO REFER

- Recurrent diabetic ketoacidosis
- Poor compliance

WHEN TO ADMIT

- Severe ketosis, hyperosmolality
- An intensive care unit or step-down unit is preferable for more severe cases

PREVENTION

- The patient should contact a provider for persistent ketonuria
- Compliance is particularly important for juvenile-onset diabetics, particularly in the teen years. Intensive family counseling may be needed
- Urine ketones should be measured with signs of infection or in insulin pump-treated patients when capillary blood glucose is persistently high

 EVIDENCE

PRACTICE GUIDELINES

- National Guideline Clearinghouse http://www.guideline.gov/summary/ summary.aspx?doc_id=3582&nbr=2808 &string=diabetic+ketoacidosis http://www.guideline.gov/summary/ summary.aspx?doc_id=3127&nbr= 2353&string=diabetic+ketoacidosis

WEB SITES

- http://www.diabetes.org/main/ application/commercewf
- http://www.cdc.gov/diabetes/
- http://www.joslin.harvard.edu/

INFORMATION FOR PATIENTS

- JAMA patient page: The ABCs of diabetes. JAMA 2002;287:2608 [PMID: 12025825]
- MEDEM http://www.medem.com/search/article_ display.cfm?path=\\TANQUERAY\M_ ContentItem&mstr=/M_ContentItem/ ZZZHMO0EQ8C.html&soc=NIH& srch_typ=NAV_SERCH

REFERENCE

- Kitabchi AE et al: Management of hyperglycemic crises in patients with diabetes. Diabetes Care 2001;24:131. [PMID: 11194218]

Umesh Masharani, MB, BS; MRCH (UK)

Diarrhea, Acute

 ## KEY FEATURES

ESSENTIALS OF DIAGNOSIS

- Defined as a stool weight of >250 g/24 h, though quantification of stool weight is necessary only in some patients with chronic diarrhea
- Increased stool frequency (>2–3 bowel movements per day) or increased liquidity of feces

GENERAL CONSIDERATIONS

- Acute diarrhea (<3 weeks) is most commonly caused by infectious agents, bacterial toxins, or drugs (Table 126, page 1308)
- Recent illnesses in family members suggests infectious diarrhea
- Ingestion of improperly stored or prepared food implicates poisoning
- Exposure to unpurified water suggests *Giardia, Cryptosporidium*, or *Cyclospora*
- Recent travel abroad suggests "traveler's diarrhea"
- Antibiotic administration suggests *Clostridium difficile* colitis
- HIV infection or sexually transmitted diseases suggest AIDS-associated diarrhea
- Proctitis and rectal discharge suggest gonorrhea, syphilis, lymphogranuloma venereum, and herpes simplex

Noninflammatory diarrhea

- Watery, nonbloody diarrhea, usually small bowel source caused by either a toxin-producing bacterium or other agents (viruses, *Giardia*)
- Prominent vomiting suggests viral enteritis or *Staphylococcus aureus* food poisoning
- Diarrhea is voluminous causing dehydration with hypokalemia and metabolic acidosis
- Fecal leukocytes are not present

Inflammatory diarrhea

- Fever and bloody diarrhea (dysentery) caused by invasion (shigellosis, salmonellosis, *Campylobacter*, or *Yersinia* infection, amebiasis, cytomegalovirus) or a toxin (*C difficile, E coli* O157:H7)
- Diarrhea small volume (<1 L/day) with left lower quadrant cramps, urgency, and tenesmus
- Fecal leukocytes usually present

 ## CLINICAL FINDINGS

SYMPTOMS AND SIGNS

- Increased stool frequency or liquidity
- Rectal discharge suggests proctitis
- Periumbilical cramps, bloating, nausea, or vomiting suggest noninflammatory diarrhea
- Fever, left lower quadrant cramps, urgency, and tenesmus suggest inflammatory diarrhea
- Physical examination may reveal abdominal tenderness, peritonitis

DIFFERENTIAL DIAGNOSIS

- Infectious: noninflammatory (nonbloody)
  - Viruses: Norwalk virus, rotavirus, adenoviruses, astrovirus, coronavirus
  - Preformed toxin (food poisoning): *S aureus, Bacillus cereus, Clostridium perfringens*
  - Toxin production: enterotoxigenic *E coli, Vibrio cholerae, Vibrio parahaemolyticus*
  - Protozoa: *Giardia lamblia, Cryptosporidium, Cyclospora, Isospora*
- Infectious: invasive or inflammatory
  - *Shigella, Salmonella, Campylobacter,* enteroinvasive *E coli, E coli* O157:H7, *Yersinia enterocolitica, C difficile* (eg, pseudomembranous colitis), *Entamoeba histolytica, Neisseria gonorrhoeae, Listeria monocytogenes*
- Associated with unprotected anal intercourse: *Neisseria gonorrhoeae,* syphilis, lymphogranuloma venereum, herpes simplex
- Noninfectious
  - Drug reaction, especially antibiotics
  - Ulcerative colitis, Crohn's disease (inflammatory)
  - Ischemic colitis (inflammatory)
  - Fecal impaction (stool may leak around impaction)
  - Laxative abuse
  - Radiation colitis (inflammatory)
  - Emotional stress

 ## DIAGNOSIS

LABORATORY TESTS

- If diarrhea worsens or persists for >7–10 days, stool should be sent for fecal leukocyte determination, stool ovum and parasite evaluation, and stool bacterial culture
- Prompt medical evaluation when
  - Signs of inflammatory diarrhea: fever (>38.5°C), bloody diarrhea, or abdominal pain
  - The passage of six or more unformed stools in 24 h
  - Profuse watery diarrhea and dehydration
  - Frail older patients
  - Immunocompromised patients (AIDS, posttransplantation)
- Stool wet mount for amebiasis in sexually active homosexuals, those with recent travel, and those whose bacterial cultures are negative
- Stool *C difficile* toxin assay if recent history of antibiotic exposure
- Stool culture with serotyping if *E coli* O157:H7 is suspected
- Three stool examinations for ova and parasites if diarrhea persists for more than 10 days
- Stool *Giardia* antigen assay if recent camping
- Rectal swab cultures for *Chlamydia, Neisseria gonorrhoeae,* and herpes simplex virus in sexually active patients with suspected proctitis

DIAGNOSTIC PROCEDURES

- In >90% of cases, acute diarrhea is mild and self-limited, and diagnostic investigation is unnecessary
- Prompt sigmoidoscopy for severe proctitis (tenesmus, discharge, rectal pain) or for suspected *C difficile* colitis, ulcerative colitis, or ischemic colitis

TREATMENT

MEDICATIONS

- Antidiarrheal agents may be used safely in mild to moderate diarrhea but should not be used in bloody diarrhea, high fever, or systemic toxicity
- Loperamide, 4 mg PO initially, followed by 2 mg after each loose stool (maximum: 16 mg/24 h)
- Bismuth subsalicylate (Pepto-Bismol), 2 tablets or 30 mL PO QID
- Anticholinergic diphenoxylate with atropine contraindicated in acute diarrhea because of the rare precipitation of toxic megacolon
- Empirical antibiotic treatment recommended with moderate to severe fever, tenesmus, or bloody stools or the presence of fecal leukocytes while the stool bacterial culture is incubating
- Fluoroquinolones (eg, ciprofloxacin 500 mg, ofloxacin 400 mg, or norfloxacin 400 mg, PO BID) for 5–7 days
- Trimethoprim-sulfamethoxazole, 160/800 mg PO BID, or erythromycin, 250–500 mg PO QID
- Metronidazole (250 mg PO TID for 7 days) when *Giardia* infection is suspected
- Specific antimicrobial treatment is recommended in shigellosis, cholera, extraintestinal salmonellosis, traveler's diarrhea, *C difficile* infection, giardiasis, amebiasis, and gonorrhea, syphilis, chlamydiosis, and herpes simplex infection
- Antibiotics not recommended in nontyphoid *Salmonella, Campylobacter, Aeromonas, Yersinia,* or *E coli* O157:H7 infection except in severe disease

THERAPEUTIC PROCEDURES

- Diet: adequate oral fluids containing carbohydrates and electrolytes; avoid high-fiber foods, fats, milk products, caffeine, and alcohol
- Rehydration: oral electrolyte solutions (eg, Pedialyte, Gatorade), or intravenous fluids (lactated Ringer's injection) with severe dehydration

 OUTCOME

WHEN TO ADMIT

- Hospitalization is required in patients with severe dehydration, toxicity, or marked abdominal pain, rebound tenderness

PREVENTION

- When traveling, eat only "peeled, packaged, and piping hot" foods

EVIDENCE

PRACTICE GUIDELINES

- DuPont HL: Guidelines on acute infectious diarrhea in adults. The Practice Parameters Committee of the American College of Gastroenterology. Am J Gastroenterol 1997;92:1962. [PMID: 9362174]
- Practice guidelines for the management of infectious diarrhea. Infectious Diseases Society of America, 2001 http://www.journals.uchicago.edu/CID/journal/issues/v32n3/001387/001387.html

WEB SITES

- CDC—Traveller's diarrhea http://www.cdc.gov/ncidod/dbmd/diseaseinfo/travelersdiarrhea_g.htm
- National Digestive Diseases Information Clearinghouse—Diarrhea http://digestive.niddk.nih.gov/ddiseases/pubs/diarrhea/index.htm

INFORMATION FOR PATIENTS

- American Academy of Family Physicians—Diarrhea http://familydoctor.org/flowcharts/534.html
- Mayo Clinic—Diarrhea http://www.mayoclinic.com/invoke.cfm?objectid=D98B8FAF-0C97-4C99-AB208D8BDF274E29

REFERENCES

- Hahn S et al: Reduced osmolarity oral rehydration solution for treating dehydration caused by acute diarrhoea in children. Cochrane Database Syst Rev 2001;(2):CD002847. [PMID: 11869639]
- Wingate D et al: Guidelines for adults on self-medication for the treatment of acute diarrhoea. Aliment Pharmacol Ther 2001;15:773. [PMID: 11380315]
- Wong CS et al: The risk of the hemolytic-uremic syndrome after antibiotic treatment of *Escherichia coli* O157 infections. N Engl J Med 2000;342:1930. [PMID: 10874060]

Kenneth R. McQuaid, MD

Diarrhea, Chronic

 KEY FEATURES

ESSENTIALS OF DIAGNOSIS

- Defined as increased stool frequency or liquidity persisting for >3 weeks
- Classified as osmotic diarrhea, secretory diarrhea, inflammatory conditions, malabsorption syndromes, motility disorders, chronic infections, and miscellaneous

GENERAL CONSIDERATIONS

- Osmotic diarrheas resolve during fasting
- Secretory diarrhea is caused by increased intestinal secretion or decreased absorption with little change in stool output during fasting
- Motility disorders are caused by abnormal intestinal motility secondary to systemic disorders or surgery due to rapid transit or to stasis of intestinal contents with bacterial overgrowth, malabsorption
- Immunocompromised patients are susceptible to *Microsporidia, Cryptosporidium,* cytomegalovirus, *Isospora belli, Cyclospora,* and *Mycobacterium avium-intracellulare* infection
- Factitious diarrhea is caused by surreptitious laxative abuse or dilution of stool

DEMOGRAPHICS

- Lactase deficiency occurs in 75% of nonwhite adults and 25% of whites; may be acquired viral gastroenteritis, medical illness, or gastrointestinal surgery

 CLINICAL FINDINGS

SYMPTOMS AND SIGNS

- Osmotic diarrheas: abdominal distension, bloating, and flatulence due to increased colonic gas production
- Secretory diarrhea: high-volume (>1 L/day) watery diarrhea, dehydration, and electrolyte imbalance
- Inflammatory conditions: abdominal pain, fever, weight loss, and hematochezia
- Malabsorption syndromes: weight loss, osmotic diarrhea, and nutritional deficiencies

DIFFERENTIAL DIAGNOSIS

Common

- Irritable bowel syndrome, lactase deficiency, parasites, caffeine, alcohol, laxative abuse

Osmotic

- Lactase deficiency
- Medications: antacids, lactulose, sorbitol, olestra
- Factitious: magnesium-containing antacids or laxatives

Secretory

- Hormonal: Zollinger-Ellison syndrome (gastrinoma), carcinoid, VIPoma, medullary thyroid carcinoma
- Laxative abuse: phenolphthalein, cascara, senna
- Villous adenoma
- Medications

Inflammatory conditions

- Inflammatory bowel disease
- Microscopic colitis (lymphocytic or collagenous)
- Cancer with obstruction and pseudodiarrhea
- Radiation colitis

Malabsorption

- Small bowel: celiac sprue, Whipple's disease, tropical sprue, eosinophilic gastroenteritis, small bowel resection, Crohn's disease
- Lymphatic obstruction: lymphoma, carcinoid, tuberculosis, *M avium-intracellulare* infection, Kaposi's sarcoma, sarcoidosis, retroperitoneal fibrosis
- Pancreatic insufficiency: chronic pancreatitis, cystic fibrosis, pancreatic cancer
- Bacterial overgrowth, eg, diabetes
- Reduced bile salts: ileal resection, Crohn's disease, postcholecystectomy

Motility disorders

- Irritable bowel syndrome
- Postsurgical: vagotomy, partial gastrectomy, blind loop with bacterial overgrowth
- Systemic disease: diabetes mellitus, hyperthyroidism, scleroderma
- Caffeine or alcohol use

Chronic infections

- Parasites: giardiasis, amebiasis, strongyloidiasis

Other

- Ischemic colitis (intestinal ischemia)
- Adrenal insufficiency

 DIAGNOSIS

LABORATORY TESTS

- Obtain complete blood cell count, serum electrolytes, liver enzymes, calcium, phosphorus, albumin, thyroid-stimulating hormone, β-carotene, and prothrombin time
- Stool osmotic gap increased in osmotic diarrheas, normal in secretory diarrhea
- Fecal fat >10 g/24 h in malabsorption syndromes
- Serological tests for celiac sprue: serum IgG and IgA antigliadin, antiendomysial antibodies, or tissue transglutaminase antibody
- Serum VIP (VIPoma), calcitonin (medullary thyroid carcinoma), gastrin (Zollinger-Ellison syndrome), and glucagon
- Urine 5-hydroxyindoleacetic acid (carcinoid), vanillmandelic acid, metanephrines (pheochromocytoma), and histamine determinations
- Fecal leukocytes implies inflammatory diarrhea
- Stool for ova and parasites (three)
- Fecal ELISA for *Giardia*-specific antigen more sensitive and specific than ova and parasite examination

IMAGING STUDIES

- Sigmoidoscopy or colonoscopy with mucosal biopsy helpful in inflammatory bowel disease and melanosis coli
- Upper endoscopy with small bowel biopsy indicated for suspected celiac sprue, Whipple's disease, and AIDS-related *Cryptosporidium, Microsporidia,* and *M avium-intracellulare* infection
- Plain abdominal radiograph
- Abdominal CT for suspected chronic pancreatitis, pancreatic cancer
- Small intestinal barium radiography in suspected Crohn's disease, small bowel lymphoma, carcinoid, and jejunal diverticula
- Somatostatin receptor scintigraphy in suspected neuroendocrine tumors

DIAGNOSTIC PROCEDURES

- Stool analysis: 24-h stool collection for weight and quantitative fecal fat

- Stool weight >300 g/24 h confirms diarrhea
- Stool weight >1000–1500 g/24 h suggests secretory diarrhea
- Fecal fat >10 g/24 h indicates a malabsorption syndrome
- Stool pH <5.6 indicates carbohydrate malabsorption
- Stool osmolality less than serum osmolality indicates factitious diarrhea
- Stool laxative screen positive in laxative abuse
- Colonic biopsy modified acid-fast staining indicated for *Cryptosporidium* and *Cyclospora*

TREATMENT

MEDICATIONS

- Loperamide: 4 mg initially, then 2 mg after each loose stool (maximum: 16 mg/day)
- Diphenoxylate with atropine: 1 tablet PO TID–QID PRN
- Codeine 15–60 mg Q 4 h; deodorized tincture of opium, 10–25 drops Q 6 h PRN, safe in most patients with chronic, intractable diarrhea
- Clonidine, 0.1–0.6 mg PO BID, or a clonidine patch, 0.1–0.2 mg/day, helpful in secretory diarrheas, diabetic diarrhea, and cryptosporidiosis
- Octreotide, 50 µg to 250 µg SQ TID, for secretory diarrheas due to neuroendocrine tumors (VIPomas, carcinoid) and in some cases of AIDS-related diarrhea
- Cholestyramine resin, 4 g PO QD–TID, in patients with bile salt–induced diarrhea secondary to intestinal resection or ileal disease

OUTCOME

COMPLICATIONS

- Dehydration
- Electrolyte abnormalities
- Malabsorption: weight loss, vitamin deficiencies

PROGNOSIS

- Cause is identifiable and treatable in almost all patients

WHEN TO ADMIT

- Secretory diarrhea with dehydration

EVIDENCE

PRACTICE GUIDELINES

- American Gastroenterological Association medical position statement: guidelines for the evaluation and management of chronic diarrhea. American Gastroenterological Association, 2001 http://www2.gastrojournal.org/scripts/om.dll/serve?action=get-media&id=a0069901461a&trueID=pdf_0069901461a&location=jgast9911606&type=pdf&name=x.pdf
- Thomas PD et al: Guidelines for the investigation of chronic diarrhoea, 2nd edition. Gut 2003;52(Suppl 5):v1. [PMID: 12801941]

WEB SITES

- American Academy of Family Physicians—Diarrhea http://familydoctor.org/flowcharts/534.html
- American Gastroenterological Association—Chronic diarrhea http://www.gastro.org/public/uptodate/topics/4974E5.htm
- CDC—Chronic diarrhea http://www.cdc.gov/ncidod/dpd/parasites/diarrhea/factsht_chronic_diarrhea.htm
- National Digestive Diseases Information Clearinghouse—Diarrhea http://digestive.niddk.nih.gov/ddiseases/pubs/diarrhea/index.htm

INFORMATION FOR PATIENTS

- Cleveland Clinic—Diarrhea http://www.clevelandclinic.org/health/health-info/docs/0100/0100.asp?index=4108
- Mayo Clinic—Diarrhea http://www.mayoclinic.com/invoke.cfm?objectid=D98B8FAF-0C97-4C99-AB208D8BDF274E29
- Uptodate—Chronic diarrhea http://patients.uptodate.com/frames.asp?page=topic.asp&file=digestiv/4974&title=Diarrhea

Kenneth R. McQuaid, MD

Diarrhea, Traveler's

 KEY FEATURES

ESSENTIALS OF DIAGNOSIS

- Usually a benign, self-limited disease occurring about a week into travel
- Prophylaxis not recommended unless there is a comorbid disease (inflammatory bowel syndrome, HIV, immunosuppressive medication)
- Single-dose therapy of a fluoroquinolone usually effective if symptoms develop

GENERAL CONSIDERATIONS

- Whenever a person travels from one country to another—particularly if the change involves a marked difference in climate, social conditions, or sanitation standards and facilities—diarrhea is likely to develop within 2–10 days
- Bacteria cause 80% of cases, with enterotoxigenic *Escherichia coli*, *Shigella* species, and *Campylobacter jejuni* being the most common pathogens. Less common are *Aeromonas*, *Salmonella*, noncholera vibrios, *Entamoeba histolytica*, and *Giardia lamblia*
- Chronic watery diarrhea may be due to amebiasis or giardiasis or, rarely, tropical sprue
- Contributory causes include unusual food and drink, change in living habits, occasional viral infections (adenoviruses or rotaviruses), and change in bowel flora

Etiology

- Most common: enterotoxigenic *E coli*, *Shigella*, *Campylobacter*
- Less common: *Aeromonas*, *Salmonella*, noncholera vibrios, *E histolytica*, *G lamblia*, adenoviruses, rotavirus
- Chronic watery diarrhea: *Entamoeba histolytica*, *G lamblia*, tropical sprue (rare)
- Associated with unprotected anal intercourse: *Neisseria gonorrhoeae*, syphilis, lymphogranuloma venereum, herpes simplex

 CLINICAL FINDINGS

SYMPTOMS AND SIGNS

- There may be up to 10 or even more loose stools per day, usually without mucus or blood
- Abdominal cramps, nausea, occasionally vomiting
- Fever is rare
- Aside from weakness and dehydration there are no systemic manifestations of infection
- The illness usually subsides spontaneously within 1–5 days, although 10% remain symptomatic for a week or longer, and in 2% symptoms persist for longer than a month

 DIAGNOSIS

LABORATORY TESTS

- In patients with fever and bloody diarrhea, stool culture may be indicated, but in most cases cultures are reserved for those who do not respond to antibiotics

TREATMENT

MEDICATIONS

- For most patients, symptomatic therapy with opioids or loperamide is all that is required provided there is no systemic illness (fever ≥39°C) or dysentery (bloody stools), in which case antimotility agents should be avoided
- Packages of oral rehydration salts to treat dehydration are available over the counter in the United States (Infalyte, Pedialyte, others) and in many foreign countries
- Loperamide (4 mg loading dose, then 2 mg after each loose stool to a maximum of 16 mg/day) with a single dose of ciprofloxacin (750 mg), levofloxacin (500 mg), or ofloxacin (300 mg) cures most cases
- If diarrhea is severe, associated with fever or bloody stools, or persists despite single-dose ciprofloxacin treatment, then 3–5 days of ciprofloxacin, 500 mg twice daily, levofloxacin, 500 mg once daily, norfloxacin, 400 mg twice daily, or ofloxacin, 300 mg twice daily, can be given
- Trimethoprim-sulfamethoxazole 160/800 mg twice daily, can be used as an alternative, but resistance is common in many areas

 OUTCOME

PROGNOSIS

- Most illnesses are short-lived and resolve without specific therapy

WHEN TO REFER

- Persistent diarrhea despite therapy

WHEN TO ADMIT

- Dehydration
- Systemic toxicity

PREVENTION

- Avoidance of fresh foods and water sources that are likely to be contaminated is recommended for travelers to developing countries, where infectious diarrheal illnesses are endemic
- Prophylaxis is recommended for those with significant underlying disease (inflammatory bowel disease, AIDS, diabetes, heart disease in the elderly, conditions requiring immunosuppressive medications) and for those whose full activity status during the trip is so essential that even short periods of diarrhea would be unacceptable
- Prophylaxis is started upon entry into the destination country and is continued for 1 or 2 days after leaving
- For stays of more than 3 weeks, prophylaxis is not recommended because of the cost and increased toxicity
- Numerous antimicrobial regimens for once-daily prophylaxis are effective, such as norfloxacin, 400 mg, ciprofloxacin, 500 mg, ofloxacin, 300 mg, or trimethoprim-sulfamethoxazole, 160/800 mg
- Bismuth subsalicylate is effective but turns the tongue and the stools black and can interfere with doxycycline absorption, which may be needed for malaria prophylaxis; it is rarely used
- Because not all travelers will have diarrhea and because most episodes are brief and self-limited, an alternative approach currently recommended is to provide the traveler with a supply of antimicrobials to be taken if significant diarrhea occurs during the trip

Diarrhea, Traveler's

 EVIDENCE

PRACTICE GUIDELINES

- National Guideline Clearinghouse http://www.guideline.gov/summary/summary.aspx?doc_id=2791&nbr=2017&string=diarrhea http://www.guideline.gov/summary/summary.aspx?doc_id=2707&nbr=1933&string=diarrhea

INFORMATION FOR PATIENTS

- Centers for Disease Control http://www.cdc.gov/ncidod/dbmd/diseaseinfo/ travelersdiarrhea_g.htm
- National Digestive Diseases Information Clearinghouse http://digestive.niddk.nih.gov/ddiseases/pubs/diarrhea/index.htm

REFERENCES

- Ansdell VE et al: Prevention and empiric treatment of traveler's diarrhea. Med Clin North Am 1999;83:945. [PMID: 10453258]
- Guerrant RL et al: Practice guidelines for the management of infectious diarrhea. Clin Infect Dis 2001;32:331. [PMID: 11170940]
- Ramzan N: Traveler's diarrhea. Gastroenterol Clin North Am 2001;30:665. [PMID: 11586551]
- Rendi-Wagner P et al: Drug prophylaxis for travelers' diarrhea. Clin Infect Dis 2002;34:628. [PMID: 11803509]

Richard A. Jacobs, MD, PhD

Digitalis Toxicity

KEY FEATURES

ESSENTIALS OF DIAGNOSIS

- Intoxication may result from acute single exposure or chronic accumulation due to accidental overmedication or renal insufficiancy
- Hyperkalemia common after acute overdose
- Many different arrhythmias can occur

GENERAL CONSIDERATIONS

- Cardiac glycosides paralyze the Na^+-K^+-ATPase pump and have potent vagotonic effects
- Intracellular effects include enhancement of calcium-dependent contractility and shortening of the action potential duration
- Digoxin and ouabain are highly tissue-bound, but digitoxin has a volume of distribution of just 0.6 L/kg, making it the only cardiac glycoside accessible to enhanced removal procedures such as hemoperfusion or repeated doses of activated charcoal

DEMOGRAPHICS

- Older age and renal impairment are associated with greater risk of accidental digoxin toxicity

CLINICAL FINDINGS

SYMPTOMS AND SIGNS

Acute overdose

- Nausea and vomiting
- Bradycardia, atrioventricular (AV) block. Junctional rhythm is common in patients with underlying atrial fibrillation
- Hyperkalemia

Chronic overingestion

- Hypokalemia and hypomagnesia are more likely, owing to concurrent diuretic treatment
- Ventricular arrhythmias (eg, ectopy, bidirectional ventricular tachycardia, or ventricular fibrillation)

DIFFERENTIAL DIAGNOSIS

- β-Blocker overdose
- Calcium channel blocker overdose
- Cardiotoxic plant or animal ingestion: oleander, foxglove, lily of the valley, rhododendron, toad venom

DIAGNOSIS

LABORATORY TESTS

- Serum digoxin level (**note:** levels drawn within 6 h of ingestion may be higher than equilibrium)
- Serum potassium (frequent measures useful as they correlate with tissue effects)

IMAGING STUDIES

- Continuous ECG monitoring

DIAGNOSTIC PROCEDURES

- Pacemaker may be needed

TREATMENT

MEDICATIONS

Emergency measures

- Treat ventricular arrhythmias initially with lidocaine (2–3 mg/kg intravenously) or phenytoin (10–15 mg/kg intravenously slowly over 30 min)
- Treat bradycardia initially with atropine (0.5–2 mg intravenously), or a transcutaneous external cardiac pacemaker

Activated charcoal

- Administer activated charcoal, 60–100 g orally or via gastric tube, mixed in aqueous slurry

Repeat-dose charcoal

- Repeated doses of activated charcoal, 20–30 g every 3–4 h, may hasten elimination of digitoxin (but not digoxin) by adsorbing drug excreted into the gut lumen ("gut dialysis")
- Sorbitol or other cathartics should *not* be used with each dose, or resulting large stool volumes may lead to dehydration or hypernatremia
- Emesis is not recommended because it may enhance vagotonic effects such as bradycardia and AV block

Specific treatment

- In severe intoxication, administer digoxin-specific antibodies [digoxin immune Fab (ovine); Digibind]
- Estimation of the Digibind dose is based on the body burden of digoxin calculated from the ingested dose or the steady-state serum digoxin concentration
  - From the ingested dose
    Number of vials = approximately 1.5 × ingested dose (mg)
  - From the serum concentration
    Number of vials = serum digoxin (ng/mL) × body weight (kg) × 10^{-2}
    Note: This is based on the equilibrium digoxin level; after acute overdose, serum levels are falsely high before tissue distribution is complete, and overestimation of the Digibind dose is likely
- Empirical dosing of Digibind may be utilized if the patient's condition is relatively stable and an underlying condition (eg, atrial fibrillation) suggests a residual level of digitalis activity. Start with one or two vials and reassess the clinical condition after 20–30 min

- **Note:** After administration of Digibind, serum digoxin levels may be falsely elevated depending on the assay technique

OUTCOME

FOLLOW-UP

- Monitor potassium levels and cardiac rhythm closely

COMPLICATIONS

- Cardiac arrest

WHEN TO ADMIT

- Symptomatic patients
- Asymptomatic patients after acute overdose, for monitoring at least several hours

PREVENTION

- Monitor renal function in elderly patients and obtain serum digoxin levels if symptoms of digoxin toxicity

EVIDENCE

PRACTICE GUIDELINES

- National Guideline Clearinghouse http://www.guideline.gov/summary/ summary.aspx?doc_id=3027&nbr=2253 &string=digitalis+toxicity

WEB SITES

- Agency for Toxic Substances and Disease Registry (ATSDR) http://www.cdc.gov/niosh/nasd/srd/ og56400.html
- Toxicology—eMedicine http://www.emedicine.com/cgi-bin/ foxweb.exe/showsection@d:/em/ga? book=emerg&sct=TOXICOLOGY

INFORMATION FOR PATIENTS

- National Institutes of Health http://www.nlm.nih.gov/medlineplus/ ency/article/000165.htm

REFERENCES

- Eddleston M et al: Acute yellow oleander (*Thevetia peruviana*) poisoning: cardiac arrhythmias, electrolyte disturbances, and serum cardiac glycoside concentrations on presentation to hospital. Heart 2000; 83(3):301. [PMID: 10677410]
- Miura T et al: Effect of aging on the incidence of digoxin toxicity. Ann Pharmacother 2000;34:427. [PMID: 10772425]
- Roever C et al: Comparing the toxicity of digoxin and digitoxin in a geriatric population: should an old drug be rediscovered? South Med J 2000;93:199. [PMID: 10701788]

Kent R. Olson, MD

Diphtheria

 KEY FEATURES

ESSENTIALS OF DIAGNOSIS

- Tenacious gray membrane at portal of entry in pharynx
- Sore throat, nasal discharge, hoarseness, malaise, fever
- Myocarditis, neuropathy
- Culture confirms the diagnosis

GENERAL CONSIDERATIONS

- An acute infection with a toxin-producing strain of *Corynebacterium diphtheriae*
- Usually attacks the respiratory tract but may involve any mucous membrane or skin wound
- The organism is spread chiefly by respiratory secretions
- Exotoxin produced by the organism is responsible for myocarditis and neuropathy. This exotoxin inhibits elongation factor, which is required for protein synthesis

DEMOGRAPHICS

- Rare in the United States and Western Europe, more likely to be encountered in persons from developing countries and those from the former Soviet Union, where vaccine programs are lacking or inadequate

 CLINICAL FINDINGS

SYMPTOMS AND SIGNS

- Nasal, laryngeal, pharyngeal, and cutaneous forms of diphtheria occur
- Nasal infection produces few symptoms other than a nasal discharge
- Laryngeal infection may lead to upper airway and bronchial obstruction
- In pharyngeal diphtheria, the most common form, a tenacious gray membrane covers the tonsils and pharynx
- Mild sore throat, fever, and malaise are followed by toxemia and prostration

DIFFERENTIAL DIAGNOSIS

- Streptococcal pharyngitis
- Oral candidiasis
- Infectious mononucleosis
- Viral pharyngitis, eg, adenovirus, herpes simplex virus
- Necrotizing gingivostomatitis (Vincent's angina, trench mouth)
- *Arcanobacterium haemolyticum* pharyngitis
- Other causes of cranial nerve or motor neuropathy, eg, myasthenia gravis, botulism, Guillain-Barré syndrome
- Myocarditis due to other causes

 DIAGNOSIS

LABORATORY TESTS

- The diagnosis is made clinically but can be confirmed by culture of the organism

TREATMENT

MEDICATIONS

- Susceptible persons exposed to diphtheria should receive a booster dose of diphtheria toxoid plus active immunization if not previously immunized, as well as a course of penicillin or erythromycin

Antitoxin

- Prepared from horse serum
- Must be given in all cases when diphtheria is suspected
- For mild early pharyngeal or laryngeal disease, the dose is 20,000–40,000 units; for moderate nasopharyngeal disease, 40,000–60,000 units; for severe, extensive, or late (3 days or more) disease, 80,000–100,000 units

Antibiotics

- Either penicillin, 250 mg orally four times daily, or erythromycin, 500 mg orally four times daily, for 14 days is effective, though erythromycin is slightly more effective in eliminating the carrier state
- Azithromycin or clarithromycin may be as effective as erythromycin

THERAPEUTIC PROCEDURES

- Removal of membrane by direct laryngoscopy or bronchoscopy may be necessary to prevent or alleviate airway obstruction

 OUTCOME

FOLLOW-UP

- The patient should be isolated until three consecutive cultures at the completion of therapy have documented elimination of the organism from the oropharynx

COMPLICATIONS

- Myocarditis and neuropathy are the most common and most serious complications
- Myocarditis causes cardiac arrhythmias, heart block, and heart failure
- The neuropathy usually involves the cranial nerves first, producing diplopia, slurred speech, and difficulty in swallowing

PROGNOSIS

- Death occurs in 5–10% of respiratory cases
- Complications and deaths are much less frequent in cutaneous diphtheria

WHEN TO REFER

- This disease must be reported to the public health authorities
- Diphtheria equine antitoxin can be obtained from the Centers for Disease Control and Prevention

WHEN TO ADMIT

- All suspected or proven cases

PREVENTION

- See Table 127 (page 1310)
- Active immunization with diphtheria toxoid is part of routine childhood immunization (usually as diphtheria-tetanus-pertussis) with appropriate booster injections
- The immunization schedule for adults is the same as for tetanus. To avoid major allergic reactions, only the "adult type" toxoid (Td) should be used
- Contacts to a case should receive erythromycin, 500 mg four times daily for 7 days, to eradicate carriage

 EVIDENCE

PRACTICE GUIDELINES

- National Guideline Clearinghouse
  http://www.guideline.gov/summary/
  summary.aspx?doc_id=3160&nbr=2386
  &string=pharyngitis
  http://www.guideline.gov/summary/
  summary.aspx?doc_id=2957&nbr=
  2183&string=pharyngitis

WEB SITES

- CDC—Division of Bacterial and Mycotic Diseases
  http://www.cdc.gov/ncidod/dbmd/
- Karolinska Institute—Directory of Bacterial Infections and Mycoses
  http://www.mic.ki.se/Diseases/c1.html

INFORMATION FOR PATIENTS

- JAMA patient page: Immunizations. JAMA 1999;282:102. [PMID: 10404918]
- Mayo Clinic
  http://www.mayoclinic.com/invoke.cfm?
  id=DS00495
- National Coalition for Adult Immunization
  http://www.nfid.org/factsheets/
  diphtadult.html

REFERENCE

- Dittmann S: Epidemic diphtheria in the Newly Independent States of the former USSR—situation and lessons learned. Int Assoc Biol Standard 1997;25:179.

Henry F. Chambers, MD

Discoid Lupus Erythematosus

 ## KEY FEATURES

ESSENTIALS OF DIAGNOSIS

- Localized red plaques, usually on the face
- Scaling, follicular plugging, atrophy, dyspigmentation, and telangiectasia of involved areas
- Histology distinctive
- Photosensitive

GENERAL CONSIDERATIONS

- Ten percent of patients with systemic lupus erythematosus (SLE) have discoid skin lesions, and 5% of patients with discoid lesions have SLE
- The disease is persistent but not life endangering unless systemic lupus intervenes, which is uncommon
- Treatment with antimalarials is effective in perhaps 60% of cases

 ## CLINICAL FINDINGS

SYMPTOMS AND SIGNS

- See Table 7 (page 1202)
- The lesions consist of dusky red, well-localized, single or multiple plaques, 5–20 mm in diameter, usually on the face; the scalp, external ears, and oral mucous membranes may be involved
- There is atrophy, telangiectasia, depigmentation, and follicular plugging
- The lesion may be covered by dry, horny, adherent scales
- On the scalp, permanent hair loss may occur

DIFFERENTIAL DIAGNOSIS

- Psoriasis
- Seborrheic dermatitis
- Acne rosacea
- Lupus vulgaris (cutaneous tuberculosis)
- Sarcoidosis
- Bowen's disease (squamous cell carcinoma in situ)
- Polymorphous light eruption
- Lichen planopilaris

 ## DIAGNOSIS

LABORATORY TESTS

- Diagnosis is based on the clinical appearance confirmed by skin biopsy in all cases

TREATMENT

MEDICATIONS

- See Table 6 (page 1199)

General measures

- Protect from sunlight; use high-SPF (>30) sunblock with UVB and UVA coverage daily
- **Caution:** Do not use any form of radiation therapy
- Avoid using drugs that are potentially photosensitizing (eg, thiazides, piroxicam) where possible

Local treatment

- High-potency corticosteroid creams applied each night and covered with airtight, thin, pliable plastic film (eg, Saran Wrap); or Cordran tape; or ultra-high-potency corticosteroid cream or ointment applied twice daily without occlusion
- Local infiltration: triamcinolone acetonide suspension, 2.5–10 mg/mL, may be injected into the lesions once a month; this should be tried before systemic therapy

Systemic treatment

- Antimalarials—**Caution:** these drugs should be used only when the diagnosis is secure, because they have been associated with flares of psoriasis, which may be in the differential diagnosis; they may also cause ocular changes, and ophthalmological evaluation is required every 6 months
- Hydroxychloroquine sulfate, 0.2–0.4 g orally daily for several months, may be effective and is often used prior to chloroquine; a 3-month trial is recommended
- Chloroquine sulfate, 250 mg daily, may be effective in some cases where hydroxychloroquine is not
- Quinacrine (Atabrine), 100 mg daily, may be the safest of the antimalarials, since eye damage has not been reported; it colors the skin yellow and is therefore not acceptable to some patients; it may be added to the above antimalarials for incomplete responses
- Isotretinoin, 1 mg/kg/day, is effective in chronic or subacute cutaneous lupus erythematosus; recurrences are prompt and predictable on discontinuation of therapy
- Thalidomide is a potent teratogen but very effective in refractory cases in doses of 50–100 mg daily

THERAPEUTIC PROCEDURES

- Monitor for neuropathy if using thalidomide
- Because of the teratogenicity of isotretinoin and thalidomide, the drugs are used with caution in women of childbearing age using effective contraception with negative pregnancy tests before and during therapy

OUTCOME

COMPLICATIONS

- Although the only morbidity may be cosmetic, this can be of overwhelming significance in more darkly pigmented patients with widespread disease
- Scarring alopecia can be prevented or lessened with close attention and aggressive therapy

PROGNOSIS

- The disease is persistent but not life endangering unless systemic lupus intervenes, which is uncommon
- Treatment with antimalarials is effective in perhaps 60% of cases

WHEN TO REFER

- If there is a question about the diagnosis, if recommended therapy is ineffective, or specialized treatment is necessary

EVIDENCE

PRACTICE GUIDELINES

- American Academy of Dermatology http://www.aadassociation.org/Guidelines/cutlupus.html

WEB SITES

- American Academy of Dermatology http://www.aad.org
- Dermatology Handbook for Family Practice from the University of Iowa http://www.vh.org/Providers/ClinRef/FPHandbook/17.html

INFORMATION FOR PATIENTS

- American Academy of Dermatology http://www.aad.org/pamphlets/
- Lupus Foundation http://www.lupus.org/education/brochures/skindisease.html

REFERENCE

- Patel P et al: Cutaneous lupus erythematosus: a review. Dermatol Clin 2002;20:373. [PMID: 12170873]

Timothy G. Berger, MD

Disseminated Intravascular Coagulation (DIC)

 KEY FEATURES

ESSENTIALS OF DIAGNOSIS

- Underlying serious illness
- Microangiopathic hemolytic anemia may be present
- Low fibrinogen, thrombocytopenia, fibrin degradation products, and prolonged prothrombin time (PT)

GENERAL CONSIDERATIONS

- If stimulus to coagulation is too great, control mechanisms are overwhelmed, leading to DIC
- Can be thought of as a consequence of circulating thrombin (normally confined to localized area)
  - Thrombin cleaves fibrinogen to fibrin, stimulates platelet aggregation, activates factors V and VIII, and releases plasminogen activator, which generates plasmin
  - Plasmin cleaves fibrin, generating fibrin degradation products, and further inactivates factors V and VIII
- Thus, excess thrombin activity produces hypofibrinogenemia, thrombocytopenia, depletion of coagulation factors, and fibrinolysis
- Caused by a number of serious illnesses: sepsis (especially with gram-negative bacteria), severe tissue injury (especially burns and head injury), obstetric complications (amniotic fluid embolus, septic abortion, retained fetus), cancer (acute promyelocytic leukemia, mucinous adenocarcinomas), and major hemolytic transfusion reactions

 CLINICAL FINDINGS

SYMPTOMS AND SIGNS

- DIC leads to both bleeding and thrombosis; bleeding is far more common, but thrombosis may dominate
- Bleeding may occur at any site; spontaneous bleeding and oozing at venipuncture sites or wounds are important clues to diagnosis
- Thrombosis most commonly manifested by digital ischemia and gangrene, but catastrophic events such as renal cortical necrosis and hemorrhagic adrenal infarction may occur
- DIC may secondarily produce microangiopathic hemolytic anemia
- Subacute DIC occurs primarily in cancer; manifested primarily as recurrent superficial and deep venous thromboses (Trousseau's syndrome)

DIFFERENTIAL DIAGNOSIS

- Severe liver disease
- Thrombotic thrombocytopenic purpura
- Sepsis-induced thrombocytopenia or anemia
- Heparin-induced thrombocytopenia
- Other microangiopathic hemolytic anemia, eg, prosthetic valve hemolysis

 DIAGNOSIS

LABORATORY TESTS

- Serum fibrinogen low (may also occur in congenital hypofibrinogenemia, severe liver disease)
- Fibrin degradation products, eg, D-dimers, elevated (may also occur in hepatic dysfunction)
- Thrombocytopenia
- PT prolonged
- When baseline fibrinogen level is markedly elevated, initial level may be normal; since half-life is approximately 4 days, declining fibrinogen level confirms DIC
- Partial thromboplastin time (PTT) may or may not be prolonged
- Microangiopathic hemolytic anemia present in ~25% of cases, and peripheral blood smear shows fragmented red blood cells
- Antithrombin III levels may be markedly depleted
- When fibrinolysis is activated, levels of plasminogen and α_2-antiplasmin may be low
- Thrombocytopenia and D-dimer elevation are usually the only abnormalities in subacute DIC
- Fibrinogen level is normal, and PTT may be normal

TREATMENT

MEDICATIONS

- Replacement therapy alone if underlying cause is rapidly reversible
- Platelet transfusion to maintain platelet count >30,000/μL
- Cryoprecipitate to replace fibrinogen, aiming for plasma fibrinogen level of 150 mg/dL
- Fresh-frozen plasma may be required for coagulation factor deficiency
- Heparin is contraindicated when any increase in bleeding is unacceptable (neurosurgical procedures)
- When DIC is producing serious clinical consequences and underlying cause not rapidly reversible, heparin may be necessary
- Heparin must be used in combination with replacement therapy to prevent an unacceptable increase in bleeding
- Heparin dose is 500–750 units per hour
- Heparin cannot be effective if antithrombin III is markedly depleted; measure antithrombin III level and if low, give fresh-frozen plasma to raise levels to >50%
- Successful heparin therapy is indicated by rising fibrinogen level; it is not necessary to prolong PTT
- Fibrin degradation products decline over 1–2 days
- Improvement in platelet count may lag by 1 week behind control of coagulopathy
- If heparin and replacement therapy does not control bleeding aminocaproic acid, 1 g IV Q hour, is added to decrease rate of fibrinolysis, raise fibrinogen level, and control bleeding
- Aminocaproic acid can *never* be used without heparin in DIC because of risk of thrombosis

THERAPEUTIC PROCEDURES

- Treatment of underlying disorder
- Mild DIC requires no specific therapy

 ## OUTCOME

PROGNOSIS

- Prognosis is that of the underlying disease

 ## EVIDENCE

PRACTICE GUIDELINES

- Bick RL: Disseminated intravascular coagulation: a review of etiology, pathophysiology, diagnosis, and management: guidelines for care. Clin Appl Thromb Hemost 2002;8:1. [PMID: 11991236]
- Taylor FB et al: Towards definition, clinical and laboratory criteria, and a scoring system for disseminated intravascular coagulation. Thromb Haemost 2001;86:1327. [PMID: 11816725]
- Toh CH et al: Current clinical practice. DIC 2002: a review of disseminated intravascular coagulation. Hematology 2003;8:65. [PMID: 12745654]

WEB SITES

- MEDLINEplus—DIC http://www.nlm.nih.gov/medlineplus/ency/article/ 000573.htm
- Merck Manual—Disseminated intravascular coagulation http://www.merck.com/pubs/mmanual/section11/chapter131/131d.htm

INFORMATION FOR PATIENTS

- Levi M et al: Disseminated intravascular coagulation. N Engl J Med 1999;341:586. [PMID: 10451465]
- Postgraduate medicine—Disseminated intravascular coagulation http://www.postgradmed.com/issues/2002/03_02/ messmore.htm

REFERENCES

- Levi M et al: Novel approaches to the management of disseminated intravascular coagulation. Crit Care Med 2000;28:S20. [PMID: 11007192]
- Schmaier AH: Disseminated intravascular coagulation. N Engl J Med 1999;341:1937. [PMID: 10610481]

Charles A. Linker, MD

Diverticulitis

 ## KEY FEATURES

ESSENTIALS OF DIAGNOSIS

- Intraabdominal infection varies from microperforation (most common) with localized paracolic inflammation to macroperforation with either abscess or generalized peritonitis
- Acute abdominal pain and fever
- Left lower abdominal tenderness and mass
- Leukocytosis

GENERAL CONSIDERATIONS

- Diverticulosis present in 25% of adults over age 40; increases with age; most asymptomatic
- Diverticulitis occurs in 10–20% of patients with diverticulosis

DEMOGRAPHICS

- Higher prevalence in societies with low fiber intake

 ## CLINICAL FINDINGS

SYMPTOMS AND SIGNS

- Abdominal pain, mild to moderate, aching, usually in the left lower quadrant
- Constipation or loose stools
- Nausea and vomiting
- Low-grade fever
- Left lower quadrant tenderness
- Palpable left lower quadrant mass
- Generalized abdominal pain and peritoneal signs in patients with free perforation

DIFFERENTIAL DIAGNOSIS

- Perforated colorectal cancer
- Infectious colitis, eg, *Campylobacter*, *Clostridium difficile*
- Inflammatory bowel disease
- Ischemic colitis
- Appendicitis
- Gynecological: pelvic inflammatory disease, tuboovarian abscess, ovarian torsion, ruptured ectopic pregnancy or ovarian cyst, mittelschmerz, endometriosis
- Urinary calculus
- Ascariasis
- Gastroenteritis

 ## DIAGNOSIS

LABORATORY TESTS

- Leukocytosis, mild to moderate
- Stool occult blood test positive

IMAGING STUDIES

- Plain abdominal films
- Barium enema, contraindicated during acute attack; perform only after resolution of clinical symptoms to document extent of diverticulosis or presence of fistula
- CT scan of the abdomen in patients who do not improve rapidly after 2–4 days of empirical therapy and to confirm diagnosis; CT indicated in severe disease to diagnose abscess

DIAGNOSTIC PROCEDURES

- Colonoscopy, contraindicated during acute attack; perform only after resolution of clinical symptoms to document extent of diverticulitis and to exclude other clinical disorders
- Sigmoidoscopy with minimal air insufflation is sometimes required in acute disease to exclude other diagnoses

TREATMENT

MEDICATIONS

- Most patients can be managed with conservative measures
- Mild diverticulitis (mild symptoms and no peritoneal signs)
  - Clear liquid diet
  - Oral antibiotics targeting both anaerobic and gram-negative bacteria, such as amoxicillin and clavulanate potassium, 875 mg/125 mg PO BID; or metronidazole, 500 mg PO TID; plus either ciprofloxacin, 500 mg PO BID, or trimethoprim-sulfamethoxazole, 160/800 mg PO BID, for 7–10 days
- Severe diverticulitis (high fevers, leukocytosis, or peritoneal signs)
  - Nothing by mouth
  - Intravenous fluids
  - Nasogastric tube suction if ileus is present
  - Intravenous antibiotics targeting both anaerobic and gram-negative bacteria, such as either single-agent therapy with a second-generation cephalosporin (eg, cefoxitin), or piperacillin-tazobactam, or ticarcillin clavulanate; or combination therapy (eg, metronidazole or clindamycin plus an aminoglycoside or third-generation cephalosporin (eg, ceftazidime, cefotaxime) for 7–10 days

SURGERY

- Surgical management is required in ~20–30% of cases
- Indications for surgery include free peritonitis and large abscesses, fistulas, or colonic obstruction
- Surgery in two stages for abscesses for which catheter drainage is not possible or helpful: diseased colon is resected, temporary colostomy of proximal colon is created, and distal colonic stump is either closed (forming a Hartmann pouch) or exteriorized as a mucous fistula; then, weeks later, colon is reconnected electively

THERAPEUTIC PROCEDURES

- Percutaneous catheter drainage of localized abdominal abscess, with subsequent single-stage elective surgical resection of diseased segment of colon

 OUTCOME

FOLLOW-UP

- Colonoscopy or barium enema 4–6 weeks after recovery from diverticulitis to diagnose extent of diverticulosis and to exclude colonic malignancy

COMPLICATIONS

- Fistula formation may involve the bladder, ureter, vagina, uterus, bowel, and abdominal wall
- Stricturing of the colon with partial or complete obstruction

PROGNOSIS

- Diverticulitis recurs in one-third
- Recurrent attacks warrant elective surgical resection

WHEN TO ADMIT

- Hospitalize patients with increasing pain, fever, or inability to tolerate oral fluids
- Hospitalize patients with severe diverticulitis and patients who are elderly or immunosuppressed or who have serious comorbid disease

PREVENTION

- High-fiber diet

 EVIDENCE

PRACTICE GUIDELINES

- Practice parameters for the treatment of sigmoid diverticulitis. American Society of Colon and Rectal Surgeons, 2000 http://www.fascrs.org/ascrspp-sd.html
- Stollman NH et al: Diagnosis and management of diverticular disease of the colon in adults. Ad Hoc Practice Parameters Committee of the American College of Gastroenterology. Am J Gastroenterol 1999;94:3110. [PMID: 10566700]
- Surgical treatment of diverticulitis. Society for Surgery of the Alimentary Tract, Inc—Medical Specialty Society, 2000 http://www.ssat.com/cgi-bin/divert.cgi? affiliation=student

WEB SITES

- National Digestive Diseases Information Clearinghouse— Diverticulosis and Diverticulitis http://digestive.niddk.nih.gov/ddiseases/ pubs/diverticulosis/index.htm
- MEDLINEplus—Diverticulitis http://www.nlm.nih.gov/medlineplus/ ency/article/000257.htm

INFORMATION FOR PATIENTS

- Cleveland Clinic—Diverticular disease http://www.clevelandclinic.org/health/ health-info/docs/2800/2824.asp? index=10352
- Mayo Clinic—Diverticulitis http://www.mayoclinic.com/invoke. cfm?id=DS00070
- National Digestive Diseases Information Clearinghouse—Colonoscopy http://digestive.niddk.nih.gov/ddiseases/ pubs/colonoscopy/index.htm

REFERENCE

- Stollman NH et al: Diagnosis and management of diverticular disease of the colon in adults. Am J Gastroenterol 1999;94:1310. [PMID: 10566700]

Kenneth R. McQuaid, MD

Dracunculiasis

 ## KEY FEATURES

ESSENTIALS OF DIAGNOSIS

- Worm can reach the skin and a blister develops, which can then ulcerate
- Most lesions are on the leg or foot
- Can be accompanied by a systemic allergic reaction

GENERAL CONSIDERATIONS

- This is an infection of connective and subcutaneous tissues by the nematode *Dracunculus medinensis*
- It occurs only in humans and is a major cause of disability
- Infection occurs by swallowing water containing the infected intermediate host, the crustacean cyclops (copepods, water fleas)
- In the human stomach, larvae escape from the crustacean and mature in subcutaneous connective tissue. After mating, the male worm dies and the gravid female (60–80 cm × 1.7–2.0 mm) moves to the surface of the body, where its head reaches the dermis and provokes a blister that ruptures on contact with water. Intermittently over 2–3 weeks, whenever the ulcer comes in contact with water, the uterus discharges great numbers of larvae, which are ingested by copepods. Most adult worms are gradually extruded; some worms retract and reemerge; and others die in the tissues, disintegrate, and may provoke a severe inflammatory reaction
- Infection does not induce protective immunity

DEMOGRAPHICS

- Since the start of the WHO eradication program, the number of infected persons has declined about 97% from over 3 million to 100,000. Endemic areas have been the Indian subcontinent; West and Central Africa north of the equator and Saudi Arabia, Iran, and Yemen. Almost all remaining cases are reported from Sudan
- All ages are affected, and prevalence may reach 60%

 ## CLINICAL FINDINGS

SYMPTOMS AND SIGNS

- Infection may be at several sites
- Patients are asymptomatic during the 9- to 14-month incubation period except in the last 1–2 weeks, when the worm reaches and becomes palpable in the skin and a blister develops around its anterior end. Several hours before the head appears at the skin surface, local erythema, burning, pruritus, and tenderness often develop at the site of emergence
- There may also be a 24-h systemic allergic reaction (pruritus, fever, nausea and vomiting, dyspnea, periorbital edema, and urticaria)
- After rupture, the tissues surrounding the ulceration frequently become indurated, reddened, and tender
- Because most lesions appear on the leg or foot, patients often must give up walking and working for days to several months
- Uninfected ulcers heal in 4–6 weeks
- The worm rarely reaches ectopic sites
- Secondary infections, including tetanus, are common. Deep "cold" abscesses may result at the sites of dying, nonemergent worms

DIFFERENTIAL DIAGNOSIS

- Cutaneous larva migrans
- Loiasis (*Loa loa* infection)
- Rat bite fever
- Gnathostomiasis
- Myiasis
- Other cause of leg ulcer, eg, venous or arterial insufficiency, bacterial pyoderma, vasculitis, pyoderma gangrenosum

 ## DIAGNOSIS

LABORATORY TESTS

- When an emerging adult worm is not visible in the ulcer or under the skin, the diagnosis may be made by detection of larvae in smears from discharging sinuses. Immersion of an ulcer in cold water stimulates larval expulsion
- Eosinophilia is usually present
- Skin and serological tests are not useful

IMAGING STUDIES

- Calcified worms can be recognized on radiographs

Dracunculiasis

 TREATMENT

MEDICATIONS

- The following drugs have an antiinflammatory effect but do not kill the adults or the larvae. This effect may alleviate symptoms, reduce duration of infection, facilitate worm removal, or expedite their spontaneous extrusion
- Metronidazole, 250 mg three times daily for 10 days, causes only minimal toxicity
- Mebendazole, 400–800 mg daily for 6 days, can be tried
- Thiabendazole, 25 mg/kg twice daily for 2–3 days after meals, frequently causes side effects, sometimes severe

SURGERY

- Preemergent female worms can sometimes be surgically removed intact under local anesthesia if not firmly embedded in deep fascia or around tendons

THERAPEUTIC PROCEDURES

- The patient should be at bed rest with the affected part elevated
- Cleanse the lesion, control secondary infection with topical antibiotics, and change dressings twice daily

Manual extraction

- Traditional extraction of emerging worms by gradually rolling them out a few centimeters each day on a small stick is still useful, especially when done along with chemotherapy and use of aseptic dressings
- The process appears to be facilitated by placing the affected part in water several times a day
- If the worm is broken during removal, however, secondary infection almost always results, leading to cellulitis, abscess formation, or septicemia

 OUTCOME

COMPLICATIONS

- Ankle and knee joint infections with resultant deformity are common complications

WHEN TO REFER

- For manual or surgical extraction

PREVENTION

- The disease is prevented by use of only noncontaminated drinking water. This can be accomplished either by preventing contamination of community water supplies through use of tube wells, hand pumps, or cisterns or treating water sources with temephos; or filtering water through nets (eg, nylon nets of 100-μm pore size); or boiling water
- All persons in an endemic area should be actively immunized against tetanus

 EVIDENCE

INFORMATION FOR PATIENTS

- Centers for Disease Control http://www.cdc.gov/ncidod/dpd/ parasites/guineaworm/factsht_ guineaworm.htm
- National Institute of Allergy and Infectious Diseases http://www.niaid.nih.gov/publications/ microbes.htm

REFERENCES

- Cairncross S, Muller R, Zagaria N: Dracunculiasis (Guinea worm disease) and the eradication initiative. Clin Microbiol Rev 2002;15:223. [PMID: 11932231]
- Centers for Disease Control and Prevention: Progress toward global dracunculiasis eradication, June 2002. MMWR Morb Mortal Wkly Rep 2002;51:810. [PMID: 12269470]

Drowning

 KEY FEATURES

ESSENTIALS OF DIAGNOSIS

- The asphyxia of drowning is usually due to aspiration of fluid
- May also result from airway obstruction caused by laryngeal spasm while the victim is gasping under water

GENERAL CONSIDERATIONS

- About 10% of victims develop laryngospasm after the first gulp and never aspirate water ("dry drowning")
- The rapid sequence of events after submersion—hypoxemia, laryngospasm, fluid aspiration, ineffective circulation, brain injury, and brain death—may take place within 5–10 min
- This sequence may be delayed for longer periods if the victim, especially a child, has been submerged in very cold water or if the victim has ingested significant amounts of barbiturates
- Immersion in cold water can also cause a rapid fall in the victim's core temperature, so that systemic hypothermia and death may occur before actual drowning

 CLINICAL FINDINGS

SYMPTOMS AND SIGNS

- Unconscious, semiconscious, or awake
- Apprehensive, restless
- Complaining of headaches or chest pain
- Vomiting is common
- Cyanosis, trismus, apnea, tachypnea, and wheezing
- A pink froth from the mouth and nose indicates pulmonary edema
- Tachycardia, arrhythmias, hypotension, cardiac arrest, and circulatory shock
- With prolonged or cold water immersion, hypothermia is likely

DIFFERENTIAL DIAGNOSIS

- Alcohol or drug intoxication
- Myocardial infarction
- Seizure
- Suicide attempt
- Head or spinal cord injury from diving
- Decompression sickness

 DIAGNOSIS

LABORATORY TESTS

- Urinalysis shows proteinuria, hemoglobinuria, and acetonuria
- Leukocytosis is usually present
- The PaO_2 is usually decreased and the $PaCO_2$ increased or decreased
- The blood pH is decreased as a result of metabolic acidosis

IMAGING STUDIES

- Chest x-rays may show pneumonitis or pulmonary edema

TREATMENT

MEDICATIONS

- Bronchospasm due to aspirated material may require use of bronchodilators
- Antibiotics should be given only when there is clinical evidence of infection—not prophylactically
- Central venous pressure (or, preferably, pulmonary artery wedge pressure) can guide the use of vascular fluid replacement, pressors, or diuretics
- Metabolic acidosis is present in 70% of near-drowning victims, but it usually corrects with adequate ventilation and oxygenation. While controversial, bicarbonate administration (1 mEq/kg) has been recommended for comatose patients

THERAPEUTIC PROCEDURES

First aid

- Immediate CPR
- Hypothermia and cervical spine injury should always be suspected
- Do *not* attempt to drain water from the victim's lungs
- The Heimlich maneuver should be used only if airway obstruction by a foreign body is suspected. The cervical spine should be immobilized if neck injury is possible
- Do *not* discontinue basic life support for seemingly "hopeless" patients until core temperature reaches 32°C. Complete recovery has been reported after prolonged resuscitation of hypothermic patients

Hospital care

- Admit all patients
- Continuous monitoring of cardiorespiratory function, serial determination of arterial blood gases, pH, renal function (serum creatinine), and electrolytes, and measurement of urinary output are required. Pulmonary edema may not appear for 24 h
- Administer oxygen immediately at the highest available concentration and maintain oxygen saturation at 90% or higher
- Endotracheal intubation and mechanical ventilation for patients unable to maintain an open airway or normal blood gases and pH
- Nasogastric intubation to remove swallowed water and prevention of aspiration

- Continuous positive airway pressure (CPAP) is the most effective means of reversing hypoxia in patients with spontaneous respirations and patent airways
- Positive end-expiratory pressure (PEEP) is also effective for treating respiratory insufficiency
- Perform serial physical examinations and chest x-rays to detect possible pneumonitis, atelectasis, and pulmonary edema
- Some near-drowning patients may progress to irreversible central nervous system damage despite apparently adequate treatment of hypoxia and shock. Mild hyperventilation to achieve a $PaCO_2$ of approximately 30 mm Hg is recommended to lower intracranial pressure
- Hypothermia—core temperature should be measured and managed as appropriate (see *Hypothermia*)

OUTCOME

FOLLOW-UP

- Keep victims of prolonged hypoxemia under close hospital observation for 2–3 days after all supportive measures have been withdrawn and clinical and laboratory findings have been stable
- Residual complications of near drowning may include intellectual impairment, convulsive disorders, and pulmonary or cardiac disease

PROGNOSIS

- Spontaneous return of consciousness often occurs in otherwise healthy individuals when submersion is very brief
- Many other patients respond promptly to immediate ventilation
- Other patients, with more severe degrees of near drowning, may have frank respiratory failure, pulmonary edema, shock, anoxic encephalopathy, cerebral edema, and cardiac arrest
- A few patients may be deceptively asymptomatic during the recovery period—only to deteriorate or die as a result of acute respiratory failure within the following 12–24 h

PREVENTION

- Avoidance of alcohol during recreational swimming or boating
- Swimming lessons early in life
- Use of personal flotation devices when boating

EVIDENCE

PRACTICE GUIDELINES

- National Guideline Clearinghouse http://www.guideline.gov/summary/summary.aspx?doc_id=3502&nbr=2728&string=drowning
- Canadian Medical Association http://mdm.ca/cpgsnew/cpgs/search/english/help/ht_drowningprevention.htm

WEB SITE

- Merck Manual—Disorder due to physical agents http://www.merck.com/pubs/mmanual/section20/sec20.htm

INFORMATION FOR PATIENTS

- American Red Cross http://www.redcross.org/services/hss/tips/healthtips/safetywater.html
- American Medical Association http://www.medem.com/medlb/article_detaillb .cfm?article_ID=ZZZ-WZQ6OBAC&sub_cat=104

REFERENCE

- Sachdeva RC: Near drowning. Crit Care Clin 1999;15:281. [PMID: 10331129]

Richard Cohen, MD, MPH
Brent R.W. Moelleken, MD, FACS

Drug Use–Related Infections

KEY FEATURES

ESSENTIALS OF DIAGNOSIS

- Common infections that occur with greater frequency in drug users: skin infections, hepatitis A, B, C, D, aspiration pneumonia, tuberculosis, pulmonary septic emboli, sexually transmitted diseases, AIDS, infective endocarditis, osteomyelitis, and septic arthritis
- Rare infections in the United States include: tetenus, malaria, and melioidosis

GENERAL CONSIDERATIONS

Skin infections

- Associated with poor hygiene and use of nonsterile technique when injecting drugs
- *Staphylococcus aureus* (including methicillin-resistant strains) and oral flora (streptococci, *Eikenella*, *Fusobacterium*, *Peptostreptococcus*) are the most common organisms, with enteric gram-negatives less common and seen in those who inject into the groin
- Cellulitis and subcutaneous abscesses occur most commonly, particularly in association with subcutaneous ("skin-popping") or intramuscular injections and the use of cocaine and heroin mixtures (probably due to ischemia)
- Myositis, clostridial myonecrosis, and necrotizing fasciitis occur infrequently but are life-threatening
- Wound botulism in association with black tar heroin occurs sporadically but often in clusters

Hepatitis

- Very common among habitual drug users
- Transmissible both by the parenteral (hepatitis B, C, and D) and by the fecal–oral route (hepatitis A)
- Multiple episodes of hepatitis with different agents can occur

Aspiration pneumonia

- Result from altered consciousness associated with drug use
- Mixed aerobic and anaerobic mouth flora are usually involved
- Complications include lung abscess, empyema, and brain abscess

Tuberculosis

- Infection with HIV has fostered the spread of tuberculosis in this population

Pulmonary septic emboli

- From venous thrombi or right-sided endocarditis

Sexually transmitted diseases

- Related to the practice of exchanging sex for drugs
- Syphilis, gonorrhea, and chancroid are the most common

AIDS

- High incidence among intravenous drug users and their sexual contacts and among the offspring of infected women

Infective endocarditis

- The organisms are most commonly *S aureus*, *Candida* (especially *Candida parapsilosis*), *Enterococcus faecalis*, other streptococci, and gram-negative bacteria (especially *Pseudomonas* and *Serratia marcescens*)
- Involvement of the right side of the heart is common, and infection of more than one valve is not infrequent
- Right-sided involvement, especially in the absence of murmurs, is often suggested by the presence of septic pulmonary emboli

Other vascular infections

- Septic thrombophlebitis
- Mycotic aneurysms resulting from direct trauma to a vessel with secondary infection most commonly occur in femoral arteries and less commonly in arteries of the neck. Aneurysms resulting from hematogenous spread of organisms frequently involve intracerebral vessels and thus are seen in association with endocarditis

Osteomyelitis and septic arthritis

- Osteomyelitis involving vertebral bodies, sternoclavicular joints, the pubic symphysis, the sacroiliac joints, and other sites usually results from hematogenous distribution of injected organisms or septic venous thrombi
- While staphylococci—often methicillin-resistant—are common organisms, *Serratia*, *Pseudomonas*, *Candida* (usually not *C albicans*), and other pathogens rarely encountered in spontaneous bone or joint disease are found

Tetanus

- Increased tetanus immunization has resulted in a decline in this disease
- Reported cases are generally when drugs are injected subcutaneously ("skin-popping")

Malaria

- Needle transmission occurs from intravenous drug users who acquired the infection in malaria-endemic areas outside the United States

Melioidosis

- This chronic pulmonary infection caused by *Burkholderia pseudomallei* is occasionally seen in debilitated drug users; most cases are reported in Asia and Australia

DEMOGRAPHICS

- There are an estimated 300,000 or more intravenous drug users in the United States

CLINICAL FINDINGS

SYMPTOMS AND SIGNS

- Those of the underlying infection

DIFFERENTIAL DIAGNOSIS

- Community-acquired pneumonia
- Endocarditis
- Complications of endocarditis, eg, pulmonary septic emboli, epidural abscess, osteomyelitis
- Skin abscess, cellulitis, myositis, necrotizing fasciitis
- Pelvic inflammatory disease
- Urinary tract infection

DIAGNOSIS

LABORATORY TESTS

- Appropriate cultures (blood, urine, and sputum)
- Complete blood cell count, liver function tests, urinalysis

IMAGING STUDIES

- Chest x-ray
- Classic radiographic findings are often absent in HIV patients with tuberculosis; any patient with infiltrates who does not respond to antibiotics is suspect
- Pain and fever precede radiographic changes of osteomyelitis and septic arthritis, sometimes by several weeks

DIAGNOSITIC PROCEDURES

- If blood cultures are positive for an organism that is an unusual cause of endocarditis, a transesophageal echocardiogram may be helpful. It is 90% sensitive in detecting vegetations and a negative study is strong evidence against endocarditis

TREATMENT

MEDICATIONS

- A common and difficult clinical problem is management of the parenteral drug user who presents with fever. In general, after obtaining appropriate cultures (blood, urine, and sputum if the chest x-ray is abnormal), empirical therapy is begun (Table 123, page 1306)
- If the chest x-ray suggests a community-acquired pneumonia (consolidation), therapy for outpatient pneumonia is begun with a second- or third-generation cephalosporin (many would add azithromycin or doxycycline to this regimen)
- If the chest x-ray suggests septic emboli (nodular infiltrates), therapy for presumed endocarditis is initiated, usually with a combination of nafcillin (or vancomycin if there is a high prevalence of methicillin-resistant *S aureus* or if enterococcus is a consideration) and gentamicin
- If the chest x-ray is normal and no focal site of infection can be found, endocarditis is presumed. While awaiting the results of blood cultures, empirical treatment with nafcillin (or vancomycin) and gentamicin is started
- If blood cultures are positive for organisms that frequently cause endocarditis in drug users (see above), endocarditis is presumed to be present and treated accordingly
- If blood cultures are positive for an organism that is an unusual cause of endocarditis, evaluation for an occult source of infection should go forward
- If blood cultures are negative and the patient responds to antibiotics, therapy should be continued for 7–14 days (oral therapy can be given once an initial response has occurred)
- In every patient, careful examination for an occult source of infection (genitourinary, dental, sinus, gallbladder, etc) should be done

 OUTCOME

COMPLICATIONS

- See the specific diagnoses

WHEN TO REFER

- For complicated infections such as endocarditis, osteomyelitis, or septic arthritis

WHEN TO ADMIT

- Complicated infections as above
- Marked systemic toxcity

PREVENTION

- Immunizations against hepatitis A and B
- Clean needle use will decrease transmission of blood-borne pathogens

 EVIDENCE

PRACTICE GUIDELINES

- National Guideline Clearinghouse http://www.guideline.gov/summary/ summary.aspx?doc_id=1680&nbr=906 &string=injection+drug+use http://www.guideline.gov/summary/ summary.aspx?doc_id=2390&nbr= 1616&string=endocarditis

INFORMATION FOR PATIENTS

- Centers for Disease Control http://www.cdc.gov/idu/hepatitis/viral_ hep_drug_use.htm
- The Mayo Clinic http://www.mayoclinic.com/invoke.cfm? id=DS00450
- American Heart Association http://www.americanheart.org/presenter. jhtml?identifier=4436

REFERENCES

- Brown PD, Levine DP: Infections in injection drug users. Infect Dis Clin North Am 2002;16:535.
- Levine DP, Brown PD: Infections in injection drug users. In: *Principles and Practice of Infectious Diseases,* ed 5. Mandell GL, Bennett JR, Dolin R (editors). Churchill Livingstone, 2000.
- Murphy EL et al: Risk factors for skin and soft-tissue abscesses among injection drug users: a case-control study. Clin Infect Dis 2001;33:35. [PMID: 11389492]

Richard A. Jacobs, MD, PhD

Dysautonomia

 KEY FEATURES

ESSENTIALS OF DIAGNOSIS

- Features may occur in isolation or combinations and include abnormalities of blood pressure, heart rate, thermoregulatory sweating, intestinal motility, sphincter control, sexual function, respiration, and ocular function

GENERAL CONSIDERATIONS

Primary neurodegenerative disorders with dysautonomia

- Primary autonomic failure
- Multisystem atrophy: constellation of parkinsonism, pyramidal signs, and cerebellar deficits; called Shy-Drager syndrome) when autonomic signs predominate
- Parkinson's disease

CNS lesions that may exhibit features of dysautonomias (usually postural hypotension)

- Spinal cord transection, other myelopathies above the T6 level (eg, due to tumor or syringomyelia), or brain stem lesions such as syringobulbia and posterior fossa tumors

Peripheral causes

- Guillain-Barré syndrome may have features of marked hypotension or hypertension or cardiac arrhythmias
- Diabetes, uremia, amyloidosis, leprosy, Chagas' disease, hepatic porphyria, botulism, the Lambert-Eaton myasthenic syndrome (the latter two may have constipation, urinary retention, and a sicca syndrome as a result of impaired cholinergic function)

 CLINICAL FINDINGS

SYMPTOMS AND SIGNS

- Syncope
- Postural hypotension
- Persistent tachycardia without other cause
- Facial flushing, hypo- or hyperhidrosis
- Vomiting, constipation, diarrhea, dysphagia, abdominal distension
- Disturbances of micturition or defecation
- Apneic episodes
- Declining night vision

DIFFERENTIAL DIAGNOSIS

- Hypovolemia
- Drugs, eg, β-blockers, calcium-channel blockers, vasodilators, diuretics
- Situational syncope, eg, micturition, defecation, cough, swallow
- Postural hypotension
  - Reduced cardiac output from volume depletion, aortic stenosis or cardiomyopathy, cardiac dysrhythmias, various medications
  - Endocrine disorders such as diabetes, Addison's disease, hypo- or hyperthyroidism, pheochromocytoma, and carcinoid syndrome

 DIAGNOSIS

LABORATORY TESTS

- Serum glucose, electrolytes, renal function
- Thryoid function tests, serum serotonin, 24-h urinary metanephrines, and 5-hydroxyindoleacetic acid
- Autonomic function tests

IMAGING STUDIES

- For those with evidence of a central lesion, imaging studies will exclude a treatable structural cause

DIAGNOSTIC PROCEDURES

- Clinical evaluation focuses on excluding reversible, nonneurological causes of symptoms
- Evaluate the Valsalva maneuver, cardiovascular response to startle, mental stress, postural change, and deep respiration, and the sudomotor (sweating) responses to warming or a deep inspiratory gasp
- Tilt-table testing may point to a neuro-cardiogenic cause of syncope
- Pharmacological studies to evaluate the pupillary responses, radiologic studies of the bladder or gastrointestinal tract, uroflowmetry and urethral pressure profiles, and recording of nocturnal penile tumescence may also be necessary in selected cases

Dysautonomia

 TREATMENT

MEDICATIONS

- Treatment may include wearing waist-high elastic hosiery, salt supplementation, sleeping in a semierect position (which minimizes the natriuresis and diuresis that occur during recumbency), and fludrocortisone (0.1–0.3 mg daily)
- Vasoconstrictor agents may be helpful and include midodrine (2.5–10 mg three times daily) and ephedrine (15–30 mg three times daily)
- Less commonly used agents are dihydroergotamine, yohimbine, and clonidine
- Refractory cases may respond to erythropoietin (epoetin alfa) or desmopressin

THERAPEUTIC PROCEDURES

- Avoid abrupt postural change, prolonged recumbency, and other precipitants (eg, straining with bowel movements)
- Medications associated with postural hypotension should be discontinued or reduced in dose
- There is no satisfactory treatment for disturbances of sweating, but an air-conditioned environment is helpful in avoiding extreme swings in body temperature
- Postprandial hypotension is helped by caffeine

 OUTCOME

WHEN TO REFER

- When the diagnosis is in question
- When symptoms do not respond to conventional therapy

EVIDENCE

PRACTICE GUIDELINES

- Gilman S et al: Consensus statement on the diagnosis of multiple system atrophy. American Autonomic Society and American Academy of Neurology. Clin Auton Res 1998;8:359.

INFORMATION FOR PATIENTS

- National Institute of Neurological Diseases and Stroke http://www.ninds.nih.gov/health_and_medical/disorders/ dysauto_doc.htm
- American Association of Neurological Surgeons http://www.neurosurgery.org/health/patient/detail.asp?DisorderID=46

REFERENCES

- Goldstein DS et al: Dysautonomias: clinical disorders of the autonomic nervous system. Ann Intern Med 2002; 137:753. [PMID: 12416949]
- Kaufmann H et al: Why do we faint? Muscle Nerve 2001;24:981. [PMID: 11439373]

Michael J. Aminoff, MD, DSc, FRCP

Dysmenorrhea

 KEY FEATURES

ESSENTIALS OF DIAGNOSIS

- **Primary dysmenorrhea** is menstrual pain associated with ovular cycles in the absence of pathological findings
- **Secondary dysmenorrhea** is menstrual pain for which an organic cause exists, such as endometriosis

GENERAL CONSIDERATIONS

Primary dysmenorrhea

- The pain usually begins within 1–2 years after the menarche and may become more severe with time
- The pain is produced by uterine vasoconstriction, anoxia, and sustained contractions mediated by prostaglandins

DEMOGRAPHICS

Primary dysmenorrhea

- The frequency of cases increases up to age 20 and then decreases with age and markedly with parity
- Fifty to 75% women are affected at some time, and 5–6% have incapacitating pain

Secondary dysmenorrhea

- It usually begins well after menarche, sometimes even as late as the third or fourth decade of life

 CLINICAL FINDINGS

SYMPTOMS AND SIGNS

Primary dysmenorrhea

- Pain is low, midline, wave-like, cramping pelvic pain often radiating to the back or inner thighs
- Cramps may last for 1 or more days and may be associated with nausea, diarrhea, headache, and flushing
- No pathological findings on pelvic examination

Secondary dysmenorrhea

- The history and physical examination commonly suggest endometriosis or pelvic inflammatory disease

DIFFERENTIAL DIAGNOSIS

- Endometriosis
- Adenomyosis (uterine endometriosis)
- Pelvic inflammatory disease
- Uterine leiomyomas (fibroids)
- Intrauterine device
- Pelvic pain syndrome
- Endometrial polyp
- Cervicitis
- Retroverted uterus
- Cervical stenosis
- Cystitis
- Interstitial cystitis

 DIAGNOSIS

IMAGING STUDIES

- MRI is the most reliable method to detect submucous myomas

DIAGNOSTIC PROCEDURES

Secondary dysmenorrhea

- Laparoscopy is often needed to differentiate endometriosis from pelvic inflammatory disease
- Submucous myomas can be detected by hysterogram, by hysteroscopy, or by passing a sound or curette over the uterine cavity during D&C

TREATMENT

MEDICATIONS

Primary dsymenorrhea

- Nonsteroidal antiinflammatory drugs (ibuprofen, ketoprofen, mefenamic acid, naproxen) are generally helpful
- Drugs should be started at the onset of bleeding to avoid inadvertent drug use during early pregnancy
- Medication should be continued on a regular basis for 2–3 days
- Ovulation can be suppressed and dysmenorrhea usually prevented by oral contraceptives

Secondary dysmenorrhea

- Periodic use of analgesics, including the nonsteroidal antiinflammatory drugs given for primary dysmenorrhea, may be beneficial
- Oral contraceptives may give relief, particularly in endometriosis
- Danazol and gonadotropin-releasing hormone agonists are effective in the treatment of endometriosis

SURGERY

- If disability is marked or prolonged, laparoscopy or exploratory laparotomy is usually warranted
- Definitive surgery depends upon the degree of disability and the findings at operation

THERAPEUTIC PROCEDURES

- Cervical stenosis may result from induced abortion, creating crampy pain at the time of expected menses with no blood flow; this is easily cured by passing a sound into the uterine cavity after administering a paracervical block

 OUTCOME

WHEN TO REFER

- The expertise of a gynecologist is frequently useful in the diagnosis and treatment of secondary dysmenorrhea

 EVIDENCE

PRACTICE GUIDELINES

- National Guideline Clearinghouse
  http://www.guideline.gov/summary/summary.aspx?doc_id=2737&nbr=1963&string=dysmenorrhea

WEB SITE

- Gynecology Handbook for Family Practitioners
  http://www.vh.org/Providers/ClinRef/FPHandbook/13.html

INFORMATION FOR PATIENTS

- University of Utah
  http://www.med.utah.edu/healthinfo/adult/gynonc/dysmen.htm
- American College of Obstetricians and Gynecologists
  http://www.medem.com/medlb/article_detaillb.cfm?article_ID=ZZZJVXZ887C&sub_cat=328

REFERENCES

- Coco AS: Primary dysmenorrhea. Am Fam Physician 1999;60:489. [PMID: 10465224]
- Wilson M et al: Dysmenorrhea. Clin Evidence 2001;6:1388

H. Trent MacKay, MD, MPH

Dyspareunia (Painful Intercourse)

 KEY FEATURES

GENERAL CONSIDERATIONS

Etiology

- Vulvovaginitis: inflammation or infection of the vagina
- Vaginismus
  - Voluntary or involuntary contraction of muscles around the introitus
  - Results from fear, pain, sexual trauma, or having learned negative attitudes toward sex during childhood
- Remnants of the hymen: a rim of hymen may remain after initial episodes of intercourse, causing pain
- Insufficient lubrication of the vagina is a frequent cause of dyspareunia in postmenopausal women
- Infection, endometriosis, tumors, or other pathological conditions: pain occurring with deep thrusting during coitus is usually due to acute or chronic infection of the cervix, uterus, or adnexa; endometriosis; adnexal tumors; or adhesions resulting from prior pelvic disease or operation
- Vulvodynia is the most frequent cause of dyspareunia in premenopausal women

 CLINICAL FINDINGS

SYMPTOMS AND SIGNS

- Questions related to sexual functioning should be asked as part of the reproductive history. Two helpful questions are, "Are you sexually active?" and "Are you having any sexual difficulties at this time?"
- During the pelvic examination, the patient should be placed in a half-sitting position and given a hand-held mirror and then asked to point out the site of pain and describe the type of pain
- Vulvovaginitis: areas of marked tenderness in the vulvar vestibule without visible inflammation
- Vulvodynia
  - A sensation of burning along with other symptoms including pain, itching, stinging, irritation, and rawness
  - Discomfort may be constant or intermittent, focal or diffuse, and experienced as either deep or superficial
  - Generally no physical findings except minimal erythema that may be associated with a subset of vulvodynia, vulvar vestibulitis

DIFFERENTIAL DIAGNOSIS

- Vulvodynia or vulvar vestibulitis
- Vaginismus
- Insufficient vaginal lubrication
- Atrophic vaginitis
- Vulvovaginitis, cervicitis, or pelvic inflammatory disease
- Endometriosis
- Lichen sclerosus
- Ovarian tumor
- Pelvic adhesions
- Remnants of the hymen

 DIAGNOSIS

DIAGNOSTIC PROCEDURES

Vulvovaginitis

- Areas of marked tenderness in the vulvar vestibule without visible inflammation occasionally show lesions resembling small condylomas on colposcopy

TREATMENT

THERAPEUTIC PROCEDURES

Vulvovaginitis

- Warty lesions on colposcopy or biopsy should be treated appropriately (see *Vaginitis*)
- Irritation from spermicides—discuss noncoital techniques to achieve orgasm until the infection subsides

Vaginismus

- Sexual counseling and education may be useful
- Self-dilation, using a lubricated finger or test tubes of graduated sizes, may help. Before coitus (with adequate lubrication) is attempted, the patient and then partner should be able to painlessly introduce two fingers into the vagina

Remnants of the hymen

- Rarely, may need manual dilation of a remaining hymen under general anesthesia
- Avoid surgery

Insufficient lubrication of the vagina

- See *Menopausal syndrome*
- For inadequate sexual arousal, sexual counseling is helpful
- Lubricants during sexual foreplay may be of use
- If lubrication remains inadequate, use estradiol vaginal ring worn continuously and replaced every 3 months Concomitant progestin therapy is not needed with the ring
- Estrogen vaginal cream

Infection, endometriosis, tumors, or other pathological conditions

- Temporarily abstain from coitus during treatment
- Consider hormonal or surgical treatment of endometriosis
- Dyspareunia from chronic pelvic inflammatory disease or extensive adhesions is difficult to treat without extirpative surgery. Couples can be advised to try coital positions that limit deep thrusting and to use manual and oral sexual techniques

Vulvodynia

- Difficult management since etiology unclear
- Surgical vestibulectomy has had success

- Antiviral, antifungal, corticosteroid, or anesthetic agents have varied success
- Pain control through behavioral therapy, biofeedback, or acupuncture has varied success
- Continuous genital burning or pain may be relieved with amitriptyline in gradually increasing doses from 10 mg/day to 75–100 mg/day

OUTCOME

WHEN TO REFER

- When symptoms persist despite first-line therapy
- For expertise in procedures

EVIDENCE

PRACTICE GUIDELINES

- National Guideline Clearinghouse http://www.guideline.gov/summary/summary.aspx?doc_id=3033&nbr=2259&string=dyspareunia

WEB SITE

- Gynecology Handbook for Family Practitioners http://www.vh.org/Providers/ClinRef/FPHandbook/13.html

INFORMATION FOR PATIENTS

- Amercian Academy of Family Physicians http://familydoctor.org/handouts/669.html
- American College of Obstetricians and Gynecologists http://www.medem.com/MedLB/article_detaillb.cfm?article_ID=ZZZ7P2WBT7C&sub_cat=2

REFERENCES

- Davis GD et al: Clinical management of vulvodynia. Clin Obstet Gynecol 1999;42:221. [PMID: 10370843]
- Masheb RM et al: Vulvodynia: an introduction and critical review of a chronic pain condition. Pain 2000;86:3. [PMID: 10779654]

H. Trent MacKay, MD, MPH

Dyspepsia

 KEY FEATURES

ESSENTIALS OF DIAGNOSIS

- Heartburn (retrosternal burning)
- Pain or discomfort centered in the upper abdomen
- Upper abdominal fullness, early satiety, burning, bloating, belching, nausea, retching, or vomiting

GENERAL CONSIDERATIONS

- Functional or "nonulcer" dyspepsia is the most common cause

DEMOGRAPHICS

- Occurs in 25% of the adult population
- Accounts for 3% of office visits

 CLINICAL FINDINGS

SYMPTOMS AND SIGNS

- Weight loss, persistent vomiting, and dysphagia warrant endoscopy or abdominal imaging
- Signs of serious disease: weight loss, organomegaly, abdominal mass, or fecal occult blood

DIFFERENTIAL DIAGNOSIS

- Peptic ulcer disease (in 15–25% of cases)
- Gastroesophageal reflux (in 20%)
- Gastritis, eg, nonsteroidal antiinflammatory drugs, alcohol, stress, *Helicobacter pylori*
- Chronic pancreatitis or pancreatic cancer
- "Indigestion" from overeating, high-fat foods, coffee
- Other drugs: aspirin, antibiotics (eg, macrolides, metronidazole), corticosteroids, digoxin, iron, theophylline, and opioids
- Gastroparesis
- Lactase deficiency
- Malabsorption
- Gastric cancer (in 1%)
- Parasitic infection, eg, *Giardia, Strongyloides, Ascaris*
- Cholelithiasis, choledocholithiasis, or cholangitis
- *H pylori* (controversial)
- Myocardial ischemia or pericarditis
- Abdominal or paraesophageal hernia
- Pregnancy
- Chronic mesenteric ischemia
- Metabolic conditions: diabetes, thyroid disease, renal insufficiency
- Intraabdominal malignancy
- Physical or sexual abuse

DIAGNOSIS

- History entails chronicity, location, and quality of the discomfort, but has limited diagnostic utility
- Under age 45 without signs of serious organic disease [dysphagia, weight loss, severe pain, vomiting, anemia, gastrointestinal (GI) bleeding]: noninvasive testing for *H pylori* (urea breath test, fecal antigen test, or serology); treat if positive
- Consider trial of proton pump inhibitors for 4–8 weeks
- If symptoms persist or recur after empirical treatment, perform esophagogastroduodenoscopy (EGD)
- Over age 45 or any age with signs of serious organic disease: upper endoscopy

LABORATORY TESTS

- Obtain complete blood cell count, serum electrolytes, liver enzymes, calcium, and thyroid-stimulating hormone

IMAGING STUDIES

- Abdominal ultrasonography indicated if pancreatic or biliary tract disease is suspected
- Upper gastrointestinal barium radiography is inferior to endoscopy

DIAGNOSTIC PROCEDURES

- Upper endoscopy indicated in all patients age >45 years with new-onset dyspepsia and in all patients with weight loss, dysphagia, recurrent vomiting, hematemesis, melena, or anemia
- Upper endoscopy helpful in reassuring patients concerned about serious underlying disease
- Noninvasive test for *H pylori*: IgG serology, fecal antigen test, or urea breath test
- Gastric emptying studies indicated for recurrent vomiting
- Ambulatory esophageal pH testing if atypical gastroesophageal reflux is suspected

Dyspepsia

TREATMENT

MEDICATIONS

- H_2-receptor antagonists or proton pump inhibitors benefit 10–20%
- H_2-receptor antagonists (ranitidine or nizatidine, 150 mg PO BID; famotidine, 20 mg PO BID; or cimetidine, 400–800 mg PO BID)
- Proton pump inhibitors (omeprazole or rabeprazole, 20 mg, lansoprazole, 30 mg, esomeprazole or pantoprazole, 40 mg PO QD)
- Antidepressants (eg, desipramine or nortriptyline, 10–50 mg PO QHS)
- Prokinetic agent, metoclopramide 10 mg PO TID, improves symptoms in up to 60%
- *H pylori* eradication therapy benefits 5–15% (see Helicobacter pylori *gastritis*)

THERAPEUTIC PROCEDURES

- Discontinue potentially offending medications if possible
- Reduce or discontinue alcohol and caffeine intake

OUTCOME

FOLLOW-UP

- Reevaluate symptoms after 4–6 weeks of empirical management; if they persist or recur, further testing with EGD, possible imaging studies

PROGNOSIS

- Half to two-thirds have functional dyspepsia, ie, no demonstrable organic cause; symptoms may be chronic

WHEN TO REFER

- Dyspepsia with signs of serious organic disease
- Chronic dyspepsia unresponsive to routine therapies

WHEN TO ADMIT

- Signs of GI bleeding
- Protracted vomiting with dehydration

EVIDENCE

PRACTICE GUIDELINES

- American Gastroenterological Association medical position statement: evaluation of dyspepsia Gastroenterology 1998;114:579. [PMID: 9496949]
- Dyspepsia. Institute for Clinical Systems Improvement—Private Nonprofit Organization, 2003 http://www.icsi.org/knowledge/detail. asp?catID=29&itemID=171
- Eisen GM et al: The role of endoscopy in dyspepsia. Gastrointest Endosc 2001; 54:815. [PMID: 11726874]

WEB SITES

- American Academy of Family Physicians—Dyspepsia http://familydoctor.org/handouts/474. html
- Digestive Diseases Foundation—Indigestion http://www.digestivedisorders.org.uk/ leaflets/indig.htm

INFORMATION FOR PATIENTS

- Cleveland Clinic—What is Indigestion? http://www.clevelandclinic.org/health/ health-info/docs/1700/1779.asp? index=7316
- Uptodate—Functional dyspepsia http://patients.uptodate.com/frames. asp?page=topic.asp&file=digestiv/ 7283&title=Dyspepsia

REFERENCES

- Soo S et al: Pharmacological interventions for non-ulcer dyspepsia. Cochrane Database Syst Rev 2000;2:CD001960. [PMID: 10796840]
- Talley NJ et al: Functional gastroduodenal disorders. Gut 1999;45(Suppl 2):II37. [PMID: 10457043]

Kenneth R. McQuaid, MD

Dystonia, Torsion

 ## KEY FEATURES

ESSENTIALS OF DIAGNOSIS

- Dystonic movements and postures
- Normal birth and developmental history. No other neurological signs
- Investigations (including CT scan or MRI) reveal no cause of dystonia

GENERAL CONSIDERATIONS

- May occur sporadically or on a hereditary basis, with autosomal dominant, autosomal recessive, and X-linked recessive modes of transmission
- The responsible gene is located at 9q34 (and has been named *DYT1*) and involves a unique mutation consisting of a GAG deletion in the dominantly inherited disorder and maps to the long arm of the X chromosome in the X-linked recessive form; the responsible gene in the autosomal recessive disorder is unknown
- Other autosomal dominant forms have also been recognized, with different or unidentified genetic loci
- Symptoms may begin in childhood or later and persist throughout life

 ## CLINICAL FINDINGS

SYMPTOMS AND SIGNS

- Onset of abnormal movements and postures in a patient with a normal birth and developmental history, no relevant past medical illness, and no other neurological signs
- Dystonic movements of the head and neck may take the form of torticollis, blepharospasm, facial grimacing, or forced opening or closing of the mouth. The limbs may also adopt abnormal but characteristic postures
- The age at onset influences both the clinical findings and the prognosis. With onset in childhood, there is usually a family history of the disorder, symptoms commonly commence in the legs, and progression is likely until there is severe disability from generalized dystonia
- In contrast, when onset is later, a positive family history is unlikely, initial symptoms are often in the arms or axial structures, and severe disability does not usually occur, although generalized dystonia may ultimately develop in some patients

DIFFERENTIAL DIAGNOSIS

- Perinatal anoxia
- Birth trauma
- Neonatal kernicterus
- Wilson's disease
- Huntington's disease
- Parkinsonism
- Sequela of encephalitis lethargica
- Neuroleptic drug therapy
- Dopa-responsive dystonia

 ## DIAGNOSIS

IMAGING STUDIES

- Investigations (including MRI or CT imaging) reveal no cause for the abnormal movements

TREATMENT

MEDICATIONS

- Idiopathic torsion dystonia usually responds poorly to drugs
- Levodopa, diazepam, baclofen, carbamazepine, amantadine, or anticholinergic medication (in high dosage) is occasionally helpful
- If not, a trial of treatment with phenothiazines or haloperidol may be worthwhile
- In each case, the dose has to be individualized, depending on response and tolerance. However, the doses of these latter drugs that are required for benefit usually lead to mild parkinsonism

THERAPEUTIC PROCEDURES

- Stereotactic thalamotomy is sometimes helpful with predominantly unilateral dystonia, especially when this involves the limbs

 OUTCOME

PROGNOSIS

- A distinct variety of dominantly inherited dystonia, mapping to a genetic locus on chromosome 14q, is remarkably responsive to levodopa
- About one-third of patients eventually become so severely disabled that they are confined to chair or bed, while another one-third are affected only mildly

 EVIDENCE

PRACTICE GUIDELINES

- Sanger TD et al: Task Force on Childhood Motor Disorders. Classification and definition of disorders causing hypertonia in childhood Pediatrics 2003;111:e89.

INFORMATION FOR PATIENTS

- National Institute of Neurological Disorders and Stroke http://www.ninds.nih.gov/health_and_medical/pubs/dystonias.htm
- Worldwide Education and Awareness for Movement Disorders http://www.mdvu.org/library/pediatric/dystonia/

REFERENCES

- Bressman SB et al: Diagnostic criteria for dystonia in DYT1 families. Neurology 2002;59:1780. [PMID: 12473770]
- Kanovsky P: Dystonia: a disorder of motor programming or motor execution? Mov Disord 2002;17:1143. [PMID: 12465050]

Michael J. Aminoff, DSc, MD, FRCP

Echinococcosis

KEY FEATURES

ESSENTIALS OF DIAGNOSIS

Cystic hydatid disease

- History of exposure to dogs associated with livestock in a hydatid-endemic region
- A liver cyst that may remain silent for 10–20 or more years until it becomes large enough to be palpable, to be visible as an abdominal swelling, or (rarely) to produce symptoms due to leakage or rupture
- Positive serological tests

GENERAL CONSIDERATIONS

- Parasitism by the larval stage of four *Echinococcus* species. *E granulosus* (cystic hydatid disease) and *E multilocularis* (alveolar hydatid disease) are the most important

Cystic hydatid disease (unilocular hydatid disease)

- There are two major strains, the pastoral and the sylvatic
- The **pastoral** strain—which is more pathogenic to humans—has a transmission cycle in which dogs are the definitive host, and sheep (usually) but cattle and other domestic livestock are intermediate hosts
- The **sylvatic**, or northern, strain is maintained in wolves and wild moose and reindeer
- Human infection occurs when eggs passed in dog feces are swallowed, penetrate the intestinal mucosa, enter the portal bloodstream, and are carried to the liver where they become hydatid cysts (65% of all cysts)
- Some larvae reach the lung (25%) and develop into pulmonary hydatids
- Infrequently, cysts form in the brain, bones, skeletal muscles, kidneys, spleen, or other tissues
- Cysts of the sylvatic strain tend to localize in the lungs
- In the liver, cysts may increase in size 1–30 mm in diameter per year and become enormous, but symptoms generally do not develop until they reach about 10 cm
- Some cysts die spontaneously; others may persist unchanged for years
- Part or all of the inner layer of hepatic and splenic cysts may calcify, which does not necessarily mean cyst death

Alveolar hydatid disease (multilocular hydatid disease)

- The life cycle involves foxes as definitive hosts and microtine rodents as intermediate hosts. Domestic dogs and cats can also become infected with the adult tapeworm when they eat infected wild rodents
- Human infection is by accidental ingestion of tapeworm eggs passed in fox or dog feces

DEMOGRAPHICS

- Endemic foci of *E granulosus* are in eastern Europe, Russia, Australia, New Zealand, India, and the United Kingdom; in North America, foci are in the western United States, the lower Mississippi valley, Alaska, and northwestern Canada
- *E multilocularis* occurs only in the northern hemisphere

CLINICAL FINDINGS

SYMPTOMS AND SIGNS

Cystic hydatid disease

- A liver cyst may remain asymtomatic for 20 or more years until it becomes large enough to produce symptoms
- Right upper quadrant mass that may be palpable and even visible
- Right upper quadrant pain, nausea, and vomiting
- Pressure effects by the cyst may result in biliary obstruction, with secondary bacterial cholangitis, cirrhosis, and portal hypertension
- A characteristic allergic clinical syndrome may follow intrabiliary extrusion of cyst contents—jaundice, biliary colic, urticaria, and a rise in the eosinophil count
- Rupture can occur into the pleural, pericardial, or peritoneal space or into the duodenum, colon, or renal pelvis
- If a cyst ruptures suddenly, anaphylaxis and death may occur

Alveolar hydatid disease

- Alveolar cysts primarily localize in the liver, where they may extend locally or metastasize to other tissues
- The larval mass has poorly defined borders and behaves like a neoplasm
- Lung involvement is rare, usually occurring by direct hepatic extension

DIFFERENTIAL DIAGNOSIS

- Amebic or pyogenic liver abscess
- Malignant or benign tumor of liver or other involved organ
- Fascioliasis (sheep liver fluke)
- Clonorchiasis (Chinese liver fluke)
- Choledocholithiasis
- Congenital liver cyst or liver cyst associated with polycystic kidney disease
- Cavitary pulmonary tuberculosis
- Cysticercosis

DIAGNOSIS

LABORATORY TESTS

- The immunoblot test is the test of choice (95% specific and 91% sensitive for liver cysts); the arc 5 test is also diagnostic. In both tests, cross-reactions can occur with *Taenia solium* cysticercosis infections
- The serological tests (ELISA and Western blot) are usually positive and differentiate *E granulosa* from *E multilocularis*
- In solitary lung cysts, false-negative serology results occur in up to 50% of infections
- Persons from whom cysts have been completely removed and carriers of dead cysts may become seronegative
- Eosinophilia is uncommon except after cyst rupture
- Liver function tests are usually normal

IMAGING STUDIES

Cystic hydatid disease

- The method of choice for liver and splenic cysts is sonography (specificity 90%) followed by CT and MRI; nearly pathognomonic is the presence within a hydatid cyst of daughter cysts; they must be distinguished, however, from blood clots within the cavity of simple cysts
- Chest films may show an elevated diaphragm when liver cysts are present
- Pulmonary cysts are best detected by chest films (calcification of the wall is rare); CT and MRI can also be done
- An intravenous urogram or bone scan may detect cysts at other sites

Alveolar hydatid disease

- X-rays show hepatomegaly and characteristic scattered areas of radiolucency, often outlined by 2- to 4-mm calcific rings

DIAGNOSTIC PROCEDURES

- Although the procedure was contraindicated, ultrasonic-guided percutaneous aspiration of hydatid cysts followed by injection of a scolicidal agent and use of oral albendazole is now used for diagnosis

TREATMENT

MEDICATIONS

Cystic hydatid disease

- Surgical resection is now partially supplanted by anthelmintic treatment
- One approach is to give albendazole to asymptomatic patients whose cysts are small and not in danger of rupture. If, after 6–9 months, the cyst has not disappeared or clearly died, it can be removed surgically
- **Albendazole,** four tablets (800 mg) daily in divided doses with meals for 3 months, is the drug of choice; continue for up to 6 months if there is a response
- Relapses occur and should be retreated
- Bone cysts are more refractory and may require a year of treatment
- Drug side effects include reversible low-grade aminotransferase elevations (15%), leukopenia to 2900/µL (2%), rare gastrointestinal symptoms (including pain at cyst sites), dizziness or headache, alopecia, rash, and pruritus. The drug is contraindicated in pregnancy
- **Praziquantel** kills protoscoleces within hydatid cysts but does not affect the germinal membrane. The drug is being evaluated as adjunctive therapy with albendazole

Alveolar hydatid disease

- Long-term drug therapy (5 years to life) for patients with nonresectable masses is with albendazole (preferred) (800 mg/day in divided doses) or with mebendazole (40 mg/kg/day in divided doses with fatty meals); the drugs inhibit growth of the parasite and have extended patient survival, but larval tissue is not completely destroyed

SURGERY

- The main surgical options available for liver cysts are partial hepatic resection, pericystectomy, and cystectomy
- Pulmonary cysts are treated by surgery plus chemotherapy

- Preoperatively, to reduce the risk of recurrence due to spillage, two drugs (taken with meals) are used for 1 month: albendazole, 10 mg/kg/day in two divided doses, and praziquantel, 25 mg/kg/day. Postoperatively, albendazole should be continued for 1 month; the additional use of praziquantel is under evaluation
- For alveolar hydatid disease, treatment is by surgical removal of the entire larval mass when possible, accompanied by drug treatment

THERAPEUTIC PROCEDURES

- Under ultrasonic guidance, percutaneous aspiration and injection of a scolicidal agent can treat accessible cysts in patients who are inoperable or refuse surgery and are not candidates for a chemotherapeutic trial. The patient should be covered with oral albendazole
- The procedure is contraindicated for cysts that communicate with the biliary tree, those that are superficially loculated, or those that have thick internal septal divisions

OUTCOME

FOLLOW-UP

- Liver function tests and complete blood cell counts should be monitored weekly when using albendazole

PROGNOSIS

- About 15% of untreated patients eventually die because of the disease or its complications
- Ninety percent of patients with nonresectable masses die within 10 years
- 25% recurrence rates after surgery

WHEN TO REFER

- All patients should be referred to a specialist with expertise in this problem

WHEN TO ADMIT

- Patients with symptomatic cysts
- Patients who will have percutaneous aspiration of cysts or surgery

PREVENTION

- In endemic areas, prevention is by prophylactic treatment of pet dogs with 5 mg/kg of praziquantel at monthly intervals to remove adult tapeworms and by health education to prevent feeding of offal to dogs

EVIDENCE

PRACTICE GUIDELINES

- Heath DD et al: Progress in control of hydatidosis using vaccination–a review of formulation and delivery of the vaccine and recommendations for practical use in control programmes. Acta Trop 2003;85(2):133.

INFORMATION FOR PATIENTS

- Centers for Disease Control http://www.cdc.gov/ncidod/dpd/ parasites/alveolarhydatid/factsht_ alveolar_hydatid.htm
- National Institutes of Health http://www.nlm.nih.gov/medlineplus/ ency/article/000676.htm

REFERENCES

- Chrieki M: Echinococcosis—an emerging parasite in the immigrant population. Am Fam Physician 2002;66:817. [PMID: 12322773]
- Ozaslan E et al: Endoscopic therapy in the management of hepatobiliary hydatid disease. J Clin Gastroenterol 2002;35:160. [PMID: 12172363]
- Yorganci K et al: Surgical treatment of hydatid cysts of the liver in the era of percutaneous treatment. Am J Surg 2002;184:63. [PMID: 12135724]

Ectopic Pregnancy

KEY FEATURES

ESSENTIALS OF DIAGNOSIS

- Amenorrhea or irregular bleeding and spotting
  - Pelvic pain, usually adnexal
  - Adnexal mass by clinical examination or ultrasound
  - Failure of serum level of human chorionic gonadotropin (hCG) to double every 48 h
- No intrauterine pregnancy on transvaginal ultrasound with serum hCG of ≥2000 mU/mL

GENERAL CONSIDERATIONS

- Occurs in about one of 150 live births, with 98% of cases being tubal pregnancies
- Implantation may also occur in the peritoneum or abdominal viscera, the ovary, and the cervix
- Undiagnosed or undetected ectopic pregnancy is the most common cause of first-trimester maternal death in the United States

DEMOGRAPHICS

- Conditions that prevent or retard migration of the fertilized ovum can predispose to ectopic implantation
- Specific risk factors are a history of infertility, pelvic inflammatory disease, ruptured appendix, and prior tubal surgery

CLINICAL FINDINGS

SYMPTOMS AND SIGNS

- 40% of cases are acute
  - Sudden onset of severe, nonradiating, intermittent lancinating lower quadrant pain
  - Backache present during attacks
  - Shock in about 10%, often after pelvic examination
  - At least two-thirds of patients give a history of abnormal menstruation
- 60% of cases are chronic
  - Blood leaks from the tubal ampulla over days
  - Persistent vaginal spotting is reported
  - A pelvic mass is palpable
  - Abdominal distension and mild paralytic ileus are often present

DIFFERENTIAL DIAGNOSIS

- Acute appendicitis
- Intrauterine pregnancy (threatened abortion)
- Pelvic inflammatory disease
- Ruptured corpus luteum cyst or ovarian follicle
- Urinary calculi
- Tuboovarian abscess
- Gestational trophoblastic neoplasia, eg, hydatidiform mole
- Shock or sepsis due to other causes

DIAGNOSIS

LABORATORY TESTS

- Complete blood cell count may show anemia and slight leukocytosis
- Serum hCG levels are lower than expected for a normal pregnancy of the same gestational age
- Serum hCG levels may rise slowly or plateau rather than double every 48 h as in viable early pregnancy or fall as in spontaneous abortion

IMAGING STUDIES

- Endovaginal ultrasound may identify the ectopic pregnancy
- An empty uterine cavity demonstrated by abdominal utrasound with an hCG of 6500 mU/mL is virtually diagnostic of an ectopic pregnancy

DIAGNOSTIC PROCEDURES

- Culdocentesis is rarely used in evaluation

Ectopic Pregnancy

 TREATMENT

MEDICATIONS

- Methotrexate (50 mg/m²) is acceptable medical therapy for early ectopic pregnancies less than 3.5 cm and unruptured, without active bleeding
- Iron supplementation may be necessary for anemia during convalescence
- All Rh-negative paitents should receive Rho(D) Ig (300 μg)

SURGERY

- Laparoscopy is the sugical procedure of choice to both confirm and permit removal of an ectopic pregnancy without need for an exploratory laparotomy
- Salpingostomy with removal of the ectopic or partial salpingectomy can usually be performed laparoscopically
- Injection of indigo carmine into the uterine cavity with flow through the contralateral tube can demonstrate its patency

 OUTCOME

COMPLICATIONS

- Tubal infertility

PROGNOSIS

- Repeat tubal pregnancy occurs in 12%
- Early ultrasound confirmation of intrauterine gestation with next pregnancy

WHEN TO REFER

- For suggestive symptoms, laboratory tests, and especially ultrasound findings that support the diagnosis

WHEN TO ADMIT

- All suspected cases of ruptured ectopic pregnancy

EVIDENCE

PRACTICE GUIDELINES

- National Guideline Clearinghouse http://www.guideline.gov/summary/summary.aspx?doc_id=3300&nbr=2526&string=ectopic+pregnancy
- ACOG practice bulletin. Medical management of tubal pregnancy Number 3, December 1998. Clinical management guidelines for obstetrician-gynecologists. American College of Obstetricians and Gynecologists. Int J Gynaecol Obstet 1999;65:97. [PMID: 10390113]

WEB SITES

- Ectopic Pregnancy Demonstration Case http://www.brighamrad.harvard.edu/Cases/bwh/hcache/94/full.html
- Guidelines, Recommendations, and Evidence-Based Medicine in Obstetrics http://matweb.hcuge.ch/matweb/endo/cours_4e_MREG/obstetrics_gynecology_guidelines.htm

INFORMATION FOR PATIENTS

- JAMA patient page: Pregnancy complications. JAMA 2001;285:1664.
- Nemours Foundation http://kidshealth.org/parent/pregnancy_newborn/pregnancy/ectopic.html

REFERENCES

- Buster J et al: Medical management of ectopic pregnancy. Clin Obstet Gynecol 1999;42:23. [PMID: 10073296]
- Hajenius PJ et al: Interventions for tubal ectopic pregnancy. Cochrane Database Syst Rev 2000;(2):CD000324. [PMID:10796710]
- Kamwendo F et al: Epidemiology of ectopic pregnancy during a 28-year period and the role of pelvic inflammatory disease. Sex Transm Infect 2000;76:28. [PMID: 10817065]
- Lipscomb GH et al: Methotrexate for treatment of ectopic pregnancy. Am J Obstet Gynecol 2002;186(6):1192. [PMID: 12066097]

William R. Crombleholme, MD

Edema, Lower Extremity

 KEY FEATURES

ESSENTIALS OF DIAGNOSIS

- History of venous thromboembolism
- Lower extremity asymmetry
- Lower extremity pain
- Lower extremity dependence
- Time course: acute or chronic edema

GENERAL CONSIDERATIONS

- Lower extremities can swell in response to increased venous or lymphatic pressures, decreased intravascular oncotic pressure, increased capillary leak, and local injury or infection
- Acute lower extremity edema: deep venous thrombosis (DVT)
- Other causes of acute edema: ruptured popliteal cyst, calf strain or trauma, cellulitis, and drug therapy with calcium channel blockers (particularly felodipine and amlodipine), thioglitazones, and minoxidil
- Chronic venous insufficiency is the most common cause of chronic lower extremity edema, affecting up to 2% of the population
- Other causes of chronic edema: postphlebitic syndrome with valvular incompetence, congestive heart failure, cirrhosis, drug therapy (as above)

 CLINICAL FINDINGS

SYMPTOMS AND SIGNS

- Assess heart, lungs, and abdomen for evidence of pulmonary hypertension (primary, or secondary to chronic lung disease), congestive heart failure (CHF), or cirrhosis
- Size of both calves should be measured 10 cm below the tibial tuberosity
- Swelling of the entire leg or swelling of one leg >3 cm more than the other suggests deep venous obstruction
- Elicit pitting and tenderness
- Chronic venous insufficiency skin findings range from hyperpigmentation and stasis dermatitis to lipodermatosclerosis and atrophie blanche to skin ulceration
- Stasis dermatitis: brawny, fibrotic skin changes
- Skin ulceration can occur, particularly in the medial malleolar area, when due to chronic venous insufficiency
- Other causes of medial malleolar skin ulceration: arterial insufficiency, vasculitis, infections (including cutaneous diphtheria), or cancer

DIFFERENTIAL DIAGNOSIS

- Cardiovascular
  - CHF (right-sided)
  - Pericardial effusion
  - Pericarditis
  - Tricuspid regurgitation
  - Tricuspid stenosis
  - Pulmonic stenosis
  - Cor pulmonale
  - Venous insufficiency (most common)
  - Venous obstruction
- Noncardiovascular
  - Cirrhosis
  - Low albumin (nephrotic syndrome, malnutrition, protein-losing enteropathy)
  - Cellulitis
  - Premenstrual fluid retention
  - Drugs (vasodilators, eg, calcium channel blockers, salt-retaining medications, eg, nonsteroidal antiinflammatory drugs, thiazolidinediones)
  - Musculoskeletal (Baker's cyst, gastrocnemius tear, compartment syndrome)
  - Lymphatic obstruction
  - Eclampsia
  - Hypothyroidism with myxedema
  - Filariasis

- Unilateral
  - DVT
  - Venous insufficiency
  - Baker's cyst
  - Cellulitis
  - Trauma
  - Lymphatic obstruction, eg, obstruction by pelvic tumor
  - Reflex sympathetic dystrophy

 DIAGNOSIS

LABORATORY TESTS

- Serum creatinine, blood urea nitrogen
- Urinalysis
- Liver tests: alkaline phosphatase, AST, GGT, total bilirubin, albumin
- Thyroid-stimulating hormone

IMAGING STUDIES

- Color duplex ultrasonography of lower extremity
- Ankle-brachial pressure index (ABPI)

DIAGNOSTIC PROCEDURES

- Consider echocardiogram

TREATMENT

THERAPEUTIC PROCEDURES

- Avoid diuretic therapy in patients with chronic venous insufficiency unless co-morbid CHF or other fluid-retaining comorbid condition
- Mechanical measures effective in chronic venous insufficiency
  - Leg elevation, above the level of the heart, for 30 min three to four times daily and during sleep; and
  - Compression therapy with stockings and devices
- Refrain from using compression therapy if there are risk factors or signs of peripheral arterial occlusive disease

 ## OUTCOME

WHEN TO REFER

- Refer to vascular surgeon:
  - Patients with chronic venous insufficiency in combination with peripheral arterial occlusive disease
  - Patients with nonhealing ulcers from chronic venous insufficiency or other causes

WHEN TO ADMIT

- Cellulitis requiring IV antibiotics
- Skin ulcers requiring grafting

 ## EVIDENCE

PRACTICE GUIDELINES

- American Medical Directors Association (AMDA): Heart failure. Columbia (MD): 2002. http://www.guidelines.gov/summary/summary.aspx?doc_id=3303&nbr=2529&string=lower+extremity+edema
- Institute for Clinical Systems Improvement—Congestive heart failure in Adults http://www.icsi.org/knowledge/detail.asp?catID=29&itemID=161

WEB SITES

- American Academy of Family Physicians (AAFP) http://familydoctor.org/
- Cleveland Clinic http://www.clevelandclinic.org/
- National Lymphedema Network http://www.lymphnet.org/

INFORMATION FOR PATIENTS

- JAMA patient page: Heart failure. JAMA 2002;287(5):676. [PMID: 11842812]
- JAMA patient page: Kidney failure. JAMA 2001;286:2898. [PMID: 11767735]
- Mayo Clinic—Thrombophlebitis http://www.mayoclinic.com/invoke.cfm?objectid=D27523B0-5309-466F-B6560F1319E7EB2D

REFERENCES

- Heit JA et al: Trends in the incidence of venous stasis syndrome and venous ulcer: a 25-year population-based study. J Vasc Surg 2001;33:1022. [PMID: 11331844]
- Valencia IC et al: Chronic venous insufficiency and venous leg ulceration. J Am Acad Dermatol 2001;44:401. [PMID: 11209109]

Ralph Gonzales, MD

Electric Shock

 KEY FEATURES

ESSENTIALS OF DIAGNOSIS

- The extent of injury is determined by the amount and type of current, the duration and area of exposure, and the pathway of the current through the body

GENERAL CONSIDERATIONS

- With alternating currents (AC) of 25–300 Hz, low voltages (<220 Hz) tend to produce ventricular fibrillation; high voltages (>1000 Hz), respiratory failure; intermediate voltages (220–1000 Hz), both
- More than 100 mA of domestic house current (AC) of 110 V at 60 Hz can cause ventricular fibrillation; DC current contact is more likely to cause asystole
- Lightning injuries differ from high-voltage electric shock injuries; lightning usually involves higher voltage, briefer duration of contact, asystole, nervous system injury, and multisystem pathological involvement
- Electrical burns are of three distinct types: flash (arcing) burns, flame (clothing) burns, and direct heating effect of tissues by the electric current

 CLINICAL FINDINGS

SYMPTOMS AND SIGNS

- The lesions are usually sharply demarcated, round or oval, painless yellow-brown areas (Joule burn) with inflammatory reaction
- Significant subcutaneous damage can be accompanied by little skin injury, particularly with larger skin surface area electrical contact
- Loss of consciousness
- With recovery there may be muscular pain, fatigue, headache, and nervous irritability
- The physical signs vary according to the action of the current
    - If the current passes through the heart or brainstem, death may occur immediately owing to ventricular fibrillation or apnea
    - Current passing through skeletal muscle can cause muscle necrosis and contractions severe enough to result in bone fracture
    - Current traversing peripheral nerves can cause acute or delayed neuropathy
    - Delayed effects can include damage to the spinal cord, peripheral nerves, bone, kidneys, and gastrointestinal tract and development of cataracts

 DIAGNOSIS

LABORATORY TESTS

- A urinalysis, serum creatine kinase (CK) and CK-MB, and an electrocardiogram should be obtained immediately

Electric Shock

 TREATMENT

THERAPEUTIC PROCEDURES

Emergency measures

- Separate victim from the electric current prior to initiation of CPR or other treatment; the rescuer must be protected
- Turn off the power, sever the wire with a dry wooden-handled ax, make a proper ground to divert the current, or separate the victim using nonconductive implements such as dry clothing

Hospital measures

- Evaluate for blunt trauma, dehydration, skin burns, hypertension, posttraumatic stress, acid-base disturbances, and neurological damage
- To counteract fluid losses and myoglobinuria due to electric shock (not lightning) burns, aggressive hydration with Ringer's lactate should seek to achieve a urine output of 50–100 mL/h

 OUTCOME

COMPLICATIONS

- Complications may occur in almost any part of the body
- Most commonly include sepsis, gangrene requiring limb amputation, or neurological, cardiac, cognitive, or psychiatric dysfunction

WHEN TO ADMIT

- Lightning or unstable electric shock victims should be hospitalized when revived and observed for shock, arrhythmia, thrombosis, infarction, sudden cardiac dilation, hemorrhage, and myoglobinuria
- Indications for hospitalization include significant arrhythmia or electrocardiographic changes, large burn, loss of consciousness, pulmonary or cardiac symptoms, or evidence of significant deep tissue or organ damage
- Extra caution is indicated when the electroshock current has followed a transthoracic route (hand to hand or hand to foot) and in patients with a cardiac history

 EVIDENCE

WEB SITE

- Merck Manual—Disorder due to physical agents http://www.merck.com/pubs/mmanual/section20/sec20.htm

INFORMATION FOR PATIENTS

- National AG Safety Database http://www.cdc.gov/nasd/docs/d000801-d000900/d000813/d000813.html
- National Institutes of Health http://www.nlm.nih.gov/medlineplus/ency/article/000053.htm

REFERENCES

- Fish RM: Electric injury, Part I: treatment priorities, subtle diagnostic factors and burns. J Emerg Med 1999;17:977. [PMID: 10595883]
- Fish RM: Electric injury, Part II: specific injuries. J Emerg Med 2000;18:27. [PMID: 10645833]

Richard Cohen, MD, MPH
Brent R.W. Moelleken, MD, FACS

Endocarditis, Infective

 KEY FEATURES

ESSENTIALS OF DIAGNOSIS

- Preexisting organic heart lesion
- Fever
- New or changing heart murmur
- Evidence of systemic emboli
- Positive blood culture
- Evidence of vegetation on echocardiography

GENERAL CONSIDERATIONS

- Important factors that determine the clinical presentation are the nature of the infecting organism; which valve is infected; and the route of infection
- More virulent organisms—*Staphylococcus aureus* in particular—tend to produce a more rapidly progressive and destructive infection. Patients are more likely to present with acute febrile illnesses, early embolization, and acute valvular regurgitation and myocardial abscess
- Viridans strains of streptococci, enterococci, and a variety of other gram-positive and gram-negative bacilli, yeasts, and fungi tend to cause a more subacute picture. Systemic and peripheral manifestations may predominate
- Many, but by no means all patients have underlying cardiac disease, which is decreasing in prevalence as a risk factor
- The initiating event is colonization of the valve by bacteria during a transient or persistent bacteremia

Native valve endocarditis

- Approximately 90% are due to either viridans streptococci (60%), *S aureus* (20%), or enterococci (5–10%). Gram-negative organisms and fungi account for a small percentage
- The microbiology in intravenous drug users differs from that of other patients. *S aureus* accounts for 60% or more of all cases and for 80–90% of cases in which the tricuspid valve is infected. Enterococci and streptococci comprise the balance in about equal proportions

Prosthetic valve endocarditis

- Early infections (ie, those occurring within 2 months after valve implantation) are commonly caused by staphylococci—both coagulase-positive and coagulase-negative—gram-negative organisms, and fungi

- Late prosthetic valve endocarditis resembles native valve endocarditis, with the majority of infections caused by streptococci, though coagulase-negative staphylococci still cause a significant proportion of cases

DEMOGRAPHICS

- Injection drug use
- Underlying valvular disease

 CLINICAL FINDINGS

SYMPTOMS AND SIGNS

- Most present with a febrile illness that has lasted several days to 2 weeks
- In the majority of cases, heart murmurs are stable, and although a changing murmur is significant diagnostically, it is the exception rather than the rule
- The characteristic peripheral lesions—petechiae (on the palate or conjunctiva or beneath the fingernails); subungual ("splinter") hemorrhages; Osler nodes (painful, violaceous raised lesions of the fingers, toes, or feet); Janeway lesions (painless erythematous lesions of the palms or soles); and Roth spots (exudative lesions in the retina)—occur in up to 20–25% of patients

DIFFERENTIAL DIAGNOSIS

- Valvular abnormality without endocarditis, eg, rheumatic heart disease, mitral valve prolapse, bicuspid or calcific aortic valve
- Flow murmur (anemia, pregnancy, hyperthyroidism, sepsis)
- Atrial myxoma
- Noninfective endocarditis, eg, systemic lupus erythematosus (Libman-Saks endocarditis), marantic endocarditis (nonbacterial thrombotic endocarditis)
- Hematuria due to other cause, eg, glomerulonephritis, renal cell carcinoma
- Acute rheumatic fever
- Vasculitis

 DIAGNOSIS

LABORATORY TESTS

- Blood culture is the most important diagnostic tool; to maximize the yield, obtain three sets of blood cultures at least 1 h apart before starting antibiotics
- In acute endocarditis, leukocytosis is common; in subacute cases, anemia of chronic disease and a normal white blood cell count are the rule
- Hematuria and proteinuria as well as renal dysfunction may result from emboli or immunologically mediated glomerulonephritis
- Clinical criteria (the Duke criteria) for the diagnosis
  - Major criteria of (1) two positive blood cultures for a typical microorganism of infective endocarditis; and (2) positive echocardiography (vegetation, myocardial abscess, or new partial dehiscence of a prosthetic valve) or a new regurgitant murmur
  - Minor criteria include (1) the presence of a predisposing condition; (2) fever >38°C; (3) embolic disease; (4) immunological phenomena (Osler nodes, Roth spots, glomerulonephritis, rheumatoid factor); (5) positive blood cultures not meeting the major criteria; and (6) a positive echocardiogram not meeting the major criteria
- A definite diagnosis is made with 80% accuracy if two major criteria, one major criterion and three minor criteria, or five minor criteria are fulfilled. If none of these criteria is met and either an alternative explanation for illness is identified or the patient has defervesced within 4 days, endocarditis is highly unlikely

IMAGING STUDIES

- The chest x-ray may show the underlying cardiac abnormality and, in right-sided endocarditis, pulmonary infiltrates
- The sensitivity of transthoracic echocardiography is between 55% and 65%; therefore, it cannot reliably rule out endocarditis but may confirm a clinical suspicion
- Transesophageal echocardiography is 90% sensitive in detecting vegetations and is particularly useful for identifying valve ring abscesses, and pulmonary and prosthetic valve endocarditis

DIAGNOSTIC PROCEDURES

- The ECG is nondiagnostic. Changing conduction abnormalities suggest myocardial abscess formation

TREATMENT

MEDICATIONS

- See Table 134 (page 1316)

SURGERY

- Valvular regurgitation resulting in acute heart failure that does not resolve promptly after institution of medical therapy is an indication for valve replacement even if active infection is present, especially if the aortic valve is involved
- Infections that do not respond to appropriate antimicrobial therapy after 7–10 days (ie, persistent fevers, positive blood cultures despite therapy) are more likely to be eradicated if the valve is replaced
- Nearly always required for fungal endocarditis and is more often necessary with gram-negative bacilli
- Infection involving the sinus of Valsalva or produces septal abscesses
- Recurrent infection with the same organism often indicates that surgery is necessary, especially with infected prosthetic valves
- Continuing embolization when the infection is otherwise responding may be an indication for surgery

 OUTCOME

FOLLOW-UP

- If infection is caused by viridans streptococci, enterococci, or coagulase-negative staphylococci, defervescence occurs in 3–4 days on average, whereas if infection is caused by *Staphylococcus aureus* or *Pseudomonas aeruginosa*, patients may remain febrile for a week or more

COMPLICATIONS

- Destruction of infected heart valves
- Myocardial abscesses leading to conduction disturbances
- Peripheral embolization
- Mycotic aneurysms
- Right-sided endocarditis, which usually involves the tricuspid valve, often leads to septic pulmonary emboli, causing infarction and lung abscesses

PROGNOSIS

- Higher morbidity and mortality associated with nonstreptococcal etiology, aortic or prosthetic valvular infection

WHEN TO REFER

- Infectious diseases consultation recommended
- Patients with signs of heart failure should be referred for surgical evaluation

WHEN TO ADMIT

- Patients with evidence of heart failure
- Patients with a nonstreptococcal etiology
- For initiation of antimicrobial therapy

PREVENTION

- Prophylactic antibiotics are given to patients with predisposing congenital or valvular anomalies who are to have any of a number of procedures (Tables 132 and 133, pages 1314 and 1315). Current recommendations are given in Table 131 (page 1313)

EVIDENCE

PRACTICE GUIDELINES

- National Guideline Clearinghouse http://www.guideline.gov/summary/summary.aspx?doc_id=2390&nbr=1616&string=endocarditis http://www.guideline.gov/summary/summary.aspx?doc_id=1472&nbr=698&string=bacteremia
- Flachskampf FA et al: Working Group on Echocardiography of the European Society of Cardiology. Guidelines from the Working Group. Recommendations for performing transesophageal echocardiography. Eur J Echocardiogr 2001;2:8.
- Olaison L, Pettersson G: Current best practices and guidelines indications for surgical intervention in infective endocarditis. Infect Dis Clin North Am 2002;16:453.

WEB SITES

- Infective Endocarditis http://edcenter.med.cornell.edu/Pathology_Cases/Vascular_Infections/VI_Summary.html
- CDC—Division of Bacterial and Mycotic Diseases http://www.cdc.gov/ncidod/dbmd/

INFORMATION FOR PATIENTS

- JAMA patient page: Endocarditis. JAMA 2002;288:128.
- American Heart Association http://www.americanheart.org/presenter.jhtml?identifier=4436 http://www.americanheart.org/presenter.jhtml?identifier=11086

REFERENCES

- Bayer AS et al: Diagnosis and management of infective endocarditis and its complications. Circulation 1998;98:2936. [PMID: 9860802]
- Olaison L et al: Enterococcal endocarditis in Sweden, 1995–1999: can shorter therapy with aminoglycosides be used? Clin Infect Dis 2002;34:159. [PMID: 11740702]

Henry F. Chambers, MD

Endometrial Cancer

 KEY FEATURES

ESSENTIALS OF DIAGNOSIS

- Abnormal bleeding is the presenting sign in 80% of cases
- Papanicolaou smear frequently negative
- After a negative pregnancy test, endometrial tissue is required to confirm the diagnosis

GENERAL CONSIDERATIONS

- Adenocarcinoma of the uterine corpus is the second most common cancer of the female genital tract

DEMOGRAPHICS

- Occurs most often in women 50–70 years of age
- History of unopposed estrogen in the past; this increased risk persists for 10 or more years after stopping the drug
- Obesity, nulliparity, diabetes, and polycystic ovaries with prolonged anovulation and the extended use of tamoxifen for the treatment of breast cancer are also risk factors

 CLINICAL FINDINGS

SYMPTOMS AND SIGNS

- Vaginal bleeding
- Obstruction of the cervix with collection of pus (pyometra) or blood (hematometra) causing lower abdominal pain may occur
- However, pain generally occurs late in the disease, with metastases or infection

DIFFERENTIAL DIAGNOSIS

- Endometrial hyperplasia or proliferation
- Uterine leiomyomas (fibroids)
- Endometrial polyp
- Cervical cancer
- Atrophic endometrium
- Adenomyosis (uterine endometriosis)
- Atrophic vaginitis
- Ovarian tumor
- Leiomyosarcoma

 DIAGNOSIS

LABORATORY TESTS

- Papanicolaou smears of the cervix occasionally show atypical endometrial cells but are an insensitive diagnostic tool

IMAGING STUDIES

- Vaginal ultrasonography may show thickness of the endometrium indicating hypertrophy and possible neoplastic change

DIAGNOSTIC PROCEDURES

- Endocervical and endometrial sampling is the only reliable means of diagnosis. Adequate specimens of each can usually be obtained during an office procedure with local anesthesia (paracervical block)
- Simultaneous hysteroscopy can localize polyps or other lesions within the uterine cavity

Staging

- Examination under anesthesia, endometrial and endocervical sampling, chest x-ray, intravenous urography, cystoscopy, sigmoidoscopy, transvaginal sonography, and MRI for extent of disease
- The staging is based on the surgical and pathological evaluation

TREATMENT

MEDICATIONS

- Advanced or metastatic endometrial adenocarcinoma may be palliated with large doses of progestins, eg, medroxyprogesterone, 400 mg intramuscularly weekly, or megestrol acetate, 80–160 mg daily orally

SURGERY

- Treatment consists of total hysterectomy and bilateral salpingo-oophorectomy. Peritoneal material for cytological examination is routinely taken

THERAPEUTIC PROCEDURES

- Preliminary external irradiation or intracavitary radium therapy is indicated if the cancer is poorly differentiated or if the uterus is definitely enlarged in the absence of myomas

OUTCOME

FOLLOW-UP

- Examination every 3-4 months for 2 years, then every 6 months

COMPLICATIONS

- Related to therapy, radiation vs surgery

PROGNOSIS

- With early diagnosis and treatment, the 5-year survival is 80–85%

WHEN TO REFER

- All patients with carcinoma of the endometrium should be referred to a gynecologist
- If invasion deep into the myometrium has occurred or if sampled preaortic lymph nodes are positive for tumor, postoperative irradiation is indicated

PREVENTION

- Prompt endometrial sampling for patients who report abnormal menstrual bleeding or postmenopausal uterine bleeding will reveal many incipient as well as clinical cases of endometrial cancer
- In comparison with the use of unopposed estrogen for menopausal therapy, there is a relative risk of endometrial cancer of 0.3% among women using continuous combined regimens of estrogen and progestin
- Younger women with chronic anovulation are at risk for endometrial hyperplasia and subsequent endometrial cancer. They can reduce the risk of hyperplasia almost completely with the use of oral contraceptives or cyclic progestin therapy

EVIDENCE

PRACTICE GUIDELINES

- National Guideline Clearinghouse http://www.guideline.gov/summary/summary.aspx?doc_id=2749&nbr=1975&string=endometrial+cancer http://www.guideline.gov/summary/summary.aspx?doc_id=3456&nbr=2682&string=endometrial+cancer

WEB SITES

- Endometrial Cancer—National Cancer Institute—CancerNet http://cancernet.nci.nih.gov/cgi-bin/srchcgi.exe?DBID=pdq&TYPE=search&UID=208+01176&ZFILE=professional&SFMT=pdq_treatment/1/0/0
- Gynecologic Cancers http://www.oncolink.com/templates/types/types.cfm?c=6

INFORMATION FOR PATIENTS

- National Institutes of Health http://www.nci.nih.gov/cancerinfo/pdq/prevention/endometrial/patient/ http://www.nci.nih.gov/cancerinfo/pdq/treatment/endometrial/patient/#Section_92
- JAMA patient page: Endometrial cancer. JAMA 2002;288:1678.
- JAMA patient page: Pap test. JAMA 1999;281:1666.

REFERENCE

- Hernandez E: Endometrial carcinoma: a primer for the generalist. Obstet Gynecol North Am 2001;28:743. [PMID: 11766149]

H. Trent MacKay, MD, MPH

Endometriosis

 KEY FEATURES

ESSENTIALS OF DIAGNOSIS

- Pelvic pain related to menstrual cycle
- Dysmenorrhea
- Dyspareunia
- Increased frequency among infertile women

GENERAL CONSIDERATIONS

- An aberrant growth of endometrium outside the uterus, particularly in the dependent parts of the pelvis and in the ovaries
- Common cause of abnormal bleeding and secondary dysmenorrhea
- Its causes, pathogenesis, and natural course are poorly understood

DEMOGRAPHICS

- The prevalence in the United States is 2% among fertile women and three- to four-fold greater than that in infertile women

 CLINICAL FINDINGS

SYMPTOMS AND SIGNS

- Aching pain tends to be constant, beginning 2–7 days before the onset of menses, and becomes increasingly severe until flow slackens
- Depending on the location and extent of the endometrial implants, infertility, dyspareunia, or rectal pain with bleeding may result
- Pelvic examination may disclose tender indurated nodules in the cul-de-sac, especially if the examination is done at the onset of menstruation

DIFFERENTIAL DIAGNOSIS

- Adenomyosis (uterine endometriosis)
- Pelvic inflammatory disease
- Uterine leiomyomas (fibroids)
- Primary dysmenorrhea
- Ovarian tumor
- Endometrial cancer
- Pelvic adhesions
- Irritable bowel syndrome
- Interstitial cystitis

 DIAGNOSIS

IMAGING STUDIES

- Ultrasound examination will often reveal complex fluid-filled masses that cannot be distinguished from neoplasms
- MRI is more sensitive and specific than ultrasound, particularly in the diagnosis of adnexal masses

DIAGNOSTIC PROCEDURES

- The clinical diagnosis of endometriosis is presumptive and is usually confirmed by laparoscopy or laparotomy
- Differentiation from bowel neoplasm depends on proctosigmoidoscopy and biopsy

TREATMENT

MEDICATIONS

- Medications are designed to inhibit ovulation over 4–9 months to prevent cyclic stimulation of endometrial implants
- The optimum duration of therapy is not known
- The gonadotropin-releasing hormone analogs such as nafarelin nasal spray, 0.2–0.4 mg twice daily, or long-acting injectable leuprolide acetate, 3.75 mg intramuscularly monthly, used for 6 months, suppress ovulation. Side effects consisting of vasomotor symptoms and bone demineralization may be relieved by "add-back" therapy with norethindrone, 5–10 mg daily
- Danazol is used for 6–9 months in the lowest dose necessary to suppress menstruation, usually 200–400 mg twice daily. Side effects are androgenic and include decreased breast size, weight gain, acne, and hirsutism
- Any of the combination oral contraceptives may be given, one daily, without interruption, for 6–12 months. Breakthrough bleeding can be treated with conjugated estrogens, 1.25 mg daily for 1 week, or estradiol, 2 mg daily for 1 week
- Medroxyprogesterone acetate, 100 mg intramuscularly every 2 weeks for four doses; then 100 mg every 4 weeks; add oral estrogen or estradiol valerate, 30 mg intramuscularly, for breakthrough bleeding. Use for 6–9 months
- Low-dose oral contraceptives can also be given cyclically; prolonged suppression of ovulation will often inhibit further stimulation of residual endometriosis, especially if taken after one of the therapies mentioned above
- Analgesics, with or without codeine, may be needed during menses. Nonsteroidal antiinflammatory drugs may be helpful

SURGERY

- The surgical treatment of moderately extensive endometriosis depends on the patient's age and symptoms and her desire to preserve reproductive function
- If the patient is under 35, resect the lesions, free adhesions, and suspend the uterus. At least 20% of patients so treated can become pregnant, although some must undergo surgery again if the disease progresses
- If the patient is over 35 years old, is disabled by pain, and has involvement of both ovaries, bilateral salpingo-oophorectomy and hysterectomy will probably be necessary
- Foci of endometriosis can be treated laparoscopically

THERAPEUTIC PROCEDURES

- The goal of medical treatment is to preserve the fertility of women wanting future pregnancies, ameliorate symptoms, and simplify future surgery or make it unnecessary

OUTCOME

PROGNOSIS

- The prognosis for reproductive function in early or moderately advanced endometriosis is good with conservative therapy
- Bilateral ovariectomy is curative for patients with severe and extensive endometriosis with pain. Following hysterectomy and oophorectomy, estrogen replacement therapy is indicated

WHEN TO REFER

- Refer to gynecologist for laparoscopic diagnosis and treatment

WHEN TO ADMIT

- Rarely necessary except in case of acute abdomen associated with a ruptured or bleeding endometrioma

EVIDENCE

PRACTICE GUIDELINES

- American Academy of Family Physicians http://www.aafp.org/afp/20000915/practice.html

WEB SITE

- Gynecology Handbook for Family Practitioners http://www.vh.org/Providers/ClinRef/FPHandbook/13.html

INFORMATION FOR PATIENTS

- American Academy of Family Physicians http://familydoctor.org/handouts/476.html
- National Institute of Child Health and Human Development http://www.nichd.nih.gov/publications/pubs/endometriosis/index.htm

REFERENCES

- Farquhar C: Endometriosis. Clin Evidence 2000;4:1058.
- Ling FW: Randomized controlled trial of depot leuprolide in patients with chronic pelvic pain and clinically suspected endometriosis. Pelvic Pain Study Group. Obstet Gynecol 1999;93:51. [PMID: 9916956]
- Olive DL et al: Treatment of endometriosis. N Engl J Med 2001;345:266. [PMID: 11474666]

H. Trent MacKay, MD, MPH

Enterobiasis

 KEY FEATURES

ESSENTIALS OF DIAGNOSIS

- Nocturnal perianal and vulvar pruritus, insomnia, irritability, restlessness
- Vague gastrointestinal symptoms
- Eggs demonstrable by cellulose tape test; worms visible on perianal skin or in stool

GENERAL CONSIDERATIONS

- Humans, the only host, can harbor a few to hundreds of worms
- The adult worms inhabit the cecum and adjacent bowel areas, lying loosely attached to the mucosa. Gravid females migrate through the anus to the perianal skin and deposit eggs in large numbers. The eggs become infective in a few hours and may then infect others or be autoinfective if transferred to the mouth by contaminated food, drink, fomites, or hands. After being swallowed, the eggs hatch in the duodenum, and the larvae migrate down to the cecum.
- Retroinfection occasionally occurs when the eggs hatch on the perianal skin and the larvae migrate through the anus into the large intestine
- The development of a mature ovipositing female from an ingested egg requires about 3–4 weeks. Eggs remain viable for 2–3 weeks outside the host
- The life span of the worm is 30–45 days

DEMOGRAPHICS

- *Enterobius vermicularis* (8–13 × 0.5 mm) is common worldwide. A second species, *Enterobius gregorii*, has been described in England

 CLINICAL FINDINGS

SYMPTOMS AND SIGNS

- Many patients are asymptomatic
- The most common and important symptom is perianal pruritus (particularly at night), due to the presence of the female worms or deposited eggs
- At night, worms may occasionally be seen near the anus. Perianal scratching may result in excoriation and impetigo. Patients sometimes report a "crawling" sensation in the anal area

DIFFERENTIAL DIAGNOSIS

- Tinea or candidiasis of the anogenital region
- Hemorrhoids
- Proctitis
- Contact dermatitis
- Strongyloidiasis
- Anal fissure
- Idiopathic anogenital pruritus

 DIAGNOSIS

LABORATORY TESTS

- Diagnosis is made by finding eggs on the perianal skin (eggs are seldom found on stool examination). The most reliable method is by applying a short strip of sealing cellulose pressure-sensitive tape (eg, Scotch Tape) to the perianal skin and then spreading the tape on a slide for low-power microscopic study; toluene is used to clear the preparation. Three such preparations made on consecutive mornings before bathing or defecation will establish the diagnosis in about 90% of cases. Before the diagnosis can be ruled out, five to seven such examinations are necessary
- Nocturnal examination of the perianal area or gross examination of stools may reveal adult worms, which should be placed in preservative, alcohol, or saline for laboratory examination
- The worms can sometimes be seen on anoscopy
- Eosinophilia is rare

TREATMENT

MEDICATIONS

- Treatment with the following drugs should be repeated at 2 and 4 weeks. Albendazole, mebendazole, and pyrantel pamoate are the drugs of choice and can be given with or without food. Albendazole and mebendazole should not be used in pregnancy. Piperazine, although effective, is not recommended because treatment requires 1 week
- **Albendazole** may reach a 100% cure rate when given as a single 400-mg dose. Abdominal pain and diarrhea are rare
- **Mebendazole** as a single 100-mg dose is also highly effective. It should be chewed for best effect. Gastrointestinal side effects are infrequent
- **Pyrantel pamoate** is highly effective, with cure rates of over 95%. It is administered as a 10-mg (base)/kg (maximum, 1 g) dose. Infrequent side effects include vomiting, diarrhea, headache, dizziness, and drowsiness. In the United States, pyrantel is available as self-medication for pinworm infection

THERAPEUTIC PROCEDURES

- Symptomatic patients should be treated, and in some situations all members of the patient's household should be treated concurrently, since for each overt case there are usually several inapparent cases. Generally, however, treatment of all nonsymptomatic cases is not necessary
- Careful washing of hands with soap and water after defecation and again before meals is important. Fingernails should be kept trimmed close and clean and scratching of the perianal area avoided. Ordinary washing of bedding will usually kill pinworm eggs; some workers recommend daily washing

 OUTCOME

COMPLICATIONS

- Rarely, worm migration—including migration through the female genital tract or into the urethra—results in ectopic inflammation (vulvovaginitis, diverticulitis, appendicitis, cystitis) or granulomatous reactions (colon, genital tract, peritoneum, and elsewhere)
- Colonic ulceration and eosinophilic colitis have been reported

PROGNOSIS

- Although annoying, the infection is benign
- Cure is readily attainable with one of several effective drugs
- Reinfection is common because of continued exposure outside the home

WHEN TO REFER

- Inability to cure the infection
- No response or progression of symptoms despite therapy

 EVIDENCE

PRACTICE GUIDELINES

- Kabani A et al: Practice guidelines for ordering stool ova and parasite testing in a pediatric population. The Alberta Children's Hospital. Am J Clin Pathol 1995;104:272.

INFORMATION FOR PATIENTS

- National Institute of Allergy and Infectious Diseases http://www.niaid.nih.gov/factsheets/ roundwor.htm
- Centers for Disease Control http://www.cdc.gov/ncidod/dpd/ parasites/pinworm/factsht_pinworm. htm

REFERENCES

- Lohiya GS et al: Epidemiology and control of enterobiasis in a developmental center. West J Med 2000;172:305. [PMID: 10832422]
- St Georgiev V: Chemotherapy of enterobiasis (oxyuriasis). Expert Opin Pharmacother 2001;2:267. [PMID: 11336585]
- Tandan T et al: Pelvic inflammatory disease associated with *Enterobius vermicularis.* Arch Dis Child 2002;86:439. [PMID: 12023182]
- Wu ML et al: *Enterobius vermicularis.* Arch Pathol Lab Med 2000;124:647. [PMID: 10747336]

Epididymitis, Acute

 ## KEY FEATURES

ESSENTIALS OF DIAGNOSIS

- Fever
- Irritative voiding symptoms
- Painful enlargement of the epididymis

GENERAL CONSIDERATIONS

- Acute epididymitis is an infectious process associated with painful enlargement of the epididymis. Fever and irritative voiding symptoms are common. In advanced states, the infection can spread to the testis. The entire scrotal contents may be painful on palpation
- Relief: supine elevation of the scrotum above the pubic symphysis (Prehn's sign)
- Two categories have different age distributions and etiological agents
- Sexually transmitted forms typically occur in men under age 40, are associated with urethritis, and result from *Chlamydia trachomatis* or *Neisseria gonorrhoeae*
- Nonsexually transmitted forms occur in older men, are associated with urinary tract infections and prostatitis, and are caused by gram-negative rods

 ## CLINICAL FINDINGS

SYMPTOMS AND SIGNS

- Symptoms follow acute physical strain, trauma, or sexual activity
- Associated symptoms of urethritis (pain at the tip of the penis and urethral discharge) or cystitis (irritative voiding symptoms)
- Pain in the scrotum may radiate along the spermatic cord or to the flank
- Fever and scrotal swelling
- Prostate tender on rectal examination

DIFFERENTIAL DIAGNOSIS

- Tumors of the testis
- Testicular torsion

 ## DIAGNOSIS

LABORATORY TESTS

- Complete blood cell count shows leukocytosis and left shift
- In sexually transmitted variety, Gram staining of a smear of urethral discharge may be gram-negative intracellular diplococci (*N gonorrhoeae*)
- White cells without visible organisms: nongonococcal urethritis, *C trachomatis*
- In nonsexually transmitted variety, urinalysis: pyuria, bacteriuria, hematuria
- Urine cultures may reveal pathogen

Epididymitis, Acute

 ## TREATMENT

MEDICATIONS

- Sexually transmitted variety: antibiotics for 21 days, treat sexual partner also
- Nonsexually transmitted variety: antibiotics for 21–28 days

THERAPEUTIC PROCEDURES

- Evaluate urinary tract to identify underlying disease
- Bed rest with scrotal elevation

 ## OUTCOME

PROGNOSIS

- Prompt treatment usually results in a favorable outcome
- Delayed or inadequate treatment may result in epididymoorchitis, decreased fertility, abscess formation

EVIDENCE

PRACTICE GUIDELINES

- 2002 national guideline for the management of epididymo-orchitis. Association for Genitourinary Medicine. Medical Society for the Study of Venereal Diseases
  http://www.agum.org.uk/ceg2002/epididymoorchitis0601.htm
- Epididymitis. Sexually transmitted diseases treatment guidelines 2002. Centers for Disease Control and Prevention
  http://www.cdc.gov/mmwr/PDF/rr/rr5106.pdf

WEB SITES

- American Academy of Family Physicians—Genital Problems in Men: Self-Care Flowcharts
  http://familydoctor.org/flowcharts/539.html
- National Institute of Allergy and Infectious Diseases—Introduction to sexually transmitted diseases
  http://www.niaid.nih.gov/factsheets/stdinfo.htm

INFORMATION FOR PATIENTS

- CDC—Gonorrhea
  http://www.cdc.gov/nchstp/dstd/Fact_Sheets/FactsGonorrhea.htm
- MEDLINEplus—Epididymitis
  http://www.nlm.nih.gov/medlineplus/ency/article/001279.htm

REFERENCES

- Barloon TJ et al: Diagnostic imaging of patients with acute scrotal pain. Am Fam Physician 1996;53:1734. [PMID: 8623698]
- Joly-Guillou ML et al: Practical recommendations for the drug treatment of bacterial infections of the male genital tract including urethritis, epididymitis and prostatitis. Drugs 1999;57:743. [PMID: 10353299]

Marshall L. Stoller, MD
Peter R. Carroll, MD

Epilepsy

 KEY FEATURES

ESSENTIALS OF DIAGNOSIS

- Recurrent seizures
- Epilepsy should not be diagnosed on the basis of a solitary seizure
- Characteristic EEG changes may occur
- Postictal confusion or focal neurological deficits may follow, and last hours

GENERAL CONSIDERATIONS

- A seizure is a transient disturbance of cerebral function due to abnormal paroxysmal brain neuronal discharge
- The most likely cause relates to the age of onset
- Idiopathic epilepsy onset is usually between the ages of 5 and 20 years
- Metabolic disorders may cause seizures. Withdrawal from alcohol or other CNS depressant drugs may be responsible. Uremia, hyponatremia, hypo- and hyperglycemia and other metabolic disorders may also be responsible
- Trauma is an important cause of seizures. Seizures in the first week after head injury do not imply that they will persist. Prophylactic anticonvulsant drugs have not been proven to reduce the incidence of posttraumatic epilepsy
- Tumors and other space-occupying lesions result in seizures that are often partial (focal), and most likely with frontal, parietal, or temporal lesions
- Vascular disease is the leading cause in patients aged 60 or older
- Alzheimer's disease and other degenerative disorders can cause seizures in later life
- Infections of the central nervous system (meningitis, encephalitis, or brain abscess) must be considered in all age groups as potentially reversible causes of seizures

DEMOGRAPHICS

- Epilepsy affects approximately 0.5% of the U.S. population

 CLINICAL FINDINGS

SYMPTOMS AND SIGNS

- See Table 93 (page 1277)
- Nonspecific prodrome in some (headache, lethargy)
- The type of aura depends on the cerebral site of origin of the seizure, eg, gustatory or olfactory hallucinations or visual hallucinations with temporal or occipital lesions
- In most patients, seizures occur unpredictably
- Fever, sleep loss, alcohol, stress, or flashing lights may precipitate seizures in some
- Clinical examination may be normal interictally unless there is a structural cause for the seizures
- Immediately postictally there may be a focal deficit (Todd's paresis) or bilateral Babinski signs
- Focal signs postictally suggest focal CNS abnormality

DIFFERENTIAL DIAGNOSIS

- Syncope
- Cardiac arrhythmia
- Stroke or transient ischemic attack
- Pseudoseizure
- Panic attack
- Migraine
- Narcolepsy

Causes of secondary seizures

- CNS vasculitis, eg, systemic lupus erythematosus
- Febrile seizures in children younger than 5 years
- Degenerative disease, eg, Alzheimer's disease
- Metabolic disorders (eg, hypoglycemia)
- Trauma
- Central nervous system infection

DIAGNOSIS

LABORATORY TESTS

- Complete blood cell count, serum glucose, liver and renal function tests, and serological tests for syphilis

IMAGING STUDIES

- Image all patients with progressive disorder and those with new onset of seizures
- Obtain an MRI if there are focal neurological symptoms or signs, focal seizures, or a focal EEG disturbance

DIAGNOSTIC PROCEDURES

- History is key, including eyewitness accounts
- The EEG is abnormal in only about 60%, but may support clinical diagnosis of epilepsy (paroxysmal spikes or sharp waves), may guide prognosis, may help classify the seizure disorder, and is important in evaluating candidates for surgical treatment
- Repeated Holter monitoring may be necessary to establish the diagnosis of cardiac arrhythmia

Epilepsy

 TREATMENT

MEDICATIONS

- Anticonvulsant drug treatment is generally not required for a single seizure unless further attacks occur or investigations reveal some underlying untreatable pathology
- Treatment with anticonvulsant drugs is generally not required for alcohol withdrawal seizures, which are self-limited
- See Table 94 (page 1278)
- The drug dose is gradually increased until seizures are controlled or side effects occur
- If seizures continue despite treatment at the maximal tolerated dose, a second drug is added and the first drug is then gradually withdrawn
- In most patients, control can be achieved with a single anticonvulsant drug
- Discontinue the medication only when the patient is seizure free for at least 3 years. Dose reduction should be gradual over a period of weeks or months. If seizures recur, treatment is reinstituted with previous drugs
- A seizure recurrence after the medication is discontinued is more likely if the patient initially failed to respond to therapy, if focal or multiple types of seizures, or if EEG abnormalities persist

SURGERY

- Operative treatment or vagal nerve stimulations are best undertaken in specialized centers

THERAPEUTIC PROCEDURES

- Advise patients to avoid situations that may be dangerous or life-threatening if they have a seizure
- State laws may require clinicians to report to the public health department any patients with seizures or other episodic lapses of consciousness

 OUTCOME

FOLLOW-UP

- Dosing should not be based simply on serum levels because some patients require levels that exceed the therapeutic range ("toxic levels") but tolerate these without ill effect
- In general, the dose of an antiepileptic agent is increased depending on clinical response, not serum drug level. The trough drug level is then measured to provide a reference point for the maximum tolerated dose
- Measure serum drug levels when another drug is added to the therapeutic regimen and to assess compliance in poorly controlled patients
- Certain antiepileptic drugs may be teratogenic. Epileptic women of childbearing potential require special care

COMPLICATIONS

- See *Status epilepticus*
- Residual encephalopathy after prolonged seizures or poor control of seizures

PROGNOSIS

- The risk of seizure recurrence varies in different series between about 30% and 70%

WHEN TO ADMIT

- Status epilepticus
- To videomonitoring unit to distinguish pseudoseizures
- If surgery is contemplated

 EVIDENCE

PRACTICE GUIDELINES

- National Guideline Clearinghouse http://www.guideline.gov/summary/ summary.aspx?doc_id=2439&nbr=1665 &string=epilepsy http://www.guideline.gov/summary/ summary.aspx?doc_id=2823&nbr= 2049&string=epilepsy
- American College of Emergency Physicians. Clinical policy for the initial approach to patients presenting with a chief complaint of seizure who are not in status epilepticus. Ann Emerg Med 1997;29:706.
- American Academy of Neurology http://www.aan.com/professionals/ practice/pdfs/gl0034.pdf

INFORMATION FOR PATIENTS

- Epilepsy Foundation http://www.epilepsyfoundation.org/ answerplace/About-Epilepsy.cfm http://www.epilepsyfoundation.org/ answerplace/faq.cfm

REFERENCES

- Alldredge BK et al: A comparison of lorazepam, diazepam, and placebo for the treatment of out-of-hospital status epilepticus. N Engl J Med 2001;345: 631. [PMID:11547716]
- Brodie MJ et al: Management of epilepsy in adolescents and adults. Lancet 2000;356:323. [PMID: 11071202]
- Wiebe S et al: A randomized, controlled trial of surgery for temporal-lobe epilepsy. N Engl J Med 2001;345:311. [PMID: 11484687]

Michael J. Aminoff, MD, DSc, FRCP

Epistaxis

 KEY FEATURES

ESSENTIALS OF DIAGNOSIS

- Bleeding from the anterior nasal cavity is by far the most common type of epistaxis encountered
- Most cases may be successfully treated by direct pressure on the bleeding site

GENERAL CONSIDERATIONS

- Bleeding from the anterior nasal cavity originates from Kiesselbach's plexus, a vascular plexus on the anterior nasal septum
- Bleeding from the posterior nasal cavity originates from the posterior half of the inferior turbinate or the top of the nasal cavity
- Predisposing factors include nasal trauma (nose picking, foreign bodies, forceful nose blowing), rhinitis, drying of the nasal mucosa from low humidity, deviation of the nasal septum, alcohol use, and antiplatelet medications

DEMOGRAPHICS

- Anterior nasal cavity bleeding is by far the most common type of epistaxis
- Only 5% of nasal bleeding originates in the posterior nasal cavity
- Less than 10% of nasal bleeding is caused by coagulopathy or tumor

 CLINICAL FINDINGS

SYMPTOMS AND SIGNS

- Bleeding from nostril or nasopharynx
- Posterior bleeding may present with hemoptysis or hemetemesis

DIFFERENTIAL DIAGNOSIS

- Nasal trauma (eg, nose picking, forceful nose blowing, foreign body)
- Allergic rhinitis or viral rhinitis
- Dry nasal mucosa
- Deviated septum
- Chronic sinusitis
- Inhaled steroids
- Cocaine use
- Alcohol use
- Antiplatelet drugs (eg, aspirin, clopidogrel)
- Thrombocytopenia
- Idiopathic thrombocytopenic purpura
- Thrombotic thrombocytopenic purpura
- Hemophilia
- Hereditary hemorrhagic telangiectasia (Osler-Weber-Rendu syndrome)
- Polycythemia vera
- Leukemia
- Wegener's granulomatosis
- Nasal tumor

 DIAGNOSIS

LABORATORY TESTS

- Laboratory assessment of bleeding parameters (platelet count, coagulation studies) may be indicated, especially in recurrent cases

TREATMENT

- Most cases of anterior epistaxis may be successfully treated by direct pressure on the bleeding site

MEDICATIONS

- Short-acting topical nasal decongestants (eg, phenylephrine, 0.125–1% solution, one or two sprays), which act as vasoconstrictors, may be helpful
- When the bleeding does not readily subside, the nose should be examined to locate the bleeding site: topical 4% cocaine [or a topical decongestant (eg, oxymetazoline) and a topical anesthetic (eg, tetracaine)] applied either as a spray or on a cotton strip serves as an anesthetic and as a vasoconstricting agent

SURGERY

Posterior nasal bleeding

- Ligation of the nasal arterial supply (internal maxillary artery and ethmoid arteries) is a possible alternative to posterior nasal packing
- Ligation of the external carotid artery may be necessary

THERAPEUTIC PROCEDURES

Anterior nasal bleeding

- Compress the nasal alae firmly for at least 10 min
- Venous pressure is reduced in the sitting position, and leaning forward lessens the swallowing of blood
- Cauterize the bleeding site with silver nitrate, diathermy, or electrocautery
- Usually anterior packing will suffice if the bleeding has not stopped

Posterior nasal bleeding

- Placement of a pack to occlude the choana before placement of a pack anteriorly
- Narcotic analgesics reduce the discomfort and elevated blood pressure caused by a posterior pack
- Endovascular embolization of the internal maxillary artery is an alternative to surgical ligation in life-threatening hemorrhage

 OUTCOME

FOLLOW-UP

- After control of the epistaxis, avoid vigorous exercise for several days
- Avoid hot or spicy foods and tobacco as they may cause vasodilation
- Once the acute episode has passed, carefully examine the nose and paranasal sinuses to rule out neoplasia
- Follow-up investigation of possible hypertension

COMPLICATIONS

- Sinusitis
- Aspiration or asphyxiation by blood

PROGNOSIS

- Generally self-limited with a good prognosis

WHEN TO REFER

- Refer to an otolaryngologist for persistent or recurrent bleeding
- If expertise in cauterization or localization of the bleeding site is needed
- For posterior nasal packing

WHEN TO ADMIT

- Because placing a nasal pack for posterior nasal bleeding is uncomfortable and because it requires oxygen supplementation to prevent hypoxia, hospitalization for several days is indicated

PREVENTION

- Avoiding nasal trauma, including nose picking
- Lubrication with petroleum jelly or bacitracin ointment
- Increased home humidity

 EVIDENCE

PRACTICE GUIDELINES

- National Guideline Clearinghouse http://www.guideline.gov/summary/ summary.aspx?doc_id=3162&nbr=2388 &string=epistaxis

WEB SITES

- Ear, Nose, and Throat Information Center http://www.netdoor.com/entinfo/
- Otolaryngology Resources on the Internet http://www.bcm.tmc.edu/oto/othersa .html

INFORMATION FOR PATIENTS

- American Academy of Otolaryngology-Head and Neck Surgery. Nosebleeds http://www.entnet.org/healthinfo/nose/ nosebleeds.cfm
- National Institutes of Health http://www.nlm.nih.gov/medlineplus/ ency/article/003106.htm

REFERENCES

- Herkner H et al: Hypertension in patients presenting with epistaxis. Ann Emerg Med 2000;35:126. [PMID: 10650229]
- Leppanen M et al: Microcatheter embolization of intractable idiopathic epistaxis. Cardiovasc Intervent Radiol 1999;22:499. [PMID: 10556410]
- Pond F et al: Epistaxis. Strategies for management. Aust Fam Physician 2000;29:933. [PMID: 11059081]
- Thaha MA et al: Routine coagulation screening in the management of emergency admission for epistaxis—is it necessary? J Laryngol Otol 2000;114:38. [PMID: 10789409]

Robert K. Jackler, MD
Michael J. Kaplan, MD

Erectile Dysfunction

 ## KEY FEATURES

ESSENTIALS OF DIAGNOSIS

- Consistent inability to maintain an erect penis with sufficient rigidity to allow sexual intercourse
- Affects 10 million American men
- Incidence is age related
- Affects ~25% of men aged >65 suffer
- Most have an organic rather than psychogenic cause

GENERAL CONSIDERATIONS

Etiology

- Loss of erections: occurs from arterial, venous, neurogenic, or psychogenic causes
- Associated with concurrent medical problems (eg, diabetes mellitus), or radical pelvic or retroperitoneal surgery
- Antihypertensive medications: centrally acting sympatholytics (methyldopa, clonidine, reserpine) can cause loss of erection, while vasodilators, α-blockers, and diuretics rarely do so
- Associated with androgen deficiency
- Loss of orgasm: if libido and erection are intact, usually of psychological origin
- Premature ejaculation: anxiety related, due to a new partner, unreasonable expectations about performance, or emotional disorders
- Loss of emission (lack of antegrade seminal fluid during ejaculation): due to retrograde ejaculation or mechanical disruption of the bladder neck (eg, after transurethral resection of the prostate)

 ## CLINICAL FINDINGS

SYMPTOMS AND SIGNS

- History: erectile dysfunction should be distinguished from problems of ejaculation, libido, and orgasm
- Degree of the dysfunction—chronic, occasional, or situational
- Timing of dysfunction
- Determine whether the patient ever has any normal erections, such as in early morning or during sleep
- Inquire about hyperlipidemia, hypertension, neurological disease, diabetes mellitus, renal failure, and adrenal and thyroid disorders
- Trauma to the pelvis or pelvic or peripheral vascular surgery
- Use of drugs, alcohol, tobacco, and recreational drugs
- Physical examination: secondary sexual characteristics
- Neurological motor and sensory examination
- Peripheral vascular examination: palpation and quantification of lower extremity pulses
- Examination of genitalia, testicles, and prostate
- Evaluate for penile scarring, plaque formation (Peyronie's disease)

 ## DIAGNOSIS

LABORATORY TESTS

- Complete blood cell count
- Urinalysis
- Lipid profile
- Serum glucose, testosterone, luteinizing hormone/follicle-stimulating hormone, and prolactin
- Serum testosterone and gonadotropin levels may help localize the site of disease

IMAGING STUDIES

- Cavernous arteries duplex ultrasound: if poor arterial inflow, perform pelvic arteriography before arterial reconstruction; if normal arterial inflow, probably venous leak
- Cavernosometry (measurement of flow required to maintain erection) and cavernosography (contrast study of the penis to determine site and extent of venous leak)

DIAGNOSTIC PROCEDURES

- Direct injection of vasoactive substances into the penis (prostaglandin E, papaverine, or a combination of drugs). Patients who respond with a rigid erection require no further vascular evaluation
- Nocturnal penile tumescence testing for frequency and rigidity in patients who fail to achieve an erection with injection of vasoactive substances

TREATMENT

MEDICATIONS

- Hormone replacement for documented androgen deficiency on endocrinological evaluation, testosterone injections (200 mg IM Q 3 weeks) or topical patches (2.5–10 mg/day) after prostate-specific antigen and digital rectal examination screening
- Alprostadil urethral suppository pellets (125, 250, 500, and 1000 µg)
- Sildenafil, 50 mg, vardenafil 5 mg, or tadalafil, 10 mg 1 h prior to anticipated sexual activity. Contraindicated in patients receiving nitroglycerin

SURGERY

- Penile prosthesis
- Rigid, malleable, hinged, or inflatable
- Vascular reconstruction
- Disorders of the arterial system: endarterectomy and balloon dilation for proximal arterial occlusion; arterial bypass procedures utilizing arterial (epigastric) or venous (deep dorsal vein) segments for distal occlusion
- Disorders of venous occlusion: ligation of certain veins (deep dorsal or emissary veins) or the crura of the corpora cavernosa

THERAPEUTIC PROCEDURES

- Vacuum constriction device: for patients with venous disorders of the penis and those who fail to achieve adequate erection with injection of vasoactive substances, use a vacuum device and rubber constriction band around proximal penis; complications rare
- Behaviorally oriented sex therapy for men with no organic dysfunction

 # OUTCOME

PROGNOSIS

- The majority of men suffering from erectile dysfunction can be managed successfully

 # EVIDENCE

PRACTICE GUIDELINES

- American Association of Clinical Endocrinologists medical guidelines for clinical practice for the evaluation and treatment of male sexual dysfunction: a couple's problem—2003 update. American Association of Clinical Endocrinologists, American College of Endocrinology, 2003 http://www.aace.com/clin/guidelines/sexdysguid.pdf
- Canadian Urological Association Guidelines Committee. Erectile dysfunction practice guidelines. Can J Urol 2002;9:1583. [PMID: 12243654]

WEB SITE

- National Kidney and Urologic Diseases Information Clearinghouse—Erectile dysfunction http://kidney.niddk.nih.gov/kudiseases/pubs/impotence/index.htm

INFORMATION FOR PATIENTS

- Cleveland Clinic—Erectile dysfunction basics http://www.clevelandclinic.org/health/health-info/docs/2900/2904.asp?index=10035
- Mayo Clinic—Erectile dysfunction http://www.mayoclinic.com/invoke.cfm?objectid=F52ADDE0-FE7E-4F9D-9ACB4F34354E023C

REFERENCES

- Goldstein I et al: Oral sildenafil in the treatment of erectile dysfunction. Sildenafil Study Group. N Engl J Med 1998;338:1397. [PMID: 9580646]
- Padma-Nathan H et al: Treatment of men with erectile dysfunction with transurethral alprostadil. Medicated Urethral System for Erection (MUSE) Study Group. N Engl J Med 1997;336:1. [PMID: 8970933]

Marshall L. Stoller, MD
Peter R. Carroll, MD

Erysipelas

 ## KEY FEATURES

ESSENTIALS OF DIAGNOSIS

- Edematous, spreading, circumscribed, hot, erythematous area, with or without vesicles or bullae
- Central face frequently involved
- Pain, chills, fever, and systemic toxicity may be striking

GENERAL CONSIDERATIONS

- A superficial form of cellulitis that occurs classically on the cheek, caused by β-hemolytic streptococci
- The disease may complicate any break in the skin that provides a portal of entry for the organism
- Erysipeloid, unlike erysipelas, is a benign bacillary infection producing redness of the skin of the fingers or the backs of the hands in fishermen and meat handlers

 ## CLINICAL FINDINGS

SYMPTOMS AND SIGNS

- See Table 7 (page 1202)
- The symptoms are pain, malaise, chills, and moderate fever
- A bright red spot appears first, very often near a fissure at the angle of the nose; this spreads to form a tense, sharply demarcated, glistening, smooth, hot area; the margin characteristically makes noticeable advances in days or even hours
- The lesion is somewhat edematous and can be pitted slightly with the finger
- Vesicles or bullae occasionally develop on the surface
- The lesion does not usually become pustular or gangrenous and heals without scar formation

DIFFERENTIAL DIAGNOSIS

- Anthrax
- Cellulitis
- Erysipeloid
- Contact dermatitis
- Herpes zoster (shingles)
- Scarlet fever
- Angioedema
- Necrotizing fasciitis
- Systemic lupus erythematosus

 ## DIAGNOSIS

LABORATORY TESTS

- Leukocytosis and an increased sedimentation rate are almost invariably present but are not specific
- Blood cultures may be positive

TREATMENT

MEDICATIONS

- Intravenous antibiotics effective against group A β-hemolytic streptococci and staphylococci are indicated for the first 48 h in all but the mildest cases
- A 7-day course is completed with penicillin VK, 250 mg, dicloxacillin, 250 mg, or a first-generation cephalosporin, 250 mg, orally four times a day
- Either erythromycin, 250 mg four times daily for 7–14 days, or clarithromycin, 250 mg twice daily for 7–14 days, is a good alternative in penicillin-allergic patients
- Quinolones have poor activity against streptococci and are not recommended

THERAPEUTIC PROCEDURES

- Place the patient at bed rest with the head of the bed elevated

 OUTCOME

COMPLICATIONS

- Unless erysipelas is promptly treated, death may result from extension of the process and systemic toxicity, particularly in the very young and in the aged

PROGNOSIS

- Erysipelas was at one time a life-threatening infection; it can now usually be quickly controlled with systemic penicillin or erythromycin therapy

WHEN TO REFER

- If there is a question about the diagnosis, if recommended therapy is ineffective, or if specialized treatment is necessary

WHEN TO ADMIT

- All but the mildest cases

 EVIDENCE

WEB SITES

- American Academy of Dermatology
  http://www.aad.org
- Dermatology Handbook for Family Practice from the University of Iowa
  http://www.vh.org/Providers/ClinRef/FPHandbook/17.html
- National Institutes of Health Medical Encyclopedia
  http://www.nlm.nih.gov/medlineplus/ency/article/000618.htm

INFORMATION FOR PATIENTS

- American Academy of Dermatology
  http://www.aad.org/pamphlets/

REFERENCES

- Baddour LM: Cellulitis syndromes: an update. Int J Antimicrob Agents 2000;14:113. [PMID: 2018804]
- Roldan YB et al: Erysipelas and tinea pedis. Mycoses 2000;43:181. [PMID: 10948816]

Timothy G. Berger, MD

Erythema Multiforme

 KEY FEATURES

ESSENTIALS OF DIAGNOSIS

- Sudden onset of symmetric erythematous skin lesions with history of recurrence
- May be macular, papular, urticarial, bullous, or purpuric
- "Target" lesions with clear centers and concentric erythematous rings or "iris" lesions may be noted in erythema multiforme minor; these are rare in drug-associated erythema multiforme major (Stevens-Johnson syndrome)
- Erythema multiforme minor on extensor surfaces, palms, soles, or mucous membranes; erythema multiforme major favors the trunk
- Herpes simplex, systemic infection or disease, and drug reactions are often associated

GENERAL CONSIDERATIONS

- An acute inflammatory skin disease due to multiple causes
- Erythema multiforme (EM) is divided clinically into minor and major types based on the clinical findings
- ~90% of cases of EM minor follow outbreaks of herpes simplex
- EM major (Stevens-Johnson syndrome) is marked by toxicity and involvement of two or more mucosal surfaces (often oral and conjunctival), is most often caused by drugs (sulfonamides, nonsteroidal antiinflammatory drugs, and anticonvulsants); visceral involvement may occur, may be serious or even fatal
- In EM major, the main differential diagnosis is toxic epidermal necrolysis, and some regard this as a variant of the same disease
- EM may also present as recurring oral ulceration, with skin lesions present in only half of the cases, and is diagnosed by oral biopsy

 CLINICAL FINDINGS

SYMPTOMS AND SIGNS

- See Table 7 (page 1202)
- Classic target lesion, most commonly seen in herpes-associated EM, consists of three concentric zones of color change, most often found acrally on the hands and feet
- Drug-associated EM is manifested by raised target-like lesions, with only two zones of color change and a central blister, or nondescript reddish or purpuric macules
- In EM major, mucous membrane ulcerations are present at two or more sites, causing pain on eating, swallowing, and urination
- Blisters are always worrisome and dictate the need for consultation
- Urticaria and drug eruptions are the chief entities that must be differentiated from EM minor
- Individual lesions of true urticaria itch, should come and go within 24 h, are usually responsive to antihistamines, and do not affect the mucosa

DIFFERENTIAL DIAGNOSIS

- EM minor: urticaria, drug eruption
- EM major in evolution
- Sweet's syndrome (acute febrile neutrophilic dermatosis)
- EM major
  - Pemphigus
  - Bullous pemphigoid
  - Drug eruptions
  - Bullous impetigo
  - Contact dermatitis
  - Dermatitis herpetiformis
  - Cicatricial pemphigoid
  - Paraneoplastic pemphigus
  - Linear IgA dermatosis
  - Pemphigus foliaceus
  - Porphyria cutanea tarda
  - Epidermolysis bullosa
  - Staph scalded skin syndrome
  - Herpes gestationis
  - Graft-versus-host disease

 DIAGNOSIS

LABORATORY TESTS

- Blood tests are unhelpful

PROCEDURES

- Skin biopsy is diagnostic (direct immunofluorescence studies are negative)

TREATMENT

MEDICATIONS

- See Table 6 (page 1199)

EM major (Stevens-Johnson)

- No good data to support the use of corticosteroids in EM major, but they are still often prescribed
- If corticosteroids are to be tried in more severe cases, they should be used early, before blistering occurs, and in moderate to high doses (prednisone, 100–250 mg) and stopped within days if there is no dramatic response; in one trial, IGIV (0.75 g/kg/day for 4 days) yielded dramatic benefit in severe cases
- Oral and topical corticosteroids are useful in the oral variant of EM
- Antistaphylococcal antibiotics are used for secondary infection, which is uncommon
- Topical therapy is not very effective in this disease
- For oral lesions, 1% diphenhydramine elixir mixed with Kaopectate or with 1% dyclonine may be used as a mouth rinse several times daily

 OUTCOME

FOLLOW-UP

- Patients who begin to blister with EM major should be seen daily

COMPLICATIONS

- EM major—extensive denudation, similar to an extensive burn

PROGNOSIS

- EM major—visceral involvement may occur, may be serious or even fatal
- EM minor usually lasts 2–6 weeks and may recur
- Immediate discontinuation of the inciting medication (before blistering) improves prognosis and reduces risk of death

WHEN TO REFER

- EM major diagnosis or suspicion

WHEN TO ADMIT

- Patients need not be admitted unless mucosal involvement interferes with hydration and nutrition; extensive denudation of skin best treated in a burn unit

 EVIDENCE

PRACTICE GUIDELINES

- American Academy of Dermatology http://www.aadassociation.org/Guidelines/cutaneousdrug.html

WEB SITES

- American Academy of Dermatology http://www.aad.org
- Dermatology Handbook for Family Practice from the University of Iowa http://www.vh.org/Providers/ClinRef/FPHandbook/17.html

INFORMATION FOR PATIENTS

- American Academy of Dermatology http://www.aad.org/pamphlets/
- American Academy of Family Physicians http://familydoctor.org/flowcharts/545.html
- National Institute of Health Medical Encyclopedia http://www.nlm.nih.gov/medlineplus/ency/article/000851.htm

REFERENCES

- Garcia-Doval I et al: Toxic epidermal necrolysis and Stevens-Johnson syndrome: does early withdrawal of causative drugs decrease the risk of death? Arch Dermatol 2000;136:323. [PMID: 10724193]
- Katta R: Taking aim at erythema multiforme. How to spot target lesions and less typical presentations. Postgrad Med 2000;107:87. [PMID: 10649667]
- Rzany B et al: Risk of Stevens-Johnson syndrome and toxic epidermal necrolysis during first weeks of antiepileptic therapy: a case-control study. Study Group of the International Case Control Study on Severe Cutaneous Adverse Reactions. Lancet 1999;353:2190. [PMID: 10392983]

Timothy G. Berger, MD

Erythema Nodosum

 KEY FEATURES

ESSENTIALS OF DIAGNOSIS

- Painful red nodules without ulceration on anterior aspects of legs
- Slow regression over several weeks to resemble contusions
- Women are predominantly affected by a ratio of 4–8:1 over men
- Some cases associated with infection or drug sensitivity

GENERAL CONSIDERATIONS

- The disease may be associated with various infections and noninfectious conditions: streptococcosis, coccidioidomycosis, other deep fungal infections, tuberculosis, *Yersinia*, syphilis, sarcoidosis, inflammatory bowel disease, pregnancy, or use of oral contraceptives or other medication

Associated conditions

- Infection: streptococcal, coccidioidomycosis, other fungal (eg, histoplasmosis, blastomycosis), tuberculosis, syphilis, *Yersinia enterocolitica*
- Other: sarcoidosis, medications (eg, oral contraceptives), inflammatory bowel disease, pregnancy, lymphoma, or leukemia

 CLINICAL FINDINGS

SYMPTOMS AND SIGNS

- See Table 7 (page 1202)
- The swellings are exquisitely tender and may be preceded by fever, malaise, and arthralgia
- They are most often located on the anterior surfaces of the legs below the knees but may occur (rarely) on the arms, trunk, and face
- The lesions, 1–10 cm in diameter, are at first pink to red; with regression, all the various hues seen in a contusion can be observed

DIFFERENTIAL DIAGNOSIS

- Erythema induratum (associated with tuberculosis)
- Nodular vasculitis
- Erythema multiforme
- Lupus panniculitis
- Poststeroid panniculitis
- Contusions or bruises
- Sweet's syndrome (acute febrile neutrophilic dermatosis)
- Subcutaneous fat necrosis (associated with pancreatitis)

 DIAGNOSIS

LABORATORY TESTS

- The histological finding of septal panniculitis is characteristic of erythema nodosum
- Evaluation of patients presenting should include a careful history and physical examination for prior upper respiratory infection or diarrheal illness, symptoms of any deep fungal infection endemic to the area, a chest x-ray, a partial protein derivative, and two consecutive ASO titers at 2- to 4-week intervals

Erythema Nodosum

TREATMENT

MEDICATIONS

- See Table 6 (page 1199)
- First identify and treat the underlying cause
- Primary therapy is with nonsteroidal antiinflammatory agents
- Saturated solution of potassium iodide, 5–15 drops three times daily, may result in prompt involution in many cases
- Side effects of potassium iodide include salivation, swelling of salivary glands, and headache
- Systemic therapy directed against the lesions themselves may include use of corticosteroids unless contraindicated by associated infection

OUTCOME

PROGNOSIS

- It usually lasts about 6 weeks and may recur
- If no underlying cause is found, only a small percentage of patients will go on to develop a significant underlying illness (usually sarcoidosis) over the next year

WHEN TO REFER

- If there is a question about the diagnosis, if recommended therapy is ineffective, or specialized treatment is necessary

EVIDENCE

WEB SITES

- American Academy of Dermatology http://www.aad.org
- Dermatology Handbook for Family Practice from the University of Iowa http://www.vh.org/Providers/ClinRef/ FPHandbook/17.html

INFORMATION FOR PATIENTS

- American Academy of Dermatology http://www.aad.org/pamphlets/
- American Osteopathic College of Dermatology http://www.aocd.org/skin/ dermatologic_diseases/erythema_ nodosum.html

REFERENCE

- Garcia-Porrua C et al: Erythema nodosum: etiologic and predictive factors in a defined population. Arthritis Rheum 2000;43:584. [PMID: 10728752]

Timothy G. Berger, MD

Esophageal Cancer

 KEY FEATURES

ESSENTIALS OF DIAGNOSIS

- Progressive solid food dysphagia
- Weight loss
- Endoscopy with biopsy establishes diagnosis

GENERAL CONSIDERATIONS

- Two histological types: squamous cell carcinoma and adenocarcinoma
- Squamous cell cancer risk factors: chronic alcohol and tobacco use, tylosis, achalasia, caustic-induced esophageal stricture, and other head and neck cancers; in some underdeveloped countries, related to HIV infection
- Half of squamous cell cancers arise in the distal third of the esophagus
- Adenocarcinoma risk factor: Barrett's metaplasia due to chronic gastro-esophageal reflux
- Most adenocarcinomas arise in the distal third of the esophagus

DEMOGRAPHICS

- Occurs usually in persons between 50 and 70 years of age
- Ratio of men to women is 3:1

 CLINICAL FINDINGS

SYMPTOMS AND SIGNS

- Solid food dysphagia (>90%)
- Odynophagia
- Significant weight loss
- Coughing on swallowing or recurrent pneumonia suggests tracheoesophageal fistula from local tumor extension
- Chest or back pain mediastinal extension
- Hoarseness suggests recurrent laryngeal nerve involvement
- Physical examination often unrevealing
- Supraclavicular or cervical lymphadenopathy hepatomegaly suggests metastatic disease

DIFFERENTIAL DIAGNOSIS

- Peptic stricture
- Achalasia
- Adenocarcinoma of gastric cardia with esophageal involvement
- Esophageal web, ring (eg, Schatzki's), or diverticulum

 DIAGNOSIS

LABORATORY TESTS

- Anemia related to chronic disease or occult blood loss
- Elevated aminotransferase or alkaline phosphatase if hepatic metastases
- Hypoalbuminemia

IMAGING STUDIES

- Chest x-rays may show adenopathy
- Barium esophagogram
- Upper endoscopy with biopsy

DIAGNOSTIC PROCEDURES

- CT of the chest and liver; endoscopic ultrasonography for staging
- TNM classification

Esophageal Cancer

 ## TREATMENT

MEDICATIONS

- Chemotherapy (cisplatin and fluo-rouracil) plus radiation therapy for patients with "curable" disease; used as neoadjuvant therapy to surgery or sometimes alone, but severe side effects

SURGERY

- Surgery alone for stage I and stage IIA cancer
- Transhiatal esophagectomy with anastomosis of the stomach to the cervical esophagus
- Transthoracic excision of the esophagus with nodal resection
- Surgery with neoadjuvant chemotherapy (cisplatin and fluorouracil) and radiation therapy for patients with stage IIB and stage III cancer

THERAPEUTIC PROCEDURES

- Palliative therapy for patients with extensive local tumor spread (T4) or distant metastases (M1), most patients with stage III and all with stage IV tumors
- Palliative therapy includes resection, radiation therapy, peroral placement of expandable, permanent wire stents, application of endoscopic laser therapy, or photodynamic therapy
- Complications of stents, perforation, migration, and tumor ingrowth, occur in 20–40%
- Photodynamic therapy employs a photo-sensitizing agent (porfimer sodium) in combination with low-power 630-nm laser irradiation delivered endoscopically
- Side effects include skin photosensitivity for 4–6 weeks and esophageal stricture

 ## OUTCOME

COMPLICATIONS

- Invasion of mediastinal structures
- Tracheoesophageal fistula

PROGNOSIS

- Overall 5-year survival is <15%
- Most patients present with advanced disease

WHEN TO REFER

- Dehydration due to dysphagea
- Palliative care

PREVENTION

- Treatment of Barrett's esophagus
- Adenocarcinoma
- Squamous cell carcinoma: eliminate cigarettes

 ## EVIDENCE

PRACTICE GUIDELINES

- Allum WH et al: Guidelines for the management of oesophageal and gastric cancer. Gut 2002;50(9Suppl 5):v1. [PMID: 12049068]
- Seitz JF et al: Carcinoma of the oesophagus. Br J Cancer 2001;84(Suppl 2):61. [PMID: 11355972]
- Wong RK et al: Combined modality radiotherapy and chemotherapy in non-surgical management of localized carcinoma of the esophagus: a practice guideline. Int J Radiat Oncol Biol Phys 2003;55:930. [PMID: 12605971]

WEB SITE

- National Cancer Institute—What you need to know about cancer of the esophagus
  http://www.cancer.gov/cancerinfo/wyntk/esophagus

INFORMATION FOR PATIENTS

- American Cancer Society—Esophageal cancer
  http://www.cancer.org/docroot/cri/content/cri_2_4_1x_what_is_esophagus_cancer_12.asp?sitearea=cri
- Cleveland Clinic—Esophageal cancer
  http://www.clevelandclinic.org/health/health-info/docs/1300/1390.asp?index=6137

REFERENCES

- Bossett JF et al: Chemoradiotherapy followed by surgery compared with surgery alone in squamous-cell cancer of the esophagus. N Engl J Med 1997;337:161. [PMID: 9219702]
- Hulscher JB et al: Extended transthoracic resection compared with limited transhiatal resection for adenocarcinoma of the esophagus. N Engl J Med 2002;347:1662. [PMID: 12444180]
- Lightdale CJ: Esophageal cancer. Am J Gastroenterol 1999;94:20. [PMID: 9934727]

Kenneth R. McQuaid, MD

Esophageal Varices

 KEY FEATURES

ESSENTIALS OF DIAGNOSIS

- Dilated submucosal veins in patients with portal hypertension
- Develop in 50% of patients with cirrhosis
- One-third develop upper gastrointestinal bleeding

GENERAL CONSIDERATIONS

- Bleeding most commonly occurs in the distal 5 cm of the esophagus
- Approximately 50% of patients with cirrhosis have esophageal varices
- One-third of patients with varices develop serious bleeding

DEMOGRAPHICS

- Portal hypertension of any cause; most commonly due to cirrhosis

 CLINICAL FINDINGS

SYMPTOMS AND SIGNS

- Acute gastrointestinal hemorrhage, usually severe, resulting in hypovolemia, postural vital signs, or shock

DIFFERENTIAL DIAGNOSIS

- Alcoholic gastritis
- Mallory-Weiss syndrome
- Portal hypertensive gastropathy
- Peptic ulcer disease
- Gastric or duodenal varices (rare)
- Vascular ectasias (angiodysplasias), eg, idiopathic arteriovenous malformation, CREST syndrome, hereditary hemorrhagic telangiectasia

 DIAGNOSIS

LABORATORY TESTS

- Complete blood cell count, platelet count, prothrombin time INR, type and cross-match, serum liver enzymes, creatinine, blood urea nitrogen

DIAGNOSTIC PROCEDURES

- Emergent upper endoscopy after the patient's hemodynamic status has been stabilized is diagnostic

 TREATMENT

MEDICATIONS

- Octreotide infusion (50-μg intravenous bolus followed by 50 μg/h) reduces splanchnic and hepatic blood flow and portal pressures
- Combined octreotide and endoscopic therapy (band ligation or sclerotherapy) is superior to either modality alone in controlling acute bleeding and early rebleeding, and it may improve survival
- Vitamin K subcutaneously
- Lactulose 30–45 mL/h PO until evacuation occurs, then reduced to 15–45 mL/h Q 8–12 h as needed to promote two or three bowel movements daily for hepatic encephalopathy
- After bleeding stops, β-blockers to reduce portal pressure: propranolol, 20 mg twice daily, or nadolol, 40 mg once daily, gradually increasing the dosage until the heart rate falls by 25% or reaches 55 beats/min
- Long-acting nitrates, such as isosorbide mononitrate, 10 mg PO QD, gradually increased to 20–40 mg PO BID as tolerated, also reduce portal pressures
- Combination therapy with isosorbide mononitrate and β-blockers may be superior and reduces side effects

SURGERY

- Emergency portal decompression
- Transvenous intrahepatic portosystemic shunts (TIPS) are indicated in the 5–10% of patients with acute variceal bleeding that cannot be controlled with pharmacological and endoscopic therapy
- TIPS can control acute hemorrhage in >90%

Esophageal Varices

- TIPS reserved for patients who have recurrent (two or more) episodes of variceal bleeding that have failed endoscopic or pharmacological therapies, gastric varices, or portal hypertensive gastropathy; in patients who are noncompliant with other therapies; in patients who live in remote locations (without access to emergency care)
- Emergency portosystemic shunt, eg, selective distal splenorenal shunt, surgery can decompress portal hypertension, but associated with a 40–60% mortality rate, seldom performed
- Liver transplantation

THERAPEUTIC PROCEDURES

- Initial management involves rapid assessment and acute resuscitation with fluids or blood products
- Transfusion of fresh frozen plasma or platelets to patients with INRs >1.8 –2.0 or with platelet counts <50,000/µL in the presence of active bleeding
- Mechanical tamponade with nasogastric tubes containing large gastric and esophageal balloons (Minnesota or Sengstaken-Blakemore tubes) provides initial control of active variceal hemorrhage in 60–90% of patients, but rebleeding occurs in 50%
- Acute endoscopic treatment with either banding or sclerotherapy arrests active bleeding in 90% of patients and reduces by half (from 70%) the chance of early recurrent bleeding
- Repeat banding at intervals of 1–2 weeks until the varices are obliterated or reduced to a small size
- Banding achieves lower rates of rebleeding, complications, and death than sclerotherapy
- Sclerotherapy involves injecting the variceal trunks with ethanolamine, tetradecyl sulfate, repeating at 3–7 days, then at 1- to 3-week intervals until the varices are obliterated
- Sclerotherapy preferred by some endoscopists for the actively bleeding patient (in whom visualization for banding may be difficult)

 OUTCOME

FOLLOW-UP

- Stenosis and thrombosis of the TIPS stents occur in the majority over time with a consequent risk of rebleeding; periodic monitoring with Doppler ultrasonography or hepatic venography
- After obliteration of varices by endoscopic banding or sclerotherapy, repeat endoscopy every 6–12 months

COMPLICATIONS

- Encephalopathy occurs in 35% after TIPS
- Hepatic failure may occur after TIPS
- Sclerotherapy complications, including chest pain, fever, bacteremia, esophageal ulceration, stricture, and perforation, occur in 20–30%
- Complications of mechanical tamponade include esophageal and oral ulcerations, perforation, aspiration, and airway obstruction

PROGNOSIS

- Mortality rate within 2 weeks after an acute bleeding episode is 30%
- Recurrent hemorrhage occurs in 70% within 1 year (half within 6 weeks)
- Mortality rate is 60% at 2 years

WHEN TO ADMIT

- All patients with variceal hemorrhage

PREVENTION

- Prophylaxis of spontaneous bacterial peritonitis: norfloxacin, 400 mg (or another quinolone) PO or per nasogastric tube BID for at least 7 days
- Risk of rebleeding is 60–80% without further therapy
- Long-term treatment with sclerotherapy or band ligation reduces rebleeding to 20–40%
- Nonselective β-adrenergic blockers (propranolol, nadolol) reduce the incidence of rebleeding comparable to that of sclerotherapy

EVIDENCE

PRACTICE GUIDELINES

- Eisen GM et al: The role of endoscopic therapy in the management of variceal hemorrhage. Gastrointest Endosc 2002;56:618. [PMID: 12397264]
- Jalan R et al: UK guidelines on the management of variceal haemorrhage in cirrhotic patients. British Society of Gastroenterology. Gut 2000;46(Suppl 3-4):III1. [PMID: 10862604]

WEB SITES

- American Academy of Family Physicians—Cirrhosis and portal hypertension http://familydoctor.org/handouts/188.html
- American Gastroenterological Association—How are the complications of cirrhosis treated? http://www.gastro.org/public/brochures/cirrhosis.html#Complications

INFORMATION FOR PATIENTS

- Cleveland Clinic—Variceal bleeding management procedures http://www.clevelandclinic.org/health/health-info/docs/1900/1930.asp?index=4721

REFERENCES

- Garcia-Tsa G: Current management of the complications of cirrhosis and portal hypertension: variceal hemorrhage, ascites, and spontaneous bacterial peritonitis. Gastroenterology 2001;120:726. [PMID: 11179247]
- Sharara A et al: Gastroesophageal variceal hemorrhage. N Engl J Med 2001;345:669. [PMID: 11547722]
- Vlachogiannakos J et al: Review article: primary prophylaxis for portal hypertensive bleeding in cirrhosis. Aliment Pharmacol Ther 2000;14:851. [PMID: 10886040]

Kenneth R. McQuaid, MD

Esophagitis, Infectious

 KEY FEATURES

ESSENTIALS OF DIAGNOSIS

- Odynophagia, dysphagia, and chest pain
- Occurs in immunosuppressed patients

GENERAL CONSIDERATIONS

- Occurs most commonly in immunosuppressed patients with AIDS, solid organ transplants, leukemia, lymphoma, and those receiving immunosuppressive drugs
- Most common pathogens: *Candida albicans*, herpes simplex, and cytomegalovirus
- *Candida* also occurs in patients who have uncontrolled diabetes mellitus and those receiving systemic corticosteroids, radiation therapy, or systemic antibiotics

 CLINICAL FINDINGS

SYMPTOMS AND SIGNS

- Odynophagia
- Dysphagia
- Substernal chest pain
- Sometimes asymptomatic (*Candida*)
- Oral thrush in 75% of patients with candidal esophagitis and 25–50% of patients with viral esophagitis
- Cytomegalovirus infection at other sites (colon and retina)
- Oral ulcers (herpes labialis) often associated with herpes simplex esophagitis

 DIAGNOSIS

DIAGNOSTIC PROCEDURES

- Endoscopy with biopsy and brushings (for microbiological and histopathological analysis)

Esophagitis, Infectious

 ## TREATMENT

MEDICATIONS

- Treatment may be empirical

Candidal esophagitis

- For patients with a normal immune system: topical nystatin, 500,000 units "swish and swallow" five times daily; clotrimazole troches, 10 mg dissolved in mouth five times daily for 7–14 days
- For immunocompromised patients (including AIDS): fluconazole, 100–200 mg PO QD
- For patients not responding to oral therapy: low-dose amphotericin B, 0.3–0.5 mg/kg/day, duration not standardized

Cytomegalovirus esophagitis

- For initial therapy: ganciclovir, 5 mg/kg IV Q 12 h for 3–6 weeks
- For patients with AIDS: continuous ganciclovir, 5 mg/kg IV daily, is required for suppressive therapy
- For patients who do not respond or cannot tolerate ganciclovir: foscarnet, 90 mg/kg IV Q 12 h for 3–6 weeks

Herpetic esophagitis

- For patients with a normal immune system: symptomatic treatment
- For immunocompromised patients: acyclovir, 200 mg PO five times daily, or 250 mg/m² IV Q 8–12 h, usually for 7–10 days; famciclovir, 250 mg PO TID; or valacyclovir, 1 g PO BID
- For nonresponders: foscarnet, 40 mg/kg IV Q 8 h for 21 days

 ## OUTCOME

PROGNOSIS

- Most patients can be effectively treated with complete symptom resolution
- Chronic suppressive therapy is sometimes required for immunocompromised patients

WHEN TO REFER

- Refer patients who do not respond to empirical therapy to a gastroenterologist for upper endoscopy, brushings, and biopsy

WHEN TO ADMIT

- Severe odynophagia with inability to take adequate oral liquids

PREVENTION

- For patients with HIV infection: immune restoration with highly active antiretroviral therapy (HAART)

 ## EVIDENCE

PRACTICE GUIDELINES

- Ouatu-Lascar R, Triadafilopoulos G: Oesophageal mucosal diseases in the elderly. Drugs Aging 1998;12:261. [PMID: 9571391]
- Vazquez JA: Therapeutic options for the management of oropharyngeal and esophageal candidiasis in HIV/AIDS patients. HIV Clin Trials 2000;1:47. [PMID: 11590489]
- Whitley RJ et al: Guidelines for the treatment of cytomegalovirus diseases in patients with AIDS in the era of potent retroviral therapy; recommendations of an international panel. Arch Intern Med 1998;158:957. [PMID: 9588429]

WEB SITES

- CDC—Dispatches http://www.cdc.gov/ncidod/eid/vol5no2/pdf/ravera.pdf
- Cleveland Clinic—Esophagitis http://www.clevelandclinic.org/health/health-info/docs/2800/2896.asp?index=10138

INFORMATION FOR PATIENTS

- MEDLINEplus—Candida esophagitis http://www.nlm.nih.gov/medlineplus/ency/article/000643.htm
- MEDLINEplus—Herpes esophagitis http://www.nlm.nih.gov/medlineplus/ency/article/000646.htm

REFERENCES

- Darouiche RO: Oropharyngeal and esophageal candidiasis in immunocompromised patients: treatment issues. Clin Infect Dis 1998;26:259. [PMID: 9502438]
- Ramanathan J et al: Herpes simplex esophagitis in the immunocompetent host: an overview. Am J Gastroenterol 2000;95:2171. [PMID: 11007213]
- Whitley RJ et al: Guidelines for the treatment of cytomegalovirus diseases in patients with AIDS in the era of potent retroviral therapy; recommendations of an international panel. Arch Intern Med 1998;158:957. [PMID: 9588429]

Kenneth R. McQuaid, MD

Falls in Elderly

KEY FEATURES

ESSENTIALS OF DIAGNOSIS

- Falls in older people are rarely due to a single cause
- Medications and alcohol use are among the most common, significant, and reversible causes of falling

GENERAL CONSIDERATIONS

Causes of falls

- Visual impairment
- Gait impairment due to
  - Podiatric disorder (ingrown nail)
  - Arthritis
  - Muscular weakness (myopathy)
  - Cerebellar ataxia (alcoholism)
  - Sensory ataxia (vitamin B_{12} deficiency, neurosyphilis)
  - Other neurological disorders (parkinsonism, Alzheimer's disease, spinal stenosis, multiple sclerosis, peripheral neuropathy)
- Environmental hazards (poor lighting, stairs, rugs, uneven floors)
- Polypharmacy (benzodiazepines, opioids, phenothiazines, vasodilators, diuretics)
- Alcohol use
- Orthostatic or postprandial hypotension
- Vertigo, presyncope, syncope, or disequilibrium
- Medical illness (pneumonia, myocardial infarction, anemia, hyponatremia)
- Other contributing factors: urinary urgency, peripheral edema, insomnia

DEMOGRAPHICS

- Thirty percent of community-dwelling elderly fall each year, including 50% of people over age 80; of those who fall 25% have serious injuries
- About 5% of falls result in fracture
- Falls are the sixth leading cause of death for older people

CLINICAL FINDINGS

SYMPTOMS AND SIGNS

Gait and balance tests

- "Up and Go Test," Romberg test, a nudge, and a 360-degree turn
  - Patient is asked to stand up from a sitting position without use of hands, walk 10 feet, turn around, walk back, and sit down
  - Is the patient able to rise from a chair without use of arms in a single, smooth attempt?
  - Is there stability immediately upon standing, or does the patient stagger?
  - Is balance maintained when the patient is pushed lightly on the sternum?
  - Is there steadiness when standing with eyes closed?
  - How is walking initiated, and does each foot swing clear of the floor and pass the opposite foot?
  - Are the steps equal?
  - Is there stopping or discontinuity between steps, or sway of the trunk, flexion of knees or back, spreading out of the arms?
  - Do the heels almost touch during the stride, or is there a wide-based gait?
  - Is a walking aid (cane, walker) necessary or being used properly?
  - Does the patient take more than 10–15 s for the "Up and Go Test"? Slower times, particularly times longer than 20 s, are often associated with other impairments in function

DIAGNOSIS

DIAGNOSTIC PROCEDURES

- Every older person should be asked about falls; many will not volunteer such information
- Review medications, including over-the-counter sleeping aids
- Examine for postural hypotension
- Examine for peripheral edema
- Ask about urinary symptoms

Falls in Elderly

 ## TREATMENT

MEDICATIONS

- Eliminate all nonessential medications that can interfere with gait, cause somnolence or urinary urgency

THERAPEUTIC PROCEDURES

- Home safety check: generally reimbursed by third-party payers, including Medicare
- For patients with repeated falls, make available phones at floor level, a portable phone, or a lightweight radio call system
- Use of an anatomically designed external hip protector reduces hip fracture risk in frail elders, but is often poorly tolerated

 ## OUTCOME

COMPLICATIONS

- Fractures, commonly of the wrist, hip, and vertebrae
- Loss of confidence and independence because of fear of repeated falls
- Chronic subdural hematoma
  - Consider in an elderly patient who presents with new neurological symptoms or signs, particularly obtundation
  - Headache is uncommonly present
- Dehydration, electrolyte imbalance, pressure sores, hypothermia, and rhabdomyolysis in patients who are unable to get up from a fall

PROGNOSIS

- Patients with a fall are at high risk of subsequent falls
- Falls are associated with a higher risk for nursing home placement
- There is a high mortality rate (approximately 20% in 1 year) in elderly women with hip fractures

WHEN TO REFER

- Refer for a home safety check any elderly individual with a history of falls or balance or gait abnormalities
- Consider referral to a physical therapist for gait assessment and training (how to get up from a fall and training with special devices)
- An interdisciplinary geriatrics assessment can be useful

PREVENTION

Screens for falls and gait impairment

- Remedy home hazards
- Perform a thorough gait assessment
- An abnormal gait may suggest remediable risk factor for falls, such as proximal muscle weakness, balance problems, or pain
- Modify factors outlined in Table 5 (page XX)
- Determine bone density and improve if needed

 ## EVIDENCE

PRACTICE GUIDELINES

- National Guideline Clearinghouse http://www.guideline.gov/summary/summary.aspx?doc_id=1808&nbr=1034&string=mobility
- American Geriatrics Society http://www.americangeriatrics.org/products/positionpapers/Falls.pdf

WEB SITES

- AARP Guide to Internet Resources on Aging http://www.aarp.org/cyber/sd1_3.htm
- Administration on Aging http://www.aoa.dhhs.gov
- Mayo Clinic—Geriatrics care pearls http://www.mayo.edu/geriatrics-rst/Pearls.html

INFORMATION FOR PATIENTS

- JAMA patient page: Fall-induced injuries. JAMA 1999;281:1962.
- American Academy of Family Physicians http://familydoctor.org/handouts/245.html
- JAMA patient page: Hip fractures. JAMA 2001;285:2814. [PMID: 11419423]

REFERENCES

- Mahoney JE: Temporal association between hospitalization and rate of falls after discharge. Arch Intern Med 2000;160:2788. [PMID: 11025789]
- Ooi WL: The association between orthostatic hypotension and recurrent falls in nursing home residents. Am J Med 2000;108:106. [PMID: 11126303]
- Tinetti ME: Clinical practice. Preventing falls in elderly persons. N Engl J Med 2003;348:42. [PMID: 12510042]

C. Bree Johnston, MD
Kenneth E. Covinsky, MD

Fatty Liver Disease, Alcoholic & Nonalcoholic

Familial Adenomatous Polyposis p. 1098. Familial Mediterranean Fever p. 1099.

KEY FEATURES

ESSENTIALS OF DIAGNOSIS

- Often asymptomatic
- Elevated aminotransferase levels and/or hepatomegaly
- Macrovesicular and/or microvesicular steatosis on liver biopsy

GENERAL CONSIDERATIONS

Alcoholic fatty liver

- Ethanol can cause hepatic steatosis (fatty liver) in the absence of malnutrition, although diets deficient in choline, methionine, and protein can contribute to alcoholic liver damage

NONALCOHOLIC STEATOHEPATITIS (NASH)

- Macrovesicular steatosis, focal infiltration by polymorphonuclear neutrophils, and Mallory's hyalin, a picture indistinguishable from alcoholic hepatitis
- Microvesicular steatosis may result in fulminant hepatic failure
- Hepatic iron overload
- Women in whom fatty liver of pregnancy develops often have a defect in fatty acid oxidation due to reduced long-chain 3-hydroxyacyl-CoA dehydrogenase activity

Etiology of NASH

- Obesity
- Diabetes mellitus
- Hypertriglyceridemia
- Cushing's syndrome
- Starvation or rapid weight loss
- Hypobetalipoproteinemia
- Total parenteral nutrition
- Corticosteroids, amiodarone, tamoxifen
- Wilson's disease
- Jejunoileal bypass
- Poisons: carbon tetrachloride, yellow phosphorus
- Microvesicular steatosis (NAFLD usually macrovesicular): Reye's syndrome, valproic acid toxicity, tetracycline, acute fatty liver of pregnancy

CLINICAL FINDINGS

SYMPTOMS AND SIGNS

- Hepatomegaly is present in 75% of patients with NASH, but the stigmata of chronic liver disease are uncommon

DIFFERENTIAL DIAGNOSIS

- Alcoholic fatty liver disease
- Hepatitis, eg, viral, alcoholic, toxic
- Cirrhosis
- Congestive heart failure
- Hepatocellular carcinoma or metastatic cancer

DIAGNOSIS

LABORATORY TESTS

- There may be mildly elevated aminotransferase and alkaline phosphatase levels
- In contrast to alcoholic liver disease, the ratio of alanine aminotransferase (ALT) to aspartate aminotransferase (AST) is almost always greater than 1 in NASH, but it decreases to less than 1 as advanced fibrosis and cirrhosis develop. An AST/ALT ratio >2 is highly suggestive of alcoholic liver disease

IMAGING STUDIES

- May be demonstrated on ultrasound, CT, or MRI

DIAGNOSTIC PROCEDURES

- Percutaneous liver biopsy is diagnostic and is the only way to assess the degree of fibrosis. The risks of the procedure must be balanced against the impact of the added information on management decisions and assessment of prognosis

Fatty Liver Disease, Alcoholic & Nonalcoholic

 ## TREATMENT

MEDICATIONS

- Ursodeoxycholic acid, 13–15 mg/kg/day, may improve liver function tests and liver histology, but the long-term benefit requires further study
- Metformin, thiazolidinediones, vitamin E, and betaine may reverse fatty liver and are under study
- Supplemental choline may reverse fatty liver associated with total parenteral nutrition

SURGERY

- Gastric bypass may be considered in patients with a body mass index >35 kg/m^2

THERAPEUTIC PROCEDURES

- Fatty liver is readily reversible with discontinuation of alcohol or treatment of other underlying conditions
- Weight loss, dietary fat restriction, and exercise can often improve liver tests and steatosis in obese patients with fatty liver, but the benefit of such measures is less clear in patients with steatohepatitis

 ## OUTCOME

COMPLICATIONS

- In patients with nonalcoholic fatty liver disease, older age, obesity, and diabetes are risk factors for advanced hepatic fibrosis and cirrhosis

PROGNOSIS

- NASH may be associated with hepatic fibrosis in 40% of cases; cirrhosis develops in 10–15%; and decompensated cirrhosis occurs in 2–5% of patients
- Hepatocellular carcinoma in cirrhosis caused by NASH can occur
- NASH may account for many cases of cryptogenic cirrhosis and can recur following liver transplantation

WHEN TO REFER

- For progressive liver diasease
- For liver biopsy

PREVENTION

- Avoid alcohol
- Maintain ideal weight
- Exercise
- Avoid hypertriglyceridemia

 ## EVIDENCE

PRACTICE GUIDELINES

- National Guideline Clearinghouse http://www.guideline.gov/summary/summary.aspx?doc_id=3491&nbr=2717&string=fatty+liver

WEB SITES

- Diseases of the Liver http://cpmcnet.columbia.edu/dept/gi/disliv.html
- Pathology Index http://www-medlib.med.utah.edu/WebPath/LIVEHTML/LIVERIDX.html

INFORMATION FOR PATIENTS

- American Liver Foundation http://www.liverfoundation.org/cgi-bin/dbs/articles.cgi?db=articles&uid=default&ID=1027&view_records=1

REFERENCES

- Angulo P: Nonalcoholic fatty liver disease. N Engl J Med 2002;346:1221. [PMID: 11961152]
- Clark JM et al: Nonalcoholic fatty liver disease. Gastroenterology 2002;122:1649. [PMID: 12016429]
- Harrison SA et al: Nonalcoholic steatohepatitis: what we know in the new millennium. Am J Gastroenterol 2002;97;2714.
- Saadeh S et al: The utility of radiological imaging in nonalcoholic fatty liver disease. Gastroenterology 2002;123:745.
- Sanyal AJ: AGA technical review on nonalcoholic fatty liver disease. Gastroenterology 2002;123:1705.

Lawrence S. Friedman, MD

Fatty Liver of Pregnancy, Acute

 KEY FEATURES

ESSENTIALS OF DIAGNOSIS

- Acute hepatic failure in the third trimester of pregnancy

GENERAL CONSIDERATIONS

- A disorder seen only in pregnancy
- Mortality of 20–30% with improved recognition and early delivery
- Etiology is unknown
- Fatty engorgement of hepatocytes demonstrable on CT of liver and on biopsy

DEMOGRAPHICS

- Usually seen after the 35th week of gestation
- More common in primigravidas and those with twins
- Incidence of 1:14,000 deliveries

 CLINICAL FINDINGS

SYMPTOMS AND SIGNS

- Gradual onset of flu-like symptoms in the third trimester of pregnancy
- Progression to abdominal pain, jaundice, encephalopathy, disseminated intravascular coagulation, and death
- Signs of hepatic failure are present on examination

DIFFERENTIAL DIAGNOSIS

- All etiologies of fulminant hepatic failure should be considered, though transaminase levels are lower (<500 U/mL) in acute fatty liver of pregnancy
- Preeclampsia may involve the liver, but does not cause jaundice and does not cause as marked an elevation of liver enzymes
- Viral hepatitis [including herpes simplex virus (HSV)]
- HELLP syndrome (hemolysis, elevated liver enzymes, low platelets)
- Viral hepatitis (including HSV)
- Choledocholithiasis
- Idiopathic cholestasis of pregnancy
- HELLP syndrome (hemolysis, elevated liver enzymes, low platelets)
- Primary biliary cirrhosis

 DIAGNOSIS

LABORATORY TESTS

- Marked elevation of alkaline phophatase
- Only moderate alanine aminotransferase and aspartate aminotransferase elevation
- Prothrombin time and bilirubin are elevated
- Leukocytosis with thrombocytopenia
- Hypoglycemia may be extreme
- Levels of toxins known to cause liver failure should be measured

IMAGING STUDIES

- Ultrasound or CT of liver

DIAGNOSTIC PROCEDURES

- Liver biopsy very rarely required

TREATMENT

MEDICATIONS

- Supportive care includes administration of glucose, platelets, and fresh frozen plasma as needed (see *Hepatic failure, acute*)

THERAPEUTIC PROCEDURES

- Diagnosis mandates immediate delivery, with vaginal delivery preferred
- A low-protein diet is needed to limit encephalopathy

 ## OUTCOME

PROGNOSIS

- Resolution of encephalopathy occurs over days
- Recurrence rates are unclear
- Most authorities advise against subsequent pregnancy, but successful outcomes have been reported

WHEN TO REFER

- When diagnosis suspected

WHEN TO ADMIT

- When diagnosis suspected

 ## EVIDENCE

PRACTICE GUIDELINES

- ACOG Committee on Obstetric Practice. ACOG practice bulletin. Diagnosis and management of preeclampsia and eclampsia. Number 33, January 2002. American College of Obstetricians and Gynecologists. Int J Gynaecol Obstet 2002;77:67. [PMID: 12094777]

WEB SITE

- Diseases of the Liver http://cpmcnet.columbia.edu/dept/gi/disliv.html

INFORMATION FOR PATIENTS

- JAMA patient page: Pregnancy complications. JAMA 2001;285:1664.
- The Liver Foundation http://www.liverfoundation.org/cgi-bin/dbs/articles.cgi?db=articles&uid=default&ID=1078&view_records=1

REFERENCE

- Castro MA et al: Reversible peripartum liver failure: a new perspective on the diagnosis, treatment, and cause of acute fatty liver of pregnancy, based on 28 consecutive cases. Am J Obstet Gynecol 1999;181:389. [PMID: 10454689]

William R. Crombleholme, MD

Fever

 KEY FEATURES

ESSENTIALS OF DIAGNOSIS

- Localizing symptoms
- Weight loss
- Joint pain
- Intravenous substance use
- Immunosuppression or neutropenia
- History of cancer
- Travel

GENERAL CONSIDERATIONS

- Fever is a regulated rise to a new "set point" of body temperature mediated by pyrogenic cytokines
- The fever pattern is of marginal value, except for the relapsing fever of malaria, borreliosis, and lymphoma, especially Hodgkin's disease
- Most febrile illnesses are due to common infections, are short lived, and are relatively easy to diagnose
- The term FUO ("fever of undetermined origin") refers to cases of unexplained fever exceeding 38.3°C on several occasions for at least 3 weeks in patients without neutropenia or immunosuppression
- In HIV-infected individuals, prolonged unexplained fever is usually due to infections with disseminated *Mycobacterium avium*, *Pneumocystis jiroveci*, cytomegalovirus, or disseminated histoplasmosis, or to lymphoma
- In the returned traveler, consider malaria, dysentery, hepatitis, and dengue fever

 CLINICAL FINDINGS

SYMPTOMS AND SIGNS

- Fever is defined as an elevated body temperature exceeding 38.3°C
- The average normal oral body temperature taken in mid morning is 36.7°C (range 36–37.4°C)
- The normal rectal or vaginal temperature is 0.5°C higher; the axillary temperature is 0.5°C lower
- Rectal is more reliable than oral temperature, particularly in mouth breathers or in tachypneic states
- The normal diurnal temperature variation is 0.5–1°C—lowest in the early morning and highest in the evening
- There is a slight sustained temperature rise following ovulation, during the menstrual cycle, and in the first trimester of pregnancy

DIFFERENTIAL DIAGNOSIS

Common causes

- Infections: bacterial, viral, rickettsial, fungal, parasitic
- Autoimmune diseases
- Central nervous system diseases: head trauma and mass lesions
- Malignant disease: renal cell carcinoma, primary or metastatic liver cancer, leukemia and lymphoma

Less common causes

- Cardiovascular diseases: myocardial infarction, thrombophlebitis, pulmonary embolism
- Gastrointestinal diseases: inflammatory bowel disease, alcoholic hepatitis, granulomatous hepatitis
- Miscellaneous diseases: drug fever, sarcoidosis, familial Mediterranean fever, tissue injury, hematoma, factitious fever

Hyperthermia

- Peripheral thermoregulatory disorders: heat stroke, malignant hyperthermia of anesthesia, and malignant neuroleptic syndrome

DIAGNOSIS

LABORATORY TESTS

- Obtain complete blood cell count with differential, urinalysis, erythrocyte sedimentation rate (ESR) or C-reactive protein level, liver tests (alkaline phosphatase, AST, GGT, total bilirubin)
- Obtain cultures of blood and urine

IMAGING STUDIES

- Chest radiography
- Abdominal ultrasound and CT scan
- Radionuclide-labeled leukocyte, gallium-67, and radiolabeled human immunoglobulin tests

DIAGNOSTIC PROCEDURES

- Temporal artery biopsy in patients aged ≥60 with elevated ESR

Fecal Incontinence p. 1100. Femoral Aneurysm p. 1101. Femoral Neuropathy p. 1101.

 Fever

 TREATMENT

MEDICATIONS

- Antipyretic therapy with aspirin or acetaminophen, 325–650 mg every 4 h
- After obtaining blood and urine cultures, empirical broad-spectrum antibiotic therapy is indicated in patients
  - Who are likely to have a clinically significant infection
  - Who are clinically unstable
  - Who have hemodynamic instability
  - Who have neutropenia (neutrophils less than 500/μL)
  - Who are asplenic (surgically or secondary to sickle cell disease)
  - Who are immunosuppressed (including individuals taking systemic corticosteroids, azathioprine, cyclosporine, or other immunosuppressive medications, and those who are HIV infected)
- If a fungal infection is suspected, add fluconazole or amphotericin B

THERAPEUTIC PROCEDURES

- Most fever is well tolerated
- When the temperature is >40°C, symptomatic treatment; >41°C emergent management of hyperthermia
- Alcohol sponges, cold sponges, ice bags, ice-water enemas, and ice baths lower body temperature in hyperthermia

 OUTCOME

PROGNOSIS

- After extensive evaluation, 25% of patients with FUO have chronic or indolent infection, 25% have autoimmune disease, 10% have malignancy; the remainder have miscellaneous other disorders or no definitive diagnosis
- Long-term follow-up of patients with initially undiagnosed FUO demonstrates that 50% become symptom-free during evaluation, 20% reach a definitive diagnosis (usually within 2 months), and 30% have persistent or recurring fever for months or years

WHEN TO REFER

- Refer patients with prolonged unexplained fever, including FUO, to expert in infectious disease

WHEN TO ADMIT

- Admit for empirical broad-spectrum antibiotic therapy patients who are likely to have a clinically significant infection, who are clinically unstable, who have hemodynamic instability, who have neutropenia, who are asplenic, or who are immunosuppressed

 EVIDENCE

PRACTICE GUIDELINES

- Hughes WT et al: Fever of Unknown Origin Guidelines: 1997 guidelines for the use of antimicrobial agents in neutropenic patients with unexplained fever. Infectious Diseases Society of America http://www.journals.uchicago.edu/IDSA/guide/SE34_551.pdf

WEB SITES

- CDC
  www.cdc.gov
- WHO
  http://www.who.int/en/
- NIH/NIAID
  http://www.niaid.nih.gov/default.htm

INFORMATION FOR PATIENTS

- Mayo Clinic Diseases and Conditions http://www.mayoclinic.com/invoke.cfm?objectid=A382B0D2-850B-434A-96D0FF7F5B318E3E
- JAMA patient page: lumbar puncture http://www.ama-assn.org/public/journals/patient/archive/jpg102302.htm
- Merck Medicus Patient Guide Report http://www.merckmedicus.com/pp/us/hcp/frame_micromedex.jsp?pg=http://merck.micromedex.com/index.asp?page=bhg

REFERENCES

- Armstrong WS et al: Human immunodeficiency virus-associated fever of unknown origin: a study of 70 patients in the United States and review. Clin Infect Dis 1999;28:341. [PMID: 10064253]
- Hopkins PM: Malignant hyperthermia: advances in clinical management and diagnosis. Br J Anaesth 2000;85:118. [PMID: 10928000]
- Mackowiak PA: Concepts of fever. Arch Intern Med 1998;158:1871. [PMID: 9759682]
- Magill AJ: Fever in the returned traveler. Infect Dis Clin North Am 1998;12:445. [PMID: 9658253]
- Pizzo PA: Fever in immunocompromised patients. N Engl J Med 1999;341:893. [PMID: 10486422]

Ralph Gonzales, MD

Fever of Unknown Origin (FUO)

KEY FEATURES

ESSENTIALS OF DIAGNOSIS

- At least 3 weeks of fever over 38.3°C on several occasions, and no diagnosis after 3 outpatient visits or 3 days of hospitalization
- **Nosocomial FUO** occurs in a hospitalized patient with fever of 38.3°C or higher on several occasions, due to a process not present or incubating at admission, in whom initial cultures are negative and the diagnosis remains unknown after 3 days of investigation
- **Neutropenic FUO** includes fever of 38.3°C or higher in a patient on several occasions with less than 500 neutrophils per milliliter in whom initial cultures are negative and the diagnosis remains uncertain after 3 days
- **HIV-associated FUO** occurs in HIV-positive patients with fever of 38.3°C or higher who have been febrile for 4 weeks or more as an outpatient or 3 days as an inpatient, in whom the diagnosis remains uncertain after 3 days of investigation with at least 2 days for cultures to incubate
- Although not usually considered separately, **FUO in solid organ transplant** recipients is a common scenario with a unique differential diagnosis (see below)

GENERAL CONSIDERATIONS

Common causes

- Most cases represent unusual manifestations of common diseases and not rare or exotic diseases—eg, tuberculosis and HIV (primary infection or opportunistic infection) are more common causes than Whipple's disease
- A thorough history—including family, occupational, social (sexual practices, use of intravenous drugs), dietary (unpasteurized products, raw meat), exposures (animals, chemicals), and travel—may give clues to the diagnosis

Age of patient

- Infections (25–40% of cases) and cancer (25–40% of cases) account for the majority of FUOs
- In the elderly (over 65 years of age), multisystem immune-mediated diseases such as temporal arteritis, polymyalgia rheumatica, sarcoidosis, rheumatoid arthritis, and Wegener's granulomatosis account for 25–30% of all FUOs

Duration of fever

- Granulomatous diseases (granulomatous hepatitis, Crohn's disease, ulcerative colitis) and factitious fever are more likely if fever has been present for 6 months or longer
- One-fourth of patients who report being febrile for 6 months or longer have no true fever. Instead, the usual normal circadian variation in temperature (temperature 0.5–1°C higher in the afternoon than in the morning) is interpreted as abnormal
- Episodic or recurrent fever patients who meet the criteria for FUO but have fever-free periods of 2 weeks or longer are similar to those with prolonged fever. Infection, malignancy, and autoimmune disorders account for only 20–25% of such fevers, whereas various miscellaneous diseases (Crohn's disease, familial Mediterranean fever, allergic alveolitis) account for another 25%. Approximately 50% remain undiagnosed but have a benign course with eventual resolution of symptoms

Immunological status

- In neutropenia, fungal infections and occult bacterial infection are important causes of FUO
- In the patient taking immunosuppressive medications (particularly organ transplant patients), cytomegalovirus infections are a frequent cause of fever, as are fungal infections, nocardiosis, *Pneumocystis jiroveci* pneumonia, and mycobacterial infections

Posttransplant

- Infections immediately after transplant often involve the transplanted organ
- Following lung transplantation, pneumonia and mediastinitis are particularly common; following liver transplantation, intraabdominal abscess, cholangitis, and peritonitis; after renal transplantation, urinary tract infections, perinephric abscesses, and infected lymphoceles
- In contrast to solid organ transplants, in bone marrow transplant patients the source of fever cannot be found in 60–70% of patients
- Most infections that occur in the first 2–4 weeks are related to the operative procedure and to hospitalization itself (wound infection, intravenous catheter infection, urinary tract infection from a Foley catheter) or are related to the transplanted organ

- Infections that occur between the first and sixth months are often related to immunosuppression. Reactivated herpes simplex, varicella-zoster, and cytomegalovirus (CMV) infections are quite common. Opportunistic infections with fungi (*Candida*, *Aspergillus*, *Cryptococcus*, *Pneumocystis*, and others), *Listeria monocytogenes*, *Nocardia*, and *Toxoplasma* are also common
- After 6 months, when immunosuppression has been reduced to maintenance levels, infections that are found in any population occur

Classification of causes of FUO

- Most patients with FUO will fit into one of five categories:
  - Infection
  - Neoplasms
  - Autoimmune disorders
  - Miscellaneous causes
  - Undiagnosed FUO
- Despite extensive evaluation, in 10–15% of patients the diagnosis remains elusive. In about 75%, the fever abates spontaneously and the clinician never knows the cause; in the remainder, more classic manifestations of the underlying disease appear

CLINICAL FINDINGS

SYMPTOMS AND SIGNS

- Document the fever in order to exclude factitious (self-induced) fever. Tachycardia, chills, and piloerection generally accompany fever
- Repeated physical examination may reveal subtle, evanescent clinical findings, such as a rash

DIFFERENTIAL DIAGNOSIS

- *Infection*: tuberculosis, endocarditis, osteomyelitis, urinary tract infection, sinusitis, occult abscess (eg, intraabdominal, dental, brain), cholangitis, primary HIV, Epstein–Barr virus, CMV, systemic mycosis, toxoplasmosis, brucellosis, Q fever, cat-scratch disease, salmonellosis, malaria
- *Neoplasm*: Hodgkin's and non-Hodgkin's lymphoma, leukemia, primary or metastatic liver cancer, renal cell carcinoma, atrial myxoma, posttransplant lymphoproliferative disease

- *Autoimmune:* adult Still's disease, systemic lupus erythematosus, cryoglobulinemia, polyarteritis nodosa, temporal (giant cell) arteritis, polymyalgia rheumatica, Wegener's granulomatosis
- *Miscellaneous causes:* drug fever, sarcoidosis, alcoholic or granulomatous hepatitis, Crohn's disease, ulcerative colitis, factitious fever, thyroiditis, hematoma, recurrent pulmonary emboli, hypersensitivity pneumonitis, familial Mediterranean fever, Whipple's disease, transplant rejection, organ ischemia and necrosis, thrombophlebitis

DIAGNOSIS

LABORATORY TESTS

- Blood culture all patients, and usually other fluids, ie, urine, sputum, stool, cerebrospinal fluid, and morning gastric aspirates (if one suspects tuberculosis), preferably when antibiotics have not been taken for several days, and hold in the laboratory for 2 weeks to detect slow-growing organisms
- Cultures on special media are requested for *Legionella, Bartonella,* or nutritionally deficient streptococci
- "Screening tests" with immunological or microbiological serologies ("febrile agglutinins") are not useful
- A single elevated titer rarely is diagnostic of an infection; a four-fold rise or fall in titer confirms a specific cause
- Direct examination of blood smears may establish a diagnosis of malaria or relapsing fever (borrelia)

IMAGING STUDIES

- Chest x-ray in all patients
- Targeted studies (eg, sinus films, gallbladder studies) are best used when symptoms, signs, or a history suggest disease in these body regions
- CT scan of the abdomen and pelvis is particularly useful for looking at the liver, spleen, and retroperitoneum. A positive CT scan often leads to a specific diagnosis. A negative CT scan is not quite as useful
- MRI is generally better than CT for lesions of the nervous system
- Ultrasound is sensitive for lesions of the kidney, pancreas, and biliary tree
- Radionuclide scans are not very helpful when used as screening tests

- A gallium scan may be more helpful than an indium-labeled white blood cell scan

DIAGNOSTIC PROCEDURES

- Echocardiography if endocarditis or atrial myxoma is being considered: transesophageal echocardiography is more sensitive than surface echocardiography for detecting valvular lesions
- Invasive procedures are often required for diagnosis
- Any abnormal finding should be aggressively evaluated: headache calls for lumbar puncture; skin from a rash should be biopsied; and enlarged lymph nodes should be aspirated or biopsied for cytology and culture
- Bone marrow aspiration with biopsy is a relatively low-yield procedure (except in HIV-positive patients, in whom mycobacterial infection is a common cause of FUO), but is low-risk and should be done if other less invasive tests have not yielded a diagnosis
- Liver biopsy will yield a specific diagnosis in 10–15% of FUO patients
- Consider laparotomy or laparoscopy in the deteriorating patient if the diagnosis is elusive despite extensive evaluation

TREATMENT

MEDICATIONS

- Therapeutic trials are indicated if a diagnosis is strongly suspected—eg, antituberculous drugs. However, if there is no clinical response in several weeks, it is imperative to stop therapy and reevaluate the patient
- In the seriously ill or rapidly deteriorating patient, empirical therapy is often given. Antituberculosis medications (particularly in the elderly or foreign-born) and broad-spectrum antibiotics are reasonable in this setting (Table 123, page 1306)
- Empirical administration of corticosteroids should be discouraged; they can suppress fever and exacerbate many infections that cause FUO

OUTCOME

WHEN TO REFER

- If patients remain symptomatic without a diagnosis after initial cultural and radiographic evaluation

WHEN TO ADMIT

- Patients who are clinically deteriorating with symptoms that are interfering with daily activity
- Progressive debilitating weight loss

EVIDENCE

PRACTICE GUIDELINES

- National Guideline Clearinghouse http://www.guideline.gov/summary/summary.aspx?doc_id=1472&nbr=698&string=fever
- Wade JC, Rubenstein EB: NCCN Fever and Neutropenia Practice Guidelines Panel. NCCN: Fever and neutropenia. Cancer Control 2001;8(6 suppl 2):16. [PMID: 11760554]

INFORMATION FOR PATIENTS

- The National Institutes of Health http://www.nlm.nih.gov/medlineplus/ency/article/003090.htm
- National Cancer Institute http://www.cancer.gov/cancerinfo/pdq/supportivecare/fever/patient

REFERENCES

- Davies GR: Fever of unknown origin. Clin Med 2001;1:177. [PMID: 11446608]
- Tal S: Fever of unknown origin in the elderly. J Intern Med 2002;242:295. [PMID: 12366602]

Richard A. Jacobs, MD, PhD

Fibrocystic Breast Disease

KEY FEATURES

ESSENTIALS OF DIAGNOSIS

- Painful, often multiple, often bilateral masses of the breasts
- Pain and size often increase premenstrually

GENERAL CONSIDERATIONS

- Most frequent lesion of the breast
- Estrogen hormone is considered a causative factor
- Encompasses a wide variety of pathological entities
- Always associated with benign changes in the breast epithelium
- Microscopic findings include cysts (gross and microscopic), papillomatosis, adenosis, fibrosis, and ductal epithelial hyperplasia
- Risk factor for breast cancer only if ductal epithelial hyperplasia is present, especially when atypia is present

DEMOGRAPHICS

- Occurs most commonly in women age 30–50
- Rare in postmenopausal women not receiving hormonal replacement therapy

CLINICAL FINDINGS

SYMPTOMS AND SIGNS

- Generally painful lump or lumps, but may be asymptomatic
- Nipple discharge may be present
- Rapid fluctuation in size of masses is common

DIFFERENTIAL DIAGNOSIS

- Breast cancer
- Fibroadenoma
- Lipoma
- Breast abscess
- Intraductal papilloma

DIAGNOSIS

IMAGING STUDIES

- Mammography may be helpful, but is often limited due to radiodensity of breast tissue in young women
- Breast ultrasonography is useful in differentiating a cystic from a solid mass

DIAGNOSTIC PROCEDURES

- Suspicious lesions should be biopsied
- Fine-needle aspiration cytology may be used, but if mass does not resolve over several months, it must be excised

TREATMENT

MEDICATIONS

- Vitamin E, 400 IU PO QD (anecdotal data)
- Danazol, 100–200 mg PO QD, for severe pain, but is rarely used due to side effects (acne, hirsutism, edema)

SURGERY

- Simple mastectomy or extensive removal of breast tissue is rarely, if ever, indicated for fibrocystic breast disease

THERAPEUTIC PROCEDURES

- Aspiration of a discrete mass suggestive of a cyst is indicated in order to alleviate pain and, more importantly, to confirm the cystic nature of the mass

OUTCOME

FOLLOW-UP

- Reexamine at intervals
- Women with proliferative or atypical epithelium on biopsy should be followed carefully by physical examination and mammography for development of breast cancer
- The patient should be advised to examine her own breasts each month just after menstruation and to inform her physician if a mass appears
- Excisional biopsy should be performed if no fluid is obtained or if fluid is bloody on aspiration, if a mass persists after aspiration, or if at any time during follow-up a persistent lump is noted

COMPLICATIONS

- Risk of breast cancer in women with proliferative or atypical changes in the epithelium is higher than in women in general

PROGNOSIS

- Exacerbations of pain, tenderness, and cyst formation may occur at any time until the menopause
- After menopause, symptoms usually subside, except in patients receiving hormone replacement therapy

PREVENTION

- Avoid trauma
- Avoid caffeine (anecdotal data)
- Wear supportive bra night and day

EVIDENCE

PRACTICE GUIDELINES

- Heisey R, Mahoney L, Watson B: Management of palpable breast lumps. Consensus guideline for family physicians. Can Fam Physician 1999;45: 1926. [PMID: 10463093]
- Zylstra S: Office management of benign breast disease. Clin Obstet Gynecol 1999;42(2):234. [PMID: 10370844]

WEB SITES

- National Women's Health Information Center
  http://www.cap.org/health_and_wellness/fact_sheets/fibrocystic.htm
- American Academy of Family Physicians
  http://familydoctor.org/flowcharts/519.html

INFORMATION FOR PATIENTS

- American Cancer Society—Benign breast conditions
  http://www.cancer.org/docroot/cri/content/cri_2_6x_benign_breast_conditions_59.asp
- University of Maryland Medicine—Benign breast conditions
  http://www.umm.edu/breast/benign.htm

REFERENCES

- Marchant DJ: Benign breast disease. Obstet Gynecol Clin North Am 2002;29:1. [PMID: 11892859]
- Morrow M: The evaluation of common breast problems. Am Fam Physician 2000;61:2371. [PMID: 10794579]
- Norlock FE: Benign breast pain in women: a practical approach to evaluation and treatment. J Am Med Womens Assoc 2002;57:85. [PMID: 11991427]

Armando E. Giuliano, MD

Filariasis

ESSENTIALS OF DIAGNOSIS

- Acute disease has irregular episodes of fever (filarial fever), with or without inflammation of lymphatics
- Elephantiasis occurs in the chronic phase as a result of interference with normal lymphatic flow

GENERAL CONSIDERATIONS

- The disease is caused by three filarial nematodes: *Wuchereria bancrofti*, *Brugia malayi*, or *Brugia timori*
- Mosquitoes become infected by ingesting microfilariae with a blood meal; at subsequent feedings, they can infect new susceptible hosts
- Over months, adult worms (females, 8–9 cm × 0.2–0.3 mm) mature and live (up to 2 decades) in or near superficial and deep lymphatics and lymph nodes and produce large numbers of viviparous circulating microfilariae, which may be seen in the blood starting 6–12 months after infection
- Pathological changes in lymph vessels are due to host immunological reactions
- Living microfilariae generally cause no lesions, with the exception of tropical pulmonary eosinophilia. Rapid death of microfilariae, however, does produce findings, and an abscess may form at the site of a dying adult worm

Tropical pulmonary eosinophilia

- Microfilariae of *W bancrofti* or *B malayi* are sequestered in the lungs but not found in the blood

DEMOGRAPHICS

- More than 80 million people are infected with lymphatic filariasis in 73 tropical and subtropical countries
- An estimated 1 million new persons are infected yearly

 CLINICAL FINDINGS

SYMPTOMS AND SIGNS

- The incubation period is generally 8–16 months in expatriates but may be longer in indigenous persons
- Many infections remain asymptomatic

Acute disease

- Episodes of fever (filarial fever), with or without inflammation of lymphatics and nodes, occur at irregular intervals and last for several days
- Characteristically, the adenolymphangitis presents as retrograde extension from the affected node (unlike ascending bacterial lymphangitis)
- With disease progression, epididymitis and orchitis as well as involvement of pelvic, abdominal, or retroperitoneal lymphatics may occur intermittently
- In travelers, allergic-like findings (hives, rashes, eosinophilia) and lymphangitis and lymphadenitis are more likely

Chronic disease

- Obstruction occurs as a result of interference with normal lymphatic flow; this includes hydrocele, scrotal lymphedema, lymphatic varices and elephantiasis, particularly of the extremities, genitals, and breasts
- Extrapulmonary manifestations include splenomegaly and moderate hepatomegaly

Occult disease

- A few persons develop occult disease, in which the classic clinical manifestations and microfilaremia are not present but microfilariae are present in the tissues

Tropical pulmonary eosinophilia

- Episodic nocturnal coughing or wheezing, dyspnea, low-grade fever, scant expectoration

DIFFERENTIAL DIAGNOSIS

- Bacterial lymphangitis
- Loiasis (*Loa loa* infection)
- Idiopathic hydrocele
- Lower extremity edema due to other cause, eg, congestive heart failure, cirrhosis, nephrotic syndrome
- Lymphoma

 DIAGNOSIS

LABORATORY TESTS

- Diagnosis of active infection is made by finding microfilariae in blood (or hydrocele fluid), a positive antigen test (available only for *W bancrofti*), or by ultrasound
- In indigenous persons, microfilariae are rare in the first 2–3 years, abundant as the disease progresses, and again rare in the obstructive stage
- In persons from nonendemic areas, inflammatory reactions may be prominent in the absence of microfilariae
- Microfilariae of *W bancrofti* are found in the blood chiefly at night (nocturnal periodicity 10 PM to 2 AM), except for a nonperiodic variety in the South Pacific. *B malayi* microfilariae are usually nocturnally periodic but in Southeast Asia may be present at all times, with a slight nocturnal rise
- Anticoagulated blood specimens are collected at times related to the periodicity of the local strain. Specimens may be stored at ambient temperatures until examined in the morning by wet film for motile larvae and by Giemsa-stained smears—thick for sensitivity and thin for specific morphology. A formalin-anionic detergent preservative can also be used. If these are negative, the blood specimens should be concentrated by the Knott concentration or membrane filtration technique
- ELISA and immunochromatographic card tests are sensitive (96–100%) and specific (nearly 100%) and are of use for amicrofilaremic persons and for daytime examination of blood. A PCR assay is available for both *W bancrofti* and *B malayi*
- Serological tests may be helpful in screening. A negative test usually rules out present or past infection, but false-positive tests occur with other filarial and helminthic infections. An indirect hemagglutination titer of 1:128 and a bentonite flocculation titer of 1:5 in combination are considered the minimum significant titers. ELISA-IgG and -IgE tests are also available
- Eosinophil counts may be elevated

Tropical pulmonary eosinophilia

- Hypereosinophilia, high filarial antibody titers and IgE levels

IMAGING STUDIES

- Live adult worms can be detected by high-frequency ultrasound of the scrotum (up to 80% of infected men) and of the female breast
- Lymphangiography and radionuclide lymphoscintigraphy may be useful imaging methods
- Diffuse miliary lesions or increased bronchovascular markings on chest films in tropical pulmonary eosinophilia

Filariasis

 TREATMENT

MEDICATIONS

- Diethylcarbamazine is the drug of choice. Cure may require multiple 12-day courses (2 mg/kg three times a day after meals, starting with small doses, and gradually increasing over 3–4 days). Adverse immunological reactions to dying microfilariae and adult worms are common. Antipyretics and analgesics may be helpful. In the United States, the drug is available only from the Parasitic Diseases Drug Service, Centers for Disease Control and Prevention, Atlanta, GA

- In areas where onchocerciasis or loiasis is also prevalent, diethylcarbamazine is often contraindicated because of the potential for severe reactions to dying microfilariae of these parasites; instead, use albendazole plus ivermectin

- During acute inflammatory episodes, it is controversial whether to treat

- Ivermectin is effective only as a microfilaricide; it is given as a single 200-μg/kg dose and repeated in 6 months. Diethylcarbamazine, however, must be given to kill the adult worms, which are the cause of the pathological features

- Albendazole (400 mg twice daily) for 3 weeks has macrofilaricidal action. The drug is free of significant side effects but should not be used in pregnancy

- Tropical pulmonary eosinophilia should be treated with diethylcarbamazine (6 mg/kg daily for 21 days)

THERAPEUTIC PROCEDURES

- General measures include rest, antibiotics for secondary infections, use of postural drainage, elastic stockings and pressure bandages for leg edema, and suspensory bandaging for orchitis and epididymitis

- Small hydroceles may benefit from a locally injected sclerosing agent, or surgery may be indicated

- To manage elephantiasis, lymphovenous shunt procedures may be useful, combined with removal of excess subcutaneous fatty and fibrous tissue, postural drainage, and physiotherapy

 OUTCOME

COMPLICATIONS

- Untreated tropical pulmonary eosinophilia can progress to chronic pulmonary fibrosis

PROGNOSIS

- The prognosis is good with treatment of early and mild cases (including low-grade lymphedema, chyluria, small hydrocele), but in advanced infection the prognosis is poor

WHEN TO REFER

- All patients should be referred to a specialist

WHEN TO ADMIT

- Debilitating filarial fever
- Progressive and disseminated disease

PREVENTION

- Mass treatment programs, in which albendazole is given once yearly with diethylcarbamazine or ivermectin, are being evaluated for their potential to interrupt lymphatic filariasis transmission

 EVIDENCE

INFORMATION FOR PATIENTS

- National Institute of Allergy and Infectious Disease http://www.niaid.nih.gov/newsroom/focuson/bugborne01/filar.htm

- Centers for Disease Control http://www.cdc.gov/ncidod/dpd/parasites/lymphaticfilariasis/factsht_lymphatic_filar.htm

REFERENCES

- Dunyo SK et al: Ivermectin and albendazole alone and in combination for the treatment of lymphatic filariasis in Ghana: follow-up after re-treatment with the combination. Trans R Soc Trop Med Hyg 2002;96:189. [PMID: 12055812]

- Ravindran B: Mass drug administration to treat lymphatic filariasis. Lancet 2002;359:1948. [PMID: 12057582]

Folliculitis

KEY FEATURES

ESSENTIALS OF DIAGNOSIS

- Itching and burning in hairy areas
- Pustules in the hair follicles

GENERAL CONSIDERATIONS

- Has multiple causes
- It may be caused by staphylococcal infection and may be more common in the diabetic
- When the lesion is deep-seated, chronic, and recalcitrant on the head and neck, it is called sycosis
- Sycosis is usually propagated by the autoinoculation and trauma of shaving; the upper lip is particularly susceptible to involvement in men
- Gram-negative folliculitis, which may develop during antibiotic treatment of acne, may present as a flare of acne pustules or nodules; *Klebsiella*, *Enterobacter*, *Escherichia coli*, and *Proteus* have been isolated from these lesions
- "Hot tub folliculitis," caused by *Pseudomonas aeruginosa*, is characterized by pruritic or tender follicular or pustular lesions occurring within 1–4 days after bathing in a hot tub, whirlpool, or public swimming pool; rarely, systemic infections may result
- Nonbacterial folliculitis may be caused by oils that are irritating to the follicle, and these may be encountered in the workplace (machinists) or at home (various cosmetics and cocoa butter or coconut oils)
- Folliculitis may also be caused by occlusion, perspiration, and rubbing, such as that resulting from tight jeans and other heavy fabrics on the upper legs
- Folliculitis on the back that looks like acne but does not respond to acne therapy may be caused by the yeast *Malassezia furfur*; this infection may require biopsy for diagnosis
- Folliculitis—so-called "steroid acne"—may be seen during topical or systemic corticosteroid therapy
- A form of sterile folliculitis called eosinophilic folliculitis consisting of urticarial papules with prominent eosinophilic infiltration is common in patients with AIDS
- Pseudofolliculitis is caused by ingrowing hairs in the beard area
  - In this entity, the papules and pustules are located at the side of and not in follicles
  - It may be treated by growing a beard, by using chemical depilatories, or by shaving with a foil-guard razor
  - Laser hair removal is dramatically beneficial in patients with pseudofolliculitis, requires limited maintenance, and can be done on patients of any skin color
  - Pseudofolliculitis is a true medical indication for such a procedure and should not be considered cosmetic

Types

- Bacterial (usually staphylococcal)
- Sycosis (chronic on head and neck)
- Gram-negative (eg, if on antibiotics for acne)
- Hot tub folliculitis (*Pseudomonas*)
- Herpes folliculitis
- Due to oils, occlusion, perspiration, or rubbing
- *M furfur* (on back) "steroid acne"
- Eosinophilic folliculitis (in AIDS)

CLINICAL FINDINGS

SYMPTOMS AND SIGNS

- The symptoms range from slight burning and tenderness to intense itching
- The lesions consist of pustules of hair follicles

DIFFERENTIAL DIAGNOSIS

- Acne vulgaris
- Miliaria (heat rash)
- Impetigo
- Tinea
- Pseudofolliculitis barbae (ingrown beard hairs)
- Hidradenitis suppurativa

DIAGNOSIS

LABORATORY TESTS

- Clinical diagnosis

TREATMENT

MEDICATIONS

- See Table 6 (page 1199)

Local measures

- Anhydrous ethyl alcohol containing 6.25% aluminum chloride (Xerac AC), applied to lesions and environs, may be helpful, especially for chronic folliculitis of the buttocks

Specific measures

- Systemic antibiotics may be tried if the skin infection is resistant to local treatment, if it is extensive or severe and accompanied by a febrile reaction, if it is complicated, or if it involves the nose or upper lip
- Extended periods of treatment (4–8 weeks or more) with antistaphylococcal antibiotics are required in some cases
- Hot tub *Pseudomonas* folliculitis virtually always resolves without treatment but may be treated with ciprofloxacin, 500 mg twice daily for 5 days
- Gram-negative folliculitis in acne patients may be treated with isotretinoin in compliance with all precautions for that medication
- Folliculitis due to *M furfur* is treated with topical 2.5% selenium sulfide, 15 min daily for 3 weeks, or with oral ketoconazole, 200 mg daily for 7–14 days
- Eosinophilic folliculitis may be treated initially by the combination of potent topical steroids and oral antihistamines; in more severe cases, treatment is with one of the following: topical permethrin (application for 12 h every other night for 6 weeks); itraconazole, 200–400 mg daily; UVB or PUVA phototherapy; or isotretinoin, 0.5 mg/kg/day for up to 5 months; a remission may be induced by some of these therapies, but chronic treatment may be required

 OUTCOME

COMPLICATIONS

- Abscess formation is the major complication of bacterial folliculitis

PROGNOSIS

- Bacterial folliculitis is occasionally stubborn and persistent, requiring prolonged or intermittent courses of antibiotics
- Steroid folliculitis is treatable by acne therapy and resolves as steroids are discontinued

WHEN TO REFER

- If there is a question about the diagnosis, if recommended therapy is ineffective, or if specialized treatment is necessary

PREVENTION

- Correct any predisposing local causes (eg, irritations of a mechanical or chemical nature)
- Control of blood glucose in diabetes may reduce the number of these infections; be sure that the water in hot tubs and spas is treated properly with chlorine
- If staphylococcal folliculitis is persistent, treatment of nasal or perineal carriage with rifampin, 600 mg daily for 5 days, or with topical mupirocin ointment 2% twice daily for 5 days, may help
- Chronic oral clindamycin, 150–300 mg/day, is also effective in preventing recurrent staphylococcal folliculitis and furunculosis

 EVIDENCE

PRACTICE GUIDELINES

- American Academy of Dermatology http://www.aadassociation.org/Guidelines/tineacapitis.html

WEB SITES

- American Academy of Dermatology http://www.aad.org
- Dermatology Handbook for Family Practice from the University of Iowa http://www.vh.org/Providers/ClinRef/FPHandbook/17.html

INFORMATION FOR PATIENTS

- American Academy of Dermatology http://www.aad.org/pamphlets/
- American Osteopathic College of Dermatology http://www.aocd.org/skin/dermatologic_diseases/folliculitis.html
- National Institutes of Health http://www.nlm.nih.gov/medlineplus/ency/article/000823.htm

REFERENCE

- Stulberg DL et al: Common bacterial skin infections. Am Fam Physician 2002;66:119. [PMID: 12126026]

Timothy G. Berger, MD

Frostbite

 ## KEY FEATURES

ESSENTIALS OF DIAGNOSIS

- Injury is due to freezing and formation of ice crystals within tissues

GENERAL CONSIDERATIONS

- Localized hypothermia, vasoconstriction, and slowed metabolism occur as temperature falls below 25°C, although oxygen demand may increase if activity continues
- Once tissue is frozen it becomes pain free

 ## CLINICAL FINDINGS

SYMPTOMS AND SIGNS

Mild cases

- Only the skin and subcutaneous tissues are involved
- The symptoms are numbness, prickling, and itching

Severe cases

- With increasing severity, deep frostbite involves deeper structures
- There may be paresthesia and stiffness
- Thawing causes tenderness and burning pain. The skin is white or yellow, loses its elasticity, and becomes immobile
- Edema, blisters, necrosis, and gangrene may appear

 ## DIAGNOSIS

IMAGING STUDIES

- MRI with magnetic resonance angiography and triple-phase bone scanning can assess the degree of involvement and distinguish viable from nonviable tissue

TREATMENT

MEDICATIONS

- A combination of ibuprofen, 200 mg four times daily, and aloe vera may prevent dermal ischemia

Antiinfective measures

- Consider tetanus prophylaxis; frostbite increases susceptibility
- Local infections may be treated with mild soaks of soapy water or povidone-iodine
- Antibiotics may be required for deep infections

THERAPEUTIC PROCEDURES

- Treat the associated systemic hypothermia (see *Hypothermia*)
- Superficial frostbite (frostnip) of extremities in the field can be treated by firm steady pressure with the warm hand (without rubbing), by placing fingers in the armpits, and, in the case of the toes or heels, by removing footwear, drying feet, rewarming, and covering with adequate dry socks or other protective footwear
- For deep frostbite, rapid thawing at temperatures slightly above body heat may significantly decrease tissue necrosis
- If there is any possibility of refreezing, the frostbitten part should not be thawed, even if this might mean prolonged walking on frozen feet
- Refreezing results in increased tissue necrosis

Rewarming

- Immerse the frozen extremity for several minutes in a moving water bath heated to 40–42°C until the distal tip of the part being thawed flushes. Water in this temperature range feels warm but not hot to the normal hand
- Dry heat (eg, stove or open fire) is more difficult to regulate and is not recommended
- After thawing has occurred and the part has returned to normal temperature (usually in about 30 min), discontinue external heat
- Victims and rescue workers should be cautioned not to attempt rewarming by exercise or thawing of frozen tissues by rubbing with snow or ice water

Protection of the part

- Avoid pressure or friction and physical therapy in the early stage. Casts, dressings, or bandages are not applied
- Keep the patient at bed rest with the affected parts elevated and uncovered at room temperature
- Protect skin blebs from physical contact
- Whirlpool therapy at 37–40°C twice daily for 15–20 min for a period of 3 or more weeks helps cleanse the skin and debrides superficial sloughing tissue

SURGERY

- Early regional sympathetic blockade can reduce symptoms; sympathectomy (within 36–72 h) is controversial. In general, other surgical intervention is to be avoided
- Amputation should not be considered until it is definitely established that the tissues are dead. Tissue necrosis (even with black eschar formation) may be quite superficial, and the underlying skin may sometimes heal spontaneously even after a period of months

 OUTCOME

FOLLOW-UP

- Gentle, progressive physical therapy to promote circulation should be instituted as tolerated

COMPLICATIONS

- Loss of fingers, toes, extremities, tip of nose
- There may be increased susceptibility to discomfort in the involved extremity upon reexposure to cold with pain, numbness, tingling, hyperhidrosis
- Cold sensitivity of the extremities and nerve conduction abnormalities may persist for years after the cold injury

PROGNOSIS

- Recovery from frostbite is most often complete

WHEN TO ADMIT

- Hypothermia
- Most cases, including all cases of deep frostbite

 EVIDENCE

PRACTICE GUIDELINES

- http://www.spartanburgems.com/ Protocol_02/frostbite.pdf

WEB SITE

- Merck Manual—Disorder due to physical agents http://www.merck.com/pubs/mmanual/ section20/sec20.htm

INFORMATION FOR PATIENTS

- Nemours Foundation http://kidshealth.org/parent/firstaid_ safe/emergencies/frostbite.html
- National Institutes of Health http://www.nlm.nih.gov/medlineplus/ ency/article/000057.htm

REFERENCE

- Murphy JV et al: Frostbite: pathogenesis and treatment. J Trauma 2000;48:171. [PMID: 10647591]

Richard Cohen, MD, MPH
Brent R.W. Moelleken, MD, FACS

Furunculosis

 KEY FEATURES

ESSENTIALS OF DIAGNOSIS

- Extremely painful inflammatory swelling based on a hair follicle that forms an abscess
- Predisposing condition (diabetes mellitus, HIV disease, injection drug use) sometimes present
- Coagulase-positive *Staphylococcus aureus* is the causative organism

GENERAL CONSIDERATIONS

- A furuncle (boil) is a deep-seated infection (abscess) involving the entire hair follicle and adjacent subcutaneous tissue
- The most common sites of occurrence are the hairy parts exposed to irritation and friction, pressure, or moisture
- Because the lesions are autoinoculable, they are often multiple
- A carbuncle consists of several furuncles developing in adjoining hair follicles and coalescing to form a conglomerate, deeply situated mass with multiple drainage points

DEMOGRAPHICS

- Predisposing cause usually not found
- However, diabetes mellitus (especially if using insulin injections), injection drug use, allergy injections, and HIV disease all increase the risk of staphylococcal infections by increasing the rate of nasal carriage

 CLINICAL FINDINGS

SYMPTOMS AND SIGNS

Furuncle

- Rounded or conical abscesses on the hairy parts exposed to irritation and friction, pressure, or moisture
- Lesions are often multiple and pain and tenderness may be prominent
- Gradually enlarges, becomes fluctuant, and then softens and opens spontaneously after a few days to 1–2 weeks to discharge a core of necrotic tissue and pus
- Infection of the soft tissue around the nails (paronychia) may be due to staphylococci when it is acute; other organisms may be involved, including *Candida* and herpes simplex (herpetic whitlow)

Carbuncle

- Consists of several furuncles in adjoining hair follicles and coalescing to form a deeply situated mass with multiple drainage points

DIFFERENTIAL DIAGNOSIS

- Inflamed sebaceous (epidermal inclusion) cyst—suddenly becomes red, tender, and expands greatly in size over one to a few days; history of prior cyst in the same location, the presence of a clearly visible cyst orifice, and the extrusion of malodorous cheesy rather than purulent material helps in the diagnosis
- Acne vulgaris
- Tinea profunda (deep tinea of hair follicle)
- Sporotrichosis
- Blastomycosis
- Hidradenitis suppurativa (recurrent tender sterile abscesses in the axillae, groin, on the buttocks, or below the breasts; presence of old scars or sinus tracts plus negative cultures suggests this diagnosis)
- Anthrax
- Tularemia

 DIAGNOSIS

LABORATORY TESTS

- Leukocytosis may occur, but a white blood cell count is rarely required
- Although *S aureus* is almost always the cause, pus should be cultured, especially in immunocompromised patients, to rule out methicillin-resistant *S aureus* or other bacteria

TREATMENT

MEDICATIONS

- Systemic antibiotics
  - Sodium dicloxacillin or cephalexin, 1 g daily in divided doses by mouth for 10 days, is usually effective
  - Erythromycin in similar doses may be used in penicillin-allergic individuals in communities with low prevalence of erythromycin-resistant staphylococci or if the particular isolate is sensitive
  - Ciprofloxacin, 500 mg twice daily, is effective against strains of staphylococci resistant to other antibiotics
- Recurrent furunculosis may be effectively treated with a combination of dicloxacillin, 250–500 mg four times daily for 2–4 weeks, and rifampin, 300 mg twice daily for 5 days, during this period
- Chronic clindamycin, 150–300 mg daily for 1–2 months, may also cure recurrent furunculosis
- Applications of topical 2% mupirocin to the nares, axillae, and anogenital areas twice daily for 5 days eliminates the staphylococcal carrier state

SURGERY

- Incision and drainage: recommended for all loculated collections; mainstay of therapy
- Use surgical incision and debridement **after** the lesions are "mature"
- It is not necessary to incise and drain an acute staphylococcal paronychia

THERAPEUTIC PROCEDURES

- Immobilize the part and avoid overmanipulation of inflamed areas
- Use moist heat to help larger lesions "localize"
- Inserting a flat metal spatula or sharpened hardwood stick into the nail fold where it adjoins the nail will release pus from a mature lesion

 OUTCOME

FOLLOW-UP

Recurrent furunculosis

- Culture of the anterior nares may identify chronic staphylococcal carriage in recurrent infections
- Family members and intimate contacts may need evaluation for staphylococcal carrier state and perhaps concomitant treatment.

PROGNOSIS

- Recurrent crops may occur for months or years

WHEN TO REFER

- If there is a question about the diagnosis, if recommended therapy is ineffective, or if specialized treatment is necessary

 EVIDENCE

WEB SITES

- American Academy of Dermatology http://www.aad.org
- Dermatology Handbook for Family Practice from the University of Iowa http://www.vh.org/Providers/ClinRef/FPHandbook/17.html

INFORMATION FOR PATIENTS

- American Osteopathic College of Dermatology http://www.aocd.org/skin/dermatologic_diseases/boils.html
- National Institutes of Health Medical Encyclopedia http://www.nlm.nih.gov/medlineplus/ency/article/001474.htm

REFERENCE

- Stulberg DL et al: Common bacterial skin infections. Am Fam Physician 2002;66:119. [PMID: 12126026]

Timothy G. Berger, MD

Gastric Cancer

 KEY FEATURES

ESSENTIALS OF DIAGNOSIS

- Dyspeptic symptoms with weight loss in patients age >40
- Iron deficiency anemia; occult blood in stools
- Abnormality on upper gastrointestinal series or endoscopy

GENERAL CONSIDERATIONS

- Gastric adenocarcinoma is the most common cancer worldwide
- Most gastric cancers arise in the antrum
- Chronic *Helicobacter pylori* gastritis is a major risk factor; however, among individuals chronically infected with *H pylori*, <1% will develop gastric carcinoma
- Other risk factors: gastric adenomas, chronic atrophic gastritis with intestinal metaplasia, pernicious anemia, and partial gastric resection >15 years previously

DEMOGRAPHICS

- Incidence in the United States has declined by two-thirds over the last 30 years
- Currently, 20,000 cases annually in the United States
- Uncommon under age 40; mean age at diagnosis is 63 years
- Men affected twice as often as women
- Incidence is higher in Latinos, African-Americans, and Asian-Americans

 CLINICAL FINDINGS

SYMPTOMS AND SIGNS

- Generally asymptomatic or nonspecific symptoms until advanced disease
- Dyspepsia, vague epigastric pain, anorexia, early satiety, and weight loss
- Acute upper gastrointestinal bleeding with hematemesis or melena
- Postprandial vomiting suggests gastric outlet obstruction
- Progressive dysphagia suggests lower esophageal obstruction
- Physical examination rarely helpful
- Gastric mass is palpated in less than 20%
- Lymphadenopathy: left supraclavicular lymph node (Virchow's node), an umbilical nodule (Sister Mary Joseph nodule)
- Rigid rectal shelf (Blumer's shelf)
- Ovarian metastases (Krukenberg tumor)

DIFFERENTIAL DIAGNOSIS

- Benign gastric ulcers
- Lymphoma
- Menetrier's disease

 DIAGNOSIS

LABORATORY TESTS

- Guaiac-positive stools
- Iron deficiency anemia or anemia of chronic disease
- Liver function test abnormalities if metastatic spread
- Serological markers (eg, carcinoembryonic antigen) not helpful

IMAGING STUDIES

- Barium upper gastrointestinal series when endoscopy is not readily available
- Upper gastrointestinal series may not detect small or superficial lesions and cannot reliably distinguish benign from malignant ulcerations
- Preoperative evaluation with abdominal CT and endoscopic ultrasonography

DIAGNOSTIC PROCEDURES

- Upper endoscopy with biopsy and cytological brushings
- Staging by TNM system
  - Stage I: T1N0, T1N1, T2N0, all M0
  - Stage II: T1N2, T2N1, T3N0, all M0
  - Stage III: T2N2, T3N1, T4N0, all M0
  - Stage IV: T4N2M0, any M1
- After preoperative staging, about two-thirds found to have localized disease (ie, stages I–III)

TREATMENT

MEDICATIONS

- Single-agent or combination chemotherapy with fluorouracil, doxorubicin, and cisplatin or mitomycin may provide palliation in up to 30%
- Patients undergoing curative resection should be considered for postoperative adjuvant chemoradiotherapy

SURGERY

- For patients with clinically localized disease (stages I–III), surgical exploration; at surgery, patients with confirmed localized disease should undergo radical surgical resection with curative intent; approximately 25% will be found to have locally unresectable tumors or peritoneal, hepatic, or distant lymph node metastases, and "curative" surgical resection is not warranted
- Palliative resection of the tumor can reduce the risk of bleeding and obstruction, lead to improved quality of life, and improve survival
- For patients with unresectable disease, gastrojejunostomy can prevent obstruction

THERAPEUTIC PROCEDURES

- Endoscopic laser or stent therapy, radiation therapy, or angiographic embolization can palliate bleeding or obstruction from unresected tumors

 OUTCOME

FOLLOW-UP

- After surgical therapy, further follow-up is determined by clinical course
- Routine follow-up not recommended

COMPLICATIONS

- Acute or chronic gastrointestinal blood loss
- Gastric outlet obstruction
- Carcinomatosis with ascites, small bowel obstruction

PROGNOSIS

- Overall long-term survival is <15%
- Survival related to tumor stage, location, and histological features
- Stage I and stage II tumors resected for cure have a >50% long-term survival
- Patients with stage III tumors have a <20% long-term survival
- Tumors of the diffuse and signet ring type have a worse prognosis than those of the intestinal type
- Tumors of the proximal stomach (fundus and cardia) have 5-year survival of <15%, a far worse prognosis than distal lesions

WHEN TO REFER

- Patients with a confirmed diagnosis of gastric adenocarcinoma should be evaluated by a general surgeon or oncologist

WHEN TO ADMIT

- Acute upper gastrointestinal bleeding
- Vomiting and dehydration

PREVENTION

- In Japan, population-based endoscopic screening is performed
- At present, population-based testing and treating of *H pylori* as a chemopreventative measure to reduce the incidence of gastric adenocarcinoma is not recommended

 EVIDENCE

PRACTICE GUIDELINES

- Earle CC et al: Neoadjuvant or adjuvant therapy for resectable gastric cancer? A practice guideline. Can J Surg 2002;45:438. [PMID: 12500920]

WEB SITES

- American Cancer Society—What are the risk factors for stomach cancer? http://www.cancer.org/docroot/cri/content/cri_2_4_2x_what_are_the_risk_factors_for_stomach_cancer_40.asp?sitearea=cri
- MD consult—Stomach Cancer http://home.mdconsult.com/das/patient/view/30939797/10002/13258.html/top?sid=203837002
- National Cancer Institute—What you need to know about stomach cancer http://www.cancer.gov/cancerinfo/wyntk/stomach

INFORMATION FOR PATIENTS

- Cleveland Clinic—Stomach cancer http://www.clevelandclinic.org/health/health-info/docs/1800/1813.asp?index=8105
- Mayo Clinic—Stomach cancer http://www.mayoclinic.com/invoke.cfm?objectid=4545F9D7-17A0-4275-9C296401969A8E11
- MEDLINEplus—Gastric cancer http://www.nlm.nih.gov/medlineplus/ency/article/000223.htm

REFERENCES

- Bonenkamp JJ et al: Extended lymphnode dissection for gastric cancer. N Engl J Med 1999;340:908. [PMID: 10089184]
- De Vivo R et al: The role of chemotherapy in the management of gastric cancer. J Clin Gastroenterol 2000;30:364. [PMID: 10875463]

Kenneth R. McQuaid, MD

Gastritis, Erosive & Hemorrhagic

 KEY FEATURES

ESSENTIALS OF DIAGNOSIS

- Hematemesis, "coffee grounds" emesis, or melena; usually not significant bleeding
- Often asymptomatic; may cause epigastric pain, anorexia, nausea, and vomiting
- Occurs most commonly in alcoholics, critically ill patients, or patients taking nonsteroidal antiinflammatory drugs (NSAIDs)

GENERAL CONSIDERATIONS

- Most common causes: drugs (especially NSAIDs), alcohol, stress due to severe medical or surgical illness, and portal hypertension ("portal gastropathy")
- Uncommon causes: caustic ingestion and radiation

DEMOGRAPHICS

- Patients using acute or chronic NSAIDs, especially aspirin
- Heavy alcohol ingestion
- Critically ill ICU patients: major risk factors are coagulopathy, mechanical ventilation, sepsis, trauma, burns, central nervous system injury, and hepatic or renal failure

 CLINICAL FINDINGS

SYMPTOMS AND SIGNS

- Often asymptomatic
- Symptoms, when they occur, include dyspepsia, anorexia, epigastric pain, nausea, and vomiting
- Upper gastrointestinal bleeding, hematemesis, "coffee grounds" emesis, or melena; bleeding is not usually hemodynamically significant

DIFFERENTIAL DIAGNOSIS

- Epigastric pain suggests peptic ulcer, gastroesophageal reflux, gastric cancer, biliary tract disease, food poisoning, viral gastroenteritis, and functional dyspepsia
- Severe pain suggests a perforated or penetrating ulcer, pancreatic disease, esophageal rupture, ruptured aortic aneurysm, gastric volvulus, and myocardial ischemia
- Upper gastrointestinal bleeding suggests peptic ulcer disease, esophageal varices, Mallory-Weiss tear, and arteriovenous malformations

 DIAGNOSIS

LABORATORY TESTS

- Hematocrit is low if significant bleeding
- Iron deficiency

IMAGING STUDIES

- Upper endoscopy for dyspepsia or upper gastrointestinal bleeding is diagnostic, demonstrating erythema, subepithelial petechiae, and erosion
- Barium upper gastrointestinal series is insensitive because abnormalities are confined to the mucosa

DIAGNOSTIC PROCEDURES

- Nasogastric tube placement reveals bloody aspirate

Gastritis, Erosive & Hemorrhagic

 ## TREATMENT

MEDICATIONS

- Stress gastritis: continuous infusions of an H_2 receptor antagonist or proton pump inhibitor to raise intragastric pH >4.0
- NSAID gastritis: empirical treatment for dyspepsia alone (without bleeding) with H_2 receptor antagonist (cimetidine 400 mg PO BID, ranitidine 150 mg PO BID, or famotidine 20 mg PO BID), or proton pump inhibitor (omeprazole 20 mg PO QD, rabeprazole 20 mg PO QD, esomeprazole 40 mg PO QD, pantoprazole 40 mg PO QD, or lansoprazole 30 mg PO QD); or change to a cyclooxygenase (COX)-2 selective agent, eg, rofecoxib
- Alcoholic gastritis: H_2 receptor antagonists or sucralfate for 2–4 weeks
- Portal hypertensive gastropathy: nonselective β-blocker (propranolol or nadolol); dose adjusted to reduce resting heart rate to <60/min

THERAPEUTIC PROCEDURES

- Portal hypertensive gastropathy: portal decompressive procedures, eg, transvenous intrahepatic portosystemic shunts, are sometimes required for acute hemorrhage

 ## OUTCOME

COMPLICATIONS

- Acute upper gastrointestinal hemorrhage
- Chronic gastrointestinal blood loss with anemia

WHEN TO REFER

- NSAID gastritis: persistent dyspepsia despite discontinuation of NSAIDs or empirical therapy should be referred for endoscopy

WHEN TO ADMIT

- NSAID gastritis: acute upper gastrointestinal (GI) hemorrhage; severe dyspepsia with concern for complicated peptic ulcer disease or alternative diagnosis
- Alcoholic gastritis: protracted vomiting and/or acute upper GI hemorrhage or signs of alcohol withdrawal
- Portal hypertensive gastropathy

PREVENTION

- Stress gastritis: prophylactic therapy warranted in high-risk ICU patients only
- H_2 receptor antagonist infusions at a dose sufficient to maintain intragastric pH >4.0
- Cimetidine (900–1200 mg), ranitidine (150 mg), or famotidine (20 mg) by continuous IV infusion over 24 h
- IV proton pump inhibitors (pantoprazole) are more expensive than H_2 receptor agonists; efficacy and optimal dosage not yet established
- NSAID gastritis: patients at high risk for NSAID-induced complications should receive cotherapy with a proton pump inhibitor and/or misoprostol, 200 μg PO QID; alternatively, a safer, COX-2 selective agent should be used (rofecoxib or celecoxib); use of low-dose aspirin negates safety of COX-2 selective agent
- High-risk patients should be tested for *Helicobacter pylori* and treated if positive

 ## EVIDENCE

PRACTICE GUIDELINES

- Chamberlain CE: Acute hemorrhagic gastritis. Gastroenterol Clin North Am 1993;22:843. [PMID: 7905865]
- Sharma P et al: Review article: *Helicobacter pylori* and reflux disease. Aliment Pharmacol Ther 2003;17:297. [PMID: 12562442]

WEB SITES

- National Digestive Diseases Information Clearinghouse—Gastritis http://digestive.niddk.nih.gov/ddiseases/pubs/gastritis/index.htm
- Mayo Clinic—Gastritis http://www.mayoclinic.com/invoke.cfm?objectid =342EF017-2230-45E3-9B6C9D069CEFA6DE

INFORMATION FOR PATIENTS

- MEDLINEplus—Acute gastritis http://www.nlm.nih.gov/medlineplus/ency/article/000240.htm
- MEDLINEplus—Chronic gastritis http://www.nlm.nih.gov/medlineplus/ency/article/000232.htm

REFERENCES

- Jung R et al: Proton-pump inhibitors for stress ulcer prophylaxis in critically ill patients. Ann Pharmacother 2002;36:1929. [PMID: 12452757]
- Wolfe MM et al: Acid suppression: optimizing therapy for gastroduodenal ulcer healing, gastroesophageal reflux disease, and stress-related erosive syndrome. Gastroenterology 2000;118(2 Suppl 1):S9. [PMID: 10868896]

Kenneth R. McQuaid, MD

Gastroesophageal Reflux Disease (GERD)

KEY FEATURES

ESSENTIALS OF DIAGNOSIS

- Heartburn exacerbated by meals, bending, or recumbency
- Endoscopy demonstrates esophageal abnormalities in <50% of patients

GENERAL CONSIDERATIONS

- Affects 20% of adults, who report at least weekly episodes of heartburn
- Up to 10% complain of daily symptoms
- Most patients have mild disease
- Up to 50% develop esophageal mucosal damage (reflux esophagitis)
- Few develop serious complications
- Uncomplicated patients treated empirically without diagnostic studies
- Investigation is required in complicated disease and those unresponsive to empirical therapy
- Pathogenesis includes
  - Relaxation or incompetence of lower esophageal sphincter
  - Hiatal hernia
  - Abnormal acid clearance (esophageal peristalsis), eg, scleroderma
  - Impaired salivation (exacerbates GERD), eg, Sjögren's syndrome, anticholinergics, radiation
  - Delayed gastric emptying (exacerbates GERD), eg, gastroparesis

DEMOGRAPHICS

- Increased in whites
- High prevalence in North America and Europe
- Chronic *Helicobacter pylori* infection may be protective in subset of patients with reduced acid secretion
- Increased in pregnancy

CLINICAL FINDINGS

SYMPTOMS AND SIGNS

- Heartburn, most often 30–60 min after meals and upon reclining, with relief from antacids
- Regurgitation—spontaneous reflux of sour or bitter gastric contents into the mouth
- Dysphagia common due to inflammation, impaired motility, or stricture
- Atypical manifestations: asthma, chronic cough, chronic laryngitis, sore throat, and noncardiac chest pain
- Gradual development of solid food dysphagia progressive over months to years suggests stricture formation
- Physical examination normal

DIFFERENTIAL DIAGNOSIS

- Peptic ulcer disease, gastritis, nonulcer dyspepsia, or cholelithiasis
- Angina pectoris
- Infectious esophagitis: *Candida*, herpes simplex virus, cytomegalovirus
- Pill-induced esophagitis
- Esophageal motility disorders, eg, achalasia, esophageal spasm, scleroderma
- Radiation esophagitis
- Zollinger-Ellison syndrome (gastrinoma) may cause severe esophagitis due to acid hypersecretion

DIAGNOSIS

LABORATORY TESTS

- Laboratory tests are normal

IMAGING STUDIES

- Upper endoscopy with biopsy
- Endoscopy reveals visible mucosal abnormalities (erythema, friability, and erosions) in 50%
- Endoscopy indicated in patients who have not responded to empirical medical management and in patients with symptoms suggesting complicated disease (dysphagia, odynophagia, occult or overt bleeding, or iron deficiency anemia), in long-standing symptoms (>5 years), in patients requiring continuous maintenance therapy, to look for Barrett's esophagus, and to differentiate peptic stricture from other benign or malignant causes of dysphagia
- Barium esophagography seldom useful; insensitive for detection of mucosal abnormalities; in patients with dysphagia, useful for detection of esophageal stricture

DIAGNOSTIC PROCEDURES

- Clinical diagnosis has sensitivity 80%, specificity 70%
- In patients with typical GERD symptoms without complications, empirical medical management recommended without diagnostic procedures
- Ambulatory esophageal pH monitoring: best study to document acid reflux, but unnecessary in most patients. Indicated
  - To document abnormal esophageal acid exposure in a patient being considered for antireflux surgery who has a normal endoscopy
  - To evaluate patients with a normal endoscopy who have reflux symptoms unresponsive to proton pump inhibitor
  - To detect association between reflux and atypical symptoms

 ## TREATMENT

MEDICATIONS

- Mild, occasional symptoms: Gaviscon alginate-antacid; other antacids provide rapid, short-term relief

Gastroesophageal Reflux Disease (GERD)

- Nonprescription H$_2$ receptor antagonists: cimetidine 200 mg, ranitidine and nizatidine 75 mg, famotidine 10 mg taken before meals may prevent symptoms; if taken after symptoms develop, symptom relief within 60 min
- Moderate symptoms: H$_2$ receptor antagonist (nizatidine 150 mg PO BID, famotidine 20 mg PO BID, or cimetidine 400–800 mg PO BID) or proton pump inhibitors (omeprazole or rabeprazole 20 mg PO QD, lansoprazole 30 mg PO QD, esomeprazole 40 mg PO QD, or pantoprazole 40 mg PO QD) for 8–12 weeks
- Promotility drugs (metoclopramide, bethanechol): reduce reflux, but side effects preclude use for reflux disease
- Severe symptoms and erosive disease: proton pump inhibitors (omeprazole 20 mg PO QD or rabeprazole 20 mg PO QD, lansoprazole 30 mg PO QD, pantoprazole 40 mg PO QD, or esomeprazole 40 mg PO QD for 8–12 weeks) produce relief and healing in >80%; given BID, they provide relief in >95%
- Patients with severe erosive esophagitis, Barrett's esophagus, or peptic stricture should be maintained on chronic proton pump inhibitor therapy
- Relapse: treated with either continuous or intermittent courses of proton pump inhibitor therapy
- Unresponsive disease: occurs in 10–20% of patients on once-daily doses of proton pump inhibitors, and in 5% of those on twice-daily doses
- Unresponsive disease: treated with higher proton pump inhibitor doses (eg, omeprazole 40 mg PO BID) or proton pump inhibitor BID (before breakfast and dinner) and a bedtime dose of an H$_2$ receptor antagonist
- Peptic stricture: chronic proton pump inhibitor therapy

SURGERY

- Surgical fundoplication produces relief in >85% of properly selected patients, 10-year success rates 60–90%
- Fundoplication may now be performed laparoscopically with low complication rates
- However, >50% of patients undergoing fundoplication require continued acid-suppression medication
- >30% develop new symptoms of dysphagia, bloating, increased flatulence, or dyspepsia

- Surgical treatment recommended for otherwise healthy patients with extra-esophageal manifestations of reflux, those with severe reflux who are unwilling to accept lifelong medical therapy, and patients with erosive disease who are intolerant of or resistant to proton pump inhibitors

THERAPEUTIC PROCEDURES

- Life-style modifications
- Reduce meal size
- Avoid bending over after meals
- Avoid lying down within 3 h after meals
- Avoid acidic foods (tomato, citrus, spicy foods, coffee) and agents that relax the lower esophageal sphincter or delay gastric emptying (fatty foods, peppermint, chocolate, alcohol, and smoking)
- Weight reduction
- Elevate the head of the bed
- Dilation of peptic stricture effective in up to 90% of symptomatic patients

 OUTCOME

FOLLOW-UP

- After discontinuation of therapy, relapse of symptoms occurs in 80% of patients within 1 year—the majority within the first 3 months
- Barrett's esophagus (intestinal metaplasia) present in up to 10% of patients with chronic reflux
- Patients with Barrett's who are operative candidates undergo endoscopic surveillance with mucosal biopsies every 3 years
- Patients with low-grade dysplasia are treated with aggressive medical management and endoscopic surveillance every 6–12 months
- For patients with high-grade dysplasia or frequent endoscopic surveillance (every 3 months) surgery is recommended; otherwise, photodynamic ablation or endoscopic mucosal resection
- Barrett's esophagus is treated long-term with proton pump inhibitors

COMPLICATIONS

- GERD: stricture formation in ~10%, acid-peptic ulceration, erosive, or hemorrhagic esophagitis; effectively treated with dilation
- Barrett's esophagus: increased annual incidence of esophageal adenocarcinoma

to 0.5% , a 40-fold risk compared to patients without Barrett's

PROGNOSIS

- Heartburn symptoms can be controlled in almost all patients with intermittent or chronic therapy
- Symptoms of regurgitation, bloating, dyspepsia may persist despite acid-reduction therapy

WHEN TO REFER

- Complicated disease: dysphagia, weight loss, fecal-occult positive stool, anemia
- Symptoms that persist despite proton pump inhibitor therapy
- Candidates for fundoplication

WHEN TO ADMIT

- Seldom required

 EVIDENCE

PRACTICE GUIDELINES

- Sampliner RE: Practice Parameters Committee of the American College of Gastroenterology. Updated guidelines for the diagnosis, surveillance, and therapy of Barrett's esophagus. Am J Gastroenterol 2002;97:1888. [PMID: 12190150]

WEB SITE

- Society of Thoracic Surgeons— Gastroesophageal reflux disease http://www.sts.org/doc/4119

INFORMATION FOR PATIENTS

- NIH Patient Education Institute— Gastroesophageal reflux disease http://www.nlm.nih.gov/medlineplus/tutorials/gerd.html

REFERENCES

- Falk GW: Barrett's esophagus. Gastroenterology 2002;122:1569. [PMID: 12016424]
- Fass R et al: Gastroesophageal reflux disease—should we adopt a new conceptual framework? Am J Gastroenterol 2002;97:1901. [PMID: 12190152]
- Spechler S et al: Long-term outcomes of medical and surgical therapies for gastroesophageal reflux disease. JAMA 2001;285:2331. [PMID: 11343480]

Kenneth R. McQuaid, MD

Gastrointestinal Bleeding, Acute Lower

 KEY FEATURES

ESSENTIALS OF DIAGNOSIS

- Hematochezia usually present
- Evaluation with colonoscopy in stable patients
- Massive active bleeding calls for evaluation with upper endoscopy, or nuclear bleeding scan, and/or angiography

GENERAL CONSIDERATIONS

- Lower gastrointestinal bleeding defined as that arising below the ligament of Treitz, ie, small intestine or colon; >95% of cases from the colon
- Lower tract bleeding is one-fourth as common as upper, tends to have a more benign course, less likely to present with shock or orthostasis (<20%) or to require transfusions (<40%)
- Spontaneous cessation in >85%, hospital mortality in <3%
- Most common cause: in patients age <50, infectious colitis, anorectal disease, and inflammatory bowel disease; in older patients, diverticulosis (50% of cases), vascular ectasias (5–10%), neoplasms (polyps or carcinoma) (10%), ischemia, radiation-induced proctitis, solitary rectal ulcer, nonsteroidal antiinflammatory drug (NSAID)-induced ulcers, small bowel diverticula, and colonic varices
- In 20% no source of bleeding can be identified
- Diverticulosis: acute, painless, large-volume maroon or bright red hematochezia occurs in 3–5%, associated with the use of NSAIDs; bleeding more commonly originates on the right side; >95% require fewer than 4 units of blood transfusion; bleeding subsides spontaneously in 80% but may recur in up to 25% of patients
- Vascular ectasias (angiodysplasias): painless bleeding ranging from melena or hematochezia to occult blood loss; bleeding most commonly originates in the cecum and ascending colon; causes: congenital, hereditary hemorrhagic telangiectasia, autoimmune disorders, typically scleroderma
- Neoplasms: benign polyps and carcinoma cause chronic occult blood loss or intermittent anorectal hematochezia
- Anorectal disease: small amounts of bright red blood noted on the toilet paper, streaking of the stool, or dripping into the toilet bowl; painless bleeding with internal hemorrhoids; pain with bleeding suggests anal fissure
- Ischemic colitis: hematochezia or bloody diarrhea associated with mild cramps; in most, the bleeding is mild and self-limited

DEMOGRAPHICS

- Lower tract bleeding is more common in older men
- Diverticular bleeding is more common in patients aged >50
- Angiodysplasia bleeding is more common in patients aged >70 and with chronic renal failure
- Ischemic colitis is most common in older patients, due to atherosclerotic disease, postoperatively after ileoaortic or abdominal aortic aneurysm surgery; in younger patients, due to vasculitis, coagulation disorders, estrogen therapy, and long-distance running

 CLINICAL FINDINGS

SYMPTOMS AND SIGNS

- Brown stools mixed or streaked with blood suggest rectosigmoid or anal source
- Painless large-volume bleeding suggests a colonic source (diverticular bleeding or vascular ectasias)
- Maroon stools suggest a right colon or small intestine source
- Black stools (melena) suggest a source proximal to the ligament of Treitz
- Bright red blood per rectum occurs uncommonly with upper tract bleeding and almost always in the setting of massive hemorrhage with shock
- Bloody diarrhea associated with cramping abdominal pain, urgency, or tenesmus suggests inflammatory bowel disease (especially ulcerative colitis), infectious colitis, or ischemic colitis

DIFFERENTIAL DIAGNOSIS

- Diverticulosis
- Vascular ectasias (angiodysplasias), eg, idiopathic arteriovenous malformation, CREST syndrome, hereditary hemorrhagic telangiectasias
- Colonic polyps
- Colorectal cancer
- Inflammatory bowel disease
- Hemorrhoids
- Anal fissure
- Ischemic colitis
- Infectious colitis
- Radiation colitis or proctitis
- NSAID-induced ulcers of small bowel or right colon

DIAGNOSIS

LABORATORY TESTS

- Complete blood cell count, platelet count, prothrombin time, partial thomboplastin time
- Serum creatinine, blood urea nitrogen
- Type and cross-match

IMAGING STUDIES

- Nuclear bleeding scans: technetium-labeled red blood cell scan
- Selective mesenteric angiography in patients with massive bleeding or positive technetium scans

DIAGNOSTIC PROCEDURES

- Nasogastic tube aspiration to exclude upper tract source
- Anoscopy
- Colonoscopy in patients in whom bleeding has ceased or in patients with moderate active bleeding immediately after rapid purge with 4–12 L polyethylene glycol solution to clear colon (rapid purge colonoscopy)
- Small intestine push enteroscopy or video capsule imaging in patients with unexplained recurrent hemorrhage of obscure origin, suspected from the small intestine
- Upper endoscopy with massive hematochezia to exclude upper gastrointestinal source

TREATMENT

MEDICATIONS

- Discontinue aspirin and other NSAIDs

SURGERY

- Surgery indicated in patients with ongoing bleeding that requires >4–6 units of blood transfusion within 24 h or >10 total units
- Limited resection of the bleeding segment of small intestine or colon, if possible
- Total abdominal colectomy with ileorectal anastomosis, otherwise

THERAPEUTIC PROCEDURES

- Therapeutic colonoscopy: high-risk lesions (eg, diverticulum with active bleeding or a visible vessel, or a vascular ectasia) can be treated endoscopically with saline or epinephrine injection, cautery (bipolar or heater probe), or application of metallic clips
- Angiography: selective mesenteric arterial infusion of vasoconstrictors (eg, vasopressin) and/or embolization of actively bleeding arteriole controls hemorrhage in >80%

OUTCOME

COMPLICATIONS

- Complications of angiography in 3–10% including atherosclerotic emboli, thrombosis, and localized bowel infarction
- Operative mortality for continuous or recurrent hemorrhage is 3–15% due to commorbid illness

PROGNOSIS

- 25% with diverticular hemorrhage have recurrent bleeding

WHEN TO ADMIT

- Patients with mild, intermittent bleeding suggesting anorectal source (blood on toilet paper, dripping in bowl) may be evaluated as outpatients
- All patients with significant hematochezia require admission

EVIDENCE

PRACTICE GUIDELINES

- Eisen GM et al: Standards of Practice Committee. An annotated algorithmic approach to acute lower gastrointestinal bleeding. Gastrointest Endosc 2001;53:859. [PMID: 11375618]

WEB SITES

- American College of Gastroenterology —Acute lower GI bleeding http://www.acg.gi.org/physicianforum/guides/acute_gibleed.html
- National Digestive Diseases Information Clearinghouse—Bleeding in the digestive tract http://digestive.niddk.nih.gov/ddiseases/pubs/bleeding/index.htm

INFORMATION FOR PATIENTS

- MEDLINEplus—Gastrointestinal bleeding http://www.nlm.nih.gov/medlineplus/ency/article/003133.htm

REFERENCES

- Bloomfeld RS et al: Endoscopic therapy of acute diverticular hemorrhage. Am J Gastroenterol 2001;96:2367. [PMID: 11515176]
- Enns R: Acute lower gastrointestinal bleeding: Part 1. Can J Gastroenterol 2001;15:509. [PMID: 11544535]
- Enns R: Acute lower gastrointestinal bleeding: Part 2. Can J Gastroenterol 2001;15:517. [PMID: 11544534]
- Gostout C: The role of endoscopy in managing lower gastrointestinal bleeding. N Engl J Med 2000;342:125. [PMID: 10631283]
- Jensen D et al: Urgent colonoscopy for the diagnosis and treatment of severe diverticular hemorrhage. N Engl J Med 2000;342:78. [PMID: 10631275]

Kenneth R. McQuaid, MD

Gastrointestinal Bleeding, Acute Upper

 KEY FEATURES

ESSENTIALS OF DIAGNOSIS

- Hematemesis (bright red blood or "coffee grounds")
- Melena in most cases; hematochezia in massive upper gastrointestinal bleeds
- Volume status to determine severity of blood loss; hematocrit is a poor early indicator of blood loss
- Endoscopy diagnostic and may be therapeutic

GENERAL CONSIDERATIONS

- Most common presentation is hematemesis or melena; hematochezia in 10% of cases
- Hematemesis is either bright red blood or brown "coffee grounds" material
- Melena develops after as little as 50–100 mL of blood loss
- Hematochezia requires a loss of >1000 mL
- Upper gastrointestinal bleeding is self-limited in 80% of cases, urgent medical therapy and endoscopic evaluation are required in the remainder
- Bleeding >48 h prior to presentation carries a low risk of recurrent bleeding
- Peptic ulcers account for ~50%
- Portal hypertension bleeding (10–20% of cases) occurs from varices (most commonly esophageal)
- Mallory-Weiss tears are lacerations of the gastroesophageal junction (5–10% of cases)
- Vascular anomalies, vascular ectasias (angiodysplasias) (7% of cases) occur in hereditary hemorrhagic telangiectasia, CREST syndrome, or sporadically, with increased incidence in chronic renal failure
- Gastric neoplasms (1% of cases)
- Erosive gastritis (<5% of cases) due to nonsteroidal antiinflammatory drugs (NSAIDs), alcohol, or severe medical or surgical illness (stress gastritis)

DEMOGRAPHICS

- 350,000 hospitalizations a year in the United States

 CLINICAL FINDINGS

SYMPTOMS AND SIGNS

- Signs of chronic liver disease implicate bleeding due to portal hypertension, but a different lesion is identified in 25–50% of patients with cirrhosis
- Dyspepsia, NSAID use, or history of previous peptic ulcer suggests peptic ulcer disease
- Heavy alcohol ingestion or retching suggests a Mallory-Weiss tear

DIFFERENTIAL DIAGNOSIS

- Hemoptysis
- Peptic ulcer disease
- Esophageal varices
- Gastric or duodenal varices (rare)
- Erosive gastritis, eg, NSAIDs, alcohol, stress
- Mallory-Weiss syndrome
- Portal hypertensive gastropathy
- Vascular ectasias (angiodysplasias), eg, idiopathic arteriovenous malformation, CREST syndrome, hereditary hemorrhagic telangiectasias
- Gastric cancer

Rare causes

- Erosive esophagitis
- Aortoenteric fistula
- Dieulafoy's lesion (aberrant gastric submucosal artery)
- Hemobilia (blood in biliary tree), eg, iatrogenic, malignancy
- Pancreatic cancer
- Hemosuccus pancreaticus (pancreatic pseudoaneurysm)

 DIAGNOSIS

LABORATORY TESTS

- Obtain complete blood cell count, platelet count, prothrombin time, partial thromboplastin time, serum creatinine, liver enzymes and serologies, and type and cross-matching for 2–4 units or more of packed red blood cells
- Hematocrit is not a reliable indicator of the severity of acute bleeding

DIAGNOSTIC PROCEDURES

- Assess hemodynamic status: systolic blood pressure; heart rate; postural hypotension
- Upper endoscopy after the patient is hemodynamically stable to identify the source of bleeding, to determine the risk of rebleeding, and to render endoscopic therapy such as cautery or injection of a sclerosant or application of a rubber band or epinephrine

TREATMENT

MEDICATIONS

- Intravenous proton pump inhibitor (omeprazole, 80-mg bolus, followed by 8 mg/h continuous infusion for 72 h) in patients admitted for active bleeding
- Oral proton pump inhibitor (omeprazole, 40 mg, or lansoprazole, 60 mg PO BID for 5 days) in patients with suspected peptic ulcer bleeding
- Octreotide, 100-μg bolus, followed by 50–100 μg/h) for bleeding related to portal hypertension

SURGERY

- Surgery is required in 5–10% with peptic ulcer disease hemorrhage that cannot be controlled with endoscopic therapy

THERAPEUTIC PROCEDURES

- Insert two 18-gauge or larger intravenous lines
- In patients without hemodynamic compromise or overt active bleeding, aggressive fluid repletion can be delayed until extent of bleeding clarified
- Patients with hemodynamic compromise should be given 0.9% saline or lactated Ringer's injection and cross-matched blood
- Nasogastric tube placed for aspiration
- Blood replacement to maintain a hematocrit of 25–30%
- In the absence of continued bleeding, the hematocrit should rise 3% for each unit of transfused packed red cells
- Transfuse blood in patients with brisk active bleeding regardless of the hematocrit
- Transfuse platelets if platelet count <50,000/μL or if impaired platelet function due to aspirin use
- Uremic patients with active bleeding should be given 1–2 doses of desmopressin (DDAVP), 0.3 μg/kg IV at 12- to 24-h intervals
- Fresh frozen plasma should be given for actively bleeding patients with a coagulopathy and an INR >1.5
- In massive bleeding, 1 unit of fresh frozen plasma should be given for each 5 units of packed red blood cells transfused
- Intraarterial embolization or vasopressin indicated (rarely) in patients with persistent bleeding from ulcers, angiomas, or Mallory-Weiss tears who have failed endoscopic therapy and are poor operative risks
- Transvenous intrahepatic portosystemic shunts (TIPS) provide effective decompression of the portal venous system and control of acute variceal bleeding and are indicated in patients in whom endoscopic modalities have failed

OUTCOME

PROGNOSIS

- Mortality rate is 10%, even higher in patients age >60
- Peptic ulcers have an overall acute mortality rate of 6–10%
- Portal hypertension has a hospital mortality rate of 15–40%; if untreated, half will rebleed during hospitalization; mortality rate of 60–80% at 1–4 years

WHEN TO REFER

- Refer to gastroenterologist for endoscopy (see below)
- Refer to surgeon for uncontrollable, life-threatening hemorrhage

WHEN TO ADMIT

- Very low risk—reliable patients without serious comorbid medical illnesses or advanced liver disease who have normal hemodynamics, no evidence of overt bleeding (hematemesis or melena) within 48 h, a negative nasogastric lavage, and normal laboratory tests do not require hospital admission and further evaluation as outpatients
- Low to moderate risk—patients are admitted after appropriate stabilization for upper endoscopy and further treatment; based on the findings may be discharged and followed as outpatients
- High risk—patients with active bleeding manifested by hematemesis or bright red blood on nasogastric aspirate, an estimated loss of >5 units of blood, persistent hemodynamic derangement despite fluid resuscitation, serious comorbid medical illness, or evidence of advanced liver disease require ICU admission

EVIDENCE

PRACTICE GUIDELINES

- Funaki B: Endovascular intervention for the treatment of acute arterial gastrointestinal hemorrhage. Gastroenterol Clin North Am 2002;31:701. [PMID: 12481726]
- Guidelines for good practice in and audit of the management of upper gastrointestinal haemorrhage. J R Coll Physicians Lond 1992;26:281. [PMID: 1404024]

WEB SITES

- American College of Gastroenterology—Effect of NSAIDS on the upper gastrointestinal tract http://www.acg.gi.org/physicianforum/gifocus/gif_nsaids.html
- American College of Gastroenterology—Understanding GI bleeding http://www.acg.gi.org/patientinfo/gibleeding/

INFORMATION FOR PATIENTS

- MD consult hematemesis http://home.mdconsult.com/das/patient/view/30939797/10002/12315.html/top?sid=203840552
- MEDLINEplus—Gastrointestinal bleeding http://www.nlm.nih.gov/medlineplus/ency/article/003133.htm

REFERENCES

- Lau JYW et al: Effect of intravenous omeprazole on recurrent bleeding after endoscopic treatment of bleeding peptic ulcers. N Engl J Med 2000;343:310. [PMID: 10922420]
- Longstreth GM et al: Successful outpatient management of acute upper gastrointestinal hemorrhage: use of practice guidelines in a large patient series. Gastrointest Endosc 1998;47:219. [PMID: 9540873]
- Van Dam J et al: Endoscopy of the upper gastrointestinal tract. N Engl J Med 1999;341:1738. [PMID: 10580074]

Kenneth R. McQuaid, MD

Giardiasis

KEY FEATURES

ESSENTIALS OF DIAGNOSIS

- Most infections are asymptomatic
- If symptomatic, there is acute or chronic diarrhea, mild to severe, with bulky, greasy, frothy, malodorous stools, free of blood and pus
- Upper abdominal discomfort, distension, excessive flatus, and lassitude
- Cysts and occasionally trophozoites in stools
- Trophozoites in duodenal fluid
- Positive immunoassays

GENERAL CONSIDERATIONS

- Protozoal infection of the upper small intestine is caused by the flagellate *Giardia lamblia* (also called *G intestinalis* and *G duodenalis*)
- The organism occurs in feces as a symmetric, heart-shaped flagellated trophozoite measuring $10–25 \times 6–12$ µm and as a cyst measuring $11–14 \times 7–10$ µm
- Only the cyst form is infectious by the oral route; trophozoites are destroyed by gastric acidity
- Humans are a reservoir for the infection; dogs, cats, beavers, and other mammals are implicated but not confirmed reservoirs or zoonotic sources of infection
- Under suitable moist, cool conditions, cysts can survive in the environment for weeks to months
- Hypogammaglobulinemia, low secretory IgA levels in the gut, achlorhydria, and malnutrition favor the development of infection
- Recent reports suggest that *Giardia* infections in AIDS may be more frequent and severe than previously thought
- Gastric giardiasis may represent reflux from the duodenum or localized infection

DEMOGRAPHICS

- The parasite occurs worldwide, especially in areas with poor sanitation
- Cysts are transmitted from fecal contamination of water or food, by person-to-person contact, or by anal-oral sexual contact. Multiple cases are common in households, children's day care centers (often the nidus for spread of organisms to the community), and mental institutions. Outbreaks occur from contamination of water supplies
- In the United States and Europe, the infection is the most common intestinal protozoal pathogen; in the United States the estimate is 100,000 to 2.5 million new infections yearly and 5000 hospital admissions

CLINICAL FINDINGS

SYMPTOMS AND SIGNS

- Many persons remain asymptomatic cyst carriers, and their infection clears spontaneously
- Syndromes include acute or chronic diarrhea and malabsorption
- The incubation period is usually 1–3 weeks but may be longer
- The illness may begin gradually or suddenly
- The acute phase may last days or weeks, but it is usually self-limited, although cyst excretion may be prolonged
- In a few patients, the disorder may become chronic and last for years
- In both the acute and chronic forms, diarrhea ranges from mild to severe; most often it is mild
- There may be no complaints other than of one bulky, loose bowel movement a day, often after breakfast
- With larger numbers of movements, the stools become increasingly watery but are usually free of blood and pus; they are frothy, malodorous, and greasy
- The diarrhea may be daily or recurrent; if recurrent, stools may be normal to mushy during intervening days, or the patient may be constipated
- Other symptoms include anorexia, nausea, vomiting, midepigastric discomfort, cramps (often after meals), belching, flatulence, borborygmi, and abdominal discomfort
- Weight loss and weakness are frequent
- Malabsorption occasionally develops in the acute or chronic stage

DIFFERENTIAL DIAGNOSIS

- Viral or bacterial gastroenteritis
- Amebiasis
- Lactase deficiency
- Irritable bowel syndrome
- Malabsorption due to other causes, eg, celiac sprue
- Laxative abuse
- Crohn's disease
- Cryptosporidiosis

DIAGNOSIS

LABORATORY TESTS

- Using stool specimens, diagnosis is by standard ova and parasite examination or by immunoassay by two methods; one for antigen (the enzyme immunoassay, sensitivity 94–100%, specificity 100%), and the other by detecting the organism using monoclonal antibody reagent (the direct fluorescent antibody assay for cysts, sensitivity and specificity of about 100%)
- Immunoassays are the preferred diagnostic method if only *Giardia* is being sought; otherwise, three stool specimens should be examined for ova and parasites. Some immunoassays require fresh or frozen stool and cannot be used with preserved specimens; additionally, some assays detect only cysts or only trophozoites
- Three stool specimens collected at intervals of 2 days or longer should be examined following concentration methods. One specimen will detect 50–75% of cases and three specimens about 90%. Unless the specimens can be submitted within an hour, they should be preserved immediately in a fixative. Purges do not increase the likelihood of finding the organism. Use of barium, antibiotics, antacids, kaolin products, or oily laxatives may temporarily (about 10 days) reduce the number of parasites
- Sometimes warranted is the search for organisms in the duodenum by the duodenal string test (Entero-Test), duodenal aspiration, endoscopic brush cytology, or duodenal biopsy (a mucosal imprint for staining should be made before sectioning)
- Tests for serum antibody are not recommended because of lack of sensitivity and specificity
- There is no eosinophilia, and the white blood cell count is normal

IMAGING STUDIES

- Radiological examination of the small bowel is usually normal

Giardiasis

TREATMENT

MEDICATIONS

- Treatment is effective with tinidazole, metronidazole, quinacrine, or furazolidone. As none of the agents cures more than 90% of infections (80% for furazolidone), retreatment with an alternative drug may be needed

- Single-dose tinidazole (not available in the United States) is the drug of choice

- All of these drugs occasionally have unpleasant side effects. The potential for carcinogenicity of furazolidone, metronidazole, and tinidazole appears negligible. Because of its rare severe toxicity, quinacrine should be used only when no other drug is available

- Tinidazole: dose of 2 g given once has cure rates of 90–100%. Adverse reactions consist of mild gastrointestinal side effects in about 10% of patients; headache and vertigo are less common

- Metronidazole dose is 250 mg three times daily for 5–7 days. It may cause gastrointestinal symptoms, headache, dizziness, a metallic taste, and candidal overgrowth, in addition to a disulfiram-like reaction in alcohol users

- Furazolidone dose is 100 mg (in suspension) four times daily for 7–10 days. Gastrointestinal symptoms, fever, headache, rash, and a disulfiram-like reaction with alcohol occur. Furazolidone can cause mild hemolysis in glucose-6-phosphate dehydrogenase-deficient persons

- Quinacrine (Mepacrine) dose is 100 mg three times daily after meals for 5–7 days. The drug has a bitter taste. Gastrointestinal symptoms, headache, and dizziness are common; harmless yellowing of the skin is infrequent. Toxic psychosis and exfoliative dermatitis are rare but may be severe. Quinacrine is contraindicated in psoriasis or in persons with a history of psychosis. Although quinacrine is not generally available in the United States, it can be obtained from a pharmacy at 800-247-9767

- Albendazole (400 mg daily for 5 days) has shown cure rates that range from 10% to 95%

- Reports with paromomycin (25–35 mg/kg/day in three divided doses for 7 days) have been mixed; because the drug is not absorbed, it has been proposed for use in pregnancy

THERAPEUTIC PROCEDURES

- Treatment of asymptomatic patients should be considered since they can transmit the infection and may occasionally become symptomatic themselves

- In selected cases, it may be best to wait a few weeks before starting treatment, as some infections will clear spontaneously. In the presence of a presumptive diagnosis but negative stool specimens, an empirical course of treatment is sometimes indicated

OUTCOME

FOLLOW-UP

- Two or more stools are analyzed weekly starting 2 weeks after therapy

- With cure, the immunoassay normally reverts to negative

COMPLICATIONS

- Extraintestinal manifestations (arthritis, anterior uveitis, urticaria) are unproven complications of giardiasis

PROGNOSIS

- With successful eradication of the infection, there are no sequelae

- Without treatment, severe malabsorption may rarely contribute to death from other causes

WHEN TO REFER

- Progressive diarrhea despite therapy

- To search for the organism in the duodenum

PREVENTION

- There is no effective chemoprophylaxis

- Since community water chlorination (0.4 mg/L) is relatively ineffective for inactivating cysts, filtration is required

- For hikers, bringing water to a boil for 1 min is adequate; halogenation with iodine or filtration with a pore size less than 1 μm can also be used. Relying on iodine halogenation is no longer recommended by the Centers for Disease Control and Prevention

- In day care centers, appropriate disposal of diapers and frequent hand washing are essential

EVIDENCE

PRACTICE GUIDELINES

- National Guideline Clearinghouse http://www.guideline.gov/summary/summary.aspx?doc_id=3065&nbr=2291&string=giardiasis http://www.guideline.gov/summary/summary.aspx?doc_id=2791&nbr=2017&string=giardiasis

INFORMATION FOR PATIENTS

- Centers for Disease Control http://www.cdc.gov/travel/diseases/giardiasis.htm

- American Academy of Family Physicians http://familydoctor.org/handouts/078.html

REFERENCES

- Aziz H et al: A comparison study of different methods used in the detection of *Giardia lamblia*. Clin Lab Sci 2001;14:150. [PMID: 11517624]

- Gardner TB et al: Treatment of giardiasis. Clin Microbiol Rev 2001;14:114. [PMID: 11148005]

Glomerulonephritis

 KEY FEATURES

ESSENTIALS OF DIAGNOSIS

- Acute renal insufficiency
- Edema
- Hypertension
- Hematuria (with or without dysmorphic red cells, red blood cell casts), and mild proteinuria

GENERAL CONSIDERATIONS

- A relatively uncommon cause of acute renal failure, ~5% of cases of intrinsic renal failure
- Acute glomerulonephritis usually signifies an inflammatory process causing renal dysfunction over days to weeks that may or may not resolve (Table 89, page 1272)
- Inflammatory glomerular lesions include mesangioproliferative, focal and diffuse proliferative, and crescentic lesions
- Rapidly progressive acute glomerulonephritis can cause permanent damage to glomeruli if not identified and treated rapidly

Causes of glomerulonephritis

- Immune complex
  - IgA nephropathy
  - Endocarditis
  - Systemic lupus erythematosus
  - Cryoglobulinemia (often associated with hepatitis C)
  - Postinfectious
  - Membranoproliferative
- Pauci-immune (ANCA⁺)
  - Wegener's granulomatosis
  - Churg-Strauss syndrome
  - Microscopic polyarteritis
- Anti-glomerular basement membrane (GBM)
  - Goodpasture's disease
  - Anti-GBM glomerulonephritis
- Other
  - Malignant hypertension
  - Hemolytic-uremic syndrome, thrombotic thrombocytopenic purpura

 CLINICAL FINDINGS

SYMPTOMS AND SIGNS

- Hypertension
- Edema first in body parts with low tissue tension such as periorbital and scrotal regions
- Dark urine

DIFFERENTIAL DIAGNOSIS

- Acute interstitial nephritis (AIN)
- Acute tubular necrosis (ATN)

DIAGNOSIS

LABORATORY TESTS

- Urinalysis dipstick: hematuria, moderate proteinuria (usually <2 g/day); microscopic: abnormal urinary sediment with cellular elements such as red cells, red cell casts, and white cells
- 24-h urine for protein excretion and creatinine clearance
- Urine creatinine clearance is an unreliable marker of glomerular filtration rate in cases of rapidly changing serum creatinine values
- Fractional excretion of sodium is usually low (<1%), unless renal dysfunction is marked
- Complement levels (C3, C4, CH50), ASO titer, anti-GBM antibody levels, ANA titers, cryoglobulins, hepatitis B surface antigen and hepatitis C virus antibody, C3 nephritic factor
- Cytoplasmic ANCA (c-ANCA) is both specific (88%) and sensitive (95%) for Wegener's
- Microscopic polyangiitis is another pauci-immune vasculitis; perinuclear ANCA (p-ANCA) is found in microscopic polyangiitis

IMAGING STUDIES

- Renal ultrasound

DIAGNOSTIC PROCEDURES

- Renal biopsy: type of glomerulonephritis can be categorized according to the immunofluorescence pattern and electron microscopy appearance
- Chest x-ray

Glomerulonephritis

TREATMENT

MEDICATIONS

- Corticosteroids in high-dose and cytotoxic agents such as cyclophosphamide, depending on the nature and severity of disease
- Antihypertensive agents
- Diuretics and salt and water restriction for fluid overload
- Angiotensin-converting enzyme inhibitors and angiotensin II receptor blockers

THERAPEUTIC PROCEDURES

- Specific therapies aimed at the underlying cause
- Plasma exchange in Goodpasture's disease, anti-GBM glomerulonephritis, and possibly dialysis

OUTCOME

FOLLOW-UP

- With nephrologist as dictated by specific disease

COMPLICATIONS

- Chronic kidney disease

WHEN TO REFER

- Any evidence of possible glomerulonephritis

WHEN TO ADMIT

- Any acute or rapidly progressive symptoms (days to weeks) may be cause for admission depending on the disease

EVIDENCE

PRACTICE GUIDELINES

- Kincaid-Smith P: Pharmacological management of membranous nephropathy. Curr Opin Nephrol Hypertens 2002;11:149. [PMID: 11856906]
- National Kidney Foundation (NKF) Kidney Disease Outcome Quality Initiative (K/DOQI) Advisory Board. K/DOQI clinical practice guidelines for chronic kidney disease: evaluation, classification, and stratification. Kidney Disease Outcome Quality Initiative. Am J Kidney Dis 2002;39(2 Suppl 2):S1. [PMID: 11904577]

WEB SITE

- National Kidney and Urologic Diseases Information Clearinghouse http://kidney.niddk.nih.gov/kudiseases/pubs/glomerular/index.htm#3

INFORMATION FOR PATIENTS

- American Academy of Family Physicians—Glomerulonephritis http://familydoctor.org/handouts/467.html
- Mayo Clinic—Glomerulonephritis http://www.mayoclinic.com/invoke.cfm?objectid=CAB55536-7CCC-44A4-832C420405FCCA39

REFERENCES

- Hricik DE et al: Glomerulonephritis. N Engl J Med 1998;339:888. [PMID: 9744974]
- Perazella MA: COX-2 inhibitors and the kidney. Hosp Pract (Off Ed) 2001;36:43. [PMID:11263799]

Suzanne Watnick, MD
Gail Morrison, MD

Goiter, Endemic

 KEY FEATURES

ESSENTIALS OF DIAGNOSIS

- Common in regions of the world with low-iodine diets
- High rate of congenital hypothyroidism and cretinism
- Goiters may become multinodular and grow to great size
- Most adults with endemic goiter are euthyroid; however, some are hypothyroid or hyperthyroid
- Impaired cognition and hearing may be subtle or severe in congenital hypothyroidism

GENERAL CONSIDERATIONS

- Up to 0.5% of iodine-deficient populations have full-blown cretinism; less severe manifestations of congenital hypothyroidism more common
- Causes: iodine deficiency (most common); certain foods (eg, sorghum, millet, maize, cassava, turnip), mineral deficiencies (selenium, iron) and water pollutants; congenital partial defects in thyroid enzyme activity
- Increase in size of thyroid nodules and emergence of new nodules in pregnancy

DEMOGRAPHICS

- ~5% of world's population have goiters
- Of these, 75% occur in areas of iodine deficiency. Such areas found in 115 countries, mostly developing nations but also in Europe, eg, in Pescopagano, Italy, 60% of adults have goiters, with hyperthyroidism in 2.9%; overt hypothyroidism in 0.2% and subclinical hypothyroidism in 3.8%, thyroid cancer in <0.1%

 CLINICAL FINDINGS

SYMPTOMS AND SIGNS

- Thyroid may become multinodular and very large
- Growth often occurs during pregnancy and may cause compressive symptoms
- Substernal goiters usually asymptomatic but can cause tracheal compression, respiratory distress, dysphagia, superior vena cava syndrome, gastrointestinal bleeding from esophageal varices, phrenic or recurrent laryngeal nerve palsy, or Horner's syndrome, or pleural or pericardial effusions (rare)
- Cerebral ischemia and stroke can result from arterial compression or thyrocervical steal syndrome
- Malignancy in <1%
- Some patients with goiter become hypothyroid; others become thyrotoxic as goiter grows and becomes more autonomous, especially if iodine added to diet
- Congenital hypothyroidism: isolated deafness, short stature, or impaired mentation

DIFFERENTIAL DIAGNOSIS

- Benign multinodular goiter
- Pregnancy (in areas of iodine deficiency)
- Graves' disease
- Hashimoto's thyroiditis
- Subacute (de Quervain's) thyroiditis
- Drugs causing hypothyroidism: lithium, amiodarone, propylthiouracil, methimazole, phenylbutazone, sulfonamides, interferon-α, iodide
- Infiltrating disease, eg, malignancy, sarcoidosis
- Suppurative thyroiditis
- Riedel's thyroiditis

 DIAGNOSIS

LABORATORY TESTS

- Serum thyroxine and thyroid-stimulating hormone (TSH) usually normal
- TSH low if multinodular goiter becomes autonomous in presence of sufficient iodine for thyroid hormone synthesis, causing hyperthyroidism
- TSH high in hypothyroidism
- Thyroid radioactive iodine uptake usually elevated, but may be normal if iodine intake has improved
- Serum levels of antithyroid antibodies usually undetectable or low
- Serum thyroglobulin often elevated

Goiter, Endemic

 TREATMENT

MEDICATIONS

- Dietary iodine supplementation (eg, addition of potassium iodide to table salt) greatly reduces prevalence of endemic goiter and cretinism but is less effective in shrinking established goiter
- Dietary iodine supplementation increases risk of autoimmune thyroid dysfunction, which may result in hypothyroidism or hyperthyroidism
- Excessive iodine intake may increase risk of goiter
- Thyroxine supplementation can shrink goiters and reduce risk of further goiter growth, but may induce hyperthyroidism in individuals with autonomous multinodular goiters; thyroxine suppression should not be started in patients with suppressed TSH levels

SURGERY

- Thyroidectomy indicated for cosmesis, compressive symptoms, or thyrotoxicosis in adults with very large multinodular goiters

PROCEDURES

- Patients may be treated with ^{131}I for large compressive goiters

 OUTCOME

FOLLOW-UP

- Partial thyroidectomy is followed by a high goiter recurrence rate in iodine-deficient geographic areas, so total thyroidectomy is preferred when surgery is indicated

COMPLICATIONS

- Initiating iodine supplementation in a geographic area causes increased frequency of hyperthyroidism in first year, followed by greatly reduced rates of toxic nodular goiter and Graves' disease thereafter
- Patients treated with ^{131}I may rarely develop Graves' disease 3–10 months after treatment
- Goiters may become multinodular and grow to great size

WHEN TO REFER

- Refer to endocrinologist for hyperthyroidism, enlarging goiter, suspicious nodules
- Refer to thyroid surgeon for thyroidectomy for cosmesis, compressive symptoms, or thyrotoxicosis in adults with very large multinodular goiters

WHEN TO ADMIT

- Thyroidectomy
- [131]I treatment

PREVENTION

- Dietary iodine supplementation started in Switzerland in 1922 with addition of potassium iodide to table salt
- Current level of supplementation in the United States is 20 mg potassium iodide per kg salt
- Iodized salt has greatly reduced incidence of endemic goiter. Unfortunately, many iodine-deficient countries have inadequate programs for iodine supplementation
- Minimum dietary requirement for iodine is about 50 µg daily; optimal iodine intake is 150–300 µg daily. Iodine sufficiency is demonstrated by urinary iodide excretion >10 µg/dL

 EVIDENCE

PRACTICE GUIDELINES

- American Association of Clinical Endocrinologists medical guidelines for clinical practice for the evaluation and treatment of hyperthyroidism and hypothyroidism. American Association of Clinical Endocrinologists, American College of Endocrinology—Medical Specialty Society, 2002 http://www.aace.com/clin/guidelines/hypo_hyper.pdf

WEB SITE

- American Association of Clinical Endocrinologists http://www.aace.com/clin/fcc/fcc-200009.php

INFORMATION FOR PATIENTS

- Merck Manual http://www.merck.com/pubs/mmanual/section1/chapter4/4c.htm
- Program Against Micronutrient Malnutrition—Emory University http://www.sph.emory.edu/PAMM/iodine.htm

REFERENCES

- Aghini-Lombardi F et al: The spectrum of thyroid disorders in an iodine-deficient community: The Pescopagano survey. J Clin Endocrinol Metab 1999;84:561. [PMID: 10022416]
- Kahaly GJ et al: Iodide induces thyroid autoimmunity in patients with endemic goitre: a randomised, double-blind, placebo-controlled trial. Eur J Endocrinol 1998;139:290. [PMID: 9758438]
- Zhao J et al: Endemic goiter associated with high iodine intake. Am J Public Health 2000;90:1633. [PMID: 11030003]

Paul A. Fitzgerald, MD

Gonococcal Infections

 KEY FEATURES

ESSENTIALS OF DIAGNOSIS

- Purulent and profuse urethral discharge, especially in men, with dysuria, yielding positive smear
- Epididymitis, prostatitis, periurethral inflammation, proctitis in men
- Cervicitis in women with purulent discharge, or asymptomatic; vaginitis, salpingitis, proctitis also occur
- Fever, rash, tenosynovitis, and arthritis with disseminated disease
- Gram-negative intracellular diplococci seen in a smear or cultured from any site, particularly the urethra, cervix, pharynx, and rectum

GENERAL CONSIDERATIONS

- Gonorrhea is caused by *Neisseria gonorrhoeae*, a gram-negative diplococcus

DEMOGRAPHICS

- Gonorrhea is most commonly transmitted during sexual activity and has its greatest incidence in the 15- to 29-year-old age group

 CLINICAL FINDINGS

SYMPTOMS AND SIGNS

Urethritis and cervicitis

- In men, there is initially burning on urination and a serous or milky discharge
- One to 3 days later, the urethral pain is more pronounced and the discharge becomes yellow, creamy, and profuse, sometimes blood tinged
- The disorder may regress and become chronic or progress to involve the prostate, epididymis, and periurethral glands with acute, painful inflammation
- Rectal infection is common in homosexual men
- Atypical sites of primary infection (eg, the pharynx) must always be considered
- Asymptomatic infection is common and occurs in both sexes
- Gonococcal infection in women often becomes symptomatic during menses. Women may have dysuria, urinary frequency, and urgency, with a purulent urethral discharge
- Vaginitis and cervicitis with inflammation of Bartholin's glands are common. Infection may be asymptomatic, with only slightly increased vaginal discharge and moderate cervicitis on examination
- Infection may remain as a chronic cervicitis. It may progress to involve the uterus and tubes with acute and chronic salpingitis and with ultimate scarring of tubes and sterility
- In pelvic inflammatory disease, anaerobes and chlamydiae often accompany gonococci

Conjunctivitis

- The most common form of eye involvement is direct inoculation of gonococci into the conjunctival sac. In adults, this occurs by autoinoculation of a person with genital infection. The purulent conjunctivitis may rapidly progress to panophthalmitis and loss of the eye unless treated promptly

DIFFERENTIAL DIAGNOSIS

- Nongonococcal urethritis, eg, *Chlamydia, Ureaplasma urealyticum*
- Septic arthritis of other bacterial cause
- Reactive arthritis (Reiter's syndrome)
- Vaginal discharge due to candidiasis, bacterial vaginosis, or trichomoniasis
- Chronic meningococcemia

 DIAGNOSIS

LABORATORY TESTS

- Gram stain of urethral discharge in men, especially during the first week after onset, typically shows gram-negative diplococci in polymorphonuclear leukocytes. Gram stain is less often positive in women
- Culture is the diagnostic gold standard, particularly when the Gram stain is negative
- A ligase chain reaction (LCR) assay that detects both *N gonorrhoeae* and *Chlamydia trachomatis* in cervical and urethral swab specimens and urine permits more rapid diagnosis of gonococcal infection. LCR also has improved sensitivity and high specificity compared with culture of swab specimens

TREATMENT

MEDICATIONS

- For urethritis or cervicitis, either ceftriaxone, 125 mg intramuscularly, or cefixime, 400 mg orally as a single dose, is the treatment of choice (availability may be a problem; cefpodoxime, 200 mg as a single dose, can be substituted, but is slightly less efficacious)
- A single oral dose of ciprofloxacin 500 mg, ofloxacin 400 mg, or levofloxacin 250 mg is also effective
- Since coexistent chlamydial infection is common, treat as well with doxycycline, 100 mg twice daily orally for 7 days, or a single 1-g oral dose of azithromycin
- Salpingitis, prostatitis, bacteremia, arthritis, and other complications due to susceptible strains in adults should be treated with penicillin G, 10 million units intravenously daily, for 5 days. Ceftriaxone, 1 g intravenously daily for 5 days, or an oral fluoroquinolone (ciprofloxacin, 500 mg twice daily, or levofloxacin, 500 mg once daily) for 5 days also are effective

THERAPEUTIC PROCEDURES

- Therapy typically is administered before antimicrobial susceptibilities are known
- All sexual partners should be treated

 ## OUTCOME

COMPLICATIONS

Disseminated disease

- Systemic complications follow the dissemination of gonococci from the primary site via the bloodstream
- Gonococcal bacteremia is associated with intermittent fever, arthralgia, and skin lesions ranging from maculopapular to pustular, which tend to be few in number and peripherally located

WHEN TO REFER

- Report to the public health department for tracing contacts
- All suspected or proven ocular gonorrhea

WHEN TO ADMIT

- Most cases of pelvic inflammatory disease (perhaps not the mild cases)
- All cases of suspected or proven disseminated disease

PREVENTION

- The condom, if properly used, can reduce the risk of infection
- Effective drugs taken in therapeutic doses within 24 h of exposure can abort an infection

 ## EVIDENCE

PRACTICE GUIDELINES

- Centers for Disease Control and Prevention. Sexually transmitted disease treatment guidelines 2002. MMWR 2002;51:No. RR-6.
- National Guideline Clearinghouse http://www.guideline.gov/summary/summary.aspx?doc_id=3031&nbr=2257&string=gonococcal+infections

WEB SITES

- CDC—Division of Bacterial and Mycotic Diseases http://www.cdc.gov/ncidod/dbmd/
- Karolinska Institute—Directory of Bacterial Infections and Mycoses http://www.mic.ki.se/Diseases/c1.html

INFORMATION FOR PATIENTS

- JAMA patient page: Sexually transmitted diseases. JAMA 1998;280:944.
- National Institute of Allery and Infectious Diseases http://www.niaid.nih.gov/factsheets/stdgon.htm

REFERENCE

- Woodward C et al: Drug treatment of common STDs: Part I. Herpes, syphilis, urethritis, chlamydia and gonorrhea. Am Fam Physician 1999;60:1387. [PMID: 10537386]

Henry F. Chambers, MD

Goodpasture's Syndrome, Pulmonary

 KEY FEATURES

ESSENTIALS OF DIAGNOSIS

- Triad of pulmonary hemorrhage, circulating anti-glomerulobasement membrane (GBM) antibody, and glomerulonephritis due to anti-GBM
- Up to one-third of patients with anti-GBM glomerulonephritis have no evidence of lung injury
- Circulating anti-GBM antibody is characteristic

GENERAL CONSIDERATIONS

- Clinical constellation of glomerulonephritis and pulmonary hemorrhage
- Idiopathic recurrent alveolar hemorrhage with rapidly progressive glomerulonephritis
- Injury mediated by anti-glomerular basement membrane (anti-GBM) antibodies
- ~5% of patients with rapidly progressive acute glomerulonephritis have anti-GBM
- Associated with influenza A infection, hydrocarbon solvent exposure, and HLA-DR2 and -B7 antigens

DEMOGRAPHICS

- Incidence in males ~6 times that in females
- Occurs most commonly in the second and third decades

 CLINICAL FINDINGS

SYMPTOMS AND SIGNS

- Usually presents with hemoptysis, though pulmonary hemorrhage may be occult
- Dyspnea, cough, hypoxemia, and bilateral pulmonary infiltrates are typical
- Iron deficiency anemia and microscopic hematuria are usually present
- Upper respiratory tract infection precedes onset in 20–60% of cases
- Possible respiratory failure
- Hypertension
- Edema

DIFFERENTIAL DIAGNOSIS

- Severe congestive heart failure (pulmonary edema and prerenal azotemia)
- Renal failure (with hypervolemia and pulmonary edema)
- Microscopic polyangiitis (polyarteritis nodosa)
- Systemic lupus erythematosus
- Henoch-Schönlein purpura
- Wegener's granulomatosis
- Legionnaire's disease
- Renal vein thrombosis with pulmonary embolism

 DIAGNOSIS

LABORATORY TESTS

- Circulating anti-GBM antibodies in serum positive in >90%
- Iron deficiency anemia
- Complement levels are normal
- Sputum contains hemosiderin-laden macrophages
- Diffusion capacity of carbon monoxide is markedly increased

IMAGING STUDIES

- Chest x-rays show shifting pulmonary infiltrates

DIAGNOSTIC PROCEDURES

- Biopsy demonstrates IgG deposits in glomeruli or alveoli

Goodpasture's Syndrome, Pulmonary

 ## TREATMENT

MEDICATIONS

- Treatment is a combination of plasma exchange therapy to remove circulating antibodies and administration of immunosuppressive drugs (steroids and cyclophosphamide) to prevent formation of new antibodies
- Give methylprednisolone, 30 mg/kg IV QD followed by oral prednisone at 1 mg/kg/day AND cyclophosphamide, 2 mg/kg/day PO

THERAPEUTIC PROCEDURES

- Plasmapheresis, performed daily for up to 2 weeks, is given in combination with the steroids and cyclophosphamide

 ## OUTCOME

FOLLOW-UP

- Anti-GBM antibody levels should decrease as the clinical course improves

COMPLICATIONS

- Renal failure
- Respiratory failure

PROGNOSIS

- Prognosis poor in patients with oliguria and a serum creatinine >6–7 mg/dL

WHEN TO REFER

- Patients should be referred to a pulmonologist, rheumatologist, or nephrologist

WHEN TO ADMIT

- Respiratory insufficiency
- Progressive or severe renal disease

 ## EVIDENCE

PRACTICE GUIDELINES

- National Guideline Clearinghouse http://www.guideline.gov/summary/summary.aspx?doc_id=2971&nbr=2197&string=vasculitis

WEB SITES

- http://www.rheumatology.org/publicati ons/primarycare/number6/hrh0034698.html

REFERENCES

- Hudson B et al: Alport's syndrome, Goodpasture's syndrome, and type IV collagen. N Engl J Med 2003;348:2543. [PMID: 12815141]
- Salama A et al: Goodpasture's disease in the absence of circulating anti-glomerular basement membrane antibodies as detected by standard techniques. Am J Kidney Dis 2002;39:1162. [PMID: 12046026]
- Shah M et al: Characteristics and outcomes of patients with Goodpasture's syndrome. South Med J 2002;95:1411. [PMID: 12597309]

Suzanne Watnick, MD
Gail Morrison, MD
Mark S. Chestnutt, MD
Thomas J. Prendergast, MD

Gouty Arthritis

 ## KEY FEATURES

ESSENTIALS OF DIAGNOSIS

- Acute onset, typically nocturnal and usually monarticular, often involving the first metatarsophalangeal joint
- Hyperuricemia in most; identification of urate crystals in joint fluid or tophi is diagnostic
- Dramatic therapeutic response to nonsteroidal antiinflammatory drugs or colchicine

GENERAL CONSIDERATIONS

- A metabolic disease of heterogeneous nature, often familial, associated with abnormal amounts of urates in the body and characterized early by a recurring acute arthritis, usually monarticular, and later by chronic deforming arthritis
- Secondary gout is related to acquired causes of hyperuricemia, eg, medication use (diuretics, cyclosporine, low-dose aspirin, and niacin), myeloproliferative disorders, multiple myeloma, hemoglobinopathies, chronic renal disease, hypothyroidism, psoriasis, sarcoidosis, and lead poisoning
- Alcohol ingestion promotes hyperuricemia by increasing urate production and decreasing the renal excretion of uric acid
- Hospitalized patients frequently suffer attacks of gout because of changes in diet (eg, inability to take oral feedings following abdominal surgery) or medications that lead either to rapid reductions or increases in the serum urate level

DEMOGRAPHICS

- Especially common in Pacific islanders, eg, Filipinos and Samoans
- Rarely caused by a specifically determined genetic aberration (eg, Lesch-Nyhan syndrome)
- 90% of patients with primary gout are men, usually over 30 years of age
- In women the onset is typically postmenopausal

 ## CLINICAL FINDINGS

SYMPTOMS AND SIGNS

- Sudden onset of arthritis, frequently nocturnal, either without apparent precipitating cause or following rapid fluctuations in serum urate levels
- The metatarsophalangeal joint (MTP) of the great toe is the most susceptible joint ("podagra"), although others, especially those of the feet, ankles, and knees, are commonly affected
- May develop in periarticular soft tissues such as the arch of the foot
- As the attack progresses, the pain becomes intense. The involved joints are swollen and exquisitely tender and the overlying skin tense, warm, and dusky red. Fever is common
- Tophi may be found in the external ears, hands, feet, olecranon, and prepatellar bursas. They are usually seen only after several attacks of acute arthritis
- Asymptomatic periods of months or years commonly follow the initial attack
- After years of recurrent severe monarthritis attacks, gout can evolve into a chronic, deforming polyarthritis of upper and lower extremities that mimics rheumatoid arthritis

DIFFERENTIAL DIAGNOSIS

Arthritis

- Cellulitis
- Septic arthritis
- Pseudogout
- Rheumatoid arthritis
- Reactive arthritis
- Osteoarthritis
- Chronic lead poisoning (saturnine gout)
- Palindromic rheumatism

Podagra

- Trauma
- Cellulitis
- Sarcoidosis
- Pseudogout
- Psoriatic arthritis
- Bursitis of first MTP joint (inflamed bunion)

Tophi

- Rheumatoid nodules
- Erythema nodosum
- Gout
- Coccidioidomycosis

- Endocarditis (Osler nodes)
- Sarcoidosis
- Polyarteritis nodosa

 ## DIAGNOSIS

LABORATORY TESTS

- The serum uric acid is elevated (>7.5 mg/dL) in 95% of patients who have serial measurements during the course of an attack. However, a single uric acid determination is normal in up to 25% of cases, so it does not exclude gout

IMAGING STUDIES

- Early in the disease, radiographs show no changes
- Later, punched-out erosions with an overhanging rim of cortical bone ("rat bite") develop. When these are adjacent to a soft tissue tophus, they are diagnostic of gout

DIAGNOSTIC PROCEDURES

- Identification of sodium urate crystals by compensated polariscopic examination of joint fluid aspirates
- Crystals are negatively birefringent and needle-like and may be found free or in neutrophils

TREATMENT

MEDICATIONS

Acute attack

- At times the pain of an acute attack may require **opioids.** Aspirin should be avoided since it aggravates hyperuricemia
- **Nonsteroidal antiinflammatory** drugs are the treatment of choice
- **Colchicine** (0.5 or 0.6 mg by mouth every hour until pain is relieved or until nausea or diarrhea appears) is also effective but is less favored, since 80% develop significant gastrointestinal side effects
- For monarticular gout, **intraarticular corticosteroid administration** (eg, triamcinolone, 10–40 mg depending on the size of the joint) is most effective
- For polyarticular gout, corticosteroids may be given intravenously (eg, methylprednisolone, 40 mg/day tapered off over 7 days) or orally (eg, prednisone, 40–60 mg/day tapered off over 7 days)

SURGERY

- Surgical excision of large tophi rarely offers mechanical improvement in selected deformities

THERAPEUTIC PROCEDURES

- Corticosteroid injections for acute monoarticular disease
- Bed rest is important and should be continued for about 24 h after the acute attack has subsided. Early ambulation may precipitate a recurrence
- Treat the acute arthritis first and hyperuricemia later, if at all. Sudden reduction of serum uric acid often precipitates further gouty arthritis

 OUTCOME

FOLLOW-UP

- Maintain uric acid level within the normal range in nontophaceous gout
- Maintain serum uric acid below 6.5 mg/dL in tophaceous gout

COMPLICATIONS

- Chronic tophaceous arthritis can occur after repeated attacks of inadequately treated acute gout
- Tophi are found in cartilage, subcutaneous and periarticular tissues, tendon, bone, the kidneys, and elsewhere
- Uric acid kidney stones are present in 5–10% of patients with gouty arthritis
- Hyperuricemia correlates highly with the likelihood of developing stones, with the risk of stone formation reaching 50% in patients with a serum urate level above 13 mg/dL
- Chronic urate nephropathy is caused by the deposition of monosodium urate crystals. Although progressive renal failure occurs in a substantial percentage of patients with chronic gout, the role of hyperuricemia in causing this outcome is controversial, because many patients with gout have numerous confounding risk factors for renal failure

PROGNOSIS

- Without treatment, the acute attack may last from a few days to several weeks, but proper treatment quickly terminates the attack
- The intervals between acute attacks vary up to years, but the asymptomatic periods often become shorter if the disease progresses

WHEN TO REFER

- Refer to a rheumatologist if patient has recurrent attacks despite treatment

WHEN TO ADMIT

- For suspected or proven superimposed septic arthritis

PREVENTION

- Asymptomatic hyperuricemia should not be treated
- Potentially reversible causes of hyperuricemia are a high-purine diet, obesity, frequent alcohol consumption, and use of certain medications (diuretics, niacin, low-dose aspirin)

- Colchicine, 0.6 mg orally QD or BID, can be used to prevent future attacks and is frequently prescribed to prevent attacks when probenecid or allopurinol is being initiated
- Two classes of drugs can lower uric acid levels in patients with frequent arthritis, tophaceous deposits, or renal damage
  - Probenicid, 1–2 g daily, is the principal uricosuric drug, which cannot be used in patients with creatinine >2 mg/dL
  - Allopurinol (100–300 mg/day based on renal function) promptly lowers plasma urate and urinary uric acid concentrations and facilitates tophus mobilization. The commonest sign of hypersensitivity to allopurinol (occurring in 2% of cases) is a pruritic rash that may progress to toxic epidermal necrolysis. Vasculitis and hepatitis are other rare complications

 EVIDENCE

PRACTICE GUIDELINES

- Pal B et al: How is gout managed in primary care? A review of current practice and proposed guidelines. Clin Rheumatol 2000;19:21. [PMID: 10752494]

INFORMATION FOR PATIENTS

- National Institute of Arthritis and Musculoskeletal and Skin Disease http://www.niams.nih.gov/hi/topics/gout/gout.htm
- American College of Foot and Ankle Surgeons http://www.acfas.org/brgoutft.html

REFERENCES

- Fam AG et al: Efficacy and safety of desensitization to allopurinol following cutaneous reactions. Arthritis Rheum 2001;44:231. [PMID: 11212165]
- Harris M et al: Effect of low dose daily aspirin on serum urate levels and urinary excretion in patients receiving probenecid for gouty arthritis. J Rheumatol 2000;27:2873. [PMID: 11128679]

David B. Hellmann, MD, FACP
John H. Stone, MD, MPH

Guillain-Barré Syndrome

 KEY FEATURES

ESSENTIALS OF DIAGNOSIS

- Acute or subacute progressive polyradiculoneuropathy
- Usually ascending, symmetric weakness
- Paresthesias are more variable

GENERAL CONSIDERATIONS

- A symmetric sensory, motor, or mixed deficit, often most marked distally
- Probably has an immunological basis, but the mechanism is unclear

DEMOGRAPHICS

- Sometimes follows infective illness, innoculations, or surgical procedures
- There is an association with preceding *Campylobacter jejuni* enteritis

 CLINICAL FINDINGS

SYMPTOMS AND SIGNS

Motor symptoms

- The main complaint is of weakness that varies widely in severity in different patients and often has a proximal emphasis and symmetric distribution
- The weakness usually begins in the legs, spreading to a variable extent but frequently involving the arms and often one or both sides of the face
- The muscles of respiration or deglutition may also be affected

Sensory symptoms

- Sensory symptoms are usually less conspicuous than motor ones, but distal paresthesias and dysesthesias are common, and neuropathic or radicular pain is present in many patients

Autonomic symptoms

- Autonomic disturbances are common, may be severe, and are sometimes life-threatening; they include tachycardia, cardiac irregularities, hypotension or hypertension, facial flushing, abnormalities of sweating, pulmonary dysfunction, and impaired sphincter control

DIFFERENTIAL DIAGNOSIS

- Chronic inflammatory demyelinating polyneuropathy (CIDP)
- Porphyria
- Diphtheritic neuropathy
- Toxic neuropathy, eg, lead, mercury, organophosphates, hexacarbon solvents
- Poliomyelitis
- Botulism
- Tick paralysis
- Spinal cord lesion
- Transverse myelitis
- West Nile virus
- Periodic paralysis syndrome

 DIAGNOSIS

LABORATORY TESTS

- The cerebrospinal fluid characteristically contains a high protein concentration with a normal cell content, but these changes may take 2 or 3 weeks to develop

DIAGNOSTIC PROCEDURES

- Electrophysiological (nerve conduction) studies may reveal marked abnormalities, which do not necessarily parallel the clinical disorder in their temporal course
- Pathological examination has shown primary demyelination or, less commonly, axonal degeneration

Guillain-Barré Syndrome

TREATMENT

MEDICATIONS

- Marked hypotension may respond to volume replacement or pressor agents
- Intravenous immunoglobulin (400 mg/kg/day for 5 days) is helpful and imposes less stress on the cardiovascular system than plasmapheresis
- Low-dose heparin to prevent pulmonary embolism should be considered
- Prednisone is ineffective and may prolong recovery time

THERAPEUTIC PROCEDURES

- Respiratory toilet and chest physical therapy help prevent atelectasis
- Plasmapheresis is of value; it is best performed within the first few days of illness and is best reserved for clinically severe or rapidly progressive cases or those with ventilatory impairment

OUTCOME

FOLLOW-UP

- Monitor spirometry: patients should be admitted to intensive care units if their forced vital capacity is declining, and intubation is considered if the forced vital capacity reaches 15 mL/kg, dyspnea becomes evident, or the oxygen saturation declines

PROGNOSIS

- Most patients eventually make a good recovery, but this may take many months, and 10–20% of patients are left with persisting disability
- Approximately 3% of patients have one or more clinically similar relapses, sometimes several years after the initial illness

WHEN TO ADMIT

- All patients should be admitted to the hospital and may need intensive care unit admission if their forced vital capacity is declining

EVIDENCE

PRACTICE GUIDELINES

- National Guideline Clearinghouse
  http://www.guideline.gov/summary/summary.aspx?doc_id=1976&nbr=1202&string=Guillain+barre
  http://www.guideline.gov/summary/summary.aspx?doc_id=2824&nbr=2050&string=Guillain+barre

WEB SITE

- Neuromuscular Disease Center
  http://www.neuro.wustl.edu/neuromuscular/

INFORMATION FOR PATIENTS

- National Institute of Neurological Disorders and Stroke
  http://www.ninds.nih.gov/health_and_medical/pubs/guillain_barre.htm
- The Mayo Clinic
  http://www.mayoclinic.com/invoke.cfm?id=DS00413

REFERENCE

- Winer JB: Guillain-Barré syndrome. Mol Pathol 2001;54:381. [PMID: 11724912]

Michael J. Aminoff, MD, DSc, FRCP

Gynecomastia

 KEY FEATURES

ESSENTIALS OF DIAGNOSIS

- Glandular enlargement of the male breast
- Often asymmetric or unilateral; may be tender
- Nipple discharge may be present
- Must be distinguished from tumors and fatty breast enlargement of obesity

GENERAL CONSIDERATIONS

Causes

- Endocrine: hyperprolactinemia of any cause, hyperthyroidism, Klinefelter's syndrome, hypogonadism
- Systemic disease: chronic liver or renal disease
- Neoplasms: testicular, adrenal, lung, liver
- Drugs (selected): alcohol, amiodarone, cimetidine, diazepam, digoxin, estrogens, finasteride, flutamide, isoniazid, ketoconazole, marijuana, omeprazole, opioids, progestins, protease inhibitors and antiretrovirals, spironolactone, testosterone, tricyclic antidepressants, eating necks of poultry that have been fed estrogen

DEMOGRAPHICS

- Common in puberty, especially in boys taller and heavier than average
- Common among elderly men
- Common in obesity
- Develops in ~50% of athletes who abuse androgens and anabolic steroids
- Family history of malignancy

 CLINICAL FINDINGS

SYMPTOMS AND SIGNS

- Breast enlargement, often asymmetric or unilateral, sometimes tender, with or without nipple discharge
- Pubertal gynecomastia: tender discoid enlargement of breast tissue beneath areola, 2–3 cm in diameter
- Testicular examination may reveal tumor

DIFFERENTIAL DIAGNOSIS

- Breast cancer
- Fatty breast enlargement of obesity
- Breast abscess (mastitis)
- Metastatic cancer, eg, prostate
- Treatment of prostate cancer with gonadotropin-releasing hormone agonists/antagonists or antiandrogens

 DIAGNOSIS

LABORATORY TESTS

- Serum prolactin elevated if gynecomastia caused by hyperprolactinemia
- Detectable serum β-human chorionic gonadotropin (hCG) implicates testicular tumor (germ cell or Sertoli cell) or other malignancy (usually lung or liver). However, low detectable levels (β-hCG <5 mU/mL) may occur in primary hypogonadism if assay cross-reacts with luteinizing hormone (LH)
- Low serum testosterone, high serum LH in primary hypogonadism
- High testosterone, high LH in partial androgen resistance
- Serum estradiol usually normal but may be increased by testicular tumors, increased β-hCG, liver disease, obesity, adrenal tumors (rare)
- Serum thyroid-stimulating hormone low in hyperthyroidism
- Karyotype (for Klinefelter's syndrome) indicated in men with persistent gynecomastia without obvious cause

IMAGING STUDIES

- Chest x-ray or lung CT if lung cancer or metastases suspected
- Testicular ultrasound if detectable β-hCG or mass on examination
- CT or MRI of abdomen/pelvis if detectable β-hCG and no mass on testicular examination or ultrasound

DIAGNOSTIC PROCEDURES

- Fine needle aspiration of suspicious masses, especially when unilateral or asymmetric, to distinguish gynecomastia from tumor or mastitis

TREATMENT

MEDICATIONS

- Treatment of underlying condition
- Discontinue potentially offending medications if possible
- Medications used to treat gynecomastia can produce adverse reactions; treat gynecomastia only if it is a troubling and persistent problem
- Tamoxifen (an antiestrogen), 10 mg PO BID, may reduce pain and breast size in >50%; relapses occur in ~28% after tamoxifen is stopped
- Danazol, 400 mg PO QD, improves gynecomastia in 40%; relapses are uncommon after danazol is stopped. Liver enzymes must be monitored

SURGERY

- Surgery is reserved for persistent or severe gynecomastia, since results are often disappointing
- Endoscopically assisted transaxillary liposuction and subcutaneous mastectomy may produce acceptable results

THERAPEUTIC PROCEDURES

- Mammography for particularly enlarged male breasts

 OUTCOME

PROGNOSIS

- Pubertal and idiopathic gynecomastia usually subside spontaneously within 1–2 years
- Drug-induced gynecomastia resolves after offending drug is discontinued

PREVENTION

- Avoidance of androgen and anabolic steroid abuse

 EVIDENCE

PRACTICE GUIDELINES

- Daniels IR et al: Gynaecomastia. Eur J Surg 2001;167:885. [PMID: 11841077]
- Dicker AP: The safety and tolerability of low-dose irradiation for the management of gynaecomastia caused by antiandrogen monotherapy. Lancet Oncol 2003;4:30. [PMID: 12517537]
- Fruhstorfer BH et al: A systematic approach to the surgical treatment of gynaecomastia. Br J Plast Surg 2003;56:237. [PMID: 12859919]

WEB SITES

- American Academy of Family Physicians—Gynecomastia: when breast form in males http://familydoctor.org/handouts/080.html
- American Society of Plastic Surgeons—Gynecomastia: male breast reduction http://www.plasticsurgery.org/public_education/procedures/Gynecomastia.cfm

INFORMATION FOR PATIENTS

- Mayo Clinic http://www.mayoclinic.com/invoke.cfm?objectid=7BB5F30F-8628-4876-B280D38A83B9965B
- MEDLINEplus—Gynecomastia http://www.nlm.nih.gov/medlineplus/ency/article/003165.htm
- University of Iowa Plastic Surgery http://www.surgery.uiowa.edu/surgery/plastic/gyneco.html

REFERENCES

- Amory JK et al: Klinefelter's syndrome. Lancet 2000;356:333. [PMID: 11071204]
- Manfredi R et al: Gynecomastia associated with highly active antiretroviral therapy. Ann Pharmacother 2001;35:438. [PMID: 11302408]
- Ting AC et al: Comparison of tamoxifen with danazol in the management of idiopathic gynecomastia. Am Surg 2000;66:38. [PMID: 10651345]

Paul A. Fitzgerald, MD

Head & Neck Cancer

 KEY FEATURES

ESSENTIALS OF DIAGNOSIS

- A firm, painless, and slowly enlarging mass is often neoplastic
- Persistent symptoms (more than 2 weeks' duration) of one or more of the following:
  - Throat pain
  - Ear pain (referred otalgia, via branches of vagus nerve that innervate both sites)
  - Change in character of voice
  - Blood in the mouth or throat
- Indirect or fiberoptic examination of the oropharynx by an experienced clinician, as well as examination and palpation of the base of the tongue and tonsillar fossae and the neck
- Regional metastatic lymphadenopathy is common at time of presentation

GENERAL CONSIDERATIONS

- A systematic intraoral, pharyngeal, and laryngeal examination (including the lateral tongue, floor of the mouth, gingiva, buccal area, palate, tonsillar fossae, and indirect or fiberoptic examination of the pharynx and larynx) and palpation of the neck for enlarged lymph nodes should be part of any head and neck examination in a patient with concerning symptoms or signs or unexplained weight loss, especially in patients over 45 who smoke tobacco or drink immoderately

DEMOGRAPHICS

- Occurs predominantly in heavy smokers and/or those with significant alcohol use
- Most common betweeen ages 50 and 70
- Incidence is 25/100,000

 CLINICAL FINDINGS

SYMPTOMS AND SIGNS

- Persistent (greater than 2 weeks) throat or ear pain (referred otalgia)
- Weight loss
- Blood in the throat or mouth
- Change in speech/voice quality (including hoarseness or dysarthria)
- Dysphagia
- Airway compromise
- Visible mass (as seen on oral examination, or indirect or fiberoptic pharyngoscopy)
- Palpable mass in base of tongue or tonsil
- Neck adenopathy (usually hard)

DIFFERENTIAL DIAGNOSIS

Oropharynx mass

- Occasionally a tumor can be misdiagnosed as a peritonsillar abscess

Laryngeal mass

- Vocal cord nodules
- Papillomas or granulomas
- Leukoplakia, as in the oral cavity, requires clarification clinically or by biopsy as judged by an experienced clinician

Oral mass

- Aphthous ulcer (canker sore, ulcerative stomatitis)
- See *Leukoplakia, erythroplakia, lichen planus*, and *oral cancer* for additional differential diagnosis

 DIAGNOSIS

LABORATORY TESTS

- Complete blood cell count, liver function tests

IMAGING STUDIES

- MRI is preferred to CT for staging
- Chest x-ray
- Chest CT may be indicated if there is concern for a second primary mass in the lung or for lung metastases

DIAGNOSTIC PROCEDURES

- Indirect or fiberoptic examination of the nasopharynx, oropharynx, hypopharynx, and larynx
- Fine needle aspiration biopsy may confirm the presence of the carcinoma and the histological type, but caution and clinical judgment should be exercised in interpreting an apparently negative result

Head & Neck Cancer

TREATMENT

MEDICATIONS

- Cisplatin as a radiosensitizer during radiation therapy
- Other chemotherapy agents including 5-fluorouracil, pacclitaxe, carboplatinol, as well as methotrexate
- Management of associated **pain** is critically important, and often includes narcotics with short (3 h) and long (8–72 h) duration of effect, nonsteroidal anti-inflammatory agents, COX-II inhibitors, and gabapentin
- See Tables 148 and 149 (pages 1329 and 1332)

SURGERY

- **Small tumors** are often best treated with a sole modality of either function-sparing surgery or radiation, depending on the site of the primary tumor
- **Large nonoropharyngeal tumors** often are best treated with surgery and postoperative irradiation

THERAPEUTIC PROCEDURES

- Treatment depends on tumor site, TNM stage, prior treatment, and patient comorbidities (such as cardiovascular and lung disease)
- There must be careful weighing of the side effects of treatment options
- **Oropharyngeal tumors** (eg, base of the tongue and tonsil fossa) are usually best treated with radiation and often concomitant chemotherapy, regardless of extent of primary and nodal disease
- **T1–2 laryngeal tumors** are usually best treated with radiation, though sometimes are amenable to endoscopic resection
- More advanced laryngeal tumors are treated with organ-presesrvation approaches that try to avoid laryngectomy
- For **unresectable recurrent disease** and distant metastases, weigh the benefits of chemotherapy and possibly palliative radiation therapy

OUTCOME

FOLLOW-UP

- Early diagnosis of recurrent squamous cell carcinoma or a new primary tumor is key to management; the incidence of second tumors is about 3–4% annually
- Commonly a patient with a prior cavity head and neck cancer is examined clinically every 4–6 weeks in the first year, every 8–10 weeks in the second year, and every 3–4 months thereafter for several additional years
- Periodic PET scans and baseline post-treatment MRIs are used by many in subsequent tumor surveillance
- Strategies for DNA or protein molecular markers are under investigation

COMPLICATIONS

- Airway compromise, requiring tracheotomy
- Bleeding may be associated with surface ulceration
- Erosion into a major artery can lead to life-threatening oral or neck hemorrhage
- Dysphagia and odynophagia may lead to weight loss, requiring a gastrostomy tube
- Failure to recognize early tumors contributes to the need for more extensive intervention, with associated greater operative risks

PROGNOSIS

- Prognosis is strongly correlated with TNM staging, including specific site of disease, extent of the primary tumor, nodal stage, and presence of distant metastases
- Overall, 65% of head and neck cancers are cured, but the prognosis ranges from better than 90% for early tongue and early larynx lesions to very poor when there is unresectable neck disease or distant metastases

WHEN TO REFER

- Specialty referral should be sought early both for diagnosis and treatment
- Indirect or fiberoptic examination of the nasopharynx, oropharynx, hypopharynx, and larynx by an otolaryngologist-head and neck surgeon should be strongly considered when there is oral erythroplakia, unexplained throat or ear pain, unexplained oral or nasal bleeding, presence of a firm neck mass, or a visible oral cavity or oropharyngeal mass

WHEN TO ADMIT

- Airway compromise, hemorrhage, dehydration
- Institution of an effective pain management regimen for severe pain

PREVENTION

- Smoking cessation and alcohol abatement programs are helpful

EVIDENCE

PRACTICE GUIDELINES

- National Guideline Clearinghouse http://www.guideline.gov/summary/summary.aspx?doc_id=2989&nbr=2215

WEB SITES

- Ear, Nose, and Throat Information Center http://www.netdoor.com/entinfo/
- Otolaryngology Resources on the Internet http://www.bcm.tmc.edu/oto/othersa.html

INFORMATION FOR PATIENTS

- American Academy of Otolaryngology. Head and neck cancer http://www.entnet.org/healthinfo/tobacco/cancer.cfm
- National Cancer Institute. Head and neck http://www.nci.nih.gov/cancer_information/xml_tab.aspx?viewid=7d080f7f-585d-40e8-bd59-13fb31481b2b&expand=Head+and+Neck

REFERENCE

- Mellott A et al: Chemoprevention in head and neck cancer. Cancer Treat Res 2001;106:221. [PMID: 11225004]

Robert K. Jackler, MD
Michael J. Kaplan, MD

Head Injury

 KEY FEATURES

ESSENTIALS OF DIAGNOSIS

- Absence of skull fracture does not exclude the possibility of severe head injury
- In many elderly patients, there may not be a known history of head trauma
- Occasionally, head injury, often trivial, precedes symptoms by several weeks

GENERAL CONSIDERATIONS

- Some guide to prognosis is provided by the mental status, since loss of consciousness for more than 1 or 2 min implies a worse prognosis than otherwise
- The degree of retrograde and posttraumatic amnesia provides an indication of the severity of injury and thus of the prognosis

DEMOGRAPHICS

- Trauma is the most common cause of death in young people, and head injury accounts for almost half of these trauma-related deaths

 CLINICAL FINDINGS

SYMPTOMS AND SIGNS

- See Table 97 (page 1280)
- Special attention should be given to the level of consciousness and extent of any brainstem dysfunction
- The clinical signs of basilar skull fracture include bruising about the orbit (raccoon sign), blood in the external auditory meatus (Battle's sign), and leakage of cerebrospinal fluid (which can be identified by its glucose content) from the ear or nose

Chronic subdural hemorrhage

- Head injury, often subtle, may precede the onset of symptoms by several weeks
- Mental changes such as slowness, drowsiness, headache, confusion, memory disturbances, personality change, or even dementia may occur
- Focal neurological deficits such as hemiparesis or hemisensory disturbance are less common

 DIAGNOSIS

IMAGING STUDIES

- See Table 97 (page 1280)
- Because injury to the spine may have accompanied head trauma, cervical spine radiographs (especially in the lateral projection) should always be obtained in comatose patients and in patients with severe neck pain or a deficit possibly related to cord compression
- CT scanning can demonstrate intracranial hemorrhage and may also provide evidence of cerebral edema and displacement of midline structures
- Skull radiographs or CT scans may provide evidence of fractures

TREATMENT

MEDICATIONS

- Measures to reduce intracranial pressure include induced hyperventilation, intravenous mannitol infusion, and intravenous furosemide; corticosteroids provide no benefit in this context
- If there is any leakage of cerebrospinal fluid, conservative treatment, with elevation of the head, restriction of fluids, and administration of acetazolamide (250 mg four times daily), is often helpful
- Antibiotics if infection occurs
- No clear evidence that prophylactic anticonvulsant therapy reduces the incidence of posttraumatic seizures

SURGERY

- Scalp lacerations and depressed or compound depressed skull fractures should be treated surgically as appropriate
- Surgical evacuation of intracranial hematomas may be needed to prevent cerebral compression and herniation
- If leakage of cerebrospinal fluid continues for more than a few days, lumbar subarachnoid drainage may be necessary

THERAPEUTIC PROCEDURES

- Simple skull fractures require no specific treatment

 ## OUTCOME

FOLLOW-UP

- If admission to the hospital is declined, family members should be given clear instructions about the need for, and manner of, checking on them at regular (hourly) intervals and for obtaining additional medical help if necessary

COMPLICATIONS

- Increased intracranial pressure from
  - Seizures
  - Dilutional hyponatremia
  - Cerebral edema
  - Intracranial hematoma requiring surgical evacuation
- Chronic subdural hemorrhage
- Normal-pressure hydrocephalus
- Posttraumatic seizure disorder
- Posttraumatic headache

PROGNOSIS

- The prognosis depends on the site and severity of brain damage

WHEN TO ADMIT

- Patients who have lost consciousness for 2 min or more following head injury should be admitted to the hospital for observation
- Patients with focal neurological deficits, lethargy, or skull fractures

 ## EVIDENCE

PRACTICE GUIDELINES

- National Guideline Clearinghouse http://www.guideline.gov/summary/summary.aspx?doc_id=2912&nbr=2138&string=head+injury http://www.guideline.gov/summary/summary.aspx?doc_id=2793&nbr=2019&string=head+injury

INFORMATION FOR PATIENTS

- JAMA patient page: Protecting against head injury. JAMA 1999;282:1010. Erratum in JAMA 2000;283:747.
- National Institute of Neurological Disorders and Stroke http://www.ninds.nih.gov/health_and_medical/disorders/tbi_doc.htm

REFERENCES

- Bavetta S, Benjamin C: Assessment and management of the head-injured patient. Hosp Med 2002;63:289. [PMID: 12066348]
- Schierhout G et al: Prophylactic antiepileptic agents after head injury: a systematic review. J Neurol Neurosurg Psychiatry 1998;64:108. [PMID: 9436738]

Michael J. Aminoff, DSc, MD, FRCP

Headache

KEY FEATURES

ESSENTIALS OF DIAGNOSIS

- Severe headache in a previously well patient is more likely than chronic headache to relate to an intracranial disorder such as hemorrhage, meningitis, or mass lesion
- Headaches worse on awakening may indicate sinusitis or intracranial mass

GENERAL CONSIDERATIONS

- Chronic headaches are commonly due to migraine, tension, or depression, but may be related to intracranial pathology
- Possibility of underlying structural lesions is important because about one-third of patients with brain tumors have a primary complaint of headache

CLINICAL FINDINGS

SYMPTOMS AND SIGNS

Tension headache

- Often pulsating or throbbing
- Bandlike pain is common
- Sense of tightness or pressure is common
- Worsens with stress and at end of day

Migraine

- Often pulsating or throbbing
- May be ocular or periorbital ice pick–like pain
- Lateralized pain is common

Cluster headache

- Ocular or ice pick–like pain
- Lateralized pain is common
- Tends to occur at the same time each day or night

Neuritic causes

- Sharp lancinating pain may be suggestive
- Pain localized to one of the divisions of the trigeminal nerve or to the pharynx and external auditory meatus, respectively, in trigeminal or glossopharyngeal neuralgia

Sinusitis-related headache

- May cause tenderness of overlying skin and bone

Ophthalmic-related headache

- Ocular or periocular pain

Intracranial mass lesion–related headache

- Typically dull or steady pain
- Pain may be worse in the morning
- Pain may be localized or general

DIFFERENTIAL DIAGNOSIS

Intracranial

- Migraine
- Cluster headache
- Brain tumor
- Subarachnoid hemorrhage
- Meningitis
- Brain abscess
- Temporal (giant cell) arteritis
- Hypertension
- Caffeine, alcohol, or drug withdrawal
- Pseudotumor cerebri
- Subdural hemorrhage
- Cerebral ischemia
- Arterial dissection (carotid or vertebral)
- Arteriovenous malformation
- Head injury
- Lumbar puncture
- Venous sinus thrombosis (intracranial venous thrombosis)
- Postlumbar puncture
- Carbon monoxide poisoning

Extracranial

- Systemic infections
- Tension headache
- Cervical arthritis
- Glaucoma
- Dental abscess
- Sinusitis
- Otitis media
- Temporomandibular joint (TMJ) syndrome
- Depression
- Somatoform disorder (somatization)
- Trigeminal neuralgia
- Glossopharyngeal neuralgia

DIAGNOSIS

LABORATORY TESTS

- Cerebrospinal fluid examination if a meningeal infection or subarachnoid hemorrhage is considered

IMAGING STUDIES

- Cranial MRI or CT scan to exclude an intracranial mass lesion in patients with
  - A progressive headache disorder
  - New onset of headache in middle or later life
  - Headaches that disturb sleep or are related to exertion
  - Headaches that are associated with neurological symptoms or a focal neurological deficit

DIAGNOSTIC PROCEDURES

- Inquire about precipitating and exacerbating factors
- Precipitating factors include recent sinusitis or hay fever, dental surgery, head injury, and symptoms suggestive of a systemic viral infection
- Alcohol is a precipitating factor for cluster headache
- Chewing as a precipitating factor is associated with TMJ dysfunction, trigeminal or glossopharyngeal neuralgia, and giant cell arteritis
- Cough-induced headache occurs with structural lesions of the posterior fossa, but a specific cause is frequently unidentifiable
- Exacerbating factors for migraine include emotional stress, fatigue, foods containing nitrite or tyramine, and menses

TREATMENT

- See specific headache disorder: tension, migraine, cluster, giant cell arteritis, posttraumatic, cough

 OUTCOME

WHEN TO REFER

- If expertise in evaluation or treatment is needed

WHEN TO ADMIT

- Depends on the underlying cause (eg, mass lesion, intracerebral bleed)

 EVIDENCE

PRACTICE GUIDELINES

- National Guideline Clearinghouse http://www.guideline.gov/summary/ summary.aspx?doc_id=3441&nbr= 2667&string=headache http://www.guideline.gov/summary/ summary.aspx?doc_id=3298&nbr= 2524&string=headache
- American Academy of Neurology http://www.aan.com/professionals/ practice/pdfs/gl0085.pdf

INFORMATION FOR PATIENTS

- JAMA patient page: Headaches. JAMA 2003;289:1462. [PMID: 12636471]
- JAMA patient page: Tension headache. JAMA 2001;285:2282. [PMID: 11368044]
- JAMA patient page: Migraine headache. JAMA 2000;284:2672. [PMID: 11185518]

REFERENCES

- Goadsby PJ: Mechanisms and management of headache. J R Coll Physicians Lond 1999;33:228. [PMID: 10402569]
- Kaniecki R: Headache assessment and management. JAMA 2003;289;1430.

Michael J. Aminoff, DSc, MD, FRCP

Headache, Acute

 KEY FEATURES

ESSENTIALS OF DIAGNOSIS

- Age >50 years
- Rapid onset with severe intensity
- History of hypertension or HIV
- Fever, hypertension
- Trauma
- Vision changes
- Neurological findings (mental status changes, motor/sensory deficits)

GENERAL CONSIDERATIONS

- In the emergency department, 1% of patients with acute headache have a life-threatening condition
- In the physician's office, the prevalence of life-threatening conditions is much lower

 CLINICAL FINDINGS

SYMPTOMS AND SIGNS

- Sudden-onset headache that reaches maximal and severe intensity within seconds or a few minutes ("thunderclap headache") suggests subarachnoid hemorrage
- Headache with uncontrolled hypertension should prompt search for other manifestations of "hypertensive urgency or emergency" [See *Hypertensive urgencies & emergencies*]
- Headache and hypertension in pregnancy may be due to preeclampsia
- Episodic headache with hypertension, palpitations, and sweats may be due to pheochromocytoma
- Physical examination should include vital signs, neurological examination, vision/fundoscopic examination, and Kernig and Brudzinski signs
- Patients ≥60 years old should be examined for scalp or temporal artery tenderness
- Diminished visual acuity suggests glaucoma, temporal arteritis, or optic neuritis
- Ophthalmoplegia or visual field defects suggest venous sinus thrombosis, tumor, or aneurysm
- Afferent pupillary defects occur with intracranial masses or optic neuritis
- Ipsilateral ptosis and miosis (Horner's syndrome) occur with carotid artery dissection
- Papilledema and/or absent retinal venous pulsation occur with elevated intracranial pressure

DIFFERENTIAL DIAGNOSIS

- Causes of headache that require immediate treatment: imminent or completed vascular events (intracranial hemorrage, thrombosis, vasculitis, malignant hypertension, arterial dissection, or aneurysm); infections (abscess; encephalitis; meningitis); intracranial masses causing intracranial hypertension; preeclampsia; and carbon monoxide poisoning

DIAGNOSIS

LABORATORY TESTS

- Cerebrospinal fluid (CSF) Gram stain, white blood cell count with differential, red blood cell count, glucose, total protein, bacterial culture, VDRL
- In suspected cases, obtain CSF polymerase chain reaction test for herpes simplex 2
- In HIV-infected patients, obtain CSF cryptococcal antigen, acid-fast bacillus stain and culture, and complement fixation and culture for coccidioidomycosis
- Erythrocyte sedimentation rate
- Urinalysis

IMAGING STUDIES

- Sinus CT or x-ray
- Noncontrast head CT immediately, followed by contrast head CT later
- In HIV-infected patients, new-onset headache warrants CT with and without contrast or MRI
- For clinical features associated with acute headache that warrant urgent or emergent neuroimaging (Table 90, page 1275)
- Perform neuroimaging prior to lumbar puncture in acute headache with abnormal neurological examination, abnormal mental status, abnormal fundoscopic examination (papilledema; loss of venous pulsations)
- Perform neuroimaging emergently in acute headache with abnormal neurological examination, abnormal mental status, "thunderclap headache"
- Perform neuroimaging urgently in acute headache with HIV infection, age >50 years (despite normal neurological examination)

DIAGNOSTIC PROCEDURES

- Lumbar puncture
- If high suspicion for subarachnoid hemorrhage or aneurysm, lumbar puncture followed by cerebral angiography

TREATMENT

- Treatment should be guided by the underlying etiology

MEDICATIONS

- Nonsteroidal antiinflammatory drugs (Table 1, page 1192)
- Opioid agonist analgesics (Table 2, page 1194)
- Clinical response to analgesics does not exclude life-threatening causes of acute headache

 OUTCOME

WHEN TO REFER

- Refer to the emergency department patients with acute headache who have
  - Age >50 years
  - Rapid onset with severe intensity
  - History of hypertension or HIV
  - Fever, hypertension
  - Trauma
  - Vision changes
  - Neurological findings (mental status changes, motor/sensory deficits)

PREVENTION

- Prophylactic treatment of migraine (Table 91, page 1275)

 EVIDENCE

PRACTICE GUIDELINES

- American College of Emergency Physicians. Clinical policy for the initial approach to adolescents and adults presenting to the emergency department with a chief complaint of headache. Ann Emerg Med 1996;821. [PMID: 8644978]
- American College of Emergency Physicians (ACEP). Clinical policy: critical issues in the evaluation and management of patients presenting to the emergency department with acute headache. http://www.acep.org/download.cfm?resource=673
- American Academy of Neurology: Migraine Headache: Evidence-based guidelines for neuroimaging in patients with acute headache http://www.aan.com/professionals/practice/guidelines.cfm

WEB SITES

- American Academy of Family Physicians (AAFP) http://familydoctor.org/
- Cleveland Clinic http://www.clevelandclinic.org/
- American Academy of Neurology http://www.aan.com/professionals/

INFORMATION FOR PATIENTS

- JAMA patient page: Temporal arteritis. JAMA 2002;287:3034. [PMID: 12064321]
- Cleveland Clinic: Diagnosing your headache: headache evaluation http://www.clevelandclinic.org/health/health-info/docs/2500/2552.asp?index=9655
- MD Consult—Headache: comprehensive version http://home.mdconsult.com/das/patient/view/30140317/10041/5473.html/top?sid=196079114

Ralph Gonzales, MD

Headache, Migraine

 KEY FEATURES

ESSENTIALS OF DIAGNOSIS

- Headache, usually pulsatile
- Nausea, vomiting, photophobia, phonophobia are common accompaniments
- May be transient neurological symptoms preceding the headache in classic migraine, typically visual disturbances
- No preceding aura is common in migraines

GENERAL CONSIDERATIONS

- The pathophysiology probably relates to serotonin and to dilation and excessive pulsation of the branches of the external carotid artery
- Focal disturbances of neurological function may precede or accompany the headaches (classic migraines) and have been attributed to constriction of branches of the internal carotid artery
- Attacks may be triggered by emotional or physical stress, lack or excess of sleep, missed meals, specific foods (eg, chocolate), alcoholic beverages, menstruation, or use of oral contraceptives

DEMOGRAPHICS

- Patients often give a family history of migraine

 CLINICAL FINDINGS

SYMPTOMS AND SIGNS

- Migrainous headaches may be lateralized or generalized, may be dull or throbbing, and are sometimes associated with anorexia, nausea, vomiting, photophobia, phonophobia, and blurring of vision

Classic migraine

- Lateralized throbbing headache that occurs episodically following its onset in adolescence or early adult life
- Visual disturbances occur quite commonly and may consist of field defects; of luminous visual hallucinations such as stars, sparks, unformed light flashes (photopsia), geometric patterns, or zigzags of light; or of some combination of field defects and luminous hallucinations (scintillating scotomas)
- Other focal disturbances such as aphasia or numbness, tingling, clumsiness, or weakness in a circumscribed distribution may also occur

Common migraine

- Headaches commonly bilateral and periorbital
- Visual disturbances and other focal neurological deficits do not occur

Basilar artery migraine

- Blindness or disturbances throughout both visual fields are accompanied or followed by dysarthria, disequilibrium, tinnitus, and perioral and distal paresthesias
- Sometimes followed by transient loss or impairment of consciousness or by a confusional state. This, in turn, is followed by a throbbing (usually occipital) headache, often with nausea and vomiting

Ophthalmoplegic migraine

- Lateralized pain, often about the eye, is accompanied by nausea, vomiting, and diplopia due to transient external ophthalmoplegia
- Ophthalmic division of the fifth nerve has also been affected in some patients

Migraine equivalent

- In rare instances, the neurological or somatic disturbance accompanying typical migrainous headaches becomes the sole manifestation of an attack ("migraine equivalent")

DIFFERENTIAL DIAGNOSIS

- Other causes of headache
- Cluster headache
- Brain tumor
- Temporal (giant cell) arteritis
- Sinusitis
- Subarachnoid hemorrhage
- Pseudotumor cerebri
- Transient ischemic attack

 DIAGNOSIS

DIAGNOSTIC PROCEDURES

- Inquire about precipitating and exacerbating factors
- Inquire about family history

Headache, Migraine

 TREATMENT

MEDICATIONS

- A simple analgesic (eg, aspirin) taken right away often provides relief, but treatment with extracranial vasoconstrictors or other drugs is sometimes necessary
  - Cafergot, a combination of ergotamine tartrate (1 mg) and caffeine (100 mg), is often particularly helpful; one or two tablets are taken at the onset of headache or warning symptoms, followed by one tablet every 30 min, if necessary, up to six tablets per attack and ten tablets per week. Alternatively, cafergot can be given rectally as suppositories (one-half to one suppository containing 2 mg of ergotamine)
  - Ergotamine tartrate can be given by inhalation (0.36 mg per puff; up to six puffs per attack) or sublingually (2 mg tablets; not more than three tablets per 24 h); or dihydroergotamine mesylate (0.5–1 mg intravenously or 1–2 mg subcutaneously or intramuscularly) may be useful in such cases. Ergotamines should be avoided during pregnancy and in those with coronary artery disease
  - Sumatriptan is a rapidly effective agent for aborting attacks when given subcutaneously by an autoinjection device (6 mg)
  - Zolmitriptan is another selective serotonin$_1$ receptor agonist that is effective for acute treatment. The optimal initial dose is 2.5 mg, and relief usually occurs within 1 h

THERAPEUTIC PROCEDURES

- Management of migraine consists of avoidance of any precipitating factors, together with prophylactic or symptomatic pharmacological treatment if necessary
- During acute attacks, many patients find it helpful to rest in a quiet, darkened room until symptoms subside

OUTCOME

COMPLICATIONS

- Very rarely, the patient may be left with a permanent neurological deficit following a migrainous attack

PREVENTION

- Prophylactic treatment may be necessary if migrainous headaches occur more frequently than two or three times a month (see Table 91, page 1275)
- Several drugs may have to be tried in turn before the headaches are brought under control. Once a drug has been found to help, it should be continued for several months
- If the patient remains headache free, the dose can then be tapered and the drug eventually withdrawn

EVIDENCE

PRACTICE GUIDELINES

- American Academy of Neurology
  http://www.aan.com/professionals/practice/pdfs/gl0085.pdf
  http://www.aan.com/professionals/practice/pdfs/gl0090.pdf
  http://www.aan.com/professionals/practice/pdfs/gl0087.pdf

INFORMATION FOR PATIENTS

- JAMA patient page: Migraine headache. JAMA 2000;284:2672. [PMID: 11185518]
- The Mayo Clinic
  http://www.mayoclinic.com/invoke.cfm?id=DS00120
  http://www.mayoclinic.com/invoke.cfm?id=AN00392

REFERENCE

- Goadsby PJ, Lipton RB, Ferrari MD: Drug therapy: migraine—current understanding and treatment. N Engl J Med 2002;346:257.

Michael J. Aminoff, MD, DSc, FRCP

Hearing Loss

 KEY FEATURES

ESSENTIALS OF DIAGNOSIS

- Three main types of hearing loss: conductive, sensory, and neural
- Most commonly due to cerumen impaction or transient auditory tube dysfunction associated with upper respiratory tract infection

GENERAL CONSIDERATIONS

Conductive loss

- Four mechanisms, each resulting in impairment of the passage of sound vibrations to the inner ear: obstruction (eg, cerumen impaction), mass loading (eg, middle ear effusion), stiffness effect (eg, otosclerosis), and discontinuity (eg, ossicular disruption)
- Generally more correctable than sensory and neural losses

Sensory loss

- Common causes include excessive noise exposure, head trauma, and systemic diseases such as diabetes mellitus

Neural hearing loss

- Occurs with lesions involving the eighth nerve, auditory nuclei, ascending tracts, or auditory cortex
- It is the least common clinically recognized cause of hearing loss
- Causes include acoustic neuroma, multiple sclerosis, and cerebrovascular disease

DEMOGRAPHICS

- Nearly 30 million Americans have impaired hearing
- For the elderly—the largest group affected—excessive noise, drugs, toxins, and heredity are the most frequent contributing factors

 CLINICAL FINDINGS

SYMPTOMS AND SIGNS

- Reduction in hearing level
- **Weber test:** a 512-Hz tuning fork is placed on the forehead or front teeth: in conductive losses, the sound appears louder in the poorer-hearing ear, whereas in sensorineural losses it radiates to the better side
- **Rinne test:** a 512-Hz tuning fork is placed alternately on the mastoid bone and in front of the ear canal: in conductive losses, bone conduction exceeds air conduction; in sensorineural losses, the opposite is true

DIFFERENTIAL DIAGNOSIS

Conductive (external or middle ear)

- Cerumen impaction (ear wax)
- Transient auditory tube dysfunction
- Acute or chronic otitis media
- Mastoiditis
- Otosclerosis
- Disruption of ossicles
- Trauma or barotrauma
- Glomus tympanicum (middle ear tumor)
- Paget's disease

Sensory

- Presbycusis (age-related)
- Excessive noise exposure
- Ménière's disease (endolymphatic hydrops)
- Labyrinthitis
- Head trauma
- Ototoxicity
- Occlusion of ipsilateral auditory artery
- Hereditary hearing loss
- Autoimmune: systemic lupus erythematosus, Wegener's granulomatosis, Cogan's syndrome
- Other systemic causes: diabetes, hypothyroidism, hyperlipidemia, renal failure, infections

Neural

- Acoustic neuroma
- Multiple sclerosis
- Cerebrovascular disease

DIAGNOSIS

DIAGNOSTIC PROCEDURES

- Formal audiometric studies are performed in a soundproofed room
- Pure-tone thresholds in decibels (dB) are obtained over the range of 250–8000 Hz (the main speech frequencies are between 500 and 3000 Hz) for both air and bone conduction
- Conductive losses create a gap between the air and bone thresholds; in sensorineural losses both air and bone thresholds are equally diminished
- The threshold of normal hearing is from 0 to 20 dB, which corresponds to the loudness of a soft whisper
- Mild hearing loss is indicated by a threshold of 20–40 dB (soft spoken voice), moderate loss by a threshold of 40–60 dB (normal spoken voice), severe loss by a threshold of 60–80 dB (loud spoken voice), and profound loss by a threshold of 80 dB (shout)
- The clarity of hearing is often impaired in sensorineural hearing loss; this is evaluated by speech discrimination testing, which is reported as percentage correct (90–100% is normal)
- The site of the lesion responsible for sensorineural loss—whether it lies in the cochlea or in the central auditory system—may be determined with auditory brainstem-evoked responses

TREATMENT

 OUTCOME

 EVIDENCE

SURGERY

- The cochlear implant—an electronic device that is surgically implanted to stimulate the auditory nerve—offers socially beneficial auditory rehabilitation to most adults with acquired deafness
- Many types of conductive hearing loss (eg, otosclerosis, tympanic membrane perforation, ossicular discontinutity) are surgically remediable

THERAPEUTIC PROCEDURES

- Hearing aids
- Assistive devices such as telephone amplifiers and infrared devices for use with TV, theaters, and auditoriums (eg, Senheiser)

WHEN TO REFER

- Every patient who complains of a hearing loss should be referred for audiological evaluation unless the cause is easily remediable (eg, cerumen impaction, otitis media)

PRACTICE GUIDELINES

- Smith PA et al: Hearing assessment in general practice, schools and health clinics: guidelines for professionals who are not qualified audiologists. Education Committee of the British Society of Audiology. Br J Audiol 2000;34:57. [PMID: 10759078]
- National Guideline Clearinghouse http://www.guideline.gov/summary/ summary.aspx?doc_id=3614&nbr=2840 &string=hearing+loss

WEB SITES

- Ear, Nose, and Throat Information Center http://www.netdoor.com/entinfo/
- Otolaryngology Resources on the Internet http://www.bcm.tmc.edu/oto/othersa. html

INFORMATION FOR PATIENTS

- American Academy of Otolaryngology-Head and Neck Surgery Hearing Health Center http://www.entlink.org/healthinfo/ hearing/hearing_health.cfm
- JAMA patient page: Adult hearing loss. JAMA 2003;289:2020. [PMID: 12697805]
- National Institutes of Health http://www.nlm.nih.gov/medlineplus/ ency/article/001045.htm

REFERENCES

- Clark GM: Cochlear implants in the third millennium. Am J Otolaryngol 1999;20:4. [PMID: 9918163]
- Klein AJ, Weber PC: Hearing aids. Med Clin North Am 1999;83:139. [PMID: 9927966]
- Morris DP et al: The common causes of hearing loss in adults. Practitioner 2000;244:70. [PMID: 10892040]

Robert K. Jackler, MD
Michael J. Kaplan, MD

Heat Exposure Syndromes

KEY FEATURES

ESSENTIALS OF DIAGNOSIS

- Four medical disorders can result: heat syncope, heat cramps, heat exhaustion, and heat stroke

GENERAL CONSIDERATIONS

Heat syncope

- Sudden unconsciousness from cutaneous vasodilation
- Typically occurs immediately following vigorous physical activity

Heat cramps

- Slow, painful muscle contractions of the skeletal muscles most heavily used
- Typically occurs immediately following vigorous physical activity
- Fluid and electrolyte depletion is cause

Heat exhaustion

- Results from prolonged strenuous activity with inadequate salt intake in a hot environment
- Characterized by dehydration, sodium depletion, or isotonic fluid loss with accompanying cardiovascular changes
- May progress to heat stroke if sweating ceases

Heat stroke

- A life-threatening medical emergency resulting from failure of the thermoregulatory mechanism
- Classic heat stroke occurs in patients with compromised homeostatic mechanisms
- Exertional heat stroke occurs in healthy persons undergoing strenuous exertion in a thermally stressful environment

DEMOGRAPHICS

- Persons at greatest risk for heat stroke are the very young, the elderly (age >65), chronically infirm, and patients receiving medications (eg, anticholinergics, antihistamines, phenothiazines) that interfere with heat-dissipating mechanisms
- Heat stroke occurs in unconditioned amateurs participating in strenuous athletic activities

CLINICAL FINDINGS

SYMPTOMS AND SIGNS

Heat syncope

- Systolic blood pressure is usually less than 100 mm Hg with a weak pulse
- The skin is typically cool and moist

Heat cramps

- Muscle spasms last 1–3 min
- The muscles are tender and there may be twitching
- The skin is moist and cool
- The victim is alert, with stable vital signs, but may be agitated and complaining of pain
- The body temperature may be normal or slightly increased

Heat exhaustion

- Prolonged symptoms and a rectal temperature over 37.8°C, increased pulse (>150% of the patient's normal) and moist skin
- Symptoms associated with heat syncope and heat cramps may be present
- The patient may be quite thirsty and weak, with central nervous system symptoms such as headache, fatigue, and, in cases due chiefly to water depletion, anxiety, paresthesias, impaired judgment, hysteria, and occasionally psychosis
- Hyperventilation secondary to heat exhaustion can lead to respiratory alkalosis

Heat stroke

- The core temperature is usually over 41°C
- Cerebral dysfunction with impaired consciousness, high fever, and absence of sweating
- The skin is hot and initially covered with perspiration. Later it dries
- The pulse is strong initially
- Blood pressure may be slightly elevated at first, but hypotension develops later
- Hyperventilation may lead to respiratory alkalosis
- Exertional heat stroke may present with sudden collapse and loss of consciousness followed by irrational behavior
- Twenty-five percent of heat stroke victims have prodromal symptoms including dizziness, weakness, nausea, confusion, disorientation, drowsiness, and irrational behavior

DIFFERENTIAL DIAGNOSIS

Heat stroke

- Neuroleptic malignant syndrome
- Malignant hyperthermia (anesthetic-associated)
- Serotonin syndrome, eg, selective serotonin reuptake inhibitors used with monoamine oxidase inhibitor
- Other drugs: anticholinergics, antihistamines, tricyclic antidepressants, monoamine oxidase inhibitors, salicylates, amphetamines, cocaine
- Thyrotoxicosis
- Prolonged seizures

DIAGNOSIS

LABORATORY TESTS

- For muscle cramps: low serum sodium, hemoconcentration, and elevated urea and creatinine may be seeen
- For heat stroke: leukocytosis, elevated BUN, hyperuricemia, hemoconcentration, acid-base abnormalities (eg, lactic acidosis), and decreased serum potassium, sodium, calcium, and phosphorus; urine is concentrated, with elevated protein, tubular casts, and myoglobinuria. Thrombocytopenia, increased bleeding and clotting times, fibrinolysis, and consumption coagulopathy may also be present. Rhabdomyolysis and myocardial, hepatic, or renal damage may be identified by elevated serum creatine kinase and aminotransferase levels and BUN and by the presence of anuria, proteinuria, and hematuria

IMAGING STUDIES

- In heat stroke, electrocardiographic findings may include ST–T changes consistent with myocardial ischemia

TREATMENT

MEDICATIONS

Heat stroke

- Chlorpromazine (25–50 mg intravenously) or diazepam (5–10 mg intravenously) can be given initially and then every 4 h to control shivering
- Antipyretics (aspirin, acetaminophen) have no effect on environmentally induced hyperthermia and are contraindicated
- Five percent dextrose in half-normal or normal saline should be administered for fluid replacement
- Fluid administration to ensure a high urine output (>50 mL/h), mannitol administration (0.25 mg/kg), and alkalinizing the urine (intravenous bicarbonate administration, 250 mL of 4%) are recommended to reduce the risk of renal failure due to rhabdomyolysis

THERAPEUTIC PROCEDURES

Heat syncope

- Place patient at recumbency in a cool place, with fluids by mouth (or intravenously if necessary)

Heat cramps

- Place patient in a cool environment and given oral saline solution (4 tsp of salt per gallon of water) to replace both salt and water. *Because of their slower absorption, salt tablets are not recommended.* The victim may have to rest for 1–3 days with continued dietary salt supplementation before returning to work or resuming strenuous activity in the heat

Heat exhaustion

- Place patient in a cool environment, provide adequate hydration (1–2 L over 2–4 h), salt replenishment—orally, if possible—and active cooling (fans, ice packs, etc) if necessary
- Physiological saline or isotonic glucose solution should be administered intravenously when oral administration is not appropriate. Intravenous 3% (hypertonic) saline may be necessary if sodium depletion is severe
- At least 24 h of rest is suggested

Heat stroke

- See *Hyperthermia*
- Aim to reduce the core temperature rapidly (within 1 h) and control the secondary effects

- Continue treatment until rectal temperature drops to 39°C
- Fluid output should be monitored by an indwelling urinary catheter

OUTCOME

FOLLOW-UP

- Because sensitivity to high environmental temperature may persist for prolonged periods following an episode of heat stroke, immediate reexposure should be avoided

COMPLICATIONS

- Hypovolemic and cardiogenic shock
- Renal failure due to rhabdomyolysis, hypokalemia, cardiac arrhythmias, disseminated intravascular coagulation, and hepatic failure
- Hypokalemia may not appear until rehydration

PROGNOSIS

- In heat stroke, morbidity or even death can result from cerebral, cardiovascular, hepatic, or renal damage

WHEN TO ADMIT

- All patients with heat syncope, exhaustion, or stroke
- Patients with heat cramps if sustained fluid and electrolyte replacement is needed

PREVENTION

- Athletic competition is not recommended when the WBGT (wet bulb globe temperature) Index exceeds 28°C
- Workers and athletes need acclimatization for hot temperatures and should drink water or balanced electrolyte fluids frequently
- Protective cooled suits have been used successfully in industry for prolonged work in environments up to 60°C

EVIDENCE

WEB SITE

- Merck Manual—Disorder due to physical agents http://www.merck.com/pubs/mmanual/section20/sec20.htm

INFORMATION FOR PATIENTS

- Centers for Disease Control http://www.bt.cdc.gov/extremeheat.htm http://www.cdc.gov/nceh/hsb/extremeheat/heatexhaustion.htm http://www.cdc .gov/nceh/hsb/extremeheat/heatstroke.htm

REFERENCE

- Khosla R et al: Heat-related illnesses. Crit Care Clin 1999;15:251. [PMID: 10331127]

Richard Cohen, MD, MPH
Brent R.W. Moelleken, MD, FACS

Helicobacter pylori Gastritis

 ## KEY FEATURES

ESSENTIALS OF DIAGNOSIS

- *Helicobacter pylori* is a spiral gram-negative rod that causes gastric mucosal inflammation

GENERAL CONSIDERATIONS

- Acute infection causes a transient illness of nausea and abdominal pain for several days associated with acute histological gastritis with polymorphonuclear neutrophils
- After these symptoms resolve, the majority progress to chronic infection with chronic, diffuse mucosal inflammation characterized by polymorphonuclear neutrophils and lymphocytes
- Eradication achieved with antibiotics in >85% leads to resolution of the chronic gastritis
- Majority of those with chronic infection are asymptomatic and suffer no sequelae, but ~15% develop a peptic ulcer
- Risk of gastric adenocarcinoma and low-grade B cell gastric lymphoma (mucosa-associated lymphoid tissue lymphoma, or MALToma) is increased 2- to 6-fold

DEMOGRAPHICS

- Infection usually acquired in childhood through person-to-person spread
- In the United States, the prevalence of infection is <10% in whites aged <30 to >50% in those aged >60
- Prevalence is higher in nonwhites and immigrants from developing countries

 ## CLINICAL FINDINGS

SYMPTOMS AND SIGNS

- Acute infection: transient epigastric pain, nausea, vomiting
- Chronic infection: usually asymptomatic; symptoms arise in patients who develop peptic ulcer disease or gastric cancer; it is controversial whether chronic infection may cause dyspepsia

DIFFERENTIAL DIAGNOSIS

- Peptic ulcer disease
- Functional or nonulcer dyspepsia
- Gastroesophageal reflux disease or hiatal hernia
- Biliary disease or pancreatitis
- Gastric or pancreatic cancer
- Viral gastroenteritis
- "Indigestion" from overeating, high-fat foods, coffee
- Angina pectoris
- In patients aged <50 with dyspepsia without signs of complications (dysphagea, weight loss, vomiting, anemia) empirical testing and treating for *H pylori* are recommended
- In patients over age 50 with chronic dyspepsia or signs of complications, endoscopy is recommended to exclude other organic disease

 ## DIAGNOSIS

LABORATORY TESTS

Noninvasive testing for *H pylori*

- Serological tests, urea breath tests, or fecal antigen tests are recommended as the most cost-effective initial tests
- Lab-based serological ELISA test has sensitivity and specificity of >90%; positive test does not necessarily imply ongoing active infection
- Rapid (office-based) serological tests have lower sensitivity and specificity (75–90%) but are less expensive and provide results within minutes
- After eradication with antibiotics, antibody levels decline to undetectable levels in 50% of patients by 12–18 months
- Fecal antigen immunoassay has sensitivity and specificity of 90%; positive test indicates active infection
- ^{13}C-urea and ^{14}C-urea breath tests have sensitivity and specificity of 90%; positive test indicates active infection
- Proton pump inhibitors significantly reduce the sensitivity of urea breath tests and fecal antigen assays (but not serological tests) and should be discontinued 14 days prior to testing

Endoscopic testing for *H pylori*

- Gastric biopsy specimens can detect *H pylori* organisms on histology and can be tested for active infection by urease production
- Urease test has sensitivity and specificity of 90%

DIAGNOSTIC PROCEDURES

- Upper endoscopy with biopsy is diagnostic

Helicobacter pylori Gastritis

 TREATMENT

MEDICATIONS

- Treat with anti–*H pylori* regimen for 10–14 days with one of the following
  - Triple-therapy: proton pump inhibitor: omeprazole 20 mg PO BID, rabeprazole 20 mg PO BID, lansoprazole 30 mg PO BID, pantoprazole 40 mg PO BID, or esomeprazole 40 mg PO QD, plus clarithromycin 500 mg PO BID, and amoxicillin 1 g PO BID *or* metronidazole 500 mg PO BID (in penicillin-allergic patients)
  - Ranitidine bismuth citrate 400 mg PO BID, plus clarithromycin 500 mg PO BID, plus amoxicillin 1g PO BID *or* tetracycline 500 mg PO BID *or* metronidazole 500 mg PO BID
  - Quadruple-therapy: proton pump inhibitor: omeprazole 20 mg PO BID, rabeprazole 20 mg PO BID, lansoprazole 30 mg PO BID, or pantoprazole 40 mg PO BID, plus bismuth subsalicylate 2 tablets PO QID, plus tetracycline 500 mg PO QID, plus metronidazole 250 mg PO QID; this regimen is recommended for patients who failed initial attempt at eradication with triple-therapy regimen
- Proton pump inhibitors should be administered before meals
- Avoid metronidazole regimens in areas of known high resistance or in patients who have failed a course of treatment that included metronidazole

 OUTCOME

FOLLOW-UP

- After antibiotic therapy, routine follow-up not recommended
- In patients with history of peptic ulcer disease with complications (bleeding) successful eradication should be confirmed with urea breath test or fecal antigen test

PROGNOSIS

- All recommended treatment regimens achieve >85% eradication
- Risk of reinfection with *H pylori* is only 1%/year

WHEN TO REFER

- Patients with persistent infection after one or two attempts at treatment should be referred to a gastroenterologist or infectious disease specialist

WHEN TO ADMIT

- Complications of *H pylori*–associated peptic ulcer disease

 EVIDENCE

PRACTICE GUIDELINES

- Howden CW et al: Guidelines for the management of *Helicobacter pylori* infection. Ad Hoc Committee on Practice Parameters of the American College of Gastroenterology. Am J Gastroenterol 1998;93:2330. [PMID: 9860388]
- Peterson WL et al: *Helicobacter pylori*-related disease: guidelines for testing and treating. Arch Intern Med 2000; 160:1285. [PMID: 10809031]

WEB SITE

- CDC—*H pylori:* the key to cure for most ulcer patients http://www.cdc.gov/ulcer/keytocure.htm

INFORMATION FOR PATIENTS

- Uptodate—*Helicobacter pylori* infection and treatment http://patients.uptodate.com/frames. asp?page=topic.asp&file=digestiv/ 8187&title=Helicobacter+pylori

REFERENCES

- Malfertheiner P et al: Current concepts in the management of *Helicobacter pylori* infection—the Maastricht 2-2000 Consensus Report. Aliment Pharmacol Ther 2002;16:167. [PMID: 11860399]
- Vaira D et al: Review article: diagnosis of *Helicobacter pylori* infection. Aliment Pharmacol Ther 2002;16(Suppl 1):16. [PMID: 11819423]

Kenneth R. McQuaid, MD

Hemochromatosis

 KEY FEATURES

ESSENTIALS OF DIAGNOSIS

- Usually diagnosed because of elevated iron saturation or serum ferritin or a family history
- Most patients are asymptomatic
- Hepatic abnormalities and cirrhosis, congestive heart failure, hypogonadism, and arthritis
- The disease is rarely recognized clinically before the fifth decade

GENERAL CONSIDERATIONS

- Autosomal recessive disease with linkage in many cases to HLA-A3
- About 85% of persons with well-established hemochromatosis are homozygous for the *C282Y* mutation
- Increased accumulation of iron as hemosiderin in the liver, pancreas, heart, adrenals, testes, pituitary, and kidneys
- Heterozygotes do not develop cirrhosis in the absence of associated disorders such as viral hepatitis or nonalcoholic fatty liver disease

DEMOGRAPHICS

- The frequency of the gene mutation averages 7% in Northern European and North American white populations, resulting in a 0.5% frequency of homozygotes (of whom 40–70% will develop iron overload and even fewer will develop clinical symptoms). By contrast, the gene mutation and hemochromatosis are uncommon in African-American and Asian-American populations

 CLINICAL FINDINGS

SYMPTOMS AND SIGNS

- The onset is usually after age 50—earlier in men than in women
- Early symptoms are nonspecific (eg, fatigue, arthralgias)

Later clinical manifestations

- Arthropathy, hepatomegaly, and evidence of hepatic insufficiency (late finding)
- Skin pigmentation (combination of slate gray due to iron and brown due to melanin, sometimes resulting in bronze color)
- Cardiac enlargement with or without heart failure or conduction defects, diabetes mellitus with its complications, and impotence in men
- Bleeding from esophageal varices
- A variant presentation in young patients is characterized by cardiac dysfunction, hypogonadotropic hypogonadism, and a high mortality rate and is not associated with the *C282Y* mutation

DIFFERENTIAL DIAGNOSIS

- Hepatomegaly due to other causes, eg, fatty liver
- Diabetes mellitus due to other causes, eg, Cushing's syndrome
- Cardiac infiltrative disease due to other causes, eg, amyloidosis, sarcoidosis
- Arthritis due to other causes, eg, rheumatoid arthritis, pseudogout
- Hyperpigmentation due to other causes, eg, hyperbilirubinemia
- Cirrhosis due to other causes

 DIAGNOSIS

LABORATORY TESTS

- Mildly abnormal liver tests [aspartate aminotransferase (AST), alkaline phosphatase], an elevated plasma iron with greater than 50% saturation of the transferrin (after an overnight fast), and an elevated serum ferritin (although a normal iron saturation and normal ferritin does not exclude the diagnosis)
- Testing for *HFE* mutations is indicated in any patient with evidence of iron overload and in siblings of patients with confirmed hemochromatosis

IMAGING STUDIES

- CT and MRI may show changes consistent with iron overload of the liver, but these techniques are not sensitive enough for screening

DIAGNOSTIC PROCEDURES

- The liver biopsy characteristically shows extensive iron deposition in hepatocytes and in bile ducts and the hepatic iron index—hepatic iron content per gram of liver converted to micromoles and divided by the patient's age—is generally greater than 1.9
- In patients who are homozygous for *C282Y*, liver biopsy is often indicated to determine whether cirrhosis is present. Biopsy can be deferred, however, in patients under age 40 in whom the serum ferritin level is <1000 μg/L, serum AST level is normal, and no hepatomegaly is present. The likelihood of cirrhosis is low in these individuals
- Liver biopsy is also indicated when iron overload is suspected even though the patient is not homozygous for *C282Y*

TREATMENT

MEDICATIONS

- The chelating agent deferoxamine is indicated for patients with hemochromatosis and anemia or in those with secondary iron overload due to thalassemia who cannot tolerate phlebotomies. The drug is administered intravenously or subcutaneously in a dose of 20–40 mg/kg/day infused over 24 h and can mobilize 30 mg of iron per day. However, treatment is painful and time consuming

SURGERY

- Liver transplantation for advanced cirrhosis associated with severe iron overload, including hemochromatosis, has been reported to lead to survival rates that are lower than those for other types of liver disease because of cardiac complications and an increased risk of infections

THERAPEUTIC PROCEDURES

- Early diagnosis and treatment in the precirrhotic phase are of great importance
- Avoid foods rich in iron (such as red meat), alcohol, vitamin C, raw shellfish, and supplemental iron
- Treatment consists initially of weekly phlebotomies of 500 mL of blood (about 250 mg of iron), continued for up to 2–3 years to achieve depletion of iron stores. This process is monitored by hematocrit and serum iron determinations. When iron store depletion is achieved (iron saturation <50% and serum ferritin level <50 µg/L), maintenance phlebotomies (every 2–4 months) are continued
- Complications of hemochromatosis—arthropathy, diabetes, heart disease, portal hypertension, and hypopituitarism—also require treatment

 ## OUTCOME

COMPLICATIONS

- Patients are at increased risk of infection with *Vibrio vulnificus, Listeria monocytogenes, Yersinia enterocolitica*, and other siderophilic organisms
- Arthropathy, diabetes, heart disease, portal hypertension, and hypopituitarism
- In patients who develop cirrhosis, there is a 15–20% incidence of hepatocellular carcinoma

PROGNOSIS

- The course of the disease is favorably altered by phlebotomy therapy. In precirrhotic patients, cirrhosis may be prevented
- Cardiac conduction defects and insulin requirements improve with treatment
- In patients with cirrhosis, varices may reverse, and the risk of variceal bleeding declines. However, cirrhotic patients must be monitored for the development of hepatocellular carcinoma

WHEN TO REFER

- All patients should be referred to a hepatologist or hematologist

PREVENTION

- Genetic testing is recommended for all first-degree family members of the proband; children of an affected person (*C282Yγ* homozygote) need to be screened only if the patient's spouse carries the *C282Yγ* or *H63D* mutation
- Screening all white men over age 30 or all adults over age 20 by measurement of the transferrin saturation or possibly the unbound iron-binding capacity has been recommended by some, but the value of screening is uncertain

 ## EVIDENCE

PRACTICE GUIDELINES

- National Guideline Clearinghouse http://www.guideline.gov/summary/summary.aspx?doc_id=3448&nbr=2674&string=hemochromatosis

WEB SITES

- Diseases of the Liver http://cpmcnet.columbia.edu/dept/gi/disliv.html
- Pathology Index http://www-medlib.med.utah.edu/WebPath/LIVEHTML/LIVERIDX.html
- Hepatic Ultrasound Images http://www.sono.nino.ru/english/hepar_en.html
- Liver Tutorials Visualization and Volume Measurement http://everest.radiology.uiowa.edu/nlm/app/livertoc/livertoc.html

INFORMATION FOR PATIENTS

- National Digestive Diseases Information Clearinghouse http://digestive.niddk.nih.gov/ddiseases/pubs/hemochromatosis/index.htm
- Mayo Clinic http://www.mayoclinic.com/invoke.cfm?id=DS00455

REFERENCES

- Bomford A: Genetics of haemochromatosis. Lancet 2002;360:1673.
- Fletcher LM et al: Excess alcohol greatly increases the prevalence of cirrhosis in hereditary hemochromatosis. Gastroenterology 2002;122:281.
- Tavill AS: Diagnosis and management of hemochromatosis. Hepatology 2001;33:1321. [PMID: 11343262]

Lawrence S. Friedman, MD

Hemolytic Uremic Syndrome

 ## KEY FEATURES

ESSENTIALS OF DIAGNOSIS

- Microangiopathic hemolytic anemia
- Thrombocytopenia
- Renal failure
- Elevated serum LDH
- Normal coagulation tests
- Absence of neurological abnormalities

GENERAL CONSIDERATIONS

- Uncommon disorder consisting of microangiopathic hemolytic anemia, thrombocytopenia, and renal failure due to microangiopathy
- Cause is unknown
- Similar to thrombotic thrombocytopenic purpura (TTP) except different vascular beds involved; pathogenesis probably similar; platelet-agglutinating factor found in plasma may be involved
- In children, hemolytic-uremic syndrome (HUS) frequently occurs after diarrheal illness due to shigella, salmonella, *Escherichia coli* strain O157:H7, or viral agents
- In adults, often precipitated by estrogen use or postpartum state
- May occur as delayed complication of autologous bone marrow or stem cell transplantation, or of cyclosporine or tacrolimus as immunosuppression in allogeneic transplantation
- Familial (hereditary) HUS: family members have recurrent episodes over several years

 ## CLINICAL FINDINGS

SYMPTOMS AND SIGNS

- Symptoms of anemia, bleeding, or renal failure
- Renal failure may or may not be oliguric
- No neurological manifestations other than those due to uremia

DIFFERENTIAL DIAGNOSIS

- Disseminated intravascular coagulation
- TTP
- Preeclampsia-eclampsia
- Vasculitis
- Acute glomerulonephritis

 ## DIAGNOSIS

LABORATORY TESTS

- Microangiopathic hemolytic anemia
- Thrombocytopenia, but often less severe than in TTP
- Peripheral blood smear should show striking red blood cell fragmentation
- LDH usually elevated out of proportion to degree of hemolysis, and Coombs test negative
- Coagulation tests normal except elevated fibrin degradation products

DIAGNOSTIC PROCEDURES

- Kidney biopsy shows endothelial hyaline thrombi in afferent arterioles and glomeruli
- Ischemic necrosis in renal cortex may occur with obstruction from intravascular coagulation

Hemolytic Uremic Syndrome

 TREATMENT

THERAPEUTIC PROCEDURES

- Treatment of choice (as in TTP): large-volume plasmapheresis with fresh-frozen replacement (exchange of up to 80 mL/kg), repeated daily until remission is achieved
- In children, HUS is almost always self-limited and requires only conservative management of acute renal failure
- In adults, high rate of permanent renal insufficiency and death without treatment

 OUTCOME

COMPLICATIONS

- Chronic renal insufficiency

PROGNOSIS

- Mortality rate of childhood form is low (<5%)
- Prognosis in adults remains unclear; without effective therapy, up to 40% have died, and 80% have had chronic renal insufficiency
- Early institution of aggressive therapy with plasmapheresis promises to be beneficial
- Survival and correction of hematological abnormalities are the rule, but restoration of renal function requires early treatment

 EVIDENCE

PRACTICE GUIDELINES

- Allford SL et al: Guidelines on the diagnosis and management of the thrombotic microangiopathic haemolytic anaemias. Br J Haematol 2003;120: 556. [PMID: 12588343]
- George JN: How I treat patients with thrombotic thrombocytopenic purpura-hemolytic uremic syndrome. Blood. 2000;96:1223. [PMID: 10942361]
- von Baeyer H: Plasmapheresis in thrombotic microangiopathy-associated syndromes: review of outcome data derived from clinical trials and open studies. Ther Apher 2002;6:320. [PMID: 12164804]

WEB SITES

- Lois Joy Galler Foundation
  http://www.loisjoygaller.org/hus.htm
- National Kidney Foundation
  http://www.kidney.org/general/atoz/content/hemolytic.html
- National Kidney and Urologic Diseases Information Clearinghouse
  http://kidney.niddk.nih.gov/kudiseases/pubs/hemolyticuremic/index.htm

INFORMATION FOR PATIENTS

- MEDLINEplus—Hemolytic uremic syndrome
  http://www.nlm.nih.gov/medlineplus/ency/article/000510.htm
- NORD—Hemolytic uremic syndrome
  http://www.rarediseases.org/search/rdbdetail_abstract.html?disname=Hemolytic%20Uremic%20Syndrome

REFERENCES

- Banatvala N et al: The United States National Prospective Hemolytic Uremic Syndrome Study: microbiologic, serologic, clinical, and epidemiologic findings. J Infect Dis 2001;183:1063. [PMID: 11237831]
- Chandler WL et al: Prothrombotic coagulation abnormalities preceding the hemolytic-uremic syndrome. N Engl J Med 2002;346:23 [PMID: 1177799]

Charles A. Linker, MD

Hemophilia A

 ## KEY FEATURES

ESSENTIALS OF DIAGNOSIS

- X-linked recessive pattern of inheritance with only males affected
- Factor VIII coagulant (VIII:C) activity low
- Factor VIII antigen normal
- Spontaneous hemarthroses

GENERAL CONSIDERATIONS

- Hemophilia A (classic hemophilia, factor VIII deficiency hemophilia) is a hereditary bleeding disorder due to deficiency of coagulation factor VIII (VIII:C)
- Factor VIII coagulant protein usually quantitatively reduced, but defective coagulant protein present by immunoassay in small number of cases
- X-linked recessive disease
- Hemophilia classified as severe if factor VIII:C levels <1%, moderate if 1–5%, and mild if levels >5%
- Families tend to breed true in severity of hemophilia
- Many hemophiliacs acquired HIV infection via factor VIII concentrate; many have developed AIDS
- HIV-associated immune thrombocytopenia may aggravate bleeding tendency

DEMOGRAPHICS

- Most common severe bleeding disorder and second most common congenital bleeding disorder, after von Willebrand's disease
- ~1 in 10,000 males affected
- Rarely, female carriers clinically affected if their normal X chromosomes are disproportionately inactivated
- Females may also be affected if they are offspring of hemophiliac father and carrier mother

 ## CLINICAL FINDINGS

SYMPTOMS AND SIGNS

- Bleeding tendency, with severity in proportion to factor VIII:C levels
- Bleeding only after major trauma or surgery in mild hemophilia
- Bleeding with mild trauma or surgery in moderately severe hemophilia
- Spontaneous bleeding in severe hemophilia
- Bleeding may occur anywhere, but most commonly into joints (knees, ankles, elbows), muscles, and gastrointestinal tract
- Spontaneous hemarthroses virtually diagnostic of hemophilia

DIFFERENTIAL DIAGNOSIS

- Hemophilia B
- von Willebrand's disease
- Disseminated intravascular coagulation
- Heparin administration
- Acquired factor deficiency or inhibitors, eg, paraproteins with anti-VIII or anti-IX activity

 ## DIAGNOSIS

LABORATORY TESTS

- Partial thromboplastin time (PTT) prolonged
- Other coagulation tests, including prothrombin time, bleeding time, and serum fibrinogen level, normal
- Factor VIII:C levels reduced, but measurements of von Willebrand factor are normal
- If plasma from a hemophiliac patient is mixed with normal plasma, PTT becomes normal; failure of PTT to normalize in such a mixing test is diagnostic of factor VIII inhibitor
- Platelet count below normal should raise suspicion of HIV-associated immune thrombocytopenia

TREATMENT

MEDICATIONS

- Infusion of factor VIII concentrates, heat-treated to reduce likelihood of HIV transmission, is standard treatment
- Recombinant factor VIII appears safe and effective, though expensive, and imposes no risk of transmitting HIV or other viruses
- Desired plasma level of factor VIII depends on bleeding severity
  - For minor bleeding, raise factor VIII:C levels to 25% with one infusion
  - For moderate bleeding (eg, deep muscle hematoma), raise level initially to 50% and maintain level >25% with repeated infusion for 2–3 days
  - For major bleeding, raise level to 100% and maintain level >50% continuously for 10–14 days
- Factor VIII concentrate dose is 60 units/kg (~4000 units for 70-kg individual); to raise level to 25% requires 1000 units; half-life of factor VIII:C is ~12 h
- To raise level to 100%, initial dose is 60 units/kg, followed by 30 units/kg Q 12 h; during surgery, verify initial rise in factor VIII levels; if levels fail to rise, suspect presence of factor VIII inhibitor
- Desmopressin, 0.3 mg/kg IV Q 24 h, may be useful in preparing patients with mild hemophilia for minor surgical procedures; causes release of factor VIII:C and raises factor VIII:C levels 2- to 3-fold for several hours
- For persistent bleeding following use of either desmopressin or factor VIII concentrate, use aminocaproic acid (EACA; Amicar), 4 g PO Q 4 h for several days
- Avoid aspirin

THERAPEUTIC PROCEDURES

- Head injuries (with or without neurological signs) are emergently treated as for major bleeding

OUTCOME

COMPLICATIONS

- Arthritis from recurrent joint bleeding
- Hepatitis B and C and HIV infection from recurrent transfusion (decreasing incidence)

PROGNOSIS

- Prognosis markedly improved by availability of factor VIII replacement
- Major limiting factor is disability from recurrent joint bleeding
- Those with hepatitis B or C or HIV have worse prognosis associated with those disorders
- ~15% develop inhibitors to factor VIII and cannot be adequately supported with factor VIII

EVIDENCE

PRACTICE GUIDELINES

- Hay CR: The 2000 United Kingdom Haemophilia Centre Doctors' Organisation (UKHCDO) inhibitor guidelines. Pathophysiol Haemost Thromb 2002;32(Suppl 1):19. [PMID: 12214141]
- Kasper CK: Hemophilia of Georgia, U.S.A. Protocols for the treatment of haemophilia and von Willebrand disease. Haemophilia 2000;6 (Suppl 1):84. [PMID: 10982273]
- United Kingdom Haemophilia Centre Doctors' Organisation: Guidelines on the selection and use of therapeutic products to treat haemophilia and other hereditary bleeding disorders. Haemophilia 2003;9:1. [PMID: 12558775]

WEB SITES

- National Heart, Lung, and Blood Institute http://www.nhlbi.nih.gov/health/public/blood/other/hemophel.htm
- National Hemophilia Foundation (NHF) www.hemophilia.org
- World Federation of Hemophilia http://www.wfh.org/ShowDoc.asp?Rubrique=28&Document=42&IndLangue=2

INFORMATION FOR PATIENTS

- Mayo Clinic—Hemophilia http://www.mayoclinic.com/invoke.cfm?id=DS00218
- MEDLINEplus—Hemophilia A http://www.nlm.nih.gov/medlineplus/ency/article/000538.htm
- National Hemophilia Foundation—Hemophilia A http://www.hemophilia.org/bdi/bdi_types1.htm

REFERENCE

- Mannucci PM et al: The hemophilias—from royal genes to gene therapy. N Engl J Med 2001;344:1773. [PMID: 11396445]

Charles A. Linker, MD

Hemophilia B

 KEY FEATURES

ESSENTIALS OF DIAGNOSIS

- X-linked recessive inheritance, with only males affected
- Factor IX coagulant activity levels low
- Spontaneous hemarthroses

GENERAL CONSIDERATIONS

- Hemophilia B (Christmas disease, factor IX hemophilia) is a hereditary bleeding disorder due to deficiency of coagulation factor IX
- Factor IX is usually quantitatively reduced, but abnormally functioning molecule is detectable immunologically in one-third of cases
- One-seventh as common as hemophilia A (factor VIII deficiency) but otherwise clinically and genetically identical

 CLINICAL FINDINGS

SYMPTOMS AND SIGNS

- Bleeding tendency, with severity in proportion to factor IX levels
- Bleeding only after major trauma or surgery in mild hemophilia
- Bleeding with mild trauma or surgery in moderately severe hemophilia
- Spontaneous bleeding in severe hemophilia
- Bleeding may occur anywhere, but most commonly into joints (knees, ankles, elbows), muscles, and gastrointestinal tract
- Spontaneous hemarthroses virtually diagnostic of hemophilia

DIFFERENTIAL DIAGNOSIS

- Hemophilia A
- vn Willebrand's disease
- Disseminated intravascular coagulation
- Heparin administration
- Acquired factor deficiency or inhibitor, eg, paraproteins with anti-VIII or anti-IX activity

 DIAGNOSIS

LABORATORY TESTS

- Partial thromboplastin time (PTT) prolonged
- Factor IX coagulant activity levels are low when measured by specific factor assays, but measurements of von Willebrand factor are normal
- Other coagulation tests, including prothrombin time, bleeding time, and serum fibrinogen level, normal
- If plasma from hemophiliac patient is mixed with normal plasma, PTT becomes normal; failure of PTT to normalize in such a mixing test is diagnostic of factor IX inhibitor
- Platelet count below normal should raise suspicion of HIV-associated immune thrombocytopenia

TREATMENT

MEDICATIONS

- Infusion of factor IX concentrates, heat treated to reduce likelihood of HIV transmission, is standard treatment
- Factor VIII concentrates are ineffective
- Factor IX concentrate dose is 80 units/kg (approximately 6000 units) to achieve 100% level; half-life is 18 h
- For major surgery, give 80 units/kg initially, followed by 40 units/kg Q 18 h; measure factor IX levels to ensure that expected levels are achieved and that factor IX inhibitor is not present
- Unlike factor VIII concentrates, factor IX concentrates contain other proteins, including activated coagulating factors that appear to contribute to risk of thrombosis with recurrent usage; more care is thus needed in deciding to use these concentrates
- Desmopressin is not useful in hemophilia B
- Avoid aspirin

 OUTCOME

COMPLICATIONS

- Risk of thrombosis with recurrent factor IX concentrate usage

PROGNOSIS

- Prognosis markedly improved by availability of factor IX replacement
- Major limiting factor is disability from recurrent joint bleeding
- Those with hepatitis B or C or HIV have worse prognosis associated with those disorders
- ~2.5% develop inhibitors to factor IX and cannot be adequately supported with factor IX

 EVIDENCE

PRACTICE GUIDELINES

- Hay CR: The 2000 United Kingdom Haemophilia Centre Doctors' Organisation (UKHCDO) inhibitor guidelines. Pathophysiol Haemost Thromb 2002;32(Suppl 1):19. [PMID: 12214141]
- Kasper CK: Hemophilia of Georgia, U.S.A. Protocols for the treatment of haemophilia and von Willebrand disease. Haemophilia 2000;6(Suppl 1):84. [PMID: 10982273]
- United Kingdom Haemophilia Centre Doctors' Organisation: Guidelines on the selection and use of therapeutic products to treat haemophilia and other hereditary bleeding disorders. Haemophilia 2003;9:1. [PMID: 12558775]

WEB SITES

- National Heart, Lung, and Blood Institute http://www.nhlbi.nih.gov/health/public/blood/other/hemophel.htm
- National Hemophilia Foundation (NHF) www.hemophilia.org
- World Federation of Hemophilia http://www.wfh.org/ShowDoc.asp?Rubrique=28&Document=42&IndLangue=2

INFORMATION FOR PATIENTS

- Mayo Clinic—Hemophilia http://www.mayoclinic.com/invoke.cfm?id=DS00218
- MEDLINEplus—Hemophilia B http://www.nlm.nih.gov/medlineplus/ency/article/000539.htm
- National Hemophilia Foundation—Hemophilia B http://www.hemophilia.org/bdi/bdi_types2.htm

REFERENCE

- Roth DA et al: Human recombinant factor IX: safety and efficacy studies in hemophilia B patients previously treated with plasma-derived factor IX concentrates. Blood 2001;98:3600. [PMID: 11739163]

Charles A. Linker, MD

Hemorrhoids

 KEY FEATURES

ESSENTIALS OF DIAGNOSIS

- Bright red blood per rectum
- Protrusion, discomfort
- Characteristic findings on external anal inspection and anoscopy

GENERAL CONSIDERATIONS

- Internal hemorrhoids are a plexus of superior hemorrhoidal veins located above the dentate line that are covered by mucosa
- External hemorrhoids arise from the inferior hemorrhoidal veins located below the dentate line and are covered with squamous epithelium of the anal canal or perianal region
- Causes include straining at stool, constipation, prolonged sitting, pregnancy, obesity, and low-fiber diet

DEMOGRAPHICS

- Prevalence increases with age
- Increased incidence with constipation with straining
- Pregnancy
- Weight-lifters

 CLINICAL FINDINGS

SYMPTOMS AND SIGNS

- Bright red blood per rectum, streaks of blood visible on toilet paper or stool to bright red blood that drips
- Rarely severe enough to result in anemia
- Mucoid discharge
- Internal hemorrhoids may gradually enlarge and protrude
- Discomfort and pain are unusual, occurring only with internal hemorrhoids when there is extensive inflammation and thrombosis of irreducible tissue, or with thrombosis of an external hemorrhoid
- External hemorrhoids readily visible on perianal inspection, or may protrude through the anus with gentle straining
- Prolapsed hemorrhoids appear as protuberant purple nodules covered by mucosa
- Thrombosed external hemorrhoid appears as an exquisitely painful, tense and bluish perianal nodule covered with skin that may be up to several centimeters in size

DIFFERENTIAL DIAGNOSIS

- Rectal prolapse
- Anal fissure
- Anal skin tag
- Perianal fistula or abscess, eg, Crohn's disease
- Infectious proctitis, eg, gonorrhea
- Anogenital warts (condyloma acuminata)
- Pruritus ani
- Proctalgia fugax or levator ani syndrome
- Lower gastrointestinal bleeding due to other cause, eg, diverticulosis, polyps, colorectal cancer

 DIAGNOSIS

DIAGNOSTIC PROCEDURES

- Anoscopy: visualization of internal hemorrhoids
- Grading
  - I. No prolapse
  - II. Prolapse with defecation spontaneously reduces
  - III. Prolapse with defecation or other times; requires manual reduction
  - IV. Permanently prolapsed mucosal tissue; visible externally

Hemorrhoids

 ## TREATMENT

SURGERY

- Surgical excision (hemorrhoidectomy) for patients with Grade IV hemorrhoids with persistent bleeding or discomfort

THERAPEUTIC PROCEDURES

- Injection sclerotherapy for symptomatic Grade I–II hemorrhoids
- Rubber band ligation for symptomatic Grade II–III hemorrhoids

Conservative measures

- High-fiber diet
- Increase fluid intake
- Application of a cotton ball tucked next to the anal opening after bowel movements for mucoid discharge
- Symptomatic relief of prolapsed hemorrhoids by suppositories (eg, Anusol with or without hydrocortisone)
- Warm sitz baths

Thrombosed external hemorrhoid

- Warm sitz baths
- Analgesics
- Ointments
- Incision to remove the clot may hasten symptomatic relief

 ## OUTCOME

FOLLOW-UP

- Bleeding usually subsides after 1–3 sessions of sclerotherapy or band ligation

COMPLICATIONS

- Sclerotherapy or rubber band ligation rarely complicated by bleeding or life-threatening pelvic cellulitis; early signs are worsening anal pain radiating to legs, or difficulty with urination

PROGNOSIS

- Recurrence is common after injection sclerosis or banding

WHEN TO REFER

- Refer to surgeon or gastroenterologist for injection sclerosis, banding, or hemorrhoidectomy

WHEN TO ADMIT

- Severe bleeding with anemia (rare)
- Incarcerated, thrombosed Grade IV internal hemorrhoids
- Pelvic cellulitis after banding or sclerotherapy

PREVENTION

- High-fiber diet
- Stool softeners to prevent straining at stool

 ## EVIDENCE

PRACTICE GUIDELINES

- Alonso-Coello P et al: Office evaluation and treatment of hemorrhoids. J Fam Pract 2003;52:366. [PMID: 12737769]
- MacRae HM et al: Comparison of hemorrhoidal treatments: a meta-analysis. Can J Surg 1997;40:14. [PMID: 9030078]
- Practice parameters for the treatment of hemorrhoids. The Standards Task Force American Society of Colon and Rectal Surgeons. Dis Colon Rectum 1993; 36:1118. [PMID: 8253007]
- Surgical management of hemorrhoids. Society for Surgery of the Alimentary Tract, Inc., 2000 http://www.ssat.com/cgi-bin/hemorr.cgi?affiliation=student

WEB SITES

- American Academy of Family Physicians—Hemorrhoids: reducing the pain and discomfort http://familydoctor.org/healthfacts/090/
- NIH Patient Education Institute—Hemorrhoid surgery http://www.nlm.nih.gov/medlineplus/tutorials/hemorrhoidsurgery.html

INFORMATION FOR PATIENTS

- Mayo Clinic—Hemorrhoids http://www.mayoclinic.com/invoke.cfm?objectid=37177394-6BD1-4401-AB747238D2AEBD84
- MEDLINEplus—Hemorrhoids http://www.nlm.nih.gov/medlineplus/ency/article/000292.htm

REFERENCES

- Berkelhammer C et al: Retroflexed endoscopic band ligation of bleeding internal hemorrhoids. Gastrointest Endosc 2002;55:532. [PMID: 11923767]
- Sardinha T et al: Hemorrhoids. Surg Clin North Am 2002;82:1153. [PMID: 12516845]

Kenneth R. McQuaid, MD

Hepatic Encephalopathy

 KEY FEATURES

ESSENTIALS OF DIAGNOSIS

- Stage 1: mild confusion, somnolence
- Stage 2: confusion
- Stage 3: stupor
- Stage 4: coma

GENERAL CONSIDERATIONS

- A state of disordered central nervous system function resulting from failure of the liver to detoxify noxious agents of gut origin because of hepatocellular dysfunction and portosystemic shunting
- Ammonia is the most readily identified toxin but is not solely responsible for the disturbed mental status
- Gastrointestinal bleeding can increase the protein in the bowel and rapidly precipitate encephalopathy. Other precipitants include constipation, alkalosis, potassium deficiency induced by diuretics, opioids, hypnotics, and sedatives; medications containing ammonium or amino compounds; paracentesis with attendant hypovolemia; hepatic or systemic infection; and portosystemic shunts (including transjugular intrahepatic portosystemic shunts)

DEMOGRAPHICS

- Alcoholic liver disease is the most common etiology of cirrhosis

 CLINICAL FINDINGS

SYMPTOMS AND SIGNS

- Metabolic encephalopathy characterized by day–night reversal, asterixis, tremor, dysarthria, delirium, drowsiness, and ultimately coma
- Symptoms occur late in liver disease except when precipitated by an acute hepatocellular insult or an episode of gastrointestinal bleeding
- Clinical diagnosis supported by asterixis, elevated serum ammonia with exclusion of other causes of delerium

DIFFERENTIAL DIAGNOSIS

- Metabolic encephalopathy, especially hyponatremia, hypoglycemia, or renal failure
- Central nervous system infection
- Altered mental status from medication effects, particularly if they are hepatically metabolized

 DIAGNOSIS

LABORATORY TESTS

- Liver function tests of advanced liver disease
- Serum and cerebrospinal fluid ammonia level is generally elevated

TREATMENT

MEDICATIONS

- Control gastrointestinal bleeding and purge blood from the gastrointestinal tract. This can be accomplished with 120 mL of magnesium citrate by mouth or nasogastric tube every 3–4 h until the stool is free of gross blood, or by administration of lactulose
- The initial dose of lactulose is 30 mL orally three or four times daily. Titrate the dose so that two or three soft stools per day are produced. When rectal use is indicated because of the patient's inability to take medicines orally, the dose is 300 mL of lactulose in 700 mL of saline or sorbitol as a retention enema for 30–60 min; it may be repeated every 4–6 h
- The ammonia-producing intestinal flora may also be controlled with neomycin sulfate, 0.5–1 g orally every 6 or 12 h for 7 days. Side effects of neomycin include diarrhea, malabsorption, superinfection, ototoxicity, and nephrotoxicity, usually only after prolonged use. Alternative antibiotics are vancomycin, 1 g orally twice daily, or metronidazole, 250 mg orally three times daily. Patients who do not respond to lactulose alone may improve with a 1-week course of an antibiotic in addition to lactulose
- Avoid opioids, tranquilizers, and sedatives metabolized or excreted by the liver
- If agitation is marked, oxazepam, 10–30 mg, which is not metabolized by the liver, may be given cautiously by mouth or by nasogastric tube
- Correct zinc deficiency, if present, with oral zinc sulfate, 600 mg/day in divided doses. Eradication of *Helicobacter pylori*, which generates ammonia in the stomach, may improve encephalopathy
- Sodium benzoate, 10 g daily, and ornithine aspartate, 9 g three times daily, may lower blood ammonia levels, but less is known about these drugs than lactulose
- Flumazenil is effective in about 30% of severe hepatic encephalopathy, but the drug is short-acting and intravenous administration is required

THERAPEUTIC PROCEDURES

- Withhold dietary protein during acute episodes
- When the patient resumes oral intake, protein intake is started at 20 g/day and increased by 10 g every 3–5 days to 60–80 g/day as tolerated, and vegetable protein is better tolerated than meat protein
- Use of special dietary supplements enriched with branched-chain amino acids is usually unnecessary except in occasional patients who are intolerant of standard protein supplements

OUTCOME

COMPLICATIONS

- Hypernatremia can develop from intensive lactulose use

WHEN TO ADMIT

- Inability to care for self or follow medical instructions

EVIDENCE

PRACTICE GUIDELINES

- Blei AT et al: Hepatic encephalopathy. Am J Gastrtoenterol 2001; 96:1968 [PMID: 11467622]

WEB SITES

- Acute Liver Failure: Case study http://path.upmc.edu/cases/case21.html
- Diseases of the Liver http://cpmcnet.columbia.edu/dept/gi/disliv.html
- Pathology Index http://www-medlib.med.utah.edu/WebPath/LIVEHTML/LIVERIDX.html
- Hepatic Ultrasound Images http://www.sono.nino.ru/english/hepar_en.html
- Liver Tutorials Visualization and Volume Measurement http://everest.radiology.uiowa.edu/nlm/app/livertoc/livertoc.html

INFORMATION FOR PATIENTS

- National Institutes of Health http://www.nlm.nih.gov/medlineplus/ency/article/000302.htm
- National Institute of Neurological Disorders and Stroke http://www.ninds.nih.gov/health_and_medical/disorders/ encephalopathy.htm

REFERENCES

- Butterworth RF: Complications of cirrhosis III. Hepatic encephalopathy. J Hepatol 2000:32:171. [PMID: 10728803]
- Ong JP: Correlation between ammonia levels and the severity of hepatic encephalopathy. Am J Med 2003;114:188.

Lawrence S. Friedman, MD

Hepatic Failure, Acute

 KEY FEATURES

ESSENTIALS OF DIAGNOSIS

- May be fulminant or subfulminant and both carry an equally poor prognosis
- Acetaminophen and idiosyncratic drug reactions are the most common causes

GENERAL CONSIDERATIONS

- In fulminant hepatic failure, encephalopathy and coagulopathy develop within 8 weeks after the onset of acute liver disease
- Subfulminant hepatic failure occurs when encephalopathy and coagulopathy appear between 8 weeks and 6 months after the onset of acute liver disease
- Acetaminophen toxicity accounts for 40% of cases. Idiosyncratic drug reactions are second
- In acute hepatic failure due to hepatitis or drug toxicity, extensive necrosis of the liver gives a typical pathological picture of acute liver atrophy

ETIOLOGY

- Acetaminophen toxicity
- Idiosyncratic drug reactions
- Poisonous mushrooms
- Viral hepatitis
- Shock
- Hyper- or hypothermia
- Budd-Chiari syndrome
- Malignancy (especially lymphomas)
- Wilson's disease
- Reye's syndrome
- Fatty liver of pregnancy and other disorders of fatty acid oxidation
- Parvovirus B19 infection

DEMOGRAPHICS

- Most cases of acute hepatic failure in the United States are caused by acute viral hepatitis, especially hepatitis B. Most of the remainder are due to hepatitis A or unknown (non-ABCDE) viruses
- In endemic areas, hepatitis D and hepatitis E cause acute hepatic failure
- Hepatitis C is a rare cause of acute hepatic failure; acute hepatitis A or B superimposed on chronic hepatitis C has a high risk of fulminant hepatitis

 CLINICAL FINDINGS

SYMPTOMS AND SIGNS

- Jaundice may be absent or minimal early
- Hepatic encephalopathy
- Coagulopathy
- Ultimately symptoms and signs of increased intracranial pressure may develop
- High risk of infection, especially with gram-positive organisms

 DIAGNOSIS

LABORATORY TESTS

- Severe hepatocellular damage (Table 57, page 1254)
- Coagulopathy
- Elevated serum ammonia
- Low factor V levels (correlate with outcome)
- In acute hepatic failure due to microvesicular steatosis (eg, Reye's syndrome), serum aminotransferase elevations may be modest (<300 units/L)

IMAGING STUDIES

- Head CT can help rule out or detect cerebral edema

460

TREATMENT

MEDICATIONS

- Prophylactic antibiotic therapy decreases the risk of infection, observed in up to 90%, but has no effect on survival and is not routinely recommended
- For suspected sepsis, broad coverage is indicated. The most frequent isolates are *Staphylococcus aureus*, *Streptococcus* species, coliforms, and, later in the course, *Candida* species
- Early administration of acetylcysteine (140 mg/kg orally followed by 70 mg/kg orally every 4 h for an additional 17 doses) is indicated for acetaminophen toxicity and improves cerebral blood flow and oxygenation in fulminant hepatic failure due to any cause. (Acetylcysteine treatment can prolong the prothrombin time leading to the erroneous perception that liver failure is worsening)
- Mannitol, 100–200 mL of a 20% solution by intravenous infusion over 10 min, may decrease cerebral edema but should be used with caution in renal failure
- The value of hyperventilation, intravenous prostaglandin E_1, and hypothermia is uncertain. Indeed, patients may already be hypothermic

SURGERY

- Early transfer to a liver transplantation center is essential

THERAPEUTIC PROCEDURES

- The treatment is directed toward correcting metabolic abnormalities. These include coagulation defects; electrolyte and acid–base disturbances; renal failure; hypoglycemia; and encephalopathy
- Hepatic-assist devices using living hepatocytes, extracorporeal whole liver perfusion, hepatocyte transplantation, and liver xenografts have shown promise. The artificial system undergoing the most extensive evaluation in the United States is the Molecular Adsorbents Recirculating System (MARS), which is based on extracorporeal albumin dialysis

OUTCOME

FOLLOW-UP

- Extradural sensors are placed to monitor intracranial pressure for impending cerebral edema
- Monitor for disseminated intravascular coagulopathy
- Monitor renal function, acid–base status

PROGNOSIS

- The mortality rate of fulminant hepatitis with severe encephalopathy is as high as 80%. The outlook is especially poor in patients younger than 10 and older than 40 years of age and in those with an idiosyncratic drug reaction
- Other adverse prognostic factors are a serum bilirubin level >18 mg/dL, INR >6.5, onset of encephalopathy more than 7 days after the onset of jaundice, and a low factor V level (<20% of normal)
- For acetaminophen-induced fulminant hepatic failure, indicators of a poor outcome (which is less common than for other causes) are acidosis (pH <7.3), INR >6.5, and azotemia (serum creatinine ≥3.4 mg/dL)
- Hyperphosphatemia (>1.2 mmol/L) and an elevated blood lactate level (>3.5 mmol/L) also predict poor survival
- Emergency liver transplantation is considered for patients with stage II to stage III encephalopathy and is associated with an 80% survival rate at 1 year. Compared with chronic hepatitis B, liver transplantation for fulminant hepatitis B is less likely to result in reinfection of the graft with hepatitis B virus

WHEN TO REFER

- Refer to a liver transplantation center early

WHEN TO ADMIT

- Any patient with acute liver disease and encephalopathy

EVIDENCE

PRACTICE GUIDELINES

- National Guideline Clearinghouse http://www.guideline.gov/summary/summary.aspx?doc_id=3449&nbr=2675&string=acute+hepatic+failure

WEB SITES

- Acute Liver Failure: Case study http://path.upmc.edu/cases/case21.html
- Diseases of the Liver http://cpmcnet.columbia.edu/dept/gi/disliv.html
- Pathology Index http://www-medlib.med.utah.edu/WebPath/LIVEHTML/LIVERIDX.html
- Hepatic Ultrasound Images http://www.sono.nino.ru/english/hepar_en.html
- Liver Tutorials Visualization and Volume Measurement http://everest.radiology.uiowa.edu/nlm/app/livertoc/livertoc.html

INFORMATION FOR PATIENTS

- American Liver Foundation http://www.liverfoundation.org/cgi-bin/dbs/articles.cgi?db=articles&uid=default&ID=1056&view_records=1
- National Institutes of Health http://www.nlm.nih.gov/medlineplus/ency/presentations/100090_1.htm

REFERENCES

- Ostapowizc G et al: Results of a prospective study of acute liver failure at 17 tertiary care centers in the United States. Ann Intern Med 2002;137:947.
- Rajvanshi P et al: Temporary support for acute liver failure. J Clin Gastroenterol 2002;35:335.

Lawrence S. Friedman, MD

Hepatic Vein Obstruction (Budd-Chiari Syndrome)

 KEY FEATURES

ESSENTIALS OF DIAGNOSIS

- Right upper quadrant pain and tenderness
- Ascites
- Imaging study showing occlusion/absence of flow in the hepatic vein(s) or inferior vena cava
- Similar picture in venoocclusive disease but major hepatic veins are patent

GENERAL CONSIDERATIONS

- Occlusion of the hepatic veins may occur from a variety of causes
- Percutaneous liver biopsy frequently shows a characteristic centrilobular congestion
- Some cytotoxic agents and pyrrolizidine alkaloids ("bush teas") may cause hepatic venoocclusive disease (occlusion of terminal venules), which mimics Budd-Chiari syndrome clinically
- Venoocclusive disease is common in patients who have undergone bone marrow transplantation, particularly those with pretransplant aminotransferase elevations or fever during cytoreductive therapy with cyclophosphamide, azathioprine, carmustine, busulfan, or etoposide or those receiving high-dose cytoreductive therapy or high-dose total body irradiation
- In India, China, and South Africa, Budd-Chiari syndrome is often the result of occlusion of the hepatic portion of the inferior vena cava, presumably due to prior thrombosis, and the clinical presentation is mild but the course is frequently complicated by hepatocellular carcinoma

Etiologies

- Caval webs
- Myeloproliferative disease, eg, polycythemia vera
- Right-sided congestive heart failure (CHF) or constrictive pericarditis
- Neoplasm compressing hepatic vein
- Paroxysmal nocturnal hemoglobinuria
- Behçet's syndrome
- Oral contraceptives or pregnancy
- Hypercoagulable state
- Post-bone-marrow transplant
- "Bush teas" (pyrrolizidine alkaloids)

 CLINICAL FINDINGS

SYMPTOMS AND SIGNS

- Tender, painful hepatic enlargement
- Jaundice; splenomegaly; and ascites
- With advanced disease, bleeding varices and hepatic coma may be evident
- Hepatopulmonary syndrome may occur

DIFFERENTIAL DIAGNOSIS

- Cholecystitis
- Shock liver
- Cirrhosis
- Hepatic congestion from right-sided CHF
- Metastatic cancer involving the liver

 DIAGNOSIS

LABORATORY TESTS

- Liver function test abnormalities are nonspecific
- Jaudice may or may not be present
- Very high alanine aminotransferase/aspartate aminotransferase (ALT/AST) (>1000) suggests occlusion of hepatic and portal veins
- Signs of decompensated liver disease (low albumin, coagulopathy) indicate poor prognosis

IMAGING STUDIES

- Hepatic imaging studies may show a prominent caudate lobe, since its venous drainage may not be occluded
- The screening test of choice is duplex Doppler ultrasonography, which has a sensitivity of 85% for detecting evidence of hepatic venous or inferior vena caval thrombosis
- Caval venography can delineate caval webs and occluded hepatic veins

TREATMENT

MEDICATIONS

- Lifelong anticoagulation and treatment of the underlying myeloproliferative disease is often required; antiplatelet therapy with aspirin and hydroxyurea may be an alternative to coumadin in myeloproliferative disorders

SURGERY

- Surgical decompression (side-to-side portacaval, mesocaval, or mesoatrial shunt) of the congested liver may be required to relieve persistent hepatic congestion
- Consider liver transplantation for cirrhosis

THERAPEUTIC PROCEDURES

- Treat ascites with fluid and salt restriction and diuretics (see *Ascites*)
- Treatable causes of Budd-Chiari syndrome should be sought
- Prompt recognition and treatment of an underlying hematological disorder may avoid the need for surgery
- Rarely, thrombolytic therapy may be attempted within 2 weeks of acute hepatic vein thrombosis
- In some cases, placement of a transjugular intrahepatic portosystemic shunt (TIPS) may be feasible, although late TIPS dysfunction is common
- Balloon angioplasty, in some cases with placement of an intravascular metallic stent, is preferred in inferior vena caval web and may be feasible when there is a short segment of thrombosis in the hepatic vein

 ## OUTCOME

COMPLICATIONS

- Liver failure
- Cirrhosis
- Spontaneous bacterial peritonitis (less common than in cirrhosis alone)

 ## EVIDENCE

WEB SITES

- Diseases of the Liver
  http://cpmcnet.columbia.edu/dept/gi/disliv.html
- Pathology Index
  http://www-medlib.med.utah.edu/WebPath/LIVEHTML/LIVERIDX.html

INFORMATION FOR PATIENTS

- National Institutes of Health
  http://www.nlm.nih.gov/medlineplus/ency/article/000239.htm
- American Liver Foundation
  http://www.liverfoundation.org/cgi-bin/dbs/articles.cgi?db=articles&uid=default&ID=1004&view_records=1

REFERENCE

- DeLeve LD et al: Toxic injury to hepatic sinusoids: sinusoidal obstruction syndrome (veno-occlusive disease). Semin Liver Dis 2002;22:27.

Lawrence S. Friedman, MD

Hepatitis A

KEY FEATURES

ESSENTIALS OF DIAGNOSIS

- Prodrome of anorexia, nausea, vomiting, malaise, aversion to smoking
- Fever, enlarged and tender liver, jaundice
- Normal to low white blood cell count; abnormal liver tests, especially markedly elevated aminotransferases
- Hepatitis can be caused by many drugs, toxic agents and viruses, and the clinical manifestations may be similar

GENERAL CONSIDERATIONS

- Transmission of hepatitis A virus (HAV) is by the fecal-oral route. The incubation period averages 30 days
- HAV is excreted in feces for up to 2 weeks before the clinical illness and rarely persists in feces after the first week of illness
- Chronic hepatitis A does not occur, and there is no carrier state

DEMOGRAPHICS

- HAV spread is favored by crowding and poor sanitation
- Common source outbreaks result from contaminated water or food

CLINICAL FINDINGS

SYMPTOMS AND SIGNS

Prodromal phase

- Onset may be abrupt or insidious, with general malaise, myalgia, arthralgia, easy fatigability, upper respiratory symptoms, and anorexia
- A distaste for smoking, paralleling anorexia, may occur early
- Nausea and vomiting are frequent, and diarrhea or constipation may occur
- Defervescence and a fall in pulse rate often coincide with the onset of jaundice
- Abdominal pain is usually mild and constant in the right upper quadrant or epigastrium, often aggravated by jarring or exertion, and rarely may be severe enough to simulate cholecystitis

Icteric phase

- Jaundice occurs after 5–10 days but may appear at the same time as the initial symptoms. Most never develop it
- With the onset of jaundice, there is often worsening of the prodromal symp-

toms, followed by progressive clinical improvement
- HAV is the only viral hepatitis that may be associated with spiking fevers
- Hepatomegaly—rarely marked—is present in over half of cases. Liver tenderness is usually present
- Splenomegaly is reported in 15% of patients, and soft, enlarged lymph nodes—especially in the cervical or epitrochlear areas—may occur

Convalescent phase

- There is an increasing sense of well-being and disappearance of symptoms

Course

- The acute illness usually subsides over 2–3 weeks with complete clinical and laboratory recovery by 9 weeks
- Clinical, biochemical, and serological recovery may be followed by one or two relapses, but recovery is the rule
- A protracted course has been reported to be associated with HLA *DRB1*1301*

DIFFERENTIAL DIAGNOSIS

- Hepatitis B, C, D (delta agent), E virus (an enterically transmitted hepatitis seen in epidemic form in Asia, North Africa, and Mexico)
- Hepatitis G virus (HGV) applies to an agent that rarely, if ever, causes frank hepatitis. Unidentified agents account for a small percentage of cases of apparent acute viral hepatitis
- A DNA virus designated the TT virus (TTV) is in up to 7.5% of blood donors and is readily transmitted by blood transfusions, but an association between this virus and liver disease has not been established. A related virus known as SEN-V has been found in 2% of U.S. blood donors, is transmitted by transfusion, and may account for some cases of transfusion-associated non-ABCDE hepatitis
- In immunocompromised and rare immunocompetent hosts, consider cytomegalovirus, Epstein–Barr virus, and herpes simplex virus

DIAGNOSIS

LABORATORY TESTS

- See Figure 3 (page 1255)
- Antibody to hepatitis A (anti-HAV) appears early in the course of the illness. Both IgM and IgG anti-HAV are detectable in serum soon after the onset
- Peak titers of IgM anti-HAV occur during the first week of clinical disease and disappear within 3–6 months
- Detection of IgM anti-HAV is an excellent test for diagnosing acute hepatitis A
- Titers of IgG anti-HAV peak after 1 month of the disease and may persist for years
- IgG anti-HAV indicates previous exposure to HAV, noninfectivity, and immunity. In the United States, about 30% of the population have serological evidence of previous infection
- The white blood cell count is normal to low, especially in the preicteric phase. Large atypical lymphocytes may occasionally be seen
- Mild proteinuria is common, and bilirubinuria often precedes the appearance of jaundice. Acholic stools are often present during the icteric phase
- Strikingly elevated aspartate or alanine aminotransferases occur early, followed by elevations of bilirubin and alkaline phosphatase; in a minority of patients, the latter persist after aminotransferase levels have normalized
- Cholestasis is occasionally marked

TREATMENT

MEDICATIONS

- If nausea and vomiting are pronounced or if oral intake is substantially decreased, intravenous 10% glucose is indicated
- Small doses of oxazepam are safe, as metabolism is not hepatic; morphine sulfate is avoided
- Corticosteroids have no benefit

THERAPEUTIC PROCEDURES

- Bed rest is recommended only for marked symptoms
- Dietary management consists of palatable meals as tolerated, without overfeeding; breakfast is usually best tolerated. Strenuous physical exertion, alcohol, and hepatotoxic agents are avoided

OUTCOME

COMPLICATIONS

- Fulminant hepatitis A is uncommon; it occurs rarely where hepatitis A occurs in chronic hepatitis C

PROGNOSIS

- In the majority, clinical recovery is complete in 3–6 weeks
- HAV does not cause chronic liver disease, though it may persist for up to 1 year, and clinical and biochemical relapses may occur before full recovery. The mortality rate is less than 0.2%

WHEN TO ADMIT

- Intractable nausea and vomiting and need for parenteral fluids
- Severe coagulopathy (eg, prothrombin time >28 s)
- Encephalopathy

PREVENTION

- Strict isolation is not necessary, but hand washing after bowel movements is required. Thorough hand washing by anyone who may contact contaminated utensils, bedding, or clothing is essential

Immune globulin

- Give immune globulin to all *close* (eg, household) personal contacts. The recommended dose, 0.02 mL/kg intramuscularly, is protective if administered during incubation

Vaccination

- Two effective inactivated hepatitis A vaccines are recommended for persons living in or traveling to endemic areas (including military personnel), patients with chronic liver disease on diagnosis, persons with clotting-factor disorders who are treated with concentrates, homosexual and bisexual men, animal handlers, illicit drug users, sewage workers, food handlers, and children and caregivers in day care centers and institutions
- Routine vaccination of all children has been recommended in states with a high incidence of hepatitis A
- HAV vaccine is effective in the prevention of secondary spread to household contacts of primary cases
- The recommended dose for adults is 1 mL (1440 ELISA units) of Havrix (GlaxoSmithKline) or 0.5 mL (50 units) of Vaqta (Merck) intramuscularly, followed by a booster dose at 6–12 months. A combined hepatitis A and B vaccine (Twinrix, GlaxoSmithKline) is available

EVIDENCE

PRACTICE GUIDELINES

- National Guideline Clearinghouse http://www.guideline.gov/summary/summary.aspx?doc_id=3454&nbr=2680&string=hepatitis http://www.guideline.gov/summary/summary.aspx?doc_id=2139&nbr=1365&string=hepatitis

WEB SITES

- Viral Hepatitis http://www.cdc.gov/ncidod/diseases/hepatitis/index.htm
- Hepatitis Information Network http://www.hepnet.com/

INFORMATION FOR PATIENTS

- National Digestive Diseases Information Clearinghouse http://digestive.niddk.nih.gov/ddiseases/pubs/viralhepatitis/index.htm
- Centers for Disease Control http://www.cdc.gov/ncidod/diseases/hepatitis/a/faqa.htm

REFERENCE

- Koff RS: Hepatitis A, hepatitis B, and combination hepatitis vaccines for immunoprophylaxis. Dig Dis Sci 2002;47:1183.

Lawrence S. Friedman, MD

Hepatitis B, Acute

 KEY FEATURES

ESSENTIALS OF DIAGNOSIS

- Prodrome of anorexia, nausea, vomiting, malaise, aversion to smoking
- Fever, tender hapatomegaly, jaundice
- Normal to low white blood cell count; abnormal liver tests, markedly elevated aminotransferases early in the course
- Liver biopsy shows hepatocellular necrosis and mononuclear infiltrate but is rarely indicated

GENERAL CONSIDERATIONS

- Hepatitis B virus (HBV) contains an inner core protein (hepatitis B core antigen, HBcAg) and outer surface coat (hepatitis B surface antigen, HBsAg)
- The incubation period is 6 weeks to 6 months (average 3 months)
- The onset of HBV is more insidious and the aminotransferase levels higher than in hepatitis A virus (HAV) infection
- Hepatitis can be caused by many drugs, toxic agents, and viruses, the clinical manifestations of which may be similar

DEMOGRAPHICS

- HBV is usually transmitted by infected blood or blood products or by sexual contact and is present in saliva, semen, and vaginal secretions
- HBsAg-positive mothers may transmit HBV at delivery; the risk of chronic infection in the infant approaches 90%
- HBV is prevalent in homosexuals and intravenous drug users, but most cases result from heterosexual transmission; the incidence has decreased by 75% since the 1980s
- Groups at risk include patients and staff at hemodialysis centers, physicians, dentists, nurses, and personnel working in clinical and pathology laboratories and blood banks
- The risk of HBV infection from a blood transfusion is less than one in 60,000 units transfused in the United States

 CLINICAL FINDINGS

SYMPTOMS AND SIGNS

Prodromal phase

- The onset may be abrupt or insidious, with malaise, myalgia, arthralgia, fatigability, upper respiratory symptoms, anorexia, and a distaste for smoking
- Nausea and vomiting, diarrhea or constipation
- Low-grade fever is generally present serum sickness may be seen
- Abdominal pain is usually mild and constant in the right upper quadrant or epigastrium
- Defervescence and a fall in pulse rate coincide with the onset of jaundice

Icteric phase

- Jaundice occurs after 5–10 days but may appear at the same time as the initial symptoms. Most never develop it
- Often worsening of the prodromal symptoms, followed by progressive clinical improvement

Convalescent phase

- Progressive sense of well-being

Course of illness

- The acute illness usually subsides over 2–3 weeks with complete clinical and laboratory recovery by 16 weeks
- In 5–10% of cases, the course may be more protracted, but less than 1% will have a fulminant course. Hepatitis B may become chronic

DIFFERENTIAL DIAGNOSIS

- Acute and chronic hepatitis ACDE
- Hepatitis G virus (HGV) rarely, if ever, causes frank hepatitis
- The TT virus (TTV), a DNA virus, is in about 8% of blood donors and is readily transmitted by blood transfusions, but an association with liver disease is not established. A related virus, SEN-V, has been found in 2% of U.S. blood donors, is transmitted by transfusion, and may account for some cases of transfusion-associated non-ABCDE hepatitis
- In immunocompromised and rare immunocompetent hosts, consider cytomegalovirus, Epstein–Barr virus, and herpes simplex virus

 DIAGNOSIS

LABORATORY TESTS

- See Figure 5 (page 1255) and Table 58 (page 1254)

HBsAg

- HBsAg appears before biochemical evidence of liver disease, and persists throughout the clinical illness; after the acute illness may be associated with chronic hepatitis
- HBsAg establishes infection with HBV and implies infectivity

Anti-HBs

- Specific antibody to HBsAg (anti-HBs) appears after clearance of HBsAg and after successful vaccination against hepatitis B
- Disappearance of HBsAg and the appearance of anti-HBs signals recovery from HBV infection, noninfectivity, and immunity

Anti-HBc

- IgM anti-HBc appears shortly after HBsAg is detected. (HBcAg alone does not appear in serum)
- Its presence in acute hepatitis indicates a diagnosis of acute hepatitis B, and it fills the serological gap when HbsAg has cleared but anti-HBs is not yet detectable; it can persist for 6 months or more and reappear during flares of chronic hepatitis B
- IgG anti-HBc also appears during acute hepatitis B but persists indefinitely
- In asymptomatic blood donors, an isolated anti-HBc with no other positive HBV serological results may represent a falsely positive result or latent infection; HBV DNA is detectable only by PCR

HBeAg

- HBeAg is found only in HBsAg-positive serum
- HBeAg indicates viral replication and infectivity
- Persistence of HBeAg in serum beyond 3 months indicates an increased likelihood of chronic hepatitis B
- Its disappearance is often followed by the appearance of anti-HBe, signifying diminished viral replication and decreased infectivity

HBV DNA

- HBV DNA in serum generally parallels the presence of HBeAg, though HBV DNA is a more sensitive and precise marker of viral replication and infectivity
- Very low levels of HBV DNA, detectable only by PCR, may persist in serum after recovery from acute hepatitis B, but the HBV DNA is bound to IgG and is rarely infectious
- Normal to low white blood cell count and large atypical lymphocytes
- Mild proteinuria is common, and bilirubinuria often precedes the appearance of jaundice. Elevated aspartate or alanine aminotransferase occurs early, followed by elevations of bilirubin and alkaline phosphatase
- Marked prolongation of the prothrombin time in severe hepatitis correlates with increased mortality

 ## TREATMENT

MEDICATIONS

- If nausea and vomiting are pronounced or oral intake is substantially decreased, give 10% glucose IV
- Small doses of oxazepam are safe, as metabolism is not hepatic; morphine sulfate is avoided
- Corticosteroids have no benefit

THERAPEUTIC PROCEDURES

- Bed rest only for severe symptoms
- Dietary management consists of palatable meals as tolerated, without overfeeding
- Strenuous physical exertion, alcohol, and hepatotoxic agents are avoided

 ## OUTCOME

COMPLICATIONS

- See *Hepatic failure, acute*
- See *Hepatitis B, chronic*

PROGNOSIS

- The risk of fulminant hepatitis is less than 1%, with a 60% mortality rate
- Following acute hepatitis B, HBV infection persists in 1–2% of immunocompetent hosts but is higher in immunocompromised hosts
- Chronic hepatitis B, particularly when HBV infection is acquired early in life and viral replication persists, confers a substantial risk of cirrhosis and hepatocellular carcinoma (up to 25–40%). Men are more at risk
- HBV may be associated with serum sickness, glomerulonephritis, and polyarteritis nodosa
- Universal vaccination of neonates in countries endemic for HBV reduces the incidence of hepatocellular carcinoma

WHEN TO ADMIT

- Intractable nausea and vomiting and need for parenteral fluids
- Encephalopathy or severe coagulopathy, which indicates impending acute hepatic failure

PREVENTION

- Strict isolation of patients is not necessary, but thorough hand washing by medical staff is essential
- Screening of donated blood for HbsAg and anti-HBc has reduced the risk of transfusion-associated hepatitis markedly. Test pregnant women for HBsAg
- Practice safe sex
- Vaccinate against HAV (after prescreening for prior immunity) in those with chronic hepatitis B

Hepatitis B immune globulin (HBIG)

- May be protective, or attenuate the severity of illness, if given within 7 days after exposure (dose is 0.06 mL/kg body weight) followed by HBV vaccine
- Use this approach after exposure to HbsAg-contaminated material via mucous membranes, breaks in the skin, and after sexual contact

Vaccination

- The current vaccines are recombinant-derived
- CDC recommends universal vaccination of infants and children (Table 127, page 1310)
- Over 90% of recipients mount protective antibody to hepatitis B
- Give 10–20 mg initially (depending on the formulation), repeated again at 1 and 6 months, but alternative schedules are approved
- Check postimmunization anti-HBs titers if need to document seroconversion
- Protection appears to be excellent even if the titer wanes—at least for 15 years—and booster reimmunization is not routinely recommended but is advised for immunocompromised persons in whom anti-HBs titers fall below 10 mIU/mL
- For vaccine nonresponders, three additional vaccine doses may elicit seroprotective anti-HBs levels in 30–50%

 ## EVIDENCE

PRACTICE GUIDELINES

- National Guideline Clearinghouse http://www.guideline.gov/summary/summary.aspx?doc_id=3454&nbr=2680&string=hepatitis http://www.guideline.gov/summary/summary.aspx?doc_id=3492&nbr=2718&string=hepatitis

WEB SITE

- The Hepatitis Information Network http://www.hepnet.com/

INFORMATION FOR PATIENTS

- JAMA patient page: Hepatitis B. JAMA 1999;282:1790.

REFERENCE

- Goldstein ST et al: Incidence and risk factors for acute hepatitis B in the United States, 1982-1988: implications for vaccination programs. J Infect Dis 2002;185:713.

Lawrence S. Friedman, MD

Hepatitis B, Chronic

 KEY FEATURES

ESSENTIALS OF DIAGNOSIS

- Chronic inflammatory reaction of the liver of more than 3–6 months' duration
- Persistently abnormal serum aminotransferase levels
- Liver biopsy shows features of chronic hepatitis, ground-glass hepatocytes

GENERAL CONSIDERATIONS

- Early in the course, hepatitis B e antigen (HbeAg) and hepatitis B virus (HBV) DNA are present in serum, indicative of active viral replications and necroinflammatory activity in the liver. These persons are at risk for progression to cirrhosis and for hepatocellular carcinoma. Low-level IgM anti-HBc is also present in about 70%
- Clinical and biochemical improvement may coincide with disappearance of HBeAg and HBV DNA from serum, appearance of anti-HBe, and integration of the HBV genome into the host genome in infected hepatocytes. If cirrhosis has not yet developed, such persons are at a lower risk for cirrhosis and hepatocellular carcinoma
- Traditional histology has been chronic persistent or chronic active hepatitis. However, more specific categorization is now possible, based on etiology; the grade of portal, periportal, and lobular inflammation (minimal, mild, moderate, or severe); and the stage of fibrosis (none, mild, moderate, severe, cirrhosis)

DEMOGRAPHICS

- Chronic hepatitis B afflicts nearly 400 million people worldwide and 1.25 million (predominantly males) in the United States

 CLINICAL FINDINGS

SYMPTOMS AND SIGNS

- See Figure 5 (page 1255)
- Clinically indistinguishable from chronic hepatitis due to other causes

DIFFERENTIAL DIAGNOSIS

- Hepatitis A, B (acute), C, D (delta), E virus (enterically transmitted in epidemic form in Asia, North Africa, and Mexico)
- Hepatitis G virus (HGV) rarely, if ever, causes frank hepatitis
- Unidentified agents account for a small number of apparent acute viral hepatitis
- TT virus (TTV), a DNA virus, is in about 8% of blood donors and is readily transmitted by blood transfusions, but an association with liver disease is not established. A related virus, SEN-V, has been found in 2% of U.S. blood donors, is transmitted by transfusion, and may account for some cases of transfusion-associated non-ABCDE hepatitis
- Autoimmune hepatitis
- α_1-Antitrypsin deficiency
- Drug-induced chronic hepatitis
- Wilson's disease
- In immunocompromised and rare immunocompetent hosts, consider cytomegalovirus, Epstein–Barr virus, and herpes simplex virus

 DIAGNOSIS

LABORATORY TESTS

- See Figure 5 (page 1255)
- In approximately 40% of cases, serum aminotransferase levels remain normal

DIAGNOSTIC PROCEDURES

- Liver biopsy may be indicated for diagnosis, staging, and predicted response to therapy

Hepatitis B, Chronic

TREATMENT

MEDICATIONS

- Treat active viral replication (HBV DNA in serum, usually with HbeAg, except with precore mutant, when HBEAg is absent and anti-HBe is present) with recombinant human interferon alfa-2b, 5 million units a day or 10 million units three times a week intramuscularly for 4 months
- Lamivudine, 100 mg orally daily as a single dose, may be used instead of interferon and is much better tolerated; it can be used in decompensated cirrhosis and may be effective in rapidly progressive hepatitis B ("fibrosing cholestatic hepatitis") following organ transplantation
- Relapse is frequent when lamivudine is stopped, and long-term treatment is associated with a high rate of viral resistance. Combined use of interferon and lamivudine offers no advantage over the use of either drug alone
- Adefovir, 10 mg orally once a day, has activity against wild-type and lamivudine-resistant HBV. Resistance to this drug has not been reported. Nephrotoxicity can develop, especially if there is underlying renal dysfunction
- Tenofovir has activity against HBV
- Nucleoside analogs are recommended for inactive HBV carriers before starting immunosuppressive therapy or cancer chemotherapy to prevent reactivation

THERAPEUTIC PROCEDURES

- Activity is modified according to symptoms; bed rest is not necessary
- The diet should be well balanced, without limitations other than sodium or protein restriction if dictated by fluid overload or encephalopathy

OUTCOME

COMPLICATIONS

- Cirrhosis
- Hepatocellular carcinoma

PROGNOSIS

- About 40% of treated patients will respond with sustained normalization of aminotransferase levels, disappearance of HBeAg and HBV DNA from serum, appearance of anti-HBe, and improved survival
- A response is most likely with an HBV DNA level under 200 pg/mL and high aminotransferase levels. Over 60% of these responders may eventually clear HBsAg from serum and liver, develop anti-HBs in serum, and be cured. Relapses are uncommon in such complete responders
- HBeAg-negative chronic hepatitis B (precore mutant) has a durable sustained response rate of only 15–25% after 12 months of interferon therapy
- The response to interferon is poor in patients with HIV coinfection and autoimmune diseases
- Lamivudine reliably suppresses HBV DNA in serum, improves liver histology in 60% of patients, and leads to normal alanine aminotransferase levels in over 40% and HBeAg seroconversion in 20% of patients after 1 year of therapy. However, 15–30% of responders experience a generally mild relapse during treatment as a result of mutation in the polymerase gene of HBV DNA that confers resistance to lamivudine. Hepatitis may recur when the drug is stopped, and long-term, perhaps indefinite treatment despite a high rate of resistance over time may be required when HBeAg seroconversion does not ensue. Rates of complete response—as well as resistance to lamivudine—increase with increasing duration of therapy

WHEN TO ADMIT

- Decompensated liver disease (eg, severe coagulopathy, variceal bleeding, severe ascites)

PREVENTION

- Strict isolation of patients is not necessary, but hand washing after bowel movements is required. Thorough hand washing by anyone who may contact contaminated utensils, bedding, or clothing is essential
- Screening of donated blood for HBsAg and anti-HBc has reduced the risk of transfusion-associated hepatitis markedly
- Pregnant women should be tested for HBsAg
- Persons with HBV should practice safe sex
- Vaccinate against HAV (after prescreening for prior immunity) in those with chronic hepatitis B

EVIDENCE

PRACTICE GUIDELINES

- National Guideline Clearinghouse http://www.guideline.gov/summary/summary.aspx?doc_id=3446&nbr=2672 &string=hepatitis http://www.guideline.gov/summary/summary.aspx?doc_id=3454&nbr= 2680&string=hepatitis

WEB SITES

- Viral Hepatitis http://www.cdc.gov/ncidod/diseases/hepatitis/index.htm
- Hepatitis Information Network http://www.hepnet.com/

INFORMATION FOR PATIENTS

- JAMA patient page: Hepatitis B. JAMA 1999;282:1790.
- American Gastroenterological Association http://www.gastro.org/public/brochures/cvh.html

REFERENCES

- Esteban R (guest ed): Advancing HBV therapy to overcome treatment challenges. Semin Liver Dis 2002; 22(suppl 1):1.
- Lok AS et al: Chronic hepatitis B. Hepatology 2001;34:1225.

Lawrence S. Friedman, MD

Hepatitis C, Acute

 KEY FEATURES

ESSENTIALS OF DIAGNOSIS

- Prodrome of anorexia, nausea, vomiting, malaise, aversion to smoking
- Fever, enlarged and tender liver, jaundice
- Normal to low white blood cell count; abnormal liver tests, especially markedly elevated aminotransferases early in the course
- Liver biopsy shows hepatocellular necrosis and mononuclear infiltrate
- Source of infection in many is unknown

GENERAL CONSIDERATIONS

- The hepatitis C virus (HCV) is a single-stranded RNA virus (hepacivirus) with properties similar to those of flavivirus. At least six major genotypes of HCV have been identified
- Coinfection is found in 30–50% of persons infected with HIV; HIV leads to more rapid progression of chronic hepatitis C to cirrhosis
- Anti-HCV is not protective, and in patients with acute or chronic hepatitis its presence in serum generally signifies that HCV is the cause

DEMOGRAPHICS

- There are more than 2.7 million HCV carriers in the United States and another 1.3 million previously exposed persons who have cleared the virus
- In the past, HCV was responsible for over 90% of cases of posttransfusion hepatitis, yet only 4% of cases of hepatitis C were attributable to blood transfusions
- Over 50% of cases are transmitted by intravenous drug use. Intranasal cocaine use and body piercing also are risk factors
- The risk of sexual and maternal–neonatal transmission is low and may be greatest in those with high circulating levels of HCV RNA. Multiple sexual partners may increase the risk of HCV infection. Transmission via breast-feeding has not been documented

 CLINICAL FINDINGS

SYMPTOMS AND SIGNS

- See Figure 4 (page 1255)
- The incubation period averages 6–7 weeks
- Clinical illness is often mild, usually asymptomatic, and characterized by waxing and waning aminotransferase elevations and a high rate (>80%) of chronic hepatitis
- Slight neurocognitive impairment has been described in patients with chronic hepatitis C
- Hepatic steatosis is a particular feature of infection with HCV genotype 3

DIFFERENTIAL DIAGNOSIS

- Hepatitis A, B, D (delta agent), E virus (an enterically transmitted hepatitis seen in epidemic form in Asia, North Africa, and Mexico)
- Hepatitis G virus (HGV) applies to an agent that rarely, if ever, causes frank hepatitis. Unidentified agents account for a small percentage of cases of apparent acute viral hepatitis
- A DNA virus designated the TT virus (TTV) is in up to 7.5% of blood donors and is readily transmitted by blood transfusions, but an association between this virus and liver disease has not been established. A related virus known as SEN-V has been found in 2% of U.S. blood donors, is transmitted by transfusion, and may account for some cases of transfusion-associated non-ABCDE hepatitis
- In immunocompromised and rare immunocompetent hosts, consider cytomegalovirus, Epstein–Barr virus, and herpes simplex virus

 DIAGNOSIS

LABORATORY TESTS

- See Figure 4 (page 1255)
- Diagnosis is based on detection of antibodies to HCV by immunoassay. The assay has moderate sensitivity (false-negatives) for the diagnosis early in the course and in healthy blood donors and low specificity (false-positives) in some persons with elevated γ-globulin levels. In these situations, a diagnosis of hepatitis C may be confirmed by use of an assay for HCV RNA and, in some cases, a supplemental recombinant immunoblot assay (RIBA) for anti-HCV
- Most RIBA-positive persons are potentially infectious, as confirmed by use of polymerase chain reaction–based tests to detect HCV RNA
- Occasional persons are found to have anti-HCV in serum, confirmed by RIBA, without HCV RNA in serum, suggesting recovery from HCV infection in the past
- In pregnant patients, serum aminotransferase levels frequently normalize despite persistence of viremia, only to increase again after delivery
- The white blood cell count is normal to low, especially in the preicteric phase. Large atypical lymphocytes may occasionally be seen
- Mild proteinuria is common, and bilirubinuria often precedes the appearance of jaundice. Acholic stools are often present during the icteric phase. Strikingly elevated aspartate or alanine aminotransferase occurs early, followed by elevations of bilirubin and alkaline phosphatase; in a minority of patients, the latter persist after aminotransferase levels have normalized
- Cholestasis is occasionally marked

TREATMENT

MEDICATIONS

- If nausea and vomiting are pronounced or if oral intake is substantially decreased, intravenous 10% glucose is indicated
- Small doses of oxazepam are safe, as metabolism is not hepatic; morphine sulfate is avoided
- Corticosteroids have no benefit

THERAPEUTIC PROCEDURES

- Bed rest is recommended only if symptoms are marked
- Dietary management consists of palatable meals as tolerated, without overfeeding; breakfast is usually best tolerated
- Strenuous physical exertion, alcohol, and hepatotoxic agents are avoided

OUTCOME

COMPLICATIONS

- HCV is a pathogenetic factor in cryoglobulinemia and membranoproliferative glomerulonephritis and may be related to lichen planus, autoimmune thyroiditis, lymphocytic sialadenitis, idiopathic pulmonary fibrosis, sporadic porphyria cutanea tarda, monoclonal gammopathies, and probably lymphoma
- The risk of type 2 diabetes mellitus may increase with chronic hepatitis C

PROGNOSIS

- In the majority, clinical recovery is complete in 3–6 weeks. Liver function returns to normal, though aminotransferase elevations persist in the majority of patients in whom chronic hepatitis C ensues
- The mortality rate is less than 1%, but the rate is higher in older people
- Fulminant hepatitis C is rare in the United States
- As many as 80% of all persons with acute hepatitis C develop chronic hepatitis, which in many cases progresses very slowly
- Cirrhosis develops in up to 30% of those with chronic hepatitis C; the risk is higher in patients coinfected with both viruses or with HIV
- Patients with cirrhosis are at risk of hepatocellular carcinoma at a rate of 3–5% per year

WHEN TO ADMIT

- Intractable nausea and vomiting and need for parenteral fluids
- Encephalopathy or severe coagulopathy indicate impending acute hepatic failure, and hospitalization is necessary

PREVENTION

- Strict isolation of patients is not necessary, but hand washing after bowel movements is required. Thorough hand washing by anyone who may contact contaminated utensils, bedding, or clothing is essential
- Testing blood for HCV has helped reduce the risk of transfusion-associated hepatitis C

EVIDENCE

PRACTICE GUIDELINES

- National Guideline Clearinghouse http://www.guideline.gov/summary/ summary.aspx?doc_id=3416&nbr=2642 &string=hepatitis http://www.guideline.gov/summary/ summary.aspx?doc_id=3454&nbr= 2680&string=hepatitis

WEB SITES

- Hepatitis C: Case study http://path.upmc.edu/cases/case17.html
- Viral hepatitis http://www.cdc.gov/ncidod/diseases/ hepatitis/index.htm
- Hepatitis Information Network http://www.hepnet.com/

INFORMATION FOR PATIENTS

- JAMA patient page: Hepatitis C. JAMA 1998;280(24):2188.
- Centers for Disease Control http://www.cdc.gov/ncidod/diseases/ hepatitis/c/faq.htm

REFERENCES

- Herrine SK: Approach to the patient with chronic hepatitis C infection. Ann Intern Med 2002;136:747.
- Jaeckel E et al: Treatment of acute hepatitis C with interferon alfa-2b. N Engl J Med 2001;345:1452.
- Lauer GM et al: Hepatitis C virus infection. N Engl J Med 2001;345:41.

Lawrence S. Friedman, MD

Hepatitis C, Chronic

 KEY FEATURES

ESSENTIALS OF DIAGNOSIS

- Chronic inflammatory reaction of the liver of more than 3–6 months' duration, demonstrated by persistently abnormal serum aminotransferase levels and characteristic histological findings
- May be made on initial presentation
- Liver biopsy shows features of chronic hepatitis, often with portal lymphoid nodules and interface hepatitis
- Source of infection often is unknown

GENERAL CONSIDERATIONS

- Chronic hepatitis has been categorized histologically as chronic persistent hepatitis and chronic active hepatitis. More specific categorization is possible, based on etiology; the grade of portal, periportal, and lobular inflammation (minimal, mild, moderate, or severe); and the stage of fibrosis (none, mild, moderate, severe, cirrhosis)
- May be the most common etiology of chronic hepatitis
- Coinfection is found in 30–50% of persons infected with HIV
- Anti-hepatitis C virus (HCV) is not protective; in chronic hepatitis its presence in serum signifies that HCV is the cause
- At least six major genotypes of HCV have been identified

DEMOGRAPHICS

- Up to 80% of patients with acute hepatitis C develop chronic hepatitis C
- There are more than 2.7 million HCV carriers in the United States and another 1.3 million previously exposed persons who have cleared the virus
- HCV was responsible for over 90% of cases of posttransfusion hepatitis; yet only 4% of cases of hepatitis C were attributable to blood transfusions
- Over 50% of cases are transmitted by intravenous drug use
- The risk of sexual and maternal–neonatal transmission is low and may be greatest in those with high circulating levels of HCV RNA. Multiple sexual partners may increase the risk of HCV infection

 CLINICAL FINDINGS

SYMPTOMS AND SIGNS

- See Figure 4 (page 1255)
- Clinically indistinguishable from chronic hepatitis due to other causes
- In approximately 40% of cases, serum aminotransferase levels are persistently normal
- Slight neurocognitive impairment has been reported

DIFFERENTIAL DIAGNOSIS

- Hepatitis A, B, C (acute) D (delta agent), E virus (an enterically transmitted hepatitis seen in epidemic form in Asia, North Africa, and Mexico)
- Hepatitis G virus (HGV) applies to an agent that rarely, if ever, causes frank hepatitis
- A DNA virus designated the TT virus (TTV) is in up to 7.5% of blood donors and is readily transmitted by blood transfusions, but an association between this virus and liver disease has not been established. A related virus known as SEN-V has been found in 2% of U.S. blood donors, is transmitted by transfusion, and may account for some cases of transfusion-associated non-ABCDE hepatitis
- In immunocompromised and rare immunocompetent hosts, consider cytomegalovirus, Epstein–Barr virus, and herpes simplex virus
- Autoimmune hepatitis
- α_1-Antitrypsin deficiency
- Drug-induced hepatitis
- Hemochromatosis
- Wilson's disease

 DIAGNOSIS

LABORATORY TESTS

- See Figure 4 (page 1255)
- Serum anti-HCV by enzyme immunoassay (EIA) is present
- In rare cases of negative EIA, HCV RNA is detected by PCR
- Hepatic steatosis (fatty liver) is a particular feature of infection with HCV genotype 3

DIAGNOSTIC PROCEDURES

- Liver biopsy is indicated in patients offered treatment for diagnosis, staging, and predicted response to therapy

 TREATMENT

MEDICATIONS

- Standard therapy is "pegylated" interferon (peginterferon) and ribavirin: two peginterferon formulations are available: Pegintron (peginterferon alfa-2b) in a dose of 1.5 mg/kg weekly, and Pegasys (peginterferon alfa-2a) in a dose of 180 mg once per week for 48 weeks
- When used with peginterferon alfa-2b, the dose of ribavirin is based on the patient's weight and may range from 800 mg to 1400 mg daily in two divided doses. When used with peginterferon alfa-2a, the daily ribavirin dose is 1000 mg or 1200 mg depending on whether the patient's weight is less than or greater than 75 kg
- Treat genotype 1a or 1b for 48 weeks if viral clearance has been achieved by 12–24 weeks
- Treat cirrhosis or a high viral level in serum (>850,000 IU/mL) for 48 weeks
- Treat genotypes 2 or 3, without cirrhosis, and with low levels of viremia (<2–3.5 × 10⁶ copies/mL) for 24 weeks with a decreased dose of ribavirin of 800 mg in a split dose
- Peginterferon alfa with ribavirin may be effective treatment for cryoglobulinemia associated with chronic hepatitis C
- Treatment of asymptomatic "chronic carriers" with normal serum aminotransferase levels is of uncertain benefit
- Coinfection of HCV and HIV may benefit from treatment of HCV if the CD4 count is not low

- Treatment with peginterferon alfa plus ribavirin is costly and side effects (flu-like symptoms) are almost universal; more serious toxicity includes psychiatric symptoms (irritability, depression), thyroid dysfunction, and bone marrow suppression
- Interferon is contraindicated with decompensated cirrhosis, profound cytopenias, severe psychiatric disorders, and autoimmune diseases
- Ribavirin should be avoided in persons over age 65 and in others in whom hemolysis could pose a risk of angina or stroke. Rash, itching, headache, cough, and shortness of breath also occur with the drug
- Lactic acidosis is a concern if also taking highly active antiretroviral therapy for HIV
- Rarely, erythropoietin and granulocyte colony-stimulating factor are used to treat therapy-induced anemia and leukopenia, respectively

THERAPEUTIC PROCEDURES

- Activity is modified according to symptoms; bed rest is not necessary
- The diet should be well balanced, without limitations other than sodium or protein restriction if dictated by fluid overload or encephalopathy
- Generally treat if less than age 70 and more than minor fibrosis on liver biopsy
- Because of high response rates to treatment with HCV genotype 2 or 3 infection, treatment may be initiated without a liver biopsy

OUTCOME

FOLLOW-UP

- Obtain a blood cell count at weeks 1, 2, and 4 after peginterferon alfa plus ribavirin therapy is started and monthly thereafter
- Patients taking ribavirin must be monitored for hemolysis, and, because of teratogenic concerns, patients must practice strict contraception until 6 months after conclusion of therapy

COMPLICATIONS

- Cryoglobulinemia and membranoproliferative glomerulonephritis
- May be related to lichen planus, autoimmune thyroiditis, lymphocytic sialadenitis, idiopathic pulmonary fibrosis, porphyria cutanea tarda, lymphoma, and monoclonal gammopathy
- Type 2 diabetes mellitus may be increased

PROGNOSIS

- Up to 80% of acute hepatitis C becomes chronic hepatitis, which in many cases progresses very slowly
- Most with persistently normal serum aminotransferase levels have mild chronic hepatitis with slow or absent progression to cirrhosis; however, cirrhosis is present in 10% of these patients
- Progression to cirrhosis occurs in 20% of affected patients after 20 years, with an increased risk in men, those who drink more than 50 g of alcohol daily, and possibly those who acquire HCV infection after age 40
- Immunosuppressed persons (hypogammaglobulinemia, HIV infection with a low CD4 count, or organ transplants receiving immunosuppressants) progress more rapidly to cirrhosis than immunocompetent persons
- Hepatocellular carcinoma develops in cirrhosis at a rate of 3–5% per year
- Peginterferon plus ribavarin probably improves survival and quality of life, are cost-effective, retard and even reverse fibrosis, and in responders may reduce the risk of hepatocellular carcinoma. Factors predicting an increased chance of response include no cirrhosis on liver biopsy (though treatment is not contraindicated by compensated cirrhosis), low serum HCV RNA levels, and infection by genotypes of HCV other than 1a, 1b, or 4

WHEN TO ADMIT

- Rarely necessary
- Only in advanced cirrhosis with decompensation

PREVENTION

- Strict isolation of patients is not necessary, but hand washing after bowel movements is required. Thorough hand washing by anyone who may contact contaminated utensils, bedding, or clothing is essential
- Testing of donated blood for HCV has helped reduce the risk of transfusion-associated hepatitis C from 10% a decade ago to about 1 in 2 million units today

EVIDENCE

PRACTICE GUIDELINES

- National Guideline Clearinghouse
  http://www.guideline.gov/summary/summary.aspx?doc_id=1518&nbr=744&string=hepatitis
  http://www.guideline.gov/summary/summary.aspx?doc_id=3454&nbr=2680&string=hepatitis

WEB SITES

- Hepatitis C: Case study
  http://path.upmc.edu/cases/case17.html
- Viral Hepatitis
  http://www.cdc.gov/ncidod/diseases/hepatitis/index.htm
- Hepatitis Information Network
  http://www.hepnet.com/

INFORMATION FOR PATIENTS

- American Gastroenterological Association
  http://www.gastro.org/public/brochures/cvh.html

REFERENCES

- Fried MW et al: Peginterferon alfa-2a plus ribavirin for chronic hepatitis C virus infection. N Engl J Med 2002; 347:975.
- Herrine SK: Approach to the patient with chronic hepatitis C infection. Ann Intern Med 2002;136:747.
- Lauer GM et al: Hepatitis C virus infection. N Engl J Med 2001;345:41.

Lawrence S. Friedman, MD

Hepatitis D (Delta)

 KEY FEATURES

ESSENTIALS OF DIAGNOSIS

- Hepatitis D virus (HDV) is a defective RNA virus that causes hepatitis only in association with hepatitis B infection
- Liver biopsy shows hepatocellular necrosis and mononuclear infiltrate but is rarely indicated

GENERAL CONSIDERATIONS

- Causes hepatitis only in the presence of hepatitis B surface antigen (HbsAg); it is cleared when the latter is cleared
- May coinfect with hepatitis B virus (HBV) or may superinfect a person with chronic hepatitis B, usually by percutaneous exposure
- Hepatitis can be caused by many drugs, toxic agents, and viruses, the clinical manifestations of which may be similar

DEMOGRAPHICS

- In the 1970s and early 1980s, HDV was endemic in some areas, such as the Mediterranean countries, where up to 80% of HBV carriers were superinfected with it. In the United States, HDV occurred primarily among intravenous drug users. However, new cases of hepatitis D are now infrequent, and cases seen today are usually from cohorts infected years ago who survived the initial impact of hepatitis D and now have inactive cirrhosis

 CLINICAL FINDINGS

SYMPTOMS AND SIGNS

- When acute hepatitis D is coincident with acute HBV infection, the infection is generally similar in severity to acute hepatitis B alone
- In chronic hepatitis B, superinfection by HDV appears to carry a worse short-term prognosis, often resulting in fulminant hepatitis or severe chronic hepatitis that progresses rapidly to cirrhosis
- Patients with long-standing chronic hepatitis D and B often have inactive cirrhosis

DIFFERENTIAL DIAGNOSIS

- Hepatitis A, B, C, E, G virus
- Unidentified agents account for a small percentage of cases of viral hepatitis
- The TT virus (TTV) is in up to 7.5% of blood donors and is readily transmitted by blood transfusions, but an association with liver disease has not been established. A related virus known as SEN-V has been found in 2% of U.S. blood donors, is transmitted by transfusion, and may account for some cases of transfusion-associated non-ABCDE hepatitis
- Cytomegalovirus, Epstein–Barr virus, and herpes simplex virus in immunocompromised and rare immunocompetent hosts
- Other causes of chronic hepatitis (see *Hepatitis B, chronic*)

 DIAGNOSIS

LABORATORY TESTS

- Diagnosis is made by detection of antibody to hepatitis D antigen (anti-HDV) or, where available, HDV RNA in serum

TREATMENT

- See Treatment of *Hepatitis B, Hepatic failure*, acute, *Cirrhosis*

 OUTCOME

COMPLICATIONS

- See *Hepatic failure, acute*
- See *Cirrhosis*

PROGNOSIS

- Threefold increased risk of hepatocellular carcinoma

WHEN TO ADMIT

- Intractable nausea and vomiting and need for parenteral fluids
- Encephalopathy or severe coagulopathy indicates impending acute hepatic failure, and hospitalization is mandatory

PREVENTION

- Hepatitis D is best prevented by prevention of hepatitis B (eg, with HBV vaccine—see *Hepatitis B*)

Hepatitis D (Delta)

 EVIDENCE

WEB SITES

- Viral Hepatitis http://www.cdc.gov/ncidod/diseases/hepatitis/index.htm
- Hepatitis Information Network http://www.hepnet.com/

INFORMATION FOR PATIENTS

- National Digestive Diseases Information Clearinghouse http://digestive.niddk.nih.gov/ddiseases/pubs/viralhepatitis/index.htm
- National Institutes of Health http://www.nlm.nih.gov/medlineplus/ency/article/000216.htm

REFERENCE

- Gaeta GB et al: Chronic hepatitis D. A vanishing disease? An Italian multicenter study. Hepatology 2000;32:824. [PMID: 11003629]

Lawrence S. Friedman, MD

Hepatitis, Alcoholic

 KEY FEATURES

ESSENTIALS OF DIAGNOSIS

- >80 g/day intake of alcohol in men and 30–40 g/day intake in women
- May present with fever, right upper quadrant pain, tender hepatomegaly, and jaundice but the patient may also be asymptomatic
- Aspartate aminotransferase (AST) is usually elevated but rarely above 300 units/L. AST is greater than alanine aminotransferase (ALT), usually by a factor of 2 or more
- Often reversible, but it is the most common precursor of cirrhosis in the United States

GENERAL CONSIDERATIONS

- Characterized by acute or chronic inflammation and parenchymal necrosis
- Can appear within a year but usually decades after onset of excessive drinking
- Many of the adverse effects of alcohol are probably mediated by the oxidative metabolite acetaldehyde, which contributes to lipid peroxidation and induction of an immune response
- Concurrent hepatitis B or C virus infection and heterozygosity for the *HFE* gene mutation for hemochromatosis increase the severity of alcoholic liver disease

DEMOGRAPHICS

- Over 80% of patients have been drinking 5 years or more before developing any liver symptoms
- The longer the duration of drinking (10–15 or more years) and the larger the alcoholic consumption, the greater the probability of developing alcoholic hepatitis and cirrhosis

 CLINICAL FINDINGS

SYMPTOMS AND SIGNS

- Can vary from asymptomatic with an enlarged liver to a critically ill individual who dies quickly
- Recent period of heavy drinking
- Anorexia and nausea
- Hepatomegaly and jaundice
- Abdominal pain and tenderness, splenomegaly, ascites, fever, and encephalopathy may be present

DIFFERENTIAL DIAGNOSIS

- Viral hepatitis
- Drug-induced hepatitis
- Cirrhosis
- Biliary tract disease
- Nonalcoholic liver disease
- Pneumonia

 DIAGNOSIS

LABORATORY TESTS

Liver panel

- AST is usually elevated up to 300 units/L, but not higher
- AST is greater than ALT, usually by a factor of 2 or more
- Serum alkaline phosphatase is generally elevated, but seldom more than three times the normal value
- Serum bilirubin is increased in 60–90% of patients

Complete blood cell count

- Anemia (usually macrocytic) may be present
- Leukocytosis with shift to the left is common with severe disease
- Leukopenia is occasionally seen and disappears after cessation of drinking
- About 10% have thrombocytopenia related to a direct toxic effect of alcohol on megakaryocyte production or to hypersplenism

Other labs

- Serum γ-glutamyl transpeptidase, carbohydrate-deficient transferrin, and mitochondrial AST may be elevated, but these tests lack both sensitivity and specificity
- The serum albumin is depressed, and the γ-globulin level is elevated in 50–75% of individuals, even in the absence of cirrhosis
- Increased transferrin saturation and hepatic iron stores are found in many due to sideroblastic anemia
- Folic acid deficiency may coexist

IMAGING STUDIES

- Imaging studies are generally not helpful in the diagnosis of alcoholic hepatitis
- Ultrasound helps exclude biliary obstruction and identifies subclinical ascites
- CT scanning with intravenous contrast or MRI may be indicated in selected cases to evaluate patients for collateral vessels, space-occupying lesions of the liver, or concomitant disease of the pancreas

DIAGNOSTIC PROCEDURES

- Liver biopsy, if done, demonstrates macrovesicular fat, polymorphonuclear neutrophil infiltration with hepatic necrosis, and Mallory bodies (alcoholic hyaline), and perivenular and perisinusoidal fibrosis. Micronodular cirrhosis may be present as well. The findings are identical to those of nonalcoholic steatohepatitis

TREATMENT

MEDICATIONS

- Give **vitamins,** particularly folic acid and thiamine; glucose administration increases the vitamin B$_1$ requirement and can precipitate Wernicke-Korsakoff syndrome if thiamine is not coadministered

Corticosteroids

- Methylprednisolone, 32 mg/day for 1 month or the equivalent, may reduce short-term mortality and either encephalopathy or a greatly elevated bilirubin concentration and prolonged prothrombin time

Experimental therapies

- Pentoxifylline—an inhibitor of tumor necrosis factor—400 mg orally three times daily for 4 weeks, may reduce 1-month mortality rates in severe disease, primarily by decreasing the risk of hepatorenal syndrome
- Other experimental therapies include propylthiouracil, oxandrolone, and S-adenosyl-l-methionine

THERAPEUTIC PROCEDURES

- Abstinence from alcohol is essential
- Provide sufficient carbohydrates and calories in anorectic patients to reduce endogenous protein catabolism, promote gluconeogenesis, and prevent hypoglycemia
- Nutritional support (40 kcal/kg with 1.5–2 g/kg as protein) improves survival in malnutrition. Use of liquid formulas rich in branched-chain amino acids does not improve survival beyond that achieved with less expensive caloric supplementation

OUTCOME

COMPLICATIONS

Alcoholic cirrhosis

- Occurs in about 10–15% of persons who consume over 50 g of alcohol (4 oz of 100-proof whiskey, 15 oz of wine, or four 12-oz cans of beer) daily for over 10 years (the risk may be lower for wine than for comparable intake of beer or spirits)
- The risk of cirrhosis is lower (5%) in the absence of other cofactors such as chronic viral hepatitis
- There are associations with polymorphisms of the genes encoding for tumor necrosis factor-α and cytochrome P-450 2E1
- Women appear to be more susceptible than men, in part because of lower gastric mucosal alcohol dehydrogenase levels

PROGNOSIS

Short term

- A prothrombin time short enough to permit liver biopsy (<3 s above control) has a 1-year mortality rate of 7%, rising to 20% if there is progressive prolongation of the prothrombin time during hospitalization
- If the prothrombin time prohibits liver biopsy, there is a 40% 1-year mortality rate
- Other unfavorable prognostic factors are hepatic encephalopathy and azotemia
- Serum bilirubin levels greater than 10 mg/dL and marked prolongation of the prothrombin time (≥6 s above control) indicate severe hepatitis with a mortality rate as high as 50%

Long term

- In the United States, the 3-year mortality rate after recovery from acute alcoholic hepatitis is 10 times that of controls
- Histologically severe disease is associated with continued excessive mortality rates after 3 years, whereas the death rate is not increased after the same period in those whose liver biopsies show only mild alcoholic hepatitis
- Complications of portal hypertension (ascites, variceal bleeding, hepatorenal syndrome), coagulopathy, following recovery from acute alcoholic hepatitis suggest a poor long-term prognosis

- The most important prognostic consideration is continued excessive drinking. A 6-month period of abstinence is generally required before liver transplantation can be considered

PREVENTION

- Abstinence from alcholol

EVIDENCE

PRACTICE GUIDELINES

- National Guideline Clearinghouse http://www.guideline.gov/summary/summary.aspx?doc_id=3520&nbr=2746&string=alcoholic+hepatitis
- American College of Gastroenterology http://www.acg.gi.org/physicianforum/guides/etolivr.html

WEB SITES

- Alcoholics Anonymous http://www.alcoholics-anonymous.org
- Diseases of the Liver http://cpmcnet.columbia.edu/dept/gi/disliv.html
- Pathology Index http://www-medlib.med.utah.edu/WebPath/LIVEHTML/LIVERIDX.html
- Hepatic Ultrasound Images http://www.sono.nino.ru/english/hepar_en.html
- Liver Tutorials Visualization and Volume Measurement http://everest.radiology.uiowa.edu/nlm/app/livertoc/livertoc.html

INFORMATION FOR PATIENTS

- JAMA patient page: Alcohol. JAMA 1999;281:1352.
- Mayo Clinic http://www.mayoclinic.com/invoke.cfm?id=HQ00200

REFERENCES

- Mathurin P et al: Corticosteroids improve short-term survival in patients with severe alcoholic hepatitis (AH): individual data analysis of the last three randomized placebo controlled double blind trials of corticosteroids in severe AH. J Hepatol 2002;36:480.
- Menon KV et al: Pathogenesis, diagnosis, and treatment of alcoholic liver disease. Mayo Clin Proc 2001;76:1021.

Lawrence S. Friedman, MD

Hepatitis, Autoimmune

 ## KEY FEATURES

ESSENTIALS OF DIAGNOSIS

- Usually young to middle-aged women
- Chronic hepatitis with high serum globulins
- Antinuclear antibody (+ANA) and/or smooth muscle antibody
- Responds to corticosteroids

GENERAL CONSIDERATIONS

- The onset is usually insidious, but up to 40% present with an acute attack of hepatitis and some cases follow a viral illness such as hepatitis A, Epstein–Barr infection, measles, or exposure to a drug or toxin such as nitrofurantoin
- There are at least three types of autoimmune hepatitis, distinguished by autoantibodies

DEMOGRAPHICS

- Though usually a disease of young women, autoimmune hepatitis can occur in either sex at any age
- Affected younger persons are often positive for HLA-B8 and -DR3; in older patients, HLA-DR4
- The principal susceptibility allele among white Americans and northern Europeans is HLA *DRB1*0301;* HLA *DRB1*0401* is a secondary but independent risk factor

 ## CLINICAL FINDINGS

SYMPTOMS AND SIGNS

- Typically, a healthy-appearing young woman with multiple spider nevi, cutaneous striae, acne, hirsutism, and hepatomegaly
- Amenorrhea may be a presenting feature
- Extrahepatic features include arthritis, Sjögren's syndrome, thyroiditis, nephritis, ulcerative colitis, and Coombs-positive hemolytic anemia

DIFFERENTIAL DIAGNOSIS

- Chronic viral hepatitis
- Primary biliary cirrhosis
- Primary sclerosing cholangitis
- Wilson's disease
- Hemochromatosis

 ## DIAGNOSIS

LABORATORY TESTS

- In classic (type I) autoimmune hepatitis, ANA or smooth muscle antibody (either or both) is detected in serum
- Serum γ-globulin levels are typically elevated (up to 5–6 g/dL), and in this setting, the enzyme immunoassay for antibody to hepatitis C virus may be falsely positive. Other antibodies, including antineutrophil cytoplasmic antibodies (ANCA), may be found
- A second type, seen more often in Europe, is characterized by circulating antibody to liver–kidney microsomes (anti-LKM1)—directed against cytochrome P-450 2D6—without anti-smooth muscle antibody or ANA. This type can be seen in patients with autoimmune polyglandular syndrome type 1
- A third variant is characterized by antibodies to soluble liver antigen/liver pancreas (anti-SLA/LP) and may represent a variant of type I autoimmune hepatitis characterized by severe disease, high relapse rate after treatment, and absence of the usual antibodies (ANA and smooth muscle antibody). Anti-SLA/LP appear to be directed against a transfer RNA complex responsible for incorporating selenocysteine into peptide chains
- The serum bilirubin is usually increased, but 20% are anicteric

TREATMENT

MEDICATIONS

- Prednisone with or without azathioprine improves symptoms and reduces hepatic inflammation. The symptomatic patients optimal for therapy have at least a 10-fold elevation of aminotransferases (or 5-fold if the serum globulins are elevated at least 2-fold), and if asymptomatic but with modest enzyme elevations, treat on clinical grounds
- Initally, give prednisone, 30 mg orally daily, or an equivalent drug with azathioprine or mercaptopurine, 50 mg/day orally. Taper prednisone after 1 week to 20 mg/day and again after 2 or 3 weeks to 15 mg/day. Ultimately, a maintenance dose of 10 mg/day is achieved

SURGERY

- Liver transplantation may be required for treatment failures, and the disease has been recognized to recur in up to one-third of transplanted livers (and rarely to develop de novo) as immunosuppression is reduced

 OUTCOME

FOLLOW-UP

- Blood cell counts are monitored weekly for the first 2 months of azathioprine therapy and monthly thereafter because of the small risk of bone marrow suppression
- The response rate to therapy with prednisone and azathioprine is 80%
- Cirrhosis does not reverse with therapy and may even develop after apparent biochemical and histological remission
- Once remission is achieved, therapy may be withdrawn, but the subsequent relapse rate is 50–90%. Relapses may again be treated in the same manner as the initial episode, with the same remission rate
- After successful treatment of a relapse, treat indefinitely with azathioprine up to 2 mg/kg and the lowest dose of prednisone needed to maintain aminotransferase levels as close to normal as possible, although another attempt at withdrawing therapy may be considered in patients remaining in remission long term (eg, ≥4 years)
- Budesonide, a corticosteroid with less toxicity than prednisone, does not appear to be effective in maintaining remission
- Nonresponders to prednisone and azathioprine may be considered for a trial of cyclosporine, tacrolimus, or methotrexate. Mycophenolate mofetil is effective when azathioprine is not tolerated or there is no response to it

COMPLICATIONS

- Concurrent primary biliary cirrhosis or primary sclerosing cholangitis occurs in up to 15% of patients with autoimmune hepatitis. Liver biopsy is indicated to help establish the diagnosis, evaluate disease severity, and determine the need for treatment

PROGNOSIS

- With azathioprine therapy, there is prompt symptomatic improvement but biochemical improvement is more gradual, with normalization of serum aminotransferase levels after several months in many cases
- Histological resolution of inflammation may require 18–24 months, the time at which repeat liver biopsy is recommended

- Failure of aminotransferase levels to normalize invariably predicts lack of histological resolution

PREVENTION

- Monitor bone density, particularly with corticosteroid use, for osteoporosis

 EVIDENCE

PRACTICE GUIDELINES

- National Guideline Clearinghouse http://www.guideline.gov/summary/ summary.aspx?doc_id=3447&nbr=2673 &string=autoimmune+hepatitis http://www.guideline.gov/summary/ summary.aspx?doc_id=3520&nbr= 2746&string=toxic+hepatitis

WEB SITES

- Diseases of the Liver http://cpmcnet.columbia.edu/dept/ gi/disliv.html
- Pathology Index http://www-medlib.med.utah.edu/ WebPath/LIVEHTML/LIVERIDX. html
- Hepatic Ultrasound Images http://www.sono.nino.ru/english/ hepar_en.html

INFORMATION FOR PATIENTS

- National Institute of Diabetes and Digestive and Kidney Diseases http://digestive.niddk.nih.gov/ddiseases/ pubs/autoimmunehep/index.htm
- National Institutes of Health http://www.nlm.nih.gov/medlineplus/ ency/article/000245.htm

REFERENCES

- Al-Khalidi JA et al: Current concepts in the diagnosis, pathogenesis, and treatment of autoimmune hepatitis. Mayo Clin Proc 2001;76:1237.
- Ben-Ari Z et al: Autoimmune hepatitis and its variant syndromes. Gut 2001; 49:589. [PMID: 11559660]
- Czaja AJ et al: Diagnosis and treatment of autoimmune hepatitis. Hepatology 2002;36:479.

Lawrence S. Friedman, MD

Hepatitis, Drug- or Toxin-Induced

 KEY FEATURES

ESSENTIALS OF DIAGNOSIS

- Drug-induced liver disease can mimic viral hepatitis, biliary tract obstruction, or other types of liver disease
- Clinicians must inquire about the use of many widely used therapeutic agents, including over-the-counter "natural" and "herbal" products in any patient with liver disease

GENERAL CONSIDERATIONS

- Drug toxicity may be categorized on the basis of pathogenesis or histological appearance

Direct hepatotoxic group

- Dose-related severity
- A latent period following exposure
- Susceptibility in all individuals. Examples include acetaminophen, alcohol, carbon tetrachloride, chloroform, heavy metals, mercaptopurine, niacin, plant alkaloids, phosphorus, tetracyclines, valproic acid, and vitamin A
- Coadministration of a second agent may increase the toxicity of the first (eg, isoniazid and rifampin, acetaminophen and alcohol)

Idiosyncratic reactions

- Reactions are sporadic, not dose- related, and occasionally associated with fever and eosinophilia
- May have genetic predisposition
- Examples include amiodarone, aspirin, carbamazepine, chloramphenicol, diclofenac, flutamide, halothane, isoniazid, ketoconazole, lamotrigine, methyldopa, oxacillin, phenytoin, pyrazinamide, quinidine, streptomycin, troglitazone (withdrawn from the market in the United States), and less commonly other thiazolidinediones, and perhaps tacrine

Cholestatic reactions

- **Noninflammatory**
- Direct effect of agent on bile secretory mechanisms: azathioprine, estrogens, or anabolic steroids containing an alkyl or ethinyl group at carbon 17, indinavir, mercaptopurine, methyltestosterone, cyclosporine
- **Inflammatory**
- Inflammation of portal areas with bile duct injury (cholangitis), often with allergic features such as eosinophilia: amoxicillin-clavulanic acid, azithromycin, chlorothiazide, chlorpromazine, chlorpropamide, erythromycin, penicillamine, prochlorperazine, semisynthetic penicillins (eg, cloxacillin), and sulfadiazine

Acute or chronic hepatitis

- Can be clinically and histologically indistinguishable from autoimmune hepatitis: aspirin, isoniazid (increased risk in HBV carriers), methyldopa, minocycline, nitrofurantoin, nonsteroidal anti-inflammatory drugs, and propylthiouracil
- Can occur with cocaine, ecstasy, efavirenz, nevirapine, ritonavir, sulfonamides, troglitazone (withdrawn from the market in the United States), zafirlukast and various herbal and alternative remedies (eg, chaparral, germander, jin bu huan, skullcap)

Other reactions

- Fatty liver: macrovesicular: alcohol, amiodarone, corticosteroids, methotrexate
- Fatty liver: microvesicular: didanosine, stavudine, tetracyclines, valproic acid, zidovudine
- Granulomas: allopurinol, quinidine, quinine, phenylbutazone, phenytoin
- Fibrosis and cirrhosis: methotrexate, vitamin A
- Peliosis hepatis (blood-filled cavities): anabolic steroids, azathioprine, oral contraceptive steroids
- Neoplasms: oral contraceptive steroids, estrogens (hepatic adenoma but not focal nodular hyperplasia); vinyl chloride (angiosarcoma)

DIFFERENTIAL DIAGNOSIS

Causes of acute hepatitis

- Viral: hepatitis A, B, C*, D (in presence of B), E, infectious mononucleosis, cytomegalovirus, herpes simplex virus, parvovirus B19
- Other infections, eg, leptospirosis, secondary syphilis, brucellosis, Q fever
- Vascular: right-sided congestive heart failure, shock liver, portal vein thrombosis, Budd-Chiari syndrome
- Metabolic: Wilson's disease, acute fatty liver of pregnancy, Reye's syndrome
- Autoimmune hepatitis
- Lymphoma or metastatic cancer

Causes of cholestasis

- Extrahepatic: choledocholithiasis, pancreatic tumor, biliary stricture, primary sclerosing cholangitis (intra- and extrahepatic)
- Intrahepatic: primary biliary cirrhosis, autoimmune cholangitis, infiltrative disease (eg, TB, sarcoidosis, lymphoma, amyloidosis), drugs

 CLINICAL FINDINGS

SYMPTOMS AND SIGNS

- Can mimic all types of liver disease

 DIAGNOSIS

DIAGNOSTIC PROCEDURES

- Inquire about the use of potentially hepatotoxic drugs or exposure to hepatotoxins

TREATMENT

MEDICATIONS

- Removing the offending agent is critical
- Corticosteroids are rarely, if ever, indicated

SURGERY

- Liver transplantation in rare instances of acute liver failure

THERAPEUTIC PROCEDURES

- Supportive treatment: see *Hepatitis*

 ## OUTCOME

FOLLOW-UP

- Monitor liver function tests until sustained improvement is seen

COMPLICATIONS

- Complications are those of liver disease of any etiology, and include hypoprothrombinemia, ascites, edema, portal hypertension, variceal bleeding, and spontaneous bacterial peritonitis

WHEN TO ADMIT

- Intractable nausea and vomiting and need for parenteral fluids
- Encephalopathy or severe coagulopathy indicates impending acute hepatic failure, and hospitalization is mandatory

 ## EVIDENCE

PRACTICE GUIDELINES

- Centers for Disease Control and Prevention (CDC); American Thoracic Society. Update: adverse event data and revised American Thoracic Society/CDC recommendations against the use of rifampin and pyrazinamide for treatment of latent tuberculosis infection–United States, 2003. MMWR 2003; 52:735.
- National Guideline Clearinghouse http://www.guideline.gov/summary/summary.aspx?doc_id=3520&nbr=2746&string=toxic+hepatitis

WEB SITES

- Diseases of the Liver http://cpmcnet.columbia.edu/dept/gi/disliv.html
- Pathology Index http://www-medlib.med.utah.edu/WebPath/LIVEHTML/LIVERIDX.html

INFORMATION FOR PATIENTS

- National Institutes of Health http://www.nlm.nih.gov/medlineplus/ency/article/000226.htm
- The National Women's Health Information Center http://www.4women.gov/faq/easyread/hepatitis-etr.htm

REFERENCES

- Bissell DM et al: Drug-induced liver injury: mechanisms and test syndromes. Hepatology 2001;33:1009.
- Hernandez LV et al: Antiretroviral hepatotoxicity in human immunodeficiency virus-infected patients. Aliment Pharmacol Ther 2001;15:1627. [PMID: 11564003]
- Ibáñez L et al: Prospective surveillance of acute serious liver disease unrelated to infectious, obstructive, or metabolic diseases: epidemiological and clinical features, and exposure to drugs. J Hepatol 2002;37:592.

Lawrence S. Friedman, MD

Hepatocellular Carcinoma

 KEY FEATURES

ESSENTIALS OF DIAGNOSIS

- Malignant neoplasms of the liver that arise from parenchymal cells are called hepatocellular carcinomas; those that originate in the ductular cells are called cholangiocarcinomas

GENERAL CONSIDERATIONS

- Hepatocellular carcinomas are associated with cirrhosis in general and hepatitis B or C in particular
- In Africa and Asia, hepatitis B is of major etiological significance; in the west and Japan hepatitis C and alcoholic cirrhosis are most common
- Other associations include hemochromatosis, aflatoxin exposure (associated with mutation of the $p53$ gene), α_1-antiprotease (α_1-antitrypsin) deficiency, and tyrosinemia
- Cirrhosis from nonalcoholic fatty liver disease is associated with hepatocellular carcinomas
- The fibrolamellar variant of hepatocellular carcinoma occurs in young women and is characterized by a distinctive histological picture, absence of risk factors, and indolent course
- Histologically, hepatocellular carcinoma is made up of cords or sheets of cells that roughly resemble the hepatic parenchyma. Blood vessels such as portal or hepatic veins are commonly involved by tumor
- Staging in the TNM classification: T0: no evidence of primary tumor; T1: solitary tumor without vascular invasion; T2: solitary tumor with vascular invasion or multiple tumors none >5 cm; T3: multiple tumors >5 cm or tumor involving a major branch or the portal or hepatic vein(s); and T4: tumor(s) with direct invasion of adjacent organs other than the gallbladder or with perforation of visceral peritoneum

DEMOGRAPHICS

- Incidence is rising in the United States and western countries because of the high prevalence of chronic hepatitis C infection

 CLINICAL FINDINGS

SYMPTOMS AND SIGNS

- May be unsuspected until there is deterioration in a cirrhotic patient who was formerly stable
- Cachexia, weakness, and weight loss are associated symptoms
- The sudden appearance of ascites, which may be bloody, suggests portal or hepatic vein thrombosis by tumor or bleeding from the necrotic tumor
- There may be a tender enlargement of the liver, with an occasionally palpable mass
- In Africa, young patients typically present with a rapidly expanding abdominal mass. Auscultation may reveal a bruit over the tumor or a friction rub when the process has extended to the surface of the liver

DIFFERENTIAL DIAGNOSIS

- Metastatic cancer
- Benign liver tumors: hemangioma, adenoma, focal nodular hyperplasia
- Pyogenic or amebic liver abscess

 DIAGNOSIS

LABORATORY TESTS

- Laboratory tests may reveal leukocytosis, as opposed to the leukopenia that is frequently encountered in cirrhotic patients
- Anemia is common, but a normal or elevated hematocrit may be found in one-third of patients from tumor elaboration of erythropoietin
- Sudden and sustained elevation of the serum alkaline phosphatase in a formerly stable patient is common
- Hepatitis B surface antigen is in most cases in endemic areas; in the United States anti-hepatitis C virus (HCV) is in up to 40% of cases
- α-Fetoprotein levels are elevated in up to 70% of patients with hepatocellular carcinoma in Western countries (though the sensitivity is lower in African-Americans); however, mild elevations are also often seen in patients with chronic hepatitis
- Serum levels of des-gamma-carboxy prothrombin are elevated in up to 90% of patients with hepatocellular carcinoma, but they may also be elevated in patients with vitamin K deficiency, chronic hepatitis, and metastatic cancer
- Cytological study of ascitic fluid rarely reveals malignant cells

IMAGING STUDIES

- Arterial-phase helical CT scanning with and without intravenous contrast or MRI are preferred for the location and vascularity of the tumor
- Ultrasound is less sensitive but is used to screen for hepatic nodules in high-risk patients
- Contrast-enhanced ultrasound has a sensitivity and specificity approaching those of arterial-phase helical CT

DIAGNOSTIC PROCEDURES

- Liver biopsy is diagnostic, though seeding of the needle tract by tumor is a potential risk ($\leq$5%), and biopsy can be deferred if imaging studies and α-fetoprotein levels are diagnostic or if surgical resection is planned

TREATMENT

MEDICATIONS

- Chemotherapy, hormonal therapy with tamoxifen, and long-acting octreotide have not been shown to prolong life
- Adaptive immunotherapy and treatment of underlying chronic viral hepatitis may lower postsurgical recurrence rates

SURGERY

- Liver transplantation may achieve a better recurrence-free survival than resection with well-compensated cirrhosis and small tumors (one tumor <5 cm or three or fewer tumors each <3 cm in diameter) but is often impractical because of the donor organ shortage; living donor liver transplantation may be considered in these cases
- Liver transplantation may be appropriate for small unresectable tumors in a patient with advanced cirrhosis, with reported 5-year survival rates of up to 75%
- Laparoscopic liver resection has been performed in selected cases

THERAPEUTIC PROCEDURES

- If disease progresses despite treatment, meticulous efforts at palliative care are essential. Patients may develop severe pain due to expansion of the liver capsule by the tumor and require concerted efforts at pain management, including opioid use
- Chemoembolization via the hepatic artery may be palliative and may prolong survival
- Injection of absolute ethanol into, radiofrequency ablation of, or cryotherapy of small tumors (<3 cm) may prolong survival; these are reasonable alternatives to surgical resection in some patients and may provide a "bridge" to liver transplantation

 OUTCOME

PROGNOSIS

- In the United States, overall 1- and 5-year survival rates for hepatocellular carcinoma are 23% and 5%, respectively
- Attempts at surgical resection are usually fruitless if concomitant cirrhosis is present and if the tumor is multifocal
- Surgical resection of solitary hepatocellular carcinomas may result in cure if liver function is preserved (Child class A or possibly B)
- Five-year survival rates rise to 56% for patients with localized resectable disease (T1, T2, T3, selected T4; N0; M0) but are virtually nil for those with localized unresectable or advanced disease

PREVENTION

- In chronic hepatitis B or cirrhosis caused by HCV or alcohol, surveillance should be considered with every 6-month α-fetoprotein testing and ultrasonography. The risk of hepatocellular carcinoma with cirrhosis is 3–5% a year

 EVIDENCE

PRACTICE GUIDELINES

- British Society of Gastroenterology http://www.bsg.org.uk/pdf_word_docs/hcc.pdf

WEB SITES

- Diagnostic and Interventional Radiology of Hepatocellular Carcinoma http://www.rad.unipi.it/works/hcc/presentation-hcc.html
- Hepatic Ultrasound Images http://www.sono.nino.ru/english/hepar_en.html
- Liver Tutorials Visualization and Volume Measurement http://everest.radiology.uiowa.edu/nlm/app/livertoc/livertoc.html

INFORMATION FOR PATIENTS

- American Cancer Society http://www.cancer.org/docroot/cri/content/cri_2_2_1x_what_is_liver_cancer_25.asp
- National Cancer Institute http://www.cancer.gov/cancerinfo/wyntk/liver

REFERENCES

- Anderson JM et al (eds): Yale University workshop on hepatocellular carcinoma. J Clin Gastroenterol 2002;35 (suppl 2):S71.
- Bruix J et al: Prognostic prediction and treatment strategy in hepatocellular carcinoma. Hepatology 2002;35:519.

Lawrence S. Friedman, MD

Herpes Simplex Virus Infections

 KEY FEATURES

ESSENTIALS OF DIAGNOSIS

- Recurrent small grouped vesicles, especially in the orolabial and genital areas
- May follow minor infections, trauma, stress, or sun exposure
- Tzanck smear is positive for multinucleated epithelial giant cells; viral cultures and direct fluorescent antibody tests are positive

GENERAL CONSIDERATIONS

- Recurrent small grouped vesicles on an erythematous base, especially in the orolabial and genital areas
- May follow minor infections, trauma, stress, or sun exposure; regional lymph nodes may be swollen and tender
- Over 85% of adults have serological evidence of herpes simplex type 1 (HSV-1) infections, most often acquired asymptomatically in childhood
- Occasionally, primary infections may be manifested as severe gingivostomatitis
- The subject may have recurrent self-limited attacks, provoked by sun exposure, orofacial surgery, fever, or a viral infection
- About 25% of the U.S. population has serological evidence of infection with herpes simplex type 2 (HSV-2)
- HSV-2 causes lesions whose morphology and natural history are similar to those caused by HSV-1 on the genitalia of both sexes; the infection is acquired by sexual contact

DEMOGRAPHICS

- In monogamous heterosexual couples where one partner has HSV-2 infection, seroconversion of the noninfected partner occurs in 10% over a 1-year period
- Up to 70% of such infections appeared to be transmitted during periods of asymptomatic shedding; uninfected female partners are at greater risk than males
- Owing to changes in sexual behavior, up to 40% of newly acquired cases of genital herpes are due to HSV-1

 CLINICAL FINDINGS

SYMPTOMS AND SIGNS

- See Table 7 (page 1202)
- The principal symptoms are burning and stinging; neuralgia may precede or accompany attacks
- The lesions consist of small, grouped vesicles that can occur anywhere but that most often occur on the vermillion border of the lips, the penile shaft, the labia, the perianal skin, and the buttocks
- Regional lymph nodes may be swollen and tender
- The lesions usually crust and heal in 1 week

DIFFERENTIAL DIAGNOSIS

- Impetigo
- Varicella (chickenpox)
- Herpes zoster (shingles)
- Scabies
- Trauma
- Genital lesions: syphilis, chancroid, lymphogranuloma venereum; Behçet's syndrome, fixed drug eruption
- Oral lesions: aphthous ulcers, herpangina (coxsackievirus), erythema multiforme, pemphigus, primary HIV infection, candidiasis, reactive arthritis, systemic lupus erythematosus, Behçet's syndrome, bullous pemphigoid

 DIAGNOSIS

LABORATORY TESTS

- Direct immunofluorescent antibody slide tests offer rapid, sensitive diagnosis; viral culture may also be helpful
- Tzanck smear is positive for multinucleated epithelial giant cells; viral cultures and direct fluorescent antibody tests are positive
- Herpes serology
  - Not used in the diagnosis of an acute genital ulcer
  - Can determine who is HSV infected and potentially infectious
  - Such testing is very useful in couples in which only one partner reports a history of genital herpes
  - Beware of laboratory variations in type of HSV serologies

Herpes Simplex Virus Infections

 ## TREATMENT

MEDICATIONS

Systemic therapy

- For first clinical episodes
  - The dosage of acyclovir is 200 mg orally five times daily (or 800 mg three times daily); of valacyclovir, 1000 mg twice daily; and of famciclovir, 250 mg three times daily. Treatment is from 7–10 days depending on the severity of the outbreak
- For recurrent herpes
  - Generally milder, does not require therapy, and when therapy is tried it is of limited benefit, with studies finding a reduction in the average outbreak by only 12–24 h
  - Recurrent herpes outbreaks may be treated with 5 days of acyclovir, 200 mg five times a day; 3 days of valacyclovir, 500 mg BID; or 5 days of famciclovir, 125 mg BID
  - For orolabial HSV, valacyclovir, 2 g BID for 1 day, is as effective as longer courses of therapy
  - The addition of a potent topical steroid three times daily reduces the duration, size, and pain of orolabial herpes treated with an oral antiviral agent
- For frequent or severe recurrences
  - Suppressive treatment will reduce outbreaks by 85% and reduces viral shedding by more than 90%
  - The recommended suppressive doses, taken continuously, are acyclovir, 400 mg twice daily; valacyclovir, 500 mg once daily; or famciclovir, 125–250 mg twice daily
  - Long-term suppression appears very safe, and after 5–7 years a substantial proportion of patients can discontinue treatment
  - It is unknown if the suppression of outbreaks and asymptomatic shedding will reduce transmission
- Local measures: topical antiviral therapy is not significantly effective

 ## OUTCOME

COMPLICATIONS

- Complications include pyoderma, eczema herpeticum, herpetic whitlow, herpes gladiatorum (epidemic herpes in wrestlers transmitted by contact), esophagitis, neonatal infection, keratitis, and encephalitis
- Recurrent attacks lasting several days

PROGNOSIS

- Recurrent attacks last several days and patients generally recover without sequelae

WHEN TO REFER

- Refractory cases not responding to oral antiviral therapy

PREVENTION

- Sunscreens are very useful adjuncts adjuncts in preventing sun-induced recurrences
- Prophylactic use of oral acyclovir may prevent recurrence; acyclovir should be started at a dosage of 200 mg five times daily beginning 24 h prior to ultraviolet light exposure, dental surgery, or orolabial cosmetic surgery; comparable doses are 500 mg twice daily for valacyclovir and 250 mg twice daily for famciclovir
- Barrier protection is not completely effective, since shedding occurs from widespread areas of the perineum not covered by condoms

 ## EVIDENCE

PRACTICE GUIDELINES

- National Guideline Clearinghouse http://www.guideline.gov/summary/ summary.aspx?doc_id=3035&nbr=2261 &string=herpes+simplex http://www.guideline.gov/summary/ summary.aspx?doc_id=3233&nbr= 2459&string=herpes+simplex

WEB SITES

- American Academy of Dermatology http://www.aad.org
- Dermatology Handbook for Family Practice from the University of Iowa http://www.vh.org/Providers/ClinRef/ FPHandbook/17.html

INFORMATION FOR PATIENTS

- The National Women's Health Center http://www.4woman.gov/faq/Easyread/ genital-etr.htm
- American Academy of Family Physicians http://familydoctor.org/healthfacts/ 091/Information for PATIENTs
- JAMA patient page: Sexually transmitted diseases. JAMA 1998;280:944.
- JAMA patient page: Genital herpes. JAMA 2001;285:3050.

REFERENCES

- Baker DA et al: Once-daily valacyclovir hydrochloride for suppression of recurrent genital herpes. Obstet Gynecol 1999;94:103. [PMID: 10289727]
- Emmert DH: Treatment of common cutaneous herpes simplex virus infections. Am Fam Physician 2000;61:1697. [PMID: 10750877]
- Wald A: New therapies and prevention strategies for genital herpes. Clin Infect Dis 1999;28(Suppl 1):S4. [PMID: 10028105]

Timothy G. Berger, MD

Herpes Zoster

 KEY FEATURES

ESSENTIALS OF DIAGNOSIS

- Pain along the course of a nerve followed by painful grouped vesicular lesions
- Involvement is unilateral; some lesions (<20) may occur outside the affected dermatome
- Lesions are usually on face or trunk
- Tzanck smear positive, especially in vesicular lesions

GENERAL CONSIDERATIONS

- An acute vesicular eruption due to the varicella-zoster virus
- It usually occurs in adults
- With rare exceptions, patients suffer only one attack
- Dermatomal herpes zoster does not imply the presence of a visceral malignancy
- Generalized disease, however, raises the suspicion of an associated immunosuppressive disorder such as Hodgkin's disease or HIV infection
- Early (within 72 h after onset) and aggressive antiviral treatment of herpes zoster reduces the severity and duration of postherpetic neuralgia

DEMOGRAPHICS

- HIV-infected patients are 20 times more likely to develop zoster, often before other clinical findings of HIV disease are present

 CLINICAL FINDINGS

SYMPTOMS AND SIGNS

- See Table 7 (page 1202)
- Pain usually precedes the eruption by 48 h or more and may persist and actually increase in intensity after the lesions have disappeared
- The lesions consist of grouped, tense, deep-seated vesicles distributed unilaterally along a dermatome
- The commonest distributions are on the trunk or face
- Up to 20 lesions may be found outside the affected dermatomes
- Regional lymph glands may be tender and swollen

DIFFERENTIAL DIAGNOSIS

- Contact dermatitis (eg, poison oak or ivy)
- Herpes simplex
- Erysipelas
- Prodromal pain mimics angina, peptic ulcer, appendicitis, biliary or renal colic

 DIAGNOSIS

LABORATORY TESTS

- Clinical
- A history of HIV risk factors and HIV testing when appropriate should be considered, especially in zoster patients under 55 years of age

TREATMENT

MEDICATIONS

- See Table 6 (page 1199)

Immunocompetent host

- Patients over age 55 should be treated with antiviral therapy; in addition, younger patients with acute moderate to severe pain may be benefited by effective antiviral therapy
- Oral famciclovir, 500 mg three times daily; valacyclovir, 1 g three times daily; or acyclovir, 800 mg five times daily; all for 7 days
- The dose of antiviral should be adjusted for renal function
- Systemic corticosteroids are effective in reducing acute pain, improving quality of life, and returning patients to normal activities much more quickly; they do not increase the risk of dissemination in immunocompetent hosts
- If not contraindicated, a tapering 3-week course of prednisone, starting at 60 mg/day, for adjunctive benefit

Immunocompromised host

- Most immunocompromised patients are candidates for antiviral therapy
- The dosage schedule is as listed above, but treatment should be continued until the lesions have completely crusted and are healed or almost healed (up to 2 weeks)
- Corticosteroids should not be given adjunctively since they increase the risk of dissemination
- Progression of disease may necessitate intravenous therapy with acyclovir, 10 mg/kg intravenously, three times daily; after 3–4 days, oral therapy may be substituted if there has been a good response to intravenous therapy; adverse effects include decreased renal function from crystallization, nausea and vomiting, and abdominal pain
- Foscarnet, administered in a dosage of 40 mg/kg two or three times daily intravenously, is indicated for treatment of acyclovir-resistant varicella-zoster virus infections

Local measures

- Calamine or starch shake lotions

Postherpetic neuralgia

- Capsaicin ointment, 0.025–0.075%, or lidocaine (Lidoderm) topical patches

- Chronic postherpetic neuralgia may be relieved by regional blocks (stellate ganglion, epidural, local infiltration, or peripheral nerve), with or without corticosteroids added to the injections
- Amitriptyline, 25–75 mg as a single nightly dose, is the first-line oral therapy beyond simple analgesics
- Gabapentin, up to 3600 mg daily (starting at 300 mg three times daily), may be added for additional pain relief

THERAPEUTIC PROCEDURES

- Nerve blocks may be important in the management of initial severe pain
- Patients should maintain good hydration, and elderly patients with reduced renal function should be followed closely

OUTCOME

COMPLICATIONS

- Sacral zoster may be associated with bladder and bowel dysfunction
- Persistent neuralgia, anesthesia or scarring of the affected area following healing, facial or other nerve paralysis, and encephalitis may occur
- Postherpetic neuralgia is most common after involvement of the trigeminal region, and in patients over 55
- Zoster ophthalmicus (V_1) can result in visual impairment

PROGNOSIS

- The eruption persists 2–3 weeks and usually does not recur
- Motor involvement in 2–3% may lead to temporary palsy
- Oral corticosteroids do not reduce the prevalence, severity, or duration of postherpetic neuralgia beyond that achieved by effective antiviral therapy

WHEN TO REFER

- Ophthalmological consultation is vital for involvement of the first branch of the trigeminal nerve

PREVENTION

- Early and aggressive antiviral therapy for postherpetic neuralgia

EVIDENCE

PRACTICE GUIDELINES

- National Guideline Clearinghouse http://www.guideline.gov/summary/summary.aspx?doc_id=1980&nbr=1206&string=herpes+zoster

WEB SITES

- American Academy of Dermatology http://www.aad.org
- Dermatology Handbook for Family Practice from the University of Iowa http://www.vh.org/Providers/ClinRef/FPHandbook/17.html

INFORMATION FOR PATIENTS

- American Academy of Dermatology http://www.aad.org/pamphlets/herpesZoster.html
- Centers for Disease Control and Prevention http://www.medem.com/search/article_display.cfm?path=\\TANQUERAY\M_ContentItem&mstr=/M_ContentItem/ZZZ729IT8FC.html&soc=CDC&srch_typ=NAV_SERCH

REFERENCES

- Alper BS et al: Does treatment of acute herpes zoster prevent or shorten postherpetic neuralgia? J Fam Pract 2000;49: 255. [PMID: 10735485]
- Dworkin RH et al: Prospects for the prevention of postherpetic neuralgia in herpes zoster patients. Clin J Pain 2000;16(2 Suppl):S90. [PMID: 10870747]
- Stankus SJ et al: Management of herpes zoster (shingles) and postherpetic neuralgia. Am Fam Physician 2000;61: 2437. [PMID: 10794584]

Timothy G. Berger, MD

Hirsutism & Virilization

 KEY FEATURES

ESSENTIALS OF DIAGNOSIS

- Menstrual disorders, hirsutism, acne
- Virilization: increased muscularity, androgenic alopecia, deepening of voice, enlargement of clitoris
- Occasionally, a palpable pelvic tumor
- Urinary 17-ketosteroids and serum dehydroepiandrosterone sulfate (DHEAS) and androstenedione elevated in adrenal disorders, variable in others
- Serum testosterone often elevated

GENERAL CONSIDERATIONS

- Major androgen is testosterone. If serum testosterone is normal, an endocrine cause for hirsuitism is extremely unlikely
- In women, circulating testosterone is normally derived from ovarian secretion (60%) and peripheral conversion from androstenedione (40%)
- Androstenedione is secreted in equal amounts by adrenals and ovaries; DHEAS secreted only by adrenals

Causes of hirsutism

- Idiopathic or familial—most women with hirsutism or androgenic alopecia have no detectable hyperandrogenism. Often hirsutism is familial and may be normal for genetic background
- Polycystic ovary syndrome—accounts for >50% of cases. Associated with amenorrhea or oligomenorrhea, anovulation, and obesity. Insulin resistance and diabetes common
- Ovarian tumor (uncommon) and adrenal carcinoma (rare)
- Steroidogenic enzyme defects
  - Baby girls with "classic" 21-hydroxylase deficiency have ambiguous genitalia and may become virilized unless corticosteroids replaced
  - 2% of adult-onset hirsutism is due to partial defect in adrenal 21-hydroxylase
  - Rare patients with hyperandrogenism and hypertension have 11-hydroxylase deficiency
  - Patients with XY karyotype and deficiency of 17α-hydroxysteroid dehydrogenase-3 or 5α-reductase-2 may present as phenotypic girls who develop virilization at puberty
- Other rare causes: acromegaly; ACTH-induced Cushing's syndrome; adrenal carcinoma, genetic cortisol resistance, maternal virilization during pregnancy

due to luteoma of pregnancy, hyperreactio luteinalis, or diffuse stromal Leydig cell hyperplasia in postmenopausal women
- Pharmacological causes: minoxidil, cyclosporine, phenytoin, anabolic steroids, diazoxide, some progestins

DEMOGRAPHICS

- Most common in women with some Mediterranean ancestry

 CLINICAL FINDINGS

SYMPTOMS AND SIGNS

- Increased sexual hair (chin, upper lip, abdomen, and chest)
- Acne due to increased sebaceous gland activity
- Menstrual irregularities, anovulation, and amenorrhea common
- Defeminization (breast size decrease, loss of feminine adipose tissue) and virilization (frontal balding, muscularity, clitoromegaly, and deepening of voice) if androgen excess is pronounced
- Virilization implicates presence of testosterone-producing neoplasm
- Hypertension seen in rare conditions with Cushing's syndrome, adrenal 11-hydroxylase deficiency, or cortisol resistance syndrome
- Clitoromegaly
- Ovarian enlargement may be cystic or neoplastic

 DIAGNOSIS

LABORATORY TESTS

- Serum androgens mainly useful to screen for rare occult adrenal or ovarian neoplasms
- Serum total testosterone and free testosterone. Some free testosterone assays are unreliable: free androgen index, analog free testosterone assay, electrochemical luminescence assay
- Serum testosterone >200 ng/dL or free testosterone >40 ng/dL indicates need for pelvic examination and ultrasound. If negative, perform adrenal CT scan
- Serum androstenedione >1000 ng/dL also implicates ovarian or adrenal neoplasm
- Milder elevations of testosterone or androstenedione are usually treated with oral contraceptives
- Markedly elevated serum DHEAS (>700 mg/dL) implies adrenal source of androgen, usually adrenal hyperplasia and rarely adrenal carcinoma. Perform adrenal CT scan
- Unclear which patients (if any) with hyperandrogenism should be screened for "late-onset" 21-hydroxylase deficiency, where baseline 17-hydroxyprogesterone is usually >300 ng/dL or stimulated level is >1000 ng/dL (30–60 min after 0.25 mg IM cosyntropin)
- Signs of Cushing's syndrome should prompt screening
- Follicle-stimulating hormone (FSH) and luteinizing hormone (LH) elevated if amenorrhea is due to ovarian failure
- LH:FSH ratio >2.0, hyperglycemia, and elevated fasting insulin level are common in polycystic ovary syndrome
- Selective venous sampling for testosterone may be required to diagnose small virilizing ovarian tumors not detected on ultrasound, MRI, or CT

IMAGING STUDIES

- Adrenal CT as described above
- Pelvic ultrasound or MRI to detect virilizing tumors of ovary
- Ultrasound shows polycystic ovaries in ~33% of normal young women, so test is not helpful in diagnosis of polycystic ovary syndrome

Hirsutism & Virilization

TREATMENT

MEDICATIONS

- Use medication if underlying cause not reversible
- Spironolactone, 50–100 mg PO BID on days 5–25 of menstrual cycle or QD if used concomitantly with oral contraceptive. Hyperkalemia or hyponatremia occur uncommonly
- Cyproterone acetate (not available in United States), 2 mg PO QD, is potent antiandrogen; usually given with oral contraceptive
- Finasteride, 5 mg PO QD, inhibits 5α-reductase, which converts testosterone to active dihydrotestosterone in skin. Modestly reduces hirsutism over 6 months—comparable results to spironolactone. Finasteride ineffective for androgenic alopecia in women
- Flutamide, 250 mg PO QD, inhibits androgen receptors and uptake. Used with oral contraceptive, likely more effective than spironolactone in improving hirsutism, acne, and male pattern baldness. Hepatotoxicity is rare
- Oral contraceptives stimulate menses, if desired, but less effective for hirsutism. Low-androgenic progestin (desogestrel, gestodene)-containing contraceptives are preferred
- Metformin, 500–1000 mg PO BID, for polycystic ovary syndrome with amenorrhea tends to restore normal menses and reduce hirsutism. Contraindicated in renal and liver disease. Does not cause hypoglycemia in nondiabetics
- Androgenic alopecia may be treated with topical minoxidil 2% solution applied BID chronically to a dry scalp. Hypertrichosis occurs in 3–5% (eg, on forehead, cheeks, upper lip, chin) and usually resolves 1–6 months after drug stopped.
- **Note: Give antiandrogen treatments only to nonpregnant women—use during pregnancy causes malformations and pseudohermaphroditism in male infants. Women should take oral contraceptives when indicated and avoid pregnancy**

SURGERY

- Resection of any testosterone-secreting ovarian or adrenal tumor
- Laparoscopic bilateral oophorectomy (if CT scan of adrenals and ovaries normal) indicated in postmenopausal women with severe hyperandrogenism, since

small hilar cell tumors of ovary may not be visible on scans

THERAPEUTIC PROCEDURES

- Treat underlying cause of hyperandrogenism if possible
- Discontinue any potentially offending drugs
- Encourage shaving, depilatories, waxing, electrolysis, or bleaching, and laser therapy for hirsutism

OUTCOME

FOLLOW-UP

- Check serum potassium and creatinine 1 month after starting spironolactone
- If testosterone elevated, follow serum testosterone during therapy or after surgery

PROGNOSIS

- Polycystic ovary syndrome: women frequently regain normal menstrual cycles with aging

EVIDENCE

PRACTICE GUIDELINES

- AACE Medical Guidelines for Clinical Practice: 2001 Hyperandrogenism http://www.aace.com/clin/guidelines/hyperandrogenism2001.pdf
- Azziz R: The evaluation and management of hirsutism. Obstet Gynecol 2003;101(5 Pt 1):995. [PMID: 12738163]
- Claman P et al: SOGC clinical practice guidelines. Hirsutism: evaluation and treatment. J Obstet Gynaecol Can 2002;24:62. [PMID: 12196888]

WEB SITES

- University of Maryland Medicine—Hirsutism http://www.umm.edu/altmed/ConsConditions/Hirsutismcc.html
- Uptodate—Patient information: Treatment of polycystic ovary syndrome http://patients.uptodate.com/frames.asp?page=topic.asp&file=endo_hor/12474

INFORMATION FOR PATIENTS

- American Academy of Family Physicians—Hirsutism http://familydoctor.org/handouts/210.html
- MEDLINEplus—Virilization http://www.nlm.nih.gov/medlineplus/ency/article/002339.htm

REFERENCES

- Bayram F et al: Comparison of high-dose finasteride (5 mg/day) versus low-dose finasteride (2.5 mg/day) in the treatment of hirsutism. Eur J Endocrinol 2002;147:467. [PMID: 12370107]
- Farquhar C et al: Spironolactone versus placebo or in combination with steroids for hirsutism and/or acne (Cochrane Review). Cochrane Database Syst Rev 2001;4:CD000194. [PMID: 11687072]
- Ibanez L et al: Treatment of hirsutism, hyperandrogenism, oligomenorrhea, dyslipidemia, and hyperinsulinism in nonobese, adolescent girls: effect of flutamide. J Clin Endocrinol Metab 2000;85:3251. [PMID: 10999817]
- Kelly CJ et al: The effect of metformin on hirsutism in polycystic ovary syndrome. Eur J Endocrinol 2002;147:217. [PMID: 12153743]
- Mercke DP et al: NIH conference. Future directions in the study and management of congenital adrenal hyperplasia due to 21-hydroxylase deficiency. Ann Intern Med 2002;136:320. [PMID: 11848730]
- Venturoli S et al: Low-dose flutamide (125 mg/day) as maintenance therapy in the treatment of hirsutism. Horm Res 2001;56:25. [PMID: 11815724]

Paul A. Fitzgerald, MD

Histoplasmosis

 KEY FEATURES

ESSENTIALS OF DIAGNOSIS

- Infection caused by *Histoplasma capsulatum*, a dimorphic fungus isolated from soil contaminated with bird or bat droppings in endemic areas
- Most patients asymptomatic; if symptomatic, respiratory illness most common
- Dissemination in profoundly immunocompromised patients

GENERAL CONSIDERATIONS

- Acute histoplasmosis frequently occurs in epidemics, often when soil containing infected bird or bat droppings is disturbed
- Infection presumably occurs by inhalation
- The organism proliferates and is carried hematogenously from lungs to other organs
- Disseminated histoplasmosis occurs rarely in patients with normal immune function
- Dissemination common in AIDS patients, usually with CD4 counts <100 cells/μL, and in other immunocompromised patients, with poor prognosis

DEMOGRAPHICS

- Endemic areas: central and eastern United States (especially Ohio River and Mississippi River valleys), eastern Canada, Mexico, Central America, South America, Africa, and southeast Asia
- Disseminated disease: most often occurs as reactivation of prior infection, but may reflect acute infection
- Chronic progressive pulmonary histoplasmosis: occurs in older patients with chronic obstructive pulmonary disease

 CLINICAL FINDINGS

SYMPTOMS AND SIGNS

- Most cases asymptomatic with no pulmonary symptoms or signs even in those who later have calcifications on chest x-ray
- Mild symptomatic illness: influenza-like illness, often lasting 1–4 days
- More severe illness: presents as atypical pneumonia, with fever, cough, and mild central chest pain for 5–15 days
- Physical examination usually normal
- Acute pulmonary histoplasmosis: marked prostration, fever, but few pulmonary complaints even when chest x-ray shows pneumonia
- Progressive pulmonary histoplasmosis
  - Fever, weight loss, and prostration
  - Dyspnea, cough
  - Oropharyngeal ulcers
  - Lymphadenopathy
  - Hepatosplenomegaly, multiorgan involvement, including adrenal glands
- Disseminated histoplasmosis in profoundly immunocompromised individuals: may be fulminant, simulating septic shock, with death ensuing rapidly without treatment

DIFFERENTIAL DIAGNOSIS

- Influenza
- Atypical pneumonia
- Coccidioidomycosis
- Tuberculosis
- Sarcoidosis
- Blastomycosis
- Pneumoconiosis, eg, silicosis
- *Pneumocystis* pneumonia
- Lymphoma (including lymphocytic interstitial pneumonitis)
- Nocardiosis

 DIAGNOSIS

LABORATORY TESTS

- Elevations of alkaline phosphatase and lactate dehydrogenase (marked) and ferritin common
- Anemia of chronic disease in chronic progressive pulmonary histoplasmosis
- Sputum culture rarely positive except in chronic pulmonary histoplasmosis
- Pancytopenia from bone marrow involvement in disseminated disease
- Blood or bone marrow cultures positive in >80% of disseminated disease in immunocompromised individuals
- Skin tests and serological tests seldom diagnostic
- Positive histoplasmin skin test reflects past infection
- In acute pulmonary histoplasmosis: screening immunodiffusion test sensitivity 50%, complement fixation titers sensitivity ~80%, combination sensitivity up to 80% in immunocompromised
- Urine antigen test: sensitivity >90% for disseminated disease in AIDS; useful to diagnose relapse
- Biopsy of affected organs with culture useful in disseminated disease

IMAGING STUDIES

- Lung and splenic calcifications on x-rays may reflect past infection
- Radiographic findings during acute illness are variable and nonspecific
- Disseminated disease in profoundly immunocompromised: chest x-ray may show a miliary pattern

TREATMENT

MEDICATIONS

- Itraconazole, 200-400 mg/day PO QD, for weeks to months for progressive pulmonary disease, and for mild to moderate nonmeningeal disseminated disease in immunocompetent or immunocompromised yields response rate of ~80%
- Amphotericin B if patient cannot take PO, failed itraconazole, has meningitis, or has severe disseminated disease and is immunocompromised. Meningitis or severe disseminated disease may require a total of ≤2.5 g of amphotericin, but once clinically stable, oral itraconazole can be substituted
- Lipid-based amphotericin B formulations appear to have reduced nephrotoxicity, allowing administration of higher doses, but are more costly
- AIDS-related histoplasmosis requires lifelong itraconazole, 200–400 mg PO QD to prevent relapse

 OUTCOME

PROGNOSIS

- Acute histoplasmosis: lasts from 1 week to 6 months but is almost never fatal
- Progressive disseminated histoplasmosis: usually fatal within 6 weeks or less; more rapidly in immunocompromised

PREVENTION

- Recurrence of AIDS-related histoplasmosis decreased with lifelong itraconazole, 200–400 mg PO QD

EVIDENCE

PRACTICE GUIDELINES

- Practice Guidelines from the Infectious Diseases Society of America http://www.journals.uchicago.edu/CID/journal/issues/v30n4/990 670/990670.web.pdf 2001
- USPHS/IDSA guidelines for the prevention of opportunistic infections in persons infected with human immunodeficiency virus. U.S. Department of Health and Human Services, Public Health Service http://aidsinfo.nih.gov/guidelines/op_infections\OI_112801.pdf

WEB SITE

- CDC http://www.cdc.gov/ncidod/dbmd/diseaseinfo/histoplasmosis_g.htm

INFORMATION FOR PATIENTS

- CDC FAQ http://www.cdc.gov/ncidod/dbmd/diseaseinfo/histoplasmosis_g.htm#What%20is%20histoplasmosis
- Cleveland Clinic—OHS http://www.clevelandclinic.org/health/health-info/docs/0900/099 8.asp?index=5635
- NIAID http://www.aegis.com/news/niaid/1994/NA941102.html

REFERENCES

- Johnson PC et al: Safety and efficacy of liposomal amphotericin B compared with conventional amphotericin B for induction therapy of histoplasmosis in patients with AIDS. Ann Intern Med 2002;137:105. [PMID: 12118965]
- Mocherla S et al: Treatment of histoplasmosis. Semin Respir Infect 2001;16:141. [PMID: 11521246]
- Wheat LJ et al: State-of-the-art review of pulmonary fungal infections. Semin Respir Infect 2002;17:158. [PMID: 12070835]

Richard J. Hamill, MD

HIV Infection

KEY FEATURES

ESSENTIALS OF DIAGNOSIS

- Risk factors: sexual contact with an infected person, parenteral exposure to infected blood by transfusion or needle sharing, perinatal exposure
- Opportunistic infections due to diminished cellular immunity—often life-threatening
- Aggressive cancers, particularly Kaposi's sarcoma and extranodal lymphoma
- Neurological manifestations: dementia, aseptic meningitis, and neuropathy

GENERAL CONSIDERATIONS

- Definition: Centers for Disease Control and Prevention AIDS case definition (Table 116, page 1296)
- Etiology: HIV-1, a retrovirus

DEMOGRAPHICS

- In 2000, ~10 million persons worldwide are infected with HIV; ~700,000 Americans are infected with HIV and ~315,000 are living with AIDS: 51% of those are gay or bisexual men; 28% are heterosexual injection drug users; 18% are heterosexual noninjection drug users; and 24% are women

CLINICAL Findings

SYMPTOMS AND SIGNS

- HIV-related infections and neoplasms affect virtually every organ
- Many HIV-infected individuals remain asymptomatic for years even without antiretroviral therapy, with a mean time of approximately 10 years between exposure and development of AIDS
- Symptoms protean and nonspecific
- Fever, night sweats, and weight loss
- Shortness of breath, cough, and fever from pneumonia
- Anorexia, nausea and vomiting, and increased metabolic rate contribute to weight loss
- Diarrhea occurs from infections with bacterial, viral, or parasitic agents
- Physical examination may be normal. Hairy leukoplakia of the tongue, disseminated Kaposi's sarcoma, and cutaneous bacillary angiomatosis are predictive; cutaneous anergy is common

- Ocular: cytomegalovirus, herpesvirus, or toxoplasmosis retinitis
- Oral: candidiasis, pseudomembranous (removable white plaques) and erythematous (red friable plaques); hairy leukoplakia; angular cheilitis; gingivitis or periodontitis; aphthous ulcers; Kaposi's sarcoma (usually on the hard palate); and warts
- Sinuses: chronic sinusitis
- Lungs: bacterial (eg, *Steptococcus pneumoniae*, *Pseudomonas aeruginosa*, *Haemophilus influenzae*), mycobacterial [eg, *Mycobacterium tuberculosis*, *M avium* complex (MAC)], fungal (eg, *Pneumocystis jiroveci*), and viral pneumonias. Noninfectious: Kaposi's sarcoma, non-Hodgkin's lymphoma, and interstitial pneumonitis
- Gastrointestinal: esophagitis (*Candida*, herpes simplex, cytomegalovirus); gastropathy and malabsorption. Enterocolitis: bacteria (*Campylobacter*, *Salmonella*, *Shigella*), viruses (cytomegalovirus, adenovirus, HIV itself), and protozoans (*Cryptosporidium*, *Entamoeba histolytica*, *Giardia*, *Isospora*, *Microsporidia*)
- Hepatic: liver infections (mycobacterial, cytomegalovirus, hepatitis B virus, hepatitis C virus) and neoplasms (lymphoma), and medication-related hepatitis
- Biliary: cholecystitis, sclerosing cholangitis, and papillary stenosis (cytomegalovirus, *Cryptosporidium*, and *Microsporidia*)
- Central nervous system: intracerebral space-occupying lesions (eg, toxoplasmosis, bacterial and nocardia abscesses, cryptococcomas, tuberculomas), HIV encephalopathy, meningitis, CNS (non-Hodgkin's) lymphoma, progressive multifocal leukoencephalopathy (PML)
- Spinal cord: HIV myelopathy
- Peripheral nervous system: inflammatory polyneuropathies, sensory neuropathies, and mononeuropathies; cytomegalovirus polyradiculopathy; transverse myelitis (herpes zoster or cytomegalovirus)
- Endocrinological: adrenal insufficiency from infection (eg, cytomegalovirus and MAC), infiltration (Kaposi's sarcoma), hemorrhage, and presumed autoimmune injury; isolated mineralocorticoid defect; thyroid function test abnormalities (high T_3, T_4, and thyroxine-binding globulin, and low reverse-T_3)
- Gynecological: vaginal candidiasis, cervical dysplasia and carcinoma, and pelvic inflammatory disease

- Malignancies: Kaposi's sarcoma, non-Hodgkin's and Hodgkin's lymphoma, primary lymphoma of the brain, cervical dysplasia and invasive cervical carcinoma, anal dysplasia and squamous cell carcinoma
- Skin: viral (herpes simplex, herpes zoster, *Molluscum contagiosum*), bacterial (*Staphylococcus* folliculitis, furuncles, bullous impetigo, dissemination with sepsis; bacillary angiomatosis caused by *Bartonella henselae* and *Bartonella quintana*), fungal (*Candida*, dermatophytes, *Malassezia furfur/Pityrosporum ovale* seborrheic dermatitis), neoplastic (Kaposi's sarcoma), and nonspecific (psoriasis, severe pruritus, xerosis) dermatitides
- Musculoskeletal: myopathy; arthritis of single or multiple joints, with or without effusions; reactive arthritis (Reiter's syndrome); psoriatic arthritis; sicca syndrome, and systemic lupus erythematosus

DIFFERENTIAL DIAGNOSIS

- Cancer, chronic infections such as tuberculosis and endocarditis, and endocrinological diseases such as hyperthyroidism; acute and chronic lung infections, diffuse interstitial pulmonary infiltrates; alcoholism, liver disease, renal dysfunction, thyroid disease, and vitamin deficiency; chronic meningitis; infectious enterocolitis, antibiotic-associated colitis, inflammatory bowel disease, and malabsorption syndromes

DIAGNOSIS

LABORATORY TESTS

- Lab findings in HIV infection (Table 117, page 1297)
- HIV antibody by enzyme-linked immunosorbent assay (ELISA), confirmed by Western blot (sensitivity >99.5%, specificity ~100%)
- ~95% of persons develop antibodies within 6 weeks after infection
- Absolute CD4 lymphocyte count: as counts decrease, risk of serious opportunistic infection over the subsequent 3–5 years increases

IMAGING STUDIES

- Tests for CNS toxoplasmosis: head CT scan, stereotactic brain biopsy
- Tests for HIV myelopathy: LP and head MRI or CT scan

DIAGNOSTIC PROCEDURES

- Tests for *P jiroveci* pneumonia: ABGs, serum LDH, chest x-ray, Wright-Giemsa stain of induced sputum, bronchoalveolar lavage
- Tests for cryptococcal meningitis: cerebrospinal fluid (CSF) culture; CSF, serum CRAG
- Tests for HIV meningitis: CSF cell count
- Tests for AIDS dementia complex, depression: neuropsychiatric testing
- Tests for myopathy: creatine kinase; muscle biopsy
- Tests for hepatic dysfunction: percutaneous liver biopsy; blood culture, biopsy of a more accessible site
- Tests for enterocolitis: stool culture and multiple ova and parasite examinations; colonoscopy and biopsy

TREATMENT

MEDICATIONS

- Fever: antipyretics
- Anorexia: megestrol acetate, 80 mg QID, or dronabinol, 2.5–5 mg TID
- Weight loss: food supplementation with high-calorie drinks; growth hormone, 0.1 mg/kg/day SQ for 12 weeks, or anabolic steroids—oxandrolone, 15–20 mg PO in 2–4 divided doses; testosterone enanthate or cypionate, 100–200 mg IM Q 2–4 weeks; or testosterone patches or gel 4–6 mg/day
- Nausea: prochlorperazine, 10 mg PO TID QAC; metoclopramide, 10 mg PO TID QAC; or ondansetron, 8 mg PO TID QAC; empiric oral antifungal agent
- Antiretroviral treatment when CD4 count <350 cells/μL (Table 120, page 1300)
- Common opportunistic infections and malignancies (Table 119, page 1298)

OUTCOME

FOLLOW-UP

- CD4 cell counts Q 3–6 months
- Viral load tests Q 3–6 months, and 1 month after change in therapy
- Health care maintenance (Table 118, page 1297)

PROGNOSIS

- The efficacy of antiretroviral treatments—especially protease inhibitors or nonnucleoside reverse transcriptase inhibitors—has improved prognosis

WHEN TO REFER

- Refer for advice regarding initiation or change of antiretroviral therapy
- Refer for management of complicated opportunistic infections

WHEN TO ADMIT

- Admit for new unexplained fever if bacterial infection requiring IV antibiotics is suspected
- Admit as indicated by acute organ system dysfunction or decline in functional status

PREVENTION

Primary prevention

- Precautions regarding sexual practices and intravenous drug use, use of perinatal HIV prophylaxis, screening of blood products, and infection control practices in the health care setting (safer sex, latex condoms, and safe needle use)

Secondary prevention

- For *P jiroveci* pneumonia when CD4 counts <200 cells/μL, a CD4 lymphocyte percentage <14%, or weight loss or oral candidiasis: trimethoprim-sulfamethoxazole, aerosolized pentamidine, or dapsone (Table 121, page 1302)
- For MAC infection when CD4 counts <75–100 cells/μL: clarithromycin (500 mg PO BID), azithromycin (1200 mg PO Q week), or rifabutin 300 mg PO QD
- For *M tuberculosis* infection when positive purified protein derivative reactions >5 mm of induration: isoniazid, 300 mg PO QD plus pyridoxine, 50 mg PO QD for 9–12 months
- For toxoplasmosis when positive IgG toxoplasma serology: trimethoprim-sulfamethoxazole (1 DS tablet PO QD), or

pyrimethamine, 25 mg PO Q week plus dapsone, 100 mg PO QD
- For cytomegalovirus in patients with CD4 counts <50 cells/μL (unless serum CMV IgG antibody test is negative): ganciclovir PO
- For cryptococcosis, candidiasis, other fungi: fluconazole, 200 mg PO QD

EVIDENCE

PRACTICE GUIDELINES

- Fauci AS et al: Guidelines for the use of antiretroviral agents in HIV-infected adults and adolescents. February 2001. www.hivatis.org.

REFERENCES

- Grabar S et al: Clinical outcome of patients with HIV-1 infection according to immunologic and virologic response after 6 months of highly active antiretroviral therapy. Ann Intern Med 2000; 133:401. [PMID: 10975957]
- Gulick RM et al: Simultaneous versus sequential initiation of therapy with indinavir, zidovudine, and lamivudine for HIV-1 infection: 100-week follow-up. JAMA 1998;280:35. [PMID: 9660361]
- Kovacs JA et al: Prophylaxis against opportunistic infections in patients with human immunodeficiency virus infection. N Engl J Med 2000;342:1416. [PMID: 10805828]

Harry Hollander, MD
Mitchell H. Katz, MD

Hoarseness, Dysphonia, & Stridor

 KEY FEATURES

ESSENTIALS OF DIAGNOSIS

- The primary symptoms of laryngeal disease are hoarseness and stridor

GENERAL CONSIDERATIONS

- Hoarseness is caused by an abnormal flow of air past the vocal cords
- Laryngitis, voice abuse, and vocal cord nodules are common causes of hoarseness

Acute hoarseness

- Acute laryngitis is thought to be viral in origin, although *Moraxella catarrhalis* and *Haemophilus influenzae* isolates from the nasopharynx occur at higher than expected frequencies

Persistent hoarseness

- Vocal cord nodules or polyps (from overuse of voice or improper use over extended periods of time) produce prolonged hoarseness
- Vocal cord polypoid changes (from vocal abuse, smoking, chemical industrial irritants, or hypothyoidism)
- Gastroesophageal reflux is a common cause of chronic hoarseness and should be considered if other causes of abnormal laryngeal airflow (such as tumor) have been excluded by laryngoscopy: less than 50% of patients have typical symptoms of heartburn and regurgitation
- In patients with a history of tobacco use, laryngeal cancer or lung cancer (leading to paralysis of a recurrent laryngeal nerve) must be strongly considered in persistent hoarseness

DEMOGRAPHICS

- Acute laryngitis is the most common cause of hoarseness

 CLINICAL FINDINGS

SYMPTOMS AND SIGNS

- The voice is "breathy" when too much air passes incompletely apposed vocal cords, as in unilateral vocal cord paralysis
- The voice is harsh when turbulence is created by irregularity of the vocal cords, as in laryngitis or a mass lesion
- Stridor, a high-pitched sound, is produced by lesions that narrow the airway
  – Airway narrowing above the vocal cords produces predominantly inspiratory stridor
  – Airway narrowing below the vocal cords produces either expiratory or mixed stridor
- In gastroesophageal reflux-induced hoarseness, the voice is usually worse in the morning and improves during the day; associated symptoms include a feeling of a lump in the throat, or an excessive desire for throat clearing

DIFFERENTIAL DIAGNOSIS

- Laryngitis
- Voice overuse
- Vocal cord nodules, polyps, or papillomas
- Intubation granulomas
- Laryngeal cancer
- Lung cancer
- Unilateral vocal cord paralysis
- Hypothyroidism
- Retrosternal goiter, thyroiditis, multinodular goiter, or thyroid carcinoma
- Gastroesophageal reflux
- Angioedema

 DIAGNOSIS

IMAGING STUDIES

- Consider chest x-ray for tumor

DIAGNOSTIC PROCEDURES

- Evaluation of an abnormal voice begins with obtaining a history of the circumstances preceding its onset and an examination of the airway
- Indirect or flexible laryngoscopy and at times videostrobolaryngoscopy
- In gastroesophageal reflux, nonresponders to medical management should undergo pH testing and manometry

TREATMENT

MEDICATIONS

- Erythromycin may reduce the severity of hoarseness and cough in acute laryngitis

Vocal cord polypoid changes

- Attention to the underlying cause may resolve the problem
- Inhaled steroid spray (eg, beclomethasone, 42 μg/spray, or dexamethasone, 84 μg/spray, two or three times a day) may hasten resolution

Gastroesophageal reflux

- Empiric trial of a proton pump inhibitor at twice-daily dosing (eg, omeprazole, 20 mg twice daily) for 2–3 months as a practical alternative to an initial pH study.
- If symptoms improve and cessation of therapy leads to reoccurrence of symptoms, resume a proton pump inhibitor at the lowest dose effective for remission, usually daily but at times on a demand basis
- H_2 receptor antagonists are generally less clinically effective

SURGERY

- Recalcitrant nodules or polyps may require excision

 ## OUTCOME

COMPLICATIONS

- In hoarseness from acute laryngitis, patients should be told to avoid vigorous use of the voice (singing, shouting) while laryngitis is present to avoid formation of vocal nodules

PROGNOSIS

Acute laryngitis

- Self-limited
- May persist for 1–2 weeks after other symptoms of upper respiratory infection have cleared

Vocal nodules

- Benign condition

WHEN TO REFER

- Refer to an otolaryngologist when hoarseness lasts longer than 2 weeks or has no obvious cause
- Refer to a speech therapist for modification of voice habits for vocal cord polyps

PREVENTION

- Prevent vocal abuse, particularly among singers
- Modification of voice habits to avoid formation of vocal cord nodules

EVIDENCE

PRACTICE GUIDELINES

- National Guideline Clearinghouse http://www.guideline.gov/summary/summary.aspx?doc_id=3147&nbr=2373&string=hoarseness http://www.guideline.gov/summary/summary.aspx?doc_id=3103&nbr=2329&string=voice+disorders
- Dejonckere PH et al: A basic protocol for functional assessment of voice pathology, especially for investigating the efficacy of (phonosurgical) treatments and evaluating new assessment techniques. Guideline elaborated by the Committee on Phoniatrics of the European Laryngological Society (ELS). Eur Arch Otorhinolaryngol 2001; 258:77. [PMID: 11307610]

WEB SITES

- Ear, Nose, and Throat Information Center http://www.netdoor.com/entinfo/
- Otolaryngology Resources on the Internet http://www.bcm.tmc.edu/oto/othersa.html

INFORMATION FOR PATIENTS

- American Academy of Otolaryngology-Head and Neck Surgery. Hoarseness. http://www.entnet.org/healthinfo/throat/hoarse.cfmhttp://www.entnet.org/healthinfo/throat/common-disorders.cfm

REFERENCES

- Garrett CG et al: Hoarseness. Med Clin North Am 1999;83:115. [PMID: 9927964]
- Hagen P et al: Dysphonia in the elderly: diagnosis and management of age-related voice changes. South Med J 1996;89:204. [PMID: 8578351]

Robert K. Jackler, MD
Michael J. Kaplan, MD

Hodgkin's Disease

 KEY FEATURES

ESSENTIALS OF DIAGNOSIS

- Painless lymphadenopathy
- Constitutional symptoms may or may not be present
- Pathological diagnosis by lymph node biopsy

GENERAL CONSIDERATIONS

- Group of cancers characterized by Reed-Sternberg cells in appropriate reactive cellular background
- Nature of the malignant cell is subject of controversy, probably B cells
- Divided into several subtypes: lymphocyte predominance, nodular sclerosis, mixed cellularity, and lymphocyte depletion
- Important feature of Hodgkin's disease: tendency to arise within single lymph node areas and spread in orderly fashion to contiguous lymph nodes
- Widespread hematogenous dissemination only late in course

DEMOGRAPHICS

- Bimodal age distribution: one peak at age 20–30 and second peak at age >50

 CLINICAL FINDINGS

SYMPTOMS AND SIGNS

- Painless lymphadenopathy (mass), commonly in neck
- Constitutional symptoms, eg, fever, weight loss, or drenching night sweats, or generalized pruritus
- Pain in involved lymph node following alcohol ingestion is an unusual symptom

DIFFERENTIAL DIAGNOSIS

- Non-Hodgkin's lymphoma
- Tuberculous lymphadenitis (scrofula)
- Cat-scratch disease
- Sarcoidosis
- Metastatic cancer
- Drug-induced pseudolymphoma (eg, phenytoin)

 DIAGNOSIS

DIAGNOSTIC PROCEDURES

- Lymph node biopsy establishes pathological diagnosis
- Staging usually clinical; laparotomy no longer routinely performed
- Staging nomenclature (Ann Arbor): stage I, one lymph node region involved; stage II, involvement of two lymph node areas on one side of diaphragm; stage III, lymph node regions involved on both sides of diaphragm; stage IV, disseminated disease with bone marrow or liver involvement
- In addition, designated stage A if there is a lack of constitutional symptoms and stage B if there is a 10% weight loss over 6 months, fever, or night sweats ("B symptoms")

TREATMENT

MEDICATIONS

- Combination chemotherapy involving doxorubicin (Adriamycin), bleomycin, vincristine, and dacarbazine (ABVD) for most patients (including all stage IIIB and IV disease)
- Shorter and more intensive regimens have produced promising results and may supplant ABVD in treatment of advanced disease
- Addition of limited chemotherapy for some patients treated with radiation appears promising

THERAPEUTIC PROCEDURES

- All patients with both localized and disseminated disease should be treated with curative intent
- Radiation therapy is initial treatment only for patients with low-risk stage IA and IIA disease
- High-dose chemotherapy with autologous stem cell transplantation is treatment of choice for relapse after initial chemotherapy

 OUTCOME

PROGNOSIS

- Excellent prognosis for stage IA or IIA disease treated by radiotherapy: 10-year survival rates >80%
- Disseminated disease (stage IIIB, IV): 5-year survival rates of 50–60%
- Prognosis is poorer in patients who are older, who have bulky disease, and who have lymphocyte depletion or mixed cellularity Hodgkin's
- Recurrent disease after initial radiotherapy may still be curable with chemotherapy
- High-dose chemotherapy with autologous stem cell transplantation for relapse offers 35–50% chance of cure if disease is still chemotherapy sensitive

 EVIDENCE

PRACTICE GUIDELINES

- Ferme C et al: French National Federation of Cancer (FNCLCC). Hodgkins disease. Br J Cancer. 2001;84(Suppl 2):55. [PMID: 11355971]
- NCCN practice guidelines for Hodgkin's disease. National Comprehensive Cancer Network. Oncology (Huntingt) 1999;13(5A):78. [PMID: 10370924]
- Prosnitz LR et al: Stage III and IV Hodgkin's disease treatment guidelines. American College of Radiology. ACR Appropriateness Criteria. Radiology 2000;215(Suppl):1257. [PMID: 11037545]

WEB SITES

- Lymphoma Research Foundation— Subtypes of Hodgkin's disease http://www.lymphoma.org/site/ PageServer?pagename=hdtypes
- NCI—Adult Hodgkin's lymphoma http://www.cancer.gov/cancerinfo/pdq/ treatment/adulthodgkins/patient/

INFORMATION FOR PATIENTS

- Mayo Clinic—Hodgkin's disease http://www.mayoclinic.com/invoke.cfm? id=DS00186
- MEDLINEplus—Hodgkin's lymphoma http://www.nlm.nih.gov/medlineplus/ ency/article/000580.htm

REFERENCES

- Ferme C et al: Intensive salvage therapy with high-dose chemotherapy for patients with advanced Hodgkin's disease in relapse or failure after initial chemotherapy: results of the Groupe d'Études des Lymphomes de l'Adulte H89 Trial. J Clin Oncol 2002;20:467. [PMID: 11786576]
- Horning SJ et al: Stanford V and radiotherapy for locally extensive and advanced Hodgkin's disease: mature results of a prospective clinical trial. J Clin Oncol 2002;20:630. [PMID: 11821442]

Charles A. Linker, MD

Hookworm Disease

KEY FEATURES

ESSENTIALS OF DIAGNOSIS

Early findings (not commonly recognized)

- Dermatitis: pruritic, erythematous, papulovesicular eruption at site of larval invasion
- Pulmonary migration of larvae: transient episodes of coughing, asthma, fever, blood-tinged sputum, marked eosinophilia

Later findings

- Intestinal symptoms: anorexia, diarrhea, abdominal discomfort
- Anemia (iron deficiency): fatigue, pallor, dyspnea on exertion, poikilonychia, heart failure
- Characteristic eggs and occult blood in the stool

GENERAL CONSIDERATIONS

- The disease, widespread in the moist tropics and subtropics and sporadically in southeastern United States, is caused by *Ancylostoma duodenale* and *Necator americanus*
- Infection is rare in regions with less than 40 inches of rainfall annually
- Humans are the only host for both species
- The worms suck blood at their attachment sites. Blood loss is proportionate to the worm burden. Over years—and depending on the host's dietary intake of iron—iron reserves can be depleted and severe anemia can result

DEMOGRAPHICS

- Probably a quarter of the world's population is infected, and in many areas the infection is a major cause of general debility, retardation of growth and development of children, and increased susceptibility to infection
- Prevalence rates can reach 80% in the humid tropics under unsanitary conditions

CLINICAL FINDINGS

SYMPTOMS AND SIGNS

Ground itch

- The first manifestation of infection
- A pruritic erythematous dermatitis, either maculopapular or vesicular, that follows skin penetration of the infective larvae
- Severity is a function of the number of invading larvae and the sensitivity of the host
- Scratching may result in secondary infection

The pulmonary stage

- Occurs when there is larval migration through the lungs
- There may be a dry cough, wheezing, blood-tinged sputum, and low-grade fever
- In heavy infections, there may be anorexia, diarrhea, vague abdominal pain, and ulcer-like epigastric symptoms
- Severe anemia may result in pallor, deformed nails, pica, and cardiac decompensation
- Marked protein loss may also occur, resulting in hypoalbuminemia, with edema and ascites

DIFFERENTIAL DIAGNOSIS

- Ascariasis
- Strongyloidiasis
- Paragonimiasis
- Tapeworm (especially *genus latum* with associated anemia)
- Tuberculosis
- Allergic bronchopulmonary aspergillosis (ABPA)
- *Mycoplasma pneumoniae* infection
- Iron-deficiency anemia due to other causes, eg, gastrointestinal malignancy

DIAGNOSIS

LABORATORY TESTS

- Diagnosis depends on demonstration of characteristic eggs in feces; a concentration method may be needed. The two species cannot be differentiated by the appearance of their eggs
- The stool usually contains occult blood. Hypochromic microcytic anemia can be severe, with hemoglobin levels as low as 2 g/dL, a low serum iron and a high iron-binding capacity, and low serum ferritin
- Eosinophilia (as high as 30–60% of a total white blood cell count reaching 17,000/μL) is usually present in the pulmonary migratory stage of infection but is not marked in the chronic intestinal stage

Hookworm Disease

TREATMENT

MEDICATIONS

- It may not be beneficial to treat light infections
- Mebendazole, pyrantel, and albendazole are highly effective drugs for treatment of both hookworm species; mebendazole or albendazole can be used to treat concurrent trichuriasis, and all three drugs can be used to treat concurrent ascariasis. The drugs are given after meals, without purges. None of the three drugs should be used in pregnancy

Pyrantel pamoate

- In *A duodenale* infections, pyrantel given as a single dose, 10 mg (base)/kg (maximum 1 g), produces cures in 75–98% of cases and a marked reduction in the worm burden in the remainder
- For *N americanus* infections, a single dose may give a satisfactory cure rate in light infection, but for moderate or heavy infection a 3-day course is necessary
- If the species is unknown, treat as for necatoriasis
- Mild and transient drowsiness and headache may occur

Mebendazole

- When mebendazole is given at a dosage of 100 mg twice daily for 3 days, cure rates for both hookworm species range from 35% to 95%
- A single 500-mg dose may be sufficient for light infections

Albendazole

- Albendazole given orally once only at a dosage of 400 mg results in the cure of 85–95% of patients with *Ancylostoma* infection and markedly reduces the worm burden in those not cured
- Because cure rates for single-dose treatments of *Necator* infection were 33–90%, treatment should be continued for 2–3 days, especially in heavy infections

Ferrous sulfate

- If anemia is present, oral ferrous sulfate and a diet high in protein and vitamins are required for at least 3 months after the anemia has been corrected in order to replace iron stores. A dosage schedule for ferrous sulfate tablets (200 mg) is one tablet three times daily for 2 months followed by one tablet daily for 4 months. Parenteral iron is rarely indicated. Blood transfusion may be necessary if anemia is severe

OUTCOME

FOLLOW-UP

- Eradication of infection is not essential, since light infections do not injure the well-nourished patient and iron loss is replaced if the patient is receiving adequate dietary iron
- Retreatment of heavy infections may be necessary at 2-week intervals until the worm burden is reduced to a low level as estimated by semiquantitative egg counts

EVIDENCE

INFORMATION FOR PATIENTS

- Centers for Disease Control http://www.cdc.gov/ncidod/dpd/parasites/hookworm/factsht_hookworm.htm
- National Institutes of Health http://www.nlm.nih.gov/medlineplus/ency/article/000629.htm

REFERENCES

- Loukas A et al: Immune responses in hookworm infections. Clin Microbiol Rev 2001;14(4):689. [PMID: 11585781]
- Utzinger J et al: Reduction in the prevalence and intensity of hookworm infections after praziquantel treatment for schistosomiasis infection. Int J Parasitol 2002;32(6):759. [PMID: 12062494]

Huntington's Disease

 ## KEY FEATURES

ESSENTIALS OF DIAGNOSIS

- Gradual onset and progression of chorea and dementia or behavioral change
- Family history of the disorder
- Responsible gene identified on chromosome 4

GENERAL CONSIDERATIONS

- Gradual onset and progression of chorea, dementia, or both
- Inherited in an autosomal dominant manner and occurs throughout the world, in all ethnic groups, with a prevalence rate of about 5 per 100,000
- The gene responsible for the disease has been located on the short arm of chromosome 4. At 4p16.3 there is an expanded and unstable CAG trinucleotide repeat
- Offspring should be offered genetic counseling. Genetic testing permits presymptomatic detection and definitive diagnosis of the disease

 ## CLINICAL FINDINGS

SYMPTOMS AND SIGNS

- Clinical onset is usually between 30 and 50 years of age
- Initial symptoms may consist of either abnormal movements or intellectual changes, but ultimately both occur
- The earliest mental changes are often behavioral, with irritability, moodiness, antisocial behavior, or a psychiatric disturbance, but a more obvious dementia subsequently develops
- The dyskinesia may initially be no more than an apparent fidgetiness or restlessness, but eventually choreiform movements and some dystonic posturing occur
- Progressive rigidity and akinesia (rather than chorea) sometimes occur in association with dementia, especially in cases with childhood onset

DIFFERENTIAL DIAGNOSIS

- Chorea developing with no family history of choreoathetosis should not be attributed to Huntington's disease, at least not until other causes of chorea have been excluded clinically and by appropriate laboratory studies
- In younger patients, self-limiting Sydenham's chorea develops after group A streptococcal infections on rare occasions
- If a patient presents solely with progressive intellectual failure, it may not be possible to distinguish Huntington's disease from other causes of dementia unless there is a characteristic family history or a dyskinesia develops
- A clinically similar autosomal dominant disorder (dentatorubral-pallidolysian atrophy), manifested by chorea, dementia, ataxia, and myoclonic epilepsy, is uncommon except in persons of Japanese ancestry. It is due to a mutant gene mapping to 12p13.31

 ## DIAGNOSIS

IMAGING STUDIES

- CT scanning usually demonstrates cerebral atrophy and atrophy of the caudate nucleus in established cases
- MRI and positron emission tomography (PET) have shown reduced glucose utilization in an anatomically normal caudate nucleus

Huntington's Disease

 TREATMENT

MEDICATIONS

- Treatment with drugs blocking dopamine receptors, such as phenothiazines or haloperidol, may control the dyskinesia and any behavioral disturbances
- Haloperidol treatment is usually begun with a dose of 1 mg once or twice daily, which is then increased every 3 or 4 days depending on the response
- Tetrabenazine, a drug that depletes central monoamines, is widely used in Europe to treat dyskinesia but is not available in the United States
- Reserpine is similar in its actions to tetrabenazine and may be helpful; the daily dose is built up gradually to between 2 and 5 mg, depending on the response
- Behavioral disturbances may respond to clozapine
- Attempts to compensate for the relative γ-aminobutyric acid (GABA) deficiency by enhancing central GABA activity or to compensate for the relative cholinergic underactivity by giving choline chloride have not been therapeutically helpful
- The therapeutic response to cysteamine (a selective depleter of somatostatin in the brain) is currently under study

 OUTCOME

PROGNOSIS

- There is no cure for Huntington's disease; progression cannot be halted; and treatment is purely symptomatic
- It usually leads to a fatal outcome within 15–20 years

WHEN TO REFER

- All patients may benefit from practitioners with particular expertise in this area
- Offspring should be offered genetic counseling

PREVENTION

- Genetic counseling is important

 EVIDENCE

PRACTICE GUIDELINES

- National Guideline Clearinghose http://www.guideline.gov/summary/ summary.aspx?doc_id=1968&nbr=1194 &string=huntingtons+disease
- International Huntington Association and the World Federation of Neurology Research Group on Huntington's Chorea. Guidelines for the molecular genetics predictive test in Huntington's disease. J Med Genet 1994;31:555.

WEB SITE

- National Institute of Neurological Disorders and Stroke http://www.ninds.nih.gov/health_and_ medical/disorders/huntington.htm

INFORMATION FOR PATIENTS

- Huntington's Disease Society of America http://www.hdsa.org/
- The Mayo Clinic http://www.mayoclinic.com/invoke.cfm? id=DS00401
- American Speech-Language-Hearing Association http://www.asha.org/speech/disabilities/ Huntington-Disease.cfm

REFERENCES

- Davies S et al: Huntington's disease. Mol Pathol 2001;54:409. [PMID: 11724916]
- Emerich DF: Neuroprotective possibilities for Huntington's disease. Expert Opin Biol Ther 2001;1:467. [PMID: 11727519]

Michael J. Aminoff, DSc, MD, FRCP

Hydatidiform Mole & Choriocarcinoma

 ## KEY FEATURES

ESSENTIALS OF DIAGNOSIS

- Uterine bleeding
- Pathological demonstration of chorio-carcinoma in samples of a pelvic or vaginal mass, or in a metastatic tumor
- Hydatidiform mole
  - Amenorrhea
  - Irregular uterine bleeding
  - Serum human chorionic gonadotropin (hCG)-β subunit >40,000 mU/mL
  - Passage of grape-like clusters of enlarged edematous villi per vagina
  - Ultrasound of uterus with characteristic "snowstorm" image and no fetus or placenta
  - Cytogenetic composition is 46, XX (85%) completely of paternal origin

GENERAL CONSIDERATIONS

- Hydatidiform mole, invasive mole, and choriocarcinoma comprise a spectrum of gestational trophoblastic neoplasia
- Partial moles generally show evidence of an embryo or gestational sac; are polypoid, slower-growing, and less symptomatic; and often present clinically as a missed abortion

DEMOGRAPHICS

- Highest rates of gestational trophoblastic neoplasia occur in some developing countries: 1/125 pregnancies in areas of Asia, 1/1500 pregnancies in the United States
- Risk factors include low socioeconomic status, a history of mole, and age below 18 or above 40

 ## CLINICAL FINDINGS

SYMPTOMS AND SIGNS

- Excessive nausea and vomiting in over one-third of patients with **hydatidiform mole**
- Uterine bleeding beginning at 6–8 weeks is usual
- In 20% of cases, the uterus appears larger than would be expected
- Intact or collapsed grape-like clusters of enlarged villi (vesicles) may be passed
- Bilaterally enlarged cystic ovaries may be palpable
- Less commonly, preeclampsia-eclampsia may develop during the second trimester
- **Choriocarcinoma** may be manifested by continued or recurrent bleeding after evacuation of a mole or following delivery, abortion, or ectopic pregnancy
- An ulcerative vaginal tumor, pelvic mass, or evidence of distant metastatic tumor may be observed
- Diagnosis is established by pathological examination of curettings or biopsy

DIFFERENTIAL DIAGNOSIS

- Similarly elevated levels of serum hCG-β subunit are seen in multiple gestation
  - Spontaneous abortion
  - Ectopic pregnancy
  - Prolapsed uterine fibroid
  - Uterine leiomyomas (fibroids), endometrial polyp, or adenomyosis (uterine endometriosis)
  - Ovarian tumor
  - Cervical neoplasm or lesion

 ## DIAGNOSIS

LABORATORY TESTS

- Serum hCG-β subunit value >40,000 mU/mL or a urinary hCG >100,000 over 24 h increases the likelihood of hydatidiform mole, though such values are occasionally seen with a normal pregnancy in multiple gestation

IMAGING STUDIES

- Ultrasound (US) has replaced all other means of preoperative diagnosis of mole
- US findings are multiple echoes indicating edematous villi within an enlarged uterus, and absent fetus and placenta
- Preoperative chest x-ray is required to evaluate for pulmonary metastases of trophoblast

TREATMENT

MEDICATIONS

- Chemotherapy is indicated for mole if malignant tissue is discovered at surgery or during follow-up examination
- For low-risk patients with a good prognosis, methotrexate, 0.4 mg/kg intramuscularly over a 5-day period, or dactinomycin, 10–12 µg/kg/day intravenously over a 5-day period, is used (see Table 148, page 1329). The side effects—anorexia, nausea and vomiting, stomatitis, rash, diarrhea, and bone marrow depression—usually are reversible in about 3 weeks and can be ameliorated by the administration of leucovorin (0.1 mg/kg)
- Repeated courses of methotrexate 2 weeks apart generally are required to destroy the trophoblast and maintain a zero chorionic gonadotropin titer, as indicated by β-hCG determination
- β-Blockers should be used preoperatively to stabilize patients who have thyrotoxicosis as a result of their mole

SURGERY

- The uterus should be emptied as soon as a mole is diagnosed, preferably by suction
- Ovarian cysts should not be resected nor ovaries removed; spontaneous regression of theca lutein cysts will occur with elimination of the mole

OUTCOME

FOLLOW-UP

- hCG levels should be negative for 1 year before conception is attempted
- In the pregnancy following a mole, hCG level should be checked 6 weeks postpartum
- Contraception should be prescribed to avoid the confusion of elevated hCG from a new pregnancy; oral contraceptive pills are preferred
- Weekly serum hCG levels are measured
- After two negative hCG levels are documented in succession, levels may be checked less frequently at intervals out to 1 year
- A plateau or rise in hCG levels mandates a repeat chest film and D&C before chemotherapy

COMPLICATIONS

- Approximately 10% of women require further treatment after evacuation of the mole; 5% develop choriocarcinoma
- hCG has minimal thyroid-stimulating hormone–like activity; at very high levels, release of T_3 and T_4 may occur and cause hyperthyroidism, which resolves promptly after resection

PROGNOSIS

- Partial moles tend to follow a benign course
- Complete moles have a greater tendency to become choriocarcinomas
- Five-year survival after courses of chemotherapy, even when metastases have been demonstrated, can be expected in at least 85% of cases of choriocarcinoma

WHOM TO REFER

- Patients with a poor prognosis should be referred to a cancer center, where multiple-agent chemotherapy probably will be given

WHEN TO ADMIT

- Patients with excessive vaginal bleeding
- Patients passing vesicular tissue
- Patients with thyrotoxicosis
- Patients with symptomatic metastatic disease

EVIDENCE

PRACTICE GUIDELINES

- Benedet JL et al: FIGO staging classifications and clinical practice guidelines in the management of gynecologic cancers. FIGO Committee on Gynecologic Oncology. Int J Gynaecol Obstet 2000;70:209. [PMID: 11041682]

WEB SITES

- Gestational Trophoblastic Disease Demonstration Case http://www.brighamrad.harvard.edu/Cases/bwh/hcache/34/full.html
- Gestational Trophoblastic Neoplasia Demonstration Case http://www.brighamrad.harvard.edu/Cases/bwh/hcache/38/full.html

INFORMATION FOR PATIENTS

- National Institutes of Health http://www.nlm.nih.gov/medlineplus/ency/article/000909.htm http://www.nlm.nih.gov/medlineplus/ency/article/001496.htm

REFERENCES

- Newlands ES et al: Recent advances in gestational trophoblastic disease. Hematol Oncol Clin North Am 1999;13:225. [PMID: 10080078]
- Seckl MJ et al: Choriocarcinoma and partial hydatidiform moles. Lancet 2000;356:36. [PMID: 10892763]

William R. Crombleholme, MD

Hyperaldosteronism, Primary

 KEY FEATURES

ESSENTIALS OF DIAGNOSIS

- Hypertension, polyuria, polydipsia, muscular weakness
- Hypokalemia, alkalosis
- Plasma and urine aldosterone levels elevated and plasma renin level low

GENERAL CONSIDERATIONS

- Aldosterone stimulates renal tubule to reabsorb sodium and excrete potassium
- Primary hyperaldosteronism may be due to unilateral adrenocortical adenoma (Conn's syndrome, 73%) or to bilateral cortical hyperplasia (27%), which may be glucocorticoid-suppressible due to an autosomal dominant genetic defect allowing ACTH stimulation of aldosterone production

DEMOGRAPHICS

- Classic hyperaldosteronism (with hypokalemia) accounts for ~0.7% of cases of hypertension
- Milder hyperaldosteronism is more frequent
- More common in women

 CLINICAL FINDINGS

SYMPTOMS AND SIGNS

- Hypertension ranging from mild to severe. Malignant hypertension rare
- Muscular weakness; episodic paralysis simulating periodic paralysis
- Fatigue and reduced stamina
- Paresthesias, sometimes with frank tetany
- Headache
- Polyuria and polydipsia
- Edema, common in secondary hyperaldosteronism, rare in primary hyperaldosteronism

DIFFERENTIAL DIAGNOSIS

- Essential hypertension
- Hypokalemic thyrotoxic periodic paralysis
- Renal vascular hypertension (hypertension and hypokalemia, but plasma renin activity is high)
- Hypokalemia due to other cause, eg, diuretics
- Secondary hyperaldosteronism (dehydration, heart failure)
- Congenital adrenal hyperplasia: 11β-hydroxylase deficiency, 17α-hydroxylase deficiency
- Cushing's syndrome
- Excessive real licorice ingestion
- Syndrome of cortisol resistance

 DIAGNOSIS

LABORATORY TESTS

- Discontinue all antihypertensives and remain off diuretics for 3 weeks
- Maintain high sodium intake (>120 mEq/day) during evaluation
- Hypokalemia, persistent even after potassium-wasting diuretics stopped
- Obtain 24-h urine aldosterone, free cortisol, and creatinine
- 24-h urine aldosterone >20 μg with low plasma renin activity (<5 μg/dL) indicates hyperaldosteronism
- 24-h urine aldosterone is <20 μg/day in rare adrenal or gonadal enzyme defects, eg, in 17α-hydroxylase (ambiguous genitalia or primary amenorrhea) or 11β-hydroxylase (virilization)
- Once hyperaldosteronism diagnosed, further testing to distinguish between resectable adrenal adenoma and nonsurgical adrenal hyperplasia
- Plasma 18-hydroxycorticosterone is >85 μg/dL with adrenal neoplasms; level <85 μg/dL is nondiagnostic
- Plasma aldosterone is measured at 8 AM while patient is supine after overnight recumbency and again after 4 h upright. With adrenal adenoma, baseline aldosterone is usually >25 ng/dL (695 pmol/L) and does not rise during upright posture. With hyperplasia, baseline aldosterone usually is <20 ng/dL and rises during upright posture

IMAGING STUDIES

- Thin-section CT suggests discrete (>1 cm diameter) adrenal adenoma in 60–80% of patients with laboratory findings suggesting adrenal adenoma

DIAGNOSTIC PROCEDURES

- Adrenal vein catheterization for aldosterone or during stimulation with cosyntropin. An adrenal vein to IVC gradient of >5:1 confirms the adrenal location of the adenoma
- Dexamethasone-suppressed adrenal scan using ^{131}I-labeled 6-iodomethyl-19-norcholesterol is recommended following CT

TREATMENT

MEDICATIONS

- Spironolactone is treatment of choice for bilateral adrenal hyperplasia
- Spironolactone therapy (lifelong) is an option for patients with unilateral adrenal adenoma (Conn's syndrome) who are poor surgical candidates
- Potassium supplements are required
- Antihypertensive medications for hypertension in bilateral adrenal hyperplasia: angiotensin receptor blockers or angiotensin-converting enzyme inhibitors preferred since they reduce renal potassium losses; thiazides aggravate potassium loss
- Low-dose dexamethasone suppression is an alternative for bilateral adrenal hyperplasia

SURGERY

- Surgical resection (laparoscopic adrenalectomy) is treatment of choice for unilateral adrenal adenoma secreting aldosterone (Conn's syndrome)
- Bilateral adrenalectomy corrects hypokalemia but not hypertension and should *not* be performed for bilateral adrenal hyperplasia

 OUTCOME

FOLLOW-UP

- Monitor electrolytes, BP, renal function

COMPLICATIONS

- Complications of chronic hypertension
- Progressive renal damage is less reversible than in essential hypertension
- Hyperkalemia and hypotension from temporary postoperative hypoaldosteronism can occur from suppression of contralateral adrenal gland following unilateral adrenalectomy for Conn's syndrome
- Surgical morbidity is 7.1%; <4.1% in major centers. Surgical mortality is rare

PROGNOSIS

- Hypertension remits after surgery in about two-thirds of cases but persists or returns despite surgery in one-third
- Prognosis much improved by early diagnosis and treatment
- Only 2% of aldosterone-secreting adrenal tumors are malignant

 EVIDENCE

PRACTICE GUIDELINES

- Foo R et al: Hyperaldosteronism: recent concepts, diagnosis, and management. Postgrad Med J 2001;77:639. [PMID: 11571370]
- Young WF Jr: Minireview: primary aldosteronism–changing concepts in diagnosis and treatment. Endocrinology 2003;144:2208. [PMID: 12746276]

WEB SITE

- MEDLINEplus— Hyperaldosteronism—primary and secondary http://www.nlm.nih.gov/medlineplus/ency/article/000330.htm

INFORMATION FOR PATIENTS

- National Adrenal Disease Foundation— Hyperaldosteronism http://www.medhelp.org/nadf/nadf9.htm

REFERENCES

- Brown MJ et al: Calcium-channel blockade can mask the diagnosis of Conn's syndrome. Postgrad Med J 1999;75:235. [PMID: 10715768]
- Harper R et al: Accuracy of CT scanning and adrenal vein sampling in the pre-operative localization of aldosterone-secreting adrenal adenomas. QJM 1999;92:643. [PMID: 10542304]
- Sawka AM et al: Primary aldosteronism: factors associated with normalization of blood pressure after surgery. Ann Intern Med 2001;135:258. [PMID: 11511140]
- Schwartz GL et al: Screening for primary aldosteronism: implications of an increased plasma aldosterone/renin ratio. Clin Chem 2002;48:1919. [PMID: 12406976]
- Ten S et al: Clinical review 130: Addison's disease 2001. J Clin Endocrinol Metab 2001;86:2909. [PMID: 11443143]
- Young WF Jr: Primary aldosteronism: management issues. Ann NY Acad Sci 2002;970:61. [PMID: 12381542]

Paul A. Fitzgerald, MD

Hypercalcemia

 KEY FEATURES

ESSENTIALS OF DIAGNOSIS

- Malignancy-associated hypercalcemia and primary hyperparathyroidism are the most common causes
- Hypercalciuria usually precedes hypercalcemia
- Hypophosphatemia suggests elevated parathyroid hormone (PTH) or parathyroid hormone–related protein (PTHrP)

GENERAL CONSIDERATIONS

- Primary hyperparathyroidism and malignancy account for 90% of all cases of hypercalcemia
- Primary hyperparathyroidism is the most common cause of hypercalcemia in ambulatory patients
- Tumor production of PTHrP is the commonest paraneoplastic endocrine syndrome, accounting for most cases of hypercalcemia in inpatients. The neoplasm is clinically apparent in nearly all cases when the hypercalcemia is detected
- Chronic hypercalcemia (over 6 months) or some manifestation such as nephrolithiasis suggests a benign cause
- Hypercalcemia can cause nephrogenic diabetes insipidus and volume depletion, which further worsen hypercalcemia

 CLINICAL FINDINGS

SYMPTOMS AND SIGNS

- Determine duration of hypercalcemia and examine for evidence for a neoplasm
- Symptoms usually occur if the serum calcium is above 12 mg/dL and tend to be more severe in acute hypercalcemia
- Constipation and polyuria occur regardless of etiology of hypercalcemia
- Stupor, coma, and azotemia may develop in severe hypercalcemia
- Polyuria is absent in familial hypocalciuric hypercalcemia
- Ventricular extrasystoles and idioventricular rhythm occur and can be accentuated by digitalis

DIFFERENTIAL DIAGNOSIS

- Increased intake or absorption
  - Milk-alkali syndrome
  - Vitamin D or A excess
- Endocrine disorders
  - Primary and secondary hyperparathyroidism
  - Renal failure
  - Acromegaly
  - Adrenal insufficiency
  - Hyperthyroidism
- Neoplastic diseases
  - Tumor production of PTHrPs (ovary, kidney, lung)
  - Multiple myeloma (osteoclast-activating factor)
- Other
  - Thiazide diuretics
  - Sarcoidosis
  - Paget's bone disease
  - Immobilization
  - Familial hypocalciuric hypercalcemia

 DIAGNOSIS

LABORATORY TESTS

- Interpretation of the serum calcium must be made in relation to the serum albumin level
- When albumin is low, serum Ca^{2+} concentration is depressed in a ratio of 0.8–1 mg of Ca^{2+} to 1 g of albumin
- The highest serum calcium levels (>15 mg/dL) generally occur in malignancy
- More than 200 mg/day of urinary calcium excretion suggests hypercalciuria; less than 100 mg/day, hypocalciuria
- Hypercalciuria from malignancy or from vitamin D therapy frequently results in hypercalcemia in case of volume depletion
- PTH and PTHrP help distinguish between malignancy-associated hypercalcemia (elevated PTHrP) and hyperparathyroidism (elevated PTH)
- Serum phosphate may or may not be low, depending on the cause
- A serum calcium × serum phosphorus product >70 markedly increases the risk of nephrocalcinosis and soft tissue calcification

IMAGING STUDIES

- The ECG can show a shortened QT interval

TREATMENT

MEDICATIONS

Emergency treatment

- Establish euvolemia to induce renal excretion of Na^+, which is accompanied by excretion of Ca^{2+}
- In dehydrated patients with normal cardiac and renal function, 0.45% saline or 0.9% saline can be given rapidly (250–500 mL/h)
- Intravenous furosemide (20–40 mg every 2 h) prevents volume overload and enhances Ca^{2+} excretion
- Thiazides can actually worsen hypercalcemia (as can furosemide if inadequate saline is given)
- In the treatment of hypercalcemia of malignancy, bisphosphonates are the mainstay of treatment. Zoledronic acid (4-mg single 15-min intravenous infusion) with adequate hydration normalizes serum calcium in 80–100% of patients in 3 days, and can be repeated as necessary to control the hypercalcemia
- See *Hyperparathyroidism*

THERAPEUTIC PROCEDURES

- In emergency cases, dialysis with low or no calcium dialysate may be needed

 OUTCOME

FOLLOW-UP

- Follow serum calcium at least after 6 months of medical therapy for hyperparathyroidism

COMPLICATIONS

- Pathologic fractures are more common in hyperthyroidism than the general population
- Renal stones
- Renal failure
- Peptic ulcer disease
- Pancreatitis
- Precipitation of calcium throughout the soft tissues
- Gestational hypercalcemia produces neonatal hypocalcemia

PROGNOSIS

- Depends on the underlying disease
- Poor prognosis in malignancy

WHEN TO REFER

- Early referral to an oncologist or nephrologist may aid in management
- Persistent hypercalcemia >10.5 mg/dL even without symptoms

WHEN TO ADMIT

- Altered mental status
- Marked dehydration and hypotension
- Severe renal insufficiency

PREVENTION

- Prevent dehydration that can further aggrevate hypercalcemia

EVIDENCE

PRACTICE GUIDELINES

- National Guideline Clearinghouse
  http://www.guideline.gov/summary/
  summary.aspx?doc_id=3639&nbr=2865
  &string=Hypercalcemia
  http://www.guideline.gov/summary/
  summary.aspx?doc_id=2361&nbr=
  1587&string=Hypercalcemia
  http://www.guideline.gov/summary/
  summary.aspx?doc_id=3099&nbr=
  2325&string=Hypercalcemia

WEB SITES

- Fluid and Electrolyte Disorders:
  MDAdvice.com
  http://www.mdadvice.com/library/ped/
  pedillsymp160.html
- National Cancer Institute
  www.nci.nih.gov

INFORMATION FOR PATIENTS

- National Institute of Osteoporosis and Related Bone Diseases
  http://www.osteo.org/newfile.
  asp?doc=p112i&doctitle=Primary+
  Hyperparathyroidism&doctype=
  HTML+Fact+Sheet
- American Association for Clinical Chemistry
  http://www.labtestsonline.org/
  understanding/analytes/calcium/
  test.html
- National Cancer Institute
  http://www.cancer.gov/cancerinfo/pdq/
  supportivecare/hypercalcemia/Patient

REFERENCES

- Body JJ: Current and future directions in medical therapy: hypercalcemia. Cancer 2000;88(12 Suppl):3054. [PMID: 10898351]
- Marx SJ: Hyperparathyroidism and hypoparathyroid disorders. N Engl J Med 2000;343:1863. [PMID: 11117980]
- Ziegler R: Hypercalcemic crisis. J Am Soc Nephrol 2001;17:S39.

Masafumi Fukagawa, MD, PhD
Kiyoshi Kurokawa, MD, MACP
Maxine A. Papadakis, MD

Hypercoagulable States

KEY FEATURES

ESSENTIALS OF DIAGNOSIS

- Thrombosis
- Erythromelalgia

GENERAL CONSIDERATIONS

- Family history usually present with congenital causes, often precipitated by trauma or pregnancy
- Acquired causes of thrombosis
  - Immobility or postoperative state
  - Cancer
  - Inflammatory disorders, eg, ulcerative colitis
  - Myeloproliferative disorder, eg, polycythemia vera, essential thrombocytosis
  - Estrogens, pregnancy
  - Heparin-induced thrombocytopenia
  - Lupus anticoagulant
  - Anticardiolipin antibodies
  - Nephrotic syndrome
  - Paroxysmal nocturnal hemoglobinuria
  - Disseminated intravascular coagulation
  - Congestive heart failure
- Congenital causes of thrombosis
  - Activated protein C resistance, eg, factor V Leiden
  - Prothrombin 20210 mutation
  - Antithrombin III deficiency
  - Protein C deficiency
  - Protein S deficiency
  - Hyperhomocystinemia
  - Dysfibrinogenemia
  - Abnormal plasminogen
- Cancer associated with increased risk of venous and arterial thrombosis
- Myeloproliferative disorders associated with high incidence of thrombosis due to qualitative platelet abnormalities
- Venous thrombosis may occur in unusual locations, eg, mesenteric, hepatic, or splenic venous beds
- Arterial thrombosis may manifest as large-vessel occlusion (stroke, myocardial infarction) or microvascular events (burning in hands and feet)
- Heparin associated with thrombocytopenia in ~10% of treatment courses; often modest and resolves spontaneously. However, thrombocytopenia may be severe and these cases are most often complicated by arterial thrombosis
- Warfarin-induced skin necrosis may occur in patients with undiagnosed protein C deficiency
  - Warfarin, by creating a vitamin K–dependent state, transiently depletes protein C (which has a short half-life) before it leads to anticoagulation
  - During this period of hypercoagulability, thrombosis of skin vessels may lead to infarction and necrosis

DEMOGRAPHICS

- Congenital hypercoagulable states often present during early adulthood rather than childhood

CLINICAL FINDINGS

SYMPTOMS AND SIGNS

- Thrombosis
- Erythromelalgia (painful redness and burning of hands) in essential thrombocytosis

DIFFERENTIAL DIAGNOSIS

- See acquired and congenital causes of thrombosis

DIAGNOSIS

LABORATORY TESTS

- Dysfibrinogenemia is diagnosed by a prolonged reptilase time
- Assays of antithrombin III, protein S, and protein C

Hypercoagulable States

 TREATMENT

MEDICATIONS

- Preoperative minidose heparin (5000 units SQ Q 8–12 h) may reduce perioperative thrombosis risk
- Heparin, 10,000 units SQ Q 12 h, may reduce thrombosis in hypercoagulable state associated with cancer
  - Low-molecular-weight heparin is more convenient, equally effective, and requires less laboratory monitoring
  - Warfarin is usually ineffective in cancer, most likely because of low-grade disseminated intravascular coagulation
- Antiplatelet therapy may be helpful for thrombosis in myeloproliferative disease, but may increase risk of bleeding
- Aspirin, 325 mg PO QD, is effective for erythromelalgia
- Warfarin is effective and given indefinitely in congenital defects such as deficiency of antithrombin III or vitamin K–dependent proteins C and S
- Warfarin-induced skin necrosis can be prevented by the use of heparin for 5–7 days until warfarin induces anticoagulation

THERAPEUTIC PROCEDURES

- Effective prophylaxis is usually available for those at increased risk of thrombosis

 OUTCOME

FOLLOW-UP

- Screen family members for congenital defects (eg, deficiency of antithrombin III or vitamin K–dependent proteins C and S)

COMPLICATIONS

- Arterial thrombosis in heparin-induced thrombocytopenia

 EVIDENCE

PRACTICE GUIDELINES

- Barger AP et al: Evaluation of the hypercoagulable state. Whom to screen, how to test and treat. Postgrad Med 2000; 108:59. [PMID: 11021259]
- Hirsh J et al: How we diagnose and treat deep vein thrombosis. Blood 2002;99: 3102. [PMID: 11964271]
- Kearon C et al: Management of patients with hereditary hypercoagulable disorders. Annu Rev Med 2000;51:169. [PMID: 10774459]

WEB SITE

- MEDLINEplus—Hypercoagulable states
  http://www.nlm.nih.gov/medlineplus/ency/article/001120.htm

INFORMATION FOR PATIENTS

- American Academy of Family Physicians—Hypercoagulation
  http://familydoctor.org/handouts/244.html
- American Heart Association—Pulmonary embolism and deep vein thrombosis
  http://circ.ahajournals.org/cgi/reprint/106/12/1436.pdf
- American Heart Association—Treatment of blood clots
  http://circ.ahajournals.org/cgi/reprint/106/20/e138.pdf
- JAMA patient page: Pulmonary embolism
  http://www.medem.com/medlb/article_detaillb.cfm?article_ID=ZZZDQHMZUIC&sub_cat=575

REFERENCES

- Federman DG et al: An update on hypercoagulable disorders. Arch Intern Med 2001;161:1051. [PMID: 11322838]
- Mann KG et al: Factor V: a combination of Dr Jekyll and Mr Hyde. Blood 2003;101:20. [PMID: 12393635]

Charles A. Linker, MD

Hyperglycemic Hyperosmolar State

KEY FEATURES

ESSENTIALS OF DIAGNOSIS

- Hyperglycemia >600 mg/dL
- Serum osmolality >310 mosm/kg
- No acidosis; blood pH above 7.3
- Serum bicarbonate >15 mEq/L
- Normal anion gap (<14 mEq/L)

GENERAL CONSIDERATIONS

- Frequently occurs with mild or occult diabetes
- Infection, myocardial infarction, stroke, or recent operation is often a precipitating event
- Drugs (phenytoin, diazoxide, glucocorticoids, and diuretics) or procedures associated with glucose loading such as peritoneal dialysis can also precipitate the syndrome
- Renal insufficiency develops from hypovolemia, leading to increasingly higher blood glucose concentrations
- Underlying renal insufficiency or congestive heart failure is common, and the presence of either worsens the prognosis

DEMOGRAPHICS

- Rarer than diabetic ketoacidosis even in older age groups
- Affects middle-aged to elderly

CLINICAL FINDINGS

SYMPTOMS AND SIGNS

- Onset may be insidious over days or weeks, with weakness, polyuria, and polydipsia
- The lack of features of ketoacidosis may retard recognition until dehydration becomes more profound than in ketoacidosis
- Fluid intake is usually reduced from inappropriate lack of thirst, nausea, or inaccessibility of fluids to bedridden patients
- Lethargy and confusion develop as serum osmolality exceeds 310 mosm/kg. Coma can occur if osmolality exceeds 320–330 mosm/kg
- Physical examination shows profound dehydration, lethargy, or coma without Kussmaul respirations

DIFFERENTIAL DIAGNOSIS

- Diabetic ketoacidosis
- Cerebrovascular accident or head trauma
- Hypoglycemia
- Sepsis
- Diabetes insipidus

DIAGNOSIS

LABORATORY TESTS

- Severe hyperglycemia (600–2400 mg/dL)
- When dehydration is less severe, dilutional hyponatremia as well as urinary sodium losses may reduce serum sodium to 120–125 mEq/L
- As dehydration progresses, serum sodium can exceed 140 mEq/L, producing serum osmolality readings of 330–440 mosm/kg
- Ketosis and acidosis are usually absent or mild
- Prerenal azotemia with serum urea nitrogen elevations over 100 mg/dL is typical

Hyperglycemic Hyperosmolar State

TREATMENT

MEDICATIONS

Saline

- Fluid replacement is paramount to correct average fluid deficits of 6–10 L
- In hypovolemia with hypotension and oliguria, initiate fluid resuscitation with isotonic 0.9% saline
- In all other cases, hypotonic (0.45%) saline is preferable because of the hyperosmolality
- As much as 4–6 L of fluid may be required in the first 8–10 h
- Once blood glucose reaches 250 mg/dL, add 5% dextrose to either water, 0.45% saline solution, or 0.9% saline solution at a rate to maintain glycemic levels of 250–300 mg/dL in order to reduce the risk of cerebral edema
- An important end point of fluid therapy is to restore urine output to 50 mL/h or more

Insulin

- Less insulin is required as compared to diabetic ketoacidotic coma
- Fluid replacement alone can reduce hyperglycemia by increasing glomerular filtration and renal excretion of glucose
- An initial dose of only 15 units intravenously and 15 units subcutaneously of regular insulin is usually quite effective, and in most cases subsequent doses need not be greater than 10–20 units subcutaneously every 4 h

Potassium

- Add potassium chloride (10 mEq/L) to initial bottles of fluids if serum potassium is not elevated. Adjust subsequent potassium replacement based on serum potassium level

Phosphate

- If severe hypophosphatemia (serum phosphate <1 mg/dL (0.35 mmol/L) develops during insulin therapy, phosphate replacement can be given as potassium salt
- To minimize the risk of tetany from an overload of phosphate replacement, an average deficit of 40–50 mmol phosphate should be replaced by intravenous infusion at a rate not to exceed 3 mmol/h. A stock solution (Abbott Laboratories) provides a mixture of 1.12 g KH_2PO_4 and 1.18 g K_2HPO_4 in a 5-mL single-dose vial representing

22 mEq potassium and 15 mmol phosphate (27 mEq); 5 mL of this stock solution in 2 L of either 0.45% saline or 5% dextrose in water, infused at 400 mL/h, will replace the phosphate at the optimal rate of 3 mmol/h and will provide 4.4 mEq of potassium per hour
- If serum phosphate remains below 0.35 mmol/L (1 mg/dL), repeat a 5-h infusion of potassium phosphate at a rate of 3 mmol/h

THERAPEUTIC PROCEDURES

- Use a flow sheet listing vital signs, time sequence of laboratory values (arterial pH, plasma glucose, acetone, bicarbonate, serum urea nitrogen, electrolytes, serum osmolality) in relation to therapy

OUTCOME

PROGNOSIS

- The overall mortality rate is more than 10 times that of diabetic ketoacidosis, because of its higher incidence in older patients and the greater dehydration
- When prompt therapy is instituted, the mortality rate can be reduced from nearly 50% to that related to the severity of coexistent disorders

WHEN TO ADMIT

- Altered mental status
- Severe volume depletion

EVIDENCE

PRACTICE GUIDELINES

- National Guideline Clearinghouse http://www.guideline.gov/summary/summary.aspx?doc_id=3582&nbr=2808&string=hyperglycemic+hyperosmolar+state
- American Diabetes Association Position Statement http://care.diabetesjournals.org/cgi/content/full/26/suppl_1/s109

WEB SITES

- CDC Diabetes Web Site http://www.cdc.gov/diabetes/
- American Association of Diabetes Educators http://www.aadenet.org/
- American Diabetes Association http://www.diabetesnet.com/ada.html

INFORMATION FOR PATIENTS

- JAMA patient page: The ABCs of diabetes. JAMA 2002;287:2608. [PMID: 12025825]
- American Diabetes Association http://www.diabetes.org/main/application/commercewf?origin=*.jsp&event=link(D4_8)

REFERENCES

- American Diabetes Association: Hyperglycemic crises in patients with diabetes mellitus. Diabetes Care 2001;24:154. [PMID: 11221603]
- Trence DL et al: Hyperglycemic crisis in diabetes mellitus type 2. Endocrinol Metab Clin North Am 2001;30:817. [PMID: 11727401]

Umesh Masharani, MB, BS; MRCH (UK)

Hyperkalemia

KEY FEATURES

ESSENTIALS OF DIAGNOSIS

- Electrocardiogram may be normal despite life-threating hyperkalemia
- Potassium release from blood cells should be ruled out in case of clotting, leukocytosis, and thrombocytosis

GENERAL CONSIDERATIONS

- Serum potassium concentration rises about 0.7 mEq/L for every decrease of 0.1 pH unit during acidosis
- In the absence of acidosis, serum potassium concentration rises about 1 mEq/L when there is a total body potassium excess of 1–4 mEq/kg. However, the higher the serum potassium concentration, the smaller the excess necessary to raise the potassium levels further
- Hyperkalemia occurs commonly in AIDS from impaired renal excretion of potassium due to the use of pentamidine or trimethoprim-sulfamethoxazole or to hyporeninemic hypoaldosteronism. There may also be an abnormality in the redistribution between intracellular and extracellular compartments
- Serious hyperkalemia is uncommon in angiotensin-converting enzyme (ACE) inhibitor-treated patients under 70 who have normal renal function. However, life-threatening hyperkalemia during combined therapy with angiotensin-converting enzyme inhibitors and spironolactone occurs

Etiology

- **Spurious**
- Leakage from erythrocytes, marked thrombocytosis or leukocytosis
- Repeated fist clenching during phlebotomy
- Specimen from arm with K^+ infusion
- **Decreased excretion**
- Renal failure
- Renal secretory defects, eg, interstitial nephritis, sickle cell disease
- Hypoaldosteronism: hyporeninism (type IV renal tubular acidosis), eg, diabetic nephropathy, heparin, AIDS; adrenal insufficiency
- Drugs that inhibit K^+ excretion (spironolactone, triamterene, ACE inhibitors, trimethoprim, nonsteroidal antiinflammatory drugs)

- **Potassium shift out of cell**
- Burns, rhabdomyolysis, hemolysis, severe infection, internal bleeding, vigorous exercise
- Metabolic acidosis
- Hypertonicity (solvent drag)
- Insulin deficiency
- Hyperkalemic periodic paralysis
- Drugs: digitalis toxicity, β-adrenergic antagonists, succinylcholine, arginine
- **Excessive intake of K^+**
- Ingestion or iatrogenic

CLINICAL FINDINGS

SYMPTOMS AND SIGNS

- Muscle weakness and, rarely, flaccid paralysis
- Abdominal distension and diarrhea may occur

DIAGNOSIS

LABORATORY TESTS

- Confirm that the hyperkalemia is genuine. Can measure plasma potassium rather than serum to avoid leakage of potassium out of cells
- Serum electrolytes and creatinine
- Consider arterial blood gas

IMAGING STUDIES

- Electrocardiography is not a sensitive method for detecting hyperkalemia, since nearly half of patients with a serum potassium level greater than 6.5 mEq/L will not manifest electrocardiographic changes

Electrocardiographic changes

- Peaked T waves
- Widening of the QRS
- Biphasic QRS–T complexes
- Inhibition of atrial depolarization despite normal conduction through usual pathways may occur
- The heart rate may be slow; ventricular fibrillation and cardiac arrest are terminal events

TREATMENT

MEDICATIONS

- See Table 81 (page 1268)
- Treatment consists of withholding potassium and giving cation exchange resin
- Emergent treatment is indicated if cardiac toxicity or muscular paralysis is present or if the hyperkalemia is severe (K^+ >6.5–7 mEq/L) even in the absence of electrocardiographic changes)

THERAPEUTIC PROCEDURES

- Hemodialysis or peritoneal dialysis may be required to remove K^+ in the presence of renal failure

OUTCOME

FOLLOW-UP

- Monitor potassium frequently (every 1–4 h) during inpatient therapy for hyperkalemia

PROGNOSIS

- Depends on the underlying condition (renal failure)
- Drug-induced hyperkalemia is generally readily reversible with therapy

WHEN TO REFER

- Refer to a nephrologist if expertise is needed for treatment, particularly for emergent treatment or to prepare for dialysis

WHEN TO ADMIT

- For serum potassium >6.0 mg/dL
- For rapidly increasing serum potassium in the setting of acutely worsening comorbid condition (eg, acute renal failure, rhabdomyolysis)

PREVENTION

- Monitor serum potassium after administration of potassium-altering drugs in patients with renal insufficiency

EVIDENCE

PRACTICE GUIDELINES

- National Guideline Clearinghouse http://www.guideline.gov/summary/summary.aspx?doc_id=3099&nbr=2325&string=hyperkalemia http://www.guideline.gov/summary/summary.aspx?doc_id=3027&nbr=2253&string=hyperkalemia

WEB SITES

- Hyperkalemia http://www.emedicine.com/emerg/topic261.htm
- Fluid and Electrolyte Disorders: MDAdvice.com http://www.mdadvice.com/library/ped/pedillsymp160.html
- National Institutes of Health http://www.nlm.nih.gov/medlineplus/ency/article/001179.htm

INFORMATION FOR PATIENTS

- JAMA patient page: Drug adherence. JAMA 1999;282:298. [PMID: 10423000]

REFERENCES

- Perazella MA: Drug-induced hyperkalemia: old culprits and new offenders. Am J Med 2000;109:307. [PMID: 10996582]
- Schepkens H et al: Life-threatening hyperkalemia during combined therapy with angiotensin-converting enzyme inhibitors and spironolactone: an analysis of 25 cases. Am J Med 2001;110:438. [PMID: 11331054]
- Schoolwerth AC et al: Renal considerations in angiotensin converting enzyme inhibitor therapy: a statement for healthcare professionals from the Council on the Kidney in Cardiovascular Disease and the Council for High Blood Pressure Research of the American Heart Association. Circulation 2001;104:1985. [PMID: 11602506]

Masafumi Fukagawa, MD, PhD
Kiyoshi Kurokawa, MD, MACP
Maxine A. Papadakis, MD

Hypernatremia

 KEY FEATURES

ESSENTIALS OF DIAGNOSIS

- Serum sodium (>145 mEq/L)
- Occurs most commonly when water intake is inadequate, as with altered mental status
- Urine osmolality helps determine whether the water loss is renal or non-renal

GENERAL CONSIDERATIONS

- An intact thirst mechanism usually prevents hypernatremia
- Excess water loss can cause hypernatremia only when adequate water intake is not possible, as with unconscious patients
- Rarely, excessive sodium intake may cause hypernatremia
- Hypernatremia in the presence of salt and water overload is uncommon but has been reported in very ill patients in the course of therapy

Etiology

- **Urine osmolality >400 mosm/kg**
- *Nonrenal losses*
- Excessive sweating, burns
- Insensible respiratory tract losses
- Diarrhea, vomiting, nasogastric suctioning, osmotic cathartics, eg, lactulose
- *Renal losses*
- Diuretics
- Osmotic diuresis, eg, hyperglycemia, mannitol, urea
- Postobstructive diuresis
- Diuretic phase of acute tubular necrosis
- *Hypertonic sodium gain*
- Salt intoxication (rare)
- Hypertonic IV fluids, tube feeds, enemas
- Primary hyperaldosteronism (hypernatremia usually mild and asymptomatic)
- **Urine osmolality <250 mosm/kg**
- Central diabetes insipidus: idiopathic, head trauma, CNS mass
- Nephrogenic diabetes insipidus: lithium, demeclocycline, prolonged urinary tract infections, interstitial nephritis, hypercalcemia, hypokalemia, congenital

 CLINICAL FINDINGS

SYMPTOMS AND SIGNS

- When dehydration exists, orthostatic hypotension and oliguria are typical findings
- Hyperthermia, delirium, and coma may be seen with severe hyperosmolality

 DIAGNOSIS

LABORATORY TESTS

- Urine osmolality >400 mosm/kg when renal water-conserving ability is functioning
- Urine osmolality <250 mosm/kg when renal water-conserving ability is impaired
- Serum osmolality invariably increased in the dehydrated state

Hypernatremia

TREATMENT

MEDICATIONS

Type of fluid for replacement

- **Hypernatremia with hypovolemia**
- Treat severe hypovolemia with isotonic (0.9%) saline to restore the volume deficit and to treat the hyperosmolality, since the osmolality of isotonic saline (308 mosm/kg) is often lower than that of the plasma
- Follow with 0.45% saline to replace any remaining free water deficit
- Milder volume deficit may be treated with 0.45% saline and 5% dextrose in water
- **Hypernatremia with euvolemia**
- Water drinking or 5% dextrose and water intravenously will result in excretion of excess sodium in the urine
- If glomerular filtration rate is decreased, diuretics will increase urinary sodium excretion but may impair renal concentrating ability, increasing the quantity of water that needs to be replaced
- **Hypernatremia with hypervolemia**
- Provide 5% dextrose in water to reduce hyperosmolality, but this will expand vascular volume
- Loop diuretics such as furosemide (0.5–1 mg/kg) should be administered intravenously to remove the excess sodium
- In severe renal insufficiency, hemodialysis may be necessary

Calculation of water deficit

- When calculating fluid replacement, both the deficit and the maintenance requirements should be added to each 24-h replacement regimen
- **Acute hypernatremia**
- In acute dehydration without much solute loss, free water loss is similar to the weight loss
- Initially, 5% dextrose in water may be employed
- As correction of water deficit progresses, therapy should continue with 0.45% saline with dextrose
- **Chronic hypernatremia**
- Water deficit is calculated to restore normal osmolality for total body water
- TBW correlates with muscle mass and therefore decreases with advancing age, cachexia, and dehydration and is lower in women than in men. Current TBW equals 0.4–0.6 of current body weight

$$\text{Volume (in L) to be replaced} = \text{Current TBW} \times \frac{[\text{Na}^+] - 140}{140}$$

THERAPEUTIC PROCEDURES

- Treatment is directed toward correcting the cause of the fluid loss and replacing water and, as needed, electrolytes
- Fluid therapy should be administered over a 48-h period, aiming for a decrease in serum sodium of 1 mEq/L/h (1 mmol/ L/h)
- Potassium and phosphate may be added as indicated by serum levels; other electrolytes are also monitored frequently

OUTCOME

COMPLICATIONS

- If hypernatremia is too rapidly corrected, the osmotic imbalance may cause water to preferentially enter brain cells, causing cerebral edema and potentially severe neurological impairment

WHEN TO REFER

- Hypernatremia >15 mEq/L

WHEN TO ADMIT

- Altered mental status
- Marked dehydation
- Hypernatremia with hypervolemia

EVIDENCE

PRACTICE GUIDELINES

- National Guideline Clearinghouse http://www.guideline.gov/summary/summary.aspx?doc_id=3305&nbr=2531&string=sodium

WEB SITES

- Dr. Rose's Peripheral Brain—Fluids and electrolytes http://faculty.washington.edu/momus/PB/fluidand.htm
- Fluid and Electrolyte Disorders: MDAdvice.com http://www.mdadvice.com/library/ped/pedillsymp160.html

INFORMATION FOR PATIENTS

- National Institutes of Health. Central pontine myelinolysis http://www.nlm.nih.gov/medlineplus/ency/article/ 000775.htm
- Serum sodium http://www.nlm.nih.gov/medlineplus/ency/article/003481.htm

REFERENCES

- Adrogue HJ et al: Hypernatremia. N Engl J Med 2000;342:1493. [PMID: 10816188]
- Kahn T: Hypernatremia with edema. Arch Intern Med 1999;159:93. [PMID: 9892337]
- Kugler JP et al: Hyponatremia and hypernatremia in the elderly. Am Fam Physician 2000;61:3623. [PMID: 10892634]

Masafumi Fukagawa, MD, PhD
Kiyoshi Kurokawa, MD, MACP
Maxine A. Papadakis, MD

Hyperparathyroidism

 ## KEY FEATURES

ESSENTIALS OF DIAGNOSIS

- Common disorder
- Patients frequently asymptomatic, hypercalcemia detected by screening
- Renal stones, polyuria, hypertension, constipation, fatigue, mental changes
- Bone pain; rarely, cystic lesions and pathological fractures
- Serum and urine calcium elevated; urine phosphate high with low or normal serum phosphate; alkaline phosphatase normal or elevated
- Elevated or high-normal serum parathyroid hormone (PTH) level

GENERAL CONSIDERATIONS

- PTH increases serum calcium and decreases serum phosphate via effects on bone osteoclastic activity and renal tubules
- PTH hypersecretion usually due to parathyroid adenoma, less commonly hyperplasia or carcinoma (rare)
- If age <30, higher incidence of multiglandular disease (36%) and carcinoma (5%) responsible for hyperparathyroidism
- In chronic renal failure, hyperphosphatemia and decreased renal vitamin D production initially decrease ionized calcium, causing stimulation of parathyroids (secondary hyperparathyroidism), which then sometimes becoming enlarged and autonomous (tertiary hyperparathyroidism). Bone disease in this setting known as "renal osteodystrophy"

DEMOGRAPHICS

- Incidence of primary hyperparathyroidism in adults is 0.1%
- More common in persons age >50
- Ratio of M:F is 1:3
- Parathyroid adenomas or hyperplasia can be familial (about 5%) or part of multiple endocrine neoplasia type 1 associated with insulinomas, gastrinomas, or pituitary tumors (MEN type 1), and MEN types 2a and 2b

 ## CLINICAL FINDINGS

SYMPTOMS AND SIGNS

- Hypercalcemia usually discovered incidentally on routine laboratory testing
- Patients may be asymptomatic
- Symptomatic patients have problems with "bones, stones, abdominal groans, psychic moans, fatigue"
- Significant bone demineralization uncommon in mild hyperparathyroidism, but osteitis fibrosa cystica may present as pathological fractures or "brown tumors" of jaw
- Bone pain and arthralgias are common
- Chronic cortical bone resorption due to excess PTH may cause diffuse demineralization, pathological fractures, or cystic bone lesions
- Polyuria and polydipsia may result from hypercalcemia-induced nephrogenic diabetes insipidus
- Calcium-containing kidney stones
- Depression, intellectual weariness, and increased sleep requirement common
- Constipation, fatigue, anemia, weight loss, muscle weakness, easy fatigability, pruritus, and paresthesias
- Anorexia, nausea, and vomiting in severe cases
- Hypertension
- Parathyroid adenomas rarely palpable; palpable mass usually a thyroid nodule
- Pancreatitis occurs in 3%
- Psychosis or even coma may accompany severe hypercalcemia
- Calcium may precipitate in corneas or soft tissue

DIFFERENTIAL DIAGNOSIS

- Hypercalcemia of malignancy
- Multiple myeloma
- Familial hypocalciuric hypercalcemia
- Vitamin D intoxication
- Sarcoidosis, tuberculosis
- Hyperthyroidism
- Vitamin D deficiency (serum 25-OH Vit D <20) can cause high serum PTH with normal serum
- High-dose glucocorticoid therapy in patients taking thiazide diuretics

 ## DIAGNOSIS

LABORATORY TESTS

- Serum calcium >10.5 mg/dL
- Elevated or high-normal PTH confirms the diagnosis. Immunoradiometric assay (IRMA) is most specific and sensitive
- Serum phosphate often low (<2.5 mg/dL)
- Serum phosphate high in secondary hyperparathyroidism (renal failure)
- Urine calcium excretion high or normal (average 250 mg/g creatinine), but low for degree of hypercalcemia
- Urine phosphate high despite low to low normal serum phosphate
- Serum alkaline phosphatase elevated only if bone disease present
- Plasma chloride and uric acid may be elevated

IMAGING STUDIES

- Preoperative imaging may be unsuccessful due to small size of gland, but if successful, may allow limited surgery; especially important if prior neck surgery
- ^{99m}Tc-sestamibi/Tc-pertechnetate subtraction scintigraphy with SPECT recommended; has sensitivity of 87%, specificity 95%
- Neck ultrasound has sensitivity of 80%
- Combination of both tests has sensitivity of 94%, but sensitivity only 55% if multiglandular disease
- MRI and CT not as sensitive as ultrasound
- MRI or ultrasound for hyperparathyroidism reveals incidental small benign thyroid nodules in ~50%
- Bone x-rays usually normal and not required, but may show demineralization, subperiosteal bone resorption (especially in radial aspects of fingers), cysts throughout skeleton, mottling of skull ("salt-and-pepper appearance"), or pathological fractures. Articular cartilage calcification (chondrocalcinosis) sometimes found
- In renal osteodystrophy, bone x-rays may show ectopic calcifications around joints or soft tissue, osteopenia, osteitis fibrosa, or osteosclerosis
- Bone densitometry of wrist, hip, and spine

TREATMENT

MEDICATIONS

- Bisphosphonates: can temporarily treat hypercalcemia and may relieve bone pain. Pamidronate, 30–90 mg IV over 2–4 h. Zoledronate, 2–4 mg IV over 15 min is also quite effective but expensive
- Propranolol may prevent adverse cardiac effects of hypercalcemia
- Glucocorticoid therapy is ineffective for hypercalcemia in hyperparathyroidism
- For secondary hyperparathyroidism of renal failure: paricalcitol, 0.04–0.1 mg/kg IV TIW after dialysis; doxercalciferol, 10 mg orally TIW after dialysis; increase to maximum of 20 mg TIW if PTH remains >400 ng/L. Hold for PTH <100 ng/L

SURGERY

- Parathyroidectomy for patients with symptomatic hyperparathyroidism, kidney stones, or bone disease
- Consider surgery in asymptomatic patients with serum calcium 1 mg/dL above the upper limit of normal with urine calcium excretion >50 mg/24 h; urine calcium excretion >400 mg/24 h; cortical bone density >2 SD below normal; age <50–60 years; difficulty ensuring medical follow-up; or pregnancy
- Minimally invasive parathyroid surgery usually sufficient if adenoma identified preoperatively; otherwise, bilateral neck exploration usually advisable
- Subtotal parathyroidectomy (3-1/2 glands removed) for patients with resistant parathyroid hyperplasia
- Keep patients hospitalized overnight
- Postoperative oral calcium and calcitriol, 0.25 mg/day orally for 2 weeks, helps prevent tetany

THERAPEUTIC PROCEDURES

- Patients with mild, asymptomatic hyperparathyroidism advised to keep active, avoid immobilization, drink adequate fluids; and avoid thiazides, large doses of vitamins D and A, calcium-containing antacids or supplements, and digitalis (hypercalcemia predisposes to toxicity)

OUTCOME

FOLLOW-UP

- Check serum calcium and albumin twice yearly, renal function and urine calcium once yearly, and bone density (distal radius) every 2 years in mild, asymptomatic hyperparathyroidism
- Postoperative calcium monitoring
- Symptomatic postoperative hypocalcemia is treated with liquid or chewable calcium carbonate and calcitriol, 0.25–1 µg PO QD
- Postoperative secondary hyperparathyroidism (PTH rising above normal while serum calcium is normal or low due to "hungry bones") occurs in ~12% and is treated with calcium and vitamin D, usually for 3–6 months
- Hyperthyroidism immediately following parathyroid surgery may require short-term propranolol

COMPLICATIONS

- Forearm and hip fractures
- UTI due to obstruction by stones may lead to renal failure and uremia
- Clouding of sensorium, renal failure, and soft tissue calcinosis from rapidly rising serum calcium
- Peptic ulcer and pancreatitis
- Pseudogout before or after surgery
- Hypercalcemia during gestation producing neonatal hypocalcemia and tetany
- In secondary hyperparathyroidism, disseminated calcification in skin, soft tissues, and arteries (calciphylaxis) can result in gangrene, arrhythmias, and respiratory failure

PROGNOSIS

- Asymptomatic mild hypercalcemia does not affect survival
- Surgical resection of sporadic parathyroid adenoma generally results in permanent cure
- Bones, despite severe cyst formation, deformity, and fracture, heal if parathyroid tumor removed
- Pancreatitis increases mortality rate
- Significant renal damage may progress even after adenoma removal
- Parathyroid carcinoma tends to invade local structures and may metastasize; repeat surgical resections and radiation therapy can prolong life

WHEN TO REFER

- Refer to parathyroid surgeon for parathyroidectomy

WHEN TO ADMIT

- Patients with severe hypercalcemia for IV hydration

PREVENTION

- Prevent renal osteodystrophy (due to secondary hyperparathyroidism in renal failure) by avoiding hyperphosphatemia

EVIDENCE

PRACTICE GUIDELINES

- Davies M et al: The management of primary hyperparathyroidism. Clin Endocrinol (Oxf) 2002;57:145. [PMID: 12153591]

WEB SITE

- Mayo Clinic—Hyperparathyroidism http://www.mayoclinic.com/invoke.cfm?id=DS00396

INFORMATION FOR PATIENTS

- American Academy of Family Physicians—Hyperparathyroidism http://familydoctor.org/handouts/251.html

REFERENCES

- Kearns AE et al: Medical and surgical management of hyperparathyroidism. Mayo Clin Proc 2002;77:87. [PMID: 11794462]
- Marx SJ: Hyperparathyroid and hypoparathyroid disorders. N Engl J Med 2000;343:1863. [PMID: 11117980]

Paul A. Fitzgerald, MD

Hyperprolactinemia

 KEY FEATURES

ESSENTIALS OF DIAGNOSIS

- Women: menstrual cycle disturbances (oligomenorrhea, amenorrhea); galactorrhea; infertility; gynecomastia
- Men: hypogonadism; decreased libido and erectile dysfunction; infertility
- Serum prolactin elevated (Table 106, page 1289)
- CT scan or MRI often demonstrates pituitary adenoma

GENERAL CONSIDERATIONS

- Prolactin's main role is to induce lactation
- During pregnancy, prolactin increases from normal (<20 ng/mL) to as high as 600 ng/mL
- Suckling stimulates continued production of prolactin
- Prolactin is mainly under inhibitory control by dopamine
- Elevated serum prolactin can be caused by numerous conditions (see Differential Diagnosis)
- Most prolactinomas are microadenomas (<1 cm in diameter) that usually do not grow, even with pregnancy or oral contraceptives
- However, macroadenomas occur and can spread into cavernous sinuses, suprasellar areas, and rarely into sinsuses by eroding the sella floor

DEMOGRAPHICS

- Prolactin-secreting pituitary tumors more common in women
- Usually sporadic but rarely familial as part of multiple endocrine neoplasia type 1 (MEN-1)

 CLINICAL FINDINGS

SYMPTOMS AND SIGNS

- Hypogonadotropic hypogonadism. Men usually have erectile dysfunction, diminished libido, sometimes gynecomastia, but never galactorrhea. Women may have oligomenorrhea or amenorrhea, infertility, galactorrhea
- Of women with secondary amenorrhea and galactorrhea, 70% have hyperprolactinemia
- Large pituitary tumors may cause headaches, visual field defects
- Pituitary prolactinomas may cosecrete growth hormone and cause acromegaly; large tumors amy cause pituitary insufficiency (hypogonadism), hypothyroidism, adrenal insufficiency, growth hormone deficiency

DIFFERENTIAL DIAGNOSIS

- See Table 106 (page 1289)

Causes of elevated prolactin

- Pregnancy, postpartum, suckling, nipple stimulation, nipple rings
- Macroprolactinemia (relatively inactive "big prolactin")
- Exercise, sleep (REM phase), stress (trauma, surgery)
- Idiopathic
- Psychotropics, cimetidine, tricyclic antidepressants, oral contraceptives, marijuana
- Prolactinoma
- Hypothyroidism
- Cirrhosis or renal failure
- Acromegaly (pituitary tumor may cosecrete prolactin and growth hormone)
- Hypothalamic disease
- Tumor near pituitary
- Systemic lupus erythematosus
- Chronic chest wall stimulation
- Multiple sclerosis, optic neuritis, spinal cord lesions

 DIAGNOSIS

LABORATORY TESTS

- Urine or serum human chorionic gonadotropin to rule out pregnancy
- Serum thyroid-stimulating hormone high if hypothyroidism is cause
- Renal and liver chemistries abnormal in renal failure or cirrhosis
- Serum calcium elevated in hyperparathyroidism (MEN-1)
- Consider assay for macroprolactinemia if asymptomatic patient with no apparent cause for hyperprolactinemia

IMAGING STUDIES

- MRI of pituitary and hypothalamus indicated for nonpregnant patients with prolactin >200 mg/dL, if headaches or visual field defects, or if persistently elevated prolactin with no discernible cause
- Small prolactinomas may be demonstrated, but clear differentiation from normal variants not always possible

Hyperprolactinemia

TREATMENT

MEDICATIONS

- Medical therapy is preferable to surgery or radiation, particularly for huge "macroprolactinomas"
- Discontinue medications known to increase prolactin, if possible, and recheck prolactin in a few weeks
- Dopamine agonists are initial treatment of choice for macroprolactinomas and to restore normal sexual function and fertility in hyperprolactinemia
- Cabergoline, 0.25 mg PO once weekly for 1 week, then 0.25 mg twice weekly for 1 week, then 0.5 mg twice weekly. Further increases may be required monthly, up to 1.5 mg twice weekly, based on serum prolactin
- Alternatives: bromocriptine (1.25–20 mg/day orally) and pergolide (0.125–2 mg/day orally)
- Quinagolide (not available in the United States) is a non–ergot-derived dopamine agonist for patients intolerant or resistant to other agents; dose: start at 0.075 mg/day PO, up to 0.6 mg/day
- Give dopamine agonists at bedtime to minimize side effects (fatigue, nausea, dizziness, and orthostatic hypotension), which usually improve with dosage reduction and continued use
- Psychiatric side effects occur, are not dose related, and may take weeks to resolve once dopamine agonist is discontinued
- Treat hypothyroidism with thyroxine
- Oral contraceptives or estrogen replacement are safe for women with microprolactinomas who have amenorrhea or wish contraception; minimal risk of stimulating adenoma enlargement
- Estrogens and testosterone can stimulate macroprolactinomas, and should not be used unless in full remission with medication or surgery

SURGERY

- Transsphenoidal resection of tumor may be urgently required for large tumors severely compromising visual fields or undergoing apoplexy
- Transsphenoidal selective resection of the pituitary adenoma is done electively for patients who do not tolerate or respond to dopamine agonists
- Craniotomy rarely indicated

THERAPEUTIC PROCEDURES

- Radiation therapy is reserved for macroadenomas that are growing despite dopamine agonist treatment
- Conventional radiation therapy most commonly used, but carries high risk of eventual hypopituitarism, and may also cause memory impairment, second tumors, and small-vessel ischemic strokes
- After radiation therapy, patients should take low-dose aspirin for life to reduce risk of stroke

OUTCOME

FOLLOW-UP

- Women with microadenomas may have dopamine agonists safely withdrawn during pregnancy
- Macroadenomas may enlarge during pregnancy; if therapy is withdrawn, they must be followed clinically and with computer-assisted visual field perimetry
- After pituitary surgery or radiation, follow serum prolactin every 3 months

COMPLICATIONS

- Macroadenomas can impair visual fields and cause hypopituitarism
- Untreated hypogonadism increases risk of osteoporosis

PROGNOSIS

- Fertility is usually promptly restored with dopamine agonists
- Discontinuing dopamine agonists after months or years usually results in reappearance of hyperprolactinemia, galactorrhea, and amenorrhea
- Nearly half—even massive tumors—shrink by >50%
- Shrinkage of pituitary adenoma occurs early, but maximum effect may take up to a year
- With dopamine agonist treatment for prolactinoma, 90% have fall in serum prolactin to ≤10% pretreatment levels; 80% achieve normal serum prolactin level

EVIDENCE

PRACTICE GUIDELINES

- Mah PM et al: Hyperprolactinemia: etiology, diagnosis, and management. Semin Reprod Med 2002;20:365. [PMID: 12536359]
- Nomikos P et al: Current management of prolactinomas. J Neurooncol 2001; 54:139. [PMID: 11761431]

WEB SITE

- American Society for Reproductive Medicine—Prolactin excess http://www.asrm.org/Patients/ FactSheets/Prolactin_Excess-Fact.pdf

INFORMATION FOR PATIENTS

- NIDDK—Prolactinoma http://www.niddk.nih.gov/health/endo/ pubs/prolact/prolact.htm
- University of Maryland Medicine— Prolactinoma—Males http://www.umm.edu/ency/article/ prolactinoma_males_symptoms_ 000337sym.htm

REFERENCES

- Pinzone JJ et al: Primary medical therapy of micro- and macroprolactinomas in men. J Clin Endocrinol Metab 2000;85:3053. [PMID: 10999785]
- Shrivastava RK et al: Giant prolactinomas: clinical management and long-term follow up. J Neurosurg 2002;97:299. [PMID: 12186457]
- Vallette-Kasic S et al: Macroprolactinemia revisited: a study on 106 patients. J Clin Endocrinol Metab 2002;87:581. [PMID: 11836289]

Paul A. Fitzgerald, MD

Hypertension, Chronic

 KEY FEATURES

ESSENTIALS OF DIAGNOSIS

- Usually asymptomatic
- Severe hypertension: occipital headache at awakening, blurry vision

GENERAL CONSIDERATIONS

- Mild to moderate hypertension nearly always asymptomatic
- Severe hypertension usually due to parenchymal renal disease, endocrine abnormalities, renal artery stenosis, drug use, or abrupt cessation of antihypertensive medications
- Table 41 (page 1235) provides classification based on blood pressure (BP) measurements

DEMOGRAPHICS

- 50 million Americans affected
- 70% are aware of their condition
- 50% of those aware are receiving treatment
- 25% of all hypertensive patients have their BP under control
- Incidence of disease increases with age
- More men than women early on
- More women than men later in life
- More common in black Americans (up to 25%)

 CLINICAL FINDINGS

SYMPTOMS AND SIGNS

- Usually asymptomatic
- Occipital headaches characteristic but uncommon
- Elevated blood pressure
- Loud A_2 on cardiac examination
- Retinal arteriolar narrowing with "silver-wiring," arteriovenous nicking
- Flame-shaped hemorrhages
- Laboratory findings usually normal
- In severe hypertension, renal dysfunction and hemolysis

DIFFERENTIAL DIAGNOSIS

Essential hypertension

- "White-coat" hypertension
- Blood pressure cuff too small

Secondary hypertension

- Adrenal: primary hyperaldosteronism, Cushing's syndrome, pheochromocytoma
- Renal: chronic renal disease, renal artery stenosis (atherosclerotic or fibromuscular dysplasia)
- Other: oral contraceptives, alcohol, nonsteroidal antiinflammatory drugs, pregnancy associated, hypercalcemia, hyperthyroidism, obstructive sleep apnea, obesity, coarctation of the aorta, acromegaly, increased intracranial pressure

 DIAGNOSIS

LABORATORY TESTS

- Hemoglobin
- Urinalysis
- Serum creatinine, blood urea nitrogen
- Serum potassium
- Fasting blood glucose
- Serum uric acid
- Electrocardiography (ECG)
- When a secondary cause is suspected, consider
  - Chest x-ray
  - Echocardiography
  - Catecholamine levels
  - Aldosterone levels
  - Urine electrolytes

TREATMENT

MEDICATIONS

- Initiation of drug therapy based on level of blood pressure, presence of target end-organ damage, and overall risk profile
- Major risk factors include smoking, dyslipidemia, diabetes mellitus, age over 60 years, and family history of cardiovascular disease
- Specific choice of pharmacotherapeutic agent should be based on other risk factors, compliance, and cost
- Diuretics: Table 43 (page 1236)
- β-Adrenergic blocking agents: Table 44 (page 1237)
- Angiotensin-converting enzyme (ACE) inhibitors and angiotensin receptor blockers: Table 45 (page 1239)
- Calcium channel-blocking agents: Table 46 (page 1241)
- α-Adrenergic blockers, vasodilators, centrally acting agents: Table 47 (page 1243)

THERAPEUTIC PROCEDURES

- Dietary changes (DASH diet): high in fruits and vegetables, low fat, low salt
- Weight reduction
- Alcohol restriction
- Salt reduction
- Adequate potassium intake
- Adequate calcium intake
- Increase physical activity
- Smoking cessation
- See Table 42 (page 1235)
- Aggressive risk factor management should be considered in all patients with hypertension
- Antihypertensive medications should be individualized: Table 48 (page 1245)
- Diabetics with hypertension should be treated aggressively, aiming for target BP <130/80, given high risk of cardiovascular events, and ACE inhibitors or angiotensin receptor blockers should be part of regimen

 OUTCOME

FOLLOW-UP

- Frequent visits until blood pressure is controlled
- Once controlled, visits can be infrequent, limited laboratory tests
- Lipid monitoring every year
- ECG every 2–4 years, depending on initial ECG

COMPLICATIONS

- Stroke
- Dementia
- Myocardial infarction
- Congestive heart failure
- Retinal vasculopathy
- Aortic dissection
- Renal disease, including proteinuria and nephrosclerosis

WHEN TO REFER

- Refer if blood pressure remains uncontrolled after three concurrent medications
- Refer if patient has uncontrolled blood pressure and symptoms and signs of end-organ damage

WHEN TO ADMIT

- Consider hospitalization if symptoms and signs of a hypertensive emergency (see *Hypertensive urgencies & emergencies*) including, in the setting of very high blood pressure, severe headache, neurological symptoms, chest pain, altered mental status, or acutely worsening renal failure

EVIDENCE

PRACTICE GUIDELINES

- McAlister FA et al: The 2001 Canadian recommendations for the management of hypertension: Part two–Therapy. Can J Cardiol 2002;18:625. [PMID: 12107420]
- Zarnke KB et al: The 2001 Canadian recommendations for the management of hypertension: Part one–Assessment for diagnosis, cardiovascular risk, causes and lifestyle modification. Can J Cardiol 2002;18:604. [PMID: 12107419]

WEB SITES

- American Society for Hypertension www.ash-us.org/
- Hypertension, Dialysis, and Clinical Nephrology, Renal Disease Electronic Journal www.hdcn.com/free.htm

INFORMATION FOR PATIENTS

- JAMA patient page: Hypertension. JAMA 2002;287:1070. [PMID: 11871440]
- American Heart Association— Understanding and controlling your blood pressure. www.americanheart.org

REFERENCES

- August P: Initial treatment of hypertension. N Engl J Med 348:620. [PMID: 12584370]
- Major outcomes in high-risk hypertensive patients randomized to angiotensin-converting enzyme inhibitor or calcium channel blocker versus diuretic. The Antihypertensive and Lipid-Lowering Treatment to Prevent Heart Attack Trial (ALLHAT) JAMA 2002;288:2981.
- The sixth report of the Joint National Committee on detection, education, and treatment of high blood pressure (JNC VI). Arch Intern Med 1997;157:2413.

Barry Massie, MD

Hypertensive Urgencies & Emergencies

 KEY FEATURES

ESSENTIALS OF DIAGNOSIS

- Important to differentiate hypertensive urgency (marked hypertension without end-organ damage) from hypertensive emergency (marked hypertension with end-organ damage)

GENERAL CONSIDERATIONS

- Hypertensive urgency usually has systolic blood pressure (BP) >220 mm Hg or diastolic BP >125 mm Hg without evidence of end-organ damage
- Hypertensive emergency defined by acute manifestations involving heart, brain, kidneys and/or retina

DEMOGRAPHICS

- Occurs in any age, gender, or racial/ethnic group
- Usually occurs in people with preexisting hypertension
- Often due to acute cessation of antihypertensive therapy
- Also occurs in setting of acute renal failure or use of high doses of sympathomimetics

 CLINICAL FINDINGS

SYMPTOMS AND SIGNS

- Symptoms depend on the end organ involved
- Headaches, irritability, confusion, and somnolence are signs of encephalopathy
- Chest pain or dyspnea occurs with cardiopulmonary involvement
- Back pain occurs with aortic dissection
- Blurry or diminished vision occurs with retinal involvement
- Cardiac examination may reveal low A_2, an S_4, or a murmur of aortic regurgitation
- Papilledema, "silver-wiring" of retinal arterioles, and flame hemorrhages are indicative of elevation of intracranial pressure
- Crackles on lung examination occur with congestive heart failure
- Hematuria, proteinuria, or other evidence of renal dysfunction
- Hemolysis
- Elevated troponin or creatine kinase (CK) occurs with myocardial damage

DIFFERENTIAL DIAGNOSIS

- Adrenal: primary hyperaldosteronism, Cushing's syndrome, pheochromocytoma
- Renal: chronic renal disease, renal artery stenosis (atherosclerotic or fibromuscular dysplasia)
- Other: oral contraceptives, alcohol, nonsteroidal antiinflammatory drugs, pregnancy associated, hypercalcemia, hyperthyroidism, obstructive sleep apnea, obesity, coarctation of the aorta, acromegaly, increased intracranial pressure

 DIAGNOSIS

LABORATORY TESTS

- Hemoglobin
- Platelet count
- Urinalysis
- Serum creatinine, blood urea nitrogen, troponin, CK
- Electrocardiography (ECG)
- Chest x-ray

DIAGNOSTIC PROCEDURES

- If central nervous system symptoms, head CT to rule out bleed
- If chest pain, echocardiogram to rule out aortic dissection
- If chest pain, renal ultrasound to rule out other causes of renal failure

TREATMENT

MEDICATIONS

Hypertensive urgency

- Goal is to relieve symptoms and bring blood pressure to reasonable level
- Clonidine, captopril, metoprolol, and hydralazine are effective oral agents
- Avoid β-blockers if cocaine use
- Avoid angiotensin-converting enzyme inhibitors if renal artery stenosis suspected
- Avoid short-acting dihydropyradine calcium channel blockers because blood pressure reduction is often precipitous

Hypertensive emergency

- Treatment goal is to reduce mean arterial pressure by 25% in 1–2 h; then to reduce BP to 160/100 over next 6–12 h
- Avoid excessive reduction in blood pressure because this can lead to coronary, cerebral, or renal hypoperfusion
- Key to pharmacological therapy is to use an agent with predictable, dose-dependent, transient effect
- Nitroprusside, labetalol, and nitroglycerin are most commonly used intravenously
- Fenoldopam, a peripheral dopamine agonist, is also effective

THERAPEUTIC PROCEDURES

- Treatment algorithm differs for hypertensive urgency and hypertensive emergency
- Goal is similar: reduce blood pressure to "safe" range without causing end-organ damage
- Table 49 (page XX) lists treatment options for hypertensive emergencies and urgencies
- In women who are pregnant or of childbearing age preeclampsia or eclampsia should be excluded; if diagnosed, proper management plans should be instituted promptly

 ## OUTCOME

FOLLOW-UP

- Patients with hypertensive urgency whose blood pressure is brought under control should be seen within 48–72 h for a recheck of blood pressure and tolerability of the antihypertensive regimen
- Patients with hypertensive emergency, once discharged from the hospital, should be followed up in 48–72 h to ensure good compliance with blood pressure medication and adequate blood pressure control

COMPLICATIONS

- Stroke
- Myocardial infarction
- Congestive heart failure
- Retinal vasculopathy
- Aortic dissection
- Renal failure

WHEN TO REFER

- Refer patients with hypertensive urgency to expert in management of severe hypertension
- Refer patients with elevated blood pressure and symptoms/signs of end-organ damage immediately for diagnostic workup and management

WHEN TO ADMIT

- Hospitalization for hypertensive urgency rarely needed

Hypertensive emergency

- Admit any patient with hypertensive emergency, in particular symptoms of encephalopathy, neurological deficits, chest pain, dyspnea, or signs of papilledema, hematuria, renal dysfunction, or ECG changes
- Usually need ICU admission for close monitoring of blood pressure and clinical symptoms and signs

 ## EVIDENCE

PRACTICE GUIDELINES

- American College of Obstetricians and Gynecologists. ACOG practice bulletin. Diagnosis and management of preeclampsia and eclampsia. Number 33, January 2002. Int J Gynaecol Obstet 2002;77:67. [PMID: 12094777]
- McAlister FA et al: The 2001 Canadian recommendations for the management of hypertension: Part two–Therapy. Can J Cardiol 2002;18:625. [PMID: 12107420]
- Zarnke KB et al: The 2001 Canadian recommendations for the management of hypertension: Part one–Assessment for diagnosis, cardiovascular risk, causes and lifestyle modification. Can J Cardiol 2002;18:604. [PMID: 12107419]

WEB SITES

- American Society for Hypertension http://www.ash-us.org/
- Hypertension, Dialysis, and Clinical Nephrology, Renal Disease Electronic Journal http://www.hdcn.com/free.htm

INFORMATION FOR PATIENTS

- JAMA patient page: Hypertension. JAMA 2002;287:1070. [PMID: 11871440]
- American Heart Association—Understanding and controlling your blood pressure. www.americanheart.org

REFERENCES

- Cherney D et al: Management of patients with hypertensive urgencies and emergencies. J Gen Intern Med 2002; 17:947. [12372930]
- Elliott WJ: Hypertensive emergencies. Crit Care Clin 2001;17:435. [PMID: 11450325]
- Phillips RA et al: Hypertensive emergencies: diagnosis and management. Prog Cardiovasc Dis 2002;45:33. [12138413]

Barry Massie, MD

Hyperthyroidism

 KEY FEATURES

ESSENTIALS OF DIAGNOSIS

- Sweating, weight loss (or gain), anxiety, loose stools, heat intolerance, irritability, fatigue, weakness, menstrual irregularity
- Tachycardia; warm, moist skin; stare; tremor
- In Graves' disease: goiter (often with bruit); ophthalmopathy
- Suppressed thyroid-stimulating hormone (TSH) in primary hyperthyroidism; increased free tetraiodothyronine (T_4) and triiodothyronine (T_3)

GENERAL CONSIDERATIONS

- Most common cause is Graves' disease, characterized by diffuse thyroid enlargement, gland hyperactivity, and antibodies against TSH receptor
- Graves' disease has familial tendency, and may be associated with other autoimmune disorders, eg, pernicious anemia, myasthenia gravis, diabetes mellitus, Addison's disease, alopecia areata, celiac disease, myasthenia gravis
- Autonomous toxic adenomas may be single (Plummer's disease) or multiple (toxic multinodular goiter)
- Subacute de Quervain's thyroiditis: possibly viral in origin, characterized by hyperthyroidism followed by hypothyroidism
- Jodbasedow disease, or iodine-induced hyperthyroidism, may occur with multinodular goiters after significant iodine intake in diet, radiographic contrast, or drugs, eg, amiodarone
- Thyrotoxicosis factitia: ingestion of excessive exogenous thyroid hormone
- Hashimoto's thyroiditis may cause transient hyperthyroidism during initial phase, and may occur postpartum
- High serum human chorionic gonadotropin levels in first 4 months of pregnancy, molar pregnancy, choriocarcinoma, and testicular malignancies may cause thyrotoxicosis

DEMOGRAPHICS

- Graves' disease is more common in women than men (8:1 ratio); onset usually between ages 20 and 40

 CLINICAL FINDINGS

SYMPTOMS AND SIGNS

- Nervousness, restlessness, heat intolerance, increased sweating, fatigue, weakness, muscle cramps, frequent bowel movements, weight loss (or gain), palpitations or angina pectoris
- Menstrual irregularities
- Stare and lid lag, tachycardia or atrial fibrillation, fine resting tremor, moist warm skin, hyperreflexia, fine hair, onycholysis, and (rarely) heart failure
- Goiter (often with a bruit) in Graves' disease. Moderately enlarged, tender thyroid in subacute thyroiditis
- Ophthalmopathy (chemosis, conjunctivitis, and mild proptosis) in 20–40% of patients with Graves' disease
- Diplopia may be due to coexistent myasthenia gravis
- Dermopathy (myxedema) in 3% of patients with Graves' disease; pretibial skin becomes erythematous, thickened, and rough
- Thyroid storm: delirium, severe tachycardia, vomiting, diarrhea, dehydration, high fever
- Hypokalemic paralysis: more common in Asian or Native American men

DIFFERENTIAL DIAGNOSIS

- General anxiety or panic disorder
- Mania
- Other hypermetabolic state, eg, cancer, pheochromocytoma
- Exophthalmos due to other cause, eg, orbital tumor
- Atrial fibrillation due to other cause
- Acute psychiatric disorders (may falsely increase serum thyroxine)
- High estrogen states, eg, pregnancy (high levels of thyroid-binding globulin increase serum total T_3 and T_4 levels; but free T_3 and free T_4 levels are normal)
- Hypopituitarism (low TSH and low free T_4)
- Subclinical hyperthyroidism (low TSH with normal free T_4)

 DIAGNOSIS

LABORATORY TESTS

- Sensitive TSH assay is the best test for thyrotoxicosis
- Serum T_3 and free T_4 usually increased
- T_4 is sometimes normal but T_3 elevated
- Hypercalcemia
- Alkaline phosphatase increased
- Anemia, neutropenia
- TSH receptor antibody (TSH-R Ab) levels high in 75% of patients with Graves' disease
- Antithyroglobulin or antithyroperoxidase (anti-TPO, antimicrosomal) antimicrosomal antibodies usually elevated in Graves' disease, but are nonspecific
- ANA and anti-double-stranded DNA antibodies usually elevated
- Erythrocyte sedimentation rate often elevated in subacute thyroiditis
- TSH elevated or normal despite thyrotoxicosis in TSH-secreting pituitary tumor
- Suppressed TSH and total T_4 >20 µg/dL or T_3 >200 ng/dL required to diagnose amiodarone-induced hyperthyroidism since high total T_4 and free T_4 are common on amiodarone

IMAGING STUDIES

- Thyroid radioactive iodine uptake and scan usually indicated for hyperthyroid patients
- High ^{123}I uptake seen in Graves' disease and toxic nodular goiter. Scan demonstrates toxic nodule or toxic multinodular goiter if present
- Low uptake characteristic of subacute thyroiditis

Hyperthyroidism

TREATMENT

MEDICATIONS

- **Graves' disease**
- Propranolol, 20 mg PO BID to start, increased until adequate response, usually 20–80 mg PO QID; improves tachycardia, tremor, diaphoresis, and anxiety of hyperthyroidism; may then use propranolol, LA, 60, 80, 120, or 160 mg PO BID. Continue until hyperthyroidism resolved
- Methimazole or propylthiouracil (thioureas) generally used for young adults, those with mild thyrotoxicosis, small goiters, or fear of radioiodine; preparing patients for surgery, and elderly patients for ^{131}I treatment
- Agranulocytosis is an uncommon but serious complication of thioureas
- Goiter occurs if patient is allowed to develop prolonged hypothyroidism on thioureas, but usually regresses rapidly with thyroid hormone replacement
- Methimazole, 10–30 mg BID, with dose reduced and given once daily as manifestations of hyperthyroidism resolve and free T_4 normalizes
- Propylthiouracil, 300-600 mg PO divided QID, with dose and frequency reduced as symptoms resolve and free T_4 normalizes
- Iodinated contrast agents [iopanoic acid (Telepaque) or ipodate sodium (Bilivist, Oragrafin)], 500 mg PO QD. Begin after thiourea commenced
- **Subacute thyroiditis**
- Propranolol for symptoms as above
- Ipodate sodium or iopanoic acid as above for 15–60 days
- **Amiodarone-induced thyrotoxicosis:** methimazole, iopanoic acid, β-blockers, prednisone
- **Hypokalemic thyrotoxic paralysis:** propranol corrects hypokalemia, even in apathetic hyperthyroidism

SURGERY

- **Graves' disease:** thyroidectomy preferred over radioiodine for pregnant women whose thyrotoxicosis not controlled with low dose thioureas, for patients aged <21 years, for patients with extremely large goiters, and those with suspected malignancy
- **Toxic solitary thyroid nodules:** partial thyroidectomy for patients aged <40, ^{131}I for those aged >40 years

THERAPEUTIC PROCEDURES

- **Graves' disease, toxic multinodular goiter**
- Radioactive iodine (^{131}I) therapy. Patients usually only on propranolol, but those with coronary disease, aged >65 years, or severe hyperthyroidism are usually first rendered euthyroid with methimazole. Contraindicated in pregnancy
- Discontinue methimazole 4 days before ^{131}I treatment; methimazole given after ^{131}I for symptomatic hyperthyroidism until euthyroid

 ## OUTCOME

FOLLOW-UP

- Check WBC periodically on thioureas, and for sore throat or febrile illness
- Follow patients clinically and with free T_4 levels every 2–3 weeks during initial treatment
- Hypothyroidism occurs commonly months to years after ^{131}I or subtotal thyroidectomy. Lifelong clinical follow-up mandatory, with TSH and free T_4 measurements when indicated

COMPLICATIONS

- Atrial fibrillation, congestive heart failure, cardiomyopathy
- Periodic hypokalemic paralysis
- Osteoporosis, hypercalcemia
- Temporary decreased libido, impotence, decreased sperm count, gynecomastia
- Diplopia or loss of vision
- Hypoparathyroidism or vocal cord palsy after thyroidectomy

PROGNOSIS

- Posttreatment hypothyroidism common, especially with ^{131}I or surgery
- Recurrence of hyperthyroidism occurs most commonly after thioureas (~50%)
- Subacute thyroiditis usually subsides spontaneously in weeks to months
- Graves' disease usually progresses, but may rarely subside spontaneously or even result in hypothyroidism
- Despite treatment, increased risk of death from cardiovascular disease, stroke, and femur fracture in women
- Mortality of thyroid storm is high
- Subclinical hyperthyroidism: prognosis is good; increased risk for bone loss

WHEN TO ADMIT

- Thyroid storm
- Hyperthyroidism-induced atrial fibrillation with severe tachycardia
- [131]I therapy or thyroidectomy

EVIDENCE

PRACTICE GUIDELINES

- AACE Medical Guidelines for Clinical Practice: Hyperthyroidism and Hypothyroidism 2002 http://www.aace.com/clin/guidelines/hypo_hyper.pdf

WEB SITE

- American Thyroid Association http://www.thyroid.org/index.php3?M_Session= 444ddf3f109e91628b84729a2dc7ca3a

REFERENCES

- Cooper DS: Antithyroid drugs in the management of patients with Graves' disease: an evidence-based approach to therapeutic controversies. J Clin Endocrinol Metab 2003;88:3474. [PMID: 12915620]
- Masiukiewicz US et al: Hyperthyroidism in pregnancy: diagnosis and treatment. Thyroid 1999;9:647. [PMID: 10447008]
- Weetman AP: Graves' disease. N Engl J Med 2000;343:1236. [PMID: 11071676]

Paul A. Fitzgerald, MD

Hypocalcemia

 ## KEY FEATURES

ESSENTIALS OF DIAGNOSIS

- Frequently mistaken for a neurological disorder
- Mainly due to insufficient action of parathyroid hormone (PTH) and/or vitamin D as well as magnesium difficiency

GENERAL CONSIDERATIONS

- Hypocalcemia implies insufficient action of PTH or active vitamin D
- The most common cause of hypocalcemia is renal failure, in which there is decreased production of active vitamin D_3 and hyperphosphatemia
- There is increased excitation of nerve and muscle cells, primarily affecting the neuromuscular and cardiovascular systems

Etiology

- **Decreased intake or absorption**
- Malabsorption
- Small bowel bypass
- Vitamin D deficit including 25-hydroxyvitamin D or 1,25-dihydroxyvitamin D
- **Increased loss**
- Alcoholism
- Chronic renal failure
- Diuretic therapy
- **Endocrine disease**
- Hypoparathyroidism
- Sepsis
- Pseudohypoparathryoidism
- Calcitonin secretion from medullary carcinoma of the thyroid
- Familial hypocalcemia
- **Physiological causes**
- Decreased serum albumin but normal ionized calcium
- Decreased end-organ response to vitamin D
- Hyperphosphatemia
- Loop diuretics

 ## CLINICAL FINDINGS

SYMPTOMS AND SIGNS

- Extensive spasm of skeletal muscle causes cramps and tetany
- Laryngospasm with stridor can obstruct the airway
- Convulsions, paresthesias of lips and extremities, and abdominal pain
- Chvostek's sign (contraction of the facial muscle in response to tapping the facial nerve anterior to the ear)
- Trousseau's sign (carpal spasm occurring after occlusion of the brachial artery with a blood pressure cuff for 3 min) is usually readily elicited
- In chronic hypoparathyroidism, cataracts and calcification of basal ganglia of the brain may appear
- Ventricular arrhythmias if there is QT prolongation

 ## DIAGNOSIS

LABORATORY TESTS

- When albumin is low, serum Ca^{2+} concentration is depressed in a ratio of 0.8–1 mg of Ca^{2+} to 1 g of albumin but the physiologically active ionized calcium is normal
- Serum phosphate is usually elevated in hypoparathyroidism or end-stage renal failure, whereas it is suppressed in early-stage renal failure or vitamin D deficiency
- Serum Mg^{2+} is commonly low, and hypomagnesemia reduces both parathyroid hormone release and tissue responsiveness to parathyroid hormone, causing hypocalcemia
- In respiratory alkalosis, total serum calcium is normal but ionized calcium is low

IMAGING STUDIES

- ECG can show prolongation of the QT interval (due to lengthened ST segment)

Hypocalcemia

 TREATMENT

MEDICATIONS

Severe, symptomatic hypocalcemia

- In the presence of tetany, arrhythmias, or seizures, calcium gluconate 10% (10–20 mL) administered intravenously over 10–15 min is indicated
- Because of the short duration of action, calcium infusion is usually required; 10–15 mg of calcium per kilogram body weight, or six to eight 10-mL vials of 10% calcium gluconate (558–744 mg of calcium), is added to 1 L of D_5W and infused over 4–6 h
- Adjust the infusion rate to maintain the serum calcium level at 7–8.5 mg/dL

Asymptomatic hypocalcemia

- Oral calcium (1–2 g) and vitamin D preparations (Table 85, page 1270) are used
- Calcium carbonate is well tolerated and less expensive than many other calcium tablets
- The low serum Ca^{2+} associated with low serum albumin concentration does not require replacement therapy
- If serum Mg^{2+} is low, therapy must include replacement of magnesium, which by itself usually will correct hypocalcemia

 OUTCOME

FOLLOW-UP

- Monitor the serum calcium level frequently (every 4–6 h) during calcium infusions for severe hypocalcemia

PROGNOSIS

- Depends on the underlying cause (eg, renal failure)

WHEN TO REFER

- Refer early to a nephrologist if renal failure is the underlying cause
- If parenteral therapy is needed

WHEN TO ADMIT

- All symptomatic patients. Intensive care unit admission may be needed
- If parenteral therapy is needed

 EVIDENCE

PRACTICE GUIDELINES

- National Guideline Clearinghouse http://www.guideline.gov/summary/summary.aspx?doc_id=3099&nbr=2325&string=hypocalcemia

WEB SITES

- Dr. Rose's Peripheral Brain—Fluids and electrolytes http://faculty.washington.edu/momus/PB/fluidand.htm
- Fluid and Electrolyte Disorders: MDAdvice.com http://www.mdadvice.com/library/ped/pedillsymp160.html

INFORMATION FOR PATIENTS

- American Association for Clinical Chemistry http://www.labtestsonline.org/understanding/analytes/calcium/test.html http://www.labtestsonline.org/understanding/analytes/pth/glance.html
- The Mayo Clinic http://www.mayoclinic.com/invoke.cfm?id=DS00280

REFERENCES

- Bushinsky DA et al: Calcium. Lancet 1998;352:306. [PMID: 9690425]
- Marx SJ: Hyperparathyroidism and hypoparathyroid disorders. N Engl J Med 2000;343:1863. [PMID: 11117980]
- Zivin JR et al: Hypocalcemia: a pervasive metabolic abnormality in the critically ill. Am J Kidney Dis 2001;7:689. [PMID: 11273867]

Masafumi Fukagawa, MD, PhD
Kiyoshi Kurokawa, MD, MACP
Maxine A. Papadakis, MD

Hypoglycemic Disorders

 KEY FEATURES

ESSENTIALS OF DIAGNOSIS

- Symptoms begin at plasma glucose levels of about 60 mg/dL and impairment of brain function at approximately 50 mg/dL
- Two types of spontaneous hypoglycemia: fasting and postprandial
- Fasting hypoglycemia is often subacute or chronic and usually presents with neuroglycopenia
- Postprandial hypoglycemia is relatively acute with symptoms of neurogenic autonomic discharge (sweating, palpitations, anxiety, tremulousness)

GENERAL CONSIDERATIONS

Fasting hypoglycemia

- Endocrine disorders, such as hypopituitarism, Addison's disease, or myxedema
- Liver malfunction, such as acute alcoholism or liver failure
- Renal failure on dialysis
- In absence of endocrine disorders, rule out hyperinsulinism from pancreatic B cell tumors or surreptitious administration of insulin (or sulfonylureas) and hypoglycemia due to non-insulin-producing extrapancreatic tumors

Postprandial (reactive) hypoglycemia

- Postprandial hypoglycemia is classified as early (within 2–3 h after a meal) or late (3–5 h after eating)
- Early, or alimentary, hypoglycemia occurs when there is a rapid discharge of ingested carbohydrate into the small bowel followed by rapid glucose absorption and hyperinsulinism
- Particularly associated with the dumping syndrome after gastrectomy
- May be functional from overactivity of the parasympathetic nervous system mediated via the vagus nerve
- Rarely, it results from defective counterregulatory responses such as deficiencies of growth hormone, glucagon, cortisol, or autonomic responses
- Alcohol-related hypoglycemia is due to hepatic glycogen depletion combined with alcohol-mediated inhibition of gluconeogenesis. Most common in malnourished alcohol abusers but can occur in anyone unable to ingest food after an acute alcoholic episode followed by gastritis and vomiting

- Factitious hypoglycemia is due to surreptitious administration of insulin or sulfonylurea

 CLINICAL FINDINGS

SYMPTOMS AND SIGNS

- Whipple's triad is characteristic of hypoglycemia regardless of the cause: a history of hypoglycemic symptoms, an associated fasting blood glucose of 40 mg/dL or less, and immediate recovery upon administration of glucose

Fasting hypoglycemia

- Healthy-appearing person with fasting hypoglycemia and confusion or abnormal behavior
- Obesity can result from overeating to relieve symptoms
- Insulinoma
- Symptoms often develop in the early morning, after missing a meal, or occasionally after exercise
- Initial CNS symptoms include blurred vision or diplopia, headache, feelings of detachment, slurred speech, and weakness
- Convulsions or coma may occur. Sweating and palpitations may not
- Personality changes vary from anxiety to psychotic behavior
- Hypoglycemic unawareness is very common

DIFFERENTIAL DIAGNOSIS

- Fasting hypoglycemia
  - Hyperinsulinism: pancreatic B cell tumor and surreptitious insulin or sulfonylureas
  - Extrapancreatic tumors
- Postprandial hypoglycemia: early hypoglycemia (alimentary)
- Postgastrectomy
- Functional (increased vagal tone): late hypoglycemia (occult diabetes)
- Delayed insulin release due to B cell dysfunction
  - Counterregulatory deficiency
  - Idiopathic
- Alcohol-related hypoglycemia
- Immunopathological hypoglycemia: antibodies to insulin receptors (which act as agonists)
- Pentamidine-induced hypoglycemia

 DIAGNOSIS

LABORATORY TESTS

- Serum insulin level of 6 μU/mL or more in the presence of blood glucose values below 40 mg/dL is diagnostic of inappropriate hyperinsulinism. Other causes of hyperinsulinemic hypoglycemia must be considered, including factitious administration of insulin or sulfonylureas
- An elevated circulating proinsulin level (above 0.2 ng/mL) in the presence of fasting hypoglycemia is characteristic of most B cell adenomas and does not occur in factitious hyperinsulinism
- In patients with epigastric distress, a history of renal stones, or menstrual or erectile dysfunction, a serum calcium, gastrin, or prolactin level may be useful in screening for MEN-1 associated with insulinoma
- Prolonged fasting up to 72 h under hospital supervision until hypoglycemia is documented
- In normal male subjects, the blood glucose does not fall below 55–60 mg/dL during a 3-day fast. In contrast, in normal premenopausal women who have fasted for only 24 h, the plasma glucose may fall normally to as low as 35 mg/dL. In these cases the women are not symptomatic, presumably owing to the development of sufficient ketonemia to supply energy needs to the brain. Insulinoma patients become symptomatic when plasma glucose drops to subnormal levels, since inappropriate insulin secretion restricts ketone formation
- A high-carbohydrate breakfast can differentiate postprandial reactive hypoglycemia from normal controls. Half of the patients with reactive hypoglycemia will have glucose levels as low as 59 mg/dL, in contrast to only 2% of controls. This test is more sensitive than a standard mixed meal

TREATMENT

MEDICATIONS

Inoperable pancreatic B cell tumors

- Diazoxide, 300–600 mg orally a day (along with a thiazide diuretic to control sodium retention)
- Glucagon
- Octreotide, 50 µg subcutaneously twice daily

SURGERY

- Surgical treatment for endocrine tumors

THERAPEUTIC PROCEDURES

Inoperable pancreatic B cell tumors

- Carbohydrate feeding every 2–3 h

Postprandial (reactive) hypoglycemia

- Frequent feedings with smaller portions of less rapidly assimilated carbohydrate combined with more slowly absorbed fat and protein

Functional alimentary hypoglycemia

- Support and mild sedation are mainstay of therapy
- Dietary manipulation is an adjunct: reduce proportion of carbohydrates in the diet, increase the frequency and reduce the size of the meals

OUTCOME

COMPLICATIONS

- Indiscriminate use and overinterpretation of glucose tolerance tests have led to an overdiagnosis of functional hypoglycemia
- As many as one-third or more of normal subjects have blood glucose levels as low as 40–50 mg/dL with or without symptoms during a 4-h glucose tolerance test

EVIDENCE

PRACTICE GUIDELINES

- National Guideline Clearinghouse
http://www.guideline.gov/summary/summary.aspx?doc_id=3127&nbr=2353&string=hypoglycemia
http://www.guideline.gov/summary/summary.aspx?doc_id=3126&nbr=2352&string=hypoglycemia

WEB SITES

- http://www.eatright.org
- http://www.diabetes.org/main/application/commercewf
- http://www.cdc.gov/diabetes/
- http://www.joslin.harvard.edu/

INFORMATION FOR PATIENTS

- National Diabetes Information Clearinghouse
http://www.niddk.nih.gov/health/diabetes/pubs/hypo/hypo.htm
- Mayo Clinic
http://www.mayoclinic.com/invoke.cfm?id=DS00198

REFERENCE

- Service FJ: Diagnostic approach to adults with hypoglycemic disorders. Endocrinol Metab Clin North Am 1999;28:519. [PMID: 10500929]

Umesh Masharani, MB, BS; MRCH (UK)

Hypogonadism, Male

 ## KEY FEATURES

ESSENTIALS OF DIAGNOSIS

- Diminished libido and erections
- Decreased growth of body hair
- Testes may be small or normal in size. Serum or free testosterone decreased
- Serum gonadotropins [luteinizing hormone (LH) and follicle-stimulating hormone (FSH)] decreased in hypogonadotropic hypogonadism (insufficient gonadotropin secretion by pituitary) and increased in hypergonadotropic hypogonadism (testicular failure)

GENERAL CONSIDERATIONS

- Caused by deficient testosterone secretion by the testes
- In hypogonadotropic form, FSH and LH deficiency may be isolated or with other pituitary abnormality

Hypogonadotropic hypogonadism

- Pituitary adenoma or hypopituitarism causing hyperprolactinemia, Cushing's syndrome, adrenal insufficiency, growth hormone excess or deficiency, thyroid hormone excess or deficiency
- Hemochromatosis
- Estrogen-secreting tumor (testicular, adrenal)
- Idiopathic
- Gonadotropin-releasing hormone agonist therapy, eg, leuprolide
- Other drugs, eg, alcohol, ketoconazole, spironolactone, marijuana
- Anorexia nervosa, cirrhosis, other serious illness, or malnutrition
- Kallmann's or Prader-Willi syndrome
- Intrathecal opioid infusion
- Congenital adrenal hypoplasia

Hypergonadotropic hypogonadism

- Male climacteric (andropause)
- Klinefelter's syndrome (47,XXY)
- Orchitis, eg, mumps, gonorrhea, tuberculosis, leprosy
- Testicular failure secondary to radiation therapy or chemotherapy
- Autoimmune, uremia, testicular trauma or torsion, lymphoma, myotonic dystrophy, androgen insensitivity

 ## CLINICAL FINDINGS

SYMPTOMS AND SIGNS

- Delayed puberty if congenital or acquired during childhood
- Decreased libido with acquired hypogonadism in most
- Erectile dysfunction, hot sweats, fatigue, or depression
- Infertility, gynecomastia, headache, or fracture
- Decreased body, axillary, beard, or pubic hair
- Loss of muscle mass and gain of weight due to increased subcutaneous fat
- Testicular size, as assessed with orchidometer (normal volume about 10–25 mL; normal length usually >6 cm), may decrease but usually remains within normal range with postpubertal hypogonadotropic hypogonadism
- In Klinefelter's syndrome, testes normal in childhood, but usually become small, firm, fibrotic, and nontender in adolescence; normal onset of puberty, variable degree of virilization, gynecomastia at puberty, tall stature with increased arm span, mental deficiency, clinodactyly, synostosis, poor social skills
- Testicular mass (Leydig cell tumor), trauma, infiltrative lesions (eg, lymphoma), or chronic infection (eg, leprosy, tuberculosis)

DIFFERENTIAL DIAGNOSIS

- Erectile dysfunction due to other cause, eg, diabetes mellitus, atherosclerosis, stroke, or drugs
- Male infertility due to other cause, eg, cryptorchism, retrograde ejaculation
- Gynecomastia due to other cause, eg, puberty, chronic liver disease, drugs, malignancy
- Hypothyroidism (may also be a cause hypogonadism)
- Depression

 ## DIAGNOSIS

LABORATORY TESTS

- Total testosterone measured nonfasting in AM is low (may be 25–50% lower, below "normal range," if fasting or drawn later in day)
- Testosterone highest at age 20–30 years, slightly lower at 30–40 years; falls gradually but progressively after age 40
- Free testosterone useful in elderly men [due to rising sex hormone-binding globulin (SHBG) with age]; best assays include equilibrium dialysis, calculated free testosterone, and non-SHBG-bound testosterone assay low. (Free androgen index, direct radioimmunoassay, and analog free testosterone assays are inaccurate)
- Check serum LH and FSH levels if low or borderline-low serum testosterone
- LH and FSH high in hypergonadotropic hypogonadism and low or inappropriately normal in hypogonadotropic hypogonadism

Hypogonadotropic hypogonadism

- Check serum prolactin: elevated in prolactinoma
- If gynecomastia, check serum androstenedione and estrone: both elevated in partial 17-ketosteroid reductase deficiency
- Check serum estradiol: elevated in cirrhosis and rare estrogen-secreting tumors (testicular Leydig cell tumor or adrenal carcinoma)
- If no clear cause for hypogonadotropic hypogonadism, check serum ferritin: elevated in hemochromatosis

Hypergonadotropic hypogonadism

- Check karyotyping or measurement of leukocyte X-inactive-specific transcriptase (XIST) by PCR for Klinefelter's syndrome

IMAGING STUDIES

- MRI of pituitary to evaluate for tumor or other lesion when no clear cause of hypogonadotropic hypogonadism
- Bone densitometry: reduced bone density in long-standing male hypogonadism

DIAGNOSTIC PROCEDURES

- Testicular biopsy is usually reserved for younger patients when reason for primary hypogonadism is unclear

Hypogonadism, Male

 ## TREATMENT

MEDICATIONS

- Testosterone replacement to reverse sexual dysfunction and muscle atrophy is usually begun when hypogonadism is confirmed and cause determined
- Screen older men for prostate cancer before initiating testosterone therapy
- Parenteral testosterone (enanthate or cypionate), 300 mg IM Q 3 weeks or 200 mg IM Q 2 weeks, usually in gluteal area, with dose adjustment per patient response
- Oral androgens, eg, methyltestosterone and fluoxymesterone, are not as effective as parenteral testosterone
- Transdermal testosterone is available in patch formulations applied QD to different nongenital skin sites: Testoderm II, 5 mg/day leaves sticky residue but causes little skin irritation; Androderm, 2.5–10 mg/day adheres more tightly but may cause skin irritation
- Topical testosterone 1% gel is available as Androgel (2.5-g and 5-g packets); starting dose is 5 g; dosage may be increased to maximum of 10 g/day if clinically indicated. Gel is applied QD to clean, dry skin of shoulders, upper arms, or abdomen, not genitals. **Note**: Hands must be washed after gel application, site allowed to dry 5 min before dressing, and clothing worn during contact with women or children
- Megestrol acetate, 20 mg PO BID, helpful for symptoms of male hypogonadism due to endocrine therapy for prostate cancer

THERAPEUTIC PROCEDURES

- Men with mosaic Klinefelter's syndrome (eg, 46XY/47XXY) may be fertile. Otherwise, infertility may be overcome by in vitro intracytoplasmic sperm injection (ICSI) into an ovum

 ## OUTCOME

FOLLOW-UP

- Follow serum testosterone if clinical response not adequate
- Follow hematocrit due to risk of polycythemia
- Reassess patient and measure serum testosterone after initiation of testosterone replacement; if inadequate clinical response or serum testosterone below normal, increase dose

COMPLICATIONS

- Osteoporosis
- Other complications of Klinefelter's syndrome include breast cancer, chronic pulmonary disease, varicosities of the legs, diabetes mellitus (8%), and impaired glucose tolerance (in an additional 19%)
- Side effects of testosterone replacement include acne, gynecomastia, aggravation of sleep apnea, reduced HDL cholesterol
- Oral androgens can cause cholestatic jaundice in 1–2%, and liver tumors or peliosis hepatis rarely with long-term use
- Megestrol acetate may cause increased appetite, weight gain, hyperglycemia, hypertriglyceridemia

PROGNOSIS

- Prognosis of hypogonadism due to pituitary lesion is that of primary disease (eg, tumor, necrosis)
- Prognosis for restoration of virility is good if testosterone replacement given

 ## EVIDENCE

PRACTICE GUIDELINES

- AACE Medical Guidelines for Clinical Practice: Hypogonadism, 2002 http://www.aace.com/clin/guidelines/hypogonadism.pdf
- Morales A et al: International Society for the Study of the Aging Male. Investigation, treatment and monitoring of late-onset hypogonadism in males. Official recommendations of ISSAM. Aging Male 2002;5:74. [PMID: 12198738]

WEB SITES

- The Pituitary Foundation http://www.pituitary.org.uk/resources/hypogon-m.htm
- Pituitary Network Association http://www.pituitary.com/disorders/hypogonadism.php

INFORMATION FOR PATIENTS

- Mayo Clinic—Hypogonadism http://www.mayoclinic.com/invoke.cfm?id=DS00300
- MEDLINEplus—hypogonadism http://www.nlm.nih.gov/medlineplus/ency/article/001195.htm

REFERENCES

- Basaria S et al: Hypogonadism and androgen replacement therapy in elderly men. Am J Med 2001;110:563. [PMID: 11343670]
- Basaria S et al: Long-term effects of androgen deprivation therapy in prostate cancer patients. Clin Endocrinol (Oxf) 2002;56:779. [PMID: 12072048]
- Daniell HW et al: Hypogonadism following prostate-bed radiation therapy for prostate carcinoma. Cancer 2001;91:1889. [PMID: 11346871]
- Howell S et al: Testosterone deficiency and replacement. Horm Res 2001;56:86. [PMID: 11786693]
- Mantovani G et al: Hypogonadotropic hypogonadism as a presenting feature of late-onset X-linked adrenal hypoplasia congenita. J Clin Endocrinol Metab 2002;87:44. [PMID: 11788621]
- Seidman SN et al: Testosterone replacement therapy for hypogonadal men with major depressive disorder: a randomized, placebo-controlled clinical trial. J Clin Psychiatry 2001;62:406. [PMID: 11465516]

Paul A. Fitzgerald, MD

Hypokalemia

KEY FEATURES

ESSENTIALS OF DIAGNOSIS

- K^+ <3.5 mEq/L
- Severe hypokalemia may induce dangerous arrhythmias and even rhabdomyolysis
- The transtubular potassium concentration gradient (TTKG) can distinguish renal from nonrenal loss of potassium

GENERAL CONSIDERATIONS

- Total potassium content of the body is 50 mEq/kg, more than 95% of which is intracellular
- A deficit of about 4–5 mEq/kg occurs for each 1 mEq/L decrement in serum potassium concentration below a level of 4 mEq/L
- Potassium shift into the cell is transiently stimulated by insulin and glucose and facilitated by β-adrenergic stimulation
- α-Adrenergic stimulation blocks potassium shift into the cell
- Aldosterone, which facilitates urinary potassium excretion through enhanced potassium secretion at the distal renal tubules, is the most important regulator of body potassium content
- Magnesium is an important cofactor for potassium uptake and for maintenance of intracellular potassium levels

Etiology: decreased potassium intake

- **Potassium shift into cell**
- Insulin excess, eg, postprandial
- Alkalosis
- β-Adrenergic agonists
- Trauma (via epinephrine release)
- Hypokalemic periodic paralysis
- **Renal potassium loss (urine K^+ >40 mEq/L)**
- *Increased aldosterone (mineralocorticoid) effects*
- Primary hyperaldosteronism
- Secondary hyperaldosteronism (dehydration, heart failure)
- Renovascular or malignant hypertension
- Cushing's syndrome
- European licorice (inhibits cortisol)
- Renin-producing tumor
- Congenital abnormality of steroid metabolism (eg, adrenogenital syndrome, 17α-hydroxylase defect)
- *Increased flow of distal nephron*
- Diuretics (furosemide, thiazides)

- Salt-losing nephropathy
- *Hypomagnesemia*
- Unreabsorbable anion
- Carbenicillin, penicillin
- *Renal tubular acidosis (type I or II)*
- Fanconi's syndrome
- Interstitial nephritis
- Metabolic alkalosis (bicarbonaturia)
- *Genetic disorder of the nephron*
- Bartter's syndrome
- Liddle's syndrome
- Hypercapnia, tetany, and rhabdomyolysis may be seen with severe hypokalemia (<2.5 mEq/L)
- **Extrarenal potassium loss (urine K^+ <20 mEq/L)**
- Vomiting, diarrhea, laxative abuse
- Villous adenoma, Zollinger-Ellison syndrome

CLINICAL FINDINGS

SYMPTOMS AND SIGNS

- Muscular weakness, fatigue, and muscle cramps are common in mild to moderate hypokalemia
- Constipation or ileus may result from smooth muscle involvement
- Flaccid paralysis, hyporeflexia

DIAGNOSIS

LABORATORY TESTS

- Urinary potassium concentration is low (<20 mEq/L) as a result of extrarenal loss and inappropriately high (>40 mEq/L) with urinary losses
- The TTKG is a simple and rapid method to evaluate net potassium secretion

$$TTKG = \frac{Urine\ K^+\ /\ Plasma\ K^+}{Urine\ osm\ /\ Plasma\ osm}$$

- Hypokalemia with a TTKG >4 suggests renal potassium loss with increased distal K^+ secretion. In such cases, plasma renin and aldosterone levels are helpful in differential diagnosis. The presence of nonabsorbed anions, including bicarbonate, also increases the TTKG

IMAGING STUDIES

- The ECG can show decreased amplitude and broadening of T waves, prominent U waves, premature ventricular contractions, and depressed ST segments

TREATMENT

MEDICATIONS

- Oral potassium is the safest way to treat mild to moderate deficiency
- All potassium formulations are easily absorbed
- Dietary potassium is almost entirely coupled to phosphate—rather than chloride—and does not correct potassium loss associated with chloride depletion, such as from diuretics or vomiting
- In the setting of abnormal renal function and mild to moderate diuretic dosage, 20 mEq/day of oral potassium is generally sufficient to prevent hypokalemia, but 40–100 mEq/day over a period of days to weeks is needed to treat hypokalemia and fully replete potassium stores
- Intravenous potassium replacement is indicated for patients with severe hypokalemia and for those who cannot take oral supplementation
- For severe deficiency, potassium may be given through a peripheral intravenous line in a concentration that should not exceed 40 mEq/L at rates of up to 40 mEq/L/h
- Coexisting magnesium and potassium depletion can result in refractory hypokalemia despite potassium repletion if there is no magnesium repletion

 OUTCOME

FOLLOW-UP

- Continuous electrocardiographic monitoring is indicated when infusing intravenous potassium for severe hypokalemia
- The serum potassium level should be checked every 3–6 h

COMPLICATIONS

- Hypokalemia increases the likelihood of digitalis toxicity. Thus, hypokalemia induced by concomitant drugs such as β_2-adrenergic agonists and diuretics may impose a substantial risk

WHEN TO REFER

- Persistent hypokalemia <3.0 mEq/L without any recent episode of gastrointestinal losses

WHEN TO ADMIT

- For severe hypokalemia (K^+ <2.5 mEq/L)
- If intravenous potassium replacement is needed
- If cardiac monitoring is necessary during potassium replacement

PROGNOSIS

- Most hypokalemia will correct with replacement after 24–72 h

 EVIDENCE

PRACTICE GUIDELINES

- National Guideline Clearinghouse http://www.guideline.gov/summary/summary.aspx?doc_id=3582&nbr=2808&string=potassium
- Cohn JN et al: New guidelines for potassium replacement in clinical practice: a contemporary review by the National Council on Potassium in Clinical Practice. Arch Intern Med 2000;160:2429.

WEB SITES

- Fluid and Electrolyte Disorders: MDAdvice.com http://www.mdadvice.com/library/ped/pedillsymp160.html
- Dr. Rose's Peripheral Brain—Fluids and electrolytes http://faculty.washington.edu/momus/PB/fluidand.htm

INFORMATION FOR PATIENTS

- National Institutes of Health http://www.nlm.nih.gov/medlineplus/ency/article/000479.htm http://www.nlm.nih.gov/medlineplus/ency/article/001101.htm

REFERENCES

- Gennari FJ: Hypokalemia. N Engl J Med 1998;339:451. [PMID: 9700180]
- Loughrey CM: Serum magnesium must also be known in profound hypokalaemia. BMJ 2002;324:1039. [PMID: 11976255]
- Rastegar A et al: Hypokalaemia and hyperkalaemia. Postgrad Med J 2001;77:759. [PMID: 11723313]
- Welfare W et al: Challenges in managing profound hypokalemia. BMJ 2002;324:269 [PMID: 11823358]

Masafumi Fukagawa, MD, PhD
Kiyoshi Kurokawa, MD, MACP
Maxine A. Papadakis, MD

Hypomagnesemia

KEY FEATURES

ESSENTIALS OF DIAGNOSIS

- **Causes neurological symptoms and arrhythmias**
- Serum concentration may not be decreased even in the presence of magnesium deficiency
- Check urinary magnesium deficiency if depletion is suspected
- Impairs release of parathyroid hormone (PTH)

GENERAL CONSIDERATIONS

- Magnesium acts directly on the myoneural junction
- Altered concentration of Mg^{2+} in the plasma usually provokes an associated alteration of Ca^{2+}
- Severe and prolonged magnesium depletion impairs secretion of PTH with consequent hypocalcemia
- Hypomagnesemia may impair end-organ response to PTH as well

Etiology

- **Diminished absorption or intake**
- Malabsorption
- Chronic diarrhea
- Laxative abuse
- Prolonged gastrointestinal suction
- Malnutrition
- Alcoholism
- Parenteral alimentation with inadequate Mg^+ content
- **Increased renal loss**
- Diuretic therapy
- Hyperaldosteronism
- Barrter's syndrome
- Hyperparathryoidism
- Hyperthyroidism
- Hypercalcemia
- Volume expansion
- Tubulointerstitial diseases
- Drugs (aminoglycoside, cisplatin, amphotericin B, pentamidine)
- **Others**
- Diabetes mellitus
- Postparathryoidectomy (hungry bone syndrome)
- Respiratory alkalosis
- Pregnancy

DEMOGRAPHICS

- Nearly half of hospitalized patients in whom serum electrolytes are ordered have unrecognized hypomagnesemia
- Common causes include use of large volumes of intravenous fluids, diuretics, cisplatin in cancer patients (with concomitant hypokalemia), and administration of nephrotoxic agents such as aminoglycosides and amphotericin B

CLINICAL FINDINGS

SYMPTOMS AND SIGNS

- Weakness, muscle cramps, and tremor
- Marked neuromuscular and central nervous system hyperirritability, with tremors, athetoid movements, jerking, nystagmus, and a positive Babinski response
- Confusion and disorientation may be prominent features
- There may be hypertension, tachycardia, and ventricular arrhythmias

DIAGNOSIS

LABORATORY TESTS

- Urinary excretion of magnesium exceeding 10–30 mg/day or a fractional excretion more than 2% indicates renal magnesium wasting
- In calculating fractional excretion of magnesium, since only 30% is protein-bound, 70% of circulating magnesium is filtered by the glomerulus
- Hypocalcemia and hypokalemia are often present
- Parathyroid hormone secretion is often suppressed

IMAGING STUDIES

- The ECG may show a prolonged QT interval, due to lengthening of the ST segment

TREATMENT

MEDICATIONS

- Intravenous fluids containing magnesium as chloride or sulfate, 240–1200 mg/day (10–50 mmol/day) during the period of severe deficit, followed by 120 mg/day (5 mmol/day) for maintenance
- Magnesium sulfate may also be given intramuscularly in a dosage of 200–800 mg/day (8–33 mmol/day) in four divided doses
- K^+ and Ca^{2+} may be required as well
- Magnesium oxide, 250–500 mg by mouth two to four times daily, is useful for repleting stores in those with chronic hypomagnesemia
- Hypokalemia and hypocalcemia of hypomagnesemia do not recover without magnesium supplementation

 OUTCOME

FOLLOW-UP

- Serum levels must be monitored and dosage of magnesium supplementation adjusted to keep the concentration from rising above 2.5 mmol/L

WHEN TO REFER

- Refer to an endocrinologist or nephrologist for consultation about repletion in the setting of marked neuromuscular symptoms or cardiac arrhythmia

WHEN TO ADMIT

- Confusion, disorientation
- Marked neuromuscular and central nervous system hyperirritability
- Need for intravenous replacement

 EVIDENCE

PRACTICE GUIDELINES

- National Guideline Clearinghouse http://www.guideline.gov/summary/summary.aspx?doc_id=3058&nbr=2284&string=hypomagnesemia

WEB SITES

- Dr. Rose's Peripheral Brain—Fluids and electrolytes http://faculty.washington.edu/momus/PB/fluidand.htm
- Fluid and Electrolyte Disorders: MDAdvice.com http://www.mdadvice.com/library/ped/pedillsymp160.html

INFORMATION FOR PATIENTS

- National Institutes of Health http://www.nlm.nih.gov/medlineplus/ency/article/000315.htm

REFERENCES

- Dacey M: Hypomagnesemic disorders. Crit Care Clin 2001;17:155. [PMID: 11219227]
- Huijgen HJ et al: Magnesium levels in critically ill patients. What should we measure? Am J Clin Pathol 2000; 114:688. [PMID: 11068541]

Masafumi Fukagawa, MD, PhD
Kiyoshi Kurokawa, MD, MACP
Maxine A. Papadakis, MD

Hyponatremia

KEY FEATURES

ESSENTIALS OF DIAGNOSIS

- Serum sodium concentration less than 130 mEq/L
- Mainly due to abnormality of water balance, and not salt balance
- Check extracellular fluid (ECF) volume and serum osmolality to assess etiology

GENERAL CONSIDERATIONS

- Implies abnormal water balance rather than abnormal sodium balance
- Hyponatremia is usually associated with abnormal serum osmolality
- An abnormal sodium balance is often associated either with volume depletion or with edema formation
- Urine sodium helps distinguish renal from nonrenal causes of hyponatremia
- Urine sodium >20 mEq/L implies renal salt wasting [diuretics, angiotensin-converting enzyme (ACE) inhibitors, mineralocorticoid deficiency, salt-losing nephropathy] and urine sodium <10 mEq/L or fractional excretion of sodium less than 1% (unless diuretics have been given) implies avid sodium retention by the kidney because of extrarenal fluid losses (vomiting, diarrhea, sweating, or third-spacing, as with ascites)

Etiology

- **Isotonic hyponatremia or pseudohyponatremia** (normal serum osmolality; artifact corrected in most U.S. labs)
- Hyperlipidemia
- Hyperproteinemia
- **Hypertonic hyponatremia** (serum osmolality >295 mosm/kg)
- Hyperglycemia
- Mannitol, sorbitol, glycerol, maltose
- Radiocontrast agents
- **Hypotonic hyponatremia** (serum osmolality <280 mosm/kg)
- *Hypovolemic*
- Extrarenal salt loss (U_{Na+} <10 mEq/L): dehydration, diarrhea, vomiting
- Renal salt loss (U_{Na+} >20 mEq/L): diuretics, ACE inhibitors, nephropathies, mineralocorticoid deficiency, cerebral sodium-wasting syndrome
- *Euvolemic*
- Syndrome of inappropriate antidiuretic hormone
- Postoperative hyponatremia
- Hypothyroidism
- Psychogenic polydipsia
- Beer potomania
- Idiosyncratic drug reaction (thiazides, ACE inhibitors)
- Endurance exercise
- *Hypervolemic* (edematous states)
- Congestive heart failure
- Liver disease
- Nephrotic syndrome (rare)
- Advanced renal failure

DEMOGRAPHICS

- Most common electrolyte abnormality observed in a general hospitalized population (about 2% of patients)

CLINICAL FINDINGS

SYMPTOMS AND SIGNS

- Frequently asymptomatic
- Symptomatic hyponatremia is usually seen with serum sodium levels less than 120 mEq/L. If symptomatic, primarily central nervous system symptoms of lethargy, weakness, confusion, delirium, and seizures
- Often symptoms are mistaken for primary neurological or metabolic disorders

DIAGNOSIS

LABORATORY TESTS

- Serum osmolality and the patient's volume status are essential to determine the etiology of hyponatremia (Figure 6, page 1269)

TREATMENT

MEDICATIONS

Hypotonic hyponatremia

- Replace lost volume with isotonic or half-normal (0.45%) saline or lactated Ringer's infusion
- The rate of correction must be adjusted to prevent permanent cerebral damage (see below)
- Corticosteroids can be used empirically if hypocortisolism is considered in the differential diagnosis

Euvolemic hyponatremia

- See *Syndrome of inappropriate antidiuretic hormone*
- Symptomatic hyponatremia
  - If there are central nervous system symptoms, hyponatremia should be rapidly treated at any level of serum sodium concentration
  - A reasonable approach is to increase the serum sodium concentration by no more than 1–2 mEq/L/h and not more than 25–30 mEq/L in the first 2 days in order to prevent central pontine myelinolysis; the rate should be reduced to 0.5–1 mEq/L/h as soon as neurological symptoms improve
  - The initial goal is to achieve a serum sodium concentration of 125–130 mEq/L, guarding against overcorrection
  - Hypertonic (eg, 3%) saline plus furosemide (0.5–1 mg/kg IV) is indicated for symptomatic hyponatremia
  - To determine how much 3% saline (513 mEq/L) to administer, obtain a spot urinary Na after a furosemide diuresis has begun. The excreted Na is replaced with 3% saline, empirically begun at 1–2 mL/kg/h and then adjusted based on urinary output and urinary sodium. For example, after furosemide, urine volume may be 400 mL/h and sodium plus potassium excretion 100 mEq/L. The excreted Na^+ is 40 mEq/h, which is replaced with 78 mL/h of 3% saline (40 mEq/h divided by 513 mEq/L)

- Asymptomatic hyponatremia
  - Restrict water intake to 0.5–1 L/day Gradual increase of serum sodium will occur over days
  - The correction rate of hyponatremia need be no more than 0.5 mEq/L/h
  - No specific treatment is needed for patients with reset osmostats
  - 0.9% saline 0.9% saline with furosemide may be used in asymptomatic patients whose serum sodium is less than 120 mEq/L. Urinary sodium and potassium losses are replaced as above
  - Demeclocycline (300–600 mg twice daily) inhibits the effect of antidiuretic hormone on the distal tubule and is useful for patients who cannot adhere to water restriction or need additional therapy. Onset of action may be 1 week, and concentrating may be permanently impaired. Therapy with demeclocycline in cirrhosis appears to increase the risk of renal failure
  - Hyponatremia occurring as part of the cerebral salt-wasting syndrome can be treated with fludrocortisone

Hypervolemic hypotonic hyponatremia

- The treatment of hyponatremia is that of the underlying condition (eg, improving cardiac output in congestive heart failure) and water restriction (to <1–2 L of water daily)
- To hasten excretion of water and salt, use of diuretics may be indicated
- Since diuretics may worsen hyponatremia, the patient must be cautioned not to increase free water intake
  - Hypertonic saline administration is dangerous in volume-overloaded states and is not routinely recommended
  - In patients with severe hyponatremia (serum sodium <110 mEq/L) and central nervous system symptoms, judicious administration of small amounts (100–200 mL) of 3% saline with diuretics may be necessary
  - Emergency dialysis should also be considered

OUTCOME

FOLLOW-UP

- If symptomatic, measure plasma sodium approximately every 4 h and observe the patient closely

COMPLICATIONS

- Central pontine myelinolysis may occur from osmotically induced demyelination due to overly rapid correction of serum sodium (an increase of more than 1 mEq/L/h, or 25 mEq/L within the first day of therapy)
- Hypoxic-anoxic episodes during hyponatremia may contribute to the demyelination

PROGNOSIS

- Premenopausal women who develop hyponatremic encephalopathy from rapidly acquired hyponatremia (eg, postoperative hyponatremia) are about 25 times more likely than postmenopausal women to die or to suffer permanent brain damage

WHEN TO REFER

- Persistent hyponatremia despite therapy

WHEN TO ADMIT

- Symptomatic hyponatremia
- Serum sodium <120 mEq/L

EVIDENCE

PRACTICE GUIDELINES

- National Guideline Clearinghouse http://www.guideline.gov/summary/summary.aspx?doc_id=3165&nbr=2391&string=hyponatremia http://www.guideline.gov/summary/summary.aspx?doc_id=3450&nbr=2676&string=hyponatremia

WEB SITES

- Fluid and Electrolyte Disorders: MDAdvice.com http://www.mdadvice.com/library/ped/pedillsymp160.html
- Dr. Rose's Peripheral Brain—Fluids and electrolytes http://faculty.washington.edu/momus/PB/fluidand.htm

INFORMATION FOR PATIENTS

- The Mayo Clinic http://www.mayoclinic.com/invoke.cfm?id=AN00621
- National Institutes of Health http://www.nlm.nih.gov/medlineplus/ency/article/000394.htm

REFERENCES

- Adrogue HJ et al: Hyponatremia. N Engl J Med 2000;342:1581.
- Cadnapaphornchai MA et al: Pathogenesis and management of hyponatremia. Am J Med 2000;109:688.
- Oster JR et al: Hyponatremia, hypoosmolality, and hypotonicity: tables and fables. Arch Intern Med 1999;159:333.

Masafumi Fukagawa, MD, PhD
Kiyoshi Kurokawa, MD, MACP
Maxine A. Papadakis, MD

Hypoparathyroidism & Pseudohypoparathyroidism

 KEY FEATURES

ESSENTIALS OF DIAGNOSIS

- Tetany, carpopedal spasms, tingling of lips and hands, muscle and abdominal cramps, psychological changes
- Positive Chvostek's sign and Trousseau's phenomenon; defective nails and teeth; cataracts
- Serum calcium low; serum phosphate high; alkaline phosphatase normal; urine calcium excretion reduced
- Serum magnesium may be low

GENERAL CONSIDERATIONS

- Parathyroid hormone (PTH) increases serum calcium and decreases serum phosphate via effects on bone osteoclastic activity and renal tubules
- Hypoparathyroidism occurs most commonly following thyroidectomy, usually transient but may be permanent
- May occur after surgical removal of parathyroid adenoma due to suppression of remaining parathyroids
- May occur in DiGeorge's syndrome, with congenital cardiac and facial anomalies
- May result from damage to gland by heavy metals, eg, copper (Wilson's disease), iron (hemochromatosis, transfusion hemosiderosis); granulomas; sporadic autoimmunity; Riedel's thyroiditis; tumors; infection; or neck irradiation (rare)
- Magnesium deficiency (malabsorption, chronic alcoholism), which prevents PTH secretion, may cause functional hypoparathyroidism
- Pseudohypoparathyroidism is characterized by hypocalcemia and high PTH levels due to renal resistance to PTH, from mutations in PTH receptor
- Pseudohypoparathyroidism may be associated with short stature, round face, obesity, short fourth metacarpals, ectopic bone formation, and mental retardation
- "Pseudopseudohypoparathyroidism" is characterized by these phenotypic abnormalities but without hypocalcemia

 CLINICAL FINDINGS

SYMPTOMS AND SIGNS

- Acute symptoms: tetany, with muscle cramps, irritability, carpopedal spasm, and convulsions; tingling of circumoral area, hands, and feet
- Chronic symptoms: lethargy, personality changes, anxiety, blurred vision due to cataracts, parkinsonism, mental retardation
- Chvostek's sign (facial muscle contraction on tapping facial nerve in front of the ear)
- Trousseau's phenomenon (carpal spasm after application of a cuff)
- Cataracts
- Nails may be thin and brittle; skin is dry and scaly, at times with candidiasis; hair loss (eyebrows)
- Deep tendon reflexes hyperactive
- Papilledema and elevated cerebrospinal fluid pressure occasionally
- Defective teeth if onset in childhood

DIFFERENTIAL DIAGNOSIS

- Pseudohypoparathyroidism (renal resistance to PTH)
- Vitamin D deficiency
- Acute pancreatitis
- Chronic renal failure
- Hypoalbuminemia
- Paresthesias or tetany due to respiratory alkalosis
- Familial hypocalcemia with hypercalciuria (normal serum PTH)

 DIAGNOSIS

LABORATORY TESTS

- Serum calcium low
- Serum phosphate high
- Alkaline phosphatase normal
- Urinary calcium low
- PTH level low
- Obtain serum magnesium: hypomagnesemia frequently accompanies hypocalcemia and may decrease parathyroid gland function
- Note: serum calcium is largely bound to albumin. If hypoalbuminemia is present, obtain ionized calcium or correct calcium level for albumin level
- Corrected Ca^{2+} = serum Ca^{2+} mg/dL + [0.8 × (4.0–albumin g/dL)]

IMAGING STUDIES

- Skull radiographs or head CT may show basal ganglia calcifications
- Bone x-rays may show increased bone density
- Other x-rays may show cutaneous calcifications

DIAGNOSTIC PROCEDURES

- Slitlamp examination may show early posterior lenticular cataract formation
- ECG shows prolonged QT interval and T wave abnormalities

TREATMENT

MEDICATIONS

Emergency treatment for acute tetany

- Ensure adequate airway
- Calcium gluconate, 10–20 mL of 10% solution IV, given *slowly* until tetany ceases. Add 10 to 50 mL of calcium gluconate 10% to 1 L of D5W or saline and give by slow IV drip; titrate to serum calcium of 8–9 mg/dL
- Oral calcium, 1–2 g daily, given as soon as possible. Liquid calcium carbonate (Titralac Plus), 500 mg/5 mL, is useful. Calcium citrate contains 21% calcium, but higher proportion is absorbed with less gastrointestinal intolerance
- Vitamin D derivatives, to be given with oral calcium, include calcitriol (1,25-dihydroxycholecalciferol), 0.25 to 4 μg PO QD; ergocalciferol (vitamin D_2), 25,000 to 150,000 units PO QD, or calcifediol (25-hydroxyvitamin D_3), 20 μg PO QD; or dihydrotachysterol, 0.125–1 mg PO QD (Table 85, page 1270)
- If hypomagnesemia is present, give $MgSO_4$ 1–2 g IV Q 6 h acutely; and magnesium oxide tablets, 600 mg 1–2 PO QD, or combined magnesium and calcium preparation (dolomite, others), chronically

Maintenance treatment

- Calcium (1–2 g/day) and vitamin D supplementation (see above) to achieve slightly low but asymptomatic serum calcium (8–8.6 mg/dL) to minimize hypercalciuria and provide margin of safety against overdosage and hypercalcemia
- Calcitriol, 0.25 μg PO QAM, titrated up to 0.5–2 μg PO QAM, to achieve near normocalcemia in patients with chronic hypocalcemia
- Avoid phenothiazines in hypocalcemia; may precipitate extrapyramidal symptoms
- Avoid furosemide; may worsen hypocalcemia

SURGERY

- Transplantation of cryopreserved parathyroid tissue from prior surgery restores normocalcemia in ~23%

 ## OUTCOME

FOLLOW-UP

- Monitor serum calcium at regular intervals (at least every 3 months)
- Monitor "spot" urine calcium to keep level <30 mg/dL if possible
- Hypercalciuria may respond to oral hydrochlorothiazide, usually given with a potassium supplement
- Hypercalcemia developing in patients with previously stable, treated hypoparathyroidism may signal new onset of Addison's disease

COMPLICATIONS

- Stridor, especially with vocal cord palsy, may cause respiratory obstruction requiring tracheostomy
- Chronic hypoparathyroidism may be associated with autoimmune diseases, eg, sprue, pernicious anemia, or Addison's disease
- Cataract formation and calcification of the basal ganglia occur in long-standing cases. Occasionally, parkinsonism or choreoathetosis develops
- Nerve root compression due to ossification of paravertebral ligaments
- Seizures in untreated patients
- Nephrocalcinosis and impaired renal function if overtreatment with calcium and vitamin D

PROGNOSIS

- Prognosis good if diagnosis made and treatment instituted promptly
- Dental changes, cataracts, and brain calcifications are permanent

WHEN TO REFER

- Refer all patients to endocrinologist for stable regimen

WHEN TO ADMIT

- Any symptomatic hypocalcemia

 ## EVIDENCE

PRACTICE GUIDELINES

- AACE Medical Guidelines for Clinical Practice: Hyperthyroidism and Hypothyroidism, 2002 http://www.aace.com/clin/guidelines/ hypo_hyper.pdf
- Guidelines for the use of radioiodine in the management of hyperthyroidism: a summary. Prepared by the Radioiodine Audit Subcommittee of the Royal College of Physicians Committee on Diabetes and Endocrinology, and the Research Unit of the Royal College of Physicians. J R Coll Physicians Lond 1995;29:464. [PMID: 8748100]
- Singer PA et al: Treatment guidelines for patients with hyperthyroidism and hypothyroidism. Standards of Care Committee, American Thyroid Association. JAMA 1995;273:808. [PMID: 7532241]

WEB SITES

- American Thyroid Association http://www.thyroid.org/index. php3?M_Session= 444ddf3f109e91628b84729a2dc7ca3a
- The Thyroid Society for Education and Research http://the-thyroid-society.org/
- Thyroid Foundation of America http://www.tsh.org

INFORMATION FOR PATIENTS

- Mayo Clinic—Hyperthyroidism http://www.mayoclinic.com/invoke.cfm? id=DS00344

REFERENCES

- Lindblom P et al: Low parathyroid hormone levels after thyroid surgery: a feasible predictor of hypocalcemia. Surgery 2002;131:515. [PMID: 12019404]
- Marx SJ: Hyperparathyroid and hypoparathyroid disorders. N Engl J Med 2000;343:1863. [PMID: 11117980]
- Thakker RV: Genetic developments in hypoparathroidism. Lancet 2001;357: 974. [PMID: 11293637]

Paul A. Fitzgerald, MD

Hypophosphatemia

KEY FEATURES

ESSENTIALS OF DIAGNOSIS

- Serious depletion of body phosphate may exist with low, normal, or high concentrations of phosphorus in serum
- May cause hypooxygenation and even rhabdomyolysis
- Reduced maximal tubular reabsorption rate of phosphate (TmP/GFR) indicates urinary phosphate loss

GENERAL CONSIDERATIONS

- Cellular uptake is stimulated by alkalemia, insulin, epinephrine, feeding, postparathryoidectomy (hungry bone syndrome), and accelerated cell proliferation
- Alcoholism
  - In acute alcohol withdrawal, increased plasma insulin and epinephrine along with respiratory alkalosis promote intracellular shift of phosphate
  - Vomiting, diarrhea, and poor dietary intake contribute to hypophosphatemia
  - Chronic alcohol use results in a decrease in the renal threshold of phosphate excretion
- Patients with chronic obstructive pulmonary disease and asthma commonly have hypophosphatemia, attributed to xanthine derivatives causing shifts of phosphate intracellularly and the phosphaturic effects of β-adrenergic agonists, loop diuretics, xanthine derivatives, and corticosteroids
- Therapy of hyperglycemia causes phosphate to accompany glucose intracellularly, and hypophosphatemia may ensue

Etiology

- **Diminished supply or absorption**
- Starvation
- Parenteral alimentation with inadequate phosphate content
- Malabsorption
- Vitamin D–resistant osteomalacia
- **Increased loss**
- Phosphaturic drugs (diuretics, theophylline, bronchodilators, corticosteroids)
- Hyperparathyroidism, hyperthyroidism
- Renal tubular acidosis (eg, monoclonal gammopathy)
- Alcoholism
- Hypokalemic nephropathy
- **Intracellular shift of phosphorus**
- Glucose administration
- Drugs (anabolic steroids, estrogen, oral contraceptives)
- Respiratory alkalosis
- Salicylate poisoning
- **Electrolyte abnormalities**
- Hypercalcemia, hypomagnesemia, metabolic alkalosis
- **Abnormal losses followed by inadequate repletion**
- Diabetes mellitus with acidosis, especially during aggressive therapy
- Recovery from starvation
- Chronic alcoholism
- Severe burns

CLINICAL FINDINGS

SYMPTOMS AND SIGNS

- With severe hypophosphatemia (1 mg/dL or less), there may be muscle weakness
- Acute, severe hypophosphatemia (0.1–0.2 mg/dL)
  - Weakness from acute hemolytic anemia
  - Infection from impaired chemotaxis of leukocytes
  - Petechial hemorrhages from platelet dysfunction
  - Rhabdomyolysis
  - Encephalopathy (irritability, confusion, dysarthria, seizures, and coma)
  - Heart failure
- Anorexia, pain in muscles and bones, and fractures can occur in chronic severe depletion

DIAGNOSIS

LABORATORY TESTS

- Spot urines with phosphate greater than 20 mg/dL suggests renal phosphate loss
- Normal TmP/GFR is 2.5-4.5 mg/dL

$$\frac{TmP}{GFR} = \frac{Serum\ Pi - (UPi \times UV)}{GFR}$$

where serum Pi = serum phosphate concentration

UPi = urine phosphate concentration

UV = urine volume

- Lower values indicate urinary phosphate loss
- Hemolytic anemia may be present
- Elevated serum creatine kinase and myoglobin in the urine from rhabdomyolysis
- Renal glycosuria and hypouricemia together with hypophosphatemia indicate Fanconi's syndrome

IMAGING STUDIES

- In chronic depletion, radiographs and biopsies of bones show changes resembling those of osteomalacia

TREATMENT

MEDICATIONS

Oral replacement

- Acute hypocalcemia can occur with parenteral administration of phosphate; therefore, when possible, oral replacement of phosphate is preferable
- Can use if the patient is asymptomatic and the serum phosphorus is >1 mg/dL
- Phosphate salts are available in skim milk [approximately 1 g (33 mmol)/L]
- Tablets or capsules of mixtures of sodium and potassium phosphate may be given to provide 0.5–1 g (18–32 mmol) per day
- Contraindications to phosphate salts include hypoparathyroidism, renal insufficiency, tissue damage and necrosis, and hypercalcemia

Intravenous replacement

- For intravenous use in asymptomatic hypophosphatemia (serum phosphorus 0.7–1 mg/dL) in patients who cannot eat, infuse 279–310 mg (9–10 mmol)/12 h until the serum phosphorus exceeds 1 mg/dL
- For symptomatic patients with severe hypophosphatemia (<0.5–1 mg/dL) who cannot eat, give intravenous phosphorus up to 1 g in 1 L of fluid over 8–12 h
- 3 g or more of phosphorus may be required over several days to replete body stores
- Be aware of potential of precipitating soft tissue calcifications with parenteral phosphorus replacement. A serum calcium × serum phosphorus product >70 markedly increases the risk of nephrocalcinosis and soft tissue calcification
- A magnesium deficit often coexists and should be treated simultaneously

THERAPEUTIC PROCEDURES

- Mild hypophosphatemia usually resolves spontaneously with treatment of the underlying cause

 OUTCOME

FOLLOW-UP

- Since the response to phosphate supplementation is not predictable, frequent monitoring of plasma and urine phosphate is necessary
- In administering phosphate-containing solutions, monitor serum calcium to guard against hypocalcemia

WHEN TO REFER

- For consultation about etiology
- If expertise in replacement is needed, particularly intravenous

WHEN TO ADMIT

- Symptomatic hypophosphatemia
- Need for parenteral replacement

PREVENTION

- Include phosphate in repletion and maintenance fluids
- For parenteral alimentation, 620 mg (20 mmol) of phosphorus is required for every 1000 nonprotein kcal to maintain phosphate balance and to ensure anabolic function. A daily ration for prolonged parenteral fluid maintenance is 620–1240 mg (20–40 mmol) of phosphorus

 EVIDENCE

PRACTICE GUIDELINES

- National Guideline Clearinghouse
  http://www.guideline.gov/summary/
  summary.aspx?doc_id=2194&nbr=1420
  &string=hypophosphatemia
  http://www.guideline.gov/summary/
  summary.aspx?doc_id=1563&nbr=789
  &string=alcoholism

WEB SITES

- Dr. Rose's Peripheral Brain—Fluids and electrolytes
  http://faculty.washington.edu/momus/
  PB/fluidand.htm
- Fluid and Electrolyte Disorders:
  MDAdvice.com
  http://www.mdadvice.com/library/ped/
  pedillsymp160.html

INFORMATION FOR PATIENTS

- National Institute on Alcoholism and Alcohol Abuse
  http://www.niaaa.nih.gov/publications/
  booklet.htm
- National Institutes of Health
  http://www.nlm.nih.gov/medlineplus/
  ency/article/000307.htm

REFERENCES

- Miller DW et al: Hypophosphatemia in the emergency department therapeutics. Am J Emerg Med 2000;18:457. [PMID: 10919539]
- Subramian R et al: Severe hypophosphatemia: pathophysiologic implications, clinical presentations, and treatment. Medicine 2000;79:1. [PMID: 10670405]

Masafumi Fukagawa, MD, PhD
Kiyoshi Kurokawa, MD, MACP
Maxine A. Papadakis, MD

Hypopituitarism

 KEY FEATURES

ESSENTIALS OF DIAGNOSIS

- Loss of one, all, or any combination of pituitary hormones
- ACTH deficiency reduces adrenal secretion of cortisol and testosterone; aldosterone secretion remains intact
- Growth hormone (GH) deficiency causes short stature in children; adults experience asthenia and increased cardiovascular mortality
- Thyroid-stimulating hormone (TSH) deficiency causes secondary hypothyroidism
- Luteinizing hormone (LH) and follicle-stimulating hormone (FSH) are secreted by the same pituitary cells and their loss causes hypogonadism in men and women
- Antidiuretic hormone deficiency results in central diabetes insipidus
- Oxytocin deficiency causes insufficient lactation in postpartum women

GENERAL CONSIDERATIONS

- Due to hypothalamic or pituitary dysfunction
- May have single or multiple hormonal deficiencies including those of anterior pituitary: growth hormone, prolactin, ACTH, TSH, LH, FSH; posterior pituitary: vasopressin (antidiuretic hormone, ADH), oxytocin
- Causes include mass lesions: pituitary adenomas, granulomas, Rathke's cleft cysts, apoplexy, metastatic carcinomas, aneurysms, brain tumors, hypophysitis, pituitary stalk inflammation
- Pituitary tumor may be part of multiple endocrine neoplasia (type 1), with tumors of parathyroid and pancreatic islets
- Hypopituitarism without mass lesions may be idiopathic, genetic, due to trauma, cranial radiation, surgery, encephalitis, hemochromatosis, autoimmune, stroke, post-CABG, chronic epidural opioid infusion, X-linked congenital adrenal hypoplasia

 CLINICAL FINDINGS

SYMPTOMS AND SIGNS

- Gonadotropin (LH and FSH) deficiency
  - Hypogonadism, delayed adolescence, infertility, decreased libido
  - Amenorrhea (women), decreased erections (men)
  - Loss of axillary, pubic, and body hair, especially with ACTH deficiency
  - Diminished beard growth (men)
  - Micropenis, cryptorchism
- TSH deficiency: fatigue, weakness, weight gain
- ACTH deficiency: symptoms of decreased cortisol with normal mineralocorticoid secretion: weakness, fatigue, weight loss, hypotension
- Growth hormone (GH) deficiency: obesity, weakness, reduced cardiac output, feelings of social isolation
- ADH deficiency: central diabetes insipidus with polyuria and polydipsia
- Oxytocin deficiency: no lactation
- Panhypopituitarism: skin is dry, pale, finely textured. Face has fine wrinkles and an apathetic countenance

DIFFERENTIAL DIAGNOSIS

- Anorexia nervosa (hypogonadotropic hypogonadism)
- Serious illness [hypogonadotropic hypogonadism, functional suppression of TSH and thyroxine (T_4)]
- Severe malnutrition (hypogonadotropic hypogonadism)
- Primary hypothyroidism causes low T_4, high prolactin
- Addison's disease
- High-dose glucocorticoids (secondary adrenal insufficiency)
- Cachexia due to other causes (eg, carcinoma, tuberculosis)
- Empty sella syndrome
- Triiodothyronine (T_3) administration can cause low TSH and low serum free T_4

 DIAGNOSIS

LABORATORY TESTS

- Serum sodium and fasting glucose may be low, potassium normal
- Low free T_4, TSH not elevated
- Low or low normal testosterone, estradiol, LH, FSH
- Elevated prolactin in prolactinoma, acromegaly, hypothalamic disease
- ACTH stimulation test: cosyntropin (synthetic ACTH analog), 0.25 mg IM or IV, normally causes cortisol to rise to >20 μg/dL in 30–60 min; ACTH deficiency causes adrenal atrophy and an abnormal response
- Baseline ACTH low or normal in secondary hypoadrenalism; ACTH high in primary adrenal disease
- Basal cortisol >19μg/dL excludes adrenal insufficiency
- Metyrapone stimulation test used if cosyntropin test is normal but pituitary adrenal insufficiency is suspected. Metyrapone, 1.5 g PO, is given at 11 PM. In hypoadrenalism, 8 AM 11-deoxycortisol <7 μg/dL and cortisol <5 μg/dL
- IGF-1 levels are normal in 50% of adults with GH deficiency, but very low levels (<84 μg/L) indicate GH deficiency except in conditions that suppress IGF-1 (malnutrition, oral estrogen, hypothyroidism, uncontrolled diabetes mellitus, liver failure)
- Screen for hemachromatosis with serum Fe, transferrin saturation, ferritin

IMAGING STUDIES

- MRI scan shows parasellar lesions
- In hemochromatosis, MRI shows hypointense anterior lobe on T1-weighted images surrounded by hyperintense cerebrospinal fluid on T2-weighted images
- In central diabetes insipidus, the posterior pituitary "bright spot" is absent on MRI T1-weighted imaging

TREATMENT

MEDICATIONS

Secondary adrenal insufficiency

- Hydrocortisone, 15 mg PO QAM and 5–10 mg PO QPM, or prednisone, 3 mg QAM and 2 mg QPM PO QD, or dexamethasone, 0.25 mg PO QD
- Fludrocortisone is rarely needed
- Give additional hydrocortisone during stress. For mild illness, doses should be doubled or tripled. For trauma or surgery, 50 mg IM or IV Q 6 h, then reduce to normal doses as stress subsides

Hypothyroidism

- Levothyroxine, 0.05–0.2 mg PO QD, for hypothyroidism only after assessment for cortisol deficiency, otherwise may precipitate adrenal crisis. Cannot rely on TSH levels

Hypogonadism

- Testosterone replacement for men
- Estrogen replacement for women
- To improve spermatogenesis, human chorionic gonadotropin (hCG), 2000–3000 units IM three times weekly, may be used with no testosterone
- If sperm count remains low, FSH injections may be added
- Clomiphene can induce ovulation

Growth hormone deficiency

- Somatotropin or somatrem (hGH) for symptomatic adults with severe growth hormone deficiency, starting at 0.2 mg (0.6 IU) SQ three times weekly or QD
- Somatotropin discontinued if no improvement in energy, mentation, or visceral adiposity within 3–6 months at maximum tolerated dosage

Hyperprolactinemia

- Hypopituitarism from prolactin-secreting pituitary tumor may be reversible with bromocriptine, cabergoline, or quinagolide or with tumor resection

Central diabetes insipidus

- Nasal desmopressin (DDAVP), 0.1 mL every 12–24 h. Oral desmopressin, 0.1 or 0.2 mg every 12–24 h. Parenteral desmopressin, 1–2 mg IV SQ every 12–24 h

SURGERY

- Transsphenoidal hypophysectomy for pituitary tumors sometimes reverses hypopituitarism

THERAPEUTIC PROCEDURES

- Radiation therapy for GH-secreting tumors, but increases risk of hypopituitarism

OUTCOME

FOLLOW-UP

- After pituitary surgery, check serum sodium frequently for 2 weeks, since postoperative hyponatremia is common
- If on somatotropin, careful monitoring for side effects including hypertension, proliferative retinopathy

COMPLICATIONS

- Mass lesions may cause visual field deficits
- Radiation therapy increases risk of small vessel ischemic strokes and second tumors
- In craniopharyngioma, 16% have diabetes insipidus preoperatively and 60% postoperatively
- Hypothalamic damage may cause morbid obesity, cognitive and emotional problems
- Growth hormone deficiency increases cardiovascular morbidity
- Rarely, acute hemorrhage occurs in large pituitary tumors (pituitary apoplexy) causing rapid loss of vision and headache, requiring emergent decompression

PROGNOSIS

- Prognosis depends on primary cause
- Patients can recover from functional hypopituitarism, eg, hypogonadism due to starvation or severe illness, ACTH suppression by glucocorticoids, TSH suppression by hyperthyroidism, or intrathecal opioids

PREVENTION

- Patients with adrenal insufficiency should wear a medical ID bracelet

EVIDENCE

PRACTICE GUIDELINES

- Arafah BM: Medical management of hypopituitarism in patients with pituitary adenomas. Pituitary 2002;5:109. [PMID: 12675508]

WEB SITE

- Mayo Clinic—Hypopituitarism http://www.mayoclinic.com/invoke.cfm?id=DS00479

INFORMATION FOR PATIENTS

- MEDLINEplus—Hypopituitarism http://www.nlm.nih.gov/medlineplus/ency/article/000343.htm

REFERENCES

- Biller BMK et al: Sensitivity and specificity of six tests for the diagnosis of adult GH deficiency. J Clin Endocrinol Metab 2002;87:2067. [PMID: 11994342]
- Vahl N et al: Continuation of growth hormone (GH) replacement in GH-deficient patients during transition from childhood to adulthood: a two-year placebo-controlled study. J Clin Endocrinol Metab 2000;85:1874. [PMID: 10843168]

Paul A. Fitzgerald, MD

Hypotension & Shock

 KEY FEATURES

ESSENTIALS OF DIAGNOSIS

- Hypotension, tachycardia, oliguria, altered mental status
- Peripheral hypoperfusion and hypoxia

GENERAL CONSIDERATIONS

- The rate of arterial blood flow is inadequate to meet tissue metabolic needs
- Shock can be classified as hypovolemic, cardiogenic, obstructive, and distributive (including septic and neurogenic)
- Hypovolemic: decreased intravascular volume resulting from loss of blood, plasma, or fluids and electrolytes; >15% blood volume loss results in hypotension, increased peripheral resistance, collapse of capillary and venous beds, and progressive tissue hypoxia
- Cardiogenic: pump failure related to myocardial infarction, myocardial contusion, cardiomyopathy, valvular regurgitation or stenosis, or arrhythmias
- Obstructive: cardiac tamponade, tension pneumothorax, and massive pulmonary embolism
- Distributive: reduction in systemic vascular resistance from sepsis, anaphylaxis, systemic inflammatory response syndrome (SIRS) produced by severe pancreatitis or burns, or acute adrenal insufficiency
- Septic: due most often to gram-negative bacteremia (*Escherichia coli, Klebsiella, Proteus,* and *Pseudomonas*); less often to gram-positive cocci and gram-negative anaerobes (*Bacteroides*)
- Neurogenic: due to traumatic spinal cord injury or effects of an epidural or spinal anesthetic; reflex vagal parasympathetic stimulation evoked by pain, gastric dilation, or fright

DEMOGRAPHICS

- Risk factors for septic shock: extremes of age, diabetes, immunosuppression, and recent urinary, biliary, or gynecological manipulation

 CLINICAL FINDINGS

SYMPTOMS AND SIGNS

- Hypotension: cool or mottled extremities and weak or absent peripheral pulses, delayed capillary refill
- Tachycardia
- Oliguria
- Bowel ischemia
- Hepatic dysfunction
- Altered mental status, increasing agitation
- Sepsis: fever, chills, hyperglycemia

 DIAGNOSIS

LABORATORY TESTS

- Check serial hematocrit, complete blood cell count, serum electrolytes, prothrombin time, partial thromboplastin time, ionized calcium, magnesium, phosphate, and cardiac enzymes
- Serum glucose to exclude hyperglycemia, reflecting insulin resistance
- Fecal occult blood test to exclude gastrointestinal hemorrhage
- Arterial blood gas determinations
- Type and cross-match, as indicated
- Urinalysis, urine culture, and blood cultures

IMAGING STUDIES

- Chest x-ray
- Electrocardiogram
- Echocardiogram
- Kidneys, ureters, and bladder x-ray or abdominal CT for abdominal pain

DIAGNOSTIC PROCEDURES

- Arterial line for continuous blood pressure measurement
- Foley catheter to measure urine output
- Central venous pressure (CVP) (right atrial pressure) or pulmonary capillary wedge pressure (PCWP) <5 mm Hg suggests hypovolemia; CVP or PCWP >18 mm Hg suggests volume overload, cardiac failure, tamponade, or pulmonary hypertension
- Pulmonary artery catheter for hemodynamic pressure measurements
- Low systemic vascular resistance (SVR) (<800 dyne $\times$ s/cm^{-5}) suggests early sepsis and neurogenic shock; high SVR (>1500 dyne $\times$ s/cm^{-5}) suggests hypovolemic and cardiogenic shock
- A high cardiac index (>4 L/min/m^2) in a hypotensive patient suggests early septic shock

TREATMENT

MEDICATIONS

- Pressor medications
  - Dopamine, >5 µg/kg/min
  - Dobutamine, 2–20 µg/kg/min
- Diuretics, thrombolytics, morphine, nitroglycerin, antiarrhythmics, and antiplatelet agents as indicated in acute myocardial infarction
- Peripheral vasoconstrictors such as epinephrine, 2–10 µg/min, or norepinephrine, 0.5–30 µg/min, in distributive or neurogenic shock
- Vasopressin (antidiuretic hormone)
- Broad-spectrum antibiotics in septic shock
- Corticosteroids in shock due to acute adrenal insufficiency
- Calcium gluconate to maintain an ionized calcium level >1.0
- Sodium bicarbonate for arterial pH <7.20

SURGERY

- Dependent on the cause of shock
- Cardiogenic shock: transcutaneous or transvenous pacing or intraaortic balloon pump, and emergent revascularization by stent angioplasty or coronary artery bypass grafting, as indicated
- Drainage or excision of source of sepsis

THERAPEUTIC PROCEDURES

- Treatment must be directed both at the manifestations of shock and at its cause
- Basic life support: airway maintenance, oxygen, cardiopulmonary resuscitation, intravenous access and fluid resuscitation with crystalloid or blood products
- Treatment is directed at maintaining a CVP of 8–12 mm Hg, a mean arterial pressure of 65–90 mm Hg, a cardiac index of 2–4 L/min/m^2, and central venous oxygen saturation of >70%

OUTCOME

PROGNOSIS

- Septic shock mortality is 40–80%

WHEN TO ADMIT

- Any patient presenting with shock

EVIDENCE

PRACTICE GUIDELINES

- Martel MJ et al: Hemorrhagic shock. J Obstet Gynaecol Can 2002;24:504. [PMID: 12196857]
- Vincent JL: International Sepsis Forum. Hemodynamic support in septic shock. Intensive Care Med 2001;27(Suppl 1):S80. [PMID: 11307372]

WEB SITES

- American College of Emergency Physicians
  http://www.acep.org/1,402,0.html
- American Thoracic Society—Common illnesses of critically ill patients
  http://www.thoracic.org/assemblies/cc/ccprimer/common.html

INFORMATION FOR PATIENTS

- JAMA patient page: CPR
  http://www.ama-assn.org/insight/spec_con/patient/pat046.pdf
- MEDLINEplus—Shock
  http://www.nlm.nih.gov/medlineplus/ency/article/000039.htm

REFERENCES

- Bernard GR et al: Efficacy and safety of recombinant human activated protein C for severe sepsis. N Engl J Med 2001; 344:699. [PMID: 11236773]
- Hochman JS et al: One-year survival following early revascularization for cardiogenic shock. JAMA 2001;285:190. [PMID: 11176812]
- Landry DW et al: The pathogenesis of vasodilatory shock. N Engl J Med 2001;345:588. [PMID: 11529214]
- Orlinsky M et al: Current controversies in shock and resuscitation. Surg Clin North Am 2001;81:1217. [PMID: 11766174]

Louis M. Messina, MD
Laura K. Pak, MD
Lawrence M. Tierney, Jr., MD

Hypothermia

 KEY FEATURES

ESSENTIALS OF DIAGNOSIS

- Systemic hypothermia is a reduction of core (rectal) body temperature below 35°C
- Oral temperatures are inaccurate; an esophageal or rectal probe that reads as low as 25°C is required

GENERAL CONSIDERATIONS

- In colder climates, elderly individuals living in inadequately heated housing are particularly susceptible
- Patients with comorbid conditions, or use of sedating or tranquilizing drugs are more vulnerable to accidental hypothermia
- Prolonged postoperative hypothermia or administration of large amounts of refrigerated stored blood (without rewarming) can cause systemic hypothermia

 CLINICAL FINDINGS

SYMPTOMS AND SIGNS

Systemic hypothermia

- Early manifestations may include weakness, drowsiness, lethargy, irritability, confusion, shivering, and impaired coordination
- The skin may appear blue or puffy
- At core temperatures below 35°C, the patient may become delirious, drowsy, or comatose and may stop breathing
- The pulse and blood pressure may be unobtainable, leading one to believe the patient is dead

Hypothermia of the extremities

- Exposure of the extremities to cold produces immediate localized vasoconstriction followed by generalized vasoconstriction
- When the skin temperature falls to 25°C, the area becomes cyanotic
- At 15°C, there is a deceptively pink, well-oxygenated appearance to the skin. Tissue damage occurs at this temperature

DIFFERENTIAL DIAGNOSIS

- Infection
- Other cause of altered mental status, eg, hypoglycemia, drugs, stroke
- Hypothyroidism
- Anorexia or malnutrition (poor fat stores)
- Adrenal insufficiency
- Burns
- Spinal cord injury

 DIAGNOSIS

LABORATORY TESTS

- Obtain complete blood cell count, prothrombin time, partial thromboplastin time, electrolytes, blood urea nitrogen, serum creatinine, liver function tests, amylase, glucose, pH, blood gases, urinalysis, and urine volume

IMAGING STUDIES

- Cardiac arrhythmias and the pathognomonic J wave of Osborn, prominent in lead II, can be seen on the electrocardiogram

TREATMENT

- See Figure 11 (page 1323)

Therapeutic Procedures

- For mild hypothermia (rectal temperature >33°C) in otherwise healthy patients, a warm bed or rapid passive rewarming with a warm bath or warm packs and blankets is usually adequate
- Moderate or severe hypothermia (core temperatures of <33°C) requires active rewarming with supportive care
- Cardiovascular support, acid-base balance, arterial oxygenation, and adequate intravascular volume should be established prior to rewarming to minimize the risk of organ infarction and "afterdrop" (recurrent hypothermia)
- Active rewarming usually includes a combination of active external and internal methods
- Aggressive rewarming should be attempted only by those experienced in the methods
- Once begun, CPR should continue until the patient has been rewarmed to at least 32°C

Active external rewarming

- Heated blankets, forced hot air, or warm baths may be used
- Rewarming by a warm bath is best done in a tub of moving water at 40–42°C, with a rate of rewarming of about 1–2°C/h. It is easier, however, to monitor the patient and to perform diagnostic and therapeutic procedures when heated blankets are used for active rewarming
- Active external warming methods may cause marked peripheral dilation that predisposes to ventricular fibrillation and hypovolemic shock
- Forced air rewarming (38–43°C) is recommended when extracorporeal blood rewarming is not available
- Antibiotics are not routinely given

Active internal (core) rewarming

- Essential for severe hypothermia
- Extracorporeal blood rewarming (cardiopulmonary, venovenous, or femorofemoral bypass) is the treatment of choice, especially in the presence of cardiac arrest
- In the absence of equipment necessary for extracorporeal rewarming, left-sided thoracotomy followed by pericardial cavity irrigation with warmed saline and cardiac massage has been effective in systemic hypothermia <28°C

- Repeated peritoneal dialysis may be employed with 2 L of warm (43°C) potassium-free dialysate solution exchanged at intervals of 10–12 min until the core temperature is raised to about 35°C
- Parenteral fluids (D_5 normal saline) should be warmed to 43°C prior to administration
- Heated, humidified air warmed to 42°C through a face mask or endotracheal tube may be administered
- Warm colonic and gastrointestinal irrigations are of less value
- Patients who are comatose or in respiratory failure should be tracheally intubated

OUTCOME

FOLLOW-UP

- Monitor cardiac rhythm
- Core temperature (esophageal preferred over rectal) should be monitored frequently during and after initial rewarming because of reports of recurrent hypothermia

COMPLICATIONS

- Metabolic acidosis, hyperkalemia, pneumonia, pancreatitis, ventricular fibrillation, hypoglycemia or hyperglycemia, coagulopathy, and renal failure may occur
- Cardiac arrhythmias may occur, especially during rewarming
- Death is usually from cardiac asystole or ventricular fibrillation

PROGNOSIS

- More than 75% of otherwise healthy patients may survive moderate or severe systemic hypothermia
- Prognosis is directly related to the severity of metabolic acidosis; if the pH is 6.6 or less, the prognosis is poor
- The prognosis is grave if there are underlying predisposing causes or if treatment is delayed
- Neuropathic sequelae such as pain, numbness, tingling, hyperhidrosis, cold sensitivity of the extremities, and nerve conduction abnormalities may persist for many years after the cold injury

PREVENTION

- "Keep warm, keep moving, and keep dry"
- Tobacco and alcohol should be avoided
- Cardiac, central vascular, or chest trauma or stimulation (catheter, cannulas, etc) should be avoided unless essential because of the risk of inducing ventricular fibrillation

EVIDENCE

PRACTICE GUIDELINES

- Durrer B et al: The medical on-site treatment of hypothermia: ICAR-MED-COM recommendation. High Alt Med Biol 2003;4:99. [PMID: 12713717]

WEB SITE

- Merck Manual—Disorders due to physical agents http://www.merck.com/pubs/mmanual/section20/sec20.htm

INFORMATION FOR PATIENTS

- The Mayo Clinic http://www.mayoclinic.com/invoke.cfm?id=DS00333
- American College of Emergency Physicians http://www.acep.org/1,205,0.html

REFERENCE

- Giesbrecht GG: Cold stress, near drowning, and accidental hypothermia: a review. Aviat Space Environ Med 2000;71:733. [PMID: 10902937]

Richard Cohen, MD, MPH
Brent R. W. Moelleken, MD, FACS

Hypothyroidism (Myxedema)

 ## KEY FEATURES

ESSENTIALS OF DIAGNOSIS

- Weakness, fatigue, cold intolerance, constipation, weight change, depression, menorrhagia, hoarseness
- Dry skin, bradycardia, delayed return of deep tendon reflexes
- Anemia, hyponatremia
- Serum free tetraiodothyronine (T_4) low
- Thyroid-stimulating hormone (TSH) elevated in primary hypothyroidism

GENERAL CONSIDERATIONS

- Severity ranges from mild, unrecognized hypothyroidism, to striking myxedema and cretinism
- Hypothyroidism due first to thyroid gland disease or second to lack of pituitary TSH
- Maternal hypothyroidism during pregnancy results in cognitive impairment in child
- Causes of hypothyroidism with goiter: Hashimoto's thyroiditis; subacute (de Quervain's) thyroiditis (after initial hyperthyroidism); Riedel's thyroiditis; iodine deficiency; genetic thyroid enzyme defects; drugs (lithium, amiodarone, propylthiouracil, methimazole, phenylbutazone, sulfonamides, interferon-α); food goitrogens in iodide-deficient areas; peripheral resistance to thyroid hormone; or infiltrating diseases
- Causes of hypothyroidism without goiter: thyroid surgery, irradiation, or radioiodine treatment; deficient pituitary TSH; severe illness
- "Subclinical" hypothyroidism, ie, clinically euthyroid individual with high TSH, normal T_4, occurs commonly in elderly women (~10% incidence)
- Amiodarone, due to high iodine content, causes clinical hypothyroidism in ~8%
- High iodine intake from other sources may also cause hypothyroidism, especially in those with underlying lymphocytic thyroiditis
- Myxedema is caused by interstitial accumulation of hydrophilic mucopolysaccharides, leading to fluid retention and lymphedema
- Hyponatremia occurs due to impaired renal tubular sodium reabsorption

 ## CLINICAL FINDINGS

SYMPTOMS AND SIGNS

- Early symptoms: fatigue, lethargy, weakness, arthralgias, myalgias, muscle cramps, cold intolerance, constipation, dry skin, headache, menorrhagia
- Late symptoms: slow speech, constipation, peripheral edema, pallor, hoarseness, decreased senses of taste, smell, and hearing, muscle cramps, aches and pains, dyspnea, weight changes (usually gain, sometimes loss), amenorrhea or menorrhagia, galactorrhea, absent sweating
- Early signs: thin, brittle nails, thinning of hair, pallor, poor turgor of mucosa, delayed return of deep tendon reflexes
- Late signs: goiter, puffiness of face and eyelids, carotenemia, thinning of outer eyebrows, tongue thickening, hard pitting edema, pleural, peritoneal, pericardial, and joint effusions
- Myxedema coma: signs of hypothyroidism and impaired mentation
- Cardiac enlargement due to pericardial effusion, bradycardia
- Hypothermia
- Pituitary enlargement due to hyperplasia of TSH-secreting cells in long-standing cases

DIFFERENTIAL DIAGNOSIS

- Chronic fatigue syndrome
- Depression
- Congestive heart failure
- Irregular vaginal bleeding due to other cause
- Anemia due to other cause
- Amyloidosis (thick tongue)
- Pituitary adenoma (may have hyperprolactinemia and pituitary often enlarged due to reversible hyperplasia of TSH-secreting cells)

 ## DIAGNOSIS

LABORATORY TESTS

- Serum TSH is increased in primary hypothyroidism but low or normal in secondary hypothyroidism (pituitary insufficiency)
- Free T_4 may be low or low normal
- Serum triiodothyronine (T_3) is not a good test for hypothyroidism
- Serum cholesterol, liver enzymes, creatine kinase, prolactin increased
- Hyponatremia
- Hypoglycemia
- Anemia (with normal or increased mean corpuscular volume)
- Thyroperoxidase or thyroglobulin antibody titers usually high in hypothyroidism due to Hashimoto's thyroiditis
- During pregnancy in women with hypothyroidism taking replacement thyroxine, check serum TSH frequently (eg, Q 1–2 months) to ensure adequate replacement

TREATMENT

MEDICATIONS

- Levothyroxine (T_4) is treatment of choice; T_4 is partially converted to T_3, the more active thyroid hormone
- Before levothyroxine started, exclude adrenal insufficiency, which would require concurrent treatment
- Levothyroxine starting dose: 50–100 μg PO QAM if no coronary disease and age <60 years; 100–150 μg PO QAM if hypothyroid during pregnancy; and 25–50 μg PO QAM if coronary disease or age >60 years. Dose titrated up by 25 μg Q 1–3 weeks until patient is euthyroid, usually at 100–250 μg QAM
- Dose of thyroxine required may increase during pregnancy or estrogen therapy
- Elevated TSH usually indicates levothyroxine underreplacement. Before increasing T_4 dosage, assess for compliance and presence of angina, diarrhea, or malabsorption
- Avoid administration of levothyroxine concurrently with binding substances, eg, iron, sucralfate, aluminum hydroxide antacids, calcium supplements, or soy milk; or with bile acid-binding resins (eg, cholestyramine)
- Suppressed TSH may indicate levothyroxine overreplacement. Assess for severe nonthyroidal illness or medications (eg, nonsteroidal antiinflammatory drugs, opioids, nifedipine, verapamil, corticosteroids)
- Amiodarone-induced hypothyroidism: treat with just enough levothyroxine to relieve symptoms
- Myxedema coma: levothyroxine sodium, 400 μg IV loading dose, then 100 μg IV QD. If hypothermic, warmed only with blankets; if hypercapnic, mechanical ventilation. Treat infections aggressively
- If adrenal insufficiency suspected, give hydrocortisone, 100 mg IV, then 25–50 mg Q 8 h
- Myxedematous patients are unusually sensitive to opiates and may develop respiratory depression with usual doses

 OUTCOME

FOLLOW-UP

- Continue levothyroxine for life; reassess dosage requirements periodically
- Surveillance for atrial arrhythmias and for osteoporosis especially in patients who require high doses of levothyroxine
- Monitor patients with subclinical hypothyroidism for subtle signs (eg, fatigue, depression, hyperlipidemia). Clinical hypothyroidism later develops in ~18%

COMPLICATIONS

- Angina pectoris, congestive heart failure; may be precipitated by too rapid thyroid replacement
- Increased susceptibility to infection
- Megacolon in long-standing hypothyroidism
- Organic psychoses with paranoid delusions ("myxedema madness")
- Adrenal crisis precipitated by thyroid replacement
- Infertility (rare), miscarriage in untreated hypothyroidism
- Sellar enlargement and TSH-secreting tumors in untreated cases
- Myxedema coma: hypothermia, hypotension, hypoventilation, hypoxia, hypercapnia, hyponatremia, convulsions and abnormal CNS signs. Often induced by underlying infection; cardiac, respiratory, or CNS illness; cold exposure; or drug use

PROGNOSIS

- Excellent prognosis with early treatment, but relapses may occur if treatment is interrupted
- Mortality rate for myxedema coma is high

WHEN TO REFER

- Difficulty titrating levothyroxine replacement to normal TSH or clinically euthyroid state
- Any patient with significant coronary disease needing levothyroxine

WHEN TO ADMIT

- Suspected myxedema coma
- Hypercapnia

EVIDENCE

PRACTICE GUIDELINES

- AACE Medical Guidelines for Clinical Practice: Hyperthyroidism and Hypothyroidism, 2002 http://www.aace.com/clin/guidelines/hypo_hyper.pdf
- Helfand M et al: Clinical guideline, part 2. Screening for thyroid disease: an update. American College of Physicians. Ann Intern Med 1998;129:144. [PMID: 9669977]

WEB SITE

- American Thyroid Association http://www.thyroid.org/patients/brochures/Hypo_brochure.pdf

INFORMATION FOR PATIENTS

- Mayo Clinic—Hypothyroidism http://www.mayoclinic.com/invoke.cfm?id=DS00353

REFERENCES

- Behnia M et al: Management of myxedematous respiratory failure: review of ventilation and weaning principles. Am J Med Sci 2000;320:368. [PMID: 11149548]
- Bunevicius R et al: Effects of thyroxine as compared with thyroxine plus triiodothyronine in patients with hypothyroidism. N Engl J Med 1999;340:424. [PMID: 9971866]
- Cooper DS: Clinical practice. Subclinical hypothyroidism. N Engl J Med 2001;345:260. [PMID: 11474665]
- Kong WM et al: A 6-month randomized trial of thyroxine treatment in women with mild subclinical hypothyroidism. Am J Med 2002;112:348. [PMID: 11904108]
- Wall CR: Myxedema coma: diagnosis and treatment. Am Fam Physician 2000;62:2485. [PMID: 11130234]
- Wiersinga WM: Thyroid hormone replacement therapy. Horm Res 2001;56:74. [PMID: 11786691]

Paul A. Fitzgerald, MD

Idiopathic Thrombocytopenic Purpura

 KEY FEATURES

ESSENTIALS OF DIAGNOSIS

- Isolated thrombocytopenia
- Other hematopoietic cell lines normal
- No systemic illness
- Spleen not palpable
- Normal bone marrow with normal or increased megakaryocytes

GENERAL CONSIDERATIONS

- Autoimmune disorder in which immunoglobulin G (IgG) autoantibody is formed that binds to platelets; unclear which antigen on platelet surface is involved
- Platelets are not destroyed by direct lysis; splenic macrophages bind to antibody-coated platelets
- Since spleen is major site of antibody production and platelet sequestration, splenectomy is highly effective therapy
- Hematologically identical to secondary thrombocytopenic purpura associated with systemic lupus erythematosus and chronic lymphocytic leukemia
- Childhood idiopathic thrombocytopenic purpura (ITP) frequently precipitated by viral infection and usually self-limited
- Adult form is usually chronic and infrequently follows viral infection
- Higher incidence with HIV infection

DEMOGRAPHICS

- Disease of young persons: peak incidence between ages 20 and 50
- 2:1 female predominance

 CLINICAL FINDINGS

SYMPTOMS AND SIGNS

- Patients are systemically well and usually not febrile
- Mucosal or skin bleeding: epistaxis, oral bleeding or hemorrhagic bullae, menorrhagia, purpura, or petechiae
- No other abnormal physical findings
- Splenomegaly should lead to consideration of an alternative diagnosis

DIFFERENTIAL DIAGNOSIS

- Thrombotic thrombocytopenic purpura
- Acute leukemia
- Myelodysplastic syndrome
- Disseminated intravascular coagulation
- Early aplastic anemia
- Drug toxicity, eg, heparin, sulfonamides, thiazides, quinine
- Alcohol abuse
- Hypersplenism
- Systemic lupus erythematosus

 DIAGNOSIS

LABORATORY TESTS

- Thrombocytopenia, which may be severe (<10,000/μL)
- Other counts are usually normal except for occasional anemia due to bleeding or associated hemolysis
- Peripheral blood smear shows normal cell morphology except for slightly enlarged platelets (megathrombocytes)
- Coexistent autoimmune hemolytic anemia (Evans's syndrome) in ~10%; associated with anemia, and peripheral smear showing reticulocytosis and spherocytes; red blood cell fragmentation should not be seen
- Coagulation studies entirely normal

DIAGNOSTIC PROCEDURES

- Bone marrow aspiration and biopsy are normal, with normal or increased number of megakaryocytes

Idiopathic Thrombocytopenic Purpura

 ## TREATMENT

MEDICATIONS

- Initial treatment: prednisone, 1–2 mg/kg/day, gradually tapered after platelet count normalizes; normal platelet count not necessary as risk of bleeding is small if platelet count is >50,000/μL
- High-dose IVIG, 1 g/kg for 1 or 2 days, rapidly raises platelet count in 90%, and platelet count rises within 1–5 days; expensive and effect lasts only 1–2 weeks, so reserved for bleeding emergencies or preparing a severely thrombocytopenic patient for surgery
- Danazol, 600 mg/day, may be used if no response to prednisone and splenectomy
- Immunosuppressive agents employed in refractory cases, eg, vincristine, azathioprine, cyclosporine, and cyclophosphamide
- Rituximab benefits some with refractory disease

SURGERY

- Splenectomy is definitive treatment; most adults ultimately undergo splenectomy
- Splenectomy indications: no initial response to prednisone or unacceptably high doses required to maintain adequate platelet count, or patient prefers surgery
- Splenectomy can be performed safely even with platelet counts <10,000/μL
- Splenectomby benefits 80% with either complete or partial remission
- ITP may recur in 10–20% of cases

THERAPEUTIC PROCEDURES

- Few adults with ITP have spontaneous remissions; most require treatment
- High-dose immunosuppression and autologous stem cell transplantation for rare patients with severe and refractory ITP
- Platelet transfusions are reserved for life-threatening bleeding and are rarely used since exogenous platelets survive no better than the patient's own (only a few hours)

 ## OUTCOME

FOLLOW-UP

- With prednisone, bleeding often diminishes within 1 day; platelet count usually begins to rise within a week, and almost always within 3 weeks
- About 80% respond to prednisone, normalizing platelet count, but thrombocytopenia usually recurs if prednisone is completely withdrawn, so the aim is to find a dose that maintains adequate platelet count (>50,000/μL)
- About 50% of patients respond to danazol

COMPLICATIONS

- Major initial concern is cerebral hemorrhage, which becomes a risk when platelet count is <5000/μL
- Fatal bleeding is rare, even at very low platelet counts

PROGNOSIS

- Prognosis for remission is good
- Disease is usually initially controlled with prednisone; splenectomy offers definitive therapy

EVIDENCE

PRACTICE GUIDELINES

- Guidelines for the investigation and management of idiopathic thrombocytopenic purpura in adults, children and in pregnancy. Br J Haematol 2003; 120:574. [PMID: 12588344]
- Idiopathic thrombocytopenic purpura: a practice guideline developed by explicit methods for the American Society of Hematology. American Society of Hematology, 2001 http://www.hematology.org/education/idiopathic.cfm

WEB SITES

- MEDLINEplus—Idiopathic thrombocytopenic purpura http://www.nlm.nih.gov/medlineplus/ency/article/ 000535.htm
- National Institute of Diabetes and Digestive and Kidney Diseases http://www.niddk.nih.gov/health/hematol/pubs/itp/itp.htm

INFORMATION FOR PATIENTS

- American Academy of Family Physicians—ITP http://familydoctor.org/handouts/113.html
- Institute of Child Health—Idiopathic thrombocytopenic purpura http://www.ich.ucl.ac.uk/factsheets/diseases_conditions/itp/

REFERENCES

- Cines DB et al: Immune thrombocytopenia purpura. N Engl J Med 2002;346:995. [PMID: 11919310]
- Portielje JE et al: Morbidity and mortality in adults with idiopathic thrombocytopenic purpura. Blood 2001;97:2549. [PMID: 113240]

Charles A. Linker, MD

Ileus, Acute Paralytic

 ## KEY FEATURES

ESSENTIALS OF DIAGNOSIS

- Precipitating factors: surgery, peritonitis, electrolyte abnormalities, severe medical illness
- Nausea, vomiting, obstipation, distension
- Minimal abdominal tenderness; decreased bowel sounds
- Plain abdominal radiography with gas and fluid distension in small and large bowel

GENERAL CONSIDERATIONS

- Neurogenic failure or loss of peristalsis in the intestine in the absence of any mechanical obstruction
- Common in hospitalized patients as a result of the following
  - Intraabdominal processes, such as recent gastrointestinal or abdominal surgery or peritoneal irritation (peritonitis, pancreatitis, ruptured viscus, hemorrhage)
  - Severe medical illness, such as pneumonia, respiratory failure requiring intubation, sepsis or severe infections, uremia, diabetic ketoacidosis, and electrolyte abnormalities (hypokalemia, hypercalcemia, hypomagnesemia, hypophosphatemia)
  - Medications, such as opioids, anticholinergics, phenothiazines

 ## CLINICAL FINDINGS

SYMPTOMS AND SIGNS

- Mild diffuse, continuous abdominal discomfort
- Nausea and vomiting
- Generalized abdominal distension
- Minimal abdominal tenderness
- No signs of peritoneal irritation
- Bowel sounds are diminished to absent

DIFFERENTIAL DIAGNOSIS

- Mechanical obstruction of small intestine or proximal colon, eg, adhesions, volvulus, Crohn's disease
- Chronic intestinal pseudoobstruction

 ## DIAGNOSIS

LABORATORY TESTS

- Obtain serum electrolytes, potassium, magnesium, phosphorus, and calcium

IMAGING STUDIES

- Plain abdominal radiography: air-fluid levels, distended gas-filled loops of small and large intestine
- Limited barium small bowel series or a CT scan can help to exclude mechanical obstruction

TREATMENT

THERAPEUTIC PROCEDURES

- Treat underlying primary medical or surgical illness
- Nasogastric suction for discomfort or vomiting
- Restrict oral intake, intravenous fluids
- Liberalize diet gradually as bowel function returns
- Minimize anticholinergic and opioid medications
- Peripheral nonopioid receptor antagonists reduce the duration of postoperative ileus; these agents are in clinical trials
- Severe or prolonged ileus requires nasogastric suction and infusion of parenteral fluids and electrolytes

 OUTCOME

FOLLOW-UP

- Return of bowel function usually heralded by return of appetite and passage of flatus
- Serial plain film radiography and/or abdominal CT warranted for persistent or worsening symptoms to distinguish from mechanical obstruction

COMPLICATIONS

- Metabolic disturbances due to prolonged nasogastric suction (hypokalemia, metabolic alkalosis)
- Delayed nutritional intake complication of prolonged postoperative immobility

PROGNOSIS

- Ileus usually resolves within 48–72 h

WHEN TO REFER

- Persistent ileus >3–5 days warrants further evaluation for underlying cause and to exclude mechanical obstruction

WHEN TO ADMIT

- All patients with ileus require admission for IV fluids

 EVIDENCE

PRACTICE GUIDELINES

- Bauer AJ et al: Ileus in critical illness: mechanisms and management. Curr Opin Crit Care 2002;8:152. [PMID: 12386517]
- Holte K et al: Postoperative ileus: progress towards effective management. Drugs 2002;62:2603. [PMID: 12466000]
- Kehlet H et al: Review of postoperative ileus. Am J Surg 2001;182(5A Suppl):3S. [PMID: 11755891]

INFORMATION FOR PATIENTS

- MEDLINEplus—Intestinal obstruction http://www.nlm.nih.gov/medlineplus/ency/article/000260.htm
- Rosen's Emergency Medicine—Small bowel obstruction http://home.mdconsult.com/das/book/30975174/view/999?sid=204180129

REFERENCES

- Kehlet H et al: Review of postoperative ileus. Am J Surg 2001;182(Suppl 5A):3S. [PMID: 11755891]
- Taguchi A et al: Selective postoperative inhibition of gastrointestinal opioid receptors. N Engl J Med 2001;345:935. [PMID: 11575284]

Kenneth R. McQuaid, MD

Immobility in Elderly

 KEY FEATURES

ESSENTIALS OF DIAGNOSIS

- Weakness, stiffness, pain, imbalance, and comorbid illness

GENERAL CONSIDERATIONS

- Although common in older people, reduced mobility is never normal
- It is an important cause of hospital-induced functional decline
- The hazards of bed rest are multiple, serious, quick to develop, and slow to reverse
- Weakness may result from disuse of muscles, malnutrition, electrolyte disturbances, anemia, neurological disorders, or myopathies
- The commonest cause of pain and stiffness is osteoarthritis, but also consider Parkinson's disease, other arthritides such as rheumatoid arthritis, and polymyalgia rheumatica
- Pain, such as painful foot problems, may immobilize the patient
- Imbalance and fear of falling are major causes of immobilization
- Imbalance often results from
  - Neurological disorders (eg, stroke, cervical myelopathy, peripheral neuropathy due to diabetes or alcohol, vestibulocerebellar abnormalities)
  - Orthostatic or postprandial hypotension
  - Drugs (eg, diuretics, antihypertensives, sedatives, neuroleptics, antidepressants)
  - Prolonged bed rest
- Psychological conditions such as severe anxiety or depression may contribute to immobilization

DEMOGRAPHICS

- Among hospitalized medical patients over 70, about 10% experience a decline in their ability to perform activities of daily living

 CLINICAL FEATURES

SYMPTOMS AND SIGNS

- Older person who is weak, stiff, has pain, or imbalance with gait
- Orthostatic or postprandial hypotension
- Depressed patients are less likely to report depressed mood and more likely to manifest somatic complaints than younger patients
- Depression and dementia frequently co-exist

 DIAGNOSIS

LABORATORY TESTS

- For a simple geriatric functional screening instrument see Table 3 (page 1196)

TREATMENT

MEDICATIONS

- For many cases of osteoarthritis, acetaminophen or glucosamine may be effective and safer than a nonsteroidal antiinflammatory drug or COX-2 inhibitor
- If depression is preventing a patient from participating in physical therapy, it may prove necessary to start with a short course of stimulant medication (eg, methylphenidate; see *Depression* or *Depression in Elderly*), at least until a more traditional antidepressant has had time to take effect

THERAPEUTIC PROCEDURES

- Reduced mobility in older people is often treatable if its causes are identified
- To minimize cardiovascular deconditioning, position patients as close to the upright position as possible, several times daily
- To reduce the risks of contracture and weakness, immediately begin range of motion and isometric and isotonic exercises while the patient is in bed
- Patients should assist with their own positioning, transferring, and self-care whenever possible
- For immobilized patients, low-dose heparin or graduated compression stockings reduce the risk of thrombosis
- Avoid restraints and discontinue invasive devices (intravenous lines, urinary catheters)
- Install handrails, lower the bed, and provide chairs of proper height with arms and rubber skid guards
- A properly fitted cane or walker may be useful
- Exercise is an effective treatment for both knee and hip osteoarthritis

OUTCOME

COMPLICATIONS

- Deconditioning of the cardiovascular system occurs within days and involves fluid shifts, decreased cardiac output, decreased peak oxygen uptake, and increased resting heart rate
- Striking changes occur in skeletal muscle, with loss of contractile velocity and strength
- Pressure sores are a serious complication; mechanical pressure, moisture, friction, and shearing forces all predispose to their development
- Thrombophlebitis and pulmonary embolism are additional serious risks
- Within days after being confined to bed, the risk of postural hypotension, falls, skin breakdown, and pulmonary embolism rises rapidly

PROGNOSIS

- Among patients who decline in their ability to do their activities of daily living (ADLs) while hospitalized, about 50% will not recover by 3 months after discharge
- Decreased ambulation and impairments in the ability to independently perform ADLs are associated with higher rates of mortality

WHEN TO REFER

- Early referral to occupational or physical therapy is essential

PREVENTION

- In hospitalized patients, bed rest orders should be avoided as much as possible
- Devices that immobilize such as Foley catheters should be withdrawn as soon as possible
- Adequate nutrition should be ensured
- The skin over pressure points should be inspected frequently, and if the patient is unable, staff should reposition the patient every 2 h

EVIDENCE

PRACTICE GUIDELINES

- http://www.guideline.gov/search/search results.aspx?Type=3&txtSearch=mobility +and+elderly&num=20
- http://www.guideline.gov/summary/ su mmary/summary.aspx?doc_id= 3103&nbr=1819&string=stroke+and+ immobility
- http://www.guideline.gov/summary/ su mmary/summary.aspx?doc_id=2593 &nbr=1819&string=stroke+and+ immobility
- http://www.guideline.gov/summary/ su mmary.aspx?doc_id=2935&nbr= 2161&string=osteoarthritis

WEB SITES

- AARP Guide to Internet Resources on Aging
  http://www.aarp.org/cyber/sd1_3.htm
- Administration on Aging
  http://www.aoa.dhhs.gov
- Mayo Clinic—Geriatrics Care Pearls
  http://www.mayo.edu/geriatrics-rst/ Pearls.html

INFORMATION FOR PATIENTS

- Medem
  http://www.fcmsdocs.org/ PublicHeathInfo/osteo.html_
  http://www.wheelchairnet.org/WCN_ ProdServ/Products/mobility.html
- American Academy of Family Physicians
  http://familydoctor.org/handouts/151. htm

REFERENCE

- van Baar ME: Effectiveness of exercise therapy in patients with osteoarthritis of the hip or knee. Arthritis Rheum 1999;42:1361. [PMID: 104032263]

C. Bree Johnston, MD
Kenneth E. Covinsky, MD

Impetigo

 KEY FEATURES

ESSENTIALS OF DIAGNOSIS

- Skin infection usually caused by *Staphylococcus aureus*
- Generally, two presentations: vesiculo-pustular type and bullous type

GENERAL CONSIDERATIONS

- A contagious and autoinoculable infection of the skin caused by staphylococci or streptococci (or both)
- Classically, two forms have been recognized: a vesiculopustular type, with thick golden-crusted lesions caused by *S aureus* or group A β-hemolytic streptococcus; and a bullous type, associated with phage group II *S aureus*
- Most cases of impetigo of either presentation now appear to be due to staphylococci

 CLINICAL FINDINGS

SYMPTOMS AND SIGNS

- See Table 7 (page 1202)
- Itching is the only symptom
- The lesions consist of macules, vesicles, bullae, pustules, and honey-colored gummy crusts that when removed leave denuded red areas
- The face and other exposed parts are most often involved
- Ecthyma is a deeper form of impetigo caused by staphylococci or streptococci, with ulceration and scarring; it occurs frequently on the legs and other covered areas

DIFFERENTIAL DIAGNOSIS

- Contact dermatitis (acute)
- Herpes simplex
- Herpes zoster (shingles)
- Tinea corporis
- Atopic dermatitis (eczema)
- Folliculitis
- Erysipelas

 DIAGNOSIS

LABORATORY TESTS

- Usually made clinically based on the appearance of the lesions
- Gram stain and culture confirm the diagnosis

Impetigo

 TREATMENT

MEDICATIONS

- Topical antibiotics are not as effective as systemic antibiotics
- Two percent mupirocin ointment (Bactroban), dispensed as 15 g and used three times daily for 10 days, may be effective for limited disease
- If the affected area is large or if there is fever or toxicity, systemic antibiotics should be given
- Dicloxacillin or cephalexin, 250 mg four times daily, is usually effective
- Erythromycin, 250 mg four times daily, is a reasonable alternative if the causative strain is sensitive

THERAPEUTIC PROCEDURES

- Crusts and weepy areas may be treated with compresses, and washcloths and towels must be segregated and washed separately

 OUTCOME

FOLLOW-UP

- Recurrent impetigo is associated with nasal carriage of *S aureus*, treated with rifampin, 600 mg daily, or intranasal mupirocin ointment twice daily for 5 days

WHEN TO REFER

- If there is a question about the diagnosis, if recommended therapy is ineffective, or specialized treatment is necessary

WHEN TO ADMIT

- Systemic toxicity

 EVIDENCE

WEB SITES

- American Academy of Dermatology http://www.aad.org
- Dermatology Handbook for Family Practice from the University of Iowa http://www.vh.org/Providers/ClinRef/FPHandbook/17.html

INFORMATION FOR PATIENTS

- Mayo Clinic http://www.mayoclinic.com/invoke.cfm?id=DS00464
- American Medical Association http://www.medem.com/medlb/article_detaillb.cfm?article_ID=ZZZYDG6G1AC&sub_cat=24

REFERENCES

- Hirschmann JV: Impetigo: etiology and therapy. Curr Clin Top Infect Dis 2002: 22:42. [PMID: 12520646]
- Levine N: Eruption on the face. Bulla formation and crusting on the forehead and nose can be easily treated. Geriatrics 2002;57:17. [PMID: 12271824]

Timothy G. Berger, MD

Infection in the Immunocompromised Host

 KEY FEATURES

ESSENTIALS OF DIAGNOSIS

- Clinical symptoms may be blunted because of immunosuppression
- Fever is often absent

GENERAL CONSIDERATIONS

Granulocytopenia

- Absolute granulocyte count below 1000/μL, and especially below 100/μL
- Increased infections with gram-negative enteric organisms, *Pseudomonas*, gram-positive cocci (particularly *Staphylococcus aureus, Staphylococcus epidermidis,* and viridans streptococci), *Candida, Aspergillus*, and other fungi such as *Trichosporon, Scedosporium, Fusarium,* and *Pseudallescheria*

Ineffective humoral immunity (eg, myeloma)

- Increased infections with encapsulated organisms such as *Haemophilus influenzae* and *Streptococcus pneumoniae*

Cellular immune deficiency

- HIV infection, lymphoreticular malignancies such as Hodgkin's disease, immunosuppressive medications
- Increased infections by a large number of organisms, such as *Listeria, Legionella, Salmonella,* and *Mycobacterium*; viruses such as herpes simplex, varicella, and cytomegalovirus (CMV); fungi such as *Cryptococcus, Coccidioides, Histoplasma,* and *Pneumocystis*; and protozoa such as *Toxoplasma*

Asplenic patients

- Increased risk of overwhelming bacteremia with encapsulated bacteria (primarily *S pneumoniae* but also *H influenzae* and *Neisseria meningitidis*)

Debilitating injury (severe burns or trauma)

- Increased infections from Foley catheters, dialysis catheters, central nervous system dysfunction (which predisposes to aspiration pneumonia and decubitus ulcers), obstructing lesions (eg, pneumonia due to an obstructed bronchus), and use of broad-spectrum antibiotics

Transplantation

- Infections immediately after transplant often involve the transplanted organ

- Lung transplantation: pneumonia and mediastinitis
- Liver transplantation: intraabdominal abscess, cholangitis, and peritonitis
- Renal transplantation: urinary tract infections, perinephric abscesses, and infected lymphoceles
- In contrast to solid organ transplants, in bone marrow transplants the source of fever cannot be found in 60–70% of patients
- Most infections that occur in the first 2–4 weeks are related to the operative procedure and to hospitalization itself (wound infection, intravenous catheter infection, urinary tract infection from a Foley catheter) or are related to the transplanted organ
- Infections that occur between the first and sixth months are often related to immunosuppression. Reactivated herpes simplex, varicella-zoster, and CMV infections are quite common. Opportunistic infections with fungi (*Candida, Aspergillus, Cryptococcus, Pneumocystis,* and others), *Listeria monocytogenes, Nocardia,* and *Toxoplasma* are also common
- After 6 months, when immunosuppression has been reduced to maintenance levels, infections that are found in any population occur

Other

- Organisms not usually pathogens in the noncompromised host may cause serious life-threatening infection in the compromised patient (eg, *S epidermidis, Corynebacterium jeikeium, Propionibacterium acnes, Bacillus* species). Therefore, interpret culture results with caution and do not disregard isolates as mere contaminants

 CLINICAL FINDINGS

SYMPTOMS AND SIGNS

- Symptoms may be subtle because of the immunosuppression
- There may be increased insulin requirements in diabetics
- Fever is often absent

DIFFERENTIAL DIAGNOSIS

- Neutropenia
  - Gram-negative enteric organisms
  - *Pseudomonas*

- Gram-positive cocci, eg, *S aureus, S epidermidis*
- Canidida
- *Aspergillus* and other fungi
- Cellular immune defect, eg, HIV, lymphoma, immunosuppressive drugs
  - Bacteria: *Listeria, Legionella, Salmonella, Mycobacterium*
  - Viruses: herpes simplex virus, varicella, CMV
  - Fungi: *Cryptococcus, Coccidioides, Histoplasma, Pneumocystis*
  - Protozoa: *Toxoplasma*
- Humoral immune defect, eg, congenital, multiple myeloma, chronic lymphocytic leukemia
  - Encapsulated organisms: *S pneumoniae, H influenzae, N meningitidis*
- Asplenia (functional or anatomic)
  - Encapsulated organisms: *S pneumoniae, H influenzae, N meningitidis*
- Noninfectious causes: transplant rejection, organ ischemia or necrosis, thrombophlebitis, and lymphoma

 DIAGNOSIS

LABORATORY TESTS

- Complete blood cell count with differential and blood cultures
- Urine and sputum cultures should be obtained if indicated clinically or radiographically
- Any focal complaints (localized pain, headache, rash) should prompt culture and imaging appropriate to the site
- If fever persists without an obvious source, evaluate for viral infection (cytomegalovirus blood cultures or antigen test), abscess (which usually occurs near previous operative sites), candidiasis involving the liver or spleen, or aspergillosis
- Toxoplasmosis serology helpful

IMAGING STUDIES

- Chest x-ray
- Other imaging tests depend on the clinical setting

DIAGNOSTIC PROCEDURES

- Sputum induction diagnoses *Pneumocystis* pneumonia in 50–80% of AIDS patients with this infection. In other situations, more invasive procedures may be required (bronchoalveolar lavage, transbronchial biopsy, or even open lung biopsy)
- Skin, liver, or bone marrow biopsy may be helpful in establishing a diagnosis

TREATMENT

MEDICATIONS

- Because infections can be rapidly progressive and life-threatening, diagnostic procedures must be done promptly, and empirical therapy is usually instituted before a specific agent has been isolated (Table 123, page 1306)
- Reduction or discontinuation of immunosuppressive medication may be necesary in life-threatening infections
- Hematopoietic growth factors (granulocyte and granulocyte-macrophage colony-stimulating factors) in prolonged neutropenia (>7 days) can reverse immunosuppression.
- The antibiotics used depend on the type of immunocompromise and site of infection

Neutropenia

- Primarily bacterial and fungal infections
- Initial treatment is often directed at gram-positive and gram-negative organisms (Table 123, page 1306)
- If the patient fails to respond, broader-spectrum antibiotics and antifungal drugs are added
- Although different antibiotic agents can be used, choices should be based on local microbiological trends

Example of one algorithm

- Initiate therapy with a fluoroquinolone active against gram-positive organisms (such as levofloxacin, gatifloxacin, or moxifloxacin) when the absolute neutrophil count falls below 500/μL
- If fever develops, cultures are obtained and vancomycin, 10–15 mg/kg every 12 h, is given (to cover methicillin-resistant *S aureus, S epidermidis*, and *Enterococcus*)
- If after 48–72 h fever continues, antifungal coverage can be increased by changing to voriconazole, 200 mg twice daily (if the patient was on fluconazole prophylaxis), and broader-spectrum antibiotics can be added sequentially. For example, to better cover *Acinetobacter, Citrobacter*, and *Pseudomonas*, the fluoroquinolone may be switched to cefipime, 2 g every 8 h intravenously; with continued fever, imipenem, 500 mg every 6 h (or meropenem, 1 g every 8 h), with or without tobramycin, 1.8 mg/kg every 8 h, may be used in place of cefipime
- If fevers persist, trimethoprim-sulfamethoxazole at 10 mg/kg/day (of trimethoprim) in three divided doses can be added to cover *Stenotrophomonas*
- Regardless of whether the patient becomes afebrile, therapy must be continued until resolution of neutropenia
- Patients with fever and neutropenia at low risk for complications (neutropenia persisting for less than 10 days, no comorbid complications requiring hospitalization, and cancer adequately treated) can be treated with oral antibiotic regimens (ciprofloxacin, 750 mg every 12 h, plus amoxicillin-clavulanic acid, 500 mg every 8 h)

Organ transplant

- For interstitial infiltrates, consider empiric treatment for *Pneumocystis* or *Legionella* species with trimethoprim-sulfamethoxazole and a macrolide
- If the patient fails to respond, add more antimicrobial agents or undertake invasive procedures to make a specific diagnosis
- By making a specific diagnosis, therapy can be specific and polypharmacy with potentially toxic agents avoided

OUTCOME

WHEN TO REFER

- Infections can be rapidly progressive and any patient who fails to respond to treatment in 2–3 days should be referred to a specialist and probably admitted to the hospital

PREVENTION

- See Table 129 (page 1312)
- Hand washing is the simplest and most effective means of decreasing nosocomial infections in *all* patients
- Invasive devices such as central and peripheral lines and Foley catheters are a potential source of infection

EVIDENCE

PRACTICE GUIDELINES

- National Guideline Clearinghouse http://www.guideline.gov/summary/ summary.aspx?doc_id=3080&nbr=2306 &string=immunocompromised

INFORMATION FOR PATIENTS

- Centers for Disease Control http://www.cdc.gov/ncidod/dpd/ parasites/cryptosporidiosis/factsht_ crypto_prevent_ci.htm http://www.cdc.gov/travel/ alteredimmun.htm

REFERENCES

- Pizzo PA: Fever in immunocompromised patients. N Engl J Med 1999; 341:893. [PMID: 10486422]
- Viscoli C: Treatment of febrile neutropenia: what is new? Curr Opin Infect Dis 2002;15:377. [PMID: 12130933]

Richard A. Jacobs, MD, PhD

Infection, Central Nervous System

KEY FEATURES

ESSENTIALS OF DIAGNOSIS

- Central nervous system infection is a medical emergency
- Immediate diagnostic steps must be instituted to establish the specific cause

GENERAL CONSIDERATIONS

- Infections can be caused by almost any infectious agent, including bacteria, mycobacteria, fungi, spirochetes, protozoa, helminths, and viruses

Etiological classification

- Central nervous system infections can be divided into several categories that are readily distinguished by cerebrospinal fluid examination as the first step toward diagnosis (Table 125, page 1307)
- Purulent meningitis
  - 18–50 years: *Streptococcus pneumoniae, Neisseria meningitidis*
  - >50 years: *S pneumoniae, N meningitidis, Listeria,* gram-negative bacilli
  - Impaired cellular immunity: *Listeria,* gram-negative bacilli, *S pneumoniae*
  - Postsurgical or posttraumatic: *S aureus, S pneumoniae,* gram-negative bacilli
- Chronic meningitis
  - TB or atypical mycobacteria
  - Fungi: *Cryptococcus, Coccidioides, Histoplasma*
  - Spirochetes: syphilis, Lyme disease, leptospirosis
  - Other: brucellosis, HIV infection
- Aseptic meningitis
  - Mumps, coxsackievirus, echoviruses
  - Infectious mononucleosis
  - Leptospirosis, syphilis, Lyme disease
- Encephalitis
- Partially treated bacterial meningitis
- Neighborhood reaction
- Noninfectious meningeal irritation
- Brain abscess
- Amebic meningoencephalitis

CLINICAL FINDINGS

SYMPTOMS AND SIGNS

- Certain symptoms and signs are common to all types of central nervous system infection: headache, fever, sensorial disturbances, neck and back stiffness, positive Kernig and Brudzinski signs, and cerebrospinal fluid abnormalities
- Although it is rare for all of these manifestations to be present in any one individual, the presence of even one should suggest the possibility of a central nervous system infection

DIFFERENTIAL DIAGNOSIS

- Subarachnoid hemorrhage
- Encephalitis
- "Neighborhood reaction" causing abnormal cerebrospinal fluid, eg, brain abscess, epidural abscess, vertebral osteomyelitis, mastoiditis, sinusitis, brain tumor
- Dural sinus thrombosis
- Noninfectious meningeal irritation: carcinomatous meningitis, sarcoidosis, SLE, drugs (eg, nonsteroidal antiinflammatory drugs, trimethoprim-sulfamethoxazole), pneumonia, shigellosis
- If fever and rash: gonococcemia, infective endocarditis, thrombotic thrombocytopenic purpura, Rocky Mountain spotted fever, viral exanthem
- Seizure due to other cause eg, febrile seizure
- Amebic meningoencephalitis (*Naegleria fowleri*)

DIAGNOSIS

LABORATORY TESTS

- See Table 125 (page 1307)
- Blood cell count, blood culture, lumbar puncture followed by careful study and culture of the cerebrospinal fluid, and a chest film
- The fluid must be examined for cell count, glucose, and protein, and a smear stained for bacteria (and acid-fast organisms when appropriate) and cultured for pyogenic organisms and for mycobacteria and fungi when indicated
- Latex agglutination tests can detect antigens of encapsulated organisms (*S pneumoniae, Haemophilus influenzae, N meningitidis,* and *Cryptococcus neoformans*) but are rarely used except for detection of *Cryptococcus* or in partially treated patients
- Polymerase chain reaction (PCR) for herpes simplex and varicella-zoster is very sensitive (>95%) and specific
- PCR to detect other organisms may not be any more sensitive than culture, but the real value is the rapidity with which results are available, ie, hours compared with days or weeks
- At present, with the exception of PCR for herpes simplex, PCR tests are performed only in reference laboratories

IMAGING STUDIES

- Since performing a lumbar puncture in the presence of a space-occupying lesion (brain abscess, subdural hematoma, subdural abscess) may result in brainstem herniation, a CT scan is performed prior to lumbar puncture if a space-occupying lesion is suspected on the basis of papilledema, coma, seizures, or focal neurological findings

TREATMENT

MEDICATIONS

- If delays are encountered in obtaining a CT scan and bacterial meningitis is suspected, blood cultures should be drawn and antibiotics and corticosteroids administered even before cerebrospinal fluid is obtained for culture to avoid delay in treatment (Table 124, page 1306)
- Antibiotics given within 4 h before obtaining cerebrospinal fluid probably do not affect culture results
- Increased intracranial pressure due to brain edema often requires treatment with hyperventilation, mannitol (25–50 g as a bolus intravenous infusion), dexamethasone (4 mg every 4–6 h)

Purulent meningitis

- Treat based on microorganisms most common for each age group (Table 124, page 1306). The identity of the causative microorganism may remain unknown for a few days
- The duration of therapy for bacterial meningitis varies depending on the etiological agent: *H influenzae* 7 days; *N meningitidis* 7 days; *S pneumoniae* 10–14 days; *L monocytogenes* 14–21 days; gram-negative bacilli 21 days
- Dexamethasone therapy is recommended for pneumococcal meningitis; 10 mg of dexamethasone administered 15–20 min before or simultaneously with the first dose of antibiotics and continued every 6 h for 4 days decreases morbidity and mortality

Brain abscess

- Therapy consists of drainage and 3–4 weeks of systemic antibiotics directed against organisms isolated
- A regimen often used includes metronidazole, 500 mg intravenously or orally every 8 h, plus ceftizoxime, 2 g intravenously every 8 h, or ceftriaxone, 2 g every 12 h
- In cases where abscesses are less than 2 cm in size, where there are multiple abscesses that cannot be drained, or if an abscess is located in an area where significant neurological sequelae would result from drainage, antibiotics for 6–8 weeks without drainage can be employed

Therapy of other types of meningitis

- See specific diagnoses

SURGERY

- Brain abscesses need drainage (excision or aspiration) if ≥4 cm in size, and systemic antibiotics

THERAPEUTIC PROCEDURES

- Treatment of cerebral edema and increased intracranial pressure may require drainage of cerebrospinal fluid by repeated lumbar puncture and placement of ventricular catheters

OUTCOME

FOLLOW-UP

- Monitor CNS pressures if extraventricular drain is in place

PROGNOSIS

- Prompt antibiotic therapy probably improves outcome in bacterial meningitis

WHEN TO ADMIT

- Acute CNS symptoms are emergencies
- All patients with meningitis, except viral, should be admitted
- Brain abscess and epidural abscess require admission

PREVENTION

Pneumococcal vaccine

- See MMWR 2000;49(No. RR-9):1.
- Recommended for patients with cerebrospinal fluid leaks
- Because of the apparent increased risk of developing pneumococcal meningitis following cochlear implants, patients receiving these implants should be vaccinated

Meningococcal vaccine

- Should be offered to asplenic patients or those with terminal complement deficiencies
- Vaccination of college freshmen living in dormitories will decrease but not eliminate risk of the disease. Should be offered to those who want to decrease their risk of the disease
- Consider for travel to epidemic or endemic regions (Nepal, sub-Saharan Africa, the "meningitis belt" from Senegal in the west to Ethiopia in the east, northern India)
- Saudi Arabia requires immunization for pilgrims to Mecca
- Although the need for revaccination has not been determined, antibody levels decline over 2–3 years, and revaccination is reasonable in 3–5 years if risk continues

EVIDENCE

PRACTICE GUIDELINES

- National Guideline Clearinghouse http://www.guideline.gov/summary/summary.aspx?doc_id=2364&nbr=1590&string=meningitis http://www.guideline.gov/summary/summary.aspx?doc_id=2666&nbr=1892&string=meningitis http://www.guideline.gov/summary/summary.aspx?doc_id=2446&nbr=1672&string=meningitis

INFORMATION FOR PATIENTS

- National Institute of Neurological Disorders and Stroke http://www.ninds.nih.gov/health_and_medical/disorders/encmenin_doc.htm
- The Mayo Clinic http://www.mayoclinic.com/invoke.cfm?id=DS00118

REFERENCES

- Attia J: The rational clinical examination. Does this adult patient have acute meningitis? JAMA 1999;282:175. [PMID: 10411200]
- Calfee DP: Brain abscess. Semin Neurol 2000;20:353. [PMID: 11051259]
- De Gans J: Dexamethasone in adults with bacterial meningitis. N Engl J Med 2002;347:1549. [PMID: 11144034]
- Hussein AS: Acute bacterial meningitis in adults. A 12-year review. Medicine (Baltimore) 2000;79:360. [PMID: 11144034]

Richard A. Jacobs, MD, PhD

Infection, Nosocomial

KEY FEATURES

ESSENTIALS OF DIAGNOSIS

- Nosocomial infections are by definition acquired during the course of hospitalization
- Hand washing is the easiest and most effective means of prevention and should be done routinely even when gloves are utilized

GENERAL CONSIDERATIONS

- Although most fevers are due to infections, about 25% of patients will have fever of noninfectious origin
- Many infections are a direct result of the use of invasive devices for monitoring or therapy such as intravenous catheters, Foley catheters, catheters placed by interventional radiology for drainage, and orotracheal tubes for ventilatory support. Early removal reduces infection
- Patients who develop nosocomial infections are often critically ill, have been hospitalized for extended periods, and have received several courses of broad-spectrum antibiotic therapy. As a result, the causative organisms are often multidrug resistant and different from those in community-acquired infections. *Staphylococcus aureus* and *S epidermidis* (a frequent cause of prosthetic device infection) may be resistant to nafcillin and cephalosporins and require vancomycin for therapy; *Enterococcus faecium* resistant to ampicillin and vancomycin; gram-negative infections caused by *Pseudomonas, Citrobacter, Enterobacter, Acinetobacter,* and *Stenotrophomonas* may be sensitive only to fluoroquinolones, carbapenems, aminoglycosides, or trimethoprim-sulfamethoxazole

DEMOGRAPHICS

- In the United States, approximately 5% of patients who enter the hospital free of infection acquire a nosocomial infection resulting in prolongation of the hospital stay, increase in cost of care, significant morbidity, and a 5% mortality rate

CLINICAL FINDINGS

SYMPTOMS AND SIGNS

- Those of the underlying disease

DIFFERENTIAL DIAGNOSIS

- Noninfectious: drug fever, postoperative atelectasis or tissue necrosis, hematoma, pancreatitis, pulmonary embolus, myocardial infarction, ischemic bowel
- Urinary tract infections
- Pneumonia
- Bacteremia, eg, indwelling catheter, wound, abscess, pneumonia, genitourinary or gastrointestinal tract
- Wound infection, eg, decubitus ulcer, *Clostridium difficile* colitis

DIAGNOSIS

LABORATORY TESTS
Reliability of culture results

- Unreliable or uninterpretable specimens are often obtained for culture that result in unnecessary use of antibiotics. The best example of this principle is the diagnosis of line-related or bloodstream infection in the febrile patient. Blood cultures from unidentified sites, a single blood culture from any site, or a blood culture through an existing line will often be positive for *S epidermidis* and will result in therapy with vancomycin. The likelihood that such a culture represents a true bacteremia is 10–20%
- Unless two separate venipuncture cultures are obtained—*not* through catheters—interpretation of results is impossible and unnecessary therapy is given
- A positive wound culture without signs of inflammation or infection, a positive sputum culture without pulmonary infiltrates on chest x-ray, or a positive urine culture in a catheterized patient without signs or symptoms of pyelonephritis are all likely to represent colonization, not infection

TREATMENT

MEDICATIONS

- When choosing antibiotics to treat the seriously ill patient, consider the previous antimicrobial therapy the patient has received as well as the "local ecology"
- It is often necessary to institute therapy with vancomycin, a carbapenem, an aminoglycoside, or a fluoroquinolone until a specific agent is isolated and sensitivities are known

OUTCOME

FOLLOW-UP

- Monitoring of high-risk areas by hospital epidemiologists detects increases in infection rates early

WHEN TO REFER

- For persistent fevers or systemic toxicity despite treatment of underlying problem

PREVENTION

- Universal precautions against potential blood-borne transmissible disease
- Hepatitis A, hepatitis B, and varicella vaccines should be considered in the appropriate setting
- Peripheral intravenous lines should be replaced every 3 days and arterial lines every 4 days
- Lines in the central venous circulation (including those placed peripherally) can be left in indefinitely and are changed or removed when they are clinically suspected of being infected, when they are nonfunctional, or when they are no longer needed
- Silver alloy–impregnated Foley catheters reduce the incidence of catheter-associated bacteriuria, and antibiotic-impregnated (minocycline plus rifampin or chlorhexidine plus silver sulfadiazine) venous catheters reduce line infections and bacteremia
- Whether the increased cost of these devices justifies their routine use should be determined by individual institutions based on local infection rates
- Attentive nursing care (positioning to prevent decubitus ulcers, wound care, elevating the head during tube feedings to prevent aspiration) is critical

EVIDENCE

PRACTICE GUIDELINES

- National Guideline Clearinghouse
  http://www.guideline.gov/summary/
  summary.aspx?doc_id=2226&nbr=1452
  &string=nosocomial
  http://www.guideline.gov/summary/
  summary.aspx?doc_id=3484&nbr=
  2710&string=nosocomial
  http://www.guideline.gov/summary/
  summary.aspx?doc_id=2573&nbr=
  1799&string=nosocomial

INFORMATION FOR PATIENTS

- National Institutes of Health
  http://www.nlm.nih.gov/medlineplus/
  ency/article/000146.htm
- National Institute of Allergy and Infectious Diseases
  http://www.niaid.nih.gov/factsheets/
  antimicro.htm

REFERENCES

- Gerberding JL et al: Emerging nosocomial infections and antimicrobial resistance. Curr Clin Top Infect Dis 1999; 19:83. [PMID: 10472481]
- Kollef MH et al: Antibiotic resistance in the intensive care unit. Ann Intern Med 2001;134:298. [PMID: 11182841]
- Lorente C et al: Prevention of infection in the intensive care unit: current advances and opportunities for the future. Curr Opin Crit Care 2002;8:461. [PMID: 12357116]
- Safdar N et al: The commonality of risk factors for nosocomial colonization and infection with antimicrobial-resistant *Staphylococcus aureus,* enterococcus, gram-negative bacilli, *Clostridium difficile,* and *Candida.* Ann Intern Med 2002;136:834. [PMID: 12044132]

Richard A. Jacobs, MD, PhD

Infertility, Female

KEY FEATURES

ESSENTIALS OF DIAGNOSIS

- Pregnancy does not result after 6–12 months of normal sexual activity without contraceptives

GENERAL CONSIDERATIONS

- About 25% of couples experience infertility at some point
- The incidence increases with age
- The male partner contributes to about one-third of cases of infertility, and a combination of male and female factors is common

CLINICAL FINDINGS

SYMPTOMS AND SIGNS

- Obtain history of sexually transmitted disease or prior pregnancies
- Discuss ill effects of cigarettes, alcohol, and other drugs on male fertility
- Prescription drugs may impair male potency
- The gynecological history should include the menstrual pattern
- The present history includes use and types of contraceptives, douches, libido, sex techniques, frequency and success of coitus, and correlation of intercourse with time of ovulation; the family history includes repeated abortions and maternal diethylstilbestrol use
- General physical and genital examinations for both partners

DIFFERENTIAL DIAGNOSIS

- Male factor (hypogonadism, varicocele, alcohol or drug use, immotile cilia syndrome)
- Polycystic ovary syndrome
- Premature ovarian failure
- Hyperprolactinemia
- Hypothyroidism
- Inadequate luteal progesterone or short luteal phase
- Endometriosis
- Uterine leiomyomas (fibroids) or polyps
- Prior pelvic inflammatory disease
- Pelvic adhesions, eg, pelvic surgery, therapeutic abortion, ectopic pregnancy, septic abortion, IUD use

DIAGNOSIS

DIAGNOSTIC PROCEDURES

- Complete blood cell count, urinalysis, cervical culture for *Chlamydia*, serological test for syphilis, rubella antibody determination, and thyroid function tests
- The woman should chart her oral basal body temperature daily on arising, record episodes of coitus and days of menstruation
- Self-performed urine tests for the midcycle luteinizing hormone (LH) surge can enhance temperature observations relating to ovulation. Coitus resulting in conception occurs during the 6-day period ending with the day of ovulation
- Before additional testing, an ejaculate for semen analysis is obtained after sexual abstinence for at least 3 days
- Semen should be examined within 1–2 h after collection. Normal semen: volume, 3 mL; concentration, 20 million sperm per milliliter; motility, 50% after 2 h; and normal forms, 60%. If the sperm count is abnormal, search for exposure to environmental and workplace toxins, alcohol or drug abuse, and hypogonadism

First testing cycle

- Perform a postcoital test just before ovulation (eg, Day 12 or 13 in an expected 28-day cycle). Preovulation timing can be enhanced by serial urinary LH tests
- Examine the patient within 6 h after coitus. The cervical mucus should be clear, elastic, and copious. A good spinnbarkeit (stretching to a fine thread 4 cm or more in length) is desirable. A small drop of cervical mucus should be obtained from within the cervical os and examined under the microscope. The presence of five or more active sperm per high-power field constitutes a satisfactory postcoital test. If no spermatozoa are found, the test should be repeated (assuming that active spermatozoa were present in the semen analysis). Sperm agglutination and sperm immobilization tests should be considered if the sperm are immotile or show ineffective tail motility
- The presence of more than three white blood cells per high-power field in the postcoital test suggests cervicitis or prostatitis. When estrogen levels are normal, the cervical mucus dried on the slide will form a fern-like pattern when viewed with a low-power microscope

- Serum progesterone should be measured at the midpoint of the secretory phase (Day 21); a level of 10–20 ng/mL confirms adequate luteal function

Second testing cycle

- Hysterosalpingography is performed using oil dye within 3 days following the menstrual period. This x-ray study will demonstrate uterine abnormalities and tubal obstruction. A repeat x-ray film 24 h later will confirm tubal patency if there is wide pelvic dispersion of the dye
- If the woman has had prior pelvic inflammation, give doxycycline, 100 mg twice daily, beginning immediately before and for 7 days after the x-ray study

Further testing

- Gross deficiencies of sperm (number, motility, or appearance) require repeat analysis. Zona-free hamster egg penetration tests evaluate the ability of the human sperm to fertilize an egg
- Obvious obstruction of the uterine tubes requires assessment for microsurgery or in vitro fertilization
- Absent or infrequent ovulation requires additional laboratory evaluation. Elevated follicle-stimulating hormone (FSH) and LH levels indicate ovarian failure causing premature menopause. Elevated LH levels in the presence of normal FSH levels confirm the presence of polycystic ovaries. Elevation of blood prolactin (PRL) levels suggests pituitary microadenoma
- Major histocompatibility antigen typing of both partners will confirm human leukocyte antigen-B locus homozygosity, found in greater numbers among infertile couples
- Ultrasound monitoring of folliculogenesis may reveal unruptured luteinized follicles
- Endometrial biopsy in the luteal phase associated with simultaneous serum progesterone levels will rule out luteal phase deficiency

Laparoscopy

- Approximately 25% of women whose basic evaluation is normal will have findings on laparoscopy explaining their infertility (eg, peritubal adhesions)

Infertility, Female

TREATMENT

MEDICATIONS

Induction of ovulation

- Clomiphene citrate. After a normal menstrual period or induction of withdrawal bleeding with progestin, give 50 mg of clomiphene orally daily for 5 days. If ovulation does not occur, increase dosage to 100 mg orally daily for 5 days. If ovulation still does not occur, the course is repeated with 150 mg daily and then 200 mg daily for 5 days, with the addition of chorionic gonadotropin, 10,000 units IM, 7 days after clomiphene

- In the presence of increased androgen production (DHEA-S >200 μg/dL), the addition of dexamethasone, 0.5 mg, or prednisone, 5 mg, at bedtime, improves the response to clomiphene. Dexamethasone should be discontinued after pregnancy is confirmed

- Bromocriptine is used only if PRL levels are elevated and there is no withdrawal bleeding following progesterone administration (otherwise, clomiphene is used). The initial dosage is 2.5 mg once daily, increased to two or three times daily in increments of 1.25 mg. The drug is discontinued once pregnancy has occurred

- Human menopausal gonadotropins (hMG) or recombinant FSH is indicated in cases of hypogonadotropism and most other types of anovulation (exclusive of ovarian failure)

- Gonadotropin-releasing hormone (GnRH)—hypothalamic amenorrhea unresponsive to clomiphene can be treated with subcutaneous pulsatile GnRH

- See *Endometriosis* for treatment

SURGERY

- Fertility can be improved with excision of ovarian tumors or ovarian foci of endometriosis, and microsurgical relief of tubal obstruction due to salpingitis

- Some cornual or fimbrial block can be relieved. Peritubal adhesions or endometriotic implants often can be treated via laparoscopy or via laparotomy

- Sperm characteristics are often improved following surgical treatment of varicocele in the man

THERAPEUTIC PROCEDURES

- Treat hypo- or hyperthyroidism. Give antibiotics for cervicitis if present. In women with abnormal postcoital tests and demonstrated antisperm antibodies causing sperm agglutination or immobilization, condom use for up to 6 months may result in lower antibody levels and improved pregnancy rates

- Women who engage in vigorous athletic training often have low sex hormone levels; fertility improves with reduced exercise and some weight gain

Inadequate transport of sperm

- Intrauterine insemination of concentrated washed sperm can bypass a poor cervical environment associated with scant or hostile cervical mucus

- For azoospermia, artificial insemination by a donor usually results in pregnancy if female function is normal

OUTCOME

PROGNOSIS

- The prognosis for normal pregnancy is good if minor disorders can be treated; it is poor if the causes of infertility are severe, untreatable, or of prolonged duration (over 3 years)

- In the absence of identifiable causes of infertility, 60% of couples will achieve a pregnancy within 3 years

- Couples with unexplained infertility who do not achieve pregnancy within 3 years should be offered ovulation induction, assisted reproductive technology, or information about adoption

WHEN TO REFER

- For induction of ovulation and procedures

EVIDENCE

PRACTICE GUIDELINES

- National Guideline Clearinghouse
http://www.guideline.gov/summary/summary.aspx?doc_id=2555&nbr=1781&string=infertility
http://www.guideline.gov/summary/summary.aspx?doc_id=2552&nbr=1778&string=infertility
http://www.guideline.gov/summary/summary.aspx?doc_id=2553&nbr=1779&string=infertility

WEB SITE

- Assisted Reproductive Technology—Centers for Disease Control and Prevention
http://www.cdc.gov/nccdphp/drh/art.htm

INFORMATION FOR PATIENTS

- American Society for Reproductive Medicine
http://www.asrm.org/Patients/faqs.html

- National Women's Health Information
http://www.4woman.gov/faq/infertility.htm

- JAMA patient page: Infertility. JAMA 1999;282(19):1888. [PMID: 10573283]

REFERENCE

- Rosene-Montella K et al: Evaluation and management of infertility in women: the internist's role. Ann Intern Med 2000; 132:973. [PMID: 10858181]

H. Trent MacKay, MD, MPH

Infertility, Male

 KEY FEATURES

GENERAL CONSIDERATIONS

- Primary infertility affects 15–20% of married couples: ~one-third of cases result from male factors, one-third from female factors, and one-third from combined factors
- Simultaneous evaluation of the female partner warranted (see *Infertility, Female*)
- Clinical evaluation is warranted following 6–12 months of unprotected intercourse

 CLINICAL FINDINGS

SYMPTOMS AND SIGNS

- History: prior testicular insults (torsion, cryptorchism, trauma), infections (mumps orchitis, epididymitis), environmental factors (excessive heat, radiation, chemotherapy), medications [anabolic steroids, cimetidine, and spironolactone may affect spermatogenesis; phenytoin may lower follicle-stimulating hormone (FSH); sulfasalazine and nitrofurantoin affect sperm motility], and drugs (alcohol, marijuana)
- Sexual habits, frequency and timing of intercourse, use of lubricants, and each partner's previous fertility experiences are important
- Loss of libido and headaches or visual disturbances
- Past medical or surgical history: thyroid or liver disease (abnormalities of spermatogenesis), diabetic neuropathy (retrograde ejaculation), radical pelvic or retroperitoneal surgery (absent seminal emission secondary to sympathetic nerve injury), or hernia repair (damage to the vas deferens or testicular blood supply)
- Physical examination: signs of hypogonadism, such as underdeveloped secondary sexual characteristics, diminished male pattern hair distribution (axillary, body, facial, pubic), eunuchoid skeletal proportions (arm span 2 inches > height; upper to lower body ratio <1.0), and gynecomastia
- Evaluate testicular size (normal size ~4.5 × 2.5 cm, volume 18 mL)
- Examine for varicocele in the standing position, with Valsalva maneuver
- Palpate the vas deferens, epididymis, and prostate

 DIAGNOSIS

LABORATORY TESTS

- Semen analysis after 72 h of abstinence (see *Infertility, Female*)
- Endocrinological evaluation: serum FSH, luteinizing hormone (LH), and testosterone
- Elevated FSH and LH and low testosterone (hypergonadotropic hypogonadism) in primary testicular failure
- Low FSH and LH and low testosterone in secondary testicular failure (hypogonadotropic hypogonadism) of hypothalmic or pituitary origin—serum prolactin should be checked

IMAGING STUDIES

- Scrotal ultrasound for varicocele
- Vasography for suspected ductal obstruction

TREATMENT

MEDICATIONS

- Genitourinary tract infections should be treated with antibiotics

Endocrine therapy

- Hypogonadotropic hypogonadism: chorionic gonadotropin, 2000 IU IM three time weekly once primary pituitary disease has been excluded or treated. If sperm counts fail to rise after 12 months, FSH/LH therapy should be initiated
- Menotropins (Pergonal), 75 IU of FSH and 75 IU of LH, 0.5–1 vial IM three time weekly

Retrograde ejaculation therapy

- α-Adrenergic agonists (eg, pseudoephedrine, 60 mg PO TID) or imipramine, 25 mg PO TID
- Collect postmasturbation urine for intrauterine insemination
- Electroejaculation in cases of absent emission

SURGERY

- Varicocele: surgical repair by scrotal, inguinal, laparoscopic, or percutaneous venographic approaches
- Ductal obstruction: operative treatment for mechanical obstruction of the ejaculatory duct is transurethral resection and unroofing of the ducts in the prostatic urethra
- For obstruction of the vas deferens, microsurgical vasovasostomy or vasoepididymostomy

THERAPEUTIC PROCEDURES

- Education
- Proper timing for intercourse
- Avoidance of spermicidal lubricants
- Removal of toxins or medications

 OUTCOME

WHEN TO REFER

- Assisted reproductive techniques: intrauterine insemination, in vitro fertilization, and gamete intrafallopian transfer

EVIDENCE

PRACTICE GUIDELINES

- Gangel EK: American Urological Association, Inc and American Society for Reproductive Medicine. AUA and ASRM produce recommendations for male infertility. American Urological Association, Inc and American Society for Reproductive Medicine. Am Fam Physician 2002;65:2589. [PMID: 12086246]
- Weidner W et al: EAU guidelines on male infertility. Eur Urol 2002;42:313. [PMID: 12361894]

WEB SITES

- MEDLINEplus—infertility http://www.nlm.nih.gov/medlineplus/ency/article/ 001191.htm
- Uptodate—Infertility in men http://patients.uptodate.com/frames.asp?page=topic.asp&file=endo_hor/8386&title=Male+infertility

INFORMATION FOR PATIENTS

- Cleveland Clinic—Male infertility treatment http://www.clevelandclinic.org/health/health-info/docs/1000/1080.asp?index=6452
- Mayo Clinic—Infertility http://www.mayoclinic.com/invoke.cfm?objectid=5B0A05CB-053F-4FD3-9BE06955A15A3CD9

REFERENCES

- Bartoov B et al: Quantitative ultramorphological analysis of human sperm: fifteen years of experience in the diagnosis and management of male factor infertility. Arch Androl 1999;43:13. [PMID: 10445101]
- McClure RD: Male infertility—realistic treatment options [editorial; comment]. J Urol 1999;161:1166. [PMID: 10081862]

Marshall L. Stoller, MD
Peter R. Carroll, MD

Influenza

 ## KEY FEATURES

ESSENTIALS OF DIAGNOSIS

- Abrupt onset of fevers, chills, malaise, cough, arthralgias, and myalgias
- Although sporadic cases do occur, most cases of influenza occur as part of epidemics or pandemics, usually in the fall or winter seasons

GENERAL CONSIDERATIONS

- An orthomyxovirus transmitted by respiratory droplets
- Three antigenic subtypes have been described: types A and B produce identical clinical symptoms, type C produces milder disease
- Pandemics usually due to type A infections with significant antigenic shift (large genetic recombination of the virus)
- Influenza is difficult to diagnose in the absence of the epidemic because it resembles other viral illnesses

DEMOGRAPHICS

- 5000–250,000 cases annually in the United States
- Incidence highest in school-age children and young adults, students, prisoners, day care and health care workers; asthmatics are at particular risk
- Complications occur most often in elderly, immunocompromised individuals

 ## CLINICAL FINDINGS

SYMPTOMS AND SIGNS

- Abrupt onset
- Fevers, chills, malaise with myalgias and headaches are common
- Nasal congestion, substernal tenderness, and nausea are not uncommon
- Fever typically lasts 3–5 days (range 1 to 7 days)
- Sore throat, cervical lymphadenopathy, and nonproductive cough are usually present
- Leukopenia is common
- Leukocytosis may be a marker of secondary complications
- Proteinuria occasionally

DIFFERENTIAL DIAGNOSIS

- Common cold
- Primary bacterial pneumonia
- Infectious mononucleosis
- Acute HIV infection
- Meningitis
- In returning tropical traveler: malaria, dengue, typhoid

 ## DIAGNOSIS

LABORATORY TESTS

- Influenza virus can be isolated from throat or nasal washings sent for tissue culture
- Direct fluorescent antibody staining of washings can also make the diagnosis, though it cannot identify subtypes

DIAGNOSTIC PROCEDURES

- Usually diagnosed clinically when characteristic symptoms are found in the setting of an epidemic

TREATMENT

MEDICATIONS

- When diagnosed early, amantadine or rimantidine can decrease the duration of symptoms and signs of influenza A but should not be used during epidemics of influenza B
- Amantadine dose reduction required in the elderly who develop CNS dysfunction
- Zanamivir (inhaled) or oseltamivir (oral) is also effective at reducing the duration and severity of symptoms, of influenza A and B but are costly and must be started within 48 h of onset of symptoms to be effective. Zanamivir is attendant with a risk of bronchospasm in asthmatics

THERAPEUTIC PROCEDURES

- Supportive measures with adequate hydration, analgesics, and rest

 OUTCOME

COMPLICATIONS

- Influenza predisposes individuals to secondary bacterial infections of the respiratory tract, especially with pneumococcus and *Staphylococcus aureus*
- Pneumonia and purulent bronchitis are frequent complications
- Reye's syndrome, a severe form of hepatic failure, occurs rarely, particularly in young children given salicylates during illness involving influenza B or varicella infections
- The pathogenesis of Reye's syndrome is unknown but aspirin use is a risk factor

PROGNOSIS

- Most patients recover fully back to baseline health within 4–7 days
- Secondary complications can lengthen the course of illness and worsen the chances of a fully recovery
- Poor outcomes usually occur in the elderly, often due to dehydration, exacerbations of comorbid conditions, or secondary complications

WHEN TO REFER

- Refer when signs of secondary complications occur

WHEN TO ADMIT

- Consider hospitalization for signs of significant secondary complications such as pneumonia or acute exacerbations of chronic bronchitis

PREVENTION

- Trivalent influenza vaccine is highly effective (85%) most years
- Vaccination is recommended for persons who are age >50 or who have heart, lung, or other chronic diseases
- Vaccine should be avoided in patients with known hypersensitivity to eggs or its components
- Vaccine is not contraindicated in patients on coumadin or corticosteroids, or in those with HIV infection
- The neuraminidase inhibitors (zanamivir or oseltamivir) can be used prophylactically for both influenza A and B
- Amantidine or rimantidine reduces the attack rate for influenza A

 EVIDENCE

PRACTICE GUIDELINES

- Prevention and control of influenza. Centers for Disease Control and Prevention, 1984 Apr (revised 2003 Apr) http://www.guideline.gov/summary/summary.aspx?doc_id=3738&nbr=2964&string=influenza+and+treatment

WEB SITE

- Centers for Disease Control and Prevention, National Center for Infectious Diseases http://www.cdc.gov/ncidod/diseases/flu/fluvirus.htm

INFORMATION FOR PATIENTS

- JAMA patient page: Immunizations. JAMA 1999;282:102. [PMID: 10404918]
- CDC FAQ http://www.cdc.gov/ncidod/diseases/flu/facts.htm

REFERENCES

- Bridges CB et al: Prevention and control of influenza. Recommendations of the Advisory Committee on Immunization Practices (ACIP). MMWR Recomm Rep 2001;50(RR-4):1. [PMID: 11334444]
- Couch RB: Influenza: prospects for control. Ann Intern Med 2000;133:992. [PMID: 11119401]
- Jefferson TO et al: Amantadine and rimantadine for preventing and treating influenza A in adults. Cochrane Database Syst Rev 2002;3:CD001169. [PMID: 12137620]
- Monto AS et al: Zanamivir prophylaxis: an effective strategy for the prevention of influenza types A and B within households. J Infect Dis 2002;186:1582. [PMID: 12447733]

Wayne X. Shandera, MD
Samuel Shelburne, MD

Insomnia

 KEY FEATURES

ESSENTIALS OF DIAGNOSIS

- Transient episodes are usually of little significance
- Stress, caffeine, physical discomfort, daytime napping, and early bedtimes are common factors
- Psychiatric disorders are often associated with persistent insomnia

GENERAL CONSIDERATIONS

Sleep physiology

- Sleep consists of two distinct states: REM (rapid eye movement) sleep, also called dream sleep, D state sleep, paradoxic sleep; and NREM (non-REM) sleep, also called S stage sleep, which is divided into stages 1, 2, 3, and 4 recognizable by different electroencephalographic patterns. Stages 3 and 4 are "delta" sleep
- **Dreaming** occurs mostly in REM and to a lesser extent in NREM sleep
- Sleep is a cyclic phenomenon, with four or five REM periods during the night accounting for about one-fourth of the total night's sleep (1 1/2–2 h)
- The first REM period occurs about 80–120 min after onset of sleep and lasts about 10 min
- Later REM periods are longer (15–40 min) and occur mostly in the last several hours of sleep. Most stage 4 (deepest) sleep occurs in the first several hours

Etiology of insomnia

- **Age-related changes** in normal sleep include an unchanging percentage of REM sleep and a marked decrease in stage 3 and stage 4 sleep, with an increase in wakeful periods during the night
- These normal changes, early bedtimes, and daytime naps play a role in the increased complaints of insomnia in older people
- Variations in sleep patterns may be due to circumstances (eg, "jet lag") or to idiosyncratic patterns ("night owls") in persons who perhaps because of different "biological rhythms" habitually go to bed late and sleep late in the morning
- Creativity and rapidity of response to unfamiliar situations are impaired by loss of sleep
- There are rare individuals who have chronic difficulty in adapting to a 24-h sleep-wake cycle (desynchronization

sleep disorder), which can be resynchronized by altering exposure to light
- **Depression** is usually associated with fragmented sleep, decreased total sleep time, earlier onset of REM sleep, a shift of REM activity to the first half of the night, and a loss of slow wave sleep
- In **manic disorders**, sleeplessness is a cardinal feature and an important early sign of impending mania in bipolar cases. Total sleep time is decreased, with shortened REM latency and increased REM activity
- Sleep-related panic attacks occur in the transition from stage 2 to stage 3 sleep in some patients with a longer REM latency in the sleep pattern preceding the attacks
- **Abuse of alcohol** may cause or be secondary to the sleep disturbance. There is a tendency to use alcohol as a means of getting to sleep without realizing that it disrupts the normal sleep cycle
- Acute alcohol intake produces a decreased sleep latency with reduced REM sleep during the first half of the night. REM sleep is increased in the second half of the night, with an increase in total amount of slow wave sleep (stages 3 and 4). Vivid dreams and frequent awakenings are common
- Chronic alcohol abuse increases stage 1 and decreases REM sleep (most drugs delay or block REM sleep), with symptoms persisting for many months after the individual has stopped drinking
- Acute alcohol or other sedative withdrawal causes delayed onset of sleep and REM rebound with intermittent awakening during the night
- **Heavy smoking** (more than a pack a day) causes difficulty falling asleep—apparently independently of the often associated increase in coffee drinking
- Excess intake near bedtime of caffeine, cocaine, and other stimulants (eg, over-the-counter cold remedies) causes decreased total sleep time—mostly NREM sleep—with some increased sleep latency
- **Sedative-hypnotics**—specifically, the benzodiazepines, which are the prescription drugs of choice to promote sleep—tend to increase total sleep time, decrease sleep latency, and decrease nocturnal awakening, with variable effects on NREM sleep
- Withdrawal causes just the opposite effects and results in continued use of the drug for the purpose of preventing withdrawal symptoms

- Antidepressants decrease REM sleep (with marked rebound on withdrawal in the form of nightmares) and have varying effects on NREM sleep
- REM sleep deprivation produces improvement in some depressions
- Persistent insomnias are also related to a wide variety of medical conditions, particularly delirium, pain, respiratory distress syndromes, uremia, asthma, and thyroid disorders
- Adequate analgesia and proper treatment of medical disorders will reduce symptoms and decrease the need for sedatives

 CLINICAL FINDINGS

SYMPTOMS AND SIGNS

- Patients may complain of difficulty getting to sleep or staying asleep, intermittent wakefulness during the night, early morning awakening, or combinations of any of these

DIFFERENTIAL DIAGNOSIS

- Acute: emotional stress, physical discomfort, jet lag
- Alcohol abuse
- Stimulants, eg, caffeine, nicotine, cocaine, pseudoephedrine
- Depression
- Poor sleep hygiene, eg, daytime naps, TV in bed
- Mania or bipolar disorder
- Medical illness, eg, chronic obstructive pulmonary disease, uremia, hyperthyroidism, hepatic encephalopathy, gastroesophageal reflux disease
- Nocturia, eg, diuretics, benign prostatic hyperplasia, incontinence, chronic heart failure
- Restless leg syndrome
- CNS disease, eg, complex partial seizures, tumor, neurosyphilis
- Medications, eg, corticosteroids, selective serotonin reuptake inhibitors, theophylline, benzodiazepine withdrawal
- Circadian rhythm disorder

DIAGNOSIS

LABORATORY TESTS

- Consider thyroid-stimulating hormone

 TREATMENT

MEDICATIONS

- There are two broad classes of treatment for insomnia, and the two may be combined: psychological (cognitive-behavioral) and pharmacological
- In situations of acute distress, such as a grief reaction, pharmacological measures may be most appropriate

Pharmacological

- These drugs are often effective for the elderly population and can be given in larger doses—twice what is prescribed for the elderly—in younger patients
  - Lorazepam (0.5 mg nightly)
  - Temazepam (7.5–15 mg nightly)
  - Zolpidem (5–10 mg nightly)
  - Zaleplon (5–10 mg nightly)
- Longer-acting agents such as flurazepam (half-life of >48 h) may accumulate in the elderly and lead to cognitive slowing, ataxia, falls, and somnolence
- In general, it is appropriate to use medications for short courses of 1–2 weeks
- Antihistamines such as diphenhydramine (25 mg nightly) or hydroxyzine (25 mg nightly) may be useful; their anticholinergic effects may produce confusion or urinary symptoms in the elderly
- Trazodone is a non–habit-forming effective sleep medication in lower than antidepressant doses (25–150 mg at bedtime). Priapism is a rare side effect requiring emergent treatment
- Triazolam is popular because of its very short duration of action. Because it has been associated with dependency, transient psychotic reactions, anterograde amnesia, and rebound anxiety, it has been removed from the market in several European countries. If used, it must be prescribed only for short periods of time

THERAPEUTIC PROCEDURES

- With primary insomnia initial efforts should be psychologically based, particularly in the elderly

Psychological

- Educate the patient regarding good sleep hygiene
  - Go to bed only when sleepy
  - Use the bed and bedroom only for sleeping and sex
  - If still awake after 20 min, leave the bedroom and return only when sleepy
  - Get up at the same time every morning regardless of the amount of sleep during the night
  - Discontinue caffeine and nicotine, at least in the evening if not completely
  - Establish a daily exercise regimen
  - Avoid alcohol as it may disrupt continuity of sleep
  - Limit fluids in the evening
  - Learn and practice relaxation techniques
- The clinician should also discuss any myths or misconceptions about sleep that the patient may hold

 OUTCOME

PREVENTION

- Discontinue use of caffeine and nicotine
- Avoid alcohol
- Regular exercise program

EVIDENCE

PRACTICE GUIDELINES

- National Guideline Clearinghouse
http://www.guideline.gov/summary/summary.aspx?doc_id=2276&nbr=1502&string=insomnia
http://www.guideline.gov/summary/summary.aspx?doc_id=2273&nbr=1499&string=insomnia
http://www.guideline.gov/summary/summary.aspx?doc_id=2275&nbr=1501&string=insomnia

WEB SITE

- Psychopharmacology Tips
http://www.dr-bob.org/tips/

INFORMATION FOR PATIENTS

- American Academy of Family Physicians
http://familydoctor.org/healthfacts/110/
- JAMA patient page: Insomnia. JAMA 1999;281:1056. [PMID: 1086442]

REFERENCES

- Morin CM et al: Behavioral and pharmacological therapies for late-life insomnia; a randomized controlled trial. JAMA 1999;281:991. [PMID: 10086433]
- Simon GE et al: Prevalence, burden and treatment of insomnia in primary care. Am J Psychiatry 1997;154:1417.

Stuart J. Eisendrath, MD
Jonathan E. Lichtmacher, MD

Insulinoma

 KEY FEATURES

ESSENTIALS OF DIAGNOSIS

- Fasting hypoglycemia, rather than post-prandial hypoglycemia
- Blood glucose <40 mg/dL in an otherwise healthy appearing person with central nervous dysfunction such as confusion or abnormal behavior
- Hypoglycemic unawareness is common

GENERAL CONSIDERATIONS

- Insulinoma is generally an adenoma of the islets of Langerhans
- Adenomas can be familial
- Ninety percent of tumors are single and benign
- Multiple benign adenomas can occur as well as malignant tumors with functional metastases
- Multiple adenomas can occur with tumors of parathyroids and pituitary [multiple endocrine neoplasia type 1 (MEN-1)]
- Rarely, B cell hyperplasia can be a cause of fasting hypoglycemia
- Patients adapt to chronic hypoglycemia by increasing their efficiency in transporting glucose across the blood–brain barrier, which masks awareness that their blood glucose is approaching critically low levels
- Counterregulatory hormonal responses as well as neurogenic symptoms such as tremor, sweating, and palpitations are blunted during hypoglycemia

 CLINICAL FINDINGS

SYMPTOMS AND SIGNS

- Whipple's triad is characteristic of hypoglycemia regardless of the cause: a history of hypoglycemic symptoms, an associated fasting blood glucose of 40 mg/dL or less, and immediate recovery upon administration of glucose
- Symptoms often develop in the early morning, after missing a meal, or occasionally after exercise
- Initial central nervous system symptoms include blurred vision or diplopia, headache, feelings of detachment, slurred speech, and weakness
- Convulsions or coma may occur
- Personality changes vary from anxiety to psychotic behavior
- Hypoglycemic unawareness is very common

DIFFERENTIAL DIAGNOSIS

- Hyperinsulinism from surreptitious insulin or sulfonylureas
- Extrapancreatic tumors
- Postprandial hypoglycemia: early hypoglycemia (alimentary)
- Postgastrectomy
- Functional (increased vagal tone): late hypoglycemia (occult diabetes)
- Delayed insulin release due to B cell dysfunction
  – Counterregulatory deficiency
  – Idiopathic
- Alcohol-related hypoglycemia
- Immunopathological hypoglycemia: antibodies to insulin receptors (which act as agonists)
- Pentamidine-induced hypoglycemia

DIAGNOSIS

LABORATORY TESTS

- Serum insulin level of 6 μU/mL or more in the presence of blood glucose values below 40 mg/dL is diagnostic of inappropriate hyperinsulinism
- An elevated circulating proinsulin level (above 0.2 ng/mL) in the presence of fasting hypoglycemia is characteristic of most B cell adenomas and does not occur in factitious hyperinsulinism
- In patients with epigastric distress, a history of renal stones, or menstrual or erectile dysfunction, a serum calcium, gastrin, or prolactin level may be useful in screening for MEN-1 associated with insulinoma
- Prolonged fasting up to 72 h under hospital supervision until hypoglycemia is documented
- In normal males, the blood glucose does not fall below 55–60 mg/dL during a 3-day fast
- In normal premenopausal women who have fasted for only 24 h, the plasma glucose may fall to as low as 35 mg/dL. However, the women are not symptomatic, owing to the development of sufficient ketonemia to supply energy needs to the brain
- Insulinoma patients become symptomatic when plasma glucose drops to subnormal levels, since inappropriate insulin secretion restricts ketone formation

IMAGING STUDIES

- Radiographic and arteriographic techniques are seldom helpful in localizing insulinomas preoperatively owing to the small size of these tumors
- Intraoperative ultrasonography and palpation is the tumor localization method of choice
- CT scan or MRI can screen for hepatic metastases
- If insulinoma is not found at the initial surgery: correlation of imaging from selective arteriography of segments of the pancreas with simultaneous hepatic vein sampling for insulin during a bolus of intraarterial calcium delivered selectively to these same pancreatic segments

TREATMENT

MEDICATIONS

- Glucagon for hypoglycemic emergencies, but its benefit may be less than for diabetic hypoglycemia because of the concomitant insulin release from the tumor
- Diazoxide, 300–600 mg daily orally, along with thiazide to control sodium retention
- Verapamil may inhibit insulin release from insulinoma cells. Use if intolerant to diazoxide
- Octreotide (50 mg of octreotide injected subcutaneously twice daily) is a synthetic analog of somatostatin. Use when surgery fails to remove the source of hyperinsulinism
- Streptozocin can decrease insulin secretion in islet cell carcinomas. Effective doses can be delivered via selective arterial catheter to decrease renal toxicity

SURGERY

- Laparoscopy using ultrasound and denucleation can be successful with a single tumor of the body or tail of the pancreas, but open surgery is necessary for tumors in the head of the pancreas

THERAPEUTIC PROCEDURES

- In islet cell carcinoma and in 5–10% of MEN-1 cases when surgical resection has not been curative, frequent feedings are necessary. Since most tumors are not responsive to glucose, carbohydrate feedings every 2–3 h are usually effective in preventing hypoglycemia

OUTCOME

COMPLICATIONS

- Irreversible brain damage from hypoglycemia
- Obesity may become a problem from frequent feeding
- Gastrointestinal upset, hirsutism, or edema from diazoxide

PROGNOSIS

- 90–95% cure at first surgical attempt for single benign adenoma when performed by a skilled surgeon
- Severe brain damage from severe prolonged hypoglycemia is irreversible
- Significant increase in survival in streptozocin-treated patients with islet cell carcinoma, with reduction in tumor mass and decrease in hyperinsulinism

WHEN TO REFER

- Refer to endocrinologist to perform inpatient 72-h fast
- Refer to skilled surgeon for resection

WHEN TO ADMIT

- For 72-h fast

EVIDENCE

INFORMATION FOR PATIENTS

- Mayo Clinic
  http://www.mayoclinic.com/invoke.cfm?id=HQ00896
- Medline Medical Encyclopedia
  http://www.nlm.nih.gov/medlineplus/ency/article/000387.htm

REFERENCES

- Boukhman MP et al: Localization of insulinomas. Arch Surg 1999;134:818. [PMID: 10443803]
- Grant CS: Surgical aspects of hyperinsulinemic hypoglycermia. Endocrinol Metab Clin North Am 1999;28:533. [PMID: 1-500930]
- Hirshberg B et al: Forty-eight-hour fast: the diagnostic test for insulinoma. J Clin Endocrinol Metab 2000;85:3222. [PMID: 10999812]

Umesh Masharani, MB, BS; MRCP (UK)

Irritable Bowel Syndrome

 KEY FEATURES

ESSENTIALS OF DIAGNOSIS

- Common chronic functional disorder characterized by abdominal pain or discomfort with alterations in bowel habits
- Limited evaluation to exclude organic causes of symptoms

GENERAL CONSIDERATIONS

- No definitive diagnostic study
- Idiopathic clinical entity characterized by some combination of chronic (>3 months) lower abdominal symptoms and bowel complaints that may be continuous or intermittent
- Abdominal discomfort or pain that has two of the following three features: relieved with defecation; onset associated with a change in frequency of stool; onset associated with a change in form (appearance) of stool
- Other symptoms include abnormal stool frequency (more than three bowel movements per day or fewer than three per week); abnormal stool form (lumpy or hard; loose or watery); abnormal stool passage (straining, urgency, or feeling of incomplete evacuation); passage of mucus; and bloating or abdominal distension
- Other somatic or psychological complaints are common

DEMOGRAPHICS

- Affects up to 20% of the adult population
- Symptoms usually begin in late teens to early 20s

 CLINICAL FINDINGS

SYMPTOMS AND SIGNS

- Symptoms for >3 months
- Subjective abdominal distension; visible distension not clinically evident
- Abdominal pain, intermittent, crampy, in the lower abdomen, relieved by defecation, worsened by stress, worse for 1–2 h after meals
- More frequent or less frequent stools with the onset of abdominal pain
- Looser stools or harder stools with the onset of pain
- Constipation, diarrhea, or alternating constipation and diarrhea
- Mucus is common
- Physical examination usually is normal
- Abdominal tenderness in the lower abdomen is common, but not pronounced; physical examination is otherwise normal

DIFFERENTIAL DIAGNOSIS

- Colonic neoplasia, inflammatory bowel disease
- Celiac disease, bacterial overgrowth, lactase deficiency, and endometriosis
- Depression and anxiety
- Sexual and physical abuse

 DIAGNOSIS

LABORATORY TESTS

- Obtain complete blood cell count, erythrocyte sedimentation rate, serum albumin, and thyroid-stimulating hormone
- Stool occult blood test
- Stool examination for ova and parasites if diarrhea

IMAGING STUDIES

- Barium enema or colonoscopy for patients aged >40–50 years

DIAGNOSTIC PROCEDURES

- Diagnosis is established with compatible symptoms and exclusion of organic disease
- Consider flexible sigmoidoscopy for patients aged <40 years
- Colonoscopy for patients aged >40–50 years

Irritable Bowel Syndrome

 ## TREATMENT

 ## OUTCOME

 ## EVIDENCE

MEDICATIONS

- Antispasmodic (anticholinergic) agents: dicyclomine, 10–20 mg PO TID–QID; hyoscyamine, 0.125 mg PO (or SL PRN), or sustained-release 0.037 mg or 0.75 mg PO BID
- Antidiarrheal agents: loperamide, 2 mg PO TID–QID, and diphenoxylate with atropine, 2.5 mg PO QID
- Fiber supplementation: bran, psyllium, methylcellulose, or polycarbophil
- Osmotic laxatives: milk of magnesia or polyethylene glycol
- Tricyclic antidepressants: nortriptyline, desipramine, imipramine, or trazodone, 25 mg QHS and increased gradually to 50–100 mg as tolerated
- Serotonin reuptake inhibitors: sertraline, 50–150 mg PO QD, or fluoxetine, 20–40 mg PO QD

THERAPEUTIC PROCEDURES

- Reassure patient
- Explain functional nature of the symptoms
- Exclude lactose intolerance by a breath hydrogen test or a trial of a lactose-free diet
- High-fiber (20–30 g/day) diet
- Behavioral modification with relaxation techniques, hypnotherapy

FOLLOW-UP

- Regular visits helpful in reducing patient anxiety and overuse of the health care system

PROGNOSIS

- Symptoms usually chronic, but episodic; majority of affected patients learn to cope with their symptoms

WHEN TO REFER

- Persistent or worsening symptoms
- Signs of organic disease (blood per rectum, positive fecal occult blood, weight loss, severe pain)
- Signs of serious psychiatric disease or physical/sexual abuse

WHEN TO ADMIT

- Patients with irritable bowel syndrome have increased rate of hospitalizations and inappropriate abdominal surgeries for abdominal pain
- ER physicians and surgeons should avoid unnecessary hospitalizations and surgeries

PRACTICE GUIDELINES

- American College of Gastroenterology Functional Gastrointestinal Disorders Task Force: Evidence-based position statement on the management of irritable bowel syndrome in North America. Am J Gastroenterol 2002;97(11 Suppl):S1. [PMID: 12425585]
- Jones J et al: British Society of Gastroenterology guidelines for the management of the irritable bowel syndrome. Gut 2000;47(Suppl 2):ii1. [PMID: 11053260]

WEB SITE

- American Academy of Family Physicians—Irritable bowel syndrome: tips on controlling tour symptoms http://familydoctor.org/healthfacts/112/

INFORMATION FOR PATIENTS

- National Digestive Diseases Information Clearinghouse—What I need to know about irritable bowel syndrome http://digestive.niddk.nih.gov/ddiseases/pubs/ibs_ez/index.htm

REFERENCES

- Camilleri M: Management of the irritable bowel syndrome. Gastroenterology 2001;120:652. [PMID: 11179242]
- Evidence-based position statement on the management of irritable bowel syndrome in North America. Am J Gastroenterol 2002;97(11 Suppl):S1. [PMID: 12425585]
- Olden K: Diagnosis of irritable bowel syndrome. Gastroenterology 2002; 122:1701. [PMID: 12016433]
- Talley NJ et al: Irritable bowel syndrome: a little understood organic disease? Lancet 2002;360:555. [PMID: 12241674]

Kenneth R. McQuaid, MD

Ischemia, Limb, Acute

 KEY FEATURES

ESSENTIALS OF DIAGNOSIS

- Causes: arterial emboli, thrombosis, or trauma
- Bruit, abnormal contralateral pulse examination, or history of secondary skin changes or intermittent claudication suggests primary arterial thrombosis
- Valvular heart disease, atrial fibrillation, or myocardial infarction suggests embolism

GENERAL CONSIDERATIONS

Arterial embolism

- 80–90% arise from the heart
- Atrial fibrillation is present in 60–70%, rheumatic heart disease in <20%
- Arterial emboli are associated with formation of thrombus in the left atrial appendage or within a postinfarct ventricular aneurysm
- Other cardiac causes: cardiac valvular prostheses and cardiac tumors (myxomas)
- Noncardiac causes: atherosclerotic lesions in proximal vessels, tumors, foreign bodies, and paradoxical emboli deriving from deep venous thrombosis in the leg
- Of emboli, 50% lodge in aortic bifurcation or the infrainguinal vessels, 30% in cerebrovascular vessels, 10% in visceral vessels, and 10% in upper extremity vessels
- Noncardiac emboli are usually small, giving rise to peripheral ulceration and digital ischemia or occasionally to a systemic illness resembling vasculitis
- Atheroemboli can also produce transient ischemic attacks, acute renal insufficiency, or bowel ischemia

Acute arterial thrombosis

- Most commonly a complication of chronic atherosclerotic occlusive disease, peripheral aneurysm, trauma, low-flow states such as hypovolemic or cardiogenic shock, or an inflammatory arteritis
- Other potential risk factors include polycythemia, dehydration, and hypercoagulable states
- Must be excluded with any knee or elbow dislocation

 CLINICAL FINDINGS

SYMPTOMS AND SIGNS

- Symptoms and signs are related to the location of the occlusion, duration of ischemia, and degree of development of collateral circulation
- Six Ps: pain, pallor, pulselessness, paresthesias, poikilothermia, and paralysis

DIFFERENTIAL DIAGNOSIS

- Musculoskeletal injury
- Shock states
- Radiculopathy

 DIAGNOSIS

LABORATORY TESTS

- Microhematuria
- Eosinophilia
- Elevated sedimentation rate
- With atheroemboli, biopsy of the infarcted tissue reveals cholesterol clefts in the small vessels under polarized light

IMAGING STUDIES

- Surface or transesophageal echocardiography to evaluate for atrial thrombus, valvular disease, patent foramen ovale, or cardiac tumor

TREATMENT

MEDICATIONS

Arterial embolism
- Heparin given immediately and continued intraoperatively

Arterial thrombosis
- Catheter-directed thrombolysis, eg, instillation of alteplase (0.5–1 mg/h), successful in 50–80% of cases, limb salvage rate 90%

SURGERY
- Treatment may include thromboendarterectomy, bypass, catheter-guided TPA thrombolysis, or a combination of these

Arterial embolism
- Acute emboli should be surgically treated
- Emergent embolectomy by balloon catheter through a small arteriotomy
- Percutaneous catheter techniques (aspiration, mechanical thrombolysis, or thrombolytic therapy)

Arterial thrombosis
- Surgical thromboendarterectomy or bypass

Arterial trauma
- Arterial thrombosis following penetrating trauma or blunt trauma requires surgical treatment

THERAPEUTIC PROCEDURES
- Acute thrombosis should be treated acutely if it causes limb-threatening symptoms and signs: rest pain, nerve or muscle dysfunction

OUTCOME

FOLLOW-UP
- Routine pulse examinations
- Ankle-brachial index

COMPLICATIONS
- Development of a compartment syndrome
- Myoglobinuria and renal failure from rhabdomyolysis
- Ischemic neuropathy

PROGNOSIS

Arterial embolism
- 5–25% risk of limb loss and 25–30% in-hospital mortality for arterial embolism

Arterial thrombosis
- Limb salvage usually possible with acute thrombosis of the iliac or superficial femoral arteries but is less likely with popliteal thrombosis
- Acute thrombosis of a popliteal aneurysm: 10–25% risk of limb loss

WHEN TO REFER
- All patients with symptoms or signs of acute limb ischemia

WHEN TO ADMIT
- All patients with symptoms and signs of limb-threatening ischemia

PREVENTION
- In atrial fibrillation, mechanical or pharmacological cardioversion may decrease the risk of further emboli
- Lifelong anticoagulation because of high frequency of recurrent emboli

EVIDENCE

PRACTICE GUIDELINES
- ACR Appropriateness Criteria for iliac angioplasty. American College of Radiology, 1999 http://www.acr.org/cgi-bin/fr?tmpl: appcrit,pdf:0999-1014_lt-iliac_ angioplasty-ac.pdf
- ACR Appropriateness Criteria for thrombolysis for lower extremity arterial and graft occlusions. American College of Radiology, 1999 http://www.guidelines.gov/summary/ summary.aspx?doc_id=2499&nbr= 1725&string=Acute+Limb+Ischemia

WEB SITES
- Society of Interventional Radiology http://www.sirweb.org/clinical/pdf/ Ischemia.pdf
- The TransAtlantic Inter-Society Consensus—Acute limb ischemia http://www.tasc-pad.org/journal/C1.pdf

INFORMATION FOR PATIENTS
- Journal of Vascular Surgery—Acute limb ischemia http://www.irexcursions.com/ALI.pdf
- MEDLINEplus—Arterial embolism http://www.nlm.nih.gov/medlineplus/ ency/article/001102.htm

REFERENCES
- Canova CR et al: Long-term results of percutaneous thrombo-embolectomy in patients with infrainguinal embolic occlusions. Int Angiol 2001;20:66. [PMID: 11342998]
- Van Cott EM et al: Laboratory evaluation of hypercoagulability with venous or arterial thrombosis. Arch Pathol Lab Med 2002;126:1281. [PMID: 12421136]

Louis M. Messina, MD
Laura K. Pak, MD
Lawrence M. Tierney, Jr., MD

Islet Cell Tumors

KEY FEATURES

ESSENTIALS OF DIAGNOSIS

- Half of pancreatic islet cell tumors are nonsecretory; patients present with weight loss, abdominal pain, or jaundice
- Secretory tumors cause a variety of manifestations depending on the hormones secreted

GENERAL CONSIDERATIONS

- Pancreatic islets cells are of several types: A cells (20%) secrete glucagon, B cells (70%) secrete insulin, D cells (5%) secrete somatostatin or gastrin, and F cells secrete pancreatic polypeptide
- Each cell type may give rise to benign or malignant neoplasms. Tumors usually present with a syndrome related to hormone hypersecretion
- Many tumors secrete two or more hormones
- Insulinomas are usually (82%) benign. May be multiple, especially in familial multiple endocrine neoplasia type 1 (MEN-1) (12% of cases). Found in pancreatic head or neck (57%), body (15%), or tail (19%), or in duodenum (9%)
- Gastrinomas secrete excessive gastrin, stimulating stomach to hypersecrete acid and causing peptic ulceration (see *Zollinger-Ellison syndrome*). Most are benign, but a minority are malignant, metastasizing to liver. Typically found in duodenum (49%), pancreas (24%), or lymph nodes (11%). Usually 5-year delay from symptom onset to diagnosis. Occur as part of MEN-1 in ~22%
- Glucagonomas are usually malignant; usually cosecrete other hormones, eg, gastrin
- Somatostatinomas and VIPomas (tumors secreting excessive vasoactive intestinal polypeptide) are very rare
- Islet cell tumors can also secrete ectopic hormones, eg, ACTH, producing Cushing's syndrome; or serotonin, producing atypical carcinoid syndrome
- Islet cell tumors may be part of MEN-1 (with pituitary and parathyroid adenomas)

CLINICAL FINDINGS

SYMPTOMS AND SIGNS

- Insulinoma: hypoglycemic symptoms
- Gastrinoma: abdominal pain (75%), diarrhea (73%), heartburn (44%), bleeding (25%), or weight loss (17%)
- Glucagonoma: diarrhea, nausea, peptic ulcer, or necrolytic migratory erythema. Weight loss and liver metastases usual at time of diagnosis. Diabetes mellitus develops in 35%
- Somatostatinoma: weight loss, diabetes mellitus, malabsorption
- VIPoma: profuse watery diarrhea, hypokalemia, acidosis (Verner-Morrison syndrome)

DIFFERENTIAL DIAGNOSIS

- Insulinoma: other cause of hypoglycemia, eg, surreptitious or excess use of insulin or sulfonylurea; liver failure; acute alcohol intoxication; sepsis; postprandial hypoglycemia (postgastrectomy, occult diabetes, idiopathic); or drugs (pentamidine, sulfamethoxazole, quinine)
- Gastrinoma: peptic ulcer disease due to other cause, eg, nonsteroidal antiinflammatory drugs, *Helicobacter pylori*; gastroesophageal reflux disease; diarrhea due to other cause; hypergastrinemia due to other cause (atrophic gastritis, gastric outlet obstruction, pernicious anemia, chronic renal failure)
- Glucagonoma or somatostatinoma: other cause of weight loss, diarrhea, or diabetes mellitus

DIAGNOSIS

LABORATORY TESTS

- Insulinoma: serum glucose low with nonsuppressed insulin; elevated proinsulin level (see *Hypoglycemic disorders*)
- Gastrinoma: serum gastrin elevated in normocalcemic patient not on a proton pump inhibitor
- Somatostatinoma: hypochlorhydria

IMAGING STUDIES

- Somatostatin receptor scintigraphy detects about 75% of noninsulinoma pancreatic cell islet tumors and their metastases
- CT and MRI also useful
- Preoperative localization for insulinomas less successful, with low sensitivities: for ultrasonography, 25%; CT, 25%; endoscopic ultrasonography, 27%; transhepatic portal vein sampling, 40%; arteriography, 45%; intraoperative palpation, 55%; intraoperative pancreatic ultrasound, 75%
- Combination of intraoperative palpation and ultrasound at surgery detects nearly all insulinomas

DIAGNOSTIC PROCEDURES

- Gastrinoma: endoscopy usually (94%) demonstrates prominent gastric folds

TREATMENT

MEDICATIONS

- Gastrinoma: high-dose proton pump inhibitors usually effective (see *Zollinger-Ellison syndrome*)
- VIPoma: octreotide improves symptoms but does not halt tumor growth. Calcitonin also may improve symptoms
- Antihormonal and anticancer chemotherapy for palliation of functioning malignant disease. Streptozocin, doxorubicin, and asparaginase produce encouraging results, especially for malignant insulinoma, but are quite toxic
- Hypoglycemia of insulinoma may be counteracted by verapamil or diazoxide
- Octreotide, a somatostatin analog, used for noninsulinoma islet cell tumor

SURGERY

- Direct resection of tumor (or tumors), which often spreads locally, is primary therapy for all islet cell neoplasms except gastrinomas
- Surgery is not usually employed for gastrinoma because of low cure rates, particularly with MEN-1
- Surgery is rarely curative for insulinomas in MEN-1, so usually reserved for dominant masses

 ## OUTCOME

COMPLICATIONS

- Pancreatic carcinoid tumors grow slowly but usually metastasize to local and distant sites, particularly to other endocrine organs

PROGNOSIS

- Surgical complication rate is ~40%; fistulas and infections occur commonly
- Extensive pancreatic resection may cause diabetes mellitus
- Overall 5-year survival higher with functional (77%) than nonfunctional (55%) tumors and higher with benign (91%) than malignant (55%) tumors
- Gastrinomas: 5-, 10-, and 20-year survival rates for gastrinomas in MEN-1 are 94%, 75%, and 58%, respectively, while survival for sporadic Zollinger-Ellison syndrome are 62%, 50%, and 31%, respectively
- Glucagonoma: median survival is 2.8 years after diagnosis

 ## EVIDENCE

PRACTICE GUIDELINES

- Aldridge MC: Islet cell tumours: surgical treatment. Hosp Med 2000;61:830. [PMID: 11211581]
- Azimuddin K et al: The surgical management of pancreatic neuroendocrine tumors. Surg Clin North Am 2001; 81:511. [PMID: 11459268]
- Mullan MH et al: Endocrine tumours of the pancreas: review and recent advances. ANZ J Surg 2001;71:475. [PMID: 11504292]

WEB SITES

- National Cancer Institute—Islet cell carcinoma http://www.cancer.gov/cancerinfo/pdq/treatment/isletcell/patient
- National Pancreas Foundation http://www.pancreasfoundation.org/index.html

INFORMATION FOR PATIENTS

- MEDLINEplus—Pancreatic islet cell tumor http://www.nlm.nih.gov/medlineplus/ency/article/000393.htm

- University of Maryland Medicine—Pancreatic islet cell tumor http://www.umm.edu/ency/article/pancreatic_islet_cell_tumor_symptoms_000393sym.htm
- Yale New Haven Health—Pancreatic islet cell tumor http://yalenewhavenhealth.org/Library/HealthGuide/IllnessConditions/topic.asp?hwid=nord716

REFERENCES

- Berger AC et al: Prognostic value of initial fasting serum gastrin levels in patients with Zollinger-Ellison syndrome. J Clin Oncol 2001;19:3051. [PMID: 11408501]
- Boukhman MP et al: Localization of insulinomas. Arch Surg 1999;134:818. [PMID: 10443803]
- Hochwald SN et al: Prognostic factors in pancreatic endocrine neoplasms: an analysis of 136 cases with a proposal for low-grade and intermediate-grade groups. Clin Oncol 2002;20:2633. [PMID: 12039924]
- Li ML et al: Gastrinoma. Curr Treat Options Oncol 2001;2:337. [PMID: 12057114]
- Matthews BD et al: Surgical experience with functioning pancreatic neuroendocrine tumors. Am Surg 2002;68:660. [PMID: 12206598]
- Shojamanesh H et al: Prospective study of the antitumor efficacy of long-term octreotide treatment in patients with progressive metastatic gastrinoma. Cancer 2002;94:331. [PMID: 11900219]

Paul A. Fitzgerald, MD

Isosporiasis

 KEY FEATURES

ESSENTIALS OF DIAGNOSIS

In immunocompetent patients

- Mild to severe diarrhea. Mucus may be present in the stool but blood is absent
- Low-grade fever, vomiting, malaise

In immunodeficient patients

- Diarrhea may be profuse
- Occasionally, severe malabsorption and weight loss
- Blood and leukocytes are seldom present
- Serological tests sometimes available

GENERAL CONSIDERATIONS

- Coccidiosis is an intracellular infection of intestinal epithelial cells by spore-forming protozoa
- The causes of coccidiosis are *Cryptosporidium parvum, Isospora belli, Cyclospora cayetanensis, Sarcocystis bovihominis,* and *S suihominis*; all but the *Sarcocystis* species complete their life cycle in a single host
- The incubation period is 7–11 days
- The infectious agents are oocysts (spores) transmitted directly from person to person or by contaminated water or food
- The *Isospora* found in humans appear to be distinct to humans only
- The organism probably requires time outside the host to sporulate and become infectious
- The pathogenesis of the diarrhea is not well understood. No enterotoxin has been identified. Voluminous secretory or malabsorption diarrhea (including vitamin B_{12}, D-xylose, and fat absorption dysfunction) can result

DEMOGRAPHICS

- The infection occur worldwide, particularly in the tropics and in regions where hygiene is poor
- Clustering occurs in days care centers and mental institutions

 CLINICAL FINDINGS

SYMPTOMS AND SIGNS

- Generally, the diarrhea caused by the coccidial and microsporidial agents is clinically indistinguishable

In immunocompetent patients

- Infection varies from no symptoms, to a mild diarrhea with flatulence and bloating, to severe and frequent watery diarrhea in which the onset may be explosive
- Mucus may be present in the stools, but there is no microscopic or gross blood
- There may be low-grade fever, malaise, anorexia, abdominal cramps, vomiting, and myalgia
- These symptoms are generally self-limited, lasting a few days to several months
- Weight loss can be marked

In immunodeficient patients

- The diarrhea can be profuse (up to 15 L daily has been reported), with cholera-like watery movements, accompanied by severe malabsorption, electrolyte imbalance, and marked weight loss; fever is uncommon
- Mucus is seen in the stools, but blood and leukocytes are seldom present
- The diarrhea may recur or persist
- Biliary tract infections can occur

DIFFERENTIAL DIAGNOSIS

- *C parvum, I belli, S bovihominis,* and *S suihominis*
- Giardiasis
- Viral gastroenteritis, eg, rotavirus
- Other traveler's diarrhea, eg, *Escherichia coli*
- Cholera
- Other causes of diarrhea in AIDS, eg, cytomegalovirus colitis

 DIAGNOSIS

LABORATORY TESTS

- Three stool specimens should be collected over 5–7 days and saved both as fresh specimens and in preservative and processed by flotation or concentration methods to detect the distinctive oocysts (differences are based on size and intracellular location)
- Diagnosis by stool examination is often difficult, for the organisms may be scanty even in the presence of significant symptoms
- Because of their buoyancy, oocysts ($20–30 \times 10–20 \ \mu m$) must be looked for just beneath the coverslip of the preparation. Confirmation is by acid-fast staining
- Serological tests are available

DIAGNOSTIC PROCEDURES

- Frequently, the diagnosis can be made only after duodenal aspiration or duodenal biopsy of multiple specimens

TREATMENT

MEDICATIONS

In immunocompetent patients

- Trimethoprim (160 mg) and sulfamethoxazole (800 mg) (TMP-SMZ) four times daily for 10 days and then twice daily for 3 weeks; or sulfadiazine, 4 g, and pyrimethamine, 35–75 mg, in four divided doses daily, plus leucovorin calcium, 10–25 mg daily, for 3–7 weeks

In immunocompromised patients

- It may be necessary to continue a maintenance dose indefinitely with TMP-SMZ three times weekly or Fansidar once weekly
- Efficacy in primary infection has also been reported for furazolidone (400 mg/day for 10 days), roxithromycin, ciprofloxacin, nitrofurantoin, metronidazole, quinacrine, pyrimethamine, albendazole with ornidazole, and diclazuril

THERAPEUTIC PROCEDURES

- Most acute infections in immunocompetent persons are self-limited and do not require treatment
- Supportive treatment for severe or chronic diarrhea includes fluid and electrolyte replacement and, in chronic cases, parenteral nutrition

 OUTCOME

WHEN TO REFER

- Persistent symptoms despite therapy, particularly in immunocompromised patients

WHEN TO ADMIT

- Profuse diarrhea causing hypotension or electrolyte imbalance

PREVENTION

- Measures to reduce exposure to these organisms are recommended for immunocompromised patients. These include reduced exposure to swimming in fresh water and boiling of drinking water (1 min) or use of a filter that removes particles over 1 μm in size

 EVIDENCE

PRACTICE GUIDELINES

- National Guideline Clearinghouse
http://www.guideline.gov/summary/summary.aspx?doc_id=3080&nbr=2306&string=cryptosporidiosis
http://www.guideline.gov/summary/summary.aspx?doc_id=2573&nbr=1799&string=cryptosporidiosis

REFERENCE

- Ambroise-Thomas P: Parasitic diseases and immunodeficiencies. Parasitology 2001;122(Suppl):S65. [PMID: 11442198]

Jaundice

 ## KEY FEATURES

ESSENTIALS OF DIAGNOSIS

- Results from accumulation of bilirubin in the body tissues; the cause may be hepatic or nonhepatic
- Hyperbilirubinemia may be due to abnormalities in the formation, transport, metabolism, and excretion of bilirubin
- Total serum bilirubin is normally 0.2–1.2 mg/dL, and jaundice may not be recognizable until levels are about 3 mg/dL

GENERAL CONSIDERATIONS

- Jaundice is caused by predominantly unconjugated or conjugated bilirubin in the serum (Table 56A, page 1253)
- In the absence of liver disease, hemolysis rarely elevates the serum bilirubin level to more than 7 mg/dL
- "Cholestasis" denotes retention of bile in the liver, and "cholestatic jaundice" implies conjugated hyperbilirubinemia from impaired bile flow

 ## CLINICAL FINDINGS

SYMPTOMS AND SIGNS

- See Table 56B (page 1253)

Unconjugated hyperbilirubinemia

- Normal stool and urine color—no bilirubin in the urine
- Mild jaundice
- Splenomegaly occurs in hemolytic disorders except in sickle cell anemia
- Abdominal or back pain may occur with acute hemolytic crises

Conjugated hyperbilirubinemia

- Hereditary cholestatic syndromes or intrahepatic cholestasis
  - May be asymptomatic
  - Intermittent cholestasis is often accompanied by pruritus, light-colored stools, and, occasionally, malaise
- Hepatocellular disease
  - Malaise, anorexia, low-grade fever, and right upper quadrant discomfort are frequent
  - Dark urine, jaundice, and, in women, amenorrhea occur
  - An enlarged, tender liver; vascular spiders; palmar erythema; ascites; gynecomastia; sparse body hair; fetor hepaticus; and asterixis may be present, depending on the cause, severity, and chronicity of liver dysfunction

Biliary obstruction

- Right upper quadrant pain, weight loss (suggesting carcinoma), jaundice, dark urine, and light-colored stools
- Symptoms and signs may be intermittent if caused by stone, carcinoma of the ampulla, or cholangiocarcinoma
- Pain may be absent early in pancreatic cancer
- Stool occult blood suggests cancer of the ampulla
- Hepatomegaly and a palpable gallbladder (Courvoisier's sign) are characteristic, but neither specific nor sensitive of pancreatic head tumor
- Fever and chills are far more common in benign obstruction and associated cholangitis

DIFFERENTIAL DIAGNOSIS

- Obstructive hepatobiliary disease [γ-glutamyl transpeptidase (GGT) elevated]
- Hepatitis, eg, viral, alcoholic, toxic
- Hemochromatosis

 ## DIAGNOSIS

LABORATORY TESTS

- Table 57 (page 1254)
- Elevated serum aspartate and alanine aminotransferase (AST, ALT) levels result from hepatocellular necrosis or inflammation, as in hepatitis; ALT is more specific for the liver than AST, but an AST level at least twice that of the ALT is typical of alcoholic liver injury
- The ALT level is greater than the AST level in nonalcoholic fatty liver disease prior to the development of cirrhosis
- An isolated elevation of serum ALT is seen in celiac disease
- Elevated alkaline phosphatase levels are seen in cholestasis or infiltrative liver disease (such as tumor or granuloma)
- Alkaline phosphatase elevations of hepatic rather than bone, intestinal, or placental origin are confirmed by concomitant elevation of GTT or 5'-nucleotidase levels

IMAGING STUDIES

- Demonstration of dilated bile ducts by ultrasonography or CT scan indicates biliary obstruction (90–95% sensitivity). Ultrasonography, CT scan, and MRI may also demonstrate hepatomegaly, intrahepatic tumors, and portal hypertension
- Spiral arterial-phase and multislice CT scanning, in which the liver is imaged during peak hepatic enhancement while the patient holds one or two breaths, improves diagnostic accuracy
- Dual-phase or triphasic spiral or multislice CT, CT arterial portography, in which imaging follows intravenous contrast infusion via a catheter placed in the superior mesenteric artery, MRI with use of ferumoxides as contrast agents, and intraoperative ultrasonography are the most sensitive techniques for detection of individual small hepatic lesions in patients eligible for resection of metastases
- Color Doppler ultrasound or contrast agents that produce microbubbles increase the sensitivity of transcutaneous ultrasound for detecting small neoplasms

- MRI is the most accurate technique for identifying isolated liver lesions such as hemangiomas, focal nodular hyperplasia, or focal fatty infiltration and for detecting hepatic iron overload
- Because of its much lower cost, ultrasonography is preferable to CT or MRI as a screening test
- Ultrasonography can detect gallstones with a sensitivity of 95%
- Magnetic resonance cholangiopancreatography (MRCP) appears to be a sensitive, noninvasive method of detecting bile duct stones, strictures, and dilation
- Endoscopic ultrasonography is the most sensitive test for detecting small lesions of the ampulla or pancreatic head and for detecting portal vein invasion by pancreatic cancer. It is also accurate in detecting or excluding bile duct stones

DIAGNOSTIC PROCEDURES

- Percutaneous liver biopsy is the definitive diagnostic method for determining the etiology and severity of the liver disease. It should be performed under ultrasound or CT guidance for suspected metastatic disease or a hepatic mass. A transjugular route can be used in patients with coagulopathy or ascites

 TREATMENT

THERAPEUTIC PROCEDURES

- Treatment of the causative etiology
- Uncomplicated obstructive jaundice responds to parenteral vitamin K
- Use endoscopic retrograde cholangiopancreatography (ERCP) or percutaneous transhepatic cholangiography (PTC) to demonstrate pancreatic or ampullary causes of jaundice, to perform papillotomy and stone extraction, or to insert a stent through an obstructing lesion

 OUTCOME

COMPLICATIONS

- Complications of ERCP include pancreatitis in 5% of cases and, less commonly, cholangitis, bleeding, or duodenal perforation after papillotomy
- Severe complications of PTC occur in 3% of cases and include fever, bacteremia, bile peritonitis, and intraperitoneal hemorrhage

EVIDENCE

PRACTICE GUIDELINES

- National Guideline Clearinghouse http://www.guideline.gov/summary/summary.aspx?doc_id=2399&nbr=1625&string=jaundice

WEB SITES

- Diseases of the Liver http://cpmcnet.columbia.edu/dept/gi/disliv.html
- Pathology Index http://www-medlib.med.utah.edu/WebPath/LIVEHTML/LIVERIDX.html

INFORMATION FOR PATIENTS

- National Institutes of Health http://www.nlm.nih.gov/medlineplus/ency/article/003243.htm

REFERENCES

- Green RM, et al: AGA technical review on the evaluation of liver chemistry tests. Gastroenterology 2002;123:1367.
- Kimmey MB (guest ed): NIH state-of-the-science conference: ERCP for diagnosis and therapy. Gastrointest Endosc 2002;56(suppl):S153.

Lawrence S. Friedman, MD

Kaposi's Sarcoma

 KEY FEATURES

ESSENTIALS OF DIAGNOSIS

- Human herpes virus 8 (HHV-8) or Kaposi's sarcoma–associated herpes virus (KSHV), is universally present in all forms of Kaposi's sarcoma
- It is a common infection in central Africa, is more common in Italy than in the United States, and is common in HIV-infected homosexual men and rare in HIV-infected hemophiliacs

GENERAL CONSIDERATIONS

- Before 1980 in the United States, this rare malignant skin lesion was seen mostly in elderly white men, had a chronic clinical course, and was rarely fatal
- Occurs endemically in an often aggressive form in young black men of equatorial Africa, but it is rare in American blacks
- The epidemiology of infection with HHV-8 or KSHV parallels the incidence of Kaposi's sarcoma in various risk groups and geographic regions
- The virus is present in the skin lesions and circulating B lymphocytes of persons with Kaposi's sarcoma but uncommonly in their normal skin

DEMOGRAPHICS

- The most common HIV-related malignancy

 CLINICAL FINDINGS

SYMPTOMS AND SIGNS

- Red, purple, or dark plaques or nodules on cutaneous or mucosal surfaces
- Commonly involves the gastrointestinal tract, but in asymptomatic patients these lesions are not sought or treated

DIFFERENTIAL DIAGNOSIS

- Bacillary angiomatosis
- Hemangioma
- Vasculitis (palpable purpura)
- Dermatofibroma
- Pyogenic granuloma
- Prurigo nodularis
- Melanoma

 DIAGNOSIS

LABORATORY TESTS

- Based on appearance of skin lesions with confirmatory biopsy
- A low sensitivity serological test is available to detect infection with HHV-8, but is not used to confirm the diagnosis

TREATMENT

MEDICATIONS

- For Kaposi's sarcoma in the elderly, palliative local therapy with intralesional chemotherapy or radiation is usually all that is required
- In the setting of iatrogenic immunosuppression, the treatment of Kaposi's sarcoma is primarily reduction of doses of immunosuppressive medications
- In AIDS-associated Kaposi's, the patient should first be given effective anti-HIV antiretrovirals (including a protease inhibitor), because in most cases this treatment alone is associated with improvement (See *HIV infection*)
- Other therapeutic options include cryotherapy or intralesional vinblastine (0.1–0.5 mg/mL) for cosmetically objectionable lesions
- Systemic chemotherapy is indicated in patients with rapidly progressive skin disease (more than 10 new lesions per month), with edema or pain, and with symptomatic visceral disease or pulmonary disease
- Liposomal doxorubicin is highly effective in controlling these cases and has considerably less toxicity—and greater efficacy—than anthracycline monotherapy or combination chemotherapeutic regimens

SURGERY

- Laser surgery for certain intraoral and pharyngeal lesions

THERAPEUTIC PROCEDURES

- Radiation therapy for accessible and space-occupying lesions

 ## OUTCOME

PROGNOSIS

- Pulmonary Kaposi's sarcoma may be life-threatening and is managed aggressively

WHEN TO REFER

- If there is a question about the diagnosis, if recommended therapy is ineffective, or specialized treatment is necessary

WHEN TO ADMIT

- Respiratory insufficiency or other signs of systemic failure

 ## EVIDENCE

PRACTICE GUIDELINES

- Masur H et al: Guidelines for preventing opportunistic infections among HIV-infected persons–2002. Recommendations of the U.S. Public Health Service and the Infectious Diseases Society of America. Ann Intern Med 2002;137 (5 Pt 2):435.

WEB SITES

- American Academy of Dermatology http://www.aad.org
- Dermatology Handbook for Family Practice from the University of Iowa http://www.vh.org/Providers/ClinRef/FPHandbook/17.html

INFORMATION FOR PATIENTS

- American Cancer Society http://www.cancer.org/docroot/cri/content/cri_2_4_1x_what_is_kaposis_sarcoma_21.asp?sitearea=cri
- National Institutes of Health http://www.nlm.nih.gov/medlineplus/ency/article/000661.htm

REFERENCES

- Antman K et al: Kaposi's sarcoma. N Engl J Med 2000;342:1027. [PMID: 10749966]
- Dezube BJ: Acquired immunodeficiency syndrome-related Kaposi's sarcoma: clinical features, staging, and treatment. Semin Oncol 2000;27:424. [PMID: 10950369]

Timothy G. Berger, MD

Larva Migrans, Visceral

 KEY FEATURES

ESSENTIALS OF DIAGNOSIS

Acute infection

- Cough, wheezing, fever
- Hepatosplenomegaly and lymphadenopathy

Ocular toxocariasis

- Most common in children
- Occurs years after the acute infection

GENERAL CONSIDERATIONS

- Most visceral larva migrans cases are due to *Toxocara canis*, an ascarid of dogs and other canids; *Toxocara cati* in domestic cats has occasionally been implicated and rarely *Belascaris procyonis* of raccoons
- The reservoir mechanism for *T canis* is latent infection in female dogs that is reactivated during pregnancy. Transmission from mother to puppies is via the placenta and milk. Most eggs passed to the environment are from puppies (2 weeks to 6 months) and lactating bitches. The life cycle of *T cati* is similar, but transplacental transmission does not occur
- Direct contact with infected animals does not produce infection, as the eggs require a 3- to 4-week extrinsic incubation period to become infective; thereafter, eggs in soil remain infective for months to years
- In humans, hatched larvae are unable to mature but continue to migrate through the tissues for up to 6 months. Eventually they lodge in various organs, particularly the lungs and liver and less often the brain, eyes, and other tissues, where they produce eosinophilic granulomas up to 1 cm in diameter

DEMOGRAPHICS

- Human infections are sporadic and probably occur worldwide
- In the United States, antibody seroprevalence is 5–7%
- Infection is generally in dirt-eating young children who ingest *T canis* or *T cati* eggs from soil or sand contaminated with animal feces, most often from puppies

 CLINICAL FINDINGS

SYMPTOMS AND SIGNS

Acute infection

- Migrating larvae may induce fever, cough, wheezing, hepatosplenomegaly, and lymphadenopathy
- Other symptoms depend on which organs are invaded, including myelitis, encephalitis, and carditis
- The acute phase may last 2–3 weeks, but resolution of all physical and laboratory findings may take up to 18 months

Ocular toxocariasis

- Generally occurs years after the acute infection
- Most cases occur in children, most commonly 5–10 years old, who present with visual impairment in one eye and sometimes leukocoria, squint, and red eye
- Other common findings are peripheral retinochoroiditis, a diffuse, painless endophthalmitis; posterior pole granuloma; and a peripheral inflammatory mass
- Uncommonly seen are an iris nodule, optic nerve granuloma, uniocular pars planitis, and a migrating retinal nematode

DIFFERENTIAL DIAGNOSIS

- Acute HIV infection
- Infectious mononucleosis
- Lymphoma
- Malaria
- Ascariasis
- Chagas' disease
- Retinoblastoma

 DIAGNOSIS

LABORATORY TESTS

Acute infection

- Leukocytosis is marked (may exceed 100,000/μL), with 30–80% due to eosinophils
- Hyperglobulinemia occurs when the liver is extensively invaded and is a useful clue in diagnosis
- An ELISA test is the most specific (92%) and sensitive (78%) serological test and may permit a presumptive diagnosis, although it does not distinguish acute from prior infection. However, rising or falling titers with twofold differences are consistent with the diagnosis
- Nonspecific isohemagglutinin titers (anti-A and anti-B) are usually greater than 1:102
- With central nervous system involvement, the cerebrospinal fluid may show eosinophils
- No parasitic forms can be found by stool examination

Ocular toxocariasis

- Generally not associated with peripheral eosinophilia, hypergammaglobulinemia, or isohemagglutinin elevation
- Serum ELISA tests may be positive, but a negative test does not rule out the diagnosis
- If doubt exists about whether a patient with a positive serum ELISA test has toxocariasis or retinoblastoma, examination of the vitreous humor for ELISA antibody and eosinophils can be helpful

IMAGING STUDIES

- In acute infection, chest radiographs may show infiltrates
- Ultrasonography may detect 1-cm hypoechoic lesions in the liver, each with a thread-like hyperechoic line
- High-resolution CT scanning of the orbit should be done for ocular symptoms

DIAGNOSTIC PROCEDURES

- Specific diagnosis can be made only by percutaneous liver biopsy or by direct biopsy of a granuloma at laparoscopy (mixed inflammatory infiltrate with numerous eosinophils), but these procedures are seldom justified and may not yield larvae

Larva Migrans, Visceral

TREATMENT

MEDICATIONS

Acute infection

- Although there is no proved specific treatment, the following drugs can be tried: albendazole (400 mg twice daily for 21 days), mebendazole (200 mg twice daily for 21 days), thiabendazole (as used in strongyloidiasis), or ivermectin
- Corticosteroids, antibiotics, antihistamines, and analgesics may be needed to provide symptomatic relief

Ocular toxocariasis

- Treatment includes oral and subconjunctival corticosteroids, and an anthelmintic drug

SURGERY

- Treatment for ocular toxocariasis includes vitrectomy for vitreous traction and laser photocoagulation

THERAPEUTIC PROCEDURES

- Treatment of symptomatic persons is primarily supportive

OUTCOME

PROGNOSIS

- Symptoms of the acute infection may persist for months but generally clear within 1–2 years
- The ultimate outcome is usually good, but permanent neuropsychological deficits have been seen
- Partial or total permanent visual impairment is rare

WHEN TO REFER

- Patients whose disease is progressive despite therapy
- All patients with ocular toxocariasis

WHEN TO ADMIT

- Progressive respiratory disaese
- Patients with central nervous system involvement or carditis

PREVENTION

- Disease in humans is best prevented by periodic treatment of puppies, kittens, and nursing dog and cat mothers, starting at 2 weeks postpartum, repeating at weekly intervals for 3 weeks and then every 6 months

EVIDENCE

INFORMATION FOR PATIENTS

- National Institutes of Health
  http://www.nlm.nih.gov/medlineplus/
  ency/article/000633.htm
- National Institute of Allergy
  http://www.niaid.nih.gov/publications/
  microbes.htm

REFERENCES

- Barisani-Asenbauer T et al: Treatment of ocular toxocariasis with albendazole. J Ocul Pharmacol Ther 2001;17:287. [PMID: 11436948]
- Hartleb M et al: Severe hepatic involvement in visceral larva migrans. Eur J Gastroenterol Hepatol 2001;13:1245. [PMID: 11711784]
- Pawlowski Z: Toxocariasis in humans: clinical expression and treatment dilemma. J Helminthol 2001;75:299. [PMID: 11818044]
- Sabrosa NA et al: Nematode infections of the eye: toxocariasis and diffuse unilateral subacute neuroretinitis. Curr Opin Ophthalmol 2001;12:450. [PMID: 11734685]

Legionnaire's Disease

 KEY FEATURES

ESSENTIALS OF DIAGNOSIS

- Patients are often immunocompromised, smokers, or have chronic lung disease
- Scant sputum production, pleuritic chest pain, toxic appearance
- Chest x-ray shows focal patchy infiltrates or consolidation
- Gram's stain of sputum shows polymorphonuclear leukocytes and no organisms

GENERAL CONSIDERATIONS

- Ranks among the three or four most common causes of community-acquired pneumonia
- Classically, this pneumonia is caused by *Legionella pneumophila*, though other species can cause identical disease
- Is more common in immunocompromised persons, in smokers, and in those with chronic lung disease
- Outbreaks have been associated with contaminated water sources, such as shower heads and faucets in patient rooms, and air conditioning cooling towers

DEMOGRAPHICS

- An estimated 8,000–18,000 cases occur each year in the United States
- Most cases are sporadic; 10–20% can be linked to outbreaks, and about 20% are nosocomial

 CLINICAL FINDINGS

SYMPTOMS AND SIGNS

- Many features of typical pneumonia, with high fevers, a toxic patient, pleurisy, and grossly purulent sputum

DIFFERENTIAL DIAGNOSIS

- Other infectious pneumonia
- Pulmonary embolism
- Aspiration pneumonia
- Myocardial infarction
- Pleurodynia (coxsackievirus)

 DIAGNOSIS

LABORATORY TESTS

- Is an atypical pneumonia, because a Gram-stained smear of sputum does not show organisms
- Culture onto charcoal-yeast extract agar or similar enriched medium is the most sensitive method (80–90% sensitivity) for diagnosis and permits identification of infections caused by species and serotypes other than *L pneumophila* serotype 1
- Dieterle's silver staining of tissue, pleural fluid, or other infected material is also a reliable method for detecting *Legionella* species
- Direct fluorescent antibody stains and serological testing are less sensitive because these will detect only *L pneumophila* serotype 1
- Serological diagnosis requires that the host respond with sufficient specific antibody production and be infected with a serotype 1 strain
- Urinary antigen tests, which are targeted for detection of *L pneumophila* serotype 1, are also less sensitive than culture

Legionnaire's Disease

 TREATMENT

MEDICATIONS

- Levofloxacin (500 mg once daily orally or intravenously), azithromycin (500 mg then 250 mg once daily, orally or intravenously), and clarithromycin (500 mg orally twice daily)—all administered for 10–14 days
- Azithromycin may be effective as a 5-day regimen
- A 21-day course of treatment and combination therapy (eg, addition of rifampin 300 mg twice daily or macrolide-fluoroquinolone) are recommended in the immunocompromised patient; improved outcome is not certain
- Tetracyclines and trimethoprim-sulfamethoxazole are used for the patient who cannot be treated with either a macrolide or a fluoroquinolone

 OUTCOME

PROGNOSIS

- Death occurs in 5–15% cases: a substantially higher proportion of fatal cases occurs during nosocomial outbreaks

WHEN TO REFER

- For progressive respiratory failure or if expertise in management is needed

WHEN TO ADMIT

- For respiratory compromise or if supportive care if needed

PREVENTION

- Improved design and maintenance of cooling towers and plumbing systems to limit the growth and spread of *Legionella* organisms
- Person-to-person transmission does not occur

EVIDENCE

PRACTICE GUIDELINES

- National Guideline Clearinghouse http://www.guideline.gov/summary/ summary.aspx?doc_id=2665&nbr= 1891&string=legionnaires

WEB SITES

- CDC—Division of Bacterial and Mycotic Diseases http://www.cdc.gov/ncidod/dbmd/
- Karolinska Institute—Directory of Bacterial Infections and Mycoses http://www.mic.ki.se/Diseases/c1.html

INFORMATION FOR PATIENTS

- JAMA patient page: Pneumonia. JAMA 2000;283:1922.
- Centers for Disease Control http://www.cdc.gov/ncidod/dbmd/ diseaseinfo/legionellosis_g.htm
- National Institute of Environmental Health Sciences http://www.niehs.nih.gov/external/faq/ legion.htm

REFERENCE

- Waterer GW et al: Legionella and community-acquired pneumonia: a review of current diagnostic tests from a clinician's viewpoint. Am J Med 2001;110:41. [PMID: 11152864]

Henry F. Chambers, MD

Leiomyoma of the Uterus

KEY FEATURES

ESSENTIALS OF DIAGNOSIS

- Irregular enlargement of the uterus (may be asymptomatic)
- Heavy or irregular vaginal bleeding, dysmenorrhea
- Acute and recurrent pelvic pain if the tumor becomes twisted on its pedicle or infarcted
- Symptoms due to pressure on neighboring organs (large tumors)

GENERAL CONSIDERATIONS

- Most common benign neoplasm of the female genital tract
- Tumor is discrete, round, firm, and often multiple, composed of smooth muscle and connective tissue
- The most convenient classification is by anatomic location:
  - Intramural
  - Submucous
  - Subserous
  - Intraligamentous
  - Parasitic (ie, deriving its blood supply from an organ to which it becomes attached)
  - Cervical
- A submucous myoma may become pedunculated and descend through the cervix into the vagina

CLINICAL FINDINGS

SYMPTOMS AND SIGNS

- In nonpregnant women, myomas are frequently asymptomatic. However, they can cause urinary frequency, dysmenorrhea, heavy bleeding (often with anemia), or other complications due to the presence of an abdominal mass. Occasionally, degeneration occurs, causing intense pain

DIFFERENTIAL DIAGNOSIS

- Adenomyosis (uterine endometriosis)
- Pregnancy
- Ovarian tumor
- Endometrial polyp
- Endometrial cancer
- Leiomyosarcoma

DIAGNOSIS

LABORATORY TESTS

- Anemia from blood loss may occur
- Rarely, polycythemia is present, presumably as a result of the production of erythropoietin by the myomas

IMAGING STUDIES

- Ultrasonography will confirm the presence of uterine myomas
- When multiple subserous or pedunculated myomas are being followed, ultrasonography is important to exclude ovarian masses
- MRI can delineate intramural and submucous myomas accurately

DIAGNOSTIC PROCEDURES

- Hysterography or hysteroscopy can confirm cervical or submucous myomas

TREATMENT

MEDICATIONS

- For marked anemia as a result of long, heavy menstrual periods, preoperative treatment with depot medroxyprogesterone acetate, 150 mg intramuscularly every 28 days, or danazol, 400–800 mg orally daily, will slow or stop bleeding, and medical treatment of anemia can be given prior to surgery
- Because the risk of surgical complications increases with the increasing size of the myoma, preoperative reduction of myoma size is desirable
- Gonadotropin-releasing hormone analogs such as depot leuprolide, 3.75 mg IM monthly, or nafarelin, 0.2–0.4 mg intranasally twice a day, are used preoperatively for 3- to 4-month periods to induce reversible hypogonadism, which temporarily reduces the size of myomas, suppresses their further growth, and reduces surrounding vascularity

SURGERY

- Emergency surgery is required for acute torsion of a pedunculated myoma
- The only emergency indication for myomectomy during pregnancy is torsion; abortion is not inevitable
- Surgical measures: available for treatment are myomectomy and total or subtotal abdominal, vaginal, or laparoscopy-assisted vaginal hysterectomy
- Myomectomy is the treatment of choice during the childbearing years
- Myomas do not require surgery on an urgent basis unless they cause significant pressure on the ureters, bladder, or bowel or severe bleeding leading to anemia or unless they are undergoing rapid growth
- Cervical myomas larger than 3–4 cm in diameter or pedunculated myomas that protrude through the cervix must be removed
- Submucous myomas can be removed using a hysteroscope and laser or resection instruments

OUTCOME

FOLLOW-UP

- Women who have small asymptomatic myomas should be examined at 6-month intervals
- Ultrasound can be used sequentially to monitor growth

COMPLICATIONS

- Infertility may be due to a myoma that significantly distorts the uterine cavity

PROGNOSIS

- Surgical therapy is curative
- Future pregnancies are not endangered by myomectomy, although cesarean delivery may be necessary after wide dissection with entry into the uterine cavity

WHEN TO REFER

- Refer to gynecologist for surgical therapy of symptomatic leiomyomata

WHEN TO ADMIT

- For acute abdomen associated with an infracted leiomyoma (rare)

EVIDENCE

PRACTICE GUIDELINES

- National Guideline Clearinghouse http://www.guideline.gov/summary/summary.aspx?doc_id=2279&nbr=1505&string=fibroids

WEB SITES

- Gynecology Handbook for Family Practitioners http://www.vh.org/Providers/ClinRef/FPHandbook/13.html

INFORMATION FOR PATIENTS

- Mayo Clinic http://www.mayoclinic.com/invoke.cfm?id=DS00078
- National Uterine Fibroids Foundation http://www.nuff.org/health_uterinefibroids.htm

REFERENCE

- Olive DL: New approaches to the management of fibroids. Obstet Gynecol Clin North Am 2000;27:669. [PMID: 10958011]

H. Trent MacKay, MD, MPH

Leishmaniasis

KEY FEATURES

ESSENTIALS OF DIAGNOSIS

- Four clinical syndromes occur
  - Visceral leishmaniasis (kala azar)
  - Cutaneous leishmaniasis
  - Mucocutaneous leishmaniasis (espundia)
  - Diffuse cutaneous leishmaniasis

GENERAL CONSIDERATIONS

- The disease is a zoonosis transmitted by bites of sand flies [phlebotomus (Old World leishmaniasis) and lutzomyia (New World leishmaniasis) species] from the wild animal reservoir (eg, rodents, Canidae, sloths, marsupials) and domestic dogs (they can die from *Leishmania infantum* infections) to humans; however, kala azar is transmitted directly from humans to humans
- Leishmaniae have two distinct forms in their life cycle. In mammalian hosts, the parasite is found in its amastigote form (Leishman-Donovan bodies, $2 \times 5\ \mu m$) within mononuclear phagocytes. When sand flies feed on an infected host, the parasitized cells are ingested with the blood meal. In the sand fly vector, the parasite converts to, multiplies, and is then transmitted during feeding as a flagellated extracellular promastigote ($10–15\ \mu m$)
- There is overlap between the four clinical syndromes, and each syndrome is caused by more than one species
- See *Leishmaniasis, visceral (kala azar)*
- See *Leishmaniasis, cutaneous*
- See *Leishmaniasis, mucocutaneous,* page 1126
- Diffuse cutaneous leishmaniasis is a state of deficient cell-mediated immunity, in which the skin lesions are generally progressive and refractory to treatment. The causative organisms are the *L mexicana* complex in the New World and *L aethiopica* in the Old World
- *Leishmania* results in lifelong latent infection
- If immunoparesis occurs, leishmaniae can become opportunistic pathogens through reactivation or new infection; in southern Europe (France, Italy, Spain, Portugal), up to 17% of people with AIDS have coinfections

DEMOGRAPHICS

- In tropical and temperate zones, an estimated 12 million persons are infected

with leishmaniasis; 1.5–2 million new cases occur yearly, of which more than 1 million are cutaneous and 500,000 visceral disease

CLINICAL FINDINGS

SYMPTOMS AND SIGNS

- Severity of infection ranges from subclinical or minimally pathological (self-curing or easily treated cutaneous lesions) to persistent, disfiguring cutaneous and mucocutaneous lesions to potentially fatal visceral disease
- See *Leishmaniasis, visceral (kala azar)*
- See *Leishmaniasis, cutaneous*
- See *Leishmaniasis, mucocutaneous,* page 1126
- In diffuse cutaneous leishmaniasis, there are widespread, leprosy-like skin lesions
- In patients with AIDS who have coinfection with *Leishmania*, splenomegaly may not occur in visceral disease

DIAGNOSIS

LABORATORY TESTS

- Definitive diagnosis is by finding the intracellular nonflagellated amastigote in Giemsa-stained biopsies from skin, mucosal lesions, liver, or lymph nodes; or from aspirates from spleen (the most sensitive site, but also a risky procedure), bone marrow, or lymph nodes; or the flagellated promastigote state in culture of these tissue
- Occasionally, the organisms are seen in mononuclear cells of Giemsa-stained smears of the buffy coat
- Culture requires up to 21 days using specialized media
- In patients with AIDS who have *Leishmania* coinfections, diagnostic criteria may be altered (*Leishmania* antibodies become undetectable and, in visceral disease, splenomegaly may not occur)
- PCR assays have high sensitivity
- Golden hamster or BALB/c mouse inoculation of the nose, footpad, or tail base may be used and requires 2–12 weeks of observation
- Serological tests (ELISA, indirect fluorescent antibody, direct agglutination, and others) and the leishmanin (Montenegro) skin test (not licensed in the United States) may facilitate diagnosis, but none is sufficiently sensitive or specific to be used alone or to speciate

DIAGNOSTIC PROCEDURES

- Specimens from skin lesions should be obtained through intact skin (cleansed with 70% alcohol) at a raised edge of an ulcer margin. Local anesthesia can be used. To obtain tissue fluid for staining, press blood out of the site with two fingers, incise a 3-mm slit, and then scrape with the blade
- When doing a biopsy, an impression smear is made, a portion is macerated for culture, and the remainder is reserved for pathological sections. For needle aspiration, sterile preservative-free saline is inserted with a 23- to 27-gauge needle; the aspirate is then cytospun at $800 \times g$ for 5 min

TREATMENT

- See *Leishmaniasis, visceral (kala azar)*
- See *Leishmaniasis, cutaneous*
- See *Leishmaniasis, mucocutaneous,* page 1126

MEDICATIONS

- The drug of choice is a pentavalent antimonial, either sodium stibogluconate or meglumine antimoniate; resistance and treatment failures are increasing in frequency
- Second-line drugs are amphotericin B and pentamidine. A lipid formulation, AmBisome, is considered by some workers to be the drug of choice for the treatment of visceral leishmaniasis
- Miltefosine, an oral drug, is approved in India for treatment of visceral leishmaniasis
- The selected drug is given on consecutive days: 28 days for visceral and mucocutaneous leishmaniasis and 20 days for cutaneous leishmaniasis. In certain regions of the world, because of resistance, longer courses are indicated. Although few side effects occur initially, they are more likely to appear with cumulative doses. Most common are gastrointestinal symptoms, fever, myalgia, arthralgia, phlebitis, and rash; hemolytic anemia, hepatitis, renal and heart damage, and pancreatitis are rare
- Therapy is discontinued if the following occur: aminotransferases three to four times normal levels or significant arrhythmias, corrected QT intervals greater than 0.50 s, or concave ST segments
- Relapses should be treated at the same dosage level for at least twice the previous duration
- In the United States, the only drug available is stibogluconate, obtainable from the Parasitic Drug Service, Centers for Disease Control and Prevention, Atlanta, GA 30333 (404-639-3670)

Paromomycin (aminosidine)

- In cutaneous leishmaniasis, topical application in various formulations has variable success that differs by region
- One ointment is paromomycin 15%/methylbenzethonium chloride 12% in soft paraffin, applied twice daily for 15 days; skin reactions may occur. The ointment cannot be used in regions of mucocutaneous leishmaniasis as it does not prevent metastatic disease

- In parenteral treatment of refractory visceral leishmaniasis, paromomycin is promising but has the potential for severe renal or otic toxicity

Miltefosine

- This alkyl phospholipid is the first oral drug for the treatment of leishmaniasis
- Approved for use in India for visceral leishmaniasis. The daily dose of 100–150 mg for 4 weeks has resulted in 95% cure rates
- Side effects include vomiting (40%), diarrhea (20%), and occasional transient elevations of serum transaminases and creatinine and urea blood nitrogen
- The drug is not recommended in pregnancy
- Preliminary reports show efficacy in cutaneous leishmaniasis

OUTCOME

FOLLOW-UP

- Patients should be monitored weekly for the first 3 weeks and twice weekly thereafter by serum chemistries, complete blood cell counts, and electrocardiography

PREVENTION

- Sand fly habitats are warm, humid microclimates, including rodent burrows, rock piles, or tree holes; these are often in sylvatic areas near forests or semiarid ecosystems. Biting is generally at twilight or at night but may occur in shaded areas during the day
- Partial protection is from permethrin applied to clothing, deet repellent, avoidance of endemic areas (especially at night), use of mosquito coils, and use of fine-mesh insecticide-impregnated nets for sleeping (may be too warm for tropical use)

WHEN TO REFER

- All patients should be referred to a clinician with expertise in this disease

EVIDENCE

PRACTICE GUIDELINES

- National Guideline Clearinghouse http://www.guideline.gov/summary/summary.aspx?doc_id=2573&nbr=1799&string=leishmaniasis http://www.guideline.gov/summary/summary.aspx?doc_id=3080&nbr=2306&string=leishmaniasis

INFORMATION FOR PATIENTS

- Centers for Disease Control http://www.cdc.gov/ncidod/dpd/parasites/leishmania/factsht_leishmania.htm
- National Institutes of Health http://www.nlm.nih.gov/medlineplus/ency/article/001386.htm

REFERENCES

- Croft SL: Monitoring drug resistance in leishmaniasis. Trop Med Int Health 2001;6:899. [PMID: 11703844]
- Croft SL et al: Chemotherapy of leishmaniasis. Curr Pharm Des 2002;8:319. [PMID: 11860369]
- Desjeux P: The increase in risk factors for leishmaniasis worldwide. Trans R Soc Trop Med Hyg 2001;95:239. [PMID: 11490989]

Leishmaniasis, Cutaneous

 KEY FEATURES

ESSENTIALS OF DIAGNOSIS

- **Old World cutaneous leishmaniasis**— moist or dry cutaneous leishmaniasis—is caused mainly by *Leishmania tropica, L major*, and *L aethiopica*
- **New World cutaneous leishmaniasis** is caused by the *L mexicana* complex

GENERAL CONSIDERATIONS

Agents of Old World cutaneous leishmaniasis

- *L tropica* is responsible for urban infections of dogs and humans
- It is found in the Middle East, India, East Africa, central Asian area of the former Soviet Union, Afghanistan, Pakistan, Turkey, Armenia, Greece, and southern France and Italy
- The incubation period is 2 months or longer, and healing is complete in 1–2 years
- *L major* infection causes lesions in dry or desert rural areas and is primarily a disease of desert rodents
- Human disease occurs in the Middle East, central Asian area of the former Soviet Union, Arabian peninsula, Afghanistan, and Africa (North, East, and sub-Saharan Africa from Senegal to Sudan and Kenya)
- *L aethiopica* infection occurs in the Ethiopian and Kenyan highlands

Agents of New World cutaneous leishmaniasis

- *L mexicana* (Texas, Oklahoma, Arizona, Mexico, Central America)
- *L amazonensis* (Amazonian basin, Venezuela, Panama)
- *L chagasi* (Central and South America)
- *L braziliensis* (Central and South America)

 CLINICAL FINDINGS

SYMPTOMS AND SIGNS

- Cutaneous swellings appear 2 weeks to several months after sand fly bites and can be single or multiple
- Depending on the leishmanial species and host immune response, lesions begin as small papules and develop into nonulcerated dry plaques or large encrusted ulcers with well-demarcated raised and indurated margins
- Satellite lesions may be present
- The lesions are painless unless secondarily infected
- Local lymph nodes may be enlarged
- Systemic symptoms are rare, but a low-grade fever of short duration may be present at the onset
- For most species, healing usually occurs spontaneously in months to 1–3 years, starting with central granulation tissue that spreads peripherally

Old World cutaneous leishmaniasis

- The lesions of *L tropica* infection tend to be single and dry, to ulcerate slowly or not at all, and to persist for a year or longer
- Leishmaniasis recidivans is a relapsing form of *L tropica* infection in which the primary lesion nearly heals, lateral spread with central healing follows, and scarring can be extensive; it is associated with hypersensitivity and a strongly positive skin test but scarce amastigotes
- Visceral involvement by *L tropica* has been reported rarely (including after troop exposure in Operation Desert Storm) and is relatively resistant to antimony treatment
- *L major* lesions are characterized by multiple, wet, rapidly ulcerating sores with crusting. Spontaneous healing is generally complete in 6–12 months
- *L aethiopica* infection can cause ulceration, rarely. Spontaneous healing is slow over several years

New World cutaneous leishmaniasis

- The lesions are usually ulcers, but vegetative, verrucous, or nodular lesions may occur also
- *L mexicana* ("chiclero's ulcer") produces destructive lesions on the ear cartilage
- Up to 80% of *L braziliensis* cutaneous lesions progress to espundia (see *Leishmaniasis, mucocutaneous,* page 1126); some *L braziliensis* complex

strains also show a chain of palpable local lymph nodes, and some *L mexicana* and South American strains can cause diffuse cutaneous leishmaniasis

DIFFERENTIAL DIAGNOSIS

- Hansen's disease (leprosy)
- Fungal infection
- Cutaneous tuberculosis
- Neoplasm
- Syphilis
- Sarcoidosis
- Yaws
- *L donovani* [see *Leishmaniasis, visceral (kala azar)*] sometimes causes cutaneous disease with visceral manifestations

DIAGNOSIS

LABORATORY TESTS

- Definitive diagnosis is made by identification of the organisms
- Microscopic examination of skin scrapings has limited sensitivity, particularly in chronic infections
- Where available after culture, species identification should be done by molecular methods
- The skin test becomes positive within 3 months and remains positive for life; false positives occur
- Serological tests are unreliable. Antibody may be undetectable or appear only at low levels after 4–6 weeks; cross-reactions occur including with leprosy

TREATMENT

MEDICATIONS

- **Old World leishmaniasis**, especially in the Middle East, is generally self-healing in about 6 months and it may be justified to withhold treatment for small, unobtrusive lesions that appear to be healing

- Parenteral sodium stibogluconate (20–28 days) should be used to treat large or multiple lesions or if the lesions are on cosmetically or functionally important areas (eg, the wrist)

- Complete healing may not be evident until weeks after the first or second course of treatment

- Amphotericin B desoxycholate and pentamidine are used for failures. Pentamidine is often effective against *L aethiopica* lesions and ketoconazole (400–600 mg/day for 4–6 weeks) against *L major* and *L (V) panamensis*

- Paromomycin ointment may also be effective against *L tropica*

- In **New World** *L mexicana* infections from Mexico and Central America, solitary nodules or ulcers in inconspicuous sites generally will heal spontaneously

- Variable success has been had with paromomycin ointment, ketaconazole, heat applications, or metronidazole (750 mg three times daily for 10 days)

- Preliminary trials with oral miltefosine (150 mg for 3–4 weeks) had reported cure rates of 94%

- Lesions on the ear, face, or hands should be treated with sodium stibogluconate but usually require only a 12- to 14-day course

- Cutaneous lesions acquired in regions of mucocutaneous leishmaniasis may be due to *L braziliensis* or *L panamensis* and should be treated with a full course of sodium stibogluconate

THERAPEUTIC PROCEDURES

- Other treatments for less severe Old World disease are physical measures (local cryotherapy or heat therapy, electrocoagulation, surgical removal) and intralesional injection of sodium stibogluconate

 OUTCOME

COMPLICATIONS

- Pyogenic complications may be followed by lymphangitis or erysipelas

- Contraction of scars can cause deformities and disfigurement, especially if lesions are on the face

Diffuse cutaneous leishmaniasis

- An uncommon complication is diffuse cutaneous leishmaniasis, caused by the *L mexicana* complex and *L aethiopica*

- It is an anergic form with nodular lesions and high parasite count

- Nonulcerating lesions resembling lepromatous leprosy occur over the entire body

- The skin test is negative, but amastigotes are abundant

- In spite of repeated doses of antimony, pentamidiine, or amphotericin, cures are rare

WHEN TO REFER

- All patients should be referred to a clinician with expertise in this disease

 EVIDENCE

PRACTICE GUIDELINES

- National Guideline Clearinghouse
  http://www.guideline.gov/summary/
  summary.aspx?doc_id=3080&nbr=2306
  &string=cryptosporidiosis
  http://www.guideline.gov/summary/
  summary.aspx?doc_id=2573&nbr=
  1799&string=cryptosporidiosis

INFORMATION FOR PATIENTS

- Centers for Disease Control
  http://www.cdc.gov/ncidod/dpd/
  parasites/leishmania/factsht_leishmania.
  htm

- National Institutes of Health
  http://www.nlm.nih.gov/medlineplus/
  ency/article/001386.htm

REFERENCES

- Alrajhi AA et al: Fluconazole for the treatment of cutaneous leishmaniasis caused by *Leishmania major*. N Engl J Med 2002;346:891. [PMID: 11907288]

- Esfandiarpour I et al: Evaluating the efficacy of allopurinol and meglumine antimoniate (Glucantime) in the treatment of cutaneous leishmaniasis. Int J Dermatol 2002;41:521. [PMID: 12207774]

- Fisher C et al: Development status of miltefosine as first oral drug in visceral and cutaneous leishmaniasis. Med Microbiol Immunol 2001;190:85. [PMID: 11770118]

- Hepburn NC: Management of cutaneous leishmaniasis. Curr Opin Infect Dis 2001;14:151. [PMID: 11979125]

Leishmaniasis, Visceral (Kala Azar)

 KEY FEATURES

ESSENTIALS OF DIAGNOSIS

- An infection of the reticuloendothelial system
- Symptoms include fever, hepatosplenomegaly, and pancytopenia
- Although humans are the major reservoir, animal reservoirs such as the dog, other canids, and rodents are important

GENERAL CONSIDERATIONS

- The disease is caused mainly by the *Leishmania donovani* complex: *L donovani* (eastern India, Bangladesh, Southeast Asia, Sudan, Ethiopia, Kenya, scattered foci in sub-Saharan Africa, the central Asian part of Russia, and northern and eastern China); *L infantum* (Mediterranean littoral, Middle East, China, central and southwestern Asia, Ethiopia, Sudan, Afghanistan, Pakistan); and *L chagasi* (South America, Central America, Mexico)
- Two other species—*L tropica* in the Middle East, the Mediterranean littoral, Kenya, India, and western Asia and *L amazonensis* in the Amazon Basin—cause visceral leishmaniasis in a few patients, generally in a milder form
- In each locale, the disease has its own peculiar clinical and epidemiological features

DEMOGRAPHICS

- More than 500,000 cases occur yearly
- Concurrent infections with HIV have been reported frequently in the Mediterranean area and some from South America

 CLINICAL FINDINGS

SYMPTOMS AND SIGNS

- The incubation period is usually 4–6 months (range: 10 days to 24 months)
- A local nonulcerating nodule at the site of the bite may precede systemic manifestations but usually is inapparent
- The onset may be acute (as early as 2 weeks after infection) or insidious
- Fever often peaks twice daily, with chills and sweats, weakness, weight loss, cough, and diarrhea
- The spleen progressively becomes huge, hard, and nontender; the liver is somewhat enlarged, and generalized lymphadenopathy is common
- Petechiae, bleeding from the nose and gums, jaundice, edema, and ascites may occur
- Hyperpigmentation, especially on the hands, feet, abdomen, and forehead, is marked in light-skinned patients
- In blacks, there may be warty eruptions or skin ulcers
- Wasting is progressive; death, often due to intercurrent infection, occurs within months to 1–2 years
- In some regions, oral and nasopharyngeal or cutaneous manifestations occur with or without visceral involvement
- In HIV-infected persons—with or without AIDS—visceral leishmaniasis can be an opportunistic infection. These patients may have a shorter duration of symptoms, no fever or splenomegaly, and a poor response to treatment

DIFFERENTIAL DIAGNOSIS

- Leukemia or lymphoma
- Cirrhosis
- Tuberculosis
- Histoplasmosis
- Infectious mononucleosis
- Brucellosis
- Malaria
- Typhoid fever
- Schistosomiasis
- African trypanosomiasis
- Tropical splenomegaly syndrome

 DIAGNOSIS

LABORATORY TESTS

- On occasion, the organism can be found in buffy coat preparations of blood, particularly obtained at night
- More commonly, the diagnosis depends on stained smears, touch preparations, culture, or animal inoculation of aspirated marrow, liver, enlarged lymph nodes, or spleen
- In immunocompetent persons, serological tests are sensitive (>90%) but false positives may occur, especially in malaria and typhoid fever
- The direct agglutination IgM test and the ELISAs become positive early; the immunofluorescent IgG test becomes positive in most persons at a titer of 1:256 or higher. After treatment, the tests remain positive for months, though in immunoincompetent persons titers may be low or undetectable
- The leishmanin skin test is always negative during active disease and becomes positive months to years after recovery. The polymerase chain reaction has excellent sensitivity and specificity
- Other characteristic findings are progressive leukopenia (seldom over 3000/µL after the first 1–2 months), with lymphocytosis and monocytosis, normochromic anemia, thrombocytopenia, and eosinophilia
- There is a marked increase in total protein up to or greater than 10 g/dL owing to an elevated IgG fraction; serum albumin is 3 g/dL or less
- Liver function tests show hepatocellular damage
- Proteinuria may be present

DIAGNOSTIC PROCEDURES

- Although splenic aspiration is the most sensitive test, because of its hazard (intraabdominal bleeding and death) it should be reserved for last and should be performed only by experienced persons; contraindications are a soft spleen in the acute phase, a prolonged prothrombin time, and platelet counts under 40,000/µL

Leishmaniasis, Visceral (Kala Azar)

 TREATMENT

MEDICATIONS

- See *Leishmaniasis*
- Sodium stibogluconate (20 mg/kg/day for 30 days, sometimes longer) is the drug of choice; however, some prefer lipid formulations of amphotericin B (AmBisome)
- Whereas Mediterranean kala azar may respond to 10–15 doses of stibogluconate (one per day), the disease in Kenya, Sudan, and India requires at least 30 days of treatment. With incomplete response or relapse, the treatment should be repeated for up to 60 days
- Failure of stibogluconate or liposomal amphotericin B should lead to use of pentamidine
- Other drugs under evaluation individually or in combination with antimony, pentamidine, or amphotericin B are allopurinol, human γ-interferon, atovaquone, and parenteral paromomycin (aminosidine)
- In Bihar, India, where the infection is becoming increasingly unresponsive to antimonials (currently 40%), liposomal amphotericin B is usually effective. Miltefosine, an oral treatment, shows high cure rates at a dosage of 100–150 mg daily for 4 weeks. Gastrointestinal side effects are frequent; the drug is contraindicated in pregnancy. It is not available in the United States

 OUTCOME

COMPLICATIONS

- Post–kala azar dermal leishmaniasis may appear after apparent cure in the Indian subcontinent and east Africa. It may simulate leprosy, as multiple hypopigmented macules or nodules develop on preexisting lesions. Erythematous patches may appear on the face. Leishmaniae are present in the skin. Antimony treatment should be tried but is often ineffective

PROGNOSIS

- Without treatment, the fatality rate reaches 90%
- Early diagnosis and treatment reduce mortality to 2–5%
- Relapses (up to 10% in India and 30% in Kenya) are most likely to occur within 6 months after completion of treatment

WHEN TO REFER

- All patients
- For splenic aspiration

 EVIDENCE

PRACTICE GUIDELINES

- National Guideline Clearinghouse http://www.guideline.gov/summary/summary.aspx?doc_id=2573&nbr=1799&string=leishmaniasis http://www.guideline.gov/summary/summary.aspx?doc_id=3080&nbr=2306&string=leishmaniasis

INFORMATION FOR PATIENTS

- Centers for Disease Control http://www.cdc.gov/ncidod/dpd/parasites/leishmania/factsht_leishmania.htm
- National Institutes of Health http://www.nlm.nih.gov/medlineplus/ency/article/001386.htm

REFERENCES

- Guerin PJ et al: Visceral leishmaniasis: current status of control, diagnosis, and treatment, and a proposed research and development agenda. Lancet Infect Dis 2002;2:494. [PMID: 12150849]
- Murray HW: Clinical and experimental advances in treatment of visceral leishmaniasis. Antimicrob Agents Chemother 2001;45:2185. [PMID: 11451673]
- Pintado V et al: HIV-associated visceral leishmaniasis. Clin Microbiol Infect 2001;7:291. [PMID: 11442562]
- Sundar S et al: Low-dose liposomal amphotericin B in refractory Indian visceral leishmaniasis: a multicenter study. Am J Trop Med Hyg 2002;66:143. [PMID: 12135284]

Leprosy

 KEY FEATURES

ESSENTIALS OF DIAGNOSIS

- Pale, anesthetic macular—or nodular and erythematous—skin lesions
- Superficial nerve thickening with associated anesthesia
- History of residence in endemic area in childhood
- Acid-fast bacilli in skin lesions or nasal scrapings, or characteristic histological nerve changes

GENERAL CONSIDERATIONS

- A chronic infectious disease caused by the acid-fast rod *Mycobacterium leprae*
- The mode of transmission probably is respiratory droplets and involves prolonged exposure in childhood
- The disease is divided into two distinct types: lepromatous and tuberculoid
- The lepromatous type occurs in persons with defective cellular immunity
- In the tuberculoid type, cellular immunity is intact and the course is more benign

DEMOGRAPHICS

- The disease is endemic in tropical and subtropical Asia, Africa, Central and South America, and the Pacific regions
- India, Myanmar, and Nepal have 70% of the cases

 CLINICAL FINDINGS

SYMPTOMS AND SIGNS

- The onset is insidious
- The lesions involve the cooler body tissues: skin, superficial nerves, nose, pharynx, larynx, eyes, and testicles
- Skin lesions may occur as pale, anesthetic macular lesions 1–10 cm in diameter; discrete erythematous, infiltrated nodules 1–5 cm in diameter; or diffuse skin infiltration
- Neurological disturbances are caused by nerve infiltration and thickening, with resultant anesthesia, and motor abnormalities
- Bilateral ulnar neuropathy is highly suggestive

Lepromatous type

- The course is progressive and malignant, with nodular skin lesions and slow, symmetric nerve involvement

Tuberculoid type

- The course is more benign and less progressive, with macular skin lesions and severe asymmetric nerve involvement of sudden onset
- Intermediate ("borderline") cases are frequent. Eye involvement (keratitis and iridocyclitis), nasal ulcers, epistaxis, anemia, and lymphadenopathy may occur

DIFFERENTIAL DIAGNOSIS

- Systemic lupus erythematosus
- Sarcoidosis
- Syphilis
- Erythema nodosum
- Erythema multiforme
- Cutaneous tuberculosis
- Vitiligo
- Scleroderma
- Mycosis fungoides
- Diffuse cutaneous leishmaniasis
- Neuropathy due to other causes, eg, amyloidosis

DIAGNOSIS

LABORATORY TESTS

- *M leprae* does not grow in artificial media but does grow in the footpads of armadillos
- The lepromatous type: abundant acid-fast bacilli in the skin lesions and a negative lepromin skin test
- The tuberculoid type: few bacilli present in the lesions and a positive lepromin skin test

DIAGNOSTIC PROCEDURES

- Laboratory confirmation requires the demonstration of acid-fast bacilli in a skin biopsy
- Biopsy of skin or of a thickened involved nerve also gives a typical histological picture

TREATMENT

MEDICATIONS

- Combination therapy is recommended for treatment of all types of leprosy
- For borderline and lepromatous cases, a three-drug regimen such as dapsone, 50–100 mg/day, clofazimine, 50 mg/day, and rifampin, 10 mg/kg/day (up to 600 mg/day), all given orally, should be used. The triple-drug combination should be administered for a minimum of 2–3 years and, ideally, until all biopsies are negative for acid-fast bacilli
- For indeterminate and tuberculoid leprosy, the dapsone-rifampin combination is recommended for 6–12 months, often followed by a course of dapsone alone for 2 or more years

OUTCOME

COMPLICATIONS

- Renal failure and hepatomegaly from secondary amyloidosis may occur with long-standing disease
- Two reactional states—erythema nodosum leprosum and reversal reactions—may occur as a consequence of therapy
- The reversal reaction
  - Typical of borderline lepromatous leprosy
  - Probably results from enhanced host immunity
  - Skin lesions and nerves become swollen and tender, but systemic manifestations are not seen
- Erythema nodosum leprosum
  - Typical of lepromatous leprosy
  - Is a consequence of immune injury from antigen-antibody complex deposition in skin and other tissues; in addition to skin and nerve manifestations, fever and systemic involvement may be seen
- Prednisone, 60 mg/day, or thalidomide, 300 mg/day (in the nonpregnant patient only), is effective for erythema nodosum leprosum. Improvement is expected within a few days after initiating prednisone, and thereafter the dose may be tapered over several weeks to avoid recurrence. Thalidomide is also tapered over several weeks to a 100-mg bedtime dose
- Erythema nodosum leprosum is usually confined to the first year of therapy, and prednisone or thalidomide can be discontinued
- Thalidomide is ineffective for reversal reactions, and prednisone, 60 mg/day, is indicated. Reversal reactions tend to recur, and the dose of prednisone should be slowly tapered over weeks to months
- Therapy for leprosy should not be discontinued during treatment of reactional states

PROGNOSIS

- In untreated cases, disfigurement due to the skin infiltration and nerve involvement may be extreme, leading to trophic ulcers, bone resorption, and loss of digits

WHEN TO REFER

- Consultation with a physician experienced in the treatment of leprosy is suggested

PREVENTION

- Elimination efforts are to reach populations that have not yet received multidrug therapy services

EVIDENCE

WEB SITES

- CDC—Division of Bacterial and Mycotic Diseases
  http://www.cdc.gov/ncidod/dbmd/
- Karolinska Institute—Directory of Bacterial Infections and Mycoses
  http://www.mic.ki.se/Diseases/c1.html

INFORMATION FOR PATIENTS

- Centers for Disease Control
  http://www.cdc.gov/ncidod/dbmd/diseaseinfo/ hansens_t.htm
- National Institutes of Health
  http://www.nlm.nih.gov/medlineplus/ency/article/001347.htm

REFERENCE

- Jacobson RR et al: Leprosy. Lancet 1999;353:655. [PMID: 10030346]

Henry F. Chambers, MD

Leptospirosis

 KEY FEATURES

ESSENTIALS OF DIAGNOSIS

- Leptospirosis is an acute and often severe infection caused by *Leptospira interrogans,* a diverse organism of 23 serogroups and over 200 serovars
- The three most common serovars are *Leptospira icterohaemorrhagiae* of rats, *Leptospira canicola* of dogs, and *Leptospira pomona* of cattle and swine
- *L icterohaemorrhagiae* causes the most severe illness
- Leptospirosis occurs worldwide, transmitted to humans by the ingestion of food and drink contaminated by the urine of the reservoir animal. The organism may also enter through minor skin lesions and probably via the conjunctiva
- The incubation period is 2–20 days

 CLINICAL FINDINGS

SYMPTOMS AND SIGNS

- Anicteric leptospirosis is the more common and milder form of the disease and is often biphasic
- Icteric leptospirosis (Weil's syndrome) (usually caused by *L icterohaemorrhagiae*) is characterized by impaired renal and hepatic function, abnormal mental status, hemorrhagic pneumonia, and hypotension
- Initial or "septicemic" phase: abrupt fever to 39–40°C, chills, abdominal pain, severe headache, and myalgias, marked conjunctival suffusion
- Following a 1- to 3-day period of improvement, the second or "immune" phase begins
- Specific antibodies appear
- A recurrence of symptoms with the onset of meningitis
- Uveitis—unilateral or bilateral
- Rash and adenopathy
- Hemorrhagic pneumonia

DIFFERENTIAL DIAGNOSIS

- Bacterial meningitis
- Influenza
- Viral hepatitis
- Yellow fever
- Dengue
- Hemorrhagic fever, eg, hantavirus
- Relapsing fever

 DIAGNOSIS

LABORATORY TESTS

- Anicteric leptospirosis: leptospires can be isolated from blood, cerebrospinal fluid, and tissues
- Leukocyte count may be normal or as high as 50,000/μL
- Urine bile, protein, casts, and red cells
- Uremia
- Elevated bilirubin and aminotransferases in 75%
- Elevated creatine kinase (>1.5 mg/dL) in 50%
- Serum creatinine is usually elevated
- Organisms may be found in the cerebrospinal fluid. The organism may be identified by darkfield examination of the patient's blood or by culture on a semisolid medium (eg, Fletcher's EMJH). Takes 1–6 weeks to become positive. May be grown from the urine
- Diagnosis is usually made by serological tests
- Agglutination tests show a 4-fold or greater rise in titer
- Indirect hemagglutination, enzyme immunosorbent assay (EIA), and ELISA tests are also available. The IgM EIA is particularly useful [positive as early as 2 days into illness, extremely sensitive and specific (93%)]
- PCR methods

IMAGING STUDIES

- Dictated by symptoms; hemorrhagic pneumonia has been described

DIAGNOSTIC PROCEDURES

- Lumbar puncture for CNS symptoms

TREATMENT

MEDICATIONS

- Severe leptospirosis: penicillin, 6 million units IV QD, is the drug of choice
- Mild to moderate leptospirosis: doxycycline, 100 mg PO BID for 7 days, is effective if started early
- Jarisch-Herxheimer reactions may occur

 OUTCOME

FOLLOW-UP

- Routine

COMPLICATIONS

- Myocarditis, aseptic meningitis, renal failure, and pulmonary infiltrates with hemorrhage
- Iridocyclitis

PROGNOSIS

- Anicteric leptospirosis is usually self-limited, lasting 4–30 days, and almost never fatal. Complete recovery is the rule
- Icteric leptospirosis has symptoms and signs that often are continuous and not biphasic, and a 5–10% mortality rate (5% for those under age 30 and 30% for those over age 60)

WHEN TO REFER

- Refer for supportive care such as dialysis

WHEN TO ADMIT

- Admit for severe liver or renal disease

PREVENTION

- Prophylaxis: doxycycline, 200 mg PO once weekly during the risk of exposure

 EVIDENCE

PRACTICE GUIDELINES

- Guidugli F et al: Antibiotics for preventing leptospirosis. Cochrane Database Syst Rev 2000;(4):CD001305. [PMID: 11034711]
- Guidugli F et al: Antibiotics for treating leptospirosis. Cochrane Database Syst Rev 2000;(2):CD001306. [PMID: 10796767]

WEB SITES

- CDC Traveler's Information on Leptospirosis http://www.cdc.gov/travel/diseases/lepto.htm
- CDC www.cdc.gov

INFORMATION FOR PATIENTS

- CDC Leptospirosis General Information http://www.cdc.gov/ncidod/dbmd/diseaseinfo/leptospirosis_g.htm
- CDC FAQ http://www.cdc.gov/ncidod/dbmd/diseaseinfo/leptospirosis_g.htm

REFERENCES

- Katz AR et al: Assessment of the clinical presentation and treatment of 353 cases of laboratory-confirmed leptospirosis in Hawaii, 1974–1998. Clin Infect Dis 2001;33:1834. [PMID: 11692294]
- Vinetz JM: Leptospirosis. Curr Opin Infect Dis 2001;14:527. [PMID: 11964872]

Richard A. Jacobs, MD, PhD

Leukemia, Acute

 ## KEY FEATURES

ESSENTIALS OF DIAGNOSIS

- Short duration of symptoms, including fatigue, fever, and bleeding
- Cytopenias or pancytopenia
- >20% blasts in bone marrow
- Blasts in peripheral blood in 90%

GENERAL CONSIDERATIONS

- A malignancy of the hematopoietic progenitor cell, which loses its ability to mature and differentiate; cells proliferate in uncontrolled fashion and replace normal bone marrow elements
- Most cases arise with no clear cause
- Radiation and some toxins (benzene) are leukemogenic; chemotherapeutic agents (procarbazine, melphalan, other alkylating agents, and etoposide) may cause leukemia
- Acute promyelocytic leukemia, characterized by chromosomal translocation t(15;17)
- Acute myelogenous leukemia (AML) usually categorized by morphology and histochemistry as acute undifferentiated leukemia (M0), acute myeloblastic leukemia (M1), acute myeloblastic leukemia with differentiation (M2), acute promyelocytic leukemia (M3), acute myelomonocytic leukemia (M4), acute monoblastic leukemia (M5), erythroleukemia (M6), or megakaryoblastic leukemia (M7)
- Acute lymphoblastic leukemia (ALL) classified by immunological phenotype as: B or T cell lineage
- Cytogenetics are single most important prognostic factor

DEMOGRAPHICS

- ALL comprises 80% of acute leukemias of childhood; peak incidence between ages 3 and 7 years
- ALL also seen in adults, causing ~20% of adult acute leukemias
- AML chiefly occurs in adults with median age at presentation of 60 years and increasing incidence with advanced age

 ## CLINICAL FINDINGS

SYMPTOMS AND SIGNS

- Clinical findings are due to replacement of normal bone marrow or infiltration of organs (skin, gastrointestinal tract, meninges)
- Gingival bleeding, epistaxis, or menorrhagia common
- Less commonly, widespread bleeding from disseminated intravascular coagulation (DIC) (in acute promyelocytic leukemia and monocytic leukemia)
- Increased susceptibility to infection with neutrophil count <500/µL; infection (eg, cellulitis, pneumonia, and perirectal infections) within days is the rule when <100/µL; death within a few hours may occur if treatment delayed; signs of infection may be absent; gram-negative bacteria or fungi (*Candida, Aspergillus*) are most common pathogens
- Gum hypertrophy
- Bone and joint pain
- Impaired circulation, causing headache, confusion, and dyspnea, with hyperleukocytosis (circulating blast count usually >200,000/µL)
- Pallor, purpura, and petechiae common
- Hepatosplenomegaly and lymphadenopathy are variable
- Bone tenderness, particularly in sternum, tibia

DIFFERENTIAL DIAGNOSIS

Acute myelogenous leukemia

- Chronic myelogenous leukemia
- Myelodysplastic syndrome ("preleukemia")
- Left-shifted bone marrow recovering from toxic insult

Acute lymphoblastic leukemia

- Chronic lymphocytic leukemia
- Lymphoma
- Hairy cell leukemia
- Atypical lymphocytosis of mononucleosis or pertussis

 ## DIAGNOSIS

LABORATORY TESTS

- Combination of pancytopenia with circulating blasts on peripheral smear
- Blasts absent from peripheral smear in up to 10% ("aleukemic leukemia")
- Serum fibrinogen low, prothrombin time prolonged, and fibrin degradation products or fibrin D-dimers present if DIC
- Blasts in cerebrospinal fluid occur with meningeal leukemia in ~5% of cases at diagnosis
- Auer rod, an eosinophilic needle-like inclusion in cytoplasm of blasts, is pathognomonic of AML
- Lack of morphological or histochemical evidence of myeloid or monocytic lineage suggests diagnosis of ALL; demonstration of characteristic surface markers by immunophenotype confirms diagnosis of ALL
- In ALL, Philadelphia chromosome t(9;22) and t(4;11), has an unfavorable prognosis
- In AML, cytogenetic studies showing t(8;21), t(15;17), and inv(16)(p13;q22) have favorable prognosis; those showing monosomy 5 and 7 and complex abnormalities are unfavorable

IMAGING STUDIES

- Chest x-ray: mediastinal mass in ALL (especially T cell)

DIAGNOSTIC PROCEDURES

- Bone marrow is hypercellular, with >20% blasts required for diagnosis of acute leukemia

TREATMENT

MEDICATIONS

Remission induction therapy

- Initial treatment goal is to produce complete remission, defined as normal peripheral blood with resolution of cytopenias, normal bone marrow with no excess blasts, and normal clinical status.
- AML: combination of an anthracycline (daunorubicin or idarubicin) plus cytarabine
- Acute promyelocytic leukemia: combination of all-*trans*-retinoic acid, a vitamin A analog that leads to terminal differentiation of acute promyelocytic leukemia cells, with anthracyclines
- ALL: combination chemotherapy including daunorubicin, vincristine, prednisone, and asparaginase

Postremission therapy

- Once in remission, postremission therapy (chemotherapy or autologous or allogeneic transplantation, depending on age, clinical status, leukemia type) is given with curative intent
- Acute promyelocytic leukemia: chemotherapy plus retinoic acid
- AML and ALL (average-risk patients): chemotherapy, autologous transplantation, or allogeneic transplantation
- Antibiotics for infection

THERAPEUTIC PROCEDURES

- AML: allogeneic transplantation is treatment of choice if no remission or high-risk cytogenetics, but cure rates only 20%
- ALL: allogeneic transplantation if adverse cytogenetics or poor responses to chemotherapy; autologous transplantation is an option in patients without a suitable donor
- Emergent leukapheresis and chemotherapy for hyperleukocytosis

 OUTCOME

FOLLOW-UP

- Repeat bone marrow

COMPLICATIONS

- Infection

PROGNOSIS

- AML: combination chemotherapy produces complete remissions in 70–80% of patients aged <60 and 40–60% of patients aged >60; postremission therapy leads to cure in 30–40% with chemotherapy, in 50% with autologous transplantation, and in 50–60% with allogeneic transplantation (for younger adults with HLA-matched siblings)
- Some AML types have better prognosis
- Acute promyelocytic leukemia: combination chemotherapy produces complete remissions in >90%; postremission chemotherapy leads to cure in 60–70%
- ALL: combination chemotherapy produces complete remissions in 80–90%

WHEN TO REFER

- Refer all patients with acute leukemia to hematologist-oncologist

WHEN TO ADMIT

- Hyperleukocytosis (leukostasis syndrome)
- With initial diagnosis

 EVIDENCE

PRACTICE GUIDELINES

- Appelbaum FR et al: National Comprehensive Cancer Network. NCCN Practice Guidelines for Acute Myelogenous Leukemia. Oncology (Huntingt) 2000;14:53. [PMID: 11195419]

WEB SITES

- JAMA patient page: Leukemia http://www.ama-assn.org/public/journals/patient/archive/pat0822.htm
- MEDLINEplus—Acute lymphocytic anemia http://www.nlm.nih.gov/medlineplus/ency/article/000541.htm

INFORMATION FOR PATIENTS

- Leukemia and Lymphoma Society, Inc. www.leukemia.org
- NCI leukemia homepage http://cancer.gov/cancerinfo/types/leukemia

REFERENCES

- Linker CA et al: Autologous stem cell transplantation for acute myeloid leukemia in first remission. Biol Blood Marrow Transplant 2000;6:50. [PMID: 10845900]
- Linker CA et al: Intensified and shortened cyclical chemotherapy for adult acute lymphoblastic leukemia. J Clin Oncol 2002; 20:2464. [PMID: 12011123]
- Tallman MS et al: Acute promyelocytic leukemia: evolving therapeutic strategies. Blood 2002;99:759. [PMID: 11806975]

Charles A. Linker, MD

Leukemia, Chronic Lymphocytic

 ## FEATURES

ESSENTIALS OF DIAGNOSIS

- Most patients asymptomatic at presentation
- Splenomegaly typical
- Lymphocytosis >5000/μL
- Mature appearance of lymphocytes
- Coexpression of CD19, CD5

GENERAL CONSIDERATIONS

- A clonal malignancy of B lymphocytes
- Usually indolent, with slowly progressive accumulation of long-lived small lymphocytes that are immunoincompetent
- Results in immunosuppression, bone marrow failure, and organ infiltration with lymphocytes
- Immunodeficiency also related to inadequate antibody production by abnormal B cells
- Prognostically useful staging system (Rai system): stage 0, lymphocytosis only; stage I, lymphocytosis plus lymphadenopathy; stage II, organomegaly; stage III, anemia; stage IV, thrombocytopenia

DEMOGRAPHICS

- Chronic lymphocytic leukemia (CLL) occurs mainly in older patients: 90% of cases occur at age >50 and median age at presentation is 65

 ## CLINICAL FINDINGS

SYMPTOMS AND SIGNS

- Incidentally discovered lymphocytosis in many
- Fatigue
- Lymphadenopathy in 80%
- Hepatomegaly or splenomegaly in 50%
- Occasionally, symptoms of hemolytic anemia or thrombocytopenia

DIFFERENTIAL DIAGNOSIS

- Atypical lymphocytosis of mononucleosis or pertussis
- Lymphoma in leukemic stage, especially mantle cell lymphoma
- Hairy cell leukemia

 ## DIAGNOSIS

LABORATORY TESTS

- Isolated lymphocytosis
- White blood cell count usually >20,000/μL and may be several hundred thousand
- Differential: usually 75–98% of circulating cells are lymphocytes
- Hematocrit and platelet count usually normal at presentation
- Autoimmune hemolytic anemia or thrombocytopenia present in 5–10%
- On peripheral smear, lymphocytes are small and mature, with condensed nuclear chromatin, and morphologically indistinguishable from normal small lymphocytes
- Larger and more immature cells in prolymphocytic leukemia (CLL variant)
- CLL is unusual in coexpressing B lymphocyte lineage marker CD19 with T lymphocyte marker CD5
- Hypogammaglobulinemia in half, becomes more common with advanced disease
- Serum protein electrophoresis: IgM paraprotein may be present in small amount

DIAGNOSTIC PROCEDURES

- Bone marrow is variably infiltrated with small lymphocytes
- Lymph node biopsy shows same pathological changes as in diffuse small cell lymphocytic lymphoma

TREATMENT

MEDICATIONS

- Fludarabine IV infusion 5 days a week once a month for 4–6 months is first-line therapy; avoid in autoimmune hemolytic anemia (may exacerbate)
- Chlorambucil, 0.6–1 mg/kg PO Q 3 weeks for ~6 months, is a convenient, well-tolerated, and usually effective alternative for older patients
- Fludarabine plus either rituximab or cyclophosphamide (or both) produces better response rates and complete response; improved remission duration or survival still uncertain
- Alemtuzumab for refractory CLL
- Prednisone for associated autoimmune hemolytic anemia or immune thrombocytopenia

SURGERY

- Splenectomy for associated autoimmune hemolytic anemia or immune thrombocytopenia

THERAPEUTIC PROCEDURES

- No specific therapy required in most cases of early indolent CLL
- Indications for treatment include progressive fatigue, symptomatic lymphadenopathy, or anemia or thrombocytopenia (symptomatic and progressive stage II disease or stage III/IV disease)
- Allogeneic transplantation potentially curative, but used only if CLL cannot be controlled by standard therapies
- Nonmyeloablative allogeneic transplantation is newer technique; may expand role of transplantation in CLL

OUTCOME

COMPLICATIONS

- Autoimmune hemolytic anemia or autoimmune thrombocytopenia in 5–10%
- Isolated lymph node transformation into aggressive large cell lymphoma (Richter's syndrome) despite stable systemic disease in ~5% of cases

PROGNOSIS

- CLL usually pursues an indolent course
- Overall, median survival is ~6 years, and 10-year survival is 25%
- Patients with stage 0 or stage I disease have median survival >10 years
- Patients with stage III or stage IV disease have median survival of <2 years
- Biological markers (eg, gene mutation status, CD38 expression, and cytogenetic abnormalities) useful in predicting outcomes of subsets of CLL patients
- Prolymphocytic leukemia, a variant of CLL, often pursues a more aggressive course

EVIDENCE

PRACTICE GUIDELINES

- Cheson BD et al: National Cancer Institute-sponsored Working Group guidelines for chronic lymphocytic leukemia: revised guidelines for diagnosis and treatment. Blood 1996;87:4990. [PMID: 8652811]
- Jacobs P et al: Chronic lymphocytic leukaemia—the haematologic basis for diagnosis and treatment. Hematology 2002;7(1):33. [PMID: 12171775]

WEB SITES

- Leukemia and Lymphoma Society, Inc. www.leukemia.org
- MEDLINEplus—Chronic lymphocytic leukemia http://www.nlm.nih.gov/medlineplus/ency/article/000532.htm
- NCI leukemia homepage http://cancer.gov/cancerinfo/types/leukemia

INFORMATION FOR PATIENTS

- Mayo Clinic—Chronic lymphocytic leukemia http://www.mayoclinic.com/invoke.cfm?objectid=8F1CFF9A-BA61-4A72-AA80F4031B87742C
- NCI—Chronic lymphocytic leukemia http://www.cancer.gov/cancerinfo/pdq/treatment/CLL/patient

REFERENCES

- Ghia P et al: The pattern of CD38 expression defines a distinct subset of chronic lymphocytic leukemia (CLL) patients at risk of disease progression. Blood 2003:101:1262. [PMID: 12406914]
- Rai KR et al: Fludarabine compared with chlorambucil as primary therapy for chronic lymphocytic leukemia. N Engl J Med 2000;343:1750. [PMID: 11114313]

Charles A. Linker, MD

Leukemia, Chronic Myelogenous

 KEY FEATURES

ESSENTIALS OF DIAGNOSIS

- Strikingly elevated white blood cell count
- Markedly left-shifted myeloid series but low percentage of promyelocytes and blasts
- Presence of Philadelphia chromosome or *bcr/abl* gene

GENERAL CONSIDERATIONS

- Myeloproliferative disorder characterized by overproduction of myeloid cells
- Associated with characteristic chromosomal abnormality, the Philadelphia chromosome, a reciprocal translocation between long arms of chromosomes 9 and 22
- Translocated portion of 9q contains *abl*, a protooncogene, which is received on 22q, at the break point cluster (bcr) site
- The fusion gene *bcr/abl* produces a novel protein that possesses tyrosine kinase activity, leading to leukemia
- Approximately 5% of cases are Philadelphia chromosome negative by light microscope cytogenetics, though molecular studies demonstrate *bcr/abl* fusion gene
- Entity formerly known as Philadelphia chromosome–negative chronic myelogenous leukemia (CML), now recognized as chronic myelomonocytic leukemia (CMML), a subtype of myelodysplasia
- "Chronic phase" of CML usually stable for years with normal bone marrow function
- Disease may progress to accelerated phase and after several years, to blast crisis
- Progression often associated with added chromosomal defects superimposed on Philadelphia chromosome
- Blast crisis CML is morphologically indistinguishable from acute leukemia

DEMOGRAPHICS

- CML occurs mainly in middle age; median age at presentation is 42 years

 CLINICAL FINDINGS

SYMPTOMS AND SIGNS

- Fatigue, night sweats, and low-grade fever
- Abdominal fullness related to splenomegaly
- Leukostasis clinical syndrome with blurred vision, respiratory distress, or priapism (rare)
- Splenomegaly (often marked)
- Sternal tenderness
- Fever in absence of infection, bone pain, and splenomegaly may mark disease acceleration
- Bleeding and infection related to bone marrow failure in blast crisis

DIFFERENTIAL DIAGNOSIS

- Reactive leukocytosis due to infection, inflammation, or cancer
- Other myeloproliferative disorder: essential thrombocytosis, polycythemia vera, or myelofibrosis

 DIAGNOSIS

LABORATORY TESTS

- Markedly elevated white blood cell (WBC) count; median WBC at diagnosis is 150,000/μL
- WBC usually >500,000/μL in rare cases of symptomatic leukostasis
- Peripheral blood smear: myeloid series left-shifted with mature forms dominating; blasts usually <5%
- Basophilia and eosinophilia may be present
- Hematocrit is usually normal at presentation
- Red blood cell (RBC) morphology normal; nucleated RBCs rarely seen
- Platelet count may be normal or elevated (sometimes strikingly elevated)
- Platelet morphology usually normal, but sometimes abnormally large forms
- The Philadelphia chromosome may be detected in peripheral blood or bone marrow
- The *bcr-abl* gene is reliably found in peripheral blood by molecular techniques
- Progressive anemia and thrombocytopenia occur in accelerated and blast phases, and percentage of blasts in blood and bone marrow increases

DIAGNOSTIC PROCEDURES

- Bone marrow aspirate and biopsy: hypercellular, with left-shifted myelopoiesis
- Myeloblasts comprise <5% of marrow cells in CML
- When blasts comprise >20% of bone marrow cells, blast phase of CML is diagnosed

TREATMENT

MEDICATIONS

- Imatinib mesylate (Gleevec), an inhibitor of tyrosine kinase activity of the *bcr-abl* oncogene, 400 mg PO QD, for chronic phase CML; well tolerated; most common toxicities are mild nausea, periorbital swelling, rash, and myalgia
- Hydroxyurea, 0.5–2.5 g PO QD, is an alternative if imatinib is not tolerated
- Hydroxyurea is given without interruption because of rapid WBC rebound and dose adjusted to keep WBC count >2000/μL and ideally near 5000/μL

THERAPEUTIC PROCEDURES

- Treatment usually not emergent even with WBC >200,000/μL
- Allogeneic bone marrow transplantation indicated if age <60 with HLA-matched sibling or if no cytogenetic response to imatinib after 6 months
- Chronic-phase disease, which recurs after allogeneic transplantation, can usually be reversed without additional chemotherapy by infusion of T lymphocytes from initial bone marrow donor
- Emergent leukapheresis is performed in conjunction with myelosuppressive therapy in rare instances of symptomatic leukostasis

OUTCOME

FOLLOW-UP

- Bone marrow cytogenetics after 6 months of imatinib treatment to assess hematological and cytogenetic remission

COMPLICATIONS

- Leukostasis clinical syndrome

PROGNOSIS

- Patients with major (<35% abnormal metaphases) or complete cytogenetic response appear to have excellent prognosis, with >95% remaining in control >2 years
- Long-term data not yet available
- In the past, median survival was 3–4 years
- With interferon-based therapies, median survival has increased to 5–6 years
- Imatinib mesylate results in hematologic control of chronic-phase disease in 98% of cases, and may lead to marked improvements in survival rates
- Allogeneic bone marrow transplantation produces overall long-term disease-free survival in 60%, and in 70–80% if patient age <40 and transplant occurs within 1 year after diagnosis
- Infusion of T lymphocytes from initial bone marrow donor in recurrent disease can produce long-term remission in 50–70%

EVIDENCE

PRACTICE GUIDELINES

- An evidence-based analysis of the effect of busulfan, hydroxyurea, interferon, and allogeneic bone marrow transplantation in treating the chronic phase of chronic myeloid leukemia. American Society of Hematology, 1999 http://www.guidelines.gov/summary/summary.aspx?doc_id=2363&nbr=1589&string=Chronic+myelogenous+leukemia
- Wetzler M: Chronic myelogenous leukemia. Cancer Control 2001;8(6 Suppl 2):44. [PMID: 11760557]

WEB SITES

- Leukemia and Lymphoma Society, Inc. www.leukemia.org
- NCI leukemia homepage http://cancer.gov/cancerinfo/types/leukemia

INFORMATION FOR PATIENTS

- MEDLINEplus—Chronic myelogenous leukemia http://www.nlm.nih.gov/medlineplus/ency/article/000570.htm
- NCI—Chronic myelogenous leukemia http://www.cancer.gov/cancerinfo/pdq/treatment/CML/patient

REFERENCES

- Kalidas M et al: Chronic myelogenous leukemia. JAMA 2001;286:895. [PMID: 11509034]
- Or R et al: Nonmyeloablative allogeneic stem cell transplantation for the treatment of chronic myeloid leukemia in first chronic phase. Blood 2003;101:441. [PMID: 12393604]
- Peggs K et al: Imatinib mesylate—the new gold standard for treatment of chronic myeloid leukemia. N Engl J Med 2003;348:1048. [PMID: 12637616]

Charles A. Linker, MD

Leukemia, Hairy Cell

 KEY FEATURES

ESSENTIALS OF DIAGNOSIS

- Pancytopenia
- Splenomegaly, often massive
- Hairy cells present on blood smear and especially in bone marrow biopsy

GENERAL CONSIDERATIONS

- Indolent cancer of B lymphocytes
- An uncommon form of leukemia

DEMOGRAPHICS

- Characteristically presents in middle-aged men
- Median age at presentation is 55 years
- Striking 5:1 male predominance

 CLINICAL FINDINGS

SYMPTOMS AND SIGNS

- Gradual onset of fatigue
- Symptoms related to markedly enlarged spleen
- Increased susceptibility to infection
- Splenomegaly almost invariably present and may be massive
- Hepatomegaly in 50% of cases
- Lymphadenopathy uncommon

DIFFERENTIAL DIAGNOSIS

- Myelofibrosis
- Chronic lymphocytic leukemia
- Waldenström's macroglobulinemia
- Non-Hodgkin's lymphoma
- Aplastic anemia
- Other cause of bone marrow infiltration, eg, metastatic cancer, infection

 DIAGNOSIS

LABORATORY TESTS

- Pancytopenia
- Anemia nearly universal
- Thrombocytopenia and neutropenia in 75% of patients
- Striking monocytopenia in nearly all, which is encountered in almost no other condition
- Peripheral blood smear: "hairy cells," with numerous characteristic cytoplasmic projections, usually present in small numbers
- Hairy cells have characteristic histochemical staining pattern, with tartrate-resistant acid phosphatase
- Hairy cells coexpress CD11c and CD22 on immunophenotyping

DIAGNOSTIC PROCEDURES

- Bone marrow aspirate: usually inaspirable (dry tap)
- Bone marrow biopsy establishes diagnosis made by characteristic morphology
- Pathological examination of spleen shows marked infiltration of red pulp with hairy cells (in contrast to usual predilection of lymphomas to involve white pulp)

TREATMENT

MEDICATIONS

- Cladribine (2-chlorodeoxyadenosine; CdA), 0.14 mg/kg daily for 7 days; relatively nontoxic; produces benefit in 95% of cases
- Treatment with pentostatin produces similar results, but more cumbersome to administer

 OUTCOME

PROGNOSIS

- Hairy cell leukemia usually indolent disorder; course dominated by pancytopenia and recurrent infections, including mycobacterial infections
- Formerly, median survival was 6 years, and only one-third survived >10 years
- Development of new therapies has changed the prognosis
- Now, most live >10 years
- With current trends in treatment, prognosis appears open-ended at this time
- Cladribine produces complete remission in >80%; response long-lasting, with few patients relapsing in first few years

 EVIDENCE

PRACTICE GUIDELINES

- Mey U et al: Advances in the treatment of hairy-cell leukaemia. Lancet Oncol 2003;4:86. [PMID: 12573350]
- Pettitt AR et al: Hairy-cell leukaemia: biology and management. Br J Haematol 1999;106:2. [PMID: 10444156]
- Seshadri P et al: Hairy cell leukemia: treatment prospects. Expert Rev Anticancer Ther 2001;1:91. [PMID: 12113139]

WEB SITES

- American Cancer Society—Treatment of hairy cell leukemia http://www.cancer.org/docroot/CRI/content/CRI_2_4_4X_Treatment_of_Hairy_Cell_Leukemia_HCL_62.asp?sitearea=
- Leukemia and Lymphoma Society, Inc. www.leukemia.org
- NCI leukemia homepage http://cancer.gov/cancerinfo/types/leukemia

INFORMATION FOR PATIENTS

- MEDLINEplus—Hairy cell leukemia http://www.nlm.nih.gov/medlineplus/ency/article/000592.htm
- NCI—Hairy cell leukemia http://newscenter.cancer.gov/cancerinfo/pdq/treatment/hairy-cell-leukemia/patient

REFERENCES

- Flinn IW et al: Long-term follow-up for remission duration, mortality, and second malignancies in hairy cell leukemia patients treated with pentostatin. Blood 2000;96:2981. [PMID: 11049974]
- Kreitman RJ et al: Efficacy of the anti-CD22 recombinant immunotoxin BL22 in chemotherapy-resistant hairy-cell leukemia. N Engl J Med 2001;345:241. [PMID: 11474661]

Charles A. Linker, MD

Leukoplakia & Erythroplakia

 KEY FEATURES

ESSENTIALS OF DIAGNOSIS

Leukoplakia

- A white lesion that, unlike oral candidiasis, cannot be removed by rubbing the mucosal surface

Erythroplakia

- Similar to leukoplakia except that it has a definite erythematous component

Oral lichen planus

- Most commonly presents as lacy leukoplakia, but may be erosive; definitive diagnosis requires biopsy

Oral cancer

- Early lesions appear as leukoplakia or erythroplakia; more advanced lesions will be larger, with invasion into tongue such that a mass lesion is palpable; ulceration may be present

GENERAL CONSIDERATIONS

Leukoplakia

- About 5% represent either dysplasia or early invasive squamous cell carcinoma
- Histologically, there is often hyperkeratoses, occurring in response to chronic irritation

Erythroplakia

- Distinction from leukoplakia is important, since about 90% of cases of erythroplakia are either dysplasia or carcinoma

Oral lichen planus

- An inflammatory pruritic disease of the skin and mucous membranes
- Mucosal lichen planus must be differentiated from leukoplakia
- Erosive oral lesions require biopsy and often direct immunofluorescence for diagnosis since lichen planus may simulate other erosive diseases
- There may be a low risk (1%) of squamous cell carcinoma arising within lichen planus

DEMOGRAPHICS

- Alcohol and tobacco use are the major etiological risk factors for oral carcinoma

 CLINICAL FINDINGS

SYMPTOMS AND SIGNS

- Intraoral examination (lateral tongue, floor of the mouth, gingiva, buccal area, palate, and tonsillar fossae) and palpation of the neck for enlarged lymph nodes in patients over 45 who smoke tobacco or drink immoderately

Leukoplakia

- Any white lesion that, unlike oral candidiasis, cannot be removed by rubbing the mucosal surface
- Usually small

Erythroplakia

- A white lesion with an erythematous component that cannot be removed by rubbing the mucosal surface

Oral lichen planus

- Lacy leukoplakia, but may be erosive
- Reticular pattern mimics candidiasis
- Erosive pattern mimics carcinoma

Oral cancer

- Early lesions appear as leukoplakia or erythroplakia; advanced lesions larger
- Invasion into tongue leads to palpable mass; ulceration may be present
- Biopsy essential for diagnosis
- Metastases to submandibular and jugulodiastric neck nodes are common

DIFFERENTIAL DIAGNOSIS

Oral leukoplakia

- Hyperkeratosis due to irritation
- Dysplasia or carcinoma
- Lichen planus
- Oral candidiasis
- Oral hairy leukoplakia

Erythroplakia

- Dysplasia or carcinoma
- Necrotizing sialometaplasia (when on hard palate)
- Ulcerative lichen planus

Oral lichen planus

- Oral cancer
- Candidiasis
- Erythema multiforme
- Pemphigus vulgaris
- Bullous pemphigoid
- Inflammatory bowel disease

 DIAGNOSIS

IMAGING STUDIES

- If squamous cell carcinoma is suspected, then metastatic evaluation of neck and imaging deep extent in oral cavity is warranted
- May include PET and MRI

DIAGNOSTIC PROCEDURES

- Any erythroplakic or enlarging leukoplakic area, and any mass lesion, should have an incisional biopsy or an exfoliative cytological examination
- Intraoral staining with 1% toluidine blue may aid in selection of the most suspicious biopsy site
- Fine-needle aspiration biopsy may be indicated if an enlarged lymph node is found

TREATMENT

MEDICATIONS

Lichen planus

- Therapy for confirmed diagnoses is management of pain
- Local and if needed systemic steroids are widely used

SURGERY

Oral cancer

- Small lesions are best treated surgically, often with a laser; if the tumor invades more than a few millimeters into the tongue then consideration of the neck is important
- Larger tumors of the oral cavity are usually treated wth resection of the primary tumor, neck dissection, and postoperative irradiation
- Reconstruction when needed is done at the time of initial surgery
  - Vascularized free flaps, with bone if needed, are commonly used
  - Myocutaneous flaps may also be used

THERAPEUTIC PROCEDURES

- Small lesions may be treated with radiation therapy (external beam, often supplemented with an implant)
- Intraoral radiation is associated with dry mouth (xerostomia) and a low risk of osteoradionecrosis of the mandible
- Use of radiation limits future treatment options as a curative dose of radiation cannot be used again within the treatment field
- Tumors of the tonsillar fossa and base of tongue are usually best treated with radiation, often with concomitant chemotherapy, reserving surgery for salvage

OUTCOME

FOLLOW-UP

- Leukoplakia, erythroplakia, lichen planus, and oral cancer require monitoring; early diagnosis of recurrent squamous cell carcinoma or a new primary lesion is key to management
- Commonly a patient with a prior malignancy is examined every 4–6 weeks in the first year, every 8–10 weeks in the second year, and every 3–4 months thereafter for several additional years; the incidence of second tumors is about 3–4% annually, likely associated with the prior use of tobacco and/or alcohol
- Periodic PET scans and baseline posttreatment MRIs are used by many in subsequent tumor surveillance

COMPLICATIONS

- Failure to recognize early tumors contributes to the need for more extensive intervention

PROGNOSIS

- Squamous cell carcinoma that invades less than 4–5 mm into the tongue has a <10% rate of nodal metastasis
- Floor of mouth and alveolar ridge are associated with neck metastases
- Base of tongue and tonsillar fossa are usually associated with nodal metastases; late distant metastases may occur in as many as 30%
- Early-stage tumors (<2 cm without nodal involvment) have cure rates above 90%

WHEN TO REFER

- Specialty referral should be sought early both for diagnosis and treatment
- Consider indirect or fiberoptic examination of the nasopharynx, oropharynx, hypopharynx, and larynx by an otolaryngologist-head and neck surgeon when there is oral erythroplakia, unexplained throat or ear pain, or unexplained oral or nasal bleeding.

PREVENTION

- Smoking cessation and alcohol abatement programs

EVIDENCE

PRACTICE GUIDELINES

- National Guideline Clearinghouse. http://www.guideline.gov/summary/summary.aspx?doc_id=3287&nbr=2513&string=leukoplakia

WEB SITES

- Ear, Nose, and Throat Information Center http://www.netdoor.com/entinfo/
- Otolaryngology Resources on the Internet http://www.bcm.tmc.edu/oto/othersa.html

INFORMATION FOR PATIENTS

- Leukoplakia Patient/Family Resources. http://unthsc-dl.slis.ua.edu/patientinfo/oral/oral-mucosa/leukoplakia.htm

REFERENCES

- Chan ES et al: Intervention for treating oral lichen planus. Cochrane Database Syst Rev 2000;CD001168. [PMID: 1079661]
- Sudbo J et al: DNA content as a prognostic marker in patients with oral leukoplakia. N Engl J Med 2001;344: 1270. [PMID: 11320386]

Robert K. Jackler, MD
Michael J. Kaplan, MD

Lichen Planus

 KEY FEATURES

ESSENTIALS OF DIAGNOSIS

- Pruritic, violaceous, flat-topped papules with fine white streaks and symmetric distribution
- Lacy lesions of the buccal mucosa
- Commonly seen along linear scratch marks (Koebner phenomenon) on anterior wrists, penis, legs
- Histopathological examination is diagnostic

GENERAL CONSIDERATIONS

- An inflammatory pruritic disease of the skin and mucous membranes characterized by distinctive papules with a predilection for the flexor surfaces and trunk
- The three cardinal findings are typical skin lesions, mucosal lesions, and histopathological features of band-like infiltration of lymphocytes and melanophages in the dermis

Oral lichen planus

- A relatively common (0.5–2% of the population) chronic inflammatory autoimmune disease
- May be difficult to diagnose clinically because of its numerous distinct phenotypic subtypes, eg, the reticular pattern may mimic candidiasis or hyperkeratosis, while the erosive pattern may mimic squamous cell carcinoma
- There is probably a low rate (1%) of squamous cell carcinoma arising within lichen planus (in addition to the possibility of clinical misdiagnosis)
- Drugs causing lichen planus–like reactions include gold, streptomycin, tetracycline, iodides, chloroquine, quinacrine, quinidine, nonsteroidal antiinflammatory drugs, phenothiazines, and hydrochlorothiazide
- Hepatitis C infection is found with greater frequency in lichen planus patients than in controls in Europe and the United States
- A benign disease, but it may persist for months or years and may be recurrent

 CLINICAL FINDINGS

SYMPTOMS AND SIGNS

- Itching is mild to severe
- The lesions are violaceous, flat-topped, angulated papules, 1–4 mm in diameter, discrete or in clusters, with very fine white streaks on the surface (Wickham's striae) on the flexor surfaces of the wrists and on the penis, lips, tongue, and buccal and vaginal mucous membranes
- In the oral mucosa lichen planus may be confused with leukoplakia
- Mucosal lichen planus in the oral, genital, and anorectal areas may be erosive and painful
- The papules may become bullous
- The disease may be generalized
- The Koebner phenomenon (appearance of lesions in areas of trauma) may be seen

DIFFERENTIAL DIAGNOSIS

- Lichenoid drug eruption
- Psoriasis
- Lichen simplex chronicus
- Secondary syphilis
- Pityriasis rosea
- Discoid lupus erythematosus
- Graft-versus-host disease
- Mucosal lesions: leukoplakia, candidiasis, erythema multiforme, pemphigus vulgaris, bullous pemphigoid, lichen sclerosus
- Lichen planus on the mucous membranes must be differentiated from leukoplakia; erosive oral lesions require biopsy and often direct immunofluorescence for diagnosis since lichen planus may simulate other erosive diseases

 DIAGNOSIS

LABORATORY TESTS

- Confirmed by biopsy showing a band-like infiltration of lymphocytes and melanophages in the dermis

TREATMENT

MEDICATIONS

Topical therapy

- See Table 6 (page 1199)
- Superpotent topical corticosteroid ointments applied twice daily are most helpful for localized disease in nonflexural areas; alternatively, high-potency corticosteroid cream or ointment may be used nightly under thin pliable plastic film
- Examples are betamethasone dipropionate in optimized vehicle, diflorasone diacetate, clobetasol propionate, and halobetasol propionate
- Tretinoin cream 0.05%: applied to mucosal lichen planus, followed by a corticosteroid ointment, may be helpful
- Topical tacrolimus: appears effective in oral and vaginal erosive lichen planus, but chronic therapy is required to prevent relapse; concern regarding absorption suggests monitoring blood counts when treating mucosal lesions

Systemic therapy

- Corticosteroids may be required in severe cases, or where the most rapid response to treatment is desired
- Unfortunately, relapse almost always occurs as the steroids are tapered
- Isotretinoin and acitretin by mouth appear to be effective in some cases of oral and cutaneous lichen planus
- Psoralens plus long-wave ultraviolet light (PUVA)

 OUTCOME

PROGNOSIS

- Benign disease, but it may persist for months or years
- May be recurrent
- Hypertrophic lichen planus and oral lesions tend to be especially persistent, and neoplastic degeneration has been described in chronically eroded lesions

WHEN TO REFER

- If there is a question about the diagnosis, if recommended therapy is ineffective, or specialized treatment is necessary

 EVIDENCE

PRACTICE GUIDELINES

- Mignogna MD et al: Clinical guidelines in early detection of oral squamous cell carcinoma arising in oral lichen planus: a 5-year experience. Oral Oncol 2001;37:262.

WEB SITES

- American Academy of Dermatology http://www.aad.org
- Dermatology Handbook for Family Practice from the University of Iowa http://www.vh.org/Providers/ClinRef/FPHandbook/17.html

INFORMATION FOR PATIENTS

- American Academy of Dermatology http://www.aad.org/pamphlets/lichen.html
- National Institutes of Health http://www.nlm.nih.gov/medlineplus/ency/article/000867.htm

REFERENCES

- Katta R: Lichen planus. Am Fam Physician 2000;61:3319. [PMID: 10865927]
- Mignogna MD et al: Oral lichen planus: different clinical features in HCV-positive and HCV-negative patients. Int J Dermatol 2000;39:134. [PMID: 10692063]

Timothy G. Berger, MD

Lichen Simplex Chronicus

KEY FEATURES

ESSENTIALS OF DIAGNOSIS

- Chronic itching
- Dry, leathery, hypertrophic, lichenified plaques appear on the neck, ankles, perineum, or almost anywhere

GENERAL CONSIDERATIONS

- A self-perpetuating scratch-itch cycle
- Intermittent itching incites the patient to scratch the lesions
- Itching may be so intense as to interfere with sleep

CLINICAL FINDINGS

SYMPTOMS AND SIGNS

- See Table 7 (page 1202)
- Lichenified lesions with exaggerated skin lines overlying a thickened, well-circumscribed scaly plaque
- Predilection for nape of neck, wrists, external surfaces of forearms, lower legs, popliteal and antecubital areas, scrotum, and vulva
- The patches are rectangular, thickened, and pigmented
- This disorder can be differentiated from plaque-like lesions such as psoriasis (redder lesions having whiter scales on the elbows, knees, and scalp and nail findings), lichen planus (violaceous, usually smaller polygonal papules), and nummular (coin-shaped) dermatitis; similar lesions are seen in chronic atopic dermatitis

DIFFERENTIAL DIAGNOSIS

- Psoriasis
- Lichen planus
- Atopic dermatitis (eczema)
- Nummular eczema (nummular dermatitis)
- Tinea corporis

DIAGNOSIS

LABORATORY TESTS

- Clinical diagnosis

TREATMENT

MEDICATIONS

- See Table 6 (page 1199)

Topical corticosteroids

- Clobetasol, halobetasol, diflorasone, and betamethasone dipropionate in augmented vehicle are effective without occlusion and are used twice daily for several weeks
- In some patients, flurandrenolide (Cordran) tape may be more effective, since it prevents scratching and rubbing of the lesion
- These superpotent steroids are probably the treatment of choice but must be used with careful follow-up to avoid local side effects
- The injection of triamcinolone acetonide suspension (5–10 mg/mL) into the lesions may occasionally be curative

THERAPEUTIC PROCEDURES

- Use of tars, such as 10% LCD (liquor carbonis detergens) in triamcinolone 0.1% ointment, or continuous occlusion with DuoDerm (occlusive flexible hydrocolloid dressing) for 7 days at a time for 1–2 months, may also be helpful; the area should be protected and the patient encouraged to become aware of when he or she is scratching

 OUTCOME

PROGNOSIS

- The disease tends to remit during treatment but may recur or develop at another site

WHEN TO REFER

- If there is a question about the diagnosis, if recommended therapy is ineffective, or specialized treatment is necessary

 EVIDENCE

WEB SITES

- American Academy of Dermatology http://www.aad.org
- Dermatology Handbook for Family Practice from the University of Iowa http://www.vh.org/Providers/ClinRef/FPHandbook/17.html

INFORMATION FOR PATIENTS

- American Academy of Family Physicians http://familydoctor.org/flowcharts/545.html

REFERENCE

- Novick CL: Unilateral, circumscribed, chronic dermatitis of the papillary-areolar complex: case report and review of the literature. Mt Sinai J Med 2001;68:321.

Timothy G. Berger, MD

Lipid Abnormalities

 ## KEY FEATURES

ESSENTIALS OF DIAGNOSIS

- Elevated serum total cholesterol or low-density lipoprotein (LDL) cholesterol, low serum high-density lipoprotein (HDL) cholesterol, or elevated serum triglycerides
- Usually asymptomatic
- In severe cases associated with metabolic abnormalities, superficial lipid deposition occurs

GENERAL CONSIDERATIONS

- Cholesterol and triglycerides are the two main circulating lipids
- Elevated levels of LDL cholesterol are associated with increased risk of atherosclerotic heart disease
- High levels of HDL cholesterol are associated with lower risk of atherosclerotic heart disease
- The exact mechanism by which LDL and HDL affect atherosclerosis is not fully delineated
- Familial genetic disorders are an uncommon, but often lethal cause, of elevated cholesterol
- Familial genetic disorders should be considered in patients who have onset of atherosclerosis in their 20s or 30s

DEMOGRAPHICS

- Nearly 20% of all adults have elevated serum total cholesterol
- More common in men than women before age 50
- More common in women than men after age 50
- More common in whites and Hispanics than among blacks
- Up to 25% of Americans have a "metabolic syndrome" that consists of a large waist circumference, elevated triglycerides, low HDL cholesterol, elevated blood pressure, and elevated serum glucose

 ## CLINICAL FINDINGS

SYMPTOMS AND SIGNS

- Usually asymptomatic
- Extremely high levels of chylomicrons or VLDL particles are associated with eruptive xanthomas
- Very high LDL levels are associated with tendinous xanthomas
- Very high triglycerides (>2000) are associated with lipemia retinalis (cream-colored vessels in the fundus)

DIFFERENTIAL DIAGNOSIS

- See Table 113 (page 1294)

Hypercholesterolemia (cholesterol, elevated)

- Idiopathic
- Hypothyroidism
- Nephrotic syndrome
- Chronic renal insufficiency
- Obstructive liver disease
- Diabetes mellitus
- Anorexia nervosa
- Cushing's syndrome
- Familial, eg, familial hypercholesterolemia
- Drugs: oral contraceptives, thiazides (short-term effect), β-blockers (short-term effect), corticosteroids, cyclosporine

Hypertriglyceridemia (triglycerides, elevated)

- Alcohol
- Obesity
- "Metabolic syndrome" (insulin resistance, low HDL)
- Diabetes mellitus
- Chronic renal insufficiency
- Lipodystrophy, eg, protease inhibitors
- Pregnancy
- Familial
- Drugs: oral contraceptives, isotretinoin, thiazides (short-term effect), β-blockers (short-term effect), corticosteroids, bile-acid binding resins

 ## DIAGNOSIS

- Screen for lipid disorders in
  - Patients with coronary heart disease, peripheral vascular disease, aortic aneurysm, or carotid artery disease
  - Men >35 years old and women >45 years old if asymptomatic or no striking family history
  - Obtain fasting serum total cholesterol, HDL cholesterol, and triglyceride levels
  - LDL cholesterol can be estimated by the following formula: LDL cholesterol = (Total cholesterol) − (HDL) − (Triglycerides/5)
- Serum thyroid-stimulating hormone to screen for hypothyroidism
- Other tests only as indicated by symptoms and signs suggestive of a secondary cause

DIAGNOSTIC PROCEDURES

- LDL cholesterol (mg/dL) is classified into 5 categories: optimal, <100; near optimal, 100–129; borderline high, 130–159; high, 160–189; very high, ≥190

TREATMENT

MEDICATIONS

- See Table 115 (page 1295)
- Choice of whether to initiate drug therapy should be based on overall risk profile and LDL cholesterol level
- LDL cholesterol threshold for treatment depends on risk factors
- Presence of CHD, diabetes, or peripheral vascular disease requires most aggressive therapy
- Presence of 2 or more risk factors, including smoking, hypertension, older age, and family history of CHD, requires treatment at LDL ≥130 mg/dL
- Presence of 1 or no risk factors requires treatment above LDL ≥160 mg/dL
- See Table 114 (page 1294)
- **HMG-CoA reductase inhibitors** (statins) have good impact on LDL, minimal impact on HDL; best data for reducing coronary events, mortality
- **Niacin** has a moderate impact on LDL, moderate impact on HDL; reduces triglycerides and has mortality benefit; high rates of intolerance, which can be improved with concomitant aspirin use
- **Bile acid binding resins** (eg, cholestyramine) have a moderate impact on LDL, minimal impact on HDL; reduce coronary events, but not mortality; mainly gastrointestinal side effects and can block the absorption of fat-soluble vitamins; safe in pregnancy
- **Fibric acid derivatives** (eg, gemfibrozil) have a moderate impact on LDL, moderate impact on HDL, and reduce triglycerides; reduce coronary events, but not mortality; side effects increased when taken with statins

THERAPEUTIC PROCEDURES

- For hypercholesterolemia, low-fat diets may produce a moderate (5–10%) decrease in LDL cholesterol
- Low-fat diet may also lower HDL cholesterol
- Substituting monounsaturated fats for saturated fats can lower LDL without affecting HDL
- In diabetics, control of hyperglycemia can improve lipid profile
- Exercise and moderate alcohol consumption can increase HDL levels
- For hypertriglyceridemia, primary therapy is dietary, including reducing alcohol, reducing fatty foods, and controlling hyperglycemia in diabetics

 OUTCOME

FOLLOW-UP

- Fasting lipid pane 3–6 months after initiation of therapy
- Annual or biannual screening depending on risk factors
- Monitoring for side effects of therapy, such as liver enzyme or myopathy in those on statins

COMPLICATIONS

- Atherosclerotic: myocardial infarction, stroke, and other vascular diseases
- Nonatherosclerotic: xanthomas and pancreatitis
- "Metabolic syndrome" patients are at increased risk of cardiovascular events
- Very high triglyceride levels (fasting TG >500 mg/dL) increase the risk of pancreatitis

WHEN TO REFER

- Refer patients with evidence of genetic disorders such as very high LDL or triglycerides to a lipid specialist

WHEN TO ADMIT

- Acute pancreatitis

EVIDENCE

- Executive summary of The Third Report of the National Cholesterol Education Program (NCEP) Expert Panel on Detection, Evaluation, and Treatment of High Blood Cholesterol in Adults. JAMA 2001; 285:2486. www.nhlbi.nih.gov/guidelines/cholesterol/index
- Lipid management in adults. Institute for Clinical Systems Improvement, 2002 http://www.icsi.org/knowledge/detail.asp?catID=29&itemID=197
- Lipid screening in adults. Institute for Clinical Systems Improvement, 2000 http://www.icsi.org/knowledge/detail.asp?catID=29&itemID=177

WEB SITES

- American Heart Association http://www.americanheart.org/presenter.jhtml?identifier=740
- American Academy of Family Physicians—Cholesterol: what you can do to lower your level http://familydoctor.org/healthfacts/029/

INFORMATION FOR PATIENTS

- American Association for Clinical Chemistry—Lipid profile http://www.labtestsonline.org/understanding/analytes/lipid/glance.html
- High blood cholesterol: What you need to know. Created by the National Cholesterol Education Program www.nhlbi.nih.gov/health/public/heart/chol/wyntk.pdf
- JAMA patient page: What you should know about cholesterol http://www.hmc.psu.edu/healthinfo/articles/cholesterol.pdf
- MEDLINEplus—Lipid disorders acquired http://www.nlm.nih.gov/medlineplus/ency/article/000403.htm

REFERENCE

- Choice of lipid-regulating drugs. Med Lett Drugs Ther 2001;43:43. [PMID: 11378632]

Robert B. Baron, MS, MD

Liver Abscess, Pyogenic

 ## KEY FEATURES

ESSENTIALS OF DIAGNOSIS

- Fever, right upper quadrant pain, jaundice
- Often in setting of biliary disease but up to 40% cryptogenic abscesses are seen on imaging study

GENERAL CONSIDERATIONS

- The liver can be invaded by bacteria via the portal vein (pylephlebitis); the common duct (ascending cholangitis); the hepatic artery, secondary to bacteremia; direct extension from an infectious process; and traumatic implantation of bacteria through the abdominal wall
- Ascending cholangitis resulting from biliary obstruction due to a stone, stricture, or neoplasm is the most common identifiable cause of hepatic abscess in the United States
- In 10% of cases, liver abscess is secondary to appendicitis or diverticulitis
- Up to 40% of abscesses have no demonstrable cause and are classified as cryptogenic. A dental source is identified in some such cases
- The most frequently encountered organisms are *Escherichia coli, Proteus vulgaris, Enterobacter aerogenes, Klebsiella pneumoniae,* and multiple anaerobic species. *Staphylococcus aureus* is usually the causative organism in chronic granulomatous disease
- Hepatic candidiasis is seen in immunocompromised patients and those with hematological malignancies
- Rarely, hepatocellular carcinoma can present as a pyogenic abscess because of tumor necrosis, biliary obstruction, and superimposed bacterial infection
- The possibility of an amebic liver abscess must always be considered

 ## CLINICAL FINDINGS

SYMPTOMS AND SIGNS

- The presentation is often insidious
- Fever is almost always present and may antedate other symptoms or signs
- Pain may be a prominent complaint and is localized to the right hypochondrium or epigastric area
- Jaundice, tenderness in the right upper abdomen, and either steady or swinging fever are the chief physical findings

DIFFERENTIAL DIAGNOSIS

- Cholecystitis
- Cholangitis
- Acute hepatitis
- Amebic liver abscess
- Appendicitis
- Right lower lobe pneumonia
- Pancreatitis
- Echinococcosis (hydatid disease)
- Liver mass, eg, hepatocellular carcinoma

 ## DIAGNOSIS

LABORATORY TESTS

- Leukocytosis with a shift to the left
- Liver function studies are nonspecifically abnormal

IMAGING STUDIES

- Chest roentgenograms usually reveal elevation of the diaphragm if the abscess is on the right side
- Ultrasound, CT, or MRI may reveal the presence of intrahepatic defects
- On MRI, characteristic findings include high signal intensity on T2-weighted images and rim enhancement
- Hepatic candidiasis is seen usually in the setting of systemic candidiasis, and on CT scan the characteristic appearance is that of multiple "bulls-eyes," but imaging studies may be negative in neutropenic patients

Liver Abscess, Pyogenic

 ## TREATMENT

MEDICATIONS

- Use antimicrobial agents (a third-generation cephalosporin and metronidazole) that are effective against coliform organisms and anaerobes
- Hepatic candidiasis often responds to intravenous amphotericin B (total dose of 2–9 g)

SURGERY

- If the abscess is at least 5 cm in diameter or the response to antibiotic therapy is not rapid, catheter or surgical (eg, laparoscopic) drainage should be undertaken
- Fungal abscesses require drainage

 ## OUTCOME

PROGNOSIS

- The mortality rate is still substantial (≥8%) and is highest in underlying biliary malignancy or severe multiorgan dysfunction
- Fungal abscesses are associated with mortality rates of up to 50%

WHEN TO ADMIT

- All patients

 ## EVIDENCE

PRACTICE GUIDELINES

- National Guideline Clearinghouse http://www.guideline.gov/summary/summary.aspx?doc_id=3258&nbr=2484&string=liver+abscess

PATIENT INFORMATION

- National Instititues of Health http://www.nlm.nih.gov/medlineplus/ency/article/000261.htm

REFERENCE

- Ng FH et al: Sequential intravenous/oral antibiotic vs. continuous intravenous antibiotic in the treatment of pyogenic liver abscess. Aliment Pharmacol Ther 2002;16:1083.

Lawrence S. Friedman, MD

Loiasis

 KEY FEATURES

ESSENTIALS OF DIAGNOSIS

- Worms make temporary appearances beneath the skin, eyes, or by Calabar swellings
- Calabar swellings are subcutaneous edematous reactions (up to 10 cm) to the worms and may migrate or be stationary

GENERAL CONSIDERATIONS

- This filarial disease is caused by infection with *Loa loa*
- The adult worms live in the subcutaneous tissues for up to 12 years
- Gravid females release microfilariae into the bloodstream, which subsequently are ingested in a blood meal by the vector-intermediate host, female chrysops species, day-biting flies. When the fly feeds again, the larval stage can infect a new host or cause superinfection
- The time to worm maturity and detection of new microfilariae is 6 months to several years

DEMOGRAPHICS

- The infection occurs in humans and monkeys in rain and swamp forest areas of West Africa from Nigeria to Angola and throughout the Congo River watershed of central Africa eastward to southwestern Sudan and western Uganda
- An estimated 3–13 million persons are infected

 CLINICAL FINDINGS

SYMPTOMS AND SIGNS

- Many infected persons are asymptomatic
- In symptomatic persons, the worms (females, 4–7 cm × 0.5 mm) are evidenced by their temporary appearance beneath the skin or conjunctiva, by unilateral edema of an extremity, or by Calabar swellings
- Natives generally have a mild form of the infection or are asymptomatic. The disease among visitors, however, is often characterized by more pronounced frequent and debilitating Calabar swellings

Calabar swellings

- Subcutaneous edematous reactions, 3–10 cm in diameter, nonpitting and nonerythematous
- At times associated with low-grade fever, local pain, and pruritus
- The swellings may migrate a few centimeters for 2–3 days or stay in place before they subside
- At irregular intervals, they recur at the same or different sites, but only one appears at a time
- When near joints, they may be temporarily disabling
- Migration across the eye may be asymptomatic or may produce pain, intense conjunctivitis, and eyelid edema
- Dying adult worms may elicit small nodules or local sterile abscesses, and dead worms may result in radiologically detectable calcification

Microfilariae

- Do not induce symptoms if in the blood
- Rarely they enter the central nervous system and may cause encephalitis, myelitis, or jacksonian seizures
- Can also induce lesions and complications in the retina, heart, lungs, kidneys, and other tissues

DIFFERENTIAL DIAGNOSIS

- Dracunculiasis
- Cutaneous larva migrans
- Gnathostomiasis
- Myiasis
- Filariasis
- Onchocerciasis (river blindness)
- Bacterial pyoderma
- Cysticercosis (with ophthalmic involvement)

 DIAGNOSIS

LABORATORY TESTS

- Specific diagnosis is made by finding characteristic microfilariae in daytime (10 AM to 4 PM) blood specimens by concentration methods; in order of increasing sensitivity, they are thick films, Knott's concentration, and Nuclepore filtration
- Presumptive diagnosis that permits treatment is based on Calabar swellings or eye migration, a history of residence in an endemic area, and marked eosinophilia (40% or greater)
- Serological tests may be positive, but cross-reactions occur with other filarial diseases and sometimes with nematode infections
- A polymerase chain reaction test, highly sensitive and specific, can detect the organism in some amicrofilaremic persons
- Natives generally are microfilaremic and serologically positive. Visitors often have more pronounced immunologically mediated findings (elevated leukocyte and eosinophil counts, hypergammaglobulinemia, increased polyclonal IgE) and frequently a positive serological test but nondetectable microfilaremia

TREATMENT

MEDICATIONS

- See specialized sources for details on proper use of **diethylcarbamazine** (drug of choice both as a micro- and macrofilaricide), since side effects to dying microfilariae may be severe, and life-threatening encephalitis can occur rarely. The dosage is 50 mg once (Day 1), 50 mg three times daily (Day 2), 100 mg three times daily (Day 3), and 3 mg/kg three times daily (Days 4–21)
- One course of treatment cures about 50% of patients; three courses, 90%
- Reactions are more likely with pretreatment microfilaria counts greater than 25/μL
- Prednisone is sometimes indicated in heavily infected persons to minimize reactions
- In the United States, diethylcarbamazine is available only from the Parasitic Diseases Drug Service, Centers for Disease Control and Prevention, Atlanta, GA 30333, telephone 404-639-3670

SURGERY

- Surgical removal of adult worms from the eye or skin is not recommended

THERAPEUTIC PROCEDURES

- Cytapheresis has been used to reduce parasite loads before starting diethylcarbamazine

 OUTCOME

COMPLICATIONS

- When ivermectin was used in treatment of 1.1 million persons with onchocerciasis in the presence of endemic loiasis, 28 neurological reactions occurred (some severe) from death of *Loa loa* microfilariae. The risk of these reactions was high when the *L loa* microfilaria load exceeded 8/μL and very high above 50/μL; albendazole at a dosage of 200 mg twice daily for 3 weeks is being evaluated as a safe way to reduce the level of *L loa* microfilariae

PROGNOSIS

- Most infections run a benign course, but some are accompanied by severe and temporarily disabling symptoms
- The prognosis is excellent with treatment

WHEN TO REFER

- Refer symptomatic patients to a specialist with expertise in this problem
- Refer all patients with ocular symptoms to an ophthalmologist

WHEN TO ADMIT

- Patients with debilitating Calabar swellings

PREVENTION

- Individual protection is facilitated by daytime use of insect repellent and by wearing light-colored clothing with long sleeves and trousers
- Diethylcarbamazine prophylaxis, 300 mg weekly, may be useful if the risk of exposure is high. It is not indicated, however, for the casual traveler or for persons who might previously have acquired any of the filarial infections

 EVIDENCE

INFORMATION FOR PATIENTS

- Centers for Disease Control http://www.guideline.gov/summary/summary.aspx?doc_id=3080&nbr=2306&string=leishmaniasis
- National Institute of Allergy and Infectious Disease http://www.niaid.nih.gov/publications/microbes.htm

REFERENCES

- Kamgno J et al: Effect of a single dose (600 mg) of albendazole on *Loa loa* microfilaraemia. Parasite 2002;9:59. [PMID: 11938697]
- Nutman TB et al: Case records of the Massachusetts General Hospital. Weekly clinicopathological exercises. Case 1-2002. A 24-year-old woman with paresthesias and muscle cramps after a stay in Africa. N Engl J Med 2002;346:115. [PMID: 11784879]

Low Back Pain

KEY FEATURES

ESSENTIALS OF DIAGNOSIS

- A precise diagnosis cannot be made in the majority of cases
- Even when anatomic defects—such as vertebral osteophytes or a narrowed disk space—are present, clinical disease cannot be assumed since such defects are common in asymptomatic patients
- The majority of patients will improve in 1–4 weeks and need no evaluation beyond the initial history and physical examination

GENERAL CONSIDERATIONS

- Exceedingly common, experienced at some time by up to 80% of the population

DEMOGRAPHICS

- Chronic low back pain from degenerative joint disease is rare before age 40

CLINICAL FINDINGS

SYMPTOMS AND SIGNS

- Radiation down the buttock and below the knee suggests a herniated disk causing nerve root irritation
- Low back pain at night, unrelieved by rest or the supine position, should suggest the possibility of malignancy
- Symptoms of large or rapidly evolving neurological deficits identify patients who need urgent evaluation for possible cauda equina tumor, epidural abscess, or, rarely, massive disk herniation
- Bilateral leg weakness (from multiple lumbar nerve root compressions) or saddle area anesthesia, bowel or bladder incontinence, or impotence (indicating sacral nerve root compressions) indicates a cauda equina process
- Pain that worsens with rest and improves with activity is characteristic of ankylosing spondylitis or other seronegative spondyloarthropathies, especially when the onset is insidious and begins before age 40
- Most degenerative back diseases produce precisely the opposite pattern, with rest alleviating and activity aggravating the pain
- Positive straight leg raising test indicates nerve root irritation. The examiner performs the test on the supine patient by passively raising the patient's leg. The test is positive if radicular pain is produced with the leg raised 60 degrees or less. The test has a specificity of 40% but is 95% sensitive with herniation at the L4–5 or L5–S1 level (the sites of 95% of disk herniations)
- The crossed straight leg sign has a sensitivity of 25% but is 90% specific for disk herniation and is positive when raising the contralateral leg reproduces the sciatica
- Disk herniation produces deficits predictable for the site involved (Table 76, page 1266)
- Deficits of multiple nerve roots suggest a cauda equina tumor, an epidural abscess, or some other important process that requires urgent evaluation and treatment
- Palpation of the spine usually does not yield diagnostic information. Point tenderness over a vertebral body may suggest osteomyelitis

DIFFERENTIAL DIAGNOSIS

- Muscular strain
- Infectious diseases (eg, osteomyelitis, epidural abscess, subacute bacterial endocarditis)
- Neoplastic disease (vertebral metastases)
- Seronegative spondylarthopathies, eg, ankylosing spondylitis
- Compression fracture
- Degenerative joint disease
- Leaking abdominal aortic aneurysm
- Renal colic
- Lumbar spinal stenosis
- Herniated disk

DIAGNOSIS

IMAGING STUDIES

- Plain x-rays are warranted promptly for suspected infection, cancer, fractures, or inflammation; selected other patients who fail to improve after 2–4 weeks of conservative therapy are also candidates
- MRI is needed urgently in any patient suspected of having an epidural mass or cauda equina tumor but not if a patient is felt to have a routine disk herniation, since most will improve over 4–6 weeks of conservative therapy

DIAGNOSTIC PROCEDURES

- If the history and physical examination do not suggest the presence of infection, cancer, inflammatory back disease, major neurological deficits, or pain referred from abdominal or pelvic disease, further evaluation can be deferred while conservative therapy is tried

TREATMENT

MEDICATIONS

- Nonsteroidal antiinflammatory drugs (NSAIDs) for analgesia, but severe pain may require opioids
- Limited evidence supports the use of "muscle relaxants" such as diazepam, cyclobenzaprine, carisoprodol, and methocarbamol. These drugs should be reserved for patients who fail NSAIDs and should also be limited to courses of 1–2 weeks

SURGERY

- Surgical consultation is needed urgently for any patient with a large or evolving neurological deficit
- Surgery for disk disease is indicated when there is documentation of herniation by some imaging procedure, a consistent pain syndrome, and a consistent neurological deficit that has failed to respond to 4–6 weeks of conservative therapy

THERAPEUTIC PROCEDURES

- All patients should be taught how to protect the back in daily activities
- Rest and back exercises, once thought to be cornerstones of conservative therapy, are now known to be ineffective for acute back pain
- Epidural corticosteroid injections can provide short-term relief of sciatica but do not improve functional status or reduce the need for surgery
- Corticosteroid injections into facet joints are ineffective for chronic low back pain

 OUTCOME

PROGNOSIS

- The great majority of patients will spontaneously improve with conservative care over 1–4 weeks

WHEN TO REFER

- Refer to neurosurgeon or orthopedist if patient has disk herniation that does not respond after 4–6 weeks of conservative therapy or sooner if patient has important neurological deficits

WHEN TO ADMIT

- Admit if symptoms and signs suggest epidural or spinal abscess, cauda equina syndrome, or new metastatic cancer

 EVIDENCE

PRACTICE GUIDELINES

- National Guideline Clearinghouse
  http://www.guideline.gov/summary/summary.aspx?doc_id=2578&nbr=1804&string=low+back+pain
  http://www.guideline.gov/summary/summary.aspx?doc_id=3498&nbr=2724&string=low+back+pain
  http://www.guideline.gov/summary/summary.aspx?doc_id=1891&nbr=1117&string=low+back+pain

INFORMATION FOR PATIENTS

- JAMA patient page: Low back pain. JAMA 1998;279:1846. [PMID: 9828721]
- American Academy of Family Physicians
  http://familydoctor.org/healthfacts/117/

REFERENCES

- Andersson GB et al: A comparison of osteopathic spinal manipulation with standard care for patients with low back pain. N Engl J Med 1999;341:1426. [PMID: 10547405]
- Browning R et al: Cyclobenzaprine and back pain. A meta-analysis. Arch Intern Med 2001;161:1613. [PMID: 11434793]
- Deyo RA et al: Low back pain. N Engl J Med 2001;344:363. [PMID: 11172169]
- Jarvik JG et al: Diagnostic evaluation of low back pain with emphasis on imaging. Ann Intern Med 2002;137:586. [PMID: 12353946]
- Vroomen PCAJ et al: Lack of effectiveness of bed rest for sciatica. N Engl J Med 1999;340:41. [PMID: 9971865]

David B. Hellmann, MD, FACP
John H. Stone, MD, MPH

Lung Cancer, Secondary

 KEY FEATURES

ESSENTIALS OF DIAGNOSIS

- Identification of a primary tumor
- Radiographic findings consistent with pulmonary metastases
- Exclusion of other diseases in the differential diagnosis for multiple pulmonary nodules

GENERAL CONSIDERATIONS

- Represent metastases from extrapulmonary malignancies
- Almost any cancer can spread to the lung, usually hematogenously via the pulmonary artery
- Lung metastases are found in 20–55% of patients dying of various cancers

 CLINICAL FINDINGS

SYMPTOMS AND SIGNS

- Symptoms are uncommon, but include cough, hemoptysis, and dyspnea in advanced cases
- Symptoms are most commonly referrable to the primary tumor

DIFFERENTIAL DIAGNOSIS

- Bronchogenic carcinoma
- Lymphoproliferative cancer
- Tuberculosis
- Lung abscess
- Granulomas (eg, tuberculous, fungal)
- Coccidioidomycosis
- Histoplasmosis
- Sarcoidosis
- Silicosis
- Coal worker's pneumoconiosis
- *Mycobacterium avium* complex
- Arteriovenous malformations
- Rheumatoid nodules
- Hamartomas
- Wegener's granulomatosis
- Methotrexate-induced

 DIAGNOSIS

LABORATORY TESTS

- Appropriate studies should be ordered in a search for the primary tumor
- Occasionally, cytological studies of pleural fluid or pleural biopsy are diagnostic
- Sputum cytology is rarely helpful

IMAGING STUDIES

- Chest CT is more sensitive than chest x-ray in detecting pulmonary metastases
- Chest x-ray usually shows multiple spherical densities with sharp margins, nearly all <5 cm
- Lesions are usually bilateral, pleural, or subpleural, and are more common in lower lung zones
- Mammography should be performed in a search for the primary tumor

DIAGNOSTIC PROCEDURES

- If a primary tumor cannot be found, tissue from lung lesions may be obtained by bronchoscopy, percutaneous biopsy, or thoracotomy

TREATMENT

SURGERY

- Resection of a solitary pulmonary nodule is often prudent in a patient with known current or prior extrapulmonary cancer
- Local resection of one or more pulmonary metastases is feasible in a few carefully selected patients

THERAPEUTIC PROCEDURES

- Management consists of treatment of the primary malignancy and any pulmonary complications

 OUTCOME

PROGNOSIS

- Overall 5-year survival in secondary lung cancer treated surgically is 20–35%

WHEN TO REFER

- All patients deserve an evaluation by a multidisciplinary lung cancer evaluation and treatment program
- For bronchoscopy or thoracotomy
- A palliative care specialist should be involved in advanced disease care

WHEN TO ADMIT

- Respiratory distress, altered mental status, pain control

 EVIDENCE

PRACTICE GUIDELINES

- National Guideline Clearinghouse
  http://www.guideline.gov/summary/
  summary.aspx?doc_id=2899&nbr=
  2125&string=lung+metastases

INFORMATION FOR PATIENTS

- National Cancer Institute
  http://cis.nci.nih.gov/fact/6_20.htm
- National Institutes of Health
  http://www.nlm.nih.gov/medlineplus/
  ency/article/000097.htm

REFERENCE

- Greelish JP et al: Secondary pulmonary malignancy. Surg Clin North Am 2000; 80:633. [PMID: 10836010]

Mark S. Chesnutt, MD
Thomas J. Prendergast, MD

Lyme Disease

KEY FEATURES

ESSENTIALS OF DIAGNOSIS

- Erythema migrans, a flat or slightly raised red lesion that expands with central clearing
- Headache or stiff neck
- Arthralgias, arthritis, and myalgias; arthritis is often chronic and recurrent
- Wide geographic distribution, with most cases in the northeast, mid-Atlantic, upper midwest, and Pacific coastal regions of the United States

GENERAL CONSIDERATIONS

- Illness caused by the spirochete *Borrelia burgdorferi* is transmitted to humans by ixodid ticks in North America, Europe, Australia, and Asia
- Ticks must feed for 24 h or longer to transmit infections
- Incidence of disease is significantly higher when tick attachment is for longer than 72 h
- The percentage of ticks infected varies on a regional basis. In the northeast and midwest, 15–65%, in the west, only 2%
- Congenital infection has been documented

DEMOGRAPHICS

- In 2000, there were 17,730 cases reported but the true incidence is not known, and overreporting remains a problem
- Most cases (over 95%) were reported from the mid-Atlantic, northeastern, and north central regions of the country
- Cases of Lyme disease reported in the midwest and southern areas are probably due to the newly discovered Lone Star tick, *Amblyomma americanum*
- Most infections occur in the spring and summer

CLINICAL FINDINGS

SYMPTOMS AND SIGNS

- Three stages: stage 1, flu-like symptoms and a typical skin rash (erythema migrans); stage 2, weeks to months later, Bell's palsy or meningitis; stage 3, months to years later, arthritis
- Great overlap; the skin, central nervous system, and musculoskeletal system can be involved early or late
- Stage 1, early localized infection: erythema migrans, fever, chills, and myalgia in about half
- Stage 2, early disseminated infection (spirochete spreads in the patient's blood or lymph): skin (in about half), cardiac (4–10% of patients), neurological (10–20%), and musculoskeletal system manifestations
- *Borrelia* lymphocytoma is a rare skin lesion
- Myopericarditis, with atrial or ventricular arrhythmias and heart block
- Headache, stiff neck
- Aseptic meningitis, Bell's palsy, or encephalitis
- Peripheral neuropathy (sensory or motor), transverse myelitis, and mononeuritis multiplex
- Conjunctivitis, keratitis
- Migratory pains in joints, muscles, and tendons, fatigue and malaise
- Stage 3, late persistent infection: musculoskeletal (up to 60%), neurological, and skin disease
- Musculoskeletal manifestations: joint and periarticular pain; frank arthritis, mainly of large joints, chronic or recurrent; and chronic synovitis
- Subacute encephalopathy (memory loss, mood changes, and sleep disturbance), axonal polyneuropathy (distal sensory paresthesias or radicular pain), rare leukoencephalitis (cognitive dysfunction, spastic paraparesis, ataxia, and bladder dysfunction)
- Acrodermatitis chronicum—lesions atrophic and sclerotic, resemble localized scleroderma

DIFFERENTIAL DIAGNOSIS

- Babesiosis
- Ehrlichiosis
- *Amblyomma americanum* (Lone Star tick) bite-related illness
- Urticaria, reaction to arthropod bite, cellulitis, erythema multiforme, granuloma annulare
- Rocky Mountain spotted fever
- Primary HIV infection
- Parvovirus B19 infection
- Rheumatic fever, Still's disease, gonococcal arthritis, sarcoidosis, systemic lupus erythematosus
- Viral meningitis
- Bell's palsy

DIAGNOSIS

LABORATORY TESTS

- Elevated sedimentation rate of >20 mm/h seen in 50% of cases and mildly abnormal liver function tests in 30%
- Mild anemia, leukocytosis, and microscopic hematuria in 10% or less
- Detection of specific antibodies to *B burgdorferi* in serum, either by indirect immunofluorescence assay (IFA) or enzyme-linked immunosorbent assay (ELISA); both false-positive and false-negative reactions occur
- A Western blot assay that can detect both IgM and IgG antibodies is used as a confirmatory test
- A two-test approach is now recommended
- PCR is very specific for detecting *Borrelia* DNA, but sensitivity is variable and depends on which body fluid is tested and which stage of disease
- Up to 85% of synovial fluid samples are PCR positive in active arthritis
- 38% of cerebrospinal fluid samples are PCR positive in acute neuroborreliosis, but only 25% are positive in chronic neuroborreliosis

DIAGNOSTIC PROCEDURES

- Diagnosis is based on both clinical manifestations and laboratory findings. A person with exposure to a potential tick habitat (within the 30 days just prior to developing erythema migrans) with erythema migrans diagnosed by a physician or at least one late manifestation of the disease and laboratory confirmation
- Positive cultures for *B burgdorferi* can be obtained early in the course of disease. Aspiration of erythema migrans lesions is positive in up to 30% of cases, 2-mm punch biopsy is positive in 50–70%, blood cultures positive in up to 50%, cerebrospinal fluid positive in 1-10%
- Peripheral neuropathy may be detected by electromyography

Lyme Disease

 ## TREATMENT

 ## OUTCOME

 ## EVIDENCE

MEDICATIONS

- See Table 137 (page 1318)
- Erythema migrans: doxycycline, 100 mg twice daily for 3–4 weeks; or amoxicillin, 500 mg three times daily for 3–4 weeks; or cefuroxime axetil, 500 mg twice daily for 3–4 weeks
- Bell's palsy: doxycycline, 100 mg twice daily for 3–4 weeks; or amoxicillin, 500 mg three times daily for 3–4 weeks
- Other central nervous system disease: ceftriaxone, 2 g IV once daily for 2–4 weeks; or penicillin G, 20 million units daily IV in 6 divided doses for 2–4 weeks; or cefotaxime, 2 g IV every 8 h for 2–4 weeks
- First-degree block (PR <0.3 s): doxycycline, 100 mg twice daily for 3–4 weeks; or amoxicillin, 500 mg three times daily for 3–4 weeks
- High-degree atrioventricular block: ceftriaxone, 2 g IV once daily for 2–4 weeks; or penicillin G, 20 million units daily IV in 6 divided doses for 2–4 weeks
- Arthritis
  - Oral: doxycycline, 100 mg twice daily for 3–4 weeks; or amoxicillin, 500 mg three times daily for 4 weeks
  - Parenteral: ceftriaxone, 2 g IV once daily for 2–4 weeks; or penicillin G, 20 million units daily IV in 6 divided doses for 2–4 weeks
- Acrodermatitis chronicum atrophicans: doxycycline, 100 mg twice daily for 3–4 weeks; or amoxicillin, 500 mg three times daily for 4 weeks

THERAPEUTIC PROCEDURES

- Tick bite: no treatment in most circumstances; observe
- If acute arthritis, need aspiration to rule out pyogenic arthritis
- If neurological symptoms, need lumbar puncture as drug and duration of therapy unique for neuroborreliosis
- If suspect peripheral neuropathy, nerve conduction studies

FOLLOW-UP

- Routine follow-up
- Complete recovery in 4–6 weeks after therapy of early disease
- Fatigue, arthralgias, mayalgias may persist for weeks or months, but do not require antimicrobial therapy
- After treatment of arthritis, arthralgias may persist and be severe; if not resolved after 3 months, retreat with antibiotics; if arthralgias still persist treat symptomatically

COMPLICATIONS

- Rarely, residual facial nerve palsy, synovitis or heart block requiring a pacemaker

PROGNOSIS

- With appropriate therapy symptoms usually resolve within 4 weeks
- The long-term outcome of adult patients with Lyme disease is not clear
- Long-term sequelae are uncommon

WHEN TO REFER

- Refer if persistent symptoms after intial appropriate therapy; usually continued symptoms are part of the natural history of the disease and not reinfection or indication for prolonged use of antibiotics

WHEN TO ADMIT

- Admit for serious complications such as high-degree heart block prevention
- Avoiding tick-infested areas, covering exposed skin, using repellents, and inspecting for ticks after exposure
- Prophylactic antibiotics following tick bites are not recommended

PRACTICE GUIDELINES

- Wormser GP et al: Practice guidelines for the treatment of Lyme disease. The Infectious Diseases Society of America. Clin Infect Dis 2000;31(Suppl 1):1. [PMID: 10982743]
- American Academy of Pediatrics. Committee on Infectious Diseases. Prevention of Lyme disease. Pediatrics 2000;105(1 Pt 1):142. [PMID: 10617720]

WEB SITES

- Lyme Disease Network http://www.lymenet.org/
- American Lyme Disease Foundation http://www.aldf.com/

INFORMATION FOR PATIENTS

- CDC Lyme Disease Home Page http://www.cdc.gov/ncidod/dvbid/lyme/index.htm

REFERENCES

- Brown SL et al: Role of serology in the diagnosis of Lyme disease. JAMA 1999;282:62. [PMID: 10404913]
- Coyle PK et al: Neurologic aspects of Lyme disease. Med Clin North Am 2002;86:261. [PMID: 11982301]
- Klempner MS et al: Two controlled trials of antibiotic treatment in patients with persistent symptoms and a history of Lyme disease. N Engl J Med 2001;345:85. [PMID: 11450676]
- Pinto DS: Cardiac manifestations of Lyme disease. Med Clin North Am 2002;86:285. [PMID: 11982302]
- Poland GA: Prevention of Lyme disease: a review of the evidence. Mayo Clin Proc 2001;76:713. [PMID: 11444404]

Richard A. Jacobs, MD, PhD

Lymphangitis & Lymphadenitis

 KEY FEATURES

ESSENTIALS OF DIAGNOSIS

- Red streak extending from an infected area toward enlarged, tender regional lymph nodes

GENERAL CONSIDERATIONS

- Lymphangitis and lymphadenitis frequently accompany a streptococcal or staphylococcal infection in the distal arm or leg
- Inciting wound can be a superficial scratch or insect bite with cellulitis, or an established abscess
- Systemic manifestations: fever, chills, tachycardia, and malaise
- If untreated, infection can progress rapidly

 CLINICAL FINDINGS

SYMPTOMS AND SIGNS

- Throbbing pain at the site of the inciting wound
- Fever of 37.8–40°C
- Chills
- Sweats
- Malaise
- Anorexia
- Regional lymph nodes significantly enlarged and tender
- Red streak extending toward regional lymph nodes

DIFFERENTIAL DIAGNOSIS

- Superficial thrombophlebitis
- Cat-scratch disease caused by *Bartonella henselae*
- Acute streptococcal hemolytic gangrene
- Superficial thrombophlebitis
- Cellulitis
- Necrotizing fasciitis
- Filariasis (acute)
- *Nocardia brasiliensis* infection

 DIAGNOSIS

LABORATORY TESTS

- Leukocytosis with a left shift
- Blood cultures often positive for *Staphylococcus* or *Streptococcus*

IMAGING STUDIES

- Consider plain film if concerned about possible retained foreign body or nectrotizing infection

TREATMENT

MEDICATIONS

- Analgesics
- Antibiotics: penicillin G, 4 million units IV every 6 h; or cefazolin, 1 every IV every 8 h; or clindamycin, 600 mg IV every 12 h

SURGERY

- Incision and drainage of abscess, excision of necrotic tissue or foreign body

THERAPEUTIC PROCEDURES

- Elevation of extremity
- Warm compresses

 OUTCOME

FOLLOW-UP

- Wound examination to determine the need for debridement or incision and drainage of an abscess

COMPLICATIONS

- Wound healing problems
- Sepsis

PROGNOSIS

- Early institution of antibiotic therapy and wound care usually controls the infection in 48–72 h
- Delayed or inadequate therapy can result in rapidly progressive infection, septicemia, and death

WHEN TO REFER

- Lymphangitis complicated by abscess, nonhealing wound, sepsis

WHEN TO ADMIT

- Signs of sepsis
- Failed outpatient management

 EVIDENCE

PRACTICE GUIDELINES

- Beltran J: MR imaging of soft-tissue infection. Magn Reson Imaging Clin North Am 1995;3:743. [PMID: 8564693]
- Ghirardelli ML et al: Diagnostic approach to lymph node enlargement. Haematologica 1999;84:242. [PMID: 10189390]
- Heller HM et al: Nodular lymphangitis: clinical features, differential diagnosis and management. Curr Clin Top Infect Dis 1994;14:142. [PMID: 8086112]

WEB SITES

- Circle of Hope—Lymphangitis http://www.lymphedemacircleofhope. org/infection.htm
- MEDLINEplus—Lymphadenitis and lymphangitis http://www.nlm.nih.gov/medlineplus/ ency/article/001301.htm
- National Lymphedema Network—What is lymphedema? http://www.lymphnet.org/whatis.html

INFORMATION FOR PATIENTS

- Cleveland Clinic—Understanding lymphedema http://www.clevelandclinic.org/health/ health-info/docs/1800/1896.asp?index= 8353
- Mayo Clinic—Painful, swollen lymph nodes (lymphadenitis) http://www.mayoclinic.com/invoke. cfm?objectid=799E8349-32F2-40FE-94FAC192833334E6
- Merck Manual—Acute lymphangitis http://www.merck.com/pubs/mmanual/ section10/chapter112/112c.htm

Louis M. Messina, MD

Laura K. Pak, MD

Lawrence M. Tierney, Jr., MD

Lymphedema

 KEY FEATURES

ESSENTIALS OF DIAGNOSIS

- Painless edema of upper or lower extremities
- Involves the dorsal surfaces of the hands and fingers or the feet and toes
- Developmental or acquired
- Unilateral or bilateral
- Edema initially pitting, with time becoming brawny and nonpitting
- No ulceration, varicosities, or stasis pigmentation
- Episodes of lymphangitis and cellulitis

GENERAL CONSIDERATIONS

- Primary lymphedema is due to congenital developmental abnormalities consisting of hypoplastic or hyperplastic changes of the proximal or distal lymphatics
- Familial lymphedema developing before age 1 is Milroy's disease; usually bilateral, it affects boys more often than girls
- Lymphedema developing during adolescence (lymphedema praecox) is unilateral; 3.5:1 female predominance
- Lymphedema after age 35 is lymphedema tarda
- Secondary lymphedema results from an inflammatory or mechanical obstruction of the lymphatics following trauma, regional lymph node resection, irradiation, bacterial or fungal infections, lymphoproliferative diseases, or filariasis

 CLINICAL FINDINGS

SYMPTOMS AND SIGNS

- Slowly progressive, painless edema
- Edema usually centered around the ankle and involves the toes and dorsum
- Hypertrophy of the limb
- Markedly thickened skin and subcutaneous tissue
- Rarely, lymphangiosarcoma or angiosarcoma (Stewart-Treves syndrome)
- Secondary fibrosis is exacerbated by superimposed episodes of acute infection

DIFFERENTIAL DIAGNOSIS

- Venous insufficiency
- Chronic venous stasis disease
- Edema secondary to congestive heart failure
- Cellulitis

 DIAGNOSIS

IMAGING STUDIES

- Venous duplex ultrasonography to exclude venous insufficiency or vascular malformations
- Lymphangiography and radioactive isotope studies if surgical reconstruction (rare)

TREATMENT

MEDICATIONS

- No effective drug therapy
- Diuretics are not recommended for long-term use but can be useful for acute exacerbation of edema secondary to infection or for coexisting venous stasis disease

SURGERY

- Primary treatment is nonsurgical
- Surgery to reduce limb bulk, either by ablative techniques (excision of excess tissue) or by physiological techniques (lymphatic reconstruction), in carefully selected cases
- Microsurgical lymphaticovenous anastomosis, though long-term efficacy is unknown

THERAPEUTIC PROCEDURES

- Meticulous skin care
- Moisturizing lotions
- Frequent leg elevation
- Manual lymphatic drainage massage
- External compression with fitted graduated (20–30 mm Hg) compression stockings
- Sequential pneumatic compression devices
- Reid sleeves for postmastectomy arm lymphedema
- Avoidance of trauma to the affected extremity

 OUTCOME

COMPLICATIONS

- Secondary infection and ulceration

PROGNOSIS

- Good with vigorous skin care regimen

WHEN TO REFER

- Refer for early intervention and counseling

WHEN TO ADMIT

- Lymphedema complicated by infection

 EVIDENCE

PRACTICE GUIDELINES

- ACR Appropriateness Criteria for unilateral upper extremity swelling and pain. American College of Radiology 1998
  http://www.acr.org/cgi-bin/fr?tmpl:appcrit,pdf:0107-112_unilateral_arm_pain_swelling_ac.pdf
- Harris SR et al: Clinical practice guidelines for the care and treatment of breast cancer: 11. Lymphedema. CMAJ 2001;164:191. [PMID: 11332311]
- Surgical management of early stage invasive breast cancer. Practice Guidelines Initiative, 2003
  http://www.cancercare.on.ca/pdf/pebc1-1f.pdf

WEB SITES

- Circle of Hope—What is lymphedema? http://www.lymphedemacircleofhope.org/lymphedema.htm
- National Lymphedema Network—What is lymphedema? http://www.lymphnet.org/whatis.html

INFORMATION FOR PATIENTS

- Cleveland Clinic—Understanding lymphedema
  http://www.clevelandclinic.org/health/health-info/docs/1800/1896.asp?index=8353
- MEDLINEplus—Lymphatic obstruction
  http://www.nlm.nih.gov/medlineplus/ency/article/001117.htm

REFERENCES

- Campisi C et al: Long-term results after lymphatic-venous anastomoses for the treatment of obstructive lymphedema. Microsurgery 2001;21:135. [PMID: 11494379]
- Ko DS et al: Effective treatment of lymphedema of the extremities. Arch Surg 1998;133:452. [PMID: 9565129]

Louis M. Messina, MD
Laura K. Pak, MD
Lawrence M. Tierney, Jr., MD

Lymphoma, Cutaneous T Cell

 KEY FEATURES

ESSENTIALS OF DIAGNOSIS

- Localized or generalized erythematous scaling plaques
- Pruritus
- Lymphadenopathy
- Distinctive histology

GENERAL CONSIDERATIONS

- A cutaneous T cell lymphoma that begins on the skin and may involve only the skin for years or decades
- Certain medications (including selective serotonin reuptake inhibitors) may produce eruptions clinically and histologically identical to those of mycosis fungoides, so this possibility must always be considered
- Lymph node enlargement may be due to benign expansion of the node (dermatopathic lymphadenopathy) or by specific involvement with mycosis fungoides

 CLINICAL FINDINGS

SYMPTOMS AND SIGNS

- See Table 6 (page 1199)
- Localized or generalized erythematous patches or plaques, usually on the trunk
- Plaques are almost always over 5 cm in diameter
- Pruritus is a frequent complaint
- The lesions often begin as nondescript or nondiagnostic patches, and it is not unusual for the patient to have skin lesions for more than a decade before the diagnosis can be confirmed
- In more advanced cases, tumors appear
- Lymphadenopathy may occur locally or widely

DIFFERENTIAL DIAGNOSIS

- Psoriasis
- Drug eruption
- Atopic dermatitis (eczema)
- Hansen's disease (leprosy)
- Tinea corporis (body ringworm)

 DIAGNOSIS

LABORATORY TESTS

- Circulating atypical cells (Sézary cells) can be detected in the blood by sensitive methods
- Eosinophilia may be present

THERAPEUTIC PROCEDURES

- The skin biopsy remains the basis of diagnosis, though at times numerous biopsies are required before the diagnosis can be confirmed

Lymphocytic Choriomeningitis p. 1128.
Lymphogranuloma Venereum p. 1128.

 ## TREATMENT

MEDICATIONS

- The treatment is complex
- Topical mechlorethamine ointment or solution, topical steroids, and PUVA are all used for early patches and plaques
- Radiation therapy for local lesions and systemic agents such as retinoids, antitumor chemotherapeutic drugs, and alpha interferon are used alone or in various combinations for more advanced disease or in patients who fail topical therapy

 ## OUTCOME

COMPLICATIONS

- Overly aggressive treatment may lead to complications and premature demise

PROGNOSIS

- Usually slowly progressive (over decades)
- Early and aggressive treatment has not been proved to cure or prevent progression of the disease
- Prognosis is better in patients with patch or plaque stage disease and worse in patients with erythroderma, tumors, and lymphadenopathy
- Survival is not reduced in patients with limited patch disease
- Elderly patients with patch and plaque stage disease commonly die of other causes

WHEN TO REFER

- All patients with suspected or proven diagnosis

 ## EVIDENCE

PRACTICE GUIDELINES

- Zelenetz AD et al: NCCN: Non-Hodgkin's lymphoma. Cancer Control 2001;8(6 Suppl 2):102.

WEB SITES

- American Academy of Dermatology http://www.aad.org
- Dermatology Handbook for Family Practice from the University of Iowa http://www.vh.org/Providers/ClinRef/FPHandbook/17.html

INFORMATION FOR PATIENTS

- American Academy of Dermatology http://www.aad.org/pamphlets/
- National Cancer Institute http://www.cancer.gov/cancerinfo/pdq/treatment/mycosisfungoides/patient# Section_3

REFERENCES

- Kim YH et al: Mycosis fungoides and the Sézary syndrome. Semin Oncol 1999;26:276. [PMID: 10375085]
- Siegel RS et al: Primary cutaneous T-cell lymphoma: review and current concepts. J Clin Oncol 2000;18:2908. [PMID: 10920140]
- van Doorn R et al: Mycosis fungoides: disease evolution and prognosis of 309 Dutch patients. Arch Dermatol 2000;136:504. [PMID: 1076864]

Timothy G. Berger, MD

Malaria

 KEY FEATURES

ESSENTIALS OF DIAGNOSIS

- History of exposure in a malaria-endemic area
- Periodic attacks of sequential chills, fever, and sweating
- Headache, myalgia, splenomegaly; anemia, leukopenia
- Characteristic parasites in erythrocytes, identified in thick or thin blood films
- Complications of *Plasmodium falciparum* malaria: cerebral findings (mental disturbances, neurological signs, convulsions), hemolytic anemia, hyperpyrexia, secretory diarrhea or dysentery, dark urine, anuria

GENERAL CONSIDERATIONS

- Four species of the genus *Plasmodium* are responsible for human malaria: *P vivax, P malariae, P ovale,* and *P falciparum*
- Transmitted from human to human by the bite of infected female mosquitoes. Transmission congenitally and by blood transfusion occurs
- The incubation period after exposure or after stopping chemoprophylaxis is, for *P falciparum*, approximately 12 days (range: 9–60 days); for *P vivax* and *P ovale*, 14 days [range: 8–27 days (initial attacks for some temperate strains may not occur for up to 8 months)]; and for *P malariae*, 30 days (range: 16–60 days)
- Untreated *P falciparum* infections can persist for up to 1.5 years but usually end in 6–8 months; *P vivax* and *P ovale* infections persist for as long as 5 years; and *P malariae* infections have lasted for as long as 50 years
- Protective immunity results from infection but decays after several years

DEMOGRAPHICS

- Annually worldwide, malaria causes clinical illness in 300 million people and results in about 2 million deaths
- About 30,000 travelers from the developed world are infected yearly, and several hundred die

 CLINICAL FINDINGS

SYMPTOMS AND SIGNS

- Typical attacks show sequentially, over 4–6 h, shaking chills (the cold stage); fever (the hot stage) to 41°C or higher; and marked diaphoresis (the sweating stage)
- Associated symptoms may include fatigue, headache, dizziness, gastrointestinal symptoms (anorexia, nausea, slight diarrhea, vomiting, abdominal cramps), myalgias, arthralgia, backache, and dry cough
- The attacks may show an every-other-day (tertian) periodicity in *P vivax, ovale,* or *falciparum* malaria or an every-third-day (quartan) periodicity in *P malariae* malaria
- Splenomegaly usually appears 4 or more days after the onset of acute symptoms; there may be mild hepatomegaly
- Between attacks, the patient feels fine
- After the primary episode, recurrences are common, each separated by a latent interval

DIFFERENTIAL DIAGNOSIS

- Influenza
- Typhoid fever
- Viral hepatitis
- Dengue
- Visceral leishmaniasis (kala azar)
- Amebic liver abscess
- Babesiosis
- Leptospirosis
- Relapsing fever

 DIAGNOSIS

LABORATORY TESTS

- Thick and thin blood films, Giemsa or Wright stained, are the mainstay of diagnosis—clinical diagnosis is only 20–60% reliable compared with microscopy
- Blood from finger sticks or from the earlobe is preferred but should be free-flowing and uncontaminated by alcohol; if venipuncture blood is used, it should be examined shortly after it is drawn to avoid changes in morphology. Specimens should be obtained at about 8-h intervals for 3 days, including during and between febrile periods
- Serological tests (ELISA and others) are not commonly used in the diagnosis of acute attacks since antibody becomes detectable only 8–10 days after onset of symptoms. Antibody persists for 10 or more years, so it does distinguish between current and past infection
- There is an ELISA and a rapid, simply accomplished dipstick format (90% specific and sensitive) sensitive only to *P falciparum*. Other tests are a quantitative buffy coat centrifugal system (does not readily differentiate the species), the polymerase chain reaction (highly sensitive and species-specific), and an indirect fluorescent antibody test (which uses the four organisms as antigens and is highly sensitive and specific)
- During paroxysms, there may be transient leukocytosis; leukopenia develops subsequently, with a relative increase in large mononuclear cells
- The number of red cells infected seldom exceeds 2% of total cells. However, in severe *P falciparum* malaria, parasitemia may reach 30% or higher; mature sexual forms disappear (sequestered in the microcirculation); hepatic function tests often become abnormal; and hemolytic jaundice, thrombocytopenia, and marked anemia with reticulocytosis may develop

 TREATMENT

MEDICATIONS

- See Table 139 (page 1329)

Antimalarial drugs

- **4-Aminoquinolines**—chloroquine, hydroxychloroquine, amodiaquine

Lymphoma, Gastric p. 1129. Macular Degeneration, Age-Related p. 1130.

Malaria

- **Diaminopyrimidines**—pyrimethamine, trimethoprim
- **Biguanides**—proguanil (chlorguanide, chlorproguanil)
- **8-Aminoquinolines**—primaquine
- **Cinchona alkaloids**—quinine, quinidine
- **Sulfonamides**—sulfadoxine, sulfadiazine, sulfamethoxazole
- **Sulfones**—dapsone
- **4-Quinoline-carbinolamines**—mefloquine
- **Antibiotics**—tetracycline, doxycycline, clindamycin
- **Others**—halofantrine, artemisinin (qinghaosu) and its derivatives, and atovaquone
- Pyrimethamine and proguanil are known as **antifolates**, since they inhibit dihydrofolate reductase of plasmodia
- **Drug combinations** used to treat chloroquine-resistant *P falciparum* malaria include Fansidar (pyrimethamine plus sulfadoxine), Maloprim (pyrimethamine plus dapsone), and Malarone (atovaquone plus proguanil)
- Seek additional information on individual drug adverse reactions, cautions, contraindications, and parasitic resistance

THERAPEUTIC PROCEDURES

Management of severe *P falciparum* malaria

- Indications for parenteral treatment are failure to ingest or retain drugs, cerebral malaria, complications, and peripheral asexual parasitemia of 5% (250,000/μL) or more
- Black urine suggests hemoglobinuria. Renal failure, metabolic acidosis, severe anemia, pulmonary edema, gram-negative sepsis, and shock may ensue
- Rehydrate cautiously, particularly in the first 24 h, since overhydration may precipitate noncardiogenic pulmonary edema. Usually, 2–3 L of fluid is needed the first day, followed by 10–20 mL/kg/day
- Early dialysis may be necessary
- Blood glucose levels should be monitored every 6 h during the acute and early convalescent period
- Treat convulsions with diazepam (0.15 mg/kg intravenously or 0.5 mg/kg rectally) or with paraldehyde (0.1 mL/kg intramuscularly from a glass syringe)

- Keep the temperature below 38.5°C using acetaminophen (paracetamol) plus tepid sponging and fanning
- Significant disseminated intravascular coagulation should be treated with fresh whole blood, clotting factors, or platelets. Transfuse fresh whole blood or packed cells for hematocrits below 20%
- Consider exchange transfusion (5–10 L) when more than 10% of red blood cells are parasitized (5% if severe dysfunction of other organs is present)

OUTCOME

FOLLOW-UP

- Blood films should be checked daily until parasitemia clears in *P falciparum*; check weekly thereafter for 4 weeks to observe for recrudescence of infection

COMPLICATIONS

From *P falciparum*

- Cerebral malaria with edema, hyperpyrexia, hemolytic anemia, noncardiogenic pulmonary edema
- Acute tubular necrosis and renal failure, which is rarely associated with blackwater fever (dark urine), most commonly due to severe hemolysis following quinine treatment
- Acute hepatopathy, with centrilobular necrosis and jaundice
- Hypoglycemia, cardiac dysrhythmias, gastrointestinal syndromes, lactic acidosis; water and electrolyte disorders

PROGNOSIS

- With prompt antimalarial treatment, the prognosis is generally good, except in *P falciparum* complications, when mortality may reach about 15%
- The prognosis is poor if more than 20% of infected red cells contain mature parasites or if more than 5% of neutrophils contain pigment. Gram-negative bacteremia may contribute to death

WHEN TO REFER

- All patients should be referred to a provider with expertise in this area

WHOM TO ADMIT

- Severe *P falciparum* malaria is a medical emergency that requires hospitalization, intensive care with monitoring of electrolytes and acid-base balance, and im-

mediate treatment without waiting for all laboratory results to be available

PREVENTION

- See Table 140 (page XX) for chemoprophylaxis
- All persons who will be exposed should receive chemoprophylaxis. (See CDC information sites below)
- When out of doors between dusk and dawn, use protective measures. Clothing should cover most of the body, and deet mosquito repellent should be applied to exposed areas every 3–4 h. To minimize the slight risk of toxic encephalopathy from deet, it should be applied sparingly and only to exposed skin and outer clothing; the Ultrathon formulation provides a reduced concentration of deet (33%) with extended protection (12 h)
- Emergency ("standby") self-treatment may be necessary when medical attention is unavailable within 24 h. Such persons may want to carry medications for self-treatment if they develop fever or flu-like symptoms (Table 139, page 1320). It is imperative that medical follow-up be sought promptly

EVIDENCE

WEB SITES

- http://www.who.int/ith/.
- http://www.cdc.gov (choose the Travelers' Health category)

INFORMATION FOR PATIENTS

- Centers for Disease Control http://www.cdc.gov/travel/malinfo.htm

REFERENCES

- Malarial Branch, Centers for Disease Control and Prevention (CDC), Atlanta, Georgia. For recorded information on prophylaxis: fax response, 888-232-3299; Internet. For additional information on prophylaxis or for management of acute attacks, phone 770-488-7788; after business hours, 404-639-2888
- Goldsmith RS: Infectious diseases: protozoal & helminthic. current Medical diagnosis and treatment. Tierney LM, McPhee SJ, Papadakis, MA (editors). McGraw-Hill, 2004

Mallory-Weiss Syndrome

 KEY FEATURES

ESSENTIALS OF DIAGNOSIS

- Defined as nonpenetrating mucosal tear at the gastroesophageal junction
- Hematemesis; usually self-limited
- Prior history of vomiting, retching, straining, lifting in 50%
- Endoscopy establishes diagnosis

GENERAL CONSIDERATIONS

- Accounts for ~5% of upper gastrointestinal bleeding

DEMOGRAPHICS

- Hiatal hernia present in majority; with vomiting, increased risk of tear
- Heavy alcohol use with vomiting or retching in 50% of patients
- Other risk factors: age, hiccups

 CLINICAL FINDINGS

SYMPTOMS AND SIGNS

- History of vomiting, retching, straining, lifting in 50%
- Hematemesis with or without melena

DIFFERENTIAL DIAGNOSIS

Other causes of hematemesis

- Hemoptysis
- Peptic ulcer disease
- Esophageal varices
- Gastric or duodenal varices (rare)
- Erosive gastritis, eg, nonsteroidal antiinflammatory drugs, alcohol, stress
- Portal hypertensive gastropathy
- Vascular ectasias (angiodysplasias)
- Gastric cancer

Rare causes

- Erosive esophagitis
- Aortoenteric fistula
- Dieulafoy's lesion (aberrant gastric submucosal artery)
- Hemobilia (blood in biliary tree), eg, iatrogenic, malignancy
- Pancreatic cancer
- Hemosuccus pancreaticus (pancreatic pseudoaneurysm)

 DIAGNOSIS

LABORATORY TESTS

- Obtain complete blood cell count, platelet count, prothrombin time, partial thromboplastin time, serum creatinine, liver enzymes and serologies, and type and cross-matching for 2–4 units or more of packed red blood cells
- Hematocrit is not a reliable indicator of the severity of acute bleeding

DIAGNOSTIC PROCEDURES

- Upper endoscopy is diagnostic: identification of a 0.5–4 cm linear mucosal tear usually located either at the gastroesophageal junction or, more commonly, just below the junction in the gastric mucosa of a hiatal hernia at the level of the diaphragm
- Assess hemodynamic status: systolic blood pressure; heart rate; postural hypotension

TREATMENT

MEDICATIONS

- Proton pump inhibitors to accelerate mucosal healing: omeprazole or rabeprazole, 20 mg PO QD, esomaprazole or pantoprazole, 40 mg PO QD

SURGERY

- Surgery with oversew of bleeding vessel rarely necessary

THERAPEUTIC PROCEDURES

- In patients without hemodynamic compromise or overt active bleeding, delay aggressive fluid repletion until extent of bleeding clarified
- For those with continuing active bleeding, insert two 18-gauge or larger intravenous lines
- Patients with hemodynamic compromise should be given 0.9% saline or lactated Ringer's injection and cross-matched blood
- Blood replacement to maintain a hematocrit of 25–30%
- In the absence of continued bleeding, the hematocrit should rise 3% for each unit of transfused packed red cells
- Transfuse blood in patients with brisk active bleeding regardless of the hematocrit
- Transfuse platelets if platelet count <50,000/μL or if impaired platelet function due to aspirin use
- Uremic patients with active bleeding should be given 1–2 doses of desmopressin (DDAVP), 0.3 μg/kg IV at 12- to 24-h intervals
- Fresh frozen plasma should be given for actively bleeding patients with a coagulopathy and an INR >1.5
- In massive bleeding, 1 unit of fresh frozen plasma for each 5 units of packed red blood cells transfused
- Endoscopic hemostatic therapy for those with continuing active bleeding
- Epinephrine 1:10,000 injection or cautery with a bipolar or heater probe coagulation device is effective in 90–95% of cases
- Angiographic arterial embolization or operative intervention is required in patients who fail endoscopic therapy

 OUTCOME

FOLLOW-UP

- None required

COMPLICATIONS

- Persistent bleeding

PROGNOSIS

- Most bleeds stop spontaneously with rapid healing of mucosal tears
- Persistent or recurrent bleeding most likely in patients with concomitant portal hypertension or coagulapathy

WHEN TO ADMIT

- All patients with significant hematemesis warrant admission
- Patients without active bleeding and without portal hypertension or coagulapathy may be discharged after 24 h
- Patients with active bleeding requiring hemostasis therapy should be observed at least 48 h

 EVIDENCE

PRACTICE GUIDELINES

- ACR Appropriateness Criteria for hematemesis. American College of Radiology, 2002 http://www.acr.org/cgi-bin/fr?tmpl: appcrit,pdf:0113-120_hematemesis-ac. pdf
- Church NI et al: Ulcers and nonvariceal bleeding. Endoscopy 2003;35:22. [PMID: 12510222]
- Savides TJ et al: Therapeutic endoscopy for nonvariceal gastrointestinal bleeding. Gastroenterol Clin North Am 2000; 29:465. [PMID: 10836190]

WEB SITE

- Yale New Haven Health—Mallory-Weiss syndrome http://yalenewhavenhealth.org/library/ healthguide/IllnessConditions/topic.asp? hwid=nord734

INFORMATION FOR PATIENTS

- Cecil Textbook of Medicine—Disease of the esophagus http://home.mdconsult.com/das/book/ 30975174/view/882?sid=204180645
- Noble: Textbok of Primary Care Medicine—Mallory-Weiss syndrome http://home.mdconsult.com/das/book/ 30975174/view/959?sid=204180645
- Robbins Pathologic Basis of Disease— The gastrointestinal tract http://home.mdconsult.com/das/book/ 30975174/view/891?sid=204180645

REFERENCE

- Kortas D et al: Mallory-Weiss tear: predisposing factors and predictors of a complicated course. Am J Gastroenterol 2001;96:2863. [PMID: 11693318]

Kenneth R. McQuaid, MD

Mania

 ## KEY FEATURES

ESSENTIALS OF DIAGNOSIS

- Mood ranging from euphoria to irritability
- Sleep disruption
- Hyperactivity
- Racing thoughts
- Grandiosity
- Variable psychotic symptoms

GENERAL CONSIDERATIONS

- Often combined with depression and may occur alone, together with mania in a mixed episode, or in cyclic fashion with depression
- In almost all cases, the manic episode is part of a broader bipolar (manic-depressive) disorder

DEMOGRAPHICS

- Spring and summer tend to be the peak periods

 ## CLINICAL FINDINGS

SYMPTOMS AND SIGNS

- A mood change characterized by elation with hyperactivity, overinvolvement in life activities, increased irritability, flight of ideas, easy distractibility, and little need for sleep
- The overenthusiastic quality of the mood and the expansive behavior initially attract others, but the irritability, mood lability with swings into depression, aggressive behavior, and grandiosity usually lead to marked interpersonal difficulties
- Activities may occur that are later regretted, eg, excessive spending, resignation from a job, a hasty marriage, sexual acting out, and exhibitionistic behavior, with alienation of friends and family
- A typical manic episode can include gross delusions, paranoid ideation of severe proportions, and auditory hallucinations usually related to some grandiose perception
- The episodes begin abruptly (sometimes precipitated by life stresses) and may last from several days to months
- Manic patients differ from schizophrenics in that the former use more effective interpersonal maneuvers, are more sensitive to the social maneuvers of others, and are more able to utilize weakness and vulnerability in others to their own advantage

DIFFERENTIAL DIAGNOSIS

- Bipolar disorder (manic-depression)
- Substance abuse, eg, cocaine
- Hypomania
- Cyclothymic disorder (depression and hypomania)
- Schizophrenia
- Hyperthyroidism
- Substance abuse, eg, cocaine, amphetamines
- Medications, eg, corticosteroids, thyroxine
- CNS disease, eg, complex partial seizures, tumor, neurosyphilis, HIV
- Personality disorder, eg, borderline, narcissistic

 ## DIAGNOSIS

LABORATORY TESTS

- Thyroid-stimulating hormone, complete blood cell count, blood urea nitrogen, serum creatinine, and serum electrolyte determinations; urinalysis

TREATMENT

MEDICATIONS

Mania due to bipolar disorder

- Acute manic or hypomanic symptoms will respond to lithium therapy after several days of treatment, but it is common to use neuroleptic drugs or high-potency benzodiazepines (eg, clonazepam) to immediately treat the excited or psychotic manic stage
- Atypical neuroleptics (olanzapine 5–20 mg QD) along with a benzodiazepine, if indicated, may be used initially to treat agitation and psychosis
- Alternatively, use haloperidol (5–10 mg PO or IM Q 2–3 h)
- Clonazepam (1–2 mg PO Q 4–6 h) may be used in lieu of or in conjunction with a neuroleptic to control acute behavioral symptoms
- Lithium (1200–1800 mg/day targeted to therapeutic serum level) is effective in acute mania or hypomania, but takes several days to take effect
- Valproic acid (750 mg/day divided and titrated to therapeutic levels) can be loaded to therapeutic levels in 2–3 days
- Carbamazepine (800–1600 mg/day) is used in patients intolerant or unresponsive to lithium
- Calcium channel blockers (verapamil) have been used in refractory patients
- Anticonvulsants such as lamotrigine (25–50 mg/day titrated slowly upward) and topiramate are beginning to be used

THERAPEUTIC PROCEDURES

Mania secondary to other conditions

- The underlying condition needs to be treated as well

OUTCOME

WHEN TO REFER

- Patients should be under the care of a psychiatrist

WHEN TO ADMIT

- Most patients with mania should be admitted for monitoring until the symptoms are brought under control

PREVENTION

- Lithium (1200–1800 mg/day targeted to therapeutic serum level) as prophylaxis can limit the frequency and severity of mood swings in 70% of patients

EVIDENCE

PRACTICE GUIDELINES

American Psychiatric Association. Practice guideline for the treatment of patients with bipolar disorder (revision). Am J Psychiatry 2002;159(4 Suppl):1. [PMID: 11958165]

- National Guideline Clearinghouse http://www.guideline.gov/summary/summary.aspx?doc_id=3302&nbr=2528&string=mania

Goodwin G et al: Evidence-based guidelines for treating bipolar disorder: recommendations from the British Association for Psychopharmacology. J Psychopharmacol 2003;1:149. [PMID: 12870562]

WEB SITES

- American Psychiatric Association http://www.psych.org/
- Internet Mental Health http://www.mentalhealth.com/t30.html
- Psychopharmacology Tips http://www.dr-bob.org/tips/
- Psychiatry On Line http://www.prior .com/psych.htm

INFORMATION FOR PATIENTS

- National Institute of Mental Health http://www.nimh.nih.gov/publicat/bipolar.cfm
- Depression and Bipolar Support Alliance http://www.dbsalliance.org/info/bipolar.html

REFERENCE

- Sato T et al: Syndromes and phenomenological subtypes underlying acute mania: a factor analytic study of 576 manic patients, Am J Psychiatry 2000;159:968.

Stuart J. Eisendrath, MD
Jonathan E. Lichtmacher, MD

Marfan's Syndrome

 ## KEY FEATURES

ESSENTIALS OF DIAGNOSIS

- Marfan's syndrome is a systemic connective tissue disease, inherited as an autosomal dominant
- Characterized by abnormalities of the skeletal system, ocular system, and cardiovascular system
- Disproportionately tall stature, thoracic deformity, and joint laxity or contractures
- Ectopia lentis and myopia
- Aortic dilation and dissection
- Mitral valve prolapse

 ## CLINICAL FINDINGS

SYMPTOMS AND SIGNS

- Wide variability in clinical presentation
- Affected patients typically are tall, with particularly long arms, legs, and digits (arachnodactyly)
- Commonly, joint dislocations and pectus excavatum
- Ectopia lentis, severe myopia, and retinal detachment
- Aortic and mitral valve regurgitation occur often from elongated chordae tendineae, which on occasion may rupture
- Mitral valve prolapse in about 85%
- Disease of the ascending aorta produces a dilated aortic root, aortic regurgitation, and aortic dissection
- Spontaneous pneumothorax
- Dural ectasia
- Striae atrophicae

DIFFERENTIAL DIAGNOSIS

- Homocystinuria due to cystathionine synthase deficiency
- Tall stature (normal)
- Aortic root disease due to other cause, eg, ankylosing spondylitis, syphilis, temporal (giant cell) arteritis, Takayasu's arteritis
- Homocystinuria (with lens dislocation)
- Ehlers-Danlos syndrome
- Idiopathic mitral valve prolapse

 ## DIAGNOSIS

LABORATORY TESTS

- No simple laboratory test
- DNA analysis can detect mutations in the fibrillin gene on chromosome 15

TREATMENT

MEDICATIONS

- Standard endocarditis prophylaxis
- Chronic β-adrenergic blockade (eg, atenolol, 1–2 mg/kg) retards the rate of aortic dilation

SURGERY

- Prophylactic replacement of the aortic root when the diameter reaches 50–55 mm (normal: <40 mm) prolongs life
- Annual orthopedic consultation for diagnosis of scoliosis

THERAPEUTIC PROCEDURES

- Regular ophthalmological surveillance to correct visual acuity and thus prevent amblyopia
- Restriction from vigorous physical exertion

OUTCOME

FOLLOW-UP

- Echocardiography at least annually to monitor aortic diameter and mitral valve function

PROGNOSIS

- Untreated, Marfan's syndrome patients commonly die in the fourth or fifth decade from aortic dissection or congestive heart failure secondary to aortic regurgitation

PREVENTION

- Prenatal and presymptomatic diagnosis for patients in whom a molecular defect in fibrillin has been found and for families in whom linkage analysis using polymorphic markers around the fibrillin gene can be performed

EVIDENCE

PRACTICE GUIDELINES

- Groenink M et al: Survival and complication free survival in Marfan's syndrome: implications of current guidelines. Heart 1999;82:499. [PMID: 10490568]

WEB SITES

- National Marfan Foundation http://www.marfan.org/
- National Institute of Arthritis and Musculoskeletal and Skin Diseases (NIAMS)/NIH http://www.niams.nih.gov/index.htm

INFORMATION FOR PATIENTS

- March of Dimes Quick Reference and Fact Sheets http://www.modimes.org/search/MsmGo.exe?grab_id=81076752&extra_arg=&page_id=853&host_id=1&query=Marfan&hiword=MARFAN+
- Questions and Answers about Marfan Syndrome, National Institute of Arthritis and Musculoskeletal and Skin Diseases (NIAMS)/NIH http://www.niams.nih.gov/hi/topics/marfan/marfan.htm

REFERENCES

- Dean JC: Management of Marfan syndrome. Heart 2002;88:97. [PMID: 12067963]
- Erkula G et al: Growth and maturation in Marfan syndrome. Am J Med Genet 2002;109:100. [PMID: 11977157]
- Gott VL et al: Replacement of the aortic root in patients with Marfan's syndrome. N Engl J Med 1999;340:1307. [PMID: 10219065]
- Pyeritz RE: The Marfan syndrome. Annu Rev Med 2000;51:481. [PMID: 10774478]

Reed E. Pyeritz, MD, PhD

Melanoma, Malignant

 KEY FEATURES

ESSENTIALS OF DIAGNOSIS

- The American Cancer Society has proposed the mnemonic "ABCD = Asymmetry, Border irregularity, Color variegation, and Diameter greater than 6 mm"
- Should be suspected in any pigmented skin lesion with recent change in appearance
- Examination with good light may show varying colors, including red, white, black, and bluish
- Borders typically irregular

GENERAL CONSIDERATIONS

- Leading cause of death due to skin disease
- Melanoma favors fair-skinned whites with a history of significant (blistering) sun exposure before the age of 18
- 10% of melanomas occur in "melanoma prone kindreds," ie, familial

Classification

- Lentigo maligna melanoma (arising on sun-exposed skin of older individuals)
- Superficial spreading malignant melanoma (the most common type, occurring in two-thirds of individuals developing melanoma, largely a disease of whites)
- Nodular malignant melanoma
- Acral lentiginous melanomas (arising on palms, soles, and nail beds); occur in nonwhites primarily); may be a difficult diagnosis because benign pigmented lesions of the hands, feet, and nails occur commonly in more darkly pigmented persons and clinicians may hesitate to biopsy the palms and especially the soles and nail beds; as a result, the diagnosis is often delayed until the tumor has become clinically obvious and histologically thick; clinicians should give special attention to new or changing lesions in these areas
- Malignant melanomas on mucous membranes
- Miscellaneous forms such as amelanotic (nonpigmented) melanoma and melanomas arising from blue nevi (rare) and congenital nevi

DEMOGRAPHICS

- One in four cases of melanoma occur before the age of 40

- Melanoma is the most common cancer of women between the ages of 25 and 29 and the second most common cause in women ages 30–34
- There are about 51,000 cases of melanoma in the United States annually, with 7800 deaths

 CLINICAL FINDINGS

SYMPTOMS AND SIGNS

- An irregular notched border where the pigment appears to be leaking into the normal surrounding skin
- Topography may be irregular, ie, partly raised and partly flat
- Color variegation, and colors such as pink, blue, gray, white, and black are indications for referral
- Bleeding and ulceration
- A mole that stands out from the patient's other moles (the "ugly duckling sign")
- A patient with a large number of moles is at increased risk for melanoma
- The history of a changing mole (evolution) is the single most important historical reason for close evaluation and possible referral
- Acral lentiginous melanomas: dark, sometimes irregularly shaped lesions on the palms and soles and new, often broad and solitary, darkly pigmented longitudinal streaks in the nails

DIFFERENTIAL DIAGNOSIS

- Acquired nevus (mole), eg, junctional nevus, compound nevus
- Seborrheic keratosis
- Lentigo, eg, solar lentigo
- Dermatofibroma
- Basal cell carcinoma (pigmented type)
- Congenital nevus
- Atypical (dysplastic) nevus
- Blue nevus
- Halo nevus
- Pyogenic granuloma
- Kaposi's sarcoma
- Pregnancy-associated darkening of nevi

 DIAGNOSIS

LABORATORY TESTS

- Skin biopsies

Melanoma, Malignant

 TREATMENT

 OUTCOME

 EVIDENCE

MEDICATIONS

- Interferon alpha and vaccine therapy may reduce recurrences in patients with high-risk melanomas

SURGERY

- Treatment consists of excision once a histological diagnosis is made
- The area is usually excised with margins dictated by the thickness of the tumor; large margins (radius ≥5 cm) are no longer indicated; thin low-risk and intermediate-risk tumors require only conservative margins of 1–3 cm; more specifically, surgical margins of 0.5 cm for melanoma in situ and 1 cm for lesions less than 1 mm in thickness are most often recommended
- Sentinel lymph node biopsy (selective lymphadenectomy) using preoperative lymphoscintigraphy and intraoperative lymphatic mapping is effective for staging melanoma patients with intermediate risk without clinical adenopathy and is recommended for all patients with lesions over 1 mm in thickness or with high-risk histological features

PROGNOSIS

- Tumor thickness is the single most important prognostic factor
- Ten-year survival rates—related to thickness in millimeters—are as follows: <0.76 mm, 96%; 0.76–1.69 mm, 81%; 1.7–3.6 mm, 57%; >3.6 mm, 31%
- With lymph node involvement, the 5-year survival rate is 30%; and with distant metastases, it is less than 10%; more accurate prognoses can be made on the basis of thickness, site, histological features, and sex of the patient
- Overall survival for melanomas in whites rose from 60% in 1960–1963 to 85% in 1983–1990, due primarily to earlier detection of lesions

WHEN TO REFER

- Any pigmented lesion with suspicious features should be referred to a dermatologist for possible biopsy

PRACTICE GUIDELINES

- National Guideline Clearinghouse http://www.guideline.gov/summary/ summary.aspx?doc_id=2741&nbr= 1967&string=melanoma
- http://www.guideline.gov/summary/ summary/summary.aspx?doc_id=2662& br=1888&string=melanoma

WEB SITES

- American Academy of Dermatology http://www.aad.org
- Dermatology Handbook for Family Practice from the University of Iowa http://www.vh.org/Providers/ClinRef/ FPHandbook/17.html

INFORMATION FOR PATIENTS

- American Academy of Dermatology http://www.aad.org/pamphlets/malmel. html
- Mayo Clinic http://www.mayoclinic.com/invoke. cfm?id=DS00439

REFERENCES

- Bafounta M et al: Is dermoscopy (epiluminescence microscopy) useful for the diagnosis of melanoma? Arch Dermatol 2001;137:1343. [PMID: 11594860]
- Balch CM et al: A new American Joint Committee on Cancer staging system for cutaneous melanoma. Cancer 2000; 88:1484. [PMID: 10717634]
- Goldstein BG et al: Diagnosis and management of malignant melanoma. Am Fam Physician 2001;63:1359. [PMID: 11310650]
- Rigel DS et al: Malignant melanoma: prevention, early detection, and treatment in the 21st century. CA Cancer J Clin 2000;50:215. [PMID: 10986965]

Timothy G. Berger, MD

Meningitis, Meningococcal

 ## KEY FEATURES

ESSENTIALS OF DIAGNOSIS

- Fever, headache, vomiting, confusion, delirium, convulsions
- Petechial rash of skin and mucous membranes
- Neck and back stiffness
- Purulent spinal fluid with gram-negative intracellular and extracellular diplococci
- Culture of cerebrospinal fluid, blood, or petechial aspiration confirms the diagnosis

GENERAL CONSIDERATIONS

- Caused by *Neisseria meningitidis* of groups A, B, C, Y, W-135, and others
- Infection is transmitted by droplets
- The clinical illness may take the form of meningococcemia (a fulminant form of septicemia) without meningitis, meningococcemia with meningitis, or predominantly meningitis
- Chronic recurrent meningococcemia with fever, rash, and arthritis can occur, particularly in those with terminal complement deficiencies

DEMOGRAPHICS

- College freshmen—particularly those living in dormitories– have been shown to have a modestly increased risk of invasive meningococcal disease

 ## CLINICAL FINDINGS

SYMPTOMS AND SIGNS

- High fever, chills, and headache; back, abdominal, and extremity pains; and nausea and vomiting are typical
- In severe cases, rapidly developing confusion, delirium, seizures, and coma occur
- Nuchal and back rigidity are typical
- A petechial rash often first appearing in the lower extremities and at pressure points is found in most cases. Petechiae may vary from pinhead-sized to large ecchymoses or even areas of skin gangrene that may later slough if the patient survives

DIFFERENTIAL DIAGNOSIS

- Meningitis due to other causes, eg, pneumococcus, *Listeria*, aseptic
- Rickettsial or echovirus infection and other bacterial infections (eg, staphylococcal infections, scarlet fever) may also produce a petechial rash
- Subarachnoid hemorrhage
- Encephalitis
- Petechial rash due to gonococcemia, infective endocarditis, thrombotic thrombocytopenic purpura, Rocky Mountain spotted fever, or viral exanthem
- "Neighborhood reaction" causing abnormal cerebrospinal fluid, eg, brain abscess, epidural abscess, vertebral osteomyelitis, mastoiditis, sinusitis, brain tumor
- Dural sinus thrombosis
- Noninfectious meningeal irritation: carcinomatous meningitis, sarcoidosis, systemic lupus erythematosus, drugs (eg, nonsteroidal antiinflammatory durgs, trimethoprim-sulfamethoxazole), pneumonia, shigellosis

 ## DIAGNOSIS

LABORATORY TESTS

- The organism is usually found by smear or culture of the cerebrospinal fluid, oropharynx, blood, or aspirated petechiae
- Prothrombin time and partial thromboplastin time are prolonged, fibrin dimers are elevated, fibrinogen is low, and the platelet count is depressed if disseminated intravascular coagulation is present

Cerebrospinal fluid analysis

- See Table 125 (page 1307)
- Typically, a cloudy or purulent fluid, with elevated pressure, increased protein, and decreased glucose content
- Usually contains more than 1000 cells/ μL, with polymorphonuclear cells predominating and containing gram-negative intracellular diplococci
- The absence of organisms in a Gram-stained smear does not rule out the diagnosis
- The capsular polysaccharide can often be demonstrated in cerebrospinal fluid or urine by latex agglutination; this is especially useful in partially treated patients, though sensitivity is only 60–80%

IMAGING STUDIES

- For neurological defects or signs of elevated intracranial pressure, MRI or CT imaging can exclude mass lesions

DIAGNOSTIC PROCEDURES

- Lumbar puncture

TREATMENT

MEDICATIONS

- See Table 123 (page 1306)
- Intravenous antimicrobial therapy should be started immediately after blood cultures are obtained in all acutely ill patients and before proceeding with imaging studies, if these are indicated
- Aqueous penicillin G is the antibiotic of choice (24 million units/24 h) in divided doses every 4 h
- In penicillin-allergic patients or those in whom pneumococcal or gram-negative meningitis is a consideration, ceftriaxone, 4 g intravenously once a day, should be used
- Chloramphenicol, 1 g every 6 h, is an alternative in the severely penicillin- or cephalosporin-allergic patient
- In critically ill patients with evidence of increased intracranial pressure, administration of dexamethasone (0.6 mg/kg/day in four divided doses) may help
- Duration of therapy: 10–14 days (with ceftriaxone a 5-day regimen has been reported to be effective)

THERAPEUTIC PROCEDURES

- Lumbar puncture should be performed in all patients with suspected meningococcal meningitis; imaging prior to lumbar puncture to rule out mass lesions is indicated if papilledema, other evidence of increased intracranial pressure, or focal neurological deficit

 OUTCOME

COMPLICATIONS

- Obtundation or deterioration in mental status may result from cerebral edema and increased intracranial pressure
- Disseminated intravascular coagulation
- Ischemic necrosis of digits, distal extremities

PROGNOSIS

- Mortality <5% with early therapy of patients with meningitis
- Meningococcemia associated with a 20% mortality

WHEN TO ADMIT

- All patients in whom meningococcal meningitis is suspected should be admitted for observation and empirical therapy

PREVENTION

- Effective polysaccharide vaccines for groups A, C, Y, and W-135 are available
- The Advisory Committee on Immunization Practices now recommends immunization with a single dose of polyvalent vaccine (active against meningococcal groups A, C, Y, and W-135) for college freshmen
- Outbreaks in closed populations are best controlled by eliminating nasopharyngeal carriage of meningococci. Rifampin is the drug of choice, in a dosage of 600 mg twice a day for 2 days. A single 500-mg oral dose of ciprofloxacin or one intramuscular 250-mg dose of ceftriaxone in adults is also effective

 EVIDENCE

PRACTICE GUIDELINES

- National Guideline Clearinghouse http://www.guideline.gov/summary/summary.aspx?doc_id=2364&nbr=1590&string=meningococcal+meningitis http://www.guideline.gov/summary/summary.aspx?doc_id=2365&nbr=1591&string=meningococcal+meningitis

WEB SITES

- CDC—Division of Bacterial and Mycotic Diseases http://www.cdc.gov/ncidod/dbmd/
- Meningococcemia Case Study http://path.upmc.edu:80/cases/case53.html

INFORMATION FOR PATIENTS

- JAMA patient page: Lumbar puncture. JAMA 2002;288:2056.
- JAMA patient page: Meningitis. JAMA 1999;281:1560.

REFERENCES

- Harrison LH et al: Risk of meningococcal infection in college students. JAMA 1999;281:1906. [PMID: 10349894]
- Peltola H: Prophylaxis of bacterial meningitis. Infect Dis Clin North Am 1999;13:685. [PMID: 10470562]

Henry F. Chambers, MD

Meningitis, Pneumococcal

 KEY FEATURES

ESSENTIALS OF DIAGNOSIS

- Fever, headache, altered mental status
- Meningismus
- Gram-positive diplococci on Gram stain of cerebrospinal fluid; counterimmuno-electrophoresis may be positive in partially treated cases

GENERAL CONSIDERATIONS

- *Streptococcus pneumoniae* is the most common cause of meningitis in adults and the second most common cause of meningitis in children over the age of 6 years
- Head trauma, with cerebrospinal fluid leaks, sinusitis, and pneumonia may precede it
- Up to 40% of infections are caused by pneumococci resistant to at least one drug and 15% are due to a strain resistant to three or more drugs

DEMOGRAPHICS

- Until 2000, *S pneumoniae* infections caused 100,000–135,000 hospitalizations for pneumonia, 6 million cases of otitis media, and 60,000 cases of invasive disease, including 3300 cases of meningitis
- Disease figures are now changing due to conjugate vaccine introduction

 CLINICAL FINDINGS

SYMPTOMS AND SIGNS

- Rapid onset, with fever, headache, and altered mentation
- Pneumonia may be present
- Compared with meningitis caused by the meningococcus, pneumococcal meningitis lacks a rash, and focal neurological deficits, cranial nerve palsies, and obtundation are more prominent features

DIFFERENTIAL DIAGNOSIS

- Meningitis due to other causes, eg, meningococcus, *Listeria*, aseptic
- Subarachnoid hemorrhage
- Encephalitis
- "Neighborhood reaction" causing abnormal cerebrospinal fluid, eg, brain abscess, epidural abscess, vertebral osteomyelitis, mastoiditis, sinusitis, brain tumor
- Dural sinus thrombosis
- Noninfectious meningeal irritation: carcinomatous meningitis, sarcoidosis, systemic lupus erythematosus, drugs (eg, nonsteroidal antiinflammatory drugs, trimethoprim-sulfamethoxazole), pneumonia, shigellosis

 DIAGNOSIS

LABORATORY TESTS

- See Table 125 (page 1307)
- The cerebrospinal fluid typically has more than 1000 white blood cells per microliter, over 60% of which are polymorphonuclear leukocytes; the glucose concentration is less than 40 mg/dL, or less than 50% of the simultaneous serum concentration; the protein usually exceeds 150 mg/dL
- Gram stain of cerebrospinal fluid shows gram-positive cocci in up to 80–90% of cases, and in untreated cases blood or cerebrospinal fluid cultures are almost always positive
- Fifty percent rate of bacteremia
- Antigen detection tests may occasionally be helpful in establishing the diagnosis in the patient who has been partially treated and in whom cultures and stains are negative

TREATMENT

MEDICATIONS

- See Tables 123 and 124 (page 1306)
- Give antibiotics as soon as the diagnosis is suspected
- If lumbar puncture must be delayed (eg, while awaiting results of an imaging study to exclude a mass lesion), ceftriaxone, 4 g, is given intravenously after blood cultures (positive in 50% of cases) have been obtained
- If gram-positive diplococci are present on the Gram stain, then vancomycin, 30 mg/kg/day intravenously in two divided doses, should be administered in addition to ceftriaxone until the isolate is confirmed not to be penicillin-resistant
- Once susceptibility to penicillin has been confirmed, penicillin, 24 million units daily in six divided doses, or ceftriaxone, 4 g/day as a single dose or as two divided doses, is recommended
- For severe penicillin allergy chloramphenicol, 50 mg/kg every 6 h, is an alternative (failures have occurred with penicillin-resistant strains)
- Duration of therapy is 10–14 days in documented cases
- The best therapy for penicillin-resistant strains is not known. Susceptibility testing is essential
- If the minimum inhibitory concentration (MIC) of ceftriaxone or cefotaxime is ≤0.5 μg/mL, single-drug therapy with either of these cephalosporins is likely to be effective; when the MIC is ≥1 μg/mL, treatment with a combination of ceftriaxone, 2 g every 12 h, plus vancomycin, 30 mg/kg/day in two divided doses, is recommended
- Give 10 mg of dexamethasone intravenously immediately prior to or concomitantly with the first dose of appropriate antibiotic and every 6 h thereafter for a total of 4 days. The anti-inflammatory activity could impair penetration of some drugs into the cerebrospinal fluid, particularly vancomycin, and cause a potential treatment failure

OUTCOME

FOLLOW-UP

- If a patient with a penicillin-resistant organism has not responded to a third-generation cephalosporin, repeat lumbar puncture is indicated to assess the bacteriological response

COMPLICATIONS

- Hearing loss
- Residual neurological deficit

PROGNOSIS

- Patients presenting with depressed levels of conciousness have a worse outcome
- Dexamethasone administered with antibiotic to adults has been associated with a 60% reduction in mortality and a 50% reduction in unfavorable outcome

WHEN TO REFER

- Consider early referral to an infectious disease specialist

WHEN TO ADMIT

- All patients with suspected bacterial meningitis

PREVENTION

- Pneumococcal vaccine recommendations (Table 127, page 1310)

EVIDENCE

PRACTICE GUIDELINES

- National Guideline Clearinghouse http://www.guideline.gov/summary/summary.aspx?doc_id=2773&nbr=1999&string=pneumococcal+meningitis

WEB SITES

- CDC—Division of Bacterial and Mycotic Diseases http://www.cdc.gov/ncidod/dbmd/
- Karolinska Institute—Directory of Bacterial Infections and Mycoses http://www.mic.ki.se/Diseases/c1.html

INFORMATION FOR PATIENTS

- JAMA patient page: Lumbar puncture. JAMA 2002;288:2056.
- JAMA patient page: Meningitis. JAMA 1999;281:1560.

REFERENCES

- de Gans J et al: Dexamethasone in adults with bacterial meningitis. N Engl J Med 2002;347:1549.
- Peltola H: Prophylaxis of bacterial meningitis. Infect Dis Clin North Am 1999;13:685. [PMID: 10470562]
- Quagliarello VJ et al: Treatment of bacterial meningitis. N Engl J Med 1997;336:708. [PMID: 9041103]
- Tunkel AR, Scheld WM: Treatment of bacterial meningitis. Curr Infect Dis Rep 2002;4:7. [PMID: 11853652]

Henry F. Chambers, MD

Menopausal Syndrome

 KEY FEATURES

ESSENTIALS OF DIAGNOSIS

- Cessation of menses due to aging or to bilateral oophorectomy
- Elevation of follicle-stimulating hormone (FSH) and luteinizing hormone (LH) levels
- Hot flushes and night sweats (in 80% of women)
- Decreased vaginal lubrication; thinned vaginal mucosa with or without dyspareunia

GENERAL CONSIDERATIONS

- Menopause denotes a 1- to 3-year period during which a woman adjusts to a diminishing and then absent menstrual flow and the physiological changes that may be associated—hot flushes, night sweats, and vaginal dryness
- Premature menopause is defined as ovarian failure and menstrual cessation before age 40; this often has a genetic or autoimmune basis
- Surgical menopause due to bilateral oophorectomy is common and can cause more severe symptoms owing to the sudden rapid drop in sex hormone levels
- Cessation of ovarian function is not associated with severe emotional disturbance or personality changes. The time of menopause often coincides with other major life changes, such as departure of children from the home, a midlife identity crisis, or divorce

DEMOGRAPHICS

- The average age at menopause in Western societies today is 51 years

 CLINICAL FINDINGS

SYMPTOMS AND SIGNS

- Menstrual cycles generally become irregular as menopause approaches
- Anovular cycles occur more often, with irregular cycle length and occasional menorrhagia
- Menstrual flow amount diminishes
- Finally, cycles become longer, with missed periods or episodes of spotting only
- When no bleeding has occurred for 1 year, the menopausal transition has occurred
- Hot flushes (feelings of intense heat over the trunk and face, with flushing of the skin and sweating)
- Hot flushes can begin before the cessation of menses and are more severe after surgical menopause
- Flushing is more pronounced late in the day, during hot weather, after ingestion of hot foods or drinks, or during periods of tension. Occurring at night, they often cause sweating and insomnia and result in fatigue on the following day
- Vaginal atrophy and decreased vaginal lubrication
- The introitus decreases in diameter
- Pelvic examination reveals pale, smooth vaginal mucosa and a small cervix and uterus
- The ovaries are not normally palpable after the menopause

DIFFERENTIAL DIAGNOSIS

- Pregnancy
- Premature ovarian failure
- Hypothyroidism or hyperthyroidism
- Hyperprolactinemia
- Polycystic ovary syndrome
- Hypothalamic amenorrhea, eg, stress, weight change, exercise
- Other endocrine causes: Cushing's syndrome, Addison's disease, androgen-secreting tumor (adrenal, ovarian), congenital adrenal hyperplasia, acromegaly
- Depression

 DIAGNOSIS

LABORATORY TESTS

- Serum FSH and LH levels are elevated
- Vaginal cytological examination will show a low estrogen effect with predominantly parabasal cells

Menopausal Syndrome

TREATMENT

MEDICATIONS

Natural menopause

- **Vasomotor Symptoms**
- Oral conjugated estrogens, 0.3 mg or 0.625 mg; estradiol, 0.5 or 1 mg; or estrone sulfate, 0.625 mg; or estradiol can be given transdermally as skin patches that are changed once or twice weekly and secrete 0.05–0.1 mg of hormone daily
- When either form of estrogen is used, add a progestin (medroxyprogesterone acetate) to prevent endometrial hyperplasia or cancer. Give estrogen on Days 1–25 of each calendar month, with 5–10 mg of medroxyprogesterone acetate added on Days 14–25. Withhold hormones from Day 26 until the end of the month, when the endometrium will be shed, producing a light, generally painless monthly period. Or give the estrogen along with 2.5 mg of medroxyprogesterone acetate daily, without stopping. This causes initial bleeding or spotting, but within a few months it produces an atrophic endometrium that will not bleed
- If the patient has had a hysterectomy, a progestin need not be used
- Explain that hot flushes will probably return if the hormone is discontinued
- When women wish to stop hormone therapy, the dose should be tapered
- In women who cannot use estrogen, megestrol acetate, 20 mg twice daily, is effective in reducing the frequency of hot flushes
- Clonidine given orally or transdermally, 100–150 µg daily, may also reduce the frequency of hot flushes, but its use is limited by side effects, including dry mouth, drowsiness, and hypotension
- **Vaginal Atrophy**
- Estradiol vaginal ring, left in place for 3 months, is suitable for long-term use. Progestin therapy to protect the endometrium is unnecessary
- Short-term use of estrogen vaginal cream will relieve symptoms of atrophy, but because of variable absorption, therapy with either systemic hormone replacement or the vaginal ring is preferable
- Testosterone propionate, 1–2%, 0.5–1 g, in a vanishing cream base used in the same manner is also effective if estrogen is contraindicated

- A bland lubricant such as unscented cold cream or water-soluble gel can be helpful at the time of coitus
- **Osteoporosis**
- Women should ingest at least 800 mg of calcium daily and 1 g of elemental calcium should be taken as a daily supplement at the time of the menopause and thereafter; calcium supplements should be taken with meals to increase their absorption. Vitamin D, 400 units/day from food, sunlight, or supplements, enhances calcium absorption
- Daily energetic walking and exercise help maintain bone mass
- **Advantages and Risks of Hormone Therapy**
- The use of long-term hormone replacement therapy for prevention is no longer indicated. Clinicians should review with women and carefully consider the risks and benefits
- Current indications for hormone therapy (estrogen and progestin) are for treatment of vasmotor symptoms, which resolve within several months to a few years

Surgical menopause

- Estrogen replacement is generally started immediately after surgery
- Conjugated estrogens 1.25 mg, estrone sulfate 1.25 mg, or estradiol, 2 mg, is given for 25 days of each month
- After age 45–50 years, this dose can be tapered to 0.625 mg of conjugated estrogens or equivalent

OUTCOME

FOLLOW-UP

- Annual visit to monitor symptoms and need for therapy
- Any bleeding after cessation of menses warrants investigation by endometrial curettage or aspiration to rule out endometrial cancer
- For women who are receiving hormone replacement therapy for vasomotor symptoms, an attempt should be made at least every 6 months to taper the dose and to discontinue therapy

COMPLICATIONS

- Dyspareunia from vaginal atrophy and decreased vaginal lubrication
- Overall health risks exceed benefits from use of combined estrogen plus progestin

for an average of 5 years. These risks include increased coronary heart disease events, cerebral vascular accidents, pulmonary emboli, invasive breast cancer, and gallbladder disease

PREVENTION

- Continued sexual activity will help prevent vaginal shrinkage

EVIDENCE

PRACTICE GUIDELINES

- National Guideline Clearinghouse http://www.guideline.gov/summary/summary.aspx?doc_id=2138&nbr=1364&string=menopause http://www.guideline.gov/summary/summary.aspx?doc_id=3464&nbr=2690&string=menopause

WEB SITE

- Menopause http://www.menopause.org/

INFORMATION FOR PATIENTS

- JAMA patient page. Perimenopause: beginning of menopause. JAMA 2003; 289:940.
- JAMA patient page. Hormone replacement therapy. JAMA 2002;288:916.

REFERENCES

- Grady D: A 60-year-old woman trying to discontinue hormone replacement therapy. JAMA 2002;28:2130. [PMID: 11966388]
- Grady D: Postmenopausal hormones—therapy for symptoms only. N Engl J Med 2003;348:1835. [PMID: 12642636]
- Rossouw JE et al: Risks and benefits of estrogen plus progestin in healthy postmenopausal women: principal results from the Women's Health Initiative randomized controlled trial. JAMA 2002; 288:321. [PMID: 12117397]
- Stephenson J: FDA orders estrogen safety warnings: agency offers guidance for HRT use. JAMA 2003;289:537. [PMID: 12578468]

H. Trent MacKay, MD, MPH

Mesothelioma

 KEY FEATURES

ESSENTIALS OF DIAGNOSIS

- Chronic progressive chest pain and dyspnea
- Pleural effusion and/or pleural thickening on chest radiographs
- Malignant cells in pleural fluid or tissue

GENERAL CONSIDERATIONS

- Primary tumors arising from the mesothelial surfaces of the pleura (80% of cases), peritoneum, pericardium, or tunica vaginalis
- 75% of pleural mesotheliomas are diffuse (usually malignant)
- Mean age at symptom onset is 60 years with time between exposure and symptoms 20–40 years

DEMOGRAPHICS

- Men outnumber women 3:1
- Malignant pleural mesothelioma is associated with asbestos exposure (70% of cases), with a lifetime risk to asbestos workers of 8%
- Cigarette smoking significantly increases the risk of bronchogenic carcinoma in asbestos workers and aggravates asbestosis, but there is no association between smoking and mesothelioma independent of asbestos
- Asbestos exposure occurs through mining, milling, manufacturing, shipyard work, insulation, brake linings, building construction and demolition, roofing materials, and other asbestos-containing products

 CLINICAL FINDINGS

SYMPTOMS AND SIGNS

- Insidious onset of shortness of breath, nonpleuritic chest pain, and weight loss
- Physical findings include dullness to percussion, diminished breath sounds, and finger clubbing in some cases
- Malignant pleural mesothelioma progresses rapidly as the tumor spreads along the pleural surface to involve the pericardium, mediastinum, and contralateral pleura
- Tumor may eventually extend beyond the thorax to involve abdominal lymph nodes and organs

DIFFERENTIAL DIAGNOSIS

- Chronic organized empyema
- Sarcoma
- Metastatic tumor to the pleura, especially adenocarcinoma
- Malignant fibrosing histiocytoma
- Other causes of pleural effusion (see *Pleural effusion*)

 DIAGNOSIS

LABORATORY TESTS

- Pleural fluid analysis often reveals a hemorrhagic exudate

IMAGING STUDIES

- Radiographic findings are nodular, irregular, unilateral pleural thickening and varying degrees of unilateral pleural effusion
- CT helps determine the extent of pleural and extrapleural involvement

DIAGNOSTIC PROCEDURES

- Thoracentesis
- Closed pleural biopsy
- Open pleural biopsy may be necessary to obtain an adequate specimen for histological diagnosis

Mesothelioma

TREATMENT

SURGERY

- Some surgeons believe that extrapleural pneumonectomy is the preferred approach for patients with early-stage disease
- Resection may offer palliative benefit in some cases

THERAPEUTIC PROCEDURES

- Treatment with surgery, radiation, chemotherapy, or a combination of methods is generally unsuccessful
- Drainage of effusions, pleurodesis, and radiation therapy may offer palliative benefit

OUTCOME

COMPLICATIONS

- Local invasion of thoracic structures with superior vena caval syndrome, hoarseness, Horner's syndrome, dysphagia
- Paraneoplastic syndrome
  - Thrombocytosis
  - Hemolytic anemia
  - Disseminated intravascular coagulopathy
  - Migratory thrombophlebitis
- Metastatic disease

PROGNOSIS

- Median survival from symptom onset ranges from 5 months in extensive disease to 16 months in localized disease
- 75% of patients are dead 1 year from diagnosis
- Most patients die of respiratory failure and complications of local extension

WHEN TO REFER

- Upon diagnosis, refer to a pulmonologist, oncologist, or possibly a thoracic surgeon who can evaluate the patient for multidisciplinary treatment

WHEN TO ADMIT

- For pleural fluid drainage
- For severe dyspnea
- For pain management

PREVENTION

- Avoidance of tobacco smoke (primary or secondary) in those with a history of asbestos exposure

EVIDENCE

PRACTICE GUIDELINES

- National Guideline Clearinghouse http://www.guideline.gov/summary/summary.aspx?doc_id=3637&nbr=2863&string=lung+cancer
- Rivera MP et al: Diagnosis of lung cancer: the guidelines. Chest 2003;123 (1 Suppl):129S.
- Detterbeck FC et al: Lung cancer. Invasive staging: the guidelines. Chest 2003;123(1 Suppl):167S.

INFORMATION FOR PATIENTS

- National Cancer Institute http://cis.nci.nih.gov/fact/6_36.htm
- National Institutes of Health http://www.nlm.nih.gov/medlineplus/ency/article/000115.htm http://www.nlm.nih.gov/medlineplus/ency/article/000116.htm

REFERENCES

- Sterman DH et al: Advances in the treatment of malignant pleural mesothelioma. Chest 2000;116:504. [PMID: 10453882]
- Sugarbaker DJ et al: Multimodality management of malignant pleural mesothelioma. Chest 1998;113 (Suppl):61S. [PMID: 9438692]

Mark S. Chesnutt, MD
Thomas J. Prendergast, MD

Mononeuropathies

KEY FEATURES

ESSENTIALS OF DIAGNOSIS

- Focal motor or sensory deficit that conforms to the territory of an individual peripheral nerve

GENERAL CONSIDERATIONS

- Injury of an individual nerve along its course
- Possible compression, angulation, or stretching of an individual nerve by neighboring anatomic structures
- Nerve affected at a point where it passes through a narrow space (entrapment neuropathy)

CLINICAL FINDINGS

SYMPTOMS AND SIGNS

- Entrapment neuropathies may result in no symptoms, in symptoms that resolve rapidly and spontaneously, or in symptoms that become progressively more disabling and distressing
- In entrapment neuropathies, the precise neurological deficit depends on the nerve involved
- Involvement of a sensory or mixed nerve commonly results in pain distal to the lesion
- Percussion of the nerve at the site of the lesion may lead to paresthesias in its distal distribution
- There are several syndromes
  - See *Carpal tunnel syndrome,* page 1082
  - See *Femoral neuropathy,* page 1101
  - See *Meralgia paresthetica,* page 1131
  - See *Ulnar neuropathy,* page 1184
- **Pronator teres syndrome** affects the anterior interosseous nerve, a motor branch of the median nerve, that arises below the elbow between the two heads of the pronator teres muscle
  - A lesion may result after trauma or from compression, eg, from a fibrous band
  - Weakness is confined to the pronator quadratus, flexor pollicis longus, and the flexor digitorum profundus to the second and third digits
- **Sciatic and common peroneal nerve palsies**
  - Most common etiology for sciatic nerve palsy is probably a misplaced deep intramuscular injection
  - Trauma to the buttock, hip, or thigh may also be responsible
  - The common peroneal nerve itself may be compressed or injured in the region of the head and neck of the fibula, eg, by sitting with crossed legs or wearing high boots
  - Common peroneal involvement causes weakness of dorsiflexion and eversion of the foot, accompanied by numbness or blunted sensation of the anterolateral aspect of the calf and dorsum of the foot
- In **tarsal tunnel syndrome** compression of the posterior tibial nerve or its branches between the bony floor and ligamentous roof of the tarsal tunnel leads to pain, paresthesias, and numbness over the bottom of the foot, especially at night, with sparing of the heel
- In **facial neuropathy**, an isolated facial palsy may occur with HIV seropositivity, sarcoidosis, Lyme disease, or most often, idiopathic (see *Bell's palsy*)

DIAGNOSIS

DIAGNOSTIC PROCEDURES

- EMG can be indispensable for the accurate localization of the focal lesion
- Entrapment neuropathy may be the sole manifestation of subclinical polyneuropathy, and this must be borne in mind and excluded by nerve conduction studies
- Peripheral nerve tumors may be distinguishable from entrapment neuropathy only by
  - Noting the presence of a mass along the course of the nerve
  - Demonstrating the precise site of the lesion with appropriate electrophysiological studies

TREATMENT

MEDICATIONS

- In some neuropathies, local infiltration of the region about the nerve with corticosteroids may be of value

SURGERY

- Surgical decompression may help when there is a progressively increasing neurological deficit or electrodiagnostic studies show evidence of partial denervation in weak muscles
- In the rare peripheral nerve tumors, symptomatic lesions are surgically removed when possible

THERAPEUTIC PROCEDURES

- When repetitive mechanical trauma is responsible, avoid by occupational adjustment or job retraining
- When acute compression is the cause such as may occur in intoxicated individuals ("Saturday night palsy"), no treatment is needed in most cases
- In chronic compressive or entrapment neuropathies, avoid aggravating factors and correct any underlying systemic conditions

 OUTCOME

PROGNOSIS

- In patients with acute compression neuropathy, complete recovery generally occurs within 2 months without treatment, presumably because the underlying pathology is demyelination
- Axonal degeneration can occur in severe cases, and then recovery takes longer and may be partial

 Mononeuropathies

 EVIDENCE

PRACTICE GUIDELINES

- National Guideline Clearinghouse http://www.guideline.gov/summary/summary.aspx?doc_id=1572&nbr=798&string=mononeuropathy

INFORMATION FOR PATIENTS

- The Mayo Clinic http://www.mayoclinic.com/invoke.cfm?id=DS00131
- National Institutes of Health http://www.nlm.nih.gov/medlineplus/ency/article/000780.htm

REFERENCE

- Aminoff MJ: Electromyography in clinical practice: clinical and electrodiagnostic aspects of neuromuscular disease, ed 3. Churchill Livingstone, 1998.

Michael J. Aminoff, MD, DSc, FRCP

Motor Neuron Disease

 KEY FEATURES

ESSENTIALS OF DIAGNOSIS

- Variable weakness and wasting of muscles without sensory changes

GENERAL CONSIDERATIONS

- There is degeneration of the anterior horn cells in the spinal cord, the motor nuclei of the lower cranial nerves, and the corticospinal and corticobulbar pathways
- Five varieties have been characterized on clinical grounds

Progressive bulbar palsy

- Bulbar involvement predominates
- Disease processes affect primarily the motor nuclei of the cranial nerves

Pseudobulbar palsy

- Bulbar involvement predominates
- Due to bilateral corticobulbar disease and thus reflects upper motor neuron dysfunction

Progressive spinal muscular atrophy

- A lower motor neuron deficit in the limbs
- Due to degeneration of the anterior horn cells in the spinal cord

Primary lateral sclerosis

- There is a purely upper motor neuron deficit in the limbs

Amyotrophic lateral sclerosis

- A mixed upper and lower motor neuron deficit is found in the limbs and bulbar muscles
- This disorder is sometimes associated with dementia or parkinsonism

DEMOGRAPHICS

- Symptoms generally begin between 30 and 60 years of age
- The disease is usually sporadic, but familial cases may occur

 CLINICAL FINDINGS

SYMPTOMS AND SIGNS

- Difficulty in swallowing, chewing, coughing, breathing, and talking (dysarthria) occur with bulbar involvement
- In progressive bulbar palsy, there is drooping of the palate, a depressed gag reflex, pooling of saliva in the pharynx, a weak cough, and a wasted, fasciculating tongue
- In pseudobulbar palsy, the tongue is contracted and spastic and cannot be moved rapidly from side to side
- Limb involvement is characterized by motor disturbances (weakness, stiffness, wasting, fasciculations) reflecting lower or upper motor neuron dysfunction
- There are no objective changes on sensory examination, though there may be vague sensory complaints
- The sphincters are generally spared

DIFFERENTIAL DIAGNOSIS

Upper motor neuron disease

- Stroke
- Space-occupying lesion
- Compressive spinal cord lesion
- Multiple sclerosis

Lower motor neuron disease

- Infections of anterior horn cells (eg, poliovirus or West Nile virus)
- Radiculopathy, plexopathy, peripheral neuropathy, and myopathy are distinguished by clinical examination
- Pure motor syndromes resembling motor neuron disease may occur in association with monoclonal gammopathy or multifocal motor neuropathies with conduction block. Multifocal motor neuropathy is distinguished by electrodiagnostic studies
- A motor neuronopathy may develop in Hodgkin's disease and has a relatively benign prognosis

 DIAGNOSIS

LABORATORY TESTS

- The serum creatine kinase may be slightly elevated but never reaches the extremely high values seen in some of the muscular dystrophies
- The cerebrospinal fluid is normal

DIAGNOSTIC PROCEDURES

- Electromyography may show changes of chronic partial denervation, with abnormal spontaneous activity in the resting muscle and a reduction in the number of motor units under voluntary control
- In patients with suspected spinal muscular atrophy or amyotrophic lateral sclerosis, the diagnosis should not be made with confidence unless such changes are found in at least three extremities
- Motor conduction velocity is usually normal but may be slightly reduced, and sensory conduction studies are also normal
- Biopsy of a wasted muscle shows the histological changes of denervation

Motor Neuron Disease

TREATMENT

MEDICATIONS

- Riluzole, 100 mg, daily reduces the presynaptic release of glutamate and may slow progression of amyotrophic lateral sclerosis
- There is otherwise no specific treatment except in patients with gammopathy, in whom plasmapheresis and immunosuppression may lead to improvement
- Multifocal motor neuropathy is treated by intravenous immunoglobulin therapy or with cyclophosphamide
- Symptomatic and supportive measures may include prescription of anticholinergic drugs (such as trihexyphenidyl, amitriptyline, or atropine) if drooling is troublesome, braces or a walker to improve mobility, and physical therapy to prevent contractures
- Spasticity may be helped by baclofen or diazepam

SURGERY

- Gastrostomy or cricopharyngomyotomy is sometimes resorted to in extreme cases of predominant bulbar involvement, and tracheostomy may be necessary if respiratory muscles are severely affected; however, in the terminal stages of these disorders, the aim of treatment should be to keep patients as comfortable as possible

THERAPEUTIC PROCEDURES

- A semiliquid diet or nasogastric tube feeding may be needed if dysphagia is severe

OUTCOME

PROGNOSIS

- The disorder is progressive, and amyotrophic lateral sclerosis is usually fatal within 3–5 years; death usually results from pulmonary infections
- Patients with bulbar involvement generally have the poorest prognosis

WHEN TO REFER

- All patients should be referred to a physician with expertise in the diagnosis and treatment of these disorders

EVIDENCE

PRACTICE GUIDELINES

- National Guideline Clearinghouse http://www.guideline.gov/summary/summary.aspx?doc_id=2819&nbr=2045&string=motor+neuron+disease

WEB SITE

- Neuromuscular Disease Center http://www.neuro.wustl.edu/neuromuscular/

INFORMATION FOR PATIENTS

- National Institute of Neurological Disorders and Stroke http://www.ninds.nih.gov/health_and_medical/disorders/ motor_neuron_diseases.htm http://www.ninds.nih.gov/health_and_medical/pubs/als.htm

REFERENCES

- Benditt JO et al: Empowering the individual with ALS at the end-of-life: disease-specific advance care planning. Muscle Nerve 2001;24:1706. [PMID: 11745983]
- Parton MJ et al: Motor neuron disease and its management. J R Coll Physicians Lond 1999;33:212. [PMID: 10402566]

Michael J. Aminoff, MD, DSc, FRCP

Mountain Sickness

 KEY FEATURES

ESSENTIALS OF DIAGNOSIS

- Mountain sickness disorders include acute mountain sickness, acute high-altitude pulmonary edema, subacute mountain sickness, and chronic mountain sickness

GENERAL CONSIDERATIONS

- Lack of sufficient time for acclimatization, increased physical activity, and varying degrees of health may be responsible for the acute, subacute, and chronic disturbances that result from hypoxia at altitudes greater than 2000 m (6560 ft)

Acute mountain sickness

- The severity correlates with altitude and rate of ascent

Acute high-altitude pulmonary edema

- This serious complication usually occurs at levels above 3000 m (9840 ft)

Acute high-altitude encephalopathy

- Appears to be an extension of the central nervous system symptoms of acute mountain sickness
- It usually occurs at elevations above 2500 m (8250 ft)
- More common in the unacclimatized
- Clinical findings are due largely to hypoxemia and cerebral edema

Subacute mountain sickness

- Occurs most frequently in unacclimatized individuals at altitudes above 4500 m (14,764 ft)

Chronic mountain sickness (Monge's disease)

- Chronic hypoxia and polycythemia in residents of high-altitude communities who have lost their acclimatization to such an environment
- May be difficult to differentiate from chronic pulmonary disease
- Uncommon condition

 CLINICAL FINDINGS

SYMPTOMS AND SIGNS

Acute mountain sickness

- Initially, headache (most severe and persistent symptom), lassitude, drowsiness, dizziness, chilliness, nausea and vomiting, dyspnea, and cyanosis
- Later, facial flushing, irritability, difficulty in concentrating, vertigo, tinnitus, visual disturbances, auditory disturbances, anorexia, insomnia, increased dyspnea and weakness on exertion, increased headaches (due to cerebral edema), palpitations, tachycardia, Cheyne-Stokes breathing, and weight loss
- More severe manifestations include pulmonary edema and encephalopathy

Acute high-altitude pulmonary edema

- Early symptoms may appear within 6–36 h
- Incessant dry cough, shortness of breath, headache, fatigue, dyspnea at rest, and chest tightness
- Later, wheezing, orthopnea, and hemoptysis may occur
- Tachycardia, mild fever, tachypnea, cyanosis, prolonged respiration, and rales and rhonchi
- Confusion or coma
- May resemble severe pneumonia

Acute high-altitude encephalopathy

- Severe headaches, confusion, truncal ataxia, staggering gait, focal deficits, nausea and vomiting, and seizures may progress to obtundation and coma
- High-altitude retinopathy can include dilated vessels, retinal hemorrhage, vitreous hemorrhage, and papilledema

Subacute mountain sickness

- Dyspnea and cough
- Dehydration, skin dryness, and pruritus

Chronic mountain sickness

- Somnolence, mental depression, hypoxemia, cyanosis, finger clubbing
- Right ventricular failure

DIFFERENTIAL DIAGNOSIS

- Migraine or tension headache
- Stroke or intracerebral bleed
- Congestive heart failure
- Alcohol or drug intoxication
- Sepsis

 DIAGNOSIS

LABORATORY TESTS

Acute high-altitude pulmonary edema

- Hypoxia
- The white cell count is often slightly elevated, but the erythrocyte sedimentation rate is usually normal
- Elevated pulmonary arterial blood pressure; normal wedge pressure

Subacute mountain sickness

- Hypoxia
- The hematocrit may be elevated

Chronic mountain sickness

- Polycythemia; hemoglobin >22 g/dL (hematocrit often >75%)
- Pulmonary function tests usually disclose alveolar hypoventilation and elevated P_{CO_2} but fail to reveal defective oxygen transport

IMAGING STUDIES

Acute high-altitude pulmonary edema

- Chest x-ray findings vary from irregular patchy infiltration in one lung to nodular densities bilaterally or with transient prominence of the central pulmonary arteries
- Transient nonspecific electrocardiographic changes, occasional right ventricular strain

Subacute and chronic mountain sickness

- There may be ECG changes of right axis deviation and right atrial and ventricular hypertrophy
- X-ray evidence of right heart enlargement and central pulmonary vessel prominence

TREATMENT

MEDICATIONS

Acute mountain sickness

- Acetazolamide, 125–250 mg every 12 h, or dexamethasone, 8 mg initially followed by 4 mg every 6 h, for as long as symptoms persist

Acute high-altitude pulmonary edema

- Nifedipine, 10 mg every 4 h, may provide symptomatic relief
- Dexamethasone, 4 mg every 6 h, may help central nervous system symptoms
- Acetazolamide, 125–250 mg every 12 h, should be administered if acute mountain sickness is suspected
- If bacterial pneumonia occurs, appropriate antibiotics should be given

Acute high-altitude encephalopathy

- Dexamethasone, 4–8 mg every 6 h

THERAPEUTIC PROCEDURES

Acute mountain sickness

- Voluntary periodic hyperventilation may relieve symptoms
- Symptoms generally clear within 24–48 h, but if the symptoms are persistent or severe, the patient must be returned to lower altitudes
- Definitive treatment is immediate descent, which is essential if reduced consciousness, ataxia, or pulmonary edema occurs
- Administration of oxygen, 1–2 L/min, will often relieve acute symptoms
- If immediate descent is not possible, portable hyperbaric chambers may provide symptomatic relief

Acute high-altitude pulmonary edema

- Rest in the semi-Fowler position (head raised) and administration of 100% oxygen by mask at a rate of 4–6 L/min for 15–30 min. To conserve oxygen, lower flow rates (2–4 L/min) may be used
- Immediate descent [at least 610 m (2000 ft)] is essential
- Recompression in a portable hyperbaric bag will temporarily reduce symptoms if immediate descent is not possible
- Treatment for acute respiratory distress syndrome may be required

Acute high-altitude encephalopathy

- Treatment is immediate descent for at least 610 m (2000 ft), continuing until symptoms improve
- Oxygen (2–4 L/min) should be administered by mask
- If immediate descent is impossible, use a portable hyperbaric chamber

Subacute mountain sickness

- Treatment consists of rest, oxygen administration, diuretics, and return to lower altitudes

Chronic mountain sickness

- Almost complete disappearance of all abnormalities eventually occurs when the patient returns to sea level

OUTCOME

PREVENTION

- Persons with symptomatic cardiac or pulmonary disease should avoid high altitudes
- Slow ascent—300 m (984 ft) per day
- Adequate rest the day before travel, reduced food intake, and avoidance of alcohol, tobacco
- Avoid unnecessary physical activity during travel
- A period of rest and inactivity for 1–2 days after arrival at high altitudes
- Acetazolamide, 125–250 mg every 12 h, beginning the day before ascent and continuing for 48–72 h at altitude, may be used as prophylaxis
- Dexamethasone, 4 mg every 12 h beginning on the day of ascent, continuing for 3 days at the higher altitude, and then tapering over 5 days, is an alternative
- Prompt medical attention with rest and high-flow oxygen if respiratory symptoms develop may prevent progression to frank pulmonary edema
- Mountaineering parties at levels of 3000 m (9840 ft) or higher should carry a supply of oxygen and equipment sufficient for several days
- An early descent of even 500 or 1000 m may result in symptomatic improvement

EVIDENCE

PRACTICE GUIDELINES

- An Advisory Committee Statement (ACS). Committee to Advise on Tropical Medicine and Travel (CATMAT). Statement on high-altitude illnesses. Can Commun Dis Rep 1998; 24:1.

WEB SITE

- Merck Manual—Disorder due to physical agents http://www.merck.com/pubs/mmanual/section20/sec20.htm

INFORMATION FOR PATIENTS

- JAMA patient page: Altitude sickness. JAMA 2002;287(17):2314. [PMID: 11998839]
- National Institutes of Health http://www.nlm.nih.gov/medlineplus/ency/article/000133.htm

REFERENCE

- Krieger BP et al: Altitude related pulmonary disorders. Crit Care Clin 1999; 15:265. [PMID: 10331128]

Richard Cohen, MD, MPH
Brent R.W. Moelleken, MD, FACS

Multiple Myeloma

 KEY FEATURES

ESSENTIALS OF DIAGNOSIS

- Bone pain, often in lower back
- Monoclonal paraprotein by serum and urine protein electrophoresis or immunoelectrophoresis
- Replacement of bone marrow by malignant plasma cells

GENERAL CONSIDERATIONS

- Malignancy of plasma cells characterized by replacement of bone marrow, bone destruction, and paraprotein formation
- Replacement of bone marrow initially causes anemia and later general bone marrow failure
- Malignant plasma cells can form tumors (plasmacytomas) that may cause spinal cord compression
- Bone involvement causes bone pain, osteoporosis, lytic lesions, pathological fractures, and hypercalcemia
- Light chain component of immunoglobulin often leads to renal failure
- Light chain components may be deposited in tissues as amyloid, worsening renal failure and causing systemic symptoms
- Failure of antibody production in response to antigen challenge makes myeloma patients especially prone to infections with encapsulated organisms, eg, *Streptococcus pneumoniae* and *Haemophilus influenzae*

DEMOGRAPHICS

- Occurs most commonly in older adults: median age at presentation is 65 years

 CLINICAL FINDINGS

SYMPTOMS AND SIGNS

- Symptoms of anemia
- Increased susceptibility to infection
- Bone pain most common in back or ribs or may present as pathological fracture, especially of femoral neck
- Symptoms of renal failure
- Neuropathy or spinal cord compression
- Pallor
- Bone tenderness
- Soft tissue masses
- Enlarged tongue, neuropathy, congestive heart failure, or hepatosplenomegaly in amyloidosis
- Fever occurs only with infection

DIFFERENTIAL DIAGNOSIS

- Monoclonal gammopathy of uncertain significance (MGUS)
- Reactive polyclonal hypergammaglobulinemia
- Waldenström's macroglobulinemia
- Metastatic cancer
- Primary hyperparathyroidism
- Lymphoma or leukemia
- Primary amyloidosis

DIAGNOSIS

LABORATORY TESTS

- Anemia nearly universal
- Red blood cell morphology normal, but rouleau formation common and may be marked
- Neutrophil and platelet counts usually normal at presentation
- Hypercalcemia
- Proteinuria
- Erythrocyte sedimentation rate elevated
- Peripheral blood smear: plasma cells rarely visible (plasma cell leukemia)
- Serum protein electrophoresis (SPEP) demonstrates paraprotein, in the majority demonstrable as a monoclonal spike in β- or γ-globulin region
- Immunoelectrophoresis (IEP) reveals this to be monoclonal protein; 60% are IgG, 25% IgA, and 15% light chains only
- Urine IEP may reveal either complete immunoglobulin or light chains in ~15% who have no demonstrable paraprotein in serum
- β_2-Microglobulin level >3 mg/L associated with poor survival
- Urinalysis may reveal proteinuria, but dipstick test (detects primarily albumin) unreliable for light chains
- Proximal renal tubular acidosis, with phosphaturia, glycosuria, uricosuria, and aminoaciduria
- Anion gap often narrow when paraprotein is cationic (70% of cases)

IMAGING STUDIES

- Bone x-rays: lytic lesions, especially in axial skeleton (skull, spine, proximal long bones, and ribs); or generalized osteoporosis
- Radionuclide bone scan: not useful in detecting bone lesions in myeloma, since usually no osteoblastic component

DIAGNOSTIC PROCEDURES

- Bone marrow biopsy: infiltration by variable numbers of plasma cells (5% to 100%); dismal outcome if bone marrow cytogenetic analysis shows deletions of chromosome 13q

Multiple Myeloma

 ## TREATMENT

 ## OUTCOME

 ## EVIDENCE

MEDICATIONS

- Combination chemotherapy with vincristine, doxorubicin (Adriamycin), and dexamethasone (VAD)
- Thalidomide and thalidomide derivatives and experimental agents CC-5013 and PS-341 (protease inhibitor) for refractory disease
- Thalidomide, berexomib (PS-341, Velcade), and the experimental agent CC-5013 (Revimid) for refractory disease
- Mobilization, hydration, and bisphosphonates for hypercalcemia
- Bisphosphonates (eg, pamidronate, 90 mg, or zoledronate, 4 mg IV Q month) to reduce pathological fractures in patients with significant bony disease

THERAPEUTIC PROCEDURES

- Observe without therapy if minimal disease or unclear whether paraproteinemia benign (MGUS) or malignant, since no advantage to early treatment of asymptomatic multiple myeloma
- Autologous stem cell transplantation in patients aged <70
- Autologous transplantation useful in relapse if disease still chemotherapy sensitive
- Allogeneic transplantation potentially curative, but role limited by unusually high mortality rate (40–50%) in myeloma patients
- Less toxic forms of allogeneic transplantation using nonmyeloablative regimens have produced encouraging results

FOLLOW-UP

- Follow height of paraprotein spike on SPEP as a useful marker for monitoring response to therapy

COMPLICATIONS

- Bony fractures
- Hypercalcemia

PROGNOSIS

- Overall, median survival for myeloma has been 3 years, but improving with new treatments
- Median survival of 5–6 years if low tumor burden: IgG spike <5 g/dL, no more than one lytic bone lesion, and no hypercalcemia or renal failure
- Median survival was 1–2 years, but now 5–6 years with early autologous stem cell transplantation for high tumor burden: IgG spike >7 g/dL, hematocrit <25%, calcium >12 mg/dL, or >3 lytic bone lesions
- Immunotherapy with allogeneic transplantation and investigational agent CC-5013 (Revimid) and PS-341 (Velcade) may improve outlook further

PRACTICE GUIDELINES

- American Society of Clinical Oncology clinical practice guidelines: the role of bisphosphonates in multiple myeloma. American Society of Clinical Oncology. 2002.
  http://www.asco.org/ac/1,1003,_ 12-002032-00_18-0024732-00_ 19-0024733-00_20-001,00.asp
- Traynor AE et al: NCCN Multiple Myeloma Practice Guidelines Panel. NCCN: Multiple myeloma. Cancer Control 2001;8(6 Suppl 2):78. [PMID: 11760563]

WEB SITES

- Multiple Myeloma Research Foundation http://www.multiplemyeloma.org/
- National Cancer Institute—What you need to know about multiple myeloma http://www.cancer.gov/cancerinfo/ wyntk/myeloma

INFORMATION FOR PATIENTS

- American Cancer Society—What is multiple myeloma? http://www.cancer.org/docroot/CRI/ content/CRI_2_4_1X_What_is_ multiple_myeloma_30.asp
- Cleveland Clinic—Multiple myeloma and plasma cell dyscrasia http://www.clevelandclinic.org/health/ health-info/docs/0300/0381.asp?index= 4413

REFERENCES

- Badros A et al: Improved outcome of allogeneic transplantation in high-risk multiple myeloma patients after nonmyeloablative conditioning. J Clin Oncol 2002;20:1295. [PMID: 11870172]
- Weber D et al: Thalidomide alone or with dexamethasone for previously untreated multiple myeloma. J Clin Oncol 2003;21:16. [PMID: 12506164]

Charles A. Linker, MD

Multiple Sclerosis

KEY FEATURES

ESSENTIALS OF DIAGNOSIS

- Episodic neurological symptoms
- Usually under 55 years of age at onset
- Single pathological lesion cannot explain clinical findings
- Multiple foci best visualized by MRI

GENERAL CONSIDERATIONS

- Pathologically, focal—often perivenular—areas of demyelination with reactive gliosis are found scattered in the white matter of the brain and spinal cord and in the optic nerves
- Should not be diagnosed unless there is evidence that two or more different regions of the central white matter have been affected at different times
- A diagnosis of clinically definite disease can be made in patients with a relapsing-remitting course and evidence on examination of at least two lesions involving different regions of the central white matter
- The diagnosis is probable in patients with multifocal white matter disease but only one clinical attack, or with a history of at least two clinical attacks but signs of only a single lesion

DEMOGRAPHICS

- Common disorder, probably an autoimmune basis, with its greatest incidence in young adults
- Much more common in persons of western European lineage who live in temperate zones. No population with a high risk for multiple sclerosis exists between latitudes 40°N and 40°S. Genetic, dietary, and climatic factors cannot account for these differences. Nevertheless, a genetic susceptibility to the disease is likely, based on twin studies, familial cases, and an association with specific HLA antigens (HLA-DR2)

CLINICAL FINDINGS

SYMPTOMS AND SIGNS

- Common initial presentation is weakness, numbness, tingling, or unsteadiness in a limb; spastic paraparesis; retrobulbar neuritis; diplopia; disequilibrium; or a sphincter disturbance such as urinary urgency or hesitancy
- Symptoms may disappear after a few days or weeks, although examination often reveals a residual deficit

Relapsing-remitting disease

- After the initial episode, it is months or years before new symptoms develop or the original ones recur
- Eventually relapses and usually incomplete remissions lead to increasing disability, with weakness, spasticity, and ataxia of the limbs, impaired vision, and urinary incontinence
- The findings on examination at this stage commonly include optic atrophy, nystagmus, dysarthria, and pyramidal, sensory, or cerebellar deficits in some or all of the limbs

Secondary progressive disease

- In some of the relapsing-remitting patients, the clinical course changes to steady deterioration, unrelated to acute relapses

Primary progressive disease

- Less common
- Symptoms steadily progress from their onset, and disability develops at a relatively early stage
- The diagnosis cannot be made unless the total clinical picture indicates involvement of different parts of the CNS at different times
- A number of factors (eg, infection, trauma) may precipitate or trigger exacerbations. Relapses are also more likely during the 2 or 3 months following pregnancy, possibly because of the increased demands and stresses that occur in the postpartum period

DIFFERENTIAL DIAGNOSIS

- Acute disseminated encephalomyelitis
- Foramen magnum lesion (Arnold-Chiari malformation)
- Progressive multifocal leukoencephalopathy
- Subacute combined degeneration of the spinal cord (B_{12} deficiency)
- Spinal cord tumor
- Vasculitis
- Neurosyphilis
- Lyme disease
- Syringomyelia
- HIV-associated myelopathy
- Human T cell lymphotropic virus-I myelopathy

DIAGNOSIS

LABORATORY TESTS

- A definitive diagnosis can never be based solely on the laboratory findings
- Lumbar puncture: there may be mild lymphocytosis or a slightly increased protein concentration in the cerebrospinal fluid, especially soon after an acute relapse. Elevated IgG in cerebrospinal fluid and discrete bands of IgG (oligoclonal bands) are present in many patients. The presence of such bands is not specific, however, since they have been found in a variety of inflammatory neurological disorders and occasionally in patients with vascular or neoplastic disorders of the nervous system

IMAGING STUDIES

- MRI of the brain or cervical cord is often helpful in demonstrating the presence of a multiplicity of lesions
- In patients presenting with myelopathy alone and in whom there is no clinical or laboratory evidence of more widespread disease, myelography or MRI may be necessary to exclude a congenital or acquired surgically treatable lesion. The foramen magnum region must be visualized to exclude the possibility of Arnold-Chiari malformation, in which part of the cerebellum and the lower brainstem are displaced into the cervical canal and produce mixed pyramidal and cerebellar deficits in the limbs

DIAGNOSTIC PROCEDURES

- The electrocerebral responses evoked by monocular visual stimulation with a checkerboard pattern stimulus, by monaural click stimulation, and by electrical stimulation of a sensory or mixed peripheral nerve have been used to detect subclinical involvement of the visual, brainstem auditory, and somatosensory pathways, respectively

TREATMENT

MEDICATIONS

- Recovery from acute relapses may be hastened by corticosteroids, but the extent of recovery is unchanged. A high dose (eg, prednisone, 60 or 80 mg) is given daily for 1 week; medication is then tapered over the following 2 or 3 weeks. Such a regimen is often preceded by methylprednisolone, 1 g intravenously for 3 days

- Long-term treatment with steroids provides no benefit and does not prevent further relapses

- In patients with relapsing-remitting or secondary progressive disease, β-interferon or daily subcutaneous administration of glatiramer acetate reduces the frequency of exacerbations

- Immunosuppressive therapy with cyclophosphamide, azathioprine, methotrexate, cladribine, or mitoxantrone may help to arrest the course of secondary progressive multiple sclerosis. The evidence of benefit is incomplete, however

- There is little evidence that plasmapheresis enhances any beneficial effects of immunosuppression in multiple sclerosis

- Intravenous immunoglobulins may reduce the clinical attack rate in relapsing-remitting disease, but the available studies are inadequate to permit treatment recommendations

THERAPEUTIC PROCEDURES

- Treatment for spasticity and for neurogenic bladder may be needed in advanced cases

- Excessive fatigue must be avoided, and patients should rest during periods of acute relapse

OUTCOME

PROGNOSIS

- At least partial recovery from acute exacerbations can reasonably be expected, but further relapses may occur without warning, and there is no means of preventing progression of the disorder. Some disability is likely to result eventually, but about half of all patients are without significant disability even 10 years after onset of symptoms

WHEN TO REFER

- If confirmation of the diagnosis is needed, or if the disease is progressive despite standard therapy

- For expertise in the use of immunotherapy

EVIDENCE

PRACTICE GUIDELINES

- Goodin DS et al: Disease modifying therapies in multiple sclerosis: subcommittee of the American Academy of Neurology and the MS Council for Clinical Practice Guidelines. Neurology 2002;58;169. [PMID 11805241]

- American Academy of Neurology http://www.aan.com/professionals/ practice/pdfs/immunizations_ms.pdf

WEB SITE

- National Institute of Neurological Disorders and Stroke http://www.ninds.nih.gov/health_and_ medical/disorders/multiple_sclerosis. htm

INFORMATION FOR PATIENTS

- National Multiple Sclerosis Society http://www.nmss.org/ http://www.nationalmssociety.org/ Brochures-Guide %20for.asp

- The Mayo Clinic http://www.mayoclinic.com/invoke.cfm? id=DS00188

REFERENCES

- Rutschmann OT: Immunization and MS: a summary of published evidence and recommendations. Neurology 2002;59:1837. [PMID: 12499473]

- Vartanian T: An examination of the results of the EVIDENCE, INCOMIN, and phase III studies of interferon beta products in the treatment of multiple sclerosis. Clin Ther 2003;25:105. [PMID: 12637114]

Michael J. Aminoff, MD, DSc, FRCP

Mushroom Poisoning

 KEY FEATURES

ESSENTIALS OF DIAGNOSIS

- Vomiting, diarrhea, and abdominal cramps after ingestion of toxic mushrooms
- Elevated hepatic transaminases and evidence of heptic dysfunction

GENERAL CONSIDERATIONS

- There are thousands of toxic mushroom species
- Ingestion of even a portion of an amatoxin-containing mushroom may be sufficient to cause death
- Cooking amatoxin-type cyclopeptides does not prevent the poisoning

 CLINICAL FINDINGS

SYMPTOMS AND SIGNS

- Amatoxin-type cyclopeptides (*Amanita phalloides, Amanita verna, Amanita virosa*, and *Galerina* species)
  - After a latent interval of 8–12 h, severe abdominal cramps and vomiting begin and progress to profuse diarrhea
  - Hepatic necrosis, hepatic encephalopathy, and frequently renal failure occur in 1–2 days
- Gyromitrin type (*Gyromitra* and *Helvella* species)
  - Toxicity is more common following ingestion of uncooked mushrooms
  - Vomiting, diarrhea, hepatic necrosis, convulsions, coma, and hemolysis may occur after a latent period of 8–12 h
- Muscarinic type (*Inocybe* and *Clitocybe* species)
  - Vomiting, diarrhea, bradycardia, hypotension, salivation, miosis, bronchospasm, and lacrimation occur shortly after ingestion
  - Cardiac arrhythmias may occur
- Anticholinergic type (*Amanita muscaria, Amanita pantherina*)
  - A variety of symptoms that may be atropine-like, including excitement, delirium, flushed skin, dilated pupils, and muscular jerking tremors
  - Symptoms begin 1–2 h after ingestion
- Gastrointestinal irritant type (*Boletus, Cantharellus*)
  - Nausea, vomiting, and diarrhea occur shortly after ingestion
- Disulfiram type (*Coprinus* species)
  - Disulfiram-like sensitivity to alcohol may persist for several days
  - Toxicity is characterized by flushing, hypotension, and vomiting after coingestion of alcohol
- Hallucinogenic (*Psilocybe* and *Panaeolus* species)
  - Mydriasis, nausea and vomiting, and intense visual hallucinations occur 1–2 h after ingestion
- *Cortinarius orellanus*
  - May cause acute renal failure due to tubulointerstitial nephritis

DIFFERENTIAL DIAGNOSIS

- Acetaminophen poisoning
- Acute viral hepatitis

 DIAGNOSIS

DIAGNOSTIC PROCEDURES

- Hepatic transaminases elevated
- Necrosis of the liver, massive and acute

Mushroom Poisoning

 ## TREATMENT

MEDICATIONS

- Emergency measures
- Administer activated charcoal for any recent ingestion

Activated charcoal

- Administer activated charcoal, 60–100 g orally or via gastric tube, mixed in aqueous slurry
- Repeated doses may be given to ensure gastrointestinal adsorption.
- After the onset of symptoms, efforts to remove the toxic agent are probably useless, especially in cases of amatoxin or gyromitrin poisoning, where there is usually a delay of 12 h or more before symptoms occur

General measures

- Amatoxin-type cyclopeptides: aggressive fluid replacement for diarrhea and intensive supportive care for hepatic failure are the mainstays of treatment. Antidote efficacy (eg, silibinin, penicillin, corticosteroids) is uncertain
- Gyromitrin type: pyridoxine, 25 mg/kg intravenously
- Muscarinic type: give atropine, 0.005–0.01 mg/kg intravenously, and repeat as needed
- Anticholinergic type: physostigmine, 0.5–1 mg intravenously, may calm extreme agitation and reverse peripheral anticholinergic manifestations, but it may also cause bradycardia, asystole, and seizures
- Gastrointestinal irritant type: treat with antiemetics and intravenous or oral fluids

THERAPEUTIC PROCEDURES

- Disulfiram type: avoid alcohol and treat alcohol reaction with fluids and supine position
- Hallucinogenic type: provide a quiet, supportive atmosphere. Diazepam or haloperidol may be used for sedation
- *Cortinarius*: provide supportive care and hemodialysis as needed for renal failure

 ## OUTCOME

PROGNOSIS

- The fatality rate of amatoxin-type cyclopeptides is about 10–20% without liver transplant
- The fatality rate of gyromitrin-type mushrooms is less than 10%
- Fatalities are rare with muscarinic type, anticholingeric type, gastrointestinal irritant type, and hallucinogenic mushrooms

WHEN TO REFER

- Liver transplant may be necessary, particularly for amatoxin-type cyclopeptides
- Contact a transplant center early

EVIDENCE

PRACTICE GUIDELINES

- National Guideline Clearinghouse http://www.guideline.gov/summary/ summary.aspx?doc_id=2707&nbr= 1933&string=mushroom+poisoning

WEB SITES

- Agency for Toxic Substances and Disease Registry (ATSDR) http://www.cdc.gov/niosh/nasd/srd/ og56400.html
- Toxicology—eMedicine http://www.emedicine.com/cgi-bin/ foxweb.exe/showsection@d:/em/ga? book=emerg&sct=TOXICOLOGY

INFORMATION FOR PATIENTS

- American Academy of Family Physicians http://familydoctor.org/handouts/129. html
- National Institutes of Health http://www.nlm.nih.gov/medlineplus/ ency/article/000003.htm

REFERENCES

- Broussard CN et al: Mushroom poisoning—from diarrhea to liver transplantation. Am J Gastroenterol 2001;96:3195. [PMID: 11721773]
- Enjalbert F et al: Treatment of amatoxin poisoning: 20-year retrospective analysis. J Toxicol Clin Toxicol 2002;40:715. [PMID 12475187]
- Yamada EG et al: Mushroom poisoning due to amatoxin. Northern California, winter 1996–1997. West J Med 1998; 169:380. [PMID: 9866444]

Kent R. Olson, MD

Myasthenia Gravis

 ## KEY FEATURES

ESSENTIALS OF DIAGNOSIS

- Fluctuating weakness of voluntary muscles, producing symptoms such as diplopia, ptosis, and difficulty in swallowing
- Activity increases weakness of affected muscles
- Short-acting anticholinesterases transiently improve the weakness

GENERAL CONSIDERATIONS

- Occurs at all ages, sometimes in association with a thymic tumor, thyrotoxicosis, rheumatoid arthritis, or lupus erythematosus
- Onset is usually insidious, but the disorder is sometimes unmasked by a coincidental infection
- Exacerbations may occur before the menstrual period and during or shortly after pregnancy
- Symptoms are due to blocks of neuromuscular transmission caused by autoantibodies binding to acetylcholine receptors
- The external ocular muscles and certain other cranial muscles, including the masticatory, facial, and pharyngeal muscles, are especially likely to be affected, and the respiratory and limb muscles may also be involved

DEMOGRAPHICS

- Commonest in young women with HLA-DR3; if thymoma is associated, older men are more commonly affected

 ## CLINICAL FINDINGS

SYMPTOMS AND SIGNS

- Patients present with ptosis, diplopia, difficulty in chewing or swallowing, respiratory difficulties, limb weakness, or some combination of these problems
- Weakness may remain localized to a few muscle groups, especially the ocular muscles, or may become generalized
- Symptoms often fluctuate in intensity during the day, and this diurnal variation is superimposed on a tendency to longer-term spontaneous relapses and remissions that may last for weeks
- Clinical examination confirms the weakness and fatigability of affected muscles
- Extraocular palsies and ptosis, often asymmetric, are common
- Pupillary responses are normal
- The bulbar and limb muscles are often weak, but the pattern of involvement is variable
- Sustained activity of affected muscles increases the weakness, which improves after a brief rest
- Sensation is normal, and there are usually no reflex changes

DIFFERENTIAL DIAGNOSIS

- Lambert-Eaton myasthenic syndrome (usually paraneoplastic)
- Botulism
- Aminoglycoside-induced neuromuscular weakness

 ## DIAGNOSIS

LABORATORY TESTS

- Elevated level of serum acetylcholine receptor antibodies has a sensitivity of 80–90%

IMAGING STUDIES

- Lateral and anteroposterior x-rays of the chest and CT scans should be obtained to demonstrate a coexisting thymoma, but normal studies do not exclude this possibility

DIAGNOSTIC PROCEDURES

- The diagnosis can generally be confirmed by the response to a short-acting anticholinesterase
- Edrophonium can be given intravenously in a dose of 10 mg (1 mL), 2 mg being given initially and the remaining 8 mg about 30 s later if the test dose is well tolerated; in myasthenic patients, there is an obvious improvement in strength of weak muscles lasting for about 5 min. Alternatively, 1.5 mg of neostigmine can be given intramuscularly, and the response then lasts for about 2 h; atropine sulfate (0.6 mg) should be available to reverse muscarinic side effects
- Electrophysiological demonstration of a decrementing muscle response to repetitive 2- or 3-Hz stimulation of motor nerves indicates a disturbance of neuromuscular transmission. Such an abnormality may even be detected in clinically strong muscles with certain provocative procedures
- Needle electromyography of affected muscles shows a marked variation in configuration and size of individual motor unit potentials, and single-fiber electromyography reveals an increased jitter, or variability, in the time interval between two muscle fiber action potentials from the same motor unit

TREATMENT

MEDICATIONS

- Medication such as aminoglycosides that may exacerbate myasthenia gravis should be avoided
- Anticholinesterase drugs provide symptomatic benefit without influencing the course of the disease
- Neostigmine, pyridostigmine, or both can be used, the dose being determined on an individual basis
- The usual dose of neostigmine is 7.5–30 mg (average, 15 mg) taken four times daily; of pyridostigmine, 30–180 mg (average, 60 mg) four times daily. Overmedication may temporarily increase weakness, which is then unaffected or enhanced by intravenous edrophonium
- Corticosteroids are indicated if there has been a poor response to anticholinesterase drugs and the patient has had thymectomy. Start while the patient is in the hospital, since weakness may initially be aggravated. The dose of corticosteroids is determined on an individual basis
- Treatment with azathioprine may also be effective. The usual dose is 2–3 mg/kg orally daily after a lower initial dose
- Early reports on the use of mycophenolate mofetil, an immunosuppressant, indicate that it may provide symptomatic relief and allow for steroid dose reduction
- In patients with major disability in whom conventional treatment is either unhelpful or contraindicated, plasmapheresis or intravenous immunoglobulin therapy may be beneficial. It may also be useful for stabilizing patients before thymectomy and for managing acute crisis

SURGERY

- Thymectomy usually leads to symptomatic benefit or remission and should be considered in all patients younger than age 60, unless weakness is restricted to the extraocular muscles
- If the disease is of recent onset and only slowly progressive, operation is sometimes delayed for a year or so, in the hope that spontaneous remission will occur

OUTCOME

COMPLICATIONS

- Aspiration pneumonia

PROGNOSIS

- The disorder follows a slowly progressive course and may have a fatal outcome owing to respiratory complications such as aspiration pneumonia

WHEN TO REFER

- Most patients with a suspected or proven diagnosis should be referred to a clinician with expertise in management of this disorder

EVIDENCE

PRACTICE GUIDELINES

- National Guideline Clearinghouse http://www.guideline.gov/summary/summary.aspx?doc_id=3347&nbr=2573&string=MYASTHENIA+GRAVIS http://www.guideline.gov/summary/summary.aspx?doc_id=1976&nbr=1202&string=MYASTHENIA+GRAVIS

INFORMATION FOR PATIENTS

- National Institute of Neurological Diseases and Stroke http://www.ninds.nih.gov/health_and_medical/pubs/myasthenia_gravis.htm
- The Mayo Clinic http://www.mayoclinic.com/invoke.cfm?id=DS00375

REFERENCES

- Palace J et al: Myasthenia gravis: diagnostic and management dilemmas. Curr Opin Neurol 2001;14:583. [PMID: 11562569]
- Vincent A et al: Myasthenia gravis. Lancet 2001;357:2122. [PMID:11445126]

Michael J. Aminoff, MD, DSc, FRCP

KEY FEATURES

ESSENTIALS OF DIAGNOSIS

- Chronic cough, sputum production, and fatigue; less commonly malaise, dyspnea, fever, hemoptysis, and weight loss
- Parenchymal infiltrates on chest radiograph, often with thin-walled cavities, that spread contiguously and often involve overlying pleura
- Isolation of nontuberculous mycobacteria in a sputum culture

GENERAL CONSIDERATIONS

- Nontuberculous mycobacteria (NTM) or "atypical" mycobacteria are ubiquitous in water and soil
- NTM may colonize the airways or appear in cultures due to environmental contamination
- Organisms are not communicable from person to person
- NTM are often resistant to most antituberculous drugs
- Complementary data are important for diagnosis, as NTM can reside or colonize airways without causing clinical disease
- *Mycobacterium avium complex* (MAC) is the most frequent cause of NTM pulmonary disease in the United States
- *M kansasii* is the second most frequent pulmonary pathogen
- Other NTM that can cause pulmonary disease are *M abscessus, M xenopi,* and *M malmoense*
- Most organisms cause a chronic progressive pulmonary infection similar to tuberculosis, but more slowly progressive
- Many patients have AIDS or preexisting lung disease
- Disseminated disease is rare in immunocompetent patients
- Disseminated MAC infection is common in patients with AIDS

 CLINICAL FINDINGS

SYMPTOMS AND SIGNS

- Chronic cough, sputum production, and fatigue
- Malaise, dyspnea, fever, hemoptysis, and weight loss are less common
- Symptoms from coexisting lung disease can confound the evaluation

DIFFERENTIAL DIAGNOSIS

- Postviral
- Bronchitis, especially in smokers
- Bronchiectasis
- Tuberculosis
- Cystic fibrosis
- Pertussis
- *Mycoplasma*
- *Chlamydia*
- Respiratory syncytial virus

 DIAGNOSIS

LABORATORY TESTS

- Diagnosis rests on recovery of the pathogen from cultures
- Bronchial washings are considered more sensitive than expectorated sputum, but their specificity for clinical disease is unknown
- Bacteriological diagnostic criteria in HIV⁻ or immunocompetent hosts requires
  - Either three positive sputum culture specimens or two positive sputum cultures and one positive acid-fast bacillus (AFB) sputum smear within a 1-year period
  - A single bronchial wash culture with a 2+ to 4+ growth, or any positive culture with a 2+ to 4+ AFB smear
- DNA probes or HPLC allow rapid species identification of NTM
- Criteria for infection in HIV-positive patients is less stringent
- Drug susceptibility testing is recommended only as follows:
  - *M kansasii* and rifampin
  - Rapid growers (*M fortuitum, abscessus,* and *chelonei*) and amikacin, doxycycline, impipenem, fluoroquinolones, clarithromycin, cefoxitin, and a sulfonamide

IMAGING STUDIES

- Chest x-ray with progressive or persistent infiltrates for 2 months, cavitary lesions, and multiple nodular densities
- Cavities are usually thin walled and with less surrounding infiltrate than seen in *M tuberculosis*
- HRCT may show multiple small nodules with or without multiple foci of bronchiectasis
- Infiltrates clear slowly

DIAGNOSTIC PROCEDURES

- Lung biopsy demonstrating NTM with granulomatous inflammation can be diagnostic

Mycobacterial Pulmonary Infections, Nontuberculous

 TREATMENT

MEDICATIONS

- See Tables 23, 24, and 122 (pages 1221, and 1303)
- *M kansasii* responds well to therapy with daily rifampin, isoniazid, and ethambutol for at least 18 months
- Treatment of immunocompromised patients is controversial and largely empirical
- Non-HIV patients with MAC pulmonary disease usually receive a combination of daily clarithromycin or azithromycin, rifampin or rifabutin, and ethambutol; streptomycin is considered for the first 2 months
- Optimal duration of therapy is unknown, but it should be continued for at least 12 months after sputum is documented negative

SURGERY

- Surgical resection is an option for progressive disease that responds poorly to chemotherapy

 OUTCOME

FOLLOW-UP

- Monitor serial chest x-rays and sputum cultures
- Follow drug-specific biochemical tests for toxicity

PROGNOSIS

- Medical treatment is initially successful in two-thirds of non-HIV patients with MAC, but relapses are common

WHEN TO REFER

- Nontuberculous mycobacterium disease other than MAC should be managed with the assistance of an infectious disease or pulmonary medicine expert

 EVIDENCE

- National Guideline Clearinghouse http://www.guideline.gov/summary/ summary.aspx?doc_id=3080&nbr= 2306&string=opportunistic+infections

INFORMATION FOR PATIENTS

- National Institutes of Health http://www.nlm.nih.gov/medlineplus/ ency/article/000640.htm
- American Medical Association http://www.medem.com/MedLB/ article_detaillb.cfm?article_ID= ZZZ06T60NAC&sub_cat=577

REFERENCES

- Anonymous: Diagnosis and treatment of disease caused by nontuberculous mycobacteria. Am J Respir Crit Care Med 1997;156(2 Part 2):S1. [PMID: 9279284]
- Holland SM: Nontuberculous mycobacteria. Am J Med Sci 2001;321:49. [PMID: 11202480]

Mark S. Chesnutt, MD
Thomas J. Prendergast, MD

Mycobacterium Infection, Atypical

 KEY FEATURES

ESSENTIALS OF DIAGNOSIS

- Lymphadenopathy and fever in disseminated disease in HIV-infected patients with CD4 <50/μL
- Pulmomary infections in patients with chronic lung disease
- Chronic pulmonary infection similar to tuberculosis in presentation: chronic productive cough, fever, weight loss
- Cervical adenopathy with mild or moderate inflammation

GENERAL CONSIDERATIONS

- About 10% of mycobacterial infections are not caused by *Mycobacterium tuberculosis* but by atypical mycobacteria
- Occur ubiquitously in the environment
- Are not communicable from person to person
- Are among the most common opportunistic infections in advanced HIV disease

Disseminated *Mycobacterium avium* infection

- *Mycobacterium avium* complex (MAC) produces asymptomatic colonization and a wide spectrum of diseases, including coin lesions, bronchitis in patients with chronic lung disease, and invasive pulmonary disease that is often cavitary and occurs in patients with underlying lung disease
- A common cause of disseminated disease in the late stages of HIV infection, when the CD4 cell count is less than 50–100/μL

Pulmonary infections

- MAC causes a chronic, slowly progressive pulmonary infection resembling tuberculosis in immunocompetent patients, who typically have underlying pulmonary disease
- *Mycobacterium kansasii* can produce clinical disease resembling tuberculosis, but the illness progresses more slowly. Most such infections occur in patients with preexisting lung disease, though 40% of patients have no known pulmonary disease

Lymphadenitis

- Most cases of lymphadenitis (scrofula) in adults are caused by *M tuberculosis* and can be a manifestation of disseminated disease

- In children, the majority of mycobacterial lymphadenitis cases are due to nontuberculous species, with *M scrofulaceum* and MAC most common

Skin and soft tissue infections

- Skin and soft tissue infections such as abscesses, septic arthritis, and osteomyelitis can result from direct inoculation or hematogenous dissemination or may occur as a complication of surgery
- *M chelonei* and *M fortuitum* are frequent causes of this type of infection
- *M marinum* infection ("swimming pool granuloma") follows exposure to nonchlorinated water

 CLINICAL FINDINGS

SYMPTOMS AND SIGNS

Disseminated *Mycobacterium avium* infection

- Persistent fever and weight loss are the most common symptoms

Pulmonary infections

- Resembles tuberculosis

Lymphadenitis

- Swollen, somewhat tender lymph node

Skin and soft tissue infections

- Most cases occur in the extremities and initially present as nodules
- Ulceration with abscess formation often follows

DIFFERENTIAL DIAGNOSIS

- Tuberculosis
- Lymphoma (disseminated disease)
- Fungal infection (cryptococcosis, histoplasmosis, coccidioidomycosis)
- Cervical lymphadenitis due to *M tuberculosis*, cat-scratch, other bacterial causes

 DIAGNOSIS

LABORATORY TESTS

Disseminated *Mycobacterium avium* infection

- The organism can usually be cultured from multiple sites, including blood, liver, lymph node, or bone marrow
- Blood culture is the preferred means of establishing the diagnosis and has a sensitivity of 98%

Pulmonary Infections

- Sputum or bronchoalveolar lavage mycobacterial culture

Lymphadenitis

- Mycobacterial culture of lymph node aspirate or surgical specimen

Skin and soft tissue infections

- Mycobacterial culture of nodule

TREATMENT

MEDICATIONS

Disseminated *Mycobacterium avium* infection

- Clarithromycin, 500 mg orally twice daily, plus ethambutol, 15 mg/kg/day as a single dose, with or without rifabutin, 300 mg/day, is the treatment of choice
- Azithromycin, 500 mg once daily, may be used instead of clarithromycin

Pulmonary infections

- Rifampin, 600 mg once daily, plus ethambutol, 15–25 mg/kg/day, plus streptomycin, 1 g intramuscularly three to five times a week for the first 4–6 months, have been used
- Inclusion of clarithromycin in the initial treatment regimen of immunocompetent patients should be strongly considered. Therapy is continued for a total of 18–24 months
- Microbiologically, *M kansasii* is similar to *M tuberculosis* and is sensitive to the same drugs except pyrazinamide, to which it is resistant. Therapy with isoniazid, ethambutol, and rifampin for 2 years (or 1 year after sputum conversion) has been highly successful

Skin and soft tissue infections

- The organisms are resistant to the usual antituberculous drugs but may be sensitive to a variety of antibiotics, including erythromycin, doxycycline, amikacin, cefoxitin, sulfonamides, imipenem, and ciprofloxacin
- Initially, parenteral drugs are given for several weeks, and this is followed by an oral regimen to which the organism is sensitive
- The duration of therapy is variable but usually continues for several months after the soft tissue lesions have healed

SURGERY

Lymphadenitis

- Unlike disease caused by *M tuberculosis*, which requires systemic therapy for 6 months, infection with nontuberculous mycobacteria can be successfully treated by surgical excision without antituberculous therapy

Skin and soft tissue infections

- Therapy includes surgical debridement along with drug therapy

OUTCOME

WHEN TO REFER

- Early referral to an infectious disease specialist if the diagnosis is in question or to an HIV specialist for treatment

WHEN TO ADMIT

- To expedite a diagnostic workup or for respiratory insufficiency

PREVENTION

- Antimicrobial prophylaxis of MAC prevents disseminated disease and prolongs survival in HIV-infected patients with CD4 counts ≤50/μL
- Single-drug regimens of clarithromycin, 500 mg twice daily, azithromycin, 1200 mg once weekly, or rifabutin, 300 mg once daily, have been shown to be effective

EVIDENCE

PRACTICE GUIDELINES

- National Guideline Clearinghouse http://www.guideline.gov/summary/summary.aspx?doc_id=3080&nbr=2306&string=atypical+mycobacterium http://www.guideline.gov/summary/summary.aspx?doc_id=2665&nbr=1891&string=mycobacterium http://www.guideline.gov/summary/summary.aspx?doc_id=1472&nbr=698&string=mycobacterium

WEB SITES

- CDC—Division of Bacterial and Mycotic Diseases http://www.cdc.gov/ncidod/dbmd/
- Karolinska Institute—Directory of Bacterial Infections and Mycoses http://www.mic.ki.se/Diseases/c1.html

INFORMATION FOR PATIENTS

- JAMA patient page: HIV/AIDS. JAMA 1999;282:606. [PMID: 10450724]
- National Institutes of Health http://www.nlm.nih.gov/medlineplus/ency/article/000640.htm

REFERENCES

- Diagnosis and treatment of disease caused by nontuberculous mycobacteria. Medical Section of the American Lung Association. Am J Respir Crit Care Med 1997;156(2 Part 2):S1. [PMID: 9279284]
- Horsburgh CR Jr: The pathophysiology of disseminated *Mycobacterium avium* complex disease in AIDS. J Infect Dis 1999;179(Suppl 3):S461. [PMID: 10099120]
- Kovacs J et al: Prophylaxis against opportunistic infection in patients with human immunodeficiency virus infection. N Engl J Med 2000;342:1416. [PMID: 10805828]

Henry F. Chambers, MD

Myelodysplastic Syndromes

 KEY FEATURES

ESSENTIALS OF DIAGNOSIS

- Cytopenias with hypercellular bone marrow
- Morphological abnormalities in two or more hematopoietic cell lines

GENERAL CONSIDERATIONS

- Group of acquired clonal disorders of hematopoietic stem cell, characterized by cytopenias, hypercellular marrow, and morphological and cytogenetic abnormalities
- "Ineffective hematopoiesis" occurs despite adequate numbers of hematopoietic stem cells
- No specific chromosomal abnormality seen, but abnormalities in chromosomes 5 and 7 common
- Causes: idiopathic (most common); postcytotoxic chemotherapy, especially mechlorethamine or procarbazine for Hodgkin's disease and melphalan for multiple myeloma or ovarian carcinoma
- May evolve into acute myelogenous leukemia (AML); has been termed "preleukemia"
- Myelodysplasia encompasses several heterogeneous syndromes
  - "Refractory anemia" (with or without ringed sideroblasts): no excess bone marrow blasts
  - "Refractory anemia with excess blasts" (RAEB): 5–19% blasts
  - Chronic myelomonocytic leukemia (CMML): proliferative syndrome including peripheral blood monocytosis >1000/μL

DEMOGRAPHICS

- Occurs most often in patients aged >60

 CLINICAL FINDINGS

SYMPTOMS AND SIGNS

- Asymptomatic, with incidentally found cytopenias
- Fatigue, infection, or bleeding related to bone marrow failure
- Wasting, fever, weight loss, and general debility
- Splenomegaly
- Pallor
- Bleeding
- Signs of infection

DIFFERENTIAL DIAGNOSIS

- AML (≥20% blasts)
- Aplastic anemia
- Anemic of chronic disease
- Vitamin B$_{12}$ or folate deficiency

 DIAGNOSIS

LABORATORY TESTS

- Anemia may be marked
- Mean cell volume is normal or increased
- Peripheral blood smear: macroovalocytes
- White blood cell count usually normal or reduced; neutropenia common
- Neutrophils may exhibit morphological abnormalities, including deficient numbers of granules, or bilobed nucleus (Pelger-Huet anomaly)
- Myeloid series may be left shifted with small numbers of promyelocytes or blasts
- Platelet count normal or reduced; hypogranular platelets may be present

DIAGNOSTIC PROCEDURES

- Bone marrow aspirate and biopsy characteristically hypercellular
- Erythroid hyperplasia common
- Signs of abnormal erythropoiesis include megaloblastic features, nuclear budding, or multinucleated erythroid precursors
- Prussian blue stain may demonstrate ringed sideroblasts
- Myeloid series often left shifted with variable increases in blasts
- Deficient or abnormal granules may be seen
- A characteristic abnormality is dwarf megakaryocytes with unilobed nucleus

TREATMENT

MEDICATIONS

- Erythropoietin 30,000 units SQ weekly, reduces red blood cell transfusion requirement in ≤20%
- Granulocyte or granulocyte-macrophage colony-stimulating factor myeloid growth factors indicated in those with severe neutropenia
- Combination of high-dose erythropoietin and myeloid growth factors produces higher response rate, but cost is prohibitive
- Azacitidine (5-azacytidine) improves both symptoms and blood counts and appears to prolong time to conversion to acute leukemia

THERAPEUTIC PROCEDURES

- Red blood cell transfusions indicated for severe anemia
- Allogeneic bone marrow transplantation in patients aged <60 with matched sibling donors produces cure in 30–50%

 OUTCOME

COMPLICATIONS

- Infection and bleeding

PROGNOSIS

- Myelodysplasia is ultimately fatal, most commonly due to infections or bleeding
- Risk of transformation to AML depends on percentage of blasts in bone marrow
- Patients with refractory anemia may survive many years, with low risk of leukemia (<10%)
- Those with excess blasts or CMML have short survivals (usually <2 years) and higher (20–50%) risk of developing acute leukemia
- Deletions of chromosomes 5 and 7 associated with poor prognosis

 EVIDENCE

PRACTICE GUIDELINES

- NCCN practice guidelines for the myelodysplastic syndromes. National Comprehensive Cancer Network. Oncology (Huntingt) 1998;12:53. [PMID: 10028503]

WEB SITES

- Mayo Clinic—Myelodysplasia http://www.mayoclinic.com/invoke.cfm?objectid=27BE5B82-A963-45C8-B7E3A112DED8E68E
- NCI—Myelodysplastic syndromes http://www.cancer.gov/cancerinfo/pdq/treatment/myelodysplastic/patient/

INFORMATION FOR PATIENTS

- American Cancer Society—Myelodysplastic syndromes http://www.cancer.org/docroot/CRI/content/CRI_2_4_3X_How_is_myelodysplastic_syndrome_diagnosed_65.asp?sitearea=
- Leukemia & Lymphoma Society http://www.leukemia-lymphoma.org/all_mat_toc.adp?item_id=54083

REFERENCES

- Castro-Malaspina H et al: Unrelated donor marrow transplantation for myelodysplastic syndromes: outcome analysis in 510 transplants facilitated by the National Marrow Donor Program. Blood 2002;99:1943. [PMID: 11877264]
- Molldrem JJ et al: Antithymocyte globulin for treatment of the bone marrow failure associated with myelodysplastic syndromes. Ann Intern Med 2002:137:156. [PMID: 12160363]
- Silverman LR et al: Randomized controlled trial of azacitidine in patients with the myelodysplastic syndrome: a study of the cancer and leukemia group B. J Clin Oncol 2002;20:2429. [PMID: 12011120]

Charles A. Linker, MD

Myocardial Infarction, Acute

 KEY FEATURES

ESSENTIALS OF DIAGNOSIS

- Sudden, but not instantaneous, development of prolonged (>30 min) anterior chest discomfort (sometimes felt as "gas" or pressure) that may produce arrhythmias, hypotension, shock, or congestive heart failure (CHF)
- Pain likely to be diminished or absent in the very elderly and long-term diabetics
- Electrocardiography: ST-segment elevation or depression, evolving Q waves, symmetric inversion of T waves
- Cardiac enzyme (CK-MB, troponin T, or troponin I) elevation
- Appearance of segmental wall motion abnormality by echocardiography

GENERAL CONSIDERATIONS

- Results from prolonged myocardial ischemia, due most often to an occlusive thrombus in a coronary artery at the site of a preexisting atherosclerotic plaque
- The location and extent of infarction depend on the anatomic distribution of the occluded vessel, the presence of additional stenotic lesions, and the adequacy of collateral circulation
- Atrioventricular (AV) block and sinus node dysfunction occur during inferior or right ventricular (RV) infarctions
- Preferred classification of infarction type is Q-wave versus non-Q-wave myocardial infarction (MI)
- Q-wave infarctions are transmural
- Non-Q-wave infarctions are predominantly subendocardial and result from incomplete occlusion or spontaneous lysis of a thrombus, often signifying the presence of additional jeopardized myocardium and associated with a higher incidence of reinfarction and recurrent ischemia
- In small infarctions, cardiac function is normal; with more extensive damage, early heart failure and hypotension (cardiogenic shock) may appear
- Consider RV infarction when patients with inferior infarction exhibit low cardiac output and raised venous pressure, confirmed by echocardiography or hemodynamic measurements

 CLINICAL FINDINGS

SYMPTOMS AND SIGNS

- Recent onset of angina or alteration in the pattern of angina or chest pressure, squeezing or "indigestion"
- Pain similar to angina in location and radiation, but more severe, usually occurs at rest, often in the early morning, builds rapidly, and is minimally responsive to nitroglycerin and even opioids
- Associated symptoms: diaphoresis, weakness, apprehensiveness, aversion to lying quietly, light-headedness, syncope, dyspnea, orthopnea, cough, wheezing, nausea and vomiting, or abdominal bloating
- ~ 20% of patients die before reaching the hospital, usually from ventricular fibrillation
- Marked bradycardia (inferior infarction) to tachycardia (increased sympathetic activity, low cardiac output, or arrhythmia)
- Blood pressure elevated (pain) to low (shock)
- Basilar rales are common and do not necessarily indicate heart failure
- Diffuse rales, wheezing, or respiratory distress usually indicate pulmonary edema and CHF
- Jugular venous distension indicates right atrial hypertension, often from right ventricular infarction or elevated left ventricular (LV) filling pressures
- Soft heart sounds may indicate LV dysfunction
- S_4 is common; S_3 indicates significant LV dysfunction
- Mitral regurgitation murmur usually indicates papillary muscle dysfunction or, rarely, rupture

DIFFERENTIAL DIAGNOSIS

- Aortic dissection, pulmonary embolism, tension pneumothorax, pericarditis, esophageal rupture

 DIAGNOSIS

LABORATORY TESTS

- Quantitative CK-MB, troponin I, and troponin T elevations as early as 4–6 h after onset; almost always abnormal by 8–12 h
- Troponins more specific than CK-MB
- Troponins may remain elevated for ≥ 5–7 days

IMAGING STUDIES

- Chest x-ray: signs of CHF, often lagging behind the clinical findings
- Echocardiography: assesses global and regional LV function, wall motion
- Doppler echocardiography: can diagnose postinfarction mitral regurgitation or ventricular septal defect
- Thallium-201 or technetium scintigraphy does not distinguish recent from old MI

DIAGNOSTIC PROCEDURES

- Angiography: can demonstrate akinesis or dyskinesis and measure ejection fraction
- Swan-Ganz hemodynamic measurements: can be invaluable in managing the complicated patient
- ST-segment elevation (>0.1 mV) in two inferior or lateral leads or two contiguous precordial leads, or with new-onset LBBB
- Q-wave MI: classic evolution of changes (hours to days) from peaked ("hyperacute") T waves, to ST-segment elevation, to Q wave development, to T wave inversion
- Non-Q-wave MI: characteristic MI presentation, elevated cardiac enzymes, and ST-segment changes (usually depression) or T wave inversion lasting ≥48 hours, *without* development of Q waves

TREATMENT

MEDICATIONS

- Aspirin, 162 mg or 325 mg PO QD, begin immediately
- Clopidogrel, 300 mg PO QD, in patients with a definite aspirin allergy
- Metoprolol, 5 mg IV Q 5 min, for up to 3 doses for a goal HR of 60
- Nitroglycerin (TNG), for chest pain to lower blood pressure, sublingually, topically, or IV if inadequate response (start 10 mg/min, then titrate up by 1 μg/kg/min over 30–60 min, higher doses PRN)
- Morphine sulfate, 4–8 mg IV, or meperidine, 50–75 mg IV, if TNG alone does not relieve pain
- Benzodiazepines for anxiety
- Thrombolytic therapy indicated in patients with >1 mm ST-segment elevations in two contiguous leads or new LBBB, and no prior CABG (see Table 39, page 1232)
- Thrombolysis is most beneficial when initiated within first 3 h, not given after 12 h of onset of chest pain
- RV MI: Treat with fluid loading, inotropic agents

THERAPEUTIC PROCEDURES

- In MI with ST-segment elevation, immediate coronary angiography and PTCA or stenting of the infarct-related artery is an alternative to thrombolysis
- In MI with cardiogenic shock, early catheterization and percutaneous or surgical revascularization is the preferred management

 ## OUTCOME

FOLLOW-UP

- For nonhypotensive patients with low ejection fractions, large infarctions, or clinical evidence of heart failure, start angiotensin-converting enzyme inhibitor on first postinfarction day; titrate and continue chronically
- Diltiazem appears to prevent reinfarction and ischemia in patients with non-Q-wave infarctions
- Patients with recurrent ischemic pain prior to discharge should undergo catheterization and, if indicated, revascularization

COMPLICATIONS

- Myocardial dysfunction, CHF, and hypotension
- Postinfarction ischemia
- Sinus bradycardia, sinus tachycardia, supraventricular premature beats, atrial fibrillation, ventricular premature beats, ventricular tachycardia, ventricular fibrillation, accelerated idioventricular rhythm, right or left bundle branch block or fascicular blocks, second- or third-degree AV block
- Rupture of a papillary muscle, interventricular septum, or LV free wall
- LV aneurysm
- Pericarditis, Dressler's syndrome
- Mural thrombi

PROGNOSIS

- Patients with a normal blood pressure, no signs of heart failure, and normal urine output have a good prognosis

WHEN TO REFER

- Obtain immediate cardiology consultation for patients with new MI

WHEN TO ADMIT

- Admit all patients with possible MI to the CCU

PREVENTION

- Control of LDL-cholesterol and blood pressure, exercise, β-blockers, and antiplatelet agents
- Cardiac rehabilitation programs and exercise training

 ## EVIDENCE

PRACTICE GUIDELINES

- Ryan TJ et al: Highlights of latest American College of Cardiology and American Heart Association Guidelines for Management of Patients with Acute Myocardial Infarction. Cardiol Rev 2002;10:35. [PMID: 11790268]
- Treatment of acute myocardial infarction. Institute for Clinical Systems Improvement, 2001 http://www.icsi.org/knowledge/detail.asp?catID=29&itemID=196

WEB SITES

- American Heart Association—Heart attack http://www.americanheart.org/presenter.jhtml?identifier=4578

INFORMATION FOR PATIENTS

- JAMA patient page: Heart attack. JAMA 1999;282(4):402. [PMID: 10432039]
- American College of Physicians—Heart attack http://familydoctor.org/handouts/291.html

REFERENCES

- Myocardial infarction redefined—a consensus document of The Joint European Society of Cardiology/American College of Cardiology Committee for the redefinition of myocardial infarction. J Am Coll Cardiol 2000;36:959. [PMID: 10987628]
- Ryan TJ: Percutaneous coronary intervention in ST-elevation myocardial infarction. Curr Cardiol Rep 2001;3:273. [PMID: 11406084]
- Zimetbaum PJ et al: Current concepts. Use of the electrocardiogram in acute myocardial infarction. N Engl J Med 2003;348:933. [PMID: 12621138]

Barry M. Massie, MD
Thomas M. Amidon, MD

Myopathies: Dermatomyositis & Polymyositis

KEY FEATURES

ESSENTIALS OF DIAGNOSIS

- Bilateral proximal muscle weakness
- Characteristic cutaneous manifestations in dermatomyositis (Gottron's papules, heliotrope rash)
- Diagnostic tests: elevated creatine kinase and other muscle enzymes, muscle biopsy, electromyography
- Increased risk of malignancy, particularly in adult dermatomyositis

GENERAL CONSIDERATIONS

- An autoimmune disease of unknown cause characterized chiefly by inflammation of muscles
- Five clinically defined subsets
  - Juvenile dermatomyositis
  - Dermatomyositis
  - Polymyositis
  - Myositis associated with malignancy
  - Myositis associated with another connective tissue disease [especially systemic lupus erythematosus (SLE)]
- Disorders of the peripheral and central nervous systems (eg, chronic inflammatory polyneuropathy, multiple sclerosis, myasthenia gravis, Eaton-Lambert disease, and amyotrophic lateral sclerosis) can produce weakness but are distinguished from inflammatory myopathies by characteristic symptoms and neurological signs and often by distinctive electromyographic abnormalities
- Inclusion body myositis can mimic polymyositis but is less responsive to treatment and has different epidemiological features
- Patients with polymyalgia rheumatica are over the age of 50 and—in contrast to patients with polymyositis—have pain but no objective weakness

DEMOGRAPHICS

- Peak incidence: fifth and sixth decades
- Women are affected twice as commonly as men
- The typical inclusion body myositis patient is white, male, and over age 50

CLINICAL FINDINGS

SYMPTOMS AND SIGNS

- Gradual and progressive muscle weakness of the proximal muscle groups of the upper and lower extremities
- Leg weakness (eg, difficulty in rising from a chair or climbing stairs) typically precedes arm symptoms
- No facial or ocular muscle weakness
- Pain and tenderness of affected muscles (25%)

In dermatomyositis

- The characteristic rash is dusky red and may appear in malar distribution mimicking the classic rash of SLE
- Erythema also occurs over other areas of the face, neck, shoulders, and upper chest and back ("shawl sign")
- Periorbital edema and a purplish (heliotrope) suffusion over the eyelids are typical signs
- Periungual erythema, dilations of nailbed capillaries, and scaly patches over the dorsum of proximal interphalangeal and metacarpophalangeal joints (Gottron's sign) are highly suggestive
- A subset of patients with polymyositis and dermatomyositis develops the "antisynthetase syndrome," a group of findings including inflammatory arthritis, Raynaud's phenomenon, interstitial lung disease, and often severe muscle disease associated with certain autoantibodies (eg, anti-Jo1 antibodies)

DIFFERENTIAL DIAGNOSIS

Muscle inflammation

- Polymyositis
- Dermatomyositis
- SLE
- Scleroderma
- Sjögren's syndrome
- Inclusion body myositis
- Trichinosis

Other causes of proximal muscle weakness

- Polymyalgia rheumatica
- Endocrine: hypothyroidism, hyperthyroidism, Cushing's syndrome
- Alcoholism
- Drugs: corticosteroids, statins, clofibrate, colchicine, chloroquine, emetine, aminocaproic acid, bretylium, penicillamine, drugs causing hypokalemia
- HIV myopathy
- Hyperparathyroidism
- Spinal stenosis
- Osteomalacia
- Mitochondrial myopathy

DIAGNOSIS

LABORATORY TESTS

- Serum levels of muscle enzymes, especially creatine kinase and aldolase, are elevated
- Antinuclear antibodies are present in many patients, and anti-Jo-1 antibodies are seen in the subset of patients that has associated interstitial lung disease

DIAGNOSTIC PROCEDURES

- Biopsy of clinically involved muscle is the only specific diagnostic test. The pathology findings in polymyositis and dermatomyositis are distinct, although both include lymphoid inflammatory infiltrates
- Electromyographic abnormalities consisting of polyphasic potentials, fibrillations, and high-frequency action potentials are helpful in establishing the diagnosis. None of the studies is specific

Myopathies: Dermatomyositis & Polymyositis

 TREATMENT

MEDICATIONS

- Most patients respond to corticosteroids: 40–60 mg or more of prednisone is required initially daily. The dose is then adjusted downward according to the response of sequentially observed serum levels of muscle enzymes
- In patients resistant or intolerant to corticosteroids, therapy with methotrexate or azathioprine may be helpful

 OUTCOME

FOLLOW-UP

- Up to one patient in four with dermatomyositis has an occult malignancy that may not be detected until months afterward in some cases
- Search for an occult malignancy should include age- and risk-appropriate cancer screening tests. If these evaluations are unrevealing, then a more invasive or extensive laboratory evaluation is probably not cost effective

COMPLICATIONS

- Hypercapnea and respiratory failure can develop from weakness of respiratory muscles
- Rhabdomyolysis with renal failure can complicate very severe muscle inflammation

PROGNOSIS

- Patients with an associated neoplasm have a poor prognosis, although remission may follow treatment of the tumor; steroids may or may not be effective in these patients

WHEN TO REFER

- Refer to a rheumatologist if patient develops respiratory weakness or rhabdomyolysis

WHEN TO ADMIT

- Admit for airway protection and urgent treatment if patient develops weakness of respiratory muscles
- Admit for rhabdomyolysis

EVIDENCE

PRACTICE GUIDELINES

- National Guideline Clearinghouse
  http://www.guideline.gov/summary/summary.aspx?doc_id=3415&nbr=2641&string=myopathy
  http://www.guideline.gov/summary/summary.aspx?doc_id=1906&nbr=1132&string=myopathy

INFORMATION FOR PATIENTS

- American Academy of Orthopaedic Surgeons
  http://orthoinfo.aaos.org/fact/thr_report.cfm?Thread_ID=266&topcategory=About%20Orthopaedics
- Arthritis Foundation
  http://www.arthritis.org/AFStore/StartRead.asp?idProduct=3327
- National Institutes of Health
  http://www.nlm.nih.gov/medlineplus/ency/article/000839.htm

REFERENCES

- Hilton-Jones D: Inflammatory muscle diseases. Curr Opin Neurol 2001;14: 591. [PMID: 11562570]
- Mastaglia FL, Zilko PJ: Inflammatory myopathies: how to treat the difficult cases. J Clin Neurosci 2003;10:99.
- Wortmann RL, DiMauro S: Differentiating idiopathic inflammatory myopathies from metabolic myopathies. Rheum Dis Clin North Am 2002;28: 759.

David B. Hellmann, MD, FACP
John H. Stone, MD, MPH

Nausea & Vomiting

 KEY FEATURES

ESSENTIALS OF DIAGNOSIS

- Nausea is a vague, intensely disagreeable sensation of sickness or "queasiness"
- Distinguished from anorexia
- Retching (spasmodic respiratory and abdominal movements) often follows
- Vomiting may or may not follow
- Vomiting should be distinguished from regurgitation, the effortless reflux of liquid or food stomach contents

GENERAL CONSIDERATIONS

- May be caused by wide variety of conditions that stimulate the vagal afferent receptors, the brainstem vomiting center, or the chemoreceptor trigger zone (Table 51, page 1249)
- May lead to serious complications, including electrolyte disturbances (hypokalemia, metabolic alkalosis), dehydration, aspiration pneumonia, Mallory-Weiss tear, and esophageal rupture

 CLINICAL FINDINGS

SYMPTOMS AND SIGNS

- Acute symptoms without abdominal pain suggest food poisoning, infectious gastroenteritis, or drugs
- Acute pain and vomiting suggest peritoneal irritation, acute gastric or intestinal obstruction, or pancreaticobiliary disease
- Persistent vomiting suggests pregnancy, gastric outlet obstruction, gastroparesis, intestinal dysmotility, psychogenic disorders, and central nervous system or systemic disorders
- Vomiting immediately after meals suggests bulimia or psychogenic causes
- Vomiting of undigested food suggests gastroparesis or a gastric outlet obstruction; physical examination reveals a succussion splash
- Inquire about neurological symptoms such as headaches, stiff neck, vertigo, and focal paresthesias or weakness

DIFFERENTIAL DIAGNOSIS

- Nausea and vomiting, causes (Table 51, page 1249)

 DIAGNOSIS

LABORATORY TESTS

- Serum electrolytes, glucose, creatinine, calcium, amylase, liver enzymes, thyroid-stimulating hormone
- Urine or serum pregnancy test

IMAGING STUDIES

- Flat and upright abdominal radiographs
- Ultrasound of abdomen or CT scan
- Barium upper gastrointestinal series
- Nuclear scintigraphic study for gastroparesis

DIAGNOSTIC PROCEDURES

- Nasogastric tube suction for patients with vomiting due to gastrointestinal obstruction, gastroparesis, ileus, or peritonitis
- Saline load test: formerly used to distinguish gastric outlet obstruction from delayed gastric emptying; this test is seldom used in era of endoscopy
- Upper endoscopy

Nausea & Vomiting

 ## TREATMENT

MEDICATIONS

- Antiemetic medications (Table 52, page 1250) given to control vomiting
- Combinations of drugs from different classes may provide better control
- Avoid antiemetic medications in pregnancy

THERAPEUTIC PROCEDURES

- For mild, self-limited, acute vomiting: no specific treatment, clear liquids and small quantities of dry foods
- For moderate to severe vomiting, nothing by mouth, give intravenous saline 0.45% solution with 20 mEq/L of potassium chloride
- Nasogastric suction for gastric decompression in patients with gastrointestinal obstruction, ileus or gastroparesis, or peritonitis

 ## OUTCOME

COMPLICATIONS

- Dehydration, hypokalemia, metabolic alkalosis, aspiration, rupture of the esophagus (Boerhaave's syndrome), and bleeding secondary to a mucosal tear at the gastroesophageal junction (Mallory-Weiss syndrome)

WHEN TO ADMIT

- Hospitalize patient for severe acute vomiting, for rehydration, evaluation, and specific therapy

PREVENTION

- Antiemetic medications (especially 5-HT$_3$ antagonists) can be given to prevent vomiting in patients undergoing chemotherapy and abdominal surgery

 ## EVIDENCE

PRACTICE GUIDELINES

- American Gastroenterological Association Medical Position Statement: Nausea and vomiting. Gastroenterology 2001;120:261. [PMID: 11208735]
- American Gastroenterological Association medical position statement: nausea and vomiting. American Gastroenterological Association, 2001 http://www2.gastrojournal.org/scripts/om.dll/serve?action=getmedia&id= a0010100261&trueID=pdf_0010100261&location=jgast0112001&type=pdf&name=x.pdf

WEB SITE

- National Digestive Diseases Information Clearinghouse—Cyclic vomiting syndrome http://digestive.niddk.nih.gov/ddiseases/pubs/cvs/index.htm

INFORMATION FOR PATIENTS

- American Academy of Family Physicians—Nausea and vomiting: self-care flowcharts http://familydoctor.org/flowcharts/529.html

REFERENCES

- Gan TJ: Postoperative nausea and vomiting—can it be eliminated? JAMA 2002;287:1233. [PMID: 11886298]
- Gralla RJ: New agents, new treatment, and antiemetic therapy. Semin Oncol 2002;29:119. [PMID: 11894022]
- Rabine J et al: Management of the patient with gastroparesis. J Clin Gastroenterol 2001;32:11. [PMID: 11154162]
- Tramer MR: A rational approach to the control of nausea and vomiting: evidence from systematic reviews. Acta Anesthesiol Scand 2001;45:4. [PMID: 11152031]

Kenneth R. McQuaid, MD

Neck Masses

KEY FEATURES

ESSENTIALS OF DIAGNOSIS

- Rapid growth and tenderness suggest an inflammatory process
- Firm, painless, and slowly enlarging masses are often neoplastic

GENERAL CONSIDERATIONS

- In young adults, most neck masses are benign (branchial cleft cyst, thyroglossal duct cyst, reactive lymphadenitis), though malignancy should always be considered (lymphoma, metastatic thyroid carcinoma)
- Lymphadenopathy is common in HIV-positive individuals, but a growing or dominant mass may well be malignant
- In adults over 40, cancer is the most common cause of persistent neck mass
- A metastasis from squamous cell carcinoma arising within the mouth, pharynx, larynx, or upper esophagus should be suspected, especially if there is a history of tobacco or significant alcohol use
- An enlarged node unassociated with an obvious infection should be further evaluated, especially if the patient has a history of smoking or alcohol use or a history of cancer

CLINICAL FINDINGS

SYMPTOMS AND SIGNS

Congenital lesions presenting as neck masses in adults

- Branchial cleft cysts
  - Usually present as a soft cystic mass along the anterior border of the sternocleidomastoid muscle
  - Usually manifest in the second or third decades of life, often when they suddenly swell or become infected
  - First branchial cleft cysts present high in the neck, sometimes just below the ear
  - A fistulous connection with the floor of the external auditory canal may be present
  - Second branchial cleft cysts, which are far more common, may communicate with the tonsillar fossa
  - Third branchial cleft cysts, which may communicate with the piriform sinus, are rare
- Thyroglossal duct cysts

  - Commonest before age 20
  - Midline neck mass, often just below the hyoid bone, that moves with swallowing

Reactive cervical lymphadenopathy

- Normal lymph nodes in the neck are usually less than 1 cm in length
- Infections involving the pharynx, salivary glands, and scalp often cause tender enlargement of neck nodes
- Enlarged nodes are common in HIV-infected persons

Tuberculous and nontuberculous mycobacterial lymphadenitis

- The usual presentation is simply single or matted nodes
- Although mycobacterial adenitis can extend to the skin and drain externally (referred to as scrofula), this late presentation is no longer common

Infectious, inflammatory, and neoplastic neck masses

- Tumor metastases
  - In older adults, 80% of firm, persistent, and enlarging neck masses are metastatic in origin
  - The great majority of these arise from squamous cell carcinoma of the upper aerodigestive tract
  - A complete head and neck examination may reveal the tumor of origin
  - Other than thyroid carcinoma, non-squamous cell metastases to the neck are infrequent
  - Although tumors not involving the head and neck seldom metastasize to the middle or upper neck, the supraclavicular region is quite often involved by lung and breast tumors
  - Infradiaphragmatic tumors, with the exception of renal cell carcinoma, rarely metastasize to the neck

Lymphoma

  - About 10% of lymphomas present in the head and neck
  - Lymphoma arising in AIDS patients is an increasing concern
  - Multiple rubbery nodes, especially in the young adult, are suggestive of this disease

DIFFERENTIAL DIAGNOSIS

- Reactive cervical lymphadenopathy (eg, pharyngitis, tuberculous lymphadenitis, cat scratch disease, Lyme disease)

- Lymphoma
- Skin abscess
- Parotitis
- Goiter or thyroiditis
- Branchial cleft cyst
- Thyroglossal duct cyst
- Metastasis from squamous cell carcinoma in mouth, pharynx, larynx, upper esophagus
- Sarcoidosis
- Metastatic thyroid carcinoma
- Autoimmune adenopathy
- Kikuchi's disease (histiocytic necrotizing lymphadenitis)

DIAGNOSIS

IMAGING STUDIES

- An MRI or PET scan prior to open biopsy may yield valuable information about a possible presumed primary site or another site for fine-needle aspiration (FNA)

DIAGNOSTIC PROCEDURES

- Common indications for FNA biopsy of a node include persistence or continued enlargement, particularly if an obvious primary tumor is not visible or palpable on physical examination

Tuberculous and nontuberculous mycobacterial lymphadenitis

- FNA is usually the best initial diagnostic approach: cytology, smear for acid-fast bacilli, culture, sensitivity test, and polymerase chain reaction (PCR) can all be done

Infectious, inflammatory, and cancerous neck masses

- Examination under anesthesia with direct laryngoscopy, esophagoscopy, and bronchoscopy is usually required to fully evaluate the tumor and exclude second primaries

Lymphoma

- FNA may be diagnostic, but open biopsy is often required

TREATMENT

SURGERY

Branchial cleft cysts

- To prevent recurrent infection and possible carcinoma, they should be completely excised, along with their fistulous tracts

Thyroglossal duct cysts

- Surgical excision is recommended to prevent recurrent infection

Reactive cervical lymphadenopathy

- Except for the occasional node that suppurates and requires incision and drainage, treatment is directed against the underlying infection

Infectious, inflammatory, and cancerous neck masses

- Treat the underlying pathology

OUTCOME

PROGNOSIS

- Prognosis is that of the underlying pathology

WHEN TO REFER

- When the diagnosis is in question or for specialized treatment, particularly for a malignancy

EVIDENCE

PRACTICE GUIDELINES

- National Guideline Clearinghouse http://www.guideline.gov/summary/summary.aspx?doc_id=2848&nbr=2074&string=cervical+lymphadenopathy
- Torsiglieri AJ Jr et al: Pediatric neck masses: guidelines for evaluation. Int J Pediatr Otorhinolaryngol 1988c;16:199. [PMID: 3235286]

WEB SITES

- Ear, Nose, and Throat Information Center http://www.netdoor.com/entinfo/
- Otolaryngology Resources on the Internet http://www.bcm.tmc.edu/oto/othersa.html
- Lymphoma of the Head and Neck Demonstration Case http://www.brighamrad.harvard.edu/Cases/bwh/hcache/47/full.html

INFORMATION FOR PATIENTS

- American Academy of Otolaryngology. Head and Neck Cancer http://www.entnet.org/healthinfo/tobacco/cancer.cfm
- National Cancer Institute. Head and Neck http://www.nci.nih.gov/cancer_information/xml_tab.aspx?viewid=7d080f7f-585d-40e8-bd59-13fb31481b2b&expand=Head+and+Neck

REFERENCES

- Amedee RG et al: Fine-needle aspiration biopsy. Laryngoscope 2001;111:1551. [PMID: 11568593]
- Ewing CA et al: Presentations of thyroglossal duct cysts in adults. Eur Arch Otorhinolaryngol 1999;256:136. [PMID: 10234482]
- Palacios E et al: Branchial cleft cyst. Ear Nose Throat J 2001;80:302. [PMID: 11393908]

Robert K. Jackler, MD
Michael J. Kaplan, MD

Neck Pain

 KEY FEATURES

ESSENTIALS OF DIAGNOSIS

- Most chronic neck pain is caused by degenerative joint disease and responds to conservative approaches

GENERAL CONSIDERATIONS

- A large group of articular and extraarticular disorders is characterized by pain that may involve simultaneously the neck, shoulder girdle, and upper extremity. Diagnostic differentiation among these disorders may be difficult

DEMOGRAPHICS

- Degeneration of cervical disks and joints may occur in adolescents but is more common after age 40

 CLINICAL FINDINGS

SYMPTOMS AND SIGNS

- Pain may be limited to the posterior neck region or, depending on the level of the symptomatic joint, may radiate segmentally to the occiput, anterior chest, shoulder girdle, arm, forearm, and hand
- Radiating pain in the upper extremity is often intensified by hyperextension of the neck and deviation of the head to the involved side
- Limitation of cervical movements is the most common objective finding
- Neurological signs depend on the extent of compression of nerve roots or the spinal cord. Compression of the spinal cord may cause long-tract involvement resulting in paraparesis or paraplegia

Acute or chronic cervical musculotendinous strain

- Cervical strain is generally caused by mechanical postural disorders, overexertion, or injury (eg, whiplash)
- Acute episodes are associated with pain, decreased cervical spine motion, and paraspinal muscle spasm, resulting in stiffness of the neck and loss of motion
- Local tenderness is often present in acute but not chronic strain

Herniated nucleus pulposus

- Rupture or prolapse of the nucleus pulposus of the cervical disks into the spinal canal causes pain that radiates to the arms at the level of C6–C7
- When intraabdominal pressure is increased by coughing, sneezing, or other movements, symptoms are aggravated, and cervical muscle spasm may often occur
- Neurological abnormalities may include decreased reflexes of the deep tendons of the biceps and triceps and decreased sensation and muscle atrophy or weakness in the forearm or hand

Arthritic disorders

- Cervical spondylosis (degenerative arthritis) is a collective term describing degenerative changes that occur in the apophysial joints and intervertebral disk joints, with or without neurological signs
- Osteoarthritis of the cervical spine is often asymptomatic but may cause diffuse neck pain, radicular pain, or myelopathy

- Myelopathy develops insidiously and is manifested by numb, clumsy hands
- Some patients also complain of unsteady walking, urinary frequency and urgency, or electrical shock sensations with neck flexion or extension (Lhermitte's sign)
- Weakness, sensory loss, and spasticity with exaggerated reflexes develop below the level of spinal cord compression

DIFFERENTIAL DIAGNOSIS

- Acute or chronic cervical musculotendinous strain
- Herniated nucleus pulposus
- Degenerative arthritides (eg, osteoarthritis)
- Inflammatory arthritides (eg, rheumatoid arthritis, ankylosing spondylitis)
- Infections (eg, meningitis, osteomyelitis)
- Cancer (eg, cervical spine metastases)

 DIAGNOSIS

IMAGING STUDIES

- Plain x-rays are often completely normal in an acute cervical strain
- In osteoarthritis, comparative reduction in height of the involved disk space is a frequent finding. The most common late x-ray finding is osteophyte formation
- Use of MRI or CT is indicated in the patient who has severe pain of unknown cause that fails to respond to conservative therapy or in the patient who has evidence of myelopathy
- MRI is more sensitive than CT in detecting disk disease, extradural compression, and intramedullary cord disease
- CT is more sensitive for demonstration of fractures

TREATMENT

MEDICATIONS

Acute or chronic cervical musculotendinous strain

- Analgesics and early mobilization (including whiplash)

Herniated nucleus pulposus

- Cervical traction, bed rest, and analgesics are usually successful for pain and radicular symptoms
- Cervical epidural steroid injections may help those who fail to improve

SURGERY

- Surgery is indicated for unremitting pain and progressive weakness from a herniated nucleus pulposus despite a full trial of conservative therapy and if a surgically correctable abnormality is identified by MRI or CT myelography. Surgical decompression achieves excellent results in 70–80% of such patients
- Surgical treatment may involve stabilization of the cervical spine when atlantoaxial subluxation occurs in patients with rheumatoid arthritis

THERAPEUTIC PROCEDURES

- Chronic pain in the zygapophysial joints resulting from whiplash injuries may benefit from percutaneous radiofrequency neurotomy

 OUTCOME

COMPLICATIONS

- Progressive degenerative disease of the cervical spine can cause cervical myelopathy with weakness and spasticity of the legs
- Serious erosive disease of joints may lead to neurological complications as sometimes occurs in rheumatoid arthritis and occasionally in ankylosing spondylitis; the usual joint involved in these disorders is the atlantoaxial joint (C1–C2)

WHEN TO REFER

- Refer to a neurosurgeon for indications described under Surgery

 EVIDENCE

PRACTICE GUIDELINES

- Gross AR et al: Clinical practice guideline on the use of manipulation or mobilization in the treatment of adults with mechanical neck disorders. Man Ther 2002;7:193. [PMID: 12419654]

INFORMATION FOR PATIENTS

- American Physical Therapy Association http://www.apta.org/brochures/NeckPain.pdf
- American Association of Neurological Surgeons http://www.neurosurgery.org/health/patient/detail.asp?DisorderID=76

REFERENCES

- Hardin J: Pain and the cervical spine. Bull Rheum Dis 2001;50:1. [PMID: 11688257]
- Hoving JL et al: Manual therapy, physical therapy, or continued care by a general practitioner for patients with neck pain. A randomized, controlled trial. Ann Intern Med 2002;136:713. [PMID: 12020139]
- Narayan P et al: Treatment of degenerative cervical disc disease. Neurol Clin 2001;19:217. [PMID: 11471766]

David B. Hellmann, MD, FACP
John H. Stone, MD, MPH

Neck Pain, Discogenic

 KEY FEATURES

ESSENTIALS OF DIAGNOSIS

- Neck pain, sometimes radiating to arms
- Restricted neck movements
- Motor, sensory, or reflex changes in arms with root involvement
- Neurological deficit in legs, gait disorder, or sphincter disturbance with cord involvement

GENERAL CONSIDERATIONS

Acute cervical disk protrusion

- Acute cervical disk protrusion leads to pain in the neck and radicular pain in the arm, exacerbated by head movement

Cervical spondylosis

- Results from chronic cervical disk degeneration, with herniation of disk material, secondary calcification, and associated osteophytic outgrowths
- One or more of the cervical nerve roots may be compressed, stretched, or angulated; and myelopathy may also develop as a result of compression, vascular insufficiency, or recurrent minor trauma to the cord

 CLINICAL FINDINGS

SYMPTOMS AND SIGNS

Acute cervical disk protrusion

- With lateral herniation of the disk, motor, sensory, or reflex changes may be found in a radicular (usually C6 or C7) distribution on the affected side (Figure 7, page 1273)
- With more centrally directed herniations, the spinal cord may also be involved, leading to spastic paraparesis and sensory disturbances in the legs, sometimes accompanied by impaired sphincter function

Cervical spondylosis

- Patients present with neck pain and restricted head movement, occipital headaches, radicular pain and other sensory disturbances in the arms, weakness of the arms or legs, or some combination of these symptoms
- Examination generally reveals that lateral flexion and rotation of the neck are limited
- A segmental pattern of weakness or dermatomal sensory loss (or both) may be found unilaterally or bilaterally in the upper limbs, and tendon reflexes mediated by the affected root or roots are depressed
- The C5 and C6 nerve roots are most commonly involved; examination frequently then reveals weakness of muscles supplied by these roots (eg, deltoids, supra- and infraspinatus, biceps, brachioradialis), pain or sensory loss about the shoulder and outer border of the arm and forearm, and depressed biceps and brachioradialis reflexes
- Spastic paraparesis may also be present if there is an associated myelopathy, sometimes accompanied by posterior column or spinothalamic sensory deficits in the legs

DIFFERENTIAL DIAGNOSIS

- A variety of congenital abnormalities may involve the cervical spine and lead to neck pain; these include hemivertebrae, fused vertebrae, basilar impression, and instability of the atlantoaxial joint
- Traumatic, degenerative, infective, and neoplastic disorders may also lead to pain in the neck
- When rheumatoid arthritis involves the spine, it tends to affect especially the cervical region, leading to pain, stiffness, and reduced mobility; displacement of vertebrae or atlantoaxial subluxation may lead to cord compression that can be life-threatening if not treated by fixation

 DIAGNOSIS

IMAGING STUDIES

Acute cervical disk protrusion

- The diagnosis is confirmed by MRI or CT myelography

Cervical spondylosis

- Plain radiographs of the cervical spine show osteophyte formation, narrowing of disk spaces, and encroachment on the intervertebral foramina, but such changes are common in middle-aged persons and may be unrelated to the presenting complaint
- CT or MRI helps to confirm the diagnosis and exclude other structural causes of the myelopathy

Neck Pain, Discogenic

 ## TREATMENT

SURGERY

Acute cervical disk protrusion

- If other measures are unsuccessful or the patient has a significant neurological deficit, surgical removal of the protruding disk may be necessary

Cervical spondylosis

- Operative treatment may be necessary to prevent further progression if there is a significant neurological deficit or if root pain is severe, persistent, and unresponsive to conservative measures

THERAPEUTIC PROCEDURES

Acute cervical disk protrusion

- In mild cases, bed rest or intermittent neck traction may help, followed by immobilization of the neck in a collar for several weeks

Cervical spondylosis

- Restriction of neck movements by a cervical collar may relieve pain

 ## OUTCOME

PROGNOSIS

- Self-limited

WHEN TO REFER

- Ergonomic consultation may improve symptoms

 ## EVIDENCE

PRACTICE GUIDELINES

- National Guideline Clearinghouse http://www.guideline.gov/summary/summary.aspx?doc_id=2803&nbr=2029&string=disc+protrusion
- Philadelphia Panel evidence-based clinical practice guidelines on selected rehabilitation interventions for neck pain. Phys Ther 2001;81:1701. [PMID: 11589644]

INFORMATION FOR PATIENTS

- JAMA patient page: Neck injuries. JAMA 2001;286:1928. [PMID: 11680473]
- American Academy of Orthopaedic Surgeons http://orthoinfo.aaos.org/fact/thr_report.cfm?Thread_ID=304&topcategory=Neck&all=all

REFERENCES

- Harris G: Managing musculoskeletal complaints with rehabilitation therapy: summary of the Philadelphia Panel evidence-based clinical practice guidelines on musculoskeletal rehabilitation interventions. J Fam Pract 2002;51:1042. [PMID: 12540330]
- Niemisto L: Radiofrequency denervation for neck and back pain. A systematic review of randomized controlled trials. Cochrane Database Syst Rev. 2003;CD004058. [PMID: 12535508]
- Schonstein E: Work conditioning, work hardening and functional restoration for workers with back and neck pain. Cochrane Database Syst Rev 2003; CD001822. [PMID: 12535416]

Michael J. Aminoff, DSc, MD, FRCP

Non-Hodgkin's Lymphoma

 ## KEY FEATURES

GENERAL CONSIDERATIONS

- Heterogeneous group of cancers of lymphocytes
- Disorders vary in clinical presentation and course from indolent to rapidly progressive
- Indolent lymphomas often disseminated at diagnosis, and bone marrow involvement frequent
- In Burkitt's lymphoma, a protooncogene c-*myc* is translocated from chromosome 8 to heavy chain locus on chromosome 14, where c-*myc* overexpression is likely related to malignant transformation
- In follicular lymphomas, translocation of possible oncogene *bcl*-2 from chromosome 8 to the heavy chain locus on chromosome 14 causes *bcl*-2 overexpression, which appears to protect the lymphoma cell against apoptosis

REAL/WHO proposed classification of lymphomas

- B cell lymphomas
  - Precursor B cell lymphoblastic lymphoma
  - Small lymphocytic lymphoma/chronic lymphocytic leukemia
  - Marginal zone lymphomas: nodal marginal zone lymphoma, extranodal MALT, splenic
  - Hairy cell leukemia
  - Follicular lymphoma
  - Mantle cell lymphoma
  - Diffuse large B cell lymphoma
  - Burkitt's lymphoma
- T cell lymphomas
  - Anaplastic large cell lymphoma
  - Peripheral T cell lymphoma
  - Mycosis fungoides

 ## CLINICAL FINDINGS

SYMPTOMS AND SIGNS

- Painless lymphadenopathy, isolated or widespread (retroperitoneal, mesenteric, and pelvic)
- Constitutional symptoms, eg, fever, drenching night sweats, or weight loss
- Extranodal sites of disease (skin, gastrointestinal tract) sometimes found on examination
- Abdominal pain or abdominal fullness in Burkitt's lymphoma because of predilection for abdomen

DIFFERENTIAL DIAGNOSIS

- Hodgkin's disease
- Metastatic cancer
- Infectious mononucleosis
- Cat-scratch disease
- Sarcoidosis
- Drug-induced pseudolymphoma (eg, phenytoin)

 ## DIAGNOSIS

LABORATORY TESTS

- Peripheral blood usually normal, but some lymphomas may present in leukemic phase
- Cerebrospinal fluid cytology shows malignant cells in some high-grade lymphomas with meningeal involvement
- Serum LDH is a useful prognostic marker and is now incorporated in risk stratification of treatment

IMAGING STUDIES

- Chest x-ray: mediastinal mass in lymphoblastic lymphoma, others
- CT scan of chest, abdomen, pelvis

DIAGNOSTIC PROCEDURES

- Needle aspiration biopsy may yield suspicious results, but lymph node biopsy (or biopsy of involved extranodal tissue) required for diagnosis and staging
- Bone marrow involvement manifested as paratrabecular lymphoid aggregates
- Staging after pathological diagnosis is established involves chest x-ray and CT of abdomen and pelvis, bone marrow biopsy, and in selected cases with high-risk morphology, lumbar puncture

Non-Hodgkin's Lymphoma

 TREATMENT

MEDICATIONS

- Chemotherapy with alkylating agents, eg, chlorambucil, 0.6–1 mg/kg Q 3 weeks, or combination chemotherapy with cyclophosphamide, vincristine, and prednisone (CVP)
- Fludarabine may produce equivalent results
- Rituximab (monoclonal antibody directed against B cell surface antigen CD20) is effective as salvage therapy for relapsed low-grade B cell lymphomas and may improve outcomes when added to initial chemotherapy
- Short-course chemotherapy [eg, three courses of cyclophosphamide, doxorubicin (hydroxydaunomycin; adriamycin), vincristine (Oncovin), and prednisone (CHOP)] plus localized radiation for localized intermediate-grade lymphomas (eg, diffuse large cell lymphoma)
- Chemotherapy with CHOP for 6–8 cycles for more advanced intermediate-grade lymphomas
- Addition of rituximab to CHOP for older patients with diffuse large cell lymphomas

THERAPEUTIC PROCEDURES

- Most indolent lymphomas are disseminated at diagnosis, but if not bulky and patient asymptomatic, no initial therapy is required; some have spontaneous remission
- Special forms of lymphoma (Burkitt's lymphoma, lymphoblastic lymphoma, mantle cell lymphoma) require individualized therapy
- Localized radiation therapy for patients who have limited indolent disease
- Radioimmunoconjugates, eg, yttrium-90 ibritumomab, which fuse anti-B cell antibodies with radiation, may produce improved results compared with antibody alone
- Allogeneic transplantation for some patients with clinically aggressive low-grade lymphomas
- Autologous stem cell transplantation early in course for high-risk lymphoma; or for intermediate-grade lymphoma that relapses after initial chemotherapy

 OUTCOME

PROGNOSIS

- Median survival with indolent lymphomas is 6–8 years; disease ultimately becomes refractory to chemotherapy
- The International Prognostic Index is widely used to categorize patients with intermediate-grade lymphoma into risk groups
- Worse prognosis if age over 60, elevated serum LDH, stage III or stage IV disease, or poor performance status
- 0–1 risk factor: 80% complete response rate to standard chemotherapy; most responses (80%) durable
- 2 risk factors: 70% complete response rate; 70% long-lasting
- More than 2 risk factors: lower response rates and poor survival with standard regimens; early treatment with high-dose therapy and autologous stem cell transplantation may improve outcome
- With relapse after initial chemotherapy, if lymphoma still partially sensitive to chemotherapy, autologous transplantation offers 50% chance of long-term salvage

EVIDENCE

PRACTICE GUIDELINES

- Pettengell R et al: Position paper on the therapeutic use of rituximab in CD20-positive diffuse large B-cell non-Hodgkin's lymphoma. Br J Haematol 2003;121:44. [PMID: 12670330]
- Zelenetz AD et al: NCCN: Non-Hodgkin's lymphoma. Cancer Control 2001;8(6 Suppl 2):102. [PMID: 11760551]

WEB SITE

- Leukemia & Lymphoma Society—Non-Hodgkin's lymphoma http://www.leukemia-lymphoma.org/all_page? item_id=7087

INFORMATION FOR PATIENTS

- NCI—What you need to know about Non-Hodgkin's lymphoma http://www.cancer.gov/cancerinfo/wyntk/non-hodgkins-lymphoma

REFERENCES

- Coiffier B et al: CHOP chemotherapy plus rituximab compared to CHOP alone in elderly patients with diffuse large-B-cell lymphoma. N Engl J Med 2002;346:235. [PMID: 11807147]
- Khouri IF et al: Nonablative allogeneic hematopoietic transplantation as adoptive immunotherapy for indolent lymphoma: low incidence of toxicity, acute graft-versus-host disease, and treatment-related mortality. Blood 2001;98:3595. [PMID: 11739162]
- Kouroukis CT et al: Chemotherapy for older patients with newly diagnosed advanced-stage, aggressive-histology non-Hodgkin lymphoma: a systematic review. Ann Intern Med 2002;136:144. [PMID: 11790067]
- Rosenwald A et al: The use of molecular profiling to predict survival after chemotherapy for diffuse large-B-cell lymphoma. N Engl J Med 2002;346:1937. [PMID: 12075054]

Charles A. Linker, MD

Obesity

 KEY FEATURES

ESSENTIALS OF DIAGNOSIS

- Excess adipose tissue, resulting in body mass index (BMI) >30
- Upper body obesity (abdomen and flank) of greater health consequence than lower body obesity (buttocks and thighs)

GENERAL CONSIDERATIONS

- More quantitative evaluation involves determination of relative weight (RW) and BMI
- RW is calculated by dividing the measured body weight by the "desirable weight" × 100 (desirable weight is the midpoint value recommended for a given height in weight tables)
- BMI more accurately reflects the presence of excess adipose tissue; it is calculated by dividing measured body weight in kilograms by the height in meters squared
- Normal: BMI = 18.5–24.9
- Overweight: BMI = 25–29.9
- Class I obesity: BMI = 30–34.9
- Class II obesity: BMI = 35–39.9
- Class III (extreme) obesity: BMI >40
- Increased abdominal circumference (>102 cm in men and >88 cm in women) or high waist/hip ratios (>1.0 in men and >0.85 in women) confers greater risk of diabetes mellitus, stroke, coronary artery disease, and early death
- Associated with significant increases in morbidity and mortality
- Surgical and obstetric risks greater
- The relative risk associated with obesity decreases with age, and weight is no longer a risk factor in adults aged >75
- 59.4% of men and 49.9% of women are overweight
- 19.9% of men and 25.1% of women are obese
- As much as 40–70% of obesity may be explained by genetic influences

 CLINICAL FINDINGS

SYMPTOMS AND SIGNS

- Degree and distribution of body fat
- Overall nutritional status
- Signs of secondary causes of obesity (hypothyroidism and Cushing's syndrome) are found in <1%

DIFFERENTIAL DIAGNOSIS

- Increased caloric intake
- Fluid retention: congestive heart failure, cirrhosis, nephrotic syndrome
- Cushing's syndrome
- Hypothyroidism
- Diabetes mellitus (type 2)
- Drugs, eg, antipsychotics, antidepressants, corticosteroids
- Insulinoma

 DIAGNOSIS

LABORATORY TESTS

- Endocrinological evaluation, including serum thyroid-stimulating hormone and dexamethasone suppression test in obese patients with unexplained recent weight gain
- Assessment for medical consequences: fasting glucose, cholesterol, and triglyceride levels, blood pressure

DIAGNOSTIC PROCEDURES

- Measurement of abdominal circumference

TREATMENT

MEDICATIONS

- Catecholaminergic or serotonergic medications are sometimes used in patients with BMI >30 or patients with BMI >27 who have obesity-related health risks
- Catecholaminergic medications include amphetamines (high abuse potential); and nonamphetamine schedule IV appetite suppressants (phentermine, diethylpropion, and mazindol); the latter are approved for short-term use only and have limited utility
- Serotonergic medications: currently unavailable; selective serotonin reuptake inhibitor antidepressants (eg, fluoxetine and sertraline) have serotonergic activity though not approved by the FDA for weight loss
- Sibutramine, 10 mg PO QD: blocks uptake of both serotonin and norepinephrine in the central nervous system; side effects include dry mouth, anorexia, constipation, insomnia, dizziness, and increased blood pressure (<5%)
- Orlistat, 120 mg PO TID with meals: reduces fat absorption in the gastrointestinal tract by inhibiting intestinal lipase; side effects include diarrhea, gas, and cramping and perhaps reduced absorption of fat-soluble vitamins

SURGERY

- Consider for patients with BMI >40, or BMI >35 if obesity-related comorbidities
- Effective surgical procedures include roux-en-Y gastric bypass (GBP) and vertical banded gastroplasty (VBG); both can be done laparoscopically
- GBP is more effective than VBG
- Surgical complications occur in up to 50%, including peritonitis due to anastomotic leak, abdominal wall hernias, staple line disruption, gallstones, neuropathy, marginal ulcers, stomal stenosis, wound infections, thromboembolic disease, nutritional deficiencies, and gastrointestinal symptoms

THERAPEUTIC PROCEDURES

- A multidisciplinary approach is recommended, including hypocaloric diets, behavior modification, aerobic exercise, and social support
- Limit foods that provide large amounts of calories without other nutrients, ie, fat, sucrose, and alcohol
- No special advantage to diets that restrict carbohydrates, advocate large amounts of protein or fats, or recommend ingestion of foods one at a time
- Plan and keep records of menus and exercise sessions, reward systems such as refundable financial contracts
- Aerobic exercise useful for long-term weight maintenance
- Severe obesity: very low-calorie diets (<800 kcal/day) for 4–6 months; side effects include fatigue, orthostatic hypotension, cold intolerance, and fluid and electrolyte disorders; less common complications include gout, gallbladder disease, and cardiac arrhythmias

 OUTCOME

COMPLICATIONS

- Hypertension, type II diabetes mellitus, hyperlipidemia, coronary artery disease, degenerative joint disease, psychosocial disability, cancers (colon, rectum, and prostate, uterus, biliary tract, breast, ovary), thromboembolic disorders, digestive tract diseases (gallstones, reflux esophagitis), skin disorders

PROGNOSIS

- Only 20% of patients will lose 20 lb and maintain the loss for >2 years; only 5% will maintain a 40-lb loss
- With very low-calorie diets, patients lose an average of 2–4 lb per week; long-term weight maintenance is less predictable and requires concurrent behavior modification and exercise
- Sibutramine, 10 mg PO QD, for 6–12 months results in average weight losses of 3–5 kg more than placebo
- Orlistat, 120 mg PO TID with meals, for up to 2 years results in 2–4 kg greater weight loss than placebo
- Both VBG and GBP lead to substantial weight loss—close to 50% of initial body weight

WHEN TO REFER

- Refer for bariatric surgery for BMI >40

WHEN TO ADMIT

- For bariatric surgery
- For complications of very low-calorie diets

EVIDENCE

PRACTICE GUIDELINES

- Clinical guidelines on the identification, evaluation, and treatment of overweight and obesity in adults. National Heart, Lung, and Blood Institute. National Institute of Diabetes and Digestive and Kidney Diseases, 1998 http://www.nhlbi.nih.gov/guidelines/obesity/ob_home.htm
- Cummings S et al: Position of the American Dietetic Association: weight management. J Am Diet Assoc 2002; 102:1145. [PMID: 12171464]

WEB SITE

- American Obesity Association http://www.obesity.org/

INFORMATION FOR PATIENTS

- Cleveland Clinic—Obesity http://www.clevelandclinic.org/health/health-info/docs/2400/2435.asp?index=9468

REFERENCES

- Choban PS et al: Bariatric surgery for morbid obesity: why, who, when, how, where, and then what? Cleve Clin J Med 2002;69:897. [PMID: 12430975]
- Glazer G: Long-term pharmacotherapy of obesity 2000. A review of safety and efficacy. Arch Intern Med 2001;161: 1814. [PMID: 11493122]
- Gokcel A et al: Evaluation of the safety and efficacy of sibutramine, orlistat and metformin in the treatment of obesity. Diabetes Obes Metab 2002;4:49. [PMID: 11874442]
- Volek JS et al: Very-low-carbohydrate weight-loss diets revisited. Cleve Clin J Med 2002;69:849. [PMID: 12430970]

Robert B. Baron, MD, MS

Onchocerciasis

 ## KEY FEATURES

ESSENTIALS OF DIAGNOSIS

- Primary findings are subcutaneous nodules that contain adult worms and skin and eye changes that result from dead or dying microfilariae
- Heavy infection leads to chronic pruritus, disfiguring skin lesions, visual impairment, and debility

GENERAL CONSIDERATIONS

- The infection is a chronic filarial disease caused by *Onchocerca volvulus*
- Humans are the only important host. The vector and intermediate host are *Simulium* flies, day biters that breed in rivers and fast-flowing streams and become infected by ingesting microfilariae with a human blood meal; at subsequent feedings, they can infect new susceptible hosts
- Female worms release motile microfilariae into the skin, subcutaneous tissues, lymphatics, and eyes; microfilariae are occasionally seen in the urine but rarely in blood or cerebrospinal fluid

DEMOGRAPHICS

- An estimated 18 million persons are infected, of whom 3–4 million have skin disease, 0.3 million are blinded, and 0.5 million are severely visually impaired
- In hyperendemic areas, more than 40% of inhabitants over 40 years of age are blind
- The infection, predominant in West Africa, also occurs in many other parts of tropical Africa and in localized areas of the southwestern Arabian peninsula, southern Mexico, Guatemala, Venezuela, Colombia, and northwestern Brazil
- The West African savanna strain is especially associated with severe blinding eye lesions

 ## CLINICAL FINDINGS

SYMPTOMS AND SIGNS

- The interval from exposure to onset of symptoms can be as long as 1–3 years

Nodules

- Adult worms, which can live for up to 14 years, typically are in fibrous subcutaneous nodules that are painless, freely movable, and 0.5–1 cm in size
- Many nodules are deep in the muscular tissues and nonpalpable

Pruritis

- May be severe, leading to skin excoriation and lichenification; other findings include pigmentary changes, papules, scaling, atrophy, pendulous skin, and acute inflammation
- May occur without skin lesions

Dermatitis

- Infected visitors, as compared with indigenous persons, may show a more prominent dermatitis despite a low to nondetectable microfiladerma or eosinophilia and an absence of nodules and eye disease

Lymphadenopathy

- There may be marked enlargement of femoral and inguinal nodes and generalized lymph node enlargement

Eye

- Microfilariae in the eye may lead to visual impairment and blindness
- Findings include itching, photophobia, anterior segment changes (limbitis, punctate and sclerosing keratitis, iritis, secondary glaucoma, cataract), and posterior segment changes (optic neuritis, optic atrophy, chorioretinitis, and other retinal findings)

DIFFERENTIAL DIAGNOSIS

- Glaucoma
- Loiasis (*Loa loa* infection)
- Gnathostomiasis
- Cysticercosis (with ophthalmic involvement)
- Sporotrichosis
- Coccidioidomycosis

 ## DIAGNOSIS

LABORATORY TESTS

- Traditional serological tests are usually positive, but cross-reactions occur with other forms of filariasis, and the tests do not distinguish current from past infection
- Immunoblot analysis of IgG_4 antibodies and an ELISA appear to be more sensitive than skin snips early in infection, but occasional cross-reactions also occur with other filarial infections
- PCR (on skin snips and urine) and antigen detection (in blood and urine) have the advantage over serology in that they are positive only in people who have active infection
- Eosinophilia (15–50%), polyclonal hypergammaglobulinemia, and elevated IgE levels are common

IMAGING STUDIES

- Ultrasound has been used to detect nonpalpable onchocercomas and to distinguish them from other lesions (lipomas, fibromas, lymph nodes, foreign body granulomas)

DIAGNOSTIC PROCEDURES

- Diagnosis is by demonstrating microfilariae in skin snips (usually obtained with a punch biopsy instrument), identifying them in the cornea or anterior chamber by slitlamp examination (after the patient has sat with head lowered between knees for 2 min) or by nodule aspiration or excision
- Skin snips placed in saline are incubated for 2–4 h before examination, or overnight for low-intensity infections
- Adult worms may be recovered in excised nodules

Onchocerciasis

 TREATMENT

MEDICATIONS

- Drug treatment is with ivermectin (a microfilaricide) as a single oral dose of 150 μg/kg given with water on an empty stomach; the patient should remain fasting for 2 more hours. The number of microfilariae in the skin diminishes markedly within 2–3 days, remains low for about 6 months, and then gradually increases; microfilariae in the anterior chamber of the eye decrease slowly in number over months, eventually disappear, and then gradually return. The optimum frequency of treatment to control symptoms and prevent disease progression remains to be determined

- To initiate treatment, three schedules have been proposed: an initial and repeat dose at 6 months, repeated doses at 3-month intervals for a year, or repeated doses at monthly intervals for a total of three doses. Thereafter, treatment is repeated at intervals of 6 months for 2 years and yearly thereafter until the adult worms die, which may take 12–15 years or longer

- With the initial treatment only, patients with microfilariae in the cornea or anterior chamber may benefit from several days of prednisone treatment (1 mg/kg/day) to avoid inflammatory eye reactions. Although single-dose ivermectin does not kill the adult worms, with repeated doses, increasing evidence suggests that the drug has a low-level macrofilaricidal action

- Adverse reactions, which are more marked with the first dose, are mild in 9% of patients and severe in 0.2%; these include edema (face and limbs), fever, pruritus, lymphadenitis, malaise, and hypotension. Ivermectin does not cause a severe reaction in the eyes or skin as occurs with diethylcarbamazine

- Ivermectin should not be used in the presence of concurrent *Loa loa* infections or pregnancy, or in patients with central nervous system diseases in which increased penetration may occur of ivermectin into the central nervous system (eg, meningitis)

- For selected patients in whom repeated ivermectin treatments do not control symptoms, suramin can be given for its macrofilaricidal action; however, because of suramin's toxicity and complex administration, it should be administered only by experts

- Doxycycline for 6 weeks has some macrofilaricidal action
- Diethylcarbamazine is no longer recommended for treatment

SURGERY

- In Latin America only, nodulectomy continues to be used for nodules on or near the head

 OUTCOME

PROGNOSIS

- With treatment, some skin and ocular lesions improve and ocular progression is prevented. The prognosis is unfavorable only for those patients who are seen for the first time with already far-advanced ocular onchocerciasis

WHEN TO REFER

- All patients should be referred to a clinician who has expertise in the diagnosis and treatment of this disease
- All patients with ocular involvement should be referred to an ophthalmologist

PREVENTION

- Mass treatment and control programs are underway since the advent of the safe drug ivermectin

EVIDENCE

INFORMATION FOR PATIENTS

- National Institute of Allergy and Imfectious Diseases http://www.niaid.nih.gov/newsroom/focuson/bugborne01/onchoc.htm
- National Institutes of Health http://www.nlm.nih.gov/medlineplus/ency/article/003040.htm

REFERENCES

- Gardon J et al: Effects of standard and high doses of ivermectin on adult worms of *Onchocerca volvulus*: a randomised controlled trial. Lancet 2002;360:203. [PMID: 12133654]
- Onchocerciasis (river blindness). Report from the eleventh InterAmerican conference on onchocerciasis, Mexico City, Mexico. Wkly Epidemiol Rec 2002; 77:249. [PMID: 12221990]
- Pennisi E: Infectious disease. New culprit emerges in river blindness. Science 2002;295:1809. [PMID: 11884722]
- Unnasch TR: River blindness. Lancet 2002;360:182. [PMID: 12133647]

Onychomycosis

 KEY FEATURES

ESSENTIALS OF DIAGNOSIS

- A trichophyton infection of one or more fingernails or toenails
- Yellowish discoloration with heaping of keratin
- Separation of the nail bed

GENERAL CONSIDERATIONS

- The species most commonly found is *Trichophyton rubrum*
- "Saprophytic" fungi may rarely (<5%) cause onychomycosis
- Onycholysis (distal separation of the nail plate from the nail bed, usually of the fingers) is caused by excessive exposure to water, soaps, detergents, alkalies, and industrial cleaning agents
- Candidal infection of the nail folds and subungual area, nail hardeners, and drug-induced photosensitivity may cause onycholysis, as may hyper- and hypothyroidism and psoriasis

 CLINICAL FINDINGS

SYMPTOMS AND SIGNS

- The nails are lusterless, brittle, and hypertrophic
- The substance of the nail is friable

DIFFERENTIAL DIAGNOSIS

- Psoriasis
- Candidal onychomycosis
- Lichen planus
- Allergy to nail polish or nail glue

 DIAGNOSIS

LABORATORY TESTS

- Laboratory diagnosis is mandatory since only 50% of dystrophic nails are due to dermatophytosis
- Portions of the nail should be cleared with 10% potassium hydroxide and examined under the microscope for hyphae
- Fungi may also be cultured

TREATMENT

MEDICATIONS

Topical treatment

- Has relatively low efficacy (10% or less), but in well-motivated patients with minimally thickened nails it can be useful
- Naftifine gel 1% or ciclopirox nail lacquer (Penlac) 8% applied twice daily may clear fingernails in 4–6 months and toenails in 12–18 months

Systemic therapy

- Is generally required for the treatment of nail onychomycosis; fingernails can virtually always be cleared, whereas toenails respond in about 60% of cases
- Fingernails
  - Uamicrosize griseofulvin, 750 mg or more daily for 6 months, is often effective
  - Treatment alternatives are itraconazole, 200 mg daily for 3 months; itraconazole, 400 mg the first 7 days of each month for 2 months; and terbinafine, 250 mg daily for 6–8 weeks
- Toenails
  - Neither griseofulvin nor ketoconazole is recommended
  - Itraconazole may be given as 200 mg daily for 3 months or 400 mg for the first 7 days of each month for 3 months for toenail onychomycosis; it is not FDA approved for treatment of toenail onychomycosis; it interacts with numerous other medications and requires gastric acid to be absorbed
- Terbinafine
  - Terbinafine, 250 mg daily for 3 months, has efficacy equal to or superior to that of itraconazole
  - About 75% of patients have significant clinical improvement, and 35–50% are cured at 1 year
  - The combination of a topical antifungal nail lacquer for 1 year and oral terbinafine for 3 months is superior to the oral agent alone, doubling the cure rate
  - Terbinafine is associated with fewer drug interactions than itraconazole (but may result in prolonged prothrombin times in patients taking warfarin)
  - Also unlike itraconazole, terbinafine is absorbed in patients with low gastric acid (those receiving H_2 blockers)

THERAPEUTIC PROCEDURES

- Difficult to treat because of the long duration of therapy required and the frequency of recurrences
- Fingernails respond more readily than toenails
- For toenails, it is in some situations best to discourage therapy and to control discomfort by paring the thickened nail plate

OUTCOME

FOLLOW-UP

- No matter which therapy is used, constant topical treatment for any coexistent tinea pedis is mandatory and should probably be continued for life to attempt to prevent recurrence

PROGNOSIS

- Once clear, fingernails often remain free of disease for years
- About 60% of patients will have substantial improvement with oral itraconazole, and 25–35% will be mycologically and clinically cured at 1 year

WHEN TO REFER

- If there is a question about the diagnosis, if recommended therapy is ineffective, or specialized treatment is necessary

EVIDENCE

PRACTICE GUIDELINES

- American Academy of Dermatology http://www.aadassociation.org/Guidelines/onychomycosis.html

WEB SITES

- American Academy of Dermatology http://www.aad.org
- Dermatology Handbook for Family Practice from the University of Iowa http://www.vh.org/Providers/ClinRef/FPHandbook/17.html

INFORMATION FOR PATIENTS

- American Academy of Family Physicians http://familydoctor.org/handouts/663.html
- The Mayo Clinic http://www.mayoclinic.com/invoke.cfm?id=DS00084

REFERENCES

- Ciclopirox (Penlac) nail lacquer for onychomycosis. Med Lett Drugs Ther 2000; 42:51. [PMID: 10859733]
- Evans EG et al: Double blind, randomised study of continuous terbinafine compared with intermittent itraconazole in treatment of toenail onychomycosis. The LION Study Group. BMJ 1999; 318:1031. [PMID: 10205099]
- Mayeaux EJ Jr: Nail disorders. Prim Care 2000;27:333. [PMID: 10815047]

Timothy G. Berger, MD

Opioid Dependency

KEY FEATURES

ESSENTIALS OF DIAGNOSIS

- Dependency is a major concern when continued use of narcotics occurs
- Withdrawal causes only moderate morbidity (similar in severity to a bout of "flu")
- Addicted patients sometimes consider themselves more addicted than they really are and may not require a withdrawal program

GENERAL CONSIDERATIONS

- The terms "opioids" and "narcotics" are used interchangeably and include a group of drugs with actions that mimic those of morphine
- The group includes natural derivatives of opium (opiates), synthetic surrogates (opioids), and a number of polypeptides, some of which have been discovered to be natural neurotransmitters
- The principal narcotic of abuse is heroin (metabolized to morphine), which is not used as a legitimate medication
- The other common narcotics are prescription drugs and differ in milligram potency, duration of action, and agonist and antagonist capabilities (Table 2, page 1194)
- The incidence of snorting and inhaling heroin ("smoking") is increasing, particularly among cocaine users

DEMOGRAPHICS

- In the United States, lifetime prevalence for heroin abuse in people aged 12 and over is approximately 1.4%

CLINICAL FINDINGS

SYMPTOMS AND SIGNS

- In mild narcotic intoxication, there are changes in mood, with feelings of euphoria; drowsiness; nausea with occasional emesis; needle tracks; and miosis
- Overdosage causes respiratory depression, peripheral vasodilation, pinpoint pupils, pulmonary edema, coma, and death

Grades of withdrawal

- Grade 0 includes craving and anxiety
- Grade 1, yawning, lacrimation, rhinorrhea, and perspiration
- Grade 2, previous symptoms plus mydriasis, piloerection, anorexia, tremors, and hot and cold flashes with generalized aching
- Grades 3 and 4, increased intensity of previous symptoms and signs, with increased temperature, blood pressure, pulse, and respiratory rate and depth
- In withdrawal from the most severe addiction, vomiting, diarrhea, weight loss, hemoconcentration, and spontaneous ejaculation or orgasm commonly occur

DIFFERENTIAL DIAGNOSIS

- Other drug dependence, eg, alcohol, amphetamines
- Underlying psychiatric disease, eg, depression, personality disorder
- Other drug withdrawal, eg, alcohol, benzodiazepines, amphetamines, cocaine
- Nausea or vomiting due to other cause
- Influenza or other viral syndrome

DIAGNOSIS

LABORATORY TESTS

- Serum or urine toxicology

Opioid Dependency

 TREATMENT

MEDICATIONS

- Treatment for withdrawal begins if grade 2 signs develop
- If a withdrawal program is necessary, use methadone, 10 mg orally (use parenteral administration if the patient is vomiting), and observe. If signs (piloerection, mydriasis, cardiovascular changes) persist for more than 4–6 h, give another 10 mg; continue to administer methadone at 4- to 6-h intervals until signs are not present (rarely more than 40 mg of methadone in 24 h)
- Divide the total amount of drug required over the first 24-h period by 2 and give that amount every 12 h
- Each day reduce the total 24-h dose by 5–10 mg. Thus, a moderately addicted patient initially requiring 30–40 mg of methadone could be withdrawn over a 4- to 8-day period
- Clonidine, 0.1 mg several times daily over a 10- to 14-day period, is both an alternative and an adjunct to methadone detoxification; it is not necessary to taper the dose
- Clonidine is helpful in alleviating cardiovascular symptoms but does not significantly relieve anxiety, insomnia, or generalized aching
- Alternative strategies include rapid and ultrarapid detoxification techniques. In rapid detoxification, withdrawal is precipitated by opioid antagonists followed by naltrexone maintenance
- Narcotic antagonists (eg, naltrexone) can be used for treatment of the patient who has been free of opioids for 7–10 days. Naltrexone blocks the narcotic "high" of heroin when 50 mg is given orally every 24 h initially for several days and then 100 mg is given every 48–72 h. Liver disorders are a major contraindication. Compliance tends to be poor, partly because of the dysphoria that can persist long after opioid discontinuance

THERAPEUTIC PROCEDURES

- Ultrarapid detoxification precipitates withdrawal with opioid antagonists under general anesthesia in a hospital and remains experimental

 OUTCOME

FOLLOW-UP

- Methadone maintenance programs are of some value in chronic recidivism. Under carefully controlled supervision, the narcotic addict is maintained on fairly high doses of methadone (40–120 mg/day) that satisfy craving and block the effects of heroin to a great degree

COMPLICATIONS

- Treatment for overdosage (or suspected overdosage) is naloxone, 2 mg intravenously
- Complications of heroin administration include infections (eg, pneumonia, septic emboli, hepatitis, and HIV infection from using nonsterile needles), traumatic insults (eg, arterial spasm due to drug injection, gangrene), and pulmonary edema

PROGNOSIS

- There is a protracted abstinence syndrome of metabolic, respiratory, and blood pressure changes over a period of 3–6 months
- The research on the impact of rapid detoxification on relapse rates, compared to more traditional methods, is limited at this time

WHEN TO REFER

- All opioid-dependent patients should be referred to an addiction specialist, unless the primary caregiver has sufficient experience with this population

WHEN TO ADMIT

- For some patients residential treatment offers the best chance for recovery. Some patients are able to enter recovery in a structured, supportive outpatient program

EVIDENCE

PRACTICE GUIDELINES

- National Guideline Clearinghouse http://www.guideline.gov/summary/ summary.aspx?doc_id=2609&nbr= 1835&string=opiate+dependency http://www.guideline.gov/summary/ summary.aspx?doc_id=855&nbr= 420&string=opioids

WEB SITE

- American Psychiatric Association http://www.psych.org/

INFORMATION FOR PATIENTS

- JAMA patient page: Drug abuse. JAMA 2000;283:1378. [PMID: 10714739]
- National Institute on Drug Abuse http://www.nida.nih.gov/Infofax/heroin. html http://www.nida.nih.gov/MOM/OP/ MOMOP1.html

REFERENCES

- Hamilton RJ et al: Complications of ultrarapid opioid detoxification with subcutaneous naltrexone pellets. Acad Emerg Med 2002;9:63. [PMID: 11772672]
- National Consensus Development panel on Effective Medical Treatment of Opiate Addiction: effective medical treatment of opiate addiction. JAMA 1998;280:1936. [PMID:9851480]

Stuart J. Eisendrath, MD
Jonathan E. Lichtmacher, MD

Osteoarthritis

 KEY FEATURES

ESSENTIALS OF DIAGNOSIS

- A degenerative disorder without systemic manifestations
- Pain relieved by rest; morning stiffness brief; articular inflammation minimal
- X-ray findings: narrowed joint space, osteophytes, increased density of subchondral bone, bony cysts

GENERAL CONSIDERATIONS

- Degeneration of cartilage and hypertrophy of bone at the articular margins
- Inflammation is usually minimal

Primary

- Most commonly affects some or all of the following—the distal interphalangeal joints and less commonly the proximal interphalangeal joints, the metacarpophalangeal and carpometacarpal joints of the thumb, the hip, the knee, the metatarsophalangeal joint of the big toe, and the cervical and lumbar spine

Secondary

- May occur in any joint as a sequela to articular injury resulting from either intraarticular or extraarticular causes
- Causes of articular injury that lead to secondary degenerative arthritis include trauma, gout, rheumatoid arthritis, hyperparathyroidism, hemochromatosis, Charcot joint

DEMOGRAPHICS

- The most common form of joint disease
- 90% of all people will have radiographic features of osteoarthritis in weight-bearing joints by age 40
- Obesity is a risk factor for knee osteoarthritis and probably for the hip

 CLINICAL FINDINGS

SYMPTOMS AND SIGNS

- Insidious onset
- Pain is made worse by activity or weight bearing and relieved by rest
- Deformity may be absent or minimal; however, bony enlargement of the interphalangeal joints is occasionally prominent: DIP (Heberden's nodes) and PIP (Bouchard's nodes)
- Coarse crepitus may often be felt in the joint
- Joint effusion and other articular signs of inflammation are mild
- Because articular inflammation is minimal and systemic manifestations are absent, degenerative joint disease should seldom be confused with other arthritides
- The distribution of joint involvement in the hands also helps distinguish osteoarthritis from rheumatoid arthritis. Osteoarthritis chiefly affects the distal and proximal interphalangeal joints and spares the wrist and metacarpophalangeal joints (except at the thumb); rheumatoid arthritis involves the wrists and metacarpophalangeal joints and spares the distal interphalangeal joints
- No systemic manifestations

DIFFERENTIAL DIAGNOSIS

- Rheumatoid arthritis
- Seronegative spondyloarthropathy, eg, psoriatic arthritis
- Gout
- Chondrocalcinosis, eg, pseudogout, Wilson's disease
- Other bone disease, eg, osteoporosis, metastatic cancer, multiple myeloma

 DIAGNOSIS

LABORATORY TESTS

- No laboratory evidence of inflammation such as elevated erythrocyte sedimentation rate

IMAGING STUDIES

- Radiographs may reveal narrowing of the joint space, sharpened articular margins, osteophyte formation and lipping of marginal bone, and thickened, dense subchondral bone, or bone cysts
- The correlation between radiographic findings and symptoms is poor

DIAGNOSTIC PROCEDURES

- Aspiration of effusions for pain relief
- Corticosteroid injections for pain relief

Osteoarthritis

 TREATMENT

MEDICATIONS

- Patients with mild disease should start with acetaminophen (2.4–4 g/day)
- Nonsteroidal antiinflammatory drugs (NSAIDs) should be considered for patients who fail to respond to acetaminophen, chondroitin sulfate, and glucosamine
- High doses of NSAIDs, as used in more inflammatory arthritides, are unnecessary

SURGERY

- Total hip and knee replacement provides excellent symptomatic and functional improvement when that joint is seriously afflicted, as indicated by severely restricted walking and pain at rest, particularly at night
- Although arthroscopic surgery for knee osteoarthritis is commonly performed, its long-term efficacy is unestablished

THERAPEUTIC PROCEDURES

- For patients with mild to moderate osteoarthritis of weight-bearing joints, a supervised walking program may result in clinical improvement of functional status without aggravating the joint pain. Weight loss can also improve the symptoms
- For patients with knee osteoarthritis and effusion, intraarticular injection of triamcinolone (20–40 mg) may obviate the need for analgesics or NSAIDs but should not be repeated more than two or three times in a year

 OUTCOME

WHEN TO REFER

- When other inflammatory arthritides cannot be confidently excluded
- For joint replacement

PROGNOSIS

- Symptoms may be quite severe and limit activity considerably (especially with involvement of the hips, knees, and cervical spine)

PREVENTION

- Weight reduction in women reduces the risk of developing symptomatic knee osteoarthritis

 EVIDENCE

PRACTICE GUIDELINES

- National Guideline Clearinghouse http://www.guideline.gov/summary/summary.aspx?doc_id=3355&nbr=2581&string=degenerative+joint+disease http://www.guideline.gov/summary/summary.aspx?doc_id=3188&nbr=2414&string=degenerative+joint+disease

INFORMATION FOR PATIENTS

- National Institute of Arthritis and Musculoskeletal and Skin Diseases http://www.niams.nih.gov/hi/topics/arthritis/oahandout.htm
- Arthritis Foundation http://www.arthritis.org/conditions/DiseaseCenter/oa.asp

REFERENCES

- Geba GP: Efficacy of rofecoxib, celecoxib, and acetaminophen in osteoarthritis of the knee. A randomized trial. JAMA 2002;287:64. [PMID: 11754710]
- Moseley JB: A controlled trial of arthroscopic surgery for osteoarthritis of the knee. N Engl J Med 2002;347:81. [PMID: 12110735]
- Pincus T: A randomized, double-blind, crossover clinical trial of diclofenac plus misoprostol versus acetaminophen in patients with osteoarthritis of the hip or knee. Arthritis Rheum 2001;44:1587. [PMID: 11465710]
- Reginster JY: Long-term effects of glucosamine sulphate on osteoarthritis progression: a randomised, placebo-controlled clinical trial. Lancet 2001; 357:251. [PMID: 11214126]

David B. Hellmann, MD, FACP
John H. Stone, MD, MPH

Osteomalacia

 KEY FEATURES

ESSENTIALS OF DIAGNOSIS

- Painful proximal muscle weakness (especially pelvic girdle); bone pain and tenderness
- Decreased bone density from diminished mineralization of osteoid
- Laboratory abnormalities may include increased alkaline phosphatase, decreased 25-hydroxyvitamin D [$25(OH)D_3$], hypocalcemia, hypocalciuria, hypophosphatemia, secondary hyperparathyroidism
- Classic radiological features may be present

GENERAL CONSIDERATIONS

- Defective mineralization of growing skeleton in children producing permanent bone deformities is known as rickets
- Defective skeletal mineralization in adults is known as osteomalacia
- Osteomalacia is caused by any condition that results in inadequate calcium or phosphate mineralization of bone
- Most common cause is deficiency of vitamin D, whose main function is to increase intestinal absorption of calcium
- Ergocalciferol (vitamin D_2) is derived from plants and used in most pharmaceutical vitamin D preparations
- Cholecalciferol (vitamin D_3) is synthesized in skin, under the influence of ultraviolet radiation
- Two sequential hydroxylations are necessary for full biological activity: first occurs in liver—to $25(OH)D_3$; second in kidney—to $1,25(OH)_2D_3$
- Some degree of vitamin D deficiency was found in 24% of postmenopausal women from 25 countries included in MORE study. Particularly common in institutionalized elderly or home-bound. May arise from insufficient sun exposure, malnutrition, malabsorption, severe nephrotic syndrome. Cholestyramine, orlistat, and anticonvulsants decrease vitamin D levels
- Dietary calcium deficiency, eg, in malnourished, elderly patients can also cause rickets and osteomalacia. Milk, especially skim milk, is a poor source of vitamin D. Breast-fed infants can develop rickets if they receive no sun exposure or vitamin D supplement
- Phosphate deficiency, eg, due to nutritional deficiency, malabsorption, phosphate-binding antacids, genetic disorders (vitamin D–resistant rickets), soft tissue tumors, renal tubular acidosis, Fanconi's syndrome, can cause osteomalacia
- Aluminum toxicity due to chronic hemodialysis with tap water dialysate or from aluminum-containing phosphate binders can cause osteomalacia
- Other causes include disorders of bone matrix, eg, hypophosphatasia (deficient alkaline phosphatase) and fibrogenesis imperfecta

 CLINICAL FINDINGS

SYMPTOMS AND SIGNS

- Initially asymptomatic in adults
- Eventually, bone pain occurs, simulating fibromyalgia
- Muscle weakness due to calcium deficiency
- Fractures with little or no trauma
- Infants and children may exhibit restlessness, interrupted sleep, bowing of legs, kyphoscoliosis, hypertrophy of epiphygeal cartilage (eg, costochondral beading)

DIFFERENTIAL DIAGNOSIS

- Osteoporosis
- Hypophosphatemia due to hyperparathyroidism
- Renal osteodystrophy
- Multiple myeloma, metastatic cancer
- Chronic hyperthyroidism

DIAGNOSIS

LABORATORY TESTS

- Alkaline phosphatase (age-adjusted) may be elevated
- $25(OH)D_3$ typically low <20 ng/mL
- Calcium or phosphate (age-adjusted) may be low
- Phosphate low in 47%
- Parathyroid hormone may be increased due to secondary hyperparathyroidism
- Urinary calcium may be low
- $1,25(OH)_2D_3$ may be low even when $25(OH)D_2$ levels are normal

IMAGING STUDIES

- Bone densitometry helps document the degree of osteopenia
- X-rays may show diagnostic features: cortical bone thinning, looser lines, stress or pathological fractures
- Whole-body MRI may be required to search for occult tumors in sporadic adult-onset hypophosphatemia, hyperphosphaturia, and low serum $1,25(OH)_2D$ levels

DIAGNOSTIC PROCEDURES

- Bone biopsy not usually necessary but is diagnostic of osteomalacia if it shows significant unmineralized osteoid

TREATMENT

MEDICATIONS

- Vitamin D deficiency treated with ergo-calciferol (D_2), 50,000 IU PO once weekly for 6–12 months, followed by at least 1000 IU PO QD. May also be given 50,000 IU PO Q 2 months
- In intestinal malabsorption, 25,000–100,000 IU of vitamin D_2 may be required daily. Some with steatorrhea respond better to 25(OH)D (calcifediol), 50–100 μg PO QD
- Oral calcium supplements with meals: calcium citrate (eg, Citracal) to provide 0.4–0.6 g elemental calcium per day; or calcium carbonate (eg, OsCal, Tums), 1–1.5 g elemental calcium per day
- Correct nutritional deficiencies in hypophosphatemic osteomalacia, discontinue aluminum-containing antacids, and give bicarbonate therapy to patients with renal tubular acidosis
- Oral phosphate supplements given chronically for X-linked or idiopathic hypophosphatemia and hyperphosphaturia, along with calcitriol, 0.25–0.5 μg PO QD, to improve impaired calcium absorption caused by oral phosphate. Consider addition of human recombinant growth hormone to reduce phosphaturia

THERAPEUTIC PROCEDURES

- Sun exposure, without SPF, stimulates vitamin D_3 production in skin, except in dark-skinned Africans

 OUTCOME

COMPLICATIONS

- Fractures

PREVENTION

- Prevention of vitamin D deficiency by adequate sunlight exposure and vitamin D supplements
- U.S. recommended daily allowance (RDA) of vitamin D is at least 10 μg (400 IU) daily. In sunlight-deprived individuals (eg, veiled women, confined patients, or residents of higher latitudes during winter), RDA should be 25 μg (1000 IU) daily
- Patients on chronic phenytoin may be treated prophylactically with vitamin D, 50,000 IU PO Q 2–4 weeks

 EVIDENCE

PRACTICE GUIDELINES

- Campbell GA: Osteomalacia: diagnosis and management. Br J Hosp Med 1990;44:332. [PMID: 2275997]
- Mawer EB et al: Vitamin D nutrition and bone disease in adults. Rev Endocr Metab Disord 2001;2:153. [PMID: 11705321] http://content.kluweronline.com/article/320630/fulltext.pdf

WEB SITES

- Oley Foundation http://www.c4isr.com/oley/lifeline/99-003.html
- The Magic Foundation http://www.magicfoundation.org/brochure/hypophosphatasia.htm

INFORMATION FOR PATIENTS

- MEDLINEplus—Osteomalacia http://www.nlm.nih.gov/medlineplus/ency/article/000376.htm
- MEDLINEplus—Rickets http://www.nlm.nih.gov/medlineplus/ency/article/000344.htm
- Tayside University Hospitals—Osteomalacia and rickets http://www.dundee.ac.uk/medicine/tayendoweb/images/osteomalacia_and_rickets.htm

REFERENCES

- Basha B et al: Osteomalacia due to vitamin D depletion: a neglected consequence of intestinal malabsorption. Am J Med 2000;108:296. [PMID: 11014722]
- De Beur SM et al: Tumors associated with oncogenic osteomalacia express genes important in bone and mineral metabolism. Bone Miner Res 2002; 17:1102. [PMID: 12054166]
- Freitag A et al: Differential diagnosis of osteoporosis. Gerontology 2002;48:98. [PMID: 11867932]
- Greenspan SL et al: The effect of thyroid hormone on skeletal integrity. Ann Intern Med 1999;130:750. [PMID: 10357695]

Paul A. Fitzgerald, MD

Osteomyelitis, Acute Pyogenic

 KEY FEATURES

ESSENTIALS OF DIAGNOSIS

- Fever and chills associated with pain and tenderness of involved bone
- Culture of blood or bone is essential for precise diagnosis
- Radiographs early in the course are typically negative

GENERAL CONSIDERATION

- Occurs as a consequence of hematogenous dissemination of bacteria, invasion from a contiguous focus of infection, or skin breakdown in the setting of vascular insufficiency
- In sickle cell anemia, *Salmonella* is the most common pathogen
- In intravenous drug users, *Staphylococcus aureus* is most common, also gram-negative infections (eg, *Pseudomonas aeruginosa* and *Serratia*)
- Contiguous focus infections are usually due to *S aureus* and *S epidermidis*

 CLINICAL FINDINGS

SYMPTOMS AND SIGNS

Hematogenous osteomyelitis

- Associated with sickle cell disease, intravenous drug users, or the elderly
- High fever, chills, and pain and tenderness of the involved bone

Osteomyelitis from a contiguous focus of infection

- Prosthetic joint replacement, decubitus ulcer, neurosurgery, and trauma are common sources of infection
- Localized signs of inflammation are usually evident, but high fever and other signs of toxicity are usually absent

Osteomyelitis associated with vascular insufficiency

- Infection originates from an ulcer or other break in the skin may appear disarmingly unimpressive
- Bone pain is often absent or muted by the associated neuropathy
- Fever is also commonly absent

DIFFERENTIAL DIAGNOSIS

- Acute hematogenous osteomyelitis should be distinguished from suppurative arthritis, rheumatic fever, and cellulitis
- More subacute forms must be differentiated from tuberculosis or mycotic infections of bone or tumors
- When osteomyelitis involves the vertebrae, it commonly traverses the disk—a finding not observed in tumor
- Cellulitis
- Septic arthritis
- Gout
- Diabetic or arterial insufficiency ulcer
- Tuberculous or mycotic bone infection
- Rheumatic fever
- Metastatic cancer
- Multiple myeloma
- Ewing's sarcoma
- Avascular necrosis

 DIAGNOSIS

LABORATORY TESTS

- Blood cultures
- Cultures from overlying ulcers, wounds, or fistulas are unreliable
- Anemia of chronic disease and a markedly elevated erythrocyte sedimentation rate (ESR) are characteristic

IMAGING STUDIES

- Early radiographic findings may include soft tissue swelling, loss of tissue planes, and periarticular demineralization of bone
- About 2 weeks after onset of symptoms, erosion and alterations of bone appear, followed by periostitis
- MRI, CT, and nuclear medicine bone scanning are more sensitive than conventional radiography

DIAGNOSTIC PROCEDURES

- One of the best bedside clues to osteomyelitis is the ability to easily advance a sterile probe through a skin ulcer to bone
- Bone biopsy for culture is essential except in those with hematogenous osteomyelitis with positive blood cultures

TREATMENT

MEDICATIONS

- Most patients require both debridement of necrotic bone and prolonged administration of antibiotics
- Traditionally, antibiotics have been administered parenterally for at least 4–6 weeks
- Oral therapy with quinolones (eg, ciprofloxacin, 750 mg twice daily) for 6–8 weeks is as effective as standard parenteral antibiotic therapy for chronic osteomyelitis with susceptible organisms
- When treating *S aureus*, quinolones are usually combined with rifampin, 300 mg twice daily

SURGERY

- Debridement of necrotic bone is usually necessary
- Revascularization of the extremity is required when osteomyelitis of a foot is accompanied by decreased perfusion due to large artery disease

 OUTCOME

FOLLOW-UP

- ESR should fall by 50% after 1 month of antibiotic therapy

COMPLICATIONS

- Inadequate treatment of bone infections results in chronic infection
- Squamous cell transformation within the chronic fistula tract

PROGNOSIS

- A good result can be expected in most cases if there is no compromise of the patient's immune system
- Progression of the disease to a chronic form may occur, especially in the lower extremities and in patients in whom circulation is impaired (eg, diabetics)

WHEN TO REFER

- Urgent consultation with a neurosurgeon or orthopedist is required for vertebral osteomyelitis associated with neurological findings

WHEN TO ADMIT

- Admit to establish the diagnosis and begin intravenous antibiotic therapy

 EVIDENCE

PRACTICE GUIDELINES

- National Guideline Clearinghouse http://www.ngc.gov/summary/summary. aspx?doc_id=2892&nbr=2118&string= osteomyelitis

INFORMATION FOR PATIENTS

- National Institutes of Health http://www.nlm.nih.gov/medlineplus/ ency/article/000437.htm
- Mayo Clinic http://www.mayoclinic.com/invoke.cfm? id=HQ00342

REFERENCES

- Carek PJ et al: Diagnosis and management of osteomyelitis. Am Fam Physician 2001;63:2413. [PMID: 11430456]
- Kothari NA et al: Imaging of musculoskeletal infections. Radiol Clin North Am 2001;39:653. [PMID: 11549164]

David B. Hellmann, MD, FACP
John H. Stone, MD, MPH

Osteoporosis

KEY FEATURES

ESSENTIALS OF DIAGNOSIS

- Symptoms range from none to severe back pain from vertebral fractures
- Spontaneous fractures often discovered incidentally on radiography; loss of height
- Low bone density usually indicates osteoporosis, but may also mean that osteomalacia is present
- Osteoporosis: bone densitometry—T score (standard deviations below young normal mean) ≤ –2.5
- Osteopenia (at risk for osteoporosis): bone densitometry T score –1.5 to –2.4
- Serum parathyroid hormone (PTH), 25-hydroxyvitamin D [$25(OH)D_3$], calcium, phosphorus, and alkaline phosphatase usually normal

GENERAL CONSIDERATIONS

- Estimated to cause 1.5 million fractures annually in the United States, mainly of the vertebrae
- Morbidity and indirect mortality rates very high
- Rate of bone formation is often normal, but bone resorption rate is increased
- Reduction in bone matrix (osteoid); remaining osteoid is mineralized, unless osteomalacia is also present
- Osteogenesis imperfecta, due to major mutation in type I collagen, results in severe osteoporosis. Spontaneous fractures occur in utero or during childhood
- Causes include estrogen (women) or androgen (men) deficiency; Cushing's syndrome (eg, glucocorticoid administration); hyperthyroidism; hyperparathyroidism; drugs (eg, alcohol, tobacco, excessive vitamin D or A, heparin); immobilization; genetic disorders (eg, aromatase deficiency, type I collagen mutations); malignancy, especially multiple myeloma; and liver disease

DEMOGRAPHICS

- Clinically evident in middle life and beyond
- Women more frequently affected than men

CLINICAL FINDINGS

SYMPTOMS AND SIGNS

- Usually asymptomatic until fractures occur
- May present as back pain of varying degrees of severity or as spontaneous fracture or collapse of a vertebra
- Loss of height is common
- Fractures of femoral neck and distal radius also common
- Once osteoporosis is identified, careful history and physical examination are required to determine its cause

DIFFERENTIAL DIAGNOSIS

- Osteomalacia or rickets
- Inadequate mineralization of existing bone matrix (osteoid)
- Osteomalacia results from inadequate calcium (usually due to vitamin D deficiency) or inadequate phosphate
- Multiple myeloma
- Metastatic cancer
- Paget's disease of bone
- Renal osteodystrophy

DIAGNOSIS

LABORATORY TESTS

- Serum calcium, phosphate, and PTH normal
- Alkaline phosphatase usually normal but may be slightly elevated, especially following fracture
- Once osteoporosis is identified, obtain serum thyroid-stimulating hormone, luteinizing hormone/follicle-stimulating hormone, testosterone (men), and $25(OH)D_3$ level

IMAGING STUDIES

- X-rays of spine and pelvis, especially femoral neck and head, the principal areas of demineralization; in skull and extremities, demineralization is less marked
- X-rays of spine commonly also show compression of vertebrae
- Bone densitometry permits screening for osteopenia in high-risk individuals and allows assessment of response to therapy
- Osteoporosis: bone densitometry—T score ≤ –2.5; osteopenia: T score –1.5 to –2.4, osteopenia
- Dual-energy x-ray absorptiometry (DEXA) can determine density of any bone, is quite accurate, and delivers negligible radiation
- CT bone densitometry is highly accurate and reproducible; however, it is more costly than DEXA and is reserved for assessing spinal bone density in patients with severe osteoporosis
- Bone densitometry screening recommended for all white and Asian women ≥55 years; all patients taking chronic prednisone; all patients with neurological disorder (eg, paraplegia); prior pathological fractures; family history of osteoporosis; alcoholism, anorexia, or malnutrition

TREATMENT

MEDICATIONS

- Supplemental calcium and vitamin D is given to prevent or treat any concurrent osteomalacia. Give calcium citrate (0.4–0.7 g elemental calcium PO QD) or calcium carbonate (1–1.5 g elemental calcium PO QD). Calcium citrate causes less gastrointestinal intolerance. Give vitamin D$_2$ 400–1000 IU PO QD
- Bisphosphonates for osteoporosis in patients taking high-dose glucocorticoids. Taken in AM with ≥8 oz water, 30–60 min before any other food or liquid. Must remain upright after taking to reduce risk of pill-induced esophagitis
- Alendronate, 10 mg PO QAM or 70 mg PO Q week; 5 mg PO QAM or 35 mg PO Q week for prevention of osteoporosis
- Risedronate, 5 mg PO QAM; or 35 mg PO Q week for treatment or prevention of osteoporosis
- All patients on bisphosphonates should receive oral calcium with evening meal and vitamin D
- Pamidronate, zoledronate IV, or nasal calcitonin-salmon (Miacalcin) if unable to tolerate bisphosphonates
- Consider estrogen or raloxifene (selective estrogen receptor modulator or SERM) for women with hypogonadism (see *Menopausal syndrome*); osteoporosis can be prevented by low-dose estrogen
- Consider teriparatide (Forteo, PTH analog) 20 µg SC QD for ≤2 years for severe osteoporosis

THERAPEUTIC PROCEDURES

- Diet adequate in protein, total calories, calcium, and vitamin D
- Discontinue or reduce doses of glucocorticoids, if possible
- High-impact physical activity (eg, jogging), stair-climbing, and weight training increase bone density
- Fall-avoidance measures
- Balance exercises can reduce fall risk
- Avoid alcohol and smoking
- Vertebroplasty, kyphoplasty are investigational procedures for pain relief following vertebral compression fractures

OUTCOME

FOLLOW-UP

- DEXA bone densitometry every 2–3 years
- Monitor patients on glucocorticoids or thiazides for development of hypercalcemia when given calcium supplements
- Reduce bisphosphonate dosage in renal insufficiency, and monitor serum phosphate

COMPLICATIONS

- Fractures common, especially femur, vertebrae, and distal radius
- Calcium supplementation for patients receiving thiazide diuretics and glucocorticoids can cause hypercalcemia; calcium taken by patients in renal failure can cause calciphylaxis
- Nasal calcitonin-salmon can cause bronchospasm and allergic reactions, rhinitis, epistaxis, back pain, and arthralgias
- Raloxifene increases the risk for thromboembolism, aggravates hot flashes, and has been associated with nausea, weight gain, depression, insomnia, leg cramps, and rash
- Estrogen replacement increases the risk for thromboembolism and myocardial infarction, breast cancer, and endometrial cancer. It has been associated with cholestatic jaundice, worsening hypertriglyceridemia, and pancreatitis. Enlargement of uterine fibroids, migraines, edema, weight changes, rash, and gastrointestinal intolerance have been reported
- Bisphosphonates (oral) can cause esophagitis, gastritis, and abdominal pain. All bisphosphonates (oral and IV) can cause myalgias and back pain
- Teriparitide may cause orthostatic hypotension, asthenia, nausea, and leg cramps; it must not be given to patients with Paget's disease

PROGNOSIS

- Bisphosphonates, calcitonin, and teriparitide can reverse osteoporosis and decrease fracture risk
- Prognosis good for preventing postmenopausal osteoporosis if estrogen therapy, raloxifene, or bisphosphonates started early and maintained for years
- Bone pain reduction may be noted within 2–4 weeks on nasal calcitonin

PREVENTION

- Diet adequate in protein, calories, calcium, and vitamin D
- Calcium and vitamin D supplements and exercise for those at risk
- Consider hormone replacement therapy for hypogonadal men and women
- Consider bisphosphonate if patient on corticosteroids >2 weeks and for prevention of osteoporosis
- Raloxifene, 60 mg PO QD, can be used by postmenopausal women in place of estrogen for osteoporosis prevention
- Give calcium supplements with meals to reduce risk of calcium oxalate nephrolithiasis

EVIDENCE

INFORMATION FOR PATIENTS

- JAMA patient page: Osteoporosis. JAMA 1999;282:1396. [PMID: 10527188]

REFERENCES

- Altkorn D et al: Treatment of postmenopausal osteoporosis. JAMA 2001;285:1415. [PMID: 11255400]
- Cauley JA et al: Effects of hormone replacement therapy on clinical fractures and height loss: The Heart and Estrogen/Progestin Replacement Study (HERS). Am J Med 2001;110:442. [PMID: 11331055]

Paul A. Fitzgerald, MD

Otitis Media, Acute

 KEY FEATURES

ESSENTIALS OF DIAGNOSIS

- Otalgia, often with an upper respiratory tract infection
- Erythema and hypomobility of tympanic membrane

GENERAL CONSIDERATIONS

- Bacterial infection of the mucosally lined air-containing spaces of the temporal bone
- Purulent material forms not only within the middle ear cleft but also within the mastoid air cells and petrous apex when they are pneumatized
- Usually precipitated by a viral upper respiratory tract infection that causes auditory tube edema, resulting in accumulation of fluid and mucus, which become secondarily infected by bacteria
- Nasotracheal intubation can cause otitis media
- The most common pathogens are *Streptococcus pneumoniae, Haemophilus influenzae,* and *Streptococcus pyogenes*
- Chronic otitis media is usually not painful except during acute exacerbations

DEMOGRAPHICS

- Most common in infants and children, though it may occur at any age
- External otitis and acute otitis media are the most common causes of earache

 CLINICAL FINDINGS

SYMPTOMS AND SIGNS

- Otalgia, aural pressure, decreased hearing, and often fever
- Typically, erythema and decreased mobility of the tympanic membrane
- Occasionally, bullae will be seen on the tympanic membrane, but these rarely indicate *Mycoplasma* infection
- When middle ear empyema is severe, the tympanic membrane can be seen to bulge outward
- In external otitis, the ear canal skin is erythematous, while in acute otitis media this generally occurs only if the tympanic membrane has ruptured, spilling purulent material into the ear canal
- Otorrhea, which persists despite topical and systemic antibiotic therapy

DIFFERENTIAL DIAGNOSIS

- Otitis externa
- Auditory (eustachian) tube dysfunction
- Mastoiditis
- Tympanosclerosis (scarred tympanic membrane)
- Referred pain: pharyngitis, sinusitis, tooth pain
- Glossopharyngeal neuralgia
- Temporomandibular joint syndrome
- Foreign body
- Cholesteatoma
- Bullous myringitis
- Herpes zoster oticus, especially when vesicles appear in the ear canal or concha

 DIAGNOSIS

LABORATORY TESTS

- Tympanocentesis and culture of middle ear fluid (see below)

DIAGNOSTIC PROCEDURE

- Clinical diagnosis

TREATMENT

MEDICATIONS

- Either amoxicillin (20–40 mg/kg/day) or erythromycin (50 mg/kg/day) plus sulfonamide (150 mg/kg/day) for 10 days
- Alternatives useful in resistant cases are cefaclor (20–40 mg/kg/day) or amoxicillin-clavulanate (20–40 mg/kg/day) combinations
- Nasal decongestants, if symptomatic
- Recurrent acute otitis media may be managed with long-term antibiotic prophylaxis: single daily doses of sulfamethoxazole (500 mg) or amoxicillin (250 or 500 mg) are given over a period of 1–3 months
- Failure of the regimen for recurrent acute otitis media is an indication for insertion of ventilating tubes

SURGERY

- Surgical drainage of the middle ear (myringotomy) is reserved for patients with severe otalgia or when complications of otitis (eg, mastoiditis, meningitis) have occurred

THERAPEUTIC PROCEDURES

- Tympanocentesis is useful for otitis media in immunocompromised patients and when infection persists or recurs despite multiple courses of antibiotics

 OUTCOME

COMPLICATIONS

- Tympanic membrane rupture
- Chronic otitis media
  - Medical treatment includes regular removal of infected debris, use of earplugs to protect against water exposure, and topical antibiotic drops for exacerbations
  - Ciprofloxacin may help to dry a chronically discharging ear when given in a dosage of 500 mg orally twice a day for 1–6 weeks
  - Definitive management is surgical in most cases
- Mastoiditis
- Meningitis
  - The most common intracranial complication of ear infection
  - In acute otitis media, it arises from hematogenous spread of bacteria, most commonly *H influenzae* and *S pneumoniae*
  - In chronic otitis media, it results either from passage of infections along preformed pathways or from direct extension
- Epidural or brain abscess (temporal lobe or cerebellum)
- Facial palsy
- Sigmoid sinus thrombosis

WHEN TO REFER

- Persistent earache demands specialty referral to exclude cancer of the upper aerodigestive tract

 EVIDENCE

PRACTICE GUIDELINES

- National Guideline Clearinghouse http://www.guideline.gov/summary/summary.aspx?doc_id=1972&nbr=1198&string=otitis+media http://www.guideline.gov/summary/summary.aspx?doc_id=3371&nbr=2597&string=otitis+media

WEB SITES

- Ear, Nose, and Throat Information Center http://www.netdoor.com/entinfo/
- Otolaryngology Resources on the Internet http://www.bcm.tmc.edu/oto/othersa.html

INFORMATION FOR PATIENTS

- JAMA patient page: Acute otitis media. JAMA 2003;290:1666. [PMID: 14506125]
- Nemours Foundation http://kidshealth.org/parent/infections/bacterial_viral/otitis_media.html
- National Institutes of Health http://www.nlm.nih.gov/medlineplus/ency/article/000638.htm

REFERENCES

- Aronovitz GH: Antimicrobial therapy of acute otitis media: review of treatment recommendations. Clin Ther 2000; 22:29. [PMID: 10688388]
- Pelton SI et al: The promise of immunoprophylaxis for prevention of acute otitis media. Pediatr Infect Dis J 1999;18:926. [PMID: 10530543]
- Pichichero ME: Acute otitis media: Part I. Improving diagnostic accuracy. Am Fam Phys 2000;61:2051. [PMID: 10779248]

Robert K. Jackler, MD
Michael J. Kaplan, MD

Otitis Media, Serous

 ## KEY FEATURES

ESSENTIALS OF DIAGNOSIS

- Blocked auditory tube remains for a prolonged period
- Resultant negative pressure will cause transudation of fluid

GENERAL CONSIDERATIONS

- Especially common in children because their auditory tubes are narrower and more horizontal in orientation than adults
- It is less common in adults, in whom it usually follows an upper respiratory tract infection or barotrauma
- In an adult with persistent unilateral serous otitis media, nasopharyngeal carcinoma must be excluded

 ## CLINICAL FINDINGS

SYMPTOMS AND SIGNS

- The tympanic membrane is dull and hypomobile
- Occasionally accompanied by air bubbles in the middle ear and conductive hearing loss

 ## DIAGNOSIS

LABORATORY TESTS

- Clinical diagnosis

Otitis Media, Serous

TREATMENT

MEDICATIONS

- A short course of oral corticosteroids (eg, prednisone, 40 mg/day for 7 days)
- Oral antibiotics (eg, amoxicillin, 250 mg orally three times daily for 7 days)
- A combination of oral corticosteroids and antibiotics
- The role of these regimens remains controversial, but they are probably of little lasting benefit

SURGERY

- When medication fails to bring relief after several months, a ventilating tube placed through the tympanic membrane may restore hearing and alleviate the sense of aural fullness

THERAPEUTIC PROCEDURES

- Similar to that for auditory tube dysfunction

OUTCOME

WHEN TO REFER

- For persistent or recurrent symptoms

PREVENTION

Plane travel

- The patient should be advised to swallow, yawn, and autoinflate frequently during descent, which may be painful if the auditory tube collapses
- Systemic decongestants (eg, pseudoephedrine, 60–120 mg) should be taken several hours before anticipated arrival time so that they will be maximally effective during descent
- Topical decongestants such as 1% phenylephrine nasal spray should be administered 1 h before arrival
- Repeated episodes of barotrauma in persons who must fly frequently may be alleviated by insertion of ventilating tubes

Scuba diving

- Problem occurs most commonly during the descent phase, when pain develops within the first 15 feet if inflation of the middle ear via the auditory tube has not occurred
- Divers must descend slowly and equilibrate in stages to avoid the development of severely negative pressures in the tympanum that may result in hemorrhage (hemotympanum) or perilymphatic fistulization, in which the oval or round window ruptures, resulting in sensory hearing loss and acute vertigo
- Emesis due to acute labyrinthine dysfunction can be very dangerous during an underwater dive
- Tympanic membrane perforation is an absolute contraindication to diving, as the patient will experience an unbalanced thermal stimulus to the semicircular canals and may experience vertigo, disorientation, and even emesis
- Individuals with only one hearing ear should be discouraged from diving because of the significant risk of otologic injury

EVIDENCE

PRACTICE GUIDELINES

- National Guideline Clearinghouse http://www.guideline.gov/summary/summary.aspx?doc_id=1972&nbr=1198&string=otitis+media
  http://www.guideline.gov/summary/summary.aspx?doc_id=3371&nbr=2597&string=otitis+media

WEB SITES

- Ear, Nose, and Throat Information Center http://www.netdoor.com/entinfo/
- Otolaryngology Resources on the Internet http://www.bcm.tmc.edu/oto/othersa.html

INFORMATION FOR PATIENTS

- National Institutes of Health http://www.nlm.nih.gov/medlineplus/ency/article/007010.htm
- National Institute on Deafness and other communication disorders http://www.nidcd.nih.gov/health/hearing/otitism.asp

REFERENCES

- Becker GD et al: Barotrauma of the ears and sinuses after scuba diving. Eur Arch Otorhinolaryngol 2001;258:159. [PMID: 11407445]
- Morris MS: Tympanostomy tubes: types, indications, techniques, and complications. Otolaryngol Clin North Am 1999;32:385. [PMID: 10393774]
- Newbegin C et al: Ear barotrauma after flying and diving. Practitioner 2000; 244:96. [PMID: 10892042]
- Slack R et al: Current management of glue ear. Practitioner 1998;242:455. [PMID: 10492959]

Robert K. Jackler, MD
Michael J. Kaplan, MD

Otitis External

 KEY FEATURES

ESSENTIALS OF DIAGNOSIS

- Erythema and edema of the ear canal skin
- Often with a purulent exudate
- Persistent external otitis in the diabetic or immunocompromised patient may evolve into osteomyelitis of the skull base, often called malignant external otitis

GENERAL CONSIDERATIONS

External otitis

- There is often a history of recent water exposure ("swimmer's ear") or mechanical trauma (eg, scratching, cotton applicators)
- Otitis externa is usually caused by gram-negative rods (eg, *Pseudomonas, Proteus*) or fungi (eg, *Aspergillus*), which grow in the presence of excessive moisture

Malignant external otitis

- Usually caused by *Pseudomonas aeruginosa*
- Osteomyelitis begins in the floor of the ear canal and may extend into the middle fossa floor, the clivus, and even the contralateral skull base

 CLINICAL FINDINGS

SYMPTOMS AND SIGNS

External otitis

- Presents with otalgia, frequently accompanied by pruritus and purulent discharge
- Examination reveals erythema and edema of the ear canal skin, often with a purulent exudate
- Manipulation of the auricle often elicits pain
- Because the lateral surface of the tympanic membrane is ear canal skin, it is often erythematous
- In contrast to acute otitis media, the tympanic membrane in otitis externa moves normally with pneumatic otoscopy
- When the canal skin is very edematous, it may be impossible to visualize the tympanic membrane

Malignant external otitis

- Presents with persistent, refractory otalgia
- Granulation tissue in ear canal
- Cranial neuropathies (especially VII, IX, X)

DIFFERENTIAL DIAGNOSIS

- Otitis media
- Skin cancer
- Traumatic auricular hematoma
- Cellulitis
- Chondritis or perichondritis
- Relapsing polychondritis
- Chondrodermatitis nodularis helicis

 DIAGNOSIS

LABORATORY TESTS

- Persistent discharge unresponsive to treatment should be cultured

IMAGING STUDIES

- Diagnosis of malignant otitis externa is confirmed by the demonstration of osseous erosion on CT and radioisotope scanning

TREATMENT

MEDICATIONS

External otitis

- Otic drops containing a mixture of aminoglycoside antibiotic and antiinflammatory corticosteroid in an acid vehicle are generally very effective (eg, neomycin sulfate, polymyxin B sulfate, and hydrocortisone)
- Drops should be used abundantly (five or more drops three or four times a day) to penetrate the depths of the canal
- In recalcitrant cases—particularly when cellulitis of the periauricular tissue has developed—oral fluoroquinolones (eg, ciprofloxacin, 500 mg twice daily for 1 week) are the drugs of choice because of their effectiveness against *Pseudomonas* species

Malignant external otitis

- Prolonged antipseudomonal antibiotic administration, often for several months

SURGERY

- Surgical debridement of infected bone is reserved for cases of malignant external otitis that have worsened despite medical therapy or when material is needed for culture

THERAPEUTIC PROCEDURES

- Fundamental to the treatment of external otitis is protection of the ear from additional moisture and avoidance of further mechanical injury by scratching
- Purulent debris filling the ear canal should be gently removed to permit entry of the topical medication
- When substantial edema of the canal wall prevents entry of drops into the ear canal, a wick is placed to facilitate entry of the medication

 OUTCOME

FOLLOW-UP

Malignant external otitis

- To avoid relapse, antibiotic therapy should be continued, even in the asymptomatic patient, until gallium scanning indicates a marked reduction in the inflammatory process

WHEN TO REFER

- Any cases of suspected malignant external otitis should be referred to an otolaryngologist

 EVIDENCE

WEB SITES

- Ear, Nose, and Throat Information Center http://www.netdoor.com/entinfo/
- Otolaryngology Resources on the Internet http://www.bcm.tmc.edu/oto/othersa.html

INFORMATION FOR PATIENTS

- American Academy of Otolaryngology-Head and Neck Surgery. Swimmer's ear http://www.entnet.org/healthinfo/ears/swimmers.cfm
- Centers for Disease Control http://www.cdc.gov/healthyswimming/swimmers_ear.htm

REFERENCES

- Holten KB et al: Management of the patient with otitis externa. J Fam Pract 2001;50:353. [PMID: 11300988]
- Roland PS: Chronic external otitis. Ear Nose Throat J 2001;80(6 Suppl):12. [PMID: 11488077]

Robert K. Jackler, MD
Michael J. Kaplan, MD

Ovarian Tumors

 KEY FEATURES

ESSENTIALS OF DIAGNOSIS

- Vague gastrointestinal discomfort
- Pelvic pressure and pain
- Many cases of early-stage cancer are asymptomatic
- Pelvic examination, CA 125, and ultrasound are mainstays of diagnosis

GENERAL CONSIDERATIONS

- Ovarian tumors are common. Most are benign, but malignant ovarian tumors are the leading cause of death from reproductive tract cancer
- The wide range of types and patterns of ovarian tumors is due to the complexity of ovarian embryology and differences in tissues of origin (Table 64, page 1258)

DEMOGRAPHICS

- In women with no family history of ovarian cancer, the lifetime risk is 1.6%, whereas a woman with one affected first-degree relative has a 5% lifetime risk. With two or more affected first-degree relatives, the risk is 7%
- Approximately 3% of women with two or more affected first-degree relatives will have a hereditary ovarian cancer syndrome with a lifetime risk of 40%
- Women with a *BRCA1* gene mutation have a 45% lifetime risk of ovarian cancer and those with a *BRAC2* mutation have a 25% risk

 CLINICAL FINDINGS

SYMPTOMS AND SIGNS

- Both benign and malignant ovarian neoplasms are either asymptomatic or experience only mild nonspecific gastrointestinal symptoms or pelvic pressure
- Early disease is typically detected on routine pelvic examination
- In advanced malignant disease, women may experience abdominal pain and bloating, and a palpable abdominal mass with ascites is often present

DIFFERENTIAL DIAGNOSIS

- Benign ovarian tumor, eg, follicle cyst, corpus luteum cyst
- Malignant ovarian tumor
- Teratoma (usually benign)
- Tuboovarian abscess
- Endometriosis
- Colon cancer
- Ectopic pregnancy
- Metastases to ovary, eg, gastrointestinal, breast

 DIAGNOSIS

LABORATORY TESTS

- An elevated serum CA 125 (>35 units) indicates a greater likelihood that an ovarian tumor is malignant
- CA 125 is elevated in 80% of women with epithelial ovarian cancer overall but in only 50% of women with early disease
- Serum CA 125 may be elevated in premenopausal women with benign disease such as endometriosis

IMAGING STUDIES

- Transvaginal sonography (TVS) is useful for screening high-risk women but has inadequate sensitivity for screening low-risk women
- Ultrasound is helpful in differentiating ovarian masses that are benign and likely to resolve spontaneously from those with malignant potential
- Color Doppler imaging may further enhance the specificity of ultrasound diagnosis

TREATMENT

MEDICATIONS

- Except for women with low-grade ovarian cancer in an early stage, postoperative chemotherapy is indicated. Several chemotherapy regimens are effective, such as the combination of cisplatin or carboplatin with paclitaxel, with clinical response rates of up to 60–70% (Table 148, page 1331)

SURGERY

Postmenopausal woman

- Most ovarian masses in postmenopausal women require surgical evaluation
- However, a postmenopausal woman with an asymptomatic unilateral simple cyst less than 5 cm in diameter and a normal CA 125 level may be followed closely with TVS. All others require surgical evaluation
- Exploratory laparotomy has been the standard approach

Ovarian cancer

- For ovarian cancer in an early stage, the standard therapy is complete surgical staging followed by abdominal hysterectomy and bilateral salpingo-oophorectomy with omentectomy and selective lymphadenectomy
- With more advanced disease, removal of all visible tumor improves survival
- For benign neoplasms, tumor removal or unilateral oophorectomy is usually performed

THERAPEUTIC PROCEDURES

Premenopausal woman

- In a premenopausal woman, an asymptomatic, mobile, unilateral, simple cystic mass less than 8–10 cm may be observed for 4–6 weeks. Most will resolve spontaneously. If the mass is larger or unchanged on repeat pelvic examination and TVS, surgical evaluation is required
- Laparoscopy may be considered for a small ovarian mass
- If malignancy is suspected, preoperative workup should include chest x-ray, evaluation of liver and kidney function, and hematological indices

OUTCOME

PROGNOSIS

- Approximately 75% of women with ovarian cancer are diagnosed with advanced disease after regional or distant metastases have become established
- The overall 5-year survival is approximately 17% with distant metastases, 36% with local spread, and 89% with early disease

WHEN TO REFER

- If a malignant ovarian mass is suspected, surgical evaluation should be performed by a gynecological oncologist

PREVENTION

- Women with a *BRCA1* gene mutation should be screened annually with TVS and CA 125 testing, and prophylactic oophorectomy is recommended by age 35 or whenever childbearing is completed because of the high risk of disease
- The benefits of such screening for women with one or no affected first-degree relatives are unproved, and the risks associated with unnecessary surgical procedures may outweigh the benefits in low-risk women

EVIDENCE

PRACTICE GUIDELINES

- National Guideline Clearinghouse http://www.guideline.gov/summary/summary.aspx?doc_id=3279&nbr=2505&string=ovarian+cancer http://www.guideline.gov/summary/summary.aspx?doc_id=2847&nbr=2073&string=ovarian+cancer

WEB SITES

- Cystic Teratoma Demonstration Case http://www.brighamrad.harvard.edu/Cases/bwh/hcache/62/full.html
- Hemorrhagic Corpus Luteum Demonstration Case http://www.brighamrad.harvard.edu/Cases/bwh/hcache/26/full.html
- Gynecologic Cancers http://www.oncolink.com/templates/types/types.cfm?c=6

INFORMATION FOR PATIENTS

- National Cancer Institute http://www.cancer.gov/cancerinfo/wyntk/ovary
- JAMA patient page: Ovarian cancer. JAMA 2002;288:406.
- National Women's Health Information Center http://www.4woman.gov/faq/Easyread/ovarian-etr.htm

REFERENCE

- Holschneider CH et al: Ovarian cancer: epidemiology, biology, and prognostic factors. Semin Surg Oncol 2000;19:3. [PMID: 10883018]

H. Trent MacKay, MD, MPH

Paget's Disease of Bone

 ## KEY FEATURES

ESSENTIALS OF DIAGNOSIS

- Often asymptomatic
- Bone pain may be first symptom
- Kyphosis, bowed tibias, large head, deafness, and frequent fractures that vary with location of process
- Serum calcium and phosphate normal; alkaline phosphatase elevated; urinary hydroxyproline elevated
- Dense, expanded bones on x-ray

GENERAL CONSIDERATIONS

- Common condition manifested by one or more bony lesions having high bone turnover and disorganized osteoid formation
- Involved bones become vascular, weak, and deformed
- Usually discovered incidentally during radiology imaging or evaluation of serum alkaline phosphatase elevation
- Familial Paget's disease is unusual but generally more severe

DEMOGRAPHICS

- Present in 1–2% of U.S. adults, especially those of Northern European ancestry; highest prevalence in Northeast United States (1.5%) and lowest in the South (0.3%)
- Usually diagnosed in patients age >40; highest prevalence is among persons aged 65 to 75 (2.3%); a rare form occurs in young people
- More common in elderly
- Slightly more common in men, with near-equal racial distribution

 ## CLINICAL FINDINGS

SYMPTOMS AND SIGNS

- Often mild and asymptomatic; only 27% symptomatic at diagnosis
- Can involve just one bone (monostotic) or multiple bones (polyostotic), particularly skull, femur, tibia, pelvis, and humerus
- Pain is usual first symptom
- Bones become soft, leading to bowed tibias, kyphosis, and frequent fractures with slight trauma
- If skull involved, patient may report headaches, increased hat size, and deafness
- Increased vascularity over involved bones causes increased warmth
- Sarcomatous change suggested by marked increase in bone pain

DIFFERENTIAL DIAGNOSIS

- Bone tumor, eg, osteosarcoma
- Multiple myeloma
- Metastatic cancer
- Fibrous dysplasia
- Osteitis fibrosa cystica (hyperparathyroidism)
- Fibrogenesis imperfecta ossium

 ## DIAGNOSIS

LABORATORY TESTS

- Serum alkaline phosphatase markedly elevated
- Serum calcium and phosphorus typically normal
- Serum calcium may be elevated, particularly if patient is at bed rest
- Urinary hydroxyproline elevated in active disease
- Sarcomatous change suggested by sudden rise in serum alkaline phosphatase

IMAGING STUDIES

- Bone radiographs show involved bones are expanded and denser than normal
- Multiple fissure fractures in long bones
- Initial lesion may be destructive and radiolucent, especially in skull ("osteoporosis circumscripta")
- Sarcomatous change suggested by appearance of new lytic lesion
- Technetium pyrophosphate bone scans helpful in delineating activity of bone lesions even before radiological changes are apparent

DIAGNOSTIC PROCEDURES

- Bone biopsy in suspected sarcomatous change

TREATMENT

MEDICATIONS

- Bisphosphonates are treatment of choice
- Therapeutic response is evidenced by normalization of serum alkaline phosphatase. Therapy is then discontinued for ~3 months or until alkaline phosphatase rises; then another cycle commenced
- Tiludronate, 400 mg PO QD for 3 months, is effective in reducing activity of bone lesions. May be taken in evening or day, but should not be taken within 2 h of meals, aspirin, indomethacin, calcium, magnesium, or aluminum-containing antacids. Esophagitis is uncommon (avoidance of recumbency after dosing not required), however, abdominal pain and nausea are common
- Alendronate, 20–40 mg PO QAM (or 70 mg PO Q week) for 3-month cycles
- Risedronate, 30 mg PO QAM for 3-month cycles
- Patient must remain upright after taking alendronate and risedronate to reduce risk of pill-induced esophagitis. Taken in AM with ≥8 oz water, at least 30–60 min before any other food or liquid
- Etidronate disodium, 5 mg/kg PO QD for 90–180 days. In severe disease, 10 mg/kg PO QD for 90 days, with rest period before subsequent course. Much less effective than other bisphosphonates
- Pamidronate, 60–120 mg IV over 2–4 h
- Nasal calcitonin-salmon (Miacalcin), 200 IU one spray QD, alternating nostrils. Used less often than bisphosphonates

THERAPEUTIC PROCEDURES

- Asymptomatic patients require no treatment unless extensive skull involvement, where prophylactic treatment may prevent deafness and stroke

 ## OUTCOME

FOLLOW-UP

- Follow alkaline phosphatase

COMPLICATIONS

- Fractures frequently occur with minimal trauma
- If patient immobilized and has excessive calcium intake, hypercalcemia and kidney stones may develop
- Vertebral collapse may lead to spinal cord compression
- Osteosarcoma may develop in long-standing lesions (rare)
- Increased vascularity may cause high-output congestive heart failure
- Arthritis frequently develops in joints adjacent to involved bone
- Extensive skull involvement may cause cranial nerve palsies. Deafness may result from entrapment of cranial nerve VIII (and from conductive hearing loss). Tinnitus and vertigo occasionally occur
- Ischemic neurological events may result form vascular "steal" phenomenon
- In severe forms, marked deformity, intractable pain, and congestive heart failure occur
- Bisphosphonates can temporarily aggravate bone pain, particularly in femur

PROGNOSIS

- Prognosis generally good
- Majority of patients treated with bisphosphonates normalize their serum alkaline phosphatase within 6 months, most maintaining this biochemical remission for several years
- Sarcomas, which occur in 1–3%, have poor prognosis
- In general, the prognosis of Paget's disease is worse the earlier in life the disease starts
- Fractures usually heal well

PREVENTION

- Prompt bisphosphonate treatment markedly reduces occurrence of complications of severe Paget's disease

 ## EVIDENCE

PRACTICE GUIDELINES

- Drake WM et al: Consensus statement on the modern therapy of Paget's disease of bone from a Western Osteoporosis Alliance symposium. Biannual Foothills Meeting on Osteoporosis, Calgary, Alberta, Canada, September 9-10, 2000. Clin Ther 2001;23:620. [PMID: 11354395]
- Lyles KW et al: A clinical approach to diagnosis and management of Paget's disease of bone. J Bone Miner Res 2001;16:1379. [PMID: 11499860]

WEB SITES

- National Osteoporosis Foundation http://www.nof.org
- The Paget Foundation http://www.paget.org/

INFORMATION FOR PATIENTS

- MEDLINEplus—Paget's Disease http://www.nlm.nih.gov/medlineplus/ency/article/000414.htm
- The National Institutes of Health Osteoporosis and Related Bone Diseases—National Resource Center—Information for patients about paget's disease of bone http://www.osteo.org/newfile.asp?doc=p110i&doctitle=Information+for+Patients+about+Paget%27s+Disease+of+Bone&doctype=HTML+Fact+Sheet

REFERENCES

- Altman RD et al: Prevalence of pelvic Paget's disease of bone in the United States. J Bone Min Res 2000;15:461. [PMID: 10750560]
- Hadjipavlou AG et al: Paget's disease of the spine and its management. Eur Spine J 2001;10:370. [PMID: 11718191]
- Lombardi A: Treatment of Paget's disease of bone with alendronate. Bone 1999; 24:59S. [PMID: 10321931]
- Schneider D et al: Diagnosis and treatment of Paget's disease of bone. Am Fam Physician 2002;65:2069. [PMID: 12046775]

Paul A. Fitzgerald, MD

Pain Disorders, Chronic

 KEY FEATURES

ESSENTIALS OF DIAGNOSIS

- Chronic complaints of pain
- Symptoms frequently exceed signs
- Minimal relief with standard treatment
- History of having seen multiple clinicians
- Frequent use of several nonspecific medications

GENERAL CONSIDERATIONS

- Components of the syndrome consist of anatomic changes, chronic anxiety and depression, anger, and an altered lifestyle
- Importance of psychological factors increases over time
- Often involves secondary gain for the patient via financial compensation or maintaining the sick role
- Clinicians unwittingly reinforce the sick role, as the nature of medical practice is to respond to complaints of illness
- It is counterproductive for the clinician to speculate whether the patient's pain is "real"
- Acceptance of the problem must precede attempts to reduce symptoms and improve function

 CLINICAL FINDINGS

SYMPTOMS AND SIGNS

- Patients often take multiple medications, stay in bed a great deal, and experience little joy in work or play
- Typically, the anatomic problem related to the pain is irreversible
- Marked decrease in pain threshold is apparent
- Chronic anxiety and depression produce heightened irritability and overreaction to stimuli
- There is often a hypochondriacal preoccupation with the body and a need for reassurance
- History of many interventions with unsatisfactory results
- Treatment failures may provoke anger, depression, and exacerbations of the chronic pain
- Relationships are impaired, including those with clinicians
- Clinicians develop covert rejection devices, such as being unavailable or making referrals to other physicians

DIFFERENTIAL DIAGNOSIS

- Somatoform disorders
- Malingering

 DIAGNOSIS

LABORATORY TESTS

- See Figure 8 (page 1281)

TREATMENT

MEDICATIONS

- Analgesics and sedatives are used only on a fixed-dose schedule to lessen their conditioning effects
- Tricyclic antidepressants and venalafaxine in doses used for depression can be helpful (see Tables 102 and 103, pages 1286 and 1287)
- Gabapentin can be helpful for neuropathic pain

THERAPEUTIC PROCEDURES

- A single clinician should direct treatment
- The physician should adopt an attitude of hopefulness for control of pain and improved function—but not for cure

Behavioral

- Behavioral approach to identify and eliminate pain reinforcers, decrease drug use, and shift focus from the pain
- Goal is to shift from a paradigm directed at biomedical cure to one of ongoing care
- Patient should discuss pain only with the physician
- Patient should be assigned self-help tasks graded toward maximal activity
- Patient should keep a self-rating chart of accomplishments and degrees of pain
- Emphasize a positive response to activities, which shift focus away from pain
- Avoid sympathy and attention to pain, which are positive reinforcers of this behavior
- Biofeedback and hypnosis

Social

- Family and significant others should be involved in care so that a physician's efforts are not undermined

Psychological

- Family therapy can help identify and eliminate "pain games" that facilitate the sick role
- Group therapy can help obtain patient involvement in care
- Individual therapy to strengthen defenses and build self-esteem

 OUTCOME

COMPLICATIONS

- Sedative and analgesic dependency
- Substance abuse
- Unemployment
- Depression

WHEN TO REFER

- Refer to a chronic pain center if specialized consultation is needed

 EVIDENCE

PRACTICE GUIDELINES

- National Guideline Clearinghouse http://www.guideline.gov/summary/summary.aspx?doc_id=2812&nbr=2038&string=chronic+pain http://www.guideline.gov/summary/summary.aspx?doc_id=2158&nbr=1384&string=chronic+pain

WEB SITES

- American Psychiatric Association http://www.psych.org/
- Internet Mental Health http://www.mentalhealth.com/t30.html
- Psychopharmacology Tips http://www.dr-bob.org/tips/
- Psychiatry On Line http://www.priory.com/psych.htm

INFORMATION FOR PATIENTS

- JAMA patient page: Managing pain. JAMA 2000;282:1778.
- American Academy of Family Physicians http://familydoctor.org/handouts/122.html
- National Institute of Neurological Disorders and stroke http://www.ninds.nih.gov/health_and_medical/disorders/chronic_pain.htm

REFERENCES

- Eisendrath SJ: Psychiatric aspects of chronic pain. Neurology 1995;45(Suppl 9):S26. [PMID: 8538883]
- Evers AW et al: Tailored cognitive-behavioral therapy in early rheumatoid arthritis for patients at risk: a randomized controlled trial. Pain 2002;100:141. [PMID: 12435467]
- Garcia-Campayo J et al: Gabapentin for the treatment of patients with somatization disorder. J Clin Psychiatry 2001;62:474. [PMID: 11465526]

Stuart J. Eisendrath, MD
Jonathan E. Lichtmacher, MD

Pancreatic Cancer

KEY FEATURES

ESSENTIALS OF DIAGNOSIS

- Obstructive jaundice (may be painless)
- Enlarged gallbladder (may be painful)
- Upper abdominal pain with radiation to back, weight loss, and thrombophlebitis are usually late manifestations

GENERAL CONSIDERATIONS

- Carcinoma is the commonest neoplasm of the pancreas. About 75% are in the head and 25% in the body and tail of the organ
- Carcinomas involving the head of the pancreas, the ampulla of Vater, the distal common bile duct, and the duodenum are considered together, because they are usually indistinguishable clinically; of these, carcinomas of the pancreas constitute over 90%. They comprise 2% of all cancers and 5% of cancer deaths
- Neuroendocrine tumors account for 2–5% of pancreatic neoplasms
- Cystic neoplasms account for only 1% of pancreatic cancers, but they are important because they are often mistaken for pseudocysts. A cystic neoplasm should be suspected when a cystic lesion in the pancreas is found in the absence of a history of pancreatitis. Whereas serous cystadenomas are benign, mucinous cystadenomas, intraductal papillary mucinous tumors, and papillary cystic neoplasms are premalignant, though their prognoses are better than the prognosis of adenocarcinoma of the pancreas
- Point mutations in codon 12 of the K-*ras* oncogene are found in 70–100%, and inactivation of the tumor suppressor genes *P16* on chromosome 9, *P53* on chromosome 17, and *DCP4* on chromosome 18 are found in 95%, 50–70%, and 50% of pancreatic cancers, respectively
- Staging by the TNM classification: Tis, carcinoma in situ; T1: tumor limited to the pancreas , ≤2 cm in greatest dimension; T2, tumor limited to the pancreas, >2 cm in greatest dimension; T3, tumor extends beyond the pancreas but without involvement of the celiac axis or the superior mesenteric artery; T4, tumor involves the celiac axis or the superior mesenteric artery

DEMOGRAPHICS

- Risk factors include age, obesity, tobacco use, chronic pancreatitis, prior abdominal radiation, and family history
- About 7–8% of pancreatic cancer patients have a a first-degree relative with pancreatic cancer, compared with 0.6% of control subjects

CLINICAL FINDINGS

SYMPTOMS AND SIGNS

- Pain is present in over 70% and is often vague, diffuse, and located in the epigastrium or left upper quadrant when the lesion is in the tail
- Radiation of pain into the back is common and sometimes predominates. Sitting up and leaning forward may afford some relief, which usually indicates extrapancreatic spread and inoperability
- Diarrhea, perhaps from maldigestion, is an occasional early symptom
- Migratory thrombophlebitis is a rare sign
- Weight loss commonly occurs late and may be associated with depression
- Occasionally acute pancreatitis is the presentation
- Jaundice is usually due to biliary obstruction in the pancreatic head
- A palpable gallbladder is indicative of obstruction by neoplasm (Courvoisier's law), but there are frequent exceptions
- A hard, fixed, occasionally tender mass may be present
- In advanced cases, a hard periumbilical (Sister Mary Joseph's) nodule may be palpable

DIFFERENTIAL DIAGNOSIS

- Choledocholithiasis
- Pancreatic pseudocyst or cystic neoplasm
- Carcinoma of the biliary tract
- Biliary stricture
- Hepatocellular carcinoma
- Primary sclerosing cholangitis
- Primary biliary cirrhosis

DIAGNOSIS

LABORATORY TESTS

- There may be mild anemia. Glycosuria, hyperglycemia, and impaired glucose tolerance or true diabetes mellitus are found in 10–20% of case
- The serum amylase or lipase level is occasionally elevated
- Liver function tests may suggest obstructive jaundice
- Steatorrhea in the absence of jaundice is uncommon
- Occult blood in the stool is suggestive of ampulla of Vater carcinoma (the combination of biliary obstruction and bleeding may give the stools a distinctive silver appearance)
- CA 19-9, with a sensitivity of 70% and a specificity of 87%, is not sensitive enough for early detection; increased values are also found in acute and chronic pancreatitis and cholangitis

IMAGING STUDIES

- With carcinoma of the head of the pancreas, the upper gastrointestinal series may show a widened duodenal loop, mucosal abnormalities in the duodenum ranging from edema to invasion, or spasm or compression
- Ultrasound is not reliable because of interference by intestinal gas
- Dual-phase spiral CT and MRI detect a mass in over 80% of cases and can delineate the extent of the tumor and allow for percutaneous fine-needle aspiration for cytological studies
- Positron emission tomography appears to be a sensitive technique for detecting pancreatic cancer and metastases

DIAGNOSTIC PROCEDURES

- Selective mesenteric arteriography may demonstrate vessel invasion by tumor, thus inoperable, but is being replaced by dual-phase spiral CT
- Endoscopic ultrasonography is useful for diagnosing pancreatic cancer and for demonstrating venous or gastric invasion. It can guide fine-needle aspiration for tissue diagnosis and tumor markers
- Endoscopic retrograde cholangiopancreatography (ERCP) may clarify an ambiguous CT or MRI study by delineating the pancreatic duct system or confirming an ampullary or biliary neoplasm

- Magnetic resonance cholangiopancreatography (MRCP) is as sensitive as ERCP in diagnosing pancreatic cancer
- Pancreatoscopy or intraductal ultrasonography can evaluate filling defects in the pancreatic duct and assess resectability of intraductal papillary mucinous tumors
- With obstruction of the splenic vein, splenomegaly or gastric varices are present, the latter delineated by endoscopy, endoscopic ultrasonography, or angiography

 TREATMENT

MEDICATIONS
- Combined irradiation and chemotherapy may be used for palliation of unresectable cancer confined to the pancreas
- Chemotherapy with fluorouracil and gemcitabine has been disappointing in metastatic pancreatic cancer, though improved response rates have been reported with gemcitabine

SURGERY
- In about 30% of cases, abdominal exploration is necessary when cytological diagnosis cannot be made or if resection is attempted
- If a mass is localized in the head of the pancreas and there is no jaundice, laparoscopy may detect tiny peritoneal or liver metastases and thereby avoid resection in about 10% of patients
- Radical pancreaticoduodenal (Whipple) resection is indicated for lesions strictly limited to the head of the pancreas, periampullary zone, and duodenum
- Surgical resection is indicated for all mucinous cystic neoplasms, symptomatic serous cystadenomas, and cystic tumors that remain undefined after helical CT, endoscopic ultrasound, and diagnostic aspiration

THERAPEUTIC PROCEDURES
- When resection is not feasible, cholecystojejunostomy or endoscopic stenting of the bile duct is performed to relieve jaundice. A gastrojejunostomy is also done if duodenal obstruction is expected to develop later; alternatively, endoscopic placement of a self-expandable duodenal stent may be feasible
- Celiac plexus nerve block or thoracoscopic splanchnicectomy may improve pain control. Photodynamic therapy is under study

 OUTCOME

PROGNOSIS
- Carcinoma of the pancreas, especially in the body or tail, has a poor prognosis. Reported 5-year survival rates range from 2% to 5%
- Lesions of the ampulla have a better prognosis, with reported 5-year survival rates of 20–40% after resection
- In carefully selected patients, resection of cancer of the pancreatic head is feasible and results in reasonable survival
- In a person whose disease progresses with treatment, meticulous efforts at palliative care are essential

PREVENTION
- In persons with a family history of pancreatic cancer, screening with spiral CT and endoscopic ultrasonography should be considered beginning 10 years before the age at which pancreatic cancer was diagnosed in a family member

Pancreatic Cancer

 EVIDENCE

PRACTICE GUIDELINES
- National Guideline Clearinghouse
http://www.guideline.gov/summary/summary.aspx?doc_id=3063&nbr=2289&string=pancreatic+cancer
http://www.guideline.gov/summary/summary.aspx?doc_id=3603&nbr=2829&string=pancreatic+cancer
http://www.guideline.gov/summary/summary.aspx?doc_id=2173&nbr=1399&string=pancreatic+cancer

WEB SITES
- Pancreatic Mass: Case Study
http://path.upmc.edu/cases/case236.html
- Pancreatic Carcinoma Demonstration Case
http://www.brighamrad.harvard.edu/Cases/bwh/hcache/27/full.html
- Islet Cell Tumor of the Pancreas Demonstration Case
http://www.brighamrad.harvard.edu/Cases/bwh/hcache/184/full.html
- Cystic and Papillary Epithelial Neoplasm of the Pancreas Demonstration Case
http://www.brighamrad.harvard.edu/Cases/bwh/hcache/159/full.html

INFORMATION FOR PATIENTS
- National Cancer Institute
http://www.cancer.gov/cancerinfo/wyntk/pancreas
- Mayo Clinic
http://www.mayoclinic.com/invoke.cfm?id=DS00357

REFERENCES
- Farrell JJ et al: Intraductal papillary mucinous tumor of the pancreas. Gastrointest Endosc 2002;55:701.
- Hunt GC et al: Assessment of EUS for diagnosis, staging, and determining resectability of pancreatic cancer: a review. Gastrointest Endosc 2002;55:232.
- Malka D et al: Risk of pancreatic adenocarcinoma in chronic pancreatitis. Gut 2002;51:849.

Lawrence S. Friedman, MD

Pancreatitis, Acute

 KEY FEATURES

ESSENTIALS OF DIAGNOSIS

- Abrupt onset of deep epigastric pain, often with radiation to the back
- Nausea, vomiting, sweating, weakness
- Abdominal tenderness, distension, fever
- Leukocytosis, elevated serum amylase
- History of previous episodes, often related to alcohol intake

GENERAL CONSIDERATIONS

- Most often due to passed gallstone, usually <5 mm in diameter, or heavy alcohol intake
- Rarely, may be the initial manifestation of a pancreatic neoplasm
- The pathogenesis may include edema or obstruction of the ampulla of Vater, resulting in bile reflux into pancreatic ducts, or direct injury to the acinar cells. Pathological changes vary from edema to necrosis, hemorrhage, and intra- and extrapancreatic fat necrosis. All or part of the pancreas may be involved

 CLINICAL FINDINGS

SYMPTOMS AND SIGNS

- There may be a history of alcohol intake or a heavy meal immediately preceding the attack, or a history of milder similar episodes or biliary colic in the past

Pain

- Severe, steady, boring epigastric pain, generally abrupt in onset
- Usually radiates into the back but may radiate to the right or left
- Often made worse by walking and lying and better by sitting and leaning forward
- The upper abdomen is tender, most often without guarding, rigidity, or rebound
- There may be distension and absent bowel sounds from paralytic ileus
- Nausea and vomiting
- Weakness, sweating, and anxiety in severe attacks
- Fever of 38.4–39°C, tachycardia, hypotension (even true shock), pallor, and cool clammy skin are often present
- Mild jaundice is common
- Occasionally, an upper abdominal mass may be palpated

- Acute renal failure (usually prerenal) may occur early in the course

DIFFERENTIAL DIAGNOSIS

- Acute cholecystitis or cholangitis
- Penetrating duodenal ulcer
- Pancreatic pseudocyst
- Ischemic bowel
- Small bowel obstruction
- Abdominal aortic aneurysm
- Kidney stone

 DIAGNOSIS

LABORATORY TESTS

- Serum amylase and lipase increase, usually in excess of three times normal, within 24 h in 90% of cases; lipase remains elevated longer than amylase
- Leukocytosis (10,000–30,000/μL), proteinuria, granular casts, glycosuria (10–20% of cases), hyperglycemia, and elevated serum bilirubin may be present
- Blood urea nitrogen (BUN) and serum alkaline phosphatase may be elevated and coagulation tests abnormal
- A serum alanine aminotransferase level of more than 80 units/L suggests biliary pancreatitis
- Decrease in serum calcium correlates well with severity of disease. Levels lower than 7 mg/dL (when serum albumin is normal) are associated with tetany
- Early hemoconcentration, hematocrit value above 47%, predicts severe disease
- An elevated C-reactive protein concentration after 48 h suggests the development of pancreatic necrosis
- The fluid amylase content is high in ascites or left pleural effusions

IMAGING STUDIES

- Plain abdominal radiographs may show gallstones, a "sentinel loop" (a segment of air-filled left upper quadrant small intestine), the "colon cutoff sign"—a gas-filled segment of transverse colon abruptly ending at the pancreatic inflammation—or linear focal atelectasis of the lower lobe of the lungs with or without pleural effusion
- CT scan can demonstrate an enlarged pancreas and pseudocysts, and can differentiate pancreatitis from other possible intraabdominal catastrophes
- Dynamic intravenous contrast-enhanced CT is of particular value after the first 3

days of severe disease to identify necrotizing pancreatitis and assess prognosis (Table 61, page 1256); avoid intravenous contrast when the serum creatinine level is >1.5 mg/dL
- Ultrasonography is less reliable, but is the initial imaging study required if gallstones are a consideration
- Endoscopic ultrasonography is useful for occult biliary disease (eg, small stones, sludge)

DIAGNOSTIC PROCEDURES

- CT-guided needle aspiration of necrotizing pancreatitis may diagnose infection
- Endoscopic retrograde cholangiopancreatography (ERCP) is generally not indicated after a first attack unless there is associated cholangitis or jaundice. However, aspiration of bile for crystal analysis may demonstrate microlithiasis in apparently idiopathic acute pancreatitis

 TREATMENT

MEDICATIONS

- Treat pain with meperidine, up to 100–150 mg intramuscularly every 3–4 h as necessary and reduce dose for severe hepatic or renal dysfunction
- No fluid or foods should be given orally until the patient is largely free of pain and has bowel sounds. Begin with clear liquids and gradually advance to a regular low-fat diet, guided by the patient's tolerance and by absence of pain
- For **severe pancreatitis** large amounts of intravenous fluids are needed to maintain intravascular volume
- Give calcium gluconate intravenously for hypocalcemia with tetany
- Infusions of fresh frozen plasma or serum albumin may be needed for coagulopathy or hypoalbuminemia
- If shock persists after adequate volume replacement (including packed red cells), pressors may be required
- Consider total parenteral nutrition (including lipids) for ileus when there will be no nutrition for at least a week. Enteral nutrition via a jejunal tube is preferable in the absence of ileus

- Imipenem (500 mg every 8 h intravenously) or possibly cefuroxime (1.5 g intravenously three times daily, then 250 mg orally twice daily), given for sterile pancreatic necrosis, may reduce the risk of pancreatic infection
- The role of intravenous somatostatin is uncertain, but octreotide is not beneficial

SURGERY

- For mild pancreatitis with cholelithiasis, cholecystostomy or cholecystectomy may be justified
- An infected pancreatic necrosis is an absolute indication for surgery
- Operation may improve survival of necrotizing pancreatitis and clinical deterioration with multiorgan failure or lack of resolution by 4–6 weeks

THERAPEUTIC PROCEDURES

- Usually a mild disease that subsides spontaneously within several days
- The pancreatic rest program includes nothing by mouth, bed rest, and nasogastric suction for moderately severe pain, vomiting, or abdominal distension
- When severe pancreatitis results from choledocholithiasis—particularly if jaundice (serum total bilirubin >5 mg/dL) or cholangitis is present—ERCP with endoscopic sphincterotomy and stone extraction is indicated

 OUTCOME

FOLLOW-UP

- Close follow-up of white blood cell count, hematocrit, serum electrolytes, serum calcium, serum creatinine, BUN, serum aspartate aminotransferase and lactate dehydrogenase (LDH), and arterial blood gases is mandatory for severely ill patients
- Cultures of blood, urine, sputum, and pleural effusion (if present) and needle aspirations of pancreatic necrosis (with CT guidance) should be obtained
- Following recovery from acute biliary pancreatitis, laparoscopic cholecystectomy is generally performed, although endoscopic sphincterotomy alone may be done

COMPLICATIONS

- Acute tubular necrosis
- Necrotizing pancreatitis

- Acute respiratory distress syndrome (ARDS); cardiac dysfunction may be superimposed
- Pancreatic abscess may develop after 6 or more weeks. It requires prompt percutaneous or surgical drainage
- Treat pancreatic infections with imipenem, 500 mg every 8 h IV
- Pseudocysts less than 6 cm in diameter often resolve spontaneously. They are multiple in 14% of cases. They may become secondarily infected and need drainage. Drainage may also help persisting pain or pancreatitis. Erosion into a blood vessel can result in a major hemorrhage into the cyst
- Pancreatic ascites may present after recovery from acute pancreatitis with absence of frank abdominal pain. Marked elevations in the ascitic protein (>3 g/dL) and amylase (>1000 units/L) levels are typical
- Chronic pancreatitis develops in about 10% of cases. Permanent diabetes mellitus and exocrine pancreatic insufficiency occur uncommonly after a single acute episode

PROGNOSIS

Ranson's criteria

- Helps assess disease severity
- When three or more of the following are present on admission, a severe course complicated by pancreatic necrosis can be predicted with a sensitivity of 60–80%: age over 55 years; white blood cell count over 16,000/μL; blood glucose over 200 mg/dL; serum LDH over 350 units/L; AST over 250 units/L
- Development of the following in the first 48 h indicates a worsening prognosis: hematocrit drop of more than 10 percentage points; BUN rise greater than 5 mg/dL; arterial P_{O_2} of less than 60 mm Hg; serum calcium of less than 8 mg/dL; base deficit over 4 mEq/L; estimated fluid sequestration of more than 6 L
- Mortality rates correlate with the number of criteria present on admission and within the first 48 h: 0–2, 1%; 3–4, 16%; 5–6, 40%; 7–8, 100%
- Severity can also be assessed using the Acute Physiology and Chronic Health (APACHE) II or III scoring system as well as the CT scan index (Table 61, page 1199)

WHEN TO REFER

- A surgeon should be consulted in all cases of severe acute pancreatitis

WHEN TO ADMIT

- The patient with severe pancreatitis requires intensive care unit care

 EVIDENCE

PRACTICE GUIDELINES

- American College of Gastroenterology http://www.acg.gi.org/physicianforum/guides/pancreas.html http://www.guideline.gov/summary/summary.aspx?doc_id=3257&nbr=2483&string=acute+pancreatitis

WEB SITE

- Acute Pancreatitis: Case study http://brighamrad.harvard.edu/Cases/bwh/hcache/28/full.html

INFORMATION FOR PATIENTS

- National Pancreas Foundation http://www.pancreasfoundation.org/acutepancreatitis.html
- National Digestive Diseases Information Clearinghouse http://digestive.niddk.nih.gov/ddiseases/pubs/pancreatitis/index.htm

REFERENCES

- Triester SL et al: Prognostic factors in acute pancreatitis. J Clin Gastroenterol 2002;34:167.
- Yadav D et al: A critical evaluation of laboratory tests in acute pancreatitis. Am J Gastroenterol 2002;97:1309.

Lawrence S. Friedman, MD

Pancreatitis, Chronic

 KEY FEATURES

ESSENTIALS OF DIAGNOSIS

- Epigastric pain, steatorrhea, weight loss, abnormal pancreatic imaging
- A mnemonic for the predisposing factors of chronic pancreatitis is TIGAR-O: toxic-metabolic, idiopathic, genetic; autoimmune, recurrent and severe acute pancreatitis, or obstructive

GENERAL CONSIDERATIONS

- Occurs most often with alcoholism (70–80% of all cases). The risk of chronic pancreatitis increases with the duration and amount of alcohol consumed, but only 5–10% of heavy drinkers develop pancreatitis
- About 2% of patients with hyperparathyroidism develop pancreatitis
- In tropical Africa and Asia, tropical pancreatitis, related in part to malnutrition, is the most common cause of chronic pancreatitis
- A stricture, stone, or tumor obstructing the pancreas can lead to obstructive chronic pancreatitis
- Rare cases of autoimmune chronic pancreatitis associated with hypergammaglobulinemia and responsive to corticosteroids have been reported
- About 10–20% of cases are idiopathic

DEMOGRAPHICS

- Genetic factors may predispose to chronic pancreatitis in some of these cases. For example, mutations of the cystic fibrosis transmembrane conductance regulator (CFTR) gene have been identified in as many as 50% of patients with idiopathic chronic pancreatitis and no other clinical features of cystic fibrosis

 CLINICAL FINDINGS

SYMPTOMS AND SIGNS

- Persistent or recurrent episodes of epigastric and left upper quadrant pain with referral to the upper left lumbar region are typical
- Anorexia, nausea, vomiting, constipation, flatulence, and weight loss are common. Abdominal signs during attacks consist chiefly of tenderness over the pancreas, mild muscle guarding, and paralytic ileus
- Attacks may last only a few hours or as long as 2 weeks; pain may eventually be almost continuous
- Steatorrhea (as indicated by bulky, foul, fatty stools) may occur late in the course

DIFFERENTIAL DIAGNOSIS

- Cholelithiasis
- Diabetes mellitus
- Malabsorption due to other causes
- Intractable duodenal ulcer
- Pancreatic cancer
- Irritable bowel syndrome

 DIAGNOSIS

LABORATORY TESTS

- Serum amylase and lipase may be elevated during acute attacks; normal amylase does not exclude the diagnosis
- Serum alkaline phosphatase and bilirubin may be elevated owing to compression of the common duct
- Glycosuria may be present
- Excess fecal fat may be demonstrated in the stool; pancreatic insufficiency may be confirmed by response to therapy with pancreatic enzyme supplements, or by a bentiromide (NBT-PABA) test or secretin stimulation test if available
- Where available, detection of decreased fecal chymotrypsin or elastase levels may be used to diagnose pancreatic insufficiency, though the tests lack sensitivity and specificity
- Vitamin B_{12} malabsorption is detectable in about 40% of patients, but clinical deficiency of vitamin B_{12} and fat-soluble vitamins is rare

IMAGING STUDIES

- Plain films show calcifications due to pancreaticolithiasis in 30% of patients
- CT may show calcifications not seen on plain films as well as ductal dilation and heterogeneity or atrophy of the gland
- Magnetic resonance cholangiopancreatography (MRCP) and endoscopic ultrasonography (with pancreatic tissue sampling) are promising diagnostic tools

DIAGNOSTIC PROCEDURES

- Endoscopic retrograde cholangiopancreatography is the most sensitive imaging study for chronic pancreatitis and may show dilated ducts, intraductal stones, strictures, or pseudocyst, but the results may be normal in patients with so-called minimal change pancreatitis
- Endoscopic ultrasonography can detect changes of chronic pancreatitis

TREATMENT

MEDICATIONS

Steatorrhea

- Treat with pancreatic supplements. A total dose of 30,000 units of lipase in capsules is given before, during, and after meals (Table 61, page 1256). Higher doses may be required in some cases. The tablets should be taken at the start of, during, and at the end of a meal
- Concurrent administration of H_2 receptor antagonists (eg, ranitidine, 150 mg twice daily), or a proton pump inhibitor (eg, omeprazole, 20–60 mg daily), or sodium bicarbonate, 650 mg before and after meals, decreases the inactivation of lipase by acid and may thereby further decrease steatorrhea
- In selected cases of alcoholic pancreatitis and in cystic fibrosis, enteric-coated microencapsulated preparations may help. However, in cystic fibrosis, high-dose pancreatic enzyme therapy has been associated with strictures of the ascending colon
- Pain secondary to idiopathic chronic pancreatitis may be alleviated by the use of pancreatic enzymes (not enteric-coated) or octreotide, 200 µg subcutaneously three times daily
- Associated diabetes should be treated

SURGERY

- Correctable coexistent biliary tract disease should be treated surgically
- Surgery may be indicated to drain persistent pseudocysts, treat other complications, or relieve pain
- When the pancreatic duct is diffusely dilated, anastomosis between the duct after it is split longitudinally and a defunctionalized limb of jejunum (modified Puestow procedure), in some cases combined with local resection of the head of the pancreas, is associated with relief of pain in 80% of cases
- In advanced cases, subtotal or total pancreatectomy may be considered as a last resort but has variable efficacy and is associated with a high rate of pancreatic insufficiency and diabetes
- Endoscopic or surgical drainage is indicated for symptomatic pseudocysts and those over 6 cm in diameter

THERAPEUTIC PROCEDURES

- A low-fat diet should be prescribed. Alcohol is forbidden because it frequently precipitates attacks. Narcotics should be avoided if possible
- When obstruction of the duodenal end of the duct can be demonstrated by endoscopic retrograde cholangiopancreatography, dilation of the duct or resection of the tail of the pancreas with implantation of duct may be successful
- Pancreatic ascites or pancreaticopleural fistulas due to a disrupted pancreatic duct can be treated with endoscopic placement of a stent across the duct
- Fragmentation of pancreatic duct stones by lithotripsy and endoscopic removal of stones from the duct, pancreatic sphincterotomy, or pseudocyst drainage may relieve pain in selected patients
- For patients with chronic pain and nondilated ducts, a percutaneous celiac plexus nerve block may be considered under either CT or endoscopic ultrasound guidance, with pain relief in approximately 50% of patients

OUTCOME

COMPLICATIONS

- Opioid addiction is common
- Brittle diabetes mellitus, pancreatic pseudocyst or abscess, cholestatic liver enzymes with or without jaundice, common bile duct stricture, steatorrhea, malnutrition, and peptic ulcer
- Pancreatic cancer develops in 4% of patients after 20 years; the risk may relate to tobacco and alcohol use

PROGNOSIS

- In many cases, it is a self-perpetuating disease characterized by chronic pain or recurrent episodes of acute pancreatitis and ultimately by pancreatic exocrine or endocrine insufficiency
- After many years, chronic pain may resolve spontaneously or as a result of surgery tailored to the cause of pain
- Over 80% of adults develop diabetes 25 years after the clinical onset of chronic pancreatitis
- The prognosis is best with recurrent acute pancreatitis caused by a remediable condition such as cholelithiasis, choledocholithiasis, stenosis of the sphincter of Oddi, or hyperparathyroidism

- In alcoholic pancreatitis, pain relief is most likely when a dilated pancreatic duct can be decompressed. In patients with disease not amenable to decompressive surgery, addiction to narcotics is a frequent outcome

PREVENTION

- Abstinence from alcohol
- Medical management of the hyperlipidemia frequently associated with the condition may prevent recurrent attacks of pancreatitis

EVIDENCE

PRACTICE GUIDELINES

- National Guideline Clearinghouse http://www.guideline.gov/summary/summary.aspx?doc_id=3068&nbr=2294&string=chronic+pancreatitis http://www.guideline.gov/summary/summary.aspx?doc_id=2167&nbr=1393&string=chronic+pancreatitis

WEB SITE

- Pancreatic Diseases http://chorus.rad.mcw.edu/index/48.html

INFORMATION FOR PATIENTS

- National Pancreas Foundation http://www.pancreasfoundation.org/chronicpancreatitis.html
- National Digestive Diseases Clearinghouse http://digestive.niddk.nih.gov/ddiseases/pubs/pancreatitis/index.htm

REFERENCES

- Cohn JA et al: Idiopathic pancreatitis related to *CFTR*: complex inheritance and identification of a modifier gene. J Invest Med 2002;50:247S. [PMID: 11726846]
- Etemad B et al: Chronic pancreatitis: diagnosis, classification, and new genetic developments. Gastroenterology 2001;120:682.

Lawrence S. Friedman, MD

Paragonimiasis

 KEY FEATURES

ESSENTIALS OF DIAGNOSIS

- Lung flukes can present with pleuritic pain and hemoptysis
- Acute cerebral infection usually presents as meningitis
- Seizures, cranial neuropathies, and meningoencephalitis can occur from chronic central nervous system infection

GENERAL CONSIDERATIONS

- Many carnivores and omnivores in addition to humans serve as reservoir hosts for the adult fluke (8–16 × 4–8 × 3–5 mm)
- Eggs reaching water, either in sputum or feces, hatch in 3–6 weeks. Released miracidia penetrate and develop in snails. Emergent cercariae encyst as metacercariae in the tissues of crabs and crayfish. Human infection results if metacercariae are ingested when the crustaceans are eaten raw or pickled
- The metacercariae excyst in the small intestine and penetrate the peritoneal cavity. Most migrate through the diaphragm and enter the peripheral lung parenchyma; some may lodge in the brain (about 1% of all cases) or at other ectopic sites
- In the lungs, the parasite becomes encapsulated by granulomatous fibrous tissue, reaching up to 2 cm in diameter. The lesion may rupture, resulting in expectoration of eggs, blood, and inflammatory cells. The prepatent period until appearance of expectorated eggs is about 6 weeks

DEMOGRAPHICS

- *Paragonimus westermani*, the lung fluke, commonly infects humans (estimated 20 million) throughout the Far East; foci are also present in West Africa, South and Southeast Asia, the Pacific Islands, Indonesia, and New Guinea

 CLINICAL FINDINGS

SYMPTOMS AND SIGNS

- Most pulmonary infections are asymptomatic
- In symptomatic cases, low-grade fever and dry cough are present initially; subsequently, pleuritic pain is common, and a rusty, blood-flecked, viscous sputum or frank hemoptysis may occur
- Acute cerebral infection is uncommon, usually manifested by meningitis
- In chronic central nervous system disease, seizures, cranial neuropathies, or meningoencephalitis may occur; death can follow
- Peritoneal cavity or the intestinal wall infection may cause abdominal pain, diarrhea or dysentery, and a palpable tumor mass
- Migratory subcutaneous nodules (a few millimeters to 1 cm in diameter) occur with about 10% of *P westermani* infections and up to 60% of *Paragonimus skrjabini* infections

DIFFERENTIAL DIAGNOSIS

- Tuberculosis
- *Mycoplasma pneumoniae* infection
- Bacterial pneumonia
- Legionnaire's disease (legionella)
- Amebic lung abscess

 DIAGNOSIS

LABORATORY TESTS

- Pulmonary disease is diagnosed by finding characteristic eggs in sputum (rusty sputum is nearly pathognomonic), feces, bronchoscopic washings, biopsy specimens, or pleural fluid; or adult flukes in subcutaneous nodules or other surgical specimens
- If eggs are not found after multiple direct sputum examinations, they may be detectable in a 24-h sputum collection processed by alkaline sodium hypochlorite concentration
- Stool examination for eggs has low sensitivity
- Serum and cerebrospinal fluid serological tests (ELISA, 99% sensitivity, 97% specificity; and immunoblot, 96% sensitivity and 99% specificity) do not differentiate active from prior infection; a newly reported IgM test may do so
- Most treated and cured patients become seronegative
- Eosinophilia (sometimes to a high level) and low-grade leukocytosis are common
- Cerebrospinal fluid may be turgid or bloody, with numerous eosinophils, and eggs may be found
- Paragonimiasis and tuberculosis must be differentiated, though chest x-ray appearance alone does not make the distinction. Since *Paragonimus* ova are destroyed by Ziehl-Neelsen stain for acid-fast bacilli, the sputum should first be examined for the eggs. The presence of a large number of eosinophils or Charcot-Leyden crystals in sputum suggests paragonimiasis

IMAGING STUDIES

- Chest films may show infiltrates, fibrosis, nodules, cavitary lesions, pleural thickening or effusion, or calcifications
- By CT, round, low-attenuation cystic lesions (5–15 mm) filled with fluid or gas are seen within the consolidation
- In acute cerebral disease, CT shows multilocular, ring-like enhancement with surrounding low-density areas
- In chronic cerebral disease, plain skull films often show round or oval-shaped calcifications, sometimes surrounded by low-density areas
- The EEG is almost always abnormal

Paragonimiasis

 TREATMENT

MEDICATIONS

Pulmonary infection

- In pulmonary paragonimiasis, praziquantel is the drug of choice (25 mg/kg after meals three times daily for 3 days, with a 4- to 6-h interval between doses)
- Bithionol is the alternative drug [30–50 mg/kg, given on alternate days for 10–15 doses (20–30 days); the daily dose should be divided into a morning and evening dose]
- For both praziquantel and bithionol, gastrointestinal symptoms, headache, and skin rashes may occur but are mild. Serial liver function tests should be done with bithionol treatment
- Bithionol is available in the United States only from the Parasitic Disease Drug Service, Centers for Disease Control, Atlanta, GA 30333
- Antibiotics may be necessary for secondary pulmonary infection
- Triclabendazole, a veterinary fasciolicide, is under investigation at a dosage of 5 mg/kg once daily for 3 days

Cerebral infection

- In the acute stage of cerebral paragonimiasis, particularly meningitis, praziquantel or bithionol may be effective
- In the chronic stage, both surgical removal of the parasites and drug usage are likely to be ineffective in diminishing neurological symptoms
- With death of parsites, severe local reactions may occur; corticosteroids should therefore be given as in cerebral cysticercosis

 OUTCOME

COMPLICATIONS

- Bronchitis, bronchiectasis, bronchopneumonia, lung abscess, fibrosis, and pleural thickening or effusion may appear

PROGNOSIS

- Cure rates of over 90% can be anticipated for both praziquantel and bithionol

WHEN TO REFER

- All patients should be referred to a clinician with expertise in the diagnosis and management of this disease

WHEN TO ADMIT

- Patients with presumed or confirmed central nervous system infection

 EVIDENCE

PRACTICE GUIDELINES

- National Guideline Clearinghouse http://www.guideline.gov/summary/ summary.aspx?doc_id=2707&nbr= 1933&string=foodborne

INFORMATION FOR PATIENTS

- Centers for Disease Control http://www.dpd.cdc.gov/dpdx/HTML/ Paragonimiasis.htm
- National Institute of Allergy and Infectious Diseases http://www.niaid.nih.gov/publications/ microbes.htm

REFERENCES

- DeFrain M, Hooker R: North American paragonimiasis: case report of a severe clinical infection. Chest 2002;121:1368. [PMID: 11948081]
- Meehan AM et al: Severe pleuropulmonary paragonimiasis 8 years after emigration from a region of endemicity. Clin Infect Dis 2002;35:87. [PMID: 12060881]

Paraphilias

 KEY FEATURES

ESSENTIALS OF DIAGNOSIS

- The excitement stage of sexual activity is associated with atypical objects or orientations
- Stimuli for excitement can be objects such as a woman's shoe, a child, instruments of torture, or incidents of aggression.

GENERAL CONSIDERATIONS

- Disorders are differentiated by the object or activity used to achieve arousal
- **Exhibitionism** is the achievement of arousal by exposing genitalia to strangers
- **Transvestism** consists of recurrent cross-dressing in a heterosexual man as a means of sexual excitation, often in masturbation foreplay
- **Voyeurism** involves attaining arousal by watching the activities of an unknowing person
- **Pedophilia** is the use of a child to achieve sexual arousal and, often, gratification
- **Incest** involves a sexual relationship with a person—usually a child—in the immediate family
- **Sexual sadism** involves inflicting pain upon the sexual object as a means of arousal
- **Sexual masochism**—erotic pleasure is achieved by being humiliated, enslaved, or physically bound or restrained
- **Necrophilia** is sexual intercourse with a dead body or the use of parts of a corpse for sexual excitation

DEMOGRAPHICS

- **Pedophilia** is seen in both sexes, but is identified more frequently in men due to social and cultural factors

 CLINICAL FINDINGS

SYMPTOMS AND SIGNS

- In exhibitionism and voyeurism, excitation often leads to masturbation as a substitute for sexual activity
- Pedophiles have difficulty in adult sexual relationships
- Male pedophiles are frequently impotent

 DIAGNOSIS

LABORATORY TESTS

- Clinical diagnosis

Paraphilias

 TREATMENT

MEDICATIONS

- Medroxyprogesterone acetate suppresses libido and is used to mute sexual behavior in men. Effects occur over 3 weeks and are reversible
- Paraphilias may respond to selective serotonin reuptake inhibitors

THERAPEUTIC PROCEDURES

Psychological

- More superficial disorders such as voyeurism are responsive to psychotherapy in a moderate percentage of cases
- Therapies focus on barriers to normal arousal patterns; as normal behaviors increase, variant behaviors will decrease

Behavioral

- Paraphilias can improve with modeling, role-playing, and conditioning

Social

- Self-help groups can facilitate adjustment to a hostile society
- Attention to family can help alleviate their guilt and accept their situation

 OUTCOME

COMPLICATIONS

- Neck binding or partial asphyxiation is often part of the sexual ritual in masochism, leading to an estimated 1000 accidental deaths annually among men
- Behaviors often persist until they conflict with the law

PROGNOSIS

- Improved when motivation for improvement comes from the patient, as opposed to the legal system

 EVIDENCE

PRACTICE GUIDELINES

- National Guideline Clearinghouse http://www.guideline.gov/summary/ summary.aspx?doc_id=3246&nbr= 2472&string=sexual+abuse

WEB SITES

- American Psychiatric Association http://www.psych.org/
- Internet Mental Health http://www.mentalhealth.com/t30.html
- Psychopharmacology Tips http://www.dr-bob.org/tips/
- Psychiatry On Line http://www.priory.com/psych.htm

INFORMATION FOR PATIENTS

- JAMA patient page: Sexual dysfunction. JAMA 1999;281:584. [PMID: 10022117]
- JAMA patient page: Sexual abuse. JAMA 1998;280:1888. [PMID: 9846790]

REFERENCES

- Reilly DR et al: Protocols for the use of cyproterone, medroxyprogesterone, and leuprolide in the treatment of paraphilia. Can J Psychiatry 2000;45:559. [PMID: 10986575]
- Speckens AE et al: Psychosexual functioning of partners of men with presumed nonorganic erectile dysfunction: cause or consequence of the disorder? Arch Sex Behav 1995;24:157. [PMID: 7794106]

Stuart J. Eisendrath, MD
Jonathan E. Lichtmacher, MD

Parkinsonism

KEY FEATURES

ESSENTIALS OF DIAGNOSIS

- Any combination of tremor, rigidity, bradykinesia, progressive postural instability
- Mild intellectual deterioration may occur

GENERAL CONSIDERATIONS

- Dopamine depletion due to degeneration of the dopaminergic nigrostriatal system leads to an imbalance of dopamine and acetylcholine
- Exposure to toxins [manganese dust, carbon disulfide, severe carbon monoxide poisoning, 1-methyl-4-phenyl-1,2,5,6-tetrahydropyridine (MPTP) for recreational purposes, neuroleptic drugs, reserpine, or metoclopramide] can lead to parkinsonism
- Postencephalitic parkinsonism is becoming increasingly rare
- Only rarely is hemiparkinsonism the presenting feature of a space-occupying lesion

DEMOGRAPHICS

- Common disorder that occurs in all ethnic groups, with an approximately equal sex distribution
- The most common variety, idiopathic Parkinson's disease (paralysis agitans), begins most often between 45 and 65 years of age
- May rarely occur on a familial basis

CLINICAL FINDINGS

SYMPTOMS AND SIGNS

- Tremor, rigidity, bradykinesia, and postural instability are the cardinal features
- Mild decline in intellectual function
- The tremor is four to six cycles per second, most conspicuous at rest, enhanced by stress, often less severe during voluntary activity; commonly confined to one limb or to one side for months or years before it becomes more generalized. It may occasionally involve the lower jaw
- Rigidity causes the flexed posture
- Bradykinesia is the most disabling symptom; a slowness of voluntary movement and a reduction in automatic movements such as swinging of the arms while walking
- The face is relatively immobile with widened palpebral fissures, infrequent blinking, and a certain fixity of facial expression
- Mild blepharoclonus
- Repetitive tapping (about twice per second) over the bridge of the nose produces a sustained blink response (Myerson's sign)
- Other findings include saliva drooling from the mouth; soft and poorly modulated voice; a variable rest tremor and rigidity in some or all of the limbs; slowness of voluntary movements; impairment of fine or rapidly alternating movements; and micrographia
- Typically no muscle weakness and no alteration in the tendon reflexes or plantar responses
- It is difficult for the patient to arise from a sitting position and begin walking
- Gait is characterized by small shuffling steps and a loss of the normal automatic arm swing; there may be unsteadiness on turning, difficulty in stopping, and a tendency to fall

DIFFERENTIAL DIAGNOSIS

- Different causes of parkinsonism
- Essential tremor
- Depression
- Wilson's disease
- Huntington's disease
- Normal pressure hydrocephalus
- Shy-Drager syndrome
- Progressive supranuclear palsy
- Cortical-basal ganglionic degeneration
- Creutzfeldt-Jakob disease

- Drugs causing parkinsonism: antipsychotics, reserpine, metoclopramide

DIAGNOSIS

DIAGNOSTIC PROCEDURES

- Diagnosis is primarily clinical

TREATMENT

MEDICATIONS

- Amantadine, usual dose (100 mg twice daily), may improve all of the clinical features of parkinsonism
- Anticholinergics are more helpful for tremor and rigidity than bradykinesia. Start with a small dose (Table 96, page 1280). Contraindicated in patients with prostatic hypertrophy, narrow-angle glaucoma, or obstructive intestinal disease; often tolerated poorly by the elderly
- Sinemet is a combination of carbidopa and levodopa in a fixed ratio (1:10 or 1:4). Start with small dose—eg, one tablet of Sinemet 25/100 (containing 25 mg of carbidopa and 100 mg of levodopa) three times daily—and gradually increase depending on the response
- Sinemet CR is a controlled-release formulation (containing 25 or 50 mg of carbidopa and 100 or 200 mg of levodopa). It is sometimes helpful in reducing fluctuations in clinical response and in reducing the frequency with which medication must be taken
- Bromocriptine and pergolide are dopamine agonists and ergot derivatives. The initial dose of bromocriptine is 1.25 mg twice daily; this is increased by 2.5 mg at 2-week intervals until benefit or side effects occur. Pergolide is similarly started in a low dose (eg, 0.05 mg daily) and built up gradually depending on the response and tolerance. Both are contraindicated in patients with mental illness or recent myocardial infarction and are best avoided in those with peripheral vascular disease or peptic ulcers as bleeding from the latter has been reported

Parkinsonism

- Pramipexole and ropinirole are two newer dopamine agonists that are not ergot derivatives. In each case, the daily dose is built up gradually. Pramipexole is started at a dosage of 0.125 mg three times daily, and the dose is doubled after 1 week and again after another week; the daily dose is then increased by 0.75 mg at weekly intervals depending on response and tolerance. Most patients require between 0.5 and 1.5 mg three times daily. Ropinirole is begun at a dosage of 0.25 mg three times daily, and the total daily dose is increased at weekly intervals by 0.75 mg until the fourth week and by 1.5 mg thereafter. Most patients require between 2 and 8 mg three times daily
- Selegiline is a monoamine oxidase B inhibitor that improves fluctuations or declining response to levodopa
- Although data are inconclusive, selegiline may arrest the progression of Parkinson's disease, which remains an important consideration for patients who are young or have mild disease
- Two catecholamine-*O*-methyltransferase inhibitors, tolcapone and entacapone, may be used as an adjunct to Sinemet when there are response fluctuations or inadequate responses
- Tolcapone is given in a dosage of 100 mg or 200 mg three times daily, and entacapone is given as 200 mg with each dose of Sinemet. With either preparation, the dose of Sinemet taken concurrently may have to be reduced by up to one-third to avoid side effects
- Entacapone is generally preferred over tolcapone because acute hepatic failure has occurred with tolcapone
- Confusion and psychotic symptoms often respond to atypical antipsychotic agents, such as olanzapine, quetiapine, risperidone, or clozapine
- Clozapine may rarely cause marrow suppression, and weekly blood cell counts are therefore necessary for patients taking it. The patient is started on 6.25 mg at bedtime and the dosage increased to 25–100 mg/day as needed. In low doses, it may also improve iatrogenic dyskinesias

SURGERY

- Thalamotomy or pallidotomy may be helpful for patients unresponsive to medical treatment or have intolerable side effects
- High-frequency bilateral stimulation of the subthalamic nuclei or globus pallidus internus may benefit all the major features of the disease, and has a lower morbidity than lesion surgery

THERAPEUTIC PROCEDURES

- Drug therapy may not be required early
- Physical and speech therapy and simple aids to daily living (eg, rails or banisters placed strategically about the home, special table cutlery with large handles, nonslip rubber table mats, and devices to amplify the voice) may help

OUTCOME

COMPLICATIONS

- Levodopa-induced dyskinesias may take any form, including chorea, athetosis, dystonia, tremor, tics, and myoclonus
- Later complications of the drug include the "on-off phenomenon," in which abrupt but transient fluctuations in the severity of parkinsonism occur unpredictably but frequently during the day. The "off" period of marked bradykinesia has been shown to relate in some instances to falling plasma levels of levodopa. During the "on" phase, dyskinesias are often conspicuous but mobility is increased
- Because of this complication, levodopa therapy should be postponed and dopamine agonists used instead, except in the elderly

WHEN TO REFER

- If expertise is needed to determine when to begin therapy
- Consultation with a practitioner with expertise in management may help when there is progressive disease despite appropriate therapy
- For physical and speech therapy

EVIDENCE

PRACTICE GUIDELINES

- Bhatia K et al: Guidelines for the management of Parkinson's disease. The Parkinson's Disease Consensus Working Group. Hosp Med 1998;59(6):469.
- Olanow CW, Koller WC: An algorithm (decision tree) for the management of Parkinson's disease: treatment guidelines. American Academy of Neurology. Neurology 1998 ;50(3 Suppl 3):S1.

INFORMATION FOR PATIENTS

- JAMA patient page: Parkinson disease. JAMA 2000;284:2012. [PMID: 11183747]
- American Association of Neurological Surgeons http://www.neurosurgery.org/health/ patient/detail.asp?DisorderID=46

REFERENCES

- Deep-Brain Stimulation for Parkinson's Disease Study Group: Deep-brain stimulation of the subthalamic nucleus or the pars interna of the globus pallidus in Parkinson's disease. N Engl J Med 2001; 345;956. [PMID: 11575287]
- Freed C et al: Transplantation of embryonic dopamine neurons for severe Parkinson's disease. N Engl J Med 2001;344;710. [PMID: 11236774]
- Miyasaki JM et al: Practice parameter: initiation of treatment for Parkinson's disease: an evidence-based review. Neurology 2002;58:11. [PMID: 11781398]

Michael J. Aminoff, MD, DSc, FRCP

Pediculosis

 KEY FEATURES

ESSENTIALS OF DIAGNOSIS

- Pruritus with excoriation
- Nits on hair shafts; lice on skin or clothes
- Occasionally, sky-blue macules (maculae ceruleae) on the inner thighs or lower abdomen in pubic louse infestation

GENERAL CONSIDERATIONS

- A parasitic infestation of the skin of the scalp, trunk, or pubic areas
- Body lice usually occur among people who live in overcrowded dwellings with inadequate hygiene facilities
- Pubic lice may be acquired by sexual transmission
- Head lice may be transmitted by shared use of hats or combs and are epidemic among children of all socioeconomic classes in elementary schools
- Head lice are very uncommon among black children
- Trench fever, relapsing fever, and typhus are transmitted by the body louse in countries where those diseases are endemic

DEMOGRAPHICS

- Adults with head lice virtually always acquire their infestation from elementary school-aged children, so a source of infection must always be sought

 CLINICAL FINDINGS

SYMPTOMS AND SIGNS

- See Table 7 (page 1202)
- Itching may be very intense in body louse infestations, and scratching may result in deep excoriations, especially over the upper shoulders, posterior flanks, and neck
- In some cases, only itching is present, with few excoriations seen
- Head lice can be found on the scalp or may be manifested as small nits resembling pussy willow buds on the scalp hairs close to the skin; they are easiest to see above the ears and at the nape of the neck
- Head and body lice are similar in appearance and are 3–4 mm long

DIFFERENTIAL DIAGNOSIS

- Head lice: seborrheic dermatitis, impetigo, hair casts (hair debris)
- Body lice: scabies, impetigo, dermatitis herpetiformis, urticaria
- Pubic lice: anogenital pruritus, scabies, atopic dermatitis (eczema)

 DIAGNOSIS

LABORATORY TESTS

- Relies on an index of suspicion and isolating the organism
- The body louse can seldom be found on the body, because the insect comes onto the skin only to feed and must be looked for in the seams of the clothing

Pediculosis

 ## TREATMENT

MEDICATIONS

- See Table 6 (page 1199)

Pubic lice

- Lindane lotion or cream (Kwell, Scabene) is used; a thin layer is applied to the infested and adjacent hairy areas; it is removed after 8 h by thorough washing
- Permethrin rinse 1% for 10 min and permethrin cream 5% applied for 8 h are effective alternatives

Head lice

- Permethrin 1% cream rinse (Nix) is the treatment of choice for head lice; it is applied to the scalp and hair and left on for 30 min to 8 h before being rinsed off; treatment should be repeated in 1 week
- Five percent permethrin lotion may be used in refractory cases
- Permethrin 1% cream (Nix) is more effective than synergized pyrethrins (RID), OTC products that are applied undiluted until the infested areas are entirely wet; after 10 min, the areas are washed thoroughly with warm water and soap and then dried
- Malathion lotion 1% (Ovide) is very effective, but it is highly volatile and flammable, so application must be done in a well-ventilated room or outdoors
- For involvement of eyelashes, petrolatum is applied thickly twice daily for 8 days, and remaining nits are then plucked off

THERAPEUTIC PROCEDURES

- Body lice are treated by disposing of the infested clothing
- Sexual contacts should be treated
- Clothes and bedclothes should be washed and dried at high temperature if possible

 ## OUTCOME

WHEN TO REFER

- If there is a question about the diagnosis, if recommended therapy is ineffective, or specialized treatment is necessary

 ## EVIDENCE

PRACTICE GUIDELINES

- National Guideline Clearinghouse
  http://www.guideline.gov/summary/
  summary.aspx?doc_id=3225&nbr=
  2451&string=pediculosis
  http://www.guideline.gov/summary/
  summary.aspx?doc_id=3452&nbr=
  2678&string=pediculosis

WEB SITES

- American Academy of Dermatology
  http://www.aad.org
- Dermatology Handbook for Family Practice from the University of Iowa
  http://www.vh.org/Providers/ClinRef/
  FPHandbook/17.html

INFORMATION FOR PATIENTS

- Centers for Disease Control and Prevention
  http://www.cdc.gov/ncidod/dpd/
  parasites/lice/factsht_body_lice.htm
- Nemours Foundation
  http://kidshealth.org/parent/infections/
  common/lice.html

REFERENCE

- Chosidow O: Scabies and pediculosis. Lancet 2000;355:819.

Timothy G. Berger, MD

Pelvic Inflammatory Disease (PID)

 ## KEY FEATURES

ESSENTIALS OF DIAGNOSIS

- Lower abdominal, adnexal, or cervical motion tenderness
- Absence of a competing diagnosis

GENERAL CONSIDERATIONS

- A polymicrobial infection of the upper genital tract associated with the sexually transmitted organisms *Neisseria gonorrhoeae* and *Chlamydia trachomatis*, endogenous organisms, including anaerobes, *Haemophilus influenzae*, enteric gram-negative rods, and streptococci
- Tuberculous salpingitis is rare in the United States but more common in developing countries; it is characterized by pelvic pain and irregular pelvic masses not responsive to antibiotic therapy. It is not sexually transmitted

DEMOGRAPHICS

- Most common in young, nulliparous, sexually active women with multiple partners
- Other risk markers include nonwhite race, douching, and smoking
- The use of oral contraceptives or barrier methods of contraception may provide significant protection

 ## CLINICAL FINDINGS

SYMPTOMS AND SIGNS

- Symtoms may include lower abdominal pain, chills and fever, menstrual disturbances, purulent cervical discharge, and cervical and adnexal tenderness
- Right upper quadrant pain (Fitz-Hugh and Curtis syndrome) may indicate an associated perihepatitis
- Diagnosis is complicated by the fact that many women have mild symptoms, not readily recognized as PID

Minimum diagnostic criteria

- Lower abdominal, adnexal, or cervical motion tenderness should be treated as PID with antibiotics unless there is a competing diagnosis such as ectopic pregnancy or appendicitis

Additional criteria

- The following criteria may be used to enhance the specificity of the diagnosis: oral temperature >38.3°C, abnormal cervical or vaginal discharge with white cells on saline microscopy, elevated erythrocyte sedimentation rate, elevated C-reactive protein, and laboratory documentation of cervical infection with *N gonorrhoeae* or *C trachomatis* awaiting results

Definitive criteria

- When the clinical or laboratory evidence is uncertain, the following criteria may be used: histopathological evidence of endometritis on endometrial biopsy, transvaginal sonography or other imaging techniques showing thickened fluid-filled tubes with or without free pelvic fluid or tuboovarian complex, and laparoscopic abnormalities consistent with PID

DIFFERENTIAL DIAGNOSIS

- Ectopic pregnancy
- Appendicitis
- Septic abortion
- Ruptured ovarian cyst or tumor
- Ovarian torsion
- Tuboovarian abscess
- Degeneration of leiomyoma (fibroid)
- Diverticulitis
- Cystitis
- Tuberculous salpingitis
- Actinomycosis with prolonged IUD use

 ## DIAGNOSIS

LABORATORY TESTS

- Abnormal cervical or vaginal discharge may show white blood cells on saline microscopy
- Endocervical culture for *N gonorrhoeae* and saline wet mount for *C trachomatis*
- Erythrocyte sedimentation rate and C-reactive protein may be elevated

IMAGING STUDIES

- Pelvic and vaginal ultrasound can differentiate ectopic pregnancy of over 6 weeks

DIAGNOSTIC PROCEDURES

- Culdocentesis will differentiate hemoperitoneum (ruptured ectopic pregnancy or hemorrhagic cyst) from pelvic sepsis (salpingitis, ruptured pelvic abscess, or ruptured appendix)
- Laparoscopy can diagnose PID, and it is imperative if the diagnosis is not certain or if the patient has not responded to antibiotic therapy after 48 h. The appendix should be visualized at laparoscopy to rule out appendicitis. Cultures obtained at the time of laparoscopy are often helpful

TREATMENT

MEDICATIONS

- Antibiotic treatment should not be delayed while awaiting culture results
- The sexual partner should be examined and treated appropriately

Inpatient regimens

- Cefoxitin, 2 g intravenously every 6 h, or cefotetan, 2 g every 12 h, plus doxycycline, 100 mg intravenously or orally every 12 h. This regimen is continued for at least 24 h after there is significant clinical improvement. Doxycycline, 100 mg twice daily, should be continued to complete a total of 14 days' therapy
- Clindamycin, 900 mg intravenously every 8 h, plus gentamicin intravenously in a loading dose of 2 mg/kg followed by 1.5 mg/kg every 8 h. This regimen is continued for at least 24 h after there is significant clinical improvement and is followed by either clindamycin, 450 mg four times daily, or doxycycline, 100 mg twice daily, to complete a total of 14 days of therapy

Outpatient regimens

- Ofloxacin, 400 mg orally twice daily for 14 days, plus metronidazole, 500 mg orally twice daily, for 14 days
- Either a single dose of cefoxitin, 2 g intramuscularly, with probenecid, 1 g orally, or ceftriaxone, 250 mg intramuscularly, plus doxycycline, 100 mg orally twice daily, for 14 days

SURGERY

- Tuboovarian abscesses may require surgical excision or transcutaneous or transvaginal aspiration
- Unilateral adnexectomy is acceptable for unilateral abscess
- Hysterectomy and bilateral salpingo-oophorectomy may be necessary for overwhelming infection or in cases of chronic disease with intractable pelvic pain

 ## OUTCOME

FOLLOW-UP

- Inpatient therapy for tuboovarian abscess should be monitored by ultrasound

COMPLICATIONS

- In spite of treatment, one-fourth of women with acute disease develop long-term sequelae, including repeated episodes of infection, chronic pelvic pain, dyspareunia, ectopic pregnancy, or infertility
- The risk of infertility increases with repeated episodes of salpingitis: it is estimated at 10% after the first episode, 25% after a second episode, and 50% after a third episode

PROGNOSIS

- Early treatment with effective antibiotcs is essential to prevent long-term sequelae
- For tuboovarian abscess, unless rupture is suspected, high-dose antibiotic therapy in the hospital is effective in 70% of cases. In 30%, there is inadequate response in 48–72 h, and surgical intervention is required

WHEN TO ADMIT

- Admit for intravenous antibiotic therapy if surgical emergencies such as appendicitis cannot be ruled out; a tuboovarian abscess; the patient is pregnant; the patient is unable to follow or tolerate an outpatient regimen; the patient has failed to respond clinically to outpatient therapy; the patient has severe illness, nausea and vomiting, or high fever; or the patient is immunodeficient (ie, has HIV infection with low CD4 counts, is taking immunosuppressive therapy, or has another immunosuppressing disease)
- Outpatient parenteral therapy is available in some settings and may be an acceptable alternative
- Patients with tuboovarian abscesses should have direct inpatient observation for at least 24 h prior to switching to outpatient parenteral therapy

 ## EVIDENCE

PRACTICE GUIDELINES

- National Guideline Clearinghouse http://www.guideline.gov/summary/ summary.aspx?doc_id=3238&nbr= 2464&string=PID

WEB SITES

- Gynecology Handbook for Family Practitioners http://www.vh.org/Providers/ClinRef/ FPHandbook/13.html
- Salpingitis Isthmica Nodosa Demonstration Case http://www.brighamrad.harvard.edu/ Cases/bwh/hcache/56/full.html

INFORMATION FOR PATIENTS

- National Women's Health Information Center http://www.4woman.gov/faq/stdpids. htm
- American College of Obstetricians and Gynecologisits http://www.medem.com/MedLB/ article_detaillb.cfm?article_ID= ZZZAB51P97C&sub_cat=9

REFERENCE

- Paavonen J: Pelvic inflammatory disease: from diagnosis to prevention. Dermatol Clin 1998;16:747. [PMID: 9891675]

H. Trent MacKay, MD, MPH

Pemphigus

KEY FEATURES

ESSENTIALS OF DIAGNOSIS

- Relapsing crops of skin bullae
- Often preceded by mucous membrane bullae, erosions, and ulcerations
- Superficial detachment of the skin after pressure or trauma variably present (Nikolsky's sign)
- Acantholysis on biopsy
- Immunofluorescence studies are confirmatory

GENERAL CONSIDERATIONS

- There are several forms of pemphigus: pemphigus vulgaris and its variant, pemphigus vegetans; and the more superficially blistering pemphigus foliaceus and its variant, pemphigus erythematosus
- An uncommon intraepidermal blistering disease occurring on skin and mucous membranes
- Caused by autoantibodies to adhesion molecules in the desmosomal complex expressed in the skin and mucous membranes
- These autoantibodies cause acantholysis, the separation of epidermal cells from each other
- The cause is unknown
- Drug-induced autoimmune pemphigus from drugs including penicillamine and captopril has been reported
- More than 95% of patients with pemphigus vulgaris are positive for HLA-DR4/DQw3 or HLA-DRw6/DQw1

DEMOGRAPHICS

- All forms may occur at any age but most commonly in middle age

CLINICAL FINDINGS

SYMPTOMS AND SIGNS

- See Table 7 (page 1202)
- An insidious onset of flaccid bullae in crops or waves
- The bullae appear spontaneously and are tender and painful when they rupture
- In pemphigus vulgaris, lesions often appear first on the oral mucous membranes, and these rapidly become erosive
- In some cases, erosions and crusts predominate over blisters
- The scalp is another site of early involvement
- Rubbing a cotton swab or finger laterally on the surface of uninvolved skin may cause easy separation of the epidermis (Nikolsky's sign)
- If the lesions become extensive, the complications of the disease lead to great toxicity and debility

DIFFERENTIAL DIAGNOSIS

- Erythema multiforme major or toxic
- Epidermal necrolysis
- Drug eruptions
- Bullous impetigo
- Contact dermatitis
- Dermatitis herpetiformis
- Bullous pemphigoid
- Cicatricial pemphigoid
- Paraneoplastic pemphigus
- Linear IgA dermatosis
- Pemphigus foliaceus
- Porphyria cutanea tarda
- Epidermolysis bullosa
- Staphylococcal scalded skin syndrome
- Herpes gestationis
- Graft-versus-host disease

DIAGNOSIS

LABORATORY TESTS

- The diagnosis is made by light microscopy and by direct and indirect immunofluorescence microscopy
- Microscopically, acantholysis is the hallmark of pemphigus, but in some patients there may be eosinophilic spongiosis initially
- Immunofluorescence microscopy shows deposits of IgG intercellularly in the epidermis; C3 and other immunoglobulins and complement components may be present on occasion
- Indirect immunofluorescence microscopy to detect circulating pemphigus antibodies is not necessary for the diagnosis, but antibody titers in some patients may correspond with disease activity and might help in management

TREATMENT

MEDICATIONS

- See Table 6 (page 1199)
- Local measures
  - In patients with limited disease, skin and mucous membrane lesions should be treated with topical corticosteroids
  - Complicating infection requires appropriate systemic and local antibiotic therapy
- Systemic measures
  - Initial therapy is with systemic steroids: prednisone, 60–80 mg daily
  - In all but the most mild cases, a steroid-sparing agent is added from the beginning, since the course of the disease is long and the steroid-sparing agents take several weeks to exert their activity
  - Azathioprine (100 mg daily) or mycophenolate mofetil (1 g twice daily) is used most frequently, the latter seeming to be the most reliable and recommended for most cases
- In refractory cases, monthly IGIV at 2 g/kg intravenously over 3 days is useful and has replaced high-dose steroids plus cyclophosphamide and pulse intravenous steroids as rescue therapy
- In pemphigus foliaceus and mild cases of pemphigus vulgaris, tetracycline, 500 mg, and nicotinamide, 500 mg, three times daily, may be tried
- Dapsone may also be tried as a steroid-sparing agent, especially in pemphigus foliaceus

THERAPEUTIC PROCEDURES

- When the disease is severe, hospitalize the patient at bed rest and provide antibiotics and intravenous feedings as indicated
- Anesthetic troches used before eating ease painful oral lesions

 OUTCOME

COMPLICATIONS

- Secondary infection is a major cause of morbidity and mortality
- Disturbances of fluid and electrolyte balance can occur owing to losses through the involved skin in severe cases

PROGNOSIS

- The course tends to be chronic in most patients, though some appear to experience remission
- Infection is the most frequent cause of death, usually from *Staphylococcus aureus* septicemia

WHEN TO REFER

- If there is a question about the diagnosis, if recommended therapy is ineffective, or specialized treatment is necessary

WHEN TO ADMIT

- For severe disease

 EVIDENCE

WEB SITES

- American Academy of Dermatology
  http://www.aad.org
- Dermatology Handbook for Family Practice from the University of Iowa
  http://www.vh.org/Providers/ClinRef/FPHandbook/17.html

INFORMATION FOR PATIENTS

- International Pemohgus Foundation
  http://www.pemphigus.org/whatisgus.html
- National Institutes of Health
  http://www.nlm.nih.gov/medlineplus/ency/article/000882.htm

REFERENCES

- Cotell S et al: Autoimmune blistering skin diseases. Am J Emerg Med 2000; 18:288. [PMID: 10830686]
- Engineer L et al: Analysis of current data on the use of intravenous immunoglobulins in management of pemphigus vulgaris. J Am Acad Dermatol 2000;43: 1049. [PMID: 11100022]
- Nousari HC et al: Pemphigus and bullous pemphigoid. Lancet 1999;354:667. [PMID: 10466686]
- Stanley JR: Understanding of the pathophysiology of pemphigus suggests innovative therapeutic approaches. Br J Dermatol 2000;142:208. [PMID: 10730750]

Timothy G. Berger, MD

Peptic Ulcer Disease

KEY FEATURES

ESSENTIALS OF DIAGNOSIS

- Peptic ulcer is a break in the gastric or duodenal mucosa, extending through the muscularis mucosae, and usually >5 mm in diameter
- Nonspecific epigastric pain in 80–90% with variable relationship to meals
- Ulcer symptoms characterized by rhythmicity and periodicity
- Ulcer complications without antecedent symptoms in 10–20%
- Of nonsteroidal antiinflammatory drug (NSAID)-induced ulcers, 30–50% are asymptomatic
- Upper endoscopy with antral biopsy for *Helicobacter pylori* is diagnostic
- Gastric ulcer biopsy or documentation of complete healing is necessary to exclude gastric malignancy

GENERAL CONSIDERATIONS

- Peptic ulcers are 5 times more common in the duodenum than in the stomach
- In the stomach, benign ulcers are most common in the antrum (60%) and at the junction of the antrum and body on the lesser curvature (25%)
- Major causes of peptic ulcer disease: NSAIDs, chronic *H pylori* infection, and acid hypersecretory states such as Zollinger-Ellison syndrome
- Up to 25% of ulcers are idiopathic
- Prevalence of *H pylori* infection in duodenal ulcer patients is ~70–75%, but only ~1 in 6 chronically infected patients develop an ulcer
- Prevalence of gastric ulcers is 10–20% and prevalence of duodenal ulcers is 2–5% in chronic NSAID users
- In NSAID users, relative risk of gastric ulcers is increased 40-fold, but risk of duodenal ulcers only slightly increased
- *H pylori* infection increases risk of NSAID-induced ulcers and complications

DEMOGRAPHICS

- In the United States, ~500,000 new cases and 4 million ulcer recurrences per year
- Incidence of duodenal ulcers is declining, while that of gastric ulcers is increasing
- Lifetime prevalence of ulcers in adults is ~10%
- Gastric ulcers are slightly more common in men than in women (1.3:1)
- Duodenal ulcers are most common between the ages of 30 and 55
- Gastric ulcers are most common between the ages of 55 and 70
- Peptic ulcers are more common in smokers

CLINICAL FINDINGS

SYMPTOMS AND SIGNS

- Epigastric pain (dyspepsia), not severe, in 80–90%
- Ulcer complications such as bleeding with no antecedent symptoms ("silent ulcers") in 20%
- Pain is relieved by food or antacids in ~50%
- Nocturnal pain that awakens the patient in two-thirds of duodenal ulcers and one-third of gastric ulcers
- Most patients have symptomatic periods lasting several weeks with intervals of months to years in which they are pain free (periodicity)
- Nausea and anorexia
- Significant vomiting and weight loss suggest gastric outlet obstruction or gastric malignancy
- Physical examination often normal
- Mild, localized epigastric tenderness to deep palpation

DIFFERENTIAL DIAGNOSIS

- Functional or nonulcer dyspepsia
- Gastritis, eg, NSAIDs, alcohol, stress, *H pylori*, pernicious anemia
- Biliary disease or pancreatitis
- Gastroesophageal reflux disease or reflux esophagitis
- "Indigestion" from overeating, high-fat foods, coffee
- Gastric or pancreatic cancer
- Angina pectoris
- Severe pain: esophageal rupture, gastric volvulus, ruptured aortic aneurysm

DIAGNOSIS

LABORATORY TESTS

- Anemia with acute blood loss from a bleeding ulcer
- Fecal occult blood test positive in one-third

- Leukocytosis suggests ulcer penetration or perforation
- Elevated serum amylase suggests ulcer penetration into the pancreas
- Fasting serum gastrin level to screen for Zollinger-Ellison syndrome

Noninvasive testing for *H pylori*

- Serological tests, urea breath test, or fecal antigen tests
- Rapid, office-based tests have lower sensitivity and specificity (75–90%)
- Laboratory-based serologic ELISA test has sensitivity and specificity of >90%; positive test does not necessarily imply ongoing active infection
- After eradication with antibiotics, antibody levels decline to undetectable levels in 50% of patients by 12–18 months
- Fecal antigen immunoassay has sensitivity and specificity of 90%; positive test indicates active infection
- ^{13}C-urea and ^{14}C-urea breath tests have sensitivity and specificity of 90%; positive test indicates active infection
- Proton pump inhibitors significantly reduce the sensitivity of urea breath tests and fecal antigen assays (but not serological tests) and should be discontinued 14 days prior to testing

Endoscopic testing for *H pylori*

- Gastric biopsy specimens can detect *H pylori* organisms on histology and can be tested for active infection by urease production
- Urease test has sensitivity and specificity of 90%

IMAGING STUDIES

- Barium upper gastrointestinal series has limited accuracy in distinguishing benign from malignant gastric ulcers

DIAGNOSTIC PROCEDURES

- Upper endoscopy better diagnostic accuracy than barium radiography
- Biopsy for the presence of malignancy and *H pylori* infection
- Duodenal ulcers are virtually never malignant and do not require biopsy
- With benign-appearing gastric ulcers, cytological brushings and biopsies of the ulcer margin reveal that 3–5% are malignant
- Nonhealing ulcers may be malignant

Peptic Ulcer Disease

 TREATMENT

MEDICATIONS

- See Table 54 (page 1251)

Peptic ulcers with active *H pylori* infection

- Acute treatment for 10–14 days with one of the following
- "Triple-therapy" regimens
  - Proton pump inhibitor before meals: omeprazole, 20 mg PO BID, rabeprazole, 20 mg PO BID, lansoprazole, 30 mg PO BID, pantoprazole, 40 mg PO BID, or esomeprazole, 40 mg PO QD plus clarithromycin, 500 mg PO BID, and amoxicillin, 1 g PO BID *or* metronidazole, 500 mg PO BID (in penicillin-allergic patients)
  - Ranitidine bismuth citrate, 400 mg PO BID, plus clarithromycin, 500 mg PO BID, plus amoxicillin, 1g PO BID *or* tetracycline, 500 mg PO BID *or* metronidazole, 500 mg PO BID
- "Quadruple-therapy" regimens
  - Proton pump inhibitor before meals: omeprazole, 20 mg PO BID, rabeprazole, 20 mg PO BID, lansoprazole, 30 mg PO BID, pantoprazole, 40 mg PO BID, or esomeprazole, 40 mg QD, plus bismuth subsalicylate, 2 tablets PO QID, plus tetracycline, 500 mg PO QID, plus metronidazole, 250 mg PO QID; recommended for patients who fail an initial attempt at eradication with triple therapy
- Continue treatment for 4–8 weeks with proton pump inhibitor: omeprazole, 20 mg PO QD, rabeprazole, 20 mg PO QD, lansoprazole, 30 mg PO QD, or pantoprazole, 40 mg PO QD or esomeprazole, 40 mg QD

Peptic ulcers with no *H pylori* infection

- Proton pump inhibitors—omeprazole or rabeprazole, 20 mg PO QD, lansoprazole, 15–30 mg PO QD, pantoprazole, 40 mg PO QD, or esomeprazole, 40 mg QD given 30 min before breakfast heals >90% of duodenal ulcers after 4 weeks and 90% of gastric ulcers after 8 weeks
- H_2 receptor antagonists may be used as a less expensive alternative to proton pump inhibitors—ranitidine, 300 mg PO QHS, nizatidine, 300 mg PO QHS, famotidine, 40 mg PO QHS, or cimetidine, 800 mg PO QHS heals 85–90% of duodenal and gastric ulcers within 6 and 8 weeks, respectively

- Chronic "maintenance" therapy indicated in patients with recurrent ulcers who either are *H pylori* negative or who have failed attempts at eradication therapy: proton pump inhibitor: omeprazole, 20 mg PO QD, rabeprazole, 20 mg PO QD, lansoprazole, 30 mg PO QD, esomeprazole, 40 mg PO QD, pantoprazole, 40 mg PO QD; or H_2 receptor antagonist: cimetidine 400–800 mg PO QHS, nizatidine or ranitidine, 150–300 mg PO QHS, famotidine, 20–40 mg PO QHS

SURGERY

- For complications of peptic ulcer disease, including perforation, penetration, gastric outlet obstruction, and bleeding that cannot be controlled with endoscopic therapy

THERAPEUTIC PROCEDURES

- Moderate alcohol intake
- Discontinue smoking
- Discontinue NSAIDs when possible

 OUTCOME

FOLLOW-UP

- Repeat biopsies after 2–3 months of therapy if gastric ulcers do not heal

COMPLICATIONS

- See *Peptic ulcer disease, complications*

PROGNOSIS

- *H pylori* not eradicated—85% of patients will have recurrence within 1 year, half of these symptomatic; after successful eradication, recurrence rates are reduced dramatically to 5–20% at 1 year

WHEN TO REFER

- Patients with persistent dyspepsia after 1–2 weeks of medical treatment
- Complications of peptic ulcer disease

WHEN TO ADMIT

- Complications of peptic ulcer disease

PREVENTION

- NSAID-induced ulcers: substitute COX-2 selective agent (celecoxib, rofecoxib) for nonselective NSAIDs
- Proton pump inhibitor: omeprazole, 20 mg PO QD, rabeprazole, 20 mg PO QD, lansoprazole, 30 mg PO QD, pan-

toprazole, 40 mg PO QD, or esomeprazole, 40 mg QD
- Misoprostol, 100–200 μg PO QID effective, but causes diarrhea in 10–20%

 EVIDENCE

WEB SITE

- MEDLINEplus—Gastric ulcer http://www.nlm.nih.gov/medlineplus/ency/article/000213.htm

REFERENCES

- Graham D: Therapy of *Helicobacter pylori*: current status and issues. Gastroenterology 2000;118:S2. [PMID: 10868895]
- Huang JQ et al: Role of *Helicobacter pylori* infection and non-steroidal anti-inflammatory drugs in peptic-ulcer disease: a meta-analysis. Lancet 2002;359:14. [PMID: 11809181]

Kenneth R. McQuaid, MD

Peptic Ulcer Disease, Complications

 ## KEY FEATURES

ESSENTIALS OF DIAGNOSIS

- Upper gastrointestinial hemorrhage, with "coffee grounds" emesis, hematemesis, melena, or hematochezia
- Perforation, with severe pain and peritonitis
- Penetration, with severe pain and pancreatitis
- Gastric outlet obstructon, with vomiting
- Emergent upper endoscopy is usually diagnostic and sometimes therapeutic

GENERAL CONSIDERATIONS

Upper gastrointestinal hemorrhage

- ~50% of upper gastrointestinal bleeding is due to peptic ulcer disease
- Bleeding occurs in 10–20% of ulcer patients
- About 80% stop bleeding spontaneously; the remainder have severe bleeding
- Overall mortality rate for ulcer bleeding is 6–10%, higher in the elderly, in those with comorbid medical problems, and in those with nosocomial bleeding, persistent hypotension or shock, bright red blood in the vomitus or nasogastric lavage fluid, or severe coagulopathy

Ulcer perforation

- Perforations develop in 5%
- May be increasing due to use of non-steroidal antiinflammatory drugs and cocaine
- Consider Zollinger-Ellison disease

Ulcer penetration

- Penetration occurs into contiguous structures such as the pancreas, liver, or biliary tree

Gastric outlet obstruction

- Occurs in 2% of patients with ulcer disease causing obstruction of pylorus or duodenum by scarring and inflammation

 ## CLINICAL FINDINGS

SYMPTOMS AND SIGNS

Upper gastrointestinal hemorrhage

- Up to 20% have no antecedent symptoms of pain
- "Coffee grounds" emesis, hematemesis, melena, or hematochezia

Ulcer perforation

- Sudden, severe abdominal pain
- Elderly or debilitated patients and those receiving chronic corticosteroid therapy may have minimal initial symptoms, presenting late with bacterial peritonitis, sepsis, and shock
- Patients appear ill, with a rigid, quiet abdomen and rebound tenderness, hypotension

Ulcer penetration

- Pain severe and constant, may radiate to the back, and is unresponsive to antacids or food
- Physical examination nonspecific

Gastric outlet obstruction

- Early satiety, vomiting, and weight loss
- Early symptoms: epigastric fullness or heaviness after meals
- Later symptoms: vomiting after eating of partially digested food contents
- Chronic obstruction may result in a grossly dilated, atonic stomach, severe weight loss, and malnutrition, dehydration
- Succussion splash in the epigastrium

DIFFERENTIAL DIAGNOSIS

- Upper gastrointestinal bleeding: bleeding esophageal varices, Mallory-Weiss tear, vascular ectasias, Dieulafoy's lesion, malignancy, aortoenteric fistula, hepatic or pancreatic lesions bleeding into pancreatobiliary system
- Severe epigastric pain: esophageal rupture, gastric volvulus, cholecystitis, acute pancreatitis, small bowel obstruction, appendicitis, ureteral colic, splenic rupture

 ## DIAGNOSIS

LABORATORY TESTS

- Upper gastrointestinal hemorrhage: anemia, positive fecal occult blood test
- Ulcer perforation: leukocytosis, and mildly elevated serum amylase
- Ulcer penetration: laboratory tests are nonspecific; mildly elevated serum amylase
- Gastric outlet obstruction: metabolic alkalosis, hypokalemia

IMAGING STUDIES

Ulcer perforation

- Upright or decubitus films of the abdomen reveal free intraperitoneal air in 75%
- Upper gastrointestinal radiography with water-soluble contrast useful
- Abdominal CT increasingly used to establish diagnosis and exclude other causes of abdominal pain

Ulcer penetration

- Barium x-ray studies and endoscopy confirm ulceration but are not diagnostic of an actual penetration

Gastric outlet obstruction

- Endoscopy is preferred diagnostic study

DIAGNOSTIC PROCEDURES

Upper gastrointestinal hemorrhage

- Nasogastric lavage demonstrates "coffee grounds" or bright red blood; lavage fluid negative for blood does not exclude active bleeding from a duodenal ulcer
- Endoscopy should be performed within 12–24 h in virtually all cases
- It is possible to predict which patients are at a higher risk of rebleeding (see When to Admit)

Gastric outlet obstruction

- Nasogastric aspiration evacuation of a large amount (>200 mL) of foul-smelling fluid establishes the diagnosis
- Saline load test

TREATMENT

MEDICATIONS

Upper gastrointestinal hemorrhage

- Antisecretory agents: intravenous proton pump inhibitors or oral proton pump inhibitors, with or without endoscopic therapy, reduce rebleeding, transfusions, and the need for further endoscopic therapy
- Octreotide (100 μg bolus; 50 μg/h) useful in patients in whom endoscopic therapy is unsuccessful in controlling bleeding

Ulcer perforation

- Initial nonoperative management for patients whose onset of symptoms is less than 12 h and whose upper gastrointestinal series with water-soluble contrast medium does not demonstrate leakage
- For patients who are poor operative candidates, fluids, nasogastric suction, antisecretory agents, and broad-spectrum antibiotics
- Up to 40% of ulcer perforations seal spontaneously
- For all others, emergency laparotomy or laparoscopy
- Postoperative treatment of *Helicobacter pylori*

Ulcer penetration

- Intravenous pantoprazole (80 mg IV bolus; 8 mg/h) until able to take oral proton pump inhibitor

Gastric outlet obstruction

- Intravenous isotonic saline and KCl, intravenous pantoprazole (80 mg IV bolus; 8 mg/h) continuous infusion, and nasogastric decompression of the stomach
- Severely malnourished patients should receive total parenteral nutrition

SURGERY

Upper gastrointestinal hemorrhage

- Patients with high-risk endoscopic lesions and those whose condition warrants ICU admission should be evaluated by a surgeon
- <10% of patients treated with hemostatic therapy require surgery

Ulcer perforation

- Closure of the perforation with an omental ("Graham") patch, at emergency laparotomy or laparoscopy

Gastric outlet obstruction

- Vagotomy and either pyloroplasty or antrectomy

THERAPEUTIC PROCEDURES

- Gastric outlet obstruction: upper endoscopy with dilation by hydrostatic balloons achieves success in two-thirds of patients; surgery for those who fail to respond

OUTCOME

PROGNOSIS

Upper gastrointestinal hemorrhage

- The risk of rebleeding or continued bleeding in ulcers with a nonbleeding visible vessel is 50%, and with active bleeding it is 80–90%
- Endoscopic therapy with injection or thermocoagulation for such lesions reduces the risk of rebleeding, the number of transfusions, and the need for subsequent surgery
- Surgical mortality for emergency ulcer bleeding is <6%

Ulcer perforation

- Surgical mortality for emergency ulcer perforation is 5%

WHEN TO ADMIT

Upper gastrointestinal hemorrhage

- Nonbleeding ulcers <2 cm in size with a base that is clean have a <5% chance of rebleeding
- Ulcers that have only a flat red or black spot have a <10% chance of significant rebleeding, those with a firmly adherent clot have a 12–33% rebleeding risk
- Patients who are hemodynamically stable with these findings

PREVENTION

- Upper gastrointestinal hemorrhage: long-term prevention of rebleeding: *H pylori* eradication; or in those with non-*H pylori*–associated ulcers, chronic bedtime dose of an H_2 antagonist or once daily dose of a proton pump inhibitor

EVIDENCE

PRACTICE GUIDELINES

- Buckley M et al: Guidelines for the management of *Helicobacter pylori*-related upper gastrointestinal diseases. Irish Helicobacter Pylori Study Group. Ir J Med Sci 1996;165(Suppl 5):1. [PMID: 8990665]

WEB SITE

- National Digestive Diseases Information Clearinghouse—*H. pylori* and peptic ulcer http://digestive.niddk.nih.gov/ddiseases/pubs/hpylori/index.htm

INFORMATION FOR PATIENTS

- JAMA patient page: Peptic ulcers http://www.ama-assn.org/public/journals/patient/archive/pat1024.htm

REFERENCES

- Donovan A et al: Perforated duodenal ulcer. Arch Surg 1998;133:1166. [PMID: 9820345]
- Jensen D et al: Randomized trial of medical or endoscopic therapy to prevent recurrent ulcer hemorrhage in patients with adherent clots. Gastroenterology 2002;123:407. [PMID: 12145792]
- Lau JY et al: Effect of intravenous omeprazole on recurrent bleeding after endoscopic treatment of bleeding peptic ulcers. N Engl J Med 2000;343:310. [PMID: 10922429]

Kenneth R. McQuaid, MD

Peritonitis, Spontaneous Bacterial

Perianal Abscess & Fistula p. 1151.

 ## KEY FEATURES

ESSENTIALS OF DIAGNOSIS

- Spontaneous bacterial infection of ascitic fluid in the absence of an apparent intraabdominal source of infection
- A history of chronic liver disease and ascites
- Fever and abdominal pain
- Neutrocytic ascites [>250 white blood cells (WBCs)/μL] with neutrophilic predominance

GENERAL CONSIDERATIONS

- Occurs with few exceptions in patients with chronic liver disease
- Affects ~20–30% of cirrhotic patients
- Most common pathogens are enteric gram-negative bacteria (*Escherichia coli, Klebsiella pneumoniae*, enterococcus) or gram-positive bacteria (*Streptococcus pneumoniae*, viridans streptococci)

DEMOGRAPHICS

- Occurs in patients with ascites secondary to portal hypertension, usually with chronic liver disease
- Patients with serum ascites total protein of <1 g/dL at increased risk

 ## CLINICAL FINDINGS

SYMPTOMS AND SIGNS

- Symptoms in 80–90%; asymptomatic in 20%
- Fever and abdominal pain present in two-thirds
- Change in mental status due to exacerbation or precipitation of hepatic encephalopathy
- Signs of chronic liver disease with ascites
- Abdominal tenderness in <50%

DIFFERENTIAL DIAGNOSIS

- Secondary bacterial peritonitis, eg, appendicitis, diverticulitis, perforated peptic ulcer, perforated gallbladder
- Peritoneal carcinomatosis
- Pancreatic ascites
- Tuberculous ascites

 ## DIAGNOSIS

LABORATORY TESTS

- Renal dysfunction, abrupt worsening of renal function
- Ascitic fluid polymorphonuclear neutrophil (PMN) count of >250 cells/μL (neutrocytic ascites) or percentage of PMNs greater than 50–70% of the ascitic fluid WBC count is presumptive evidence of bacterial peritonitis
- Ascitic fluid Gram stain is insensitive
- Ascitic fluid cultures should be obtained by inoculating count blood culture bottles at the bedside
- 10–30% of patients with neutrocytic ascites have negative ascitic bacterial cultures ("culture-negative neutrocytic ascites"), but are presumed nonetheless to have bacterial peritonitis and treated empirically
- Blood cultures occasionally are positive, helping to identify the organism when ascitic fluid is sterile

IMAGING STUDIES

- Abdominal ultrasound helpful in locating optimal site for paracentesis

DIAGNOSTIC PROCEDURES

- Abdominal paracentesis

Peritonitis, Spontaneous Bacterial

TREATMENT

MEDICATIONS

- Patients with neutrocytic ascites are presumed infected and should be started—regardless of symptoms—on antibiotics
- Empirical therapy usually employs a third-generation cephalosporin, such as cefotaxime, 2 g IV Q 8–12 h (depending on renal function)
- If enterococcus infection is suspected, ampicillin is added
- Recommended duration of antibiotic is 5 days or until the ascites fluid PMN count decreases to <250 cells/μL
- Intravenous albumin, 1.5 g/kg on Day 1 and Day 3, is recommended to reduce the development of renal failure and mortality

SURGERY

- Liver transplant is the most effective treatment for spontaneous bacterial peritonitis

OUTCOME

FOLLOW-UP

- Repeat paracentesis at 5 days after start of antibiotic therapy if there is persistent fever, pain, or clinical deterioration

COMPLICATIONS

- Renal failure develops in up to 40% of patients and is a major cause of death

PROGNOSIS

- Mortality of spontaneous bacterial peritonitis exceeds 30%, but if recognized and treated early, mortality is <10%
- Causes of death include liver failure, hepatorenal syndrome, or bleeding complications

WHEN TO REFER

- Patients failing to improve within 3–5 days of initial therapy
- Patients with possible secondary peritonitis, ie, ascites infected by an intraabdominal infection (appendicitis, diverticulitis); should be considered in patients with ascites total protein <1 g/dL, glucose <50 mg/dL, or LDH > upper limit of normal for serum
- Secondary peritonitis should also be considered in patients with polymicrobial infection and patients with high ascitic neutrophil counts (>10,000/μL)

WHEN TO ADMIT

- Symptomatic patients require admission with intravenous antibiotics
- Selected asymptomatic patients may be treated with oral antibiotics with close follow-up

PREVENTION

- Up to 70% of patients who survive an episode of spontaneous bacterial peritonitis will have another episode within 1 year
- Secondary prophylaxis is recommended with norfloxacin, 400 mg PO QD; ciprofloxacin, 750 mg PO once weekly; or trimethoprim-sulfamethoxazole, 1 double-strength tablet PO QD
- Secondary prophylaxis reduces the rate of recurrent infections to <20%
- Primary prophylaxis is also recommended in patients with no history of spontaneous bacterial peritonitis but who are at increased risk of infection

due to low-protein ascites (total ascitic protein <1 g/dL)
- Suggested regimens are ciprofloxacin, 750 mg PO Q week or Septra DS, one tablet PO 5 days per week

EVIDENCE

PRACTICE GUIDELINES

- Mowat C et al: Review article: spontaneous bacterial peritonitis—diagnosis, treatment and prevention. Aliment Pharmacol Ther 2001;15:1851. [PMID: 11736714]
- Soares-Weiser K et al: Evidence based case report. Antibiotic treatment for spontaneous bacterial peritonitis. BMJ 2002;324:100. [PMID: 11786457]

WEB SITE

- Family Practice Handbook—Ascites and spontaneous bacterial peritonitis http://www.vh.org/adult/provider/ familymedicine/FPHandbook/ Chapter05/18-5.html

INFORMATION FOR PATIENTS

- MEDLINEplus—Peritonitis, spontaneous http://www.nlm.nih.gov/medlineplus/ ency/article/000648.htm

REFERENCES

- Garcia-Tsao G: Current management of the complications of cirrhosis and portal hypertension: variceal hemorrhage, ascites, and spontaneous bacterial peritonitis. Gastroenterology 2001;1220: 726. [PMID: 11179247]
- Rimola A et al: Diagnosis, treatment and prophylaxis of spontaneous bacterial peritonitis: a consensus document. J Hepatol 2000;32:142. [PMID: 10673079]
- Soares-Weiser K et al: Evidence based case report. Antibiotic treatment for spontaneous bacterial peritonitis. BMJ 2002;324:100. [PMID: 11786457]

Kenneth R. McQuaid, MD

Personality Disorders

 ## KEY FEATURES

ESSENTIALS OF DIAGNOSIS

- Long history dating back to childhood
- Recurrent maladaptive behavior
- Low self-esteem and lack of confidence
- Minimal introspective ability with a tendency to blame others for all problems
- Major difficulties with interpersonal relationships or society
- Depression with anxiety when maladaptive behavior fails

GENERAL CONSIDERATIONS

- Personality results from the interaction of a genetic substrate with personal drives and outside influences
- Classification of disorder subtypes depends on the predominant symptoms and their severity
- The most severe disorders are those that bring the patient into greatest conflict with society and tend to be classified as antisocial or borderline

Types of personality disorders

- Paranoid
- Schizoid (introverted, withdrawn)
- Obsessive-compulsive
- Histrionic (dependent, immature, seductive, egocentric, emotionally labile)
- Schizotypal (socially isolated, suspicious, eccentric behaviors)
- Narcissistic
- Avoidant (fear rejection, low self-esteem)
- Dependent (passive, unable to make decisions, poor self-esteem)
- Antisocial (selfish, callous, promiscuous, impulsive)
- Borderline (impulsive, unstable and intense relationships, affective instability, suicidal)

 ## CLINICAL FINDINGS

SYMPTOMS AND SIGNS

- See Table 100 (page 1284)

DIFFERENTIAL DIAGNOSIS

- Anxiety disorder, eg, general anxiety disorder
- Major depressive disorder
- Psychotic disorder, eg, schizophrenia
- Substance abuse
- Bipolar disorder
- Personality change due to medical illness, eg, CNS tumor, stroke

 ## DIAGNOSIS

LABORATORY TESTS

- These are mainly clinical diagnoses

IMAGING STUDIES

- Consider head CT if there is an abrupt personality change

TREATMENT

MEDICATIONS

- Antipsychotics may be required for short periods when conditions have temporarily decompensated into transient psychoses. Options include
  - Haloperidol, 2–5 mg PO Q 3–4 h
  - Olanzapine, 2.5–10 mg/day
  - Risperidone, 0.5–2 mg/day with lorazepam, 1–2 mg PO Q 4 h
- Carbamazepine, 400–800 mg daily in divided doses decreases severity of behavioral dyscontrol
- Antidepressants have improved anxiety, depression, and sensitivity to rejection in some borderline patients
- Selective serotonin reuptake inhibitors may have a role in reducing aggressive behavior in impulsive aggressive patients

THERAPEUTIC PROCEDURES

Social

- Day hospitals, halfway houses, and self-help communities use peer pressure to modify self-destructive behavior

Behavioral

- Operant and aversive conditioning use reinforcement and punishment to change behavior
- Dialectical behavioral therapy uses a cognitive-behavioral model to address self-awareness, interpersonal functioning, affective lability, and reactions to stress

Psychological

- Best conducted in group settings and helpful when specific behaviors need to be improved
- Individual therapy should initially be supportive, to restabilize and mobilize defenses
- Long-term introspective therapy may be warranted if the patient has the ability to observe his or her own behavior

 OUTCOME

COMPLICATIONS

- Up to 80% of hospitalized borderline patients make a suicide attempt at some time during treatment
- Drug abuse is frequent among borderline patients

PROGNOSIS

- Antisocial and borderline categories have a guarded prognosis
- Patients with poor outcomes are more likely to have a hisory of parental abuse and a family history of mood disorder
- Mild schizoid or passive-aggressive tendencies have a better prognosis

WHEN TO REFER

- When patient distress or second psychotic illness is present

WHEN TO ADMIT

- Hospitalization is rarely indicated except in cases of suicidal risk

 EVIDENCE

PRACTICE GUIDELINES

- National Guideline Clearinghouse
  http://www.guideline.gov/summary/
  summary.aspx?doc_id=3055&nbr=
  2281&string=personality+disorders
  http://www.guideline.gov/summary/
  summary.aspx?doc_id=1407&nbr=
  665&string=personality+disorders
  http://www.guideline.gov/summary/
  summary.aspx?doc_id=2972&nbr=
  2198&string=PTSD

WEB SITE

- American Psychiatric Association
  http://www.psych.org/

INFORMATION FOR PATIENTS

- National Institutes of Health
  http://www.nlm.nih.gov/medlineplus/
  ency/article/000939.htm

REFERENCES

- Schultz S et al: Olanzapine safety and efficacy in patients with borderline personality disorder and comorbid dysthymia. Biol Psychiatry 1999;46: 1429. [PMID: 10578457]
- Swenson CR et al: Implementing dialectical behavioral therapy. Psychiatr Serv 2002;53:171.

Stuart J. Eisendrath, MD
Jonathan E. Lichtmacher, MD

Pertussis, *Bordetella*

 ## KEY FEATURES

ESSENTIALS OF DIAGNOSIS

- Predominantly in infants under age 2 years
- Adults are an important reservoir of infection
- Two-week prodromal catarrhal stage of malaise, cough, coryza, and anorexia
- Paroxysmal cough ending in a high-pitched inspiratory "whoop"
- Absolute lymphocytosis, often striking; culture confirms diagnosis

GENERAL CONSIDERATIONS

- An acute infection of the respiratory tract caused by *Bordetella pertussis*, a gram-negative coccobacillus
- Infection is transmitted by respiratory droplets
- Neither immunization nor disease confers lasting immunity to pertussis
- Adults are an important reservoir of this highly contagious disease
- The diagnosis often is not considered in adults, who may not have atypical presentation. Cough persisting more than 2 weeks is suggestive of pertussis

DEMOGRAPHICS

- This disease causes high morbidity and mortality in many countries
- In the United States, 5000–7000 cases are reported each year
- Incidence of pertussis has increased steadily since the 1980s

 ## CLINICAL FINDINGS

SYMPTOMS AND SIGNS

- Symptoms of classic pertussis last about 6 weeks and are divided into three consecutive stages
- The catarrhal stage is characterized by its insidious onset, with lacrimation, sneezing, and coryza, anorexia, and malaise, and a hacking night cough that tends to become diurnal
- The paroxysmal stage is characterized by bursts of rapid, consecutive coughs followed by a deep, high-pitched inspiration (whoop)
- The convalescent stage usually begins 4 weeks after onset of the illness with a decrease in the frequency and severity of paroxysms of cough

DIFFERENTIAL DIAGNOSIS

- Viral or bacterial pneumonia
- Asthma
- Other causes of chronic cough in adults, eg, postnasal drip, gastroesophageal reflux disease, tuberculosis, *Mycobacterium avium* complex
- Bronchiolitis, eg, respiratory syncytial virus (children)
- Croup (children)

 ## DIAGNOSIS

LABORATORY TESTS

- The white blood cell count is usually 15,000–20,000/μL (rarely, as high as 50,000/μL or more), 60–80% of which are lymphocytes
- The diagnosis is established by isolating the organism from nasopharyngeal culture. A special medium (eg, Bordet-Gengou agar) must be requested

TREATMENT

MEDICATIONS

- Erythromycin, 500 mg four times a day orally for 10 days, shortens the duration of carriage. It also may diminish the severity of coughing paroxysms
- Azithromycin, 500 mg orally for 3 days, or clarithromycin, 500 mg orally twice daily for 7 days, is probably as effective as erythromycin and likely to be better tolerated
- Active immunization with pertussis vaccine is recommended for all infants, usually combined with diphtheria and tetanus toxoids (DTP) (Table 127, page 1310)

 OUTCOME

WHEN TO REFER

- Pertussis is a disease that should be reported to the public health authorities

WHEN TO ADMIT

- Adults must be admitted if respiratory insufficiency (eg, hypoxia) is present

PREVENTION

- Immunizations (Table 127, page 1310)
- Pertussis vaccine is recommended for all infants, combined with DTP
- Infants and susceptible adults with significant exposure should receive prophylaxis with erythromycin (40 mg/kg/day, up to 2 g/day, for 10 days)
- Booster doses of pertussis vaccine have not been recommended after age 6 except in outbreaks

 EVIDENCE

PRACTICE GUIDELINES

- National Guideline Clearinghouse
  http://www.guideline.gov/summary/
  summary.aspx?doc_id=839&nbr=60&st
  ring=pertussis
  http://www.guideline.gov/summary/
  summary.aspx?doc_id=3376&nbr=
  2602&string=pertussis

WEB SITES

- CDC—Division of Bacterial and Mycotic Diseases
  http://www.cdc.gov/ncidod/dbmd/
- Karolinska Institute—Directory of Bacterial Infections and Mycoses
  http://www.mic.ki.se/Diseases/c1.html

INFORMATION FOR PATIENTS

- JAMA patient page: Immunizations. JAMA 1999;282:102. [PMID: 10404918]
- American Medical Association
  http://www.medem.com/medlb/article_
  detaillb.cfm?article_ID=
  ZZZPWVII1AC&sub_cat=286

REFERENCES

- Cherry JD: Epidemiological, clinical, and laboratory aspects of pertussis in adults. Clin Infect Dis 1999;28(Suppl 2):S112. [PMID: 10447028]
- Hewlett EL: A commentary on the pathogenesis of pertussis. Clin Infect Dis 1999;28(Suppl 2):S94. [PMID: 10447025]

Henry F. Chambers, MD

Pharyngitis & Tonsillitis

 KEY FEATURES

ESSENTIALS OF DIAGNOSIS

- Sore throat
- Fever
- Anterior cervical adenopathy
- Tonsillar exudate
- Focus is to treat group A β-hemolytic streptococcus infection to prevent rheumatic sequaelae

GENERAL CONSIDERATIONS

- Group A β-hemolytic streptococci (*Streptococcus pyogenes*) are the most common bacterial cause of exudative pharyngitis
- Transmission is by droplets of infected secretions
- The main concern is to determine whether the etiology is group A β-hemolytic streptococcal infection (GABHS), because of the complications of rheumatic fever and glomerular nephritis
- A second public health policy concern is to reduce the extraordinary cost (both in dollars and in the development of antibiotic-resistant *Streptococcus pneumoniae* in the United States associated with unnecessary and unrecommended antibiotic use
- Group A streptococci producing erythrogenic toxin may cause scarlet fever rashes in susceptible persons
- About one-third of patients with infectious mononucleosis have secondary streptococcal tonsillitis, requiring treatment
- Ampicillin should routinely be avoided if mononucleosis is suspected because it induces a rash

DEMOGRAPHICS

- Pharyngitis and tonsillitis account for over 10% of all office visits to primary care clinicians and 50% of outpatient antibiotic use

 CLINICAL FINDINGS

SYMPTOMS AND SIGNS

- **Centor diagnostic criteria**
  - Fever over 38°C
  - Tender anterior cervical adenopathy
  - Lack of a cough
  - Pharyngotonsillar exudate
- Sore throat may be severe, with odynophagia, tender adenopathy, and a scarlatiniform rash
- Hoarseness, cough, and coryza are not suggestive of this disease
- Marked lymphadenopathy and a shaggy white-purple tonsillar exudate, often extending into the nasopharynx, suggest mononucleosis, especially if present in a young adult

DIFFERENTIAL DIAGNOSIS

- Viral pharyngitis
- Epstein–Barr virus/infectious mononucleosis
- Primary HIV infection
- Candidiasis
- Necrotizing ulcerative gingivostomatitis (Vincent's fusospirochetal disease)
- Retropharyngeal abscess
- Diphtheria
- *Neisseria gonorrhoeae*
- Mycoplasma
- Anaerobic streptococci
- *Corynebacterium haemolyticum*
- Epiglottitis

 DIAGNOSIS

LABORATORY TESTS

- The presence of the four Centor diagnostic criteria strongly suggests GABHS, and some would treat regardless of laboratory results
- When three of the four are present, laboratory sensitivity of rapid antigen testing exceeds 90%
- When only one criterion is present, GABHS is unlikely
- The sensitivity of current GABHS rapid antigen tests is now excellent, exceeding 90% in appropriately selected patients
- Routine throat cultures are not needed
- Leukocytosis with neutrophil predominance is common

 TREATMENT

MEDICATIONS

- A single injection of benzathine penicillin or procaine penicillin, 1.2 million units, is optimal treatment, but the injections are painful; if compliance is an issue, it may be the best choice
- Analgesics and antiinflammatory agents, such as aspirin or acetaminophen

Oral antibiotics

- Penicillin V potassium (250 mg orally three times daily or 500 mg twice daily for 10 days) or cefuroxime axetil (250 mg orally twice daily for 5–10 days) is effective
- The efficacy of a 5-day regimen of penicillin V appears to be similar to that of a 10-day course, with a 94% clinical response rate and an 84% eradication rate
- Erythromycin (500 mg orally four times a day) or azithromycin (500 mg once daily for 3 days) can be used for the penicillin-allergic patient

Pharyngitis & Tonsillitis

- Macrolides are less effective than penicillins
  - The prevalence of macrolide resistance among strains of group A streptococci may be as high as 25–40%
  - Macrolides are considered second-line agents because of the risk of treatment failure
- Macrolide-resistant strains almost always are susceptible to clindamycin (a 10-day course of 300 mg three times a day orally), which is an alternative for serious infections
- Cephalosporins are somewhat more effective than penicillin in producing bacteriological cures; 5-day administration has been successful for cefpodoxime and cefuroxime

For treatment failures

- Second course of treatment with the same drug
- Alternatives to penicillin include cefuroxime and other cephalosporins, dicloxacillin (which is β-lactamase resistant), and amoxicillin with clavulanate
- Erythromycin resistance—with failure rates of about 25%—is an increasing problem
- In cases of severe penicillin allergy, cephalosporins should be avoided as the cross-reaction is common (8% or more)

SURGERY

- Patients with recurrent abscesses should have their tonsils removed

THERAPEUTIC PROCEDURES

Treatment strategies based on the four Centor criteria

- Test with GABHS rapid antigen tests patients who satisfy two or more criteria, and treat only those with positive results
- Test with current GABHS rapid antigen tests patients who satisfy two or three criteria, and treat those with positive results and all patients who satisfy all four criteria without testing them
- Or test nobody and treat all who satisfy three or four criteria

Ancillary treatment

- Salt water gargling may be soothing
- In severe cases, anesthetic gargles and lozenges (eg, benzocaine) may provide additional symptomatic relief

OUTCOME

FOLLOW-UP

- Patients who have had rheumatic fever should be treated with a continuous course of antimicrobial prophylaxis (erythromycin, 250 mg orally twice daily, or penicillin G, 500 mg orally daily) for at least 5 years

COMPLICATIONS

- Low (10–20%) incidence of treatment failures (positive culture after treatment despite symptomatic resolution) and recurrences

Suppurative

- Sinusitis, otitis media, mastoiditis, peritonsillar abscess, and suppuration of cervical lymph nodes

Nonsuppurative

- Rheumatic fever may follow recurrent episodes of pharyngitis beginning 1–4 weeks after the onset of symptoms
- Glomerulonephritis follows a single infection with a nephritogenic strain of streptococcus group A (eg, types 4, 12, 2, 49, and 60), more commonly on the skin than in the throat, and begins 1–3 weeks after the onset of the infection
- Toxic shock syndrome
- Scarlet fever

WHEN TO REFER

- Peritonsillar abscess

WHEN TO ADMIT

- Occasionally, odynophagia is so intense that hospitalization for intravenous hydration and antibiotics is necessary
- Suspected or known epiglottitis

PROGNOSIS

- Streptococcal pharyngitis usually resolves after a week
- Spontaneous resolution of symptoms without treatment still leaves the risk of rheumatic complications

EVIDENCE

PRACTICE GUIDELINES

- National Guideline Clearinghouse http://www.guideline.gov/summary/summary.aspx?doc_id=3160&nbr=2386&string=pharyngitis http://www.guideline.gov/summary/summary.aspx?doc_id=2957&nbr=2183&string=pharyngitis http://www.guideline.gov/summary/summary.aspx?doc_id=1841&nbr=1067&string=tonsillitis

WEB SITES

- Ear, Nose, and Throat Information Center http://www.netdoor.com/entinfo/
- Otolaryngology Resources on the Internet http://www.bcm.tmc.edu/oto/othersa.html

INFORMATION FOR PATIENTS

- JAMA patient page: Strep throat. JAMA 2000;284:2964. [PMID: 11147992]
- American Academy of Otolaryngology-Head and Neck Surgery. Sore throat http://www.entlink.org/healthinfo/throat/sore_throat.cfm

REFERENCES

- Cooper RJ et al: Principles of appropriate antibiotic use for acute pharyngitis in adults: background. Ann Intern Med 2001;134:509. [PMID: 11255530]
- Gonzales R et al: Principles of appropriate antibiotic use for treatment of acute respiratory tract infections in adults: background, specific aims, and methods. Ann Intern Med 2001;134:479. [PMID: 11255524]
- Neuner JM et al: Diagnosis and management of adults with pharyngitis. Ann Intern Med 2003;139:113

Robert K. Jackler, MD
Michael J. Kaplan, MD

Pheochromocytoma

 KEY FEATURES

ESSENTIALS OF DIAGNOSIS

- "Attacks" of headache, perspiration, palpitations
- Hypertension, frequently sustained but often paroxysmal, especially during surgery or obstetric delivery
- Attacks of nausea, abdominal pain, chest pain, weakness, dyspnea, tremor, visual disturbance
- Anxiety, tremor, weight loss, or heat intolerance
- Elevated urinary catecholamines or metanephrines. Normal serum tetraiodothyronine (T_4) and thyroid-stimulating hormone (TSH)

GENERAL CONSIDERATIONS

- Hypertension caused by excessive secretion of norepinephrine or neuropeptide Y
- Tumor located in either or both adrenals or anywhere along sympathetic chain
- "Rule of tens": 10% in children; 10–15% familial; 10% without hypertension; 10% extraadrenal, and of those, 10% extraabdominal, location; 10% bilateral adrenal location (more frequent in familial cases); 10% metastatic at diagnosis. Metastases later discovered in another 5%
- Familial pheochromocytomas bilateral (70%) and associated with calcitonin-secreting medullary thyroid carcinoma and hyperparathyroidism (MEN-2a); medullary thyroid carcinoma and syndrome of multiple mucosal neuromas (MEN-2b); neurofibromatosis (Recklinghausen's disease); von Hippel-Lindau disease (hemangiomas of retina and CNS; pancreatic cysts; renal cysts, adenomas and carcinomas); islet cell tumors (rare)

DEMOGRAPHICS

- Pheochromocytomas rare, found in <0.3% of hypertensive patients
- Incidence higher with moderate to severe hypertension
- Annually, ~2 cases per million population diagnosed clinically, but 250–1300 cases per million in autopsy series, indicating most cases are not diagnosed during life

CLINICAL FINDINGS

SYMPTOMS AND SIGNS

- Some normotensive and asymptomatic
- Typically causes attacks of severe headache (80%), perspiration (70%), and palpitations (60%)
- May cause anxiety (50%), sense of impending doom, or tremor (40%)
- Hypertension in 90%; paroxysms of severe hypertension in 50%
- Vasomotor changes during attack include mottled cyanosis and facial pallor; facial flushing may occur as attack subsides
- May have angina, abdominal pain, vomiting, increased appetite, and weight loss
- May have cardiac enlargement; postural tachycardia, postural hypotension; mild elevation of basal body temperature
- Retinal hemorrhage or cerebrovascular hemorrhage occurs occasionally
- Other possible findings: psychosis or confusion, seizures, hyperglycemia, bradycardia, constipation, paresthesias, Raynaud's phenomenon, pulmonary edema and heart failure, syncope, abdominal discomfort due to mass
- Pheochromocytomas may secrete other peptides causing Cushing's syndrome (ACTH), erythrocytosis (erythropoietin), or hypercalcemia (parathyroid-related peptide; PTHrP)

DIFFERENTIAL DIAGNOSIS

- Other cause of secondary hypertension, eg, primary hyperaldosteronism, Cushing's syndrome, renal artery stenosis
- Panic attacks
- Thyrotoxicosis
- Acute intermittent porphyria
- Carcinoid syndrome
- Paroxysmal tachycardia
- Preeclampsia-eclampsia

DIAGNOSIS

LABORATORY TESTS

- TSH, free T_4, and triiodothyronine (T_3) normal
- WBC and glucose elevations common
- A 24-h urine specimen is collected with acid preservative and assayed for total and fractional catecholamines, metanephrines, and creatinine
- 24-h urine or "spot" urine: usually >2.2 μg total metanephrine per mg creatinine and >135 μg total catecholamines per gram creatinine
- Urinary total metanephrines has test sensitivity of 97%. Urine vanillylmandelic acid (VMA) has sensitivity of 89%. VMA not usually required
- Some drugs, foods, medical conditions, and stress interfere with assays
  - Drugs: acetaminophen, amphetamines, bronchodilators, captopril, cocaine, contrast media (meglumine, acetrizoate, or diatrizoate), cimetidine, codeine, decongestants, levodopa, labetalol, metoclopramide
  - Foods: bananas, caffeine, coffee
  - Conditions: acute illness, vigorous exercise, severe emotion, carcinoid, brain lesions, renal failure
- ~10% of hypertensive patients have misleadingly elevated level of tests
- High plasma and urine catecholamine and metanephrine levels during or following attack are sensitive tests for pheochromocytoma associated with paroxysmal hypertension. Proper collection essential
- Serum chromogranin A elevated in 90% and can serve as tumor marker
- Genetic testing for patients or relatives suspected of having von Hippel-Lindau disease, MEN-2a or -2b, or familial paraganglioma

IMAGING STUDIES

- Thin-section CT of adrenals. Glucagon and IV contrast agents should not be used during scanning, since they can provoke hypertensive crisis; especially with uncontrolled hypertension
- MRI does not require IV contrast; lack of radiation during pregnancy
- CT and MRI have sensitivity of ~90% for adrenal pheochromocytoma and 95% for adrenal tumors >0.5 cm
- Incidental adrenal adenomas (2–4% of scans) can be misleading
- If no adrenal tumor found, CT scan extended to abdomen, pelvis, and chest
- Whole-body ^{123}I metaiodobenzylguanidine (MIBG) scan can localize tumors with 85% sensitivity and 99% specificity
- Drugs reducing MIBG uptake by pheochromocytoma: tricyclic antidepressants, cyclobenzaprine (for 6 weeks); amphetamines, phenylpropanolamine, phenothiazines, haloperidol, thiothixene, diet pills, nasal decongestants, cocaine (for 2 weeks); selective serotonin reuptake inhibitors (for an unknown duration)

TREATMENT

MEDICATIONS

- Preoperative α-adrenergic blockade: phenoxybenzamine, 10 mg PO Q 12 h, increasing about every 3 days until hypertension controlled. Usual maintenance dose is 20–60 mg PO BID. Optimal blockade achieved when supine BP <160/90 mm Hg and standing BP >80/45 mm Hg
- Calcium channel blockers also effective and better tolerated than α-blockers
- Propranolol, 10–40 mg PO QID, to control tachycardia and other arrhythmias after BP is controlled
- Maintain BP control at least 4–7 days or until optimal cardiac status established
- Preoperative autotransfusion and generous intraoperative IV fluid reduces risk of postresection hypotension
- Postoperative shock treated with IV saline or colloid and high doses of IV norepinephrine
- Metyrosine, 250 mg PO QID, increase daily by increments of 250–500 mg to maximum 4 g/day to reduce catecholamine synthesis for inoperable or metastatic tumors
- Combination chemotherapy (eg, cyclophosphamide, vincristine, and dacarbazine) for metastatic pheochromocytomas

SURGERY

- Laparoscopic removal of tumor or tumors is treatment of choice
- Open laparotomy for large tumors
- Nicardipine, 2–6 μg/kg/min, or nitroprusside, 0.5–10 μg/kg/min, continuous IV infusion, for severe intraoperative hypertension
- Atenolol (1 mg boluses), esmolol, or lidocaine IV for tachyarrhythmias

THERAPEUTIC PROCEDURES

- ^{131}I-MIBG for metastatic pheochromocytomas

OUTCOME

FOLLOW-UP

- Recheck urinary catecholamine levels 2 weeks after surgery to exclude multiple or metastatic tumors
- Check ^{131}I-MIBG whole-body scan 2–3 months postop
- Thereafter, recheck symptoms and BP regularly
- Lifetime clinical surveillance for recurrence or metastases required
- Follow chromogranin A if elevated before surgery

COMPLICATIONS

- Complications of severe hypertension
- Catecholamine-induced cardiomyopathy
- Sudden death from cardiac arrhythmia
- Hypertensive crises with sudden blindness or stroke
- Decongestants, bladder catheterization, needle biopsy, anesthesia, intubation, unopposed β-blockade, and surgical manipulation of tumor may induce hypertensive paroxysms
- Metyrosine causes CNS side effects and crystalluria; hydration must be ensured

PROGNOSIS

- Malignancy determined by whether metastases are present or develop
- Complete cure is usually achieved if tumor is successfully removed before irreparable cardiovascular damage
- In about 25%, hypertension persists or returns in spite of successful surgery
- Surgical mortality rate <3%
- Death may occur from hypertensive crisis induced by intravenous contrast, glucagons, or needle biopsy
- Patients with metastatic pheochromocytoma have 5-year survival rate of 50%; however, prolonged survival does occur

PREVENTION

- D₅W infusion postoperatively to prevent hypoglycemia

EVIDENCE

PRACTICE GUIDELINES

- Bravo EL: Pheochromocytoma: an approach to antihypertensive management. Ann NY Acad Sci 2002;970:1. [PMID: 12381537]

INFORMATION FOR PATIENTS

- National Cancer Institute— Pheochromocytoma http://www.cancer.gov/cancerinfo/pdq/treatment/pheochromocytoma/patient/

REFERENCES

- Lenders JW et al: New advances in the biochemical diagnosis of pheochromocytoma: moving beyond catecholamines. Ann NY Acad Sci 2002;970:29. [PMID: 12381539]
- Walther MM: New therapeutic and surgical approaches for sporadic and hereditary pheochromocytoma. Ann NY Acad Sci 2002;970:41. [PMID: 12381540]

Paul A. Fitzgerald, MD

Photodermatitis

 KEY FEATURES

ESSENTIALS OF DIAGNOSIS

- Painful or pruritic erythema, edema, or vesiculation on sun-exposed surfaces: the face, neck, hands, and "V" of the chest
- Inner upper eyelids spared, as is the area under the chin

GENERAL CONSIDERATIONS

- Acute or chronic inflammatory skin reaction due to hypersensitivity to sunlight or other sources of actinic rays, photosensitization of the skin by certain drugs, or idiosyncrasy to actinic light as seen in some constitutional disorders, including the porphyrias and many hereditary disorders (phenylketonuria, xeroderma pigmentosum, and others)
- Contact photosensitivity may occur with perfumes, antiseptics, and other chemicals
- Photodermatitis is manifested most commonly as phototoxicity—a tendency for the individual to sunburn more easily than usual—or, more rarely, as photoallergy, a true immunological reaction that often presents with papular or vesicular lesions

Etiology

- Medications: phenothiazines, sulfones, chlorothiazides, griseofulvin, sulfonylureas, nonsteroidal antiinflammatory drugs, antibiotics (eg, tetracycline)
- Systemic disease: systemic lupus erythematosus, porphyria cutanea tarda, variegate porphyria
- Polymorphous light eruption (idiopathic)

 CLINICAL FINDINGS

SYMPTOMS AND SIGNS

- See Table 7 (page 1202)
- Acute inflammatory skin reaction, which if severe enough, is accompanied by pain, fever, gastrointestinal symptoms, malaise, and even prostration, but this is very rare
- Erythema, edema, and possibly vesiculation and oozing on exposed surfaces
- Peeling of the epidermis and pigmentary changes often result
- Inner upper eyelids spared, as is the area under the chin
- The lips are commonly involved in hereditary polymorphous light eruption, a disorder seen in persons of Native American descent

DIFFERENTIAL DIAGNOSIS

- Contact dermatitis

 DIAGNOSIS

LABORATORY TESTS

- The key to diagnosis is localization of the rash to photoexposed areas, though these eruptions may become generalized with time to involve even photoprotected areas
- Blood and urine tests are not helpful in diagnosis unless porphyria cutanea tarda is suggested by the presence of blistering, scarring, milia (white cysts 1 –2 mm in diameter) and skin fragility of the dorsal hands, and facial hypertrichosis

TREATMENT

MEDICATIONS

- Drugs should be suspected in cases of photoallergy even if the particular medication (such as hydrochlorothiazide) has been used for months

Local measures

- Mid-potency to high-potency topical steroids are of limited benefit in phototoxic reactions but may help in polymorphous light eruption and photoallergic reactions

Systemic measures

- Aspirin may have some value for fever and pain of acute sunburn, as prostaglandins appear to play a pathogenetic role in the early erythema
- Systemic corticosteroids in doses as described for acute contact dermatitis may be required for severe photosensitivity reactions
- Immunosuppressives may be indicated for severe photosensitivity, such as azathioprine, in the range of 50–150 mg/day; or cyclosporine, 3–5 mg/kg/day

THERAPEUTIC PROCEDURES

- When the eruption is vesicular or weepy, treatment is similar to that of any acute dermatitis, using cooling and soothing wet dressing

 OUTCOME

PROGNOSIS

- The most common phototoxic reactions are usually benign and self-limiting except when the burn is severe or when it occurs as an associated finding in a more serious disorder
- Polymorphous light eruption and some cases of photoallergy can persist for years

WHEN TO REFER

- If there is a question about the diagnosis, if recommended therapy is ineffective, or specialized treatment is necessary

PREVENTION

- While sunscreens are useful agents in general and should be used by persons with photosensitivity, patients may react to such low amounts of energy that sunscreens alone may not be sufficient
- Sunscreens with an SPF of 30–50, usually containing avobenzone (Parasol 1789), titanium dioxide, and micronized zinc oxide, are especially useful in patients with photoallergic dermatitis

EVIDENCE

PRACTICE GUIDELINES

- National Guideline Clearinghouse http://www.guideline.gov/summary/summary.aspx?doc_id=1308&nbr=557&string=photodermatitis

WEB SITES

- American Academy of Dermatology http://www.aad.org
- Dermatology Handbook for Family Practice from the University of Iowa http://www.vh.org/Providers/ClinRef/FPHandbook/17.html

INFORMATION FOR PATIENTS

- American Academy of Dermatology http://www.aad.org/Kids/sunsafety.html
- Centers for Disease Control and Prevention http://www.cdc.gov/ChooseYourCover/qanda.htm

REFERENCES

- Millard TP et al: Photodermatoses in the elderly. Clin Geriatr Med 2001;17:691,vi.
- Roelandts R: The diagnosis of photosensitivity. Arch Dermatol 2000;136:1152.

Timothy G. Berger, MD

Pityriasis Rosea

 KEY FEATURES

ESSENTIALS OF DIAGNOSIS

- Oval, fawn-colored, scaly eruption following cleavage lines of trunk
- Herald patch precedes eruption by 1–2 weeks
- Occasional pruritus

GENERAL CONSIDERATIONS

- Common mild, acute inflammatory disease that is 50% more common in females
- The eruption usually lasts 4–8 weeks and heals without scarring

DEMOGRAPHICS

- Young adults are principally affected, mostly in the spring or fall

 CLINICAL FINDINGS

SYMPTOMS AND SIGNS

- See Table 7 (page 1202)
- Diagnosis is made by finding one or more classic lesions
- The lesions consist of oval, fawn-colored plaques up to 2 cm in diameter; the centers of the lesions have a crinkled or "cigarette paper" appearance and a collarette scale, ie, a thin bit of scale that is bound at the periphery and free in the center
- Only a few lesions in the eruption may have this characteristic appearance
- Lesions follow cleavage lines on the trunk (so-called Christmas tree pattern), and the proximal portions of the extremities are often involved
- Herald patch precedes eruption by 1–2 weeks
- Pruritus, if present, is usually mild
- Variants that affect the flexures (axillae and groin), so-called inverse pityriasis rosea, and papular variants, especially in black patients, also occur

DIFFERENTIAL DIAGNOSIS

- Secondary syphilis
- Tinea corporis (body ringworm)
- Seborrheic dermatitis
- Tinea versicolor (pityriasis versicolor)
- Lichen planus
- Psoriasis
- Nummular eczema
- Drug eruption
- Viral exanthem

 DIAGNOSIS

LABORATORY TESTS

- Based on appearance of skin lesions
- A serological test for syphilis should be performed if at least a few perfectly typical lesions are not present and especially if there are palmar and plantar or mucous membrane lesions or adenopathy, features that are suggestive of secondary syphilis
- Tinea corporis may present with red, slightly scaly plaques, but rarely are there more than a few lesions of tinea corporis compared to the many lesions of pityriasis rosea; a scraping of scale for a KOH test will rapidly make the diagnosis of tinea

TREATMENT

 OUTCOME

 EVIDENCE

MEDICATIONS

- See Table 6 (page 1199)
- The most effective management consists of daily UVB treatments for a week, or prednisone as used for contact dermatitis; topical steroids of medium strength (triamcinolone 0.1%) may also be used if pruritus is bothersome
- Oral erythromycin for 14 days was reported to clear 73% of patients within 2 weeks (compared with none of the patients on placebo)

THERAPEUTIC PROCEDURES

- Often requires no treatment
- In Asians, Hispanics, or blacks, in whom lesions may remain hyperpigmented for some time, more aggressive management may be indicated

WHEN TO REFER

- If there is a question about the diagnosis, if recommended therapy is ineffective, or if specialized treatment is necessary

WEB SITES

- American Academy of Dermatology
  http://www.aad.org
- Dermatology Handbook for Family Practice from the University of Iowa
  http://www.vh.org/Providers/ClinRef/FPHandbook/17.html

INFORMATION FOR PATIENTS

- American Academy of Dermatology
  http://www.aad.org/pamphlets/pityrias.html
- National Institutes of Health
  http://www.nlm.nih.gov/medlineplus/ency/article/000871.htm

REFERENCES

- Blauvelt A: Skin diseases associated with human herpesvirus 6, 7, and 8 infection. J Investig Dermatol Symp Proc 2001;6:197.
- Eslick GD: Atypical pityriasis rosea or psoriasis guttata? Early examination is the key to a correct diagnosis. Int J Dermatol 2002;41:788.

Timothy G. Berger, MD

Plague

 KEY FEATURES

ESSENTIALS OF DIAGNOSIS

- History of exposure to rodents in endemic area
- Sudden onset of high fever, malaise, muscular pains, and prostration
- Axillary or inguinal lymphadenitis (bubo)
- Bacteremia, pneumonitis, and meningitis may occur
- Positive smear and culture from bubo and positive blood culture

GENERAL CONSIDERATIONS

- An infection of wild rodents with *Yersinia pestis*, a small bipolar-staining gram-negative rod
- It is transmitted among rodents and to humans by the bites of fleas or from contact with infected animals
- If a plague victim develops pneumonia, the infection can be transmitted by droplets to other individuals
- The incubation period is 2–10 days
- Because of its extreme virulence, its potential for dissemination and person-to-person transmission, and efforts to develop the organism as an agent of biowarfare, plague bacillus is considered a high-priority agent for bioterrorism
- Following the flea bite, the organisms spread through the lymphatics to the lymph nodes, which become greatly enlarged (bubo). They may then reach the bloodstream to involve all organs

DEMOGRAPHICS

- It is endemic in California, Arizona, Nevada, and New Mexico

 CLINICAL FINDINGS

SYMPTOMS AND SIGNS

- The onset is sudden, with high fever, malaise, tachycardia, intense headache, and severe myalgias
- The patient appears profoundly ill. Delirium may ensue
- If pneumonia develops, tachypnea, productive cough, blood-tinged sputum, and cyanosis also occur
- Signs of meningitis may develop
- A pustule or ulcer at the site of inoculation and lymphangitis may be observed
- Axillary, inguinal, or cervical lymph nodes become enlarged and tender and may suppurate and drain
- With hematogenous spread, the patient may rapidly become toxic and comatose, with purpuric spots (black plague) appearing on the skin
- Primary plague pneumonia is a fulminant pneumonitis with bloody, frothy sputum and sepsis

DIFFERENTIAL DIAGNOSIS

- Tularemia
- Lymphadenopathy of extremity due to bacterial infection
- Genital lymphadenopathy due to lymphogranuloma venereum, syphilis
- Typhoid fever
- Influenza
- Rickettsial disease, eg, epidemic typhus, Q fever
- Anthrax
- Other bacterial pneumonia
- Hantavirus pulmonary syndrome
- Sepsis due to other causes

 DIAGNOSIS

LABORATORY TESTS

- The plague bacillus may be found in smears from aspirates of buboes examined with Gram's stain
- Cultures from bubo aspirate or pus and blood are positive but may grow slowly
- In convalescing patients, an antibody titer rise may be demonstrated by agglutination tests

TREATMENT

MEDICATIONS

- Therapy should be started immediately once plague is suspected
- Either streptomycin (the agent with which there is greatest experience), 1 g every 12 h intravenously, or gentamicin, administered as a 2 mg/kg loading dose, then 1.7 mg/kg every 8 h intravenously, is effective
- Alternatively, doxycycline, 100 mg twice daily orally or intravenously, may be used
- The duration of therapy is 10 days

THERAPEUTIC PROCEDURES

- Patients with plague pneumonia are placed in strict respiratory isolation

OUTCOME

PROGNOSIS

- Pneumonia or meningitis is usually fatal

WHEN TO REFER

- All suspected cases should be referred to an infectious disease specialist
- All cases must be reported to the public health authorities

WHEN TO ADMIT

- All suspected or known cases

PREVENTION

- Drug prophylaxis may provide temporary protection for persons exposed to plague, particularly by the respiratory route. Tetracycline hydrochloride, 500 mg orally once or twice daily for 5 days, is effective
- The efficacy of plague vaccines—both live and killed—is not clearly established

EVIDENCE

PRACTICE GUIDELINES

- National Guideline Clearinghouse http://www.guideline.gov/summary/summary.aspx?doc_id=2983&nbr=2209&string=plague

WEB SITES

- CDC—Division of Bacterial and Mycotic Diseases http://www.cdc.gov/ncidod/dbmd/
- Karolinska Institute—Directory of Bacterial Infections and Mycoses http://www.mic.ki.se/Diseases/c1.html

INFORMATION FOR PATIENTS

- CDC Bioterrorism http://www.bt.cdc.gov/agent/plague/index.asp
- National Insitute of Allergy and Infectious Diseases http://www.niaid.nih.gov/factsheets/plague.htm

REFERENCE

- Koornhof HJ et al: Yersiniosis. II: The pathogenesis of *Yersinia* infections. Eur J Clin Microbiol Infect Dis 1999;18:87. [PMID: 10219573]

Henry F. Chambers, MD

Pleural Effusion

 KEY FEATURES

ESSENTIALS OF DIAGNOSIS

- May be asymptomatic; chest pain seen in the setting of pleuritis, trauma, or infection
- Dyspnea is common with large effusions
- Dullness to percussion and decreased breath sounds over the effusion
- Radiographic evidence of pleural effusion
- Diagnostic findings on thoracentesis

GENERAL CONSIDERATIONS

- Pleural fluid is produced at 0.01 mL/kg/body weight/h; a normal volume in the pleural space is 5–15 mL
- Transudative effusions (see Laboratory Tests) occur in the absence of pleural disease; 90% of cases result from congestive heart failure
- Exudative effusions are most commonly due to pneumonia (parapneumonic effusions) and malignancy (malignant effusions)
- Analysis of pleural fluid allows for identification of the pathophysiological process leading to accumulation of pleural fluid
  - Increased production due to increased hydrostatic or decreased oncotic pressures (transudates)
  - Increased production due to abnormal capillary permeability (exudates)
  - Decreased lymphatic clearance of fluid (exudates)
  - Infection in the pleural space (empyema)
  - Bleeding into the pleural space (hemothorax)
- A definitive diagnosis is made through cytology or identification of causative organism in 25% of cases
- In 50–60% of cases, classification of the effusion leads to a presumptive diagnosis

 CLINICAL FINDINGS

SYMPTOMS AND SIGNS

- Dyspnea, cough, or chest pain with respirations
- Symptoms are more common in patients with underlying cardiopulmonary disease
- Large effusions are more likely to be symptomatic
- Bronchial breath sounds and egophony above the effusion are caused by compressive atelectasis
- Massive effusions may cause contralateral shift of the trachea and bulging of intercostal spaces
- A pleural friction rub indicates infarction or pleuritis

DIFFERENTIAL DIAGNOSIS

- Atelectasis
- Chronic pleural thickening
- Lobar consolidation
- Subdiaphragmatic process
- Table 36 (page 1230)

DIAGNOSIS

LABORATORY TESTS

- See Table 37 (page 1231)
- Pleural fluid should be sent for protein, glucose, LDH, cell count, Gram stain, and culture
- Grossly purulent fluid signifies empyema; Gram stain and culture are confirmatory
- Exudates have one of the following
  - Pleural fluid protein/serum protein >0.5
  - Pleural fluid LDH/serum LDH >0.6
  - Pleural fluid LDH more than two-thirds upper limit of normal serum LDH
- Transudates lack any of these features
- Hemothorax is defined as a pleural fluid hematocrit/peripheral hematocrit ratio >0.5
- Elevated pleural fluid amylase suggests pancreatitis, pancreatic pseudocyst, adenocarcinoma of the lung, or esophageal rupture
- Pleural fluid triglyceride level >100 mg/dL suggests disruption of the thoracic duct

- Pleural fluid cytology has a sensitivity of 50–65% for detecting malignancy
- Repeat cytological examination, followed by thoracoscopy or video-assisted thoracoscopic surgery (VATS), is indicated if suspicion is high and cytology is negative

IMAGING STUDIES

- Chest x-rays can detect as little as 175–200 mL of pleural fluid on a frontal and 75–100 mL on a lateral view
- Chest CT can identify as little as 10 mL of pleural fluid
- Lateral decubitus chest films can determine if blind thoracentesis may be performed; a minimum 1 cm of fluid must be seen for the procedure to be done safely
- Ultrasonography should be used to safely guide thoracentesis of small effusions

DIAGNOSTIC PROCEDURES

- Diagnostic paracentesis should be performed for any new pleural effusion without apparent cause
- Pleural biopsy should be performed in cases of suspected tuberculous effusion
- Pleural fluid culture is only 44% sensitive for tuberculous effusion; culture and histological examination of pleural tissue increases this to 70–90%

Pleural Effusion

TREATMENT

MEDICATIONS

- Appropriate antibiotics for pleural infections (see Tables 122 and 123, pages 1303 and 1306)

SURGERY

- Thoracotomy may be required in hemothorax to control hemorrhage, remove clot, and treat complications
- Chest tube insertion (tube thoracostomy)
  - Rarely indicated for transudates
  - May be useful in malignant effusions
  - Indicated for some complicated parapneumonic effusions and empyema

THERAPEUTIC PROCEDURES

- Therapeutic thoracentesis: transient benefit for dyspnea in transudative effusions
- Pleurodesis involves placing an irritant into the pleural space to obliterate it by producing adhesions; side effects are pain and fever; premedication is necessary
  - Doxycycline is 70–75% effective
  - Talc is 90% effective
  - Rarely indicated for transudates
  - Often used for recurrent malignant effusions
- Intrapleural fibrinolysis: streptokinase, 250,000 U or urokinase 100,000 U in 100 mL of saline can improve drainage of empyema or complicated parapneumonic effusions with loculations

Transudative effusions

- Treatment is directed at the underlying cause
- Therapeutic thoracentesis may offer only transient relief from dyspnea
- Tube thoracostomy and pleurodesis are rarely indicated

Malignant effusion

- Systemic therapy may address the underlying malignancy
- Repeated thoracentesis or chest tube insertion (tube thoracostomy) may be needed as local therapy to relieve symptoms related to the effusion itself
- Pleurodesis can reduce reaccumulation of fluid

Parapneumonic effusion

- Simple effusions (free-flowing, sterile) will resolve with treatment of the pneumonia and do not require drainage
- Complicated effusions should be drained via chest tube if fluid analysis reveals pH <7.2 or glu <60; drainage should be considered for pH 7.2–7.3 or LDH >1000 mg/dL
- Empyema should be drained via chest tube

Hemothorax

- If small-volume and stable, observation is adequate
- All other cases should be treated with immediate drainage via a large-bore chest tube

OUTCOME

FOLLOW-UP

- Serial chest x-rays to ensure resolution

COMPLICATIONS

- Fibrothorax can occur if hemothorax is not evacuated

PROGNOSIS

- Depends on the etiology of the effusion

WHEN TO REFER

- All large effusions, exudative effusions, and complicated transudative effusions should be evaluated with the assistance of a pulmonologist

WHEN TO ADMIT

- For large-volume thoracentesis, chest tube placement, or complicated closed pleural biopsy

EVIDENCE

PRACTICE GUIDELINES

- Antony VB et al: American Thoracic Society Guidelines: Management of malignant pleural effusions. Am J Respir Crit Care Med 2000;162:1987. [PMID: 11069845]
- Colice GL et al: Medical and surgical treatment of parapneumonic effusions: an evidence-based guideline. Chest 2000;118:1158. [PMID: 11035692]

INFORMATION FOR PATIENTS

- National Institutes of Health http://www.nlm.nih.gov/medlineplus/ency/article/000086.htm
- Mayo Clinic http://www.mayoclinic.com/invoke.cfm?id=DS00244

REFERENCE

- Muthuswamy P et al: Clinical problem-solving. The effusion that would not go away. N Engl J Med 2001;345:756. [PMID: 11547746]

Mark S. Chesnutt, MD

Thomas J. Prendergast, MD

Pneumocystis Pneumonia

KEY FEATURES

ESSENTIALS OF DIAGNOSIS

- *Pneumocystis carinii* is a fungus found in lungs of many domesticated and wild mammals and *P jiroveci* in humans worldwide
- Infection causes pneumonia, with fever, dyspnea, nonproductive cough
- Bibasilar crackles on auscultation in many cases, others have no findings
- Bilateral diffuse interstitial disease without hilar adenopathy on chest x-ray
- Reduced partial pressure of oxygen
- *P jiroveci* in sputum, bronchoalveolar lavage fluid, or lung tissue

GENERAL CONSIDERATIONS

- Based on serology, asymptomatic infections occur at a young age in most persons

DEMOGRAPHICS

- Most common in patients with AIDS, also occurs in patients with cancer, severe malnutrition, or immunosuppressive or radiation therapy (eg, for organ transplants, cancer)
- Mode of transmission unknown but likely airborne
- *Pneumocystis* pneumonia occurs in up to 80% of AIDS patients not on prophylaxis, usually at CD4 cell counts <200/μL
- Infection outside of the lungs is rare, unless patient is receiving aerosolized pentamidine prophylaxis
- In non-AIDS patients on immunosuppressives, symptoms often begin when corticosteroids are tapered or discontinued

CLINICAL FINDINGS

SYMPTOMS AND SIGNS

- Fever, tachypnea, shortness of breath, and cough, usually nonproductive
- Normal lung examination or bibasilar crackles; findings may be slight compared to degree of illness and chest x-ray abnormality
- Spontaneous pneumothorax may occur if patient had previous episodes or received aerosolized pentamidine prophylaxis
- In AIDS: fever, fatigue, and weight loss may occur for weeks or months before pulmonary symptoms

DIFFERENTIAL DIAGNOSIS

- Bacterial pneumonia
- Tuberculosis
- Coccidioidomycosis
- Histoplasmosis
- Cytomegalovirus
- Kaposi's sarcoma
- Lymphoma (including lymphocytic interstitial pneumonitis)
- Pulmonary embolism

DIAGNOSIS

LABORATORY TESTS

- Lactate dehydrogenase elevation sensitive but not specific
- Lymphopenia with low CD4 count common
- Arterial blood gases show hypoxemia and hypocapnia
- Serological tests not helpful
- Culture not possible
- Specimens of induced sputum can be stained to demonstrate cysts
- If induced sputum is negative and suspicion is high, diagnostic specimens may be obtained by bronchoalveolar lavage (sensitivity 86–97%) or, if necessary, by transbronchial lung biopsy (sensitivity 85–97%)
- PCR for *P jiroveci* appears sensitive but does not provide more rapid diagnosis

IMAGING STUDIES

- Chest x-ray usually shows diffuse "interstitial" infiltrates, but early in infection, these may be heterogeneous, miliary, or patchy; may also show diffuse or focal consolidation, cystic changes, nodules, or cavitation within nodules
- Pleural effusions not seen
- Chest x-ray normal in 5–10%
- Upper lobe infiltrates common if patient received aerosolized pentamidine prophylaxis
- Pulmonary function tests (PFTs) show reduced vital capacity, total lung capacity, and diffusing capacity
- Gallium lung scanning shows diffuse uptake. While sensitivity is high (>95%), specificity is low (20–40%), so test usually obtained only if high suspicion and normal chest x-ray and PFTs

DIAGNOSTIC PROCEDURES

- Fine-needle aspiration and open lung biopsy are infrequently done

Pneumocystis Pneumonia

TREATMENT

MEDICATIONS

- If disease suspected clinically, start empiric therapy while work-up proceeds
- For mild to moderate pneumocytosis in AIDS and non-AIDS patients: oral trimethoprim-sulfamethoxazole (TMP-SMZ)
- If vomiting or intractable diarrhea: IV TMP-SMZ
- Dose based on TMP: 20 mg/kg (12–15 mg/kg may decrease side effects with the same efficacy) PO or IV QD divided TID or QID for 14–21 days
- Hypersensitivity to sulfonamide common in AIDS
- Symptoms persist for 4–6 days after starting treatment, and sometimes worsen transiently during the first 3–5 days
- If PaO$_2$ on admission <70 mm Hg: add prednisone 40 mg BID for 5 days, then 40 mg QD for 5 days, then 20 mg QD until therapy complete
- If patient requires fluid restriction or has history of sulfonamide hypersensitivity: pentamidine, 3 mg/kg IV/IM QD for 14–21 days
- For mild to moderate disease in patient who does not tolerate TMP-SMZ or pentamidine: atovaquone, 750 mg PO TID for 21 days
- Other alternatives: clindamycin, 600 mg PO TID, plus primaquine, 15 mg PO QD; dapsone, 100 mg PO QD, plus trimethoprim, 15 mg/kg/day PO divided TID; or trimetrexate, 45 mg/m^2 IV QD, plus high-dose leucovorin (salvage therapy)

OUTCOME

PROGNOSIS

- Without treatment, mortality of pneumocytosis is nearly 100%
- Early treatment reduces mortality to 10–20% in AIDS and to 30–50% in other immunodeficient patients
- Recurrence is common without prophylaxis

PREVENTION

- Primary prophylaxis if CD4 <200/ μL, CD4 lymphocyte percentage <14%, or weight loss or oral candidiasis
- Secondary prophylaxis if history of pneumocytosis until durable response to HAART and CD4 >250/μL
- First-line prophylaxis: TMP-SMZ 1 double-strength tablet PO 3 times weekly or QD. Hypersensitivity common, but if mild may be able to treat through it
- Alternative: dapsone, 50–100 mg PO QD or 100 mg PO 2–3 times weekly. Check glucose-6-phosphate dehydrogenase level prior to start, and methemoglobin level at 1 month
- Alternative: aerosolized pentamidine, 300 mg Q month. Predisposes to apical pneumocytosis, extrapulmonary pneumocytosis, and pneumothorax

EVIDENCE

PRACTICE GUIDELINES

- 2001 USPHS/IDSA guidelines for the prevention of opportunistic infections in persons infected with human immunodeficiency virus. U.S. Department of Health and Human Services, Public Health Service http://aidsinfo.nih.gov/guidelines/op_infections\OI_112801.pdf
- Infectious Diseases Society of America— Summary of the guidelines for preventing opportunistic infections among hematopoietic stem cell transplant recipients http://www.journals.uchicago.edu/CID/journal/issues/v33n2/001547/001547.web.pdf

WEB SITES

- AIDS Info by the USDHHS http://aidsinfo.nih.gov/
- Project Inform— www.projectinform.org/

INFORMATION FOR PATIENTS

- CDC http://www.cdc.gov/hiv/pubs/brochure/pcpb.htm
- JAMA patient page: HIV infection: the basics. JAMA 2002;288:268. [PMID: 12123237]
- MEDLINEplus http://www.nlm.nih.gov/medlineplus/ency/article/000671.htm

REFERENCE

- Trikalinos TA et al: Discontinuation of *Pneumocystis carinii* prophylaxis in patients infected with human immunodeficiency virus: a meta-analysis and decision analysis. Clin Infect Dis 2001;33:1901. [PMID: 11692302]

Richard J. Hamill, MD

Pneumonia, Anaerobic, & Lung Abscess

 KEY FEATURES

ESSENTIALS OF DIAGNOSIS

- History of or predisposition to aspiration
- Indolent symptoms, including fever, weight loss, malaise
- Poor dentition
- Foul-smelling purulent sputum (in many patients)
- Infiltrate in dependent lung zone, with single or multiple areas of cavitation or pleural effusion

GENERAL CONSIDERATIONS

- Nocturnal aspiration of small amounts of oropharyngeal secretions is typically not pathological
- Larger aspirations may cause nocturnal asthma, chemical pneumonitis, bronchiectasis, mechanical obstruction, and pleuropulmonary infection
- Predisposing factors include drug or alcohol use, seizures, anesthesia, central nervous system disease, or trachea or nasogastric tubes
- Periodontal disease and poor oral hygiene are associated with a greater likelihood of pleuropulmonary infection
- Disease usually occurs in dependent lung zones
- Most infections include multiple anaerobic bacteria: *Prevotella melaninogenica,* peptostreptococcus, *Fusobacterium nucleatum,* and *Bacteroides*

DEMOGRAPHICS

- Risk factors are poor dentition, heavy alcohol use, and aspiration

 CLINICAL FINDINGS

SYMPTOMS AND SIGNS

- Onset is insidious; necrotizing pneumonia, abscess, or empyema may be apparent at presentation
- Constitutional symptoms of fever, malaise, and weight loss are common
- Cough with foul-smelling expectorant suggests anaerobic infection
- Poor dentition is typical
- Patients are rarely edentulous; this finding suggests an obstructing bronchial lesion

DIFFERENTIAL DIAGNOSIS

- Other causes of cavitary lung disease: tuberculosis, fungal infection, bronchogenic cancer, pulmonary infarction, Wegener's granulomatosis, cavitary bacterial pneumonia
- Fungal infection, eg, histoplasmosis
- Bronchiectasis

 DIAGNOSIS

LABORATORY TESTS

- Culture of expectorated sputum is not useful due to contamination with oral flora

IMAGING STUDIES

- The chest x-ray in a lung abscess will show a thick-walled cavity surrounded by consolidation, occasionally with an air-fluid level
- Necrotizing pneumonia demonstrates multiple areas of cavitation within an area of consolidation
- Empyema is characterized by purulent pleural fluid and may accompany the findings of abscess or necrotizing pneumonia
- Ultrasonography may identify loculations or help localize fluid for safe thoracentesis

DIAGNOSTIC PROCEDURES

- Thoracentesis with pleural fluid analysis should be performed on all effusions

TREATMENT

MEDICATIONS

- Clindamycin (600 mg IV Q 8 h, then 300 mg PO Q 6 h after initial improvement)
- Amoxicillin-clavulanate (875 mg PO Q 12 h)
- Penicillin (amoxicillin 500 mg PO TID or penicillin G 1–2 million U IV Q 4–6 h) plus metronidazole 500 mg PO or IV Q 8–12 h
- Therapy should be continued until the chest x-ray improves, usually for a month or more

SURGERY

- Open pleural drainage is sometimes needed due to loculations associated with a parapneumonic effusion

THERAPEUTIC PROCEDURES

- Thoracentesis
- Anaerobic pleuropulmonary infection requires drainage with a thoracostomy tube for empyema

OUTCOME

FOLLOW-UP

- Monitor chest x-ray; if it does not improve, consider other etiologies

COMPLICATIONS

- Sepsis
- Parapneumonic effusion
- Empyema with loculations and/or pleural scarring and the need for surgical decortication via thoracotomy

PROGNOSIS

- Excellent with appropriate antimicrobial therapy

WHEN TO REFER

- Refer to infectious disease expert, pulmonary specialist, or thoracic surgeon if no response to antibiotic therapy or concern about the presence of another process (eg, cancer)

WHEN TO ADMIT

- Hypoxia
- Severe malnutrition
- Marked systemic symptoms

PREVENTION

- Good dental hygiene

EVIDENCE

PRACTICE GUIDELINES

- National Guideline Clearinghouse
  http://www.guideline.gov/summary/
  summary.aspx?doc_id=3351&nbr=
  2577&string=aspiration+pneumonia
  http://www.guideline.gov/summary/
  summary.aspx?doc_id=2665&nbr=
  1891&string=aspiration+pneumonia

INFORMATION FOR PATIENTS

- National Institutes of Health
  http://www.nlm.nih.gov/medlineplus/
  ency/article/000121.htm
- American Lung Association
  http://www.lungusa.org/diseases/
  lungpneumoni.html

REFERENCES

- Levinson ME: Anaerobic pleuropulmonary infection. Curr Opin Infect Dis 2001;14:187. [PMID: 11979131]
- Mansharamani N: Lung abscess in adults: clinical comparison of immunocompromised to non-immunocompromised patients. Respir Med 2002; 96:178. [PMID: 11905552]

Mark S. Chesnutt, MD
Thomas J. Prendergast, MD

Pneumonia, Community-Acquired

 KEY FEATURES

ESSENTIALS OF DIAGNOSIS

- Symptoms and signs of an acute lung infection: fever or hypothermia, cough with or without sputum, dyspnea, chest discomfort, sweats or rigors
- Bronchial breath sounds or rales are frequent auscultatory findings
- Parenchymal infiltrate on chest radiograph
- Occurs outside of the hospital or less than 48 h after admission in a patient who has not been hospitalized or residing in a long-term care facility for 14 days or more before the onset of symptoms

GENERAL CONSIDERATIONS

- Defined as beginning outside the hospital or being diagnosed within 48 h of admission
- The most deadly infectious disease in the United States and the sixth leading cause of death overall
- Mortality is 14% among hospitalized patients and 1% among outpatients
- Prospective studies fail to identify the cause in 40–60% of cases, though bacteria are more commonly identified than viruses
- The most common bacterial pathogens are *Streptococcus pneumoniae* (two-thirds of cases), *Haemophilus influenzae, Mycoplasma pneumoniae, Chlamydia pneumoniae, Staphylococcus aureus, Neisseria meningitidis, Moraxella catarrhalis,* and *Klebsiella pneumoniae*
- Common viral causes include influenza, respiratory syncytial virus, adenovirus, and parainfluenza virus
- Assessment of epidemiological risk factors may help in diagnosing pneumonia due to *Chlamydia psittaci* (psittacosis), *Coxiella burnetii* (Q fever), *Francisella tularensis* (tularemia), endemic fungi (blastomyces, coccidioides, histoplasma), and sin nombre virus (hantavirus pulmonary syndrome)

 CLINICAL FINDINGS

SYMPTOMS AND SIGNS

- Acute or subacute onset of fever, cough with or without sputum, and dyspnea
- Rigors, sweats, chills, pleurisy, and chest discomfort are common
- Fatigue, anorexia, headache, myalgias, and abdominal pain can be present
- Physical findings include fever or hypothermia, tachypnea, tachycardia, and mild oxygen desaturation
- Altered breath sounds or rales are common
- Dullness to percussion may be present with a parapneumonic effusion

DIFFERENTIAL DIAGNOSIS

- Bacterial pneumonia
- Viral pneumonia
- Aspiration pneumonia
- *Pneumocystis jiroveci* pneumonia
- Bronchitis
- Lung abscess
- Tuberculosis
- Pulmonary embolism
- Myocardial infarction
- Sarcoidosis
- Lung neoplasm
- Hypersensitivity pneumonitis
- Bronchiolitis, BOOP

 DIAGNOSIS

LABORATORY TESTS

- See Table 19 (page 1218)
- Gram stain and culture of sputum are controversial, but recommended in hospitalized patients
- Preantibiotic blood cultures are generally recommended for hospitalized patients
- Arterial blood gas, complete blood cell count, and a comprehensive metabolic panel are recommended for all hospitalized patients
- HIV serology should be considered in hospitalized patients

IMAGING STUDIES

- Chest x-ray can confirm the diagnosis and detect associated lung diseases
- Findings range from patchy airspace infiltrates to diffuse alveolar or interstitial infiltrates
- Clearing of infiltrates can take 6 weeks

DIAGNOSTIC PROCEDURES

- Sputum induction is reserved for patients who cannot provide expectorated samples or may have *Pnuemocystis carinii* or *Mycobacterium tuberculosis* pneumonia
- Thoracentesis with pleural fluid analysis should be performed in all patients with effusions

Pneumonia, Community-Acquired

 TREATMENT

MEDICATIONS

- See Table 19 (page 1218)
- Outpatient therapy
  - Macrolides: clarithromycin, 500 mg BID, azithromycyin, 500 mg initially, then 250 mg QD for 4 days
  - Doxycycline, 100 mg BID
  - Fluoroquinolones with enhanced *S pneumoniae,* activity: gatifloxacin, 400 mg QD, levofloxacin, 500 mg QD, or moxifloxacin 400 mg QD
  - Alternatives are erythromycin, amoxicillin-clavulanate, and some second- or third-generation cephalosporins
- Hospitalized patients on a general medical ward
  - Extended-spectrum β-lactam (ceftriaxone or cefotaxime) with a macrolide (clarithromycin or azithromycin) if *H influenzae* suspected
  - Fluoroquinolones with enhanced *S pneumoniae* activity (gatifloxicin, levofloxacin, moxifloxacin)
  - β-Lactam/β-lactamase inhibitor (ampicillin-sulbactam or piperacillin-tazobactam) with a macrolide
- Patients in intensive care unit
  - Macrolide or fluoroquinolone plus an extended-spectrum cephalosporin or β-lactam/β-lactamase inhibitor
  - Penicillin-allergic patients may receive a fluoroquinolone with or without clindamycin
  - Suspected aspiration pneumonia should be treated with fluoroquinolone with or without clindamycin, metronidazole, or β-lactam/β-lactamase inhibitor
- Patients with cystic fibrosis or bronchiectasis should receive empiric antipseudomonal therapy
- Duration of therapy
  - Influenced by the severity of illness, the etiological agent, response to therapy, and other medical problems
  - For *S pneumoniae* treat for 72 h after the patient becomes afebrile
  - 2 weeks is minimum for pneumonia due to *S aureus, P aeruginosa, Klebsiella,* anaerobes, *M pneumoniae, C pneumoniae,* or *Legionella,* treat for a minimum of 2 weeks

 OUTCOME

FOLLOW-UP

- Chest x-ray 6 weeks after therapy

COMPLICATIONS

- Parapneumonic effusion—simple or complicated
- Empyema
- Sepsis
- Respiratory failure and/or ARDS
- Pneumotocele
- Lung abscess
- Focal bronchiectasis

PROGNOSIS

- Excellent with appropriate antimicrobial and supportive care

WHEN TO REFER

- Extensive disease and/or seriously ill
- Progression of disease or failure to improve on antibiotics

WHEN TO ADMIT

- The PORT score stratifies patients by mortality and can assist in decisions regarding admission (Tables 20 and 21, pages 1220)

PREVENTION

- Polyvalent pneumococcal vaccine
  - Can prevent or lessen the severity of pneumococcal infections
  - Indications are age >65 or any chronic illness increasing the risk of community-acquired pneumonia
- Influenza vaccine
  - Effective at preventing primary influenza pneumonia and secondary bacterial pneumonia
  - Given annually to patients who are >65, are residents of chronic care facilities, have cardiopulmonary disease, or were recently hospitalized with chronic metabolic disorders
- Hospitalized patients who would benefit from vaccine should receive it in hospital
- Pneumococcal and influenza vaccines can be given simultaneously and are not contraindicated immediately after a pneumonia

 EVIDENCE

PRACTICE GUIDELINES

- Bartlett JG et al: Practice guidelines for the management of community-acquired pneumonia in adults. Clin Infect Dis 2000;31:347. [PMID: 10987697]
- Niederman MS et al: Guidelines for the management of adults with community-acquired pneumonia. Diagnosis, assessment of severity, antimicrobial therapy, and prevention. Am J Respir Crit Care Med 2001;163:1730. [PMID: 11401897]

INFORMATION FOR PATIENTS

- American Lung Association http://www.lungusa.org/diseases/lungpneumoni.html
- National Institute on Aging http://www.nia.nih.gov/health/agepages/pneum.htm

REFERENCES

- Metlay JP et al: Testing strategies in the initial management of patients with community-acquired pneumonia. Ann Intern Med 2003;138:109. [PMID: 12529093]
- Singh N et al: Rational empiric antibiotic prescription in the ICU. Chest 2000;117:1496. [PMID: 10807841]

Mark S. Chesnutt, MD
Thomas J. Prendergast, MD

Pneumonia, Hospital-Acquired

 KEY FEATURES

ESSENTIALS OF DIAGNOSIS

- Occurs more than 48 h after admission to the hospital and excludes any infection present at the time of admission
- At least two of the following: fever, cough, leukocytosis, purulent sputum
- New or progressive parenchymal infiltrate on chest radiograph
- Especially common in patients requiring intensive care or mechanical ventilation

GENERAL CONSIDERATIONS

- Second most common form of hospital-acquired infection
- Leading cause of deaths due to nosocomial infections
- Mortality rates range from 20 to 50%
- Highest morbidity and mortality occur in ICU and mechanically ventilated patients
- Most common organisms are *Pseudomonas aeruginosa, Staphylococcus aureus, Enterobacter, Klebsiella pneumoniae,* and *Escherichia coli*
- Anaerobic organisms, when isolated, are commonly part of a polymicrobial flora
- Colonization of the pharynx with bacteria is the most important step in pathogenesis and is promoted by instrumentation, contamination, and patient factors
- Increased gastric pH leading to bacterial overgrowth has been suggested as a possible risk factor

 CLINICAL FINDINGS

SYMPTOMS AND SIGNS

- Presentation is nonspecific, but includes the findings seen in community-acquired pneumonia
- Fever, leukocytosis, purulent sputum, or a new or progressive infiltrate on chest x-ray is usually seen

DIFFERENTIAL DIAGNOSIS

- Congestive heart failure
- Atelectasis
- Aspiration
- Acute respiratory distress syndrome
- Pulmonary thromboembolism
- Pulmonary hemorrhage
- Drug reactions

 DIAGNOSIS

LABORATORY TESTS

- Blood cultures identify the pathogen in up to 20% of cases
- Arterial blood gases help define illness severity and the need for supplemental oxygen
- Complete blood cell count and chemistry tests are not helpful in identifying the etiological agent, but can assist in determining illness severity and complications
- Examination of sputum and sputum cultures is controversial, but may be useful in guiding antibiotic therapy
- Direct fluorescent antibody staining for *Legionella* can be helpful when this organism is suspected
- Sputum stains and cultures for mycobacteria and fungi may be diagnostic

IMAGING STUDIES

- X-ray findings are nonspecific and range from patchy infiltrates to lobar consolidation to diffuse alveolar or interstitial infiltrates
- Progression of infiltrates and lack of improvement during antibiotic therapy are poor prognostic signs and may put the diagnosis in question

DIAGNOSTIC PROCEDURES

- Thoracentesis with pleural fluid analysis is indicated for any effusion
- Endotracheal aspiration and fiberoptic bronchoscopy with lavage or use of a protected specimen brush are used most commonly in patients with ventilator-associated pneumonia (VAP)
- A recent trial using quantitative culture of bronchoalveolar lavage or protected specimen brush samples in suspected VAP reduced antibiotic use, shortened the duration of organ dysfunction, and decreased mortality

Pneumonia, Hospital-Acquired

 TREATMENT

 OUTCOME

 EVIDENCE

MEDICATIONS

- See Table 123 (page 1306)
- Treatment is usually empirical and should be started as soon as the diagnosis is suspected
- Initial regimens should be broad and tailored to the specific clinical setting
- No consensus regimens exist, but guidelines separate patients by disease severity
- Mild to moderate disease with early onset (<5 days after hospitalization) or without unusual risk factors
  - Second-generation cephalosporin or nonantipseudomonal third-generation cephalosporin or
  - Combination of a β-lactam/β-lactamase inhibitor
- Severe, late onset (>5 days after hospitalization), or with ICU-acquired disease or VAP
  - Combination of antibiotics against *P aeruginosa*, *Acinetobacter*, and *Enterobacter* species
  - Include aminoglycoside or fluoroquinolone plus one of the following: antipseudomonal penicillin, antipseudomonal cephalosporin, imipenem-cilastin, or aztreonam
  - Vancomycin is added for concern for methicillin-resistant *S aureus* (patients with head trauma, coma, diabetes, renal failure, or ICU stay)
  - Anaerobic coverage with clindamycin, or a β-lactam/β-lactamase inhibitor is added for patients with aspiration, recent thoracoabdominal surgery, or airway obstruction
  - Macrolide is added where there is risk for *Legionella* (patients on high-dose steroids)
- Duration of therapy should be individualized, but at least 14–21 days for gram-negative bacterial pneumonia

COMPLICATIONS

- Parapneumonic effusion—simple or complicated
- Empyema
- Sepsis
- Respiratory failure and/or ARDS
- Pneumotocele
- Lung abscess
- Focal bronchiectasis

PROGNOSIS

- Mortality rates range from 20 to 50%, and are highest in mechanically ventilated patients

WHEN TO REFER

- Extensive disease
- Seriously ill patient, particularly in the setting of comorbid conditions (eg, liver disease)
- Progression of disease or failure to improve on antibiotics

PREVENTION

- Sucralfate use for gastric ulcer prophylaxis (rather than H_2-receptor antagonists or proton-pump inhibitors) may reduce the incidence of VAP

PRACTICE GUIDELINES

- National Guideline Clearinghouse http://www.guideline.gov/summary/summary.aspx?doc_id=2718&nbr=1944&string=hospital+pneumonia

INFORMATION FOR PATIENTS

- National Institutes of Health http://www.nlm.nih.gov/medlineplus/ency/article/000146.htm
- American Lung Association http://www.lungusa.org/diseases/lungpneumoni.html

REFERENCES

- Arozullah AM et al: Development and validation of a multifactorial risk index for predicting postoperative pneumonia after major noncardiac surgery. Ann Intern Med 2001;135:847. [PMID: 11712875]
- Fagon JY et al: Invasive and noninvasive strategies for management of suspected ventilator-associated pneumonia. A randomized trial. Ann Intern Med 2000; 132:621. [PMID: 10766680]
- Morehead RS et al: Ventilator-associated pneumonia. Arch Intern Med 2000; 160:1926 [PMID: 10888967]

Mark S. Chesnutt, MD
Thomas J. Prendergast, MD

Pneumonia, Idiopathic Fibrosing Interstitial

 KEY FEATURES

ESSENTIALS OF DIAGNOSIS

- Progressive dyspnea and cough
- Diffuse dry rales on ausculation of the chest
- Restrictive ventilatory defect and abnormal gas exchange
- Bibasilar, peripheral interstitial fibrosis on chest x-ray or CT
- Exclusion of known causes of interstitial lung disease

GENERAL CONSIDERATIONS

- Formerly known as idiopathic pulmonary fibrosis (IPF) or in Britain as cryptogenic fibrosing alveolitis
- Historically, diagnosis was based on clinical and radiographic criteria, with lung biopsy uncommon
- Several histological patterns once grouped together as IPF are now recognized to be associated with different natural histories and responses to therapy
- Evaluation must first identify patients whose disease is truly idiopathic; most identifiable causes of interstitial lung diseases are infectious, drug-related, or due to exposures, or associated with other medical conditions
- A specific diagnosis allows providers to give accurate information on natural history and to distinguish patients most likely to benefit from treatment
- See Table 29 (page 1225)

DEMOGRAPHICS

- Age range usually 40–70 years old
- Slight male predominance
- More common in cigarette smokers than nonsmokers

 CLINICAL FINDINGS

SYMPTOMS AND SIGNS

- Insidious dry cough and exertional dyspnea lasting months
- Diffuse, fine late inspiratory crackles on ascultation of the lungs
- Clubbing is present at the time of diagnosis in 25–50%

DIFFERENTIAL DIAGNOSIS

- Bronchiolitis obliterans with organizing pneumonia (BOOP)
- Interstitial lung disease due to infection (eg, fungal, viral, *Pneumocystis jiroveci* pneumonia, tuberculosis)
- Drug-induced fibrosis, eg, amiodarone, bleomycin
- Sarcoidosis
- Pneumoconiosis
- Hypersensitivity pneumonitis
- Asbestosis
- See Table 28 (page 1224)

 DIAGNOSIS

LABORATORY TESTS

- To exclude other etiologies
  - ANA, RF
  - Erythrocyte sedimentation rate
  - Aldolase, anti-Jo-1 antibody

IMAGING STUDIES

- Chest x-ray and HRCT classically demonstrate low lung volumes and diffuse, patchy fibrosis with pleural-based honeycombing

DIAGNOSTIC PROCEDURES

- Transbronchial biopsy cannot be used to definitively diagnose usual interstitial pneumonitis, though it may exclude it by confirming an alternative diagnosis
- Restrictive physiology with decreased diffusing capacity on pulmonary function testing

TREATMENT

MEDICATIONS

- Treatment is controversial: no randomized study has demonstrated that treatment improves survival

 ## OUTCOME

FOLLOW-UP

- Serial pulmonary function tests and assessment of gas exchange

COMPLICATIONS

- Hypoxemia requiring oxygen therapy
- Respiratory failure

PROGNOSIS

- Median survival approximately 3 years, depending on stage at presentation

WHEN TO REFER

- All patients should be evaluated by a pulmonologist at the time of diagnosis to assist with diagnosis, consider treatment options, and evaluate for lung transplantation

WHEN TO ADMIT

- Progressive respiratory failure

EVIDENCE

PRACTICE GUIDELINES

- American Thoracic Society: Idiopathic pulmonary fibrosis: diagnosis and treatment. International consensus statement. American Thoracic Society (ATS), and the European Respiratory Society (ERS). Am J Respir Crit Care Med 2000;161(2 Pt 1):646.

INFORMATION FOR PATIENTS

- American Lung Association http://www.lungusa.org/diseases/pulmfibrosis.html
- National Heart, Lung, and Blood Institute http://www.nhlbi.nih.gov/health/public/lung/other/idiopath.htm

REFERENCES

- American Thoracic Society/Respiratory Society International Multidisciplinary Consensus Classification of the Idiopathic Interstitial Pneumonias. Am J Respir Crit Care Med 2002;165:277. [PMID: 11790668]
- Gross TJ et al: Idiopathic pulmonary fibrosis. N Engl J Med 2001;345:517. [PMID: 11519507]
- Idiopathic pulmonary fibrosis: diagnosis and treatment. American Thoracic Society International consensus statement. Am J Respir Crit Care Med 2000;161:646. [PMID: 10673212]
- Katzenstein AL et al: Idiopathic pulmonary fibrosis: clinical relevance of pathologic classification. Am J Respir Crit Care Med 1998;157:1301. [PMID: 9563754]

Mark S. Chesnutt, MD
Thomas J. Prendergast, MD

Pneumonia, Pneumococcal

 KEY FEATURES

ESSENTIALS OF DIAGNOSIS

- Productive cough, fever, rigors, dyspnea, early pleuritic chest pain
- Consolidating lobar pneumonia on chest x-ray
- Lancet-shaped gram-positive diplococci on Gram stain of sputum

GENERAL CONSIDERATIONS

- The most common cause of community-acquired pyogenic bacterial pneumonia
- Alcoholism, HIV infection, sickle cell disease, splenectomy, and hematological disorders are predisposing factors
- Up to 40% of infections are caused by pneumococci resistant to at least one drug and 15% are due to a strain resistant to three or more drugs

DEMOGRAPHICS

- Until 2000, *Streptococcus pneumoniae* infections caused 100,000–135,000 hospitalizations for pneumonia, 6 million cases of otitis media, and 60,000 cases of invasive disease, including 3300 cases of meningitis
- Disease figures are now changing due to conjugate vaccine introduction

 CLINICAL FINDINGS

SYMPTOMS AND SIGNS

- High fever, productive cough, occasionally hemoptysis, and pleuritic chest pain
- Rigors can occur within the first few hours of infection
- Bronchial breath sounds are an early sign
- Differentiating pneumococcal from other bacterial pneumonias is not possible clinically or radiographically because of significant overlap in presentations

DIFFERENTIAL DIAGNOSIS

- Pneumonia due to other causes, eg, *Haemophilus influenzae*, influenza
- Aspiration pneumonia or lung abscess
- Pulmonary embolism
- Myocardial infarction
- Acute exacerbation of chronic bronchitis
- Acute bronchitis
- Hypersensitivity pneumonitis

 DIAGNOSIS

LABORATORY TESTS

- A good-quality sputum sample (less than 10 epithelial cells and more than 25 polymorphonuclear leukocytes per high-power field) shows gram-positive diplococci in 80–90% of cases
- Blood cultures are positive in up to 25% of selected cases and much more commonly so in HIV-positive patients

IMAGING STUDIES

- Chest x-ray shows findings of consolidation, often with a lobar distribution, infiltrates, pleural effusion

TREATMENT

MEDICATIONS

- Initial antimicrobial therapy of pneumonia is empirical pending isolation and identification of the causative agent (Table 19, page 1218)

Outpatient

- Amoxicillin, 750 mg twice daily for 7–10 days
- Alternatives are azithromycin, one 500 mg dose on the first day and 250 mg for the next 4 days; clarithromycin, 500 mg twice daily for 10 days; or doxycycline, 100 mg twice daily for 10 days

Inpatient

- Aqueous penicillin G (susceptible strains), 2 million units intravenously every 4 h
- Ceftriaxone, 1 g intravenously every 24 h
- For highly penicillin-resistant strain, vancomycin, 1 g every 12 h
- Fluoroquinolones with enhanced gram-positive activity (eg, levofloxacin, 500 mg once daily; moxifloxacin, 400 mg once daily; or gatifloxacin, 400 mg once daily) are effective oral alternatives

THERAPEUTIC PROCEDURES

- Pleural effusions developing after initiation of antimicrobial therapy usually are sterile, and thoracentesis need not be performed if the patient is otherwise improving
- Thoracentesis is indicated for an effusion present prior to initiation of therapy and in the patient who has not responded to antibiotics after 3–4 days

OUTCOME

FOLLOW-UP

- Repeat chest x-ray 6–8 weeks after treatment to ensure resolution of infiltrate

COMPLICATIONS

- Parapneumonic (sympathetic) effusion is common and may cause recurrence or persistence of fever
- Empyema occurs in 5% or less of cases and is differentiated from sympathetic effusion by the presence of organisms on Gram-stained fluid or positive pleural fluid cultures

- Pneumococcal pericarditis (rare)
- Pneumococcal arthritis (rare)
- Pneumococcal endocarditis usually involves the aortic valve and often occurs in association with meningitis and pneumonia

PROGNOSIS

- The mortality rate remains high in the setting of advanced age, multilobar disease, severe hypoxemia, extrapulmonary complications, and bacteremia

WHEN TO REFER

- Early referral to a pulmonologist for management of seriously ill patients

WHEN TO ADMIT

- The Pneumonia Patient Outcomes Research Team (PORT) model can be used along with clinical judgment in the initial decision on whether to hospitalize a patient (Tables 20 and 21, pages 1220)
- Patients under 50 years old without comorbid conditions or physical examination abnormalities listed in Table 20 (page 1120) have the lowest risk

PREVENTION

Pneumococcal vaccine

- Contains purified polysaccharide from 23 of the most common strains of *S pneumoniae*, which cause 90% of bacteremic episodes in the United States
- Is about 60–70% effective in preventing bacteremic disease in immunocompetent patients
- Is about 50% effective in preventing bacteremic disease in patients with underlying diseases (not severely compromised) and only about 10% effective in immunocompromised patients
- Current recommendations
  - Table 127 (page 1310)
  - Patients at increased risk of developing severe pneumococcal disease, especially asplenic patients and those with sickle cell disease
  - Chronic illnesses (eg, cardiopulmonary disease, alcoholism, renal disease, cancer)
  - All individuals over 65 years of age
  - Elderly individuals with unknown immunization status should be immunized once

- Revaccination
  - Recommended every 5 years, regardless of age, for those with the highest risk of fatal pneumococcal disease (eg, asplenic patients, nephrotic syndrome or renal failure, HIV, leukemia, lymphoma, myeloma, immunosuppressive medications, transplant patients)
  - 65 years of age if primary vaccine was at least 5 years before
- High-risk individuals previously immunized with the 14-valent vaccine

EVIDENCE

PRACTICE GUIDELINES

- National Guideline Clearinghouse http://www.guideline.gov/summary/summary.aspx?doc_id=2665&nbr=1891&string=pneumococcal+pneumonia http://www.guideline.gov/summary/summary.aspx?doc_id=2773&nbr=1999&string=pneumococcal+pneumonia

WEB SITES

- CDC—Division of Bacterial and Mycotic Diseases http://www.cdc.gov/ncidod/dbmd/
- Karolinska Institute—Directory of Bacterial Infections and Mycoses http://www.mic.ki.se/Diseases/c1.html

INFORMATION FOR PATIENTS

- JAMA patient page: Pneumonia. JAMA 2000;283:1922.
- JAMA patient page: Immunizations. JAMA 1999;282:102. [PMID: 10404918]

REFERENCE

- Whitney CG, Schaffner W, Butler JC: Rethinking recommendations for use of pneumococcal vaccines in adults. Clin Infect Dis 2001;33:662. [PMID: 11486289]

Henry F. Chambers, MD

Pneumonitis, Hypersensitivity

 KEY FEATURES

ESSENTIALS OF DIAGNOSIS

- A link between symptoms and exposure may be obtained from work or environmental history
- Antigen can be microbial agents, animal proteins, or chemical sensitizers
- Presentation can be acute or a subacute illness

GENERAL CONSIDERATIONS

- A nonatopic, nonasthmatic allergic pulmonary disease
- Manifested mainly as occupational disease where exposure to an inhaled organic agent leads to acute and eventually chronic pulmonary disease

Etiology

- See Table 35 (page 1230)
- Farmer's lung (moldy hay)
- "Humidifier" lung (contaminated humidifier, heating, or air conditioning)
- Bird fancier's lung ("pigeon breeder's disease")
- Bagassosis (moldy sugar cane fiber)
- Sequoiosis (moldy redwood sawdust)
- Maple bark stripper's disease
- Mushroom picker's disease (moldy compost)
- Suberosis (moldy cork dust)
- Detergent worker's lung (enzyme additives)

 CLINICAL FINDINGS

SYMPTOMS AND SIGNS

- Acute illness characterized by malaise, chills, fever, cough, dyspnea, and nausea 4–8 h after exposure
- Bibasilar crackles, tachypnea, tachycardia, and (occasionally) cyanosis are found
- Subacute illness occurs in 15% of cases and is characterized by insidious onset of chronic cough and progressive dyspnea, anorexia, and weight loss

DIFFERENTIAL DIAGNOSIS

- Sarcoidosis
- Asthma
- Atypical pneumonia
- Collagen vascular disease, eg, systemic lupus erythematosus
- Idiopathic pulmonary fibrosis
- Lymphoma

 DIAGNOSIS

LABORATORY TESTS

- Pulmonary function studies show a restrictive pattern with decreased diffusion capacity
- Leukocytosis with a left shift
- Arterial blood gas shows hypoxemia
- Hypersensitivity pneumonitis antibody panels are available and may reveal precipitating antibodies to the offending allergen in serum

IMAGING STUDIES

- Chest x-ray classically shows small nodular densities sparing the apices and bases
- Pulmonary fibrosis may be found with repeated exposure to the offending agent

DIAGNOSTIC PROCEDURES

- Bronchoscopy with bronchoalveolar lavage
- Surgical lung biopsy is occasionally necessary

Pneumonitis, Hypersensitivity

 TREATMENT

MEDICATIONS

- Corticosteroids (prednisone, 0.5 mg/kg/day, tapered over 4–6 weeks) are typically used despite the lack of a placebo-controlled trial

THERAPEUTIC PROCEDURES

- Identification of the offending agent with removal or avoidance
- Change in occupation is often unavoidable

 OUTCOME

FOLLOW-UP

- Monitor serial chest x-rays and pulmonary function tests

COMPLICATIONS

- Progressive pulmonary fibrosis and respiratory failure

PROGNOSIS

- Good if diagnosed early and offending agent is avoided

WHEN TO REFER

- For assistance in diagnosis, treatment, and follow-up

WHEN TO ADMIT

- Hypoxemic respiratory failure

EVIDENCE

INFORMATION FOR PATIENTS

- American Academy of Family Physicians http://familydoctor.org/handouts/134.html
- National Institutes of Health http://www.nlm.nih.gov/medlineplus/ency/article/000109.htm

REFERENCES

- Glazer CS et al: Clinical and radiologic manifestations of hypersensitivity pneumonitis. J Thorac Imaging 2002;17:261. [PMID: 12362065]
- Hayakawa H et al: Clinicopathological features of chronic hypersensitivity pneumonitis. Respirology 2002;7:359. [PMID: 12421245]

Mark S. Chesnutt, MD
Thomas J. Prendergast, MD

Pneumothorax, Spontaneous

 ## KEY FEATURES

ESSENTIALS OF DIAGNOSIS

- Acute onset of uilateral chest pain and dyspnea
- Minimal physical findings in mild cases; unilateral chest expansion, decreased tactile fremitus, hyper-resonance, diminished breath sounds may occur
- Mediastinal shift, cyanosis, and hypotension are seen in tension pneumothorax
- Presence of pleural air on chest radiograph

GENERAL CONSIDERATIONS

- Traumatic pneumothorax occurs as a result of penetrating or blunt trauma
- Iatrogenic pneumothorax may follow procedures such as central line placement or transbronchial biopsy
- Tension pneumothorax usually occurs in the setting of penetrating trauma, lung infection, cardiopulmonary resuscitation, or positive-pressure ventilation
- Spontaneous pneumothorax occurs in the absence of trauma and is classified as either secondary (complicating pre-existing lung disease) or primary (in the absence of prior lung disease)
- Risk factors for secondary pneumothorax include chronic obstructive pulmonary disease (COPD), asthma, cystic fibrosis, tuberculosis, prior pneumocystis pneumonia, menstruation (catemenial pneumothorax), and many interstitial lung diseases

DEMOGRAPHICS

- Primary pneumothorax affects mainly tall, thin males between 10 and 30 years of age
- Family history and smoking may be contributing factors in primary spontaneous pneumothorax

 ## CLINICAL FINDINGS

SYMPTOMS AND SIGNS

- Chest pain ranges from minimal to severe
- Dyspnea is almost always present
- Symptoms usually begin at rest and resolve within 24 h, even if the pneumothorax persists
- In the setting of COPD or asthma, patients may present with life-threatening respiratory failure
- Diminished breath sounds, decreased tactile fremitus, and decreased movement of the chest are often seen with large pneumothoraces
- Physical findings may be absent in small (<15%) pneumothoraces
- Tension pneumothorax should be suspected if marked tachycardia, mediastinal or tracheal shift, or hypotension is present
- Crepitus may be found over the chest wall and adjacent structures

DIFFERENTIAL DIAGNOSIS

- Emphysematous bleb mimicking loculated pneumothorax
- Myocardial infarction
- Pneumonia
- Pulmonary embolus
- Pneumomediastinum can be caused by rupture of the esophagus or bronchus
- Upper respiratory tract infection
- Rib fracture
- Pericarditis
- Mesothelioma

 ## DIAGNOSIS

LABORATORY TESTS

- Arterial blood gas usually reveals hypoxemia and acute respiratory alkalosis
- QRS axis and precordial T wave changes may mimic acute myocardial infarction in left-sided pneumothorax

IMAGING STUDIES

- A visceral pleural line on chest x-ray is diagnostic; an expiratory film will increase sensitivity
- Secondary pleural effusion can occur
- Supine patients may demonstrate the "deep sulcus sign"—an abnormally radiolucent costophrenic angle
- Large amounts of subpleural air with contralateral mediastinal shift are present in tension pneumothorax

Pneumonitis, Nonspecific Interstitial p. 1156.
Pneumonitis, Radiation p. 1157.

Pneumothorax, Spontaneous

 ## TREATMENT

MEDICATIONS

- Symptomatic treatment for cough and chest pain is appropriate
- Supplemental oxygen may increase the rate of reabsorption of pleural air
- Reliable patients with small (<15%), primary pneumothoraces may be observed

SURGERY

- Simple aspiration of pleural air through a small-bore catheter can be performed for large or progressive pneumothoraces
- Placement of a small-bore chest tube (7F–14F) attached to a one-way Heimlich valve protects against development of a tension pneumothorax and may permit observation from home
- Chest tube placement (tube thoracostomy) may be indicated for secondary, large, or tension pneumothorax, as well as for patients with severe symptoms or mechanically ventilated patients
- Thoracoscopy or open thoracotomy for removal of blebs or pleurodesis may be indicated in recurrent primary pneumothorax, failed tube thoracostomy

THERAPEUTIC PROCEDURES

- Pleurodesis is indicated in recurrent or refractory cases

 ## OUTCOME

FOLLOW-UP

- Serial chest x-rays should be obtained at 24-h intervals
- Chest tubes may be removed when the air leak subsides

COMPLICATIONS

- Tension pneumothorax, which may be life-threatening
- Pneumomediastinum and subcutaneous emphysema

PROGNOSIS

- 50% recurrence rate in smokers
- 30% risk of recurrence in spontaneous pneumothorax treated with observation or chest tube placement
- Recurrence following surgical therapy is less common

WHEN TO ADMIT

- Large, severely symptomatic, or progressive primary pneumothorax
- Secondary pneumothorax

PREVENTION

- Smokers should be counseled to quit
- Future exposure to high altitudes, unpressurized flight, and scuba diving should be avoided

 ## EVIDENCE

PRACTICE GUIDELINES

- National Guideline Clearinghouse http://www.guideline.gov/summary/summary.aspx?doc_id=3102&nbr=2328&string=pneumothorax
- Henry M et al: BTS guidelines for the management of spontaneous pneumothorax. Thorax 2003;58(Suppl 2):ii39.

INFORMATION FOR PATIENTS

- The Mayo Clinic http://www.mayoclinic.com/invoke.cfm?id=HQ01228
- American Lung Association http://www.lungusa.org/diseases/pneumothorax.html

REFERENCES

- Light RW: Manual aspiration: the preferred method for managing primary spontaneous pneumothorax? Am J Respir Crit Care Med 2002;165:1202. [PMID: 11991864]
- Sahn SA et al: Spontaneous pneumothorax. N Engl J Med 2000;342:868. [PMID: 10727592]
- Weissberg D et al: Pneumothorax. Chest 2000;117:1279. [PMID: 10807811]

Mark S. Chesnutt, MD
Thomas J. Prendergast, MD

Polyarteritis Nodosa & Microscopic Polyangiitis

 KEY FEATURES

ESSENTIALS OF DIAGNOSIS

- Microscopic polyangiitis (MPA) may involve small blood vessels (capillaries, arterioles, venules) as well as medium-sized vessels
- Classic polyarteritis nodosa (PAN) involves only medium-sized vessels (but substantial overlap occurs)
- Clinical findings depend on the arteries involved
- Common symptoms of both disorders include fever and other constitutional symptoms, abdominal pain, livedo reticularis, mononeuritis multiplex, anemia, and an elevated sedimentation rate
- Classic PAN is often associated with hypertension but spares the lung
- Ten to 30% of PAN are associated with hepatitis B or C

Etiology

- Idiopathic
- Hepatitis B or C
- Drugs, eg, propylthiouracil, hydralazine, allopurinol, penicillamine, sulfasalazine

GENERAL CONSIDERATIONS

- PAN is a medium-sized necrotizing arteritis with a predilection for involving peripheral nerves, mesenteric vessels (including renal arteries), heart, and brain but the capability of involving most organs
- MPA is a nongranulomatous vasculitis involving small blood vessels; it is often associated with antineutrophil cytoplasmic antibodies (ANCAs) that produce a perinuclear p-ANCA pattern on immunofluorescence testing and are directed against myeloperoxidase, a constituent of neutrophil granules

 CLINICAL FINDINGS

SYMPTOMS AND SIGNS

- Insidious onset, with fever, malaise, weight loss
- Pain in the extremities is often a prominent early feature caused by arthralgia, myalgia (particularly affecting the calves), or neuropathy
- Mononeuritis multiplex (most common: foot-drop)
- Microscopic polyangiitis: pulmonary hemorrhage and glomerulonephritis
- PAN, skin: livedo reticularis, subcutaneous nodules, and skin ulcers
- PAN involvement of the renal arteries leads to a renin-mediated hypertension
- PAN seldom involves the lung
- Abdominal pain—particularly diffuse periumbilical pain precipitated by eating—is common to both polyarteritis nodosa and microscopic polyangiitis. Nausea and vomiting are frequently associated
- Infarction compromises the function of major viscera and may lead to acalculous cholecystitis or appendicitis
- Some patients present dramatically with an acute abdomen caused by mesenteric vasculitis and gut perforation or with hypotension resulting from rupture of a microaneurysm in the liver, kidney, or bowel

DIFFERENTIAL DIAGNOSIS

- Wegener's granulomatosis
- Churg-Strauss syndrome
- Endocarditis
- Cryoglobulinemia
- Cholesterol atheroembolic disease
- Other systemic causes of peripheral neuropathy, eg, rheumatoid arthritis, diabetes mellitus, amyloidosis, sarcoidosis, multiple myeloma
- Other causes of mesenteric ischemia, eg, embolism, atherosclerosis

DIAGNOSIS

LABORATORY TESTS

- The sedimentation rate is almost always elevated, often strikingly so
- Leukocytosis is common
- Three-fourths of patients with MPA are ANCA positive (usually with antibodies directed against myeloperoxidase, causing a p-ANCA pattern on immunofluorescence testing)
- Patients with classic PAN are ANCA negative
- Serological tests for hepatitis B or C are positive in 10–30% of patients with polyarteritis nodosa
- MPA: hematuria, proteinuria, and red blood cell casts in the urine

IMAGING STUDIES

- Mesenteric angiogram revealing microaneurysms is diagnostic

DIAGNOSTIC PROCEDURES

- Biopsies of symptomatic sites (eg, nerve, muscle, lung, or kidney) have high sensitivities and specificities
- The diagnosis of both of these disorders requires confirmation with either a tissue biopsy or, in the case of polyarteritis nodosa, an angiogram
- Patients suspected of having polyarteritis nodosa—eg, on the basis of mesenteric ischemia or new-onset hypertension occurring in the setting of a systemic illness—may be diagnosed by the angiographic finding of aneurysmal dilations in the renal, mesenteric, or hepatic arteries

Polyarteritis Nodosa & Microscopic Polyangiitis

 ## TREATMENT

MEDICATIONS

- For polyarteritis nodosa, corticosteroids in high doses (up to 60 mg of prednisone daily) may control fever and constitutional symptoms and heal vascular lesions
- Pulse methylprednisolone (eg, 1 g intravenously daily for 3 days) may be necessary for patients who are critically ill at presentation
- Immunosuppressive agents, especially cyclophosphamide, appear to improve the survival of patients when given with steroids
- In microscopic polyangiitis, patients are more likely to require cyclophosphamide because of the urgency in treating pulmonary hemorrhage and glomerulonephritis

 ## OUTCOME

COMPLICATIONS

- Mesenteric vasculitis can cause bowel ischemia with bleeding or perforation

PROGNOSIS

- Without treatment, the 5-year survival rate in these disorders is poor—on the order of 20%
- With appropriate therapy, remissions are possible in many cases and the 5-year survival rate has improved to 60–90%
- Relapses may occur in both disorders—approximately 35% among patients with microscopic polyangiitis and perhaps less in those with polyarteritis nodosa

WHEN TO REFER

- Refer to a rheumatologist to assist with establishing the diagnosis and planning therapy

WHEN TO ADMIT

- Admit for therapy whenever the patient develops new visceral complications such as bowel ischemia, cardiomyopathy, or rapidly progressive neuropathy

 ## EVIDENCE

INFORMATION FOR PATIENTS

- Johns Hopkins University http://vasculitis.med.jhu.edu/typesof/polyarteritis.html
- National Institutes of Health http://www.nlm.nih.gov/medlineplus/ency/article/001438.htm
- Cleveland Clinic Foundation http://www.clevelandclinic.org/arthritis/treat/facts/vasculitis.htm

REFERENCES

- Bonsib SM: Polyarteritis nodosa. Semin Diagn Pathol 2001;18:14. [PMID: 11296989]
- Jennette JC et al: Microscopic polyangiitis (microscopic polyarteritis). Semin Diagn Pathol 2001;18:3. [PMID: 11296991]
- Stone JH: Polyarteritis nodosa. JAMA 2002; 288(13):1632.

David B. Hellmann, MD, FACP
John H. Stone, MD, MPH

KEY FEATURES

ESSENTIALS OF DIAGNOSIS

- Chronic anovulation
- Infertility
- Elevated plasma testosterone and luteinizing hormone (LH) values and a reversed follicle-stimulating hormone (FSH) /LH ratio
- Hirsutism (in 70% of patients)

GENERAL CONSIDERATIONS

- The primary lesion is unknown
- There is a steady state of elevated estrogen (estrone), androgen, and LH levels rather than the fluctuating levels in ovulating women
- Increased estrone comes from conversion of androgens to estrone in body fat or from excessive levels of androgens seen in some women of normal weight. High estrone levels may cause suppression of pituitary FSH and a relative increase in LH
- Constant LH stimulation of the ovary results in anovulation, multiple cysts, and theca cell hyperplasia with excess androgen output
- The polycystic ovary has a thickened, pearly white capsule and may not be enlarged

DEMOGRAPHICS

- Affects 2–5% of women of reproductive age

 CLINICAL FINDINGS

SYMPTOMS AND SIGNS

- Hirsutism (70% of cases), obesity (40%), and virilization (20%)
- Amenorrhea (50% of cases) and abnormal uterine bleeding (20%); 20% have normal menstruation
- Women are generally infertile, although they may ovulate occasionally

DIFFERENTIAL DIAGNOSIS

- Hypothalamic amenorrhea, eg, stress, weight change, exercise
- Obesity
- Hypothyroidism
- Hyperprolactinemia
- Premature ovarian failure
- Cushing's syndrome
- Congenital adrenal hyperplasia
- Androgen-secreting tumor (adrenal, ovarian)
- Pregnancy

 DIAGNOSIS

LABORATORY TESTS

- Check FSH, LH, prolactin, thyroid-stimulating hormone, testosterone, and dehydroepiandrosterone sulfate (DHEAS) when amenorrhea has persisted for 6 months

IMAGING STUDIES

- Pelvic ultrasound may document polycystic ovaries (not necessary for diagnosis)

Polycystic Ovary Syndrome (Persistent Anovulation)

 TREATMENT

MEDICATIONS

- If the patient wishes to become pregnant, clomiphene or other drugs can be employed for ovulatory stimulation. The addition of dexamethasone, 0.5 mg at bedtime, to a clomiphene regimen may increase the likelihood of ovulation by suppression of ACTH and circulating adrenal androgens

- For women who are unresponsive to clomiphene, 3- to 6-month courses of metformin, 500 mg three times daily, may bring resumption of regular cycles and ovulation. This agent reduces the hyperinsulinemia and hyperandrogenemia seen with polycystic ovary syndrome

- If the patient does not desire pregnancy, medroxyprogesterone acetate, 10 mg/day for the first 10 days of each month, should be given. This will ensure regular shedding of the endometrium so that hyperplasia will not occur. If contraception is desired, a low-dose combination oral contraceptive can be used; this is also useful in controlling hirsutism, for which treatment must be continued for 6–12 months before results are seen

- Dexamethasone, 0.5 mg each night, is helpful in women with excess adrenal androgen secretion. If hirsutism is severe, some patients will elect to have a hysterectomy and bilateral oophorectomy followed by estrogen replacement therapy. Spironolactone, an aldosterone antagonist, is also useful for hirsutism in doses of 25 mg three or four times daily

THERAPEUTIC PROCEDURES

- In obese patients with polycystic ovaries, weight reduction is often effective; a decrease in body fat will lower the conversion of androgens to estrone and thereby help to restore ovulation

- Hirsutism may be managed with epilation and electrolysis

 OUTCOME

FOLLOW-UP

- In long-term anovular patients over age 35, it is wise to search for an estrogen-stimulated cancer with mammography and endometrial aspiration

PROGNOSIS

- Women have insulin resistance and hyperinsulinemia when infused with glucose and are at increased risk of early-onset type 2 diabetes mellitus

- Women have an increased long-term risk of cancer of the breast and endometrium because of unopposed estrogen secretion

WHEN TO REFER

- If expertise in diagnosis is needed

- If the patient is having infertility problems

 EVIDENCE

PRACTICE GUIDELINES

- National Guideline Clearinghouse http://www.guideline.gov/summary/summary.aspx?doc_id=2847&nbr=2073&string=polycystic+ovary+syndrome

- American College of Obstetricians and Gynecologists. ACOG Practice Bulletin. Clinical Management Guidelines for Obstetrician-Gynecologists: number 41, December 2002. Obstet Gynecol 2002; 100:1389.

WEB SITE

- Gynecology Handbook for Family Practitioners http://www.vh.org/Providers/ClinRef/FPHandbook/13.html

INFORMATION FOR PATIENTS

- Nemours Foundation http://kidshealth.org/teen/sexual_health/girls/pcos.html

- American Academy of Family Physicians http://familydoctor.org/handouts/620.html

REFERENCES

- Guzick DS (editor): Polycystic ovarian syndrome. Obstet Gynecol Clin North Am 2001;28:1. [PMID: 11292997–11293007]

- Moghetti P et al: Metformin effects on clinical features, endocrine and metabolic profiles, and insulin sensitivity in polycystic ovarian syndrome: a randomized, double-blind, placebo-controlled 6-month trial, followed by open, long-term clinical evaluation. J Clin Endocrinol Metab 2000;85:139. [PMID: 10634377]

H. Trent MacKay, MD, MPH

Polymyalgia Rheumatica & Giant Cell Arteritis

 KEY FEATURES

ESSENTIALS OF DIAGNOSIS

- Giant cell arteritis is characterized by headache, jaw claudication, polymyalgia rheumatica, visual abnormalities, and a markedly elevated erythrocyte sedimentation rate (ESR)
- The hallmark of polymyalgia rheumatica is pain and stiffness in shoulders and hips

GENERAL CONSIDERATIONS

- Polymyalgia rheumatica and giant cell arteritis probably represent a spectrum of one disease and frequently coexist
- The important difference between the two conditions is that polymyalgia rheumatica alone does not cause blindness and responds to low-dose (10–20 mg/day) prednisone therapy, whereas giant cell arteritis can cause blindness and large artery complications and requires high-dose therapy (40–60 mg/day)

DEMOGRAPHICS

- Both affect patients over age 50
- Giant cell arteritis is more common in northern Europeans and their descendants

 CLINICAL FINDINGS

SYMPTOMS AND SIGNS

Polymyagia rheumatica

- Pain and stiffness of the shoulder and pelvic girdle areas
- Fever, malaise, and weight loss
- Anemia and a markedly elevated sedimentation rate are almost always present
- Muscle pain much greater than muscle weakness

Giant cell arteritis

- Headache, scalp tenderness, visual symptoms, jaw claudication, or throat pain
- The temporal artery is usually normal on physical examination but may be nodular, enlarged, tender, or pulseless
- Blindness results from occlusive arteritis of the posterior ciliary branch of the ophthalmic artery; the ischemic optic neuropathy of giant cell arteritis may produce no funduscopic findings for the first 24–48 h after the onset of blindness
- Asymmetry of pulses in the arms, a murmur of aortic regurgitation, or bruits heard near the clavicle resulting from subclavian artery stenoses identify an affected aorta or its major branches
- Forty percent of patients with giant cell arteritis have nonclassic symptoms at presentation, chiefly respiratory tract problems (most frequently dry cough), mononeuritis multiplex (most frequently with painful paralysis of a shoulder), or fever of unknown origin
- The fever can be as high as 40°C and is frequently associated with rigors and sweats
- Unexplained head or neck pain in an older patient may signal the presence of giant cell arteritis

DIFFERENTIAL DIAGNOSIS

Polymyalgia rheumatica

- Rheumatoid arthritis
- Polymyositis
- Chronic infection, eg, endocarditis
- Multiple myeloma
- Malignancy
- Fibromyalgia
- Polyarteritis nodosa

Giant cell (temporal) arteritis

- Migraine
- Glaucoma
- Takayasu's arteritis
- Uveitis
- Carotid plaque with embolic amaurosis fugax
- Trigeminal neuralgia

 DIAGNOSIS

LABORATORY TESTS

- An elevated ESR, with a median result of about 65 mm/h, occurs in more than 90% of patients with polymyalgia rheumatica or giant cell arteritis
- Most patients also have a mild normochromic, normocytic anemia and thrombocytosis

IMAGING STUDIES

- Role of ultrasonography of temporal arteries is controversial
- Angiography is helpful in the subset of patients that has large-artery disease (especially subclavian artery)

DIAGNOSTIC PROCEDURES

- Temporal artery biopsy
- Diagnostic findings of giant cell arteritis may still be present 2 weeks (or even considerably longer) after starting corticosteroids
- An adequate biopsy specimen (2 cm in length) is essential, because the disease may be segmental

TREATMENT

MEDICATIONS

Polymyalgia rheumatica

- Prednisone, 10–20 mg/day; if no dramatic improvement within 72 h, the diagnosis should be revisited

Giant cell arteritis

- The urgency of early diagnosis and treatment in giant cell arteritis relates to the prevention of blindness
- When a patient has symptoms and findings suggestive of temporal arteritis, therapy with prednisone, 60 mg daily, is initiated immediately
- Prednisone should be continued in a dosage of 60 mg/day for 1–2 months before tapering

 ## OUTCOME

FOLLOW-UP

- Course is monitored by a composite of the patient's symptoms and laboratory markers of inflammation (ie, hematocrit, ESR, and C-reactive protein)
- In adjusting the dosage of steroid, the erythrocyte sedimentation rate is a useful but not absolute guide to disease activity. A common error is treating the ESR rather than the patient
- Within 1–2 months after beginning treatment, the patient's symptoms and laboratory abnormalities will resolve
- Disease flares are common (50% or more) as prednisone is tapered
- The total duration of treatment varies considerably but ranges from 6 months to more than 2 years

COMPLICATIONS

- Blindness; once blindness develops, it is usually permanent
- Thoracic aortic aneurysms occur 17 times more frequently in patients with giant cell arteritis than in normal individuals

PROGNOSIS

- Impact on survival appears small

WHEN TO REFER

- Refer to a rheumatologist to establish the diagnosis, plan therapy, and monitor treatment
- Consult an ophthalmologist for visual changes

WHEN TO ADMIT

- Admit for evaluation and high-dose intravenous methylprednisolone if patient acutely develops visual loss

 ## EVIDENCE

PRACTICE GUIDELINES

- National Guideline Clearinghouse http://www.guideline.gov/summary/summary.aspx?doc_id=1906&nbr=1132&string=fibromyalgia http://www.guideline.gov/summary/summary.aspx?doc_id=3415&nbr=2641&string=fibromyalgia
- American Academy of Family Physicians http://www.aafp.org/afp/20000401/2061.html

INFORMATION FOR PATIENTS

- National Institute of Arthritis and Musculoskeletal and Skin Diseases http://www.niams.nih.gov/hi/topics/polymyalgia/index.htm
- Cleveland Clinic Foundation http://www.clevelandclinic.org/arthritis/treat/facts/polymyalgia.htm

REFERENCES

- Evans JM et al: Polymyalgia rheumatica and giant cell arteritis. Rheum Dis Clin North Am 2000;26:493. [PMID: 10989509]
- Jover JA et al: Combined treatment of giant cell arteritis with methotrexate and prednisone. Ann Intern Med 2001; 134:106. [PMID: 11177313]
- Salvarani C et al: Is duplex ultrasonography useful for the diagnosis of giant cell arteritis? Ann Intern Med 2002;137: 232.
- Salvarani C et al: Polymyalgia rheumatica and giant cell arteritis. N Engl J Med 2002;347:261.
- Smetana GW et al: Does this patient have temporal arteritis? JAMA 2002; 287:92. [PMID: 11754714]

David B. Hellmann, MD, FACP
John H. Stone, MD, MPH

Polyneuropathies

KEY FEATURES

ESSENTIALS OF DIAGNOSIS

- Weakness, sensory disturbances, or both in the extremities
- Pain sometimes common
- Depressed or absent tendon reflexes
- May be family history of neuropathy
- May be history of systemic illness or toxic exposure

GENERAL CONSIDERATIONS

- Categorized as axonal or demyelinating as distinguished by neurophysiological findings
- The cause is suggested by the history, mode of onset, and predominant clinical manifestations
- In about half of cases, no specific cause can be established; of these, slightly less than half are found to be heredofamilial

Inherited neuropathies

- Charcot-Marie-Tooth disease
- Dejerine-Sottas disease (HMSN type III)
- Friedreich's ataxia
- Refsum's disease (HMSN type IV)
- Porphyria
  - Motor symptoms usually occur first, and weakness is often most marked proximally and in the upper limbs
  - Sensory symptoms and signs may be proximal or distal in distribution
  - Autonomic involvement is sometimes pronounced
  - Neuropathy is axonal in type

Neuropathies associated with systemic and metabolic disorders

- Diabetes mellitus
  - Symmetric sensory or mixed polyneuropathy
  - Asymmetric motor radiculoneuropathy or plexopathy (diabetic amyotrophy)
  - Thoracoabdominal radiculopathy
  - Autonomic neuropathy
  - Isolated lesions of individual nerves may occur singly or in any combination
- Uremia
  - Symmetric sensorimotor polyneuropathy
  - Tends to affect the lower limbs more than the upper limbs
  - More marked distally than proximally

- Alcoholism and nutritional deficiency (thiamine and B_{12})
  - Axonal distal sensorimotor polyneuropathy
  - Frequently accompanied by painful cramps, muscle tenderness, and painful paresthesias
  - Often more marked in legs than arms
  - Symptoms of autonomic dysfunction may be conspicuous
  - A similar distal sensorimotor polyneuropathy is a well-recognized feature of beriberi (thiamine deficiency)
  - In vitamin B_{12} deficiency, distal sensory polyneuropathy may develop but is usually overshadowed by CNS manifestations
- Paraproteinemias, especiallly multiple myeloma, but also with macroglobulinemia and cryoglobulinemia
  - A gradual onset, progressive, symmetric sensorimotor neuropathy
  - Often accompanied by pain and dysesthesias in the limbs
  - Carpal tunnel syndrome may be seen in generalized amyloidosis

Neuropathies associated with infectious and inflammatory diseases

- Leprosy
  - Sensory disturbances from involvement of intracutaneous nerves
  - Motor deficits result from involvement of superficial nerves where their temperature is lowest, eg, the ulnar nerve in the region proximal to the olecranon groove
- AIDS
  - Chronic symmetric sensorimotor axonal polyneuropathy with normal cerebrospinal fluid (CSF) findings
  - Progressive polyradiculopathy or radiculomyelopathy that leads to leg weakness and urinary retention (CSF may show mononuclear pleocytosis and increased protein and low glucose concentrations); cytomegalovirus is responsible in at least some cases
  - An inflammatory demyelinating polyradiculoneuropathy with weakness more obvious distally than proximally and depressed or absent tendon reflexes (CSF shows an increased cell count and protein concentration)
- Lyme borreliosis
- Sarcoidosis
- Polyarteritis
- Rheumatoid arthritis

Critical illness neuropathy (axonal)

- Initial manifestation may be difficulty in weaning from a mechanical ventilator
- In more advanced cases, there is wasting and weakness of the extremities and loss of tendon reflexes
- Sensory abnormalities are relatively inconspicuous
- Good prognosis if patients recover from the underlying critical illness

Other neuropathies

- Toxic neuropathies
- Neuropathies associated with malignant diseases (see Table 151, page 1340)
- Acute idiopathic polyneuropathy (Guillain-Barré syndrome)
- Chronic inflammatory polyneuropathy

CLINICAL FINDINGS

SYMPTOMS AND SIGNS

- Weakness
- Sensory disturbance
- Pain

DIAGNOSIS

LABORATORY TESTS

- Complete blood cell count and sedimentation rate, serum protein electrophoresis, determination of plasma urea and electrolytes, liver and thyroid function tests, tests for rheumatoid factor and antinuclear antibody, HBsAg determination, a serological test for syphilis, fasting blood glucose level, urinary heavy metal levels, CSF examination, and chest radiography
- These tests should be ordered selectively, as guided by symptoms and signs

DIAGNOSTIC PROCEDURES

- In axonal neuropathies, nerve conduction velocity is normal or reduced only mildly and needle electromyography (EMG) shows denervation in affected muscles
- In demyelinating neuropathies, conduction may be slowed considerably, or even blocked completely, without EMG signs of denervation
- Cutaneous nerve biopsy may help establish a precise diagnosis (eg, polyarteritis, amyloidosis)

TREATMENT

MEDICATIONS

- Neuropathic pain may respond to simple analgesics such as aspirin
- Narcotics or narcotic substitutes may be necessary for severe hyperpathia or pain induced by minimal stimuli, but their use should be avoided as far as possible
- Episodic stabbing pains may respond to phenytoin, carbamazepine, gabapentin, or tricyclic antidepressants
- Postural hypotension is often helped by wearing waist-high elastic stockings and sleeping in a semierect position at night
  - Fludrocortisone reduces postural hypotension, but doses as high as 1 mg/day are sometimes necessary in diabetics and may lead to recumbent hypertension
  - Midodrine, an α-agonist, is sometimes helpful in a dose of 2.5–10 mg three times daily
- Impotence and diarrhea are difficult to treat
- A flaccid neuropathic bladder may respond to parasympathomimetic drugs such as bethanechol chloride, 10–50 mg three or four times daily

THERAPEUTIC PROCEDURES

- Treatment of the underlying cause

 OUTCOME

WHEN TO REFER

- If the diagnosis is uncertain
- For specialized diagnostic tests or for nerve biopsy
- For physical therapy

PREVENTION

- Physical therapy helps prevent contractures, and splints can maintain a weak extremity in a position of useful function
- Anesthetic extremities must be protected from injury
- To guard against burns, patients should check the temperature of water and hot surfaces with a portion of skin having normal sensation, measure water temperature with a thermometer, or use cold water for washing or lower the temperature setting of their hot-water heaters
- Shoes should be examined frequently for grit or foreign objects in order to prevent pressure lesions
- Patients should avoid leaning on elbows or sitting with crossed legs for lengthy periods
- The use of a frame or cradle to reduce contact with bedclothes may be helpful for pain or dysesthesias

 EVIDENCE

PRACTICE GUIDELINES

- National Guideline Clearinghouse http://www.guideline.gov/summary/ summary.aspx?doc_id=3550&nbr= 2776&string=polyneuropathy

INFORMATION FOR PATIENTS

- Beth Israel Medical Center http://stoppain.org/pain_medicine/ polyneuropathy.html
- The Mayo Clinic http://www.mayoclinic.com/invoke.cfm? id=DS00131

REFERENCES

- Jensen PG et al: Management of painful diabetic neuropathy. Drugs Aging 2001; 18;737.
- Manji H: Neuropathy in HIV infection. Curr Opin Neurol 2000;13;589. [PMID: 11073368]
- Saperstein DS et al: Clinical spectrum of chronic acquired demyelinating polyneuropathies. Muscle Nerve 2001; 24;311. [PMID: 11353415]
- Wicklund MP et al: Paraproteinemic neuropathy. Curr Treat Options Neurol 2001;3:147. [PMID: 11180752]

Michael J. Aminoff, MD, DSc, FRCP

Polyps, Colonic & Small Intestinal

 KEY FEATURES

ESSENTIALS OF DIAGNOSIS

- Discrete mass lesions that are flat or protrude into the intestinal lumen
- Most commonly sporadic, may be inherited as part of familial polyposis syndrome
- Three major pathological groups: mucosal neoplastic (adenomatous) polyps, mucosal nonneoplastic polyps (hyperplastic, juvenile polyps, hamartomas, inflammatory polyps), and submucosal lesions (lipomas, lymphoid aggregates, carcinoids, pneumatosis cystoides intestinalis)
- Nonneoplastic mucosal polyps have no malignant potential; adenomatous polyps do
- Of polyps removed at colonoscopy, over 70% are adenomatous; most of the remainder are hyperplastic; distinguished by histology

GENERAL CONSIDERATIONS

- Adenomatous polyps are tubular, villous, or tubulovillous; sessile or pedunculated
- >95% of adenocarcinoma arise from adenomas
- Small adenomas (<1 cm) have a low risk of being malignant; larger adenomas (>1 cm) have a much higher risk (>10%) of harboring malignancy or high-grade dysplasia

DEMOGRAPHICS

- Adenomatous polyps are present in 35% of adults aged >50 years

 CLINICAL FINDINGS

SYMPTOMS AND SIGNS

- Usually asymptomatic
- Chronic occult blood loss may lead to iron deficiency anemia
- Large polyps may ulcerate, resulting in intermittent hematochezia

DIFFERENTIAL DIAGNOSIS

- Colorectal cancer
- Nonneoplastic polyp, eg, hyperplastic, inflammatory
- Submucosal polyp, eg, lipoma, lymphoid aggregate
- Other causes of occult gastrointestinal bleeding, eg, arteriovenous malformation, inflammatory bowel disease

 DIAGNOSIS

LABORATORY TESTS

- Fecal occult blood tests detect <40% of adenomas >1 cm in diameter

IMAGING STUDIES

- Barium enema, whether single- or double-contrast, has unacceptably low sensitivity (~50%) and specificity for the detection of colorectal polyps
- Spiral CT colonography ("virtual colonoscopy") detects over 80–90%

DIAGNOSTIC PROCEDURES

- Flexible sigmoidoscopy: about one-half to one-third of colonic adenomas are within the reach of the flexible sigmoidoscope
- Colonoscopy is best means of detecting and removing adenomatous polyps

Polyps, Colonic & Small Intestinal

 ## TREATMENT

SURGERY

- Primary surgical resection may be required for large (>2–3 cm) sessile polyps
- Malignant polyps are adenomas that appear grossly benign at endoscopy but on histological assessment are found to contain cancer
- Malignant polyps (termed "favorable") are adequately treated by polypectomy alone if the polyp is completely excised, well differentiated, margin is not involved, and no vascular or lymphatic invasion
- Risk of residual cancer or nodal metastasis is 0.3% for pedunculated malignant polyps and 1.5% for sessile malignant polyps
- Surgical resection for "unfavorable" malignant polyps

THERAPEUTIC PROCEDURES

- Colonoscopic polypectomy is possible for most polyps, particularly pedunculated polyps

 ## OUTCOME

FOLLOW-UP

- Periodic colonoscopic surveillance is recommended to detect "metachronous" adenomas
- In high-risk patients, colonoscopy is recommended at 3 years after the initial colonoscopy and polypectomy; in low-risk patients, at 5 years
- Excision site of "favorable" malignant polyps should be checked in 3 months for residual tissue

COMPLICATIONS

- Complications of colonoscopic polypectomy include perforation in 0.2%, bleeding in 1%

PREVENTION

- Nonsteroidal antiinflammatory drugs (NSAIDs), aspirin, and COX-2 selective NSAIDs may decrease the incidence of colorectal adenomas and the progression to cancer; due to their other side effects, routine prophylaxis with these agents is not currently recommended

 ## EVIDENCE

PRACTICE GUIDELINES

- Management of colonic polyps and adenomas. Society for Surgery of the Alimentary Tract, Inc., 2000 http://www.ssat.com/cgi-bin/polyps.cgi?affiliation=student
- Polyp guideline: diagnosis, treatment, and surveillance for patients with colorectal polyps. American College of Gastroenterology, 2000 http://www-east.elsevier.com/ajg/issues/9511/ajg3434fla.htm

WEB SITE

- American Society for Gastrointestinal Endoscopy—Understanding polyps and their treatment http://www.asge.org/gui/patient/polyps_brochure.asp

INFORMATION FOR PATIENTS

- American Society of Colon and Rectal Surgeons—Polyps of the colon & rectum http://www.fascrs.org/brochures/polyps.html
- National Institute of Diabetes and Digestive and Kidney Diseases—What I need to know about colon polyps http://digestive.niddk.nih.gov/ddiseases/pubs/colonpolyps_ez/index.htm

REFERENCES

- Bond JH: Polyp guideline: diagnosis, treatment, and surveillance for patients with colorectal polyps. Practice Parameters Committee of the American College of Gastroenterology. Am J Gastroenterol 2000;95:3053. [PMID: 11095318]
- Lieberman D et al: Use of colonoscopy to screen asymptomatic adults for colorectal cancer. N Engl J Med 2000; 343:162. [PMID: 10900274]

Kenneth R. McQuaid, MD

Pompholyx (Dyshidrotic Eczema)

 KEY FEATURES

ESSENTIALS OF DIAGNOSIS

- "Tapioca" vesicles of 1–2 mm on the palms, soles, and sides of fingers, associated with pruritus
- Vesicles may coalesce to form multiloculated blisters
- Scaling and fissuring may follow drying of the blisters
- Appearance in the third decade, with lifelong recurrences

GENERAL CONSIDERATIONS

- "Dyshidrotic eczema" is a misnomer, suggesting that the vesicles of this condition are related to eccrine sweat ducts and sweating, which they are not
- An extremely common form of hand dermatitis, preferably called pompholyx (Gr "bubble") or vesiculobullous dermatitis of the palms and soles
- Patients often have an atopic background and report flares with stress
- In Scandinavia, women with contact allergy to nickel and pompholyx appear to flare when given oral challenges with nickel; nickel-free diets have given variable results; the chelator disulfiram has been reported to cause a 25% improvement in one controlled study in nickel-sensitive patients, and oral cromolyn sodium has also been shown to be of benefit
- Patients with widespread dermatitis due to any cause may develop pompholyx-like eruptions as a part of an autoeczematization response

 CLINICAL FINDINGS

SYMPTOMS AND SIGNS

- See Table 7 (page 1202)
- Small clear vesicles stud the skin at the sides of the fingers and on the palms or soles; they look like the grains in tapioca
- Lesions may be associated with intense itching
- Later, the vesicles dry and the area becomes scaly and fissured

DIFFERENTIAL DIAGNOSIS

- Vesicular tinea
- Contact dermatitis
- Tinea pedis with dermatophytid reaction of palms
- Scabies
- Nonsteroidal antiinflammatory drugs

 DIAGNOSIS

LABORATORY TESTS

- Unroofing the vesicles and scraping the blister roof for a KOH examination will reveal hyphae in cases of bullous tinea, which may be confused with pompholyx

TREATMENT

MEDICATIONS

- See Table 6 (page 1199)
- Topical corticosteroids help some patients dramatically
- Systemic steroids should be avoided in this chronic condition
- A high-potency topical steroid used early in the attack may help abort the flare and ameliorate pruritus
- Topical steroids can effectively treat the scaling and fissuring that are seen after the vesicular phase

THERAPEUTIC PROCEDURES

- Patients respond to PUVA therapy using topical psoralen and UVA light

OUTCOME

PROGNOSIS

- For most patients, the disease is an inconvenience
- For some, vesiculobullous hand eczema can be incapacitating

WHEN TO REFER

- If there is a question about the diagnosis, if recommended therapy is ineffective, or specialized treatment is necessary

PREVENTION

- Avoid anything that irritates the skin; patients should wear cotton gloves inside vinyl gloves when doing dishes or other wet chores, use long-handled brushes instead of sponges, and use a hand cream after washing the hands
- If a history of nickel allergy (rashes with costume jewelry or from watchbands) is obtained, nickel-free diets may be considered

EVIDENCE

WEB SITES

- American Academy of Dermatology http://www.aad.org
- Dermatology Handbook for Family Practice from the University of Iowa http://www.vh.org/Providers/ClinRef/FPHandbook/17.html

INFORMATION FOR PATIENTS

- National Institutes of Health http://www.nlm.nih.gov/medlineplus/ency/article/000832.htm

REFERENCE

- Swartling C et al: Treatment of dyshidrotic hand dermatitis with intradermal botulinum toxin. J Am Dermatol 2002:47:667. [PMID: 12399757]

Timothy G. Berger, MD

Porphyria Cutanea Tarda

 KEY FEATURES

ESSENTIALS OF DIAGNOSIS

- Noninflammatory blisters on sun-exposed sites, especially the dorsal surfaces of the hands
- Hypertrichosis, skin fragility
- Associated liver disease
- Elevated urine porphyrins

GENERAL CONSIDERATIONS

- The most common type of porphyria
- Cases are sporadic or hereditary
- The disease is associated with ingestion of certain medications (eg, estrogens), and liver disease from alcoholism or hepatitis C
- Most patients improve with treatment

 CLINICAL FINDINGS

SYMPTOMS AND SIGNS

- See Table 7 (page 1202)
- Painless blistering and fragility of the skin of the dorsal surfaces of the hands
- Facial hypertrichosis and hyperpigmentation are common

DIFFERENTIAL DIAGNOSIS

- Pseudoporphyria: dialysis, medications (tetracycline, nonsteroidal antiinflammatory drugs)
- Contact dermatitis
- Scabies
- Tinea manuum
- Atopic dermatitis (eczema)

 DIAGNOSIS

LABORATORY TESTS

- Urinary uroporphyrins are elevated two- to five-fold above coproporphyrins
- There may be abnormal liver function tests, evidence of hepatitis C infection, increased liver iron stores, and hemochromatosis gene mutations

Porphyria Cutanea Tarda

 TREATMENT

MEDICATIONS

- Phlebotomy without oral iron supplementation at a rate of one unit every 2–4 weeks will gradually lead to improvement
- Very low-dose antimalarials (as low as 200 mg of hydroxychloroquine twice weekly) will increase the excretion of porphyrins, improving the skin disease; treatment is continued until the patient is asymptomatic; urine porphyrins may be monitored

THERAPEUTIC PROCEDURES

- Stopping all triggering medications and substantially reducing or stopping alcohol consumption may alone lead to improvement

 OUTCOME

COMPLICATIONS

- Sclerodermoid skin lesions may develop on the trunk, scalp, and face

PROGNOSIS

- Most patients improve with treatment

WHEN TO REFER

- If there is a question about the diagnosis, if recommended therapy is ineffective, or if specialized treatment is necessary

PREVENTION

- The wavelength of light triggering the lesions is beyond that absorbed by sunscreens, which for that reason are ineffective
- Barrier sun protection with clothing is required

 EVIDENCE

WEB SITES

- American Academy of Dermatology
  http://www.aad.org
- Dermatology Handbook for Family Practice from the University of Iowa
  http://www.vh.org/Providers/ClinRef/FPHandbook/17.html

INFORMATION FOR PATIENTS

- National Digestive Diseases Information Clearinghouse
  http://digestive.niddk.nih.gov/ddiseases/pubs/porphyria/index.htm
- Iron Disorders Institute
  http://www.irondisorders.org/disorders/pct/index.htm

REFERENCES

- Bulaj ZJ et al: Hemochromatosis genes and other factors contributing to the pathogenesis of porphyria cutanea tarda. Blood 2000;95:1565. [PMID: 10688809]
- Rich MW: Porphyria cutanea tarda. Don't forget to look at the urine. Postgrad Med 1999;105:208. [PMID: 10223097]

Timothy G. Berger, MD

Porphyria, Acute Intermittent

 KEY FEATURES

ESSENTIALS OF DIAGNOSIS

- Unexplained abdominal crisis, generally in young women
- Acute central or peripheral nervous system dysfunction
- Recurrent psychiatric illnesses
- Hyponatremia
- Porphobilinogen in the urine during an attack

GENERAL CONSIDERATIONS

- Acute intermittent porphyria is caused by deficiency of porphobilinogen deaminase activity, leading to increased excretion of aminolevulinic acid and porphobilinogen in the urine
- Genetics: mutation in the porphobilinogen deaminase gene
- Inherited as an autosomal dominant
- It remains clinically silent in the majority of patients who carry the trait
- Characteristic abdominal pain may be due to abnormalities in autonomic innervation in the gut
- Cutaneous photosensitivity is absent
- Attacks precipitated by numerous factors, including drugs and intercurrent infections
- Hyponatremia, due to inappropriate release of antidiuretic hormone and gastrointestinal loss of sodium

DEMOGRAPHICS

- Usually presents in adulthood and has serious consequences
- Women usually develop clinical illness
- Symptoms beginning in the teens or 20s, but in rare cases after menopause

 CLINICAL FINDINGS

SYMPTOMS AND SIGNS

- Intermittent abdominal pain of varying severity, sometimes simulating an acute abdome
- Absence of fever and leukocytosis
- Complete recovery between attacks
- Autonomic neuropathy
- Peripheral neuropathy, symmetric or asymmetric, mild or profound
- Central nervous system manifestations include seizures, psychosis, and abnormalities of the basal ganglia

DIFFERENTIAL DIAGNOSIS

- Acute abdominal pain due to other cause, eg, appendicitis, peptic ulcer disease, cholecystitis, diverticulitis, ruptured ectopic pregnancy, familial Mediterranean fever
- Polyneuropathy due to other cause
- Guillain-Barré syndrome
- Lead or other heavy metal poisoning
- Psychosis due to other cause
- Syndrome of inappropriate antidiuretic hormone due to other cause
- Dark urine due to other cause, eg, alkaptonuria

 DIAGNOSIS

LABORATORY TESTS

- Hyponatremia, often profound
- Freshly voided urine is of normal color but may turn dark upon standing in light and air
- Urine porphobilinogen increased during an acute attack

TREATMENT

MEDICATIONS

- Analgesics
- Intravenous glucose
- High-carbohydrate intake, a minimum of 300 g of carbohydrate per day PO or IV
- Hematin up to 4 mg/kg IV QD or BID
- Adverse consequences of hematin therapy include phlebitis and coagulopathy

THERAPEUTIC PROCEDURES

- High-carbohydrate diet diminishes the number of attacks
- Withdrawal of the inciting agent

OUTCOME

FOLLOW-UP

- EKG
- Electrolytes
- Glucose
- Mental status

PROGNOSIS

- Acute attacks may be life-threatening and require prompt diagnosis

WHEN TO REFER

- Genetic counseling

WHEN TO ADMIT

- Abdominal crisis
- Marked hyponatremia
- Acute CNS dysfunction

PREVENTION

- Avoidance of factors known to precipitate attacks, especially drugs (Table 144, page 1326)
- Starvation diets must be avoided

EVIDENCE

WEB SITES

- American Porphyria Foundation
  http://www.porphyriafoundation.com
- Canadian Porphyria Foundation
  http://www.cpf-inc.ca/

INFORMATION FOR PATIENTS

- American Porphyria Foundation—AIP, HCP, VP, & ADP Brochure
  http://www.porphyriafoundation.com/aip.html
- Canadian Porphyria Foundation—AIP information sheet
  http://www.cpf-inc.ca/AIP.htm
- MEDLINEplus Medical Encyclopedia: Porphyria
  http://www.nlm.nih.gov/medlineplus/ency/article/001208.htm
- The Porph Forum
  http://members.tripod.com/~theaipforum/

REFERENCES

- Badminton MN et al: Management of acute and cutaneous porphyries. Int J Clin Pract 2002;56:272. [PMID: 12074210]
- Desnick RJ et al: Inherited porphyrias. In: Emery and Rimoin's principles and practice of medical genetics, ed 4. Rimoin DL et al (editors). Churchill Livingstone, 2002.
- Grandchamp B: Acute intermittent porphyria. Semin Liver Dis 1998;18:17. [PMID: 9516674]
- Sassa S et al: Molecular aspects of the inherited porphyrias. J Intern Med 2000;247:169. [PMID: 10692079]

Reed E. Pyeritz, MD, PhD

Postherpetic Neuralgia

 KEY FEATURES

ESSENTIALS OF DIAGNOSIS

- Past history of herpes zoster (shingles)
- Occurrence of pain for months or years in the same dermatomal distribution as was affected by the herpes zoster

GENERAL CONSIDERATIONS

- Herpes zoster (shingles) is due to infection of the nervous system by varicella-zoster virus
- About 15% of patients who develop shingles suffer from postherpetic neuralgia. This complication seems especially likely to occur in the elderly, when the rash is severe, and when the first division of the trigeminal nerve is affected

 CLINICAL FINDINGS

SYMPTOMS AND SIGNS

- Severe pain, sometimes burning or tingling and quite disabling, occurs in areas of prior shingles

DIFFERENTIAL DIAGNOSIS

- Temporomandibular joint
- Dental disturbance
- Giant cell arteritis
- Sinusitis and ear infection
- Glaucoma (pain usually localized to the periorbital region)
- Angina pectoris

 DIAGNOSIS

DIAGNOSTIC PROCEDURES

- A history of shingles and the presence of cutaneous scarring resulting from shingles aid in the diagnosis

TREATMENT

MEDICATIONS

- The incidence of postherpetic neuralgia may be reduced by the treatment of shingles with oral acyclovir or famciclovir, but this is disputed (see *Herpes zoster*)
- Systemic corticosteroids do not help
- Management of the established complication is essentially medical
- If simple analgesics fail to help, a trial of a tricyclic drug (eg, amitriptyline, up to 100–150 mg/day) in conjunction with a phenothiazine (eg, perphenazine, 2–8 mg/day) is often effective
- Other patients respond to carbamazepine (up to 1200 mg/day), phenytoin (300 mg/day), or gabapentin (up to 3600 mg/day)
- Topical application of capsaicin cream (eg, Zostrix, 0.025%) may also be helpful, perhaps because of depletion of pain-mediating peptides from peripheral sensory neurons

 OUTCOME

PREVENTION

- Early treatment of zoster

 EVIDENCE

PRACTICE GUIDELINES

- National Guideline Clearinghouse
  http://www.guideline.gov/summary/
  summary.aspx?doc_id=3500&nbr=
  2726&string=postherpetic+neuralgia

INFORMATION FOR PATIENTS

- The Mayo Clinic
  http://www.mayoclinic.com/invoke.cfm?
  id=DS00277
- Beth Israel Medical Center
  http://stoppain.org/pain_medicine/
  shingles.html

REFERENCES

- Alper BS et al: Does treatment of acute herpes zoster prevent or shorten postherpetic neuralgia? J Fam Pract 2000;49: 255. [PMID: 10735485]
- Rice AS et al: Gabapentin in postherpetic neuralgia: a randomized, double blind, placebo controlled study. Pain 2001;94;215. [PMID: 11690735]

Michael J. Aminoff, DSc, MD, FRCP

Posttraumatic Stress Disorder

 KEY FEATURES

ESSENTIALS OF DIAGNOSIS

- A syndrome characterized by "reexperiencing" a traumatic event (eg, rape, severe burns, military combat), along with decreased responsiveness and avoidance of current events associated with the trauma
- Alcohol and other drugs are commonly used in self-treatment

GENERAL CONSIDERATIONS

- Included among the anxiety disorders in *DSM-IV*
- The symptoms may be precipitated or exacerbated by events that are a reminder of the original stress
- Symptoms frequently arise after a long latency period (eg, child abuse can result in later-onset posttraumatic stress syndrome)

 CLINICAL FINDINGS

SYMPTOMS AND SIGNS

- Physiological hyperarousal, which includes startle reactions, intrusive thoughts, illusions, overgeneralized associations, sleep problems, nightmares, dreams about the precipitating event, impulsivity, difficulties in concentration, and hyperalertness

DIFFERENTIAL DIAGNOSIS

- Anxiety disorders
- Affective disorders
- Personality disorders exacerbated by stress
- Somatic disorders with psychic overlay

 DIAGNOSIS

LABORATORY TESTS

- Thyroid-stimulating hormone
- Complete blood cell count
- Toxicology screen (if suspected)
- Glucose

TREATMENT

MEDICATIONS

- Early treatment of anxious arousal with β-blockers (eg, propranolol, 80–160 mg daily) may lessen the peripheral symptoms of anxiety (eg, tremors, palpitations) and help prevent the development of the disorder
- Antidepressant drugs—particularly selective serotonin reuptake inhibitors (SSRIs)—in full dosage are helpful in ameliorating depression, panic attacks, sleep disruption, and startle responses in chronic PTSD. Sertraline is FDA approved for this purpose
- Antiseizure medications such as carbamazepine (400–800 mg daily) will often mitigate impulsivity and difficulty with anger management
- Benzodiazepines (Table 101, page 1285) such as clonazepam (1–4 mg daily) will reduce anxiety and panic attacks when used in adequate dosage, but dependency problems are a concern, particularly when the patient has had such problems in the past

THERAPEUTIC PROCEDURES

- The therapeutic approach is to facilitate the normal recovery that was blocked at the time of the trauma. Therapy at that time should be brief and simple (catharsis and working through of the traumatic experience), expecting quick recovery and promoting a sense of mastery and acceptance over the traumatic event
- Early cognitive-behavioral interventions can also speed recovery
- Treatment initiated later, when symptoms have crystallized, includes programs for cessation of alcohol and other drug abuse, group and individual psychotherapy, and improved social support systems
- Psychological debriefing in a single session, once considered a mainstay in prevention of PTSD, is under scrutiny

 OUTCOME

PROGNOSIS

- The sooner the symptoms arise after the initial trauma and the sooner therapy is initiated, the better the prognosis
- Resolution may be delayed if others' responses to the patient's difficulties are thoughtlessly harmful or if the secondary gains outweigh the advantages of recovery
- The longer the symptoms persist, the worse the prognosis

WHEN TO REFER

- Marital problems are a major area of concern, and it is important that the clinician have available a dependable referral source when marriage counseling is indicated

 EVIDENCE

PRACTICE GUIDELINES

- National Guideline Clearinghouse http://www.guideline.gov/summary/summary.aspx?doc_id=815&nbr=314&string=PTSD http://www.guideline.gov/summary/summary.aspx?doc_id=1902&nbr=1128&string=PTSD

WEB SITES

- American Psychiatric Association http://www.psych.org/
- Internet Mental Health http://www.mentalhealth.com/t30.html
- National Center for Posttraumatic Stress Disorder http://www. ncptsd.org
- Posttraumatic stress disorder alliance http://www.ptsdalliance.org

INFORMATION FOR PATIENTS

- JAMA patient page: Posttraumatic stress disorder. JAMA 2001;286:630.
- National Institute of Mental Health http://www.nimh.nih.gov/anxiety/ptsdri1.cfm
- American Psychiatric Association http://www.medem.com/medlb/article_detaillb.cfm?article_ID=ZZZS560CT7C&sub_cat=47

REFERENCES

- Brady K et al: Efficacy and safety of sertraline treatment of posttraumatic stress disorder, a randomised control trial. JAMA 2000;283:1837.
- Pitman RK et al: Pilot study of secondary prevention of PTSD with propranolol. Biol Psychiatry 2002;51:189.

Stuart J. Eisendrath, MD
Jonathan E. Lichtmacher, MD

Preeclampsia & Eclampsia

 KEY FEATURES

ESSENTIALS OF DIAGNOSIS

- Preeclampsia
  - Blood pressure of ≥140 mm Hg systolic or ≥90 mm Hg diastolic after 20 weeks' gestation
  - Proteinuria of ≥0.3 g in 24 h
- Severe preeclampsia
  - Blood pressure of ≥160 mm Hg systolic or ≥110 mm Hg diastolic
  - Proteinuria ≥5 g in 24 h or 4+ on dipstick
  - Oliguria of <500 mL in 24 h
  - Thrombocytopenia
  - Hemolysis elevated liver enzymes low platelets (HELLP)
  - Pulmonary edema
- Fetal growth restriction

GENERAL CONSIDERATIONS

- Cause is unknown, but an immunological cause is suspected
- The only cure is delivery of the fetus and placenta
- Uncontrolled eclampsia is a significant cause of maternal death
- Use of diuretics, dietary changes, aspirin, and vitamin-mineral supplements have not been shown to be effective
- Early diagnosis is the key to treatment
- Many cases are asymptomatic early
- 5% of women with preeclampsia progress to eclampsia

DEMOGRAPHICS

- Occurs in 7% of pregnant women in the United States
- Higher incidence in primiparas
- Other risk factors are multiple gestations, chronic hypertension, diabetes, renal disease, collagen-vascular and autoimmune disease, and gestational trophoblastic disease

 CLINICAL FINDINGS

SYMPTOMS AND SIGNS

- See Table 69 (page 1262)
- Hypertension, proteinuria, and edema are classically required for the diagnosis, but presentation varies greatly
- Can occur any time after 20 weeks' gestation and up to 6 weeks postpartum
- Severity can be assessed with reference to the six sites where disease has its effects: CNS, kidneys, liver, hematological and vascular systems, and the fetal placental unit
- Few complaints are present in mild disease; antepartum fetal testing is reassuring
- Symptoms are dramatic and persist in severe disease; thrombocytopenia may progress to disseminated intravascular coagulation

DIFFERENTIAL DIAGNOSIS

- Essential hypertension or other cause of secondary hypertension
- Chronic renal failure or proteinuria due to other cause
- Primary seizure disorder
- Thrombotic thrombocytopenic purpura
- Other cause of abdominal pain, eg, cholecystitis, appendicitis, acute fatty liver of pregnancy
- Gallbladder and pancreatic disease
- Hemolytic uremic syndrome

 DIAGNOSIS

LABORATORY TESTS

- See Table 69 (page 1262)
- Platelet count is over 100,000 in mild to moderate disease
- Thrombocytopenia seen in severe disease
- Hemolysis, elevated liver enzymes, and low platelets describe the HELLP syndrome
- Hyperuricemia is helpful in diagnosis, as in pregnancy, it is seen only with gout, renal failure, or preeclampsia-eclampsia

Preeclampsia & Eclampsia

TREATMENT

MEDICATIONS

- Sedatives and opiates should be avoided, as they interfere with fetal assessment
- Two doses of steroids (betamethasone, 12 mg or dexamethasone, 16 mg) 12–24 h apart should be given if fetal immaturity is present
- Diazepam (5–10 mg) or magnesium sulfate (4 g bolus, then 2–3 g/h unless abnormal renal function is present) is used to stop seizures
- Hydralazine, 5–10 mg IV every 20 min, nifedipine 10 mg SL or PO, or labetalol, 10–20 mg IV every 20 min can be used
- Oxytocin may be used to induce or augment labor
- Magnesium sulfate infusion should be continued postpartum until preeclampsia-eclampsia begins to resolve (1–7 days), as indicated by the onset of diuresis (100–200 mL/h)
- Antihypertensive therapy is used if diastolic blood pressure >110, with a target of 90–100

SURGERY

- Cesarean section is reserved for the usual fetal indications or when rapid delivery is needed
- Regional anesthesia or analgesia is acceptable

THERAPEUTIC PROCEDURES

- Nonstress and stress fetal testing or a biophysical profile should be obtained initially and then serially to confirm fetal well-being
- Daily fetal kick counts can be recorded by the mother
- Amniocentesis should be considered to evaluate lung maturity if hospitalization occurs at 30–37 weeks

Preeclampsia

- Disease of any severity at 36 weeks or later is managed by delivery
- Prior to 36 weeks, severe disease requires delivery except in cases of extreme fetal prematurity
- Bed rest is the cornerstone of therapy for mild to moderate preeclampsia; it may be attempted at home or in the hospital depending on the degree of organ system involvement
- Epigastric pain, thrombocytopenia, and visual disturbances are strong indications for delivery

Eclampsia

- Seizing patients are placed on their side to increase placental blood flow and avoid aspiration
- Maternal and fetal status determine the method of delivery

OUTCOME

FOLLOW-UP

- Blood pressure, reflexes, proteinuria, and fetal monitoring are required regularly in hospitalized patients
- Blood cell count, electrolytes, proteinuria, and liver enzymes should be checked every 1–2 days in hospitalized patients
- 24-h urine protein and creatinine clearance on admission and as indicated
- Magnesium levels are checked every 4–6 h and infusions titrated to serum levels of 4–6 mEq/L
- Urine output is checked hourly in severe disease or eclampsia
- Patients on magnesium infusions are followed for signs of toxicity such as loss of deep tendon reflexes or respiratory depression; calcium gluconate can be used for reversal

WHEN TO ADMIT

- Moderate or severe preeclampsia or an unreliable home situation warrants hospitalization

EVIDENCE

PRACTICE GUIDELINES

- ACOG Committee on Practice Bulletins. ACOG Practice Bulletin. Chronic hypertension in pregnancy. Obstet Gynecol 2001;98:suppl 177. [PMID: 11508256]
- National Guideline Clearinghouse http://www.guideline.gov/summary/summary.aspx?doc_id=1478&nbr=704&string=eclampsia
- ACOG Committee on Obstetrics Practice. ACOG practice bulletin. Diagnosis and management of preeclampsia and eclampsia. Number 33, January 2002. American College of Obstetricians and Gynecologists. Int J Gynaecol Obstet 2002;77:67. [PMID: 12094777]

WEB SITES

- Guidelines, Recommendations, and Evidence-Based Medicine in Obstetrics http://matweb.hcuge.ch/matweb/endo/cours_4e_MREG/obstetrics_gynecology_guidelines.htm
- Clinical Guidelines in Obstetrics and Gynecology http://www.rcog.org.uk/guidelines.asp?PageID=105

INFORMATION FOR PATIENTS

- JAMA patient page: Pregnancy complications. JAMA 2001;285:1664.
- American Academy of Family Physicians http://familydoctor.org/handouts/064.html

REFERENCE

- Lain KY et al: Contemporary concepts of the pathogenesis and management of pre-eclampsia. JAMA 2002;287:3183. [PMID:12076198]

William R. Crombleholme, MD

Pregnancy

 KEY FEATURES

ESSENTIALS OF DIAGNOSIS

- Amenorrhea, weight gain, nausea and vomiting, and breast changes
- Positive pregnancy test

GENERAL CONSIDERATIONS

- Prompt diagnosis of pregnancy allows early prenatal care and avoidance of harmful activities or exposures
- In the event of an unwanted pregnancy, early diagnosis allows for counseling regarding adoption or termination

 CLINICAL FINDINGS

SYMPTOMS AND SIGNS

- No symptoms or signs are diagnostic
- Amenorrhea, weight gain
- Nausea and vomiting
- Breast tenderness and tingling
- Urinary frequency and urgency
- "Quickening" (perception of the first fetal movement) is noted at about 18 weeks' gestation
- Signs
  - Breast changes, abdominal enlargement, and cyanosis of the vagina and cervical portio (week 7)
  - Softening of the cervix (week 7)
  - Generalized enlargement and softening of the corpus (post-week 8)
  - Uterine fundus is palpable above the pubic symphysis by 12–15 weeks from last menstrual period
  - Fundus reaches the umbilicus by 20–22 weeks
  - Fetal heart tones heard by Doppler at 10 to 12 weeks

DIFFERENTIAL DIAGNOSIS

- Myomas can be confused with a gravid uterus
- A midline ovarian tumor may displace a nonpregnant uterus
- Ectopic pregnancies may show lower levels of human chorionic gonadotropin (hCG) that level off or fall
- Premature menopause

 DIAGNOSIS

LABORATORY TESTS

Diagnostic tests

- All urine or blood pregnancy tests rely on detection of placental hCG and are accurate at the time of a missed period or shortly after it
- Laboratory and home assays use monoclonal antibodies specific for hCG
- hCG levels increase shortly after implantation, double every 48 h, peak at 50–75 days, and fall in second and third trimesters

Screening at the time of diagnosis

- Urinalysis, culture of a mid-stream urine sample, complete blood cell count (CBC), serological test for syphilis, rubella antibody titer, blood group and Rh type, atypical antibody screening, and hepatitis B surface antigen testing are recommended
- HIV testing should be encouraged
- Cervical cultures for *Neisseria gonorrhoea* and *Chlamydia*, as well as Pap smear, are indicated
- Testing for abnormal hemoglobins should be done in patients at risk for sickle cell or thalassemia traits
- Tuberculosis skin testing is recommended for high-risk groups
- Tay-Sachs screening is offered to Jewish women with Jewish partners
- Cystic fibrosis screening should be offered
- Hepatitis C screening should be offered to mothers at high risk

Screening during pregnancy

- Maternal serum α-fetoprotein (AFP) is offered to all women to screen for neural tube defects and is mandatory in some states (16–20 weeks)
- hCG and estriol levels are combined with AFP (triple screen) for detection of fetal Down's syndrome
- Screening for gestational diabetes by checking glucose 1 h post a 50-g glucose load (26–28 weeks)
- 3-h glucose tolerance test follows up an abnormal 1-h glucose load test
- Repeat Rh testing for negative patients [28 weeks, though result is not required before Rho(D) Ig is given]
- CBC to evaluate for anemia of pregnancy (28–32 weeks)

- Repeat tests for syphilis, HIV, and cervical cultures in at-risk patients (36 weeks to delivery)
- Screening for group B streptococcal (GBS) colonization can be done by rectovaginal culture at 35–37 weeks
  - If negative, no prophylaxis is given
  - Intrapartum prophylaxis with penicillin or clindamycin is given if screening cultures are positive
  - Patients with risk factors for GBS or who deliver at less than 37 weeks receive intrapartum prophylaxis
  - Patients without a culture at 35–37 weeks receive prophylaxis only for a history of GBS bacteriuria or prior GBS disease in an infant, intrapartum fevers, or membrane rupture >18 h

IMAGING STUDIES

- X-rays should be avoided unless essential and approved by a physician
- Fetal ultrasound for accurate dating and to evaluate fetal anatomy is usually done at 18–20 weeks' gestation
- In multiple pregnancies, ultrasound is repeated every 4 weeks to identify discordant growth

TREATMENT

MEDICATIONS

- Prenatal vitamins with iron and folic acid are indicated
- Medications should not be taken unless prescribed or authorized by the patient's provider (Tables 68 and 71, pages 1261 and 1263)
- Penicillin (5 MU followed by 2.5 MU Q 4 h until deliver), or clindamycin (900 mg IV Q 8 h) are given for prophylaxis of Group B streptococcal infection with susceptible isolates

THERAPEUTIC PROCEDURES

- Genetic counseling with the option of chorionic villous sampling or amniocentesis should be offered to women 35 or older at delivery, a family history of congenital abnormalities, or previous child with a metabolic disease, chromosomal abnormality, or neural tube defect

OUTCOME

FOLLOW-UP

- Prenatal visits should be scheduled
  - Every 4 weeks from 0–28 weeks
  - Every 2 weeks from 28–36 weeks
  - Weekly from 36 weeks to delivery

COMPLICATIONS

- Fetal alcohol syndrome: no safe level of alcohol intake has been established for pregnancy
- Cigarette smoking increases risk of abruptio placentae, placenta previa, and premature rupture of the membranes
- Premature delivery and lower birth weights are more common in children born to smokers
- Maternal cocaine, amphetamine, and opioid use in pregnancy is associated with numerous complications

WHEN TO REFER

- If the practitioner has no training or experience in prenatal care

WHEN TO ADMIT

- For any major medical or pregnancy-related complication

PREVENTION

- Hepatitis B vaccination for women with potential occupational exposure or household contacts
- Live virus immunizations (measles, rubella, varicella, yellow fever) are contraindicated during pregnancy
- Influenza vaccine is indicated in all women who will be in their second or third trimester during "flu season"
- Decrease caffeine intake
- Avoid ingestion of raw meat, all tobacco, alcohol, and recreational drugs, exposure to environmental tobacco smoke, excessive heat, hot tubs, and saunas, and handling of cat feces or litter
- Exercise should be mild to moderate, with heart rate kept below 140 bpm

EVIDENCE

PRACTICE GUIDELINES

- National Guideline Clearinghouse
  http://www.guideline.gov/summary/
  summary.aspx?doc_id=3442&nbr=
  2668&string=prenatal+care
  http://www.guideline.gov/summary/
  summary.aspx?doc_id=3497&nbr=
  2723&string=pregnancy
  http://www.guideline.gov/summary/
  summary.aspx?doc_id=2951&nbr=
  2177&string=pregnancy

WEB SITES

- Clinical Guidelines in Obstetrics and Gynecology
  http://www.rcog.org.uk/guidelines.asp?
  PageID=105
- Guidelines, Recommendations, and Evidence-Based Medicine in Obstetrics
  http://matweb.hcuge.ch/matweb/endo/
  cours_4e_MREG/obstetrics_
  gynecology_guidelines.htm
- Obstetric Ultrasound
  http://www.ob-ultrasound.net

INFORMATION FOR PATIENTS

- JAMA patient page: Birth labor. JAMA 2002;288:1432.
- JAMA patient page: Delivering a healthy infant. JAMA 2002;287:1604.
- Patient-Oriented Materials for Pregnancy and Beyond
  http://www.noah-health.org/english/
  pregnancy/pregnancy.html

REFERENCES

- Haertsch M et al: What is recommended for healthy women during pregnancy? A comparison of seven prenatal clinical practice guideline documents. Birth 1999;26:24. [PMID: 10352052]
- Koren G et al: Drugs in pregnancy. N Engl J Med 1998;338:1128. [PMID: 9545362]
- Schrag SJ et al: Group B streptococcal disease in the era of intrapartum antibiotic prophylaxis. N Engl J Med 2000; 342:15. [PMID: 10620644]

William R. Crombleholme, MD

Premenstrual Syndrome

KEY FEATURES

ESSENTIALS OF DIAGNOSIS

- Recurrent, variable cluster of troublesome physical and emotional symptoms that develops during the 7–14 days before the onset of menses
- Symptoms subside when menstruation occurs
- In about 10% of affected women, the syndrome may be severe

GENERAL CONSIDERATIONS

- The pathogenesis is still uncertain. Psychosocial factors may play a role
- Suppression of ovulation with an oral contraceptive is sometimes helpful, but the patient often complains that she still has premenstrual syndrome

DEMOGRAPHICS

- Intermittently affects about one-third of all premenopausal women, primarily those 25–40 years of age

CLINICAL FINDINGS

SYMPTOMS AND SIGNS

- Women may not experiences all the symptoms or signs at one time
- Bloating
- Breast pain
- Ankle swelling
- A sense of increased weight
- Skin disorders
- Irritability, aggressiveness, depression, inability to concentrate, libido change, lethargy, and food cravings

DIFFERENTIAL DIAGNOSIS

- Depression
- Premenstrual dysphoric disorder
- Endometriosis
- Uterine leiomyomas (fibroids)
- Pregnancy
- Anxiety disorder
- Hypothyroidism

DIAGNOSIS

DIAGNOSTIC PROCEDURES

- Careful evaluation of the patient
- History of symptoms

Premenstrual Syndrome

 TREATMENT

MEDICATIONS

- Serotonin reuptake inhibitors such as fluoxetine, 20 mg/day, are effective in relieving tension, irritability, and dysphoria with few side effects
- Luteal-phase administration of danazol, 200 mg/day on cycle Days 14–28, is effective in reducing symptoms of mastalgia. Other symptoms are not affected by this low-dose therapy
- Suppression of ovarian function with a gonadotropin-releasing hormone (GnRH) agonist diminishes all symptoms during therapy. "Add-back therapy" to provide the hormones suppressed by the GnRH agonist with low-dose estrogen and progestin may allow extended use of a GnRH agonist

THERAPEUTIC PROCEDURES

- Current treatment methods are mainly empirical
- Provide support for the emotional and physical distress
- Advise the patient to keep a daily diary of all symptoms for 2–3 months to help in evaluating the timing and characteristics of the syndrome. If her symptoms occur throughout the month rather than in the 2 weeks before menses, she may be depressed or may have other emotional problems in addition to premenstrual syndrome
- A diet emphasizing complex carbohydrates can be recommended. Foods high in sugar content and alcohol should be avoided to minimize reactive hypoglycemia. Use of caffeine should be minimized whenever tension and irritability predominate
- Vitamin B_6, up to 100 mg/day, may be beneficial in the treatment of premenstrual symptoms and premenstrual depression. At this dosage level, neurological side effects are rare
- A program of regular conditioning exercise, such as jogging, can decrease depression, anxiety, and fluid retention

 OUTCOME

PROGNOSIS

- Symptom-specific therapy is usually helpful in ameliorating symptoms

 EVIDENCE

WEB SITE

- Gynecology Handbook for Family Practitioners http://www.vh.org/Providers/ClinRef/FPHandbook/13.html

INFORMATION FOR PATIENTS

- Mayo Clinic http://www.mayoclinic.com/invoke.cfm?id=DS00134
- American Academy of Family Physicians http://familydoctor.org/healthfacts/141/

REFERENCES

- Grady-Weliky TA: Clinical practice. Premenstrual dysphoric disorder. N Engl J Med 2003;348:433. [PMID: 12556546]
- Kessel B: Premenstrual syndrome, advances in diagnosis and treatment. Obstet Gynecol Clin North Am 2000;27:625. [PMID: 10958008]
- Wyatt KM et al: Efficacy of vitamin B_6 in the treatment of premenstrual syndrome: systematic review. BMJ 1999; 318:1375. [PMID: 10334745]

H. Trent MacKay, MD, MPH

Prostate Cancer

 KEY FEATURES

ESSENTIALS OF DIAGNOSIS

- Prostatic induration on digital rectal examination or elevation of prostate-specific antigen (PSA)
- Most often asymptomatic
- Rarely: systemic symptoms (weight loss, bone pain)

GENERAL CONSIDERATIONS

- Most common cancer detected in American men
- Second leading cause of cancer-related death
- In 2001, 198,000 new cases of prostate cancer, about 31,500 deaths
- At autopsy, >40% of men aged >50 years have prostatic carcinoma, most often occult
- Incidence increases with age: autopsy incidence ~30% of men aged 60–69 versus 67% in men aged 80–89 years
- Risk factors: black race, men with a family history of prostatic cancer, history of high dietary fat intake, and perhaps men who have undergone vasectomy
- A 50-year-old American man has a lifetime risk of 40% for latent cancer, of 9.5% for clinically apparent cancer, and of 2.9% for death from prostatic cancer

 CLINICAL FINDINGS

SYMPTOMS AND SIGNS

- Focal nodules or areas of induration within the prostate on digital rectal examination (DRE)
- Obstructive voiding symptoms
- Lymph node metastases
- Lower extremity lymphedema
- Back pain or pathological fractures
- Rarely, signs of urinary retention (palpable bladder) or neurological symptoms as a result of epidural metastases and cord compression

 DIAGNOSIS

LABORATORY TESTS

- Elevations in serum PSA (normal <4 ng/mL)
- PSA correlates with the volume of both benign and malignant prostatic tissue
- 18–30% of men with PSA 4.1–10 ng/mL have prostatic cancer
- Age-specific PSA reference ranges exist
- Most organ-confined cancers have PSA levels <10 ng/mL
- Advanced disease (seminal vesicle invasion, lymph node involvement, or occult distant metastases) have PSA levels >40 ng/mL
- Elevations in serum urea nitrogen or creatinine in patients in urinary retention or those with ureteral obstruction due to locally or regionally advanced prostatic cancers
- Elevations in alkaline phosphatase or hypercalcemia in patients with bony metastases
- Disseminated intravascular coagulation (DIC) in patients with advanced prostatic cancers

IMAGING STUDIES

- Transrectal ultrasound (TRUS): most prostatic cancers are hypoechoic
- MRI of the prostate
- Positive predictive value for detection of both capsular penetration and seminal vesicle invasion is similar for both TRUS and MRI

DIAGNOSTIC PROCEDURES

- Prostatic biopsy
  - TRUS-guided biopsy from the apex, mid portion, and base of the prostate. Done in men who have an abnormal DRE or an elevated PSA. Systematic rather than only lesion-directed biopsies are recommended.
  - Fine-needle aspiration biopsies should be considered in patients at an increased risk of bleeding.
- Majority of prostatic cancers are adenocarcinomas

 TREATMENT

MEDICATIONS

- Adrenal
  - Ketoconazole, 400 mg TID (adrenal insufficiency, nausea, rash, ataxia)

- Aminoglutethimide, 250 mg QID (adrenal insufficiency, nausea, rash, ataxia)
- Glucocorticoids: prednisone, 20–40 mg QD (gastrointestinal bleeding, fluid retention)
- Pituitary, hypothalamus
  - Estrogens, 1–3 mg QD (gynecomastia, hot flushes, thromboembolic disease, erectile dysfunction)
  - Luteinizing hormone-releasing hormone (LHRH) agonists, monthly or 3-monthly depot injection (erectile dysfunction, hot flushes, gynecomastia, rarely anemia)
- Prostate cell
  - Antiandrogens: flutamide, 250 mg TID, or bicalutamide, 50 mg QD (no erectile dysfunction when used alone; nausea, diarrhea)
- Testis
  - Orchiectomy (gynecomastia, hot flushes, impotence)
  - Ketoconazole for patients with advanced prostatic cancer who present with spinal cord compression, bilateral ureteral obstruction, or DIC
  - Complete androgen blockade by combining an antiandrogen with use of an LHRH agonist or ochiectomy

THERAPEUTIC PROCEDURES

- Patients need to be advised of all treatment options (including surveillance), benefits, risks, and limitations
- For minimal capsular penetration, standard irradiation or surgery
- For locally extensive cancers, including seminal vesicle and bladder neck invasion, combination therapy (androgen deprivation combined with surgery or irradiation)
- Androgen deprivation for metastatic disease
- Localized disease
  - Optimal form of treatment controversial
  - Selected patients may be candidates for surveillance; patients with an anticipated survival of >10 years should be considered for treatment with radical prostatectomy, radiation therapy
- Radical prostatectomy
  - For stages T1 and T2 prostatic cancers, local recurrence is uncommon after radical prostatectomy; organ-confined cancers rarely recur; cancers locally extensive (capsular penetration, seminal vesicle invasion) have higher

local (10–25%) and distant (20–50%) relapse rates
  - Adjuvant therapy (radiation for patients with positive surgical margins or androgen deprivation for lymph node metastases)
- Radiation therapy: external beam radiotherapy and transperineal implantation of radioisotopes
- Morbidity is limited; survival with localized cancers is 65% at 10 years
- Newer techniques of radiation (implantation, conformal therapy using three-dimensional reconstruction of CT-based tumor volumes, heavy particle, charged particle, and heavy charged particle) improve local control rates
- Brachytherapy, the implantation of permanent or temporary radioactive sources (palladium, iodine, or iridium)

 OUTCOME

FOLLOW-UP

- Surveillance alone may be appropriate for patients who are older and have very small and well-differentiated cancers

PREVENTION

Screening for prostatic cancer

- Screening tests currently available include DRE, PSA testing, TRUS
- Detection rates of DRE vary from 1.5% to 7%
- TRUS has low specificity (and therefore high biopsy rate). TRUS increases the detection rate very little when compared with the combined use of DRE and PSA testing
- With PSA testing, 2–2.5% of men older than age 50 have prostatic cancer compared with a rate of 1.5% using DRE screening alone. However, PSA is not specific for cancer
- Age-specific reference ranges for PSA have been established and increase specificity: for men aged 40–49 years, PSA reference range is <2.5 ng/mL; for men 50–59, <3.5 ng/mL; for men 60–69, <4.5 ng/mL; for men 70–79, <6.5 ng/mL
- PSA velocity (serial measurement of PSA), PSA density (serum PSA/volume of the prostate as measured by ultrasound), and PSA transition zone density (the zone of the prostate that undergoes enlargement during development of benign prostatic hyperplasia)

- Free and protein-bound PSA levels can be measured: cancer patients have a lower percentage of free serum PSA
- PSA testing should be performed yearly in men with a normal DRE and a PSA >2.5 ng/mL and biennially in those with a normal DRE and serum PSA <2.5 ng/mL

 EVIDENCE

PRACTICE GUIDELINES

- Prostate specific antigen (PSA): best practice policy. American Urological Association, Inc., 1999 http://www.cancernetwork.com/journals/oncology/o0002e.htm

WEB SITE

- American Foundation for Urologic Disease—Prostate cancer resource guide http://www.afud.org/pca/pcaindex.html

INFORMATION FOR PATIENTS

- Cleveland Clinic—Prostate cancer http://www.clevelandclinic.org/health/health-info/docs/1900/1932.asp?index=8634

REFERENCES

- Barry MJ et al: Outcomes for men with clinically nonmetastatic prostate carcinoma managed with radical prostatectomy, external beam radiotherapy, or expectant management: a retrospective analysis. Cancer 2001;91:2302. [PMID: 11413519].
- Koppie TM et al: Patterns of treatment of patients with prostate cancer initially managed with surveillance: results from The CaPSURE database. Cancer of the Prostate Strategic Urological Research Endeavor. J Urol 2000;164:81. [PMID: 10840429]
- Labrie F: Screening and early hormonal treatment of prostate cancer are accumulating strong evidence and support [see comments]. Prostate 2000;43:215. [PMID: 10797496]

Marshall L. Stoller, MD
Peter R. Carroll, MD

Prostatitis, Acute Bacterial

 KEY FEATURES

ESSENTIALS OF DIAGNOSIS

- Fever
- Irritative voiding symptoms
- Perineal or suprapubic pain
- Exquisite tenderness common on rectal examination
- Positive urine culture

GENERAL CONSIDERATIONS

- Usual causative agents: *Escherichia coli* and *Pseudomonas*
- Less common: *Enterococcus*

 CLINICAL FINDINGS

SYMPTOMS AND SIGNS

- Perineal, sacral, or suprapubic pain
- Fever
- Irritative voiding complaints
- Obstructive symptoms
- Urinary retention
- Exquisitely tender prostate

DIFFERENTIAL DIAGNOSIS

- Acute pyelonephritis
- Epididymitis
- Diverticulitis
- Urinary retention from benign or malignant prostatic enlargement
- Acute bacterial prostatitis
  – Fever: +
  – Urinalysis: +
  – Expressed prostatic secretions: contraindicated
  – Bacterial culture: +
- Chronic bacterial prostatitis
  – Fever: –
  – Urinalysis: –
  – Expressed prostatic secretions: +
  – Bacterial culture: +
- Nonbacterial prostatitis
  – Fever: –
  – Urinalysis: –
  – Expressed prostatic secretions: +
  – Bacterial culture: –
- Prostatodynia
  – Fever: –
  – Urinalysis: –
  – Expressed prostatic secretions: –
  – Bacterial culture: –

 DIAGNOSIS

LABORATORY TESTS

- Complete blood cell count: leukocytosis and a left shift
- Urinalysis: pyuria, bacteriuria, hematuria
- Urine culture: positive

TREATMENT

MEDICATIONS

- IV ampicillin and an aminoglycoside until afebrile for 24–48 h, then PO quinolone for 4–6 weeks
- Ampicillin, IV 1 g q6h, and gentamicin, IV 1 mg/kg q8h for 21 days
- Ciprofloxacin, PO 750 mg q12h for 21 days
- Ofloxacin, PO 200–300 mg q12h for 21 days
- Trimethoprim-sulfamethoxazole, PO 160/800 mg q12h for 21 days—increasing resistance noted (up to 20%)

THERAPEUTIC PROCEDURES

- Suprapubic drainage if urinary retention
- Urethral catheterization or instrumentation is contraindicated
- Prostatic massage is contraindicated

 OUTCOME

FOLLOW-UP

- Posttreatment urine culture
- Posttreatment examination of expressed prostatic secretions after completion of therapy

PROGNOSIS

- With effective treatment, chronic bacterial prostatitis is rare

 EVIDENCE

PRACTICE GUIDELINES

- 2002 national guideline for the management of prostatitis. Association for Genitourinary Medicine. Medical Society for the Study of Venereal Diseases, 2002. http://www.agum.org.uk/ceg2002/prostatitis0601.htm
- Naber KG et al: EAU guidelines for the management of urinary and male genital tract infections. Urinary Tract Infection (UTI) Working Group of the Health Care Office (HCO) of the European Association of Urology (EAU). Eur Urol 2001;40:576. [PMID: 11752870]

WEB SITES

- American Urological Association—Causes and management of prostatitis http://www.urologyhealth.org/search/index.cfm?topic=115&search=Cystitis%20AND%20acute&searchtype=and
- National Institute on Aging—Prostate problems http://www.nia.nih.gov/health/agepages/prostate.htm
- National Kidney and Urologic Diseases Information Clearinghouse—What I need to know about prostate problems http://kidney.niddk.nih.gov/kudiseases/pubs/prostate_ez/index.htm

INFORMATION FOR PATIENTS

- Cleveland Clinic—Prostatitis http://www.clevelandclinic.org/health/health-info/docs/1900/1962.asp?index=8527
- Mayo Clinic—Prostatitis http://www.mayoclinic.com/invoke.cfm?objectid= 8754C233-295A-4871-BB6EAE0904F9233A

REFERENCE

- Lummus WE et al: Prostatitis. Emerg Med Clin North Am 2001;19:691. [PMID: 11554282]

Marshall L. Stoller, MD
Peter R. Carroll, MD

Prostatitis, Chronic Bacterial

 KEY FEATURES

ESSENTIALS OF DIAGNOSIS

- Irritative voiding symptoms
- Perineal or suprapubic discomfort, often dull and poorly localized
- Positive expressed prostatic secretions and culture

GENERAL CONSIDERATIONS

- Although chronic bacterial prostatitis may evolve from acute bacterial prostatitis, many men have no history of acute infection
- Most common: gram-negative rods
- Less common: *Enterococcus*

 CLINICAL FINDINGS

SYMPTOMS AND SIGNS

- Variable, some patients are asymptomatic, most have irritative voiding symptoms, low back and perineal pain
- Many report a history of urinary tract infections
- Physical examination often unremarkable; prostate may feel normal, boggy, or indurated

DIFFERENTIAL DIAGNOSIS

- Chronic urethritis, cystitis, perianal disease

 DIAGNOSIS

- Culture secretions or postprostatic massage urine specimen

LABORATORY TESTS

- Urinalysis: normal unless a secondary cystitis is present
- Expressed prostatic secretions: >10 leukocytes/hpf, especially lipid-laden macrophages

TREATMENT

MEDICATIONS

- Antiinflammatory agents (indomethacin, ibuprofen)
- Quinolones, trimethoprim-sulfamethoxazole, carbenicillin, erythromycin, or cephalexin, for 6–12 weeks

Regimens

- Ciprofloxacin, 250–500 mg every 12 h; orally, 1–3 months
- Ofloxacin, 200–400 mg every 12 h; orally, 1–3 months
- Trimethoprim-sulfamethoxazole, 160/800 mg every 12 h [increasing resistance noted (up to 20%)]; orally, 1–3 months

THERAPEUTIC PROCEDURES

- Hot sitz baths

 ## OUTCOME

PROGNOSIS

- Difficult to cure
- Symptoms and recurrent urinary tract infections can be controlled by suppressive antibiotic therapy

 ## EVIDENCE

PRACTICE GUIDELINES

- Gurunadha Rao Tunuguntla HS et al: Management of prostatitis. Prostate Cancer Prostatic Dis 2002;5:172. [PMID: 12496977]
- Schaeffer AJ et al: Overview summary statement. Diagnosis and management of chronic prostatitis/chronic pelvic pain syndrome (CP/CPPS). Urology 2002; 60(6 Suppl):1. [PMID: 12521576]

WEB SITE

- American Urological Association—Causes and management of prostatitis http://www.urologyhealth.org/search/index.cfm?topic=115&search=Cystitis%20AND%20acute&searchtype=and

INFORMATION FOR PATIENTS

- Cleveland Clinic—Prostatitis http://www.clevelandclinic.org/health/health-info/docs/1900/1962.asp?index=8527
- MEDLINEplus—Chronic prostatitis http://www.nlm.nih.gov/medlineplus/ency/article/000523.htm

REFERENCES

- Litwin MS et al: The National Institutes of Health chronic prostatitis symptom index: development and validation of a new outcome measure. Chronic Prostatitis Collaborative Research Network. J Urol 1999;162:369. [PMID: 10411041]
- Nickel JC et al: Research guidelines for chronic prostatitis: consensus report from the first National Institutes of Health International Prostatitis Collaborative Network. Urology 1999;54:229. [PMID: 10443716]

Marshall L. Stoller, MD
Peter R. Carroll, MD

Prostatodynia

 ## KEY FEATURES

GENERAL CONSIDERATIONS

- Prostatodynia is a noninflammatory disorder that affects young and middle-aged men and has variable causes, including voiding dysfunction and pelvic floor musculature dysfunction

 ## CLINICAL FINDINGS

SYMPTOMS AND SIGNS

- Variable, no history of urinary tract infections; hesitancy and interruption of flow; lifelong history of voiding difficulty
- Physical examination is unremarkable, except increased anal sphincter tone and periprostatic tenderness may be observed

DIFFERENTIAL DIAGNOSIS

- Acute cystitis, other prostatitis syndromes
- Acute bacterial prostatitis
  - Fever: +
  - Urinalysis: +
  - Expressed prostatic secretions: contraindicated
  - Bacterial culture: +
- Chronic bacterial prostatitis
  - Fever: –
  - Urinalysis: –
  - Expressed prostatic secretions: +
  - Bacterial culture: +
- Nonbacterial prostatitis
  - Fever: –
  - Urinalysis: –
  - Expressed prostatic secretions: +
  - Bacterial culture: –
- Prostatodynia
  - Fever: –
  - Urinalysis: –
  - Expressed prostatic secretions: –
  - Bacterial culture: –

 ## DIAGNOSIS

LABORATORY TESTS

- Urinalysis: normal
- Expressed prostatic secretions: normal numbers of leukocytes

DIAGNOSTIC PROCEDURES

- Urodynamic testing: dysfunctional voiding (detrusor contraction without urethral relaxation, high urethral pressures, spasms of the urinary sphincter); indicated in patients failing empiric trials of α-blockers or anticholinergics

TREATMENT

MEDICATIONS

- α-Blocking agents: terazosin, 1–10 mg PO QD; or doxazosin, 1–8 mg PO QD
- Anticholinergics
- Diazepam

THERAPEUTIC PROCEDURES

- Biofeedback techniques
- Sitz baths

 OUTCOME

PROGNOSIS

- Variable depending on the specific cause

 EVIDENCE

PRACTICE GUIDELINES

- Gurunadha Rao Tunuguntla HS et al: Management of prostatitis. Prostate Cancer Prostatic Dis 2002;5:172. [PMID: 12496977]
- Nickel JC: Practical approach to the management of prostatitis. Tech Urol 1995;1:162. [PMID: 9118386]
- Thin RN: The chronic prostatitis syndromes. J R Army Med Corps 1997;143:155. [PMID: 9403823]

WEB SITES

- American Urological Association— Causes and management of prostatitis http://www.urologyhealth.org/search/index.cfm?topic=115&search=Cystitis%20AND%20acute&searchtype=and
- National Institute on Aging—Prostate problems http://www.nia.nih.gov/health/agepages/prostate.htm
- National Kidney and Urologic Diseases Information Clearinghouse—What I need to know about prostate problems http://kidney.niddk.nih.gov/kudiseases/pubs/prostate_ez/index.htm

INFORMATION FOR PATIENTS

- Cleveland Clinic—Prostatitis http://www.clevelandclinic.org/health/health-info/docs/1900/1962.asp?index=8527
- Mayo Clinic—Prostatitis http://www.mayoclinic.com/invoke.cfm?objectid= 8754C233-295A-4871-BB6EAE0904F9233A
- MEDLINEplus—Nonbacterial prostatitis http://www.nlm.nih.gov/medlineplus/ency/article/000524.htm

REFERENCE

- Nickel JC et al: Prevalence of prostatitis-like symptoms in a population based study using the National Institutes of Health chronic prostatitis symptom index. J Urol 2001;165:842. [PMID: 11176483]

Marshall L. Stoller, MD
Peter R. Carroll, MD

Pruritus, Anogenital

 KEY FEATURES

ESSENTIALS OF DIAGNOSIS

- Itching, chiefly nocturnal, of the anogenital area
- Examination is highly variable, ranging from no skin findings to excoriations and inflammation of any degree, including lichenification

GENERAL CONSIDERATIONS

- May be due to intertrigo, psoriasis, lichen simplex chronicus, or seborrheic or contact dermatitis (from soaps, colognes, douches, contraceptives, and perhaps scented toilet tissue)
- May be due to irritating secretions, as in diarrhea, leukorrhea, or trichomoniasis, or to local disease (candidiasis, dermatophytosis, erythrasma)
- Uncleanliness may be at fault
- In pruritus ani, hemorrhoids are often found, and leakage of mucus and bacteria from the distal rectum onto the perianal skin may be important in cases in which no other skin abnormality is found
- In women, pruritus ani by itself is rare, and pruritus vulvae does not usually involve the anal area, though anal itching will usually spread to the vulva
- In men, pruritus of the scrotum is most commonly seen in the absence of pruritus ani
- When all possible known causes have been ruled out, the condition is diagnosed as idiopathic or essential pruritus—by no means rare

 CLINICAL FINDINGS

SYMPTOMS AND SIGNS

- The only symptom is itching, which is chiefly nocturnal
- Physical findings are usually not present, but there may be erythema, fissuring, maceration, lichenification, excoriations, or changes suggestive of candidiasis or tinea

DIFFERENTIAL DIAGNOSIS

- Idiopathic
- Intertrigo
- Psoriasis
- Hemorrhoids
- Lichen simplex chronicus
- Seborrheic dermatitis
- Contact dermatitis
- Candidiasis
- Tinea
- Erythrasma
- Irritants: diarrhea, vaginal discharge
- Lichen sclerosis et atrophicus
- Pinworm

 DIAGNOSIS

LABORATORY TESTS

- Urinalysis and blood glucose testing may lead to a diagnosis of diabetes mellitus
- Microscopic examination or culture of tissue scrapings may reveal yeasts or fungi
- Stool examination may show pinworms

Pruritus, Anogenital

 TREATMENT

MEDICATIONS

General measures

- Treating constipation, preferably with high-fiber management (psyllium), may help

Local measures

- Pramoxine cream or lotion or hydrocortisone-pramoxine (Pramosone), 1% or 2.5% cream, lotion, or ointment, is helpful in managing pruritus in the anogenital area; the ointment or cream should be applied after a bowel movement
- Potent fluorinated topical corticosteroids may lead to atrophy and striae if used for more than a few days and should in general be avoided; this includes combinations with antifungals
- The use of strong steroids on the scrotum may lead to persistent severe burning on withdrawal of the drug
- Soaks with aluminum subacetate solution, 1:20, are of value if the area is acutely inflamed and oozing
- Affected areas may be painted with Castellani's solution, Balneol Perianal Cleansing Lotion, or Tucks premoistened pads, ointment, or cream (all Tucks preparations contain witch hazel) may be very useful for pruritus ani

THERAPEUTIC PROCEDURES

- Instruct the patient to use very soft or moistened tissue or cotton after bowel movements and to clean the perianal area thoroughly with cool water if possible
- Women should use similar precautions after urinating
- Instruct the patient regarding the harmful and pruritus-inducing effects of scratching
- Underclothing should be changed daily

 OUTCOME

PROGNOSIS

- Although benign, anogenital pruritus may be persistent and recurrent

WHEN TO REFER

- If there is a question about the diagnosis, if recommended therapy is ineffective, or specialized treatment is necessary

PREVENTION

- Instruct the patient in proper anogenital hygiene after treating systemic or local conditions

EVIDENCE

PRACTICE GUIDELINES

- National Guideline Clearinghouse
  http://www.guideline.gov/summary/summary.aspx?doc_id=3392&nbr=2618&string=intertrigo
  http://www.guideline.gov/summary/summary.aspx?doc_id=2670&nbr=1896&string=intertrigo
  http://www.guideline.gov/summary/summary.aspx?doc_id=3388&nbr=2614&string=lichen
- American Academy of Dermatology
  http://www.aadassociation.org/Guidelines/contderm.html

WEB SITES

- American Academy of Dermatology
  http://www.aad.org
- Dermatology Handbook for Family Practice from the University of Iowa
  http://www.vh.org/Providers/ClinRef/FPHandbook/17.html

INFORMATION FOR PATIENTS

- American Academy of Dermatology
  http://www.aad.org/pamphlets/
- American Academy of Family Physicians
  http://familydoctor.org/flowcharts/532.html

REFERENCE

- Vincent C: Anorectal pain and irritation: anal fissure, levator syndrome, proctalgia fugax, and pruritus ani. Prim Care 1999;26:53. [PMID: 9922294]

Timothy G. Berger, MD

Pseudotumor Cerebri

 KEY FEATURES

ESSENTIALS OF DIAGNOSIS

- Headache, worse on straining
- Visual obscurations or diplopia may occur
- Level of consciousness may be impaired
- Other deficits depend on cause of intracranial hypertension or on herniation syndrome
- Examination reveals papilledema

GENERAL CONSIDERATIONS

- Pseudotumor cerebri is a diagnosis of exclusion in the setting of elevated intracranial pressure and normal cerebrospinal fluid
- Thrombosis of the transverse venous sinus as a noninfectious complication of otitis media or chronic mastoiditis is one cause, and sagittal sinus thrombosis may lead to a clinically similar picture
- Other causes include chronic pulmonary disease, endocrine disturbances such as hypoparathyroidism or Addison's disease, vitamin A toxicity, and the use of tetracycline or oral contraceptives
- Cases have also followed withdrawal of corticosteroids after long-term use

DEMOGRAPHICS

- Most patients are young women who are frequently obese

 CLINICAL FINDINGS

SYMPTOMS AND SIGNS

- Symptoms include headache, diplopia, and other visual disturbances due to papilledema and abducens nerve dysfunction
- Examination reveals papilledema and some enlargement of the blind spots, but patients otherwise look well. Abducens palsy is common

DIFFERENTIAL DIAGNOSIS

- Venous sinus thrombosis
- Dural arteriovenous malformation
- Space-occupying lesion, eg, brain tumor
- Meningitis
- Systemic hypertension
- Migraine
- Glaucoma
- Associated conditions: hypoparathyroidism, Addison's disease, chronic pulmonary disease
- Associated drugs: vitamin A, tetracycline, minocycline, oral contraceptives, corticosteroid withdrawal, isotretinoin, danazol

 DIAGNOSIS

LABORATORY TESTS

- Lumbar puncture confirms the presence of intracranial hypertension, but the cerebrospinal fluid is normal

IMAGING STUDIES

- Investigations reveal no evidence of a space-occupying lesion, and the CT scan shows small or normal ventricles
- MR venography can help to detect thrombosis of the transverse venous sinus and sagittal sinus thrombosis

Pseudotumor Cerebri

 TREATMENT

MEDICATIONS

- Acetazolamide (250 mg orally three times daily) reduces formation of cerebrospinal fluid and can be initial therapy
- Oral corticosteroids (eg, prednisone, 60–80 mg daily) may also be necessary
- Any specific cause of pseudotumor cerebri requires appropriate treatment
  - Hormone therapy should be initiated if there is an underlying endocrine disturbance
  - Discontinue the use of tetracycline, oral contraceptives, or vitamin A
  - If corticosteroid withdrawal is responsible, the medication should be reintroduced and then tapered more gradually

SURGERY

- If medical treatment fails to control the intracranial pressure, surgical placement of a lumboperitoneal or other shunt—or subtemporal decompression or optic nerve sheath fenestration—should be undertaken to preserve vision

THERAPEUTIC PROCEDURES

- Obese patients should be advised to lose weight
- Repeated lumbar puncture to lower the intracranial pressure by removal of cerebrospinal fluid is effective on a short-term basis, but pharmacological approaches to treatment are also necessary

 OUTCOME

FOLLOW-UP

- Treatment is monitored by checking visual acuity and visual fields, funduscopic appearance, and pressure of the cerebrospinal fluid

COMPLICATIONS

- Untreated pseudotumor cerebri can lead to secondary optic atrophy and permanent visual loss

PROGNOSIS

- Discontinuing the use of tetracycline, oral contraceptives, or vitamin A will allow for resolution of pseudotumor cerebri due to these agents
- In many instances. no specific cause is found, and the disorder remits spontaneously after several months

WHEN TO REFER

- All patients benefit from specialist referral to exclude specific causes and specialized care to monitor treatment response with visual acuity and field checks, and funduscopic examination

WHEN TO ADMIT

- Patients in need of surgical placement of a device to reduce intracranial hypertension

EVIDENCE

INFORMATION FOR PATIENTS

- http://www.djo.harvard.edu/meei/PI/pse udotcereb.html
- National Institute of Neurological Diseases and Stroke http://www.ninds.nih.gov/health_and_medical/disorders/pseudotumorcerebri_doc.htm
- National Institutes of Health http://www.nlm.nih.gov/medlineplus/ency/article/000351.htm

REFERENCES

- Friedman DI et al: Diagnostic criteria for idiopathic intracranial hypertension. Neurology 2002;59:1492. [PMID: 12455560]
- Krajewski KJ: Idiopathic intracranial hypertension: pseudotumor cerebri. Optometry 2002;73:546. [PMID: 12387561]

Michael J. Aminoff, DSc, MD, FRCP

Psittacosis

 KEY FEATURES

ESSENTIALS OF DIAGNOSIS

- Fever, chills, and cough; headache common
- Atypical pneumonia with slightly delayed appearance of signs of pneumonitis
- Contact with infected bird (psittacine, pigeons, many others) 7–15 days previously
- Isolation of chlamydiae or rising titer of complement-fixing antibodies

GENERAL CONSIDERATIONS

- Etiological agent is *Chlamydia psittaci*, a bacterium
- Infection is acquired by inhaling dried secretions from infected birds (parrots, parakeets, pigeons, chickens, ducks, and many others), which may or may not appear ill
- The incubation period is 6 to 19 days
- The history may be difficult to obtain if the patient acquired infection from an illegally imported bird

 CLINICAL FINDINGS

SYMPTOMS AND SIGNS

- The onset is usually rapid, with fever, chills, myalgia, dry cough, and headache
- Signs include temperature–pulse dissociation, dullness to percussion, and rales
- Pulmonary findings may be absent early
- Dyspnea and cyanosis may occur later
- Endocarditis, which is culture negative, may occur

DIFFERENTIAL DIAGNOSIS

- Other atypical pneumonia (eg, viral pneumonia, *Mycoplasma pneumoniae*, *Chlamydia pneumoniae*)
- Unusual presentations of typical bacterial pneumonia
- Hypersensitivity pneumonitis
- Other cause of culture-negative endocarditis

 DIAGNOSIS

LABORATORY TESTS

- The diagnosis is usually made serologically
- Acute and convalescent serology demonstrating a rise in titer of complement-fixing antibidy
- Antibodies appear during the second week
- Antibody response may be suppressed by early chemotherapy

IMAGING STUDIES

- The radiographic findings are those of atypical pneumonia, which tends to be interstitial and diffuse in appearance, though consolidation can occur
- Psittacosis is indistinguishable from other bacterial or viral pneumonias by radiography

TREATMENT

MEDICATIONS

- Doxycycline 100 mg orally every 12 h or intravenously every 12 h, for 14–21 days
- Macrolides are also effective

OUTCOME

COMPLICATIONS

- Endocarditis, hepatitis, and neurological complications may occasionally occur
- Severe pneumonia requiring intensive care support may also occur
- Fatal cases have been reported

PROGNOSIS

- Excellent with early treatment

WHEN TO REFER

- Early referral to an infectious disease specialist for severe disease may aid in management

WHEN TO ADMIT

- Respiratory compromise
- Rapidly deteriorating clinical course
- Suspected or proven endocarditis

PREVENTION

- Traceback of infected birds to distributors and breeders often is not possible because of limited regulation of the pet bird industry

EVIDENCE

PRACTICE GUIDELINES

- Centers for Disease Control and Prevention. Compendium of measures to control *Chlamydia psittaci* infection among humans (psittacosis) and pet birds (avian chlamydiosis), 2000. MMWR Recomm Rep 2000;49 (RR-8):3.

WEB SITES

- CDC—Division of Bacterial and Mycotic Diseases http://www.cdc.gov/ncidod/dbmd/
- Karolinska Institute—Directory of Bacterial Infections and Mycoses http://www.mic.ki.se/Diseases/c1.html

INFORMATION FOR PATIENTS

- National Institutes of Health http://www.nlm.nih.gov/medlineplus/ency/article/000088.htm

REFERENCE

- Elliott JH: Psittacosis. A flu like syndrome. Aust Fam Physician 2001; 30:739. [PMID: 11681143]

Henry F. Chambers, MD

Psoriasis

 KEY FEATURES

ESSENTIALS OF DIAGNOSIS

- Silvery scales on bright red, well-demarcated plaques, usually on the knees, elbows, and scalp
- Nail findings include pitting and onycholysis (separation of the nail plate from the bed)
- Mild itching (usually)
- May be associated with psoriatic arthritis
- Histopathology is not often useful and can be confusing

GENERAL CONSIDERATIONS

- A common benign, acute or chronic inflammatory skin disease based on a genetic predisposition
- Injury or irritation of normal skin tends to induce lesions of psoriasis at the site (Koebner's phenomenon)
- Psoriasis has several variants—the most common is the plaque type

 CLINICAL FINDINGS

SYMPTOMS AND SIGNS

- See Table 7 (page XX)
- There are often no symptoms, but itching may occur
- Although psoriasis may occur anywhere, examine the scalp, elbows, knees, palms and soles, and nails
- The lesions are red, sharply defined plaques covered with silvery scales; the glans penis and vulva may be affected; occasionally, only the flexures (axillae, inguinal areas) are involved
- Fine stippling ("pitting") in the nails is highly suggestive
- Psoriatics often have a pink or red intergluteal fold
- There may be associated seronegative arthritis, often involving the distal interphalangeal joints
- Eruptive (guttate) psoriasis consisting of myriad lesions 3–10 mm in diameter occurs occasionally after streptococcal pharyngitis
- Plaque type or extensive erythrodermic psoriasis with abrupt onset may accompany HIV infection

DIFFERENTIAL DIAGNOSIS

- Atopic dermatitis (eczema)
- Contact dermatitis
- Nummular eczema (discoid eczema, nummular dermatitis)
- Tinea
- Candidiasis
- Intertrigo
- Seborrheic dermatitis
- Pityriasis rosea
- Secondary syphilis
- Pityriasis rubra pilaris
- Onychomycosis (nail findings)
- Cutaneous features of reactive arthritis
- Cutaneous T cell lymphoma (mycosis fungoides)

 DIAGNOSIS

DIAGNOSTIC PROCEDURES

- The combination of red plaques with silvery scales on elbows and knees, with scaliness in the scalp or nail findings, is diagnostic
- Psoriasis lesions are well demarcated and affect extensor surfaces—in contrast to atopic dermatitis, with poorly demarcated plaques in flexural distribution
- In body folds, scraping and culture for *Candida* and examination of scalp and nails will distinguish psoriasis from intertrigo and candidiasis

TREATMENT

MEDICATIONS

- See Table 6 (page 1199)

Limited disease (mild to moderate)

- Topical steroid cream or ointment
  - Restrict the highest-potency steroids to 2–3 weeks of twice-daily use; then three or four times on weekends or switch to a midpotency corticosteroid
  - Rarely induces a lasting remission
- Calcipotriene ointment 0.005%, a vitamin D analog, is used twice daily
  - It is the second most commonly used topical treatment (after topical steroids)
  - Substitute calcipotriene once the topical steroids have controlled the lesions; once- or twice-daily calcipotriene is then continued chronically
  - It usually cannot be applied to the groin or the face because of irritation
  - Incompatible with many topical steroids; it must be applied at a different time
- Tazarotene gel
  - A topical retinoid for mild to moderate plaque psoriasis is available in 0.05% and 0.1% formulations; the 0.05% is less effective when used once-daily
  - It is more expensive than calcipotriene and more irritating
  - May be applied with topical steroids
  - Anthralin may be used, but is irritating and may stain the skin
- Oclusion alone clears isolated plaques in 30–40% patients
  - Duoderm is placed on the lesions and left undisturbed for a minimum of 5 days, up to 7 days and then replaced; responses may be seen within several weeks
- For the scalp
  - Start with a tar shampoo, daily
  - For thick scales, use 6% salicylic acid gel (eg, Keralyt), P & S solution (phenol, mineral oil, and glycerin), or oil-based fluocinolone acetonide 0.01% (Derma-Smoothe/FS) under a shower cap at night, and shampoo in the morning
  - In order of increasing potency, triamcinolone 0.1%, or fluocinolone, betamethasone dipropionate, fluocinonide or amcinonide, and clobetasol are available in solution form for use on the scalp twice daily
- Psoriasis in the body folds

- Potent steroids cannot be used
- Tacrolimus (protopic 0.1% or 0.03%) ointment or pimecrolimus (Elidel 1%) cream applied BID can be effective in intertriginous psoriasis (but not plaques type); burning may complicate and may be avoided by applying mild steroid (hydrocortisone 1% to 2.5%) BID for the week of treatment

Moderate to severe disease (more than 30% of the body surface)

- Parenteral corticosteroids should not be used because of possible induction of pustular lesions
- Methotrexate is very effective in doses up to 25 mg once weekly
- Acitretin, a synthetic retinoid, is most effective for pustular psoriasis at 0.5–1 mg/kg/day, but it also improves erythrodermic and plaque types and psoriatic arthritis; liver enzymes and serum lipids must be checked periodically; because acitretin is a teratogen women must wait at least 3 years after completing treatment before considering pregnancy
- Cyclosporine dramatically improves psoriasis in severe cases
- Systemic immunomodulators (etanercept, alefacept) can be effective

THERAPEUTIC PROCEDURES

- Moderate to severe disease
  - The treatment of choice is narrow-band UVB light exposure three times weekly; clearing usually occurs around 7 weeks, and maintenance may be needed since relapses are frequent
  - Severe disease unresponsive to ultraviolet light may be treated in a psoriasis day care center with the Goeckerman regimen, using crude coal tar for many hours and exposure to UVB light; this offers the best chance for prolonged remissions
  - PUVA (psoralen plus ultraviolet A) may be effective even if standard UVB treatment has failed; may be used with other therapy, eg, acitretin

OUTCOME

COMPLICATIONS

- Treatment with calcipotriene may result in hypercalcemia
- Long-term use of PUVA is associated with an increased risk of skin cancer (especially squamous cell carcinoma and perhaps melanoma)

PROGNOSIS

- The course tends to be chronic and unpredictable, and the disease may be refractory to treatment

WHEN TO REFER

- If there is a question about the diagnosis, if recommended therapy is ineffective, or specialized treatment is necessary

EVIDENCE

PRACTICE GUIDELINES

- American Academy of Dermatology http://www.aadassociation.org/Guidelines/psoriasis.html
- National Guideline Clearinghouse http://www.guideline.gov/summary/summary.aspx?doc_id=3388&nbr=2614&string=psoriasis
- Spuls PI et al: The development of practice guidelines for the treatment of severe plaque form psoriasis. Arch Dermatol 1998;134:1591.

WEB SITE

- American Academy of Dermatology http://www.aad.org

INFORMATION FOR PATIENTS

- American Academy of Dermatology http://www.aad.org/Kids/psoriasis.html
- National Institute of Arthritis and Musculoskeletal and Skin Diseases http://www.niams.nih.gov/hi/topics/psoriasis/psoriafs.htm

REFERENCES

- Lebwohl M et al: Treatment of psoriasis. Part 1. Topical therapy and phototherapy. J Am Acad Dermatol 2001;45:487. [PMID: 11568737]
- Lebwohl M et al: Treatment of psoriasis. Part 2. Systemic therapies. J Am Acad Dermatol 2001;45:649. [PMID: 11606913]
- Mason J et al: Topical preparations for the treatment of psoriasis: a systematic review. Br J Dermatol 2002;146:351. [PMID: 11952534]
- Pardasani AG et al: Treatment of psoriasis: an algorithm-based approach for primary care physicians. Am Fam Physician 2000;61:725. [PMID: 10695585]

Timothy G. Berger, MD

Psoriatic Arthritis

 ## KEY FEATURES

ESSENTIALS OF DIAGNOSIS

- Psoriasis precedes onset of arthritis in 80% of cases
- Arthritis usually asymmetric, with "sausage" appearance of fingers and toes
- Resembles rheumatoid arthritis; rheumatoid factor is negative
- Sacroiliac joint involvement common; ankylosis of the sacroiliac joints may occur

GENERAL CONSIDERATIONS

Patterns or subsets of arthritis accompanying psoriasis

- Joint disease that resembles rheumatoid arthritis with symmetric polyarthritis
- An oligoarticular form that may lead to considerable destruction of the affected joints
- Predominant involvement of the distal interphalangeal joints; pitting of the nails and onycholysis are frequently associated
- A severe deforming arthritis (arthritis mutilans) with marked osteolysis
- A spondylitic form in which sacroiliitis and spinal involvement predominate; 50% of these patients are HLA-B27 positive

DEMOGRAPHICS

- Arthritis is at least five times more common in patients with severe skin disease than in those with only mild skin findings

 ## CLINICAL FINDINGS

SYMPTOMS AND SIGNS

- Although psoriasis usually precedes the onset of arthritis, arthritis precedes or occurs simultaneously with the skin disease in approximately 20% of cases
- May be a single patch of psoriasis (typically hidden in the scalp, gluteal cleft, or umbilicus)
- Nail pitting, a residue of previous psoriasis, is sometimes the only clue

DIFFERENTIAL DIAGNOSIS

- Rheumatoid arthritis
- Gout
- Osteoarthritis
- Other causes of sacroiliitis: reactive arthritis (Reiter's syndrome), ankylosing spondylitis, inflammatory bowel disease

 ## DIAGNOSIS

LABORATORY TESTS

- Elevation of the sedimentation rate
- Rheumatoid factor is not present

IMAGING STUDIES

- Radiographic findings are most helpful in distinguishing the disease from other forms of arthritis
- There are marginal erosions of bone and irregular destruction of joint and bone, which, in the phalanx, may give the appearance of a sharpened pencil ("pencil-in-cup")
- Fluffy periosteal new bone may be marked, especially at the insertion of muscles and ligaments into bone. Such changes will also be seen along the shafts of metacarpals, metatarsals, and phalanges
- Asymmetric sacroiliitis

TREATMENT

MEDICATIONS

- Nonsteroidal antiinflammatory drugs (NSAIDs) are usually sufficient for mild cases
- Corticosteroids are less effective in psoriatic arthritis than in other forms of inflammatory arthritis
- In resistant cases, methotrexate may be helpful
- For cases with disease that is refractory to methotrexate, etanercept or infliximab is usually effective for both arthritis and psoriatic skin disease
- Successful treatment of the skin lesions (eg, by PUVA therapy) commonly—though not invariably—is accompanied by an improvement in peripheral articular symptoms

THERAPEUTIC PROCEDURES

- Treatment regimens are symptomatic

 OUTCOME

COMPLICATIONS

- Fusion of peripheral or spinal joints

PROGNOSIS

- Generally better than rheumatoid arthritis, but severe cases occur

WHEN TO REFER

- Refer when joint disease does not respond to NSAIDs or when skin disease is severe

 EVIDENCE

PRACTICE GUIDELINES

- American Academy of Dermatology
http://www.aadassociation.org/Guidelines/psoriasis.html
- American College of Rheumatology
http://www.rheumatology.org/research/guidelines/refer/refer.html

INFORMATION FOR PATIENTS

- Arthritis Foundation
http://www.arthritis.org/conditions/diseasecenter/juvenilepsoriaticarthritis.asp
- National Institutes of Health
http://www.nlm.nih.gov/medlineplus/ency/article/000413.htm

REFERENCES

- Gladman DD: Current concepts in psoriatic arthritis. Curr Opin Rheumatol 2002;14:361.
- Mease PJ et al: Etanercept in the treatment of psoriatic arthritis and psoriasis: a randomized trial. Lancet 2000;356: 385. [PMID: 10972371]

David B. Hellmann, MD, FACP
John H. Stone, MD, MPH

Pulmonary Embolism

 KEY FEATURES

ESSENTIALS OF DIAGNOSIS

- Predisposition to venous thrombosis, usually of the lower extremities
- Usually either dyspnea, chest pain, hemoptysis, or syncope
- Tachypnea and a widened alveolar–arterial PO_2 difference
- Characteristic defects on ventilation-perfusion lung scan, spiral CT scan of the chest, or pulmonary angiogram

GENERAL CONSIDERATIONS

- Cause of an estimated 50,000 deaths annually in the United States and the third most common cause of death in hospitalized patients
- Majority of cases are not recognized antemortem: <10% with fatal emboli receive specific treatment
- Pulmonary thromboembolism (PE) and deep venous thrombosis (DVT) are manifestations of the same disease, with the same risk factors
  - Immobility (bed rest, stroke, obesity)
  - Hyperviscosity (polycythemia)
  - Increased central venous pressures (low cardiac output, pregnancy)
  - Vessel damage (prior DVT, orthopedic surgery, trauma)
  - Hypercoagulable states, either acquired or inherited
- Pulmonary thromboemboli most often originate in deep veins of the major calf muscles
- 50–60% of patients with proximal lower extremity DVT will develop PE; 50% of these events are asymptomatic
- Hypoxemia results from vascular obstruction leading to dead space ventilation, right-to-left shunting, and decreased cardiac output

Pulmonary embolisms

- Fat embolism
- Air embolism
- Amniotic fluid embolism
- Septic embolism (eg, endocarditis)
- Tumor embolism (eg, renal cell carcinoma)
- Foreign body embolism (eg, talc in IV drug use)
- Parasite egg embolism (schistosomiasis)

 CLINICAL FINDINGS

SYMPTOMS AND SIGNS

- See Table 30 (page 1226)
- Clinical findings depend on the size of the embolus and the patient's preexisting cardiopulmonary status
- Dyspnea occurs in 75–85% and pain in 65–75% of patients
- Tachypnea is the only sign reliably found in more than 50% of patients
- 97% of patients in the PIOPED study had at least one of the following: dyspnea, tachypnea, or chest pain with breathing

DIFFERENTIAL DIAGNOSIS

- Myocardial infarction (heart attack)
- Pneumonia
- Pericarditis
- Congestive heart failure
- Pleuritis (pleurisy)
- Pneumothorax
- Pericardial tamponade

 DIAGNOSIS

LABORATORY TESTS

- ECG is abnormal in 70% of patients; sinus tachycardia and nonspecific ST-T changes are the most common findings
- Acute respiratory alkalosis, hypoxemia, and widened arterial–alveolar O_2 gradient (A–a DO_2), but these findings are not diagnostic (Table 30, page 1226)
- A normal D-dimer level by the ELISA assay virtually rules out DVT (sensitivity is 97%); however, many hospitals use a less-sensitive latex-agglutination assay

IMAGING STUDIES

Chest x-ray

- The most frequent findings are atelectasis, infiltrates, and pleural effusions; Westermark's sign is focal oligemia with a prominent central pulmonary artery; Hampton's hump is a pleural-based area of increased intensity from intraparenchymal hemorrhage
- Lung scanning (V/Q scan): a "normal" scan can exclude PE; a "high probability" scan is sufficient to make the diagnosis in most cases; "indeterminate" scans are common and do not further refine clinical pretest probabilities

- Helical CT arteriography is supplanting V/Q scanning as the initial diagnostic study
  - It requires administration of intravenous radiocontrast dye but is otherwise noninvasive
  - It is very sensitive for the detection of thrombus in the proximal pulmonary arteries but less so in the segmental and subsegmental arteries
- Venous thrombosis studies: venous ultrasonography is the test of choice in most centers; diagnosing DVT establishes the need for treatment and may preclude invasive testing in cases where there is a high suspicion for PE
- In the setting of a nondiagnostic V/Q scan, negative serial DVT studies over 2 weeks predict a low risk (<2%) of subsequent DVT over the next 6 weeks
- Pulmonary angiography is the reference standard for the diagnosis of PE
  - It is invasive, but safe—minor complications in <5%
  - Its role in the diagnosis of PE is controversial, but it is generally used when there is a high clinical probability and negative noninvasive studies
- MRI is a primary research tool for the diagnosis of PE
- Integrated approach: Figure 2 (page 1227)

Pulmonary Embolism

TREATMENT

MEDICATIONS

- See Tables 33 and 34 (pages 1230)
- Anticoagulation regimen consists of unfractionated heparin (UFH) followed by warfarin to maintain the INR 2.0–3.0 for a total of 6 months
- Compared with UFH, low-molecular-weight heparins (LMWH) are easier to dose, require no monitoring, have similar hemorrhage rates, and are at least as effective
- LMWH enables home-based therapy in selected patients
- Warfarin is contraindicated in pregnancy; LMWH can be used instead
- Guidelines for the duration of full anticoagulation
  - 6 months for an initial episode with a reversible risk factor
  - 12 months after an initial, idiopathic episode
  - 6–12 months to indefinitely in patients with irreversible risk factors or recurrent disease
- Low-dose anticoagulation
- New data support the use of long-term low-intensity warfarin (INR 1.5–2.0) after full anticoagulation is completed
- Thrombolytic therapy accelerates resolution of thrombi when compared to heparin, but does not improve mortality
- Thrombolytics carry a 10-fold greater risk of intracranial hemorrhage compared with heparin (0.2–2.1%)
- Thrombolytics are indicated in patients who are hemodynamically unstable while on heparin
- Venal caval interruption (IVC filters) may be indicated where there is a significant contraindication to anticoagulation or where recurrence occurs despite adequate anticoagulation
- IVC filters decrease the short-term incidence of PE, but increase the rate of recurrent DVT

SURGERY

- Pulmonary embolectomy is an emergency procedure with a high mortality rate performed at few centers

THERAPEUTIC PROCEDURES

- Catheter devices that fragment and extract thrombus have been used on small numbers of patients

- Platelet counts should be monitored for the first 14 days of UFH due to the risk of immune-mediated thrombocytopenia
- Warfarin has interactions with many drugs

OUTCOME

COMPLICATIONS

- Immune-mediated thrombocytopenia in 3% of patient on UFH
- The major complication of anticoagulation with heparin is hemorrhage; risk of any hemorrhage is 0–7%, 0–2% for fatal hemorrhage
- The risk of hemorrhage on warfarin is 3–4% per patient year, but correlates with INR
- Approximately 1% of patients have chronic thromboembolic pulmonary hypertension; selected patients may benefit from pulmonary endarterectomy

PROGNOSIS

- Overall prognosis depends on the underlying disease rather than on the thromboembolic event
- Death from recurrent PE occurs in only 3% of cases; 6 months of anticoagulation therapy reduces the risk of recurrent thrombosis and death by 80–90%
- Perfusion defects resolve in most survivors

WHEN TO REFER

- All patients evaluated for or diagnosed with a PE should be evaluated by an expert (typically a pulmonologist, hematologist, or internist)

WHEN TO ADMIT

- Patients with an acute PE should be admitted for stabilization, initiation of therapy, evaluation of cause of PE, and education

PREVENTION

- See Tables 31 and 32 (pages 1228 and 1229)

EVIDENCE

PRACTICE GUIDELINES

- National Guideline Clearinghouse
  http://www.guideline.gov/summary/summary.aspx?doc_id=2592&nbr=1818&string=pulmonary+embolism
  http://www.guideline.gov/summary/summary.aspx?doc_id=2381&nbr=1607&string=pulmonary+embolism

INFORMATION FOR PATIENTS

- JAMA patient page: Pulmonary embolism. JAMA 2003;290:2828. [PMID: 14657080]
- Mayo Clinic
  http://www.mayoclinic.com/invoke.cfm?id=DS00429

REFERENCES

- Ridker PM et al: Long-term, low-intensity warfarin therapy for the prevention of recurrent venous thromboembolism. N Engl J Med 2003. [PMID: 14658125]
- Van Strijen MJL et al: Single-detector helical computed tomography as the primary diagnostic test in suspected pulmonary embolism: a multicenter clinical management study of 510 patients. Ann Intern Med 2003;138:307. [PMID: 12585828]
- The PIOPED Investigators: Value of the ventilation/perfusion scan in acute pulmonary embolism. Results of the prospective investigation of pulmonary embolism diagnosis (PIOPED). JAMA 1990;263:2753. [PMID: 2332918]

Mark S. Chesnutt, MD
Thomas J. Prendergast, MD

Pulmonary Hypertension

 KEY FEATURES

ESSENTIALS OF DIAGNOSIS

- Dyspnea, fatigue, chest pain, and exertional syncope
- Narrow splitting of second heart sound with loud pulmonary component; findings of right ventricular hypertrophy and cardiac failure in advanced disease
- Hypoxemia and increased wasted ventilation on pulmonary function tests
- ECG evidence of right ventricular strain or hypertrophy and right atrial enlargement
- Enlarged central pulmonary arteries on chest x-ray

GENERAL CONSIDERATIONS

- The normal pulmonary circulation is unique in that it has low pressure and resistance, but high flow
- Pulmonary hypertension is present when pulmonary artery pressure rises to a level inappropriate for cardiac output
- Pulmonary hypertension is self-perpetuating, introducing changes in pulmonary vessels that further narrow the vascular bed, increasing pressures
- Primary (idiopathic) pulmonary hypertension is a rare disorder of young and middle-aged women

Etiology of secondary pulmonary hypertension

- Chronic pulmonary embolism
- Chronic obstructive pulmonary disease (COPD)
- Interstitial lung disease
- Scleroderma
- Left to right intracardiac shunt
- Drugs: fenfluramine, dexfenfluramine, phentermine, bleomycin, amiodarone, talc (via IV drug use)
- Pulmonary venoocclusive disease
- Valve disease: mitral stenosis, mitral regurgitation, aortic stenosis
- Left-sided heart failure
- Atrial myxoma
- Polycythemia vera
- Cirrhosis with portal hypertension
- HIV
- Schistosomiasis
- Sickle cell disease

 CLINICAL FINDINGS

SYMPTOMS AND SIGNS

- In its early stages, symptoms are due primarily to the underlying disease
- Progressive dyspnea
- Dull retrosternal chest pain
- Fatigue and exertional syncope
- Narrow splitting of S_2, accentuation of P_2, and a systolic click may be heard
- Tricuspid and pulmonic insufficiency with signs of right ventricular failure and cor pulmonale are found in advanced disease

DIFFERENTIAL DIAGNOSIS

- Primary pulmonary hypertension
- Secondary pulmonary hypertension
- Cor pulmonale (right heart failure due to pulmonary disease)
- Congestive heart failure
- Right-sided valve disease
- Mitral stenosis

 DIAGNOSIS

LABORATORY TESTS

- Polycythemia is found in cases resulting from chronic hypoxemia
- ECG findings consist of right axis deviation, right ventricular hypertrophy, right ventricular strain, or right atrial enlargement
- Routine pulmonary function tests are typically unrevealing, but can show a reduction in the single breath diffusion capacity
- HIV tests, collagen vascular serological studies, and liver function tests can help rule out selected secondary causes

IMAGING STUDIES

- Chest x-rays may show pulmonary artery dilation; right atrial and ventricular enlargement can be seen in advanced cases
- "Pruning" of peripheral pulmonary arteries can be seen on chest x-ray in cases associated with COPD
- Echocardiography can be used to estimate pulmonary artery systolic pressure, as well as give information about cardiac valvular disease
- Ventilation-perfusion scanning can identify cases due to chronic thromboemboli

DIAGNOSTIC PROCEDURES

- Right heart catheterization allows for precise hemodynamic measurements and identifies postcapillary disease, intracardiac shunting, or thromboembolic disease
- Polysomnography may be required to exclude ventilatory disorders
- Open-lung biopsy may be required to diagnose pulmonary venoocclusive disease

Pulmonary Hypertension

 TREATMENT

MEDICATIONS

- Supplemental oxygen for at least 15 h/day has been shown to slow the progression of pulmonary hypertension due to COPD
- Inhaled nitric oxide is effective in lowering pulmonary pressures transiently in patients with asthma and ARDS
- Anticoagulation has been used in cases of unknown etiology, since multiple small emboli may be responsible
- Vasodilator therapy has been disappointing in both primary and secondary disease
- Continuous long-term prostacyclin infusion may confer benefit in selected cases of secondary disease
- Diuretics along with salt restriction help treat cor pulmonale
- Digitalis use in cor pulmonale is controversial

SURGERY

- Single- or double-lung transplant may be performed on patients with end-stage disease; 2-year survival is 50%

THERAPEUTIC PROCEDURES

- Phlebotomy for patients with hematocrit >60% will reduce blood viscosity

 OUTCOME

FOLLOW-UP

- Periodic reassessment of pulmonary artery pressures to determine progression and/or response to thearpy

COMPLICATIONS

- Cor pulmonale

PROGNOSIS

- Depends on the severity of the underlying disease
- Disease due to a fixed obliteration of the pulmonary vascular bed responds poorly to therapy

WHEN TO REFER

- When considering the diagnosis or therapeutic options

WHEN TO ADMIT

- For initiation of vasodilator therapy
- For carefully monitored diuresis
- For debilitating peripheral edema

 EVIDENCE

PRACTICE GUIDELINES

- National Guideline Clearinghouse http://www.guideline.gov/summary/summary.aspx?doc_id=3145&nbr=2371&string=pulmonary+hypertension
- British Cardiac Society Guidelines and Medical Practice Committee, and approved by the British Thoracic Society and the British Society of Rheumatology: Recommendations on the management of pulmonary hypertension in clinical practice. Heart 2001;86(Suppl 1):11.

INFORMATION FOR PATIENTS

- American Heart Association http://circ.ahajournals.org/cgi/reprint/106/24/e192.pdf
- Centers for Disease Control http://www.cdc.gov/cvh/fs-pulmonary_hypertension.htm

REFERENCES

- Fedullo PF et al: Chronic thromboembolic pulmonary hypertension. N Engl J Med 2001;345:1465. [PMID: 11794196]
- Hoeper MM et al: New treatments for pulmonary arterial hypertension. Am J Respir Crit Care Med 2002;165:1209. [PMID: 11991870]
- Krowka MJ: Pulmonary hypertension: diagnostics and therapeutics. Mayo Clin Proc 2000;75:625. [PMID: 10852424]

Mark S. Chesnutt, MD
Thomas J. Prendergast, MD

Pulmonary Nodule, Solitary

 KEY FEATURES

ESSENTIALS OF DIAGNOSIS

- An isolated, <3 cm rounded opacity on chest radiograph that is outlined by normal lung and not associated with infiltrate, atelectasis, or adenopathy

GENERAL CONSIDERATIONS

- Most are asymptomatic and represent an unexpected radiographic finding
- Associated with a 10–68% risk of malignancy
- Most benign nodules are infectious granulomas; benign neoplasms such as hamartomas account for 5% of solitary nodules
- Symptoms alone rarely establish etiology, but can be used with radiographic data to assess the probability of malignancy
- The goal of evaluation is to determine the probability of malignancy in any nodule in order to justify resection or biopsy versus observation

DEMOGRAPHICS

- Malignant nodules are rare in persons under age 30
- Above age 30, risk for malignancy increases with age
- Smokers are at increased risk, with the likelihood of cancer increasing with the number of daily cigarettes
- A history of malignancy increases the likelihood that a nodule represents cancer

 CLINICAL FINDINGS

SYMPTOMS AND SIGNS

- Solitary nodules are discovered incidentally on radiographic studies

DIFFERENTIAL DIAGNOSIS

- Granulomatous disease
- Benign neoplasm
- Bronchogenic carcinoma
- Granuloma (tuberculous, fungal)
- Lung abscess
- Hamartoma
- Metastatic cancer
- Arteriovenous malformation
- Resolving pneumonia
- Rheumatoid nodule
- Pulmonary infarction
- Carcinoid
- Pseudotumor (loculated fluid in a fissure)

 DIAGNOSIS

LABORATORY TESTS

- Sputum cytology is highly specific, but insensitive for detecting malignant nodules

IMAGING STUDIES

- Comparison with prior radiographic studies allows estimation of doubling time: rapid doubling time (<30 days) suggests infection; slow doubling time (<465 days) suggests benignity
- HRCT for any nodule
- Increasing size on CT scan correlates with malignancy: 1% malignancy rate for 2–5 mm; 33% for 11–20 mm; 80% for 21–45 mm
- CT features suggesting malignancy
  - Spiculations or a peripheral halo
  - Sparse stippled or eccentric calcifications
  - Thick-walled (>16 mm) cavitary lesions
- CT features associated with benign processes
  - Smooth, well-defined margins
  - Dense central or laminar calcifications
- Positron emission tomography (PET) is highly sensitive (85–95%) and specific (70–85%) for detecting malignant nodules and is incorporated in many diagnostic algorithms with HRCT

DIAGNOSTIC PROCEDURES

- In patients with a high probability of malignancy, biopsies rarely yield a specific benign diagnosis
- Bronchoscopy yields a diagnosis in 10–80%, depending on the size and location of the nodule; complications are rare
- Transthoracic needle aspiration (TTNA) has a diagnostic yield of 50–97%, with a 30% risk of pneumothorax
- Video-assisted thoracoscopic surgery (VATS) is used for initial evaluation of intermediate risk nodules; frozen sections can direct treatment in the operating room

Pulmonary Nodule, Solitary

 TREATMENT

SURGERY

- Surgical resection via open thoracotomy or VATS is indicated for proven malignancies, nodules likely to be malignant, and certain intermediate risk nodules

THERAPEUTIC PROCEDURES

- A probability of malignancy should be assigned to each nodule based on clinical and radiographic features
- Watchful waiting is appropriate for patients with low probability (<8%) of malignancy (<age 30, lesions stable for >2 years, benign calcification pattern)
- Resection is indicated for patients with a high probability (>70%) of malignancy and no contraindications to surgery
- Optimal management of patients with an intermediate probability (8–70%) of malignancy is controversial; bronchoscopy, transthoracic needle biopsy, VATS, PET scan, and contrast-enhanced HRCT are used

 OUTCOME

FOLLOW-UP

- Patients being followed for a nodule with a low probability of malignancy should get chest x-rays every 3 months for 1 year, then every 6 months for 1 year

WHEN TO REFER

- For specialized diagnostic procedures such as bronchoscopy, transthoracic needle aspiration, or thoracoscopic surgery

 EVIDENCE

PRACTICE GUIDELINES

- National Guideline Clearinghouse
  http://www.guideline.gov/summary/
  summary.aspx?doc_id=3638&nbr=
  2864&string=solitary+pulmonary+
  nodule
  http://www.guideline.gov/summary/
  summary.aspx?doc_id=2570&nbr=
  1796&string=solitary+pulmonary+
  nodule

INFORMATION FOR PATIENTS

- National Institutes of Health
  http://www.nlm.nih.gov/medlineplus/
  ency/article/000071.htm
- American Medical Association
  http://www.medem.com/MedLB/
  article_detaillb.cfm?article_ID=
  ZZZ06T60NAC&sub_cat=577

REFERENCES

- Gould MK et al: Accuracy of positron emission tomography for diagnosis of pulmonary nodules and mass lesions. A meta-analysis. JAMA 2001;285:914. [PMID: 11180735]
- Gurney JW: Determining the likelihood of malignancy in solitary pulmonary nodules with Bayesian analysis. Part I. Theory. Radiology 1993;186:405. [PMID: 8421743]
- Lacasse Y et al: Transthoracic needle aspiration biopsy for the diagnosis of localised pulmonary lesions: a meta-analysis. Thorax 1999;54:884. [PMID: 10491450]
- Ost D et al: Evaluation and management of the solitary pulmonary nodule. Am J Respir Crit Care Med 2000; 162:782. [PMID: 10988081]

Mark S. Chestnutt, MD
Thomas J. Prendergast, MD

Pyelonephritis, Acute

 ## KEY FEATURES

ESSENTIALS OF DIAGNOSIS

- Fever
- Flank pain
- Irritative voiding symptoms
- Positive urine culture

GENERAL CONSIDERATIONS

- Acute pyelonephritis is an infectious inflammatory disease involving the kidney parenchyma and renal pelvis.
- Most common causative agents: *Escherichia coli*, *Proteus*, *Klebsiella*, *Enterobacter*, and *Pseudomonas*
- Less common: *Enterococcus faecalis* and *Staphylococcus aureus*

 ## CLINICAL FINDINGS

SYMPTOMS AND SIGNS

- Fever; flank pain; shaking chills; urgency, frequency, dysuria; nausea, vomiting, diarrhea; tachycardia; costovertebral angle tenderness

DIFFERENTIAL DIAGNOSIS

- Appendicitis, cholecystitis, pancreatitis, or diverticulitis; lower lobe pneumonia; acute epididymitis; prostatitis

 ## DIAGNOSIS

LABORATORY TESTS

- Complete blood cell count: leukocytosis and a left shift
- Urinalysis: pyuria, bacteriuria, hematuria, white blood cell casts
- Urine (and sometimes blood) culture positive

IMAGING STUDIES

- Renal ultrasound (in complicated cases) to evaluate for hydronephrosis from stone or other obstruction

Pyelonephritis, Acute

 ## TREATMENT

MEDICATIONS

- Inpatients: IV ampicillin and an amino-glycoside until afebrile for 24 h, then PO antibiotics for 3 weeks
- Outpatients: quinolones or nitrofuran-toin

Regimens

- Ampicillin, 1 g q6h, and gentamicin, 1 mg/kg q8h IV for 21 days
- Ciprofloxacin, 750 mg q12h PO for 21 days
- Ofloxacin, 200–300 mg q12h PO for 21 days
- Trimethoprim-sulfamethoxasole, 160/800 mg q12h PO for 21 days [increasing resistance noted (up to 20%)]

SURGERY

- Nephrostomy drainage if ureteral obstruction

THERAPEUTIC PROCEDURES

- Fevers for ≤72 h; failure to respond warrants ultrasound to exclude complications
- Catheter drainage if urinary retention

 ## OUTCOME

FOLLOW-UP

- Follow-up urine cultures after completion of treatment

PROGNOSIS

- With prompt diagnosis and treatment, good prognosis
- Complicating factors, underlying renal disease, and increasing patient age, less favorable

WHEN TO ADMIT

- Admit if severe infections or complicating factors; obtain urine and blood cultures

EVIDENCE

PRACTICE GUIDELINES

- Bass PF 3rd et al: Urinary tract infections. Prim Care 2003;30:41. [PMID: 12838910]

WEB SITES

- American College of Obstetricians and Gynecologists—Urinary tract infections http://www.medem.com/MedLB/article_detaillb.cfm?article_ID=ZZZ1LJ5770D&sub_cat=2008
- National Kidney and Urologic Diseases Information Clearinghouse—Pyelonephritis (Kidney Infection) in Adults http://kidney.niddk.nih.gov/kudiseases/pubs/pyelonephritis/index.htm

INFORMATION FOR PATIENTS

- Mayo Clinic—Urinary tract infection http://www.mayoclinic.com/invoke.cfm?objectid=364657CC-439E-4166-843C62403DD3A8D9

REFERENCES

- Proceedings of the 5th International Symposium on Clinical Evaluation of Drug Efficacy in Urinary Tract Infection and of the Urinary Tract Infections Symposia of the Commission for Treatment of Urinary Tract Infection of the International Society of Chemotherapy, 29 June–3 July1997, Sydney, Australia. Int J Antimicrob Agents 1999;11:183. [PMID: 10465618]
- Talan DA et al: Comparison of ciprofloxacin (7 days) and trimethoprim-sulfamethoxazole (14 days) for acute uncomplicated pyelonephritis in women: a randomized trial. JAMA 2000;283:1583. [PMID: 10735395]

Marshall L. Stoller, MD
Peter R. Carroll, MD

Radiation Reactions

 KEY FEATURES

ESSENTIAL OF DIAGNOSIS

- Damage depends on
  - The quantity of radiation delivered to the body
  - The dose rate
  - The organs exposed
  - The type of radiation (x-rays, neutrons, γ-rays, α or β particles)
  - The duration of exposure
  - The energy transfer from the radioactive wave or particle to the exposed tissue

GENERAL CONSIDERATIONS

- The National Committee on Radiation Protection has established the maximum permissible radiation exposure for occupationally exposed workers over age 18 as 0.1 rem per week for the whole body (but not to exceed 5 rem per year) and 1.5 rem per week for the hands
- For purposes of comparison, routine chest x-rays deliver 0.1–0.2 rem

Radiation terminology

- A rad is the unit of absorbed dose
- A rem is the unit of any radiation dose to body tissue in terms of its estimated biological effect
- Roentgen (R) refers to the amount of radiation dose delivered to the body
- For x-ray or γ-ray radiation, rems, rads, and roentgens are virtually the same
- For particulate radiation from radioactive materials, these terms may differ greatly (eg, for neutrons, 1 rad equals 10 rems)
- In the Système International (SI) nomenclature, the rad has been replaced by the gray (Gy), and 1 rad equals 0.01 Gy = 1 cGy
- The SI replacement for the rem is the Sievert (Sv), and 1 rem equals 0.01 Sv

 CLINICAL FINDINGS

SYMPTOMS AND SIGNS

Skin and mucous membranes

- Erythema, epilation, destruction of fingernails, or epidermolysis

Hematopoietic tissues

- Damage to the blood-forming organs may vary from transient depression of one or more blood elements to complete destruction

Cardiovascular system

- Pericarditis with effusion or constrictive pericarditis may occur after a period of months or even years
- Myocarditis is less common
- Smaller vessels (the capillaries and arterioles) are more readily damaged than larger blood vessels

Reproductive effects

- In males, small single doses of radiation (200–300 cGy) cause temporary aspermatogenesis, and larger doses (600–800 cGy) may cause permanent sterility
- In females, single doses of 200 cGy may cause temporary cessation of menses, and 500–800 cGy may cause permanent castration
- Moderate to heavy irradiation of the embryo in utero results in injury to the fetus (eg, mental retardation) or in embryonic death and abortion

Respiratory tract

- High or repeated moderate doses of radiation may cause pneumonitis, often delayed for weeks or months

Mouth, pharynx, esophagus, and stomach

- Mucositis with edema and painful swallowing of food may occur within hours or days after exposure
- Gastric secretion may be inhibited by high doses of radiation

Intestines

- Inflammation and ulceration may follow moderately large doses of radiation

Endocrine glands and viscera

- Hepatitis and nephritis may be delayed effects of therapeutic radiation
- The normal thyroid, pituitary, pancreas, adrenals, and bladder are relatively resistant to low or moderate doses of radiation; parathyroid glands are especially resistant

Nervous system

- The brain and spinal cord are much more sensitive to acute exposures than the peripheral nerves

Systemic reaction (radiation sickness)

- Anorexia, nausea, vomiting, weakness, exhaustion, lassitude, and in some cases prostration may occur, singly or in combination
- Dehydration, anemia, and infection may follow

 DIAGNOSIS

LABORATORY TESTS

- Serial lymphocyte counts are useful for dose estimation and monitoring of the clinical impact of exposure

TREATMENT

MEDICATIONS

- Ondansetron, 8 mg orally twice or three times daily, for nausea and vomiting
- Alternatives include chlorpromazine, 25–50 mg given deeply intramuscularly every 4–6 h as necessary or 10–25 mg orally every 4–6 h as necessary; and dimenhydrinate, 50–100 mg, or perphenazine, 4–8 mg, 1 h before and 1 and 4 h after radiation therapy has been recommended
- Blood and platelet transfusions, blood stem cell transplantation, bone marrow transplants, antibiotics, fluid and electrolyte maintenance, and other supportive measures may be useful
- Recombinant hematopoietic growth factors (filgrastim and sargramostim or molgramostim) can accelerate hematopoietic recovery

THERAPEUTIC PROCEDURES

- Particulate or radioisotope exposures should be decontaminated in designated confined areas
- For many radioisotopes, chelation, blocking, or dilution therapy is indicated
- Treatment of systemic reactions is symptomatic and supportive

 ## OUTCOME

COMPLICATIONS

- Skin scarring, atrophy, and telangiectasis; cataract, dry eye syndrome, retinopathy; neuropathy, myelopathy, cerebral injury; obliterative endarteritis, coronary artery disease, pericarditis; thyroid disease; pulmonary fibrosis, hepatitis, intestinal stenosis, and nephritis
- Neoplastic disease, including leukemia and cancers of the skin, breast, lung, and thyroid, is increased after exposed to radiation at relatively low doses (<0.2 Gy)
- High-dose radon exposure is associated with an increased risk of lung cancer. Association of ionizing radiation with several other cancers is not well quantified
- Prenatal irradiation may increase the risk of congenital abnormalities and childhood cancer
- Carcinogenesis from low-dose (<10 rem) exposure to adults has not been demonstrated

PROGNOSIS

- Death after acute lethal radiation exposure is due to hematopoietic failure, gastrointestinal mucosal damage, central nervous system damage, widespread vascular injury, or secondary infection
- Four hundred to 600 cGy of x-ray or γ-ray radiation applied to the entire body at one time may be fatal within 60 days; death is usually due to hemorrhage, anemia, and infection secondary to hematopoietic injury
- Levels of 1000–3000 cGy to the entire body destroy gastrointestinal mucosa; this leads to toxemia and death within 2 weeks
- Total-body doses above 3000 cGy cause widespread vascular damage, cerebral anoxia, hypotensive shock, and death within 48 h

 ## EVIDENCE

PRACTICE GUIDELINES

- National Guideline Clearinghouse http://www.guideline.gov/summary/summary.aspx?doc_id=3089&nbr=2315&string=radiation+exposure http://www.guideline.gov/summary/summary.aspx?doc_id=3209&nbr=2435&string=radiation+exposure

WEB SITE

- Radiation Health Effects Resource: Ionizing Radiation Health Effects (RadEFX) http://radefx.bcm.tmc.edu/ionizing/ionizing.htm_

INFORMATION FOR PATIENTS

- National Institutes of Health http://www.nih.gov/health/chip/od/radiation/
- U.S. Environmental Protection Agency http://www.epa.gov/radiation/understand/health_effects.htm

REFERENCE

- Reeves GI: Radiation injuries. Crit Care Clin 1999;15:457. [PMID: 10331137]

Richard Cohen, MD, MPH
Brent R.W. Moelleken, MD, FACS

Rape

 KEY FEATURES

ESSENTIALS OF DIAGNOSIS

- Women neither secretly want to be raped nor do they expect, encourage, or enjoy rape
- Rape is always a terrifying experience in which most victims fear for their lives
- The rapist is usually a hostile man who uses sexual intercourse to terrorize and humiliate a woman

GENERAL CONSIDERATIONS

- Rape, or sexual assault, is legally defined in different ways in various jurisdictions
- Clinicians and emergency room personnel who deal with rape victims should be familiar with the laws pertaining to sexual assault in their own state
- From a medical and psychological viewpoint, it is essential that persons treating rape victims recognize the nonconsensual and violent nature of the crime
- Penetration may be vaginal, anal, or oral and may be by the penis, hand, or a foreign object
- The absence of genital injury does not imply consent by the victim
- The assailant may be unknown to the victim or, more frequently, may be an acquaintance or even the spouse
- "Unlawful sexual intercourse," or statutory rape, is intercourse with a female before the age of majority even with her consent

DEMOGRAPHICS

- About 95% of reported rape victims are women
- Rape involves severe physical injury in 5–10% of cases

 CLINICAL FINDINGS

SYMTOMS AND SIGNS

- Each patient will react differently to this personal crisis

Rape trauma syndrome

- Immediate or acute
  - Shaking, sobbing, and restless activity may last from a few days to a few weeks
  - The patient may experience anger, guilt, or shame or may repress these emotions
  - Reactions vary depending on the victim's personality and the circumstances of the attack
- Late or chronic
  - Problems related to the attack may develop weeks or months later
  - The life-style and work patterns of the individual may change
  - Sleep disorders or phobias often develop
  - Loss of self-esteem can in rare cases lead to suicide

 DIAGNOSIS

LABORATORY TESTS

- Culture the vagina, anus, or mouth (as appropriate) for *Neisseria gonorrhoeae* and *Chlamydia*. Perform a Papanicolaou smear of the cervix, a wet mount for *Trichomonas vaginalis*, a baseline pregnancy test, and VDRL test. A confidential test for HIV antibody can be obtained if desired by the patient and repeated in 2–4 months if initially negative. Repeat the pregnancy test if the next menses is missed, and repeat the VDRL test in 6 weeks. Obtain blood (10 mL without anticoagulant) and urine (100 mL) specimens if there is a history of forced ingestion or injection of drugs or alcohol

DIAGNOSTIC PROCEDURES

- The clinician who first sees the alleged rape victim should be empathetic. Begin with a statement such as, "This is a terrible thing that has happened to you. I want to help"
- Secure written consent from the patient, guardian, or next of kin for gynecological examination and for photographs if they are likely to be useful as evidence. If police are to be notified, do so, and obtain advice on the preservation and transfer of evidence
- Obtain and record the history in the patient's own words. The sequence of events, ie, the time, place, and circumstances, must be included. Note the date of the last menstrual period, whether or not the woman is pregnant, and the time of the most recent coitus prior to the sexual assault. Note the details of the assault such as body cavities penetrated, use of foreign objects, and number of assailants
- Note whether the victim is calm, agitated, or confused (drugs or alcohol may be involved). Record whether the patient came directly to the hospital or whether she bathed or changed her clothing. Record findings but do not issue even a tentative diagnosis lest it be erroneous or incomplete
- Have the patient disrobe while standing on a white sheet. Hair, dirt, and leaves; underclothing; and any torn or stained clothing should be kept as evidence. Scrape material from beneath fingernails and comb pubic hair for evidence. Place all evidence in separate clean paper bags or envelopes and label carefully

Rape

- Examine the patient, noting any traumatized areas that should be photographed. Examine the body and genitals with a Wood light to identify semen, which fluoresces; positive areas should be swabbed with a premoistened swab and air-dried in order to identify acid phosphatase. Colposcopy can be used to identify small areas of trauma from forced entry, especially at the posterior fourchette
- Perform a pelvic examination, explaining all procedures and obtaining the patient's consent before proceeding gently with the examination. Use a narrow speculum lubricated with water only. Collect material with sterile cotton swabs from the vaginal walls and cervix and make two air-dried smears on clean glass slides. Wet and dry swabs of vaginal secretions should be collected and refrigerated for subsequent acid phosphatase and DNA evaluation. Swab the mouth (around molars and cheeks) and anus in the same way, if appropriate. Label all slides carefully. Collect secretions from the vagina, anus, or mouth with a premoistened cotton swab, place at once on a slide with a drop of saline, and cover with a coverslip. Look for motile or nonmotile sperm under high, dry magnification, and record the percentage of motile forms
- Perform appropriate laboratory tests
- Transfer clearly labeled evidence, eg, laboratory specimens, directly to the clinical pathologist in charge or to the responsible laboratory technician, in the presence of witnesses (never via messenger), so that the rules of evidence will not be breached

TREATMENT

MEDICATIONS

- Give analgesics or sedatives if indicated
- Administer tetanus toxoid if deep lacerations contain soil or dirt particles
- Give ceftriaxone, 125 mg intramuscularly, to prevent gonorrhea. In addition, give metronidazole, 2 g as a single dose, and doxycycline, 100 mg twice daily for 7 days to treat chlamydial infection. Incubating syphilis will probably be prevented by these medications, but the VDRL test should be repeated 6 weeks after the assault

THERAPEUTIC PROCEDURES

- Prevent pregnancy by using one of the methods discussed in *Contraception, emergency*, if necessary
- Vaccinate against hepatitis B
- Consider HIV prophylaxis
- Make sure the patient and her family and friends have a source of ongoing psychological support

OUTCOME

FOLLOW-UP

- Clinicians and emergency room personnel who deal with rape victims should work with community rape crisis centers whenever possible to provide ongoing support and counseling

COMPLICATIONS

- All victims suffer some psychological aftermath
- Some rape victims may acquire sexually transmissible disease or become pregnant

EVIDENCE

PRACTICE GUIDELINES

- National Guideline Clearinghouse
http://www.guideline.gov/summary/summary.aspx?doc_id=3050&nbr=2276&string=rape
http://www.guideline.gov/summary/summary.aspx?doc_id=3082&nbr=2308&string=rape

INFORMATION FOR PATIENTS

- National Women's Health Information Center
http://www.4woman.gov/faq/sexualassault.htm
- American Academy of Family Physicians
http://familydoctor.org/handouts/314.html

REFERENCE

- Linden JA: Sexual assault. Emerg Med Clin North Am 1999;17:685. [PMID: 10516847]

H. Trent MacKay, MD, MPH

Rash, Drug

 KEY FEATURES

ESSENTIALS OF DIAGNOSIS

- Usually, abrupt onset of widespread, symmetric erythematous eruption
- May mimic any inflammatory skin condition
- Constitutional symptoms (malaise, arthralgia, headache, and fever) may be present

GENERAL CONSIDERATIONS

- Only a minority of cutaneous drug reactions result from allergy
- True allergic drug reactions involve prior exposure, an "incubation" period, reactions to doses far below the therapeutic range, restriction to a limited number of syndromes (anaphylactic and anaphylactoid, urticarial, vasculitic, etc), and reproducibility
- Amoxicillin, trimethoprim-sulfamethoxazole, and ampicillin or penicillin are the commonest causes of urticarial and maculopapular reactions
- Toxic epidermal necrolysis and Stevens-Johnson syndrome are most commonly produced by sulfonamides and anticonvulsants
- Phenolphthalein, pyrazolone derivatives, tetracyclines, nonsteroidal antiinflammatory drugs, trimethoprim-sulfamethoxazole, and barbiturates are the major causes of fixed drug eruptions

DEMOGRAPHICS

- Rashes are among the most common adverse reactions to drugs and occur in 2–3% of hospitalized patients

 CLINICAL FINDINGS

SYMPTOMS AND SIGNS

- The onset is usually abrupt, with bright erythema and often severe itching, but may be delayed
- Fever and other constitutional symptoms may be present
- The skin reaction usually occurs in symmetric distribution
- Table 8 (page 1203) summarizes the types of skin reactions, their appearance and distribution, and the common offenders in each case

DIFFERENTIAL DIAGNOSIS

- Viral exanthem
- Early erythema multiforme major
- Other causes of erythema nodosum eg, infection, sarcoidosis
- Atopic dermatitis (eczema)
- Secondary syphilis
- Systemic lupus erythematosus
- Acute HIV infection
- Scarlet fever
- Toxic shock syndrome
- Lichen planus

 DIAGNOSIS

LABORATORY TESTS

- Routinely ordered blood work is of no value in the diagnosis of drug eruptions

DIAGNOSTIC PROCEDURES

- Skin biopsies may be helpful in making the diagnosis
- Observation after discontinuation, which may be a slow process, helps establish the diagnosis
- Rechallenge, though of theoretical value, may pose a danger to the patient and is best avoided

TREATMENT

MEDICATIONS

General Measures

- Antihistamines may be of value in urticarial and angioneurotic reactions
- Epinephrine 1:1000, 0.5–1 mL intravenously or subcutaneously should be used as an emergency measure
- In severe cases, corticosteroids may be used at doses similar to those used for acute contact dermatitis

THERAPEUTIC PROCEDURES

- Systemic manifestations are treated as they arise (eg, anemia, icterus, purpura)
- The varieties and stages of dermatitis are treated according to the major dermatitis present

 OUTCOME

COMPLICATIONS

- Some cutaneous drug reactions may be associated with a clinical complex involving other organs (complex drug reactions); most common is an infectious mononucleosis-like illness and hepatitis associated with administration of anticonvulsants

PROGNOSIS

- Drug rash usually disappears upon withdrawal of the drug and proper treatment

WHEN TO REFER

- If there is a question about the diagnosis, if recommended therapy is ineffective, or if specialized treatment is necessary

WHEN TO ADMIT

- Extensive blistering eruptions resulting in erosions and superficial ulcerations demand hospitalization and nursing care as for burn patients

 EVIDENCE

PRACTICE GUIDELINES

- American Academy of Dermatology
  http://www.aadassociation.org/
  Guidelines/cutaneousdrug.html

WEB SITES

- American Academy of Dermatology
  http://www.aad.org
- Dermatology Handbook for Family Practice from the University of Iowa
  http://www.vh.org/Providers/ClinRef/
  FPHandbook/17.html

INFORMATION FOR PATIENTS

- American Academy of Dermatology
  http://www.aad.org/pamphlets/
- Mayo Clinic
  http://www.mayoclinic.com/
  invoke.cfm?id=HQ01195

REFERENCE

- Kim NY: Pigmentary diseases. Med Clin North Am 1998;82:1185. [PMID: 9769800]

Timothy G. Berger, MD

Rash, Heat

 KEY FEATURES

ESSENTIALS OF DIAGNOSIS

- Burning, itching, superficial aggregated small vesicles, papules, or pustules on covered areas of the skin, usually the trunk
- More common in hot, moist climates
- Rare forms associated with fever and even heat prostration

GENERAL CONSIDERATIONS

- An acute dermatitis that occurs most commonly on the trunk and intertriginous areas
- A hot, moist environment is the most frequent cause; bedridden febrile patients are susceptible
- Plugging of the ostia of sweat ducts occurs, with consequent ballooning and ultimate rupture of the sweat duct, producing an irritating, stinging reaction
- Increase in numbers of resident aerobes, notably cocci, apparently plays a role

 CLINICAL FINDINGS

SYMPTOMS AND SIGNS

- See Table 7 (page 1202)
- The usual symptoms are burning and itching
- In severe cases, fever, heat prostration, and even death may result
- The lesions consist of small, superficial, red, thin-walled, discrete but closely aggregated vesicles (miliaria crystallina), papules (miliaria rubra), or vesicopustules or pustules (miliaria pustulosa)
- The reaction occurs most commonly on covered areas of the skin

DIFFERENTIAL DIAGNOSIS

- Folliculitis
- Drug eruption

 DIAGNOSIS

LABORATORY TESTS

- Clinical diagnosis

TREATMENT

MEDICATIONS

- See Table 6 (page 1199)
- Triamcinolone acetonide, 0.1% in Sarna lotion, or a mid-potency corticosteroid in a lotion or cream—but not ointment—base, should be applied two to four times daily
- Secondary infections (superficial pyoderma) are treated with dicloxacillin, 250 mg four times daily by mouth
- Anticholinergic drugs given by mouth may be helpful in severe cases, eg, glycopyrrolate, 1 mg twice daily

 OUTCOME

PROGNOSIS

- Usually a mild disorder, but severe forms (tropical anhidrosis and asthenia) result from interference with the heat-regulating mechanism

WHEN TO REFER

- If there is a question about the diagnosis, if recommended therapy is ineffective, or if specialized treatment is necessary

PREVENTION

- Use of an antibacterial preparation such as chlorhexidine prior to exposure to heat and humidity may help prevent the condition
- Susceptible persons should avoid exposure to hot, humid environments

 EVIDENCE

WEB SITES

- American Academy of Dermatology http://www.aad.org
- Dermatology Handbook for Family Practice from the University of Iowa http://www.vh.org/Providers/ClinRef/FPHandbook/17.html

INFORMATION FOR PATIENTS

- American Academy of Pediatrics http://www.medem.com/medlb/article_detaillb.cfm?article_ID=ZZZG8JSV8EC&sub_cat=25

REFERENCE

- Wenzel FG et al: Nonneoplastic disorders of the eccrine glands. J Am Acad Dermatol 1998;38:1.

Timothy G. Berger, MD

Raynaud's Disease & Phenomenon

KEY FEATURES

ESSENTIALS OF DIAGNOSIS

- Episodic bilateral digital pallor, cyanosis, and rubor
- Precipitated by cold or emotional stress; relieved by warmth

GENERAL CONSIDERATIONS

- An episodic vasospastic disorder characterized by digital color change (white-blue-red) with exposure to cold or emotional stress
- Called Raynaud's disease if symptoms persist for >3 years without evidence of an associated disease
- Called Raynaud's phenomenon if associated with autoimmune diseases, myeloproliferative disorders, multiple myeloma, cryoglobulinemia, myxedema, macroglobulinemia, or arterial occlusive disease
- Occurs in 10% of the general population
- Other vasospastic disorders, eg, variant angina and migraine headache, are common in patients with Raynaud's

DEMOGRAPHICS

- 70–80% of patients are women
- Raynaud's disease usually appears first between ages 15 and 45, almost always in women

CLINICAL FINDINGS

SYMPTOMS AND SIGNS

- Mild discomfort, paresthesias, numbness, and trace edema often accompany the color changes
- The affected extremities may be entirely normal between attacks
- Raynaud's disease is symmetric
- Raynaud's phenomenon infrequently involves the feet and toes
- Raynaud's disease is benign and entirely reversible
- Raynaud's phenomenon may progress to atrophy of the terminal fat pads and development of fingertip gangrene

DIFFERENTIAL DIAGNOSIS

- Neurogenic thoracic outlet syndrome or carpal tunnel syndrome
- Frostbite, ergotamine toxicity, and chemotherapeutic agents
- Bleomycin and vincristine chemotherapy
- Atherosclerosis, Buerger's disease, embolic disease, repetitive motion injury
- Vasospasm with contrast injection
- Acrocyanosis
- Livedo reticularis

DIAGNOSIS

LABORATORY TESTS

- Complete blood cell count
- Autoimmune workup, if suspected

IMAGING STUDIES

- Conventional digital angiography is indicated only in cases of tissue loss or to rule out atheroemboli, atherooclusive disease, or arterial trauma

DIAGNOSTIC PROCEDURES

- Diagnosis is based on clinical criteria

Raynaud's Disease & Phenomenon

 TREATMENT

MEDICATIONS

- Aspirin
- Vasodilators
- Nifedipine, sustained-release 30 mg PO QD, or diltiazem, sustained-release 30 mg PO QD
- Fluoxetine, 20 mg PO QD
- Discontinue oral contraceptives, β-blockers, and ergotamine

SURGERY

- Bypass surgery for severe Raynaud's phenomenon associated with reconstructible arterial occlusive disease
- Sympathectomy for unreconstructible occlusive disease or pure vasospastic disease refractory to medical management

THERAPEUTIC PROCEDURES

- Warmth and protection of the hands
- Moisturizing lotion
- Smoking cessation
- Stress management

 OUTCOME

PROGNOSIS

- Raynaud's disease usually benign
- Raynaud's phenomenon prognosis is that of the associated disease

WHEN TO REFER

- Raynaud's syndrome with tissue loss
- Severe arterial insufficiency from atheroocclusive disease

PREVENTION

- Avoidance of cold exposure
- Stress reduction

 EVIDENCE

PRACTICE GUIDELINES

- Drug therapy for peripheral vascular disease. A national clinical guideline. Scottish Intercollegiate Guidelines Network, 1998 http://www.sign.ac.uk/ pdf/sign27.pdf
- Eberhardt RT et al: Drug treatment of peripheral vascular disease. Heart Dis 2000;2:62. [PMID: 11728242]

WEB SITES

- National Heart, Lung, and Blood Institute—Raynaud's phenomenon http://www.nhlbi.nih.gov/health/ public/blood/other/raynaud.htm
- Uptodate—Raynaud's phenomenon http://patients.uptodate.com/frames. asp?page=topic.asp&file=arth_rhe/ 6020&title=Raynauds+disease

INFORMATION FOR PATIENTS

- Cleveland Clinic—Raynaud's phenomenon http://www.clevelandclinic.org/ health/ health-info/docs/3100/3132.asp? index=9849
- Mayo Clinic—Raynaud's disease http://www.mayoclinic.com/invoke.cfm? objectid=BEC8E664-5EE6-41C1-8955642FA71A0EEF
- MEDLINEplus—Raynaud's phenomenon http://www.nlm.nih.gov/medlineplus/ ency/article/000412.htm

REFERENCES

- Coleiro B et al: Treatment of Raynaud's phenomenon with the selective serotonin reuptake inhibitor fluoxetine. Rheumatology (Oxford) 2001;40:1038. [PMID: 11561116]
- Pache M et al: Cold feet and prolonged sleep-onset latency in vasospastic syndrome. Lancet 2001;358:125. [PMID: 11463418]

Louis M. Messina, MD
Laura K. Pak, MD
Lawrence M. Tierney, Jr., MD

Reflex Sympathetic Dystrophy

 KEY FEATURES

ESSENTIALS OF DIAGNOSIS

- Burning or aching pain in an injured extremity more severe than would be expected given the inciting trauma
- Localized vasomotor instability

GENERAL CONSIDERATIONS

- Occurs equally in all age groups and both sexes
- Can involve either the arms or the legs
- Causes include trauma, closed fractures, simple lacerations, burns, operative procedures, and myocardial infarction

 CLINICAL FINDINGS

SYMPTOMS AND SIGNS

- Early stages: pain, tenderness, and hyperesthesia localized to the injured area; extremity is warm, dry, swollen, and red or slightly cyanotic; with time, muscle spasm and joint stiffness limit mobility; the nails may become ridged
- Advanced stages: pain is more diffuse, nocturnal pain; extremity is cool, clammy, and intolerant of temperature changes
- Patient concerned to avoid external stimuli
- Pain and disuse lead to loss of function

DIFFERENTIAL DIAGNOSIS

- Acute limb ischemia
- Thoracic outlet syndrome
- Nerve root compression or radiculopathy

 DIAGNOSIS

IMAGING STUDIES

- Bone radiographs: asymmetric osteopenia more severe than anticipated from immobility alone

TREATMENT

MEDICATIONS

- Diazepam, 2 mg PO BID; or alprazolam, 0.125–0.25 mg PO QD
- Opioids
- Gabapentin

SURGERY

- Sympathectomy
- Implantable spinal cord biostimulator devices have had limited success

THERAPEUTIC PROCEDURES

- Early physical therapy involving active and passive exercises
- Protection from further injury
- Avoidance of irritating stimuli
- Sympathetic (stellate ganglion or lumbar) blocks

 OUTCOME

COMPLICATIONS

- Chronic pain syndrome
- Disability

PROGNOSIS

- Good with early diagnosis and appropriate intervention

WHEN TO REFER

- Signs and symptoms of reflex sympathetic dystrophy

WHEN TO ADMIT

- Intractable pain

PREVENTION

- Avoid trauma to peripheral nerves during surgery
- Following injury to an extremity, splinting and adequate analgesia, followed by early mobilization

 EVIDENCE

PRACTICE GUIDELINES

- Greipp ME: Complex regional pain syndrome—type I: research relevance, practice realities. J Neurosci Nurs 2003;35:16. [PMID: 12789717]
- Turner-Stokes L: Reflex sympathetic dystrophy—a complex regional pain syndrome. Disabil Rehabil 2002;24:939. [PMID: 12523947]

WEB SITES

- National Institute of Neurological Disorders and Stroke—Reflex sympathetic dystrophy syndrome http://www.ninds.nih.gov/health_and_medical/disorders/reflex_sympathetic_dystrophy.htm
- Reflex Sympathetic Dystrophy Syndrome Association of America—Clinical Practice Guidelines: reflex sympathetic dystrophy & complex regional pain syndrome http://www.rsds.org/cpgeng.htm

INFORMATION FOR PATIENTS

- Mayo Clinic—Complex regional pain syndrome http://www.mayoclinic.com/invoke.cfm?objectid=8F3237C2-D7C0-4063-AE87DC86D78085FE
- MEDLINEplus—Complex regional pain syndrome http://www.nlm.nih.gov/medlineplus/ency/article/007184.htm

REFERENCES

- Kemmler MA et al: Impact of spinal cord stimulation on sensory characteristics in complex regional pain syndrome type 1: a randomized trial. Anesthesiology 2001;95:72. [PMID: 11465587]
- Wasner G et al: Vascular abnormalities in reflex sympathetic dystrophy (CPRS 1): mechanisms and diagnostic value. Brain 2001;124:587. [PMID: 11222458]

Louis M. Messina, MD
Laura K. Pak, MD
Lawrence M. Tierney, Jr., MD

Renal Artery Stenosis

 KEY FEATURES

ESSENTIALS OF DIAGNOSIS

- Produced predominantly by atherosclerotic occlusive disease (80–90% of patients) or fibromuscular dysplasia (10–15%)
- Patients with occlusive disease have common risk factors for atherosclerosis, lesions are focal proximal or ostial calcific plaques, "spillover" aortic disease
- Patients with fibromuscular dysplasia are usually women 30–50 years of age with distal renal artery disease that often extends into the branch vessels in a classic "string of beads" pattern of alternating stenoses and dilations

GENERAL CONSIDERATIONS

- Of patients with hypertension ~5% have renal artery stenosis
- In patients aged >60 years with diastolic blood pressure >105 mm Hg and serum creatinine >2 mg/dL, 70% have renovascular disease
- In hypertensive children aged <5 years with hypertension, 80% have renovascular disease
- Consider renal artery stenosis in patients with poorly controlled or acutely worsening hypertension on three or more antihypertensive medications, particularly when presenting in conjunction with renal insufficiency, lateral abdominal bruit, or noncardiogenic "flash" pulmonary edema, and in patients with a history of acute renal failure when starting an angiotensin-converting enzyme (ACE) inhibitor
- Renal artery stenosis is noted in as many as 45% of patients undergoing angiography for aortoiliac occlusive disease
- Suspect in patients with rapidly progressive renal insufficiency and no evidence of obstructive uropathy or intrinsic renal disease (no proteinuria, no polycystic disease)

 CLINICAL FINDINGS

SYMPTOMS AND SIGNS

- Hypertension, often severe and refractory to antihypertensive medications
- Lateral abdominal bruit

DIFFERENTIAL DIAGNOSIS

- Essential hypertension
- Hypertensive nephrosclerosis
- Primary hyperaldosteronism
- Cushing's syndrome
- Coarctation of the aorta

 DIAGNOSIS

LABORATORY TESTS

- Serum creatinine >2 mg/dL
- Urinalysis: no proteinuria

IMAGING STUDIES

- Initial screening tests: duplex ultrasound, captopril renal scintigraphy, and MRA, each of which has sensitivity and specificity >90%
- Ultrasound and MRA can assess renal size, cortical thickness, and presence of infarcts, but can miss small accessory renal arteries, which when diseased can contribute to renovascular hypertension
- Angiography: indicated for treatment by percutaneous angioplasty and stenting or surgery

Renal Artery Stenosis

 TREATMENT

MEDICATIONS

- Antihypertensive drug therapy, individualizing (Table 49, page 1247)
- α-Adrenoreceptor blocking agents, sympatholytic agents, and vasodilator agents (Table 48, page 1245)
- β-Adrenergic blocking agents (Table 45, page 1239)
- Calcium channel-blocking agents (Table 47, page 1246)
- Diuretics (Table 44, page 1237)
- Hypertensive emergencies and urgencies (Table 50, page 1248)
- Avoid ACE inhibitors and ACE receptor blockers

SURGERY

- For hypertension refractory to aggressive medical management or renal artery stenosis with progressive renal failure or sudden-onset noncardiogenic pulmonary edema
- For patients with lesions refractory to angioplasty, complex lesions extending into the branch vessels, or concomitant aortic disease requiring surgical reconstruction
- Superior long-term patency
- Transaortic renal endarterectomy, renal artery bypass, or extraanatomic (hepatorenal, splenorenal, or iliorenal) bypass
- Nephrectomy for patients with renovascular hypertension and irreversible renal atrophy
- Endarterectomy and aortorenal bypass have 5-year patency >80%, beneficial blood pressure response in 70–90%, and improvement or stabilization in renal function in 70–80%

THERAPEUTIC PROCEDURES

- Endovascular treatment (angioplasty and stenting) for focal, proximal, nonostial plaques that do not extend into the branch vessels
- Angioplasty alone effective for fibromuscular dysplasia
- Primary stenting for stenoses in renal arteries >6 mm yields improved patency over angioplasty alone

 OUTCOME

FOLLOW-UP

- Careful blood pressure monitoring

COMPLICATIONS

- Renal failure

PROGNOSIS

- The long-term patency of renal artery stents is yet undefined, but a 20–44% restenosis rate from intimal hyperplasia is noted at 6–36 months
- Overall, 3–13% of initially stented patients ultimately require surgery

WHEN TO REFER

- Renal artery stenosis with poorly controlled hypertension or renal insufficiency

WHEN TO ADMIT

- Malignant hypertension

PREVENTION

- Antilipidemic, antihypertensive therapy to prevent atherosclerosis

EVIDENCE

PRACTICE GUIDELINES

- Martin LG et al: Standards of Practice Committee. Quality improvement guidelines for angiography, angioplasty, and stent placement in the diagnosis and treatment of renal artery stenosis in adults. J Vasc Interv Radiol 2002;13: 1069. [PMID: 12427805]
- Procedure guideline for diagnosis of renovascular hypertension. Society of Nuclear Medicine, Inc, 1999 http://www.snm.org/pdf/Renal2.pdf

WEB SITE

- American Osteopathic Association— Hypertension and renal artery stenosis http://www.aoa-net.org/Publications/ JAOA/Supplements/1000jaff.pdf

INFORMATION FOR PATIENTS

- American Osteopathic Association— Hypertension and renal artery stenosis http://www.aoa-net.org/Publications/ JAOA/Supplements/1000jaff.pdf
- Ohio State University Medical Center— Renal artery stenosis http://www.acs.ohio-state.edu/units/ osuhosp/patedu/ Materials/PDFDocs/ dis-cond/general/ ren-art.pdf

REFERENCES

- Paty PS et al: Is prosthetic renal artery reconstruction a durable procedure? An analysis of 489 bypass grafts. J Vasc Surg 2001;34:127. [PMID: 11436085]
- Safian R: Renal-artery stenosis. N Engl J Med 2001;344:431. [PMID: 11172181]
- van de Ven PJ et al: Arterial stenting and balloon angioplasty in ostial atherosclerotic renovascular disease: a randomised trial. Lancet 1999;353:282. [PMID: 9929021]

Louis M. Messina, MD
Laura K. Pak, MD
Lawrence M. Tierney, Jr., MD

Renal Cell Carcinoma

 KEY FEATURES

ESSENTIALS OF DIAGNOSIS

- Gross or microscopic hematuria
- Flank pain or mass in some patients
- Systemic symptoms such as fever, weight loss may be prominent
- Solid renal mass on imaging

GENERAL CONSIDERATIONS

- ~2.3% of all adult cancers
- In 2001, ~30,800 cases of renal cell carcinoma and ~12,100 deaths in the United States

DEMOGRAPHICS

- Peak incidence in sixth decade of life
- Male-to-female ratio = 2:1
- Cause is unknown
- Risk factor: cigarette smoking
- Familial: von Hippel-Lindau syndrome
- Association with dialysis-related acquired cystic disease

 CLINICAL FINDINGS

SYMPTOMS AND SIGNS

- Hematuria (gross or microscopic) in 60% of cases
- Flank pain or an abdominal mass in ~30%
- Triad of flank pain, hematuria, and mass in ~10–15%, often a sign of advanced disease
- Symptoms of metastatic disease (cough, bone pain) in ~20–30% at presentation
- Often detected incidentally

DIFFERENTIAL DIAGNOSIS

- Angiomyolipomas (fat density usually visible by CT)
- Transitional cell cancers of the renal pelvis (more centrally located, involvement of the collecting system, positive urinary cytology reports)
- Adrenal tumors (superoanterior to the kidney) and oncocytomas
- Renal abscesses

 DIAGNOSIS

LABORATORY TESTS

- Hematuria in 60%
- Paraneoplastic syndromes
- Erythrocytosis from increased erythropoietin production in ~5% (anemia far more common)
- Hypercalcemia in 10%
- Stauffer's syndrome, a reversible syndrome of hepatic dysfunction

IMAGING STUDIES

- Renal mass on intravenous urography, ultrasound, or CT scan

DIAGNOSTIC PROCEDURES

- CT scanning is the most valuable imaging test; it confirms character of the mass, stages the lesion
- Chest radiographs for pulmonary metastases
- Bone scans for large tumors, bone pain, elevated alkaline phosphatase levels
- MRI and duplex Doppler ultrasonography can assess for the presence and extent of tumor thrombus within the renal vein or vena cava in selected patients

TREATMENT

MEDICATIONS

- For metastatic renal cell carcinoma, no effective chemotherapy is available
- Vinblastine yields short-term partial response rates of 15%
- Biological response modifiers: α-interferon yields partial response rate of 15–20% and interleukin-2, partial response rate of 15–35%

SURGERY

- Radical nephrectomy for localized renal cell carcinoma
- Partial nephrectomy for patients with a small cancer, single kidney, bilateral lesions, or significant medical renal disease

THERAPEUTIC PROCEDURES

- Cell type and histological pattern do not affect treatment
- Patients with metastatic disease usually should be considered for palliative therapy with surgery followed by systemic therapy—biological response modifiers

 OUTCOME

PROGNOSIS

- For patients with solitary resectable metastases, radical nephrectomy with resection of the metastasis has resulted in 5-year disease-free survival rates of 15–30%

 EVIDENCE

PRACTICE GUIDELINES

- Mickisch G et al: Guidelines on renal cell cancer. Eur Urol 2001;40:252. [PMID: 11684839]
- Whang YE et al: Renal cell carcinoma. Curr Opin Oncol 2003;15:213. [PMID: 12778014]

WEB SITES

- American Cancer Society—What is kidney cancer (renal cell carcinoma)? http://www.cancer.org/docroot/cri/content/cri_2_4_1x_what_is_kidney_cancer_22.asp?sitearea=cri
- National Cancer Institute—What you need to know about kidney cancer http://www.cancer.gov/cancerinfo/wyntk/kidney

INFORMATION FOR PATIENTS

- Cleveland Clinic—Renal cell cancer http://www.clevelandclinic.org/health/health-info/docs/1400/1437.asp?index=6176
- Mayo Clinic—Kidney cancer http://www.mayoclinic.com/invoke.cfm?objectid=162FE2ED-4D6F-4BB4-9DF39A9952A1A2EA

REFERENCES

- Chan DY et al: Laparoscopic radical nephrectomy: cancer control for renal cell carcinoma. J Urol 2001;166:2095. [PMID: 11696714].
- Figlin RA: Renal cell carcinoma: management of advanced disease. J Urol 1999;161:381. [PMID: 9915408]
- Mickisch GH et al: Radical nephrectomy plus interferon-alfa-based immunotherapy compared with interferon alfa alone in metastatic renal-cell carcinoma: a randomised trial. Lancet 2001;358:966. [PMID: 11583750]

Marshall L. Stoller, MD
Peter R. Carroll, MD

Renal Failure, Acute

 KEY FEATURES

ESSENTIALS OF DIAGNOSIS

- Defined as a sudden decrease in renal function, resulting in an inability to maintain fluid and electrolyte balance and to excrete nitrogenous wastes
- Sudden increase in blood urea nitrogen (BUN) or serum creatinine
- Oliguria often associated
- Symptoms and signs depend on cause

GENERAL CONSIDERATIONS

- 5% of hospital admissions and 30% of ICU admissions have acute renal failure
- 25% of hospitalized patients develop acute renal failure
- Serum creatinine concentration can typically increase 1–1.5 mg/dL daily
- Three categories of acute renal failure: prerenal azotemia, intrinsic renal failure, and postrenal azotemia

 CLINICAL FINDINGS

SYMPTOMS AND SIGNS

- Nausea, vomiting
- Malaise
- Hypertension
- Pericardial friction rub, effusions, and cardiac tamponade
- Arrhythmias
- Rales
- Abdominal pain and ileus
- Bleeding secondary to platelet dysfunction
- Encephalopathy, altered sensorium, asterixis, seizures
- Oliguria, defined as urine output <500 mL/day

DIFFERENTIAL DIAGNOSIS

Prerenal azotemia

- Dehydration
- Hemorrhage, eg, gastrointestinal bleeding
- Congestive heart failure
- Renal artery stenosis including fibromuscular dysplasia
- Nonsteroidal antiinflammatory drugs (NSAIDs), angiotensin-converting enzyme inhibitors

Postrenal azotemia

- Obstruction, eg, benign prostatic hyperplasia, bladder tumor

Intrinsic renal disease

- Acute tubular necrosis
  - Toxins: NSAIDs, antibiotics, contrast, multiple myeloma, rhabdomyolysis, hemolysis, chemotherapy, hyperuricemia, cyclosporine
  - Ischemia, eg, prolonged prerenal azotemia
- Acute glomerulonephritis
  - Immune complex: IgA nephropathy, endocarditis, systemic lupus erythematosus (SLE), cryoglobulinemia, postinfectious, membranoproliferative
  - Pauci-immune (ANCA⁺): Wegener's granulomatosis, Churg-Strauss syndrome, microscopic polyarteritis
  - Anti-glomerular basement membrane (GBM): Goodpasture's disease, anti-GBM glomerulonephritis
  - Other: malignant hypertension, thrombotic thrombocytopenic purpura
- Acute interstitial nephritis
  - Drugs: β-lactams, sulfa, diuretics, NSAIDs, rifampin, phenytoin, allopurinol
  - Infections: *Streptococcus*, leptospirosis, cytomegalovirus, histoplasmosis, Rocky Mountain spotted fever
  - Immune: SLE, Sjögren's syndrome, sarcoidosis, cryoglobulinemia

DIAGNOSIS

LABORATORY TESTS

- Serum creatinine and BUN elevated
- BUN/creatinine ratio >20:1 in prerenal and postrenal azotemia, and acute glomerulonephritis; <20:1 in acute tubular necrosis and acute interstitial nephritis
- Hyperkalemia
- Anion gap metabolic acidosis
- Hyperphosphatemia
- Hypocalcemia
- Anemia
- Fractional excretion of sodium (FE_{Na}) is useful index in classification
- FE_{Na} = clearance of Na^+/GFR = clearance of Na^+/creatinine clearance
- FE_{Na} = (urine Na^+/plasma Na^+)/(urine Cr/plasma Cr) × 100
- FE_{Na} low (<1%) in prerenal azotemia, acute glomerulonephritis; high (>1%) in acute tubular necrosis; variable in postrenal azotemia, acute interstitial nephritis

IMAGING STUDIES

- Bladder ultrasonography
- CT or MRI if retroperitoneal fibrosis from tumor or radiation suspected
- Renal ultrasound to exclude obstruction

DIAGNOSTIC PROCEDURES

- ECG: peaked T waves, PR prolongation, and QRS widening in hyperkalemia, long QT interval with hypocalcemia

TREATMENT

THERAPEUTIC PROCEDURES

- Prerenal azotemia: treatment depends on cause; maintenance of euvolemia, attention to serum potassium, avoidance of nephrotoxic drugs
- Postrenal azotemia: relief of obstruction if present
- Intrinsic renal failure: treatment depends on cause (see *Tubular necrosis, acute*); hold offending agents
- Catheters or stents to treat obstruction
- Bladder catheterization if hydroureter and hydronephrosis are present with an enlarged bladder on ultrasound
- Hemodialysis, peritoneal dialysis: indications include
  - Uremic symptoms such as pericarditis, encephalopathy, or coagulopathy
  - Fluid overload unresponsive to diuresis
  - Refractory hyperkalemia
  - Severe metabolic acidosis (pH <7.20)
  - Neurological symptoms such as seizures or neuropathy

 OUTCOME

WHEN TO REFER

- Persistence of acute renal failure for 2–4 weeks

WHEN TO ADMIT

- Significant acid–base, fluid, or electrolyte abnormalities or uremia

 EVIDENCE

PRACTICE GUIDELINES

- DuBose TD Jr et al: Acute renal failure in the 21st century: recommendations for management and outcomes assessment. Am J Kidney Dis 1997;29:793. [PMID: 9159318]

WEB SITE

- National Kidney and Urologic Diseases Information Clearinghouse http://kidney.niddk.nih.gov/kudiseases/pubs/glomerular/index.htm#3

INFORMATION FOR PATIENTS

- MD Consult–Acute renal failure http://home.mdconsult.com/das/patient/view/30707629/10002/13771.html/top?sid=201563461

REFERENCES

- Albright RC Jr: Acute renal failure: a practical update. Mayo Clin Proc 2001;76:67. [PMID:11155415
- Holt SG et al: Pathogenesis and treatment of renal dysfunction in rhabdomyolysis. Intensive Care Med 2001;27:803. [PMID:11430535]
- Mehta R et al: Diuretics, mortality, and nonrecovery of renal function in acute renal failure. JAMA 2002;288:2547. [PMID: 12444861]
- Sauret JM et al: Rhabdomyolysis. Am Fam Physician 2002;65:907. [PMID: 11898964]
- Singri N et al: Acute renal failure. JAMA 2003;289:747. [PMID: 12585954]

Suzanne Watnick, MD
Gail Morrison, MD

Renal Failure, Chronic

 KEY FEATURES

ESSENTIALS OF DIAGNOSIS

- Progressive azotemia over months to years
- Symptoms and signs of uremia when nearing end-stage disease
- Hypertension in the majority
- Isosthenuria and broad casts in urinary sediment are common
- Bilateral small kidneys on ultrasound are diagnostic

GENERAL CONSIDERATIONS

- Major causes (>50% of cases) are diabetes mellitus and hypertension
- Glomerulonephritis, cystic diseases, and other urological diseases account for another 20–25%, unknown causes (~15%) (Table 87, page 1271)
- Rarely reversible
- Progressive decline in renal function

 CLINICAL FINDINGS

SYMPTOMS AND SIGNS

- Symptoms develop slowly and are non-specific
- Asymptomatic until renal failure is far advanced [glomerular filtration rate (GFR) <10–15 mL/min]
- Fatigue, weakness, and malaise
- Gastrointestinal complaints such as anorexia, nausea, vomiting, a metallic taste in the mouth, and hiccups
- Neurological irritability, difficulty in concentrating, insomnia, restless legs, and twitching
- Pruritus
- Decreased libido, menstrual irregularities
- Chest pain from pericarditis
- Renal osteodystrophy (osteitis fibrosa cystica), osteomalacia, and adynamic bone disease

DIFFERENTIAL DIAGNOSIS

- See Table 88 (page 1272)

 DIAGNOSIS

LABORATORY TESTS

- Serum creatinine and blood urea nitrogen (BUN) elevated; evidence of previously elevated creatinine and BUN, abnormal prior urinalyses help to differentiate between acute and chronic renal failure
- Plot of the inverse of serum creatinine ($1/S_{Cr}$) versus time if 3 or more prior measurements are available helps to estimate time to end-stage renal disease
- Anemia
- Platelet dysfunction, bleeding time prolongation
- Metabolic acidosis
- Hyperphosphatemia, hypocalcemia
- Hyperkalemia
- Isosthenuria
- Urinary sediment: broad waxy casts

IMAGING STUDIES

- Renal ultrasound for anatomic abnormalities, kidney size, and echogenicity

DIAGNOSTIC PROCEDURES

- Possible renal biopsy

TREATMENT

MEDICATIONS

- Acute hyperkalemia: calcium chloride or gluconate IV, insulin administration with glucose IV, bicarbonate IV, and ion exchange resin (sodium polystyrene sulfonate) PO or PR, cardiac monitoring
- Chronic hyperkalemia: dietary potassium restriction, sodium polystyrene sulfonate, 15–30 g PO QD in juice or sorbitol
- Acid–base disorders: sodium bicarbonate, calcium bicarbonate, or sodium citrate 20–30 mmol/day divided into 2 doses, titrated to maintain serum bicarbonate at >20 mEq/L
- Hypertension: salt and water restriction, weight loss, decreased salt diet (4–6 to 2 g/day), angiotensin-converting enzyme (ACE) inhibitors or angiotensin II receptor blockers (if serum potassium and GFR permit), calcium channel-blocking agents, diuretics, and β-blocking agents; clonidine, hydralazine, minoxidil as adjunctive drugs
- Congestive heart failure: salt and water restriction, loop diuretics; avoid ACE inhibitors if serum creatinine >3 mg/dL
- Anemia
  - Recombinant erythropoietin (epoetin alfa), 50 units/kg (3000–4000 units/dose) once or twice a week IV or SQ
  - Ferrous sulfate, 325 mg QD–TID if the serum ferritin is <100 ng/mL or if iron saturation is <20–25%
- Coagulopathy: dialysis
  - Desmopressin, 25 mg IV Q 8–12 h for 2 doses for surgery
  - Conjugated estrogens, 0.6 mg/kg diluted in 50 mL of 0.9% sodium chloride infused over 30–40 min QD, or 2.5–5 mg PO QD for 5–7 days; effect lasts several weeks
- Renal osteodystrophy, osteomalacia
  - Dietary phosphorus restriction
  - Oral phosphorus/binding agents such as calcium carbonate or calcium acetate given in divided doses three or four times daily with meals titrated to a serum calcium of 10 mg/dL and serum phosphorus of 4.5 mg/dL
  - Vitamin D or vitamin D analogs (if iPTH >2–3 × normal), serum phosphate <7 mg/dL and calcium <11 mg/dL
  - Calcitriol 0.25–0.5 mg QD or QOD

SURGERY

- Renal transplantation

THERAPEUTIC PROCEDURES

- Hemodialysis, peritoneal dialysis: indications include
  - Uremic symptoms such as pericarditis, encephalopathy, or coagulopathy
  - Fluid overload unresponsive to diuresis
  - Refractory hyperkalemia
  - Severe metabolic acidosis (pH <7.20)
  - Neurological symptoms such as seizures or neuropathy
- Dialysis Outcomes Quality Initiative (DOQI) guidelines: begin dialysis in nondiabetics at GFR of 10 mL/min or serum creatinine of 8 mg/dL, in diabetics at GFR of 15 mL/min or serum creatinine of 6 mg/dL

Diet

- Protein restriction to <1 g/kg/day, and if beneficial, to <0.6 g/kg/day
- Salt restriction to ≤2 g/day of sodium for nondialysis patient approaching end-stage renal disease
- Water restriction to <1–2 L /day of fluid
- Potassium restriction to <60–70 mEq/day
- Phosphorus restriction to <5–10 mg/kg/day
- Magnesium-containing laxatives and antacids contraindicated

OUTCOME

FOLLOW-UP

- Check serum creatinine and potassium within 9–10 days if ACE inhibitors used

PROGNOSIS

- Mortality is higher for patients on dialysis than for age-matched controls; annual mortality rate is 22.4 deaths per 100 patient years
- Common causes of death: cardiac dysfunction (48%), infection (15%), cerebrovascular disease (6%), and malignancy (4%)

WHEN TO REFER

- When GFR 60 mL/min for comanagement

WHEN TO ADMIT

- Congestive heart failure, pericarditis
- Severe acid–base or electrolyte disturbances or uremia

EVIDENCE

PRACTICE GUIDELINES

- Barrett BJ et al: Clinical practice guidelines for the management of anemia coexistent with chronic renal failure. J Am Soc Nephrol 1999;10(Suppl 13): S292. [PMID: 10425612]

WEB SITE

- National Kidney and Urologic Diseases Information Clearinghouse http://kidney.niddk.nih.gov/kudiseases/pubs/glomerular/index.htm#3

REFERENCES

- Barry JM: Current status of renal transplantation. Patient evaluations and outcomes. Urol Clin North Am 2001;28: 677. [PMID: 11791486]
- McCarthy JR: A practical approach to the management of patients with chronic renal failure. Mayo Clin Proc 1999;74:269. [PMID: 10089997]
- Ramanathan V et al: Renal transplantation. Semin Nephrol 2001;21:213. [PMID: 112457820]
- Ruggenenti P et al: Progression, remission, regression of chronic renal diseases. Lancet 2001;357:1601. [PMID: 11377666]

Suzanne Watnick, MD
Gail Morrison, MD

Rhabdomyolysis

 KEY FEATURES

ESSENTIALS OF DIAGNOSIS

- Necrosis of skeletal muscle
- Can be encountered in a wide variety of clinical settings, alone or in concert with other disorders of muscle

GENERAL CONSIDERATIONS

- Rhabdomyolysis is generally seen with concomitant myopathy, though the term rhabdomyolysis refers only to a test abnormality
- Commonly due to a syndrome of crush injury to muscle, associated with myoglobinuria, renal insufficiency, markedly elevated creatine kinase (CK) levels, and, frequently, multiorgan failure as a consequence of other complications of the trauma

Causes

- Crush injury
- Prolonged immobility, eg, drug overdose, exposure, hypothermia
- Statin use
- Myositis, eg, polymyositis, dermatomyositis
- Seizure
- Strenuous exercise or heat stroke
- Hypokalemia or hypophosphatemia
- Severe volume contraction
- Acute alcoholic intoxication (rare)

 CLINICAL FINDINGS

SYMPTOMS AND SIGNS

- Often there is little evidence for muscle injury on external examination of these patients—and specifically, neither myalgia nor myopathy is present
- Can be associated with myopathy (objective weakness of muscle) or myalgias (pain in the muscle)

DIFFERENTIAL DIAGNOSIS

- Myopathy without muscle necrosis or elevated creatine phosphokinase, eg, endocrine causes of hyperthyroidism, Cushing's syndrome
- Other cause of myalgia, eg, influenza
- Polymyalgia rheumatica
- A simple intramuscular injection may cause some elevation of CK

 DIAGNOSIS

LABORATORY TESTS

- Elevated serum CK is the biochemical indicator of skeletal muscle necrosis
- A urinary dipstick testing positive for blood (due to myoglobinuria) in the absence of red blood cells in the sediment
- Elevations of alanine aminotransferase and lactate dehydrogenase may be present, and may have been obtained for other reasons, such as suspected liver disease or hemolysis. When these tests are disproportionately elevated, confirm that they are not of muscle origin with a CK determination

Rhabdomyolysis

 TREATMENT

 OUTCOME

EVIDENCE

MEDICATIONS

- Vigorous fluid resuscitation
- Mannitol 100 mg IV QD for 3 days
- Alkalinization of the urine with 2 ampules of sodium bicarbonate in 1 L D5 ½ normal saline

COMPLICATIONS

- Renal insufficiency due to myoglobinuria is caused by tubular damage resulting from filtered myoglobin and is nearly always associated with hypovolemia

PROGNOSIS

- Renal insufficiency is usually reversible with hydration. The role of urine alkalinization is unproven

PRACTICE GUIDELINES

- American Academy of Family Physicians http://www.aafp.org/afp/20020301/907.html

INFORMATION FOR PATIENTS

- National Institutes of Health http://www.nlm.nih.gov/medlineplus/ency/article/000473.htm

REFERENCES

- Holt SG et al: Pathogenesis and treatment of renal dysfunction in rhabdomyolysis. Intensive Care Med 2001;27:803. [PMID: 11430535]
- Vanholder R et al: Rhabdomyolysis. J Am Soc Nephrol 2000;1:1553. [PMID: 10906171]
- Warren JD et al: Rhabdomyolysis: a review. Muscle Nerve 2002; 25:332.

David B. Hellmann, MD, FACP
John H. Stone, MD, MPH

Rheumatoid Arthritis

 KEY FEATURES

ESSENTIALS OF DIAGNOSIS

- Prodromal systemic symptoms of malaise, fever, weight loss, and morning stiffness
- Onset usually insidious and in small joints; progression is centripetal and symmetric; deformities common
- Radiographic findings: juxtaarticular osteoporosis, joint erosions, and narrowing of the joint spaces
- Rheumatoid factor usually present
- Extraarticular manifestations: subcutaneous nodules, pleural effusion, pericarditis, lymphadenopathy, splenomegaly with leukopenia, and vasculitis

GENERAL CONSIDERATIONS

- A chronic systemic inflammatory disease of unknown cause, chiefly affecting synovial membranes of multiple joints
- The pathological findings in the joint include chronic synovitis with pannus formation. The pannus erodes cartilage, bone, ligaments, and tendons

DEMOGRAPHICS

- Female patients outnumber males almost 3:1
- Usual age at onset is 20–40 years

 CLINICAL FINDINGS

SYMPTOMS AND SIGNS

- The onset of articular signs of inflammation is usually insidious
- Prodromal symptoms of malaise, weight loss, and vague periarticular pain or stiffness
- Characteristically symmetric joint swelling with associated stiffness, warmth, tenderness, and pain
- Stiffness persisting for over 30 min is prominent in the morning and subsides during the day
- Proximal interphalangeal and metacarpophalangeal (MCP) joints of the fingers as well as the wrists, knees, ankles, and toes are most often involved
- Entrapment syndromes are not unusual—particularly entrapment of the median nerve at the carpal tunnel of the wrist
- Twenty percent of patients have subcutaneous nodules, most commonly over bony prominences but also in the bursas and tendon sheaths
- After months or years, deformities may occur; the most common are ulnar deviation of the fingers, boutonniere deformity (hyperextension of the distal interphalangeal joint with flexion of the proximal interphalangeal joint), "swan-neck" deformity (flexion of the distal interphalangeal with extension of the proximal interphalangeal joint), and valgus deformity of the knee
- Dryness of the eyes, mouth, and other mucous membranes is found, especially in advanced disease

Ocular manifestations

- Episcleritis, scleritis, peripheral ulcerative keratitis
- In severe cases, the corneal melt syndrome of scleromalacia perforans

DIFFERENTIAL DIAGNOSIS

- Gout with tophi (mistaken for nodules)
- Systemic lupus erythematosus
- Parvovirus B19 infection
- Osteoarthritis or inflammatory osteoarthritis
- Septic arthritis
- Polymyalgia rheumatica
- Hemochromatosis (MCP and wrist joints)
- Adult Still's disease
- Lyme disease
- Rheumatic fever
- Rubella arthritis
- Hepatitis B or C
- Palindromic rheumatism
- Hypertrophic pulmonary osteoarthropathy (paraneoplastic)
- Systemic vasculitis, especially polyarteritis nodosa, mixed cryoglobulinemia, and antineutrophil cytoplasmic antibody-associated vasculitides

 DIAGNOSIS

LABORATORY TESTS

- Rheumatoid factor, an IgM antibody directed against the Fc fragment of IgG, is present in the sera of more than 75% of patients
- During both the acute and chronic phases, the erythrocyte sedimentation rate and the γ-globulins (most commonly IgM and IgG) are typically elevated
- A moderate hypochromic normocytic anemia is common
- The white blood cell count is normal or slightly elevated, but leukopenia may occur, often in the presence of splenomegaly (eg, Felty's syndrome)
- The platelet count is often elevated, roughly in proportion to the severity of overall joint inflammation
- Joint fluid examination is valuable, reflecting abnormalities that are associated with varying degrees of inflammation (see Tables 74 and 75, page 1266)

IMAGING STUDIES

- X-ray changes are the most specific for rheumatoid arthritis. X-rays, however, are not sensitive in that most of those taken during the first 6 months are read as normal
- The earliest changes occur in the wrists or feet and consist of soft tissue swelling and juxtaarticular demineralization. Later, diagnostic changes of uniform joint space narrowing and erosions develop

Rheumatoid Arthritis

TREATMENT

MEDICATIONS

- Nonsteroidal antiinflammatory drugs (NSAIDs) are the first-line drugs. They have analgesic and antiinflammatory effects but do not prevent erosions or alter the progression of the disease
- Cyclooxygenase (COX)-2 inhibitors are just as effective and less likely to cause clinically significant upper gastrointestinal hemorrhage or ulceration
- Disease-modifying antirheumatic drugs (DMARDs) should be started as soon as the diagnosis is certain
- Methotrexate is the treatment of choice for patients who fail to respond to NSAIDs. Methotrexate is generally well tolerated and often produces a beneficial effect in 2–6 weeks
- Tumor necrosis factor inhibitors work faster than methotrexate and may replace that drug as the remitting agent of first choice
- Hydroxychloroquine is useful for patients with mild disease
- Corticosteroids usually produce an immediate and dramatic antiinflammatory effect, and they may slow the rate of bony destruction
- Corticosteroids may be used on a short-term basis to tide patients over acute disabling episodes, to facilitate other treatment measures (eg, physical therapy), or to manage serious extra-articular manifestations (eg, pericarditis, perforating eye lesions)
- Corticosteroids may also be indicated for active and progressive disease that does not respond favorably to conservative management and when there are contraindications to or therapeutic failure of other agents
- Leflunomide, a pyrimidine synthesis inhibitor, is also FDA approved for treatment of rheumatoid arthritis (RA)
- Anakinra, a recombinant form of human interleukin-1 receptor antagonist, may be given to adult patients who have failed one or more DMARDs

SURGERY

- Long-standing, severe, erosive disease may benefit from joint replacements
- Hips, knees, shoulders, and metacarpophalangeal joints may benefit from replacement in cases of advanced destruction

THERAPEUTIC PROCEDURES

- Nonpharmacological: physical therapy, occupational therapy, joint rest, exercise, splinting, heat and cold, assist devices, and splints
- Intraarticular corticosteroids (triamcinolone, 10–40 mg) may be helpful if one or two joints are the chief source of difficulty

OUTCOME

FOLLOW-UP

- Frequent follow-up early after diagnosis to ensure appropriate patient education and response to treatment
- Patients on DMARDs require monitoring of blood cell counts, hepatic and renal function every 6–8 weeks

COMPLICATIONS

- Joint destruction
- Rheumatoid vasculitis (eg, skin ulcers, vasculitic neuropathy, pericarditis)
- Osteoporosis
- Cushing's syndrome from corticosteroids

PROGNOSIS

- Patients who present with polyarthritis that appears to be (but probably is not) RA experience remission 50–75% within 2 years
- Patients whose joint symptoms persist beyond 2 years die, on average, 10–15 years earlier than people without RA
- Patients who have polyarthritis lasting more than 12 weeks are at greatest risk for persistent disease and are candidates for aggressive therapy

WHEN TO REFER

- Progressive disease despite therapy
- Refer early to a physical or occupational therapist

WHEN TO ADMIT

- Admission is sometimes required at diagnosis to exclude other entities
- Superimposed septic arthritis
- Rheumatoid vasculitis
- Severe ocular inflammatory disease (eg, impending corneal melt)

EVIDENCE

PRACTICE GUIDELINES

- American College of Rheumatology http://www.rheumatology.org/research/guidelines/ra-mgmt/ra-mgmt.html http://www.rheumatology.org/research/guidelines/ra-drug/ra-drug.html

WEB SITE

- http://www.arthritis.org

INFORMATION FOR PATIENTS

- National Institute of Arthritis and Musculoskeletal and Skin Diseases http://www.niams.nih.gov/hi/topics/arthritis/rahandout.htm
- Arthritis Foundation http://www.arthritis.org/conditions/DiseaseCenter/ra.asp

REFERENCES

- Keane J et al: Tuberculosis associated with infliximab, a tumor necrosis factor a neutralizing agent. N Engl J Med 2001;345:1098. [PMID: 11596589]
- Kremer JM: Concominant leflunomide therapy in patients with active rheumatoid arthritis despite stable doses of methotrexate. Ann Intern Med 2002; 137:726.
- Lipsky PE et al: Infliximab and methotrexate in the treatment of rheumatoid arthritis. N Engl J Med 2000;343:1594. [PMID: 11096166]
- van Everdingen AA: Low-dose prednisone therapy for patients with early active rheumatoid arthritis: clinical efficacy, disease-modifying properties, and side effects. A randomized, double-blind, placebo-controlled clinical trial. Ann Intern Med 2002;136:1. [PMID: 11777359]

David B. Hellmann, MD, FACP
John H. Stone, MD, MPH

Rhinitis, Allergic

 ## KEY FEATURES

ESSENTIALS OF DIAGNOSIS

- Seasonal occurrence of watery eyes, sneezing, itchy nose and eyes
- An inflammatory response orchestrated by an allergen-specific IgE antibody
- Eosinophilia of nasal secretions and occasionally of bood
- Skin tests usually of little value

GENERAL CONSIDERATIONS

- "Hay fever" symptoms are similar to those of viral rhinitis but are usually persistent and show seasonal variation and are not associated with constitutional symptoms of fever or myalgia
- Nasal symptoms are often accompanied by eye irritation (allergic conjunctivitis), which causes pruritus, erythema, and excessive tearing
- Up to 40% of patients manifest lower respiratory symptoms: cough, wheezing, chest tightness, or dyspnea
- Can be associated with eczematous dermatitis, pruritis

 ## CLINICAL FINDINGS

SYMPTOMS AND SIGNS

- Physical examination may reveal inflamed, edematous, or even pale boggy nasal mucosa
- The mucosa of the turbinates is usually pale or violaceous because of venous engorgement; this is in contrast to the erythema of viral rhinitis
- Nasal polyps, which are yellowish boggy masses of hypertrophic mucosa, may be seen

DIFFERENTIAL DIAGNOSIS

- Viral rhinitis (common cold)
- Viral conjunctivitis
- Vasomotor rhinitis (eg, cold air or irritant-induced)
- Acute or chronic sinusitis
- Rhinitis medicamentosa (drug-induced rhinitis)
- Nasal polyposis
- Foreign body
- Wegener's granulomatosis

 ## DIAGNOSIS

LABORATORY TESTS

- Usually a clinical diagnosis
- Confirmation of IgE-mediated hypersensitivity to aeroallergens is occasionally indicated
- Allergy skin tests or radioallergosorbent tesing (RAST) or enzyme-linked immunosobent assay (ELISA) are available to detect specific IgE

TREATMENT

MEDICATIONS

- The choice of medications is guided by the predominant symptoms (Table 72, page 1264)

Intranasal corticosteroid sprays

- Mainstay of treatment
- More effective—and frequently less expensive—than nonsedating antihistamines
- There may be a delay in onset of relief of 1–2 weeks
- May also shrink nasal polyps, thereby providing an improved nasal airway and delaying or eliminating the indications for endoscopic sinus surgery
- Beclomethasone (42 μg/spray twice daily each nostril), flunisolide (25 μg/spray twice daily each nostril), mometasone furoate (200 μg once daily per nostril), and fluticasone propionate (200 μg once daily per nostril); the latter two synthetic glucocorticoids appear to have higher topical potencies and lipid solubility and reduced systemic bioavailability, suggesting possible practical advantages

Over-the-counter antihistamines

- Loratidine, 10 mg once a day (less sedating than other OTC antihistamines)
- Brompheniramine or chlorpheniramine (4 mg orally every 6–8 h, or 8–12 mg orally every 8–12 h as a sustained-release tablet)
- Clemastine (1.34–2.68 mg orally twice daily)

Oral H$_1$ receptor antagonists

- Cetirizine (10 mg orally once daily), fexofenadine (60 mg orally twice daily or 120 mg once daily); fexofenadine appears to be nonsedating and cetirizine mildly sedating; ebastine (10–20 mg orally once daily) and misolastine (10 mg once daily)
- H$_1$ receptor antagonist antihistamine nasal sprays include levocabastine (0.2 mg twice daily) and azelastine (two sprays per nostril, 1.1 mg/day)

Anticholinergic agents

- Intranasal anticholinergic agents such as ipratropium bromide 0.03% (42 μg per nostril three times daily) sprays when rhinorrhea is a major symptom
- Intranasal cromolyn spray prior to the onset of seasonal symptoms

Sympathomimetics

- Particularly effective for nasal symptoms, but prolonged topical use may lead to rebound vasodilation, called rhinitis medicamentosa

Immunotherapy

- Repeated long-term injection of allergen is an effective method for reducing or eliminating symptoms and signs of allergic disorders
- Recommended for patients with severe allergic rhinitis who respond poorly to medications or whose allergens are not avoidable
- Unequivocally effective in allergic rhinitis and allergic conjunctivitis

 OUTCOME

WHEN TO REFER

- Moderate to severe cases, when avoidance measures, antihistamine administration, and nasal corticosteroids do not adequately control symptoms
- Associated persistent asthma
- Recurrent sinusitis
- Nasal polyposis

PREVENTION

- Allergen avoidance is most important, including staying indoors when pollen counts are high, avoiding pets, and reducing indoor dust and mold
- Maintaining an allergen-free environment by covering pillows and mattresses with plastic covers, substituting synthetic materials (foam mattress, acrylics) for animal products (wool, horsehair) and removing dust-collecting household fixtures (carpets, drapes, bedspreads, wicker) is worth the attempt to help more troubled patients
- Air purifiers and dust filters (such as Bionair models) may also aid in maintaining an allergen-free environment

Rhinitis, Allergic

 EVIDENCE

PRACTICE GUIDELINES

- National Guidelines Clearinghouse http://www.guideline.gov/summary/summary.aspx?doc_id=3373&nbr=2599&string=allergic+rhinitis http://www.guideline.gov/summary/summary.aspx?doc_id=1876&nbr=1102&string=allergic+rhinitis
- American Academy of Family Physicians http://www.aafp.org/afp/20021201/practice.html

WEB SITES

- Allergy, Asthma, and Immunology Online http://allergy.mcg.edu
- American Academy of Allergy, Asthma and Immunology http://www.aaaai.org

INFORMATION FOR PATIENTS

- JAMA patient page: Seasonal allergic rhinitis. JAMA 2001;286:3038.
- American Academy of Allergy, Asthma and Immunology http://www.medem.com/search/article_display.cfm?path=\\TAN QUERAY\M_ContentItem&mstr=/M_ContentItem/ZZZDF2LJZ6C.html&soc=ACAAI&srch_typ=NAV_SERCH

REFERENCES

- Corren J: Intranasal corticosteroids for allergic rhinitis: how do different agents compare? J Allergy Clin Immunol 1999;104(4 Part 1):S144. [PMID: 10518811]
- Hadley JA: Evaluation and management of allergic rhinitis. Med Clin North Am 1999;83:13. [PMID: 9927957]

Jeffrey L. Kishiyama, MD
Daniel C. Adelman, MD
Michael J. Kaplan, MD

Rosacea

 KEY FEATURES

ESSENTIALS OF DIAGNOSIS

- A chronic facial disorder of middle-aged and older people
- A vascular component (erythema and telangiectasis) and a tendency to flush easily
- An acneiform component (papules and pustules) may also be present
- A glandular component accompanied by hyperplasia of the soft tissue of the nose (rhinophyma)

GENERAL CONSIDERATIONS

- Rosacea is usually a lifelong affliction, so maintenance therapy is required
- A chronic facial disorder of middle-aged and older people

 CLINICAL FINDINGS

SYMPTOMS AND SIGNS

- See Table 7 (page 1202)
- The cheeks, nose, and chin—at times the entire face—may have a rosy hue
- No comedones
- Inflammatory papules are prominent, and there may be pustules
- Associated seborrhea may be found
- The patient often complains of burning or stinging with episodes of flushing
- It is not uncommon for patients to have associated ophthalmic disease, including blepharitis and keratitis

DIFFERENTIAL DIAGNOSIS

- Acne vulgaris
- Seborrheic dermatitis
- Topical steroid use
- Perioral dermatitis
- Systemic lupus erythematosus
- Carcinoid
- Dermatomyositis
- Rosacea is distinguished from acne by age, the presence of the vascular component, and the absence of comedones
- The rosy hue of rosacea is due to inflammation and telangiectases and generally will pinpoint the diagnosis
- Topical steroids can change trivial dermatoses of the face into perioral dermatitis and steroid rosacea

 DIAGNOSIS

LABORATORY TESTS

- Clinical diagnosis

Rosacea

 TREATMENT

MEDICATIONS

- See Table 6 (page 1199)
- Medications are directed only at the inflammatory papules and pustules and the erythema that surrounds them

Local therapy

- Metronidazole, 0.75% gel applied twice daily or 1% cream once daily, is the topical treatment of choice
- If metronidazole is not tolerated, topical clindamycin (solution, gel, or lotion) used twice daily is effective
- Erythromycin as described above may be helpful (see *Acne vulgaris*)
- Five to eight weeks of treatment may be needed for significant response

Systemic therapy

- Tetracycline or erythromycin, 250 or 500 mg orally twice daily on an empty stomach, should be used when topical therapy is inadequate
- Minocycline or doxycycline, 50–100 mg daily to twice daily, may work in refractory cases
- Isotretinoin may succeed where other measures fail; a dosage of 0.5–1 mg/kg/day orally for 12–28 weeks is recommended
- Metronidazole, 250 mg twice daily for 3 weeks, may be worth trying but is seldom required; side effects are few, though metronidazole may produce a disulfiram-like effect when the patient ingests alcohol

SURGERY

- The only satisfactory treatment for the telangiectasias is laser surgery
- Rhinophyma (soft tissue and sebaceous hyperplasia of the nose) responds to surgical debulking

 OUTCOME

PROGNOSIS

- Tends to be a stubborn and persistent process
- It can usually be controlled adequately

WHEN TO REFER

- If there is a question about the diagnosis, if recommended therapy is ineffective, or if specialized treatment is necessary

 EVIDENCE

WEB SITES

- American Academy of Dermatology http://www.aad.org
- Dermatology Handbook for Family Practice from the University of Iowa http://www.vh.org/Providers/ClinRef/FPHandbook/17.html

INFORMATION FOR PATIENTS

- American Academy of Dermatology http://www.aad.org/pamphlets/rosacea.html
- National Institute for Arthritis and Musculoskeletal and Skin Diseases http://www.niams.nih.gov/hi/topics/rosacea/rosacea.htm

REFERENCES

- Thiboutot DM: Acne and rosacea. New and emerging therapies. Dermatol Clin 2000;18:63. [PMID: 10626112]
- Zuber TJ: Rosacea. Prim Care 2000;27:309. [PMID: 10815045]

Timothy G. Berger, MD

Salicylate Poisoning

 KEY FEATURES

ESSENTIALS OF DIAGNOSIS

- Tachypnea, altered mental status
- Metabolic acidosis
- Typical arterial blood gases reveal respiratory alkalosis and metabolic acidosis
- Elevated salicylate level diagnostic

GENERAL CONSIDERATIONS

- Salicylates (aspirin, methyl salicylate, etc) are found in a variety of over-the-counter and prescription medications
- Salicylates uncouple cellular oxidative phosphorylation, resulting in anaerobic metabolism and excessive production of lactic acid and heat, and they also interfere with several Krebs cycle enzymes
- A single ingestion of more than 200 mg/kg of salicylate is likely to produce significant acute intoxication
- Poisoning may also occur as a result of chronic excessive dosing over several days
- Although the half-life of salicylate is 2–3 h after small doses, it may increase to 20 h or more in patients with intoxication

 CLINICAL FINDINGS

SYMPTOMS AND SIGNS

- Acute ingestion often causes nausea and vomiting, occasionally with gastritis
- Moderate intoxication causes hyperpnea (deep and rapid breathing), tachycardia, and tinnitus
- Serious intoxication may result in agitation, confusion, coma, seizures, cardiovascular collapse, pulmonary edema, hyperthermia, and death

DIFFERENTIAL DIAGNOSIS

- Other causes of anion gap acidosis, eg, alcoholic ketoacidosis, metformin toxicity, isoniazid poisoning, iron poisoning, methanol or ethylene glycol toxicity, carbon monoxide poisoning
- Acetaminophen poisoning (common co-ingestion)

 DIAGNOSIS

LABORATORY TESTS

- Diagnosis is suspected in any patient with metabolic acidosis and is confirmed by measuring the stat serum salicylate level
- Patients with levels greater than 100 mg/dL (1000 mg/L) after an acute overdose are more likely to have severe poisoning
- Patients with subacute or chronic intoxication may suffer severe symptoms with levels of only 60–70 mg/dL
- The arterial blood gas typically reveals a respiratory alkalosis with an underlying metabolic acidosis
- Anion gap metabolic acidosis
- The prothrombin time is often elevated owing to salicylate-induced hypoprothrombinemia

Salicylate Poisoning

 TREATMENT

MEDICATIONS

Emergency and supportive measures

- Administer activated charcoal, 60–100 g orally or via gastric tube, mixed in aqueous slurry
- Repeated doses may be given to ensure gastrointestinal adsorption or to enhance elimination of the drug. Do not use for comatose or convulsing patients unless it can be given by gastric tube and the airway is protected by a cuffed endotracheal tube
- Gastric lavage and extra doses of activated charcoal may be needed in patients who ingest more than 10 g of aspirin. The desired ratio of charcoal to aspirin is about 10:1 by weight; while this cannot always be given as a single dose, it may be administered over the first 24 h in divided doses every 2–4 h
- Treat metabolic acidosis with intravenous sodium bicarbonate. This is critical because acidosis (acidemia, pH <7.40) promotes greater entry of salicylate into cells, worsening toxicity

Specific treatment

- Alkalinization of the urine enhances renal salicylate excretion by trapping the salicylate anion in the urine. Add 100 meq (two ampules) of sodium bicarbonate to 1 L of 5% dextrose in 0.2% saline, and infuse intravenously at a rate of about 150–200 mL/h
- Unless the patient is oliguric, add 20–30 mEq of potassium chloride to each liter of intravenous fluid
- Patients who are volume depleted often fail to produce an alkaline urine (paradoxical aciduria) unless potassium is given

THERAPEUTIC PROCEDURES

- Hemodialysis may be lifesaving and is indicated for patients with severe metabolic acidosis, markedly altered mental status, or significantly elevated salicylate levels [>100–120 mg/dL (1000–1200 mg/L) after acute overdose or >60–70 mg/dL (600–700 mg/L) with subacute or chronic intoxication]

 OUTCOME

FOLLOW-UP

- Monitor serum salicylate level every 2 h initially to determine if it is continuing to rise
- Patients with massive ingestion (eg, >100 tablets) may have delayed absorption and require prolonged observation until levels fall into normal range

COMPLICATIONS

- Intubation and controlled ventilation may cause sudden and severe deterioration in patients with marked respiratory alkalosis, if the P_{CO_2} rises and the pH is allowed to fall

WHEN TO ADMIT

- Suicidal ingestion
- History of massive ingestion with rising levels
- Evidence of significant intoxication (altered mental status, metabolic acidosis, elevated salicylate level)

PROGNOSIS

- Good if blood pH is maintained above 7.4 and hemodialysis is promptly performed in patients with serious toxicity

 EVIDENCE

PRACTICE GUIDELINES

- Position statement and practice guidelines on the use of multi-dose activated charcoal in the treatment of acute poisoning. American Academy of Clinical Toxicology; European Association of Poisons Centres and Clinical Toxicologists. J Toxicol Clin Toxicol 1999;37:731.

INFORMATION FOR PATIENTS

- American Association of Poison Control Centers http://www.1-800-222-1222. info/poisonCenter/home.asp
- The Mayo Clinic http://www.mayoclinic.com/invoke.cfm?id=HQ01263

REFERENCES

- Chan TY: Ingestion of medicated oils by adults: the risk of severe salicylate poisoning is related to the packaging of these products. Hum Exp Toxicol 2002;21:171. [PMID: 12099617]
- Cohen DL et al: Chronic salicylism resulting in noncardiogenic pulmonary edema requiring hemodialysis. Am J Kidney Dis 2000;36:E20. [PMID: 10977813]
- Higgins RM et al: Alkalinization and hemodialysis in severe salicylate poisoning: comparison of elimination techniques in the same patient. Clin Nephrol 1998; 50:178. [PMID: 9776422]

Kent R. Olson, MD

Sarcocystosis

 KEY FEATURES

ESSENTIALS OF DIAGNOSIS

- Mild, protracted diarrhea
- Subcutaneous swelllings over the sites of muscle involvement, associated with erythema, tenderness, fever, eosinophilia

GENERAL CONSIDERATIONS

- The causes of coccidiosis are *Cryptosporidium parvum, Isospora belli, Cyclospora cayetanensis, Sarcocystis bovihominis,* and *S suihominis*
- *Sarcocystis* is a two-host coccidian. Human disease occurs as two syndromes, both rare: an enteric infection in which humans are the definitive host and a muscle infection in which humans are an intermediate host
- In the enteric form, sporocysts (9–16 μm) passed in human feces are not infective for humans but must be ingested by cattle or pigs. Humans become infected by eating poorly cooked beef or pork containing oocysts of *S bovihominis* or *S suihominis*, respectively. Organisms enter intestinal epithelial cells and are transformed into oocysts that release sporocysts into the feces
- The muscle form results when humans ingest sporocysts in feces from an infected carnivore that has eaten prey that harbored sarcocysts. The sporocysts liberate sporozoites that invade the intestinal wall and are disseminated to skeletal muscle
- Although the small bowel is the usual location of infection, other sites can be involved

DEMOGRAPHICS

- The muscle form occurs worldwide, particularly in the tropics and in regions where hygiene is poor
- The intestinal form has been reported only from Asia

 CLINICAL FINDINGS

SYMPTOMS AND SIGNS

- Generally, the forms of diarrhea caused by the coccidial and microsporidial agents are clinically indistinguishable from each other
- The intestinal infection is often asymptomatic or causes mild but protracted diarrhea; an eosinophilic necrotizing enteritis has been reported
- In the muscle form, there is subcutaneous and muscular inflammation lasting several days to 2 weeks and the finding of swellings at these sites, sometimes associated with local erythema, tenderness and myalgia, fever, and eosinophilia
- Sarcocysts are often asymptomatic and are found incidentally at autopsy in cardiac muscle

DIFFERENTIAL DIAGNOSIS

- *Isospora belli, Cyclospora cayetanensis,* and *Sarcocystis*
- Giardiasis
- Viral gastroenteritis, eg, rotavirus
- Other traveler's diarrhea, eg, *Escherichia coli*
- Cryptosporidiosis
- Other causes of diarrhea in AIDS, eg, cytomegalovirus colitis
- Trichinosis

 DIAGNOSIS

LABORATORY TESTS

- Diagnosis is by stool examination for oocysts and by biopsy of subcutaneous lesions

TREATMENT

MEDICATIONS

- No antibiotic treatment is consistently successful; sulfadiazine and tinidazole can be tried

THERAPEUTIC PROCEDURES

- Most acute infections in immunocompetent persons are self-limited and do not require treatment

 OUTCOME

WHEN TO REFER

- Refer all confirmed or suspected cases with protracted diarrhea, particularly in immunocompromised patients
- Refer all cases of sarcocyst muscle disease

 EVIDENCE

INFORMATION FOR PATIENTS

- Department of Natural Resources, Michigan http://www.michigan.gov/dnr/0,1607, 7-153-10370_12150_ 12220-27272–,00.html

REFERENCES

- Ambroise-Thomas P: Parasitic diseases and immunodeficiencies. Parasitology 2001;122(Suppl):S65. [PMID: 11442198]
- Arness MK et al: An outbreak of acute eosinophilic myositis attributed to human *Sarcocystis* parasitism. Am J Trop Med Hyg 1999;61:548. [PMID: 10548287]

Sarcoidosis

 ## KEY FEATURES

ESSENTIALS OF DIAGNOSIS

- Symptoms related to the lung, skin, eyes, peripheral nerves, liver, kidney, heart, and other tissues
- Demonstration of noncaseating granulomas in biopsy specimen
- Exclusion of other granulomatous disorders

GENERAL CONSIDERATIONS

- A systemic disease of unknown etiology
- Granulomatous inflammation of the lungs is present in 90% of cases

DEMOGRAPHICS

- Highest incidence in North American blacks and northern European whites
- Among blacks, women are more frequently affected than men
- Disease onset is usually in the third or fourth decade

 ## CLINICAL FINDINGS

SYMPTOMS AND SIGNS

- Malaise, fever, and insidious dyspnea
- Symptoms referable to the skin, eyes, peipheral nerves, liver, kidney, or heart may also prompt initial evaluation
- Some patients are asymptomatic and are diagnosed after abnormal findings are noted on a chest x-ray
- Crackles are uncommon on chest examination
- Erythema nodosum, parotid gland enlargement, hepatosplenomegaly, and lymphadenopathy may be noted
- Myocardial sarcoidosis is found in 5% of patients and can lead to restrictive cardiomyopathy, arrhythmias, and conduction disturbances

DIFFERENTIAL DIAGNOSIS

- Other granulomatous diseases must be excluded
- Tuberculosis
- Lymphoma (including lymphocytic interstitial pneumonitis)
- Histoplasmosis
- Coccidioidomycosis
- Idiopathic pulmonary fibrosis
- Pneumoconiosis (especially berylliosis)
- Syphilis

 ## DIAGNOSIS

LABORATORY TESTS

- Leukopenia
- Elevation of erythrocyte sedimentation rate
- Hypercalcemia in 5%, hypercalciuria in 20%
- Angiotensin-converting enzyme (ACE) levels are commonly elevated in active disease; this finding is neither sensitive nor specific enough to be of diagnostic value
- Pulmonary function tests may show obstruction or restriction, with diminished diffusion capacity

IMAGING STUDIES

- Radiographic findings are variable
  - Hilar adenopathy alone (stage I)
  - Hilar adenopathy with parenchymal involvement (stage II)
  - Parenchymal involvement alone (stage III)
- Parenchymal involvement usually manifests as diffuse reticular infiltrates, but focal infiltrates, acinar shadows, nodules, and rare cavitation are seen
- Pleural effusion occurs in <10% of patients

DIAGNOSTIC PROCEDURES

- Biopsy demonstrating noncaseating granulomas is required for diagnosis
- Easily accessible biopsy sites include lymph nodes, skin lesions, or salivary glands
- Transbronchial biopsy has a yield of 75–90%
- Bronchoalveolar lavage is usually characterized by an increase in lymphocytes with a high CD4/CD8 ratio; this may be used to follow disease activity, but not for diagnosis
- Some experts believe biopsy is unnecessary in stage I disease with a presentation highly suggestive of sarcoidosis

TREATMENT

MEDICATIONS

- Corticosteroids (prednisone, 0.5-1.0 mg/kg/day) are indicated for constitutional symptoms, hypercalcemia, iritis, arthritis, central nervous system involvement, cardiac involvement, hepatitis, cutaneous lesions other than erythema nodosum, and symptomatic pulmonary lesions
- Long-term therapy is usually required over months to years
- Immunosuppressive drugs and cyclosporine have been tried when benefits of steroid therapy have been exhausted

 OUTCOME

FOLLOW-UP

- At a minimum, yearly physical examination, pulmonary function studies, chemistry panel, ophthalmological evaluation, chest x-ray, and EKG

COMPLICATIONS

- Hemoptysis
- Pneumothorax
- Mycetoma formation in lung cavities
- Respiratory failure in advanced disease

PROGNOSIS

- 20% of patients with lung involvement suffer irreversible lung impairment, with progressive fibrosis, bronchiectasis, and cavitation
- Outlook is best for patients with stage I disease, worse with radiographic parenchymal involvement
- Erythema nodosum is associated with a good outcome
- Death from pulmonary insufficiency occurs in about 5% of patients

 EVIDENCE

PRACTICE GUIDELINES

- Costabel U, Hunninghake GW: ATS/ERS/WASOG statement on sarcoidosis. Sarcoidosis Statement Committee. American Thoracic Society. European Respiratory Society. World Association for Sarcoidosis and Other Granulomatous Disorders. Eur Respir J 1999;14(4):735.

INFORMATION FOR PATIENTS

- National Heart, Lung, and Blood Institute http://www.nhlbi.nih.gov/health/ public/lung/other/sarcoidosis/index.htm
- American Medical Association http://www.ama-assn.org/public/ journals/patient/archive/jpg031302.htm

REFERENCE

- Statement on sarcoidosis. American Thoracic Society International consensus statement. Am J Respir Crit Care Med 1999;160:736. [PMID: 10430755]

Mark S. Chesnutt, MD
Thomas J. Prendergast, MD

Scabies

 ## KEY FEATURES

ESSENTIALS OF DIAGNOSIS

- Generalized very severe itching
- Pruritic vesicles and pustules in "runs" or "galleries," especially on finger webs and the heels of the palms and in wrist creases
- Mites, ova, and brown dots of feces visible microscopically
- Red papules or nodules on the scrotum and on the penile glans and shaft are pathognomonic

GENERAL CONSIDERATIONS

- Caused by *Sarcoptes scabiei*
- Usually spares the head and neck (though these areas may be involved in the elderly, and in patients with AIDS)
- Usually acquired through the bedding of an infested individual or by other close contact

 ## CLINICAL FINDINGS

SYMPTOMS AND SIGNS

- See Table 7 (page 1202)
- Itching is almost always present and can be quite severe
- Lesions are more or less generalized excoriations with small pruritic vesicles, pustules, and "runs" or "burrows" in the web spaces and on the heels of the palms, wrists, elbows, and around the axillae
- Often, burrows are found only on the feet, as they have been scratched off in other locations
- The burrow appears as a short irregular mark, 2–3 mm long and the width of a hair
- Characteristic lesions may occur on the nipples in females and as pruritic papules on the scrotum or penis in males
- Pruritic papules may be seen over the buttocks

DIFFERENTIAL DIAGNOSIS

- Pediculosis (lice)
- Atopic dermatitis (eczema)
- Contact dermatitis
- Arthropod bites (insect bites)
- Urticaria
- Dermatitis herpetiformis

 ## DIAGNOSIS

LABORATORY TESTS

- The diagnosis should be confirmed by microscopic demonstration of the organism, ova, or feces in a mounted specimen, best done on unexcoriated lesions from interdigital webs, wrists, elbows, or feet
- A bit of immersion oil is placed on the lesion and a No. 15 blade is used to scrape the lesion flat
- Diagnosis can also be confirmed in most cases with the burrow ink test: apply ink to the burrow and then do a very superficial shave biopsy by sawing off the burrow with a No. 15 blade, painlessly and bloodlessly; the mite, ova, and feces can be seen under the light microscope

TREATMENT

MEDICATIONS

- Goal is to treat mites and control the dermatitis, which can last months after eradication of the mites, with mid-potency topical steroids (0.1% triamcinolone cream)
- Treatment consists mainly of disinfestations; add systemic antibiotics if secondary pyoderma is present
- Permethrin 5% cream; treat with a single application for 8–12 h; may repeat in 1 week
- Resistance to permethrin is rare
- Crotamiton cream or lotion: an alternative, applied in the same way as permethrin but is used nightly for 4 nights; it is far less effective if used for only 48 h
- Benzyl benzoate: a lotion or emulsion in strengths from 20% to 35% and used as generalized applications (from collarbones down) overnight for two treatments 1 week apart
- The USP formula is 275 mL benzyl benzoate (containing 5 g of triethanolamine and 20 g of oleic acid) in water to make 1000 mL; it is cosmetically acceptable, clean, and not overly irritating
- Treatment failures: most are due to incorrect use or incomplete treatment of the housing unit
- Repeat treatment with permethrin once weekly for 2 weeks, with reeducation regarding the method and extent of application
- Pregnant patients: treat only if they have documented scabies; use permethrin 5% cream once for 12 h—or 5% or 6% sulfur in petrolatum applied nightly for 3 nights from the collarbones down
- Immunocompetent treatment failures: ivermectin in a dose of 200 μg/kg effective in about 75% of cases with one dose and 95% of cases with two doses 2 weeks apart
- In immunosuppressed hosts and those with crusted (hyperkeratotic) scabies: multiple doses of ivermectin (every 2 weeks for two or three doses) plus topical therapy with permethrin once or twice weekly may be effective when topical treatment and oral therapy alone fail
- Persistent pruritic postscabietic papules: may be treated with mid- to high-potency steroids or with intralesional triamcinolone acetonide (2.5–5 mg/mL)

THERAPEUTIC PROCEDURES

- Bedding and clothing should be laundered or cleaned or set aside for 14 days in plastic bags
- Must treat all persons in a family or institutionalized group

OUTCOME

WHEN TO REFER

- If there is a question about the diagnosis, if recommended therapy is ineffective, or if specialized treatment is necessary

EVIDENCE

PRACTICE GUIDELINES

- National Guideline Clearinghouse
  http://www.guideline.gov/summary/summary.aspx?doc_id=3047&nbr=2273&string=scabies

WEB SITES

- American Academy of Dermatology
  http://www.aad.org
- Dermatology Handbook for Family Practice from the University of Iowa
  http://www.vh.org/Providers/ClinRef/FPHandbook/17.html

INFORMATION FOR PATIENTS

- Centers for Disease Control and Prevention
  http://www.niams.nih.gov/hi/topics/rosacea/rosacea.htm
- National Institutes of Health
  http://www.nlm.nih.gov/medlineplus/ency/article/000830.htm

REFERENCES

- Chosidow O: Scabies and pediculosis. Lancet 2000;355:819. [PMID: 10711939]
- Parish LC et al: The saga of ectoparasitoses: scabies and pediculosis. Int J Dermatol 1999;38:432. [PMID: 10397581]

Timothy G. Berger, MD

Schistosomiasis

KEY FEATURES

ESSENTIALS OF DIAGNOSIS

- Exposure to infection in an endemic area

Acute phase

- Abrupt onset (2–6 weeks postexposure) of abdominal pain, weight loss, headache, malaise, chills, fever, myalgia, diarrhea (sometimes bloody), dry cough, hepatomegaly, and eosinophilia

Chronic phase

- Either diarrhea, abdominal pain, blood in stool, hepatomegaly or hepatosplenomegaly, and bleeding from esophageal varices (*Schistosoma mansoni* or *Schistosoma japonicum* infection); or terminal hematuria, urinary frequency, and urethral and bladder pain (*Schistosoma haematobium* infection)
- Depending on species, characteristic eggs in feces, urine, or scrapings or biopsy of rectal or bladder mucosa

GENERAL CONSIDERATIONS

- The disease is caused mainly by three blood flukes (trematodes): *S mansoni*, which causes intestinal schistosomiasis, is widespread in Africa and occurs in the Arabian peninsula, South America, and the Caribbean; vesical (urinary) schistosomiasis, caused by *S haematobium*, is found throughout the Middle East and Africa; and Asiatic intestinal schistosomiasis, due to *S japonicum*, is important in China and the Philippines
- Except for the allergic response in the acute syndrome (see below), the disease is primarily due to delayed hypersensitivity
- The life span of the worms ranges from 5 to 30 years or more

DEMOGRAPHICS

- Infects more than 200 million persons worldwide, induces severe consequences in 20 million persons annually, resulting in up to 200,000 deaths
- In the United States, an estimated 400,000 immigrants are infected, but transmission does not occur because appropriate snail intermediate hosts are absent

CLINICAL FINDINGS

SYMPTOMS AND SIGNS

- Although a large proportion of infected persons have light infections (<100 eggs per gram of feces) and are asymptomatic, an estimated 50–60% have symptoms and 5–10% advanced organ damage
- Cercarial dermatitis produces a localized itchy erythematous or petechial rash to macules and papules that last up to 5 days

Acute schistosomiasis (Katayama fever)

- Primarily an allergic response to the developing schistosomes and may occur with the three schistosomes (rare with *S haematobium*)
- The incubation period is 2–7 weeks; the severity of illness ranges from mild to (rarely) life-threatening
- In addition to fever, malaise, urticaria, diarrhea (sometimes bloody), myalgia, dry cough, leukocytosis, and marked eosinophilia, the liver and spleen may be temporarily enlarged
- The patient again becomes asymptomatic in 2–8 weeks

Chronic schistosomiasis

- This stage begins 6 months to several years after infection
- In *S mansoni* and *S japonicum* infections, findings include diarrhea, abdominal pain, irregular bowel movements, blood in the stool, a hard enlarged liver, and splenomegaly
- With subsequent slow progression over 5–15 years or longer, the following may appear: anorexia, weight loss, weakness, polypoid intestinal tumors, and features of portal and pulmonary hypertension
- Immune complex glomerulonephritis may occur
- In *S haematobium* infection, early symptoms of urinary tract disease are frequency and dysuria, followed by terminal hematuria and proteinuria

DIFFERENTIAL DIAGNOSIS

- *Acute*
  - Amebiasis
  - Bacterial dysentery, eg, *Shigella*, *Salmonella*
  - Viral hepatitis
  - Typhoid fever
  - Malaria
- *Chronic*
  - Typhoid fever
  - Visceral leishmaniasis
  - Lymphoma
  - Amebiasis
  - Portal hypertension due to other causes, eg, cirrhosis, portal vein thrombosis
  - Hematuria due to other causes, eg, urinary tract infections, renal cell carcinoma

DIAGNOSIS

LABORATORY TESTS

- Screening is by testing for eggs (ova) and occult blood in feces and urine (the excretion of which may be irregular and require repeated testing), for protein and leukocytes in urine, and by serology
- Definitive diagnosis is by finding characteristic live eggs in excreta or mucosal biopsy
- In *S haematobium* infection, eggs may be found in the urine or, less frequently, in the stools. Eggs are sought in urine specimens collected between 9 AM and 2 PM or in 24-h collections. They are processed either by examination of the sediment or preferably by membrane filtration
- In *S mansoni* and *S japonicum* infections, eggs may be found in stool specimens by direct examination, but concentration with a method such as the Kato-Katz quantitative method is often necessary; heavy infections are those with counts over 400 eggs per gram
- ELISA, immunoblot, and other tests are used in screening and may detect some egg-negative or ectopic infections
- Early in acute schistosomiasis, stool examination may be negative (examinations should be repeated for at least 6 months) but serological tests positive
- Anemia is common. Eosinophilia, common during the acute stage, usually is absent in the chronic stage

IMAGING STUDIES

- In *S mansoni* and *S japonicum* infections, barium swallow, esophagoscopy, barium enema or colonoscopy, chest x-ray, or an ECG may be indicated. Ultrasound examination of the liver may show the pathognomonic pattern of periportal fibrosis and replaces the need for liver biopsy
- In advanced *S haematobium* disease, cystoscopy may show "sandy patches," ulcers, and areas of squamous metaplasia; lower abdominal plain films may show calcification of the bladder wall or ureters. Sonography is considered the imaging technique of choice but may fail to show the calcification. CT—which may demonstrate pathognomonic "turtleback" calcifications—intravenous pyelography, and retrograde cystography and pyelography may be useful

DIAGNOSTIC PROCEDURES

- If stool eggs are not found, biopsy may be necessary. Specimens should be examined as crush preparations between two glass slides and also examined histologically

TREATMENT

MEDICATIONS

- Treatment should be given only if live ova are identified
- Praziquantel can be used to treat all species; alternative drugs of choice are oxamniquine for *S mansoni* and metrifonate for *S haematobium*
- The praziquantel dosage is 20 mg/kg—give twice in 1 day for *S haematobium* and *S mansoni* and three times in 1 day for *S japonicum* and *S mekongi*. The dosages should be given at 4- to 6-h intervals with water after a meal. The drug should not be used in pregnancy
- Oxamniquine is highly effective only in *S mansoni* infections. For strains in the western hemisphere and western Africa, a dose of 15 mg/kg is given once. Some recommend 40–60 mg/kg/day in two or three divided doses for 2–3 days in all of Africa and in the Arabian peninsula. When divided doses are needed, they are separated by 6-8 h. The drug is contraindicated in pregnancy

SURGERY

- In selected instances, surgery may be indicated for removal of polyps and for obstructive uropathy

THERAPEUTIC PROCEDURES

- For bleeding esophageal varices, sclerotherapy is the treatment of choice

OUTCOME

FOLLOW-UP

- After treatment, periodic laboratory follow-up for continued passage of eggs is essential, starting at 3 months and continuing at intervals for 1 year; if found, viability should be determined, since dead eggs are passed for some months

COMPLICATIONS

- Portal hypertension with contracted liver, splenomegaly, pancytopenia, esophageal varices
- Pulmonary hypertension with cor pulmonale and edema due to right heart failure
- Large bowel stricture, granulomatous masses, colonic polyposis, and persistent *Salmonella* infection may occur
- Transverse myelitis, epilepsy, or optic neuritis may result from collateral circulation of eggs or ectopic worms
- Sequelae of *S haematobium* infection include bladder polyp formation, cystitis, chronic *Salmonella* infection, pyelitis, pyelonephritis, urolithiasis, hydronephrosis due to ureteral obstruction, renal failure, and death. Severe liver, lung, genital, or neurological disease is rare
- Bladder cancer has been associated with vesicular schistosomiasis

PROGNOSIS

- Cure rates with praziquantel of 85% and higher are achieved at 6 months for *S haematobium*, *S mansoni*, and *S japonicum* infections, with marked reduction in egg counts (>90%) in those not cured
- In advanced disease with extensive involvement of the intestines, liver, bladder, or other organs, the outlook is poor even with treatment

WHEN TO REFER

- All patients with chronic schistosomiasis

WHEN TO ADMIT

- In areas where cysticercosis may coexist with a schistosomal infection being treated with praziquantel, treatment is best conducted in a hospital to monitor for death of cysticerci, which may be followed by neurological complications

EVIDENCE

PRACTICE GUIDELINES

- National Guideline Clearinghouse
http://www.guideline.gov/summary/
summary.aspx?doc_id=2284&nbr=
1510&string=schistosomiasis

INFORMATION FOR PATIENTS

- Centers for Disease Control
http://www.cdc.gov/ncidod/dpd/
parasites/schistosomiasis/factsht_
schistosomiasis.htm
- National Institutes of Health
http://www.nlm.nih.gov/medlineplus/
ency/article/001321.htm

REFERENCES

- Ghoneim MA: Bilharziasis of the genitourinary tract. BJU Int 2002;89 (Suppl 1):22. [PMID: 11876729]
- Ross AG et al: Schistosomiasis. N Engl J Med 2002;346:1212. [PMID: 11961151]

Schizophrenia

KEY FEATURES

ESSENTIALS OF DIAGNOSIS

- Social withdrawal, usually slowly progressive, often with deterioration in personal care
- Loss of ego boundaries, with inability to perceive oneself as a separate entity
- Loose thought associations, often with slowed thinking or overinclusive and rapid shifting from topic to topic
- Absorption in inner thoughts and frequent sexual or religious preoccupations
- Auditory hallucinations, often of a derogatory nature
- Delusions, frequently of a grandiose or persecutory nature
- Symptoms of at least 6 months' duration

Frequent additional signs

- Flat affect and rapidly alternating mood shifts irrespective of circumstances
- Hypersensitivity to environmental stimuli, with feelings of enhanced sensory awareness
- Variable behavior incongruent with the external environment
- Concrete thinking with inability to abstract; inappropriate symbolism
- Impaired concentration worsened by hallucinations and delusions
- Depersonalization: behaving like a detached observer of one's own actions

GENERAL CONSIDERATIONS

- Massive disruption of thinking, mood, and overall behavior, as well as poor filtering of stimuli
- Origin believed to have genetic, environmental, and neurotransmitter pathophysiological components
- Schizophrenic disorders subdivided into types by prominent phenomena
  - *Disorganized (hebephrenic)*: incoherence and incongruous or silly affect
  - *Catatonic*: psychomotor disturbance or either excitement or rigidity
  - *Paranoid*: persecutory or grandiose delusions, and hallucinations
  - *Undifferentiated*: lack of symptoms specific enough to fit other types
  - *Residual*: for persons with a history of clear schizophrenia, but who presently exhibit only milder signs without overt psychosis

CLINICAL FINDINGS

SYMPTOMS AND SIGNS

- A history of a major disruption in the individual's life may precede gross psychotic deterioration
- Gradual decompensation usually predates the acute episode
- "Positive" symptoms
  - Delusions are often paranoid, involving perceived threat from others
  - Hallucinations are typically auditory
- "Negative" symptoms
  - Diminished sociability
  - Restricted affect
  - Impoverished speech
- Appearance: may be bizarre, though usually patients are just mildly unkempt
- Motor activity: generally reduced, though a broad spectrum is seen
- Social function: marked withdrawal, disturbed interpersonal relationships
- Speech: neologisms (made-up words or phrases) and echolalia (repetition of others' words), and verbigeration (repetition of senseless words or phrases)
- Affect: flat, occasionally inappropriate
- Mood: depression present in most cases, less apparent during acute psychosis
- Thought content: varies from paucity of ideas to rich delusions

DIFFERENTIAL DIAGNOSIS

- Schizophrenia should be distinguished from other psychoses
  - *Delusional disorders* are characterized by nonbizarre delusions with minimal impairment on daily life
  - *Schizoaffective disorders* fail to fit within the definitions of either schizophrenia or affective disorders
  - *Schizophreniform disorders* have a duration of less than 6 months, but more than 1 week
  - *Brief psychotic disorders* result from psychological stress, last less than 1 week, and have a much better prognosis
  - *Late life psychosis* occurs after age 60 and is accompanied by cognitive impairment
  - *Atypical psychoses* describes psychotic symptoms arising from a cause that may be apparent only later
  - Clues are precipitous onset and a good premorbid history

- Manic episodes
- Obsessive-compulsive disorder
- Psychotic depression
- Drug intoxication and abuse
- Thyroid, adrenal, and pituitary disorders
- Complex partial seizures and temporal lobe dysfunction may produce psychotic symptoms
- Drug toxicities, particularly overdoses of typical antipsychotics, can produce catatonia

DIAGNOSIS

LABORATORY TESTS

- Tests to rule out metabolic deficiencies; endocrine disorders may be appropriate
- Toxicology screen

IMAGING STUDIES

- Ventricular enlargement and cortical atrophy on CT have been correlated with chronicity, cognitive impairment, and poor response to neuroleptics
- Decreased frontal lobe activity on positron emission tomography scan has been associated with negative symptoms
- MRI can exclude temporal lobe disorders

TREATMENT

MEDICATIONS

- See Tables 102 and 103 (pages 1286 and 1287)
- Typical neuroleptics (phenothiazines, thioxanthenes, butyrophenones, dihydroindolones, dibenzoxazepines, and benzisoxazoles)
- Newer, atypical neuroleptics (clozapine, risperidone, olanzapine, quetiapine, ziprasidone, and aripiprazole)
- Atypical agents cause less tardive dyskinesia and extrapyramidal symptoms
- Atypical agents are more effective than typical agents on negative symptoms
- Antidepressant drugs may be used with antipsychotics if significant depression is present
- Resistant cases may require addition of lithium, carbamazepine, or valproate
- Addition of benzodiazepine can resolve catatonic symptoms and allow a lower neuroleptic dose

THERAPEUTIC PROCEDURES

Social

- Board and care homes with experienced staff can improve functioning and limit hospitalizations
- Nonresidential self-help groups (Recovery, Inc.) should be utilized
- Vocational rehabilitation and work agencies (Goodwill Industries, Inc.) can provide structured work situations

Psychological

- Need for psychotherapy varies markedly with patient status and history
- Insight-oriented psychotherapy is often counterproductive
- Cognitive-behavioral therapy with medication management may be efficacious
- Family therapy may alleviate the patient's stress and assist relatives in coping

Behavioral

- Music from portable players with headphones can divert attention from auditory hallucinations

OUTCOME

FOLLOW-UP

- Clozapine: 1% risk of agranulocytosis; weekly WBC for 6 months, then every other week thereafter and weekly for 1 month after discontinuation
- Ziprasidone can cause QT prolongation; pretreatment ECG and cardiac risk factor screen are necessary
- Quetiapine: associated with cataracts; ophthalmological examination at initiation and biannually

COMPLICATIONS

- Neuroleptic malignant syndrome is uncommon but serious side effect of neuroleptics
- Tardive dyskinesia may occur after chronic use of neuroleptics
- Anticholinergic and adrenergic side effects are more frequent with low-potency neuroleptics
- Extrapyramidal symptoms are seen with high-potency neuroleptics
- Olanzapine has been associated with significant weight gain with case reports of type 2 diabetes

PROGNOSIS

- For removal of positive symptoms, prognosis is excellent in most patients
- Negative symptoms are more difficult to treat
- Prognosis is guarded when psychosis is associated with a history of serious drug abuse, due to likely CNS damage
- Life expectancy is 20% shorter in schizophrenics, mostly due to higher mortality among young patients

WHEN TO ADMIT

- Gross disorganization
- Risk of self-harm or harm to others

EVIDENCE

PRACTICE GUIDELINES

- National Guideline Clearinghouse
  http://www.guideline.gov/summary/summary.aspx?doc_id=2904&nbr=2130&string=schizophrenia
  http://www.guideline.gov/summary/summary.aspx?doc_id=3017&nbr=2243&string=schizophrenia

WEB SITES

- American Psychiatric Association
  http://www.psych.org/
- Internet Mental Health
  http://www.mentalhealth.com/t30.html
- Psychopharmacology Tips
  http://www.dr-bob.org/tips/
- Psychiatry On Line
  http://www.priory.com/psych.htm

INFORMATION FOR PATIENTS

- JAMA patient page: Schizophrenia. JAMA 2001;286:494.
- National Institute of Mental Health
  http://www.nimh.nih.gov/publicat/schizoph.htm

REFERENCES

- Eisendrath SJ, Chamberlain J: Psychiatry in the critical care unit. In: Current diagnosis and treatment in critical care, ed 2. Bongard FS, Sue DY (editors). Appleton & Lange, 2002.
- Glassman AH et al: Antipsychotic drugs: prolonged QTc interval, torsade de pointes, and sudden death. Am J Psychiatry 2001;158:1774. [PMID: 11691681]
- Kane JM et al: Efficacy and safety of aripiprazole and haloperidol versus placebo in patients with schizophrenia and schizoaffective disorder. J Clin Psychiatry 2002;63:763.
- Rector NA et al: Cognitive behavioral therapy for schizophrenia: an empirical review. J Nerv Ment Dis 2001;189:278. [PMID: 11379970]

Stuart J. Eisendrath, MD
Jonathan E. Lichtmacher, MD

Scleroderma (Systemic Sclerosis)

 ## KEY FEATURES

ESSENTIALS OF DIAGNOSIS

- Diffuse thickening of skin, with telangiectasia and areas of increased pigmentation and depigmentation
- Raynaud's phenomenon in 90% of patients
- Systemic features of dysphagia, hypomotility of gastrointestinal tract, pulmonary fibrosis, and cardiac and renal involvement
- Positive test for antinuclear antibodies nearly universal

GENERAL CONSIDERATIONS

- A chronic disorder characterized by diffuse fibrosis of the skin and internal organs
- Two forms of systemic sclerosis are generally recognized: limited (80% of patients) and diffuse (20%)
- Microchimerism (long-term persisting cells from pregnancy) could be involved in the pathogenesis
- Patients presenting with systemic sclerosis or an eosinophilic fasciitis-like syndrome should be asked about tryptophan use, which is banned by the Food and Drug Administration

Eosinophilic fasciitis

- A rare disorder presenting with skin changes that resemble diffuse systemic sclerosis
- The inflammatory abnormalities, however, are limited to the fascia rather than the dermis and epidermis.
- Unlike in systemic sclerosis, patients have peripheral blood eosinophilia, absence of Raynaud's phenomenon, a good response to prednisone, and an increased risk of developing aplastic anemia

DEMOGRAPHICS

- Symptoms usually appear in the third to sixth decades
- Women are affected about four times as frequently as men

 ## CLINICAL FINDINGS

SYMPTOMS AND SIGNS

- Most frequently, skin involvement precedes visceral involvement
- Polyarthralgia and Raynaud's phenomenon (present in 90% of patients) are early manifestations
- With time the skin becomes thickened and hidebound, with loss of normal folds
- Telangiectasia, pigmentation, and depigmentation are characteristic
- Ulceration about the fingertips and subcutaneous calcification are seen
- Dysphagia from esophageal dysfunction (abnormalities in motility and later from fibrosis) is common
- Fibrosis and atrophy of the gastrointestinal tract cause hypomotility, and malabsorption results from bacterial overgrowth
- Diffuse pulmonary fibrosis and pulmonary vascular disease are reflected in low diffusing capacity and decreased lung compliance
- Cardiac abnormalities include pericarditis, heart block, myocardial fibrosis, and right heart failure secondary to pulmonary hypertension
- Systemic sclerosis renal crisis, resulting from obstruction of smaller renal blood vessels, indicates a grave prognosis

DIFFERENTIAL DIAGNOSIS

- Several conditions classified as "localized" sclerosis may mimic systemic morphea and limited systemic sclerosis. These disorders are generally limited to the skin (typically in a localized fashion) and are associated with excellent prognoses
- Eosinophilic fasciitis
- Eosinophilic-myalgia syndrome (due to tryptophan use)
- Overlap syndrome ("mixed connective tissue disease")
- Raynaud's disease
- Morphea
- Amyloidosis
- Graft-versus-host disease
- Cryoglobulinemia

 ## DIAGNOSIS

LABORATORY TESTS

- Antinuclear antibody tests are nearly always positive (Tables 73 and 79, pages 1265 and 1267)
- The scleroderma antibody (SCL-70) directed against topoisomerase III is found in one-third of patients with diffuse systemic sclerosis and in 20% of those with CREST syndrome
- Anticentromere antibody is seen in 50% of those with CREST syndrome and in 1% of individuals with diffuse systemic sclerosis
- Elevation of the sedimentation rate is unusual
- Mild anemia is often present
- Proteinuria and cylindruria appear in association with renal involvement

Scleroderma (Systemic Sclerosis)

TREATMENT

MEDICATIONS

- Severe Raynaud's syndrome may respond to calcium channel blockers, eg, long-acting nifedipine, 30–120 mg/day, or to losartan, 50 mg/day
- Intravenous iloprost, a prostacyclin analog that causes vasodilation and platelet inhibition, is moderately effective in healing digital ulcers
- Intravenous prostaglandins (epoprostenol or PGE_2) or a subcutaneous protacyclin analogue (treprostinil) may be effective in pulmonary hypertension. An endothelin-1 antagonist, bosentan, improves symptoms and exercise tolerance in pulmonary hypertension
- Esophageal reflux can be reduced using antacids, H_2 blockers, and proton pump inhibitors (eg, omeprazole, 20–40 mg/day)
- Malabsorption due to bacterial overgrowth also responds to antibiotics, eg, tetracycline, 500 mg four times daily
- The hypertensive crises associated with systemic sclerosis renal crisis must be treated early and aggressively (in the hospital) with angiotensin-converting enzyme inhibitors, eg, captopril, 37.5–75 mg/day in three divided doses
- Prednisone has little or no role in the treatment of scleroderma
- Cyclophosphamide, a drug with many important side effects, may improve severe interstitial lung disease

SURGERY

- Digital sympathectomy may provide at least temporary relief in severe digital ischemia

THERAPEUTIC PROCEDURES

- Treatment is symptomatic and supportive

OUTCOME

COMPLICATIONS

- End-stage renal disease and often death from the malignant hypertension associated with scleroderma renal crisis
- Pulmonary hypertension
- Pulmonary fibrosis
- Profound gastrointestinal hypomotility and bacterial overgrowth
- Digital loss

PROGNOSIS

- Patients with CREST syndrome have a much better prognosis than those with diffuse disease, in large part because patients with limited disease do not develop renal failure or interstitial lung disease
- The 9-year survival rate in scleroderma averages approximately 40%
- The prognosis tends to be worse in those with diffuse scleroderma, in blacks, in males, and in older patients

WHEN TO REFER

- Patients should be managed in consultation with a rheumatologist

WHEN TO ADMIT

- Scleroderma renal crisis
- Advanced pulmonary hypertension

EVIDENCE

PRACTICE GUIDELINES

- Drake LA et al: Guidelines of care for scleroderma and sclerodermoid disorders. American Academy of Dermatology. J Am Acad Dermatol 1996;35:609.

INFORMATION FOR PATIENTS

- National Institute of Arthritis and Musculoskeletal and Skin Diseases http://www.niams.nih.gov/hi/topics/scleroderma/scleroderma.htm
- American College of Dermatology http://www.rheumatology.org/patients/factsheet/scler.html

REFERENCES

- LeRoy EC et al: Criteria for the classification of early systemic sclerosis. J Rheumatol 2001;28:1573. [PMID: 11469464]
- Rubin LJ et al: Bosentan therapy for pulmonary arterial hypertension. N Engl J Med 2002;346:896.
- Sule SD et al: Update on management of scleroderma. Bull Rheum Dis 2000; 49:1. [PMID: 11286150]
- White B: Evaluation and management of pulmonary fibrosis in scleroderma. Curr Rheumatol Rep 2002;4:108.
- Wigley FM: When is scleroderma really scleroderma? J Rheumatol 2001;28: 1471. [PMID: 11469447]
- Wigley FM: Raynaud's phenomenon. N Engl J Med 2002;347:1001.

David B. Hellmann, MD, FACP
John H. Stone, MD, MPH

Sclerosing Cholangitis, Primary

KEY FEATURES

ESSENTIALS OF DIAGNOSIS

- Males, aged 20–50 years old
- Often associated with ulcerative colitis
- Progressive jaundice, itching, and other features of cholestasis
- Diagnosis based on characteristic cholangiographic findings
- 10% risk of cholangiocarcinoma

GENERAL CONSIDERATIONS

- Characterized by a diffuse inflammation of the biliary tract leading to fibrosis and strictures of the biliary system
- Associated with the histocompatible antigens HLA-B8 and -DR3 or -DR4, suggesting that genetic factors may play an etiological role
- Antineutrophil cytoplasmic antibodies (ANCA), with fluorescent staining characteristics and target antigens distinct from those found in patients with Wegener's granulomatosis or vasculitis, are found in 70% of patients
- In patients with AIDS, sclerosing cholangitis may result from infections caused by cytomegalovirus (CMV), *Cryptosporidium,* or microsporum
- Occasional patients have clinical and histological features of both sclerosing cholangitis and autoimmune hepatitis. Even more rarely, an association with chronic pancreatitis (sclerosing pancreaticocholangitis) is seen, and this entity is often responsive to corticosteroids
- The diagnosis is difficult to make after biliary surgery or intrahepatic artery chemotherapy, which may result in bile duct injury
- Primary sclerosing cholangitis must be distinguished from idiopathic adulthood ductopenia, a rare disorder affecting young to middle-aged adults who manifest cholestasis resulting from loss of interlobular and septal bile ducts yet who have a normal cholangiogram

DEMOGRAPHICS

- The disease is most common in men aged 20–40 and is closely associated with ulcerative colitis (and occasionally Crohn's colitis), which is present in approximately two-thirds of patients; however, only 1–4% of patients with ulcerative colitis develop clinically significant sclerosing cholangitis
- As in ulcerative colitis, smoking is associated with a decreased risk of primary sclerosing cholangitis

CLINICAL FINDINGS

SYMPTOMS AND SIGNS

- Clinically, primary sclerosing cholangitis presents as progressive obstructive jaundice, frequently associated with malaise, pruritus, anorexia, and indigestion
- Occasional patients have clinical and histological features of both sclerosing cholangitis and autoimmune hepatitis

DIFFERENTIAL DIAGNOSIS

- Primary biliary cirrhosis
- Choledocholithiasis
- Cancer of pancreas or biliary tree
- Biliary stricture
- Drug-induced cholestasis, eg, chlorpromazine
- Inflammatory bowel disease complicated by cholestatic liver disease
- Idiopathic adulthood ductopenia
- *Clonorchis sinensis* (Chinese liver fluke)
- *Fasciola hepatica* (sheep liver fluke)
- Sclerosing cholangitis due to CMV, cryptosporidiosis, microsporidiosis (in AIDS)

DIAGNOSIS

LABORATORY TESTS

- Patients may be diagnosed in the presymptomatic phase because of an elevated alkaline phosphatase level
- ANCA, serum antinuclear, anticardiolipin, and antithyroperoxidase antibodies and rheumatoid factor may be present

IMAGING STUDIES

- The diagnosis is generally made by endoscopic retrograde cholangiography (ERCP); increasingly, magnetic resonance cholangiography is being used as a noninvasive diagnostic approach but is less sensitive than ERCP for visualizing the intrahepatic ducts. Biliary obstruction by a stone or tumor should be excluded

DIAGNOSTIC PROCEDURES

- The disease may be confined to small intrahepatic bile ducts, in which case ERCP is normal and the diagnosis is suggested by liver biopsy
- Liver biopsy is needed for staging, which is based on the degree of inflammation and fibrosis

Sclerosing Cholangitis, Primary

 ## TREATMENT

MEDICATIONS

- Treatment with corticosteroids and broad-spectrum antimicrobial agents provides inconsistent results
- Episodes of acute bacterial cholangitis may be treated with ciprofloxacin
- Ursodeoxycholic acid in standard doses (10–15 mg/kg/day) may improve liver function test results but does not appear to alter the natural history. However, high-dose ursodeoxycholic acid (20 mg/kg/day) may reduce cholangiographic progression and liver fibrosis

SURGERY

- In patients without cirrhosis, surgical resection of a dominant bile duct stricture may lead to longer survival than endoscopic therapy by decreasing the subsequent risk of cholangiocarcinoma
- For patients with cirrhosis and clinical decompensation, liver transplantation is the procedure of choice

THERAPEUTIC PROCEDURES

- Careful endoscopic evaluation of the biliary tree may permit balloon dilation of localized strictures. If there is a major stricture, short-term placement of a stent may relieve symptoms and improve biochemical abnormalities with sustained improvement after the stent is removed
- Repeated balloon dilation of a recurrent dominant bile duct stricture may improve survival. However, long-term stenting may increase the rate of complications such as cholangitis

 ## OUTCOME

COMPLICATIONS

- Complications of chronic cholestasis, such as osteoporosis and malabsorption of fat-soluble vitamins, may occur
- Cholangiocarcinoma may complicate the course in at least 10% of cases and may be difficult to diagnose by cytological examination or biopsy because of false-negative results. A serum CA 19-9 level >100 units/mL is suggestive but not diagnostic of cholangiocarcinoma

PROGNOSIS

- Survival averages 10 years once symptoms appear
- Adverse prognostic markers are older age, higher serum bilirubin and aspartate aminotransferase levels, lower albumin levels, and a history of variceal bleeding
- Actuarial survival rates with liver transplantation are as high as 85% at 3 years, but rates are much lower once cholangiocarcinoma has developed. Following transplantation, patients have an increased risk of nonanastomotic biliary strictures and—in those with ulcerative colitis—colon cancer
- Patients who are unable to undergo liver transplantation will ultimately require high-quality palliative care
- When the disease is confined to small intrahepatic bile ducts, the survival is longer and there is a lower rate of cholangiocarcinoma than with involvement of the large ducts

WHEN TO REFER

- All patients

PREVENTION

- In patients with ulcerative colitis, primary sclerosing cholangitis is an independent risk factor for the development of colorectal dysplasia and cancer, and strict adherence to a colonoscopic surveillance program is advisable

 ## EVIDENCE

PRACTICE GUIDELINES

- Lee Y-M et al: Management of primary sclerosing cholangitis. Am J Gastroenterol 2002;97:528.
- National Guideline Clearinghouse http://www.guideline.gov/summary/summary.aspx?doc_id=2967&nbr=2193&string=cholangitis http://www .guideline.gov/summary/summary.aspx?doc_id=3449&nbr=2675&string=cholangitis

WEB SITE

- Endoscopic Retrograde Cholangiopancreatography (ERCP) http://www.surgery.wisc.edu/patient/patient_hbp_ercp.html

INFORMATION FOR PATIENTS

- National Digestive Diseases Information Clearinghouse http://digestive.niddk.nih.gov/ddiseases/pubs/primarysclerosingcholangitis/index.htm
- National Institutes of Health http://www.nlm.nih.gov/medlineplus/ency/article/000285.htm

REFERENCES

- Bergquist A et al: Hepatic and extrahepatic malignancies in primary sclerosing cholangitis. J Hepatol 2002;36:321.
- Björnsson E et al: Patients with small duct primary sclerosing cholangitis have a favourable long-term prognosis. Gut 2002;51:731.
- Soetikno RM et al: Increased risk of colorectal neoplasia in patients with primary sclerosing cholangitis and ulcerative colitis: a meta-analysis. Gastrointest Endosc 2002;56:48.

Lawrence S. Friedman, MD

Serum Sickness (Immune Complex Disease)

 KEY FEATURES

ESSENTIALS OF DIAGNOSIS

- Fever, pruritus, and arthropathy
- Reaction is delayed in onset, usually 7–10 days, when specific IgG antibodies are generated against the allergen
- Immune complexes found circulating in serum or deposited in affected tissues

GENERAL CONSIDERATIONS

- Serum sickness reactions occur when immune complexes formed by the binding of drugs or heterologous serum to antibodies; these complexes deposit in the vascular endothelium and produce immune-mediated tissue injury
- The reaction occurs 7–10 days after exposure, when specific IgG antibodies are generated against the allergen
- The commonly affected organs include skin (urticaria, vasculitis), joints (arthritis), and kidney (nephritis)

 CLINICAL FINDINGS

SYMPTOMS AND SIGNS

- Usually a self-limited illness, but can be a severe vasculitis
- Constitutional symptoms are common
- Fever
- Urticaria
- Arthritis
- Nephritis

DIFFERENTIAL DIAGNOSIS

- Infection
- Autoimmune hypersensitivity
- Vasculitis
- Systemic lupus erythematosus (SLE)
- Rheumatoid arthritis (RA)

 DIAGNOSIS

LABORATORY TESTS

- The specific IgG antibody may be present in sufficient quantity in serum to be detected by the precipitin-in-gel method; ELISA will detect antibodies present in lesser amounts
- Decreased C3, C4, or CH50 is nonspecific evidence of immune complex disease
- Immune complexes can be detected circulating in serum or deposited in affected tissues
- Increased erythrocyte sedimentation rate
- Red blood cell casts if nephritis is present

Serum Sickness (Immune Complex Disease)

 TREATMENT

MEDICATIONS

- Aspirin or nonsteroidal antiinflammatory drugs for fever and arthritis
- Antihistamines and topical steroids for dermatitis
- Systemic corticosteroids are used for systemic vasculitis manifesting as glomerulonephritis or neuropathy

 OUTCOME

PROGNOSIS

- Good to excellent if inciting antigen is identified and withdrawn (eg, drug, serum, etc)

WHEN TO REFER

- To an allergist for assistance in identifying inciting agent(s)
- To a rheumatologist if autoimmune disorder is suspected (eg, SLE, RA, or vasculitis)

PREVENTION

- Avoid known inciting agents

 EVIDENCE

PRACTICE GUIDELINES

- Joint Task Force on Practice Parameters, the American Academy of Allergy, Asthma and Immunology, and the Joint Council of Allergy, Asthma and Immunology: Executive summary of disease management of drug hypersensitivity: a practice parameter. Ann Allergy Asthma Immunol 1999;83(6 Pt 3):665.

WEB SITES

- National Institutes of Health www.nih.gov/niams/healthinfo
- American Academy of Allergy, Asthma and Immunology http://www.aaaai.org
- American College of Rheumatology http://www.acr.org

INFORMATION FOR PATIENTS

- JAMA patient page: Allergies. JAMA 2000;283:424.[PMID: 10647806]
- American College of Allergy, Asthma and Immunology http://www.medem.com/search/article_display.cfm?path=\\TANQUERAY\M_ContentItem&mstr=/M_ContentItem/ZZZEA5MS2BC .html&soc=Medem_ACAAI&srch_typ=NAV_SERCH

REFERENCES

- Cuellar ML: Drug-induced vasculitis. Curr Rheumatol Rep 2002;4:55. [PMID: 11798983]
- Fiorentino DF: Cutaneous vasculitis. J Am Acad Dermatol 2003;48:311. [PMID: 12637912]
- Venzor J: Urticarial vasculitis. Clin Rev Allergy Immunol 2002; 23:201. [PMID: 12221865]

Jeffrey L. Kishiyama, MD
Daniel C. Adelman, MD

Sexual Dysfunction

 KEY FEATURES

ESSENTIALS OF DIAGNOSIS

- Large category of vasocongestive and orgasmic disorders
- Often involve problems of sexual adaptation, education, and technique

GENERAL CONSIDERATIONS

- Two common conditions in men are erectile dysfunction and ejaculation disturbances
- In women, the two most common forms are vaginismus and frigidity

Erectile dysfunction

- The inability to achieve an erection adequate for satisfactory intercourse
- Causes can be psychological, physiological, or both
- A history of occasional erections—especially nocturnal tumescence—can demonstrate a psychological origin

Ejaculation disturbances

- Ejaculation control is an acquired behavior that is minimal in adolescence and increases with experience
- Sexual ignorance, anxiety, guilt, depression, and relationship problems may interfere with learning control
- Interference with the sympathetic nerve distribution through surgery or trauma can be responsible

Vaginismus

- Conditioned response in which a spasm of the perineal muscles occurs if there is any stimulation of the area
- The desire is to avoid penetration

Frigidity

- Characterized by a general lack of sexual responsiveness
- Sexual activity varies from avoidance to an occasional orgasm
- Poor sexual techniques, early traumatic sexual experiences, and marital problems may be uncovered as causes
- Organic causes include conditions causing dyspareunia, pelvic pathology, mechanical obstruction, and neurological deficits

 CLINICAL FINDINGS

SYMPTOMS AND SIGNS

Erectile dysfunction

- Often will be mentioned only after direct questioning
- Patients will sometimes use the term "impotence" to describe premature ejaculation

Ejaculation disturbances

- Patients may not relate symptoms without direct questions regarding their sex lives

Frigidity

- Difficulty in experiencing erotic sensation and lack of vasocongestive response
- Should be differentiated from orgasmic dysfunction, in which varying degrees of difficulty are experienced in achieving orgasm

DIFFERENTIAL DIAGNOSIS

- Depression or anxiety
- Underlying medical condition, eg, diabetes, peripheral vascular disease, hyperprolactinemia, hypogonadism
- Dyspareunia or chronic pelvic pain
- Drugs or substance use, eg, selective serotonin reuptake inhibitors (SSRIs), tricyclic antidepressants, alcohol

 DIAGNOSIS

DIAGNOSTIC PROCEDURES

Erectile Dysfunction

- Depression must be ruled out
- Workup must differentiate between anatomic, endocrine, neurological, and psychological causes
- Even if an irreversible cause is identified, this knowledge may help the patient to accept the condition

Other conditions

- Clinical diagnosis

Sexual Dysfunction

 TREATMENT

MEDICATIONS

Erectile dysfunction

- Sildenafil (25–100 mg), vardenafil (2.5–20 mg), or tadalafil (5–20 mg) 1 h prior to intercourse) is useful
- Sildenafil, vardenafil, and tadalafil must not be used concurrently with nitrates due to a risk of hypotension leading to sudden death

Ejaculation disturbances

- SSRIs have been effective, due to their common effect in delaying ejaculation

THERAPEUTIC PROCEDURES

- Anxiety and guilt about parental injunctions against sex may contribute to sexual dysfunction

Erectile dysfunction

- The effect of this problem on relationships must be considered and addressed

Ejaculation disturbances

- Psychotherapy is best suited to cases where interpersonal or intrapsychic problems predominate
- A combined behavioral-psychological approach is most effective

Vaginismus

- Responds well to desensitization with graduated Hegar dilators along with relaxation techniques
- Masters and Johnson have used behavioral approaches in all of the sexual dysfunctions, with concomitant supportive psychotherapy and with improvement of the communication patterns of the couple

Frigidity

- Organic causes (conditions causing dyspareunia, pelvic pathology, mechanical obstruction, and neurological deficits) and contributing intrapersonal issues must be uncovered and addressed
- As with other psychosexual disorders, behavioral approaches with supportive psychotherapy and improved communication within couples can be effective

 OUTCOME

PREVENTION

- The proximity of other people (eg, mother-in-law) in a household is frequently an inhibiting factor in sexual relationships. Some social engineering may alleviate the problem

EVIDENCE

PRACTICE GUIDELINES

- National Guideline Clearinghouse http://www.guideline.gov/summary/summary.aspx?doc_id=3725&nbr=2951&string=sexual+dysfunction http://www.guideline.gov/summary/summary.aspx?doc_id=2577&nbr=1803&string=sexual+dysfunction

WEB SITE

- American Psychiatric Association http://www.psych.org/

INFORMATION FOR PATIENTS

- http://www.medem.com/MedLB/article_detaillb.cfm?article_ID=ZZZSAC20NAC&sub_cat=2
- American College of Obstetricians and Gynecologists http://www.medem.com/MedLB/article_detaillb.cfm?article_ID=ZZZ7P2WBT7C&sub_cat=2

INFORMATION FOR PATIENTS

- JAMA patient page: Sexual dysfunction. JAMA 1999;281:584.
- JAMA patient page: Sexual abuse. JAMA 1998;280:1888.

REFERENCES

- Boyce EG et al: Sildenafil citrate, a therapeutic update. Clin Ther 2001;23:2. [PMID: 11219477]
- Speckens AE et al: Psychosexual functioning of partners of men with presumed nonorganic erectile dysfunction: cause or consequence of the disorder? Arch Sex Behav 1995;24:157.

Stuart J. Eisendrath, MD
Jonathan E. Lichtmacher, MD

Sexually Transmitted Diseases

 KEY FEATURES

GENERAL CONSIDERATIONS

- The commonest sexually transmitted diseases are gonorrhea, syphilis, condyloma acuminatum, chlamydial genital infections, herpesvirus genital infections, *Trichomonas* vaginitis, chancroid, granuloma inguinale, scabies, louse infestation, and bacterial vaginosis (among lesbians)
- Shigellosis, hepatitis A, B, and C, amebiasis, giardiasis, cryptosporidiosis, salmonellosis, and campylobacteriosis may also be transmitted by sexual (oral–anal) contact, especially in homosexual males
- Homosexual contact is a typical method of transmission of HIV, though bidirectional heterosexual transmission is occurring more commonly
- In most infections caused by sexually tranmitted bacteria, spirochetes, chlamydiae, viruses, or protozoal agents, early lesions occur on genitalia or other sexually exposed mucous membranes; however, wide dissemination may occur, and involvement of nongenital tissues and organs may mimic many noninfectious disorders
- All sexually transmitted diseases have subclinical or latent phases that play an important role in long-term persistence of the infection or in its transmission from infected (but largely asymptomatic) persons to other contacts

Sexual assault

- The risk of developing a sexually transmitted disease following a sexual assault has not been established
- Victims of assault have a high baseline rate of infection (*Neisseria gonorrhoeae* 6%, *Chlamydia trachomatis* 10%, *Trichomonas vaginalis* 15%, and bacterial vaginosis 34%), and the risk of acquiring infection as a result of the assault is significant but is often lower than the preexisting rate (*N gonorrhoeae* 6–12%, *C trachomatis* 4–17%, *T vaginalis* 12%, syphilis 0.5–3%, and bacterial vaginosis 19%)
- Although seroconversion to HIV has been reported following sexual assault when this was the only known risk, this risk is felt to be low. The likelihood of HIV transmission from anal or vaginal receptive intercourse when the source is known to be HIV positive is 1–3 per 1000
- Victims should be evaluated within 24 h after the assault

 CLINICAL FINDINGS

SYMPTOMS AND SIGNS

- See individual diseases

 DIAGNOSIS

LABORATORY TESTS

- Simultaneous infection by several different agents is common, and any person with a sexually transmitted disease should be tested for syphilis; a repeat study should be done in 3 months if negative, since seroconversion is delayed after primary infection
- Laboratory examinations are of particular importance in the diagnosis of asymptomatic patients during the subclinical or latent phases of sexually transmitted diseases

Sexual assault

- Victims should be evaluated within 24 h after the assault and cultures for *N gonorrhoeae and C trachomatis* (if culture is not available, nonculture tests, such as nucleic acid amplification tests, are acceptable)
- If the test is positive, it must be confirmed with a second test using a different target sequence
- Vaginal secretions are cultured and examined for *Trichomonas*
- If a discharge is present, if there is itching, or if secretions are malodorous, a wet mount should be examined for *Candida* and bacterial vaginosis
- A blood sample should be obtained for immediate serological testing for syphilis, hepatitis B, and HIV

TREATMENT

MEDICATIONS

Sexual assault

- The usefulness of presumptive therapy is controversial
- If therapy is given, a reasonable regimen would be hepatitis B vaccination (without hepatitis B immune globulin, the first dose given at the initial evaluation and follow-up doses at 1–2 months and 4–6 months) and one dose of ceftriaxone, 125 mg intramuscularly, plus metronidazole, 2 g orally as a single dose, plus doxycycline, 100 mg orally twice daily for 7 days, or azithromycin, 1 g orally as a single dose. In premenopausal women, azithromycin should be used instead of doxycycline until the pregnancy status is determined; if the pregnancy test is positive, metronidazole should be given only after the first trimester
- Because prophylactic antiretroviral therapy for HIV has not been studied in this setting, firm recommendations cannot be made and the decision to institute therapy should be individualized. If therapy is given, it should be prompt, and certainly no later than 72 h

THERAPEUTIC PROCEDURES

- As a rule, sexual partners should be treated simultaneously to avoid prompt reinfection

 OUTCOME

FOLLOW-UP

Sexual assault

- Follow-up examination for sexually transmitted disease after an assault should be repeated within 1–2 weeks, since concentrations of infecting organisms may not have been sufficient to produce a positive culture at the time of initial examination
- If prophylactic treatment was given, tests should be repeated only if the victim has symptoms
- If prophylaxis was not administered, the individual should be seen in 1 week so that any positive tests can be treated
- Follow-up serological testing for syphilis and HIV infection should be performed in 6, 12, and 24 weeks if the initial tests are negative

 EVIDENCE

PRACTICE GUIDELINES

- Centers for Disease Control and Prevention: Sexually transmitted diseases treatment guidelines 2002. MMWR Recomm Rep 2002;51(RR-6):1. [PMID: 12184549]
- National Guideline Clearinghouse http://www.guideline.gov/summary/summary.aspx?doc_id=3242&nbr=2468&string=STDs

INFORMATION FOR PATIENTS

- National Institute of Allergy and Infectious Diseases http://www.niaid.nih.gov/factsheets/stdinfo.htm
- American Academy of Family Physicians http://familydoctor.org/healthfacts/165/

REFERENCE

- Bamberger JD: Post-exposure prophylaxis for human immunodeficiency virus (HIV) infection following sexual assault. Am J Med 1999;106:323-326. [PMID: 10190382]

Richard A. Jacobs, MD, PhD

Shigellosis

 KEY FEATURES

ESSENTIALS OF DIAGNOSIS

- Diarrhea, often with blood and mucus
- Crampy abdominal pain, high fevers, and systemic toxicity
- White blood cells in stools; organism isolated on stool culture

GENERAL CONSIDERATIONS

- *Shigella* dysentery is a common disease, often self-limited and mild but occasionally serious
- Food-borne illness
- *Shigella sonnei* is the leading cause in the United States, followed by *Shigella flexneri*
- *Shigella dysenteriae* causes the most severe form of the illness
- There has been a rise in strains resistant to multiple antibiotics

DEMOGRAPHICS

- Residence in or travel to a foreign country
- Men who have sex with men at higher risk
- Exposure to contaminated food, especially in outbreak setting
- Approximately 450,000 cases (mostly due to *S sonnei*) occur in the United States each year
- In the developing world, *S flexneri* predominates

 CLINICAL FINDINGS

SYMPTOMS AND SIGNS

- Table 126 (page 1308)
- The illness usually starts abruptly, with diarrhea, lower abdominal cramps, and tenesmus
- The diarrheal stool often is mixed with blood and mucus
- Systemic symptoms are fever, chills, anorexia and malaise, and headache
- The abdomen is tender
- Temporary disaccharidase deficiency may follow the diarrhea

DIFFERENTIAL DIAGNOSIS

- Invasive diarrhea due to other bacteria: *Salmonella*, *Campylobacter*, enteroinvasive *Escherichia coli*, *Yersinia enterocolitica*
- Amebic dysentery
- *Clostridium difficile* colitis
- Inflammatory bowel disease
- Viral gastroenteritis

 DIAGNOSIS

LABORATORY TESTS

- See Table 136 (page 1318)
- The stool shows many leukocytes and red cells
- Stool culture is positive for shigellae in most cases, but blood cultures grow the organism in less than 5% of cases

DIAGNOSTIC PROCEDURES

- Sigmoidoscopic examination reveals an inflamed, engorged mucosa with punctate, sometimes large areas of ulceration

TREATMENT

MEDICATIONS

- Ciprofloxacin (contraindicated in pregnancy), 500 mg twice daily or levofloxacin, 500 mg once daily for 3 days
- Trimethoprim-sulfamethoxazole, one double-strength tablet twice a day for 3 days (relegated to second-line therapy because of increasing drug resistance)
- Azithromycin, 500 mg on Day 1 then 250 mg daily for 4 days

THERAPEUTIC PROCEDURES

- Treatment of dehydration and hypotension is lifesaving in severe cases

 OUTCOME

COMPLICATIONS

- Temporary disaccharidase deficiency may follow the diarrhea
- Reactive arthritis (Reiter's) is an uncommon complication, usually occurring in HLA-B27 individuals infected by *Shigella*
- Hemolytic-uremic syndrome can occur after *S dysenteriae* type 1 infection

PROGNOSIS

- Complete recovery is the norm, although it may be several months before bowel habits are entirely normal

WHEN TO REFER

- If management consultation is needed

WHEN TO ADMIT

- Severe dehydration requiring parenteral fluid replacement

PREVENTION

- Wash hands with soap carefully and frequently, especially after going to the bathroom, after changing diapers, and before preparing foods or beverages
- Dispose of soiled diapers properly
- Disinfect diaper changing areas after using them
- Persons with diarrheal illness should not prepare food for others
- Travelers in the developing world should "boil it, cook it, peel it, or forget it"
- Avoid drinking pool water

 EVIDENCE

PRACTICE GUIDELINES

- National Guideline Clearinghouse http://www.guideline.gov/summary/ summary.aspx?doc_id=2791&nbr= 2017&string=diarrhea http://www.guideline.gov/summary/ summary.aspx?doc_id=2707&nbr=1933 &string=diarrhea

WEB SITES

- CDC—Division of Bacterial and Mycotic Diseases http://www.cdc.gov/ncidod/dbmd/
- Karolinska Institute—Directory of Bacterial Infections and Mycoses http://www.mic.ki.se/Diseases/c1.html

INFORMATION FOR PATIENTS

- JAMA patient page: Preventing dehydration from diarrhea. JAMA 2001; 185:362.
- JAMA patient page: Food-borne illnesses. JAMA 1999;281:1866. [PMID: 10340376]
- Centers for Disease Control http://www.cdc.gov/ncidod/dbmd/ diseaseinfo/ shigellosis_g.htm

REFERENCES

- Ashkenazi S et al: Growing antimicrobial resistance of *Shigella* isolates. J Antimicrob Chemother 2003;51:427. [PMID: 12562716]
- Khan WA et al: Treatment of shigellosis: V. Comparison of azithromycin and ciprofloxacin. A double-blind, randomized, controlled trial. Ann Intern Med 1997;126:697. [PMID: 9139555]

Henry F. Chambers, MD

Sickle Cell Anemia

 KEY FEATURES

ESSENTIALS OF DIAGNOSIS

- Irreversibly sickled cells on peripheral blood smear
- Positive family history and lifelong personal history of hemolytic anemia
- Recurrent painful episodes
- Hemoglobin S is major hemoglobin seen on electrophoresis

GENERAL CONSIDERATIONS

- Autosomal recessive disorder in which abnormal hemoglobin leads to chronic hemolytic anemia with numerous clinical consequences
- Single DNA base change leads to amino acid substitution of valine for glutamine in sixth position on β-globin chain
- Abnormal tetramer designated hemoglobin S can form polymers that damage red blood cell (RBC) membrane
- Polymer formation and early membrane damage reversible but with repeated sickling, RBCs damaged beyond repair and become irreversibly sickled
- Sickling increased by increased RBC hemoglobin S concentration, RBC dehydration, acidosis, and hypoxemia
- Sickling retarded markedly by hemoglobin F; high hemoglobin F levels associated with more benign course
- Patients with heterozygous genotype (hemoglobin AS) have sickle cell trait
- Acute painful episodes due vasoocclusion by sickled RBCs occur spontaneously or are provoked by infection, dehydration, or hypoxia

DEMOGRAPHICS

- Hemoglobin S gene carried in 8% of African-Americans
- Sickle cell anemia occurs in 1 birth in 400 in African-Americans
- Onset during first year of life, when hemoglobin F levels fall

 CLINICAL FINDINGS

SYMPTOMS AND SIGNS

- Chronic hemolytic anemia produces jaundice, pigment (calcium bilirubinate) gallstones, splenomegaly, and poorly healing ulcers over the lower tibia
- Anemia may be life-threatening during hemolytic or aplastic crises
- Hemolytic crises result from splenic sequestration of sickled cells (primarily in childhood, before spleen has infarcted) or with coexistent disorders such as glucose-6-phosphate dehydrogenase deficiency
- Aplastic crises occur when bone marrow compensation is reduced by infection or folate deficiency
- Acute painful episodes, commonly in bones and chest, last hours to days and produce low-grade fever
- Acute vasoocclusion may cause priapism and strokes due to sinus thrombosis
- Repeated vasoocclusion affects heart (cardiomegaly, hyperdynamic precordium, systolic murmurs); liver; bone (ischemic necrosis, staphylococcal or salmonella osteomyelitis); spleen (infarction, asplenia); and kidney (infarction of renal medullary papillae, renal tubular concentrating defects, and gross hematuria)
- Retinopathy, blindness
- Increased susceptibility to infection due to hyposplenism, complement defects
- Hepatomegaly, nonpalpable spleen in adults
- Sickle cell trait: most often, no symptoms or signs; acute vasoocclusion occurs only under extreme conditions
- May have episodes of gross hematuria or renal tubular defect causing inability to concentrate urine

DIFFERENTIAL DIAGNOSIS

- Other sickle cell syndromes: sickle cell trait, sickle thalassemia, or hemoglobin SC disease
- Osteomyelitis
- Hematuria due to other cause
- Acute rheumatic fever
- Gaucher's disease (bone pain crises)

 DIAGNOSIS

LABORATORY TESTS

- Serum indirect bilirubin, LDH, elevated; serum haptoglobin low
- Hematocrit usually 20–30%
- Reticulocyte count elevated
- Peripheral blood smear: irreversibly sickled cells comprise 5–50% of RBCs; reticulocytosis (10–25%); nucleated RBCs; Howell-Jolly bodies and target cells
- White blood cell count characteristically elevated to 12,000–15,000/μL; thrombocytosis may occur
- Screening test for sickle hemoglobin positive
- Hemoglobin electrophoresis confirms diagnosis
- Sickle cell anemia (homozygous S): hemoglobin S usually comprises 85–98% of hemoglobin and no hemoglobin A is present; hemoglobin F levels variably increased
- Sickle cell trait: complete blood cell count and peripheral blood smear normal; hemoglobin electrophoresis shows that hemoglobin S comprises ~40% of hemoglobin

IMAGING STUDIES

- Chest x-ray in acute chest syndrome
- Bone x-rays show characteristic abnormalities
- CT shows hepatomegaly and absence of spleen

TREATMENT

 OUTCOME

 EVIDENCE

MEDICATIONS

- Folic acid, 1 mg PO QD
- Hydroxyurea, 500–750 mg PO QD, increases hemoglobin F levels and reduces frequency of painful crises in patients whose quality of life is disrupted by frequent pain crises; long-term safety uncertain, concern exists about potential for secondary malignancies

THERAPEUTIC PROCEDURES

- Prenatal diagnosis and genetic counseling should be made available to those with personal or family history
- No specific treatment is available for sickle cell anemia
- Pneumococcal vaccination reduces incidence of infections
- Acute painful episodes: identify precipitating factors and treat infections if present; maintain good hydration, and administer oxygen if hypoxic
- Sickle cell trait: no treatment necessary; genetic counseling appropriate
- Transfusions for aplastic or hemolytic crises
- Exchange transfusion primarily indicated for treatment of intractable pain crises, priapism, and stroke
- Allogeneic bone marrow transplantation under investigation as possible curative option for severely affected young patients

COMPLICATIONS

- Sickle cell anemia becomes a chronic multisystem disease, with death from organ failure
- Acute chest syndrome

PROGNOSIS

- With improved supportive care, average life expectancy is now between ages 40 and 50

PRACTICE GUIDELINES

- Ballas SK: Sickle cell anaemia: progress in pathogenesis and treatment. Drugs 2002;62:1143. [PMID: 12010077]
- Ballas SK: Sickle cell disease: current clinical management. Semin Hematol 2001;38:307. [PMID: 11605165]
- Rees DC et al: General Haematology Task Force by the Sickle Cell Working Party. Guidelines for the management of the acute painful crisis in sickle cell disease. Br J Haematol 2003;120:744. [PMID: 12614204]

WEB SITES

- Georgia Comprehensive Sickle Cell Center at Grady Health System http://www.scinfo.org/
- MEDLINEplus—Sickle cell anemia http://www.nlm.nih.gov/medlineplus/ency/article/000527.htm

INFORMATION FOR PATIENTS

- Mayo Clinic—Sickle cell anemia http://www.mayoclinic.com/invoke.cfm?id=DS00324
- Nemours Foundation http://kidshealth.org/parent/medical/heart/sickle_cell_anemia.html

REFERENCES

- Vichinsky EP et al: Causes and outcomes of the acute chest syndrome in sickle cell disease. National Acute Chest Syndrome Study Group. N Engl J Med 2000;342:1855. [PMID: 10861320]
- Walters MC et al: Impact of bone marrow transplantation for symptomatic sickle cell disease: an interim report. Blood 2000;95:1918. [PMID: 10706855]

Charles A. Linker, MD

Sinusitis, Acute

 KEY FEATURES

ESSENTIALS OF DIAGNOSIS

- Pain is usually unilateral over the maxillary sinus or toothache-like
- Symptoms usually last for more than a week
- Change of secretions from mucoid to purulent green or yellow
- Occasional visible swelling or erythema over a sinus

GENERAL CONSIDERATIONS

- Diseases that swell the nasal mucous membrane, such as viral or allergic rhinitis, are usually the underlying cause
- Usually is a result of impaired mucociliary clearance and obstruction of the osteomeatal complex, resulting in the accumulation of mucous secretion in the sinus cavity that becomes secondarily infected by bacteria
- The typical pathogens are the same as those that cause acute otitis media: *Streptococcus pneumoniae*, other streptococci, *Haemophilus influenzae*, and, less commonly, *Staphylococcus aureus* and *Moraxella catarrhalis*
- About 25% of healthy asymptomatic individuals may, if sinus aspirates are cultured, harbor these bacteria
- Discolored nasal discharge and poor response to decongestants suggest sinusitis

DEMOGRAPHICS

- Uncommon compared with viral rhinitis, but still affects over 14% of the population
- The prevalence of nosocomial sinusitis is as high as 40% in critically ill intubated patients

 CLINICAL FINDINGS

SYMPTOMS AND SIGNS

- Maxillary sinusitis
  - Pain and pressure over the cheek
  - Pain may refer to the upper incisor and canine teeth
  - May result from dental infection, and tender teeth should be carefully examined for abscess
- Ethmoid sinusitis
  - Usually accompanied by maxillary sinusitis; the symptoms of maxillary sinusitis generally predominate
  - Pain and pressure over the high lateral wall of the nose that may radiate to the orbit
  - Periorbital cellulitis may be present
- Sphenoid sinusitis
  - Usually seen in the setting of pansinusitis
  - The patient may complain of a headache "in the middle of the head" and often points to the vertex
  - Sixth nerve palsy may occur as the abducens nerve courses just lateral to the sinus
- Frontal sinusitis
  - Usually pain and tenderness of the forehead
  - This is most easily elicited by palpation of the orbital roof just below the medial end of the eyebrow
  - Palpation here is more accurate than percussion of the supraorbital area or forehead

DIFFERENTIAL DIAGNOSIS

- Upper respiratory tract infection
- Viral rhinitis
- Allergic rhinitis
- Nasal polyposis
- Dental abscess
- Rhinocerebral mucormycosis
- Otitis media
- Pharyngitis
- Dacryocystitis
- Paranasal sinus cancer

 DIAGNOSIS

LABORATORY TESTS

- It is usually possible to make the diagnosis on clinical grounds alone

IMAGING STUDIES

- Routine radiographs are not cost effective; they may be helpful when clinically based criteria are difficult to evaluate
  - Sinus x-rays can show soft tissue density without bone destruction
  - An air-fluid level may also be seen
- Coronal CT scans are reasonably sensitive, but not specific; sinus abnormalities can be seen in the majority of patients with an upper respiratory tract infection, while only 2% develop bacterial sinusitis
- Sinusitis is a clinical diagnosis for which CT may be helpful in confirming, denying, or monitoring

Sinusitis, Acute

 TREATMENT

MEDICATIONS

- Antibiotic use is the most cost-effective treatment
- For symptom improvement, use oral or nasal decongestants (or both)—eg, oral pseudoephedrine, 30–120 mg per dose, up to 240 mg/day; nasal oxymetazoline, 0.05%, or xylometazoline, 0.05–0.1%, one or two sprays in each nostril every 6–8 h for up to 3 days
- Amoxicillin (500 mg orally three times a day), possibly with clavulanate (125 mg three times a day)
- Trimethoprim-sulfamethoxazole (TMP-SMZ 4 mg/kg TMP and 20 mg/kg SMZ twice daily; available as tablets with 80 or 160 mg TMP and 160 or 800 mg SMZ)
- Cephalexin (250–500 mg orally four times a day)
- Cefuroxime (250 mg orally twice daily)
- Cefaclor (250 mg orally three times a day)
- Cefixime (400 mg orally daily)
- Quinolones, such as ciprofloxacin (500 mg twice daily), levofloxacin (500 mg once daily), moxifloxacin (400 mg once daily), and sparfloxacin (200 mg once daily after an initial dose of 400 mg)
- Macrolides, such as azithromycin (500 mg once daily, possibly for only 3 days) or clarithromycin (500 mg orally twice daily, for 14 days)

 OUTCOME

COMPLICATIONS

- Mucocele; treatment is surgical
- Osteomyelitis requires prolonged antibiotics as well as removal of necrotic bone; the frontal sinus is most commonly affected, with bone involvement suggested by a tender puffy swelling of the forehead
- Cavernous sinus thrombosis
- Meningitis
- Epidural and intraparenchymal brain abscesses

PROGNOSIS

- Two-thirds of untreated patients will improve symptomatically within 2 weeks

WHEN TO REFER

- Recurrent sinusitis or sinusitis that does not appear to respond clinically warrants evaluation by a specialist
- Any complication of sinusitis

 EVIDENCE

PRACTICE GUIDELINES

- Antimicrobial treatment guidelines for acute bacterial rhinosinusitis. Sinus and Allergy Health Partnership. Otolaryngol Head Neck Surg 2000;123(1 Part 2):5. [PMID: 10887346]
- Benninger MS et al: Diagnosis and treatment of uncomplicated acute bacterial rhinosinusitis: summary of the Agency for Health Care Policy and Research evidence-based report. Otolaryngol Head Neck Surg 2000; 122:1. [PMID: 10629474]
- Brooks I et al: Medical management of acute bacterial sinusitis. Recommendations of a clinical advisory committee on pediatric and adult sinusitis. Ann Otol Rhinol Laryngol 2000; 182(Suppl):2. [PMID: 10823486]

WEB SITES

- Ear, Nose, and Throat Information Center http://www.netdoor.com/entinfo/
- Otolaryngology Resources on the Internet http://www.bcm.tmc.edu/oto/othersa.html

INFORMATION FOR PATIENTS

- Sinusitis, NIAID Fact Sheet http://www.niaid.nih.gov/factsheets/sinusitis.htm
- American Academy of Family Physicians http://familydoctor.org/handouts/686.html

REFERENCES

- Gwaltney JM Jr: Acute community acquired bacterial sinusitis: to treat or not to treat. Can Respir J 1999;6(Suppl A):46A. [PMID: 10202234]
- Piccirillo JF et al: Impact of first-line vs second-line antibiotics for the treatment of acute uncomplicated sinusitis. JAMA 2001;286:1849. [PMID: 11597286]
- Williams JW Jr et al: Antibiotics for acute maxillary sinusitis. Cochrane Database Syst Rev 2000:CD000243. [PMID: 10796515]

Robert K. Jackler, MD
Michael J. Kaplan, MD

Sjögren's Syndrome

 KEY FEATURES

ESSENTIALS OF DIAGNOSIS

- Dryness of eyes and dry mouth (sicca components) are the most common features; they occur alone or in association with rheumatoid arthritis or other connective tissue disease
- Rheumatoid factor and other autoantibodies common
- Increased incidence of lymphoma

GENERAL CONSIDERATIONS

- Chronic autoimmune dysfunction of exocrine glands in many areas of the body
- Dryness of the eyes, mouth, and other areas covered by mucous membranes
- Frequently associated with a rheumatic disease, most often rheumatoid arthritis
- Also associated with systemic lupus erythematosus (SLE), primary biliary cirrhosis, scleroderma, polymyositis, Hashimoto's thyroiditis, polyarteritis, and interstitial pulmonary fibrosis
- Keratoconjunctivitis sicca results from inadequate tear production caused by lymphocyte and plasma cell infiltration of the lacrimal glands

Associated conditions

- Rheumatoid arthritis
- SLE
- Primary biliary cirrhosis
- Scleroderma
- Polymyositis
- Hashimoto's thyroiditis
- Polyarteritis nodosa
- Idiopathic pulmonary fibrosis

DEMOGRAPHICS

- The disorder is predominantly a disease of women, in a ratio of 9:1
- Greatest incidence between age 40 and 60 years

 CLINICAL FINDINGS

SYMPTOMS AND SIGNS

- Ocular burning, itching, ropy secretions, and impaired tear production during crying
- Parotid enlargement, which may be chronic or relapsing, develops in one-third of patients
- Dryness of the mouth (xerostomia) leads to difficulty in speaking and swallowing and to severe dental caries
- There may be loss of taste and smell
- Systemic manifestations include dysphagia, pancreatitis, pleuritis, obstructive lung disease (in the absence of smoking), neuropsychiatric dysfunction, and vasculitis
- Renal tubular acidosis (type I, distal) occurs in 20% of patients. Chronic interstitial nephritis, which may result in impaired renal function, may be seen

DIFFERENTIAL DIAGNOSIS

- Sicca complex associated with other autoimmune disease, eg, sarcoidosis, rheumatoid arthritis, SLE, scleroderma
- Other causes of dry mouth or eyes, eg, anticholinergics, mumps, irradiation, seasonal allergies, irritation from smoking

 DIAGNOSIS

LABORATORY TESTS

- Rheumatoid factor is found in 70% of patients
- Antibodies against the cytoplasmic antigens SS-A and SS-B (also called Ro and La, respectively) are often present (Tables 73 and 79, pages 1265 and 1267)
- When SS-A antibodies are present, extraglandular manifestations are far more common.

DIAGNOSTIC PROCEDURES

- Lip biopsy is the only specific diagnostic technique and has minimal risk; if lymphoid foci are seen in accessory salivary glands, the diagnosis is confirmed
- Biopsy of the parotid gland should be reserved for patients with atypical presentations such as unilateral gland enlargement
- The Schirmer test, which measures the quantity of tears secreted

TREATMENT

MEDICATIONS

- Pilocarpine (5 mg four times daily) and the acetylcholine derivative cevimeline (30 mg three times daily) are helpful for severe xerostomia
- Atropinic drugs and decongestants decrease salivary secretions and should be avoided

THERAPEUTIC PROCEDURES

- Treatment is symptomatic and supportive
- Artificial tears applied frequently will relieve ocular symptoms and avert further desiccation
- Sipping water frequently or using sugar-free gums and hard candies usually relieves dry mouth symptoms
- A program of oral hygiene is essential in order to preserve dentition

 ## OUTCOME

COMPLICATIONS

- A spectrum of lymphoproliferation ranging from benign to malignant may be found
- Malignant lymphomas and Waldenström's macroglobulinemia occur nearly 50 times more frequently than can be explained by chance alone in primary Sjögren's syndrome

PROGNOSIS

- Usually benign and consistent with a normal life span
- Prognosis is mainly influenced by the nature of the associated disease
- The patients (3–10% of the total Sjögren's population) at greatest risk of developing lymphoma have severe dryness, marked parotid gland enlargement, splenomegaly, vasculitis, peripheral neuropathy, anemia, and mixed monoclonal cryoglobulinemia

 ## EVIDENCE

PRACTICE GUIDELINES

- Johns Hopkins University http://www.hopkins-arthritis.som.jhmi.edu/edu/acr/acr.html#sjogrens

Information for PATIENTs

- National Institute of Arthritis and Musculoskeletal and Skin Diseases http://www.niams.nih.gov/hi/topics/sjogrens/index.htm
- National Institute of Neurological Disorders and Stroke http://www.ninds.nih.gov/health_and_medical/disorders/sjogrens_doc.htm

REFERENCES

- Carsons S: A review and update of Sjögren's syndrome: manifestations, diagnosis, and treatment. Am J Manag Care 2001;7(14 Suppl):S433. [PMID: 11605978]
- Fox RI et al: Use of muscarinic agonists in the treatment of Sjögren's syndrome. Clin Immunol 2001;101:249.
- Garcia-Carrasco M: Primary Sjögren syndrome: clinical and immunologic disease patterns in a cohort of 400 patients. Medicine 2002;81:270. [PMID: 12169882]
- Ramos-Casals M: Primary Sjögren syndrome: hematologic patterns of disease expression. Medicine 2002;81:281. [PMID: 12169883]

David B. Hellmann, MD, FACP
John H. Stone, MD, MPH

Sleep Apnea, Obstructive

 KEY FEATURES

ESSENTIALS OF DIAGNOSIS

- Daytime somnolence or fatigue
- A history of loud snoring with witnessed apneic events
- Overnight polysomnography demonstrates apneic episodes with hypoxemia

GENERAL CONSIDERATIONS

- Upper airway obstruction results from a loss of pharyngeal muscle tone during sleep
- Patients with narrowed upper airways are predisposed to the condition
- Ingestion of alcohol or sedatives before sleep and nasal obstruction from any cause may precipitate or worsen the condition
- Cigarette smoking and hypothyroidism are risk factors

DEMOGRAPHICS

- Most patients are obese, middle-aged men

 CLINICAL FINDINGS

SYMPTOMS AND SIGNS

- Patients complain of daytime somnolence or fatigue, morning sluggishness, or cognitive impairment
- Recent weight gain, headaches, and impotence may be present
- Bed partners usually report loud cyclical snoring and witnessed apneas with restlessness and thrashing movements during sleep
- Systemic hypertension is usually present
- Physical examination may show evidence of pulmonary hypertension with cor pulmonale
- Oropharyngeal narrowing due to excessive soft tissue may be seen
- A short, thick neck is common
- Bradyarrhythmias may occur during sleep
- Tachyarrhythmias may be seen once airflow is reestablished following an apneic episode

DIFFERENTIAL DIAGNOSIS

- Central sleep apnea
- Mixed sleep apnea
- Obesity-hypoventilation syndrome (Pickwickian syndrome)
- Narcolepsy
- Alcohol or sedative abuse
- Depression
- Hypothyroidism
- Seizure disorder

 DIAGNOSIS

LABORATORY TESTS

- Erythrocytosis is common
- Thyroid-stimulating hormone should be checked

DIAGNOSTIC PROCEDURES

- Overnight polysomnography is essential to make the diagnosis
- Apneic episodes are defined as breath cessation for 10 s or more
- Hypopnea is defined as a decrement in airflow with a drop in oxyhemoglobin saturation of 4% or more
- An otolaryngological examination should be performed
- Screening with home nocturnal pulse oximetry has a high negative predictive value if no desaturations are seen

Sleep Apnea, Obstructive

 TREATMENT

MEDICATIONS

- Pharmacological therapy is not successful

SURGERY

- Uvulopalatopharyngoplasty, the resection of pharyngeal tissue and removal of a portion of the soft palate and uvula, is helpful in approximately half of selected patients
- Nasal septoplasty is performed if gross nasal septal deformity is present
- Tracheostomy is the definitive therapy, but is reserved for life-threatening, refractory cases

THERAPEUTIC PROCEDURES

- Weight loss and avoidance of alcohol and hypotic medications are initial steps
- 10–20% weight loss may be curative
- Nasal continuous positive airway pressure (CPAP) is curative in many patients
- Polysomnography is often necessary to determine the level of CPAP (usually 5–15 mm Hg) required
- Prosthetic devices inserted into the mouth to prevent pharyngeal occlusion can be modestly effective, but compliance is limiting

 OUTCOME

COMPLICATIONS

- Cor pulmonale
- Life-threatening cardiac arrhythmias
- Systemic hypertension

PROGNOSIS

- Only 75% of patients continue to use CPAP after 1 year

WHEN TO REFER

- For a sleep study

 EVIDENCE

PRACTICE GUIDELINES

- National Guideline Clearinghouse http://www.guideline.gov/summary/summary.aspx?doc_id=3181&nbr=2407&string=obstructive+sleep+apnea

  http://www.guideline.gov/summary/summary.aspx?doc_id=2932&nbr=2158&string=obstructive+sleep+apnea

INFORMATION FOR PATIENTS

- National Institute of Neurological Disorders and Stroke http://www.ninds.nih.gov/health_and_medical/disorders/sleep_apnea.htm
- American Medical Association http://www.medem.com/medlb/article_detaillb.cfm?article_ID=ZZZWT155MNC&sub_cat=593

REFERENCES

- Exar EN et al: The upper airway resistance syndrome. Chest 1999;115:1127. [PMID: 10208219]
- Fogel RB et al: Obstructive sleep apnea. Adv Intern Med 2000;45:351. [PMID: 10635055]
- Garrigue S et al: Benefit of atrial pacing in sleep apnea syndrome. N Engl J Med 2002;346:404. [PMID: 11832528]
- Wright J et al: Continuous positive airways pressure for obstructive sleep apnea. Cochrane Database Syst Rev 2000;2:CD001106. [PMID: 10796595]
- Yap WS et al: Central sleep apnea and hypoventilation syndrome. Curr Treat Options Neurol 2001;3:51. [PMID: 11123858]

Mark S. Chesnutt, MD
Thomas J. Prendergast, MD

Small Intestinal Neoplasms

 KEY FEATURES

ESSENTIALS OF DIAGNOSIS

- Acute gastrointestinal bleeding with hematochezia or melena or chronic gastrointestinal blood loss resulting in fatigue and iron deficiency anemia

GENERAL CONSIDERATIONS

- Benign and malignant tumors of the small intestine are rare
- Often no symptoms or signs
- Obstruction due to luminal narrowing or intussusception
- Benign tumors include single or multiple polyps, lipomas, benign stromal tumors (leiomyomas)
- Villous adenomas occur most commonly in the periampullary region of the duodenum and carry a high risk for invasive cancer
- Malignant small bowel tumors are extremely rare
- Adenocarcinoma occurs most commonly in the duodenum or proximal jejunum
- Ampullary carcinoma incidence is increased >200-fold in patients with familial adenomatous polyposis
- Nonampullary adenocarcinoma of the small intestine: 80% have metastasized at the time of diagnosis
- Lymphoma may arise primarily in the gastrointestinal tract or involve it secondarily in disseminated disease
- In the United States, primary lymphoma accounts for 5% of all lymphomas and 20% of small bowel malignancies
- Lymphoma occurs most commonly in the distal small intestine
- Majority are non-Hodgkin's intermediate or high-grade B cell lymphomas; T cell lymphomas occur in celiac sprue
- In the Middle East, lymphomas occur in immunoproliferative small intestinal disease
- Carcinoid tumors account for one-third of small intestinal tumors; >95% of gastrointestinal carcinoids occur in the rectum, appendix, or small intestine (especially ileum)
- Carcinoid tumors derive from neuroendocrine cells and secrete serotonin or its precursors
- Most are malignant, though many behave in an indolent fashion
- Even small carcinoid tumors may metastasize, usually extension to the local lymph nodes and to the liver
- Carcinoid syndrome occurs in <10% of patients and only in patients with hepatic metastasis; caused by tumor secretion of hormonal mediators

DEMOGRAPHICS

- Multiple small bowel polyps may suggest intestinal polypsis syndrome
- Hamartomas: Peutz-Jeghers syndrome, juvenile polypsis
- Adenomas or periampullary adenoma: familial adenomatous polypsis

 CLINICAL FINDINGS

SYMPTOMS AND SIGNS

- Benign stromal tumors: most are asymptomatic, some may ulcerate and cause acute or chronic bleeding or obstruction
- Malignant small bowel tumors: anemia, bleeding, obstruction, or evidence of metastatic disease
- Nonampullary adenocarcinoma of the small intestine: obstruction, acute or chronic bleeding, or weight loss
- Ampullary carcinoma: jaundice due to bile duct obstruction or bleeding
- Primary lymphoma: abdominal pain, weight loss, nausea and vomiting, distension, anemia, and occult blood in the stool
- Carcinoid tumors: most asymptomatic; if symptomatic, usually with carcinoid syndrome with cramps, flushing, diarrhea, cyanosis, or bronchospasm, cardiac right-sided valvular lesions; intussusception with obstruction rare

DIFFERENTIAL DIAGNOSIS

- Crohn's disease

Benign polyps

- Mucosal polyps: adenomas, hamartomas, hyperplastic
- Lipoma
- Benign stromal tumor (leiomyoma)

Malignant lesions

- Adenocarcinoma
- Lymphoma (primary or secondary)
- Carcinoid
- Malignant stromal tumor (leiomyosarcoma)
- Kaposi's sarcoma

 DIAGNOSIS

LABORATORY TESTS

- Alpha heavy chains in the serum in 70% of patients with lymphoma occurring in immunoproliferative small intestinal disease
- Hypoalbuminemia secondary to protein-losing enteropathy in lymphoma
- Urinary 5-hydroxyindoleacetic acid >10 mg/24 h and serum serotonin elevated in carcinoid tumors

IMAGING STUDIES

- Barium radiographic studies, either enteroclysis or a small bowel series, for diagnosis or small bowel tumors, primary lymphoma
- Chest and abdominal CT help to determine stage of primary lymphoma
- Abdominal CT for carcinoid tumors, hepatic metastases
- Somatostatin receptor scintigraphy positive in >90% of hepatic metastases from carcinoid tumors
- Echocardiogram for carcinoid heart disease

DIAGNOSTIC PROCEDURES

- Enteroscopy to visualize and biopsy small intestinal tumors
- Endoscopic, percutaneous, or laparoscopic biopsy establishes the diagnosis of primary intestinal lymphoma
- Bone marrow biopsy, and, in some cases, lymphangiography for staging of primary lymphoma
- Proctoscopy: rectal carcinoids usually detected incidentally as submucosal nodules usually <1 cm in size during proctoscopy
- Appendectomy: appendiceal carcinoids <2 cm in size are identified in 0.3%

TREATMENT

MEDICATIONS

- Role of adjuvant chemotherapy in primary lymphoma is unclear
- Systemic chemotherapy with or without radiation therapy for primary lymphoma with extensive disease
- Octreotide, 150–500 μg subcutaneously three times daily, inhibits serotonin secretion, providing dramatic relief of symptoms in 90% for a median period of 1 year

SURGERY

- Surgical or endoscopic excision of benign tumors recommended
- Surgical excision of benign stromal tumors
- Surgical resection of ampullary carcinoma is curative in up to 40%
- Resection of nonampullary adenocarcinoma for control of symptoms
- Resection of primary intestinal lymphoma for stage IE disease
- Surgical debulking for stage III or IV disease
- Local excision or simple appendectomy for carcinoid tumors for palliation of obstructive symptoms
- More extensive cancer resection operation is warranted for carcinoid tumors >2 cm in size since they are associated with metastasis in >20% of appendiceal and ~10% of rectal carcinoids
- Resection of hepatic metastases for refractory carcinoid syndrome, diarrhea

THERAPEUTIC PROCEDURES

- Hepatic artery occlusion and chemotherapy in hepatic metastases

OUTCOME

FOLLOW-UP

- Periodic surveillance of periampullary region villous adenomas by endoscopic retrograde cholangiopancreatography or endoscopic ultrasound

COMPLICATIONS

- Cardiac right-sided valvular lesions are a late manifestation of metastatic carcinoid tumors

PROGNOSIS

- Carcinoid tumors: overall 5-year survival rate is 50%
- Carcinoid tumors: for disease confined to the small intestine, local excision cures >85%; for resectable disease with lymph node involvement, 5-year disease-free survival is 80%, but by 25 years, only 25% are disease free

EVIDENCE

PRACTICE GUIDELINES

- De Franco A et al: Imaging of small bowel tumors. Rays 2002;27:35. [PMID: 12696273]
- Kariv R et al: Malignant tumors of the small intestine—new insights into a rare disease. Isr Med Assoc J 2003;5:188. [PMID: 12725140]
- Miettinen M et al: Gastrointestinal stromal tumors (GISTs): definition, occurrence, pathology, differential diagnosis and molecular genetics. Pol J Pathol 2003;54:3. [PMID: 12817876]

WEB SITES

- MEDLINEplus—Small bowel resection http://www.nlm.nih.gov/medlineplus/ency/article/002943.htm
- National Cancer Institute—Small intestine cancer http://www.cancer.gov/cancerinfo/pdq/treatment/smallintestine/patient
- University of Alabama—Intestinal Neoplasms http://cchs-dl.slis.ua.edu/clinical/oncology/gastrointestinal/instestinal.html

INFORMATION FOR PATIENTS

- Cleveland Clinic—Small intestine cancer http://www.clevelandclinic.org/health/health-info/docs/1400/1446.asp?index=6225
- Columbia University of Physicians and Surgeons—Gastrointestinal cancers http://cpmcnet.columbia.edu/texts/guide/hmg17_0010.html#17.35

REFERENCES

- Gill S et al: Small intestinal neoplasms. J Clin Gastroenterol 2001;33:267. [PMID: 11588539]
- Kulke M et al: Carcinoid tumors. N Engl J Med 1999;340:858. [PMID: 10080850]

Kenneth R. McQuaid, MD

Smallpox & Vaccinia

 KEY FEATURES

ESSENTIALS OF DIAGNOSIS

- Prodromal high fever
- Eruption progressing from papules to vesicles to pustules, then crusts
- All lesions in the same stage
- Face and distal extremities (including palms and soles) favored

GENERAL CONSIDERATIONS

- Reintroduction of vaccination for first-responder and military population because of bioterrorist threat
- The incubation period for smallpox averages 12 days (7–17 days)
- Immunization with vaccinia is not recommended for persons with eczema, in whom widespread vaccinia (eczema vaccinatum) may result, with lesions resembling those of smallpox
- Exposure to a recently vaccinated person may lead to generalized disease in persons with certain skin diseases
- Prior vaccination does not prevent generalized vaccinia, but previously vaccinated individuals have milder disease
- Progression of the primary inoculation site to a large ulceration occurs in persons with systemic immune deficiency, with a possible fatal outcome

 CLINICAL FINDINGS

SYMPTOMS AND SIGNS

- See Table 7 (page 1202)

Smallpox

- **Prodrome:** abrupt onset of high fever, severe headaches, and backaches, with the infected person appearing quite ill
- **Infectious phase:** appearance of an enanthem, followed in 1–2 days by a skin eruption
  - Lesions begin as macules, progressing to papules, then pustules, and finally crusts over 14–18 days
  - The face is affected first, followed by the upper extremities, the lower extremities, and trunk, completely evolving over 1 week
  - Lesions are relatively monomorphous, especially in each anatomic region
- All lesions in same stage of development differentiates rash from varicella

Vaccinia

- Inoculation with vaccinia produces a papular lesion on day 2–3 that progresses to an umbilicated papule by day 4 and a pustular lesion by the end of the first week
- The lesion collapses centrally, and crusts, with the crust eventually detaching up to a month after the inoculation

DIFFERENTIAL DIAGNOSIS

- Generalized varicella zoster virus (VZV) infection
- Generalized herpes simplex virus (HSV)

 DIAGNOSIS

LABORATORY TESTS

- Direct fluorescent antibody testing for HSV and VZV are first-line diagnostic tests to differentiate VZV, HSV, vaccinia, and smallpox
- Smallpox is a clinical diagnosis but viral infection can be confirmed by electron microscopy, antigen detection, and PCR

TREATMENT

MEDICATIONS

- No specific and proven antiviral therapy for vaccinia or smallpox
- Vaccinia immune globulin is used to treat eczema vaccinatum and progressive vaccinia
- Cidofovir may have some activity against these poxviruses

THERAPEUTIC PROCEDURES

- Strict respiratory and contact isolation crucial
- Patient should be immunized if in early stage of disease
- No antiviral therapy clearly effective
- Supportive care critical
- CDC should be contacted immediately in the event of suspect case(s)

OUTCOME

COMPLICATIONS

- Serious complications in about 5/100,000 persons include encephalitis, progressive vaccinia, and eczema vaccinatum

PROGNOSIS

- Generalized vaccinia may be fatal

WHEN TO ADMIT

- Until the diagnosis is confirmed, strict isolation of the patient is indicated

PREVENTION

- U.S. vaccination campaign voluntary, focusing on first responders and military personnel

EVIDENCE

WEB SITES

- Centers for Disease Control: Anthrax and other bioterrorism-related issues http://www.bt.cdc.gov/
- American Academy of Dermatology http://www.aad.org
- Dermatology Handbook for Family Practice from the University of Iowa http://www.vh.org/Providers/ClinRef/FPHandbook/17.html

INFORMATION FOR PATIENTS

- American Academy of Dermatology http://www.aad.org/pamphlets/

REFERENCES

- Breman J et al: Diagnosis and management of smallpox. N Engl J Med 2002; 346:1300. [PMID: 11923491]
- Mack T: A different view of smallpox and vaccination. N Engl J Med 2003; 348:460. [PMID: 12496354]
- Sepkowitz K: How contagious is vaccinia? N Engl J Med 2003;348:439. [PMID: 12496351]

Timothy G. Berger, MD

Somatoform Disorders

 ## KEY FEATURES

ESSENTIALS OF DIAGNOSIS

- Physical symptoms involving one or more organ systems
- Symptoms are not intentional
- Subjective complaints exceed objective findings
- Correlation between symptom development and psychosocial stress

GENERAL CONSIDERATIONS

- This diagnostic grouping includes conversion disorder, somatization disorder, pain disorder associated with psychological factors, and hypochondriasis
- It is difficult to discern whether the psychosocial distress seen in these conditions has caused or is the result of a chronic disease
- Vulnerability in an organ system and exposure to family members with somatization problems are thought to interact in the development of symptoms

DEMOGRAPHICS

- *Conversion disorder* is more common in lower socioeconomic classes and certain cultures
- *Somatization disorder* usually occurs before age 30 and is 10 times more common in women

 ## CLINICAL FINDINGS

SYMPTOMS AND SIGNS

- A precipitating emotional event often precedes somatic symptoms
- In *conversion disorder*, psychic conflict is converted into physical symptoms. The somatic symptom is typically paralysis, and the affected organ system may have symbolic meaning (eg, arm paralysis in marked anger)
- In *somatization disorder*, multiple physical complaints are referable to several organ systems. Anxiety, panic disorder, and depression are often present. Preoccupation with medical and surgical issues often precludes other life activities. Patients have often undergone multiple surgeries and have evidence of long-standing symptoms. Multiple symptoms that frequently change and have eluded diagnosis by three or more physicians support this diagnosis
- In *pain disorder associated with psychological factors*, patients have a long history of complaints of severe pain not consonant with anatomic and clinical signs. Exacerbations and remission of complaints correlate with psychogenic factors
- Patients with *hypochondriasis* have a fear of disease and preoccupation with the body. They exhibit perceptual amplification and heightened responsiveness. Family members who served as a role model for hypochondriacal behavior may be a clue to the diagnosis

DIFFERENTIAL DIAGNOSIS

- *Depression* must be considered in any patient with a condition judged to be somatoform
- *Factitious disorders*, which differ from this grouping in that symptom production is intentional
- Intoxication states

 ## DIAGNOSIS

DIAGNOSTIC PROCEDURES

- In *conversion disorder* with pseudo-seizures, video-EEG may be necessary to rule out epilepsy
- Since all somatoform disorders are diagnoses of exclusion, a workup sufficient to rule out physical illness is required

Somatoform Disorders

 TREATMENT

MEDICATIONS

- Drugs should not be prescribed in place of frequent appointments

THERAPEUTIC PROCEDURES

Behavioral

- Biofeedback can be helpful in training patients to recognize symptoms and learn countermaneuvers that provide relief

Psychological

- Psychological intervention by the primary clinician should focus on pragmatic changes
- Analytic approaches focused on exploration of early experiences often fail, as patients do not relate these to their current distress
- Group therapy sometimes allows ventilation, improves coping, and focuses on interpersonal adjustment
- *Conversion disorder* is sometimes helped by hypnosis or amobarbital interviews

Social

- Family members should attend appointments to learn how best to live with the patient
- Peer support groups can encourage patients to accept and live with their problem
- Communication with employers may be necessary to encourage long-term interest in the employee/patient

 OUTCOME

FOLLOW-UP

- Regular appointments are helpful. These should be brief and not symptom contingent
- Care should be consolidated under a primary clinician, with consultants for evaluation only
- Ongoing reevaluation is important. Somatoform disorders may coexist with physical illness, which can be overlooked

PROGNOSIS

- Intervention is most successful when instituted before chronicity develops

EVIDENCE

PRACTICE GUIDELINES

- National Guideline Clearinghouse http://www.guideline.gov/summary/summary.aspx?doc_id=1407&nbr=665&string=somatoform+disorder

WEB SITES

- American Psychiatric Association http://www.psych.org/
- Internet Mental Health http://www.mentalhealth.com/t30.html
- Psychopharmacology Tips http://www.dr-bob.org/tips/
- Psychiatry On Line http://www.priory.com/psych.htm

INFORMATION FOR PATIENTS

- National Institutes of Health http://www.nlm.nih.gov/medlineplus/ency/article/000922.htm

REFERENCES

- Eisendrath SJ: Factitious physical disorders. West J Med 1994;160:177. [PMID: 8169474]
- Eisendrath SJ et al: Somatization disorders: effective management in primary care. J Musculoskel Med 1997;4:47.
- Yeung A: Somatoform disorders. West J Med 2001;176:253.

Stuart J. Eisendrath, MD
Jonathan E. Lichtmacher, MD

Spasticity

 KEY FEATURES

ESSENTIALS OF DIAGNOSIS

- The term "spasticity" is commonly used for an upper motor neuron deficit, but it properly refers to an increase in resistance to passive movement that affects different muscles to a different extent

GENERAL CONSIDERATIONS

- It is often a major complication of stroke, cerebral or spinal injury, static perinatal encephalopathy, and multiple sclerosis
- Spasticity may be exacerbated by decubitus ulcers, urinary or other infections, and nociceptive stimuli

 CLINICAL FINDINGS

SYMPTOMS AND SIGNS

- A velocity-dependent increase in resistance to passive movement that affects different muscles to a different extent
- Is not uniform in degree throughout the range of a particular movement
- Is commonly associated with other features of pyramidal deficit

 DIAGNOSIS

DIAGNOSTIC PROCEDURES

- Diagnosis made clinically

TREATMENT

MEDICATIONS

- Drug management is important, but treatment may increase functional disability when increased extensor tone is providing additional support for patients with weak legs
- Dantrolene weakens muscle contraction by interfering with the role of calcium. It is best avoided in patients with poor respiratory function or severe myocardial disease. Treatment is begun with 25 mg once daily, and the daily dose is built up by 25-mg increments every 3 days, depending on tolerance, to a maximum of 100 mg four times daily. Side effects include diarrhea, nausea, weakness, hepatic dysfunction (which may rarely be fatal, especially in women older than 35), drowsiness, light-headedness, and hallucinations
- Lioresal is an effective drug for treating spasticity of spinal origin and painful flexor (or extensor) spasms. The maximum recommended daily dose is 80 mg; treatment is started with a dose of 5 or 10 mg twice daily and then built up gradually
  - Side effects include gastrointestinal disturbances, lassitude, fatigue, sedation, unsteadiness, confusion, and hallucinations
  - Diazepam may modify spasticity by its action on spinal interneurons and perhaps also by influencing supraspinal centers, but effective doses often cause intolerable drowsiness and vary with different patients
- Tizanidine, a centrally acting α_2-adrenergic agonist, is as effective as these other agents but is probably better tolerated. The daily dose is built up gradually, usually to 8 mg taken three times daily. Side effects include sedation, lassitude, hypotension, and dryness of the mouth
- Motor-point blocks by intramuscular phenol have been used to reduce spasticity selectively in one or a few important muscles and may permit return of function in patients with incomplete myelopathies
- Intramuscular administration of botulinum toxin may also be helpful
- Intrathecal injection of phenol or absolute alcohol may be helpful in more severe cases, but greater selectivity can be achieved by nerve root or peripheral nerve neurolysis. These procedures should not be undertaken until the spasticity syndrome is fully evolved, ie, only after about 1 year or so, and only if long-term drug treatment either has not been helpful or carries a significant risk to the patient

SURGERY

- In patients with severe spasticity and limited use of the legs, a surgically implanted lioresal pump may provide significant relief and improve hygiene
- A number of surgical procedures, eg, adductor or heel cord tenotomy, may help in the management of spasticity and facilitate patient management
- For example, obturator neurectomy is helpful in patients with marked adductor spasms that interfere with personal hygiene or cause gait disturbances
- Posterior rhizotomy reduces spasticity, but its effect may be short-lived, whereas anterior rhizotomy produces permanent wasting and weakness in the muscles that are denervated

 ## OUTCOME

WHEN TO REFER

- Refer early to a physical therapist

PREVENTION

- Physical therapy with appropriate stretching programs is important during rehabilitation after the development of an upper motor neuron lesion and in subsequent management of the patient. The aim is to prevent joint and muscle contractures and perhaps to modulate spasticity

 ## EVIDENCE

PRACTICE GUIDELINES

- National Guideline Clearinghouse http://www.guideline.gov/summary/summary.aspx?doc_id=1968&nbr=1194&string=movement+disorders
- Bhatia K et al: Guidelines for the management of Parkinson's disease. The Parkinson's Disease Consensus Working Group. Hosp Med 1998;59:469.

INFORMATION FOR PATIENTS

- Worldwide Education and Awareness for Movement Disorders http://www.wemove.org/spa/
- National Institutes of Health http://www.nlm.nih.gov/medlineplus/ency/article/003297.htm

REFERENCE

- Auff E et al: Clinical applications of botulinum toxin type A. Eur J Neurol 1999;6:Suppl 4.

Michael J. Aminoff, DSc, MD, FRCP

Spinal Cord Tumors, Primary & Metastatic

 KEY FEATURES

ESSENTIALS OF DIAGNOSIS

- Pain, especially with extradural lesions
- Weakness, sensory disturbances, and reflex changes below the level of the lesion
- Bladder, bowel, and sexual dysfunction may occur

GENERAL CONSIDERATIONS

- Approximately 10% of spinal tumors are intramedullary
- Ependymoma is the most common type of intramedullary tumor; the remainder are other types of glioma
- Extramedullary tumors may be extradural or intradural in location
- Among the primary extramedullary tumors, neurofibromas and meningiomas are relatively common, benign, and may be intra- or extradural
- Carcinomatous metastases, lymphomatous or leukemic deposits, and myeloma are usually extradural
- Prostate, breast, lung, and kidney are common primary sites for metastases

 CLINICAL FINDINGS

SYMPTOMS AND SIGNS

- Tumors may lead to spinal cord dysfunction by direct compression, by ischemia secondary to arterial or venous obstruction, and, in the case of intramedullary lesions, by invasive infiltration
- Symptoms usually develop insidiously
- Pain with extradural lesions; characteristically aggravated by coughing or straining; may be radicular, localized to the back, or felt diffusely in an extremity; and may be accompanied by motor deficits, paresthesias, or numbness, especially in the legs; often precedes specific neurological symptoms in case of epidural metastases
- Sphincter disturbances may occur
- Localized spinal tenderness
- Segmental lower motor neuron deficit or dermatomal sensory changes (or both) may be found at the level of the lesion, while an upper motor neuron deficit and sensory disturbance are found below it

DIFFERENTIAL DIAGNOSIS

- Primary tumor, eg, ependymoma, meningioma, neurofibroma
- Lymphoma, leukemia, multiple myeloma
- Metastases, eg, cancer of the prostate, breast, lung, kidney
- Cervical or lumbar disk disease
- Multiple sclerosis
- Tuberculosis (Pott's disease)

 DIAGNOSIS

LABORATORY TESTS

- Cerebrospinal fluid removed at myelography is often xanthochromic and contains a greatly increased protein concentration with normal cell content and glucose concentration

IMAGING STUDIES

- Findings on plain radiography are commonly abnormal with metastatic deposits
- MRI or CT myelography may be necessary to identify and localize the site of cord compression
- The combination of known tumor elsewhere in the body, back pain, and either abnormal plain films of the spine or neurological signs of cord compression is an indication to perform MRI or CT on an urgent basis
- Some clinicians proceed to spinal MRI or myelography based solely on new back pain in a cancer patient; if a complete block is present at lumbar myelography, a cisternal myelogram is performed to determine the upper level of the block and the possibility of block higher in the cord

Spinal Cord Tumors, Primary & Metastatic

TREATMENT

MEDICATIONS

- Dexamethasone in high dosage (eg, 25 mg four times daily for 3 days, followed by rapid tapering of the dosage, depending on response) to reduce cord swelling and relieve pain

SURGERY

- Intramedullary tumors are treated by decompression and surgical excision (when feasible) and by irradiation; prognosis depends on the cause and severity of cord compression before it is relieved
- Surgical decompression for epidural metastases is reserved for tumors that are unresponsive to irradiation or have previously been irradiated and for cases with an uncertain diagnosis

THERAPEUTIC PROCEDURES

- Epidural spinal metastases are treated with irradiation, irrespective of cell type; long-term outlook is poor, but radiation treatment may delay the onset of major disability

OUTCOME

PROGNOSIS

- Depends on the underlying lesion

WHEN TO ADMIT

- All patients

EVIDENCE

PRACTICE GUIDELINES

- American Society for Interventional and Therapeutic Neuroradiology: Embolization of spinal arteriovenous fistulae, spinal arteriovenous malformations, and tumors of the spinal axis. AJNR Am J Neuroradiol 2001;22(8 Suppl):S28.
- National Guideline Clearinghouse http://www.guideline.gov/summary/summary.aspx?doc_id=3639&nbr=2865&string=spinal+tumors http://www.guideline.gov/summary/summary.aspx?doc_id=1897&nbr=1123&string=back+pain

INFORMATION FOR PATIENTS

- National Institutes of Health http://www.nlm.nih.gov/medlineplus/ency/article/001403.htm
- American Cancer Society http://www.cancer.org/docroot/cri/content/cri_2_4_4x_treatment_of_specific_types_of_brain_and_spinal_cord_tumors_3.asp?sitearea=cri

REFERENCES

- Major PP: Efficacy of bisphosphonates in the management of skeletal complications of bone metastases and selection of clinical endpoints. Am J Clin Oncol 2002;25(6 Suppl 1):S10.
- Shiff D: Spinal cord compression. Neurol Clin 2003;21:67.
- Sundaresan N: Surgery for solitary metastases of the spine: rationale and results of treatment. Spine 2002;27:1802. [PMID: 12195075]

Michael J. Aminoff, MD, DSc, FRCP

Spinal Cord Vascular Diseases

 ## KEY FEATURES

ESSENTIALS OF DIAGNOSIS

- Sudden onset of back or limb pain and neurological deficit in limbs
- Motor, sensory, or reflex changes in limbs depending on level of lesion
- Imaging studies distinguish between infarct and hematoma

GENERAL CONSIDERATIONS

Infarction of the spinal cord

- Rare and occurs only in the anterior spinal artery territory (which supplies the anterior two-thirds of the cord), because this artery is supplied by only a limited number of feeders
- Infarction usually from interrupted flow in one or more of these feeders, eg, with aortic dissection, aortography, polyarteritis, or severe hypotension, or after surgical resection of the thoracic aorta
- Infarcts are usually caudal because the anterior spinal artery receives numerous feeders in the cervical region

Epidural or subdural hemorrhage

- Occurs in association with bleeding disorders, anticoagulant drugs, trauma or lumbar puncture; epidural hemorrhage
- May also be related to a vascular malformation or tumor deposit

Arteriovenous malformation of the spinal cord

- Congenital lesions that present with spinal subarachnoid hemorrhage or myeloradiculopathy
- Most malformations are in the thoracolumbar region and are extramedullary
- Cervical arteriovenous malformations lead to symptoms and signs in the arms and are intramedullary

 ## CLINICAL FINDINGS

SYMPTOMS AND SIGNS

Infarction of the spinal cord

- Acute onset of flaccid, areflexic paraplegia that evolves after a few days or weeks into a spastic paraplegia with extensor plantar responses
- Dissociated sensory loss, with impairment of appreciation of pain and temperature but preservation of vibration and position sense

Epidural or subdural hemorrhage

- Sudden severe back pain followed by an acute compressive myelopathy necessitating urgent CT or MRI and surgical evacuation

Arteriovenous malformation of the spinal cord

- Motor and sensory disturbances in the legs and sphincter disorders
- Pain in the legs or back is often severe
- Examination reveals an upper, lower, or mixed motor deficit in the legs
- Sensory deficits are also present and are usually extensive, although occasionally they are confined to radicular distribution

DIFFERENTIAL DIAGNOSIS

- Primary tumor, eg, ependymoma, meningioma, neurofibroma
- Lymphoma, leukemia, multiple myeloma
- Metastases, eg, cancer of the prostate, breast, lung, kidney
- Cervical or lumbar disk disease
- Epidural abscess
- Multiple sclerosis
- Tuberculosis (Pott's disease)

 ## DIAGNOSIS

LABORATORY TESTS

Imaging Studies

- Urgent imaging (CR or MRI) is indicated for epidural or subdural hemorrhage
- Spinal MRI may not detect an arteriovenous malformation, and negative findings do not exclude the diagnosis. Myelography is a good screening test
- In arteriovenous malformation of the spinal cord, myelography (performed with the patient prone and supine) can show serpiginous filling defects due to enlarged vessels. Selective spinal arteriography confirms the diagnosis

TREATMENT

SURGERY

- Epidural or subdural hemorrhage: urgent surgical evacuation is indicated
- Arteriovenous malformations of the spinal cord that are posterior to the cord can be treated by ligation of feeding vessels and excision of the fistulous anomaly or by embolization procedures

THERAPEUTIC PROCEDURES

- Infarction of the spinal cord: treatment is symptomatic

 OUTCOME

PROGNOSIS

- Delay in treatment of an arteriovenous malformation of the spinal cord may lead to increased and irreversible disability or to death from recurrent subarachnoid hemorrhage

WHEN TO ADMIT

- All patients

 EVIDENCE

PRACTICE GUIDELINES

- National Guideline Clearinghouse http://www.guideline.gov/summary/ summary.aspx?doc_id=2451&nbr= 1677&string=epidural+hematoma
- American Society for Interventional and Therapeutic Neuroradiology: Embolization of spinal arteriovenous fistulae, spinal arteriovenous malformations, and tumors of the spinal axis. AJNR Am J Neuroradiol 2001;22(8 Suppl):S28.

WEB SITE

- Neuromuscular Disease Center http://www.neuro.wustl.edu/ neuromuscular/

INFORMATION FOR PATIENTS

- National Institute of Neurological Diseases and Stroke http://www.ninds.nih.gov/health_and_ medical/disorders/spinal_infarction.htm http://www.ninds.nih.gov/health_and_ medical/pubs/arteriovenous.htm

REFERENCE

- Goodin DS: Neurological complications of aortic disease and surgery. In: Neurology and general medicine, ed 3. Aminoff MJ (editor). Churchill Livingstone, 2001.

Michael J. Aminoff, DSc, MD, FRCP

Spinal Trauma

 KEY FEATURES

ESSENTIALS OF DIAGNOSIS

- History of trauma followed immediately or after a variable interval by an acute neurological deficit
- Signs of myelopathy on examination

GENERAL CONSIDERATIONS

- While spinal cord damage may result from whiplash injury, severe injury usually relates to fracture-dislocation causing compression or deformity of the cord either cervically or in the lower thoracic and upper lumbar regions
- Extreme hypotension following injury may also lead to cord infarction

 CLINICAL FINDINGS

SYMPTOMS AND SIGNS

Total cord transaction

- Immediate flaccid paralysis and loss of sensation below the level of the lesion
- Reflex activity is lost for a variable period; urinary and fecal retention
- As reflex function returns, spastic paraplegia or quadriplegia develops, with hyperreflexia and extensor plantar responses, but a flaccid atrophic (lower motor neuron) paralysis may be found depending on the segments of the cord affected
- The bladder and bowels regain some reflex function, permitting urine and feces to be expelled at intervals
- As spasticity increases, flexor or extensor spasms (or both) of the legs become troublesome, especially if the patient develops bed sores or a urinary tract infection
- Paraplegia with the legs in flexion or extension may eventually result

Lesser degrees of injury

- Mild limb weakness, distal sensory disturbance, or both
- Sphincter function may be impaired, urinary urgency and urgency incontinence being especially common. A unilateral cord lesion leads to an ipsilateral motor disturbance with accompanying impairment of proprioception and contralateral loss of pain and temperature appreciation below the lesion (Brown-Séquard's syndrome)
- A central cord syndrome may lead to a lower motor neuron deficit and loss of pain and temperature appreciation, with sparing of posterior column functions
- A radicular deficit may occur at the level of the injury—or, if the cauda equina is involved, there may be evidence of disturbed function in several lumbosacral roots

DIFFERENTIAL DIAGNOSIS

- The history of the preceding trauma distinguishes the disorder from other causes of nontraumatic myelopathy

 DIAGNOSIS

DIAGNOSTIC PROCEDURES

- Obtain history of trauma

TREATMENT

MEDICATIONS

- Early treatment with high doses of corticosteroids (eg, methylprednisolone, 30 mg/kg by intravenous bolus, followed by 5.4 mg/kg/h for 23 h) can improve neurological recovery if commenced within 8 h after injury

SURGERY

- If there is cord compression, decompressive laminectomy and fusion

THERAPEUTIC PROCEDURES

- Immobilization
- Anatomic realignment of the spinal cord by traction and other orthopedic procedures is important

 OUTCOME

FOLLOW-UP

- Subsequent care of the residual neurological deficit—paraplegia or quadriplegia—requires treatment of spasticity and care of the skin, bladder, and bowels

COMPLICATIONS

- Decubiti
- Urinary tract infection
- Renal calculi
- Depression
- Pneumonia

WHEN TO ADMIT

- All patients (to a spinal trauma center, if available)

 EVIDENCE

PRACTICE GUIDELINES

- National Guideline Clearinghouse
  http://www.guideline.gov/summary/summary.aspx?doc_id=2964&nbr=2190&string=spinal+trauma
  http://www.guideline.gov/summary/summary.aspx?doc_id=850&nbr=394&string=spinal+trauma
  http://www.guideline.gov/summary/summary.aspx?doc_id=1677&nbr=903&string=spinal+trauma

INFORMATION FOR PATIENTS

- Paralyzed Veterans of America
  http://www.pva.org/NEWPVASITE/publications/pdf/IntroSCI.pdf
- American Association of Neurological Surgeons
  http://www.neurosurgery.org/health/patient/detail.asp?DisorderID=42

REFERENCE

- Gimenez y Robotta M et al: Strategies for regeneration and repair in spinal cord traumatic injury. Prog Brain Res 2002;137:191 [PMID: 12440369]

Michael J. Aminoff, DSc, MD, FRCP

Squamous Cell Carcinoma

 KEY FACTORS

ESSENTIALS OF DIAGNOSIS

- Nodule, ulcer, or patch usually on sun-exposed sites or in the genital area

GENERAL CONSIDERATIONS

- Squamous cell carcinoma (SCC) usually occurs subsequent to prolonged sun exposure on exposed parts in fair-skinned individuals who sunburn easily and tan poorly
- It may arise from an actinic keratosis

DEMOGRAPHICS

- SCC is about 20% as common as basal cell carcinoma

 CLINICAL FINDINGS

SYMPTOMS AND SIGNS

- The lesions appear as small red, conical, hard nodules that occasionally ulcerate; they are not as distinctive as basal cell carcinomas and are more easily misdiagnosed clinically
- Since cutaneous SCC may metstasize, palpate draining nodes at affected area

DIFFERENTIAL DIAGNOSIS

- Actinic keratosis
- Basal cell carcinoma
- Seborrheic keratosis
- Warts
- Keratoacanthomas resemble squamous cell carcinoma histologically and for all practical purposes should be treated as though they were skin cancers

 DIAGNOSIS

DIAGNOSTIC PROCEDURES

- The diagnosis is made by biopsy

Squamous Cell Carcinoma

 ## TREATMENT

SURGERY

- The preferred treatment of squamous cell carcinoma is excision
- Fresh tissue microscopically controlled excision (Mohs) is recommended for high-risk lesions (lips, temples, ears, nose) and for recurrent tumors

THERAPEUTIC PROCEDURES

- Electrodesiccation and curettage and x-ray radiation may be used for some lesions
- Some keratoacanthomas respond to intralesional injection of fluorouracil or methotrexate, but they must be excised if they do not

 ## OUTCOME

FOLLOW-UP

- Follow-up must be more frequent and thorough than for basal cell carcinoma, starting at every 3 months, with careful examination of lymph nodes
- In addition, palpation of the lips is essential to detect hard or indurated areas that represent early squamous cell carcinoma; all such cases must be biopsied
- Multiple SCCs are very common on the sun-exposed skin of organ transplant patients because of the host's immunosuppressed state; the tumors begin to appear after 5 years of immunosuppression

COMPLICATIONS

- The frequency of metastasis is not precisely known, though metastatic spread is said to be less likely with SCC arising out of actinic keratoses than with those that arise de novo
- In actinically induced SCCs, rates of metastasis are estimated from retrospective studies to be 3–7%
- SCCs, of the lip, oral cavity, tongue, and genitalia have much higher rates of metastasis and require special management

PROGNOSIS

- Tumor aggressiveness correlates with the size of the lesion, duration, location, origin, and degree of anaplasia
- Tumors of the scalp, eyelids, nose, ears and lips invade subcutaneous tissues and have a greater risk of subclinical tumor extension

WHEN TO REFER

- If there is a question about the diagnosis, if recommended therapy is ineffective, or specialized treatment is necessary

PREVENTION

- Sun protection and avoidance

 ## EVIDENCE

PRACTICE GUIDELINES

- National Guideline Clearinghouse http://www.guideline.gov/summary/summary.aspx?doc_id=3391&nbr=2617&string=squamous+cell+carcinoma
- American Acadmey of Dermatology http://www.aadassociation.org/Guidelines/cutaneoussquamous.html

WEB SITES

- American Academy of Dermatology http://www.aad.org
- Dermatology Handbook for Family Practice from the University of Iowa http://www.vh.org/Providers/ClinRef/FPHandbook/17.html

INFORMATION FOR PATIENTS

- American Academy of Dermatology http://www.aad.org/pamphlets/ http://www.aad.org/pamphlets/sqamous.html
- JAMA patient page: Skin cancer. JAMA 1999;281:676. [PMID: 10029132]

REFERENCE

- Garner KL et al: Basal and squamous cell carcinoma. Prim Care 2000;27:447. [PMID: 10815054]

Timothy G. Berger, MD

Status Epilepticus

KEY FEATURES

ESSENTIALS OF DIAGNOSIS

- Occurrence of two or more convulsions with recovery of consciousness between attacks
- A fixed and enduring epileptic condition (for 30 min or more)

GENERAL CONSIDERATIONS

- Status epilepticus is a medical emergency
- Most common cause is poor compliance with the anticonvulsant drug; others include alcohol withdrawal, intracranial infection or neoplasms, stroke, metabolic disorders, and drug overdose
- Mortality rate of convulsive status may be as high as 20%, with a high incidence of neurological and mental sequelae
- Prognosis relates to the length of time between onset of status epilepticus and start of effective treatment

CLINICAL FINDINGS

SYMPTOMS AND SIGNS

- Status epilepticus may be manifested in two clinical subtypes
  - Tonic-clonic convulsive status epilepticus
  - Nonconvulsive status epilepticus is characterized by fluctuating abnormal mental status, confusion, impaired responsiveness, and automatism. It has two subtypes: absence (petit mal) and complex partial status epilepticus

DIFFERENTIAL DIAGNOSIS

- Seizure due to hypoglycemia, electrolyte abnormality, alcohol withdrawal, cocaine, bacterial meningitis, herpes encephalitis, brain tumor, CNS vasculitis
- Syncope
- Cardiac arrhythmia
- Stroke or transient ischemic attack
- Pseudoseizure
- Panic attack
- Migraine
- Narcolepsy

DIAGNOSIS

LABORATORY TESTS

- Electroencephalography (EEG) is essential both in establishing the diagnosis of nonconvulsive status epilepticus and its two subtypes

TREATMENT

MEDICATIONS

- See Table 94 (page 1278)
- Initial treatment with intravenous lorazepam or diazepam is usually helpful regardless of the type of status epilepticus, but phenytoin, phenobarbital, carbamazepine, and other drugs are also needed

Initial management

- Maintenance of the airway and 50% dextrose (25–50 mL) intravenously in case of hypoglycemia
- If seizures continue, give 10 mg diazepam intravenously over 2 min, and repeat after 10 min if necessary; hypotension and respiratory depression may occur
- Alternatively, give 4 mg intravenous bolus of lorazepam, repeat once after 10 min if necessary—effective in halting seizures for a brief period but occasionally causes respiratory depression
- Also give phenytoin (18–20 mg/kg) intravenously at 50 mg/min for initiation of longer seizure control
  - The drug is best injected directly but can also be given in saline; it precipitates if injected into glucose-containing solutions
  - Because arrhythmias may develop during rapid administration of phenytoin, electrocardiographic monitoring is prudent. Phenytoin may cause hypotension, especially if diazepam has also been given
  - In the United States, injectable phenytoin has been replaced by fosphenytoin, which is rapidly and completely converted to phenytoin following intravenous administration
  - No dosing adjustments are necessary because fosphenytoin is expressed in terms of phenytoin equivalents (PE); fosphenytoin is less likely to cause reactions at the infusion site, can be given with all common intravenous solutions, and may be administered at a faster rate (150 mg PE/min). It is also more expensive

If seizures continue

- Phenobarbital is then given in a loading dose of 10–20 mg/kg intravenously by slow or intermittent injection (50 mg/min). Respiratory depression and hypotension are common complications and should be anticipated

- If these measures fail, general anesthesia with ventilatory assistance and neuromuscular junction blockade may be required
- Alternatively, intravenous midazolam may control refractory status epilepticus; the suggested loading dose is 0.2 mg/kg, followed by 0.05–0.2 mg/kg/h

OUTCOME

FOLLOW-UP

- After status epilepticus is controlled, an oral drug program for the long-term management of seizures is started, and investigations into the cause of the disorder are pursued

WHEN TO REFER

- Many patients can benefit from the expertise of a neurologist

WHEN TO ADMIT

- All patients until seizure control is obtained

EVIDENCE

PRACTICE GUIDELINES

- Appleton R et al: The treatment of convulsive status epilepticus in children. The Status Epilepticus Working Party, Members of the Status Epilepticus Working Party. Arch Dis Child 2000;83:415.

INFORMATION FOR PATIENTS

- National Institute of Neurological Disorders and Stroke http://www.ninds.nih.gov/health_and_ medical/disorders/epilepsy.htm
- Epilepsy Foundation http://www.epilepsyfoundation.org/ answerplace/About-Epilepsy.cfm

REFERENCES

- Alldredge BK et al: A comparison of lorazepam, diazepam, and placebo for the treatment of out-of-hospital status epilepticus. N Engl J Med 2001;345: 631. [PMID: 11547716]
- Benbadis SR et al: Advances in the treatment of epilepsy. Am Fam Physician 2001;64:91. [PMID: 11456438]
- Kwan P et al: The mechanisms of action of commonly used antiepileptic drugs. Pharmacol Ther 2001;90:21. [PMID: 11448723]
- Wu YW et al: Incidence and mortality of generalized convulsive status epilepticus in California. Neurology 2002; 58:1070. [PMID: 11940695]

Michael J. Aminoff, DSc, MD, FRCP

Stress & Adjustment Disorders

 ## KEY FEATURES

ESSENTIALS OF DIAGNOSIS

- Anxiety or depression clearly secondary to an identifiable stress
- Subsequent symptoms of anxiety or depression commonly elicited by similar stress of lesser magnitude
- Alcohol and other drugs are commonly used in self-treatment

GENERAL CONSIDERATIONS

- Stress exists when the adaptive capacity of the individual is overwhelmed by events
- The event may be an insignificant one objectively considered, and even favorable changes (eg, promotion and transfer) requiring adaptive behavior can produce stress
- For each individual, stress is subjectively defined, and the response to stress is a function of each person's personality and physiological endowment
- The causes of stress are different at different ages—eg, in young adulthood, the sources of stress are found in the marriage or parent-child relationship, the employment relationship, and the struggle to achieve financial stability; in the middle years, the focus shifts to changing spousal relationships, problems with aging parents, and problems associated with having young adult offspring who themselves are encountering stressful situations; in old age, the principal concerns are apt to be retirement, loss of physical capacity, major personal losses, and thoughts of death
- Maladaptive behavior in response to stress is called adjustment disorder, with the major symptom specified (eg, "adjustment disorder with depressed mood")

 ## CLINICAL FINDINGS

SYMPTOMS AND SIGNS

- Common subjective responses are fear (of repetition of the stress-inducing event), rage (at frustration), guilt (over aggressive impulses), and shame (over helplessness)
- Acute and reactivated stress may be manifested by restlessness, irritability, fatigue, increased startle reaction, and a feeling of tension
- Inability to concentrate, sleep disturbances (insomnia, bad dreams), and somatic preoccupations often lead to self-medication, most commonly with alcohol or other central nervous system depressants

DIFFERENTIAL DIAGNOSIS

- Anxiety disorders
- Affective disorders
- Personality disorders exacerbated by stress
- Somatic disorders with psychic overlay

 ## DIAGNOSIS

DIAGNOSTIC PROCEDURES

- Obtain history
- Identify precipitating sources of stress

Still's Disease, Adult p. 1174. Storage Pool
Disease p. 1175. Streptococcal, Group A
Infections p. 1175.

Stress & Adjustment Disorders

 ## TREATMENT

MEDICATIONS

- Judicious use of sedatives (Table 101, page 1285) (eg, lorazepam, 1–2 mg orally daily) for a limited time and as part of an overall treatment plan can provide relief

THERAPEUTIC PROCEDURES

Behavioral

- Stress reduction techniques include immediate symptom reduction (eg, rebreathing in a bag for hyperventilation) or early recognition and removal from a stress source before full-blown symptoms appear
- It is often helpful for the patient to keep a daily log of stress precipitators, responses, and alleviators
- Relaxation and exercise techniques are also helpful in reducing the reaction to stressful events

Social

- While it is not easy for the patient to make necessary changes (or they would have been made long ago), it is important for the clinician to establish the framework of the problem, since the patient's denial system may obscure the issues
- Clarifying the problem allows the patient to begin viewing it within the proper context and facilitates the sometimes difficult decisions the patient eventually must make (eg, change of job or relocation of adult dependent offspring)

Psychological

- Prolonged in-depth psychotherapy is seldom necessary in cases of isolated stress response or adjustment disorder
- Supportive psychotherapy with an emphasis on the here and now and strengthening of existing defenses is a helpful approach

 ## OUTCOME

PROGNOSIS

- Return to satisfactory function after a short period is part of the clinical picture of this syndrome
- Resolution may be delayed if others' responses to the patient's difficulties are thoughtlessly harmful or if the secondary gains outweigh the advantages of recovery
- The longer the symptoms persist, the worse the prognosis

 ## EVIDENCE

PRACTICE GUIDELINES

- National Guideline Clearinghouse http://www.guideline.gov/summary/summary.aspx?doc_id=1503&nbr=729&string=adjustment+disorder http://www.guideline.gov/summary/summary.aspx?doc_id=1407&nbr=665&string=adjustment+disorder

WEB SITES

- American Psychiatric Association http://www.psych.org/
- Internet Mental Health http://www.mentalhealth.com/t30.html
- Psychopharmacology Tips http://www.dr-bob.org/tips/
- Psychiatry On Line http://www.priory.com/psych.htm

INFORMATION FOR PATIENTS

- American Academy of Family Physicians http://familydoctor.org/healthfacts/167/
- National Cancer Institute http://www.cancer.gov/cancerinfo/pdq/supportivecare/adjustment/patient

REFERENCES

- Brady K et al: Efficacy and safety of sertraline treatment of posttraumatic stress disorder, a randomised control trial. JAMA 2000;283:1837.
- Pitman RK et al: Pilot study of secondary prevention of PTSD with propranolol. Biol Psychiatry 2002;51:189.

Stuart J. Eisendrath, MD
Jonathan E. Lichtmacher, MD

Stroke, Intracerebral Hemorrhage

 KEY FEATURES

ESSENTIALS OF DIAGNOSIS

- Hypertension is the usual etiology
- Usually occurs suddenly and without warning, often during activity

GENERAL CONSIDERATIONS

Hypertensive intracerebral hemorrhage

- Spontaneous intracerebral hemorrhage in patients with no angiographic evidence of an associated vascular anomaly (eg, aneurysm or angioma) is usually due to hypertension
- Likely pathological basis is microaneurysms that develop on perforating vessels 100–300 μm in diameter in hypertensive patients
- Occurs most frequently in the basal ganglia and less commonly in the pons, thalamus, cerebellum, and cerebral white matter
- Extension into the ventricular system or subarachnoid space may cause signs of meningeal irritation

Other causes

- May occur with hematological and bleeding disorders (eg, leukemia, thrombocytopenia, hemophilia, or disseminated intravascular coagulation), anticoagulant therapy, liver disease, cerebral amyloid angiopathy, and primary or secondary brain tumors
- Bleeding from an intracranial aneurysm or arteriovenous malformation is primarily into the subarachnoid space, but it may also be partly intraparenchymal
- In some cases, no specific cause for cerebral hemorrhage can be identified

 CLINICAL FINDINGS

SYMPTOMS AND SIGNS

Hemorrhage into the cerebral hemisphere

- Consciousness is initially lost or impaired in about one-half of patients
- Vomiting is frequent at the onset, and headache is sometimes present
- Focal symptoms and signs follow, depending on the site of the bleed
- With hypertensive hemorrhage, there is generally a rapidly evolving neurological deficit with hemiplegia or hemiparesis
- A hemisensory disturbance occurs with more deeply placed lesions
- With lesions of the putamen, loss of conjugate lateral gaze may be present
- With thalamic hemorrhage, there may be a loss of upward gaze, downward or skew deviation of the eyes, lateral gaze palsies, and pupillary inequalities

Cerebellar hemorrhage

- Sudden onset of nausea and vomiting, disequilibrium, headache, and loss of consciousness that may terminate fatally within 48 h
- Less commonly, the onset is gradual and episodic or slowly progressive, suggesting an expanding cerebellar lesion
- Onset and course can be intermediate
  - Lateral conjugate gaze palsies to the side of the lesion
  - Small reactive pupils
  - Contralateral hemiplegia; peripheral facial weakness
  - Ataxia of gait, limbs, or trunk
  - Periodic respiration
  - Or some combination of these findings

DIFFERENTIAL DIAGNOSIS

- Ischemic stroke
- Subarachnoid hemorrhage
- Space-occupying lesion, eg, brain tumor
- Subdural or epidural hemorrhage

 DIAGNOSIS

LABORATORY TESTS

- A complete blood cell count, platelet count, bleeding time, prothrombin and partial thromboplastin times, and liver and renal function tests may reveal a predisposing cause
- Lumbar puncture is contraindicated because it may cause herniation in patients with a large hematoma

IMAGING STUDIES

- CT scanning (without contrast) is important in confirming hemorrhage and for determining the size and site of the hematoma
- CT is superior to MRI for detecting intracranial hemorrhage of less than 48 h duration
- If the patient's condition permits further intervention, cerebral angiography may reveal an aneurysm or arteriovenous malformation

TREATMENT

SURGERY

- In cerebellar hemorrhage, prompt surgical evacuation of the hematoma is appropriate
- Decompression is helpful when a superficial hematoma in cerebral white matter is causing mass effect and herniation

THERAPEUTIC PROCEDURES

- In noncerebellar hemorrhage, neurological management is generally conservative and supportive, either in cases of profound deficit with associated brainstem compression or more localized deficits
- The treatment of underlying structural lesions or bleeding disorders depends on their nature

 OUTCOME

PROGNOSIS

- Surgery for cerebellar hemorrhage may lead to complete resolution of the clinical deficit
- Untreated cerebellar hemorrhage can spontaneously deteriorate with a fatal outcome from brainstem herniation

WHEN TO ADMIT

- All patients

 EVIDENCE

PRACTICE GUIDELINES

- National Guideline Clearinghouse http://www.guideline.gov/summary/ summary.aspx?doc_id=3103&nbr= 2329&string=stroke
- American Academy of Neurology http://www.aan.com/professionals/ practice/pdfs/gl0097.pdf

WEB SITE

- Cerebrovascular Accident http://rehab.educ.ucalgary.ca/courses/ core/301.03/Cardiovascular/ cva-overview.html

INFORMATION FOR PATIENTS

- JAMA patient page: Stroke. JAMA 1999;281:1146. [PMID: 10188669]
- National Institute of Neurological Disorders and Stroke http://www.ninds.nih.gov/health_and_ medical/disorders/stroke.htm
- The Mayo Clinic http://www.mayoclinic.com/invoke.cfm? id=DS00150

REFERENCE

- Hill MD et al: Rate of stroke recurrence in patients with primary intracerebral hemorrhage. Stroke 2000;31:123. [PMID: 10625726]

Michael J. Aminoff, DSc, MD, FRCP

Stroke, Ischemic

 KEY FEATURES

ESSENTIALS OF DIAGNOSIS

- Thrombotic or embolic occlusion of a major vessel leads to cerebral infarction
- The resulting deficit depends on the particular vessel involved and the extent of any collateral circulation

GENERAL CONSIDERATIONS

- Strokes are traditionally subdivided into infarcts (thrombotic or embolic) and hemorrhages, but clinical distinction may not be possible
- A previous stroke is a risk factor for a subsequent stroke

DEMOGRAPHICS

- The third leading cause of death in the United States, despite a general decline in the incidence of stroke in the last 30 years

 CLINICAL FINDINGS

SYMPTOMS AND SIGNS

- See Table 92 (page 1276)
- Onset is usually abrupt, and there may then be very little progression except that due to brain swelling
- Clinically, must examine the heart for arrhythmia or murmur, and check for carotid and subclavian bruits
- In hemiplegia of pontine origin, the eyes often deviate to the paralyzed side, whereas in a hemispheric lesion, the eyes commonly deviate away from the hemiplegic side

Carotid circulation

- Ophthalmic artery occlusion is symptomless in most, but may produce *amaurosis fugax*—sudden and brief loss of vision in one eye
- Anterior cerebral artery occlusion distal to junction with anterior communicating artery causes weakness and cortical sensory loss in the contralateral leg and sometimes mild proximal arm weakness; may see contralateral grasp reflex, paratonic rigidity, and abulia (lack of initiative) or frank confusion; urinary incontinence is common
- Middle cerebral artery occlusion
  - Contralateral hemiplegia, hemisensory loss, and homonymous hemianopia (ie, bilaterally symmetric loss of vision in half of the visual fields), with the eyes deviated to the side of the lesion; if the dominant hemisphere is involved, global aphasia is also present
  - May be impossible to distinguish from occlusion of the internal carotid artery
  - May also see considerable swelling of the hemisphere, leading to drowsiness, stupor, and coma
- Occlusions of different branches of the middle cerebral artery cause more limited findings
  - Anterior main division occlusion: expressive dysphasia, contralateral paralysis and loss of sensations in the arm, the face, and, to a lesser extent, the leg
  - Posterior branch occlusion: receptive (Wernicke's) aphasia and a homonymous visual field defect

Vertebrobasilar circulation

- Posterior cerebral artery occlusion may lead to thalamic syndrome of sensory loss, ipsilateral facial, ninth and tenth cranial nerve lesions, limb ataxia and numbness, and Horner's syndrome, combined with contralateral sensory loss of the limb
- Occlusion of both vertebral arteries or the basilar artery: coma with pinpoint pupils, flaccid quadriplegia, sensory loss, and variable cranial nerve abnormalities
- Partial basilar artery occlusion: diplopia, visual loss, vertigo, dysarthria, ataxia, weakness or sensory disturbances in some or all of the limbs, and discrete cranial nerve palsies
- Occlusion of any major cerebellar artery
  - Vertigo, nausea, vomiting, nystagmus, ipsilateral limb ataxia, and contralateral spinothalamic sensory loss in the limbs
  - Massive cerebellar infarction may lead to coma, tonsillar herniation, and death

DIFFERENTIAL DIAGNOSIS

- Hypoglycemia
- Transient ischemic attack
- Intracerebral hemorrhage or other mass lesion (eg, tumor)
- Focal seizure (Todd's paralysis)
- Migraine
- Peripheral causes of vertigo (Ménière's disease)

 DIAGNOSIS

LABORATORY TESTS

- Complete blood cell count, sedimentation rate, blood glucose, and serological tests for syphilis
- Antiphospholipid antibodies, serum lipids, and homocysteine
- ECG to help exclude a cardiac arrhythmia or recent myocardial infarction that might be a source of embolization
- Blood cultures if endocarditis is suspected

IMAGING STUDIES

- A CT scan of the head (without contrast) will exclude cerebral hemorrhage, but may not distinguish between a cerebral infarct and tumor
- CT scanning is preferable to MRI in the acute stage because it is quicker and hemorrhage is not easily detected by MRI in the first 48 h
- In selected patients, carotid duplex studies, MRI and MR angiography, and conventional angiography may also be necessary
- Diffusion-weighted MRI is more sensitive than standard MRI in detecting cerebral ischemia
- Echocardiography if heart disease is suspected

DIAGNOSTIC PROCEDURES

- Holter monitoring if paroxysmal cardiac arrhythmia suspected

TREATMENT

MEDICATIONS

Anticoagulants

- If the CT shows no hemorrhage, and there is a cardiac source of embolization, start intravenous heparin while warfarin is introduced for a target INR of 2–3 for the prothrombin time
- Some physicians prefer to wait for 2 or 3 days before initiating anticoagulant treatment after the CT scan is repeated and there is no evidence of hemorrhagic transformation

Thrombolytics

- Intravenous thrombolytic therapy with recombinant tissue plasminogen activator (0.9 mg/kg to a maximum of 90 mg, with 10% given as a bolus over 1 min and the remainder over 1 h) is effective in reducing the neurological deficit in selected patients without CT evidence of intracranial hemorrhage when administered within 3 h after onset of ischemic stroke, but later administration has not been proven effective or safe
- Recent hemorrhage, increased risk of hemorrhage (eg, treatment with anticoagulants), arterial puncture at a noncompressible site, and systolic pressure above 185 mm Hg or diastolic pressure above 110 mm Hg are among the contraindications to this treatment

THERAPEUTIC PROCEDURES

- Early management consists of general supportive measures
- Avoid lowering the blood pressure of hypertensive patients within 2 weeks of stroke, as ischemic areas may be further compromised—unless the systolic pressure exceeds 200 mm Hg, in which case it can be lowered gradually to 170 –200 mm Hg and then, after 2 weeks, reduced further
- Physical therapy with early mobilization and active rehabilitation are important
- Occupational therapy may improve morale and motor skills, while speech therapy may be beneficial in patients with expressive dysphasia or dysarthria

OUTCOME

PROGNOSIS

- The prognosis for survival after cerebral infarction is better than after cerebral or subarachnoid hemorrhage
- Loss of consciousness after a cerebral infarct implies a poorer prognosis than otherwise
- The extent of the infarct governs the potential for rehabilitation

PREVENTION

- Patients who have had a cerebral infarct are at risk for further strokes and for myocardial infarcts
- Statin therapy to lower serum lipid levels may reduce this risk
- Antiplatelet therapy with aspirin, 325 mg a day, reduces the recurrence rate by 30% among patients without a cardiac cause for the stroke who are not candidates for carotid endarterectomy. Nevertheless, the cumulative risk of recurrence of noncardioembolic stroke is still 3–7% annually
- A 2-year comparison did not show benefit of warfarin (INR 1.4–2.8) over aspirin (325 mg daily), and higher doses of warfarin should be avoided as they lead to an increased incidence of major bleeding

EVIDENCE

PRACTICE GUIDELINES

- American Stroke Association/American Academy of Neurology Joint Report: Anticoagulants and antiplatelet agents in acute ischemic stroke. Stroke 2002;33: 1934.
- American Academy of Neurology http://www.aan.com/professionals/ practice/pdfs/gl0017.pdf

WEB SITES

- Acute Cerebral Infarction Demonstration Case http://www.brighamrad.harvard. edu/Cases/bwh/hcache/93/full.html
- Cerebrovascular Accident http://rehab.educ.ucalgary.ca/courses/ core/301.03/Cardiovascular/ cva-overview.html
- Carotid Artery Stenosis Demonstration Case http://www.brighamrad.harvard.edu/ Cases/bwh/hcache/6/full.html

INFORMATION FOR PATIENTS

- JAMA patient page: Stroke. JAMA 1999;281:1146. [PMID: 10188669]
- The Mayo Clinic http://www.mayoclinic.com/invoke.cfm? id=DS00150

REFERENCES

- Albers GW et al: Intravenous tissue-type plasminogen activator for treatment of acute stroke: the Standard Treatment with Alteplase to Reverse Stroke (STARS) study. JAMA 2000;283:1145. [PMID: 10703776]
- Caplan LR: Treatment of patients with stroke. Arch Neurol 2002;59:703. [PMID: 12020249]
- Mohr JP et al: A comparison of warfarin and aspirin for the prevention of recurrent ischemic stroke. N Engl J Med 2001;345:1444. [PMID: 11794192]
- Powers WJ: Oral anticoagulant therapy for the prevention of stroke. N Engl J Med 2001;345:1493. [PMID: 11794201]

Michael J. Aminoff, MD, DSc, FRCP

Strongyloidiasis

KEY FEATURES

ESSENTIALS OF DIAGNOSIS

- Pruritic dermatitis at sites of larval penetration
- Diarrhea, epigastric pain, nausea, malaise, weight loss
- Cough, rales, transient pulmonary infiltrates
- Eosinophilia; characteristic larvae in stool specimens, duodenal aspirate, or sputum
- Hyperinfection syndrome: severe diarrhea, bronchopneumonia, ileus

GENERAL CONSIDERATIONS

- Infection is caused by *Strongyloides stercoralis* (2–2.5 × 30–50 mm)
- Major symptoms result from adult parasitism, principally in the duodenum and jejunum, or from larval migration through pulmonary and cutaneous tissues
- The primary host is humans
- The parasite is uniquely capable of maintaining its life cycle both within humans and in soil. Infection occurs when filariform larvae in soil penetrate the skin, enter the bloodstream, and are carried to the lungs and ascend the bronchial tree to the glottis. The larvae are then swallowed and carried to the duodenum and upper jejunum, where they mature to the adult stage
- Recrudescence of a chronic asymptomatic infection may occur with the immunosuppression; exacerbation may lead to the hyperinfection syndrome
- In the hyperinfection syndrome, autoinfection is greatly increased, resulting in a marked increase in the intestinal worm burden and in massive dissemination of filariform larvae to the lungs and most other tissues, where they can cause local inflammatory reactions and granuloma formation

DEMOGRAPHICS

- Endemic in tropical and subtropical regions; although the prevalence is generally low, in some areas disease rates exceed 25%
- Total world prevalence is 60 million
- In the United States, highest infection rates are found in immigrants from endemic areas, in parts of Appalachia (up to 4%), and in southeastern areas; Puerto Rico is also an endemic area
- Multiple infections in households are common, and prevalence may be high in mental institutions (2–4%)
- The infection is prevalent among immunosuppressed persons

CLINICAL FINDINGS

SYMPTOMS AND SIGNS

- Up to 30% are asymptomatic
- The time from larval penetration of the skin until their appearance in the feces is 3–4 weeks
- The acute syndrome is uncommon, in which cutaneous symptoms, usually of the feet, are followed by pulmonary and then intestinal symptoms
- Most present with chronic symptoms (continuous or with irregular exacerbations) that can persist for life

Skin manifestations

- In acute infection in sensitized patients, there may be focal edema, inflammation, petechiae, serpiginous or urticarial tracts, and intense itching
- In chronic infections, both stationary urticaria and larva currens occur, characterized by transient eruptions that migrate in serpiginous tracts

Intestinal manifestations

- Symptoms range from mild to severe, the most common being diarrhea, abdominal pain, and flatulence
- Anorexia, nausea, vomiting, and pruritus ani may be present; with increasing severity, fever and malaise may appear
- Diarrhea may alternate with constipation, and in severe cases the feces contain mucus and blood
- Malabsorption or a protein-losing enteropathy can result from a large worm burden

Pulmonary manifestations

- With migration of larvae through the lungs, symptoms may be limited to a dry cough and low-grade fever, dyspnea, wheezing, and hemoptysis may occur; asthma is rare
- Bronchopneumonia, bronchitis, pleural effusion, and miliary abscesses can develop; the cough may be productive of an odorless, mucopurulent sputum

Hyperinfection syndrome

- Intense dissemination of filariform larvae to the lungs and other tissues can result in pleural effusion, pericarditis and myocarditis, hepatic granulomas, cholecystitis, purpura, nephrotic syndrome, ulcerating lesions at all levels of the gastrointestinal tract, central nervous system involvement, paralytic ileus, perforation and peritonitis, gram-negative septicemia and meningitis (due to larval carriage of enterobacteria from the colon), cachexia, shock, and death

DIFFERENTIAL DIAGNOSIS

- Hookworm disease
- Ascariasis
- Giardiasis
- Amebiasis
- Acute eosinophilic pneumonia (Löffler's syndrome)
- Tropical pulmonary eosinophilia (*Wuchereria bancrofti*, *Brugia malayi*)
- Peptic ulcer disease
- Cutaneous larva migrans

DIAGNOSIS

LABORATORY TESTS

Detection of eggs and larva

- Eggs are seldom found in feces
- Diagnosis requires finding the larval stages in feces or duodenal fluid. Four to six specimens, some unpreserved, should be collected at 2-day intervals or longer (the number of larvae in feces varies from day to day)
- Since the sensitivity of direct microscopic examination of one specimen is about 30%, it is essential that one-half of the specimens be processed, unpreserved, in the Baermann concentration or agar plate culture methods, the sensitivities of which are high

Serological and hematological findings

- In chronic low-grade intestinal strongyloidiasis, the white blood cell count is often normal, with a slightly elevated percentage of eosinophils. However, with increasing larval migration, eosinophilia may reach 50% and leukocytosis 20,000/μL

Strongyloidiasis

Immunocompromised patients

- Eosinophilia may not be seen. Mild anemia may be present
- Serum IgE immunoglobulins may be elevated
- An ELISA is sensitive (85%) and specific (97%), as is Western blot, but cross-reactions can occur with the filaria and other helminthic infections. A positive test indicates current or past infection

Hyperinfection

- There may be hypoproteinemia, malabsorption, abnormal liver function, and extensive pulmonary opacities. Filariform larvae may appear in the urine. Eosinopenia, when present, is thought to be an unfavorable prognostic sign

IMAGING STUDIES

- Small bowel x-rays may show inflammation, prominent mucosal folds, bowel dilation, delayed emptying, or ulcerative duodenitis
- In chronic infections, the findings can resemble nontropical and tropical sprue, or there may be narrowing, rigidity, and diminished peristalsis
- During pulmonary migration of larvae, chest films are normal or show fine miliary nodules or changing patches of pneumonitis, abscess, or effusion

DIAGNOSTIC PROCEDURES

- The diagnosis can sometimes be made by finding larvae in mucus obtained by the duodenal string test or by duodenal intubation and aspiration
- Duodenal biopsy is seldom indicated but will confirm the diagnosis in most. Rarely, larvae are found in sputum or bronchial washings during the pulmonary phase or in urine

TREATMENT

MEDICATIONS

- Treatment should continue until the parasite is eradicated
- In concurrent infection with hookworm, strongyloidiasis, or ascariasis, eradicate the latter infections first

Ivermectin

- The drug of choice

- The dosage is 200 μg/kg; give a second dose within several days
- Cure rates range from 82% to 95%
- In the hyperinfection syndrome in immunocompromised patients, it may be necessary to prolong treatment or change to thiabendazole

Thiabendazole

- An oral dose of 25 mg/kg (maximum, 1.5 g per dose) is given after meals twice daily for 2–3 days. Repeat the course in 2 weeks
- A 5- to 7-day (or longer) course is needed for disseminated infections; side effects become severe
- Side effects, including headache, weakness, vomiting, vertigo, and decreased mental alertness, occur in 30% of patients and may be severe. Erythema multiforme and Stevens-Johnson syndrome can occur. The side effects can be lessened if the drug is taken after meals

Albendazole

- Albendazole is given at a dosage of 400 mg twice daily for 3–7 days and repeated in 1 week; cure rates in several studies ranged from 38% to 95%
- Albendazole is less effective than ivermectin

OUTCOME

FOLLOW-UP

- Multiple stool examinations should be done at weekly intervals, preferably by the Baermann concentration method
- In selected instances, to control infections that cannot be eradicated, once-monthly treatments can be tried with a 1-day dose of ivermectin or 2-day course of thiabendazole

PROGNOSIS

- Favorable except in the hyperinfection syndrome and in infections associated with debilitating diseases

WHEN TO REFER

- Immunocompromised patients
- Disseminated disease

WHEN TO ADMIT

- Patients with the hyperinfection syndrome
- Severe pulmonary symptoms

EVIDENCE

PRACTICE GUIDELINES

- National Guideline Clearinghouse http://www.guideline.gov/summary/summary.aspx?doc_id=3258&nbr=2484&string=strongyloides

INFORMATION FOR PATIENTS

- Centers for Disease Control http://www.dpd.cdc.gov/dpdx/HTML/Strongyloidiasis.htm

REFERENCES

- Loutfy MR et al: Serology and eosinophil count in the diagnosis and management of strongyloidiasis in a non-endemic area. Am J Trop Med Hyg 2002;66:749. [PMID: 12224585]
- Zaha O et al: Efficacy of ivermectin for chronic strongyloidiasis: two single doses given 2 weeks apart. J Infect Chemother 2002;8:94. [PMID: 11957127]

Stupor & Coma

KEY FEATURES

ESSENTIALS OF DIAGNOSIS

- The stuporous patient is unresponsive except when subjected to repeated vigorous stimuli
- The comatose patient is unarousable and unable to respond to external events or inner needs, although reflex movements and posturing may be present

GENERAL CONSIDERATIONS

- Coma is a major complication of serious central nervous system disorders
- Abrupt onset of coma suggests subarachnoid hemorrhage, brainstem stroke, intracerebral hemorrhage, or acute herniation syndrome, whereas a slower onset and progression occur with other structural or mass lesions
- A metabolic cause is likely with a preceding intoxicated state or agitated delirium

Intracranial causes

- Anoxic brain injury or head trauma
- Ischemic stroke or intracerebral hemorrhage
- Subarachnoid hemorrhage
- Meningitis or encephalitis
- Brainstem hemorrhage, infarct, or mass
- Mass lesion causing brainstem compression
- Subdural hematoma
- Seizure

Metabolic causes

- Hypoglycemia
- Diabetic ketoacidosis
- Hyperglycemic hyperosmolar state
- Drugs, eg, alcohol, opioids, sedatives, antidepressants, salicylates
- Uremic or hepatic encephalopathy
- Hypernatremia or hyponatremia
- Hypercalcemia
- Hypothermia
- Heat stroke
- Myxedema
- Carbon monoxide poisoning

CLINICAL FINDINGS

SYMPTOMS AND SIGNS

- On examination, attention is paid to the behavioral response to painful stimuli, the pupils and their response to light, the position of the eyes and their movement in response to passive movement of the head and ice-water caloric stimulation, and the respiratory pattern

Response to painful stimuli

- Purposive limb withdrawal from painful stimuli implies that sensory pathways from and motor pathways to the stimulated limb are functionally intact
- Unilateral absence of responses to stimuli to both sides of the body implies a corticospinal lesion; bilateral absence suggests brainstem involvement, bilateral pyramidal tract lesions, or psychogenic unresponsiveness
- Decorticate posturing with lesions of the internal capsule and rostral cerebral peduncle, decerebrate posturing with dysfunction or destruction of the midbrain and rostral pons

Pupils

- Hypothalamic disease processes may lead to unilateral Horner's syndrome; bilateral diencephalic involvement or destructive pontine lesions to small but reactive pupils
- Ipsilateral pupillary dilation with no response to light occurs with compression of the third cranial nerve, eg, with uncal herniation
- The pupils are slightly smaller than normal but responsive to light in many metabolic encephalopathies; however, they may be fixed and dilated following overdosage with atropine, scopolamine, or glutethimide, and pinpoint (but responsive) with opiates
- Pupillary dilation for several hours following cardiopulmonary arrest implies a poor prognosis

Eye movements

- Conjugate deviation of the eyes to the side suggests the presence of an ipsilateral hemispheric lesion or a contralateral pontine lesion
- A mesencephalic lesion leads to downward conjugate deviation
- Dysconjugate ocular deviation in coma implies a structural brainstem lesion (or preexisting strabismus)

Oculomotor responses to passive head turning

- In response to brisk rotation, flexion, and extension of the head, conscious patients with open eyes do not exhibit contraversive conjugate eye deviation (doll's-head eye response) unless there is voluntary visual fixation or bilateral frontal pathology
- With cortical depression in lightly comatose patients, a brisk doll's-head eye response is seen
- With brainstem lesions, this oculocephalic reflex becomes impaired or lost, depending on the lesion site

Oculovestibular reflex

- Tested by caloric stimulation using irrigation with ice water. In normal subjects, jerk nystagmus is elicited for about 2 or 3 min, with the slow component toward the irrigated ear
- In unconscious patients with an intact brainstem, the fast component of the nystagmus disappears, so that the eyes tonically deviate toward the irrigated side for 2–3 min before returning to their original position. With impairment of brainstem function, the response is perverted and disappears
- In metabolic coma, oculocephalic and oculovestibular reflex responses are preserved, at least initially

Respiratory patterns

- Cheyne-Stokes respiration may occur with bihemispheric or diencephalic disease or in metabolic disorders
- Hyperventilation occurs with lesions of the brainstem tegmentum
- Apneustic breathing (prominent end-inspiratory pauses) suggests damage at the pontine level
- Atactic breathing (completely irregular pattern, with deep and shallow breaths occurring randomly): associated with lesions of the lower pons and medulla

DIFFERENTIAL DIAGNOSIS

- Brain death
- Persistent vegetative state
- Locked-in syndrome

DIAGNOSIS

LABORATORY TESTS

- Blood is drawn for serum glucose, electrolyte, and calcium levels; arterial blood gases; liver and renal function tests; and toxicological studies as indicated

IMAGING STUDIES

- CT scan to identify a structural lesion

DIAGNOSTIC PROCEDURES

- The diagnostic workup of the comatose patient must proceed concomitantly with management
- Lumbar puncture (if CT scan reveals no structural lesion) to exclude subarachnoid hemorrhage or meningitis

 TREATMENT

MEDICATIONS

- Dextrose 50% (25 g), naloxone (0.4–1.2 mg), and thiamine (50 mg) are given intravenously

THERAPEUTIC PROCEDURES

- Treatment of coma depends on underlying cause

Emergency measures

- Supportive therapy for respiration or blood pressure is initiated
- In hypothermia, all vital signs may be absent; all such patients should be rewarmed before the prognosis is assessed
- The patient is positioned on one side with the neck partly extended, dentures removed, and secretions cleared by suction; if necessary, the patency of the airways is maintained with an oropharyngeal airway

 OUTCOME

WHEN TO ADMIT

- Admit all patients to an ICU

PROGNOSIS

- In coma due to cerebral ischemia and hypoxia, the absence of pupillary light reflexes at the time of initial examination implies little chance of regaining independence; by contrast, preserved pupillary light responses, the development of spontaneous eye movements (roving, conjugate, or better), and extensor, flexor, or withdrawal responses to pain at this early stage imply a relatively good prognosis

 EVIDENCE

PRACTICE GUIDELINES

- National Guideline Clearinghouse http://www.guideline.gov/summary/summary.aspx?doc_id=3103&nbr=2329&string=stupor http://www.guideline.gov/summary/summary.aspx?doc_id=3582&nbr=2808&string=coma http://www.guideline.gov/summary/summary.aspx?doc_id=2793&nbr=2019&string=coma

INFORMATION FOR PATIENTS

- National Institute of Neurological Disorders and Stroke http://www.ninds.nih.gov/health_and_medical/disorders/coma_doc.htm

REFERENCE

- Malik K, Hess DC: Evaluating the comatose patient. Rapid neurologic assessment is key to appropriate management. Postgrad Med 2002;111:38. [PMID: 11868313]

Michael J. Aminoff, MD, DSc, FRCP

Subarachnoid Hemorrhage

 KEY FEATURES

ESSENTIALS OF DIAGNOSIS

- Sudden severe headache
- Signs of meningeal irritation usually present
- Obtundation or coma is common
- Focal deficits frequently absent

GENERAL CONSIDERATIONS

- 5–10% of strokes are due to subarachnoid hemorrhage
- Hemorrhage is usually from rupture of an aneurysm or arteriovenous malformation
- No specific cause found in 20% of cases
- See Table 92 (page 1276)

 CLINICAL FINDINGS

SYMPTOMS AND SIGNS

- Sudden onset of headache with severity never experienced previously by the patient
- May be followed by nausea and vomiting and loss or impairment of consciousness (transient or progress to coma and death)
- Patient is often confused and irritable and may show other symptoms of an altered mental status
- Nuchal rigidity and other signs of meningeal irritation seen, except in deeply comatose patients
- Focal neurological deficits may be present and may suggest the site of the underlying lesion

DIFFERENTIAL DIAGNOSIS

- Meningitis
- Migraine
- Intracerebral hemorrhage
- Ischemic stroke

 DIAGNOSIS

IMAGING STUDIES

- CT scan should be performed immediately to confirm that hemorrhage has occurred and to search for its source
- CT is faster and more sensitive in detecting hemorrhage in the first 24 h than MRI
- CT may rarely be normal in patients with suspected hemorrhage; if so, cerebrospinal fluid must be examined for blood or xanthochromia before the possibility of subarachnoid hemorrhage is discounted

DIAGNOSTIC PROCEDURES

- Cerebral arteriography helps to determine the source of bleeding; performed when the patient's condition has stabilized and surgery is feasible
- Bilateral carotid and vertebral arteriography are necessary because aneurysms are often multiple, while arteriovenous malformations may be supplied from several sources
- MR angiography may also permit visualization of vascular anomalies but is less sensitive than conventional arteriography

TREATMENT

MEDICATIONS

- Phenytoin to prevent seizures

SURGERY

- Causal lesion is treated surgically or by interventional radiology

THERAPEUTIC PROCEDURES

- Major aim is to prevent further hemorrhages
- Conscious patients are confined to bed, advised against exertion or straining, treated symptomatically for headache and anxiety, and given laxatives or stool softeners
- Lower blood pressure gradually for severe hypertension, but not below a diastolic level of 90 mm Hg

OUTCOME

PROGNOSIS

- Approxmately 20% of patients with aneurysms will have further bleeding within 2 weeks and 40% within 6 months
- The greatest risk of further aneurysmal hemorrhage is within a few days of the initial bleed, thus early obliteration (within 2 days) is preferred

WHEN TO ADMIT

- All patients

PREVENTION

- See Intracranial aneurysm

EVIDENCE

PRACTICE GUIDELINES

- National Guideline Clearinghouse
  http://www.guideline.gov/summary/summary.aspx?doc_id=3122&nbr=2348&string=subarachnoid+hemorrhage
  http://www.guideline.gov/summary/summary.aspx?doc_id=3298&nbr=2524&string=subarachnoid+hemorrhage

WEB SITES

- 3-D Visualization of Brain Aneurysms
  http://everest.radiology.uiowa.edu/nlm/app/aneur/brain/aneur.html
- Cerebrovascular Accident
  http://rehab.educ.ucalgary.ca/courses/core/301.03/Cardiovascular/cva-overview.html

INFORMATION FOR PATIENTS

- National Institutes of Health
  http://www.nlm.nih.gov/medlineplus/ency/article/000701.htm
- Brain Aneurysm Basics
  http://www.bafound.org/subarachnoid hemorrhage .htm

REFERENCES

- Johnston SC et al: Which unruptured cerebral aneurysms should be treated? A cost-utility analysis. Neurology 1999; 52:1806. [PMID: 10371527]
- Polin RS et al: Efficacy of transluminal angioplasty for the management of symptomatic cerebral vasospasm following aneurysmal subarachnoid hemorrhage. J Neurosurg 2000;92:284. [PMID: 10659016]
- Wardlaw JM et al: The detection and management of unruptured intracranial aneurysms. Brain 2000;123:205. [PMID: 10648430]

Michael J. Aminoff, DSc, MD, FRCP

Syndrome of Inappropriate Antidiuretic Hormone (SIADH)

 KEY FEATURES

ESSENTIALS OF DIAGNOSIS

- Serum sodium concentration less than 130 mEq/L
- Hypotonic, euvolemic hyponatremia

GENERAL CONSIDERATIONS

- Hyponatremia occurs from abnormal water balance rather than abnormal sodium balance
- Retention of electrolyte-free water because of impaired excretion and inappropriate ADH excess results in hyponatremia and low serum osmolality
- Patterns of abnormal ADH secretion
  - Random secretion (eg, carcinomas)
  - Reset osmostat (eg, elderly, pulmonary diseases)
  - Leak of ADH (eg, basilar skull fractures)

Etiology

- **Central nervous system disorders**
- Head trauma
- Stroke
- Subarachnoid hemorrhage
- Hydrocephalus
- Brain tumor
- Encephalitis
- Guillain-Barré syndrome
- Meningitis
- Acute psychosis
- Acute intermittent porphyria
- **Pulmonary lesions**
- Tuberculosis
- Bacterial pneumonia
- Aspergillosis
- Bronchiectasis
- Neoplasms
- Positive-pressure ventilation
- **Malignancies**
- Bronchogenic carcinoma
- Pancreatic carcinoma
- Prostatic carcinoma
- Renal cell carcinoma
- Adenocarcinoma of colon
- Thymoma
- Osteosarcoma
- Malignant lymphoma
- Leukemia

- **Drugs**
- *Increased ADH production*
- Antidepressants: tricyclics, monoamine oxidase inhibitors, selective serotonin reuptake inhibitors
- Antineoplastics: cyclophosphamide, vincristine
- Carbamazepine
- Methylenedioxymethamphetamine (MDMA; Ecstasy)
- Clofibrate
- Neuroleptics: thiothixene, thioridazine, fluphenazine, haloperidol, trifluoperazine
- *Potentiated ADH action*
- Carbamazepine
- Chlorpropamide, tolbutamide
- Cyclophosphamide
- Nonsteroidal antiinflammatory drugs
- Somatostatin and analogs
- **Others**
- Postoperative
- Pain
- Stress
- AIDS
- Pregnancy (physiological)
- Hypokalemia

DEMOGRAPHICS

- Most common cause of hyponatremia in hospitalized patients

 CLINICAL FINDINGS

SYMPTOMS AND SIGNS

- Frequently asymptomatic
- Symptoms usually seen with serum sodium levels less than 120 mEq/L
- If symptomatic, primarily central nervous system symptoms of lethargy, weakness, confusion, delirium, and seizures
- Often symptoms are mistaken for primary neurological or metabolic disorders

 DIAGNOSIS

LABORATORY TESTS

- See Figure 6 (page 1199)
- Decreased osmolality (<280 mosm/kg) with inappropriately increased urine osmolality (>150 mosm/kg)
- Low blood urea nitrogen (BUN) (<10 mg/dL) and hypouricemia (<4 mg/dL), which are not only dilutional but result from increased urea and uric acid clearances in response to the volume-expanded state
- A high BUN suggests a volume-contracted state, which excludes a diagnosis of SIADH

Syndrome of Inappropriate Antidiuretic Hormone (SIADH)

 TREATMENT

MEDICATIONS

Symptomatic hyponatremia

- If there are central nervous system symptoms, hyponatremia should be rapidly treated at any level of serum sodium concentration
- Increase the serum sodium concentration by no more than 1–2 mEq/L/h and not more than 25–30 meq/L in the first 2 days in order to prevent central pontine myelinolysis
- The rate should be reduced to 0.5–1 mEq/L/h as soon as neurologic symptoms improve
- The initial goal is to achieve a serum sodium concentration of 125–130 mEq/L, guarding against overcorrection
- Hypertonic (eg, 3%) saline plus furosemide (0.5–1 mg/kg intravenously) is indicated for symptomatic hyponatremia
  - To determine how much 3% saline (513 mEq/L) to administer, obtain a spot urinary Na after a furosemide diuresis has begun
  - The excreted Na is replaced with 3% saline, empirically begun at 1–2 mL/kg/h, and then adjusted based on urinary output and urinary sodium. For example, after furosemide, urine volume may be 400 mL/h and sodium plus potassium excretion 100 mEq/L. The excreted Na^+ is 40 mEq/h, which is replaced with 78 mL/h of 3% saline (40 mEq/h divided by 513 mEq/L)

Asymptomatic hyponatremia

- In asymptomatic hyponatremia, the correction rate need be no more than 0.5 mEq/L/h
  - Restrict water intake to 0.5–1 L/day
  - 0.9% saline with furosemide may be used when serum sodium is less than 120 mEq/L. Urinary sodium and potassium losses are replaced as above
  - Demeclocycline (300–600 mg twice daily) inhibits the effect of ADH on the distal tubule and is useful for patients who cannot adhere to water restriction or need additional therapy. Onset of action may be 1 week, and concentrating may be permanently impaired. Therapy with demeclocycline in cirrhosis appears to increase the risk of renal failure
  - Selective vasopressin V2 antagonist

- Oral selective V2 antagonists may be available for treatment of SIADH in the near future

 OUTCOME

FOLLOW-UP

- If symptomatic, measure plasma sodium approximately every 4 h and observe the patient closely

COMPLICATIONS

- Central pontine myelinolysis may occur from osmotically induced demyelination due to overly rapid correction of serum sodium (an increase of more than 1 meq/L/h, or 25 meq/L within the first day of therapy)
- Hypoxic-anoxic episodes during hyponatremia may contribute to the demyelination

PROGNOSIS

- Associated with underlying cause of SIADH
- Premenopausal women who develop hyponatremic encephalopathy from rapidly acquired hyponatremia (eg, postoperative hyponatremia) are about 25 times more likely than postmenopausal women to die or to suffer permanent brain damage

WHEN TO ADMIT

- Symptomatic hyponatremia
- Serum sodium <120 meq/L

 EVIDENCE

PRACTICE GUIDELINES

- National Guideline Clearinghouse
  http://www.guideline.gov/summary/summary.aspx?doc_id=3639&nbr=2865&string=SIADH

WEBSITES

- Dr. Rose's Peripheral Brain—Fluids and electrolytes
  http://faculty.washington.edu/momus/PB/fluidand.htm
- Fluid and Electrolyte Disorders:
  MDAdvice.com
  http://www.mdadvice.com/library/ped/pedillsymp160.html

INFORMATION FOR PATIENTS

- National Institutes of Health
  http://www.nlm.nih.gov/medlineplus/ency/article/000394.htm
  http://www.nlm.nih.gov/medlineplus/ency/article/000314.htm

REFERENCES

- Adrogue HJ et al: Hyponatremia. N Engl J Med 2000;342:1581.
- Cadnapaphornchai MA et al: Pathogenesis and management of hyponatremia. Am J Med 2000;109:688.
- Izzedine H et al: Angiotensin-converting enzyme inhibitor-induced syndrome of inappropriate secretion of antidiuretic hormone: case report and review of the literature. Clin Pharmacol Ther 2002; 71:503. [PMID: 12087354]
- Oster JR et al: Hyponatremia, hypoosmolality, and hypotonicity: tables and fables. Arch Intern Med 1999;159:333.

Masafumi Fukagawa, MD, PhD
Kiyoshi Kurokawa, MD, MACP
Maxine A. Papadakis, MD

Syphilis

 KEY FEATURES

ESSENTIALS OF DIAGNOSIS

- Syphilis is a complex infectious disease caused by *Treponema pallidum*, a spirochete capable of infecting almost any organ or tissue in the body and causing protean clinical manifestations
- Transmission occurs most frequently during sexual contact; sites of inoculation are usually genital but may be extragenital

GENERAL CONSIDERATIONS

- The risk of syphilis after unprotected sex with an individual with early syphilis is ~30–50%
- Syphilis can be transferred from mother to fetus after the tenth week of pregnancy (congenital syphilis)
- Two major clinical stages: early (infectious) syphilis and late syphilis are separated by a symptom-free latent period. During early latency the infectious stage is liable to recur
- Early (infectious) syphilis includes the primary lesions (chancre and regional lymphadenopathy); secondary lesions (commonly involving skin and mucous membranes, occasionally bone, central nervous system, or liver); relapsing lesions during early latency; and congenital lesions
- Late syphilis consists of so-called benign (gummatous) lesions involving skin, bones, and viscera; cardiovascular disease (principally aortitis); and central nervous system and ocular syndromes

DEMOGRAPHICS

- Between 1985 and 1990, there was a dramatic increase in infectious syphilis
- In 1998, a syphilis elimination program began targeting high-risk populations—women of childbearing age, sexually active teens, drug users, inmates of penal institutions, persons with multiple sexual partners or those who have sex with prostitutes—and emphasizing screening, early treatment, contact tracing, and condom use. A decrease in the number of primary and secondary cases was reported in 2001 (6103 cases) compared with 1998 (7035 cases)

 CLINICAL FINDINGS

SYMPTOMS AND SIGNS

Primary

- Painless ulcer (chancre) on genitalia, perianal area, rectum, pharynx, tongue, lip, or elsewhere 2–6 weeks after exposure
- Nontender enlargement of regional lymph nodes

Secondary, early latent

- Generalized maculopapular skin rash
- Mucous membrane lesions, including patches and ulcers
- Weeping papules (condylomas) in moist skin areas
- Generalized nontender lymphadenopathy
- Fever
- Meningitis, hepatitis, osteitis, arthritis, iritis

Late latent ("hidden")

- No physical signs

Late (tertiary)

- Infiltrative tumors of skin, bones, liver (gummas)
- Aortitis, aneurysms, aortic regurgitation
- Central nervous system disorders, including meningovascular and degenerative changes, paresthesias, shooting pains, abnormal reflexes, dementia, or psychosis

DIFFERENTIAL DIAGNOSIS

- Primary syphilis (genital ulcer): herpes simplex virus, chancroid, granuloma inguinale, lymphogranuloma venereum, trauma, neoplasm
- Secondary syphilis: rash, genital warts
- Tertiary syphilis: other causes of aortic root disease, other chronic meningitis

 DIAGNOSIS

LABORATORY TESTS

- Serological testing, microscopic detection of *T pallidum* in lesions, and other examinations (biopsies, lumbar puncture, x-rays) for evidence of tissue damage
- HIV test at the time of diagnosis

Nontreponemal antigen tests

- Most common are the VDRL and rapid plasma reagin (RPR)
- VDRL and RPR generally become positive 4–6 weeks after infection, or 1–3 weeks after a primary lesion. These serological tests are not highly specific
- False-positive reactions are frequent in connective tissue diseases, infectious mononucleosis, malaria, HIV, febrile diseases, leprosy, intravenous drug use, infective endocarditis, old age, hepatitis C viral infection, and pregnancy
- False-negative results when very high antibody titers are present (the prozone phenomenon)
- RPR titers are often higher than VDRL titers and thus are not comparable
- Titers are used to assess adequacy of therapy

Treponemal antibody tests

- The fluorescent treponemal antibody absorption (FTA-ABS) helps determine whether a positive nontreponemal antigen test is indicative of syphilis or false-positive
- Because of its greater sensitivity, the FTA-ABS test is also of value when there is clinical evidence of syphilis but the nontreponemal serological test is negative. The test is positive in most patients with primary syphilis and in virtually all with secondary syphilis
- The FTA-ABS test may revert to negative with adequate therapy
- False-positive FTA-ABS tests occur in systemic lupus erythematosus, Lyme disease, and hypergammaglobulinemia
- The *T pallidum* hemagglutination (TPHA) test and the particle agglutination test (TPPA) are comparable in sensitivity and specificity

DIAGNOSTIC PROCEDURES

- In primary and secondary syphilis, *T pallidum* may be shown by darkfield microscopic examination of fresh exudate from lesions or aspirated from regional lymph nodes
- Immunofluorescent staining for *T pallidum* of dried smears of fluid taken from early lesions may be helpful
- Cerebrospinal fluid (CSF) findings in neurosyphilis include elevation of total protein, lymphocytic pleocytosis, and a positive cerebrospinal fluid VDRL
- CSF may, however, be completely normal
- CSF VDRL may be negative in 30–70% of cases of neurosyphilis
- Cerebrospinal fluid FTA-ABS is controversial

 TREATMENT

MEDICATIONS

- For primary and secondary syphilis: benzathine penicillin G, 2.4 million units IM once
- For late latent syphilis or latent syphilis of unknown duration: benzathine penicillin G, 2.4 million units IM × 3 at 7 day intervals
- For neurosyphilis: aqueous penicillin G, 18–24 million units IV QD (3–4 million units Q 4 h or as a continuous infusion) for 10–14 days
- For patients allergic to penicillin, doxycycline, 100 mg PO BID for 14 days or tetracycline, 500 mg PO QID for 14 days, for infectious syphilis. In syphilis of more than 1-year duration or of unknown duration, treat for 28 days
- Preliminary data suggest azithromycin, 2 g PO once or ceftriaxone 1 g QD IM or IV for 8–10 days, is efficacious against infectious syphilis. Ceftriaxone, 2 g QD IM or IV for 10–14 days, can be used for neurosyphilis
- Patients with gonorrhea and exposure to syphilis should be treated with separate regimens effective against both diseases

 OUTCOME

FOLLOW-UP

- Syphilis patients must abstain from sexual activity until rendered noninfectious by antibiotic therapy
- Primary, secondary, early latent syphilis—reexamine clinically and serologically at 6 and 12 months (at 3, 6, 9, 12, and 24 months if HIV infected). If nontreponemal antibody titers fail to decrease 4-fold by 6 months, an HIV test should be repeated; a lumbar puncture should be considered; and if careful follow-up cannot be ensured, treatment should be repeated with 2.4 million units of benzathine penicillin IM weekly for 3 weeks
- In latent syphilis—repeat serologies at 6, 12, and 24 months. If titers increase 4-fold or if initially high titers (>1:32) fail to decrease 4-fold by 12–24 months, an HIV test and lumbar puncture (LP) should be performed and retreatment given
- In neurosyphilis—repeat LP every 6 months. If CSF cell count has not decreased by 6 months or is not normal at 2 years, a second course of treatment is given

COMPLICATIONS

- The Jarisch-Herxheimer reaction, fever and aggravation of the clinical picture, may be prevented or modified by simultaneous administration of antipyretics or corticosteroids

PROGNOSIS

- Late syphilis may be highly destructive and permanently disabling and may lead to death. If no treatment, about one-third of people infected with syphilis will undergo spontaneous cure, about one-third will remain in the latent phase throughout life, and about one-third will develop serious late lesions

WHEN TO REFER

- Refer if uncertain about interpretation of serologies, need for LP, or optimal therapy, or if patient has severe penicillin allergy

WHEN TO ADMIT

- Admit for complications (stroke, meningoencephalitis, dementia, etc) or for careful observation for Jarish-Herxheimer reaction

PREVENTION

- Avoidance of sexual contact
- Latex condoms
- Abortive penicillin therapy 2.4 million units of procaine penicillin G intramuscularly

 EVIDENCE

PRACTICE GUIDELINES

- UK National Guidelines—Medical Society for the Study of Venereal Diseases—-Late syphilis http://www.mssvd.org.uk/PDF/CEG2001/late%20$%20final%20b%2031%2012%2002.pdf

WEB SITE

- CDC—National Center for HIV, STD and TB Prevention—Division of Sexually Transmitted Diseases http://www.cdc.gov/nchstp/dstd/SyphilisInfo.htm

INFORMATION FOR PATIENTS

- JAMA patient page: Syphilis. JAMA 2000;284:520. [PMID: 10939892]

REFERENCE

- 2002 guidelines for treatment of sexually transmitted diseases. MMWR Recomm Rep 2002;51(RR-6):1. [PMID: 12184549]

Richard A. Jacobs, MD, PhD

Systemic Lupus Erythematosus

 KEY FEATURES

ESSENTIALS OF DIAGNOSIS

- Occurs mainly in young women
- Rash over areas exposed to sunlight
- Joint symptoms in 90% of patients
- Multiple system involvement
- Depression of hemoglobin, white blood cells, platelets
- Antinuclear antibody with high titer to native DNA

GENERAL CONSIDERATIONS

- An inflammatory autoimmune disorder that affects multiple organ systems
- The clinical course is marked by spontaneous remission and relapses

DEMOGRAPHICS

- 85% of patients are women
- Occurs in 1:1000 white women but in 1:250 black women

 CLINICAL FINDINGS

SYMPTOMS AND SIGNS

- Fever, anorexia, malaise, and weight loss
- Most patients have skin lesions at some time; the characteristic "butterfly" rash affects fewer than half of patients
- Alopecia is common
- Raynaud's phenomenon, present in about 20% of patients, often antedates other features of the disease
- Joint symptoms, with or without active synovitis, occur in over 90% of patients and are often the earliest manifestation. The arthritis is seldom deforming
- Ocular manifestations include conjunctivitis, photophobia, transient or permanent monocular blindness, and blurring of vision
- Pulmonary manifestations include pleurisy, pleural effusion, bronchopneumonia, pneumonitis, and restrictive lung disease
- Cardiac involvement includes pericarditis, myocarditis, cardiac arrhythmias. The typical verrucous endocarditis of Libman-Sacks is usually clinically silent but occasionally can produce acute or chronic valvular incompetence—most commonly mitral regurgitation—and can serve as a source of emboli
- Mesenteric vasculitis occasionally occurs in systemic lupus erythematosus (SLE)

and may closely resemble polyarteritis nodosa, including the presence of aneurysms in medium-sized blood vessels. Abdominal pain (particularly postprandial), ileus, peritonitis, and perforation may result

- Neurological complications include psychosis, organic brain syndrome, seizures, peripheral and cranial neuropathies, transverse myelitis, and strokes. Severe depression and psychosis are sometimes exacerbated by the administration of large doses of corticosteroids
- Several forms of glomerulonephritis may occur, including mesangial, focal proliferative, diffuse proliferative, and membranous

DIFFERENTIAL DIAGNOSIS

- Drug-induced lupus (Table 77, page 1267). Procainamide, hydralazine, and isoniazid are most often associated
- Four features of drug-induced lupus separate it from SLE: the sex ratio is nearly equal; nephritis and central nervous system features are not ordinarily present; hypocomplementemia and antibodies to native DNA are absent; and the clinical features and most laboratory abnormalities often revert toward normal when the offending drug is withdrawn
- Scleroderma
- Rheumatoid arthritis
- Inflammatory myopathy, especially dermatomyositis
- Rosacea
- Vasculitis, eg, polyarteritis nodosa
- Endocarditis
- Lyme disease

 DIAGNOSIS

LABORATORY TESTS

- SLE is characterized by the production of many different autoantibodies (Tables 73, 79, and 80, pages 1265, 1267, and 1268)
- Antinuclear antibody tests are sensitive but not specific for systemic lupus—ie, they are positive in virtually all patients with lupus but are positive also in many patients with nonlupus conditions such as rheumatoid arthritis, hepatitis, and interstitial lung disease
- Antibodies to double-stranded DNA and to Sm are specific for systemic lupus but not sensitive, since they are present in only 60% and 30% of patients, respectively
- Depressed serum complement—a finding suggestive of disease activity—often returns toward normal in remission
- Three types of antiphospholipid antibodies occur (Table 80, page 1268). The first causes the biological false-positive tests for syphilis; the second is the lupus anticoagulant, which is a risk factor for venous and arterial thrombosis and miscarriage; anticardiolipin antibodies are the third type of antiphospholipid antibodies
- Abnormality of urinary sediment is almost always found in association with renal lesions. Red blood cells, with or without casts, and mild proteinuria are frequent

DIAGNOSTIC PROCEDURES

- The diagnosis can be made with reasonable probability if 4 of the 11 criteria set forth in Table 78 (page 1267) are met. These criteria should be viewed as rough guidelines that do not supplant clinical judgment in the diagnosis of SLE
- Renal biopsy is useful in deciding whether to treat with cyclophosphamide, and to rule out end-stage renal disease that may no longer benefit from treatment

Systemic Lupus Erythematosus

 TREATMENT

MEDICATIONS

- Skin lesions often respond to the local administration of corticosteroids
- Minor joint symptoms can usually be alleviated by rest and nonsteroidal antiinflammatory drugs (NSAIDs)
- Antimalarials (hydroxychloroquine) may be helpful in treating lupus rashes or joint symptoms that do not respond to NSAIDs
- Corticosteroids are required for the control of certain serious complications, such as thrombocytopenic purpura, hemolytic anemia, myocarditis, pericarditis, convulsions, and nephritis
- Immunosuppressive agents such as cyclophosphamide, chlorambucil, and azathioprine are used in cases resistant to corticosteroids. Cyclophosphamide improves renal survival. Overall patient survival, however, is no better than in the prednisone-treated group
- Systemic steroids are not usually given for minor arthritis, skin rash, leukopenia, or the anemia associated with chronic disease

THERAPEUTIC PROCEDURES

- Avoid sun exposure and use sunscreen

 OUTCOME

COMPLICATIONS

- Thrombocytopenic purpura
- Hemolytic anemia
- Myocarditis
- Pericarditis
- Convulsions
- Nephritis

PROGNOSIS

- 10-year survival rate exceeds 85%
- In most patients, the illness pursues a relapsing and remitting course
- In some patients, the disease pursues a virulent course, leading to serious impairment of vital structures such as lung, heart, brain, or kidneys, and the disease may lead to death
- Accelerated atherosclerosis attributed, in part, to corticosteroid use, has been responsible for a rise in late deaths due to myocardial infarction

WHEN TO REFER

- Most patients should be followed in consultation with a rheumatologist and often a nephrologist

WHEN TO ADMIT

- Severe renal disease
- Pulmonary insufficiency
- Cardiac involvement
- Central nervous system disease
- Acute abdominal pain

 EVIDENCE

PRACTICE GUIDELINES

- Guidelines for referral and management of systemic lupus erythematosus in adults. American College of Rheumatology Ad Hoc Committee on Systemic Lupus Erythematosus Guidelines. Arthritis Rheum 1999; 42:1785. [PMID: 10513791]
- National Guideline Clearinghouse http://www.guideline.gov/summary/ summary.aspx?doc_id=3390&nbr= 2616&string=Lupus

INFORMATION FOR PATIENTS

- National Institute of Arthritis and Musculoskeletal and Skin Diseases http://www.niams.nih.gov/hi/topics/ lupus/slehandout/index.htm
- Lupus Foundation of America http://www.lupus.org/education/faq. html

REFERENCES

- Gordon C: Long-term complications of systemic lupus erythematosus. Rheumatology 2002;41:1095.
- Ho A et al: A decrease in complement is associated with increased renal and hematologic activity in patients with systemic lupus erythematosus. Arthritis Rheum 2001;44:2350. [PMID: 11665976]
- Illei GG et al: Combination therapy with pulse cyclophosphamide plus pulse methylprednisolone improves long-term renal outcome without adding toxicity in patients with lupus nephritis. Ann Intern Med 2001;135:248. [PMID: 11511139]
- Karim MY et al: Mycophenolate mofetil for systemic lupus erythematosus refractory to other immunosuppressive agents. Rheumatology 2002;41:876.
- Levine JS et al: The antiphospholipid syndrome. N Engl J Med 2002;346:752.

David B. Hellmann, MD, FACP
John H. Stone, MD, MPH

Takayasu's Arteritis

 ## KEY FEATURES

ESSENTIALS OF DIAGNOSIS

- Polyarteritis with predilection for the branches of the aortic arch
- Segmental stenoses, occlusions, and aneurysms
- Elevated sedimentation rate

GENERAL CONSIDERATIONS

- A rare polyarteritis of unknown cause

DEMOGRAPHICS

- Predominantly affects Asian women age <40

 ## CLINICAL FINDINGS

SYMPTOMS AND SIGNS

- Clinical presentations depend on the stage of disease (early "inflammatory" or late "occlusive") and the vessels involved
- Early stages: fever, myalgias, arthralgias, and pain over the involved artery
- Later stages: syncope, dizziness, amaurosis fugax, stroke, angina, pulmonary hypertension, and claudication
- Hypertension in >25% related to renal artery stenosis or aortic coarctation
- Vascular bruits, diminished peripheral pulses, or asymmetric blood pressure measurements

DIFFERENTIAL DIAGNOSIS

- Atheroocclusive disease
- Giant cell arteritis

 ## DIAGNOSIS

LABORATORY TESTS

- Leukocytosis
- Elevated sedimentation rate

IMAGING STUDIES

- Angiography shows combined occlusive and aneurysmal disease; the subclavian artery, descending thoracic aorta, renal artery, carotid artery, and mesenteric arteries are most commonly involved, but the ascending and abdominal aorta and the vertebral, coronary, pulmonary, iliac, and brachial arteries can also be affected
- MRA or CTA used for routine surveillance

TREATMENT

MEDICATIONS

- Early, active stage: corticosteroids, eg, prednisone, 1 mg/kg PO QD
- Cytotoxic agents may be added if steroids are ineffective

SURGERY

- Surgical or percutaneous intervention if disease indolent and clinical scenario warrants treatment
- Surgical indications are similar to those for arterial stenoses and aneurysms of other etiologies
- Percutaneous angioplasty or stenting can be done for short-segment stenoses, but there is a high recurrence rate

THERAPEUTIC PROCEDURES

- Histological examination of the resected artery shows nonspecific transmural inflammation or chronic fibrosis

 OUTCOME

COMPLICATIONS

- Stroke
- Renal insufficiency
- Limb loss

PROGNOSIS

- Good if diagnosed and treated early

WHEN TO REFER

- Symptoms, signs, and diagnosis of Takayasu's arteritis

WHEN TO ADMIT

- Takayasu's arteritis with complication

Takayasu's Arteritis

 EVIDENCE

PRACTICE GUIDELINES

- Sabbadini MG et al: Takayasu's arteritis: therapeutic strategies. J Nephrol 2001; 14(6):525. [PMID: 11783609]
- Weyand CM et al: Medium- and large-vessel vasculitis. N Engl J Med. 2003; 349:160. [PMID: 12853590]

WEB SITES

- MEDLINEplus—Takayasu arteritis http://www.nlm.nih.gov/medlineplus/ ency/article/001250.htm
- Takayasu's Arteritis Foundation International http://www.takayasu.org/
- Takayasu's Arteritis Association http://www.takayasus.com/

INFORMATION FOR PATIENTS

- Cleveland Clinic—Takayasu arteritis http://www.clevelandclinic.org/health/ health-info/docs/1700/1738.asp? index=7097
- NIH—Patient Education Institute: Vasculitis http://www.nlm.nih.gov/medlineplus/ tutorials/vasculitis.html
- Johns Hopkins Vasculitits Center— Takayasu arteritis http://vasculitis.med.jhu.edu/typesof/ takayasu.html
- Uptodate—Overview of vasculitis http://patients.uptodate.com/frames. asp?page=topic.asp&file=arth_rhe/ 4492&title=Takayasu+arteritis

REFERENCE

- Johnston SL et al: Takayasu arteritis: a review. J Clin Pathol 2002;55:481. [PMID: 12101189]

Louis M. Messina, MD
Laura K. Pak, MD
Lawrence M. Tierney, Jr., MD

Tapeworm Infection, Beef

 KEY FEATURES

ESSENTIALS OF DIAGNOSIS

- Generally asymptomatic
- Patients often discover segments of the tapeworm in clothing or stool

GENERAL CONSIDERATIONS

- Six tapeworms infect humans frequently
- The large tapeworms are *Taenia saginata* (the beef tapeworm, up to 25 m in length), *Taenia solium* (the pork tapeworm, 7 m), and *Diphyllobothrium latum* (the fish tapeworm, 10 m)
- The small tapeworms are *Hymenolepis nana* (the dwarf tapeworm, 25–40 mm), *Hymenolepis diminuta* (the rodent tapeworm, 20–60 cm), and *Dipylidium caninum* (the dog tapeworm, 10–70 cm)
- Humans are the only definitive host of *T saginata* and *T solium*
- An adult tapeworm consists of a head (scolex), a neck, and a chain of individual segments (proglottids) in which eggs form in mature segments
- Humans are infected by eating raw or undercooked beef containing viable cysticerci, *Cysticercus bovis*. In the human intestines, the cysticercus develops into an adult worm

DEMOGRAPHICS

- Four of the six tapeworms occur worldwide; the pork and fish tapeworms have more limited distribution
- The infection occurs in most countries with beef husbandry but is highly endemic in parts of the Far East, central and eastern Africa, and the central Asian area of the former Soviet Union
- Gravid segments of *T saginata* in the human intestine detach themselves from the chain and are passed in feces to soil. When proglottids or eggs are ingested by grazing cattle or other domesticated bovines, the eggs hatch to release embryos that encyst in muscle as cysticerci.

 CLINICAL FINDINGS

SYMPTOMS AND SIGNS

- Large tapeworms are generally asymptomatic
- Occasionally, vague gastrointestinal symptoms (eg, nausea, diarrhea, abdominal pain) and systemic symptoms (eg, fatigue, hunger, dizziness) have been attributed to the infections
- Vomiting of proglottid segments or obstruction of the bile duct, pancreatic duct, or appendix is rare

DIFFERENTIAL DIAGNOSIS

- Pork, fish, dwarf, rodent, or dog tapeworms
- Chronic fatigue syndrome
- Chronic hepatitis
- Irritable bowel syndrome
- Amebiasis
- Ascariasis
- Enterobiasis (pinworm, mostly children)
- Hookworm disease
- Strongyloidiasis
- Celiac sprue or tropical sprue
- Pernicious anemia (*D latum*)

 DIAGNOSIS

LABORATORY TESTS

- Serological tests are not available

DIAGNOSTIC PROCEDURES

- Infection is often discovered by the patient finding segments in stool, clothing, or bedding
- To determine the species, proglottid segments are either flattened between glass slides and examined microscopically for anatomic detail or differentiated by enzyme electrophoresis of glucose phosphate isomerase
- Eggs are only infrequently present in stools, but the perianal cellophane tape test, as used to diagnose pinworm, is sometimes useful in detecting *T saginata* eggs. However, *Taenia* eggs look alike and do not permit species differentiation except by specialized methods

TREATMENT

MEDICATIONS

- Praziquantel in a single dose of 10 mg/kg achieves cure rates of about 99%. At this dose, side effects are minimal
- With a single dose of four tablets (2 g) of niclosamide (not available in the United States), cure rates over 90% can be anticipated. The drug is given in the morning before the patient has eaten. The tablets *must be chewed thoroughly* and swallowed with water. Eating may be resumed in 2 h. The drug usually produces no side effects
- Pre- and posttreatment purges are not used for either drug

 OUTCOME

FOLLOW-UP

- A disintegrating worm is usually passed within 24–48 h of treatment. Since efforts are not generally made to recover and identify the scolex, cure can be presumed only if regenerated segments have not reappeared 3–5 months later
- If it is preferred that parasitic cure be established immediately, the head (scolex) must be found in posttreatment stools; a laxative is given 2 h after treatment, and stools must be collected in a preservative for 24 h. To facilitate examination, toilet paper must be disposed of separately

PROGNOSIS

- Excellent with therapy

WHEN TO REFER

- For assistance in making the diagnosis
- Inability to clear the infection

PREVENTION

- *C bovis* is killed by cooking at 56°C or freezing at −10°C for 5 days. Pickling is not adequate

 EVIDENCE

PRACTICE GUIDELINES

- National Guideline Clearinghouse http://www.guideline.gov/summary/summary.aspx?doc_id=2707&nbr=1933&string=foodborne

INFORMATION FOR PATIENTS

- National Institutes of Health http://www.nlm.nih.gov/medlineplus/ency/article/001391.htm
- The Mayo Clinic http://www.mayoclinic.com/invoke.cfm?id=ID00002

REFERENCE

- Hoberg EP: Taenia tapeworms: their biology, evolution and socioeconomic significance. Microbes Infect 2002;4:859. [PMID: 12270733]

Tapeworm Infection, Dwarf

 KEY FEATURES

ESSENTIALS OF DIAGNOSIS

- Infection may be asymptomatic
- Can cause nonspecific gastrointestinal symptoms of nausea, diarrhea, pain, and weight loss

GENERAL CONSIDERATIONS

- Six tapeworms infect humans frequently
- The large tapeworms are *Taenia saginata* (the beef tapeworm, up to 25 m in length), *Taenia solium* (the pork tapeworm, 7 m), and *Diphyllobothrium latum* (the fish tapeworm, 10 m)
- The small tapeworms are *Hymenolepis nana* (the dwarf tapeworm, 25–40 mm), *Hymenolepis diminuta* (the rodent tapeworm, 20–60 cm), and *Dipylidium caninum* (the dog tapeworm, 10–70 cm)
- An adult tapeworm consists of a head (scolex), a neck, and a chain of individual segments (proglottids) in which eggs form in mature segments. The scolex is the attachment organ and generally lodges in the upper part of the small intestine
- Multiple infections are the rule for small tapeworms and may occur for *D latum*; however, it is rare for a person to harbor more than one or two of the taeniae

Dwarf tapeworm

- *H nana* is the most common cestode
- It can reach high prevalence, particularly in children, in regions of the world with poor fecal hygiene and in closed institutions worldwide
- Humans are the definitive host of *H nana*; rodent-adapted strains occur in rodents
- The life cycle is unusual in that both larval and adult stages are found in the human intestine, internal autoinfection can occur, and generally there is no intermediate host
- Transmission usually results from eggs transferred directly from human to human (the eggs are immediately infective) but sometimes involves fomites, water, or food or the swallowing of fleas

Rodent tapeworm

- *H diminuta* is a common parasite of rodents. Many arthropods (eg, rat fleas, beetles, and cockroaches) serve as intermediate hosts
- Humans—most commonly young children—are infected by accidentally swal-

lowing the infected arthropods, usually in cereals or stored products

Dog tapeworm

- *D caninum* infection generally occurs in young children in close association with infected dogs or cats
- Transmission results from swallowing the infected intermediate hosts, ie, fleas or lice

 CLINICAL FINDINGS

SYMPTOMS AND SIGNS

- Light infections are generally asymptomatic
- Heavy infections, particularly with *H nana*, may cause diarrhea, abdominal pain, anorexia, vomiting, weight loss, and irritability

DIFFERENTIAL DIAGNOSIS

- Chronic fatigue syndrome
- Chronic hepatitis
- Irritable bowel syndrome
- Amebiasis
- Ascariasis
- Enterobiasis (pinworm, mostly children)
- Hookworm disease
- Strongyloidiasis
- Celiac sprue or tropical sprue
- Pernicious anemia (*D latum*)

 DIAGNOSIS

LABORATORY TESTS

- *H nana* and *H diminuta* infections are diagnosed by finding characteristic eggs in feces; proglottids are usually not seen
- *D caninum* infection is diagnosed by detection of proglottids (the size of melon seeds) in feces or after their active migration through the anus
- Serological tests are not available

TREATMENT

MEDICATIONS

H nana

- Praziquantel, the drug of choice, produces 95% cure rates with a single 25-mg/kg dose
- Niclosamide (not available in the United States), the alternative drug, produces cure rates of 75% when given at a single dosage of four tablets (2 g) for 5–7 days; some workers repeat the course 5 days later. The drug is given in the morning before the patient has eaten. The tablets *must be chewed thoroughly* and swallowed with water. Eating may be resumed in 2 h. The drug usually produces no side effects

H diminuta and *D caninum*

- Treatment is with niclosamide or praziquantel in dosages as for *H nana*. Cure rates are not established

 OUTCOME

WHEN TO REFER

- For persistent or progressive infection despite treatment

 EVIDENCE

PRACTICE GUIDELINES

- National Guideline Clearinghouse
http://www.guideline.gov/summary/
summary.aspx?doc_id=2791&nbr=
2017&string=animal+borne

INFORMATION FOR PATIENTS

- Centers for Disease Control
http://www.dpd.cdc.gov/dpdx/HTML/
Taeniasis.htm
- National Institutes of Health
http://www.nlm.nih.gov/medlineplus/
ency/article/001391.htm

REFERENCE

- Hoberg EP: Taenia tapeworms: their biology, evolution and socioeconomic significance. Microbes Infect 2002;4:859. [PMID: 12270733]

Tapeworm Infection, Fish

 KEY FEATURES

ESSENTIALS OF DIAGNOSIS

- One of six tapeworms that commonly infects humans
- Infections are generally asymptomatic but occasionally there can be nonspecifc gastrointestinal discomfort
- Macrocytic megaloblastic anemia can develop

GENERAL CONSIDERATIONS

- Six tapeworms infect humans frequently. The large tapeworms are *Taenia saginata* (the beef tapeworm, up to 25 m in length), *Taenia solium* (the pork tapeworm, 7 m), and *Diphyllobothrium latum* (the fish tapeworm, 10 m). The small tapeworms are *Hymenolepis nana* (the dwarf tapeworm, 25–40 mm), *Hymenolepis diminuta* (the rodent tapeworm, 20–60 cm), and *Dipylidium caninum* (the dog tapeworm, 10–70 cm). Four of the six tapeworms occur worldwide; the pork and fish tapeworms have more limited distribution
- An adult tapeworm consists of a head (scolex), a neck, and a chain of individual segments (proglottids) in which eggs form in mature segments. The scolex is the attachment organ and generally lodges in the upper part of the small intestine
- Multiple infections are the rule for small tapeworms and may occur for *D latum*; however, it is rare for a person to harbor more than one or two of the taeniae
- Eggs passed in human feces that reach fresh water are taken up first by crustaceans that in turn are eaten by fish, both of which are intermediate hosts
- Human infection results from eating raw or inadequately cooked brackish or freshwater fish, including salmon
- Nonhuman reservoir hosts include dogs, bears, and other fish-eating mammals
- Some persons (mostly Scandinavian residents) who harbor the fish tapeworm develop a macrocytic megaloblastic anemia accompanied by thrombocytopenia and mild leukopenia. Gastric acidity is normal. The anemia is a result of the worm's competing with the host for vitamin B_{12}

DEMOGRAPHICS

- *D latum* is found in temperate and subarctic lake regions

 CLINICAL FINDINGS

SYMPTOMS AND SIGNS

- Large tapeworm infections are generally asymptomatic
- Occasionally, vague gastrointestinal symptoms (eg, nausea, diarrhea, abdominal pain) and systemic symptoms (eg, fatigue, hunger, dizziness) have been attributed to the infections
- Vomiting of proglottid segments or obstruction of the bile duct, pancreatic duct, or appendix is rare
- If B_{12} deficiency develops, clinical findings are indistinguishable from those of pernicious anemia. They include glossitis, dyspnea, tachycardia, and neurological findings (numbness, paresthesias, disturbances of coordination, impairment of vibration and position sense, and dementia)

DIFFERENTIAL DIAGNOSIS

- Beef, pork, dwarf, rodent, or dog tapeworm
- Chronic fatigue syndrome
- Chronic hepatitis
- Irritable bowel syndrome
- Amebiasis
- Ascariasis
- Enterobiasis (pinworm, mostly children)
- Hookworm disease
- Strongyloidiasis
- Celiac sprue or tropical sprue
- Pernicious anemia (*D latum*)

 DIAGNOSIS

LABORATORY TESTS

- Diagnosed by finding characteristic operculated eggs in stool; repeat examinations and concentration may be necessary
- Proglottids are occasionally vomited or passed in feces; their internal morphology is diagnostic
- The presence of hydrochloric acid in the stomach differentiates tapeworm anemia from pernicious anemia; in both conditions, the Schilling test is abnormal

TREATMENT

MEDICATIONS

- Praziquantel in a single dose of 10 mg/kg achieves cure rates of about 99%. At this dose, side effects are minimal
- With a single dose of four tablets (2 g) of niclosamide (not available in the United States), cure rates over 90% can be anticipated. The drug is given in the morning before the patient has eaten. The tablets *must be chewed thoroughly* and swallowed with water. Eating may be resumed in 2 h. Niclosamide usually produces no side effects
- Pre- and posttreatment purges are not used for either drug
- The anemia and neurological manifestations respond to vitamin B_{12} as used in treatment of pernicious anemia

 OUTCOME

FOLLOW-UP

- A disintegrating worm is usually passed within 24–48 h of treatment. Since efforts are not generally made to recover and identify the scolex, cure can be presumed only if regenerated segments have not reappeared 3–5 months later
- If it is preferred that parasitic cure be established immediately, the head (scolex) must be found in posttreatment stools; a laxative is given 2 h after treatment, and stools must be collected in a preservative for 24 h. To facilitate examination, toilet paper must be disposed of separately

WHEN TO REFER

- If confirmation of the diagnosis is needed or if symptoms are progressive despite therapy
- If there is difficulty distinguishing tapeworm-induced B_{12} deficiency from pernicious anemia

 EVIDENCE

INFORMATION FOR PATIENTS

- National Institute of Allergy and Infectious Diseases http://www.niaid.nih.gov/factsheets/foodbornedis.htm
- Centers for Disease Control http://www.cdc.gov/ncidod/dpd/parasites/taenia/default.htm

REFERENCE

- Hoberg EP: Taenia tapeworms: their biology, evolution and socioeconomic significance. Microbes Infect 2002;4:859. [PMID: 12270733]

Tapeworm Infection, Pork

 KEY FEATURES

ESSENTIALS OF DIAGNOSIS

- Generally asymptomatic
- Can cause nonspecific gastrointestinal symptoms of nausea, diarrhea, and pain

GENERAL CONSIDERATIONS

- Six tapeworms infect humans frequently
- The large tapeworms are *Taenia saginata* (the beef tapeworm, up to 25 m in length), *Taenia solium* (the pork tapeworm, 7 m), and *Diphyllobothrium latum* (the fish tapeworm, 10 m
- The small tapeworms are *Hymenolepis nana* (the dwarf tapeworm, 25–40 mm), *Hymenolepis diminuta* (the rodent tapeworm, 20–60 cm), and *Dipylidium caninum* (the dog tapeworm, 10–70 cm)
- Humans are the only definitive host of *T solium*
- An adult tapeworm consists of a head (scolex), a neck, and a chain of individual segments (proglottids) in which eggs form in mature segments
- Gravid segments of *T solium* in the human intestine detach themselves from the chain and are passed in feces to soil. When pigs ingest human feces containing proglottids and eggs, the eggs hatch to release embryos that encyst in muscle as cysticerci. Humans become infected when they eat undercooked pork containing viable *C cellulosae*. In the human intestines, the *Cysticercus* develops into an adult worm
- Humans are the intermediate host when they become infected with the larval (*Cysticercus*) stage by accidentally ingesting eggs in human feces; the eggs are immediately infectious (see *Cysticercosis*)
- Transmission of eggs may occur as a result of autoinfection (hand to mouth), direct person-to-person transfer, ingestion of food or drink contaminated by eggs, or (rarely) regurgitation of proglottids into the stomach

DEMOGRAPHICS

- The pork tapeworm is particularly prevalent in Mexico, Latin America, the Iberian Peninsula, the Slavic countries, Africa, Southeast Asia, India, and China
- In the United States and Canada, human infection is rare, usually encountered in persons infected abroad; cysticercosis in hogs is uncommon

 CLINICAL FINDINGS

SYMPTOMS AND SIGNS

- Large tapeworms are generally asymptomatic
- Occasionally, vague gastrointestinal symptoms (eg, nausea, diarrhea, abdominal pain) and systemic symptoms (eg, fatigue, hunger, dizziness) have been attributed to the infections
- Vomiting of proglottid segments or obstruction of the bile duct, pancreatic duct, or appendix is rare

DIFFERENTIAL DIAGNOSIS

- Beef, fish, dwarf, rodent, and dog tapeworm
- Chronic fatigue syndrome
- Chronic hepatitis
- Irritable bowel syndrome
- Amebiasis
- Ascariasis
- Enterobiasis (pinworm, mostly children)
- Hookworm disease
- Strongyloidiasis
- Celiac sprue or tropical sprue
- Pernicious anemia (*D latum*)

 DIAGNOSIS

LABORATORY TESTS

- Infection is often discovered by the patient finding segments in stool, clothing, or bedding
- To determine the species, proglottid segments are either flattened between glass slides and examined microscopically for anatomic detail or differentiated by enzyme electrophoresis of glucose phosphate isomerase
- Serological tests are not available

TREATMENT

MEDICATIONS

- Praziquantel in a single dose of 10 mg/kg achieves cure rates of about 99%. At this dose, side effects are minimal
- With a single dose of four tablets (2 g) of niclosamide (not available in the United States), cure rates over 90% can be anticipated. The drug is given in the morning before the patient has eaten. The tablets *must be chewed thoroughly* and swallowed with water. Eating may be resumed in 2 h. The drug usually produces no side effects
- Neither drug kills eggs released from disintegrating segments; therefore, to avoid the theoretical possibility of cysticercosis from hatching eggs, give a moderate purgative 2–3 h after treatment to rapidly eliminate segments and eggs from the bowel. Instruct the patient about the need after defecation for careful washing of the hands and perianal area and for careful disposal of feces for 4 days after therapy
- A pretreatment purge is not used for either drug

 OUTCOME

FOLLOW-UP

- A disintegrating worm is usually passed within 24–48 h of treatment. Since efforts are not generally made to recover and identify the scolex, cure can be presumed only if regenerated segments have not reappeared 3–5 months later
- If it is preferred that parasitic cure be established immediately, the head (scolex) must be found in posttreatment stools; a laxative is given 2 h after treatment, and stools must be collected in a preservative for 24 h. To facilitate examination, toilet paper must be disposed of separately

WHEN TO REFER

- For persistent disease despite appropriate therapy

PREVENTION

- *C cellulosae* is killed by cooking at 65°C or freezing at −20°C for 12 h. Pickling is not adequate
- Because the prognosis is often poor in cerebral cysticercosis, *T solium* infections must be immediately eradicated

 EVIDENCE

PRACTICE GUIDELINES

- National Guideline Clearinghouse http://www.guideline.gov/summary/summary.aspx?doc_id=2707&nbr=1933&string=pork

INFORMATION FOR PATIENTS

- Centers for Disease Control http://www.dpd.cdc.gov/dpdx/HTML/Taeniasis.htm
- National Institutes of Health http://www.nlm.nih.gov/medlineplus/ency/article/001391.htm

REFERENCE

- Hoberg EP: Taenia tapeworms: their biology, evolution and socioeconomic significance. Microbes Infect 2002;4:859. [PMID: 12270733]

Testicular Cancer

 ## KEY FEATURES

ESSENTIALS OF DIAGNOSIS

- Commonest neoplasm in men aged 20–35
- Typical presentation as a patient-identified painless nodule
- Orchiectomy necessary for diagnosis

GENERAL CONSIDERATIONS

- Rare, 2–3 new cases per 100,000 males in the United States each year
- 90–95% of all primary testicular tumors are germ cell tumors (seminoma and nonseminoma), remainder are nongerminal neoplasms (Leydig cell, Sertoli cell, gonadoblastoma)
- Lifetime probability of developing testicular cancer is 0.2% for an American white male
- Slightly more common on the right than on the left, bilateral in 1–2%
- Cause unknown
- History of unilateral or bilateral cryptorchism
- Risk of development of malignancy is highest for the intraabdominal testis (1:20) and lower for the inguinal testis (1:80)
- Orchiopexy does not alter the malignant potential of the cryptorchid testis; it does facilitate examination and tumor detection
- 5–10% of these tumors occur in the contralateral, normally descended testis

 ## CLINICAL FINDINGS

SYMPTOMS AND SIGNS

- Most common symptom: painless enlargement of the testis
- Sensation of heaviness
- Acute testicular pain from intratesticular hemorrhage in ~10%
- Symptoms relating to metastatic disease, such as back pain (retroperitoneal metastases), cough (pulmonary metastases), or lower extremity edema (vena cava obstruction), in 10%
- Asymptomatic at presentation in 10%
- Physical examination: testicular mass or diffuse enlargement of the testis in the majority of cases
- Secondary hydroceles in 5–10%
- Supraclavicular adenopathy
- Retroperitoneal mass
- Gynecomastia in 5% of germ cell tumors

DIFFERENTIAL DIAGNOSIS

- Epidermoid cyst

 ## DIAGNOSIS

LABORATORY TESTS

- Human chorionic gonadotropin, α-fetoprotein, and lactate dehydrogenase
- Liver function tests
- 24-h urine creatinine clearance

IMAGING STUDIES

- Scrotal ultrasound

Testicular Cancer

TREATMENT

SURGERY

- Radical orchiectomy by inguinal exploration with early vascular control of the spermatic cord structures
- Scrotal approaches and open testicular biopsies should be avoided

Seminomas

- Stage I and IIa (retroperitoneal disease <10 cm in diameter) seminomas treated by radical orchiectomy and retroperitoneal irradiation have 5-year disease-free survival rates of 98% and 92–94%, respectively. Stage IIb (>10 cm retroperitoneal involvement) and stage III seminomas are treated with primary chemotherapy (etoposide and cisplatin or cisplatin, etoposide, and bleomycin). Among stage III patients, 95% will attain a complete response following orchiectomy and chemotherapy

Nonseminomas

- Up to 75% of stage A nonseminomas are cured by orchiectomy alone
- Modified retroperitoneal lymph node dissections have been designed to preserve the sympathetic innervation for ejaculation
- Selected patients may be offered surveillance: tumor is confined within the tunica albuginea; tumor does not demonstrate vascular invasion; tumor markers normalize after orchiectomy; radiographic imaging shows no evidence of disease (chest x-ray and CT); and reliable patient
- Surveillance is done monthly for the first 2 years and bimonthly in year 3: tumor markers at each visit, and chest x-ray and CT every 3–4 months. Majority of relapses occur within the first 8–10 months. With rare exceptions, patients who relapse can be cured by chemotherapy or surgery. The 5-year disease-free survival rate for stage A is 96% to 100%; for low-volume stage B disease, it is 90%
- Patients with bulky retroperitoneal disease (>3 cm nodes) or metastases are treated with primary cisplatin-based combination chemotherapy following orchiectomy (etoposide and cisplatin or cisplatin, etoposide, and bleomycin)
- For a residual mass greater than 3 cm, resection is mandatory
- If tumor markers fail to normalize following primary chemotherapy, salvage chemotherapy is required (cisplatin, etoposide, bleomycin, ifosfamide)

OUTCOME

PROGNOSIS

- Patients with bulky retroperitoneal or disseminated disease treated with primary chemotherapy followed by surgery have a 5-year disease-free survival rate of 55–80%

EVIDENCE

PRACTICE GUIDELINES

- Laguna MP et al: EAU guidelines on testicular cancer. Eur Urol 2001;40:102. [PMID: 11528185]
- [No authors listed] NCCN practice guidelines for testicular cancer. National Comprehensive Cancer Network. Oncology (Huntingt) 1998;12:417. [PMID: 10028524]
- Segal R et al: Surveillance programs for early stage non-seminomatous testicular cancer: a practice guideline. Can J Urol 2001;8:1184. [PMID: 11268306]

WEB SITES

- American Cancer Society—What is testicular cancer?
  http://www.cancer.org/docroot/cri/content/cri_2_4_1x_what_is_testicular_cancer_41.asp?sitearea=cri
- National Cancer Institute—questions and answers about testicular cancer
  http://cis.nci.nih.gov/fact/6_34.htm
- Testicular Cancer Resource Center
  http://tcrc.acor.org/

INFORMATION FOR PATIENTS

- Mayo Clinic—Testicular cancer
  http://www.mayoclinic.com/invoke.cfm?objectid=91B1CB36-2B25-4B93-8FB60CFCAC19B62D
- MEDLINEplus—Testicular cancer
  http://www.nlm.nih.gov/medlineplus/ency/article/001288.htm

REFERENCES

- Heidenreich A et al: Organ-sparing surgery for malignant germ cell tumor of the testis. J Urol 2001;166:2161. [PMID: 11696727].
- Sweeney CJ et al: Results and outcome of retroperitoneal lymph node dissection for clinical stage I embryonal carcinoma–predominant testis cancer. J Clin Oncol 2000;18:358. [PMID: 10637250]

Marshall L. Stoller, MD
Peter R. Carroll, MD

Tetanus

 KEY FEATURES

ESSENTIALS OF DIAGNOSIS

- History of wound and possible contamination
- Jaw stiffness followed by spasms of jaw muscles (trismus)
- Stiffness of the neck and other muscles, dysphagia, irritability, hyperreflexia
- Finally, painful convulsions precipitated by minimal stimuli

GENERAL CONSIDERATIONS

- Caused by the neurotoxin tetanospasmin elaborated by *Clostridium tetani*
- Spores of this organism are ubiquitous in soil. When introduced into a wound, spores may germinate
- Tetanospasmin interferes with neurotransmission at spinal synapses of inhibitory neurons
- Minor stimuli result in uncontrolled spasms, and reflexes are exaggerated
- Most cases occur in unvaccinated individuals
- Persons at risk are the elderly, migrant workers, newborns, and injection drug users, who may acquire the disease through subcutaneous injections

 CLINICAL FINDINGS

SYMPTOMS AND SIGNS

- The first symptom may be pain and tingling at the site of inoculation, followed by spasticity of the muscles nearby
- Stiffness of the jaw, neck stiffness, dysphagia, and irritability are other early signs
- Hyperreflexia develops later, with spasms of the jaw muscles (trismus) or facial muscles and rigidity and spasm of the muscles of the abdomen, neck, and back
- Painful tonic convulsions precipitated by minor stimuli are common
- Spasms of the glottis and respiratory muscles may cause acute asphyxia
- The patient is awake and alert throughout the illness. The sensory examination is normal. The temperature is normal or only slightly elevated
- Urinary retention and constipation may result from spasm of the sphincters
- Respiratory arrest and cardiac failure are late, life-threatening events

DIFFERENTIAL DIAGNOSIS

- Meningitis
- Rabies
- Tetany due to hypocalcemia
- Strychnine poisoning
- Neuroleptic malignant syndrome
- Trismus due to peritonsillar abscess

 DIAGNOSIS

LABORATORY TESTS

- The diagnosis is made clinically

TREATMENT

MEDICATIONS

- Passive immunization should be used in nonimmunized individuals and those whose immunization status is uncertain whenever a wound is contaminated or likely to have devitalized tissue
- Tetanus immune globulin, 250 units, is given intramuscularly. Active immunization with tetanus toxoid should be started concurrently
- Table 128 (page 1131) provides a guide to prophylactic management
- Penicillin, 20 million units daily, is given to all patients—even those with mild illness—to eradicate toxin-producing organisms

THERAPEUTIC PROCEDURES

- Minimal stimuli can provoke spasms, so the patient should be placed at bed rest and monitored under the quietest conditions possible
- Sedation, paralysis with curare-like agents, and mechanical ventilation are often necessary to control tetanic spasms

 OUTCOME

COMPLICATIONS

- Respiratory arrest
- Pneumonia

PROGNOSIS

- High mortality rates are associated with a short incubation period, early onset of convulsions, and delay in treatment
- Contaminated lesions about the head and face are more dangerous than wounds on other parts of the body
- The overall mortality rate is about 40%, but this can be reduced with ventilator management

WHEN TO REFER

- For confirmation of the disease, refer to an infectious disease specialist
- For the specialized treatment of the neuromuscular symptoms, refer to a neurologist

WHEN TO ADMIT

- Any patient in whom there is clinical suspicion of the disease
- Intensive care unit may be needed

PREVENTION

- Tetanus is completely preventable by active immunization
- For primary immunization of adults, tetanus toxoid is administered as two doses 4–6 weeks apart, with a third dose 6–12 months later. Booster doses are given every 10 years or at the time of major injury if it occurs more than 5 years after a dose (Table 127, page 1310)

 EVIDENCE

PRACTICE GUIDELINES

- National Guideline Clearinghouse http://www.guideline.gov/summary/summary.aspx?doc_id=3502&nbr=2728&string=tetanus http://www.guideline.gov/summary/summary.aspx?doc_id=3353&nbr=2579&string=tetanus

WEB SITES

- CDC—Division of Bacterial and Mycotic Diseases http://www.cdc.gov/ncidod/dbmd/
- Karolinska Institute—Directory of Bacterial Infections and Mycoses http://www.mic.ki.se/Diseases/c1.html

INFORMATION FOR PATIENTS

- JAMA patient page: Immunizations. JAMA 1999;282:102.
- Mayo Clinic http://www.mayoclinic.com/invoke.cfm?id=DS00227

REFERENCE

- Hsu SS et al: Tetanus in the emergency department: a current review. J Emerg Med 2001;20:357. [PMID: 11348815]

Henry F. Chambers, MD

Thalassemia

 ## KEY FEATURES

ESSENTIALS OF DIAGNOSIS

- Microcytosis out of proportion to degree of anemia
- Positive family history or lifelong personal history of microcytic anemia
- Abnormal red blood cell (RBC) morphology with microcytes, acanthocytes, and target cells
- In β-thalassemia, elevated levels of hemoglobin A2 or F

GENERAL CONSIDERATIONS

- Hereditary disorders characterized by reduction in synthesis of globin chains (α or β), causing reduced hemoglobin synthesis and eventually, hypochromic microcytic anemia
- Normal adult hemoglobin primarily hemoglobin A, a tetramer of two α-chains and two β-chains ($\alpha_2\beta_2$)
- α-Thalassemia syndromes determined by number of functional α-globin genes
  - Normal (four α-globin genes)
  - Silent carrier (three α-globin genes, normal hematocrit)
  - α-Thalassemia minor or trait [two α-globin genes, hematocrit 32–40%, mean cell volume (MCV) 60–75]
  - Hemoglobin H disease (one α-globin gene, hematocrit 22–32%, MCV 60-70)
  - Hydrops fetalis (0 α-globin genes)
- β-Thalassemia: reduced β-globin chain synthesis results in relative increase in percentages of hemoglobins A2 and F compared to hemoglobin A, as β-like globins (γ and δ) substitute for missing β-chains
- With reduced β-chains, excess α-chains precipitate, causing hemolysis; bone marrow becomes hyperplastic, resulting in bony deformities, osteopenia, and pathological fractures

DEMOGRAPHICS

- α-Thalassemia occurs primarily in persons from southeast Asia and China, and, less commonly, in blacks
- β-Thalassemia affects persons of Mediterranean origin (Italian, Greek) and to lesser extent Chinese, other Asians, and blacks

 ## CLINICAL FINDINGS

SYMPTOMS AND SIGNS

- α-Thalassemia silent carriers are asymptomatic
- α-Thalassemia trait: clinically normal with mild microcytic anemia
- Hemoglobin H disease: chronic hemolytic anemia of variable severity, pallor, and splenomegaly
- Hydrops fetalis: fetal death
- Heterozygous for β-thalassemia (thalassemia minor): mild microcytic anemia
- Homozygous for mild β-thalassemia (thalassemia intermedia): chronic hemolytic anemia
- Homozygous for major β-thalassemia (thalassemia major): severe anemia requiring transfusion; growth failure; bony deformities (abnormal facial structure, pathological fractures); hepatosplenomegaly and jaundice

DIFFERENTIAL DIAGNOSIS

- Iron deficiency anemia (thalassemia has lower MCV, normal iron studies, more normal RBC count, more abnormal peripheral blood smear at modest levels of anemia)
- Other hemoglobinopathy, eg, sickle thalassemia, hemoglobin C disorders
- Sideroblastic anemia
- Anemia of chronic disease

 ## DIAGNOSIS

LABORATORY TESTS

α-Thalassemia trait

- Mild anemia (hematocrit 28-40%) with strikingly low MCV (60–75 fL)
- RBC count normal or increased
- Peripheral blood smear mildly abnormal: microcytes, hypochromia, occasional target cells, acanthocytes
- Reticulocyte count and iron studies normal
- Hemoglobin electrophoresis: no increase in percentage of hemoglobins A2 or F and no hemoglobin H (thus usually a diagnosis of exclusion)

Hemoglobin H disease

- Variably severe hemolytic anemia (hematocrit 22–32%) with remarkably low MCV (60–70 fL)
- Peripheral blood smear markedly abnormal: hypochromia, microcytosis, target cells, poikilocytosis
- Reticulocyte count elevated
- Hemoglobin electrophoresis: shows hemoglobin H comprises 10–40% of the hemoglobin

β-Thalassemia minor

- Mild anemia (hematocrit 28–40%) with MCV 55–75 fL
- RBC count normal or increased
- Peripheral blood smear mildly abnormal: hypochromia, microcytosis, target cells, basophilic stippling
- Reticulocyte count normal or slightly elevated
- Hemoglobin electrophoresis: elevated hemoglobin A2 to 4–8% and occasionally elevated hemoglobin F to 1–5%

β-Thalassemia major

- Severe anemia (hematocrit sometimes <10% without transfusion)
- Peripheral blood smear bizarre: severe poikilocytosis, hypochromia, microcytosis, target cells, basophilic stippling, nucleated RBCs
- Hemoglobin electrophoresis: little or no hemoglobin A, variable amounts of hemoglobin A2, and major hemoglobin present is hemoglobin F

TREATMENT

MEDICATIONS

- Mild thalassemias (α-thalassemia trait or β-thalassemia minor) usually require no treatment and should be identified to avoid repeated evaluations for iron deficiency and inappropriate administration of supplemental iron
- α-Thalassemia trait and thalassemia intermedia may require transfusion during infection or other stress
- Hemoglobin H disease: folate supplementation; avoid medicinal iron and oxidative drugs such as sulfonamides
- Severe thalassemia: regular transfusions and folate supplementation

SURGERY

- Splenectomy indicated if hypersplenism causes marked increase in transfusion requirement

THERAPEUTIC PROCEDURES

- Prenatal diagnosis and genetic counseling should be offered
- Blood transfusions as above
- Allogeneic bone marrow transplantation for β-thalassemia major in children who have not yet experienced iron overload and chronic organ toxicity

 OUTCOME

COMPLICATIONS

- Bony deformities, osteopenia, and pathological fractures in β-thalassemia
- Complications of blood transfusions as below
- Splenomegaly may result from chronic hemolysis

PROGNOSIS

- Mild thalassemia (α-thalassemia trait or β-thalassemia minor): normal life expectancy
- Thalassemia intermedia: may develop transfusional iron overload; patients survive into adulthood but with hepatosplenomegaly and bony deformities
- β-Thalassemia major
  - Clinical course modified significantly by transfusion therapy, but transfusional iron overload causes heart failure, cirrhosis, and endocrinopathies, usually after >100 units
  - Death from cardiac failure usually occurs between ages 20 and 30
  - Long-term survival is >80% in cases undergoing allogeneic bone marrow transplantation

PREVENTION

- Deferoxamine routinely given as iron-chelating agent to avoid or postpone hemosiderosis in transfusion-dependent patients; low-iron diet may also help

 EVIDENCE

PRACTICE GUIDELINES

- Dumars KW et al: Practical guide to the diagnosis of thalassemia. Council of Regional Networks for Genetic Services (CORN). Am J Med Genet 1996;62:29. [PMID: 8779321]
- Lo L et al: Thalassemia: current approach to an old disease. Pediatr Clin North Am 2002;49:1165. [PMID: 12580361]

WEB SITES

- Childrens Hospital Oakland—Thalassemia http://www.thalassemia.com/medical/definition.shtml
- Cooley's Anemia Foundation, Inc. What is thalassemia http://cooleysanemia.org/sections.php?sec=1&tab=6&sub=49&cooleys_sess=9302841ca25676bb456daea8f6d06f83
- Thalassemia Foundation of Canada—FAQ http://www.thalassemia.ca/ faq.html

INFORMATION FOR PATIENTS

- March of Dimes—Thalassemia http://www.marchofdimes.com/professionals/681_1229.asp
- Mayo Clinic—Thalassemia http://www.mayoclinic.com/invoke.cfm?objectid=DB830EF9-0BCA-4FE0-963AC966F187099C
- MEDLINEplus—Thalassemia http://www.nlm.nih.gov/medlineplus/ency/article/000587.htm

REFERENCES

- Aessopos A et al: Cardiac involvement in thalassemia intermedia: a multicenter study. Blood 2001;97:3411. [PMID: 11369631]
- Chui D et al : Hemoglobin H disease: not necessarily a benign disorder. Blood 2003;101:791. [PMID: 12393486]

Charles A. Linker, MD

Thoracic Aortic Aneurysm

 KEY FEATURES

GENERAL CONSIDERATIONS

- Aneurysms of the thoracic aorta account for fewer than 10% of aortic aneurysms
- Causes: medial degeneration, chronic dissection, vasculitis, and collagen-vascular disease (Marfan's syndrome or Ehlers-Danlos syndrome), trauma, syphilis (rare)
- Type 1 extends from the left subclavian artery to the renal arteries, type 2 from the left subclavian artery to the iliac bifurcation, type 3 from the midthoracic to the infrarenal region, and type 4 from the diaphragmatic hiatus to the infrarenal region
- The prevalence of each type is roughly equal, but type 4 aneurysms have the lowest operative mortality (2–5%) and lowest risk of postoperative neurological deficits

 CLINICAL FINDINGS

SYMPTOMS AND SIGNS

- Most are asymptomatic and discovered incidentally
- Substernal, back, or neck pain
- Dyspnea, stridor, or a brassy cough from pressure on the trachea
- Dysphagia from pressure on the esophagus
- Hoarseness from pressure on the left recurrent laryngeal nerve
- Neck and arm edema from external compression of the superior vena cava
- Aortic regurgitation murmur with aneurysms of the ascending aorta

DIFFERENTIAL DIAGNOSIS

- Lung neoplasm
- Thymoma
- Cyst
- Substernal goiter

 DIAGNOSIS

LABORATORY TESTS

- Preoperative evaluation: electrocardiogram, creatinine, complete blood count, and type and cross-match

IMAGING STUDIES

- CT scan and MRI/MRA
- Aortography: to assess involvement of the arch vessels, coronary arteries, and aortic valve

Thoracic Aortic Aneurysm

 TREATMENT

MEDICATIONS
- Antihypertensives to control blood pressure
- β-Blockers to slow aneurysmal growth

SURGERY
- Indications for surgical treatment: new aortic insufficiency, presence of symptoms, rapid expansion, or size >6 cm in good risk surgical candidates
- Open surgical replacement with synthetic graft; sometimes requires left heart bypass

THERAPEUTIC PROCEDURES
- Endovascular repair reduces cardiopulmonary risk, but the location of the aneurysm (proximity to arch vessels or spinal arteries) may preclude endovascular repair
- Endovascular treatment remains experimental

 OUTCOME

FOLLOW-UP
- CT scan every 6–8 months

COMPLICATIONS
- Surgical complications
- Pulmonary complications
- Injury to recurrent laryngeal nerve, phrenic nerve, carotid and subclavian arteries
- Spinal cord paraplegia

PROGNOSIS
- Surgical morbidity and mortality are higher than with abdominal aortic aneurysms
- 30-day operative mortality is 8–20% with repair of type 1 and type 2 aneurysms
- 5-year survival for patients with unrepaired thoracic aneurysms >6 cm is 20–25%

WHEN TO REFER
- Aneurysm diameter greater than 4.5 cm

WHEN TO ADMIT
- Symptomatic or ruptured aneurysm for elective repair when 6.0 cm or greater

PREVENTION
- Cardiovascular risk factor assessment and modification
- Smoking cessation

EVIDENCE

PRACTICE GUIDELINES
- Diagnosis of chest pain. Institute for Clinical Systems, 2001 http://www.icsi.org/knowledge/detail.asp?catID=29&itemID=169
- Eggebrecht H et al: Interventional management of aortic dissection. Herz 2002;27:539. [PMID: 12378400]
- Veith FJ et al: Guidelines for development and use of transluminally placed endovascular prosthetic grafts in the arterial system. Endovascular Graft Committee. J Vasc Surg 1995;21:670. [PMID: 7707571]

WEB SITES
- American Heart Association http://www.americanheart.org/presenter.jhtml?identifier=8458
- MEDLINEplus—Thoracic aortic aneurysm http://www.nlm.nih.gov/medlineplus/ency/article/001119.htm

INFORMATION FOR PATIENTS
- Cleveland Clinic—Aneurysm http://www.clevelandclinic.org/health/health-info/docs/0300/0391.asp?index=3930
- Mayo Clinic—Aortic aneurysm http://www.mayoclinic.com/invoke.cfm?objectid=FE3FE459-7D1E-405F-95E9339CD2E974B8

REFERENCES
- Chuter TAM et al: Multi-branched stent-graft for type III thoracoabdominal aortic aneurysm. J Vasc Interv Radiol 2001;12:391. [PMID: 11287522]
- Elefteriades JA: Natural history of thoracic aortic aneurysms: indications for surgery, and surgical versus nonsurgical risks. Ann Thorac Surg 2002;74:S1877. [PMID: 12440685]

Louis M. Messina, MD
Laura K. Pak, MD
Lawrence M. Tierney, Jr., MD

Thoracic Outlet Syndrome

 KEY FEATURES

ESSENTIALS OF DIAGNOSIS

- Subdivided into neurogenic, venous, and arterial types, depending on which structures are compressed in the interscalene triangle or costoclavicular space
- Neurogenic: most common (>90%), often the most difficult to diagnose and treat; history of whiplash trauma or repetitive upper extremity activity, particularly overhead activity
- Venous: also called Paget-Schroetter syndrome or effort thrombosis; involves external compression of the subclavian vein by the first rib, anterior scalene muscle, clavicle, and costocoracoid ligament; often a history of repetitive upper arm exercises or clavicular fracture
- Arterial: least common; compression of the subclavian artery between the anterior and middle scalene muscles produces subclavian artery aneurysms, which result in digital ischemia due to atheroemboli; arm claudication less common

 CLINICAL FINDINGS

SYMPTOMS AND SIGNS

Neurogenic

- Supraclavicular and anterior chest wall burning pain
- Segmental pain and paresthesias of the arm in an ulnar nerve distribution
- Weakness of the intrinsic muscles of the hand
- Thenar or hypothenar muscle wasting (rare)
- Physical examination: supraclavicular tenderness, positive brachial plexus tension testing
- Positive Adson test
- Positive Roos test
- Positive Tinel sign
- Electrophysiological testing usually negative

Venous

- Presents as acute unilateral arm edema, axillary fullness, hand cyanosis, and enlarged shoulder and chest wall collateral veins

Arterial

- Positive Wylie-Allen test, arm heaviness/tiredness with activity, digital ischemia or splinter hemorrhage secondary to emboli

DIFFERENTIAL DIAGNOSIS

- Other cause of brachial plexus neuropathy
- Neck disorder, eg, osteoarthritis, herniated disk, tumor
- Shoulder osteoarthritis
- Reflex sympathetic dystrophy
- Carpal tunnel syndrome

 DIAGNOSIS

LABORATORY TESTS

- With thrombosis of vein, obtain plasma levels of antithrombin III, factor V Leiden, anticardiolipin antibody, fibrinogen, proteins C and S, lupus anticoagulant, homocysteine and prothrombin gene mutation

IMAGING STUDIES

- Neurogenic: chest film for cervical rib
- Venous: positional venography
- Arterial: angiography

TREATMENT

MEDICATIONS
- Analgesics
- Muscle relaxants

SURGERY

Neurogenic
- Surgical resection of the hypertrophied anterior and middle scalene muscles, brachial plexus neurolysis, and resection of bony abnormalities in severe refractory cases

Venous
- Anterior scalene and first rib resection with venolysis. If axillary-subclavian vein thrombosis, preoperative thrombolysis followed immediately by surgery with intraoperative angioplasty of any residual venous stenosis, or surgical thrombectomy

Arterial
- Removal of anterior and middle scalene muscles, resection of the aneurysm with polytetrafluoroethylene interposition graft

THERAPEUTIC PROCEDURES

Neurogenic
- Physical therapy: Edgelow Neurovascular Entrapment Self-Treatment (ENVEST) program
- Transcutaneous electrical nerve stimulation

OUTCOME

COMPLICATIONS
- Loss of function
- Chronic venous stasis disease
- Ischemic ulceration

PROGNOSIS
- Neurogenic: after surgery symptoms return within 1 year in as many as 25% of patients
- Venous: prognosis is excellent with appropriate treatment

WHEN TO REFER
- Any suspected arterial or venous thoracic outlet syndrome
- Neurogenic thoracic outlet syndrome refractory to a dedicated course of medical treatment

WHEN TO ADMIT
- Acute venous occlusion
- Digital ischemia

PREVENTION
- Ergonomic workplace

EVIDENCE

PRACTICE GUIDELINES
- Novak CB: Thoracic outlet syndrome. Clin Plast Surg 2003;30:175. [PMID: 12737351]
- Surgery for thoracic outlet syndrome (TOS). Washington State Department of Labor and Industries, 1999 http://www.guidelines.gov/summary/summary.aspx?doc_id=1900&nbr=1126&string=Thoracic+Outlet+Syndrome.

WEB SITES
- American Academy of Orthopaedic Surgeons—Thoracic outlet syndrome http://orthoinfo.aaos.org/fact/thr_report.cfm?Thread_ID=206&topcategory=Shoulder
- MEDLINEplus—Thoracic outlet syndrome http://www.nlm.nih.gov/medlineplus/ency/article/001434.htm

INFORMATION FOR PATIENTS
- Cleveland Clinic—Thoracic outlet syndrome http://www.clevelandclinic.org/health/health-info/docs/1300/1355 .asp?index=6123
- Mayo Clinic—Thoracic outlet syndrome http://www.mayoclinic.com/invoke.cfm?objectid=51E8E5FD-9ACA-4DAA-8DF2586D5F34C061

REFERENCES
- Alexrod DA et al: Outcomes after surgery for thoracic outlet syndrome. J Vasc Surg 2001;33:1220. [PMID: 11389421]
- Pascarelli EF et al: Understanding work-related upper-extremity disorders: clinical findings in 485 computer users, musicians, and others. J Occup Rehabil 2001;11:1. [PMID: 11706773]

Louis M. Messina, MD
Laura K. Pak, MD
Lawrence M. Tierney, Jr., MD

Thromboangiitis Obliterans (Buerger's Disease)

 KEY FEATURES

ESSENTIALS OF DIAGNOSIS

- An episodic and segmental inflammatory and thrombotic process of the peripheral arteries and veins
- Presents with claudication, rest pain
- Linked to tobacco use
- Episodic, with quiescent periods lasting weeks, months, or years

GENERAL CONSIDERATIONS

- Cause is unknown
- History of cold sensitivity or Raynaud's phenomenon
- Characterized by occlusion of distal arteries, producing claudication, rest pain, and tissue necrosis
- Associated with migratory superficial segmental thrombophlebitis; affected vein shows inflammatory infiltrate in the vessel wall, microabscesses, thrombus, or recanalization with perivascular fibrosis
- Clinical course is usually episodic, with acute exacerbations followed by remissions

DEMOGRAPHICS

- Most commonly occurs in men age <40 who smoke, particularly those of Eastern European or Asian background
- <20% of affected patients are women

 CLINICAL FINDINGS

SYMPTOMS AND SIGNS

- Intermittent claudication typically begins in the arch of the foot and progresses to the calf
- Rest pain and diminished sensation from ischemic neuropathy in >70% of patients
- No pathognomonic signs
- Proximal pulses are normal; distal pulses are diminished or absent
- Affected digits may be pale, cyanotic, or erythematous
- Ulcers, typically located at the nail margins, in 75% of patients
- Allen test positive
- May have concomitant thrombophlebitis

DIFFERENTIAL DIAGNOSIS

- Limb ischemia due to emboli or atherosclerotic occlusive disease
- Autoimmune disorders: Raynaud's disease, polyarteritis nodosa, systemic lupus erythematosus, antiphospholipid antibody syndrome, Takayasu's arteritis
- Rare: ergotamine intoxication, cannabis arteritis, hypothenar hammer syndrome

 DIAGNOSIS

LABORATORY TESTS

- Obtain complete blood cell count, prothrombin time, partial thromboplastin time, sedimentation rate, antinuclear antibody, lupus anticoagulant, rheumatoid factor, anticentromere antibody, and antiphospholipid antibody

IMAGING STUDIES

- Angiography: involvement of distal arteries with sparing of proximal arteries, segmental appearance with skip areas, no vascular calcification, and extensive collateralization via tortuous "corkscrew" vessels
- Peripheral ultrasound or angiography and echocardiography are done to exclude an embolic source

DIAGNOSTIC PROCEDURES

- Diagnosed by biopsy of affected vein

TREATMENT

MEDICATIONS

- Nonsteroidal antiinflammatory medications and opioids for pain control
- Aspirin, 325 mg PO QD, or other antiplatelet agents
- Calcium channel blockers
- Iloprost and vascular endothelial growth factor (VEGF) are investigational agents

SURGERY

- Sympathectomy is indicated for relief of intractable rest pain and healing of refractory ulcers, often in conjunction with digital amputation
- Amputation is reserved for patients with wet gangrene or severe rest pain

THERAPEUTIC PROCEDURES

- Smoking cessation, elimination of chewing tobacco and marijuana, and avoidance of nicotine replacement and exposure to second-hand smoke
- Local wound care: limited debridement, appropriate dressings, and intravenous antibiotics for cellulitis
- Moisturization of nonulcerated skin
- Lamb's wool between the toes, heel protectors, sheepskin-lined boots (Rooke boots)
- Supplemental oxygen by nasal cannula, hyperbaric oxygen

 OUTCOME

COMPLICATIONS

- Gangrene
- Cellulitis
- Amputation/limb loss

PROGNOSIS

- Prognosis dependent on smoking cessation
- More than 90% of patients who quit smoking avoid amputation

WHEN TO REFER

- Refer patients with symptoms and signs of Buerger's disease to a vascular surgeon

WHEN TO ADMIT

- Limb-threatening ischemia

PREVENTION

- Tobacco cessation and nicotine avoidance

 EVIDENCE

PRACTICE GUIDELINES

- Borner C et al: Long-term follow-up of thromboangiitis obliterans. Vasa 1998;27:80. [PMID: 9612110]
- Szuba A: Thromboangiitis obliterans. An update on Buerger's disease. West J Med 1998;168:255. [PMID: 9584663]

WEB SITES

- Columbia University College of Physicians and Surgeons—Buerger's disease
  http://cpmcnet.columbia.edu/texts/guide/hmg16_0005.html
- Johns Hopkins Vasculitis Center—Buerger's disease
  http://vasculitis.med.jhu.edu/typesof/buergers.html
- University of Michigan Health Center—Buerger's disease
  http://www.med.umich.edu/1libr/aha/umcirc08.htm

INFORMATION FOR PATIENTS

- Mayo Clinic—Buerger's disease
  http://www.mayoclinic.com/invoke.cfm?objectid=91D74792-B1CA-4B8C-97A6F3CCBAFA655F
- MEDLINEplus—Thromboangiitis obliterans
  http://www.nlm.nih.gov/medlineplus/ency/article/000172.htm
- Merck Manual—Thromboangiitis obliterans
  http://www.merck.com/pubs/mmanual/section16/chapter212/212c.htm

REFERENCE

- Olin JW: Current concepts: thromboangiitis obliterans (Buerger's disease). N Engl J Med 2000;343:864. [PMID: 10995867]

Louis M. Messina, MD
Laura K. Pak, MD
Lawrence M. Tierney, Jr., MD

Thrombophlebitis, Superficial Veins

 KEY FEATURES

ESSENTIALS OF DIAGNOSIS

- Induration, redness, and tenderness along a superficial vein
- Often a history of recent intravenous line or trauma
- No significant swelling of the extremity

GENERAL CONSIDERATIONS

- May occur spontaneously in patients with varicose veins, in pregnant or post-partum women, or with thromboangiitis obliterans or Behçet's disease
- May occur after trauma or after intravenous infusion
- Migratory superficial thrombophlebitis may occur in abdominal cancer such as carcinoma of the pancreas (Trousseau's syndrome)
- Long saphenous vein and its tributaries are most often involved
- Superficial thrombophlebitis is associated with occult deep vein thrombosis in ~20% of cases
- Pulmonary emboli are rare unless there is extension of clot into the deep veins

 CLINICAL FINDINGS

SYMPTOMS AND SIGNS

- Dull pain in the region of the involved vein
- Induration, redness, and tenderness
- Dilated, thrombosed superficial veins
- No edema or deep calf tenderness
- Chills and high fever suggest septic or suppurative phlebitis

DIFFERENTIAL DIAGNOSIS

- Deep vein thrombosis
- Cellulitis
- Lymphangitis
- Erythema nodosum
- Erythema induratum (associated with tuberculosis)
- Panniculitis

 DIAGNOSIS

LABORATORY TESTS

- Blood culture: in septic thrombophlebitis, the causative organism is often *Staphylococcus* or a gram-negative rod
- Complete blood cell count

IMAGING STUDIES

- Ultrasound to rule out deep venous thrombosis and assess extent of superficial thrombosis

TREATMENT

MEDICATIONS

- Nonsteroidal antiinflammatory drugs
- Septic thrombophlebitis requires IV antibiotics for 7- to 10-day course
- Anticoagulation for rapidly progressing disease or extension into the deep system

SURGERY

- Excision of the involved vein indicated for symptoms that persist over 2 weeks, or for recurrent phlebitis
- Immediate excision of an infected vein if the patient becomes septic

THERAPEUTIC PROCEDURES

- Ambulation
- Warm compresses
- Limb elevation

OUTCOME

PROGNOSIS

- Course is generally benign and brief
- Prognosis depends on the underlying pathological process
- Phlebitis of a saphenous vein occasionally extends to the deep veins, which may cause chronic venous insufficiency, limb edema, and pulmonary emboli

WHEN TO REFER

- Suspected deep venous thrombosis
- Septic thrombophlebitis
- Recurrent thrombophlebitis
- Thrombophlebitis in suprageniculate greater saphenous vein

WHEN TO ADMIT

- Septic thrombophlebitis

EVIDENCE

PRACTICE GUIDELINES

- Guex JJ: Thrombotic complications of varicose veins. A literature review of the role of superficial venous thrombosis. Dermatol Surg 1996;22:378. [PMID: 8624665]
- Kalodiki E et al: Superficial thrombophlebitis and low-molecular-weight heparins. Angiology 2002;53:659. [PMID: 12463618]
- Venous thromboembolism. Institute for Clinical Systems Improvement, 2002 http://www.icsi.org/knowledge/detail. asp?catID=29&itemID=202

WEB SITES

- MEDLINEplus—Superficial thrombophlebitis http://www.nlm.nih.gov/medlineplus/ ency/article/000199.htm
- Merck Manual—Superficial thrombophlebitis http://www.merck.com/pubs/ mmanual_home2/sec03/ch036/ch036c. htm
- Society of Interventional Radiology— Vascular diseases diagnosis http://www.sirweb.org/patPub/vascular Diagnosis.shtml

INFORMATION FOR PATIENTS

- Mayo Clinic—Thrombophlebitis http://www.mayoclinic.com/invoke.cfm? id=DS00223

REFERENCE

- Belcaro G et al.: Superficial thrombophlebitis of the legs: a randomized, controlled, follow-up study. Angiology 1999;50:523. [PMID: 10431991]

Louis M. Messina, MD
Laura K. Pak, MD
Lawrence M. Tierney, Jr., MD

Thrombotic Thrombocytopenic Purpura

 ## KEY FEATURES

ESSENTIALS OF DIAGNOSIS

- Thrombocytopenia
- Microangiopathic hemolytic anemia
- Normal coagulation tests
- Elevated serum lactate dehydrogenase (LDH)

GENERAL CONSIDERATIONS

- Uncommon syndrome characterized by microangiopathic hemolytic anemia, thrombocytopenia, noninfectious fever, neurological disorders, and renal insufficiency
- Markedly elevated serum LDH
- Pathogenesis appears to be deficiency of a von Willebrand factor–cleaving protease, in some cases due to antibody against the protease
- Occasionally precipitated by estrogen use, pregnancy, drugs, or infections (eg, HIV)

DEMOGRAPHICS

- Occurs primarily in young adults between age 20 and 50
- Slight female predominance

 ## CLINICAL FINDINGS

SYMPTOMS AND SIGNS

- Fever may be present
- Pallor and symptoms of anemia
- Purpura, petechiae, and bleeding
- Neurological symptoms and signs, including headache, confusion, aphasia, and alterations in consciousness from lethargy to coma, may wax and wane over minutes; hemiparesis and seizures with more advanced disease
- Abdominal pain and tenderness due to pancreatitis

DIFFERENTIAL DIAGNOSIS

- Disseminated intravascular coagulation
- Hemolytic uremic syndrome
- Preeclampsia–eclampsia
- Meningitis
- Evan's syndrome (idiopathic thrombocytopenic purpura with autoimmune hemolytic anemia)

 ## DIAGNOSIS

LABORATORY TESTS

- Peripheral smear shows microangiopathic changes with fragmented red blood cells (RBCs) (schistocytes, helmet cells, triangle forms)
- Anemia is universal and may be marked
- Usually marked reticulocytosis and occasional circulating nucleated RBCs
- Thrombocytopenia is invariably present and may be severe
- Increased indirect bilirubin and occasionally hemoglobinemia and hemoglobinuria from hemolysis; methemalbuminemia may impart brown color to plasma
- LDH markedly elevated in proportion to severity of hemolysis; Coombs test negative
- Coagulation tests (prothrombin time, partial thromboplastin time, fibrinogen) normal unless ischemic tissue damage causes secondary disseminated intravascular coagulation
- Elevated fibrin degradation products may be seen, as in other acutely ill patients
- Renal insufficiency, with abnormal urinalysis

DIAGNOSTIC PROCEDURES

- Pathologically, may see thrombi in capillaries and small arteries, with no evidence of inflammation

Thrombotic Thrombocytopenic Purpura

TREATMENT

MEDICATIONS

- Prednisone and antiplatelet agents [aspirin (325 mg PO TID) and dipyridamole (75 mg PO TID)] have been used in addition to plasmapheresis, but their role is unclear
- Management of refractory patients who do not respond to plasmapheresis or have rapid recurrences is controversial
- Combination of splenectomy, corticosteroids, and dextran used with success
- Immunosuppression (eg, cyclophosphamide) also effective

SURGERY

- Splenectomy may be indicated for refractory disease
- Splenectomy during remission may prevent subsequent relapses

THERAPEUTIC PROCEDURES

- Emergent large-volume plasmapheresis is the treatment of choice for thrombotic thrombocytopenic purpura: 60–80 mL/kg of plasma removed and replaced with fresh-frozen plasma, continued daily until complete remission; optimal duration of plasmapheresis after remission unknown

OUTCOME

PROGNOSIS

- With plasmapheresis, formerly dismal prognosis has dramatically changed; 80–90% now recover completely
- Neurological abnormalities are usually reversed
- Most complete responses are durable, but 20% of cases are chronic and relapsing

EVIDENCE

PRACTICE GUIDELINES

- Allford SL et al: Guidelines on the diagnosis and management of the thrombotic microangiopathic haemolytic anaemias. Br J Haematol 2003;120:556. [PMID: 12588343]
- Rock GA: Management of thrombotic thrombocytopenic purpura. Br J Haematol 2000;109:496. [PMID: 10886194]
- von Baeyer H: Plasmapheresis in thrombotic microangiopathy-associated syndromes: review of outcome data derived from clinical trials and open studies. Ther Apher 2002;6:320. [PMID: 12164804]

WEB SITE

- Baylor Health Care System—TTP support group http://www.bhcs.com/library/healthguide/selfhelp/topic.asp?hwid=shc29ttp

INFORMATION FOR PATIENTS

- American College of Physicians—Treatment of refractory thrombotic thrombocytopenic purpura http://www.annals.org/issues/v138n2/fpdf/200301210-00004.pdf
- MEDLINEplus—Thrombotic thrombocytopenic purpura http://www.nlm.nih.gov/medlineplus/ency/article/000552.htm

REFERENCES

- Moake JL: Thrombotic microangiopathies. N Engl J Med 2002;347:589. [PMID: 12192020]
- Zheng X et al: Remission of chronic thrombocytopenic purpura after treatment with cyclophosphamide and rituximab. Ann Intern Med 2003;138:105. [PMID: 12529092]

Charles A. Linker, MD

Thyroid Cancer

KEY FEATURES

ESSENTIALS OF DIAGNOSIS

- Painless swelling in region of thyroid
- Thyroid function tests usually normal
- Past history of head-neck radiation
- Positive thyroid needle aspiration

GENERAL CONSIDERATIONS

- Most thyroid cancers are microscopic and indolent. Larger thyroid cancers require treatment

Papillary carcinoma

- Pure papillary or mixed papillary-follicular carcinoma is most common thyroid malignancy (76%)
- Childhood head-neck radiation or nuclear fallout exposure (eg, Chernobyl accident) imparts increased lifelong risk
- May be familial (3%) or associated with Cowden's disease (multiple hamartomas of skin and mucous membranes and high incidence of breast cancer) or adenomatous polyposis coli
- Least aggressive thyroid malignancy, but spreads via thyroid lymphatics, becoming multifocal in 60% and involving both lobes in 30%. ~80% have microscopic metastases to cervical lymph nodes. 15% of adults and 60% of youths have palpable lymph nodes

Follicular carcinoma

- Second most common thyroid malignancy (16% of thyroid cancers); generally more aggressive than papillary carcinoma
- Metastases commonly found in neck lymph nodes, bone, and lungs

Medullary thyroid carcinoma

- 4% of thyroid cancers
- One-third sporadic, one-third familial, one-third associated with multiple endocrine neoplasia (MEN) type 2
- Early local metastases usually present, and late metastases may appear in bones, lungs, adrenals, or liver
- Peptides (eg, serotonin, ACTH, corticotropin-releasing hormone) can cause symptoms and serve as tumor markers

Anaplastic thyroid carcinoma

- 1% of thyroid cancers
- Older patient with rapidly enlarging mass in a multinodular goiter

- Most aggressive thyroid carcinoma; metastasizes early to surrounding lymph nodes and distant sites

Other thyroid malignancies

- 3% of thyroid cancers
- Lymphoma; metastatic bronchogenic, breast, and renal carcinomas, melanoma

DEMOGRAPHICS

- Incidence of papillary and follicular thyroid carcinomas increases with age
- Female/male ratio is 3:1
- 40 cases per million population diagnosed clinically, but 13% have microscopic thyroid cancer at autopsy in the United States

CLINICAL FINDINGS

SYMPTOMS AND SIGNS

- Thyroid cancer usually presents as a palpable, firm, nontender nodule, but can arise from multinodular goiter
- Larger cancers can cause neck discomfort, dysphagia, or hoarseness
- ~3% present with metastasis, usually to local lymph nodes but sometimes to distant sites such as bone or lung
- Metastatic differentiated thyroid carcinoma may secrete enough thyroxine to produce thyrotoxicosis
- Medullary thyroid carcinoma causes flushing and diarrhea (30%) and fatigue; ~5% develop Cushing's syndrome
- Anaplastic or long-standing tumors can produce hoarseness related to recurrent laryngeal nerve palsy from pressure or invasion of surrounding tissues

DIFFERENTIAL DIAGNOSIS

- Benign thyroid nodule, eg, adenoma, cyst
- Subacute thyroiditis
- Benign multinodular goiter
- Lymphadenopathy due to other cause
- Metastasis from head and neck cancer
- Lymphoma

DIAGNOSIS

LABORATORY TESTS

- Serum thyroid-stimulating hormone (TSH), free tetraiodothyronine (T_4) generally normal unless concomitant thyroiditis; metastatic follicular carcinoma may secrete enough thyroxine to suppress TSH
- Serum thyroglobulin level high in most metastatic papillary and follicular tumors; useful marker for recurrent or metastatic disease except if antithyroglobulin Ab present. Assay serum thyroglobulin level preoperatively, postoperatively when hypothyroid (before ^{131}I therapy) or during TRH, and when euthyroid
- Serum calcitonin level frequently elevated in medullary thyroid carcinoma, but nonspecific test; obtain preoperatively as useful marker for recurrent or metastatic disease
- Serum carcinoembryonic antigen (CEA) levels usually elevated with medullary carcinoma; obtain preoperatively as useful marker for recurrent or metastatic disease
- Genetic testing of siblings and children of patients with medullary carcinoma for *RET* protooncogene mutations, which occur in MEN-2 and familial medullary thyroid carcinoma

IMAGING STUDIES

- ^{131}I or ^{123}I thyroid scan: useful in diagnosis of follicular carcinomas
- Neck ultrasound: aids in determining size and location of malignancy and neck metastases. More sensitive than neck palpation; especially useful if prior known metastases, persistent elevation in serum thyroglobulin, or detectable levels of antithyroglobulin antibodies
- Chest x-ray (CXR) or CT scan may demonstrate metastases, but iodinated contrast greatly reduces effectiveness of radioiodine scanning and therapy. Medullary carcinoma in thyroid, nodes, and liver may calcify, but lung metastases rarely do
- Positron emission tomography scan and MRI to detect metastases

DIAGNOSTIC PROCEDURES

- Fine needle aspiration biopsy for clinically suspicious nodules

944

TREATMENT

MEDICATIONS

- Levothyroxine, 0.05–0.1 mg PO QD, immediately after thyroidectomy and continued for life; dose adjusted to produce mild suppression of serum TSH without causing thyrotoxicosis

SURGERY

- Surgical removal is treatment of choice for thyroid carcinomas
- Subtotal thyroidectomy for adults aged <45 with single tumor <1 cm
- Surgical resection of metastases to brain (radiation or radioactive iodide therapy ineffective), and of bulky recurrent tumor in neck region
- Total thyroidectomy for medullary thyroid carcinoma; repeated neck dissections often required over time
- Prophylactic total thyroidectomy, ideally at age 6 years, in persons found to have *RET* protooncogene mutations
- Local resection, combined with radiation therapy, for anaplastic thyroid carcinoma

THERAPEUTIC PROCEDURES

- Radioactive ^{131}I therapy: outpatient doses of 30–50 mCi ^{131}I for patients with radioiodine uptake in thyroid bed; inpatient doses of 125–200 mCi ^{131}I for patients with evidence of metastases. Lithium may improve efficacy in metastases with poor radioiodine uptake
- Patients are allowed to become hypothyroid before ^{131}I treatment, since high TSH levels stimulate uptake of ^{131}I into tumor
- External beam radiation therapy for bone metastases

 OUTCOME

FOLLOW-UP

- Monitor serum TSH, and adjust thyroxine dose (as above)
- Performing whole-body ^{131}I or ^{123}I scan at 2–4 months after total or near-total thyroidectomy will detect ~65% of metastases
- Perform another ^{131}I or ^{123}I whole-body scan ~6–12 months after the postoperative scan and check serum thyroglobulin measurement while hypothyroid
- Follow serum thyroglobulin levels
- Two successive whole-body scans negative for metastases are required for tentative diagnosis of remission
- Follow serum calcitonin and CEA periodically after surgery for medullary carcinoma
- Surveillance of family of patients with medullary thyroid carcinoma

COMPLICATIONS

- Local or distant metastases, including occult lung metastases in 10–15%
- Medullary carcinomas may secrete serotonin and prostaglandins, producing flushing and diarrhea; or ACTH or corticotropin-releasing hormone, causing Cushing's syndrome. Coincident pheochromocytoma and hyperparathyroidism may occur in MEN-related cases
- Permanent hypothyroidism, possible hypoparathyroidism, and vocal cord palsy after radical neck surgery
- Immediate autotransplantation of incidentally resected parathyroids into neck muscles reduces postoperative hypoparathyroidism

PROGNOSIS

- Prognosis for papillary (and follicular) carcinoma is generally excellent
- Palpable lymph node metastases in papillary thyroid cancer do not increase mortality, but do increase risk of local recurrence
- Prognosis worsened by follicular instead of papillary carcinoma, older age, male sex, bone or brain metastases, large pulmonary metastases, and lack of ^{131}I uptake into metastases
- Brain metastases (in 1%) reduce median survival to 12 months; prognosis improved by surgical resection

- Mortality increased 2-fold by 10 years and 3-fold by 25 years in patients not receiving ^{131}I ablation
- Prognosis for medullary thyroid carcinoma is variable: 5-year survival is 82%; 10-year survival rate is 69%
- Prognosis for anaplastic thyroid carcinoma is poor: 1-year survival rate is ~10%; 5-year survival is ~5%

WHEN TO ADMIT

- Admit for thyroidectomy for at least 1 day postoperatively to monitor for late bleeding, airway problems, and tetany
- Admit for high-dose ^{131}I therapy

 EVIDENCE

PRACTICE GUIDELINES

- AACE Medical Guidelines for Clinical Practice: 2001 Thyroid carcinoma http://www.aace.com/clin/guidelines/thyroid_carcinoma.pdf

WEB SITE

- American Thyroid Association—Thyroid cancer http://www.thyroid.org/patients/brochures/ThyroidCancer_brochure.pdf

REFERENCES

- Alzahrani AS et al: 123I isotope as a diagnostic agent in the follow-up of patients with differentiated thyroid cancer: comparison with post 131I therapy whole body scanning. J Clin Endocrinol Metab 2001;86:5294. [PMID: 11701695]
- Kebebew E et al: Total thyroidectomy or thyroid lobectomy in patients with low-risk differentiated thyroid cancer: surgical decision analysis of a controversy using a mathematical model. World J Surg 2000;24:1295. [PMID: 11038197]
- Thieblemont C et al: Primary thyroid lymphoma is a heterogeneous disease. J Clin Endocrinol Metab 2002;87:105. [PMID:11788631]
- Vitale G et al: Current approaches and perspectives in the therapy of medullary thyroid carcinoma. Cancer 2001;91: 1797. [PMID: 11335906]

Paul A. Fitzgerald, MD

Thyroid Nodules & Multinodular Goiter

KEY FEATURES

ESSENTIALS OF DIAGNOSIS

- Single or multiple thyroid nodules commonly found with careful thyroid examinations
- Thyroid function tests are mandatory
- Thyroid biopsy for single or dominant nodules or if history of head-neck radiation
- Ultrasound examination sometimes useful for biopsy and follow-up
- Clinical follow-up is required

GENERAL CONSIDERATIONS

- Palpable enlargement of the thyroid (goiter) may be diffuse or nodular
- Most patients with goiter are euthyroid, but many have hypothyroidism or hyperthyroidism
- Causes of diffuse and multinodular goiters include benign multinodular goiter, iodine deficiency, pregnancy (in areas of iodine deficiency), Graves' disease, Hashimoto's thyroiditis, subacute thyroiditis, or infections
- Causes of solitary thyroid nodule include benign adenoma, colloid nodule, cyst, primary thyroid malignancy or (less frequently) metastatic neoplasm
- Risk of malignancy higher if history of head-neck radiation; family history of thyroid cancer; or personal history of another malignancy

DEMOGRAPHICS

- Goiter found in 4% of North American adults
- Incidence of goiter higher in iodine-deficient geographic areas (see *Goiter, endemic*)

CLINICAL FINDINGS

SYMPTOMS AND SIGNS

- Most small thyroid nodules are asymptomatic and discovered incidentally on physical or radiological examination
- Graves' disease, toxic multinodular goiter, hyperfunctioning nodules, and subacute thyroiditis can cause hyperthyroidism (eg, sweating, weight loss, anxiety, loose stools, heat intolerance, tachycardia, tremor)
- Hashimoto's thyroiditis may cause goiter and hypothyroidism (eg, fatigue, cold intolerance, constipation, weight gain, depression, dry skin, delayed return of deep tendon reflexes)
- Thyroid nodules or multinodular goiter can grow and cause cosmetic embarrassment, discomfort, hoarseness, or dysphagia. Large retrosternal multinodular goiters can cause dyspnea due to tracheal compression
- Malignancy is suggested by hoarsesness or vocal cord paralysis; nodules in men or young women; nodule that is solitary, firm, large, or adherent to trachea or strap muscles; enlarged lymph nodes; distant metastases
- Benign nodules suggested by older women; soft nodule; multinodular goiter

DIFFERENTIAL DIAGNOSIS

- Benign multinodular goiter
- Iodine-deficient goiter
- Pregnancy (in areas of iodine deficiency)
- Graves' disease
- Hashimoto's thyroiditis
- Subacute (de Quervain's) thyroiditis
- Drugs causing hypothyroidism: lithium, amiodarone, propylthiouracil, methimazole, phenylbutazone, sulfonamides, interferon-α, iodide
- Infiltrating disease, eg, malignancy, sarcoidosis
- Suppurative thyroiditis
- Riedel's thyroiditis
- Nonthyroid neck mass, eg, lymphadenopathy, lymphoma, branchial cleft cyst

DIAGNOSIS

LABORATORY TESTS

- Obtain thyroid-stimulating hormone (TSH) (sensitive assay) and free thyroxine (FT_4); results may show hypothyroidism or hyperthyroidism
- Antithyroperoxidase antibodies or antithyroglobulin antibodies usually very high in Hashimoto's thyroiditis

IMAGING STUDIES

- Neck ultrasound indicated for most patients with thyroid nodules, to accurately determine nodule size and consistency and whether palpable nodule is part of a multinodular goiter, and to follow nodules
- Solid nodules often malignant; cystic nodules usually benign
- Neck ultrasound preferred over CT and MRI because of accuracy
- Radioactive iodine (RAI; ^{123}I or ^{131}I) scans have limited utility in evaluation of thyroid nodules

DIAGNOSTIC PROCEDURES

- Fine-needle aspiration (FNA) biopsy of suspicious nodules (thyroiditis frequently coexists with malignancy); for cystic nodules, cytological examination of centrifuged supernatant increases diagnostic yield
- FNA biopsy success is increased by ultrasound guidance
- Of thyroid FNA biopsies, ~70% are benign, 10% follicular neoplasm (suspicious cytology), 5% malignant, and 15% nondiagnostic. Among patients with follicular neoplasm (suspicious), ~20–40% harbor malignancy, with higher risk in young patients and if nodules fixed or >3 cm
- Cytology should be done on cystic fluid obtained at FNA. Cystic nodules yielding serous fluid are usually benign, those yielding bloody fluid have higher chance of malignancy. Repeat FNA biopsy if cytology nondiagnostic and nodule remains palpable
- Nonpalpable nodules (found on neck CT, MRI, or ultrasound) require FNA only if >1.5 cm or history of head-neck radiation

TREATMENT

MEDICATIONS

- Levothyroxine, 0.05–0.2 mg PO QD if elevated TSH
- Thyroxine not required to suppress small nodules, unless TSH elevated
- Consider levothyroxine, 0.05–0.1 mg QD, "suppression" of nodules >2 cm, if TSH elevated or normal. Avoid if baseline TSH is low suggesting autonomous thyroid hormone secretion, since levothyroxine will be ineffective and may cause thyrotoxicosis
- Long-term levothyroxine suppression of TSH tends to keep nodules from enlarging and limits development of new nodules, but few existing nodules actually shrink
- Levothyroxine suppression best for younger patients; may increase risk for angina and arrhythmia in patients with cardiovascular disease; causes small loss of bone density in many post-menopausal women not on estrogen replacement

SURGERY

- Surgical resection indicated for solitary nodule with history of head-neck radiation due to malignancy risk
- Surgical resection of toxic adenoma cures hyperthyroidism
- Excision of multinodular goiters causing compressive symptoms

PROCEDURES

- Aspiration of cystic nodule with fluid sent for cytology. Multiple aspirations may be required because cysts tend to recur
- Regular careful clinical evaluation and thyroid palpation or ultrasound examinations in all patients
- Periodic bone densitometry in patients who are on levothyroxine suppression and at risk for osteoporosis

OUTCOME

FOLLOW-UP

- Regular periodic palpation of all thyroid nodules and rebiopsy if growth occurs
- Monitor patients on levothyroxine suppression for atrial arrhythmias and osteoporosis

PROGNOSIS

- Benign nodules usually persist or grow slowly; they may involute. Malignant transformation is rare
- Prognosis of malignant nodules depends on histology (see *Thyroid cancer*)
- Multinodular goiters tend to persist or grow slowly, even in iodine-deficient areas where iodine repletion usually does not shrink established goiters
- Patients with small incidentally discovered nonpalpable thyroid nodules are at very low risk for malignancy; nonpalpable thyroid nodules >1 cm diameter are benign in 98.4% of cases; even those with malignancy have little morbidity and mortality

EVIDENCE

PRACTICE GUIDELINES

- Lawrence W Jr et al: Diagnosis and management of patients with thyroid nodules. J Surg Oncol 2002;80:157. [PMID: 12115799]
- Lewinski A: The problem of goitre with particular consideration of goitre resulting from iodine deficiency (II): management of non-toxic nodular goitre and of thyroid nodules. Neuroendocrinol Lett 2002;23:356. [PMID: 12195241]

WEB SITES

- American Cancer Society http://www.cancer.org/downloads/CRI/Thyroid%20Cancer%20_PDF_.pdf
- American Thyroid Association—Thyroid nodule http://www.thyroid.org/patients/brochures/Nodules_brochure.pdf

INFORMATION FOR PATIENTS

- Mayo Clinic—Thyroid nodule http://www.mayoclinic.com/invoke.cfm?objectid=6014E6CA-8B4E-49B0-ACA1FC378D888DAE
- Uptodate—Patient information: Thyroid nodules http://patients.uptodate.com/frames.asp?page=topic.asp&file=endo_hor/11828

REFERENCES

- Alexander EK et al: Assessment of non-diagnostic ultrasound-guided fine needle aspirations of thyroid nodules. J Clin Endocrinol Metab 2002;87:4924. [PMID: 12414851]
- Kim EK et al: New sonographic criteria for recommending fine-needle aspiration biopsy of nonpalpable solid nodules of the thyroid. AJR Am J Roentgenol 2002;178:687. [PMID: 11856699]
- Mittendorf EA et al: The results of ultrasound-guided fine-needle aspiration biopsy for evaluation of nodular thyroid disease. Surgery 2002;132:648. [PMID: 12407349]
- Nabriski D et al: Clinical relevance of non-palpable thyroid nodules as assessed by ultrasound-guided fine needle aspiration biopsy. J Endocrinol Invest 2003;26:61. [PMID: 12602536]
- Wemeau JL et al: Effects of thyroid-stimulating hormone suppression with levothyroxine in reducing the volume of solitary thyroid nodules and improving extranodular nonpalpable changes: a randomized, double-blind, placebo-controlled trial by the French Thyroid Research Group. J Clin Endocrinol Metab 2002;87:4928. [PMID: 12414852]

Paul A. Fitzgerald, MD

Thyroiditis

 KEY FEATURES

ESSENTIALS OF DIAGNOSIS

- Swelling of thyroid gland, sometimes causing pressure symptoms in acute and subacute forms; painless enlargement or rubbery firmness in chronic form
- Thyroid function tests variable
- Serum antithyroid antibody tests often positive: antithyroperoxidase, antimicrosomal, antithyroglobulin Ab

GENERAL CONSIDERATIONS

- Classification: chronic lymphocytic ("Hashimoto's") thyroiditis due to autoimmunity; subacute thyroiditis (de Quervain's thyroiditis, granulomatous thyroiditis, and giant cell thyroiditis); suppurative thyroiditis; and Riedel's thyroiditis
- Hashimoto's thyroiditis most common thyroid disorder in the United States
- Frequency of Hashimoto's thyroiditis increased by dietary iodine supplementation; certain drugs (eg, amiodarone, interferon-α) may induce thyroid autoantibodies
- May be associated with other autoimmune diseases, eg, diabetes mellitus, pernicious anemia, adrenal insufficiency (Schmidt's syndrome), other endocrine deficiencies (autoimmune polyglandular failure syndrome), inflammatory bowel disease, celiac disease; usually, concurrent with Graves' disease
- Postpartum thyroiditis is a form of autoimmune thyroiditis accompanied by transient hyperthyroidism followed by hypothyroidism
- Thyroiditis commonly occurs in patients with hepatitis C
- Suppurative thyroiditis is rare, caused by pyogenic organisms, usually during systemic infection
- Riedel's thyroiditis: rarest form

DEMOGRAPHICS

- Hashimoto's thyroiditis is often familial and is 6 times more common in women than men
- Subacute thyroiditis usually affects young and middle-aged women
- Riedel's thyroiditis usually found in middle-aged or elderly women

 CLINICAL FINDINGS

SYMPTOMS AND SIGNS

Hashimoto's thyroiditis

- Thyroid gland usually diffusely enlarged, firm, and finely nodular. One lobe may be asymmetrically enlarged, raising concerns about neoplasm
- Neck tightness; pain and tenderness not usually present
- Thyroiditis often progresses to hypothyroidism, which is usually permanent; uncommonly, thyroiditis causes transient thyrotoxicosis
- Rarely, a hypofunctioning gland may become hyperfunctioning with onset of coexistent Graves' disease
- Depression and chronic fatigue
- About one-third of patients have mild dry mouth (xerostomia) or dry eyes (keratoconjunctivitis sicca) related to Sjögren's syndrome
- May have diplopia due to coexistent myasthenia gravis
- May have manifestations of other autoimmune diseases listed above
- 40% of women and 20% of men exhibit focal thyroiditis at autopsy

Subacute thyroiditis

- Acute, usually painful, thyroid enlargement, with dysphagia. May have malaise or signs of thyrotoxicosis
- If no pain, called "silent thyroiditis"
- May persist for weeks or months

Suppurative thyroiditis

- Severe pain, tenderness, redness, and fluctuation around thyroid gland

Riedel's thyroiditis

- Usually causes hypothyroidism
- Enlargement often asymmetric; gland is stony hard and adherent to neck structures, causing dysphagia, dyspnea, pain, and hoarseness

DIFFERENTIAL DIAGNOSIS

- Benign multinodular goiter
- Iodine-deficient (endemic) goiter
- Graves' disease
- Thyroid cancer
- Other malignancies (eg, lymphoma)

DIAGNOSIS

LABORATORY TESTS

- Thyroid-stimulating hormone (TSH) level is elevated if thyroiditis causes hypothyroidism, suppressed if it causes hyperthyroidism
- Serum-free tetraiodotyronine (T_4) usually elevated in acute and subacute thyroiditis with hyperthyroidism; normal or low in the chronic forms
- Hashimoto's thyroiditis: antithyroperoxidase levels increased in 95%; antithyroglobulin antibodies increased in 60% (very nonspecific)
- Thyroid autoantibodies also found in other types of thyroiditis, and mildly elevated titers found in 13% of asymptomatic women and 3% of asymptomatic men. Only 1% of the population has antibody titers >1:6400
- Subacute thyroiditis: erythrocyte sedimentation rate markedly elevated and antithyroid antibodies low

IMAGING STUDIES

- Radioiodine scan and uptake usually not required; characteristically very low in initial, hyperthyroid phase of subacute thyroiditis, distinguishing it from Graves' disease
- Radioiodine uptake may be high with an uneven scan in chronic thyroiditis, with enlargement of the gland, and low in Riedel's thyroiditis
- Ultrasound of thyroid helps distinguish thyroiditis from multinodular goiter or thyroid nodules that are suspicious for malignancy

DIAGNOSTIC PROCEDURES

- Biopsy may be required to distinguish asymmetric thyroiditis from carcinoma

TREATMENT

MEDICATIONS

Hashimoto's thyroiditis

- Levothyroxine given in usual doses (50–200 μg PO QD) if hypothyroidism or large goiter present
- In one study, selenium selenite (200 μg PO QD for 3 months) reduced serum antithyroperoxidase levels by 49%, versus 10% reduction with placebo
- If thyroid gland only minimally enlarged and patient euthyroid (normal TSH), do not administer levothyroxine but follow patient until hypothyroidism develops

Subacute thyroiditis

- Aspirin is drug of choice and is continued for several weeks
- Propranolol, 10–40 mg PO Q 6 h, for thyrotoxic symptoms
- Iodinated contrast agents promptly normalize triiodothyronine (T_3) levels and dramatically improve thyrotoxic symptoms. Sodium ipodate (Oragrafin, Bilivist) or iopanoic acid (Telepaque) given 500 mg PO QD until free T_4 normalizes
- Transient hypothyroidism treated with thyroxine, 50–100 μg PO QD, if symptomatic

Suppurative thyroiditis

- Antibiotics

Riedel's thyroiditis

- Tamoxifen, 10 mg PO BID, usually induces partial to complete remissions within 3–6 months, and must be continued for years
- Short-term glucocorticoid treatment may be added for relief of pain and compression symptoms

SURGERY

- Suppurative thyroiditis requires surgical drainage when fluctuation is marked
- For Riedel's thyroiditis, surgery usually fails to permanently alleviate compression and is difficult due to dense fibrous adhesions

 OUTCOME

FOLLOW-UP

- Euthyroid patients with Hashimoto's thyroiditis must be followed long-term as hypothyroidism may develop years later

COMPLICATIONS

- Hashimoto's thyroiditis may lead to hypothyroidism or transient thyrotoxicosis
- Subacute and chronic thyroiditis can be complicated by dyspnea and, in Riedel's struma, vocal cord palsy from pressure on neck structures
- Riedel's thyroiditis usually occurs with other manifestations of multifocal systemic fibrosis syndrome, eg, retroperitoneal fibrosis, fibrosing mediastinitis
- Perimenopausal women with high antithyroperoxidase levels are at risk for depression independent of thyroid hormone levels
- Graves' disease may develop
- Carcinoma or lymphoma may be associated with chronic thyroiditis and must be considered if uneven painless enlargements continue in spite of treatment
- Hashimoto's thyroiditis may be associated with other autoimmune disorders

PROGNOSIS

- Hashimoto's thyroiditis has an excellent prognosis, as it either remains stable for years or progresses slowly to hypothyroidism, which is easily treated
- Subacute thyroiditis may smolder for months; spontaneous remissions and exacerbations are common
- Postpartum thyroiditis usually resolves with return to normal thyroid function

 EVIDENCE

PRACTICE GUIDELINES

- Pearce EN et al: Thyroiditis. N Engl J Med. 2003;348:2646. [PMID: 12826640]
- Slatosky J et al: Thyroiditis: differential diagnosis and management. Am Fam Physician 2000;61:1047. Erratum in Am Fam Physician 2000;62:318. [PMID: 10706157]

WEB SITES

- American Association of Clinical Endocrinologists http://www.aace.com
- American Thyroid Association http://www.thyroid.org/patients/brochures/FunctionTests_brochure.pdf
- Mayo Clinic—Subacute thyroiditis http://www.mayoclinic.com/invoke.cfm?objectid=7574A58E-05DE-4E78-9058AE99AB5C6829

INFORMATION FOR PATIENTS

- MEDLINEplus—Chronic thyroiditis http://www.nlm.nih.gov/medlineplus/ency/article/000371.htm
- MEDLINEplus—Painless thyroiditis http://www.nlm.nih.gov/medlineplus/ency/article/000388.htm
- MEDLINEplus—Subacute thyroiditis http://www.nlm.nih.gov/medlineplus/ency/article/000375.htm

REFERENCES

- Dang AH et al: Lithium-associated thyroiditis. Endocr Pract 2002;8:232. [PMID: 12113638]
- Lazarus JH et al: Postpartum thyroiditis. Autoimmunity 2002;35:169. [PMID: 12389641]

Paul A. Fitzgerald, MD

Tinea Corporis or Tinea Circinata

 KEY FEATURES

ESSENTIALS OF DIAGNOSIS

- Ring-shaped lesions with an advancing scaly border and central clearing or scaly patches with a distinct border
- On exposed skin surfaces or the trunk
- Microscopic examination of scrapings or culture confirms the diagnosis

GENERAL CONSIDERATIONS

- The lesions are often on exposed areas of the body such as the face and arms
- All species of dermatophytes may cause this disease, but *Trichophyton rubrum* is the most common pathogen, usually representing extension onto the trunk or extremities of tinea cruris, pedis, or manuum
- Body ringworm usually responds promptly to conservative topical therapy or to griseofulvin by mouth within 4 weeks

 CLINICAL FINDINGS

SYMPTOMS AND SIGNS

- See Table 7 (page 1202)
- Ring-shaped lesions with an advancing scaly border and central clearing or scaly patches with a distinct border
- Location: on exposed skin surfaces or the trunk
- Itching may be present
- A history of exposure to an infected cat may occasionally be obtained, usually indicating microsporum infection

DIFFERENTIAL DIAGNOSIS

- Psoriasis
- Impetigo
- Seborrheic dermatitis
- Secondary syphilis
- Pityriasis rosea
- Erythema multiforme
- Nummular eczema (discoid eczema, nummular dermatitis)
- Granuloma annulare
- Bacterial folliculitis
- Discoid lupus erythematosus

 DIAGNOSIS

DIAGNOSTIC PROCEDURES

- Hyphae can be demonstrated by removing a peripheral scale and examining it microscopically using KOH
- The diagnosis may be confirmed by culture

TREATMENT

MEDICATIONS

- See Table 6 (page 1199)

Local measures

- Antifungal creams: miconazole, 2% cream; clotrimazole, 1% solution, cream, or lotion; ketoconazole, 2% cream; econazole, 1% cream or lotion; sulconazole, 1% cream; oxiconazole, 1% cream; ciclopirox, 1% cream; naftifine, 1% cream or gel; butenafine cream; and terbinafine, 1% cream
- Miconazole, clotrimazole, butenafine, and terbinafine are available OTC
- Allylamines (especially terbinafine and butenafine) require shorter courses and lead to the most rapid response and prolonged remissions
- In general, use of betamethasone-clotrimazole (Lotrisone) does not justify the expense

Systemic measures

- Griseofulvin (ultramicrosize), 250–500 mg twice daily, is used; typically, only 2–4 weeks of therapy are required
- Itraconazole as a single week-long pulse of 200 mg once daily is also effective in tinea corporis
- Terbinafine, 250 mg daily for 1 month, is an alternative

THERAPEUTIC PROCEDURES

- Treatment should be continued for 1–2 weeks after clinical clearing

OUTCOME

PROGNOSIS

- Body ringworm usually responds promptly to conservative topical therapy or to griseofulvin by mouth within 4 weeks

WHEN TO REFER

- If there is a question about the diagnosis, if recommended therapy is ineffective, or if specialized treatment is necessary

EVIDENCE

PRACTICE GUIDELINES

- American Academy of Dermatology
  http://www.aadassociation.org/
  Guidelines/tineacruris.htm

WEB SITES

- American Academy of Dermatology
  http://www.aad.org
- Dermatology Handbook for Family Practice from the University of Iowa
  http://www.vh.org/Providers/ClinRef/
  FPHandbook/17.html

INFORMATION FOR PATIENTS

- National Instiues of Health Medical Encyclopedia
  http://www.nlm.nih.gov/medlineplus/
  ency/article/000877.htm
- American Medical Association
  http://www.medem.com/search/article_
  display .cfm?path=\\TANQUERAY\
  M_ContentItem&mstr=/M_Content
  Item/ZZZ8W2QJU9C.html&soc=
  AMA&srch_typ=NAV_SERCH

REFERENCE

- Crawford F et al: Topical treatments for fungal infections of the skin and nails of the foot. Cochrane Database Syst Rev 2000(2):CD001434. [PMID: 10796792]

Timothy G. Berger, MD

Tinea Cruris

 KEY FEATURES

ESSENTIALS OF DIAGNOSIS

- Marked itching in intertriginous areas, usually sparing the scrotum
- Peripherally spreading, sharply demarcated, centrally clearing erythematous lesions
- May have associated tinea infection of feet or toenails
- Laboratory examination with microscope or culture confirms diagnosis

GENERAL CONSIDERATIONS

- Must be distinguished from other lesions involving the intertriginous areas, such as candidiasis, seborrheic dermatitis, intertrigo, psoriasis of body folds ("inverse psoriasis"), erythrasma, and rarely tinea versicolor

 CLINICAL FINDINGS

SYMPTOMS AND SIGNS

- See Table 7 (page 1202)
- Typical lesions are erythematous and sharply demarcated, with central clearing and active, spreading scaly peripheries
- Marked itching in intertriginous areas, usually sparing the scrotum
- May have associated tinea infection of feet or toenails
- The area may be hyperpigmented on resolution

DIFFERENTIAL DIAGNOSIS

- Erythrasma is best diagnosed with Wood's light—a brilliant coral-red fluorescence is seen
- Candidiasis
- Seborrheic dermatitis
- Intertrigo
- Psoriasis of body folds ("inverse psoriasis")
- Tinea versicolor (pityriasis versicolor)

 DIAGNOSIS

LABORATORY TESTS

- Hyphae can be demonstrated microscopically in potassium hydroxide preparations
- The organism may be cultured readily
- Tinea cruris must be distinguished from other lesions involving the intertriginous areas, such as candidiasis, seborrheic dermatitis, intertrigo, psoriasis of body folds ("inverse psoriasis"), erythrasma, and rarely tinea versicolor
- Candidiasis is generally bright red and marked by satellite papules and pustules outside of the main border of the lesion; *Candida* typically involves the scrotum
- Tinea versicolor can be diagnosed by the KOH preparation
- Seborrheic dermatitis also often involves the face, sternum, and axillae
- Intertrigo tends to be more red, less scaly, and present in obese individuals in moist body folds with less extension onto the thigh
- Inverse psoriasis is characterized by distinct plaques; other areas of typical psoriatic involvement should be checked, and the KOH examination will be negative

TREATMENT

MEDICATIONS

- See Table 6 (page 1199)

General measures

- Drying powder [eg, miconazole nitrate (Zeasorb-AF])] should be dusted into the involved area in patients with excessive perspiration or occlusion of skin due to obesity

Local measures

- See preparations listed in *Tinea corporis*
- There is great variation in expense, with miconazole, clotrimazole, and terbinafine available OTC and usually at a lower price
- Terbinafine cream is curative in over 80% of cases after once-daily use for 7 days

Systemic measures

- Griseofulvin ultramicrosize is reserved for severe cases; give 250–500 mg orally twice daily for 1–2 weeks
- Itraconazole, 200 mg daily, or terbinafine, 250 mg daily, for 1 week, are also effective

THERAPEUTIC PROCEDURES

- Underwear should be loose fitting

 OUTCOME

WHEN TO REFER

- If there is a question about the diagnosis, if recommended therapy is ineffective, or if specialized treatment is necessary

 EVIDENCE

PRACTICE GUIDELINES

- American Academy of Dermatology http://www.aadassociation.org/ Guidelines/tineacruris.htm

WEB SITES

- American Academy of Dermatology http://www.aad.org
- Dermatology Handbook for Family Practice from the University of Iowa http://www.vh.org/Providers/ClinRef/ FPHandbook/17.html

INFORMATION FOR PATIENTS

- American Medical Association http://www.medem.com/search/article_ display.cfm?path=\\TANQUERAY\M_ ContentItem&mstr=/M_ContentItem/ ZZZ8W2QJU9C.html&soc= AMA&srch_typ=NAV_SERCH
- National Institutes of Health Medical Encyclopedia http://www.nlm.nih.gov/medlineplus/ ency/article/000876.htm

REFERENCE

- Crawford F et al: Topical treatments for fungal infections of the skin and nails of the foot. Cochrane Database Syst Rev 2000(2):CD001434. [PMID: 10796792]

Timothy G. Berger, MD

Tinea Manuum & Pedis

 KEY FEATURES

ESSENTIALS OF DIAGNOSIS

- Most often presenting with asymptomatic scaling
- May progress to fissuring or maceration in toe web spaces
- Itching, burning, and stinging of interdigital webs, palms, and soles seen occasionally; deep vesicles in inflammatory cases
- The fungus is shown in skin scrapings examined microscopically or by culture of scrapings

GENERAL CONSIDERATIONS

- An extremely common acute or chronic dermatosis
- Certain individuals appear to be more susceptible than others
- Most infections are caused by *Trichophyton* species
- Interdigital tinea pedis is the most common cause of leg cellulitis in healthy individuals

 CLINICAL FINDINGS

SYMPTOMS AND SIGNS

- See Table 7 (page 1202)
- Most often presents with asymptomatic scaling that may progress to fissuring or maceration in toe web spaces
- Itching, burning, and stinging of interdigital webs, palms, and soles seen occasionally; deep vesicles in inflammatory cases
- Tinea pedis has several presentations that vary with the location
- On the sole and heel, may appear as chronic noninflammatory scaling, occasionally with thickening and cracking of the epidermis; this may extend over the sides of the feet in a "moccasin" distribution
- Often appears as a scaling or fissuring of the toe webs, perhaps with sodden maceration
- There may be grouped vesicles distributed anywhere on the soles or palms, generalized exfoliation of the skin of the soles, or nail involvement in the form of discoloration and thickening and crumbling of the nail plate

DIFFERENTIAL DIAGNOSIS

- Erythrasma
- Psoriasis
- Contact dermatitis
- Dyshidrosis (pomphylox)
- Scabies
- Pitted keratolysis
- Tinea pedis must be differentiated from other skin conditions involving the same areas, such as
  - Interdigital erythrasma (use Wood's light)
  - Psoriasis: repeated fungal cultures should be negative
- Contact dermatitis (from shoes) will often involve the dorsal surfaces and will respond to topical or systemic corticosteroids

 DIAGNOSIS

LABORATORY TESTS

- The KOH preparation is usually positive
- As the web spaces become more macerated, the KOH preparation and fungal culture are less often positive because bacterial species begin to dominate

TREATMENT

MEDICATIONS

Local measures

- See Table 6 (page 1199)
- Macerated stage—treat with aluminum subacetate solution soaks for 20 min twice daily
- Broad-spectrum antifungal creams and solutions (containing imidazoles or ciclopirox instead of tolnaftate and haloprogin) will help combat diphtheroids and other gram-positive organisms present at this stage and alone may be adequate therapy
- If topical imidazoles fail, try 1 week of once-daily allylamine treatment (terbinafine or butenafine)
- Dry and scaly stage—use any of the agents listed in *Tinea corporis*
- The addition of urea 10% lotion or cream (Carmol) under an occlusive dressing may increase the efficacy of topical treatments in thick ("moccasin") tinea of the soles

Systemic measures

- Griseofulvin should be used only for severe cases or those recalcitrant to topical therapy
- Itraconazole, 200 mg daily for 2 weeks or 400 mg daily for 1 week, or terbinafine, 250 mg daily for 2–4 weeks, may be used in refractory cases

THERAPEUTIC PROCEDURES

- Socks should be changed frequently, and absorbent nonsynthetic socks are preferred

 OUTCOME

FOLLOW-UP

- The use of powders containing antifungal agents (eg, Zeasorb-AF) or chronic use of antifungal creams may prevent recurrences, which occur commonly

WHEN TO REFER

- If there is a question about the diagnosis, if recommended therapy is ineffective, or if specialized treatment is necessary

PREVENTION

- The essential factor in prevention is personal hygiene
- Wear open-toed sandals if possible; use of rubber or wooden sandals in community showers and bathing places is often recommended
- Careful drying between the toes after showering is essential; a hair dryer used on low setting may be used

 EVIDENCE

PRACTICE GUIDELINES

- American Academy of Dermatology http://www.aadassociation.org/ Guidelines/gltineacruris.html

WEB SITES

- American Academy of Dermatology http://www.aad.org
- Dermatology Handbook for Family Practice from the University of Iowa http://www.vh.org/Providers/ClinRef/ FPHandbook/17.html

INFORMATION FOR PATIENTS

- American Academy of Dermatology http://www.aad.org/education/ tineainfect.htm
- American Academy of Family Physicians http://familydoctor.org/handouts/ 316.html

REFERENCE

- Crawford F et al: Topical treatments for fungal infections of the skin and nails of the foot. Cochrane Database Syst Rev 2000(2):CD001434. [PMID: 10796792]

Timothy G. Berger, MD

Tinea Versicolor

 ## KEY FEATURES

ESSENTIALS OF DIAGNOSIS

- Pale macules with fine scales that will not tan, or hyperpigmented macules
- Velvety, tan, pink, whitish, or brown macules that scale with scraping
- Central upper trunk the most frequent site
- Yeast and short hyphae observed on microscopic examination of scales

GENERAL CONSIDERATIONS

- Mild, superficial *Malassezia furfur* infection of the skin (usually of the trunk)
- Patients often first notice that involved areas will not tan, causing hypopigmentation
- High recurrence rate after treatment

 ## CLINICAL FINDINGS

SYMPTOMS AND SIGNS

- See Table 7 (page 1202)
- Lesions are asymptomatic, with occasional itching
- The lesions are velvety, tan, pink, white, or brown macules that vary from 4–5 mm in diameter to large confluent areas
- The lesions initially do not look scaly, but scales may be readily obtained by scraping the area
- Lesions may appear on the trunk, upper arms, neck, face, and groin

DIFFERENTIAL DIAGNOSIS

- Seborrheic dermatitis
- Pityriasis rosea
- Postinflammatory pigmentary change (eg, acne, atopic dermatitis)
- Secondary syphilis
- Vitiligo
- Hansen's disease (leprosy)
- Vitiligo usually presents with periorificial lesions or lesions on the tips of the fingers; vitiligo (and not tinea versicolor) is characterized by total depigmentation, not just a lessening of pigmentation

 ## DIAGNOSIS

LABORATORY TESTS

- Large, blunt hyphae and thick-walled budding spores ("spaghetti and meatballs") may be seen under the 10× objective when skin scales have been cleared in 10% KOH
- Fungal culture is not useful

TREATMENT

MEDICATIONS

- See Table 6 (page 1199)

Topical treatments

- Selenium sulfide lotion 2.5%, which may be applied from neck to waist daily and left on for 5–15 min for 7 days; this treatment is repeated weekly for a month and then monthly for maintenance

- Ketoconazole shampoo lathered on the chest and back and left on for 5 min may also be used weekly for maintenance

- Tinver lotion (contains sodium thiosulfate) is effective

- Sulfur-salicylic acid soap or shampoo (Sebulex) or zinc pyrithrone–containing shampoos used on a continuing basis may be effective prophylaxis

Systemic therapy

- Ketoconazole, 200 mg daily orally for 1 week or 400 mg as a single oral dose, results in short-term cure of 90% of cases; patients should be instructed not to shower for 8 to 12 h after taking ketoconazole, because it is delivered in sweat to the skin; the single dose may not work in more hot and humid areas

THERAPEUTIC PROCEDURES

- Stress to the patient that the raised and scaly aspects of the rash are being treated; the alterations in pigmentation may take months to fade or fill in

- Irritation and odor from these agents are common complaints from patients

 OUTCOME

COMPLICATIONS

- More protracted therapy with ketoconazole carries a small but finite risk of drug-induced hepatitis for a completely benign disease

PROGNOSIS

- Relapses are common: without maintenance therapy, recurrences will occur in over 80% of "cured" cases over the subsequent 2 years

WHEN TO REFER

- If there is a question about the diagnosis, if recommended therapy is ineffective, or if specialized treatment is necessary

EVIDENCE

PRACTICE GUIDELINES

- American Academy of Dermatologists http://www.aadassociation.org/ Guidelines/superpityriasis.html

WEB SITES

- American Academy of Dermatology http://www.aad.org
- Dermatology Handbook for Family Practice from the University of Iowa http://www.vh.org/Providers/ClinRef/ FPHandbook/17.html

INFORMATION FOR PATIENTS

- American Academy of Dermatology http://www.aad.org/pamphlets/tineav. html
- American Academy of Family Physicians http://familydoctor.org/flowcharts/545. html

REFERENCE

- Crawford F et al: Topical treatments for fungal infections of the skin and nails of the foot. Cochrane Database Syst Rev 2000(2):CD001434. [PMID: 10796792]

Timothy G. Berger, MD

Tourette's Syndrome

 KEY FEATURES

ESSENTIALS OF DIAGNOSIS

- Multiple motor and phonic tics
- Symptoms begin before age 21 years
- Tics occur frequently for at least 1 year
- Tics vary in number, frequency, and nature over time

GENERAL CONSIDERATIONS

- The diagnosis of the disorder is often delayed for years, the tics being interpreted as psychiatric illness or some other form of abnormal movement. Patients are thus often subjected to unnecessary treatment before the disorder is recognized

DEMOGRAPHICS

- Tics are noted first in childhood, generally between the ages of 2 and 15

 CLINICAL FINDINGS

SYMPTOMS AND SIGNS

- Motor tics are the initial manifestation in 80% of cases and most commonly involve the face, whereas in the remaining 20%, the initial symptoms are phonic tics
- All patients ultimately develop a combination of different motor and phonic tics
- Motor tics occur especially about the face, head, and shoulders (eg, sniffing, blinking, frowning, shoulder shrugging, head thrusting)
- Phonic tics commonly consist of grunts, barks, hisses, throat-clearing, coughs, etc, but sometimes also of verbal utterances including coprolalia (obscene speech)
- There may be echolalia (repetition of the speech of others), echopraxia (imitation of others' movements), and palilalia (repetition of words or phrases)
- Some tics may be self-mutilating in nature, such as nail-biting, hair-pulling, or biting of the lips or tongue
- Obsessive-compulsive behaviors are commonly associated and may be more disabling than the tics themselves
- In addition to obsessive-compulsive behavior disorders, psychiatric disturbances may occur because of the associated cosmetic and social embarrassment

DIFFERENTIAL DIAGNOSIS

- Wilson's disease

 DIAGNOSIS

DIAGNOSTIC PROCEDURES

- Examination usually reveals no abnormalities other than the tics

Tourette's Syndrome

 TREATMENT

MEDICATIONS

- Clonazepam (in a dose that depends on response and tolerance) or clonidine (2–5 μg/kg/day) may be helpful, and avoids some of the long-term extrapyramidal side effects of haloperidol
- Haloperidol is started in a low daily dose (0.25 mg) that is gradually increased (by 0.25 mg every 4 or 5 days) until there is maximum benefit with a minimum of side effects or until side effects limit further increments. A total daily dose of between 2 and 8 mg is usually optimal, but higher doses are sometimes necessary
- Phenothiazines, such as fluphenazine (2–15 mg daily), have been used, but patients unresponsive to haloperidol are usually unresponsive to these as well
- Pimozide, an oral dopamine-blocking drug related to haloperidol, may be helpful in patients who cannot tolerate or have not responded to haloperidol. Treatment is started with 1 mg daily and the daily dose increased by 1–2 mg every 10 days; the average dose is between 7 and 16 mg daily
- Treatment with risperidone, calcium channel blockers, tetrabenazene, or clomipramine has yielded mixed results

THERAPEUTIC PROCEDURES

- Treatment is symptomatic and may need to be continued indefinitely

 OUTCOME

PROGNOSIS

- The disorder is chronic, but the course may be punctuated by relapses and remissions

WHEN TO REFER

- When the diagnosis is uncertain
- For expertise in management, particularly if patients do not respond to conventional therapy

 EVIDENCE

PRACTICE GUIDELINES

- Tourette Syndrome Association http://www.tsa-usa.org/research/guidetodiagnosis.html

INFORMATION FOR PATIENTS

- Tourette Syndrome Association http://www.tsa-usa.org/what_is/Faqs.html
- National Institute of Neurological Disorders and Stroke http://www.ninds.nih.gov/health_and_medical/pubs/tourette_syndrome.htm

REFERENCE

- Jankovic J: Tourette's syndrome. N Engl J Med 2001;345;1184. [PMID 11642235]

Michael J. Aminoff, MD, DSc, FRCP

Toxoplasmosis in the Immunocompetent Patient

 ## KEY FEATURES

ESSENTIALS OF DIAGNOSIS

Acute primary infection

- Fever, malaise, headache, lymphadenopathy (especially cervical), myalgia, arthralgia, stiff neck, sore throat; occasionally, rash, hepatosplenomegaly, retinochoroiditis, confusion; in various combinations
- Positive serological tests with high and rising IgG and IgM
- Isolation of *Toxoplasma gondii* from blood or body fluids; tachyzoites in histological sections of tissue or cytological preparations of body fluids

GENERAL CONSIDERATIONS

- *T gondii*, an obligate intracellular protozoan, is found worldwide in humans and many species of animals and birds. The cat is the definitive host
- The parasite exists in three forms: the **trophozoite** (tachyzoite) (3×7 μm) is the rapidly proliferating form in tissues that causes acute disease. The **cyst**, containing viable bradyzoites, is the latent form that can persist indefinitely as a chronic infection, particularly in muscle and nerve tissue. The **oocyst** is the form passed only in the feces of the cat family. The oocysts, which contain infective sporozoites, are infectious within 12 h to several days after passage and can remain infective in moist soil for weeks or months
- Human infection results from ingestion of cysts in raw or undercooked meat; from ingestion of oocysts in contaminated food or water, by careless handling of contaminated cat litter, or from soil by soil-eating children; from transplacental transmission of trophozoites; or rarely, from direct inoculation of trophozoites, as in blood transfusion

DEMOGRAPHICS

- Antibody prevalence rates range from less than 5% in some parts of the world (absence of cats and minimal ingestion of meat) to 15–29% in the United States and over 80% in France

 ## CLINICAL FINDINGS

SYMPTOMS AND SIGNS

- Over 80% of primary infections are asymptomatic
- The incubation period for symptomatic persons is 1–2 weeks
- Generally, on recovery, both asymptomatic and symptomatic infections persist as chronic latent (cyst) infections

Primary infection in the immunocompetent host

- Most symptomatic infections are acute, mild, febrile multisystem illnesses that resemble infectious mononucleosis
- Lymphadenopathy, usually nontender, particularly of the head and neck, is the most common finding
- Other features in various combinations are malaise, myalgia, arthralgia, headache, sore throat, and maculopapular or urticarial rash
- Hepatosplenomegaly may occur
- Rarely, severe cases are complicated by pneumonitis, meningoencephalitis, hepatitis, myocarditis, and retinochloroditis
- Symptoms may fluctuate, but most patients recover spontaneously within a few weeks

Congenital infection

- Congenital transmission occurs only as a result of infection in a nonimmune (usually asymptomatic) woman during pregnancy

Retinochoroiditis

- Develops gradually weeks to years after congenital infection (generally bilateral) or as an acquired infection in a young child (generally unilateral)
- The inflammatory process may persist for weeks to months in focally necrotic retinal lesions
- Visual defects are accompanied by pain and photophobia
- Rarely, progression may result in glaucoma and blindness

DIFFERENTIAL DIAGNOSIS

- Normal host
  - Infectious mononucleosis
  - Cytomegalovirus infection
  - Acute HIV infection
  - Lymphoma
  - Sarcoidosis
  - Tuberculosis
  - Cat-scratch disease
- Immunocompromised
  - CNS lymphoma or metastatic cancer
  - Bacterial brain abscess
  - Fungal brain abscess, eg, *Aspergillus*, histoplasma
  - Cryptococcoma
  - Tuberculoma
  - *Nocardia* brain abscess

 ## DIAGNOSIS

LABORATORY TESTS

- Diagnosis depends principally on serological tests
- Diagnosis is occasionally made from tissue (blood, bone marrow aspirates, cerebrospinal fluid sediment, sputum, and other tissues or body fluids or placental tissue) either by demonstration of trophozoites or characteristic histology, isolation of the organism in mice (more sensitive) or in tissue culture (more rapid, 3–6 days), or amplification of *T gondii* DNA by polymerase chain reaction

Serological tests

- Serological tests can be done on blood, cerebrospinal fluid, aqueous humor, and other body fluids
- The ELISA, immunosorbent, and immunofluorescent assay tests separate IgM and IgG antibody.
- IgM antibody appears 1–2 weeks after start of infection, reaches a peak at 6–8 weeks, and then gradually declines over 18 months. As IgM antibody can persist for 5 years or longer, a positive finding does not necessarily represent recent infection; however, a negative finding does rule out acute infection
- IgG antibody appears within 1–2 weeks, peaks in 1–2 months, and may persist at high titers for years and at low levels for life. When positive, it reliably indicates present or past infection; when negative, it reliably rules out any infection

Acute infection in immunocompetent patients

- Test initially for IgG antibody, which reliably establishes the presence or absence of infection

Toxoplasmosis in the Immunocompetent Patient

- The diagnosis is established by seroconversion from negative to positive or by a fourfold rise in serological titers by any test
- A presumptive diagnosis is based on a single IgM titer of over 1:64 and a very high IgG titer (>1:1000). Confirmatory testing should always be done, preferably in a reference laboratory

Toxoplasmic retinochoroiditis

- This is usually associated with stable, usually low IgG titers and no IgM antibody. If IgG antibody in aqueous humor is higher than in the serum, the diagnosis is suspected

OTHER LABORATORY FINDINGS

- Leukocyte counts are normal or reduced, often with lymphocytosis or monocytosis with rare atypical cells, but there is no heterophil antibody

IMAGING STUDIES

- Chest radiographs may show interstitial pneumonia

TREATMENT

MEDICATIONS

- The treatment of choice is pyrimethamine, 25–100 mg once daily, plus either trisulfapyrimidines (4–6 g/day in four divided doses) or sulfadiazine, 1–1.5 g four times daily; continue this treatment for 3–4 weeks
- Folinic acid (leucovorin), 10–25 mg with each dose of pyrimethamine, should be given concurrently to avoid bone marrow suppression
- Patients should be screened for a history of sulfonamide sensitivity. To prevent crystal-induced nephrotoxicity, good urine output should be maintained; alkalinization with sodium bicarbonate may also be useful
- Pyrimethamine side effects include headache and gastrointestinal symptoms
- Clindamycin (600 mg four times daily) may be a useful alternative drug; because it concentrates in the choroid, it is also used in the treatment of ocular disease
- Atovaquone (750 mg three or four times daily), dapsone, other macrolides, and immunotherapy are under evaluation
- The lymphadenopathic form of toxoplasmosis is usually not treated unless findings are severe or persist or there is

overt visceral disease. If treatment is started, it should continue for 3–4 weeks and then be reassessed. Serological tests are not useful for evaluating the response to treatment
- Since most episodes of retinochoroiditis are self-limited, opinions vary on indications for and type of treatment
- In toxoplasmosis in pregnancy, spiramycin is given at a dosage of 3 g daily in four divided doses for 3–4 weeks (see specialized texts for detail)

OUTCOME

FOLLOW-UP

- Platelet and white blood cell counts should be performed at least twice weekly while taking pyrimethamine

PROGNOSIS

- The outlook in immunocompetent adults is excellent and chronic asymptomatic infection is usually benign

WHEN TO REFER

- All patients with retinochoroiditis
- Progressive or unresponsive disease on therapy

WHEN TO ADMIT

- Stiff neck, confusion

PREVENTION

- Freezing of meat to −20°C for 2 days or heating to 60°C for 4 min kills cysts in tissues
- Hands, kitchen surfaces, and cooking utensils must be thoroughly cleaned after contact with raw meat
- Children's play areas should be protected from cat (and dog) feces. Indoor cats should be fed only dry, canned, or cooked meet. Litter boxes should be changed daily, as freshly deposited oocysts are not infective for 48 h

EVIDENCE

PRACTICE GUIDELINES

- National Guideline Clearinghouse http://www.guideline.gov/summary/summary.aspx?doc_id=2277&nbr=1503&string=toxoplasmosis http://www.guideline.gov/summary/summary.aspx?doc_id=3080&nbr=2306&string=toxoplasmosis

INFORMATION FOR PATIENTS

- Center for the Evaluation of Risks to Human Reproduction http://cerhr.niehs.nih.gov/genpub/topics/toxoplasmosis2-ccae.html
- Centers for Disease Control http://www.cdc.gov/ncidod/dpd/parasites/toxoplasmosis/factsht_toxoplasmosis.htm

REFERENCES

- Derouin F: Anti-toxoplasmosis drugs. Curr Opin Investig Drugs 2001;2:1368. [PMID: 1890349]
- Kopecky D et al: Knowledge-based interpretation of toxoplasmosis serology test results including fuzzy temporal concepts—the Toxonet system. Medinfo 2001;10(Part 1):484. [PMID: 11604787]
- Luder CG et al: Toxoplasmosis: a persisting challenge. Trends Parasitol 2001;17:460. [PMID: 11587941]
- Montoya JG: Laboratory diagnosis of *Toxoplasma gondii* infection and toxoplasmosis. J Infect Dis 2002;185(Suppl 1):S73. [PMID: 11865443]

Toxoplasmosis in the Immunocompromised Patient

 KEY FEATURES

ESSENTIALS OF DIAGNOSIS

- Central nervous system mass lesions; retinochoroiditis, pneumonitis, myocarditis less common; sometimes other findings as above
- Positive IgG titers moderately high; IgM antibody usually absent. Tissue diagnosis as above

GENERAL CONSIDERATIONS

- *Toxoplasma gondii*, an obligate intracellular protozoan, is found worldwide in humans and many species of animals and birds. The cat is the definitive host
- The parasite exists in three forms: the **trophozoite** (tachyzoite) (3×7 mm) is the rapidly proliferating form in tissues that causes acute disease. The **cyst**, containing viable bradyzoites, is the latent form that can persist indefinitely as a chronic infection, particularly in muscle and nerve tissue. The **oocyst** is the form passed only in the feces of the cat family. The oocysts, which contain infective sporozoites, are infectious within 12 h to several days after passage and can remain infective in moist soil for weeks or months
- Human infection results from ingestion of cysts in raw or undercooked meat; from ingestion of oocysts in contaminated food or water, by careless handling of contaminated cat litter, or from soil by soil-eating children; from transplacental transmission of trophozoites; or rarely, from direct inoculation of trophozoites, as in blood transfusion

DEMOGRAPHICS

- Antibody prevalence rates range from less than 5% in some parts of the world (absence of cats and minimal ingestion of meat) to 15–29% in the United States and over 80% in France

 CLINICAL FINDINGS

SYMPTOMS AND SIGNS

- Over 80% of primary infections are asymptomatic
- The incubation period for symptomatic persons is 1–2 weeks
- Generally, on recovery, both asymptomatic and symptomatic infections persist as chronic latent (cyst) infections

Reactivated disease in the immunologically compromised host

- Reactivated toxoplasmosis occurs in patients with AIDS, cancer, or those given immunosuppressive drugs
- The infection may present in specific organs (brain, lungs, and eye most commonly, but also heart, skin, gastrointestinal tract, and liver) or as disseminated disease
- Between 30% and 50% of AIDS patients seropositive for past *Toxoplasma* infection will develop meningeal (uncommon), mass (single or multiple), or diffuse intracerebral *Toxoplasma* lesions, associated with clinical findings of fever, headache, altered mental status, seizures, and focal (or, infrequently, nonfocal) neurological deficits

DIFFERENTIAL DIAGNOSIS

- Normal host
  - Infectious mononucleosis
  - Cytomegalovirus infection
  - Acute HIV infection
  - Lymphoma
  - Sarcoidosis
  - Tuberculosis
  - Cat-scratch disease
- Immunocompromised
  - CNS lymphoma or metastatic cancer
  - Bacterial brain abscess
  - Fungal brain abscess, eg, *Aspergillus*, histoplasma
  - Cryptococcoma
  - Tuberculoma
  - *Nocardia* brain abscess

 DIAGNOSIS

LABORATORY TESTS

- Diagnosis depends principally on serological tests
- Diagnosis is occasionally made from tissue (blood, bone marrow aspirates, cerebrospinal fluid sediment, sputum, and other tissues or body fluids or placental tissue) either by demonstration of trophozoites or characteristic histology, isolation of the organism in mice (more sensitive) or in tissue culture (more rapid, 3–6 days), or amplification of *T gondii* DNA by polymerase chain reaction

Serological tests

- Serological tests can be done on blood, cerebrospinal fluid, aqueous humor, and other body fluids
- The ELISA, immunosorbent, and immunofluorescent assay tests separate IgM and IgG antibody
- IgM antibody appears 1–2 weeks after start of infection, reaches a peak at 6–8 weeks, and then gradually declines over 18 months. As IgM antibody can persist for 5 years or longer, a positive finding does not necessarily represent recent infection; however, a negative finding does rule out acute infection
- IgG antibody appears within 1–2 weeks, peaks in 1–2 months, and may persist at high titers for years and at low levels for life. When positive, it reliably indicates present or past infection; when negative, it reliably rules out any infection

Recrudescent infection in immunosuppressed patients

- Antibody titers cannot be depended on, since most patients have IgG titers that reflect past infection, significant rises are infrequent, and IgM antibody is rare
- Absence of IgG does not rule out the diagnosis of central nervous system or chorioretinitis toxoplasmosis
- The cerebrospinal fluid may show mild pleocytosis (predominantly lymphocytes and monocytes), elevated protein, and normal glucose
- In AIDS patients, *Toxoplasma* can sometimes be isolated from the blood or in cerebrospinal fluid (Wright-Giemsa stain or by PCR amplification)
- The diagnosis is presumed if the patient responds to empirical antibiotic treatment after a suggestive brain MRI is obtained

IMAGING STUDIES

- Chest radiographs may show interstitial pneumonia
- In HIV-infected persons, cerebral toxoplasmosis typically appears as multiple lesions with a predilection for the basal ganglion by MRI (the more sensitive test) or CT scan (typically: multiple, isodense or hypodense, ring-enhancing mass lesions)

 TREATMENT

MEDICATIONS

- Immunocompromised patients with active infection (primary or recrudescent) must be treated (Table 119, page 1298)
- Therapy should continue for 4–6 weeks after cessation of symptoms—which may require up to a 6-month course, to be followed by drug prophylaxis as long as immunosuppression persists
- In HIV-infected persons, acute toxoplasmosis must be treated followed by continued prophylaxis; if there is positive IgG *Toxoplasma* serology but no symptoms, prophylaxis is desirable
- For prophylaxis, treat with trimethoprim-sulfamethoxazole (one double-strength tablet daily) or a combination of pyrimethamine, 25 mg orally once a week, plus dapsone, 100 mg orally daily

 OUTCOME

PROGNOSIS

- In immunosuppressed patients, the disease is usually fatal if untreated; improvement occurs with early treatment, but recrudescence is common

WHEN TO REFER

- Refer to a clinician with expertise in this field

WHEN TO ADMIT

- Central nervous system symptoms
- Respiratory compromise

PREVENTION

- Freezing of meat to −20°C for 2 days or heating to 60°C for 4 min kills cysts in tissues
- Hands, kitchen surfaces, and cooking utensils must be thoroughly cleaned after contact with raw meat
- Children's play areas should be protected from cat (and dog) feces
- Indoor cats should be fed only dry, canned or cooked meet. Litter boxes should be changed daily, as freshly deposited oocysts are not infective for 48 h

 EVIDENCE

PRACTICE GUIDELINES

- National Guideline Clearinghouse
  http://www.guideline.gov/summary/summary.aspx?doc_id=2277&nbr=1503&string=toxoplasmosis
  http://www.guideline.gov/summary/summary.aspx?doc_id=3080&nbr=2306&string=toxoplasmosis

INFORMATION FOR PATIENTS

- Centers for Disease Control
  http://www.cdc.gov/ncidod/dpd/parasites/toxoplasmosis/factsht_toxoplasmosis.htm

REFERENCES

- Derouin F: Anti-toxoplasmosis drugs. Curr Opin Investig Drugs 2001;2:1368. [PMID: 11890349]
- Julander I et al: Polymerase chain reaction for diagnosis of cerebral toxoplasmosis in cerebrospinal fluid in HIV-positive patients. Scand J Infect Dis 2001;33:538. [PMID: 11515766]
- Kopecky D et al: Knowledge-based interpretation of toxoplasmosis serology test results including fuzzy temporal concepts—the Toxonet system. Medinfo 2001;10(Part 1):484. [PMID: 11604787]
- Montoya JG: Laboratory diagnosis of *Toxoplasma gondii* infection and toxoplasmosis. J Infect Dis 2002;185(Suppl 1):S73. [PMID: 11865443]

Transient Ischemic Attack

KEY FEATURES

ESSENTIALS OF DIAGNOSIS

- Focal neurological deficit of acute onset
- Clinical deficit resolves completely within 24 h

GENERAL CONSIDERATIONS

- Focal, ischemic, cerebral neurological deficits that last for less than 24 h (usually less than 1–2 h)
- Embolization is an important etiology; a source may be apparent in the heart or a major extracranial artery to the head
- Embolization may explain why separate attacks may affect different parts of the territory supplied by the same vessel

Cardiac embolic sources

- Rheumatic heart disease, mitral valve disease, cardiac arrhythmia, infective endocarditis, atrial myxoma, and mural thrombi after MI
- Atrial septal defects and patent foramen ovale may permit emboli from the veins to reach the brain ("paradoxical emboli")

Cerebrovascular sources

- An ulcerated plaque on a major artery to the brain may be a source of emboli
- In the anterior circulation, atherosclerotic changes occur most commonly near the carotid bifurcation extracranially, and may cause a bruit
- Other (less common) abnormalities of blood vessels that may cause transient ischemic attacks (TIAs): fibromuscular dysplasia, which affects particularly the cervical internal carotid artery; atherosclerosis of the aortic arch; inflammatory arterial disorders such as giant cell arteritis, systemic lupus erythematosus, polyarteritis, and granulomatous angiitis; and meningovascular syphilis
- Hypotension may reduce cerebral blood flow and rarely cause a TIA if a major extracranial artery to the brain is markedly stenosed
- The subclavian steal syndrome may lead to transient vertebrobasilar ischemia from stenosis or occlusion of one subclavian artery proximal to the source of the vertebral artery
- Hematological causes: polycythemia, sickle cell disease, and hyperviscosity

DEMOGRAPHICS

- Proper treatment of TIAs can help prevent strokes

- About 30% of patients with stroke have a history of TIAs
- Risk of stroke is highest within one month after a TIA and then progressively declines
- Incidence of stroke is not related to the number or duration of individual TIAs but is increased in patients with hypertension or diabetes

CLINICAL FINDINGS

SYMPTOMS AND SIGNS

- Symptoms vary markedly among patients, but tend to be consistent in a given individual
- Onset abrupt, and recovery often occurs within a few minutes
- If the TIA is in the carotid territory, common symptoms are weakness and heaviness of the contralateral arm, leg, or face, singly or in combination
- Numbness or paresthesias may occur either as sole manifestation or with motor deficits
- There may be dysphasia, or monocular visual loss in the eye contralateral to affected limbs
- During an attack, examination may reveal flaccid weakness with pyramidal distribution, sensory changes, hyperreflexia or an extensor plantar response on the affected side, dysphasia, or any combination of these
- Examination reveals no neurological abnormality, but a carotid bruit or cardiac abnormality may be present
- Vertebrobasilar TIA may have vertigo, ataxia, diplopia, dysarthria, dimness or blurring of vision, perioral numbness and paresthesias, and weakness or sensory complaints on one, both, or alternating sides of the body
- Drop attacks due to bilateral leg weakness, without headache or loss of consciousness, may occur, in relation to head movements
- Attacks may occur intermittently, and stop spontaneously
- Findings in the subclavian steal syndrome may include a bruit in the supraclavicular fossa, unequal radial pulses, and a difference of 20 mm Hg or more between the systolic blood pressures in the arms

DIFFERENTIAL DIAGNOSIS

- Stroke
- Hypoglycemia
- Focal seizure (Todd's paralysis)
- Syncope
- Migraine
- Peripheral causes of vertigo (eg, Ménière's disease)

DIAGNOSIS

LABORATORY TESTS

- Complete blood cell count, fasting blood glucose and serum cholesterol and homocysteine, serological test for syphilis
- Blood cultures if endocarditis is suspected

IMAGING STUDIES

- Chest x-ray
- CT scan of the head will exclude cerebral hemorrhage or a rare tumor masquerading as a TIA
- Carotid duplex ultrasonography for detecting significant stenosis of the internal carotid artery
- MR angiography may reveal stenotic lesions of large vessels but is less sensitive than conventional arteriography
- Patients with vertebrobasilar TIA are treated medically and are not subjected to arteriography unless there is clinical evidence of stenosis in carotid or subclavian arteries
- Echocardiography with bubble contrast is performed if a cardiac source is likely

DIAGNOSTIC PROCEDURES

- ECG
- Holter monitoring if a paroxysmal cardiac arrhythmia is suspected
- Assessment for hypertension, heart disease, hematological disorders, diabetes mellitus, hyperlipidemia, and peripheral vascular disease

Transient Ischemic Attack

TREATMENT

MEDICATIONS

Embolization from the heart

- Anticoagulants should be started immediately, unless contraindicated
- The fear of causing hemorrhage into a previously infarcted area is misplaced, since there is a far greater risk of further embolism to the cerebral circulation if treatment is withheld
- Use IV heparin (loading dose of 5000–10,000 units of standard molecular weight heparin, and maintenance infusion of 1000–2000 units/h depending on the partial thromboplastin time) while warfarin sodium is introduced
- Warfarin is more effective than aspirin in reducing the incidence of cardioembolic events, but when its use is contraindicated, aspirin (325 mg daily) may be used in nonrheumatic atrial fibrillation

Embolization from the cerebrovascular system

- In presumed or angiographically verified atherosclerotic changes in the extracranial or intracranial cerebrovascular circulation, antithrombotic medication is prescribed
- Treatment with aspirin, 325 mg daily, significantly reduces the frequency of TIA and stroke
- Dipyridamole added to aspirin does not offer any advantage over aspirin alone
- In patients intolerant of aspirin, clopidogrel may be used
- There is no convincing evidence that anticoagulant drugs are of value

SURGERY

- When there is a surgically accessible high-grade stenosis (70–99% in luminal diameter) on the side appropriate to carotid ischemic attacks and there is relatively little atherosclerosis elsewhere in the cerebrovascular system, carotid endarterectomy reduces the risk of ipsilateral carotid stroke, especially when TIAs are of recent onset (<2 months)
- Surgery is not indicated for mild stenosis (<30%); its benefits are unclear with severe stenosis plus diffuse intracranial atherosclerotic disease
- Surgical extracranial-intracranial arterial anastomosis is generally not helpful in TIAs associated with stenotic lesions of the distal internal carotid or the proximal middle cerebral arteries

THERAPEUTIC PROCEDURES

- Treatment is to prevent further TIAs and stroke
- Cigarette smoking should be stopped, and cardiac sources of embolization, hypertension, diabetes, hyperlipidemia, arteritis, or hematological disorders should be treated appropriately

OUTCOME

PROGNOSIS

- In general, carotid TIAs are more likely than vertebrobasilar TIAs to be followed by stroke
- The stroke risk is greater in patients older than 60 years, in diabetics, or after TIAs that last longer than 10 min and with symptoms or signs of weakness, speech impairment, or gait disturbance

WHEN TO REFER

- If CT scan is normal, no cardiac source of embolization, and patient is a good operative risk, refer for possible endarterectomy

PREVENTION

- Anticoagulation of atrial fibrillation (except lone atrial fibrillation)
- Control of hypertension
- Control of lipids

EVIDENCE

PRACTICE GUIDELINES

- National Guideline Clearinghouse http://www.guideline.gov/summary/summary.aspx?doc_id=3103&nbr=2329&string=transient+ischemic+attack
- Albers GW et al: AHA Scientific Statement. Supplement to the guidelines for the management of transient ischemic attacks: a statement from the Ad Hoc Committee on Guidelines for the Management of Transient Ischemic Attacks, Stroke Council, American Heart Association. Stroke 1999; 30:2502.

WEB SITES

- Transient Ischemic Attacks http://path.upmc.edu/cases/case114.html
- Carotid Artery Stenosis Demonstration Case http://www.brighamrad.harvard.edu/Cases/bwh/hcache/6/full.html

INFORMATION FOR PATIENTS

- JAMA patient page: Stroke. JAMA 1999;281:1146. [PMID: 10188669]
- National Institute of Neurological Disorders and Stroke http://www.ninds.nih.gov/health_and_medical/disorders/tia_doc.htm
- American Heart Association http://www.americanheart.org/presenter.jhtml?identifier=4781

REFERENCES

- Johnston SC et al: Transient ischemic attack. N Engl J Med 2002;347:1687. [PMID: 12444184]
- Kelly J et al: Transient ischaemic attacks: under-reported, over-diagnosed, under-treated. Age Ageing 2001;30:379. [PMID: 11709374]

Michael J. Aminoff, MD, DSc, FRCP

Trichinosis

 KEY FEATURES

ESSENTIALS OF DIAGNOSIS

- History of ingestion of raw or inadequately cooked pork, boar, or bear

First week

- Diarrhea, cramps, malaise

Second week to 1–2 months

- Muscle pain and tenderness, fever, periorbital and facial edema, conjunctivitis
- Eosinophilia and elevated serum enzymes; positive serological tests; larvae in muscle biopsy

GENERAL CONSIDERATIONS

- Caused worldwide by *Trichinella spiralis*. Four other species also identified
- Infection is usually acquired by eating viable encysted larvae in uncooked pork. In some cases, the source of infection is the flesh of dogs (East Asia), horses (France), or wild animals, particularly bears, walruses, bush pigs, foxes, or cougars (United States)
- The adult worms (2–3.6 mm × 75–90 mm) survive for up to about 6 weeks
- In the natural cycle, larvae develop into adult worms in the intestines when a carnivore ingests parasitized muscle

DEMOGRAPHICS

- The disease is present wherever pork is eaten but is a greater problem in many temperate areas than in the tropics
- In the United States, there has been a marked reduction in prevalence in pigs (rates in commercial pork are nil to 0.01%) and in incidence in humans

 CLINICAL FINDINGS

SYMPTOMS AND SIGNS

- The incubation period is 2–7 days (range: 12 h to 28 days)
- Findings range from asymptomatic to a mild short-lasting febrile illness to a severe multisystem illness that in rare cases is fatal

Intestinal stage

- When present, malaise, diarrhea, and abdominal cramps persist for 1–7 days; nausea and vomiting may occur
- Fever is rare

Muscle invasion stage

- This begins at the end of the first week and lasts about 6 weeks
- Findings include fever (low-grade to marked); muscle pain and tenderness, edema, and spasm; periorbital and facial edema; sweating; photophobia and conjunctivitis; weakness; pain on swallowing; dyspnea, coughing, and hoarseness; nail and subconjunctival hemorrhages; and rashes
- The most frequently parasitized muscles are the masseters, tongue, diaphragm, intercostal muscles, and extraocular, laryngeal, paravertebral, nuchal, deltoid, pectoral, gluteus, biceps, and gastrocnemius. Meningitis, encephalitis, myocarditis, bronchopneumonia, nephritis, and peripheral and cranial nerve disorders

Convalescent stage

- This generally begins in the second month but in severe infections may not begin before 3 months or longer
- Vague muscle pains for months
- Permanent muscular atrophy can occur

DIFFERENTIAL DIAGNOSIS

- Eosinophilia-myalgia syndrome
- Eosinophilic fasciitis
- Dermatomyositis
- Influenza
- Polyarteritis nodosa
- Viral gastroenteritis
- Polymyalgia rheumatica
- Fibromyalgia
- Sarcocystosis

DIAGNOSIS

LABORATORY TESTS

- Elevated serum muscle enzymes (creatine kinase, lactate dehydrogenase, aspartate aminotransferase)
- There may be a marked hypergammaglobulinemia
- Absence of an elevated sedimentation rate is a useful diagnostic clue
- Leukocytosis and eosinophilia appear during the second week. The proportion of eosinophils rises to a maximum of 20–90% in the third or fourth week and then slowly declines to normal over the next few months
- Serological tests can detect most clinically manifest cases but are not sufficiently sensitive to detect low-level infections. Circulating antigen can be detected about 2 weeks after infection in heavily infected persons and in 3–4 weeks in light infections
- More than one antibody test should be used and then repeated to observe for seroconversion or for a rising titer. The bentonite flocculation (BF) test (positive titer, ≥1:5) is highly sensitive and is considered nearly 100% specific. It becomes positive in the third or fourth week, and reaches a maximum titer at about 2 months, and generally reverts to negative in 2–3 years. The immunofluorescence test (positive titer >16) is also highly sensitive, though less specific than the BF test; it may become positive in the second week. The IgM and IgG ELISAs are also showing high sensitivity and specificity
- Adult worms may be looked for in feces, though they are seldom found. In the second week, there are occasional larvae in blood, duodenal washings, and, rarely, in centrifuged spinal fluid

IMAGING STUDIES

- Chest films during the acute phase may show disseminated or localized infiltrates
- Late calcification of muscle cysts cannot be detected radiologically

Trichinosis

DIAGNOSTIC PROCEDURES

- Confirmation of the diagnosis is by detection of larvae in muscle biopsies
- In the third to fourth weeks, biopsy of skeletal muscle (approximately 1 cm³) may be definitive (particularly gastrocnemius and pectoralis), preferably at a site of swelling or tenderness or near tendinous insertions. Portions of the specimen should be examined microscopically by compression between glass slides, by digestion, and by preparation of multiple histological sections. If the biopsy is done too early, larvae may not be detectable. Myositis even in the absence of larvae is a significant finding

 ## TREATMENT

MEDICATIONS

Intestinal phase

- Albendazole is the drug of choice in a dosage of 400 mg twice daily for 10 days
- Mebendazole is an alternative drug at a dosage of 200–300 mg three times daily for 3 days, followed by 400–500 mg three times daily for 10 days
- A third alternative drug is thiabendazole at a dosage of 25 mg/kg (maximum, 1.5 g per dose) twice daily after meals for 3–7 days; side effects, sometimes severe, are common
- Corticosteroids are contraindicated in the intestinal phase

Muscle invasion phase

- In this stage, severe infections require hospitalization and high doses of corticosteroids (40–60 mg/day for 1–2 days), followed by lower doses for several days or weeks to control symptoms. However, because corticosteroids may suppress the inflammatory response to adult worms, they should be used only when symptoms are severe
- Although specific drug treatment has not been shown to be effective in the muscle invasion stage, albendazole, mebendazole, or thiabendazole can be tried

THERAPEUTIC PROCEDURES

- Treatment is principally supportive, since in most cases recovery is spontaneous without sequelae

 ## OUTCOME

FOLLOW-UP

- Antibody tests should be repeated to observe for seroconversion or for a rising titer

COMPLICATIONS

- Granulomatous pneumonitis
- Encephalitis
- Cardiac failure

PROGNOSIS

- Death is rare—sometimes within 2–3 weeks in overwhelming infections, more often in 4–8 weeks from a major complication such as cardiac failure or pneumonia

WHEN TO ADMIT

- Patients with severe muscle infections

PREVENTION

- The disease has been significantly reduced where public health measures prevent feeding of uncooked garbage to hogs and by animal inspections
- The chief safeguard is adequate cooking of pork to 77°C or by freezing meat at −17°C for 20 days (longer if meat is over 15 cm thick). *T nativa* in game is often relatively resistant to freezing
- Low doses of γ-irradiation are effective in killing larvae

EVIDENCE

PRACTICE GUIDELINES

- National Guideline Clearinghouse http://www.guideline.gov/summary/summary.aspx?doc_id=2707&nbr=1933&string=foodborne
- Gamble HR et al: International Commission on Trichinellosis: recommendations on methods for the control of *Trichinella* in domestic and wild animals intended for human consumption. Vet Parasitol 2000;93:393.

INFORMATION FOR PATIENTS

- Centers for Disease Control http://www.cdc.gov/ncidod/dpd/parasites/trichinosis/factsht_trichinosis.htm
- National Institutes of Health http://www.nlm.nih.gov/medlineplus/ency/article/000631.htm

REFERENCES

- Bruschi F et al: New aspects of human trichinellosis: the impact of new *Trichinella* species. Postgrad Med J 2002;78:15. [PMID: 11796866]
- Kociecka W: Trichinellosis: human disease, diagnosis and treatment. Vet Parasitol 2000;93:365. [PMID: 11099848]
- Vojnikovic B et al: Severe trichinellosis cured with pulse doses of glucocorticoids. Coll Antropol 2001;25 (Suppl):131. [PMID: 11817004]
- Watt G et al: Blinded, placebo-controlled trial of antiparasitic drugs for trichinosis myositis. J Infect Dis 2000;182:371. [PMID: 10882628]

Trichuriasis

 KEY FEATURES

ESSENTIALS OF DIAGNOSIS

- Light to moderate infections are generally asymptomatic
- Heavy infections can cause dysentery and blood loss in the stool
- The *Trichuris* dysentery syndrome is marked dysentery, anemia, rectal prolapse, clubbing of fingers, and growth stunting

GENERAL CONSIDERATIONS

- The slender worms, 30–50 mm in length, attach by means of their anterior whip-like end to the mucosa of the large intestine, particularly to the cecum
- Eggs are passed in the feces but require 2–4 weeks for larval development after reaching the soil before becoming infective; thus, person-to-person transmission is not possible
- Infections are acquired by ingestion of the infective egg. The larvae hatch in the small intestine and mature in the large bowel but do not migrate through the tissues

DEMOGRAPHICS

- *Trichuris trichiura* is a common intestinal parasite of humans throughout the world, particularly in the subtropics and tropics
- Persons of all ages are affected

 CLINICAL FINDINGS

SYMPTOMS AND SIGNS

- Light (fewer than 10,000 eggs per gram of feces) to moderate infections rarely cause symptoms
- Heavy infections (30,000 or more eggs per gram of feces) may be accompanied by abdominal cramps, tenesmus, diarrhea, distension, flatulence, and nausea and vomiting
- With persistent dysentery and blood loss into the stool, the *Trichuris* dysentery syndrome can appear, which is accompanied by anemia, rectal prolapse, clubbing of fingers, growth stunting, and possibly cognitive defects
- Adult worms are sometimes seen in stools
- Invasion of the appendix, with resulting appendicitis, is rare

DIFFERENTIAL DIAGNOSIS

- Lactase deficiency
- Giardiasis
- Tapeworm, eg, *Hymenolepis nana*
- Hookworm disease (with iron deficiency anemia)
- Strongyloidiasis
- Celiac sprue or tropical sprue

 DIAGNOSIS

LABORATORY TESTS

- Diagnosis is by identification of characteristic eggs and, sometimes, adult worms in stools
- Eosinophilia (5–20%) is common with all but light infections
- Charcot-Leyden crystals may be seen in stool
- Severe iron deficiency anemia may be present with heavy infections

TREATMENT

MEDICATIONS

- Patients with asymptomatic light infections do not require treatment
- For those with heavier or symptomatic infections, give mebendazole or albendazole. Thiabendazole should *not* be used because it is not effective and because it is potentially toxic
- Iron replacement may be needed for anemia

Albendazole

- A single oral dose of 400 mg has resulted in cure rates of 33–90%, with marked reduction in egg counts in those not cured
- Daily treatment for 3 days improves cure rates
- Albendazole should not be used in pregnancy

Mebendazole

- A dosage of 100 mg twice daily before or after meals for 3 days results in cure rates of 60–80%, with marked reduction in ovum counts in the remaining patients
- There may be an advantage for the tablets to be chewed before swallowing
- In mild disease, a 500-mg dose may be sufficient, whereas in severe trichuriasis a longer course of treatment (up to 6 days) or a repeat course will often be necessary
- Gastrointestinal side effects from the drug are rare
- The drug is contraindicated in pregnancy

OUTCOME

PROGNOSIS

- The prognosis is excellent with treatment

EVIDENCE

INFORMATION FOR PATIENTS

- National Institutes of Health
  http://www.nlm.nih.gov/medlineplus/ency/article/001364.htm
- Centers for Disease Control
  http://www.dpd.cdc.gov/dpdx/HTML/Trichuriasis.htm

REFERENCES

- Crompton DW et al: Nutritional impact of intestinal helminthiasis during the human life cycle. Annu Rev Nutr 2002; 22:35. [PMID: 12055337]
- Pedersen S et al: Whipworm-nutrition interaction. Trends Parasitol 2001;17 (10):470. [PMID: 11642259]

Trigeminal Neuralgia

 KEY FEATURES

ESSENTIALS OF DIAGNOSIS

- Brief episodes of stabbing facial pain
- Pain is in the territory of the second and third division of the trigeminal nerve
- Pain exacerbated by touch

GENERAL CONSIDERATIONS

- Trigeminal neuralgia ("tic douloureux") is most common in middle and later life
- It affects women more frequently than men

 CLINICAL FINDINGS

SYMPTOMS AND SIGNS

- Momentary episodes of sudden lancinating facial pain
- Commonly arises near one side of the mouth and then shoots toward the ear, eye, or nostril on that side
- The pain may be triggered by touch, movement, drafts, and eating. To prevent further attacks, many patients try to hold the face still
- Symptoms remain confined to the distribution of the trigeminal nerve (usually the second or third division) on one side only
- Neurological examination shows no abnormality unless trigeminal neuralgia is symptomatic of some underlying lesion, such as multiple sclerosis or a brainstem neoplasm

DIFFERENTIAL DIAGNOSIS

- Atypical facial pain
  - Especially common in middle-aged women
  - Generally a constant burning pain that may have a restricted distribution at onset but soon spreads to the rest of the face on the affected side and sometimes involves the other side, the neck, or the back of the head as well
- Temporomandibular joint dysfunction
  - Occurs with malocclusion, abnormal bite, or faulty dentures
  - May be tenderness of the masticatory muscles, and an association between pain onset and jaw movement
  - Diagnosis requires dental examination and x-rays
- Giant cell arteritis—may have pain on mastication
- Sinusitis and ear infections
- Glaucoma
- Multiple sclerosis
- Brainstem tumor
- Dental caries or abscess
- Otitis media
- Glossopharyngeal neuralgia
- Postherpetic neuralgia

 DIAGNOSIS

IMAGING STUDIES

- CT scans and cerebral MRIs are normal in patients with classic trigeminal neuralgia

DIAGNOSTIC PROCEDURES

- The characteristic features of the pain in trigeminal neuralgia usually distinguish it from other causes of facial pain
- In a young patient presenting with trigeminal neuralgia, multiple sclerosis must be suspected even if there are no other neurological signs. In such circumstances, findings on evoked potential testing, head MRI, and examination of cerebrospinal fluid may be corroborative

Trigeminal Neuralgia

TREATMENT

MEDICATIONS

- Carbamazepine is most helpful (monitor blood cell counts and liver function tests)
- Phenytoin is second choice (Table 94, page 1278)
- Baclofen (10–20 mg three or four times daily) may be helpful, alone or in combination with carbamazepine or phenytoin
- Gabapentin may relieve pain in patients refractory to conventional therapy and those with multiple sclerosis; up to 2400 mg/day is given in divided doses

SURGERY

- Surgical exploration, radiofrequency rhizotomy, and gamma radiosurgery should be reserved for specialized centers

OUTCOME

PROGNOSIS

- Spontaneous remissions for several months or longer may occur
- As the disorder progresses the episodes of pain become more frequent, remissions become shorter and less common, and a dull ache may persist between the episodes of stabbing pain

EVIDENCE

PRACTICE GUIDELINES

- National Guideline Clearinghouse http://www.guideline.gov/summary/ summary.aspx?doc_id=3500&nbr= 2726&string=trigeminal+neuralgia

INFORMATION FOR PATIENTS

- The Mayo Clinic http://www.mayoclinic.com/invoke.cfm? id=DS00446
- National Institute of Neurological Disorders and Stroke http://www.ninds.nih.gov/health_and_ medical/disorders/trigemin_doc.htm

REFERENCES

- Kondziolka DE et al: Stereotactic radiosurgery for the treatment of trigeminal neuralgia. Clin J Pain 2002;18;42. [PMID: 11803302]
- Sindrup SH et al: Pharmacotherapy of trigeminal neuralgia. Clin J Pain 2002; 18;22. [PMID: 11803299]

Michael J. Aminoff, DSc, MD, FRCP

Trypanosomiasis, African (*T b gambiense*)

 KEY FEATURES

ESSENTIALS OF DIAGNOSIS

- History of exposure to tsetse flies with bite lesion usually absent
- Hemolymphatic-stage symptoms usually absent. Trypanosomes in blood or lymph node aspirates; positive serology

Meningoencephalitic stage

- Insomnia
- Motor and sensory disorders, abnormal reflexes
- Somnolence to coma
- Trypanosomes and increased white blood cells and protein in cerebrospinal fluid

GENERAL CONSIDERATIONS

- Caused by *Trypanosoma brucei gambiense* [see also *Trypanosomiasis, African (T b rhodesiense)*]. Both are hemoflagellates
- The organisms are transmitted by bites of tsetse flies (glossina species), which inhabit shaded areas along rivers
- Humans are the principal mammalian host; it is uncertain if there is an animal reservoir, but domestic animals can be infected
- Trypanosomes ingested in a blood meal undergo a developmental period of 18–35 days in the fly; when the fly feeds again on a new mammalian host, the infective stage is injected

DEMOGRAPHICS

- Found in moist sub-Saharan savanna and riverine forests of west and central Africa up to the eastern Rift Valley
- About 50,000 deaths occur yearly
- Of new infections yearly, approximately 100,000 are Gambian but only several hundred are Rhodesian

 CLINICAL FINDINGS

SYMPTOMS AND SIGNS

- There is generally a long asymptomatic period in which chancres are rare and the hemolymphatic stage may be absent or may go unnoticed; when symptoms do manifest after weeks to years, they are often initially mild and ignored by the patient

The hemolymphatic (early) stage

- Fever, headache, joint pains, and malaise may recur at irregular intervals corresponding to waves of parasitemia
- Between febrile episodes there are symptom-free periods
- Transient rashes may appear, often pruritic and papular or circinate
- Examination may reveal mild enlargement of the liver and spleen

The meningoencephalitic (late) stage

- This stage appears only months after infection
- With progression, death occurs in up to several years
- Insomnia, anorexia, personality changes, apathy, and headaches are the early findings
- A variety of motor or tonus disorders may develop, including tremors and disturbances of speech, gait, and reflexes; somnolence appears late
- The patient becomes severely emaciated and, finally, comatose
- Death often results from secondary infection

DIFFERENTIAL DIAGNOSIS

- *Trypanosoma brucei rhodesiense* infection
- Malaria
- Influenza and pneumonia
- Infectious mononucleosis
- Leukemia or lymphoma
- Arbovirus encephalitis
- Wilson's disease
- Psychosis due to other causes, eg, neurosyphilis

DIAGNOSIS

LABORATORY TESTS

- Anemia, increased sedimentation rate, thrombocytopenia, and increased serum globulin are common
- Eosinophilia is not seen
- Definitive diagnosis requires identifying motile organisms in wet films and after Giemsa or Wright's staining of thin and thick blood films; or aspirates of bite lesions, lymph nodes, or bone marrow; or of cerebrospinal fluid
- Because the number of trypanosomes in blood fluctuates (they may be undetectable 3 of 5 days but are more common during febrile periods), multiple anticoagulated specimens should be examined daily for as long as 15 days
- Other diagnostic tests with blood are intraperitoneal inoculation of rodents (sensitive but only effective for *T b rhodesiense*), culture, Millipore filtration, and DEAE-cellulose anion exchange centrifugation

Cerebrospinal fluid

- Cerebrospinal fluid is clear and shows an increase in pressure, lymphocytes, and protein
- Large eosinophilic plasma cells (Mott cells) are rarely seen but are considered pathognomic
- With progression of the disease, the parasite is more likely to be found in cerebrospinal fluid than in blood or lymph nodes
- To detect the organism, the fluid should be examined within 20 min (to avoid parasitic lysis) and centrifuged twice (doubles sensitivity), inoculated into an experimental animal, and cultured

Antibody detection assays

- Several antibody detection assays are used epidemiologically and for case finding for Gambian infections
- False-positive results can be due to animal trypanosomes that are noninfectious to humans
- A field-adapted card agglutination test (sensitivity about 96%, specificity high) detects circulating and cerebrospinal fluid antigen. Positive results of these antigen and antibody tests should be followed by parasitic confirmatory testing

- Circulating IgM antibody becomes positive about 12 days after infection; its titers may fluctuate or be undetectable during brief periods of excess antigen, and a negative test does not rule out infection
- In late central nervous system disease, though both circulating antibody and parasitemia may fall below detectable levels, serological tests of the cerebrospinal fluid (including IgM) may prove useful

DIAGNOSTIC PROCEDURES

- If present, only soft lymph nodes should be selected for aspiration (25-gauge needle); after the node is gently kneaded, the aspirate is examined immediately for motile organisms

TREATMENT

MEDICATIONS

- Because all of the drugs used (except eflornithine) are highly toxic (mortality during drug treatment can reach 5–10%), specific detection of the organism rather than immunoassays is a prerequisite for treatment

The hemolymphatic stage

- The drug of choice is intravenous suramin [100–200 mg (test dose), then 1 g on Days 1, 3, 7, 14, and 21]
- Alternative drugs of choice are intravenous eflornithine (400 mg/kg/day in four divided doses for 14 days, followed by 300 mg/kg/day orally for 3–4 weeks; cure rate 97%) or pentamidine (4 mg/kg/day intramuscularly for 7–10 days; cure rate 93%)

The meningoencephalitic stage

- In central nervous system involvement, use melarsoprol and eflornithine, rather than suramin and pentamidine, which do not adequateliy cross the blood-brain barrier
- Drug of choice is intravenous melarsoprol, 2–3.6 mg/kg/day for 3 days; after 1 week, 3.6 mg/kg for 3 days; repeat after 10–21 days. Relapse rates for infections, formerly low (5–8%), have markedly increased
- Melarsoprol causes a reactive encephalopathy in up to 20% of patients; corticosteroids may prevent this
- Alternative treatments are eflornithine (as above) or intravenous tryparsamide,

30 mg/kg (maximum: 2 g) every 5 days for 12 injections, plus intravenous suramin, 100–200 mg (test dose), followed by 10 mg/kg every 5 days for 12 injections; the treatment may be repeated in 1 month
- Systemic eflornithine is highly effective and associated with only mild toxicity in early and late *T b gambiense* infections
- Eflornithine is expensive, and its continued availability (from WHO) is uncertain. In the United States, eflornithine has been approved for topical use to remove facial hair; suramin and melarsoprol are available only from the CDC Drug Service, Centers for Disease Control and Prevention, Atlanta, GA

OUTCOME

FOLLOW-UP

- Proper follow-up to ensure detection of the encephalitic stage requires initial cerebrospinal fluid examination, repeat studies at intervals during treatment, 3 months after treatment, and then at 6-month intervals for 2 years

PROGNOSIS

- Most patients—even those with advanced disease—recover following treatment
- Relapses are uncommon (about 2%)
- When therapy is started late, irreversible brain damage or death is common
- Most persons will die if untreated

WHEN TO REFER

- Diagnosis and treatment are best done by a specialist

WHEN TO ADMIT

- All patients who are in a presumed or confirmed meningoencephalitic stage

PREVENTION

- Individual prevention should include wearing long sleeves and trousers, avoiding dark-colored clothing, and using mosquito nets while sleeping. Repellents have no effect
- Pentamidine is used in chemoprophylaxis (controversial). One intramuscular injection (4 mg/kg, maximum 300 mg) protects for 3–6 months. It may suppress early symptoms, resulting in late recognition of the disease. The drug is toxic and should be used only for per-

sons at high risk (ie, those with constant, heavy exposure to tsetse flies in areas with known transmission of Gambian disease)
- Performing serological tests every 6 months during exposure and for 3 years afterward is the safest method for detecting the disease at an early stage

EVIDENCE

INFORMATION FOR PATIENTS

- Centers for Disease Control http://www.cdc.gov/ncidod/dpd/ parasites/trypanosomiasis/factsht_ wa_trypanosomiasis.htm
- National Institutes of Health http://www.nlm.nih.gov/medlineplus/ ency/article/001362.htm

REFERENCES

- Burchmore RJ et al: Chemotherapy of human African trypanosomiasis. Curr Pharm Des 2002;8:256. [PMID: 11860365]
- Legros D et al: Treatment of human African trypanosomiasis—present situation and needs for research and development. Lancet Infect Dis 2002;2:437. [PMID: 12127356]
- Lejon V et al: Stage determination and follow-up in sleeping sickness. Med Trop (Mars) 2001;61:355. [PMID: 11803826]

Trypanosomiasis, African (*T b rhodesiense*)

 KEY FEATURES

ESSENTIALS OF DIAGNOSIS

- History of exposure to tsetse flies

Hemolymphatic stage

- Irregular fevers, headaches, joint pains, malaise, pruritus, papular skin rash, edemas
- Posterior cervical or generalized lymphadenopathy; hepatosplenomegaly
- Anemia, weight loss
- Trypanosomes in blood or lymph node aspirates; positive serology

Meningoencephalitic stage

- Insomnia, motor and sensory disorders, abnormal reflexes, somnolence to coma
- Trypanosomes and increased white blood cells and protein in cerebrospinal fluid

GENERAL CONSIDERATIONS

- Caused by *Trypanosoma brucei rhodesiense* and *Trypanosoma brucei gambiense* [see *Trypanosomiasis, African* (T b gambiense)], both hemoflagellates
- The organisms are transmitted by bites of tsetse flies (glossina species), which inhabit shaded areas along rivers
- Trypanosomes ingested in a blood meal undergo a developmental period of 18–35 days in the fly; when the fly feeds again on a new mammalian host, the infective stage is injected

DEMOGRAPHICS

- *T b rhodesiense* occurs to the east of the Rift Valley in the savannah of east and southeast Africa and along the shores of Lake Victoria
- *T b rhodesiense* infection is primarily a zoonosis of game animals; humans are infected sporadically
- About 50,000 deaths occur yearly
- Of new infections yearly, approximately 100,000 are Gambian but only several hundred Rhodesian
- Among visitors to the East African game parks, infections are rare, with about one case a year appearing in the United States

 CLINICAL FINDINGS

SYMPTOMS AND SIGNS

- Infections go through the following three stages, which are virulent, and untreated patients die within weeks to a year
- There is is a local pruritic, painful inflammatory reaction (3–10 cm) with regional lymphadenopathy that appears about 48 h after the tsetse fly bite and lasts 2–4 weeks

The hemolymphatic (early) stage

- High fever, severe headache, joint pains, and malaise recur at irregular intervals corresponding to waves of parasitemia
- Between febrile episodes there are symptom-free periods that last up to 2 weeks
- Transient rashes may appear, often pruritic and papular or circinate
- Examination reveals mild enlargement of the liver and spleen, and edema (peripheral, pleural, ascites, etc)
- Nodes of the posterior cervical group (Winterbottom's sign) may be enlarged
- With progression of the disease, there is weight loss and debilitation
- Myocardial involvement may appear early, and the patient may succumb to myocarditis before meningoencephalitic signs appear

The meningoencephalitic (late) stage

- This stage appears within a few weeks or months of onset
- Insomnia, anorexia, personality changes, apathy, and headaches are the early findings
- A variety of motor or tonus disorders may develop, including tremors and disturbances of speech, gait, and reflexes; somnolence appears late
- The patient becomes severely emaciated and, finally, comatose. Death often results from secondary infection

DIFFERENTIAL DIAGNOSIS

- *Trypanosoma brucei gambiense* infection
- Influenza and pneumonia
- Malaria
- Infectious mononucleosis
- Leukemia or lymphoma
- Arbovirus encephalitis
- Wilson's disease
- Psychosis due to other causes, eg, neurosyphilis

 DIAGNOSIS

LABORATORY TESTS

- Anemia, increased sedimentation rate, thrombocytopenia, and increased serum globulin are common. Eosinophilia is not seen
- Definitive diagnosis requires identifying motile organisms in wet films and after Giemsa or Wright staining of thin and thick blood films; of aspirates of bite lesions, lymph nodes, or bone marrow; or of cerebrospinal fluid. Because the number of trypanosomes in blood fluctuates (they may be undetectable 3 out of 5 days but are more common during febrile periods), multiple anticoagulated specimens should be examined daily for as many as 15 days using 10–15 mL for centrifugation; the trypanosomes are concentrated in the buffy coat
- Other diagnostic tests with blood are intraperitoneal inoculation of rodents, culture, Millipore filtration, and DEAE-cellulose anion-exchange centrifugation
- Cerebrospinal fluid is clear and shows an increase in pressure, lymphocytes, and protein. Large eosinophilic plasma cells (Mott cells) are rarely seen but are considered pathognomic
- With progression of the disease, the parasite is more likely to be found in cerebrospinal fluid than in blood or lymph nodes. To detect the organism, the fluid should be examined within 20 min (to avoid parasitic lysis) and centrifuged twice (doubles sensitivity), inoculated into an experimental animal, and cultured
- Several antibody detection assays are available. False-positive results can be due to animal trypanosomes that are noninfectious to humans. A field-adapted card agglutination test (sensitivity about 96%, specificity high) detects circulating and cerebrospinal fluid antigen. Positive results of these antigen and antibody tests should be followed by parasitic confirmatory testing
- Circulating IgM antibody becomes positive about 12 days after infection; its titers may fluctuate or be undetectable during brief periods of excess antigen, and a negative test does not rule out infection

- In late central nervous system disease, though both circulating antibody and parasitemia may fall below detectable levels, serological tests of the cerebrospinal fluid (including IgM) may prove useful

DIAGNOSTIC PROCEDURES

- Only soft lymph nodes should be selected for aspiration (25-gauge needle); after the node is gently kneaded, the aspirate is examined immediately for motile organisms

 TREATMENT

MEDICATIONS

- Because all of the drugs used (except eflornithine) are highly toxic (mortality during drug treatment can reach 5–10%), specific detection of the organism rather than immunoassays is a prerequisite for treatment

Early disease, the hemolymphatic stage

- The drug of choice is intravenous suramin [100–200 mg (test dose), then 1 g on Days 1, 3, 7, 14, and 21]
- Alternative drug of choice is pentamidine (4 mg/kg/day intramuscularly for 7–10 days; cure rate 93%)

Late disease with central nervous system involvement

- In central nervous system involvement, use melarsoprol, rather than suramin and pentamidine, which do not adequately cross the blood-brain barrier
- Drug of choice is intravenous melarsoprol, 2–3.6 mg/kg/day for 3 days; after 1 week, 3.6 mg/kg for 3 days; repeat after 10–21 days
- Melarsoprol causes a reactive encephalopathy in up to 20% of patients; corticosteroids may prevent this
- Systemic eflornithine should not be used, as its efficacy is inconsistent
- Suramin and melarsoprol are available only from the CDC Drug Service, Centers for Disease Control and Prevention, Atlanta, GA

 OUTCOME

FOLLOW-UP

- Proper follow-up to ensure detection of the encephalitic stage requires initial cerebrospinal fluid examination, repeat studies at intervals during treatment, 3 months after treatment, and then at 6-month intervals for 2 years

PROGNOSIS

- Most patients—even those with advanced disease—recover following treatment. Relapses are uncommon (about 2%)
- When therapy is started late, irreversible brain damage or death is common
- Most persons with African trypanosomiasis will die if untreated

WHEN TO REFER

- Diagnosis and treatment are best done by a specialist

WHEN TO ADMIT

- All patients with suspected or confirmed meningoencephalitic disease

PREVENTION

- Individual prevention in endemic areas should include wearing long sleeves and trousers, avoiding dark-colored clothing, and using mosquito nets while sleeping. Repellents have no effect
- Pentamidine should not be used in chemoprophylaxis

 EVIDENCE

PRACTICE GUIDELINES

- Centers for Disease Control http://www.cdc.gov/ncidod/dpd/parasites/trypanosomiasis/factsht_ea_trypanosomiasis.htm
- National Institute of Allergy and Infectious Diseases http://www.niaid.nih.gov/publications/microbes.htm

REFERENCES

- Burchmore RJ et al: Chemotherapy of human African trypanosomiasis. Curr Pharm Des 2002;8:256. [PMID: 11860365]
- Legros D et al: Treatment of human African trypanosomiasis—present situation and needs for research and development. Lancet Infect Dis 2002;2:437. [PMID: 12127356]
- Lejon V et al: Stage determination and follow-up in sleeping sickness. Med Trop (Mars) 2001;61:355. [PMID: 11803826]

Trypanosomiasis, American (Chagas' Disease)

 KEY FEATURES

ESSENTIALS OF DIAGNOSIS

Acute stage

- Inflammatory lesion at site of inoculation; prolonged fever, tachycardia, hepatosplenomegaly, lymphadenopathy, myocarditis
- Parasites in peripheral blood, positive serological tests

Chronic stage

- Heart failure with cardiac arrhythmias
- In some regions, dysphagia, severe constipation, and radiological evidence of megaesophagus or megacolon
- Positive xenodiagnosis or hemoculture, positive serological tests; abnormal ECG

GENERAL CONSIDERATIONS

- Caused by *Trypanosoma cruzi*, a protozoan parasite of humans and wild and domestic animals found in wild animals and in humans from southern South America to southern United States
- The disease is often acquired in childhood; the proportion of infected persons increases with age
- In many countries in South America, Chagas' disease is the most important cause of heart disease
- The organism has a predilection for myocardium, smooth muscle, and central nervous system glial cells

DEMOGRAPHICS

- An estimated 16 million people are infected, mostly in rural areas, resulting in about 45,000 deaths yearly
- In the United States, less than 10 instances of local transmission have been confirmed
- A large number of immigrants to the United States from endemic areas of Latin America (particularly Central America) are infected (estimated 50,000–100,000)
- A few infections following blood transfusion have been reported

 CLINICAL FINDINGS

SYMPTOMS AND SIGNS

- Up to 70% of infected persons remain asymptomatic despite lifelong infection

Acute stage

- Seen principally in children
- Lasts 2–4 months and leads to death in up to 10% of cases
- The earliest findings are at the site of inoculation either in the eye—Romaña's sign (unilateral bipalpebral edema, conjunctivitis, local lymphadenopathy)—or in the skin—a chagoma (furuncle-like lesion with local lymphadenopathy)
- Subsequent findings include fever, malaise, headache, hepatomegaly, mild splenomegaly, and generalized lymphadenopathy
- Acute myocarditis may lead to biventricular failure, but arrhythmias are rare
- Meningoencephalitis is limited to young children and is often fatal

Latent stage (indeterminate phase)

- This asymptomatic stage may last 10 to 30 years but the serological tests and sometimes parasitological examination confirm the presence of the infection

Chronic stage

- Usually manifested by cardiac disease in the third and fourth decades of life, characterized by arrhythmias, congestive heart failure (often with prominent right-sided findings), ventricular aneurysms, and systemic or pulmonary embolization originating from mural thrombi. Valvular lesions are absent. Sudden cardiac arrest in young adults may occur and is attributed to ventricular fibrillation
- Megacolon and megaesophagus occur in some areas of Chile, Argentina, and Brazil; findings include dysphagia, regurgitation, constipation, sigmoid volvulus, and parotid gland hypertrophy. Megasyndromes can also affect the urinary tract
- In immunosuppressed persons—including infrequently in AIDS patients and transplant recipients—latent Chagas' disease may reactivate. Common findings are cardiomyopathy and brain lesions indistinguishable from cerebral toxoplasmosis

DIFFERENTIAL DIAGNOSIS

- Acute stage: malaria, rheumatic fever, African trypanosomiasis
- Myocarditis due to other causes, eg, coxsackie, Rocky Mountain spotted fever, toxoplasmosis, drugs
- Arrhythmia or congestive heart failure due to other causes, eg, sick sinus syndrome, coronary artery disease
- Toxic megacolon due to inflammatory bowel disease or *Clostridium difficile*–associated colitis
- Idiopathic achalasia

DIAGNOSIS

LABORATORY TESTS

- Laboratory tests will identify most acute and congenital cases and up to 40% of chronic ones
- In the **acute phase**, the organism may be found as motile trypanosomes in anticoagulated blood; as Giemsa-stained trypanosomes in anticoagulated blood used to prepare thin and thick or buffy coat films; or by blood culture or animal inoculation. Occasionally, amastigotes can be found in tissue aspirates or biopsies of chagomas or lymph nodes by direct examination, staining, or culture
- In the **chronic phase**, the organism is rarely found directly, but may be detected by culture, animal inoculation, or xenodiagnosis. The latter consists of permitting uninfected laboratory-reared bugs of the local major vector to feed on the patients and then examining their intestinal contents for trypanosomes
- In **both acute and chronic** infection, blood should also be cultured using appropriate media and inoculated into laboratory mice or rats 3–10 days old
- *Trypanosoma rangeli*, a nonpathogenic blood trypanosome also found in humans in Central America and northern South America, must not be mistaken for *T cruzi* trypomastogotes

- Several highly sensitive IgG serological tests (hemagglutination inhibition, complement fixation, ELISA, Western blot, immunofluorescence, others) are available. However, up to three of these tests should be done because false negative (including some cases of depressed immune response) and false positive tests are common. The latter may occur in other infections, including leishmaniasis, malaria, syphilis, and *T rangeli* infection, and in autoimmune diseases. For ELISA and immunofluorescent tests, sensitivity is 93–98% and specificity (excluding leishmaniasis) is 99%
- IgM antibodies are elevated early in the acute stage but are replaced by IgG antibodies as the disease progresses. Maximum titers are reached in 3–4 months; thereafter, titers can remain positive at a low level for life. In chronic infections, when circulating organisms are difficult to find, the polymerase chain reaction and recombinant DNA methods often assess effectiveness of chemotherapy (clearance of parasites), whereas the serological tests do not

IMAGING STUDIES

- Right bundle branch block and arrhythmias are the most significant electrocardiographic abnormalities
- In certain regions of South America, radiological examination may show megaesophagus, megacolon, or cardiac enlargement with characteristic apical aneurysms

 ## TREATMENT

MEDICATIONS

- Treatment is indaequate because the two drugs used, nifurtimox and benznidazole, are potentially toxic, must be used for a long period, and are ineffective in chronic infection
- Treatment is indicated in acute infection (regardless of the time since infection) but not in latent infection and is controversial in the chronic stage
- Nifurtimox is given orally in daily doses of 8–10 mg/kg in four divided doses after meals for 90–120 days. It generally produces gastrointestinal complaints, weight loss, tremors, and peripheral neuropathy. Hallucinations, pulmonary infiltrates, and convulsions are rare. In the United States, nifurtimox is available only from the Parasitic Disease Drug

Service, Centers for Disease Control, Atlanta, GA
- Benznidazole—not available in the United States—is given at a dosage of 5 mg/kg/day for 60 days. Its side effects include granulocytopenia, rash, and peripheral neuropathy. The drug is better tolerated by children
- In the chronic stage, digoxin is not well tolerated. The most effective antiarrhythmic drug is amiodarone. Cardiac pacemakers are used for atrioventricular block. Amiodarone and angiotensin-converting enzyme inhibitors may result in better survival in selected patients

 ## OUTCOME

COMPLICATIONS

- Chronic disease complications, including cardiac disease and sudden cardiac arrest
- Megacolon and megaesophagus, constipation, sigmoid volvulus, and parotid gland hypertrophy. Megasyndromes can also affect the urinary tract

PROGNOSIS

- Adults with chronic heart disease may die of the disease
- The use of nifurtimox and benznidazole reduces the duration and severity of infection, but cure is achieved in only about 70% of patients. In the chronic phase, although parasitemia may disappear in up to 70% of patients, treatment does not alter the serological reaction, cardiac function, or progression of the disease

WHEN TO REFER

- All patients should be referred to an infectious disease specialist
- Refer to a cardiologist for either acute or chronic cardiac disease
- Refer to a gastroenterologist for any megasyndromes

PREVENTION

- In South America, a major eradication program based on improved housing, use of residual pyrethroid insecticides, and screening of blood donors has achieved striking reductions in infections in children
- In endemic areas, blood should not be used for transfusion unless at least two serological tests are negative; otherwise, blood can be treated with gentian violet to kill the parasites

 ## EVIDENCE

PRACTICE GUIDELINES

- National Guideline Clearinghouse http://www.guideline.gov/summary/summary.aspx?doc_id=3303&nbr=2529&string=heart+failure

INFORMATION FOR PATIENTS

- Centers for Disease Control http://www.cdc.gov/ncidod/dpd/parasites/chagasdisease/factsht_chagas_disease.htm
- National Institutes of Health http://www.nlm.nih.gov/medlineplus/ency/article/001372.htm

REFERENCES

- Umezawa ES et al: Chagas' disease. Lancet 2002;359:627. [PMID: 11867143]
- Urbina JA: Specific treatment of Chagas disease: current status and new developments. Curr Opin Infect Dis 2001; 14(6):733. [PMID: 11964893]

Tuberculosis in HIV

 ## KEY FEATURES

ESSENTIALS OF DIAGNOSIS

- Fatigue, weight loss, fever, night sweats, and cough
- Pulmonary infiltrates on chest radiograph, most often apical
- Positive tuberculin skin test reaction (most cases)
- Acid-fast bacilli on smear of sputum or sputum culture positive for *Mycobacterium tuberculosis* (MTB)

GENERAL CONSIDERATIONS

- Latent tuberculosis infection (LTBI) occurs when bacilli are contained within granulomata, the typical response to infection in immunocompetent persons
- LTBI is nontransmissible, but may become active disease if a host's immune function becomes impaired
- Reactivation occurs within 2 years in up to 50% of HIV⁺ patients with LTBI
- Nonadherence is a major cause of treatment failure, disease transmission, and development of drug resistance

DEMOGRAPHICS

- HIV increases the risk of reactivation disease
- Risk factors for drug resistance include immigration from a region with drug-resistant tuberculosis; close contact with a patient infected with drug-resistant tuberculosis; unsuccessful prior therapy; and patient noncompliance

 ## CLINICAL FINDINGS

SYMPTOMS AND SIGNS

- Cough is the most common symptom
- Blood-streaked sputum is common, frank hemoptysis is rare
- Slowly progressive constitutional symptoms include malaise, anorexia, weight loss, fever, and night sweats
- Patients appear chronically ill and malnourished
- Chest examination is nonspecific; posttussive apical rales are classic
- Extrapulmonary disease is especially common, often with lymphadenitis or miliary disease
- Atypical presentations are becoming more common

DIFFERENTIAL DIAGNOSIS

- Pneumonia or lung abscess
- Lung cancer
- Lymphoma
- *Mycobacterium avium* complex (or other nontuberculous mycobacteria)
- Sarcoidosis
- Fungal infection, eg, histoplasmosis
- Endocarditis
- Nocardiosis

 ## DIAGNOSIS

LABORATORY TESTS

- Tuberculin skin test (Table 22, page 1220)
- Definitive diagnosis depends on recovery of *M tuberculosis* from cultures or identification with DNA or RNA amplification techniques
- Three consecutive first AM sputum samples are advised
- Cultures on solid media to identify *M tuberculosis* may require 12 weeks; liquid medium culture systems can identify growth in several days
- DNA fingerprinting with restriction fragment-length polymorphism analysis can identify individual strains
- Pleural fluid cultures for tuberculosis are positive in only 25% of effusions

IMAGING STUDIES

- In early HIV disease, the radiographic features resemble those without HIV disease
- Atypical radiographic features are seen in late HIV infection: lower lung, diffuse or miliary infiltrates, pleural effusions, and hilar and lymph node involvement

DIAGNOSTIC PROCEDURES

- Sputum induction is required for patients unable to voluntarily produce a sample
- Bronchoscopy may be considered in smear-negative patients in whom there is a high suspicion of disease

TREATMENT

MEDICATIONS

- See Tables 23 and 24 (page 1221)
- Patients with HIV disease and tuberculosis respond best when the HIV infection is treated concurrently; in some cases, prolonged antituberculous therapy may be warranted
- Multiple drugs to which the organism is susceptible are used
- At least two new drugs are added when treatment failure is suspected
- When a twice- or thrice-weekly regimen is used, dosages are increased (Table 24, page 1221)
- Coadminister pyridoxine, 10–50 mg/day
- Treatment is similar to treatment of tuberculosis in HIV-negative patients, with the following additional considerations
  - Directly observed therapy (DOT) is indicated for all HIV⁺ patients
  - Longer duration of therapy
  - Awareness of drug interactions between rifampin or rifabutin and protease inhibitors or nonnucleoside reverse transcriptase inhibitors used to treat HIV
  - Pyridoxine should be given to all HIV⁺ patients on isoniazid to reduce nervous system side effects

Extrapulmonary disease

- In most cases, regimens effective for pulmonary disease are adequate
- Nine months of therapy for miliary, meningeal, bone, or joint involvement
- Corticosteroids reduce complications of tuberculous pericarditis and meningitis

SURGERY

- Early debridement and drainage are recommended for skeletal involvement

THERAPEUTIC PROCEDURES

- Needle biopsy of the pleura reveals granulomatous inflammation in 60% of patients with tuberculous pleural effusions
- Culture of three pleural biopsy specimens combined with microscopic examination increases the diagnostic yield to 90%
- Complete blood cell count, lung function tests, blood urea nitrogen, and creatinine should be checked at baseline

- Visual acuity and red-green color vision testing is recommended before initiating ethambutol
- Audiometry should be performed prior to streptomycin therapy
- Routine monitoring for evidence of drug toxicity is not recommended

OUTCOME

FOLLOW-UP

- Monthly visits are recommended for outpatients
- Monthly sputum smears and cultures should be done until documented negative
- Patients with negative sputum after 2 months of therapy should have smear and culture repeated at the end of therapy
- Patients with multidrug-resistant tuberculosis (MDRTB) should have sputum smear and culture monthly throughout therapy
- Chest x-ray is recommended on conclusion of successful therapy
- Patients whose cultures do not turn negative or have persistent symptoms after 3 months of therapy should be evaluated for MDRTB

COMPLICATIONS

- Development of drug resistance

WHEN TO REFER

- All cases of drug-resistant TB
- All cases of TB in HIV⁺ patients
- DOT is recommended for all patients with MDRTB and those receiving twice- or thrice-weekly therapy

WHEN TO ADMIT

- Patients who are incapable of self-care or likely to expose susceptible individuals to tuberculosis
- Hospitalization is not necessary for initial therapy in most patients
- Hospitalized patients require isolation in an appropriately ventilated room until three sputums from different days are negative for MTB organisms

PREVENTION

- Despite a negative purified protein derivative (PPD) skin test, HIV⁺ patients who are close contacts of patients with

active MTB should receive 12 months of preventive therapy (see *Tuberculosis, latent infection*)
- HIV⁺ patients with positive PPD skin tests but without active MTB should be treated (see *Tuberculosis, latent infection*)
- All suspected and confirmed cases of MTB should be reported to local and state public health authorities

EVIDENCE

PRACTICE GUIDELINES

- Horsburgh CR et al: Practice guidelines for the treatment of tuberculosis. Clin Infect Dis 2000;31:633. [PMID: 11017808]
- National Guideline Clearinghouse http://www.guideline.gov/summary/summary.aspx?doc_id=3080&nbr=2306&string=tuberculosis+and+hiv

WEB SITE

- Centers for Disease Control and Prevention's Division of Tuberculosis Elimination http://www.cdc.gov/nchstp/tb/

INFORMATION FOR PATIENTS

- American Lung Association http://www.lungusa.org/diseases/tbhivfac.html
- Centers for Disease Control http://www.cdc.gov/hiv/pubs/brochure/oi_tb.htm

REFERENCE

- American Thoracic Society/Centers for Disease Control and Prevention/Infectious Diseases Society of America: Treatment of tuberculosis. Am J Respir Crit Care Med 2003;167:603.

Mark S. Chesnutt, MD
Thomas J. Prendergast, MD

Tuberculosis, Bones & Joints

 KEY FEATURES

ESSENTIALS OF DIAGNOSIS

- In most cases, a single site of bone or joint is infected
- Spine—especially lower thoracic—or knee are the most common sites
- Chest x-ray abnormal in less than half

GENERAL CONSIDERATIONS

- Infection of the musculoskeletal system is caused by hematogenous spread from a primary lesion in the respiratory tract
- It may occur shortly after primary infection or may be seen years later as a disease reactivation
- Tuberculosis of the thoracic or lumbar spine (Pott's disease) usually occurs in the absence of extraspinal infection
- Tuberculosis of peripheral joints is almost always monarticular, with the knee the most common site

DEMOGRAPHICS

- A disease of children, the elderly, or those with HIV infection

 CLINICAL FINDINGS

SYMPTOMS AND SIGNS

- Onset is generally insidious without systemic symptoms
- Pain may be mild at onset, is usually worse at night, and may be accompanied by stiffness
- As the disease process progresses, limitation of joint motion becomes prominent because of muscle contractures and joint destruction
- Symptoms of pulmonary tuberculosis may also be present
- Local findings during the early stages may be limited to tenderness, soft tissue swelling, joint effusion, and increase in skin temperature about the involved area
- Abscess formation with spontaneous drainage externally leads to sinus formation
- Progressive destruction of bone in the spine may cause a gibbus deformity

DIFFERENTIAL DIAGNOSIS

- All subacute and chronic infections (bacterial, fungal) of bone
- Gonococcal arthritis
- Mycotic bone infection
- Pyogenic osteomyelitis or septic arthritis
- Rheumatoid arthritis
- Sporotrichosis
- Metastatic cancer
- Osseous dysplasia

 DIAGNOSIS

LABORATORY TESTS

- Recovery of the acid-fast organism from joint fluid, pus, or tissue specimens

IMAGING STUDIES

- The earliest changes are soft tissue swelling and distension of the joint capsule by the effusion
- Subsequently, bone atrophy causes thinning of the trabecular pattern, narrowing of the cortex, and enlargement of the medullary canal
- As joint disease progresses, destruction of cartilage, both in the spine and in peripheral joints, is manifested by narrowing of the joint cleft and focal erosion of the articular surface, especially at the margins
- With spinal tuberculosis, CT scanning is helpful in demonstrating paraspinal soft tissue extensions of the infection (eg, psoas abscess, epidural extension)

DIAGNOSTIC PROCEDURES

- Biopsy of the bony lesion, synovium, or a regional lymph node may demonstrate the characteristic histopathological picture of caseating necrosis and giant cells

TREATMENT

MEDICATIONS

- See Tuberculosis
- Four drugs: isoniazid, 300 mg/day; rifampin, 600 mg/day; pyrazinamide, 25 mg/kg/day; and ethambutol, 15 mg/kg/day
- If the isolate is sensitive to isoniazid and rifampin, the ethambutol can be stopped, with the pyrazinamide maintained for 2 months. Isoniazid and rifampin are continued for a total of 6 months

SURGERY

- Surgical debridement is indicated for recurrent joint effusions and other indicators of poor clinical response to antituberculous medications

OUTCOME

COMPLICATIONS

- Destruction of bones or joints may occur in a few weeks or months if adequate treatment is not provided
- Deformity due to joint destruction, abscess formation with spread into adjacent soft tissues, and sinus formation are common

EVIDENCE

PRACTICE GUIDELINES

- National Guideline Clearinghouse http://www.guideline.gov/summary/ summary.aspx?doc_id=2663&nbr= 1889&string=tuberculosis
- Infectious Diseases Society of America http://www.journals.uchicago.edu/ CID/journal/issues/v31n3/000549/ 000549.web.pdf
- Centers for Disease Control http://www.cdc.gov/mmwr/preview/ mmwrhtml/rr5211a1.htm

INFORMATION FOR PATIENTS

- National Institutes of Health http://www.nlm.nih.gov/medlineplus/ ency/article/000417.htm
- American Academy of Family Physicians http://familydoctor.org/handouts/ 185.html

REFERENCE

- Turgut M: Spinal tuberculosis (Pott's disease): its clinical presentation, surgical management, and outcome. A survey study on 694 patients. Neurosurg Rev 2001;24:8. [PMID: 11339471]

David B. Hellmann, MD, FACP
John H. Stone, MD, MPH

Tuberculosis, Latent Infection

 KEY FEATURES

ESSENTIALS OF DIAGNOSIS

- A positive tuberculin skin test
- No evidence of active infection with tuberculosis
- A history (knowingly or not) of exposure to *Mycobacterium tuberculosis* (MTB)

GENERAL CONSIDERATIONS

- Targeted skin testing is used to identify persons at high risk for tuberculosis (TB) and who would benefit from treatment of latent tuberculosis infection (LTBI)
- LTBI describes patients who have been infected with *M tuberculosis*, but do not have active disease
- Individuals with LTBI have contained, but not eradicated infection
- The importance of identifying and treating LTBI is to prevent reactivation disease
- LTBI is nontransmissible, but may become active disease if a host's immune function becomes impaired
- Without preventive therapy, 10% of patients with LTBI will have reactivation during their lifetime, with 50% of cases occurring within 2 years of primary infection
- Reactivation occurs within 2 years in up to 50% of HIV⁺ patients with LTBI
- 2–10 weeks are required for primary infection to manifest an immune response to skin testing
- Persons who have bacillus Calmette-Guérin (BCG) may have a positive purified protein derivative (PPD) tuberculin test for the rest of their lives

 CLINICAL FINDINGS

SYMPTOMS AND SIGNS

- Patients are asymptomatic; the disease is uncovered by screening with the tuberculin skin test
- Any pulmonary or constitutional symptoms should prompt an evaluation for active disease prior to prophylactic treatment

DIFFERENTIAL DIAGNOSIS

- Vaccine BCG

 DIAGNOSIS

LABORATORY TESTS

- All patients with risk factors should be tested for HIV

IMAGING STUDIES

- Chest x-ray is required to rule out active pulmonary tuberculosis

DIAGNOSTIC PROCEDURES

- The Mantoux test is the preferred skin test (Table 22, page 1220)
  - 0.1 mL of PPD containing 5 tuberculin units is injected intradermally on the volar forearm
  - Transverse width in millimeters of induration at 48–72 h is measured
- False-positive tuberculin skin test reactions occur in patients previously vaccinated against MTB with BCG
- Prior vaccination with BCG does not alter the interpretation of the tuberculin skin test
- False-negative tests may result from improper technique, concurrent infections, malnutrition, advanced age, immunosuppression of any kind, and fulminant MTB infection
- Due to waning immunity, some patients with LTBI may have a negative skin test many years after exposure
- Two-step testing or "boosting"
  - Performed to reduce the likelihood that a boosted reaction will later be misinterpreted as a recent infection in individuals who will be tested repeatedly (health care workers)
  - A second test is performed 1–3 weeks after a negative test
  - If negative, the patient is uninfected or anergic; if positive, a "boosted reaction" is likely
- Anergy testing is not recommended to distinguish a true-negative test from anergy

Tuberculosis, Latent Infection

 ## TREATMENT

MEDICATIONS

- Treatment substantially reduces the risk that infection will progress to active disease
- Patients suspected of having active disease should be treated with multidrug regimens until the diagnosis is confirmed or excluded
- Exposed persons who are skin-test negative and HIV negative may be observed without treatment or treated for 6 months
- Isoniazid (INH)
  - 9 months treatment (≥270 doses within 12 months)
  - 300 mg QD or 15 mg/kg twice weekly
  - Coadministration of pyridoxine, 10–50 mg/day, for patients at risk of INH neuropathy (diabetes, uremia, malnutrition, alcoholism, HIV infection, pregnancy, seizure disorder)
  - INH plus pyridoxine is appropriate for pregnant or lactating women
- Rifampin/pyrazinamide (RIF/PZA)
  - 2 months (≥60 doses within 3 months)
  - 10 mg/kg/day RIF to maximum of 600 mg/day and 15–20 mg/day PZA to maximum of 2 g/day
- Rifampin
  - 4-month regimen (≥120 doses over 4 months)
  - Used for patients who cannot receive INH or PZA
- Contacts of persons with INH-resistant, RIF-sensitive MTB should receive RIF/PZA or RIF regimens
- Contacts of persons with multidrug- resistant TB (MDRTB) should receive two drugs to which the organism is sensitive
- HIV[+] contacts should be treated for 12 months

THERAPEUTIC PROCEDURES

- It is not necessary to routinely monitor liver function tests unless there are abnormalities at baseline or there are clinical reasons to obtain the measurements

 ## OUTCOME

FOLLOW-UP

- All contacts of persons with MDRTB should be followed for 2 years regardless of treatment
- Patients being treated for LTBI should be seen monthly to evaluate for evidence of active TB, hepatitis, and adherence to treatment

COMPLICATIONS

- Development of active TB
- Drug toxicity

PROGNOSIS

- Almost all properly treated patients with TB can be cured
- Relapse rates are <5% with current regimens
- Treatment failure is most commonly due to nonadherence

WHEN TO REFER

- HIV[+] patients receiving antiretroviral therapy should be referred to TB and HIV experts if they are to receive rifampin therapy

PREVENTION

- Close contacts of patients with active TB should be retested 10–12 weeks after a negative test
- Despite a negative skin test, close contacts of patients with TB should consider treatment if they are immunosuppressed

 ## EVIDENCE

PRACTICE GUIDELINES

- Horsburgh CR et al: Practice guidelines for the treatment of tuberculosis. Clin Infect Dis 2000;31:633. [PMID: 11017808]
- National Guideline Clearinghouse http://www.guideline.gov/summary/summary.aspx?doc_id=4004&nbr=3134&string=latent+tuberculosis http://www.guideline.gov/summary/summary.aspx?doc_id=2663&nbr=1889&string=tuberculosis

INFORMATION FOR PATIENTS

- Centers for Disease Control http://www.cdc.gov/nchstp/tb/faqs/qa.htm
- National Institute of Allergy and Infectious Disease http://www.niaid.nih.gov/factsheets/tb.htm

REFERENCES

- American Thoracic Society and The Centers for Disease Control and Prevention: Diagnostic standards and classification of tuberculosis in adults and children. Am J Respir Crit Care Med 2000;161(4 Part 1):1376. [PMID: 10764337]
- American Thoracic Society and The Centers for Disease Control and Prevention: Targeted tuberculin testing and treatment of latent tuberculosis infection. Am J Respir Crit Care Med 2000;161(4 Part 2):S221. [PMID: 10764341]
- American Thoracic Society/Centers for Disease Control and Prevention/Infectious Diseases Society of America: Treatment of tuberculosis. Am J Respir Crit Care Med 2003;167:603.

Mark S. Chesnutt, MD
Thomas J. Prendergast, MD

Tuberculosis, Pulmonary

 KEY FEATURES

ESSENTIALS OF DIAGNOSIS

- Fatigue, weight loss, fever, night sweats, and cough
- Pulmonary infiltrates on chest radiograph, most often apical
- Positive tuberculin skin test reaction (most cases)
- Acid-fast bacilli on smear of sputum or sputum culture positive for *Mycobacterium tuberculosis* (MTB)

GENERAL CONSIDERATIONS

- **Primary infection** occurs with inhalation of airborne droplets containing viable tubercle bacilli and subsequent lymphangitic and hematogenous spread before immunity develops
- **Progressive primary tuberculosis** occurs in 5% of cases, with pulmonary and constitutional symptoms
- **Latent tuberculosis infection** (LTBI) occurs when bacilli are contained within granulomata
- LTBI is nontransmissible, but may become active disease if a host's immune function becomes impaired
- Up to one-third of new urban cases are from primary infection acquired by person-to-person transmission
- Resistance to one or more drugs is seen in 15% of tuberculosis patients in the United States and is increasing
- Nonadherence is a major cause of treatment failure, disease transmission, and development of drug resistance

DEMOGRAPHICS

- Infects 20–40% of the world population annually (3 million deaths)
- Occurs disproportionately among malnourished, homeless, and marginally housed individuals
- Gastrectomy, silicosis, diabetes mellitus, HIV, and immunosuppressive drugs increase the risk of reactivation
- Risk factors for drug resistance include immigration from regions with drug-resistant tuberculosis; close contact with patients infected with drug-resistant tuberculosis; unsuccessful prior therapy; and patient noncompliance with treatment

 CLINICAL FINDINGS

SYMPTOMS AND SIGNS

- Cough is the most common symptom
- Blood-streaked sputum is common, frank hemoptysis is rare
- Slowly progressive constitutional symptoms include malaise, anorexia, weight loss, fever, and night sweats
- Patients appear chronically ill
- Chest examination is nonspecific; posttussive apical rales are classic
- Atypical presentations are becoming more common, usually among the elderly and HIV⁺ patients

DIFFERENTIAL DIAGNOSIS

- Pneumonia or lung abscess
- Lung cancer or lymphoma
- *Myobacterium avium* complex (or other nontuberculous mycobacteria)
- Sarcoidosis
- Fungal infection, eg, histoplasmosis
- Endocarditis
- Silicosis or asbestosis
- Nocardiosis

 DIAGNOSIS

LABORATORY TESTS

- Tuberculin skin test (Table 22, page 1220)
- Definitive diagnosis is on *M tuberculosis* culture or identification with DNA or RNA amplification techniques
- Three consecutive first AM sputum samples are advised
- Cultures on solid media may require 12 weeks; liquid medium culture systems can identify growth in several days
- DNA fingerprinting with restriction fragment-length polymorphism analysis can identify individual strains
- Pleural fluid cultures are positive in only 25% of tuberculous effusions

IMAGING STUDIES

Chest x-ray

- In primary disease, there may be homogeneous infiltrates, hilar and paratracheal lymph node enlargement, and/or segmental atelectasis; cavitation may be seen with progressive disease
- In reactivation disease, there may be fibrocavitary apical disease, nodules, and infiltrates, usually in apical or posterior segments of upper lobes, but in other locations in 30% of cases, more commonly in elderly patients
- Miliary pattern (diffuse small nodular densities) reflects hematological or lymphangitic spread
- Ghon (calcified primary focus) and Ranke (calcified primary focus with calcified hilar lymph node) complexes represent healed primary infection

DIAGNOSTIC PROCEDURES

- Sputum induction is required for patients unable to voluntarily produce a sample
- Bronchoscopy may be considered in smear-negative patients in whom there is a high suspicion of disease
- Needle biopsy of the pleura reveals granulomatous inflammation in 60% of tuberculous pleural effusions; culture of three pleural biopsy specimens combined with microscopic examination increases the diagnostic yield to 90%

TREATMENT

MEDICATIONS

- See dosages in Table 24 (page 1221)
- Multiple drugs to which the organism is susceptible are used; at least two new drugs are added when treatment failure is suspected; when a twice- or thrice-weekly regimen is used, dosages are increased (Tables 23 and 24, page 1221)
- Coadminister pyridoxine, 10–50 mg/day, for patients at risk of isoniazid neuropathy (diabetes, uremia, malnutrition, alcoholism, HIV infection, pregnancy, seizure disorder)

For HIV⁻ patients

- Six- rather than 9-month regimen
- Daily isoniazid (INH), rifampin (RIF), and pyrazinamide (PZA) for 2 months
- Ethambutol (EMB) or streptomycin is added where prevalence of INH resistance is 4% or higher
- If isolate is RIF and INH sensitive, continue these two drugs for 4 months
- Therapy is continued for at least 3 months beyond documentation of sputum cultures negative for MTB
- Directly observed therapy (DOT) regimens

- INH/RIF/PZA plus EMB or strepto-mycin daily for 2 months, then INH/RIF 2–3 times/week for 4 months if susceptibility is demonstrated
- INH/RIF/PZA plus EMB or strepto-mycin daily for 2 weeks, then 2 times/week for 6 weeks, then INH/RIF 2 times/week for 4 months if susceptibility is demonstrated
- INH/RIF/PZA plus EMB or strepto-mycin 3 times/week for 6 months

Drug-resistant TB

- MTB resistant only to INH can be treated with 6 months of RIF/PZA plus EMB or streptomycin or 12 months of RIF/EMB
- Treatment requires individualized daily treatment with DOT under an experienced clinician
- Most strains have at least INH or RIF resistance and require three drugs to which susceptibility is proven
- The three-drug regimen is continued until negative cultures are documented; a two-drug regimen is continued for another 12–24 months

Pregnant or lactating women

- INH, RIF, and EMB, with EMB excluded if INH resistance is unlikely
- The teratogenicity of PZA is unknown and streptomycin is contraindicated due to a risk of congenital deafness
- Pyridoxine should be given with INH
- Breast-feeding is not contraindicated

Extrapulmonary disease

- In most cases, regimens effective for pulmonary disease are adequate
- 9 months of therapy for miliary, meningeal, bone, or joint involvement
- Corticosteroids reduce occurrence of tuberculous pericarditis and meningitis

SURGERY

- Early debridement and drainage are recommended for skeletal involvement

OUTCOME

FOLLOW-UP

- Complete blood cell counts, lung function tests, and renal function should be checked at baseline
- Visual acuity and red-green color vision testing is recommended before initiating EMB and audiometry should be performed prior to streptomycin
- Routine monitoring for evidence of drug toxicity should be considered
- Monthly visits are recommended for outpatients with monthly sputum smears and cultures until documented negative
- If sputum is negative after 2 months of therapy, repeat smear and culture at the end of therapy
- Patients with multidrug-resistant tuberculosis (MDRTB) should have sputum smear and culture monthly throughout therapy
- Chest x-ray is recommended on conclusion of successful therapy
- Patients whose cultures do not turn negative or have persistent symptoms after 3 months of therapy should be evaluated for MDRTB

COMPLICATIONS

- Development of drug resistance

PROGNOSIS

- Without preventive therapy, 10% of patients with LTBI will have reactivation during their lifetime, with 50% of cases occurring within 2 years of primary infection
- Almost all properly treated patients with tuberculosis can be cured; relapse rates are less than 5% with current regimens
- The main cause of treatment failure is nonadherence to therapy

WHEN TO REFER

- All cases of drug-resistant TB
- DOT is recommended with MDRTB and those receiving twice- or thrice-weekly therapy

WHEN TO ADMIT

- Patients who are incapable of self-care or likely to expose susceptible individuals to tuberculosis
- Hospitalization is not necessary for initial therapy in most patients

- Hospitalized patients require isolation in an appropriately ventilated room until three sputums from different days are negative for MTB organisms

PREVENTION

- Vaccine bacillus Calmette-Guérin (BCG) was developed from an attenuated strain of *M bovis*
- BCG not recommended in the United States due to its variable effectiveness, the low prevalence of TB infection, and the interference of the vaccine with determination of LTBI
- All suspected and confirmed cases of MTB should be reported to local and state public health authorities

EVIDENCE

PRACTICE GUIDELINES

- American Thoracic Society, Centers for Disease Control and Prevention, Infectious Diseases Society of America: Treatment of tuberculosis. Am J Respir Crit Care Med 2003;167:603. [PMID: 12588714]

WEB SITE

- CDC's Division of Tuberculosis Elimination http://www.cdc.gov/nchstp/tb/

INFORMATION FOR PATIENTS

- National Institute of Allergy and Infectious Disease http://www.niaid.nih.gov/publications/pubTB/TBEnglish06.pdf

REFERENCES

- Blumberg HM: American Thoracic Society, Centers for Disease Control and Prevention, Infectious Diseases Society of America: Treatment of tuberculosis. Am J Respir Crit Care Med 2003; 167:603. [PMID: 12588714]
- Small PM et al: Management of tuberculosis in the United States. N Engl J Med 2001;345:189. [PMID: 11463015]

Mark S. Chesnutt, MD
Thomas J. Prendergast, MD

Tuberculous Meningitis

 KEY FEATURES

ESSENTIALS OF DIAGNOSIS

- Gradual onset of listlessness, irritability, and anorexia
- Headache, vomiting, and seizures common
- Cranial nerve abnormalities typical
- Tuberculous focus may be evident elsewhere
- Cerebrospinal fluid shows several hundred lymphocytes, low glucose, and high protein

GENERAL CONSIDERATIONS

- Caused by rupture of a meningeal tuberculoma resulting from earlier hematogenous seeding of tubercle bacillus from a pulmonary focus, or may be a consequence of miliary spread

 CLINICAL FINDINGS

SYMPTOMS AND SIGNS

- The onset is usually gradual, with listlessness, irritability, anorexia, and fever, followed by headache, vomiting, convulsions, and coma
- In older patients, headache and behavioral changes are prominent early symptoms. Nuchal rigidity and cranial nerve palsies occur as the meningitis progresses
- Evidence of active tuberculosis elsewhere or a history of prior tuberculosis is present in up to 75% of patients
- The tuberculin skin test is usually (not always) positive

DIFFERENTIAL DIAGNOSIS

- May be confused with any other type of meningitis, but the gradual onset, the predominantly lymphocytic pleocytosis of the spinal fluid, and evidence of tuberculosis elsewhere often point to the diagnosis
- Chronic lymphocytic meningitis due to fungi (cryptococcus, coccidioides, histoplasma), brucellosis, leptospirosis, syphilis, Lyme disease, HIV infection, neurocysticercosis
- Carcinomatous meningitis
- Sarcoidosis
- Subdural hematoma

 DIAGNOSIS

LABORATORY TESTS

- The spinal fluid is frequently yellowish, with increased pressure, 100–500 cells/mL (predominantly lymphocytes, though neutrophils may be present early during infection), increased protein, and decreased glucose (Table 125, page 1307)
- Acid-fast stains of cerebrospinal fluid usually are negative, and cultures also may be negative in 15–25% of cases

IMAGING STUDIES

- Chest x-ray often reveals abnormalities compatible with tuberculosis but may be normal

TREATMENT

MEDICATIONS

- Presumptive diagnosis followed by early, empirical antituberculous therapy is essential for survival and to minimize sequelae
- Even if cultures are not positive, a full course of therapy is warranted if the clinical setting is suggestive of tuberculous meningitis
- Regimens that are effective for pulmonary tuberculosis (but adminstered for 12 months) are effective also for tuberculous meningitis (Table 24, page 1221)
- Rifampin, isoniazid, and pyrazinamide all penetrate into cerebrospinal fluid well
- The penetration of ethambutol is more variable, but therapeutic concentrations can be achieved, and the drug has been successfully used for meningitis
- Some authorities recommend the addition of corticosteroids for patients with focal deficits or altered mental status. Dexamethasone, 0.15 mg/kg four times daily for 1–2 weeks, then discontinued in a tapering regimen over 4 weeks, may be used

 OUTCOME

COMPLICATIONS

- Result from inflammatory exudate primarily involving the basilar meninges and arteries
  - Chronic brain syndrome
  - Seizure disorders
  - Cranial nerve palsies
  - Stroke
  - Obstructive hydrocephalus

PROGNOSIS

- High morbidity and mortality associated with stupor, coma, focal neurological deficits

WHEN TO REFER

- Consultation with a physician experienced in the treatment of tuberculosis is recommended

WHEN TO ADMIT

- Recommended for all suspected cases for initial evaluation and treatment

 EVIDENCE

PRACTICE GUIDELINES

- Tuberculous Meningitis http://www.guideline.gov/summary/ summary.aspx?doc_id=2157&nbr= 1383&string=tuberculous+meningitis

WEB SITES

- CDC—Division of Bacterial and Mycotic Diseases http://www.cdc.gov/ncidod/dbmd/
- National Tuberculosis Center http://www.umdnj.edu/ntbcweb/
- Pathology of Tuberculosis http://telpath2.med.utah.edu/WebPath/ TUTORIAL/MTB/MTB.html

INFORMATION FOR PATIENTS

- JAMA patient page: Lumbar puncture. JAMA 2002;288:2056.
- JAMA patient page: Tuberculosis. JAMA 2000;283:2060.
- JAMA patient page: Meningitis. JAMA 1999;281:1560.

REFERENCE

- Bidstrup C et al: Tuberculous meningitis in a country with a low incidence of tuberculosis: still a serious disease and a diagnostic challenge. Scand J Infect Dis 2002;34:811. [PMID: 12578148]

Henry F. Chambers, MD

Tubular Necrosis, Acute

 ## KEY FEATURES

ESSENTIALS OF DIAGNOSIS

- Acute renal failure
- Fractional excretion of sodium (FE_{Na}) >1%
- Urine sediment with pigmented granular casts and renal tubular epithelial cells

GENERAL CONSIDERATIONS

- Acute renal failure due to tubular damage
- Accounts for 85% of intrinsic acute renal failure
- Two major causes are ischemia and nephrotoxin exposure
- Ischemic acute renal failure occurs in prolonged hypotension or hypoxemia such as dehydration, shock, sepsis, and following major surgical procedures
- Nephrotoxin exposure includes both exogenous and endogenous

Exogenous nephrotoxins

- Aminoglycosides
- Vancomycin, acyclovir, and several cephalosporins
- Amphotericin B
- Radiographic contrast media
- Cyclosporine
- Antineoplastics, such as cisplatin and organic solvents, and heavy metals (mercury, cadmium, and arsenic)

Endogenous nephrotoxins

- Uric acid, paraproteins
- Myoglobinuria as a consequence of rhabdomyolysis
- Hemoglobinuria, massive intravascular hemolysis
- Hyperuricemia
- Bence Jones protein

 ## CLINICAL FINDINGS

SYMPTOMS AND SIGNS

- See Renal failure, acute

DIFFERENTIAL DIAGNOSIS

- Prerenal azotemia, eg, dehydration
- Postrenal azotemia, eg, benign prostatic hyperplasia
- Other renal causes of acute renal failure
  - Acute glomerulonephritis: immune complex (eg, IgA nephropathy), pauci-immune (eg, Wegener's granulomatosis), anti-glomerular basement membrane disease
  - Acute interstitial nephritis: drugs (eg, β-lactams), infections (eg, *Streptococcus*), immune (eg, systemic lupus erythematosus)

 ## DIAGNOSIS

LABORATORY TESTS

- Serum creatinine (Cr) and blood urea nitrogen (BUN) elevated
- BUN/creatinine ratio <20:1 in acute tubular necrosis
- Hyperkalemia
- Anion gap metabolic acidosis
- Hyperphosphatemia
- Urinalysis: urine may be brown with pigmented granular casts or "muddy brown" casts; renal tubular epithelial cells and epithelial cell casts
- FE_{Na} = clearance of Na^+/GFR = clearance of Na^+/creatinine clearance = (urine Na^+/plasma Na^+)/(urine Cr/plasma Cr) × 100
- FE_{Na} high (>1%) in acute tubular necrosis

IMAGING STUDIES

- Renal ultrasound

DIAGNOSTIC PROCEDURES

- Renal biopsy is rarely indicated

TREATMENT

MEDICATIONS

- Loop diuretics in large doses (eg, furosemide, 20–160 mg PO or 0.4–0.6 mg/kg/h increasing to a maximum of 1 mg/kg/h IV BID)
- Thiazide, eg, chlorothiazide, 500 mg IV Q 8–12 h
- Phosphate-binding agents
  - Aluminum hydroxide, 500 mg PO TID with meals
  - Calcium carbonate, 500–1500 mg PO TID with meals, calcium acetate, 667 mg 2–4 tabs PO TID with meals, or sevelamer, 800–1600 mg PO TID with meals

THERAPEUTIC PROCEDURES

- Dietary protein restriction of 0.6 g/kg/day
- Nutritional support
- Avoid volume overload
- Avoid hyperkalemia
- Avoid magnesium-containing antacids and laxatives
- Hemodialysis, peritoneal dialysis: indications include
  - Uremic symptoms such as pericarditis, encephalopathy, or coagulopathy
  - Fluid overload unresponsive to diuresis
  - Refractory hyperkalemia
  - Severe metabolic acidosis (pH <7.20)
  - Neurological symptoms such as seizures or neuropathy

 OUTCOME

COMPLICATIONS

- Loop diuretics in large doses may cause deafness

PROGNOSIS

- Nonoliguric acute tubular necrosis has a better outcome
- Mortality from acute renal failure is 20–50% in medical illness and up to 70% in a surgical setting
- Increased mortality with advanced age, severe underlying disease, and multisystem organ failure
- Leading causes of death are infections, fluid and electrolyte disturbances, and worsening of underlying disease

WHEN TO REFER

- Rapidly rising BUN/Cr

WHEN TO ADMIT

- Decompensation from: acute renal failure; volume overload; hyperkalemia; uremic symptoms

PREVENTION

- Montior patients closely with rising serum creatinine after radiographic contrast media

 EVIDENCE

PRACTICE GUIDELINES

- Abernethy VE, Lieberthal W: Acute renal failure in the critically ill patient. Crit Care Clin 2002;18:203. [PMID: 12053831]
- Esson ML et al: Diagnosis and treatment of acute tubular necrosis. Ann Intern Med 2002;137:744. [PMID: 12416948]

WEB SITE

- National Kidney and Urologic Diseases Information Clearinghouse http://kidney.niddk.nih.gov/kudiseases/pubs/glomerular/index.htm#3

INFORMATION FOR PATIENTS

- PENN State—Acute renal failure http://www.hmc.psu.edu/healthinfo/a/acuterenalfailure.htm
- Robert Wood Johnson Hospital Hamilton—Acute tubular necrosis http://www.rwjhamilton.org/Atoz/Encyclopedia/article/000512.asp

REFERENCES

- Albright RC Jr: Acute renal failure: a practical update. Mayo Clin Proc 2001; 76:67. [PMID:11155415]
- Murphy SW et al: Contrast nephropathy. J Am Soc Nephrol 2000;11:177. [PMID: 10616853]
- Nissenson AR: Acute renal failure: definition and pathogenesis. Kidney Int 1998;66(Suppl):S7. [PMID: 9573567]
- Perazella MA: Crystal-induced acute renal failure. Am J Med 1999;106:459. [PMID: 10225250]
- Vanholder R et al: Rhabdomyolysis. J Am Soc Nephrol 2000;11:1553. [PMID: 10906171]

Suzanne Watnick, MD
Gail Morrison, MD

Tularemia

 KEY FEATURES

ESSENTIALS OF DIAGNOSIS

- History of contact with rabbits, other rodents, and biting arthropods (eg, ticks in summer) in endemic area
- Fever, headache, nausea, and prostration
- Papule progressing to ulcer at site of inoculation
- Enlarged regional lymph nodes
- Serological tests or culture of ulcer, lymph node aspirate, or blood confirm the diagnosis

GENERAL CONSIDERATIONS

- An infection of wild rodents—particularly rabbits and muskrats—with *Francisella* (*Pasteurella*) *tularensis*
- Usually acquired by contact with animal tissues (eg, trapping muskrats, skinning rabbits), from ticks, or from biting flies
- Risk factors for pneumonic tularemia include lawn-mowing and brush-cutting, underscoring the potential for probable aerosol transmission of the organism
- The incubation period is 2–10 days
- *F tularensis* has been classified as a high-priority agent for potential bioterrorism use because of its virulence and relative ease of dissemination

 CLINICAL FINDINGS

SYMPTOMS AND SIGNS

- Infection often produces a local lesion and widespread organ involvement but may be entirely asymptomatic
- Fever, headache, and nausea begin suddenly
- A local lesion—a papule at the site of inoculation—develops and soon ulcerates
- The local lesion may be on the skin of an extremity or in the eye
- Regional lymph nodes may become enlarged and tender and may suppurate
- Pneumonia may develop from hematogenous spread of the organism or may be primary after inhalation of infected aerosols, which are responsible for human-to-human transmission
- Following ingestion of infected meat or water, an enteric form may be manifested by gastrointestinal symptoms, stupor, and delirium
- Hematogenous spread may produce meningitis, perisplenitis, pericarditis, pneumonia, and osteomyelitis
- In any type of involvement, the spleen may be enlarged and tender and there may be nonspecific rashes, myalgias, and prostration

DIFFERENTIAL DIAGNOSIS

- Anthrax
- Cat-scratch disease
- Infectious mononucleosis
- Plague
- Typhoid fever
- Lymphoma
- Rickettsial disease, eg, epidemic typhus, Q fever
- Rat-bite fever
- Meningococcemia
- Sporotrichosis
- Herpes simplex virus conjunctivitis

 DIAGNOSIS

LABORATORY TESTS

- Culturing the organism from blood or infected tissue requires special media. For this reason and because cultures of *F tularensis* may be hazardous to laboratory personnel, the diagnosis is usually made serologically
- A positive agglutination test (>1:80) develops within 2 weeks and may persist for several years
- Culture of ulcer, lymph node aspirate, or blood confirms the diagnosis

TREATMENT

MEDICATIONS

- Streptomycin, 7.5–10 mg/kg intramuscularly or intravenously every 12 h for 7–10 days
- Chloramphenicol, 50–100 mg/kg/day, is indicated for meningitis

OUTCOME

COMPLICATIONS

- Hematogenous spread may produce meningitis, perisplenitis, pericarditis, pneumonia, and osteomyelitis

WHEN TO REFER

- Early referral to an infectious disease specialist may aid in management

WHEN TO ADMIT

- Serious cases
- Any complications from hematogenous spread

EVIDENCE

PRACTICE GUIDELINES

- National Guideline Clearinghouse http://www.guideline.gov/summary/ summary.aspx?doc_id=2981&nbr= 2207&string=tularemia

WEB SITES

- CDC—Division of Bacterial and Mycotic Diseases http://www.cdc.gov/ncidod/dbmd/
- Karolinska Institute—Directory of Bacterial Infections and Mycoses http://www.mic.ki.se/Diseases/c1.html

INFORMATION FOR PATIENTS

- National Institutes of Health http://www.nlm.nih.gov/medlineplus/ ency/article/000856.htm
- National Institute of Allergy and Infectious Diseases http://www.niaid.nih.gov/factsheets/ tularemia.htm

REFERENCE

- Feldman KA et al: An outbreak of primary pneumonic tularemia on Martha's Vineyard. N Engl J Med 2001;345: 1601. [PMID: 11757506]

Henry F. Chambers, MD

Typhoid Fever

 KEY FEATURES

ESSENTIALS OF DIAGNOSIS

- Gradual onset of malaise, headache, sore throat, cough, and either diarrhea or constipation
- Rose spots, relative bradycardia, splenomegaly, and abdominal distension and tenderness
- Leukopenia; blood, stool, and urine culture positive for *Salmonella*

GENERAL CONSIDERATIONS

- The term "typhoid fever" applies when *Salmonella enterica* subspecies *enterica* serotype typhi is the cause of enteric fever accompanied by bacteremia
- Enteric fever generally refers to a typhoidal type illness caused by serotypes other than typhi
- Infection is transmitted by consumption of contaminated food or drink
- Infection begins when organisms cross the intestinal mucosa. Bacteremia occurs, and the infection then localizes principally in the lymphoid tissue of the small intestine (particularly within 60 cm of the ileocecal valve). Peyer's patches become inflamed and may ulcerate, with involvement greatest during the third week of disease
- The incubation period is 5–14 days

DEMOGRAPHICS

- 400 cases per year in the United States, mostly among travelers
- An estimated 21 million cases of typhoid fever and 200,000 deaths occur worldwide

 CLINICAL FINDINGS

SYMPTOMS AND SIGNS

Prodromal stage

- Increasing malaise, headache, cough, and sore throat
- Often with abdominal pain and constipation, while the fever ascends in a stepwise fashion
- During the early prodrome, physical findings are few
- There may be marked constipation

Later stage

- After about 7–10 days, the fever reaches a plateau and the patient is much more ill, appearing exhausted and often prostrated
- Marked constipation may develop into "pea soup" diarrhea
- Splenomegaly, abdominal distension and tenderness, relative bradycardia, dicrotic pulse, and occasionally meningismus appear
- The rash (rose spots) commonly appears during the second week of disease. The individual spot, found principally on the trunk, is a pink papule 2–3 mm in diameter that fades on pressure. It disappears in 3–4 days

DIFFERENTIAL DIAGNOSIS

- Brucellosis
- Tuberculosis
- Infective endocarditis
- Q fever and other rickettsial infections
- Other cause of acute diarrhea
- Viral hepatitis
- Lymphoma
- Adult Still's disease
- Malaria

DIAGNOSIS

LABORATORY TESTS

- Best diagnosed by isolation of the organism from blood culture, which is positive in the first week of illness in 80% of patients who have not taken antibiotics
- Cultures of bone marrow occasionally are positive when blood cultures are not
- Stool culture is not reliable because it may be positive in gastroenteritis without typhoid fever

Typhoid Fever

TREATMENT

MEDICATIONS

- Ciprofloxacin, 500 mg orally twice daily or 400 mg intravenously twice daily for 5–7 days
- Ceftriaxone, 2 g intravenously once daily for 10–14 days
- Azithromycin, 1 g orally for 5 days
- Dexamethasone (3 mg/kg over 30 min intravenously, then 1 mg/kg every 6 h for 8 doses) reduces mortality in patients with severe typhoid fever (eg, those with delirium, coma, shock)
- Many strains are resistant to ampicillin and chloramphenicol; resistance to trimethoprim-sulfamethoxazole is increasing

OUTCOME

FOLLOW-UP

- Follow-up examination, with blood cultures for fever, as relapse can occur

COMPLICATIONS

- Complications occur in about 30% of untreated cases and account for 75% of all deaths
- Intestinal hemorrhage, manifested by a sudden drop in temperature and signs of shock followed by dark or fresh blood in the stool, or intestinal perforation, accompanied by abdominal pain and tenderness, is most likely to occur during the third week

PROGNOSIS

- Mortality rate is about 2% in treated cases
- With complications, the prognosis is poor
- Relapses occur in 5–10% cases; these are treated the same as primary infection
- A residual carrier state frequently persists in spite of chemotherapy

WHEN TO REFER

- Report to the public health department to trace contacts or carriers
- Refer early to an infectious disease specialist

WHEN TO ADMIT

- For intravenous antibiotics or supportive care

PREVENTION

- Immunization is not always effective but should be provided for household contacts of a typhoid carrier, for travelers to endemic areas, and during epidemic outbreaks
- A multiple-dose oral vaccine and a single-dose parenteral vaccine are available
- Adequate waste disposal and protection of food and water supplies from contamination are important public health measures to prevent salmonellosis
- Carriers must not be permitted to work as food handlers

EVIDENCE

PRACTICE GUIDELINES

- National Guideline Clearinghouse http://www.guideline.gov/summary/ summary.aspx?doc_id=3180&nbr= 2406&string=typhoid+fever http://www.guideline.gov/summary/ summary.aspx?doc_id=2791&nbr= 2017&string=typhoid+fever

WEB SITES

- CDC—Division of Bacterial and Mycotic Diseases http://www.cdc.gov/ncidod/dbmd/
- Karolinska Institute—Directory of Bacterial Infections and Mycoses http://www.mic.ki.se/Diseases/c1.html

INFORMATION FOR PATIENTS

- Centers for Disease Control http://www.cdc.gov/ncidod/dbmd/ diseaseinfo/ typhoidfever_g.htm
- National Institutes of Health http://www.nlm.nih.gov/medlineplus/ ency/article/001332.htm

REFERENCE

- Parry CM et al: Typhoid fever. N Engl J Med 2002;347:1770. [PMID: 12456854]

Henry F. Chambers, MD

Ulcerative Colitis

 KEY FEATURES

ESSENTIALS OF DIAGNOSIS

- Bloody diarrhea
- Lower abdominal cramps and fecal urgency
- Anemia, low serum albumin
- Negative stool cultures
- Sigmoidoscopy is key to diagnosis

GENERAL CONSIDERATIONS

- Idiopathic inflammatory condition that involves the mucosal surface of the colon, resulting in diffuse friability and erosions with bleeding
- In 50% of cases, disease is confined to the rectosigmoid region (proctosigmoiditis); 30% extend to the splenic flexure (left-sided colitis); <20% extend more proximally (extensive colitis)
- Most affected patients experience periods of symptomatic flare-ups and remissions

DEMOGRAPHICS

- More common in nonsmokers and former smokers, severity may worsen in patients who stop smoking
- Appendectomy at age <20 reduces risk

 CLINICAL FINDINGS

SYMPTOMS AND SIGNS

- Bloody diarrhea
- Cramps, abdominal pain
- Fecal urgency and tenesmus
- Abdominal tenderness, rebound tenderness
- Bright red blood on digital rectal examination

Mild disease

- Diarrhea infrequent
- Rectal bleeding and mucus intermittent
- Fecal urgency and tenesmus
- Left lower quadrant cramps, relieved by defecation
- No significant abdominal tenderness

Moderate disease

- Diarrhea more severe with frequent bleeding
- Abdominal pain and tenderness
- Mild fever

Severe disease

- >6–10 bloody bowel movements per day
- Signs of hypovolemia and impaired nutrition
- Abdominal pain and tenderness

Fulminant disease

- Rapid progression of symptoms and signs of severe toxicity (hypovolemia, hemorrhage requiring transfusion, and abdominal distension with tenderness) over 1–2 weeks in fulminant colitis

Toxic megacolon

- Colonic dilation of >6 cm on plain films with signs of toxicity in <2%, heightens risk of perforation

Extracolonic manifestations

- Occur in 25% of cases
- Erythema nodosum, pyoderma gangrenosum
- Episcleritis
- Thromboembolic events
- Oligoarticular, nondeforming arthritis
- Sclerosing cholangitis, with risk of cholangiocarcinoma

DIFFERENTIAL DIAGNOSIS

- Infectious colitis: *Salmonella, Shigella, Campylobacter,* amebiasis, *Clostridium difficile,* enteroinvasive *Escherichia coli,* cytomegalovirus (in AIDS)
- Ischemic colitis
- Crohn's disease
- Diverticular disease
- Colon cancer
- Antibiotic-associated diarrhea or pseudomembranous colitis
- Infectious proctitis: gonorrhea, chlamydia, herpes, syphilis
- Radiation colitis or proctitis

 DIAGNOSIS

LABORATORY TESTS

- Obtain hematocrit, erythrocyte sedimentation rate, and serum albumin
- Anemia in moderate to severe disease
- Hypoalbuminemia in moderate to severe disease
- Antineutrophil cytoplasmic antibodies with perinuclear staining (p-ANCA) in 50–70%; sometimes useful to distinguish from Crohn's disease in patients with indeterminate colitis
- Stools for bacterial (including *C difficile*) culture, ova and parasites

IMAGING STUDIES

- Plain abdominal radiographs
- Barium enema is of little utility and may precipitate toxic megacolon

DIAGNOSTIC PROCEDURES

- Sigmoidoscopy establishes diagnosis
- Colonoscopy should not be performed in patients with severe disease because of the risk of perforation, but after improvement colonoscopy is recommended to determine extent of disease, and for cancer surveillance

 TREATMENT

MEDICATIONS

Mild to moderate colitis

- Mesalamine, 800 mg PO TID (Asacol), or 1 g PO QID (Pentasa), balsalazide, 2.25 g PO TID, or sulfasalazine, 500 mg PO BID and increased gradually over 1–2 weeks to 2 g PO BID; 50–75% improve
- Folic acid 1 mg PO QD should be given to all patients taking sulfasalazine
- Corticosteroid therapy to patients who fail to improve after 2–3 weeks
- Hydrocortisone foam or enemas (80–100 mg BID), or prednisone, 20–30 mg twice daily, taper after 2 weeks by no more than 5 mg/week, slower tapering after 15 mg/day
- Antidiarrheal agents (eg, loperamide, 2 mg, diphenoxylate with atropine, 1 tablet, or tincture of opium, 8–15 drops up to four times daily), but should not be given in the acute phase of illness

Distal colitis

- Mesalamine suppository, 500 mg PR BID for proctitis, and as an enema 4 g PR QHS for proctosigmoiditis, for 3–12 weeks; 75% of patients improve
- Hydrocortisone suppository or foam for proctitis and hydrocortisone enema (80–100 mg) for proctosigmoiditis; less effective

Ulcerative Colitis

Severe colitis

- Corticosteroid therapy improves 50–75%
- Methylprednisolone, 48–64 mg, or hydrocortisone 300 mg, in 3 divided doses
- Hydrocortisone enema, 100 mg BID as a drip over 30 min
- Immunosuppressive agents
- Cyclosporine, 4 mg/kg/day IV, improves 60–75% of patients with severe colitis that is not improving after 7–10 days of intravenous steroids

Fulminant colitis and toxic megacolon

- Broad-spectrum antibiotics targeting anaerobes and gram-negative bacteria
- Mercaptopurine or azathioprine long-term therapy for patients with severe steroid-resistant colitis

Maintenance therapy

- Sulfasalazine, 1–1.5 g PO BID; olsalazine, 500 mg PO BID; and mesalamine, 800 mg PO TID (Asacol) or 500 mg PO QID (Pentasa) reduces relapse rate from 75% to <33%
- For distal colitis: mesalamine suppositories (500 mg PO QD) or oral mesalamine, balsalazide, or sulfasalazine reduces the relapse rate from 80–90% to <20% within 1 year

Refractory disease

- Mercaptopurine or azathioprine
- Infliximab (5 mg/kg) single IV infusion

SURGERY

- Total proctocolectomy with ileostomy (standard ileostomy, continent ileostomy, or ileoanal anastomosis) required in 25% of patients
- Indications for surgery include patients with severe disease (eg, severe hemorrhage) who fail to improve after 7–10 days of corticosteroid or cyclosporine therapy; perforation; refractory disease requiring chronic steroids to control symptoms; fulminant colitis or toxic megacolon that worsens or fails to improve within 48–72 h; dysplasia or carcinoma on surveillance colonoscopic biopsies

THERAPEUTIC PROCEDURES

Mild to moderate colitis

- Regular diet
- Limit intake of caffeine and gas-producing vegetables
- Fiber supplements (eg, psyllium, 3.4 g PO BID; methylcellulose, 2 g PO BID; bran powder, 1 tbsp PO BID)

Severe colitis

- Discontinue all oral intake, total parenteral nutrition
- Avoid opioid and anticholinergic agents
- Restore circulating volume with fluids and blood
- Correct electrolyte abnormalities

Fulminant colitis and toxic megacolon

- Nasogastric suction, roll patients from side to side and onto the abdomen

OUTCOME

COMPLICATIONS

- Toxic megacolon
- Colon cancer
- Sclerosing cholangitis with risk of cholangiocarcinoma

PROGNOSIS

- Lifelong disease characterized by exacerbations and remissions
- In most patients, disease is readily controlled by medical therapy without need for surgery
- Majority never require hospitalization
- Surgery results in complete cure of the disease

WHEN TO REFER

- Patients with severe or refractory disease requiring immunomodulatory therapy

WHEN TO ADMIT

- Hospitalize patients with severe colitis

PREVENTION

- Colon cancer in ~0.5–1% per year of patients who have had colitis for >10 years
- Colonoscopy with multiple random mucosal biopsies recommended every 1–2 years in patients with extensive colitis, beginning 8–10 years after diagnosis
- Folic acid, 1 mg PO QD, decreases risk of colon cancer

EVIDENCE

PRACTICE GUIDELINES

- Wexner SD et al: Practice parameters for the treatment of mucosal ulcerative colitis—supporting documentation. The Standards Practice Task Force. The American Society of Colon and Rectal Surgeons. Dis Colon Rectum 1997; 40:1277. [PMID: 9369100]

WEB SITE

- MEDLINEplus—Ulcerative Colitis http://www.nlm.nih.gov/medlineplus/ulcerativecolitis.html

INFORMATION FOR PATIENTS

- National Digestive Diseases Information Clearinghouse—Ulcerative colitis http://digestive.niddk.nih.gov/ddiseases/pubs/colitis/index.htm

REFERENCES

- Chey W et al: Infliximab therapy for refractory ulcerative colitis. Am J Gastroenterol 2001;96:2373. [PMID: 11513177]
- D'Haens G et al: Intravenous cyclosporine versus intravenous corticosteroids as single therapy for severe attacks of ulcerative colitis. Gastroenterology 2001;120:1323. [PMID: 11313301]
- Gionchetti P et al: Review article: treatment of mild to moderate ulcerative colitis and pouchitis. Aliment Pharmacol Ther 2002;16(Suppl 4):13. [PMID: 12047254]

Kenneth R. McQuaid, MD

Urinary Incontinence

 KEY FEATURES

GENERAL CONSIDERATIONS

- Urinary incontinence is the involuntary loss of urine
- Urinary continence depends on both bladder and sphincteric mechanisms; dysfunction of either component may result in incontinence
- Most common in older patients
- Prevalence 5–15% in the community, >50% in long-term care facilities

Classification

- **Total incontinence**: uncontrolled loss of urine at all times and in all positions. Results when sphincteric efficiency is lost (previous surgery, nerve damage, cancerous infiltration) or when an abnormal connection between the urinary tract and the skin exists that bypasses the urinary sphincter (vesicovaginal or ureterovaginal fistulas)
- **Stress incontinence:** loss of urine associated with activities that increase intra-abdominal pressure (coughing, sneezing, lifting, exercising), though not in the supine position, results from urethral sphincteric insufficiency due to laxity of the pelvic floor musculature—in multiparous women or after pelvic surgery
- **Urge incontinence:** loss of urine that is preceded by a strong, unexpected urge to void, unrelated to position or activity, results from detrusor hyperreflexia or sphincter dysfunction due to inflammatory conditions or neurogenic disorders of the bladder
- **Overflow incontinence:** loss of urine in patients with chronic urinary retention results from the chronically distended bladder receiving an additional increment of urine, so that intravesical pressure just exceeds the outlet resistance, allowing a small amount of urine to dribble out

 CLINICAL FINDINGS

SYMPTOMS AND SIGNS

- The history permits subclassification into one of four categories of incontinence
- Physical examination is done to exclude fistula for cases of total incontinence, neurological abnormalities in cases of urge incontinence (spasticity, flaccidity, rectal sphincter tone, bulbocavernosus reflex), or distended bladder in cases of overflow incontinence

 DIAGNOSIS

LABORATORY TESTS

- Urinalysis and urine culture to exclude urinary tract infection. Serum creatinine to exclude renal dysfunction
- Cystograms to demonstrate fistula sites and descensus of the bladder neck (descent of bladder neck more than 1.5 cm on straining view) in cases of stress incontinence. Postvoid residual urine volume assessed by urethral catheterization or ultrasonography

DIAGNOSTIC PROCEDURES

- History, supplemented with a voiding diary

Special tests

- Urodynamic evaluation can assess both bladder and sphincteric function. Indicated in patients with moderate to severe incontinence, those suspected of having neurological disease, and those with urge incontinence when infection and neoplasm have been excluded
- Cystometry to assess bladder capacity, accommodation, sensation, voluntary control, contractility, and response to pharmacological intervention. Normal adult bladder capacity = 350–500 mL. Decreased capacity occurs in incontinence, infections, interstitial cystitis, radiation damage, upper motor neuron lesions, and postoperative changes. Increased bladder capacity occurs with chronic urinary tract obstruction, lower motor neuron lesions, and sensory neuropathies
- Urethral profilometry, electromyography, or combined video studies to assess sphincteric function

Urinary Incontinence

 TREATMENT

MEDICATIONS

- Urge incontinence: effective agents include anticholinergic medications (oxybutinin, 5–15 mg/day, or tolterodine, 2–4 mg/day) or tricyclic antidepressants (imipramine, 25–75 mg PO at bedtime)

SURGERY

- Total incontinence: congenital defects and acquired lesions require surgical correction. Sphincter injuries following prostatectomy may be managed by surgical reconstruction
- Stress incontinence: the bladder neck descends below the midportion of the pubic symphysis. Surgical treatment centers on placing the bladder neck into an appropriate anatomical location, allowing increased intraabdominal pressure to be transmitted to the bladder and bladder neck

THERAPEUTIC PROCEDURES

- Overflow incontinence: placement of a urethral catheter in the acute setting. Further treatment must address the underlying disease

 OUTCOME

PROGNOSIS

- Surgery is usually corrective for stress incontinence

EVIDENCE

PRACTICE GUIDELINES

- Urinary incontinence. American Medical Directors Association, 2001 http://www.guidelines.gov/summary/summary.aspx?doc_id=1812&nbr=1038&string=urinary+incontinence

WEB SITES

- National Institute on Aging—Urinary incontinence http://www.nia.nih.gov/health/agepages/urinary.htm
- National Kidney and Urologic Diseases Information Clearinghouse—Urinary incontinence in women http://kidney.niddk.nih.gov/kudiseases/pubs/uiwomen/index.htm

INFORMATION FOR PATIENTS

- American Academy of Family Physicians—Urinary incontinence: embarrassing but treatable http://familydoctor.org/healthfacts/189/

REFERENCES

- Andersson KE: Drug therapy for urinary incontinence. Baillieres Best Pract Res Clin Obstet Gynaecol 2000;14:291. [PMID: 10897323]
- Jackson S et al: The effect of oestrogen supplementation on post-menopausal urinary stress incontinence: a double-blind placebo-controlled trial. Br J Obstet Gynaecol 1999;106:711. [PMID: 10428529]
- Knapp PM Jr: Identifying and treating urinary incontinence: the crucial role of the primary care physician. Postgrad Med 1998;103:279. [PMID: 9553601]
- Schmidt RA et al: Sacral nerve stimulation for treatment of refractory urinary urge incontinence. Sacral Nerve Stimulation Study Group. J Urol 1999;162:352. [PMID: 10411037]

Marshall, L. Stoller, MD
Peter R. Carroll, MD

Urinary Incontinence in Elderly

 KEY FEATURES

ESSENTIALS OF DIAGNOSIS

- Delirium is the most common cause of transient or potentially reversible incontinence
- Detrusor overactivity (urge incontinence) is the most common cause of established incontinence

GENERAL CONSIDERATIONS

Transient causes (the mnemonic "DIAPPERS")

- Delirium (most common cause in hospitalized patients)
- Infection (symptomatic urinary tract infection)
- Atrophic urethritis and vaginitis
- Pharmaceuticals [eg, potent diuretics, anticholinergics, psychotropics, opioid analgesics, α-blockers (in women), α-agonists (in men), and calcium channel blockers]
- Psychological factors (severe depression with psychomotor retardation)
- Excess urine output (diuretics, excess fluid intake, hyperglycemia and peripheral edema and its associated nocturia)
- Restricted mobility (see *Immobility in elderly*)
- Stool impaction

Established causes

- Detrusor overactivity (urge incontinence)
  - Uninhibited bladder contractions that cause leakage
  - Most common cause of established geriatric incontinence, accounting for two-thirds of cases; usually idiopathic
- Urethral incompetence (stress incontinence)
- Urethral obstruction
- Detrusor underactivity (overflow incontinence)

 CLINICAL FINDINGS

SYMPTOMS AND SIGNS

- Atrophic urethritis and vaginitis: vaginal mucosal friability, erosions, telangiectasia, petechiae, or erythema
- Detrusor overactivity (urge incontinence): women complain of urinary leakage after the onset of an intense urge to urinate that cannot be forestalled
- Urethral incompetence (stress incontinence): urinary loss occurs with laughing, coughing, or lifting heavy objects
- Urethral obstruction: dribbling incontinence after voiding, urge incontinence due to detrusor overactivity (which coexists in two-thirds of cases), or overflow incontinence due to urinary retention
- Detrusor underactivity (overflow incontinence): urinary frequency, nocturia, and frequent leakage of small amounts

 DIAGNOSIS

LABORATORY TESTS

- Review medications
- Check urinalysis for infection
- Consider tests for hyperglycemia, hypercalcemia, diabetes insipidus

IMAGING STUDIES

- Ultrasonography can determine postvoid residual
- Renal ultrasound to exclude hydronephrosis in men whose postvoiding residual urine exceeds 150 mL, particularly if the incontinence developed suddenly
- In older men for whom surgery is planned, urodynamic confirmation of obstruction is strongly advised

DIAGNOSTIC PROCEDURES

- To test for stress incontinence, have the patient relax her perineum and cough vigorously (a single cough) while standing with a full bladder
  - Instantaneous leakage indicates stress incontinence if urinary retention has been excluded by postvoiding residual determination using ultrasound
  - A delay of several seconds or persistent leakage suggests the problem is caused by an uninhibited bladder contraction induced by coughing
- Because detrusor overactivity may be due to bladder stones or tumor, the abrupt onset of otherwise unexplained urge incontinence—especially if accompanied by perineal or suprapubic discomfort or sterile hematuria—should be investigated by cystoscopy and cytological examination of the urine
- An elevated postvoiding residual urine (generally over 450 mL) distinguishes detresor underactivity from detrusor overactivity and stress incontinence, but only urodynamic testing differentiates it from urethral obstruction in men

TREATMENT

MEDICATIONS

Transient causes

- Discontinue all anticholinergic agents or substitute with less anticholinergic effects (eg, sertraline instead of desipramine)

Established causes

- Detrusor overactivity: oxybutynin (2.5–5 mg three or four times daily), long-acting oxybutynin (5–15 mg daily), or tolterodine (1–2 mg twice daily) may reduce episodes of incontinence; watch for delirium, dry mouth, or urinary retention
- Urethral incompetence (stress incontinence): topical or oral estrogens are helpful only if atrophic vaginitis with urethral irritation is present
- Urethral obstruction: for prostatic obstruction without retention, treatment with α-blocking agents (eg, terazosin, 1–10 mg daily; prazosin, 1–5 mg orally twice daily; tamsulosin, 0.4–0.8 mg daily) may relieve symptoms
- Detrusor underactivity: antibiotics (only for symptomatic upper urinary tract infection or as prophylaxis against recurrent symptomatic infections with intermittent catheterization)

THERAPEUTIC PROCEDURES

Established causes

- Detrusor overactivity
  - The cornerstone is behavioral therapy
  - Patients are instructed to void every 1–2 h while awake (increased by 30 min until the interval is 4–5 h)
  - Pelvic floor exercises, behavioral approaches, and biofeedback can be extremely helpful
  - In refractory cases, where intermittent catheterization is feasible, the physician may choose to induce urinary retention with a bladder relaxant and have the patient empty the bladder three or four times daily
- Urethral incompetence (stress incontinence)
  - Pelvic muscle and pelvic floor exercises are effective for mild to moderate stress incontinence; they can be combined with biofeedback, electrical stimulation, or vaginal cones
  - A pessary or a tampon (for women with vaginal stenosis)

- Urethral obstruction
  - For the nonoperative candidate, use an intermittent or indwelling catheter
- Detrusor underactivity
  - Augmented voiding techniques (eg, double voiding, suprapubic pressure)
  - Intermittent or indwelling catheterization

SURGERY

- Although a last resort, surgery is the most effective treatment for stress incontinence, resulting in a cure rate of 75–85% even in older women
- Surgical decompression is the most effective treatment for urethral obstruction, especially in the setting of urinary retention

OUTCOME

COMPLICATIONS

- The most important complication is restriction of social activity
- In immobile patients, incontinence increases the risk for pressure ulcers

PROGNOSIS

- Some incontinence resolves spontaneously
- In most patients, treatment of exacerbating factors, and pharmacological and nonpharmacological treatments can substantially reduce the severity

WHEN TO REFER

- Refer to a multidisciplinary incontinence clinic or geriatrician if there is no response to first-line measures

PREVENTION

- Weight loss may be beneficial

EVIDENCE

PRACTICE GUIDELINES

- Urinary incontinence in adults: acute and chronic management. Clinical Practice Guideline, No. 2, 1996 update. United States Department of Health and Human Services. Public Health Service, AHCPR. Publication No. 96-0682.
- National Guidelines Clearinghouse http://www.guideline.gov/summary/summary.aspx?doc_id=1812&nbr=1038&string=urinary+incontinence

WEB SITE

- NGC: Urinary incontinence http://www.guideline.gov/FRAMESETS/guideline_fs.asp?guideline=001038&sSearch_string=urinary+incontinence

INFORMATION FOR PATIENTS

- JAMA patient page: Stress incontinence. JAMA 2003;290:426. [PMID: 12865384]

REFERENCE

- Burgio KL: Behavioral vs drug treatment for urge urinary incontinence in older women: a randomized, controlled trial. JAMA 1998;280:1995. [PMID: 9863850]

C. Bree Johnston, MD
Kenneth E. Covinsky, MD

Urinary Stone Disease

 KEY FEATURES

ESSENTIALS OF DIAGNOSIS

GENERAL CONSIDERATIONS

- 240,000–720,000 Americans per year
- Males > females (4:1)
- Initial presentation predominates in the third and fourth decades
- Incidence is greatest during hot summer months
- Geographic factors (high humidity and elevated temperatures); diet (sodium and protein intake, excess intake of oxalate and purines); fluid intake; and genetic factors (cystinuria; distal renal tubular acidosis) contribute to urinary stone formation
- Five major types of urinary stones: calcium oxalate, calcium phosphate, struvite, uric acid, and cystine
- Most urinary stones contain calcium (85%) and are radiopaque; uric acid stones are radiolucent
- **Hypercalciuric calcium nephrolithiasis** (>200 mg/24 h) can be caused by absorptive, resorptive, and renal disorders (Table 86, page 1271)
  - Absorptive hypercalciuria is secondary to increased absorption of calcium at the level of the small bowel, predominantly in the jejunum, and can be further subdivided into types I, II, and III. Type I absorptive hypercalciuria is independent of calcium intake. There is increased urinary calcium on a regular or even a calcium-restricted diet. Type II absorptive hypercalciuria is diet dependent. Type III absorptive hypercalciuria is secondary to a renal phosphate leak, which results in increased vitamin D synthesis and secondarily increased small bowel absorption of calcium
  - Resorptive hypercalciuria is secondary to hyperparathyroidism. Hypercalcemia, hypophosphatemia, hypercalciuria, and an elevated serum parathyroid hormone level are found
  - Renal hypercalciuria occurs when the renal tubules are unable to efficiently reabsorb filtered calcium, and hypercalciuria and secondary hyperparathyroidism result
- **Hyperuricosuric calcium nephrolithiasis** is secondary to dietary excesses or uric acid metabolic defects
- **Hyperoxaluric calcium nephrolithiasis** is usually due to primary intestinal disorders, including chronic diarrhea, inflammatory bowel disease, or steatorrhea
- **Hypocitraturic calcium nephrolithiasis** may be secondary to chronic diarrhea, type I (distal) renal tubular acidosis, chronic hydrochlorothiazide treatment, or idiopathic
- **Uric acid calculi:** contributing factors include low urinary pH, hyperuricemia, myeloproliferative disorders, malignancy with increased uric acid production, abrupt and dramatic weight loss, and uricosuric medications
- **Struvite calculi** (magnesium-ammonium-phosphate, "staghorn" calculi) occur with recurrent urinary tract infections with urease-producing organisms, including *Proteus, Pseudomonas, Providencia,* and, less commonly, *Klebsiella,* staphylococci, and *Mycoplasma*
- **Cystine calculi**

 CLINICAL FINDINGS

SYMPTOMS AND SIGNS

- Colicky pain in the flank, usually severe
- Nausea and vomiting
- Patients constantly moving—in sharp contrast to those with an acute abdomen
- Pain episodic and radiates anteriorly over the abdomen
- With stone in the ureter, pain may be referred into the ipsilateral testis or labium
- With stone at the ureterovesical junction, marked urinary urgency and frequency
- Stone size does not correlate with the severity of the symptoms

 DIAGNOSIS

LABORATORY TESTS

- Urinalysis: microscopic or gross (~10%) hematuria. Absence of microhematuria does not exclude urinary stones
- Urinary pH: persistent urinary pH <5.0 is suggestive of uric acid or cystine stones; persistent pH >7.5 is suggestive of a struvite stone

Metabolic evaluation

- Stone analysis on recovered stones
- Uncomplicated first-time stone formers: serum calcium, phosphate, electrolytes, and uric acid
- Recurrent stone formers or patients with a family history of stone disease: 24-h urine collection on a random diet for volume, urinary pH, and calcium, uric acid, oxalate, phosphate, and citrate excretion
- To subcategorize patients: a second 24-h urine collection on a restricted calcium (400 mg/day) and sodium (100 mEq/day) diet is undertaken, if necessary
- Serum parathyroid hormone and calcium load tests

IMAGING STUDIES

- Plain film of the abdomen and renal ultrasound will diagnose most stones
- Plain film of the abdomen: radiopaque stones
- Abdominal ultrasonography: stones at the ureterovesical junction can be imaged if patient has a full bladder
- Otherwise, transvaginal or transrectal ultrasonography
- Spiral CT sensitivity exceeds that of ultrasound or intravenous urography
- Intravenous urography is indicated when the diagnosis remains uncertain

TREATMENT

MEDICATIONS

- **Type I absorptive hypercalciuria:** cellulose phosphate, 10–15 g in 3 divided doses given with meals to decrease bowel absorption of calcium. Follow-up metabolic surveillance every 6–8 months to exclude hypomagnesemia, secondary hyperoxaluria, and recurrent calculi. Thiazide therapy can decrease renal calcium excretion
- **Type II absorptive hypercalciuria:** decreasing calcium intake by 50% (approximately 400 mg QD). There is no specific medical therapy
- **Type III absorptive hypercalciuria:** orthophosphates (0.5 g TID) to inhibit vitamin D synthesis
- **Renal hypercalciuria:** thiazides (effective long-term)
- **Hyperuricosuric calcium nephrolithiasis:** dietary purine restrictions or allopurinol, 300 mg PO QD (or both)
- **Hyperoxaluric calcium nephrolithiasis:** measures to curtail the diarrhea or steatorrhea, oral calcium supplements with meals, oral ascorbic acid supplements, and encouraging increased fluid intake
- **Hypocitraturic calcium nephrolithiasis:** potassium citrate, 20 mEq PO TID.
- **Uric acid calculi:** potassium citrate 20 mEq PO TID to increase urinary pH above 6.5. Patients should monitor their urinary alkalinization with Nitrazine pH paper. If hyperuricemia is present, allopurinol, 300 mg QD
- **Struvite calculi:** percutaneous nephrolithotomy, with appropriate perioperative antibiotics. Postoperative irrigation through nephrostomy tubes to eliminate small fragments. Acetohydroxamic acid, an effective urease inhibitor, is poorly tolerated
- **Cystine calculi:** difficult to manage medically. Prevention by increased fluid intake, alkalinization of the urine above pH 7.5 (monitored with Nitrazine pH paper), penicillamine and tiopronin

SURGERY

- **Resorptive hypercalciuria:** surgical resection of the adenoma
- **Infection with ureteral obstruction:** a medical emergency requiring both prompt drainage by a ureteral catheter or a percutaneous nephrostomy tube, and antibiotics

- **Ureteral stones:** stones <6 mm in diameter will usually pass spontaneously. Conservative observation with appropriate pain medications for up to 6 weeks
  - Therapeutic intervention required if spontaneous passage does not occur
  - Indications for earlier intervention include severe pain unresponsive to medications, fever, persistent nausea and vomiting requiring intravenous hydration
  - Distal ureteral stones—either ureteroscopic stone extraction or in situ extracorporeal shock wave lithotripsy (ESWL) under anesthesia
  - Proximal and midureteral stones can be treated with ESWL or ureteroscopic extraction, and a double-J ureteral stent to ensure adequate drainage
- **Renal stones:** conservative observation for patients presenting without pain, urinary tract infections, or obstruction. Intervention if calculi become symptomatic or grow in size. For renal stones <3 cm, treat by ESWL. For stones in the inferior calix or those >3 cm, treat by percutaneous nephrolithotomy. Perioperative antibiotics as indicated by preoperative urine cultures

THERAPEUTIC PROCEDURES

- Forced intravenous fluid diuresis is not productive and exacerbates pain

OUTCOME

PREVENTION

- Increased fluid intake (doubling previous fluid intake) to reduce stone recurrence. Patients are encouraged to ingest fluids during meals, 2 h after each meal, prior to going to sleep in the evening and during the night

EVIDENCE

PRACTICE GUIDELINES

- Sandhu C et al: Urinary tract stones–Part II: current status of treatment. Clin Radiol 2003;58:422. [PMID: 12788311]

WEB SITES

- NIH—Patient Education Institute Kidney Stones http://www.nlm.nih.gov/medlineplus/tutorials/kidneystones.html

INFORMATION FOR PATIENTS

- Cleveland Clinic—Kidney stones http://www.clevelandclinic.org/health/health-info/docs/0000/0046.asp?index=4349

REFERENCE

- Kosar A et al: Comparative study of long-term stone recurrence after extracorporeal shock wave lithotripsy and open stone surgery for kidney stones. Int J Urol 1999;6:125. [PMID: 10226822]

Marshall L. Stoller, MD
Peter R. Carroll, MD

Urticaria & Angioedema

 KEY FEATURES

ESSENTIALS OF DIAGNOSIS

- Eruptions of evanescent wheals or hives
- Itching is usually intense but may on rare occasions be absent
- Special forms of urticaria have special features (dermographism; cholinergic, solar, or cold urticaria)
- Most incidents are acute and self-limited over a period of 1–2 weeks
- Chronic urticaria (episodes lasting >6 weeks) may have an autoimmune basis

GENERAL CONSIDERATIONS

- The most common causes of acute urticaria are foods, viral infections, and medications
- Nonallergic causes of urticaria: drugs, eg, atropine, pilocarpine, morphine, and codeine; arthropod bites, eg, insect bites and bee stings; physical factors such as heat, cold, sunlight, and pressure; and neurogenic factors such as in cholinergic urticaria induced by exercise, excitement, hot showers
- Allergic causes of urticaria: penicillins, aspirin, and other medications; inhalants, eg, feathers and animal danders; ingestion of shellfish, tomatoes, or strawberries; injections of sera and vaccines; external contactants, eg, various chemicals and cosmetics; and infections such as hepatitis
- Chronic urticaria (episodes lasting >6 weeks) may have an autoimmune basis; the cause is often not found
- Autoimmune thyroid disease may coexist, but treatment of the thyroid disease does not improve the urticaria
- Physical forms of urticaria have special features (dermographism; cholinergic, solar, or cold urticaria)

DEMOGRAPHICS

- Chronic uritcaria is most common in young adult women

 CLINICAL FINDINGS

SYMPTOMS AND SIGNS

- See Table 7 (page 1202)
- Lesions are itchy red swellings of a few millimeters to many centimeters
- The morphology of the lesions may vary over a period of minutes to hours
- Individual lesions in true urticaria last less than 24 h, and often only 2–4 h
- Angioedema is involvement of deeper vessels, with swelling of the lips, eyelids, palms, soles, and genitalia in association with more typical lesions
- Angioedema is no more likely than urticaria to be associated with systemic complications such as laryngeal edema or hypotension
- In cholinergic urticaria, triggered by a rise in core body temperature (hot showers, exercise), wheals are 2–3 mm in diameter with a large surrounding red flare

DIFFERENTIAL DIAGNOSIS

- Vasculitis
- Erythema multiforme
- Contact dermatitis (eg, poison oak or ivy)
- Cellulitis

 DIAGNOSIS

LABORATORY TESTS

- Laboratory studies are not likely to be helpful in the evaluation of acute or chronic urticaria unless there are suggestive findings in the history and physical examination
- Quantitative immunoglobulins, cryoglobulins, cryofibrinogens, and antinuclear antibodies are often sought in urticaria but are rarely found
- Liver tests may be elevated, since a serum sickness–like prodrome, with urticaria, may be associated with acute hepatitis B infection

DIAGNOSTIC PROCEDURES

- In patients with individual slightly purpuric lesions that persist past 24 h, a skin biopsy may help exclude urticarial vasculitis

TREATMENT

MEDICATIONS

- H₁ antihistamines
  - Hydroxyzine, 10 mg twice daily to 25 mg three times daily to even 100 mg three times daily, may be very useful if tolerated; giving hydroxyzine as one dose of 50–75 mg at night may reduce sedation and other side effects
  - Cyproheptadine, 4 mg four times daily, may be useful for cold urticaria
- Add "nonsedating" or less sedating antihistamines if the generic sedating antihistamines are not effective
  - Fexofenadine is given in a dosage of 60 mg twice a day
  - Loratadine in a dosage of 10 mg/day is similar to the other H₁ antihistamines in effectiveness
  - Cetirizine, a metabolite of hydroxyzine may be sedating (13% of patients) and is given in a dosage of 10 mg/day
  - Doxepin (a tricyclic antidepressant), 25 mg three times daily, or, more commonly, 25–75 mg at bedtime, can be very effective in chronic urticaria; it has anticholinergic side effects
- H₂ antihistamines in combination with H₁ blockers may be helpful in patients with symptomatic dermatographism
- Adjuvants
  - Calcium channel blockers (used for at least 4 weeks)
  - Terbutaline, 1.25–2.5 mg three times daily
  - Colchicine, 0.6 mg twice daily
  - Danazol
  - Warfarin
  - Systemic steroids in a dose of about 40 mg daily will usually suppress acute and chronic urticaria; however, the use of corticosteroids is rarely indicated
  - Topical treatment is rarely rewarding

 ## OUTCOME

PROGNOSIS

- Acute urticaria usually lasts only a few days to 6 weeks
- Half of patients whose urticaria persists for more than 6 weeks will have it for years

WHEN TO REFER

- If there is a question about the diagnosis, if recommended therapy is ineffective, or if specialized treatment is necessary

 ## EVIDENCE

PRACTICE GUIDELINES

- Joint Task Force on Practice Parameters in Allergy, Asthma and Immunology http://www.jcaai.org/Param/Urticaria.htm

WEB SITES

- American Academy of Dermatology http://www.aad.org
- Dermatology Handbook for Family Practice from the University of Iowa http://www.vh.org/Providers/ClinRef/FPHandbook/17.html

INFORMATION FOR PATIENTS

- American Academy of Dermatology http://www.aad.org/pamphlets/Urticaria.html
- American Academy of Allergy, Asthma, and Immunology http://www.allergy.mcg.edu/advice/urtic.html

REFERENCES

- Black AK et al: Antihistamines in urticaria and angioedema. Clin Allergy Immunol 2002;17:249. [PMID: 12113219]
- Cha YJ et al: Angioedema due to losartan. Ann Pharmacother 1999;33:936. [PMID: 10492494]
- Grattan CE et al: Chronic urticaria. J Am Acad Dermatol 2002;46:657. [PMID: 12004303]
- Kaplan AP: Diagnostic tests for urticaria and angioedema. Clin Allergy Immunol 2000;15:111. [PMID: 10943290]

Timothy G. Berger, MD

Vaginal Bleeding, Abnormal Premenopausal

 ## KEY FEATURES

ESSENTIALS OF DIAGNOSIS

- Blood loss of over 80 mL per cycle
- Excessive bleeding, often with the passage of clots, may occur at regular menstrual intervals (**menorrhagia**) or irregular intervals (**dysfunctional uterine bleeding**)
- Etiology most commonly dysfunctional uterine bleeding on a hormonal basis

GENERAL CONSIDERATIONS

- Average normal menstrual bleeding lasts 4 days (range, 2–7 days), with a mean blood loss of 40 mL
- Bleeding cycles less than 21 days apart are likely anovular
- Blood loss of over 80 mL per cycle is abnormal and frequently produces anemia
- **Ovulation bleeding**, a single episode of spotting between regular menses, is quite common. Heavier or irregular intermenstrual bleeding warrants investigation
- **Anovulatory bleeding** (dysfunctional uterine bleeding) is usually caused by overgrowth of endometrium due to estrogen stimulation without adequate progesterone to stabilize growth

DEMOGRAPHICS

- Anovulation associated with high estrogen levels commonly occurs in teenagers, in women aged late 30s to late 40s, and in extremely obese women or those with polycystic ovary syndrome

 ## CLINICAL FINDINGS

SYMPTOMS AND SIGNS

- Obtain
  - A careful description of the duration and amount of flow, related pain, and relationship to the last menstrual period (LMP). The presence of blood clots or the degree of inconvenience caused by the bleeding may be more useful indicators
  - A history of pertinent illnesses
  - A history of all medications taken in the past month
- Perform a careful pelvic examination to look for pregnancy, uterine myomas, adnexal masses, or infection

DIFFERENTIAL DIAGNOSIS

- Ovulation bleeding (spotting episode between menses)
- Anovulatory cycle (dysfunctional uterine bleeding)
- Polycystic ovary syndrome (type of anovulatory cycle)
- Pregnancy
- Ectopic pregnancy
- Spontaneous abortion
- Uterine leiomyomas (fibroids)
- Endometrial polyp
- Cervicitis or pelvic inflammatory disease
- Adenomyosis (uterine endometriosis)
- Cervical cancer
- Cervical polyp
- Endometrial hyperplasia
- Endometrial cancer
- Hypothyroidism
- Hyperprolactinemia
- Diabetes mellitus
- Bleeding disorder, eg, von Willebrand's disease

 ## DIAGNOSIS

LABORATORY TESTS

- Cervical smears as needed for cytological and culture studies
- Complete blood cell count, sedimentation rate, and glucose levels
- Pregnancy test
- Thyroid function and blood clotting should be considered
- Tests for ovulation in cyclic menorrhagia include basal body temperature records, serum progesterone measured 1 week before the expected onset of menses, and analysis of an endometrial biopsy specimen for secretory activity shortly before the onset of menstruation

IMAGING STUDIES

- Ultrasound can evaluate endometrial thickness or diagnose intrauterine or ectopic pregnancy or adnexal masses
- Endovaginal ultrasound with saline infusion sonohysterography can diagnose endometrial polyps or subserous myomas
- MRI can definitively diagnose submucous myomas and adenomyosis

DIAGNOSTIC PROCEDURES

- In women over age 35 perform endometrial sampling to rule out endometrial hyperplasia or carcinoma prior to initiation of hormonal therapy for dysfunctional uterine bleeding
- If cancer of the cervix is suspected, colposcopically directed biopsies and endocervical curettage are indicated as first steps
- Hysteroscopy can visualize endometrial polyps, submucous myomas, and exophytic endometrial cancers. It is useful immediately before D&C

Vaginal Bleeding, Abnormal Premenopausal

TREATMENT

MEDICATIONS

Dysfunctional uterine bleeding

- Usually can be treated with progestins, which stabilize endometrial growth
- Give medroxyprogesterone acetate, 10 mg/day, or norethindrone acetate, 5 mg/day, for 10–14 days starting on Day 15 of the cycle, following which withdrawal bleeding (medical curettage) occurs
- Repeat treatment for several cycles and reinstitute if amenorrhea or dysfunctional bleeding recurs
- In women who are bleeding actively, any combination oral contraceptive can be given four times daily for 1 or 2 days followed by two pills daily through Day 5 and then one pill daily through Day 20; after withdrawal bleeding occurs, pills are taken in the usual dosage for three cycles

Heavy bleeding

- For intractable heavy bleeding, danazol, 200 mg four times daily, is sometimes used to create an atrophic endometrium
- Alternatively, a gonadotropin-releasing hormone agonist such as depot leuprolide, 3.75 mg IM monthly, or nafarelin, 0.2–0.4 mg intranasally twice daily, can be used for up to 6 months to create a temporary cessation of menstruation by ovarian suppression
- IV conjugated estrogens, 25 mg every 4 h for three or four doses, can be used, followed by oral conjugated estrogens, 2.5 mg daily, or ethinyl estradiol, 20 μg daily, for 3 weeks, with the addition of medroxyprogesterone acetate, 10 mg daily for the last 10 days of treatment, or a combination oral contraceptive daily for 3 weeks. This will thicken the endometrium and control the bleeding

Menorrhagia

- Nonsteroidal antiinflammatory drugs in the usual antiinflammatory doses will often reduce blood loss in menorrhagia—even that associated with an IUD
- Prolonged use of a progestin, as in a minipill, in injectable contraceptives, or in the therapy of endometriosis, can also lead to intermittent bleeding, sometimes severe. In this instance, the endometrium is atrophic and fragile. If bleeding occurs, it should be treated with estrogen as follows: ethinyl estradiol, 20 μg/day for 7 days, or conjugated estrogens, 1.25 mg/day for 7 days

THERAPEUTIC PROCEDURES

- Discuss stressful situations that may contribute to anovulation, such as prolonged emotional turmoil or excessive use of drugs or alcohol
- If the abnormal bleeding is not controlled by hormonal treatment, a D&C is necessary to check for incomplete abortion, polyps, submucous myomas, or endometrial cancer
- D&C is usually not necessary in women under age 40
- Endometrial ablation through the hysteroscope with laser photocoagulation or electrocautery is an option; this technique is designed to reduce or prevent any future menstrual flow

OUTCOME

FOLLOW-UP

- Monitor for the development of iron-deficiency anemia

WHEN TO REFER

- Refer if bleeding does not stop with first-line therapy or if expertise is needed with a procedure

EVIDENCE

PRACTICE GUIDELINES

- National Guideline Clearinghouse
  http://www.guideline.gov/summary/summary.aspx?doc_id=2279&nbr=1505&string=uterine+bleeding
  http://www.guideline.gov/summary/summary.aspx?doc_id=2556&nbr=1782&string=uterine+bleeding

WEB SITE

- Gynecology Handbook for Family Practitioners
  http://www.vh.org/Providers/ClinRef/FPHandbook/13.html

PATIENT INFORMATION

- American College of Obstetricians and Gynecologists
  http://www.medem.com/MedLB/article_detaillb.cfm?article_ID=ZZZOQCEN97C&sub_cat=9
- Mayo Clinic
  http://www.mayoclinic.com/invoke.cfm?id=HO00159

REFERENCES

- Farquhar CM et al: An evaluation of the risk factors for endometrial hyperplasia in premenopausal women with abnormal menstrual bleeding. Am J Obstet Gynecol 1999;181:525. [PMID: 10486458]
- Pasqualotto EB et al: Accuracy of preoperative diagnostic tools and outcome of hysteroscopic management of menstrual dysfunction. J Am Assoc Gynecol Laparosc 2000;7:201. [PMID: 10806263]

H. Trent MacKay, MD, MPH

Vaginal Bleeding, Postmenopausal

 KEY FEATURES

ESSENTIALS OF DIAGNOSIS

- Vaginal bleeding that occurs 6 months or more following cessation of menstrual function
- Bleeding is usually painless
- Bleeding may be a single episode of spotting or profuse bleeding for days or months

GENERAL CONSIDERATIONS

- The most common causes are atrophic endometrium, endometrial proliferation or hyperplasia, endometrial or cervical cancer, and administration of estrogens without added progestin

DEMOGRAPHICS

- Postmenopausal
- Obesity
- Nulliparity
- Diabetes
- History of anovulation
- Tamoxifen therapy

 CLINICAL FINDINGS

SYMPTOMS AND SIGNS

- Uterine bleeding is usually painless, but pain will be present if the cervix is stenotic, if bleeding is severe and rapid, or if infection or torsion or extrusion of a tumor is present
- The vulva and vagina should be inspected for areas of bleeding, ulcers, or neoplasms

DIFFERENTIAL DIAGNOSIS

- Atrophic endometrium
- Endometrial hyperplasia or proliferation
- Endometrial cancer
- Atrophic vaginitis
- Perimenopausal bleeding
- Endometrial polyp
- Unopposed exogenous estrogen
- Cervical cancer
- Uterine leiomyomas (fibroids)
- Trauma
- Bleeding disorder
- Cervical polyp
- Cervical ulcer
- Vaginal cancer
- Vulvar cancer

 DIAGNOSIS

LABORATORY TESTS

- A cytological smear of the cervix and vaginal pool should be taken

IMAGING STUDIES

- Transvaginal sonography should be used to measure endometrial thickness. A measurement of 4 mm or less indicates a very low likelihood of hyperplasia or endometrial cancer

DIAGNOSTIC PROCEDURES

- If the endometrial thickness by transvaginal sonography is greater than 4 mm, endocervical curettage and endometrial aspiration should be performed, preferably in conjunction with hysteroscopy

TREATMENT

MEDICATIONS

- Treat simple endometrial hyperplasia with cyclic progestin therapy (medroxy-progesterone acetate, 10 mg/day, or norethindrone acetate, 5 mg/day) for 21 days of each month for 3 months
- A repeat D&C or endometrial biopsy should be performed, and if tissues are normal and estrogen replacement therapy is reinstituted, a progestin should be prescribed in a cyclic or continuous regimen

SURGERY

- Aspiration curettage (with polypectomy if indicated) will frequently be curative
- If endometrial hyperplasia with atypical cells or carcinoma of the endometrium is found, hysterectomy is necessary

 ## OUTCOME

FOLLOW-UP

- Annual visit for pelvic examination and transvaginal sonography

COMPLICATIONS

- Endometrial cancer
- Complex hyperplasia with atypia has a high risk of becoming adenocarcinoma of the endometrium and requires hysterectomy

WHEN TO REFER

- Refer for hysteroscopy by gynecologist

PREVENTION

- Avoidance of unopposed estrogen therapy
- Weight reduction
- Simple endometrial hyperplasia responds well to medical therapy

 ## EVIDENCE

PRACTICE GUIDELINES

- National Guideline Clearinghouse
http://www.guideline.gov/summary/summary.aspx?doc_id=2564&nbr=1790&string=abnormal+uterine+bleeding
http://www.guideline.gov/summary/summary.aspx?doc_id=2749&nbr=1975&string=menopause+and+bleeding

WEB SITE

- Gynecology Handbook for Family Practitioners
http://www.vh.org/Providers/ClinRef/FPHandbook/13.html

INFORMATION FOR PATIENTS

- American College of Obstetricians and Gynecologists
http://www.medem.com/MedLB/article_detaillb.cfm?article_ID=ZZZOQCEN97C&sub_cat=9
http://www.medem.com/MedLB/article_detaillb.cfm?article_ID=ZZZ7Z2GWQMC&sub_cat=9

REFERENCE

- Gull B et al: Transvaginal ultrasonography in women with postmenopausal bleeding: is it always necessary to perform an endometrial biopsy? Am J Obstet Gynecol 2000;185:509. [PMID: 10739500]

H. Trent MacKay, MD, MPH

Vaginitis

 ## KEY FEATURES

ESSENTIALS OF DIAGNOSIS

- Vaginal irritation, pruritus, pain, or unusual discharge

GENERAL CONSIDERATIONS

- Inflammation and infection of the vagina are common
- Results from a variety of pathogens, allergic reactions to vaginal contraceptives or other products, or the friction of coitus
- The normal vaginal pH is 4.5 or less, and *Lactobacillus* is the predominant organism
- At the time of the midcycle estrogen surge, clear, elastic, mucoid secretions from the cervical os are often profuse
- In the luteal phase and during pregnancy, vaginal secretions are thicker, white, and sometimes adherent to the vaginal walls
- These normal secretions can be confused with vaginitis by concerned women

Candida albicans

- Pregnancy, diabetes, and use of broad-spectrum antibiotics or corticosteroids predispose to *Candida* infections
- Heat, moisture, and occlusive clothing also contribute to the risk

Trichomonas vaginalis

- This protozoal flagellate infects the vagina, Skene's ducts, and lower urinary tract in women and the lower genitourinary tract in men
- It is transmitted through coitus

Bacterial vaginosis

- This condition is considered to be a polymicrobial (overgrowth of *Gardnerella* and other anaerobes) and is not sexually transmitted

Condylomata acuminata (genital warts)

- Caused by various types of the human papillomavirus
- Sexually transmitted
- Pregnancy and immunosuppression favor growth

 ## CLINICAL FINDINGS

SYMPTOMS AND SIGNS

- Take a careful history
  - Onset of the last menstrual period
  - Recent sexual activity
  - Use of contraceptives, tampons, or douches
  - Vaginal burning, pain, pruritus
  - Profuse or malodorous discharge
- The physical examination: careful inspection of the vulva and speculum examination of the vagina and cervix

Candida albicans

- Pruritus
- Vulvovaginal erythema
- White curd-like discharge that is not malodorous

Trichomonas vaginalis

- Pruritus and a malodorous frothy, yellow-green discharge
- Diffuse vaginal erythema and red macular lesions on the cervix in severe cases

Bacterial vaginosis

- Increased malodorous discharge without obvious vulvitis or vaginitis
- Discharge is grayish, frothy

Condylomata acuminata

- Warty growths on the vulva, perianal area, vaginal walls, or cervix
- Vulvar lesions: obviously wart-like
- Fissures may be at the fourchette
- Vaginal lesions may show diffuse hypertrophy or a cobblestone appearance
- These lesions may be related to dysplasia and cervical cancer

DIFFERENTIAL DIAGNOSIS

- Normal vaginal discharge
- Bacterial vaginosis
- *Trichomonas* vaginitis
- *Candida* vulvovaginitis
- Atrophic vaginitis
- Genital warts (condyloma acuminata)
- Friction from intercourse
- Reaction to douches, tampons, condoms, soap

 ## DIAGNOSIS

LABORATORY TESTS

- The cervix is cultured for *Gonococcus* or *Chlamydia* if applicable
- The vaginal pH is frequently greater than 4.5 in infections due to trichomonads (pH of 5.0–5.5) and bacterial vaginosis
- Examine a specimen of vaginal discharge microscopically
  - In a drop of 0.9% saline solution (wet mount) to search for motile organisms with flagella (trichomonads) and epithelial cells covered with bacteria to such an extent that cell borders are obscured (clue cells)
  - In a drop of 10% potassium hydroxide to search for the filaments and spores of *Candida* and an amine-like "fishy" odor of *Trichomonas*
- Cultures with Nickerson's medium may be used if *Candida* is suspected but not demonstrated
- Vaginal cultures are generally not useful in diagnosis

DIAGNOSTIC PROCEDURES

- Vulvar or cervical lesions of condylomata acuminata may be visible by colposcopy only after pretreatment with 4% acetic acid, when they appear whitish, with prominent papillae

TREATMENT

MEDICATIONS

Candida albicans

- The short-term cure rates are similar with all listed regimens
- Three-day regimens
  - Butoconazole (2% cream, 5 g)
  - Clotrimazole (two 100-mg vaginal tablets)
  - Terconazole (0.8% cream, 5 g, or 80 mg suppository)
  - Miconazole (200-mg vaginal suppository) once daily
- Seven-day regimens
  - Clotrimazole (1% cream or 100-mg vaginal tablet)
  - Miconazole (2% cream, 5 g, or 100-mg vaginal suppository)
  - Terconazole (0.4% cream, 5 g) once daily
- Single-dose regimens
  - Clotrimazole (500-mg tablet)
  - Tioconazole ointment (6.5%, 5 g)
  - Fluconazole, 150 mg orally
- Fourteen-day regimens: nystatin (100,000 unit vaginal tablet once daily)
- Recurrent candidal vulvovaginitis: ketoconazole, 100 mg orally once daily for up to 6 months

Trichomonas vaginalis

- Recommend treatment of both partners
  - Metronidazole, 2 g, single dose
  - For treatment failure in the absence of reexposure, retreat with metronidazole, 500 mg twice a day for 7 days
  - If this is not effective, metronidazole susceptibility testing can be arranged with the CDC

Bacterial vaginosis

- Metronidazole, 500 mg orally twice daily for 7 days
- Clindamycin vaginal cream (2%, 5 g), once daily for 7 days
- Metronidazole gel (0.75%, 5 g), twice daily for 5 days
- Metronidazole, 2 g orally as a single dose
- Clindamycin, 300 mg orally twice daily for 7 days

Condylomata acuminata

- For vulvar warts
  - Podophyllum resin 25% in tincture of benzoin (do not use during pregnancy or on bleeding lesions). Wash off after 2–4 h
  - 80–90% trichloroacetic or bichloroacetic acid. Apply carefully to avoid the surrounding skin
- Freezing with liquid nitrogen
- Patient-applied regimens include podofilox 0.5% solution or gel and imiquimod 5% cream
- Vaginal warts may be treated with cryotherapy with liquid nitrogen, trichloroacetic acid, or podophyllum resin
- Interferon is not recommended for routine use

THERAPEUTIC PROCEDURES

- Routine examination of sex partners is not necessary for the management of genital warts. However, partners may wish to be examined for detection and treatment of genital warts and other STDs

Condylomata acuminata

- Vulvar warts: freezing with cryoprobe and electrocautery
- Vaginal warts: extensive warts may require treatment with CO_2 laser under anesthesia

OUTCOME

FOLLOW-UP

- Examination for pelvic infection

EVIDENCE

PRACTICE GUIDELINES

- National Guideline Clearinghouse http://www.guideline.gov/summary/summary.aspx?doc_id=3034&nbr=2260&string=vaginitis http://www.guideline.gov/summary/summary.aspx?doc_id=3032&nbr=2258&string=vaginitis http://www.guideline.gov/summary/summary.aspx?doc_id=2670&nbr=1896&string=vaginitis

WEB SITE

- Gynecology Handbook for Family Practitioners http://www.vh.org/Providers/ClinRef/FPHandbook/13.html

INFORMATION FOR PATIENTS

- American Social Health Association http://www.ashastd.org/stdfaqs/vaginitis.html
- National Institute of Allergy and Infectious Diseases http://www.niaid.nih.gov/factsheets/stdvag.htm
- JAMA patient page: Papillomavirus. JAMA 2002;287:2452. [PMID: 12004891]
- AMA patient page: Sexually transmitted diseases. JAMA 1998; 280:944. [UI: 98410698]

REFERENCE

- Egan ME: Diagnosis of vaginitis. Am Fam Physician 2000;62:1095. [PMID: 10997533]

H. Trent MacKay, MD, MPH

Varicella & Herpes Zoster

KEY FEATURES

ESSENTIALS OF DIAGNOSIS

- Fever and malaise before visible skin lesions (varicella)
- Pain before onset of skin lesions in a dermatome (herpes zoster)
- Typical incubation period of 2–3 weeks between exposure and clinical onset

GENERAL CONSIDERATIONS

- Chickenpox is spread by inhalation of infective droplets or by contact with skin lesions

DEMOGRAPHICS

- Disease manifestation include either chickenpox (varicella), which occurs typically in children, and shingles (zoster), which occurs more commonly in elderly or immunocompromised individuals

CLINICAL FINDINGS

SYMPTOMS AND SIGNS

Varicella (chickenpox)

- Fever and malaise mild in children, marked in adults
- Vesicular eruptions often first involve oropharynx
- Rash involves face, scalp, and trunk and then moves out to the extremities
- Lesions erupt over 1–5 days so all stages of eruption present simultaneously
- Vesicles and pustules are superficial, elliptical, with slightly serrated borders
- Multinucleated giant cells on Tzanck smear of materials from vesicle bases

ZOSTER (SHINGLES)

- Pain is often severe and precedes the lesions
- Lesions follow any nerve route distribution (thoracic and lumbar most common)
- Vesicular skin lesions resemble varicella
- Lesions on tip of nose indicate potential ophthalmic involvement
- Facial palsy, vertigo, tinnitus, deafness, or external ear lesions suggest geniculate ganglion involvement

DIFFERENTIAL DIAGNOSIS

Varicella (chickenpox)

- Herpes simplex (cold or fever sore; genital herpes)
- Herpes zoster (shingles)
- Contact dermatitis
- Scabies
- Atopic dermatitis (eczema) (acute)
- Miliaria (heat rash)
- Photodermatitis
- Smallpox
- Rickettsialpox
- Hand, foot, and mouth disease

HERPES ZOSTER (SHINGLES)

- Contact dermatitis (eg, poison oak or ivy)
- Herpes simplex
- Varicella (chickenpox)
- Erysipelas
- Prodromal pain mimics angina, peptic ulcer, appendicitis, biliary or renal colic

DIAGNOSIS

LABORATORY TESTS

- Leukopenia often present in varicella
- Zoster symptoms and signs often highly characteristic, not requiring further diagnostic testing
- When diagnosis remains in doubt, direct fluorescent antibody (DFA) testing, viral culture, and polymerase chain reaction (PCR) testing can be helpful

DIAGNOSTIC FINDINGS

- Most patients with a history of exposure and clinical symptoms and signs of varicella do not need further diagnostic testing

TREATMENT

 OUTCOME

 EVIDENCE

MEDICATIONS

- Acyclovir or related drugs can reduce the duration and severity of chickenpox or zoster infection, especially when started early, but is seldom needed in immunocompetent patients
- Acyclovir may reduce the likelihood and/or severity of postherpetic neuralgia
- Acyclovir usually indicated in immunocompromised patients with systemic varicella infection
- Foscarnet may be useful in acyclovir-resistant varicella, especially in those on chronic acyclovir therapy
- Prevention: varicella immunoglobulin is effective in preventing chickenpox in exposed individuals
- Vaccination, with live, attenuated virus, is 85% effective at preventing disease and 95% effective at preventing serious complications
- Adults should receive a second vaccine dose 1–2 months after the first dose
- Postherpetic neuralgia: initial treatment with acyclovir and corticosteroids may reduce the incidence and severity
- Once established, pain may be treated with tricyclic antidepressants, lidocaine patches, and antiepileptics such as carbamazepine and gabapentin

THERAPEUTIC PROCEDURES

- Isolate patients with active vesicles or pneumonia from seronegative patients

COMPLICATIONS

Varicella (chickenpox)

- Interstitial pneumonia more common in adults than children
- Ischemic strokes, though uncommon, may be due to an associated vasculitis
- Hepatitis occurs in 0.1%
- Encephalitis, characterized by ataxia, nystagmus, and even death, is rare (0.025%)
- Reye's syndrome may occur in conjunction with aspirin use usually in children
- Congenital malformations occur with first-trimester infections

SHINGLES (ZOSTER)

- Skin lesions beyond the dermatome, visceral lesions, and encephalitis occur in immunocompromised individuals
- Postherpetic neuralgia occurs in 60–70% of elderly patients; corticosteroids are controversial but may be of some benefit when tapered over 21 days for prevention of postherpetic neuralgia

PROGNOSIS

- Total duration of varicella from onset of symptoms to disappearance of crusts usually ≤2 weeks
- Zoster symptoms and lesions usually resolve within 6 weeks

WHEN TO REFER

- Refer patients with synchronous progression of the lesions, which raises the concern for smallpox, to local health department and infectious disease experts for confirmation

WHEN TO ADMIT

- Consider hospitalization for signs of visceral involvement, especially pulmonary involvement. Varicella pneumonia can be lethal, especially in adults

PRACTICE GUIDELINES

- General recommendations on immunization: recommendations of the Advisory Committee on Immunization Practices (ACIP) and the American Academy of Family Physicians (AAFP). American Academy of Family Physicians; Centers for Disease Control and Prevention, 2002 http://www.guideline.gov/summary/summary.aspx?doc_id=3180&nbr=2406&string=varicella+and+treatment

WEB SITE

- National Institute of Allergy and Infectious Diseases, National Institutes of Health http://www.niaid.nih.gov/

INFORMATION FOR PATIENTS

- Web MD varicella http://my.webmd.com/content/healthwise/129/32072
- NIAID Facts About Shingles (Varicella-Zoster Virus) http://www.niaid.nih.gov/factsheets/shinglesfs.htm

REFERENCES

- Ampofo K et al: Persistence of immunity to live attenuated varicella vaccine in healthy adults. Clin Infect Dis 2002; 34:774. [PMID: 11830801]
- Gnann JW Jr et al: Herpes zoster. N Engl J Med 2002;347:340. [PMID: 12151472]
- Hall S et al: Second varicella infections: are they more common than previously thought? Pediatrics 2002;109:1068. [PMID: 12042544]

Wayne X. Shandera, MD
Samuel Shelburne, MD

Varicose Veins

 KEY FEATURES

ESSENTIALS OF DIAGNOSIS

- Dilated, tortuous superficial veins in the lower extremities
- May be asymptomatic or associated with fatigue, aching discomfort, thrombosis, bleeding, or localized pain
- Edema, pigmentation, and ulceration suggest concomitant venous stasis disease

GENERAL CONSIDERATIONS

- Abnormally dilated veins in the legs produced by venous reflux and valvular incompetence
- Long saphenous vein and its tributaries most commonly involved; short saphenous vein may also be affected
- Primary varicosities: inherited vein wall or valve defect
- Secondary varicosities: valve damage following thrombophlebitis, trauma, deep venous thrombosis, arteriovenous fistula, pregnancy, or pelvic tumor
- With long-standing disease, the skin may develop secondary changes such as fibrosis, chronic edema, and skin pigmentation and atrophy
- Risk factors: female gender, pregnancy, family history, prolonged standing, and history of phlebitis

DEMOGRAPHICS

- Occur in 15% of adults
- Increased frequency after pregnancy

 CLINICAL FINDINGS

SYMPTOMS AND SIGNS

- Dull, aching heaviness, fatigue, worsened by standing
- Itching from eczematoid dermatitis
- Dilated, tortuous, elongated veins, visible when the patient is standing
- Smaller, flat, blue-green reticular veins, telangiectasias, and spider veins
- Signs of chronic venous insufficiency: brownish pigmentation and thinning of the skin above the ankle, edema, fibrosis, scaling dermatitis, and ulceration

DIFFERENTIAL DIAGNOSIS

- Klippel-Trenaunay syndrome: varicose veins, limb hypertrophy, and a cutaneous birthmark (portwine stain or venous malformation)

 DIAGNOSIS

IMAGING STUDIES

- Duplex ultrasonography detects location of incompetent valves; helpful preoperatively

DIAGNOSTIC PROCEDURES

- Brodie-Trendelenburg test positive

TREATMENT

SURGERY

- Indications: disabling pain, recurrent superficial thrombophlebitis, erosion of the overlying skin with bleeding, and manifestations of chronic venous insufficiency (particularly ulceration)
- Varicose vein excision (stab avulsion) combined with high ligation of the saphenofemoral junction or ligation of perforator branches
- Stripping of the entire saphenous system rarely required

THERAPEUTIC PROCEDURES

- Periodic leg elevation
- Regular exercise
- Knee-high or thigh-high elastic graduated (20–30 mm Hg) compression stockings
- Compression bandages (Ace wrap or Unna boot) when complicated by ulceration
- Compression sclerotherapy: injection of 23.4% hypertonic saline or 2.5% sodium morrhuate and compression stockings

 OUTCOME

COMPLICATIONS

- Ulceration, bleeding, chronic stasis dermatitis, superficial venous thrombosis, and thrombophlebitis

PROGNOSIS

- Recurrence rate is ~10%
- Even after adequate treatment, secondary tissue changes may not regress

PREVENTION

- Continued use of compression stockings, leg elevation, and exercise

EVIDENCE

PRACTICE GUIDELINES

- Guidelines of care for sclerotherapy treatment of varicose and telangiectatic leg veins. American Academy of Dermatology. J Am Acad Dermatol 1996;34:523. [PMID: 8609276]
- Baccaglini U et al: Sclerotherapy of varicose veins of the lower limbs. Consensus paper. North American Society of Phlebology. Dermatol Surg 1996; 22:883. [PMID: 9246172]

WEB SITES

- NIH—Patient Education Institute: Varicose Veins—Sclerotherapy http://www.nlm.nih.gov/medlineplus/ tutorials/ varicoseveins.html
- Society of Interventional Radiology— Vascular diseases diagnosis http://www.sirweb.org/patPub/ vascularDiagnosis.shtml

INFORMATION FOR PATIENTS

- Cleveland Clinic—Varicose vein ligation/stripping http://www.clevelandclinic.org/health/ health-info/docs/2500/2588.asp? index=9561
- MEDLINEplus—Varicose veins http://www.nlm.nih.gov/medlineplus/ ency/article/001109.htm

REFERENCES

- Belcaro G et al: Endovascular sclerotherapy, surgery, and surgery plus sclerotherapy in superficial venous incompetence: a randomized, 10 year follow-up trial— final results. Angiology 2000;51:529. [PMID: 10917577]
- Bradbury A et al: The relationship between lower limb symptoms and superficial and deep venous reflux on duplex ultrasonography: the Edinburgh Vein Study. J Vasc Surg 2000;32:921. [PMID: 11054224]

Louis M. Messina, MD
Laura K. Pak, MD
Lawrence M. Tierney, Jr., MD

Vascular Disease, Peripheral

 KEY FEATURES

ESSENTIALS OF DIAGNOSIS

- Peripheral vascular disease (PVD) is a common cause of disability
- A predictor of cardiovascular morbidity and mortality

GENERAL CONSIDERATIONS

- Type 1 disease affects about 10–15% of patients with PVD and is limited to the aorta and common iliac arteries
- Type 2 disease (~25% of patients) involves the aorta and common iliac and external iliac arteries
- Type 3 disease (~60–70% of patients) involves the aorta and iliac, femoral, popliteal, and tibial arteries
- High incidence of coexisting cerebrovascular and coronary artery disease
- ~30% have severe triple-vessel coronary artery disease

DEMOGRAPHICS

- Risk factors for type 1 disease: younger men and middle aged women who are heavy smokers or who have hyperlipidemia
- Risk factors for type 2 and type 3 disease: older age, male gender, diabetes, hypertension, hypercholesterolemia

 CLINICAL FINDINGS

SYMPTOMS AND SIGNS

- Claudication, rest pain, and gangrene
- Male erectile dysfunction with occlusive disease of the iliac arteries
- Leriche's syndrome: a triad of bilateral hip and buttock claudication, erectile dysfunction, and absent femoral pulses
- Claudication is pain, numbness, or weakness in the calves, thighs, or buttocks produced by walking and completely relieved after rest
- Ischemic rest pain is typically described as pain across the dorsum of the foot with elevation and relieved with dependency; it implies severe arterial insufficiency and impending limb loss
- Absent or weak femoral pulse or the presence of an iliac or femoral bruit suggests inflow disease
- Normal femoral pulse but diminished or absent popliteal pulse is indicative of superficial femoral artery stenosis or occlusion
- Normal femoral and popliteal pulses but nonpalpable dorsalis pedis or posterior tibial pulse indicate tibial disease
- The ratio of ankle to brachial systolic blood pressures (ankle-brachial index, or ABI) is useful in gauging the degree of arterial insufficiency
- A normal ABI is 1.0
- Claudication occurs at ABI <0.8
- Rest pain and nonhealing ulcers occur at ABI <0.4
- A toe-brachial index (TBI) can be used in diabetic or renal failure patients when tibial arteries are calcified and noncompressible
- A penile-brachial index (PBI) can be used when vasogenic impotence is suspected; significant arterial disease is suggested by a PBI <0.6
- Index measurements can be used to monitor progression of disease and to assess the effect of therapeutic intervention
- Atrophy of the skin, subcutaneous tissues, and muscles, elevation pallor, dependent rubor, hair loss, and coolness of the skin indicate advanced ischemia
- Ulcers over pressure points

DIFFERENTIAL DIAGNOSIS

- Musculoskeletal disorder
- Lumbar spinal stenosis or nerve root compression (neurogenic or pseudoclaudication)
- Venous disease
- Peripheral neuropathy
- Nocturnal leg cramps
- Arterial embolism
- Thromboangiitis obliterans (Buerger's disease)
- Polyarteritis nodosa
- For popliteal artery occlusion with unilateral claudication in a young, healthy person consider popliteal artery entrapment, trauma, compression by Baker's cyst, popliteal adventitial cystic disease
- Reflex sympathetic dystrophy
- Raynaud's disease

 DIAGNOSIS

IMAGING STUDIES

- Radiographs of the lower leg and foot to rule out osteomyelitis underlying an infected ulcer or to identify calcification of potential runoff vessels
- Duplex ultrasound used for diagnosis and in routine follow-up of infrainguinal bypass grafts to screen for graft stenoses
- Gadolinium-enhanced MRA in patients with severe renal insufficiency or contrast allergy
- Angiography indicated for percutaneous endovascular treatment or in preparation for surgical intervention

TREATMENT

MEDICATIONS

- Pentoxifylline, 400 mg PO TID, unclear efficacy
- Cilostazol, 100 mg PO BID; side effects of headache, dizziness in ~20%, and contraindicated in patients with heart failure
- Propionyl-L-carnitine, 1000 mg PO BID
- Ginkgo biloba extract, 120 mg PO QD, but may increase risk of bleeding
- Aspirin, 325 mg PO QD

- Clopidogrel, 75 mg PO QD, or warfarin dosed to maintain an INR of 2.0–3.0 reserved for patients with unreconstructible disease or for postoperative patients perceived to have a higher risk of graft thrombosis due to a hypercoagulable state, suboptimal conduit, or poor distal runoff
- Sildenafil, 25–50 mg 30 min to 4 h prior to sexual activity for male erectile dysfunction

SURGERY

- Local wound care and debridement for ulcers
- Percutaneous or open surgery considered for good-risk patients with short-distance (<2 blocks) claudication that impairs their ability to work or perform activities of daily living, or development of rest pain or gangrene
- Medical management is optimized preoperatively
- Consider stress testing or coronary angiography preoperatively

Open surgery

- Aortobifemoral bypass grafting done with a bifurcated polytetrafluoroethylene or Dacron graft anastomosed end-to-end with the infrarenal abdominal aorta and end-to-side to each common femoral artery has an 80% 10-year patency rate
- Axillary-femoral or femoral-femoral bypass graft done for high-risk patients has a lower 10-year patency rate of 50%
- Autogenous greater saphenous vein can be used as the bypass conduit for infrainguinal occlusive disease with a 5-year patency rate of 75–80%
- Thomboendarterectomy is an alternative to bypass for short-segment lesions in larger arteries in type 1 disease
- Long-segment closed superficial femoral artery endarterectomy combined with distal stenting is an alternative to femoral popliteal bypass in high-risk surgical patients with suboptimal veins
- Lumbar sympathectomy is reserved for symptomatic patients with unreconstructable disease
- Iliac artery revascularization is done for male erectile dysfunction

THERAPEUTIC PROCEDURES

- Blood pressure control, tobacco cessation, and lipid-lowering medications
- Initiation of a daily exercise program

Endovascular techniques

- Stent angioplasty of common iliac artery stenoses with self-expanding (Wall) stents or balloon-expandable (Palmaz) stents has a 3-year patency rate of 70–80%
- Angiography and/or stenting of distal lesions (external iliac or infrainguinal arteries) is not as successful: 3-year primary patency rate of 55–60%; the lesions most amenable to this treatment are discrete, short-segment (<5 cm long), concentric lesions in noncalcified large-diameter vessels

OUTCOME

FOLLOW-UP

- Serial pulse examination and ABIs
- Duplex ultrasound surveillance is advised at 6-month intervals to detect stenotic, or "threatened," grafts before they progress to occlusion

COMPLICATIONS

- Operative complications for open aortic surgery: myocardial infarction or arrhythmia, renal insufficiency, bowel ischemia, impotence or retrograde ejaculation, and blue toe syndrome
- Late complications: graft thrombosis, graft infection, and aortoduodenal fistula
- Angiogram complications: hematoma, pseudoaneurysm, arteriovenous fistula, retroperitoneal hemorrhage, arterial occlusion, dissection or rupture, distal emboli, contrast nephropathy
- Operative mortality is 2–5% for open aortic surgery and 1–3% for infrainguinal bypass

PROGNOSIS

- Of patients with claudication 25% will eventually develop ischemic rest pain or ulceration, 10% will require amputation; 5-year survival of 50%
- 5-year patency rate for infrainguinal saphenous vein grafts is 60–80%

WHEN TO REFER

- Life-style limiting short distance claudication
- Rest pain
- Ischemic ulceration

WHEN TO ADMIT

- Limb-threatening ischemia

EVIDENCE

PRACTICE GUIDELINES

- Cardella JF et al: Optimal resources for the examination and endovascular treatment of the peripheral and visceral vascular systems. AHA Intercouncil report on peripheral and visceral angiographic and interventional laboratories. Circulation 1994;89:1481. [PMID: 8124831]
- Drug therapy for peripheral vascular disease. A national clinical guideline. Scottish Intercollegiate Guidelines Network, 1998 http://www.sign.ac.uk/pdf/sign27.pdf

WEB SITES

- American Heart Association—Peripheral vascular disease http://www.americanheart.org/presenter.jhtml?identifier= 4692
- MEDLINEplus—Arteriosclerosis of the extremities http://www.nlm.nih.gov/medlineplus/ency/article/000170.htm

INFORMATION FOR PATIENTS

- JAMA patient page: Peripheral arterial disease http://www.ama-assn.org/public/journals/patient/archive/pat0919.htm

REFERENCES

- Hiatt WR: Medical treatment of peripheral arterial disease and claudication. N Engl J Med 2001;344:1608. [PMID: 11372014]
- Muradin GSR et al: Balloon dilation and stent implantation for treatment of femoropopliteal arterial disease: meta-analysis. Radiology 2001;221:137. [PMID: 11568332]

Louis M. Messina, MD
Laura K. Pak, MD
Lawrence M. Tierney, Jr., MD

Venous Insufficiency, Chronic

 ## KEY FEATURES

ESSENTIALS OF DIAGNOSIS

- History of varicose veins, phlebitis, or leg injury
- Early sign: ankle edema
- Late signs: varicosities, pigmentation, stasis dermatitis, and induration from fibrosis of the subcutaneous tissue and skin, and ulceration

GENERAL CONSIDERATIONS

- Causes: deep venous thrombosis (most common), leg trauma, varicose veins, obstruction of the pelvic veins, or congenital or acquired arteriovenous fistula or venous anomaly

 ## CLINICAL FINDINGS

SYMPTOMS AND SIGNS

- Progressive edema of the leg with dull aching discomfort
- Varicosities often present
- Stasis dermatitis, brownish pigmentation, brawny induration, and ulceration
- Thin, shiny, atrophic, and cyanotic skin
- Cellulitis
- Weeping dermatitis
- Venous stasis ulcers

DIFFERENTIAL DIAGNOSIS

- Congestive heart failure
- Chronic renal disease, nephrotic syndrome
- Cirrhosis
- Hypoalbuminemia
- Lymphedema
- Other causes of chronic leg ulcers, eg, autoimmune diseases (Felty's syndrome), arterial insufficiency, sickle cell anemia, erythema induratum, and fungal infections

 ## DIAGNOSIS

LABORATORY TESTS

- Electrolytes, albumin, complete blood cell count

IMAGING STUDIES

- Venous ultrasound to rule out deep venous thrombosis

Venous Insufficiency, Chronic

 TREATMENT

MEDICATIONS

- Unna boot, semipermeable hydrophilic foam dressing, or calcium alginate dressing for weepy ulcers
- Systemic antibiotics and topical antifungal agents (eg, clotrimazole 1% cream or miconazole 2% cream) for active infection
- Zinc oxide ointment with ichthammol, 3%, QD or BID for chronic dermatitis

SURGERY

- Wide debridement and skin grafting in combination with open or endoscopic ligation of incompetent saphenous and perforating veins
- Venous reconstructive surgery is rarely indicated

THERAPEUTIC PROCEDURES

Acute care

- Bed rest with leg elevation, and wet saline compresses for acute weeping dermatitis
- Deep venous thrombosis prophylaxis and external compression

Chronic care

- Intermittent periodic elevation of the legs during the day and elevation of the legs at night (kept above the level of the heart with pillows under the mattress); avoidance of long periods of sitting or standing; knee- or thigh-high graduated compression stockings (20–30 mm Hg); regular exercise
- Wet-to-dry normal saline, hydrogel, silvadine, or Promogran dressings plus Ace wrap compression, or an Unna boot or wound vac for venous ulcerations

 OUTCOME

COMPLICATIONS

- Cellulitis
- Limb loss

PROGNOSIS

- Recurrent venous stasis ulcers and progressive stasis changes of the skin are not uncommon

WHEN TO REFER

- Nonhealing wound
- Progression of venous stasis disease

WHEN TO ADMIT

- Sepsis
- Refractory cellulitis
- Threatened limb loss

PREVENTION

- Early and aggressive management of acute deep venous thrombosis
- Surgical treatment (eg, sclerosis or stripping) of varicose veins

 EVIDENCE

PRACTICE GUIDELINES

- Classification and grading of chronic venous disease in the lower limbs. A consensus statement. Ad Hoc Committee, American Venous Forum. J Cardiovasc Surg (Torino) 1997;38:437. [PMID: 9358799]
- The care of patients with chronic leg ulcer. A national clinical guideline. Scottish Intercollegiate Guidelines Network, 1998 http://www.guideline.gov/summary/summary.aspx?doc_id=2901&nbr=2127&string=Chronic+Venous+Insufficiency
- Vanscheidt W et al: Guidelines for testing drugs for chronic venous insufficiency. Vasa 2000;29:274. [PMID: 11141651]

WEB SITES

- Clinical Digital Libraries project—Chronic venous insufficiency clinical resources http://capstoneclinic-dl.slis.ua.edu/clinical/cardiology/cardiovascular/pvd/venous/chronic-venous-insufficiency.html
- MEDLINEplus—Venous Insufficiency http://www.nlm.nih.gov/medlineplus/ency/article/000203.htm
- National Lymphedema Network—When it's not lymphedema http://www.lymphnet.org/lymphlink1099.html

INFORMATION FOR PATIENTS

- Penn State—Chronic venous insufficiency http://www.hmc.psu.edu/healthinfo/c/chronicvenous.htm

REFERENCE

- Mohr DN et al: The venous stasis syndrome after deep venous thrombosis or pulmonary embolism: a population-based study. Mayo Clin Proc 2000; 75:1249. [PMID: 11126832]

Louis M. Messina, MD
Laura K. Pak, MD
Lawrence M. Tierney, Jr., MD

Venous Stasis Ulcers

 KEY FEATURES

ESSENTIALS OF DIAGNOSIS

- Past history of varicosities, thrombophlebitis, or postphlebitic syndrome
- Irregular ulceration, often on the medial aspect of the lower legs above the malleolus
- Edema of the legs, varicosities, hyperpigmentation, and red and scaly areas (stasis dermatitis) and scars from old ulcers support the diagnosis

GENERAL CONSIDERATIONS

- Patients at risk may have a history of venous insufficiency, either with obvious varicosities or with a past history of thrombophlebitis, or with immobility of the calf muscle group (paraplegics, etc)
- Red, pruritic patches of stasis dermatitis often precede ulceration
- Because venous insufficiency is the most common cause of lower leg ulceration, testing of venous competence is a required part of the evaluation even when no changes of venous insufficiency are present

 CLINICAL FINDINGS

SYMPTOMS AND SIGNS

- Classically, chronic edema is followed by a dermatitis, which is often pruritic; these changes are followed by hyperpigmentation, skin breakdown, and eventually sclerosis of the skin of the lower leg
- The ulcer base may be clean, but it may have a yellow fibrin eschar that often requires surgical treatment
- Ulceration is often on the *medial* aspect of the lower legs above the malleolus
- Edema of the legs, varicosities, hyperpigmentation, and red and scaly areas (stasis dermatitis) and scars from old ulcers support the diagnosis
- Ulcers that appear on the feet, toes, or above the knees are atypical for venous stasis—consider other diagnoses

DIFFERENTIAL DIAGNOSIS

- Venous insufficiency
- Arterial insufficiency (arterial ulcer)
- Stasis dermatitis
- Bacterial pyoderma (eg, infected wound or bite)
- Trauma
- Diabetic ulcer
- Pressure ulcer
- Vasculitis
- Pyoderma gangrenosum
- Skin cancer
- Infection (eg, mycobacterial, fungal, tertiary syphilis, leishmaniasis, amebiasis)
- Sickle cell anemia
- Embolic disease (including cholesterol emboli)
- Cryoglobulinemia
- Calciphylaxis

 DIAGNOSIS

LABORATORY TESTS

- Thorough evaluation of the patient's vascular system (including measurement of the ankle-brachial index) is essential

IMAGING STUDIES

- Doppler ultrasound is usually sufficient (except in the diabetic) to elucidate the cause of most vascular cases of lower leg ulceration

TREATMENT

MEDICATIONS

Cleaning of the ulcer

- The patient is instructed to clean the base with saline or cleansers such as Saf-clens or Cara-klenz daily
- Once the base is clean
  - The ulcer is treated with metronidazole gel to reduce bacterial growth and odor
  - Any red dermatitic skin is treated with a medium- to high-potency steroid ointment
  - The ulcer is then covered with an occlusive hydroactive dressing (Duoderm or Cutinova) or a polyurethane foam (Allevyn) followed by an Unna zinc paste boot, changed weekly

Systemic therapy

- Pentoxifylline, 400 mg three times daily administered with compression accelerates healing
- Zinc supplementation is occasionally beneficial in patients with low serum zinc levels
- If cellulitis accompanies the ulcer, systemic antibiotics are recommended

SURGERY

- A curette or small scissors can be used to remove the yellow fibrin eschar, under local anesthesia if the areas are very tender
- Grafting for severe or nonhealing ulcers
  - Full- or split-thickness grafts often do not take, and pinch grafts (small shaves of skin laid onto the bed) may be more effective
  - Cultured epidermal cell grafts—or Apligraf, a bilayered skin construct—may accelerate wound healing, but they are very expensive

 OUTCOME

PROGNOSIS

- The ulcer should begin to heal within weeks, and healing should be complete within 2–3 months

WHEN TO REFER

- If there is a question about the diagnosis, if recommended therapy is ineffective, or if specialized treatment is necessary

PREVENTION

- Elevation of an edematous leg above the heart for more than 2 h two times a day
- Compression stockings to reduce edema
  - Compression should achieve a pressure of 30 mm Hg below the knee and 40 mm Hg at the ankle
  - The stockings should not be used in patients with arterial insufficiency with an ankle-brachial pressure index less than 0.7
  - Pneumatic sequential compression devices may be of great benefit

 EVIDENCE

PRACTICE GUIDELINES

- National Guideline Clearinghouse http://www.guideline.gov/summary/summary.aspx?doc_id=2901&nbr=2127&string=leg+ulcers

WEB SITES

- American Academy of Dermatology http://www.aad.org
- Dermatology Handbook for Family Practice from the University of Iowa http://www.vh.org/Providers/ClinRef/FPHandbook/17.html

INFORMATION FOR PATIENTS

- American Academy of Dermatology http://www.aad.org/pamphlets/
- National Institutes of Health Medical Encyclopedia http://www.nlm.nih.gov/medlineplus/ency/article/000834.htm

REFERENCES

- Jull AB et al: Oral pentoxifylline for treatment of venous leg ulcers. Cochrane Database Syst Rev 2000(2):CD001733. [PMID: 10796661]
- McMullin GM: Improving the treatment of leg ulcers. Med J Aust 2001; 175:375. [PMID: 11700817]

Timothy G. Berger, MD

Vertigo

KEY FEATURES

ESSENTIALS OF DIAGNOSIS

- Either a sensation of motion when there is no motion or an exaggerated sense of motion in response to a given bodily movement
- Cardinal symptom of vestibular disease
- Must differentiate peripheral from central etiologies of vestibular dysfunction

GENERAL CONSIDERATIONS

- Etiologies of vestibular disorders can be determined based on the duration of symptoms (seconds, hours, days, months) and whether auditory symptoms are present (Table 11, page 1210)
- Vertigo can occur as a side effect of anticonvulsants (eg, phenytoin), antibiotics (eg, aminoglycosides, doxycycline, metronidazole), hypnotics (eg, diazepam), analgesics (eg, aspirin), and tranquilizing drugs or of alcohol

Endolymphatic hydrops (Meniere's syndrome)

- Results from distension of the endolymphatic compartment of the inner ear; the primary lesion appears to be in the endolymphatic sac, which filters and excretes endolymph
- Although a precise cause of hydrops cannot usually be established, two causes are syphilis and head trauma
- Episodic vertigo resembling Ménière's syndrome but without accompanying auditory symptoms is known as recurrent vestibulopathy
  - The pathogenic mechanism of this symptom complex is usually unknown, though a few patients suffer from a variant of migraine and others develop the classic syndrome of endolymphatic hydrops

CLINICAL FINDINGS

SYMPTOMS AND SIGNS

- See Table 11 (page 1210)
- Perform a Romberg test, evaluate gait, and observe for nystagmus

Peripheral vestibulopathy

- Vertigo is usually of sudden onset, may be so severe that the patient is unable to walk or stand, and is frequently accompanied by nausea and vomiting
- Tinnitus and hearing loss may be associated and provide support for a otologic origin
- **Nystagmus** is usually horizontal with a rotary component; the fast phase usually beats away from the diseased side
- Visual fixation tends to inhibit nystagmus except in very acute peripheral lesions or with central nervous system disease
- Positioning nystagmus can be induced with the **Nylen-Bárány** and the **Fukada tests**; these maneuvers are of limited use when the patient is able to visually fixate, but this may be overcome by making observations in the dark by means of an electronystagmographic recording
- For the **Nylen-Bárány test**, the patient is put in a sitting position on the examination table with the head turned to the right and quickly lowered to the supine position with the head extending over the edge and placed 30 degrees lower than the body; watch for nystagmus for 30 s; repeat with the head turned to the left; perform the maneuver without turning the head
- The **Fukada test**, in which the patient walks in place with eyes closed, is useful for detecting subtle defects; a positive response is observed when the patient rotates, usually toward the side of the diseased labyrinth
- Typically with **"positional vertigo"** symptoms develop several seconds following a head movement (latency period) and subside within 10–60 s; constant repetition of the positional change leads to habituation
- In central lesions there is no latent period, fatigability, or habituation of the signs and symptoms
- **Ménière's syndrome** consists of episodic vertigo, usually lasting 1–8 h; low-frequency sensorineural hearing loss, often fluctuating; tinnitus, usually low-tone and "blowing" in quality; and a sensation of aural pressure

- Symptoms wax and wane as the endolymphatic pressure rises and falls
- Caloric testing reveals loss or impairment of thermally induced nystagmus on the involved side
- In **labyrinthitis**, there is an acute onset of continuous, usually severe vertigo lasting several days to a week, hearing loss, and tinnitus
  - During the recovery period (several weeks) rapid head movements may bring on transient vertigo
  - Hearing may return to normal or remain permanently impaired in the involved ear

Central vestibulopathy

- Vertigo tends to develop gradually, often becoming progressively more severe and debilitating
- Nystagmus is not always present but can occur in any direction and may be dissociated in the two eyes; it is often nonfatigable, vertical rather than horizontal in orientation, without latency, and unsuppressed by visual fixation

DIFFERENTIAL DIAGNOSIS

- Imbalance
- Light-headedness
- Syncope

DIAGNOSIS

LABORATORY TESTS

- Electronystagmography is useful in differentiating central from peripheral causes of vertigo

IMAGING STUDIES

- The evaluation of central audiovestibular dysfunction usually requires MRI of the brain

Venous Thrombosis, Intracranial p. 1186. Ventricular Septal Defect p. 1186.

Vertigo

TREATMENT

MEDICATIONS

- The most common drug classes employed, the antihistamines, anticholinergics, and sedative-hypnotics, should be used only for patients with prominent nausea and vomiting and are best tapered and halted when symptoms are resolved, usually within 1–2 weeks
- In acute severe vertigo, vestibular suppressants such as diazepam, 2.5–5 mg sublingually, orally, or intravenously, may abate an attack
- Relief from nausea and vomiting usually requires an antiemetic delivered intramuscularly or by rectal suppository
- Less severe vertigo may often be alleviated with antihistamines such as meclizine, 25 mg, or cyclizine or dimenhydrinate, 25–50 mg, PO Q 6 h
- Scopolamine, administered in low dosage transdermally (0.5 mg/day), has proved beneficial in recurrent vertigo, although side effects (dry mouth, blurred vision, urinary obstruction) often limit its utility (one-half or even one-fourth of a patch may still help without producing side effects)
- A combination of drugs may help if a single drug fails
- In Ménière's disease, treatment is intended to lower endolymphatic pressure; a low-salt diet (<2 g sodium daily), at times supplemented by hydrochlorothiazide, 50–100 mg daily, adequately controls symptoms in the majority of patients
- Prednisone has been used for clusters refractory to diuretics, low-salt diet, and vestibular suppressants

SURGERY

- Surgical remedies are reserved for those who remain substantially disabled despite a prolonged and varied trial of medical therapy and exercises
- Selective section of the vestibular portion of the eighth nerve brings relief of vertigo in over 90% of such patients
- Surgical removal of the semicircular canals (labyrinthectomy) is also highly effective but is appropriate only for patients with little or no hearing in the involved ear

THERAPEUTIC PROCEDURES

- Bed rest may reduce the severity of acute vertigo

- In chronic or recurrent vertigo, physical activity should be encouraged once nausea and vomiting have resolved
- In general, patients should be instructed to repeatedly perform maneuvers that provoke vertigo—up to the point of nausea or fatigue—in an effort to habituate them
- Patients refractory to conventional therapy may benefit from a formal rehabilitation program under the guidance of a physical therapist
- A series of head maneuvers (theoretically intended to reposition free-floating otolithic particles) may help in the management of **positioning vertigo;** these are as effective as vestibular habituation exercises and are less time consuming
- Some refractory patients will benefit from selective chemical destruction of the vestibular hair cell population by infusion of ototoxins (eg, gentamicin) transtympanically into the middle ear; results in patients with Ménière's syndrome have been impressive, with about 80–90% of patients relieved of severe vertigo

OUTCOME

WHEN TO REFER

- Audiological evaluation, caloric stimulation, electronystagmography, CT scan or MRI, and brainstem auditory evoked potential studies are indicated in patients with persistent vertigo or when central nervous system disease is suspected
- For patients with recalcitrant vertigo or clusters of attacks, specialty referral may be useful

EVIDENCE

PRACTICE GUIDELINES

- National Guideline Clearinghouse http://www.guideline.gov/summary/ summary.aspx?doc_id=2440&nbr= 1666&string=vertigo

WEB SITES

- Ear, Nose, and Throat Information Center http://www.netdoor.com/entinfo/
- Otolaryngology Resources on the Internet http://www.bcm.tmc.edu/oto/othersa. html

INFORMATION FOR PATIENTS

- American Academy of Otolaryngology http://www.entnet.org/healthinfo/ balance/dizziness.cfm
- Mayo Clinic http://www.mayoclinic.com/invoke. cfm?id=DS00435

REFERENCES

- Furman JM et al: Benign paroxysmal positional vertigo. N Engl J Med 1999;341:1590. [PMID: 10564690]
- Thai-Van H et al: Ménière's disease: pathophysiology and treatment. Drugs 2001;61:1089. [PMID: 11465871]

Robert K. Jackler, MD
Michael J. Kaplan, MD

Visceral Artery Insufficiency

 ## KEY FEATURES

ESSENTIALS OF DIAGNOSIS

- Chronic intestinal ischemia: epigastric or periumbilical pain, bloating or diarrhea, and food avoidance (diagnosis of exclusion)
- Acute intestinal ischemia: severe epigastric and periumbilical abdominal pain and a high leukocyte count

GENERAL CONSIDERATIONS

- Chronic intestinal ischemia results from atherosclerotic occlusive lesions at the origins of the superior mesenteric, celiac, and inferior mesenteric arteries
- Acute intestinal ischemia may result from embolic occlusion of a visceral branch of the abdominal aorta, generally in patients with mitral valvular disease, atrial fibrillation, or left ventricular mural thrombus; thrombosis of an atherosclerotic mesenteric vessel; or low flow or shock state due to cardiac failure or arterial spasm induced by ergot or cocaine intoxication; or postcoarctectomy syndrome
- Emboli are responsible for almost half of cases
- Celiac axis compression syndrome: stenosis of the celiac artery caused by external compression of the arcuate ligament may cause chronic mesenteric ischemia
- Mesenteric vein occlusion causes 5–15% of cases of acute mesenteric ischemia
- Risk factors for mesenteric vein occlusion: hypercoagulable state (malignancy; protein C, protein S, or antithrombin III deficiency; presence of anticardiolipin or antiphospholipid antibody; polycythemia vera), intra-abdominal sepsis, previous splenectomy or portal angiography or sclerotherapy, portal hypertension, and cirrhosis

DEMOGRAPHICS

- Almost 30% of patients with peripheral vascular disease have asymptomatic occlusive disease of the mesenteric arteries

 ## CLINICAL FINDINGS

SYMPTOMS AND SIGNS

- Chronic mesenteric ischemia: epigastric or periumbilical postprandial pain, often accompanied by bloating or diarrhea, and, at later stages, food avoidance (sitophobia), resulting in weight loss
- Acute mesenteric ischemia: sudden onset of severe epigastric and periumbilical abdominal pain, acidosis and hypotension, with minimal appreciable findings on abdominal examination except abdominal distension
- Ischemic colitis: bouts of crampy lower abdominal pain and mild—often bloody—diarrhea

DIFFERENTIAL DIAGNOSIS

- Peptic ulcer disease
- Gastroesophageal reflux
- Bowel obstruction
- Pancreatitis
- Irritable bowel syndrome
- Malignancy

 ## DIAGNOSIS

LABORATORY TESTS

- Obtain complete blood cell count and electrolytes
- Arterial blood gas if suspect acidosis
- Hypercoagulable workup may be indicated for mesenteric vein thrombosis

IMAGING STUDIES

- Visceral angiography indicated in any person over 45 years of age who appears chronically ill, with risk factors for arterial occlusive disease, and no other identifiable cause for abdominal symptoms
- Mesenteric artery thrombosis from atheroocclusive disease causes occlusion at the origin of the vessel
- Emboli most often lodge within the superior mesenteric artery at the first jejunal branch
- With shock or arterial spasm, vessels are pruned but patent
- Mesenteric vein occlusion: contrast-enhanced abdominal CT scan or arterial portography

DIAGNOSTIC PROCEDURES

- Ischemic colitis: colonoscopy reveals segmental inflammatory changes, most prominent in the watershed areas of the rectosigmoid junction and splenic flexure

Visceral Artery Insufficiency

 TREATMENT

MEDICATIONS

- Long-term anticoagulation for mesenteric vein thrombosis
- Broad-spectrum antibiotics for acute mesenteric ischemia
- Catheter-directed thrombolytics (alteplase, 0.5–1 mg/h) for thrombotic disease or vasodilators (papaverine, 30–60 mg/h) for nonocclusive disease
- Perioperative nutritional supplementation

SURGERY

- Surgical or endovascular management is directed toward restoration of antegrade visceral arterial flow
- Chronic mesenteric ischemia: transaortic endarterectomy and mesenteric artery bypass
  - A 5–9% mortality rate and a 10–25% recurrence rate at long-term follow-up
  - A higher recurrence rate with stenting of short-segment lesions; these patients require routine angiographic follow-up
- Acute mesenteric ischemia: emergent laparotomy indicated for patients with embolic disease, acidosis, hemodynamic instability, or severe or progressive abdominal pain.
  - Surgical options include thromboembolectomy or bypass, and resection of any nonviable bowel
  - Second-look operation if any bowel is of questionable viability
- Celiac axis compression syndrome: division of the arcuate ligament combined with mesenteric reconstruction for multivessel occlusive disease; yields variable postoperative results
- Ischemic colitis: conservative management is usually adequate; surgery indicated for progressive symptoms or stricture formation

 OUTCOME

COMPLICATIONS

- Bowel infarction
- Intraabdominal sepsis

PROGNOSIS

- Mortality approaches 80% in acute bowel infarction

WHEN TO REFER

- Symptoms and signs of acute or chronic mesenteric ischemia

WHEN TO ADMIT

- Acute mesenteric ischemia

 EVIDENCE

PRACTICE GUIDELINES

- Moneta GL: Screening for mesenteric vascular insufficiency and follow-up of mesenteric artery bypass procedures. Semin Vasc Surg 2001;14:186. [PMID: 11561279]
- Trompeter M et al: Non-occlusive mesenteric ischemia: etiology, diagnosis, and interventional therapy. Eur Radiol 2002;12:1179. Epub 2001 Dec 21. [PMID: 11976865]

WEB SITES

- Albany Medical Center—Acute mesenteric ischemia http://www.amc.edu/Vascular/vas_visceral_info.htm#Acute
- University of Kansas—Vascular surgery: chronic mesenteric ischemia http://www.kumc.edu/vsurg/dean.htm

INFORMATION FOR PATIENTS

- Mayo Clinic—Mesenteric ischemia http://www.mayoclinic.com/invoke.cfm?objectid=61253DCD-5CF2-4204-83572DEB6DD0CB89
- MEDLINEplus—Mesenteric artery ischemia http://www.nlm.nih.gov/medlineplus/ency/article/001156.htm

REFERENCES

- Kasirajan K et al: Chronic mesenteric ischemia: open surgery versus percutaneous angioplasty and stenting. J Vasc Surg 2001;33:63. [PMID: 11137925]
- Klotz S et al: Diagnosis and treatment of nonocclusive mesenteric ischemia after open heart surgery. Ann Thorac Surg 2001;72:1583. [PMID: 11722048]

Louis M. Messina, MD
Laura K. Pak, MD
Lawrence M. Tierney, Jr., MD

Vitamin B$_{12}$ Deficiency

 KEY FEATURES

ESSENTIALS OF DIAGNOSIS

- Macrocytic anemia
- Macroovalocytes and hypersegmented neutrophils on peripheral blood smear
- Serum vitamin B$_{12}$ level <100 pg/mL

GENERAL CONSIDERATIONS

- All vitamin B$_{12}$ comes from diet (foods of animal origin)
- After ingestion, vitamin B$_{12}$ bound to intrinsic factor, a protein secreted by gastric parietal cells
- Vitamin B$_{12}$-intrinsic factor complex is absorbed in terminal ileum by cells with specific receptors for the complex; it is then transported through plasma and stored in the liver
- Liver stores are sufficient that vitamin B$_{12}$ deficiency develops only >3 years after vitamin B$_{12}$ absorption ceases
- Causes of vitamin B$_{12}$ deficiency
  - Decreased intrinsic factor production: pernicious anemia (most common cause of B$_{12}$ deficiency), gastrectomy
  - Dietary deficiency (seen only in vegans)
  - Competition for B$_{12}$ in gut: blind loop syndrome, fish tapeworm (rare)
  - Decreased ileal B$_{12}$ absorption: surgical resection, Crohn's disease, metformin
  - Pancreatic insufficiency
  - *Helicobacter pylori* infection
  - Transcobalamin II deficiency (rare)
- Pernicious anemia is associated with atrophic gastritis and other autoimmune diseases, eg, immunoglobulin A (IgA) deficiency, polyglandular endocrine failure syndromes

DEMOGRAPHICS

- Pernicious anemia is hereditary, though rare clinically before age 35

 CLINICAL FINDINGS

SYMPTOMS AND SIGNS

- Megaloblastic anemia, which may be severe
- Pallor and mild icterus
- Glossitis and vague gastrointestinal disturbances, eg, anorexia, diarrhea
- Neurological manifestations: peripheral neuropathy usually occurs first; then subacute combined degeneration of the spinal cord affecting posterior columns, causing difficulty with position and vibration sensation and balance; then, in advanced cases, central nervous system, causing dementia or other neuropsychiatric changes
- Decreased vibration and position sensation
- Neurological manifestations occasionally precede hematological changes; patients with suspicious neurological symptoms and signs should be evaluated for vitamin B$_{12}$ deficiency despite normal mean cell volume (MCV) and absence of anemia

DIFFERENTIAL DIAGNOSIS

- Folic acid deficiency (other cause of megaloblastic anemia)
- Myelodysplastic syndrome (other cause of macrocytic anemia with abnormal morphology)
- Other cause of peripheral neuropathy, ataxia, or dementia

 DIAGNOSIS

LABORATORY TESTS

- Anemia of variable severity; hematocrit may be as low as 10–15%
- MCV strikingly elevated: 110–140 fL; may be normal if coexistent thalassemia or iron deficiency
- Serum vitamin B$_{12}$ level low, usually <100 pg/mL (normal 150–350 pg/mL), establishes diagnosis
- Serum methylmalonic acid or homocysteine level elevations can confirm diagnosis when serum vitamin B$_{12}$ level is borderline
- Peripheral blood smear: macro-ovalocytes characteristic; hypersegmented neutrophils with mean lobe count >4, or ≥1 six-lobed neutrophils; anisocytosis and poikilocytosis
- Reticulocyte count reduced
- Pancytopenia present in severe cases
- Serum lactate dehydrogenase (LDH) elevated and indirect bilirubin modestly increased

DIAGNOSTIC PROCEDURES

- Schilling test used to document decreased absorption of oral vitamin B$_{12}$ characteristic of pernicious anemia
- Vitamin B$_{12}$, 1000 mg given IM to saturate transport proteins, then radiolabeled vitamin B$_{12}$ given PO, and 24-h urine collected to determine how much vitamin B$_{12}$ is absorbed and excreted; abnormal excretion of <3% occurs with impaired absorption of oral vitamin B$_{12}$
- In second stage of Schilling test (done 2 months after vitamin B$_{12}$ replacement), radiolabeled vitamin B$_{12}$ is given with intrinsic factor; in pernicious anemia low absorption should normalize
- Bone marrow morphology is characteristic: marked erythroid hyperplasia, megaloblastic changes in erythroid series, and giant metamyelocytes in myeloid series

Vitamin B₁₂ Deficiency

 TREATMENT

MEDICATIONS

- Vitamin B_{12}, 100 μg IM QD for 1 week, then Q week for 1 month, then Q month for life, for pernicious anemia
- Oral cobalamin, 1000 μg PO QD, may be tried instead of parenteral therapy but must be continued indefinitely
- Antibiotics if vitamin B_{12} deficiency is caused by bacterial overgrowth in a blind loop
- Pancreatic enzymes if deficiency is due to pancreatic insufficiency
- Anthelmintic agent if deficiency is due to fish tapeworm
- **Note**: Large doses of folic acid may produce hematological responses in cases of vitamin B_{12} deficiency but allow neurological damage to progress

 OUTCOME

FOLLOW-UP

- Pernicous anemia is a lifelong disorder; if patients discontinue monthly therapy, the vitamin deficiency will recur
- Brisk reticulocytosis occurs 5–7 days after therapy, and the hematological picture normalizes in 2 months
- How frequently: check hematocrit
- Follow serum vitamin B_{12} level

COMPLICATIONS

- Nervous system complications include subacute combined degeneration of the spinal cord, psychosis, and dementia
- Atrophic gastritis seen in pernicious anemia is associated with increased risk of gastric carcinoma
- Hypokalemia may complicate the first several days of parenteral vitamin B_{12} therapy in pernicious anemia, particularly if anemia is severe

PROGNOSIS

- Patients with pernicious anemia respond to parenteral vitamin B_{12} therapy with immediate improvement in sense of well-being
- Nervous system manifestations are reversible if they are of relatively short duration (<6 months) but may be permanent if treatment is not initiated promptly

 EVIDENCE

PRACTICE GUIDELINES

- Dharmarajan TS et al: Vitamin B_{12} deficiency. Recognizing subtle symptoms in older adults. Geriatrics 2003;58:30, 37. [PMID: 12650116]
- Lane LA et al: Treatment of vitamin B_{12}-deficiency anemia: oral versus parenteral therapy. Ann Pharmacother 2002;36:1268. [PMID: 12086562]
- Oh R et al: Vitamin B_{12} deficiency. Am Fam Physician 2003;67:979. PMID: 12643357

WEB SITES

- MEDLINEplus—Pernicious anemia http://www.nlm.nih.gov/medlineplus/ency/article/000569.htm
- NIH—Vitamin B_{12} http://www.cc.nih.gov/ccc/supplements/vitb12.html

INFORMATION FOR PATIENTS

- American Family Physician. Information from your family doctor. Vitamin B_{12}. Am Fam Physician 2003;67:993. PMID: 12643358
- Mayo Clinic—Vitamin deficiency anemia http://www.mayoclinic.com/invoke.cfm?objectid=2BC66873-33D3-4F88-9FCFFA3261CA58AE& section=3
- University of Maryland Medicine Megaloblastic (Pernicious) Anemia http://www.umm.edu/blood/aneper.htm

REFERENCE

- Kaptan K et al: Helicobacter pylori—is it a novel causative agent in vitamin B_{12} deficiency? Arch Intern Med 2000; 160:1349. [PMID: 10809040]

Charles A. Linker, MD

von Willebrand's Disease

 KEY FEATURES

ESSENTIALS OF DIAGNOSIS

- Family history with autosomal dominant pattern of inheritance
- Bleeding time prolonged, either at baseline or after challenge with aspirin
- Factor VIII antigen or ristocetin cofactor levels reduced
- Factor VIII coagulant activity levels reduced in some patients

GENERAL CONSIDERATIONS

- Most common congenital disorder of hemostasis
- Autosomal dominant transmission
- Characterized by deficient or defective von Willebrand factor (vWF), a protein that mediates platelet adhesion
- Platelets adhere to subendothelium via vWF, which binds to platelet receptor composed of glycoprotein Ib (missing in Bernard-Soulier syndrome)
- Platelet aggregation normal in von Willebrand's disease
- vWF has separate function protecting from degradation factor VIII coagulant protein (factor VIII:C, deficient in hemophilia A); may thus secondarily cause coagulation disturbance because of deficient factor VIII:C levels, but coagulopathy is rarely severe
- Subtypes of von Willebrand's disease
  - Type I (80% of cases): quantitative decrease in vWF
  - Type IIa: qualitative abnormality prevents multimer formation; only small multimers present that cannot mediate platelet adhesion
  - Type IIb: qualitative abnormality causes rapid clearance of functional large multimeric forms
  - Type III: rare autosomal recessive disorder in which vWF nearly absent
  - Pseudo-von Willebrand disease: rare disorder in which platelet binds large vWF multimers with excessive avidity, causing their clearance from plasma

DEMOGRAPHICS

- Common disorder affecting both men and women

 CLINICAL FINDINGS

SYMPTOMS AND SIGNS

- Mild bleeding in most cases
- Rarely as severe as hemophilia, and spontaneous hemarthroses do not occur
- Mucosal bleeding usually (epistaxis, gingival bleeding, menorrhagia), but gastrointestinal bleeding may occur
- Incisional bleeding usually occurs after surgery or dental extractions
- Bleeding tendency is exacerbated by aspirin
- Bleeding tendency decreases during pregnancy or estrogen use

DIFFERENTIAL DIAGNOSIS

- Other qualitative platelet disorders, eg, uremia, aspirin use, Glanzmann's thrombasthenia
- Thrombocytopenia
- Hemophilia
- Waldenström's macroglobulinemia

 DIAGNOSIS

LABORATORY TESTS

- Platelet number and morphology normal
- Bleeding time usually (not always) prolonged; measure whenever diagnosis is considered because it correlates most closely with clinical bleeding
- When bleeding time is normal in von Willebrand's disease, it will be prolonged markedly by aspirin; normal persons prolong their bleeding time to a minor extent with aspirin but rarely out of the normal range
- In the most common form of von Willebrand's disease (type I), vWF plasma levels are reduced, as measured by factor VIII antigen or by ristocetin cofactor activity
- When factor VIII antigen is reduced, may also see a decrease in factor VIII coagulant (factor VIII:C) levels; when factor VIII:C levels <25%, partial thromboplastin time is prolonged
- Platelet aggregation studies with standard agonists (ADP, collagen, thrombin) are normal, but platelet aggregation in response to ristocetin may be subnormal
- In difficult cases, it may be helpful to perform a direct assay of the multimeric composition of vWF

von Willebrand's Disease

 TREATMENT

MEDICATIONS

- Desmopressin, 0.3 μg/kg IV × 1, is useful for mild type I von Willebrand's disease
  - vWF levels usually rise 2- to 3-fold in 30–90 min, apparently via release of stored vWF from endothelial cells
  - Can be given only every 24 h as stores of vWF become depleted
- Desmopressin is not effective in type IIa von Willebrand's disease, in which no endothelial stores are present
- Desmopressin may be harmful in type IIb, leading to thrombocytopenia and increased bleeding
- Factor VIII concentrate, eg, Humate-P (Armour), 20–50 units/kg depending on disease severity, is treatment of choice if factor replacement is required; some (not all) of these products contain functional vWF and do not transmit HIV or hepatitis
- ε-Aminocaproic acid (EACA; Amicar) is useful as adjunctive therapy during dental procedures; after either cryoprecipitate or desmopressin, 4 g orally every 4 h to reduce the likelihood of bleeding

THERAPEUTIC PROCEDURES

- In mild bleeding disorder, no treatment is routinely given other than aspirin avoidance
- In preparation for surgical or dental procedures, measure bleeding time as the best indicator of bleeding likelihood; prophylactic therapy may be reasonably withheld if the procedure is minor and bleeding time is normal

 OUTCOME

PROGNOSIS

- Prognosis is excellent
- In most cases, bleeding disorder is mild, and replacement therapy is effective in more serious cases

 EVIDENCE

PRACTICE GUIDELINES

- Federici AB et al: Subcommittee on von Willebrand Factor. Acquired von Willebrand syndrome: data from an international registry. Thromb Haemost 2000;84:345. [PMID: 10959711]
- United Kingdom Haemophilia Centre Doctors' Organisation: Guidelines on the selection and use of therapeutic products to treat haemophilia and other hereditary bleeding disorders. Haemophilia 2003;9:1. [PMID: 12558775]

WEB SITES

- Mayo Clinic—Von Willebrand's disease http://www.mayoclinic.com/invoke.cfm?objectid=5E0ED3F5-02FB-4258-A88D5ACBBE6A534C
- MEDLINEplus—Von Willebrand's disease http://www.nlm.nih.gov/medlineplus/ency/article/000544.htm

INFORMATION FOR PATIENTS

- National Heart, Lung, and Blood Institute http://www.nhlbi.nih.gov/health/prof/blood/other/hemophilia/backgrou.htm
- National Hemophilia Foundation—Von Willebrand's disease http://www.hemophilia.org/bdi/bdi_types3.htm

REFERENCES

- Mannucci PM et al: Treatment of von Willebrand disease with a high-purity factor VIII/von Willebrand factor concentrate: a prospective, multicenter study. Blood 2002;99:450. [PMID: 11781224]
- Sadler JE et al: Impact, diagnosis and treatment of von Willebrand disease. Thromb Haemost 2000;84:160. [PMID: 10959685]

Charles A. Linker, MD

Vulvar Cancer

 KEY FEATURES

ESSENTIALS OF DIAGNOSIS

- History of genital warts
- History of prolonged vulvar irritation, with pruritus, local discomfort, or slight bloody discharge
- Biopsy is necessary to make the diagnosis

GENERAL CONSIDERATIONS

- The vast majority of cancers of the vulva are squamous lesions; basal cell carcinomas are also found
- Several subtypes (particularly 16, 18, and 31) of the human papillomavirus have been identified in some but not all vulvar cancers
- As with squamous cell lesions of the cervix, a grading system of vulvar intraepithelial neoplasia (VIN) from mild dysplasia to carcinoma in situ has been established

DEMOGRAPHICS

- Usually occurs in women over 50 years of age
- The likelihood that a superimposed vulvar cancer will develop in a woman with a nonneoplastic epithelial disorder (vulvar dystrophy) ranges from 1% to 5%

 CLINICAL FINDINGS

SYMPTOMS AND SIGNS

- Early lesions may suggest or include nonneoplastic epithelial disorders
- Late lesions appear as a mass, an exophytic growth, or a firm, ulcerated area in the vulva

DIFFERENTIAL DIAGNOSIS

- Chronic granulomatous lesions (eg, lymphogranuloma venereum, syphilis), condylomas, hidradenoma, or neurofibroma
- Genital warts (condyloma acuminata)
- Lichen sclerosus
- Lichen planus
- Ulcer: herpes simplex virus, chancroid, syphilis, granuloma inguinale, lymphogranuloma venereum, Behçet's syndrome
- Hidradenitis suppurativa
- Vulvar intraepithelial neoplasia
- Psoriasis
- Paget's disease
- Papillary hidradenoma
- Bartholin's cyst or abscess

 DIAGNOSIS

LABORATORY TESTS

- Pathological examination of biopsies of lesion(s)

IMAGING STUDIES

- Preoperative colposcopy of vulva, vagina and cervix
- Pelvic CT to rule out lymphadenopathy

DIAGNOSTIC PROCEDURES

- Biopsy is essential for the diagnosis and should be performed with any localized atypical vulvar lesion, including white patches
- Multiple skin-punch specimens can be taken in the office under local anesthesia, with care to include tissue from the edges of each lesion sampled
- Lichen sclerosus and other associated leukoplakic changes in the skin should be biopsied

Vulvar Cancer

TREATMENT

MEDICATIONS

- A 7:3 combination of betamethasone and crotamiton is particularly effective for itching
- After an initial response, fluorinated steroids should be replaced with hydrocortisone because of their skin atrophying effect
- For lichen sclerosus, apply clobetasol propionate cream 0.05% twice daily for 2–3 weeks, then once daily until symptoms resolve. Application one to three times a week can be used for long-term maintenance therapy

SURGERY

In situ carcinoma

- In situ squamous cell carcinoma of the vulva and small, invasive basal cell carcinoma of the vulva should be excised with a wide margin
- If the squamous carcinoma in situ is extensive or multicentric, laser therapy or superficial surgical removal of vulvar skin may be required. In this way, the clitoris and uninvolved portions of the vulva may be spared. Skin grafting may be necessary, but mutilating vulvectomy is avoided

Invasive carcinoma

- Invasive carcinoma confined to the vulva without evidence of spread to adjacent organs or to the regional lymph nodes will necessitate radical vulvectomy and inguinal lymphadenectomy if the patient is able to withstand surgery
- Debilitated patients may be candidates for palliative irradiation only

OUTCOME

FOLLOW-UP

- Examination every 3 months for 2 years postoperatively, then every 6 months for an additional 3 years

COMPLICATIONS

- Depends on extent of surgery
- Wound infection
- Wound breakdown
- Lymphedema may occur as a late complication in up to 30%

PROGNOSIS

- Basal cell carcinomas very seldom metastasize, and carcinoma in situ by definition has not metastasized. With adequate excision, the prognosis for both lesions is excellent
- Patients with invasive vulvar carcinoma 3 cm in diameter or less without inguinal lymph node metastases who can sustain radical surgery have about a 90% chance of a 5-year survival. If the lesion is greater than 3 cm and has metastasized, the likelihood of 5-year survival is less than 25%

WHEN TO REFER

- All patients with invasive vulvar carcinoma should be referred to a gynecological oncologist

PREVENTION

- Careful examination of the vulva for premalignant lesions at all gynecological examinations

EVIDENCE

PRACTICE GUIDELINES

- National guideline on the management of vulval conditions. Int J STD AIDS 2002;13:411.
- Practice guidelines: vulvar cancer. Society of Gynecologic Oncologists Clinical Practice Guidelines. Oncology (Huntingt) 1998;12:275.

WEB SITES

- Vaginal Cancer—National Cancer Institute—CancerNet http://cancernet.nci.nih.gov/ cgi-bin/srchcgi.exe?DBID =pdq&TYPE=search&UID=208+ 01055&ZFILE=professional& SFMT=pdq_treatment/1/0/0
- Vulvar Cancer—National Cancer Institute—CancerNet http://cancernet.nci.nih.gov/ cgi-bin/srchcgi.exe?DBID= pdq&TYPE=search&UID=208+ 01038&ZFILE=professional& SFMT=pdq_treatment/1/0/0
- Gynecologic Cancers http://www.oncolink.com/templates/ types/types.cfm?c=6

INFORMATION FOR PATIENTS

- American College of Obstetricians and Gynecologists http://www.medem.com/MedLB/ article_detaillb.cfm?article_ID=ZZZB9 W29EQC&sub_cat=263
- Mayo Clinic http://www.mayoclinic.com/invoke.cfm? id=AN00448

REFERENCES

- Nash JD et al: Vulvar cancer. Surg Oncol Clin North Am 1998;7:335. [PMID: 9537980]
- Thomas E et al: Premalignant vulval disorders. Clin Evidence 2000;4:1115.

H. Trent MacKay, MD, MPH

Waldenström's Macroglobulinemia

 ## KEY FEATURES

ESSENTIALS OF DIAGNOSIS

- Symptoms nonspecific: splenomegaly common on examination
- Monoclonal immunoglobulin M (IgM) paraprotein
- Infiltration of bone marrow by plasmacytic lymphocytes
- Absence of lytic bone disease

GENERAL CONSIDERATIONS

- Malignant disease of B cells that appear to be hybrid of lymphocytes and plasma cells
- Cells characteristically secrete IgM paraprotein, and this macroglobulin causes many clinical manifestations

DEMOGRAPHICS

- Occurs mainly in patients aged 60–79

 ## CLINICAL FINDINGS

SYMPTOMS AND SIGNS

- Insidious fatigue related to anemia
- Mucosal or gastrointestinal bleeding related to engorged blood vessels and platelet dysfunction with hyperviscosity syndrome (usually when viscosity >4 times that of water)
- Nausea, vertigo, or visual disturbances; or alterations in consciousness from mild lethargy to stupor and coma with hyperviscosity syndrome
- Symptoms of cold agglutinin disease or peripheral neuropathy from IgM paraprotein
- Hepatosplenomegaly or lymphadenopathy may be present
- Retinal vein engorgement
- Purpura may be present
- Bone tenderness absent

DIFFERENTIAL DIAGNOSIS

- Monoclonal gammopathy of uncertain significance
- Multiple myeloma
- Chronic lymphocytic leukemia
- Lymphoma

 ## DIAGNOSIS

LABORATORY TESTS

- Anemia nearly universal, and rouleau formation common
- White blood cell cell and platelet count usually normal
- Peripheral blood smear: abnormal plasmacytic lymphocytes usually in small numbers
- Serum protein electrophoresis (SPEP) demonstrates monoclonal IgM spike in β- or γ-globulin region
- Serum viscosity usually increased above normal (>1.4–1.8 times viscosity of water)
- No strict correlation between paraprotein concentration and serum viscosity
- Positive Coombs, cold agglutinin or cryoglobulin tests may be positive due to IgM paraprotein
- If macroglobulinemia is suspected but SPEP shows only hypogammaglobulinemia, repeat SPEP while maintaining blood at 37°C, since paraprotein may precipitate at room temperature
- No evidence of renal failure

IMAGING STUDIES

- Bone x-rays: normal

DIAGNOSTIC PROCEDURES

- Bone marrow aspiration and biopsy: characteristic infiltration by the plasmacytic lymphocytes

TREATMENT

MEDICATIONS

- Chemotherapy with chlorambucil, cyclophosphamide, or fludarabine
- Cladribine
- Rituximab (monoclonal antibody)

THERAPEUTIC PROCEDURES

- Emergent plasmapheresis for marked hyperviscosity syndrome (stupor or coma)
- Plasmapheresis alone periodically for some patients
- Autologous stem cell transplantation in younger patients with more aggressive disease

 OUTCOME

PROGNOSIS

- Median survival rate is 3–5 years; some patients may survive 10 years or longer

 EVIDENCE

PRACTICE GUIDELINES

- Anagnostopoulos A et al: Autologous and allogeneic stem cell transplantation in Waldenstrom's macroglobulinemia: review of the literature and future directions. Semin Oncol 2003;30:286. [PMID: 12720154]
- Gertz MA et al: Treatment recommendations in Waldenstrom's macroglobulinemia: consensus panel recommendations from the Second International Workshop on Waldenstrom's Macroglobulinemia. Semin Oncol 2003;30:121. [PMID: 12720120]

WEB SITES

- International Waldenstrom's macroglobulinemia Foundation http://www.iwmf.com/
- Research fund for Waldenstrom http://www.waldenstromsresearch.org/whatis.htm

INFORMATION FOR PATIENTS

- ACS—Treatment of Waldenstrom's macroglobulinemia http://www.cancer.org/docroot/CRI/content/CRI_2_4_4X_Treatment_of_Waldenstroms_Macroglobulinemia_32.asp
- MEDLINEplus—Macroglobulinemia of Waldenstrom http://www.nlm.nih.gov/medlineplus/ency/article/000588.htm
- NCI—Waldenstrom's macroglobulinemia http://cis.nci.nih.gov/fact/6_4.htm

REFERENCES

- Dimopoulos MA et al: Waldenström's macroglobulinemia: clinical features, complications, and management. J Clin Oncol 2000;18:214. [PMID: 10623712]
- Dimopoulos MA et al: Treatment of Waldenström's macroglobulinemia with rituximab. J Clin Oncol 2002;20:2327. [PMID: 11981004]

Charles A. Linker, MD

Warts

 KEY FEATURES

ESSENTIALS OF DIAGNOSIS

- Verrucous papules anywhere on the skin or mucous membranes, usually no larger than 1 cm in diameter
- Prolonged incubation period (average 2–18 months); spontaneous "cures" are frequent (50%)
- "Recurrences" (new lesions) are frequent

GENERAL CONSIDERATIONS

- Caused by human papillomaviruses (HPVs)
- Especially in genital warts, simultaneous infection with numerous wart types is common
- Genital HPVs are divided into low-risk and high-risk types depending on the likelihood of their association with cervical and anal cancer

 CLINICAL FINDINGS

SYMPTOMS AND SIGNS

- There are usually no symptoms
- Tenderness on pressure occurs with plantar warts; itching occurs with anogenital warts
- Occasionally a wart will produce mechanical obstruction (eg, nostril, ear canal, urethra)
- Warts vary widely in shape, size, and appearance
- Flat warts are most evident under oblique illumination
- Subungual warts may be dry, fissured, and hyperkeratotic and may resemble hangnails or other nonspecific changes
- Plantar warts resemble plantar corns or calluses

DIFFERENTIAL DIAGNOSIS

- Non-genital warts
  - Actinic keratosis
  - Squamous cell carcinoma
  - Molluscum contagiosum
  - Seborrheic keratosis
  - Skin tag (acrochordon)
  - Nevus
  - Verrucous zoster (in AIDS)
- Genital warts (condyloma acuminata)
  - Secondary syphilis (condyloma lata)
  - Psoriasis
  - Seborrheic keratosis
  - Molluscum contagiosum
  - Bowenoid papulosis and squamous cell carcinoma
  - Lichen planus
  - Pearly penile papules
  - Skin tag (acrochordon)

 DIAGNOSIS

LABORATORY TESTS

- Clinical diagnosis

DIAGNOSTIC PROCEDURES

- Biopsy may be necessary for definitive diagnosis

TREATMENT

MEDICATIONS

Liquid nitrogen

- Apply to achieve a thaw time of 20–45 s; two freeze-thaw cycles are used every 2–4 weeks for several visits
- Scarring will occur if used incorrectly
- May cause permanent depigmentation in darkly pigmented individuals
- It is useful on dry penile warts and on filiform warts on the face and body

Keratolytic agents and occlusion

- Any of the following salicylic acid products may be used against common warts or plantar warts: Occlusal, Trans-Ver-Sal, and Duofilm
- Plantar warts may be treated by applying a 40% salicylic acid plaster (Mediplast) after paring; the plaster may be left on for 5–6 days, then removed, the lesion pared down, and another plaster applied; it may take months to eradicate
- Chronic occlusion alone with water-impermeable tape (duct tape, adhesive tape) for months may be effective

Podophyllum resin

- Paint each anogenital wart carefully (protecting normal skin) every 2–3 weeks with 25% podophyllum resin (podophyllin) in compound tincture of benzoin
- Avoid use in pregnancy
- The purified active component of the resin, podofilox, is available for use at home twice daily three consecutive days a week for cycles of 4–6 weeks; it is less irritating and more effective than podophyllum resin
- May need multiple cycles of treatment

Imiquimod

- A 5% cream of this local interferon inducer can clear external genital warts, particularly in women
- Treatment is once-daily on 3 alternate days per week; response may take up to 12 weeks; recurrences may occur
- There is less pregnancy risk than with podophyllum resin and appears to be the "patient-administered" treatment of choice in women
- In men, the more rapid response, lower cost, and similar efficacy make podophyllotoxin the initial treatment of

choice, with imiquimod used for recurrences or refractory cases
- May be used to treat superficial flat warts

Other agents

- Bleomycin diluted to 1 unit/mL injected into plantar and common warts; do not use on digital warts because of the potential complications of Raynaud's phenomenon, nail loss, and terminal digital necrosis
- Cimetidine, 35–50 mg/kg daily, for younger patients with common warts
- Apply aquaric acid dibutylester 0.2–2% directly to the warts from once weekly to five times weekly to induce a mild contact dermatitis; most warts clear over 10–20 weeks
- Injection of candida antigen may be used in the same way

Retinoids

- Tretinoin (Retin-A) cream or gel applied topically twice daily may be effective for facial or beard flat warts
- Extensive warts may remit after 4–8 weeks of oral retinoids

THERAPEUTIC PROCEDURES

Operative removal

- For genital warts, snip biopsy (scissors) removal followed by light electrocautery is more effective than cryotherapy but does scar

Laser therapy

- The CO_2 laser effectively treats recurrent warts, periungual warts, plantar warts, and condylomata acuminata
- It leaves open wounds that must fill in with granulation tissue over 4–6 weeks and is best reserved for warts resistant to other modalities

Physical modalities

- Soaking warts in hot (42.2°C) water for 10–30 min daily for 6 weeks can result in dramatic involution

OUTCOME

PROGNOSIS

- Development of new lesions is common
- Warts may disappear spontaneously or may be unresponsive to treatment

WHEN TO REFER

- If there is a question about the diagnosis, if recommended therapy is ineffective, or if specialized treatment is necessary

PREVENTION

- The use of condoms may reduce transmission of genital warts
- A person with flat warts should be educated about the infectivity of warts and advised not to scratch the areas
- Using an electric shaver may prevent autoinoculation

EVIDENCE

PRACTICE GUIDELINES

- National Guideline Clearinghouse http://www.guideline.gov/summary/summary.aspx?doc_id=3240&nbr=2466&string=warts

WEB SITE

- American Academy of Dermatology http://www.aad.org

INFORMATION FOR PATIENTS

- American Academy of Dermatology http://www.aad.org/Kids/warts.html
- American Academy of Family Physicians http://familydoctor.org/handouts/209.html

REFERENCE

- Gibbs S: Local treatments for cutaneous warts: systematic review. BMJ 2002; 325:461. [PMID: 12202325]
- Wiley DJ: External genital warts: diagnosis, treatment and prevention. Clin Infect Dis 2002;35(Suppl 2):S210. [PMID: 12353208]

Timothy G. Berger, MD

Wegener's Granulomatosis

 KEY FEATURES

ESSENTIALS OF DIAGNOSIS

- Triad of upper respiratory tract disease, lower respiratory disease, and glomerulonephritis
- Suspect this diagnosis whenever mundane respiratory systems (eg, nasal congestion, sinusitis) are refractory to usual treatment
- Pathology defined by the triad of small vessel vasculitis, granulomatous inflammation, and necrosis
- Cytoplasmic antineutophil cytoplasmic antibody (c-ANCA) pattern of immunofluorescence has moderate sensitivity and excellent specificity if confirmed by an enzyme immunoassay for antibodies to proteinase-3
- 10% of patients have a perinuclear (p)-ANCA pattern on immunofluorescence testing for ANCA, caused by antibodies to myeloperoxidase
- Renal disease often rapidly progressive

GENERAL CONSIDERATIONS

- The disease presents as vasculitis of small arteries, arterioles, and capillaries, necrotizing granulomatous lesions of both upper and lower respiratory tract, and glomerulonephritis

DEMOGRAPHICS

- Annual incidence of 10 per million
- Occurs most commonly in the fourth and fifth decades of life
- Affects men and women with equal frequency

 CLINICAL FINDINGS

SYMPTOMS AND SIGNS

- Usually develops over 4–12 months
- Fever, malaise, and weight loss
- 90% of patients present with upper or lower respiratory tract symptoms or both
- Upper respiratory tract symptoms can include nasal congestion, sinusitis, otitis media, mastoiditis, inflammation of the gums, or stridor due to subglottic stenosis
- Physical examination can be remarkable for congestion, crusting, ulceration, bleeding, and even perforation of the nasal mucosa
- The lung is affected initially in 40% and eventually in 80%, with symptoms including cough, dyspnea, and hemoptysis
- Renal involvement (75%) may be subclinical until renal insufficiency is advanced
- Other early symptoms can include unilateral proptosis (from pseudotumor), red eye from scleritis, arthritis, purpura, and dysesthesia due to neuropathy
- Destruction of the nasal cartilage with "saddle nose" deformity occurs late
- Patients are at high risk for venous thrombotic events (deep venous thrombosis, pulmonary embolus)

DIFFERENTIAL DIAGNOSIS

- Polyarteritis nodosa
- Microscopic polyangiitis
- Churg-Strauss syndrome
- Chronic sinusitis
- Goodpasture's disease
- Systemic lupus erythematosus
- Sarcoidosis

 DIAGNOSIS

LABORATORY TESTS

- The cytoplasmic pattern of immunofluorescence (c-ANCA), caused by antibodies to proteinase-3, a constituent of neutrophil granules, has a high specificity (>90%)
- In the setting of active disease, the sensitivity of c-ANCA is also reasonably high (≥70%)
- The p-ANCA pattern is caused by antibodies to myeloperoxidase and is much less specific. Approximately 10–25% of patients with classic Wegener's granulomatosis have p-ANCA
- The urinary sediment in the renal disease invariably contains red cells, with or without white cells, and red cell casts

IMAGING STUDIES

- Chest CT is more sensitive than chest radiography for infiltrates, nodules, masses, and cavities

PROCEDURES

- ANCA testing does not eliminate the need in most cases for confirmation of the diagnosis by tissue biopsy
- The full range of pathological changes is usually evident only on thoracoscopic lung biopsy. Histological features include vasculitis, granulomatous inflammation, geographic necrosis, and acute and chronic inflammation
- Renal biopsy discloses a segmental necrotizing glomerulonephritis with multiple crescents (characteristic but not diagnostic)

Wegener's Granulomatosis

 ## TREATMENT

MEDICATIONS

- Prednisone and oral cyclophosphamide
- Methotrexate, 20–25 mg/week, is a reasonable substitute for oral cyclophosphamide in patients who do not have immediately life-threatening disease

THERAPEUTIC PROCEDURES

- Early treatment is crucial in preventing renal failure and may be lifesaving

 ## OUTCOME

FOLLOW-UP

- Complete blood cell count every 2 weeks for patients on daily cyclophosphamide

COMPLICATIONS

Permanent disease-related complications

- Suffered by 85% of patients
- End-stage renal disease
- Decreased hearing
- Visual impairment
- Subglottic stenosis
- Saddle-nose deformity

Permanent treatment-related complications

- Suffered by 40% of patients
- Multitudinous effects of corticosteroids
- Cyclophosphamide
  - Bone marrow hypoplasia
  - Secondary malignancy (bladder, leukemia)
  - Hemorrhagic cystitis
  - Infertility

PROGNOSIS

- Without treatment it is invariably fatal, most patients surviving less than a year after diagnosis
- Remissions have been induced in up to 75% of patients treated with cyclophosphamide and prednisone, though half of these patients eventually suffer disease recurrences

WHEN TO REFER

- All patients should be followed with a rheumatologist. Other subspecialty consultations may be appropriate

WHEN TO ADMIT

- Alveolar hemorrhage
- Rapidly progressive glomerulonephritis

 ## EVIDENCE

WEB SITE

- http://vasculitis.med.jhu.edu

REFERENCES

- Regan MJ et al: Treatment of Wegener's granulomatosis. Rheum Dis Clin North Am 2001;27:863. [PMID: 11723769]
- Stone JH: The WGET Research Group. Limited versus severe Wegener's granulomatosis: baseline data from the Wegener's granulomatosis etanercept trial. Arthritis Rheum 2003;48:2299.

David B. Hellmann, MD, FACP
John H. Stone, MD, MPH

Weight Loss & Malnutrition in Elderly

 ## KEY FEATURES

ESSENTIALS OF DIAGNOSIS

- Unintended weight loss exceeding 5% in 1 month or 10% in 6 months
- Failure to thrive

GENERAL CONSIDERATIONS

- Undernutrition affects substantial numbers of elderly persons and often precedes hospitalization for "failure to thrive"
- "Failure to thrive"
  - A syndrome lacking a consensus definition but generally represents a constellation of weight loss, weakness, and progressive functional decline
  - The label is typically applied when some triggering event—loss of social support, a bout of depression or pneumonia, the addition of a new medication—pulls a struggling elderly person below the threshold of successful independent living
- Poor fitting dentures or oral health problems may contribute to nutritional problems, particularly in those with dementia
- Total caloric needs are reduced by about 30% in the elderly, but protein needs may be increased

DEMOGRAPHICS

- Risk factors for malnutrition include chronic disease, functional impairment, and depression

 ## CLINICAL FINDINGS

SYMPTOMS AND SIGNS

- A 10% loss of weight suggests severe malnutrition
- A loss of 5% suggests moderate malnutrition
- Subcutaneous tissue loss can be best evaluated in the subscapular, suprailiac, and triceps skinfolds
- A body mass index under 22 should raise concern about significant malnutrition

DIFFERENTIAL DIAGNOSIS

Medical

- Chronic heart, lung disease
- Dementia
- Oral problems (eg, poor denture fit)
- Dysphagia
- Mesenteric ischemia
- Cancer
- Diabetes
- Hyperthryoidism

Psychological

- Alcoholism
- Depression
- Social isolation
- Limited funds
- Problems with shopping or food preparation
- Inadequate assistance with feeding

Drug-related

- Nonsteroidal antiinflammatory drugs
- Antiepileptics
- Digoxin
- Selective serotonin reuptake inhibitors

 ## DIAGNOSIS

LABORATORY TESTS

- Laboratory studies are intended to uncover an occult metabolic or neoplastic cause
- Useful laboratory studies include complete blood cell count, serum chemistries (including glucose, thyroid-stimulating hormone, creatinine, calcium), urinalysis

IMAGING STUDIES

- Chest x-ray
- Further imaging (eg, mammography, colonoscopy) as dictated by the clinical presentation

TREATMENT

THERAPEUTIC PROCEDURES

- Aim for a caloric intake of about 25 kcal/kg, based on ideal body weight
- Nutritional supplements may lead to weight gain; use of instant breakfast powder in whole milk (for those who can tolerate dairy products) is a less costly alternative
- For those who have lost the ability to feed themselves, assiduous hand feeding may allow maintenance of weight
- Artificial nutrition and hydration ("tube feeding") is an alternative, but it deprives the patient of the taste and texture of food as well as the social milieu typically associated with mealtime
- If the patient makes repeated attempts to pull out the tube during a trial of artificial nutrition, the treatment burden becomes substantial, and the utility of tube feeding should be reconsidered
- Megestrol acetate has not been shown to increase body mass in the elderly

 ## OUTCOME

FOLLOW-UP

- Patients with malnutrition are at higher risk for death, functional decline, and nursing home placement

COMPLICATIONS

- Hospitalized patients with malnutrition are more likely to experience multiple life-threatening complications

PROGNOSIS

- Though commonly employed, there is no evidence that tube feeding prolongs life in patients with end-stage dementia

WHEN TO REFER

- Early involvement of a nutritionist may be helpful
- Consider dental or denture evaluation

WHEN TO ADMIT

- Malnutrition is rarely an indication for admission in and of itself
- The threshold for admission should be lower when a malnourished patient presents with an acute illness such as pneumonia

 ## EVIDENCE

PRACTICE GUIDELINES

- National Guidelines Clearinghouse http://www.guideline.gov/summary/summary.aspx?doc_id=3304
- American Academy of Family Physicians http://www.aafp.org/afp/20020215/640.html

WEB SITES

- AARP Guide to Internet Resources on Aging http://www.aarp.org/cyber/sd1_3.htm
- Administration on Aging http://www.aoa.dhhs.gov
- Merck Manual of Geriatrics http://www.merck.com/pubs/mm_geriatrics/contents.htm

INFORMATION FOR PATIENTS

- JAMA patient page: healthy diet. JAMA 2000;283:2198. [PMID: 10791513]
- Federal nutrition.gov http://www.info.gov.hk/elderly/english/healthinfo/selfhelptips/common-e.htm

REFERENCES

- Covinsky KE: The relationship between clinical assessments of nutritional status and adverse outcomes in older hospitalized medical patients. J Am Geriatr Soc 1999;47:532. [PMID: 10323645]
- Finucane TE: Tube feeding in patients with advanced dementia: a review of the evidence. JAMA 1999;282:1365. [PMID: 10527184]

C. Bree Johnston, MD
Kenneth E. Covinsky, MD

Weight Loss, Involuntary

 KEY FEATURES

ESSENTIALS OF DIAGNOSIS

- Decreased caloric intake
- Fever
- Change in bowel habits
- Secondary confirmation (eg, changes in clothing size)
- Substance abuse
- History of age-appropriate cancer screening

GENERAL CONSIDERATIONS

- Body weight is determined by a person's caloric intake, absorptive capacity, metabolic rate, and energy losses
- Involuntary weight loss is clinically significant when it exceeds 5% or more of usual body weight over a 6- to 12-month period
- Often indicates serious physical or psychological illness
- Most common causes are cancer (~30% of cases), gastrointestinal disorders (~15%), and dementia or depression (~15%).
- In approximately 15–25% of cases, no cause for the weight loss can be found

 CLINICAL FINDINGS

SYMPTOMS AND SIGNS

- History should include medication profile and 24-h diet recall
- Night sweats, cough, breast mass, constipation, hematochezia, bone pain suggest cancer
- Nausea, vomiting, diarrhea, abdominal pain suggest gastrointestinal disease
- Anhedonia, sleep disorder, suicidal ideation, recent psychosocial stressors suggest depression
- Memory loss, wandering, isolation suggest dementia
- Physical examination for evidence of cancer

DIFFERENTIAL DIAGNOSIS

Medical

- Malignancy
- Gastrointestinal disorders, eg, malabsorption, pancreatic insufficiency, peptic ulcer
- Hyperthyroidism
- Chronic heart, lung, or renal disease
- Uncontrolled diabetes mellitus
- Mesenteric ischemia (ischemic bowel)
- Dysphagia
- Anorexia due to azotemia
- Hypercalcemia
- Tuberculosis
- Subacute bacterial endocarditis

Psychosocial

- Depression
- Dementia
- Alcoholism
- Anorexia nervosa
- Loss of teeth, poor denture fit
- Social isolation
- Poverty
- Inability to shop or prepare food

Drug-related

- Nonsteroidal antiinflammatory drugs
- Antiepileptics
- Digoxin
- Selective serotonin reuptake inhibitors

 DIAGNOSIS

LABORATORY TESTS

- Obtain complete blood cell count
- Serologic tests
- Serum thyroid-stimulating hormone
- Urinalysis
- Fecal occult blood tests

IMAGING STUDIES

- Chest x-ray
- Upper gastrointestinal series and/or abdominal CT scan
- When these tests are normal, more definitive gastrointestinal investigation (eg, tests for malabsorption; endoscopy) and cancer screening (eg, Pap smear, mammography, prostate-specific antigen)

DIAGNOSTIC PROCEDURES

- If initial diagnostic workup is unrevealing, follow-up is preferable to further diagnostic testing

TREATMENT

MEDICATIONS

- Appetite stimulants (mild to moderate effectiveness): corticosteroids, progestational agents, dronabinol, and serotonin antagonists
- Anabolic agents: growth hormone and testosterone derivatives
- Anticatabolic agents: omega-3 fatty acids, pentoxifylline, hydrazine sulfate, and thalidomide

THERAPEUTIC PROCEDURES

- Treatment of the underlying disorder
- Consultation with dietician
- Caloric supplementation to achieve intake of 30–40 kcal/kg/day
- Oral feeding is preferred, but temporary nasojejunal tube, or permanent cutaneous gastric or jejunal tube may be necessary

 OUTCOME

PROGNOSIS

- Rapid unintentional weight loss is predictive of morbidity and mortality
- Mortality rates at 2-year follow-up: 8% for unexplained involuntary weight loss, 19% for weight loss due to nonmalignant disease, and 79% for weight loss due to malignant disease

 EVIDENCE

PRACTICE GUIDELINES

- American Medical Directors Association http://www.guidelines.gov/summary/summary.aspx?doc_id=3304&nbr=2530&string=malnutrition

WEB SITES

- NIH www.nih.gov
- National Nutrition Summit: Information Resources (CBM 2000-3) http://www.nlm.nih.gov/pubs/cbm/nutritionsummit.html

INFORMATION FOR PATIENTS

- MEDLINEplus Medical Encyclopedia http://www.nlm.nih.gov/medlineplus/ency/article/003107.htm
- http://home.mdconsult.com/das/patient/view/29691814/10002/2001.html/top?sid=191869237

REFERENCES

- Gazewood JD et al: Diagnosis and management of weight loss in the elderly. J Fam Pract 1998;47:19. [PMID: 9673603]
- Lankisch P et al: Unintentional weight loss: diagnosis and prognosis. The first prospective follow-up study from a secondary referral centre. J Intern Med 2001;249:41. [PMID: 11168783]
- Poehlman ET et al: Energy expenditure, energy intake, and weight loss in Alzheimer disease. Am J Clin Nutr 2000;71:650S. [PMID: 10681274]

Ralph Gonzales, MD

Whipple's Disease

 KEY FEATURES

 CLINICAL FINDINGS

 DIAGNOSIS

ESSENTIALS OF DIAGNOSIS

- Multisystemic disease
- Fever, lymphadenopathy, arthralgias
- Malabsorption
- Duodenal biopsy with PAS-positive macrophages with characteristic bacillus

GENERAL CONSIDERATIONS

- Rare multisystemic illness caused by infection with the bacillus *Tropheryma whippelei*
- Source of infection is unknown, but no cases of human-to-human spread have been documented

DEMOGRAPHICS

- May occur at any age but most commonly affects white men in the fourth to sixth decades

SYMPTOMS AND SIGNS

- Clinical manifestations are protean
- Arthralgias or a migratory, nondeforming arthritis in 80%
- Gastrointestinal symptoms in 75% include abdominal pain, diarrhea, and variable malabsorption with distension, flatulence, and steatorrhea
- Weight loss in almost all patients
- Protein-losing enteropathy with hypoalbuminemia and edema
- Intermittent low-grade fever in >50%
- Chronic cough
- Generalized lymphadenopathy
- Myocardial involvement: congestive failure or valvular regurgitation
- Ocular: uveitis, vitritis, keratitis, retinitis, and retinal hemorrhages
- CNS involvement in ~10%: dementia, lethargy, coma, seizures, myoclonus, or hypothalamic signs
- Cranial nerve findings: ophthalmoplegia or nystagmus
- Physical examination
  - Low-grade fever
  - Hypotension (late)
  - Lymphadenopathy in 50%
  - Heart murmurs
  - Peripheral joint inflammation, swelling
  - Neurological findings
  - Hyperpigmentation on sun-exposed areas in up to 40%

DIFFERENTIAL DIAGNOSIS

- Malabsorption due to other cause, eg, celiac or tropical sprue
- Inflammatory bowel disease
- Sarcoidosis
- Reactive arthritis (Reiter's syndrome)
- Systemic vasculitis
- Infective endocarditis
- Intestinal lymphoma
- Familial Mediterranean fever
- Behçet's syndrome
- Intestinal *Mycobacterium-avium intracellulare* (in AIDS)

LABORATORY TESTS

- PCR to confirm the diagnosis by demonstrating the presence of 16S ribosomal RNA of *T whippelei* in blood, cerebrospinal fluid, vitreous fluid, synovial fluid, or cardiac valves; sensitivity of 97%, specificity of 100%

DIAGNOSTIC PROCEDURES

- Endoscopic biopsy of the duodenum demonstrates infiltration of the lamina propria with PAS-positive macrophages that contain gram-positive, non–acid-fast bacilli, and dilatation of the lacteals
- Biopsy of other involved organs or lymph nodes for histological evaluation of the involved tissues may be necessary

Whipple's Disease

TREATMENT

MEDICATIONS

- Trimethoprim-sulfamethoxazole (1 double-strength tablet PO BID for 1 year) is recommended as first-line therapy
- Alternatives: ceftriaxone or chloramphenicol

THERAPEUTIC PROCEDURES

- Prolonged treatment for at least 1 year is required
- After antibiotic treatment, repeat biopsies for PCR; negative results predict a low likelihood of clinical relapse

OUTCOME

FOLLOW-UP

- Patients must be followed closely after treatment for recurrence

COMPLICATIONS

- Some neurological signs may be permanent

PROGNOSIS

- Antibiotic therapy results in a dramatic clinical improvement within several weeks
- Complete response within 1–3 months
- Relapse may occur in up to one-third of patients after discontinuation of treatment
- If untreated, the disease is fatal

EVIDENCE

PRACTICE GUIDELINES

- Marth T: The diagnosis and treatment of Whipple's disease. Curr Allergy Asthma Rep 2001;1:566. [PMID: 11892086]
- Marth T et al: Whipple's disease. Lancet 2003;361:239. [PMID: 12547551]

WEB SITES

- MEDLINEplus—Whipple's Disease http://www.nlm.nih.gov/medlineplus/ency/article/000209.htm
- National Digestive Diseases Information Clearinghouse—Whipple's disease http://digestive.niddk.nih.gov/ddiseases/pubs/whipple/index.htm
- NINDS Whipple's Disease Information Page http://www.ninds.nih.gov/health_and_medical/disorders/whipples.htm

INFORMATION FOR PATIENTS

- Cleveland Clinic—Whipple's disease http://www.clevelandclinic.org/health/health-info/docs/1200/1236.asp?index=5958
- Mayo Clinic—Whipple's disease http://www.mayoclinic.com/invoke.cfm?objectid=6FFA88B7-C3EB-447D-B72CF3351578FEF4
- Medical College of Wisconsin—Whipple's disease http://healthlink.mcw.edu/article/930591431.html

REFERENCES

- Raoult D et al: Cultivation of the bacillus of Whipple's disease. N Engl J Med 2000;342:620. [PMID: 10699161]
- Ratnaike RN: Whipple's disease. Postgrad Med J 2000;76:760. [PMID: 11085766]

Kenneth R. McQuaid, MD

Wilson's Disease

 KEY FEATURES

ESSENTIALS OF DIAGNOSIS

- Characterized by excessive deposition of copper in the liver and brain
- Rare autosomal recessive disorder that usually occurs between the first and third decades
- Serum ceruloplasmin, the plasma copper-carrying protein, is low. Urinary excretion of copper is high

GENERAL CONSIDERATIONS

- The genetic defect, localized to chromosome 13, affects a copper-transporting adenosine triphosphatase (ATP7B) in the liver and leads to oxidative damage of hepatic mitochondria
- Over 200 different mutations in the Wilson disease gene have been identified, making genetic diagnosis impractical
- The major physiological aberration is excessive absorption of copper from the small intestine and decreased excretion of copper by the liver, resulting in increased tissue deposition, especially in the liver, brain, cornea, and kidney

DEMOGRAPHICS

- Adolescents and young adults

 CLINICAL FINDINGS

SYMPTOMS AND SIGNS

- Consider the diagnosis in any child or young adult with hepatitis, splenomegaly with hypersplenism, hemolytic anemia, portal hypertension, and neurological or psychiatric abnormalities; also consider in persons under 40 years of age with chronic or fulminant hepatitis
- Hepatic involvement may range from elevated liver tests (although the alkaline phosphatase may be low) to cirrhosis and portal hypertension
- The neurological manifestations are related to basal ganglia dysfunction and include a resting, postural, or kinetic tremor and dystonia of the bulbar musculature with resulting dysarthria and dysphagia
- Psychiatric features include behavioral and personality changes and emotional lability
- The pathognomonic sign is the brownish or gray-green Kayser-Fleischer ring, which represents fine pigmented granular deposits in Descemet's membrane in the cornea close to the endothelial surface. The ring is usually most marked at the superior and inferior poles of the cornea. It can frequently be seen with the naked eye and almost invariably by slit lamp examination. It may be absent in patients with hepatic manifestations only but is usually present in those with neuropsychiatric disease

DIFFERENTIAL DIAGNOSIS

- Acute hepatitis
- Cholestasis
- Acute hepatic failure
- Chronic hepatitis
- Cirrhosis
- Hepatomegaly
- Other cause of hepatitis, fulminant hepatic failure, or cirrhosis, eg, viral, toxins, hemochromatosis
- Tremor due to other causes, eg, Parkinson's disease, essential tremor
- Dementia due to other causes, eg, Huntington's disease
- Behavior change due to other medical illness, eg, neurosyphilis, brain tumor

 DIAGNOSIS

LABORATORY TESTS

- Increased urinary copper excretion (>100 µg/24 h) or low serum ceruloplasmin levels (<20 µg/dL), and elevated hepatic copper concentration (>250 µg/g of dry liver). However, increased urinary copper and low serum ceruloplasmin levels are not specific for Wilson's disease
- In equivocal cases (when the serum ceruloplasmin level is normal), the diagnosis may require demonstration of low radiolabeled copper incorporation into ceruloplasmin or urinary copper determination after a penicillamine challenge

DIAGNOSTIC PROCEDURES

- Liver biopsy may show acute or chronic hepatitis or cirrhosis and is used to quantify hepatic copper

TREATMENT

MEDICATIONS

- Oral penicillamine (0.75–2 g/day in divided doses) is the drug of choice, making possible urinary excretion of chelated copper. Add pyridoxine, 25–50 mg per week, since penicillamine is an antimetabolite of this vitamin
- If penicillamine treatment cannot be tolerated because of gastrointestinal, hypersensitivity, or autoimmune reactions, consider the use of trientine, 250–500 mg three times a day
- Oral zinc acetate, 50 mg three times a day, promotes fecal copper excretion and may be used as maintenance therapy after decoppering with a chelating agent or as first-line therapy in presymptomatic or pregnant patients
- Ammonium tetrathiomolybdate has shown promise as initial therapy for neurological Wilson's disease
- Treatment should continue indefinitely
- Once the serum nonceruloplasmin copper level is within the normal range, the dose of chelating agent can be reduced to the minimum necessary for maintaining that level

SURGERY

- Liver transplantation is indicated for fulminant hepatitis (often after plasma exchange as a stabilizing measure), end-stage cirrhosis, and, in selected cases, intractable neurological disease

THERAPEUTIC PROCEDURES

- Early treatment to remove excess copper is essential before it can produce neurological or hepatic damage
- Early in the treatment phase, restrict dietary copper (shellfish, organ foods, and legumes)

OUTCOME

FOLLOW-UP

- Serum nonceruloplasmin copper
- Urine copper

COMPLICATIONS

- Fulminant hepatitis and cirrhosis
- Renal calculi, the Fanconi defect, renal tubular acidosis, hypoparathyroidism, and hemolytic anemia may occur

PROGNOSIS

- The prognosis is good if effective treatment occurs before liver or brain damage
- The disease may stabilize with treatment in cirrhosis

PREVENTION

- Family members, especially siblings, require screening with serum ceruloplasmin, liver function tests, and slit-lamp examination

EVIDENCE

PRACTICE GUIDELINES

- National Guideline Clearinghouse http://www.guideline.gov/summary/summary.aspx?doc_id=3520&nbr=2746&string=hepatolenticular+degeneration
- Roberts EA et al: A practice guideline on Wilson disease. Hepatology. 200337:1475.

WEB SITES

- Diseases of the Liver http://cpmcnet.columbia.edu/dept/gi/disliv.html
- Pathology Index http://www-medlib.med.utah.edu/WebPath/LIVEHTML/LIVERIDX.html
- Hepatic Ultrasound Images http://www.sono.nino.ru/english/hepar_en.html
- Liver Tutorials Visualization and Volume Measurement http://everest.radiology.uiowa.edu/nlm/app/livertoc/livertoc.html

INFORMATION FOR PATIENTS

- National Digestive Diseases Information Clearinghouse http://digestive.niddk.nih.gov/ddiseases/pubs/wilson/index.htm
- National Institute of Neurological Disorders and Stroke http://www.ninds.nih.gov/health_and_medical/disorders/wilsons_doc.htm

REFERENCE

- Emre S et al: Orthotopic liver transplantation for Wilson's disease: a single-center experience. Transplantation 2001; 72:1232. [PMID: 11602847]

Lawrence S. Friedman, MD

Zollinger-Ellison Syndrome

 KEY FEATURES

ESSENTIALS OF DIAGNOSIS

- Peptic ulcer disease severe and atypical
- Gastric acid hypersecretion
- Diarrhea common, relieved by nasogastric suction
- Most cases are sporadic; 25% with multiple endocrine neoplasia (MEN) type 1

GENERAL CONSIDERATIONS

- Caused by gastrin-secreting gut neuroendocrine tumors (gastrinomas), which result in hypergastrinemia and acid hypersecretion
- Gastrinomas cause <1% of peptic ulcer disease
- Primary gastrinomas may arise in the pancreas (25%), duodenal wall (45%), or lymph nodes (5–15%), other locations (20%)
- Most gastrinomas are solitary or multifocal nodules that are potentially resectable; 25% are small multicentric gastrinomas associated with MEN 1 that are more difficult to resect
- Gastrinomas are malignant in less than two-thirds; one-third have already metastasized to the liver at initial presentation
- Screening for Zollinger-Ellison syndrome with fasting gastrin levels indicated for patients with ulcers that are refractory to standard therapies, giant ulcers (>2 cm), ulcers located distal to the duodenal bulb, multiple duodenal ulcers, frequent ulcer recurrences, ulcers associated with diarrhea, ulcers occurring after ulcer surgery, ulcers with complications, ulcers with hypercalcemia or a family histories of ulcers, and ulcers not related to *Helicobacter pylori* or nonsteroidal antiinflammatory drugs (NSAIDs)

 CLINICAL FINDINGS

SYMPTOMS AND SIGNS

- Peptic ulcers in >90%, usually solitary and in proximal duodenal bulb, but may be multiple or in distal duodenum
- Isolated gastric ulcers do not occur
- Gastroesophageal reflux symptoms
- Diarrhea, steatorrhea, and weight loss (in ~33%) secondary to pancreatic enzyme inactivation

DIFFERENTIAL DIAGNOSIS

- Peptic ulcer disease due to other cause, eg, NSAIDs, *H pylori*
- Gastroesophageal reflux disease, esophagitis, gastritis, pancreatitis, or cholecystitis
- Diarrhea due to other cause
- Other gut neuroendocrine tumor: carcinoid, insulinoma, VIPoma, glucagonoma, somatostatinoma
- Hypergastrinemia due to other cause: atrophic gastritis, gastric outlet obstruction, pernicious anemia, chronic renal failure

DIAGNOSIS

LABORATORY TESTS

- Fasting serum gastrin concentration increased (>150 pg/mL) in patients not taking H_2 receptor antagonists for 24 h or proton pump inhibitor for 6 days
- Obtain serum calcium, parathyroid hormone, prolactin, leutinizing hormone-follicle-stimulating hormone, and growth hormone level in all patients with Zollinger-Ellison syndrome to exclude MEN 1
- Gastric pH of >3.0 implies hypochlorhydria and excludes gastrinoma

IMAGING STUDIES

- CT, MRI, and transabdominal ultrasound have sensitivity of <50–70% for hepatic metastases and 35% for primary tumors
- Somatostatin receptor scintigraphy (SRS) has high sensitivity (> 90%) for detecting hepatic metastases, much lower sensitivity the primary tumor
- Endoscopic ultrasonography (EUS) is indicated in patients with negative SRS, has sensitivity of >90% for tumors of the pancreatic head and ~50% for tumors in the duodenal wall or adjacent lymph nodes
- Combination of SRS and EUS can localize >90% of primary gastrinomas preoperatively

DIAGNOSTIC PROCEDURES

- Secretin stimulation test distinguishes Zollinger-Ellison syndrome from other causes of hypergastrinemia
- Secretin, 2 units/kg IV, produces a rise in serum gastrin of >200 pg/mL within 2–30 min in 85% of patients with gastrinoma

Zollinger-Ellison Syndrome

 TREATMENT

MEDICATIONS

- Proton pump inhibitors (omeprazole, rabeprazole, pantoprazole, esomeprazole, or lansoprazole), 40–120 mg/day, titrated to achieve a basal acid output of <10 mEq/h for metastatic disease

SURGERY

- Primary resection of gastrinoma at laparotomy for localized disease
- Preoperative studies and intraoperative palpation and sonography allow successful localization and resection in the majority of cases
- Surgical resection of isolated hepatic metastases

 OUTCOME

COMPLICATIONS

- In patients with unresectable disease, complications of gastric acid hypersecretion can be prevented in almost all cases by sufficient titration of proton pump inhibitors
- Treatment options for metastatic disease include interferon, octreotide, combination therapy, and chemoembolization

PROGNOSIS

- 15-year survival of patients without liver metastases at initial presentation is >80%
- 10-year survival of patients with hepatic metastases is 30%

WHEN TO REFER

- All patients with Zollinger-Ellison syndrome should be referred to a gastrointestinal surgeon with expertise in evaluation and management

 EVIDENCE

PRACTICE GUIDELINES

- Cheer SM et al: Pantoprazole: an update of its pharmacological properties and therapeutic use in the management of acid-related disorders. Drugs 2003; 63:101. [PMID: 12487624]
- Li ML et al: Gastrinoma. Curr Treat Options Oncol 2001;2:337. [PMID: 12057114]
- Quan C et al: Management of peptic ulcer disease not related to *Helicobacter pylori* or NSAIDs. Am J Gastroenterol 2002;97:2950. [PMID: 12492176]

WEB SITES

- MEDLINEplus—Zollinger-Ellison syndrome
  http://www.nlm.nih.gov/medlineplus/ency/article/000325.htm
- National Digestive Diseases Information Clearinghouse—Zollinger-Ellison syndrome
  http://digestive.niddk.nih.gov/ddiseases/pubs/zollinger/index.htm

INFORMATION FOR PATIENTS

- Cleveland Clinic—Zollinger-Ellison syndrome
  http://www.clevelandclinic.org/health/health-info/docs/1200/1238.asp?index=5956
- Florida State University College of Medicine—Zollinger-Ellison syndrome
  http://fsumed-dl.slis.ua.edu/clinical/gastroenterology/upper/stomachdisorders/zollinger.html
- Mayo Clinic—Zollinger-Ellison syndrome
  http://www.mayoclinic.com/invoke.cfm?objectid=00895C9E-1914-4475-86F645783A952DE7

REFERENCE

- Li ML et al: Gastrinoma. Curr Treat Options Oncol 2001;2:337. [PMID: 12057114]

Kenneth R. McQuaid, MD

A–Z
in Brief

Abortion, Recurrent

 KEY FEATURES

- Defined as loss of three or more previable (< 500 g) pregnancies in succession
- Women with three previous unexplained losses have a 70–80% chance of carrying a subsequent pregnancy to viability

 CLINICAL FINDINGS

- Occurs in 0.4–0.8% of all pregnancies
- Clinical findings are similar to those in spontaneous abortion

 DIAGNOSIS

- Preconception therapy aims to detect maternal or paternal defects contributing to abortion; these are found in about 50% of couples
- Polycystic ovaries, thyroid abnormalities, and diabetes should be ruled out
- Hypercoagulable states should be ruled out
- Endometrial tissue should be examined to determine the adequacy of its response to hormones in the postovulatory phase
- Hysteroscopy or hysterography can exclude or uterine abnormalities
- Chromosomal analysis of partners identifies balanced translocations in 5% of couples

 TREATMENT

- Early prenatal care and frequent office visits are routine
- Complete bed rest is justified only for bleeding or pain
- Empiric sex steroid therapy is contraindicated

William R. Crombleholme, MD

Acetaminophen Overdose

 KEY FEATURES

- Toxic dose: > 200 mg/kg or 7 g (acute) or more than 4–6 g/day (chronic)
- Nausea, vomiting early after acute ingestion
- Hepatic necrosis evident after 24–36 h
- Fulminant hepatic failure can occur

 CLINICAL FINDINGS

- Early: nausea and vomiting
- After 24 h: elevated transaminases, evidence of hepatic dysfunction and fulminant hepatic failure
- Massive overdose can cause coma, hypotension, metabolic acidosis

 DIAGNOSIS

- Elevated serum acetaminophen level (> 150 mg/L at 4 h or 75 mg/L at 8 h)
- Chronic excessive dosing may produce only moderately elevated levels
- Elevated hepatic transaminases, prothrombin time/INR, bilirubin
- Metabolic acidosis, encephalopathy indicate poor prognosis

 TREATMENT

- Oral activated charcoal (if given within 2–3 h of acute ingestion)
- Oral *N*-acetylcysteine (NAC), 140 mg/kg loading dose, followed by 70 mg/kg q4h
- Traditional US oral regimen: 72 h
- UK/Europe: IV NAC for 20 h
- Alternate oral treatment end point: may stop NAC if no evident liver injury at 36 h after ingestion
- Fulminant liver failure may require emergency liver transplantation

Kent R. Olsen, MD

Acidosis, Respiratory

 KEY FEATURES

- Acute compensation is an increase in serum HCO_3 of 1 mEq/L per 10 mm Hg increase in P_{CO_2}, and for chronic respiratory acidosis, an increase in serum HCO_3^- of 3.5 mEq/L per 10 mm Hg increase in P_{CO_2}

 CLINICAL FINDINGS

- Acutely, somnolence, confusion, myoclonus, asterixis
- Increased intracranial pressure (papilledema, pseudotumor cerebri)
- Coma from CO_2 narcosis

 DIAGNOSIS

- Low arterial pH, increased P_{CO_2}
- In the chronic state, HCO_3 may be elevated along with hypochloremia from NH_4^+ and Cl^- renal loss (Table 82)

 TREATMENT

- Administer naloxone, 0.04–2 mg IV for possible drug overdose
- For all forms of respiratory acidosis, treatment is to improve ventilation

Masafumi Fukagawa, MD, PhD, FJSIM
Kiyoshi Kurokawa, MD, MACP
Maxine A. Papadakis, MD

Acrocyanosis

KEY FEATURES

- An uncommon vasospastic disorder characterized by persistent cyanosis of the hands and feet and, to a lesser degree, the forearms and legs
- Associated with arteriolar vasoconstriction combined with dilation of the subcapillary venous plexus of the skin
- Worse in cold weather; does not completely disappear during warm
- Occurs primarily in women, most common in the teens and 20s; may improve with advancing age or during pregnancy

CLINICAL FINDINGS

- Symmetric coldness, sweating, slight edema, cyanotic discoloration of the hands or feet
- Peripheral pulses are normal
- Pain, trophic lesions, and disability do not occur

DIAGNOSIS

- Characteristic clinical picture

TREATMENT

- Avoidance of cold exposure

Louis M. Messina, MD
Laura K. Pak, MD
Lawrence M. Tierney, Jr, MD

Actinic Keratosis

KEY FEATURES

- Actinic keratoses are considered premalignant, but only 1:1000 lesions/yr progress to become squamous cell carcinomas

CLINICAL FINDINGS

- Actinic keratoses are small (0.2–1 cm) patches—flesh-colored, pink, or slightly hyperpigmented—that feel like sandpaper and are tender when the finger is drawn over them
- They occur on sun-exposed parts of the body in persons of fair complexion

DIAGNOSIS

- Clinical
- Differential diagnosis includes squamous cell carcinoma, Bowen's disease (squamous cell carcinoma in situ), nonpigmented seborrheic keratosis, psoriasis, seborrheic dermatitis, seborrheic keratosis, Paget's disease. See differential diagnosis for *Scaly lesions*

TREATMENT

- Liquid nitrogen is a rapid, effective method of eradication. The lesions crust and disappear in 10–14 days
- An alternative treatment is the use of 0.5%–5% fluorouracil cream (new 0.5% formulation, Carac). This agent may be rubbed into the lesions morning and night until they become red and sore, crusted, and eroded (usually 2–3 weeks), and then it is stopped. Alternately, 5-fluorouracil 0.5% cream once daily for 4–6 weeks

Timothy G. Berger, MD

Adenovirus Infections

KEY FEATURES

- More than 40 types, which produce a variety of clinical syndromes
- Usually self-limited except in immunosuppressed hosts

CLINICAL FINDINGS

- Common cold
- Nonstreptococcal exudative pharyngitis
- Lower respiratory tract infections
- Epidemic keratoconjunctivitis
- Hemorrhagic cystitis
- Acute gastroenteritis
- Disseminated disease in transplant recipients

DIAGNOSIS

- Can be cultured from appropriate specimens when definitive diagnosis is desired

TREATMENT

- Disease usually self-limited
- Immunocompromised patients often treated with ribavirin, although efficacy unclear
- Vaccine against certain strains used in military personnel to prevent outbreaks

Wayne X. Shandera, MD
Samuel Shelburne, MD

Alkalosis, Respiratory

 KEY FEATURES

- Symptoms in acute respiratory alkalosis are related to decreased cerebral blood flow
- Causes include the following:
  - Hyperventilation syndrome
  - Hypoxia, including severe anemia
  - CNS-mediated disorders (anxiety hyperventilation, cerebrovascular accident, infection, trauma, tumor, pharmacological and hormonal stimulation [salicylates, nicotine, xanthines], pregnancy [progesterone], hepatic failure, septicemia, recovery from metabolic acidosis, heat exposure)
  - Pulmonary disease
  - Mechanical overventilation

 CLINICAL FINDINGS

- Acutely, light-headedness, anxiety, paresthesias, numbness about the mouth, and a tingling sensation in the hands and feet
- Tetany in severe alkalosis from a fall in ionized calcium
- In chronic cases, findings are those of the responsible condition
- Elevated arterial blood pH, with low P_{CO_2}
- Serum bicarbonate is decreased in chronic respiratory alkalosis. Although serum HCO_3^- is frequently below 15 mEq/L in metabolic acidosis, it is unusual to see such a low level in respiratory alkalosis, and its presence implies a superimposed (noncompensatory) metabolic acidosis

 TREATMENT

- Treatment is directed toward the underlying cause
- In acute hyperventilation syndrome from anxiety, rebreathing into a paper bag increases P_{CO_2}. Sedation may be necessary if the process persists
- Rapid correction of chronic respiratory alkalosis may result in metabolic acidosis as P_{CO_2} is increased in the setting of previous compensatory decrease in HCO_3^-

Masafumi Fukagawa, MD, PhD, FJSIM
Kiyoshi Kurokawa, MD, MACP
Maxine A. Papadakis, MD

Alkaptonuria

 KEY FEATURES

- Alkaptonuria is caused by a recessively inherited deficiency of the enzyme homogentisic acid oxidase
- Homogentisic acid accumulates slowly in cartilage throughout the body, leading to degenerative joint disease of the spine and peripheral joints

 CLINICAL FINDINGS

- Back pain; difficult to distinguish from ankylosing spondylitis
- On radiograph sacroiliac joints are not fused
- Examination shows slight darkish-blue color below the skin in areas overlying cartilage, such as in the ears, called "ochronosis"
- In some patients, more severe hyperpigmentation in the sclera, conjunctiva, and cornea
- Accumulation of metabolites in heart valves can lead to aortic or mitral stenosis
- Predisposition to coronary artery disease

 DIAGNOSIS

- Homogentisic acid is present in large amounts in the urine, which turns black spontaneously on exposure to air
- Quantitative analysis of homogentisic acid in urine or plasma 3

 TREATMENT

- Nonsteroidal antiinflammatory drugs for arthritis
- Although the syndrome causes considerable morbidity, life expectancy is reduced only modestly

Reed E. Pyeritz, MD, PhD

Allergic Bronchopulmonary Aspergillosis (ABPA)

 KEY FEATURES

- Also known as allergic bronchopulmonary mycosis
- A bronchopulmonary hypersensitivity disorder caused by allergy to fungal antigens
- Seen in atopic asthmatics aged 20–40, usually in response to *Aspergillus* species

 CLINICAL FINDINGS

- Dyspnea, wheezing, cough, brown-flecked sputum
- Relapses after therapy are common
- Complications include bronchiectasis, hemoptysis, and pulmonary fibrosis

 DIAGNOSIS

- Primary criteria: (1) history of asthma, (2) peripheral eosinophilia, (3) immediate skin reactivity, or (4) precipitating antibodies to *Aspergillus* antigen, (5) elevated serum IgE, (6) pulmonary infiltrates, (7) central bronchiectasis
- Secondary criteria: *Aspergillus* in sputum, a history of brown-flecked sputum, or delayed skin reactivity to *Aspergillus* antigen
- Presence of primary criteria 1–6 makes diagnosis almost certain

 TREATMENT

- Prednisone, 0.5–1 mg/kg/day, for at least 2 mo, then careful tapering
- Itraconazole, 200 mg QD to BID, may be added for steroid-dependent patients
- Bronchodilators are helpful

Mark S. Chesnutt, MD
Thomas J. Prendergast, MD

Amenorrhea, Primary

 KEY FEATURES

- Menarche ordinarily occurs between 11 and 15 yr (average age in US, 12.7 yr)
- Primary amenorrhea is failure of any menses to appear
- Evaluation recommended at age 14 if no menarche or breast development or if height in lowest 3%; recommended at age 16 if no menarche
- Causes of primary amenorrhea:
  - Hypothalamic-pituitary (low-normal FSH): idiopathic delayed puberty; pituitary tumor; hypothalamic amenorrhea (eg, stress, weight change, exercise); anorexia nervosa; hypothyroidism; Cushing's syndrome; GnRH or gonadotropin deficiency (eg, Kallmann's syndrome or craniopharyngioma)
  - Hyperandrogenism (low-normal FSH): adrenal tumor or adrenal hyperplasia; polycystic ovary syndrome; ovarian tumor; exogenous androgenic steroids
  - Ovarian causes (high FSH): gonadal dysgenesis (Turner's syndrome); autoimmune ovarian failure; ovarian enzyme deficiencies (rare)
  - Pseudohermaphroditism (high LH): testosterone synthesis defect, complete androgen resistance (testicular feminization)
  - Anatomic defect (normal FSH): vaginal agenesis, absent uterus, atrophic endometrium, imperforate hymen
  - Pregnancy (high hCG)

 CLINICAL FINDINGS

- Nausea, amenorrhea, breast engorgement, weight gain suggest pregnancy
- Headaches or visual field abnormalities suggest pituitary or hypothalamic tumor
- Obesity and short stature suggest Cushing's syndrome
- Hirsutism, virilization, and acne suggest excessive testosterone
- Short stature suggests growth hormone or thyroid hormone deficiency
- Short stature and gonadal dysgenesis indicate Turner's syndrome
- Tall stature suggests eunuchoidism or gigantism
- Anosmia suggests Kallmann's syndrome

- Perform external pelvic and rectal examination to assess for hymenal patency and presence of a uterus

 DIAGNOSIS

- Check serum FSH, LH, prolactin, testosterone, TSH, free T_4, and pregnancy test
- Check serum electrolytes and further hormonal evaluation if patient is virilized or hypertensive.
- Obtain MRI of hypothalamus and pituitary if low-normal FSH and LH, especially if high prolactin
- Consider karyotyping to diagnose XO-XX mosaicism if normal uterus and high FSH without classic features of Turner's syndrome

 TREATMENT

- Treatment directed at underlying cause
- Hormone replacement therapy for females with permanent hypogonadism
- See *Secondary amenorrhea & menopause*

Paul A. Fitzgerald, MD

Anaerobic Infections, Bacteremia & Endocarditis

 KEY FEATURES

- Anaerobic bacteremia usually originates from the GI tract, the oropharynx, decubitus ulcers, or the female genital tract. Endocarditis resulting from anaerobic and microaerophilic streptococci and bacteroides (rare) originates from the same sites

 CLINICAL FINDINGS

- Related to site of original and metastatic infection

 DIAGNOSIS

- Culture of blood and affected tissues

 TREATMENT

- Most cases of anaerobic or microaerophilic streptococcal endocarditis can be effectively treated with 12–20 million units of penicillin G daily for 4–6 weeks, but optimal therapy of other types of anaerobic bacterial endocarditis must rely on laboratory guidance. Metronidazole, 500 mg IV q8h, should be used if *Bacteroides* sp is identified

Henry F. Chambers, MD

Anaerobic Infections, Central Nervous System

KEY FEATURES

- Common cause of brain abscess, subdural empyema, or septic CNS thrombophlebitis
- The organisms reach CNS by direct extension from sinusitis, otitis, or mastoiditis or by hematogenous spread from chronic lung infections

CLINICAL FINDINGS

- Various neurological deficits

DIAGNOSIS

- CT scan
- Culture of infected tissue

TREATMENT

- Antimicrobial therapy (eg, penicillin, 20 million units IV, in combination with metronidazole, 500–750 mg IV q8h) is an important adjunct to surgical drainage. Duration of therapy is 6–8 weeks
- Some small multiple brain abscesses can be treated with antibiotics alone without surgical drainage

Henry F. Chambers, MD

Anaerobic Infections, Chest

KEY FEATURES

- Frequently occur in the setting of poor oral hygiene and periodontal disease, aspiration of saliva (which contains 10^8 anaerobic organisms per milliliter in addition to aerobes)
- May lead to necrotizing pneumonia, lung abscess, and empyema
- Polymicrobial infection is the rule. Anaerobes—particularly *P melaninogenica,* fusobacteria, and peptostreptococci—are frequently isolated etiological agents

CLINICAL FINDINGS

- Fever, productive cough, night sweats, weight loss
- Poor dentition (frequently)

DIAGNOSIS

- Pleural fluid culture
- CXR
- CT scan

TREATMENT

- Clindamycin, 600 mg IV once, followed by 300 mg PO q6–8h, is the treatment of choice
- Penicillin, 2 million units IV q4h, followed by amoxicillin, 750–1000 mg PO q12h, is a reasonable alternative
- These infections respond slowly. A duration of 3–4 weeks or more of antimicrobial therapy is typical

Henry F. Chambers, MD

Anaerobic Infections, Intra-Abdominal

KEY FEATURES

- In the colon there are up to 10^{11} anaerobes per gram of content, predominantly *B fragilis*, clostridia, and peptostreptococci
- These organisms play a central role in most intra-abdominal abscesses (diverticulitis, appendicitis, or perirectal abscess) and may also participate in hepatic abscess and cholecystitis
- The bacteriology of these infections includes anaerobes as well as enteric gram-negative rods and, on occasion, enterococci

CLINICAL FINDINGS

- Related to infected organ

DIAGNOSIS

- Exam, labs, and CT scan

TREATMENT

- Therapy should be directed both against anaerobes and gram-negative aerobes
- Antibiotics that are reliably active against *B fragilis* include metronidazole, chloramphenicol, imipenem, ampicillin-sulbactam, ticarcillin-clavulanic acid, piperacillin-tazobactam
- Table 135, page 1317 summarizes the antibiotic regimens for management of moderate to moderately severe infections (eg, patient hemodynamically stable, good surgical drainage possible or established, low APACHE score, no multiple-organ failure) and severe infections (eg, major peritoneal soilage, large or multiple abscesses, patient hemodynamically unstable), particularly if drug-resistant organisms are suspected

Henry F. Chambers, MD

Anaerobic Infections, Skin & Soft Tissue

 KEY FEATURES

- Usually occur after trauma, with inadequate blood supply, in association with diabetes, or after surgery and are most common in areas contaminated by oral or fecal flora
- Several terms (eg, bacterial synergistic gangrene, synergistic necrotizing cellulitis, necrotizing fasciitis, nonclostridial crepitant cellulitis) have been used to classify these infections. Although there are some differences in microbiology among them, their differentiation on clinical grounds alone is difficult
- All are mixed infections caused by aerobic and anaerobic organisms

 CLINICAL FINDINGS

- There may be progressive tissue necrosis and a putrid odor

 DIAGNOSIS

- Surgical exploration

 TREATMENT

- Broad-spectrum antibiotics active against both anaerobes and gram-positive and gram-negative aerobes (eg, piperacillin-tazobactam or vancomycin plus metronidazole plus gentamicin or tobramycin) should be instituted empirically and modified by culture results (Tables 122, page 1303, 123, page 1306, 135, page 1317)
- Require aggressive surgical débridement of necrotic tissue for cure

Henry F. Chambers, MD

Anaerobic Infections, Upper Respiratory Tract

 KEY FEATURES

- *Prevotella melaninogenica* and anaerobic spirochetes are commonly involved in periodontal infections
- These organisms, fusobacteria, and peptostreptococci may cause chronic sinusitis, peritonsillar abscess, chronic otitis media, and mastoiditis

 CLINICAL FINDINGS

- Related to infected organ

 DIAGNOSIS

- Culture
- CT scan

 TREATMENT

- Tables 122, page 1305, 123, page 1306
- Oral anaerobic organisms have been uniformly susceptible to penicillin, but there has been a trend of increasing penicillin resistance, usually resulting from β-lactamase production
- Penicillin, 1–2 million units IV q4h (if parenteral therapy is required) or 0.5 g orally QID for less severe infections, or clindamycin, 600 mg IV q8h or 300 mg PO q6h, can be used
- Indolent, established infections (eg, mastoiditis or osteomyelitis) may require prolonged courses of therapy (eg, 4–6 weeks or longer)

Henry F. Chambers, MD

Anal Cancer

 KEY FEATURES

- Carcinoma of the anus is relatively rare: only 1–2% of all cancers of the large intestine and anus
- Squamous cancers (keratinizing, transitional cell, and cloacogenic; 80%); the rest are adenocarcinomas (20%)
- Increased incidence among people practicing receptive anal intercourse, those with a history of other sexually transmitted diseases, and those with HIV infection
- Human papillomavirus (HPV) infection in > 80%
- Increased risk in combined HIV and HPV infection

 CLINICAL FINDINGS

- Anal bleeding, pain, and local tumor

 DIAGNOSIS

- Anoscopy and biopsy establish diagnosis
- MR scan and endoluminal ultrasonogram for staging

 TREATMENT

- Local excision for small superficial lesions of the perianal skin
- Combined-modality therapy for tumors invading the sphincter or rectum: external radiation with simultaneous chemotherapy (fluorouracil and either mitomycin or cisplatin)
- Local control achieved in 80% of patients
- Radical surgery (abdominoperineal resection) for patients who fail chemotherapy and radiation therapy
- 5-yr survival rate is 60–70% for localized (stages I–III) disease and >25% for metastatic (stage IV) disease

Kenneth R. McQuaid, MD

Anal Fissures

 KEY FEATURES

- Linear or rocket-shaped ulcers usually <5 mm
- Occur most commonly in the posterior midline, 10% anteriorly
- Arise from trauma during defecation

 CLINICAL FINDINGS

- Severe, tearing pain during defecation followed by throbbing discomfort
- May lead to constipation because of fear of recurrent pain
- Mild associated hematochezia
- Chronic fissures fibrosis and a skin tag at the outermost edge (sentinel pile)

 DIAGNOSIS

- Diagnosis confirmed by visual inspection of the anal verge while gently separating the buttocks
- Digital and anoscopic examinations may cause severe pain and may not be possible

 TREATMENT

- Fiber supplements
- Sitz baths
- Hydrocortisone 1% ointment
- Topical nitroglycerin 0.2–0.5% ointment applied by cotton swab to the anus and anal canal BID for 6–8 weeks heals up to 80% of patients with chronic anal fissure
- Botulinum toxin (20 units) injection into the internal anal sphincter heals 90%
- Partial lateral internal sphincterotomy is effective for chronic or recurrent fissures but may be complicated by minor fecal incontinence

Kenneth R. McQuaid, MD

Anemia of Chronic Disease

 KEY FEATURES

- Many chronic systemic diseases associated with mild or moderate anemia (eg, chronic infection or inflammation, cancer, liver disease)
- Anemia of chronic renal failure has different pathophysiology (reduced erythropoietin) and is usually more severe
- Largely caused by sequestration of iron within reticuloendothelial system
- Decreased dietary intake of folate or iron common in ill patients, causing coexistent folate or iron deficiency. Many also have ongoing GI bleeding. Hemodialysis patients regularly lose both iron and folate during dialysis

 CLINICAL FINDINGS

- Symptoms of anemia, which is usually modest
- Suspect diagnosis in patients with known chronic diseases

 DIAGNOSIS

- Hematocrit usually > 25% (except in renal failure); if < 25%, evaluate for coexistent iron deficiency or folic acid deficiency
- Mean corpuscular volume usually normal or slightly low
- Red blood cell morphology nondiagnostic; reticulocyte count neither strikingly reduced nor increased
- Low serum iron, low transferrin saturation
- Normal or increased serum ferritin; serum ferritin < 30 μg/L suggests coexistent iron deficiency
- Normal or increased bone marrow iron stores

 TREATMENT

- In most cases, no treatment necessary
- Purified recombinant erythropoietin (eg, 30,000 units SC every week) effective for anemia of renal failure, AIDS, cancer, rheumatoid arthritis
- In renal failure, optimal response to erythropoietin requires adequate dialysis
- Erythropoietin is very expensive; used only when patient is transfusion dependent or when quality of life clearly improved by hematological response

Charles A. Linker, MD

Anemia, Hemolytic

 KEY FEATURES

- Anemia present only when RBC survival is extremely short or ability of bone marrow to compensate is impaired for some second reason
- Absence of RBC production causes hematocrit to fall ~3% points per week; if fall is faster, suspect blood loss or hemolysis
- Hemolytic anemia can be classified as:

  1. Coombs positive (immune) hemolytic anemia: autoimmune, drugs, infection, lymphoproliferative disease, Rh or ABO incompatibility

  2. Coombs negative hemolytic anemia: intrinsic red cell disease

  – Abnormal hemoglobin: sickle cell disease, thalassemia, methemoglobinemia

  – Membrane defect: hereditary spherocytosis, hereditary elliptocytosis, paroxysmal nocturnal hemoglobinuria

  – Enzyme defect: G6PD deficiency, pyruvate kinase deficiency

  3. Coombs negative hemolytic anemia: extrinsic disease

  – Microangiopathic hemolytic anemia: thrombotic thrombocytopenic purpura, hemolytic uremic syndrome, disseminated intravascular coagulation, prosthetic valve hemolysis, metastatic adenocarcinoma, vasculitis, malignant hypertension, HELLP syndrome

  – Splenic sequestration

  – Infection: *Plasmodium, Clostridium, Borrelia*

  – Burns

 CLINICAL FINDINGS

- Symptoms of anemia
- Jaundice, pigment (calcium bilirubinate) gallstones, and cholecystitis in chronic hemolysis
- Palpable spleen

 DIAGNOSIS

- Serum haptoglobin level may be low
- Reticulocytosis usually present, unless second disorder (infection, folate deficiency) is superimposed on hemolysis
- Transient hemoglobinemia occurs if intravascular hemolysis

- Hemoglobinuria occurs when capacity for reabsorption of hemoglobin by renal tubular cells is exceeded
- Urine hemosiderin test positive; indicates prior intravascular hemolysis
- Hemoglobinemia and methemalbuminemia if severe intravascular hemolysis
- Indirect bilirubin elevated, total bilirubin elevated to ≥ 4 mg/dL
- Serum lactate dehydrogenase levels strikingly elevated in microangiopathic hemolysis; may be elevated in other hemolytic anemias

 TREATMENT

- Treatment of the underlying cause
- Folic acid, 1 mg PO QD
- Transfusions may be needed

Charles A. Linker, MD

Anemia, Sideroblastic

 KEY FEATURES

- Heterogeneous group of disorders in which reduced hemoglobin synthesis occurs because of failure to incorporate heme into protoporphyrin to form hemoglobin
- Iron accumulates, particularly in mitochondria
- Sometimes represents stage in evolution of a generalized bone marrow disorder (myelodysplasia) that may terminate in acute leukemia
- Other causes include chronic alcoholism and lead poisoning

 CLINICAL FINDINGS

- Symptoms of anemia; no other specific clinical features

 DIAGNOSIS

- Anemia usually moderate, hematocrit 20–30%
- Mean corpuscular volume usually normal or slightly increased, but occasionally low, leading to confusion with iron deficiency
- Peripheral blood smear characteristically shows dimorphic population of RBCs: 1 normal and 1 hypochromic
- Coarse basophilic stippling of RBCs and serum lead level elevated in lead poisoning
- Bone marrow iron stain shows generalized increase in iron stores and ringed sideroblasts (RBCs with iron deposits encircling the nucleus) and marked erythroid hyperplasia (resulting from ineffective erythropoiesis)
- Serum iron and transferrin saturation high

 TREATMENT

- Occasionally, transfusion required for severe anemia
- Erythropoietin therapy not usually effective

Charles A. Linker, MD

Angiitis of the CNS, Primary

 KEY FEATURES

- Small and medium-sized vasculitis limited to the brain and spinal cord

 CLINICAL FINDINGS

- Biopsy-proved cases have predominated in men who present with a history of weeks to months of headaches, encephalopathy, and multifocal strokes
- Systemic symptoms and signs are absent

 DIAGNOSIS

- MRI of the brain is almost always abnormal
- Spinal fluid often reveals a mild lymphocytosis and a modest increase in protein level
- Angiograms classically reveal a "string of beads" pattern produced by alternating segments of arterial narrowing and dilation
- However, neither MRI nor angiogram appearance is specific for vasculitis
- Definitive diagnosis requires a compatible clinical picture; exclusion of infection, neoplasm, or metabolic disorder or drug exposure (eg, cocaine) that can mimic primary angiitis of the central nervous system; and a positive brain biopsy
- Many patients who fit this clinical profile (stroke, HA, but no encephalopathy) and have disease diagnosed by angiography (but not biopsy) probably have vasospasm rather than true vasculitis
- Routine laboratory tests are usually normal

 TREATMENT

- Usually improve with prednisone therapy
- May require cyclophosphamide

David B. Hellmann, MD, FACP
John H. Stone, MD, MPH

Angina Pectoris, Unstable

 KEY FEATURES

- Accelerating or "crescendo" pattern of angina pectoris (see *Angina pectoris*)
- Worse prognosis than stable angina because more likely to progress to myocardial infarction
- Unstable new-onset angina, if exertional and responsive to rest and medication, is not associated with poor prognosis

 CLINICAL FINDINGS

- Angina occurs at rest or with less exertion than previously
- Lasts longer
- Is less responsive to medication

 DIAGNOSIS

- Most patients with unstable angina manifest ECG changes during pain: ST-segment depression, T wave flattening, or inversion
- ST-segment elevation is more ominous and has to be considered and treated as myocardial infarction until proven otherwise
- Possible left ventricular dysfunction during pain and for a period afterward
- See *Angina pectoris* for other symptoms and signs

 TREATMENT

- Hospitalization, bed rest, telemetry, and supplemental oxygen
- Rule out myocardial infarction with three serial cardiac enzymes (troponin I, troponin T, and CK-MB) q6–8 h and follow-up ECGs
- Cardiology consultation as soon as possible
- Benzodiazepine sedation if anxiety is present
- **Aspirin** (first-line therapy): 325 mg immediately, and then once daily
- **Heparin** (first-line therapy) if symptoms have occurred within the past 24 hours, are stuttering, or are unremitting
- **Low-molecular-weight heparin** (eg, enoxaparin 1mg/kg subcutaneously q12 h, slightly superior to IV heparin
- Clopidogrel (300-mg loading dose, then 75 mg/day) is sometimes added as third agent

- **Nitrates** (first-line therapy): sublingual, oral, or topical nitroglycerin initially, but continuous drip if pain persists or recurs
  – Continuous BP monitoring required
  – Start at 10 μg/min, titrate up to 1 μg/kg/min over 30–60 minutes, increasing to higher doses if needed
- **Opioids,** intravenous for unrelieved pain and pulmonary congestion
- **β-blockers** (first-line therapy) oral or intravenous for more rapid effect
  – For example, metoprolol 5-mg doses × 3 at 5-min intervals), unless overt heart failure
  – Titrate up for goal heart rate of 60/min as tolerated by blood pressure
- Reduce systolic blood pressure to 100–120 with nitroglycerin and β-blockers, except in patients with severe hypertension previously
- Institute early exercise or pharmacologic stress testing or coronary arteriography
- If continued pain despite above medications, fluctuating ST-segment depression, or positive cardiac enzymes, consider GIIb/IIIa receptor blockers (eg, tirofiban, 0.4 mg/kg/min for 30 min, then 0.1 μg/kg/min) pending emergent arteriography
- Thrombolytics do not have a role in unstable angina without ST-segment elevation

Barry Massie, MD
Thomas Amidon, MD

Angiostrongyliasis Costaricensis

 KEY FEATURES

- The helminth causes an eosinophilic ileocolitis, has been identified in humans (predominantly children) in Mexico, Central America, Venezuela, Brazil, and USA
- The known geographic range of the parasite in rodents (the definitive host) extends from northern South America to Texas
- Infection occurs from ingestion of the larvae in the intermediate host (slugs, snails) or from food contaminated by larvae in slug or snail mucus
- In humans, the larvae mature in the mesenteric vessels

 CLINICAL FINDINGS

- The inflammatory response to adult worms, larvae, and eggs can be severe, resulting in a marked eosinophilic granulomatous reaction and vasculitis and ischemic necrosis of the intestine
- Most cases involve the ileocecal region, appendix, ascending colon, regional nodes
- Findings include fever, right lower quadrant abdominal pain and a mass, leukocytosis, and eosinophilia
- Some patients have relapsing symptoms that can continue for months
- Bowel complications include perforation, bleeding, incomplete or complete obstruction, and infarction. The intraabdominal mass can mimic tumor

 DIAGNOSIS

- Neither eggs or larvae are passed in stool; diagnosis is made by agglutination serological test

 TREATMENT

- There is no specific treatment; albendazole, thiabendazole, or mebendazole can be tried (as above). Operative treatment is frequently necessary

Ankle Sprains

 KEY FEATURES

- Most involve the lateral ligament complex, particularly the anterior talofibular ligament

 CLINICAL FINDINGS

- Varus sprains include a spectrum of severity, ranging from slight loss of function to prompt swelling, prominent pain, and inability to bear weight
- Tenderness and marked swelling are typically present
- Hemorrhage from torn ligaments and damaged peroneal muscle tendons may cause substantial ecchymosis

 DIAGNOSIS

- Stability of the anterior talofibular and calcaneofibular ligaments should be assessed with the "anterior drawer" sign: With the foot held in slight plantar flexion, the examiner cups the patient's heel with one hand and the patient's shin with the other. The examiner then applies gentle anterior force in the plane of the patient's foot. Excessive anterior motion of the foot constitutes a positive test (grade III sprain). (Grades I and II correspond to mild to moderate injuries)
- Plain radiographs exclude bony injury

 TREATMENT

- RICE (*r*est, *i*ce, *c*ompression, *e*levation)
- Early application of a compression dressing is essential to control swelling and provide stability to the joint
- Weight bearing should be minimal, with liberal use of crutches
- Patients should be informed that symptoms from lateral ankle sprains may take weeks or months to resolve, and that this period will be prolonged by premature attempts to bear weight on the injured ankle
- Surgical repairs of ruptured lateral ligaments provide excellent outcomes but are usually necessary only in cases of chronically unstable joints

David B. Hellmann, MD, FACP
John H. Stone, MD, MPH

Anorectal Infections

 KEY FEATURES

- Proctitis is inflammation of the distal 15 cm of rectum
- Most cases of proctitis are sexually transmitted, especially by anal-receptive intercourse
- Proctocolitis is inflammation that extends above the rectum to the sigmoid colon or more proximally caused by *Campylobacter, Entamoeba histolytica, Shigella*, and enteroinvasive *Escherichia coli*
- Causes include *Neisseria gonorrhoeae, Treponema pallidum* (syphilis), *Chlamydia trachomatis*, herpes simplex virus type 2 (HSV-2), human papillomavirus (HPV)
- Venereal warts (condylomata acuminata) caused by HPV occur in up to 50% of homosexual men

 CLINICAL FINDINGS

- Proctitis: anorectal discomfort, tenesmus, constipation, and discharge
- Gonorrhea proctitis: itching, burning, tenesmus, and mucopurulent discharge
- Complications of untreated gonorrheal infections include strictures, fissures, fistulas, and perirectal abscesses
- Anal syphilis: asymptomatic, chancre, or proctitis
- In primary syphilis, chancre may mimic a fissure, fistula, or ulcer; in secondary syphilis, condylomata lata, foul-smelling mucous discharge, and inguinal lymphadenopathy
- *C trachomatis* causes proctitis similar to gonorrhea or lymphogranuloma venereum, proctocolitis with fever and bloody diarrhea, painful perianal ulcerations, anorectal strictures and fistulas, and inguinal lymphadenopathy (buboes)
- HSV-2 proctitis: severe pain, itching, constipation, tenesmus, urinary retention, and radicular pain; small vesicles or ulcers in the perianal area or anal canal
- Venereal warts noted on the perianal skin and within the anal canal; otherwise asymptomatic
- Higher rate of HPV progression to high-grade dysplasia or anal cancer in HIV-positive individuals

 DIAGNOSIS

- Gonorrhea proctitis: blind swab of the anal canal has sensitivity of < 60%
- Obtain Gram's stain and culture from the rectum during anoscopy, cultures from the urethra and pharynx in men, and cultures from the cervix in women
- Dark-field microscopy of scrapings from the chancre or condylomata diagnostic in anal syphilis
- Serum VDRL positive in 75% of primary and in 99% of secondary cases
- Culture of rectal discharge or rectal biopsy for *C trachomatis* has sensitivity of > 80%
- Sigmoidoscopy in HSV-2 shows vesicular or ulcerative lesions in the distal rectum
- Diagnosis by viral culture or HSV-2 antigen detection assays of vesicular fluid

 TREATMENT

- Cefixime, 400 mg PO once, eftriaxone, 250 mg IM once, or ciprofloxacin, 500 mg PO once, for *N gonorrhoeae*
- Doxycycline, 100 mg PO BID for 10 days, or ofloxacin, 300 mg PO BID for 10 days, for *C trachomatis*
- Benzathine penicillin G, 2.4 million units IM once, or doxycycline, 100 mg PO BID for 2 weeks, for *T pallidum*
- Acyclovir, 400 mg PO 5 times daily for 5–10 days, for HSV-2
- Chronic suppressive therapy for patients with AIDS and recurrent relapses
- Podophyllum resin applied topically for small perianal warts from HPV; CO_2 laser surgery or cryosurgery for anal lesions; higher relapse rate after therapy in HIV-positive individuals
- Examine and treat patient's sexual partners
- Surveillance anoscopy every 3–6 mo in HIV-positive individuals

Kenneth R. McQuaid, MD

Antiarrhythmic Agent Overdose

 ### KEY FEATURES

- Quinidine, disopyramide, and procainamide are class Ia antiarrhythmic agents, and flecainide is a class Ic agent

 ### CLINICAL FINDINGS

- Arrhythmias, syncope, hypotension, and widening of the QRS complex on the ECG (> 100–120 ms)
- With type Ia drugs, a lengthened QT interval and atypical or polymorphous ventricular tachycardia (torsades de pointes) may occur

 ### DIAGNOSIS

- Blood levels of quinidine and procainamide (and active metabolite NAPA) are generally available from hospital lab
- ECG monitoring for QRS and QT interval prolongation

 ### TREATMENT

- Administer activated charcoal, 60–100 g PO or via gastric tube, mixed in aqueous slurry for ingestions within 1 h. Do not use for comatose or convulsing patients unless they are endotracheally intubated
- Consider gastric lavage for recent (1 h) large ingestions. Consider whole bowel irrigation for ingestion of sustained-release formulations
- Perform continuous cardiac monitoring
- Treat cardiotoxicity (hypotension, QRS interval widening) with IV boluses of sodium bicarbonate, 50–100 mEq
- Torsades de pointes ventricular tachycardia may be treated with IV magnesium or overdrive pacing

Kent R. Olsen, MD

Antipsychotic Agent Overdose

 ### KEY FEATURES

- Chlorpromazine and related drugs are used as antiemetics and antipsychotic agents and as potentiators of analgesic and hypnotic drugs

 ### CLINICAL FINDINGS

- Drowsiness, orthostatic hypotension common, especially with agents that have α-blocking properties
- Larger doses can cause obtundation, miosis, severe hypotension, tachycardia, convulsions, coma
- Prolongation of QRS or QT intervals (or both) and ventricular arrhythmias may occur (particularly with thioridazine)
- With therapeutic or toxic doses, an acute extrapyramidal dystonic reaction similar to Parkinson's disease, with spasmodic contractions of the face and neck muscles, extensor rigidity of the back muscles, carpopedal spasm, and motor restlessness can be seen
- Severe rigidity accompanied by hyperthermia and metabolic acidosis (neuroleptic malignant syndrome) may occasionally occur and is life-threatening

 ### DIAGNOSIS

- Clinical

 ### TREATMENT

- Administer activated charcoal and consider gastric lavage for large ingestions
- Treat hypotension with fluids and pressor agents. Hypotension and cardiac arrhythmias associated with widened QRS intervals with thioridazine poisoning may respond to IV sodium bicarbonate as used for tricyclic antidepressants
- Treat hyperthermia and maintain cardiac monitoring
- For extrapyramidal signs, give diphenhydramine, 0.5–1 mg/kg IV, or benztropine mesylate, 0.01–0.02 mg/kg IM. Continue with oral doses for 1–2 days
- Bromocriptine, 2.5–7.5 mg PO daily, may treat mild or moderate neuroleptic malignant syndrome. Dantrolene, 2–5 mg/kg IV, can lessen muscle contractions

Kent R. Olsen, MD

Aortic Regurgitation

 ### KEY FEATURES

- Nonrheumatic causes are more common than rheumatic heart disease
- Nonrheumatic causes include bicuspid valves, infective endocarditis, hypertension, cystic medial necrosis, Marfan's syndrome, aortic dissection, ankylosing spondylitis, Reiter's syndrome, and syphilis

 ### CLINICAL FINDINGS

- High-pitched, decrescendo diastolic murmur along the left sternal border
- Hyperactive, enlarged left ventricle
- Wide pulse pressure with peripheral signs
- Usually slowly progressive and asymptomatic until middle age, although onset may sometimes be rapid, as in infective endocarditis or myocardial infarction
- Exertional dyspnea and fatigue are the most frequent symptoms, but paroxysmal nocturnal dyspnea and pulmonary edema may also occur
- May present with left-sided failure or chest pain
- Coronary artery disease and syncope are less common than in aortic stenosis

 ### DIAGNOSIS

- ECG: left ventricular hypertrophy
- CXR: left ventricular dilation
- Echo-Doppler confirms the diagnosis and estimates severity
- Serial assessments of left ventricular size and function are critical in determining the timing for valve replacement
- Cardiac catheterization can help quantify severity and is used preoperatively to evaluate the coronary and aortic root anatomy

 ### TREATMENT

- Surgery is often urgently required in rapid-onset regurgitation (even with active infection)
- Vasodilators (eg, hydralazine, nifedipine, and angiotensin-converting enzyme inhibitors) may be used transiently for preoperative stabilization
- In chronic cases, vasodilators can reduce the severity of regurgitation as well as postpone surgery in asymptomatic patients

- Surgery is usually indicated once aortic regurgitation causes symptoms
- Surgery is also indicated for those who have an ejection fraction < 45–50% or who exhibit progressive deterioration of left ventricular function irrespective of symptoms
- Operative mortality is usually 3–5%

Barry Massie, MD
Thomas Amidon, MD

Aortic Stenosis

 ## KEY FEATURES

- Most commonly caused by progressive valvular calcification (sclerosis precedes stenosis)
- Increasingly common with age
- Most common valve lesion requiring surgery in developed countries
- Much more frequent in men, smokers, and hypertensives

 ## CLINICAL FINDINGS

- Delayed and diminished carotid pulses
- Soft, absent, or paradoxically split S_2
- Harsh systolic murmur, sometimes with thrill along left sternal border, often radiating to the neck; may be louder at apex in older patients
- In adults, usually asymptomatic until middle or old age
- Left ventricular hypertrophy progresses over time
- Patients may present with left ventricular failure, angina pectoris, or syncope
- Syncope, typically exertional, may be due to arrhythmias (usually ventricular tachycardia, sometimes sinus bradycardia), hypotension, or decreased cerebral perfusion

 ## DIAGNOSIS

- ECG: usually shows left ventricular hypertrophy
- CXR fluoroscopy: calcified valve
- Echo-Doppler is usually diagnostic
- Cardiac catheterization is the definitive diagnostic procedure and should be performed in most patients to exclude concomitant coronary artery disease
- Stenosis must be distinguished from supravalvular and outflow obstruction of the left ventricular infundibulum

 ## TREATMENT

- After onset of heart failure, angina, or syncope, the mortality rate without surgery is 50% in 3 yr
- Surgery is indicated for all symptomatic patients, including those with left ventricular dysfunction
- Surgical mortality rate is 2–5%, higher (10%) with age >75, substantially higher with left ventricular dysfunction, severe coronary disease, or prior myocardial infarction
- Except in adolescents, balloon valvuloplasty should be reserved only for poor surgical candidates or as an intermediate procedure to stabilize high-risk patients before surgery

Barry M. Massie, MD
Thomas M. Amidon, MD

Aphthous Ulcer

 KEY FEATURES

- Canker sore or ulcerative stomatitis
- Large or persistent areas of ulcerative stomatitis may be secondary to erythema multiforme or drug allergies, acute herpes simplex, pemphigus, pemphigoid, bullous lichen planus, Behçet's disease, or inflammatory bowel disease
- Cause remains uncertain, although an association with human herpesvirus 6 has been suggested

 CLINICAL FINDINGS

- Very common and easy to recognize
- Found on nonkeratinized mucosa (eg, buccal and labial mucosa and not gingiva or palate)
- May be single or multiple, are usually recurrent, and appear as small (usually 1–2 mm but sometimes 1–2 cm), round painful ulcerations with yellow-gray fibrinoid centers surrounded by red halos
- The painful stage lasts 7–10 days; healing is completed in 1–3 weeks

 DIAGNOSIS

- Based on clinical appearance
- Squamous cell carcinoma may occasionally present in this fashion. When the diagnosis is not clear, incisional biopsy is indicated

TREATMENT

- Topical steroids (triamcinolone acetonide, 0.1%, or fluocinonide ointment, 0.05%) in an adhesive base (Orabase-Plain) provide symptomatic relief
- Other topical therapies are diclofenac 3% in hyaluronan 2.5%, doxymycine-cyanoacrylate, mouthwashes containing the enzymes amyloglucosidase and glucose oxidase, and amlexanox 5% oral paste
- A 1-week tapering course of prednisone (40–60 mg/day) can be used

Robert K. Jackler, MD
Michael J. Kaplan, MD

Arbovirus Encephalitides

 KEY FEATURES

- Arthropod-borne viruses
- St. Louis and California encephalitides common in US
- West Nile encephalitis identified in 1999; now present in much of US
- Disease in US tends to occur in outbreaks during periods of mosquito proliferation

 CLINICAL FINDINGS

- Age-dependent; residual neurological deficits more likely in the elderly
- Fevers, sore throat, stiff neck, nausea, vomiting, lethargy, coma
- Signs of meningeal irritation, tremors, cranial nerve palsies are common
- CSF: elevated protein and opening pressure and lymphocytosis
- Motor weakness common in West Nile infection

 DIAGNOSIS

- Clinical symptoms, with history of mosquito or other vector exposure
- Lymphocytopenia
- PCR assays may be diagnostic
- West Nile: serum and CSF IgM ELISA confirm the diagnosis

 TREATMENT

- Vigorous supportive measures
- Prevention: mosquito control measures

Wayne X. Shandera, MD
Samuel Shelburne, MD

Arsenic Poisoning

 KEY FEATURES

- Found in some pesticides and industrial chemicals

 CLINICAL FINDINGS

- Symptoms usually appear within 1 h after ingestion but may be delayed as long as 12 h
- Abdominal pain, vomiting, watery diarrhea, and skeletal muscle cramps
- Profound dehydration and shock may occur
- In chronic poisoning, symptoms can be vague but often include those of peripheral sensory neuropathy

 DIAGNOSIS

- Urinary arsenic levels may be falsely elevated after certain meals (eg, seafood) that contain large quantities of relatively nontoxic organic arsenic

 TREATMENT

EMERGENCY MEASURES

- Perform gastric lavage and administer 60–100 g of activated charcoal

ANTIDOTE

- For symptomatic patients or those with massive overdose, give dimercaprol injection (BAL), 10% solution in oil, 3–5 mg/kg IM q4–6h for 2 days. The side effects include nausea, vomiting, headache, and hypertension
- Follow dimercaprol with oral penicillamine, 100 mg/kg/day in 4 divided doses (maximum, 2 g/day), or succimer (DMSA), 10 mg/kg q8h for 1 week
- Consult a medical toxicologist or regional poison control center for advice regarding chelation

Kent R. Olsen, MD

Arthritis & Inflammatory Bowel Diseases

 ### KEY FEATURES

- One fifth of patients with inflammatory bowel disease have arthritis
- Second most common extraintestinal manifestation (after anemia)

 ### CLINICAL FINDINGS

- Two distinct forms of arthritis occur. The first is peripheral arthritis—usually a nondeforming asymmetric oligoarthritis of large joints—in which the activity of the joint disease parallels that of the bowel disease. The second is a spondylitis that is indistinguishable by symptoms or x-ray film from ankylosing spondylitis and follows a course independent of the bowel disease. About 50% of these patients are HLA-B27-positive
- About two-thirds of patients with Whipple's disease experience arthralgia or arthritis, most often an episodic, large-joint polyarthritis. The arthritis usually precedes GI manifestations by years and resolves as the diarrhea develops

 ### DIAGNOSIS

- Clinical
- Differential diagnosis includes reactive arthritis (Reiter's syndrome), ankylosing spondylitis, psoriatic arthritis, Whipple's disease

 ### TREATMENT

- Controlling the intestinal inflammation usually eliminates the peripheral arthritis
- Spondylitis often requires NSAIDs, which need to be used cautiously because they may activate the bowel disease in a few patients

David B. Hellmann, MD, FACP
John H. Stone, MD, MPH

Arthritis in Sarcoidosis

 ### KEY FEATURES

- May occur early (within 6 mo of onset of symptoms) or late
- Often associated with erythema nodosum
- Rarely deforming

 ### CLINICAL FINDINGS

- Early arthritis usually begins in one or both ankles and can additively involve knees, wrists, and hands
- Early arthritis is strongly associated with erythema nodosum and often produces more periarticular swelling than frank joint swelling
- Axial skeleton spared
- Late arthritis is less severe and less widespread
- Dactylitis (sausage digit) may occur in association with overlying cutaneous sarcoidosis
- Commonly self-limited, resolving after several weeks or months and rarely resulting in chronic arthritis, joint destruction, or significant deformity
- Often associated with erythema nodosum

 ### DIAGNOSIS

- Contingent on demonstration of other extra-articular manifestations of sarcoidosis and biopsy evidence of non-caseating granulomas
- In chronic arthritis, radiographs show typical changes in the bones of the extremities with intact cortex and cystic changes

 ### TREATMENT

- Usually symptomatic and supportive
- A short course of corticosteroids may be effective in severe and progressive joint disease
- Colchicine may be of value

David B. Hellmann, MD, FACP
John H. Stone, MD, MPH

Arthritis, Viral

 ### KEY FEATURES

- Arthritis may be a manifestation of many viral infections
- Generally mild and of short duration, terminating without lasting ill effects

 ### CLINICAL FINDINGS

- Mumps arthritis may occur in the absence of parotitis
- Rubella arthritis, which occurs more commonly in adults than in children, may appear immediately before, during, or soon after the disappearance of the rash. Its usual polyarticular and symmetric distribution mimics that of rheumatoid arthritis
- In adults, polyarthritis may follow infection with human parvovirus B19
- Transient polyarthritis may be associated with type B hepatitis and typically occurs before the onset of jaundice; it may occur in anicteric hepatitis as well
- Hepatitis C infection may be associated with chronic polyarthralgia or polyarthritis that mimics rheumatoid arthritis

 ### DIAGNOSIS

- Viral serologies

 ### TREATMENT

- NSAIDs are the mainstay of treatment for most forms of viral arthritis
- Symptoms secondary to hepatitis C virus may respond to interferon-α if the virological response is good

David B. Hellmann, MD, FACP
John H. Stone, MD, MPH

Asbestosis

 KEY FEATURES

- A nodular interstitial fibrosis occurring in workers chronically exposed to asbestos fibers
- Cigarette smoking increases the prevalence of pleural and parenchymal changes and markedly increases the incidence of lung carcinoma

 CLINICAL FINDINGS

- Inexorably progressive dyspnea, inspiratory crackles
- Clubbing and cyanosis are present in some cases
- Lower lungs are involved more than upper lungs
- Pulmonary function tests show restrictive dysfunction and reduced diffusing capacity

 DIAGNOSIS

- Radiographic features include interstitial fibrosis, thickened pleura, and calcified pleural plaques on lateral chest walls and diaphragm
- High-resolution CT is the best imaging method

 TREATMENT

- No specific treatment

Mark S. Chesnutt, MD
Thomas J. Prendergast, MD

Ascites, Malignant

 KEY FEATURES

- Two-thirds of cases are due to peritoneal carcinomatosis, from adenocarcinomas of the ovary, uterus, pancreas, stomach, colon, lung, or breast
- One-third of cases are due to lymphatic obstruction or portal hypertension from hepatocellular carcinoma or diffuse hepatic metastases

 CLINICAL FINDINGS

- Nonspecific abdominal discomfort and weight loss
- Increased abdominal girth
- Nausea or vomiting caused by partial or complete intestinal obstruction

 DIAGNOSIS

- Abdominal CT useful to demonstrate primary malignancy or hepatic metastases but seldom confirms diagnosis of peritoneal carcinomatosis
- Paracentesis demonstrates low serum ascites–albumin gradient (<1.1 mg/dL), increased total protein (>2.5 g/dL), and elevated WBC (often both neutrophils and mononuclear cells but with a lymphocyte predominance)
- Ascitic fluid cytology is positive in 95%
- Laparoscopy is diagnostic in patients with negative cytology

 TREATMENT

- Diuretics not useful in controlling ascites
- Periodic large-volume paracentesis for symptomatic relief
- Intraperitoneal chemotherapy sometimes used
- Prognosis is extremely poor: only 10% survival at 6 mo
- Ovarian cancer is an exception; with surgical debulking and intraperitoneal chemotherapy, long-term survival is possible

Kenneth R. McQuaid, MD

Aspergillosis

 KEY FEATURES

- *Aspergillus fumigatus* is the usual cause of aspergillosis, although many species of *Aspergillus* cause disease
- These fungi often colonize burn eschar and debris in the external ear canal
- Clinical illness results from abnormal immune response or tissue invasion, which can occur in immunocompetent adults
- Life-threatening invasive aspergillosis usually occurs in profound immunodeficiency, particularly prolonged severe neutropenia
- Allergic bronchopulmonary aspergillosis (ABPA) occurs in asthmatics and sometimes in cystic fibrosis

 CLINICAL FINDINGS

- ABPA:
  - Asthmatics or cystic fibrosis patients develop worsening bronchospasm
  - Waxing and waning course with gradual improvement but may cause saccular bronchiectasis and end-stage fibrotic lung disease
- In immunocompetent patients, aspergillosis causes:
  - Chronic sinusitis
  - Aspergillomas, colonization of preexisting pulmonary cavities, found incidentally by CXR or symptomatic with hemoptysis
- In immunocompromised patients, invasive aspergillosis causes:
  - Pulmonary disease, leading to severe necrotizing pneumonia
  - Pleuritic chest pain, reflecting tissue infarction
  - Ulcerative tracheobronchitis that coexists with parenchymal pulmonary disease in AIDS patients
  - Hematogenous dissemination to CNS, skin, and other organs

 DIAGNOSIS

- ABPA:
  - Fleeting pulmonary infiltrates, eosinophilia, high IgE levels, and *Aspergillus* precipitins in the blood
  - Aspergillomas of the lung seen on CXR or CT

- Invasive aspergillosis:
  - CXR initially shows patchy infiltration, then severe necrotizing pneumonia
  - Elevated serum lactate dehydrogenase (resulting from tissue infarction)
  - Blood cultures of very low yield
  - Unlike in ABPA, serological tests have low sensitivity
  - Detection of galactomannan by ELISA has sensitivity of 89% and specificity of 98% for invasive disease, although multiple determinations may be needed
  - Isolation of *Aspergillus* from pulmonary secretions does not necessarily imply invasive disease
  - Mainstay of diagnosis is biopsy demonstration of *Aspergillus* in tissue as branched septate hyphae, although specimens do not invariably grow the organism

 ## TREATMENT

- ABPA: for acute exacerbations, prednisone, 1 mg/kg/day PO tapered slowly over several months; itraconazole, 200 mg PO qd for 16 weeks appears to improve pulmonary function and decrease steroid requirements
- Sinus disease: long-term antifungal therapy (eg, itraconazole, 200 mg PO BID for weeks to months) and surgical débridement
- Aspergillomas: if, symptomatic, surgical resection; itraconazole may yield some benefit; intracavitary amphotericin B and bronchoscopic removal have little success
- Invasive aspergillosis:
  - Reversal of any correctable immunosuppression
  - Early diagnosis and high-dose amphotericin B when diagnosis likely or proven
  - Increase amphotericin dose rapidly to 0.8–1.5 mg/kg/day IV as tolerated for several weeks, then use doses of 0.6 mg/kg/day until clinical resolution
  - Itraconazole, 200–400 PO or IV qd, has activity against *Aspergillus* and is used for less severe disease or as a follow-up to amphotericin B therapy
  - Lipid formulations of amphotericin B have less nephrotoxicity, allowing administration of higher doses, but are more costly
  - Caspofungin acetate, 70 mg IV load, then 50 mg qd IV, is approved for invasive aspergillosis in patients refractory to or intolerant of other treatments. Caspofungin may be added to amphotericin B in critically ill patients not responding to amphotericin B
  - Surgical resection of invasive pulmonary aspergillosis warrants further study after promising results in neutropenic patients
  - Mortality rate of pulmonary or disseminated disease in immunocompromised patients is >50%

Richard Hamill, MD

Aspiration of Gastric Contents, Acute

 ## KEY FEATURES

- Also known as Mendelson's syndrome, it is one of the most common causes of ARDS
- Severity depends on the characteristics and amount of gastric contents; more severe injury is caused by more acidic pH

 ## CLINICAL FINDINGS

- Abrupt onset of respiratory distress with cough, wheezing, and fever
- Hypoxemia and bibasilar crackles may be noted immediately
- CXR demonstrates infiltrates in dependent lung zones within hours
- Fever and leukocytosis occur even in absence of bacterial superinfection
- Secondary pulmonary infection occurs in 25% of patients, usually after 2–3 days
- Hypotension secondary to alveolar injury and intravascular volume depletion is common

 ## DIAGNOSIS

- History of aspiration or condition known to predispose to it
- Sudden onset of respiratory distress with hypoxia and typical radiographic features
- Exclusion of other cardiopulmonary conditions causing hypoxia and infiltrates

 ## TREATMENT

- Acute treatment consists of airway protection and supplemental oxygen, with ventilatory support as needed
- No evidence supports routine use of corticosteroids or prophylactic antibiotics

Mark S. Chesnutt, MD
Thomas J. Prendergast, MD

Aspiration of Gastric Contents, Chronic

 KEY FEATURES

- May result from primary disorders of the larynx or esophagus

 CLINICAL FINDINGS

- Chronic cough
- Nocturnal asthma or symptoms
- Interstitial lung disease
- Bronchiectasis
- Recurrent lung infections

 DIAGNOSIS

- Ambulatory monitoring of esophageal pH detects pathological reflux
- Esophagogastroscopy and barium swallow may be necessary to rule out esophageal disease
- Swallowing evaluation by a speech pathologist

 TREATMENT

- Elevation of the head of the bed, cessation of smoking, weight reduction, avoidance of caffeinated products and alcohol, and acid suppressive therapy (eg, proton pump inhibitors; see *Gastroesophageal reflux disease*)
- Metoclopramide may be helpful in some patients
- Nissen fundoplication for pathological reflux despite medical therapy
- Speech–swallowing therapy

Mark S. Chesnutt, MD
Thomas J. Prendergast, MD

Asthma, Occupational

 KEY FEATURES

- Estimated 2–5% of all asthma cases are related to occupation

 CLINICAL FINDINGS

- Dyspnea, wheezing, and cough, which correlate with the workplace
- Patients will often report feeling better in the evenings or during weekends and vacations

 DIAGNOSIS

- Requires a high index of suspicion and a careful history of work exposures
- Spirometry before and after exposure to the implicated substance
- Peak flow measurements at and outside of the workplace
- Bronchial provocation testing is helpful in some cases

 TREATMENT

- Bronchodilators
- Avoidance of further exposure to the offending agent

Mark S. Chesnutt, MD
Thomas J. Prendergast, MD

Atrial Fibrillation

 KEY FEATURES

- Irregularly irregular heart rhythm
- Untreated, the atrial rate is 400–600 bpm; the ventricular response is irregular, ranging from 80–180 bpm
- The most common chronic arrhythmia, affecting nearly 10% of individuals older than 80
- Rarely life threatening
- If the ventricular rate is rapid enough, it can precipitate hypotension, myocardial ischemia, or myocardial dysfunction
- Propensity for stroke from embolization of an atrial thrombus

 CLINICAL FINDINGS

- Irregularly irregular pulse
- Often occurs paroxysmally before becoming the established rhythm
- Older or inactive individuals may have relatively few symptoms; however, some patients are made uncomfortable by the irregular rhythm
- In patients with heart disease, rheumatic disease, and other valvular heart disease, dilated cardiomyopathy, atrial septal defect, hypertension, coronary heart disease, and thyrotoxicosis can cause attacks
- In patients with normal hearts, pericarditis, chest trauma, thoracic or cardiac surgery, pulmonary disease, electrolyte disturbances, acute alcohol excess or withdrawal, and medications such as theophylline and β-adrenergic agonists can cause attacks

 DIAGNOSIS

- ECG: lack of normal P waves and an irregular, rapidly fluctuating baseline; irregular ventricular rhythm, with heart rate usually 80–180 bpm
- Echocardiography: visualization of fibrillating atria with irregular ventricular contractions
- Echocardiography recommended in patients with newly diagnosed atrial fibrillation who do not have an obvious, easily correctable cause
- Ambulatory ECG monitoring or event recorders are indicated when paroxysmal atrial fibrillation is suspected
- Obtain thyroid-stimulating hormone to exclude thyrotoxicosis

TREATMENT

- Up to two-thirds of patients experiencing a first episode will spontaneously revert to sinus rhythm within 24 h
- If atrial fibrillation persists or has been present for >1 week, spontaneous conversion is unlikely, and management consists of rate control and anticoagulation
- Rate control is defined as ventricular rate of 50–100 bpm with usual daily activities, and not exceeding 120 bpm except with moderate to strenuous activity
- Conventional rate-control agents used singly or, in younger adults, often in combination, include digoxin, β-blockers, and calcium channel blockers (Table 40, page 1233)
- In patients with heart failure, coronary artery disease, or ongoing ischemia, β-blockers (metoprolol or esmolol) are preferred
- If hypertension is present or β-blockers are contraindicated, calcium channel blockers are effective (diltiazem or verapamil)
- Amiodarone is a useful adjunct when rate control with other agents is incomplete or contraindicated or when cardioversion is anticipated
- Do not use digoxin, verapamil, or β-blockers if atrial fibrillation is associated with a known or suspected accessory pathway
- Urgent electrical cardioversion is indicated in patients with shock or severe hypotension, pulmonary edema, or ongoing myocardial infarction or ischemia, even if atrial fibrillation has been present for > 48 h
- Elective electrical or pharmacological cardioversion is recommended in patients with an initial episode of recent onset when there is an identifiable precipitating factor and in those who remain symptomatic despite aggressive efforts at rate control
- If cardioversion is planned and the duration of atrial fibrillation exceeds 2–3 days or is unknown, perform a transesophageal echocardiography to exclude an atrial thrombus and attempt electrical cardioversion while the patient remains sedated
- If thrombus is present, delay cardioversion until after 3–4 weeks of therapeutic warfarin anticoagulation (INR of 2–3)
- Use heparin while awaiting therapeutic warfarin anticoagulation in atrial fibrillation with mitral stenosis, a history of embolic events, or demonstrated thrombus on transesophageal echocardiography
- After cardioversion, maintain therapeutic anticoagulation for at least 1–6 mo
- Patients with paroxysmal or persistent atrial fibrillation who fail to convert should be anticoagulated indefinitely, except for "lone atrial fibrillation" (age younger than 60 and no associated heart disease, hypertension, atherosclerotic vascular disease, or diabetes)
- Atrial fibrillation is considered refractory if it causes persistent symptoms or limits activity despite vigorous efforts at rate control and cardioversion. In such cases, consider radiofrequency atrioventricular node ablation and permanent pacing

Barry M. Massie, MD
Thomas M. Amidon, MD

Atrial Flutter

 KEY FEATURES

- Ectopic impulse formation occurs at atrial rates of 250–350/min, with transmission of every second, third, or fourth impulse through the AV node to the ventricles
- Atrial flutter is less common than fibrillation
- Occurs most often in chronic obstructive pulmonary disease (COPD) and less commonly with rheumatic or coronary heart disease, congestive heart failure, atrial septal defect, or surgically repaired congenital heart disease
- Ventricular rate control is attempted as in atrial fibrillation but is much more difficult to achieve
- Risk of systemic embolization is slightly increased

 CLINICAL FINDINGS

- Regular pulse with heart rate between 250–350 bpm
- Symptoms include anxiety, shortness of breath, light-headedness
- Physical examination may show findings of COPD

 DIAGNOSIS

- ECG: characteristic atrial flutter waves transmitted in a regular 2:1, 3:1, or 4:1 pattern to the ventricles

 TREATMENT

- Initially, digoxin, a β-blocker, or a calcium channel blocker (Table 40, page 1233) is used for rate control; conversion to sinus rhythm may result
- If not, ibutilide converts atrial flutter to sinus rhythm in ~50–70% of patients within 60–90 min
- Electrical cardioversion (25–50 J) is effective in ~90% of patients
- Precardioversion anticoagulation is not necessary for atrial flutter of < 48 h duration except in the setting of mitral valve disease
- Anticoagulation is prudent in chronic atrial flutter, particularly because transient periods of atrial fibrillation are common in these patients
- In chronic atrial flutter, rate control is often difficult. Amiodarone is the drug of choice

- In patients refractory to drug therapy, consider radiofrequency ablation of a possible atypical reentry circuit

Barry M. Massie, MD
Thomas M. Amidon, MD

Atrial Septal Defect

 KEY FEATURES

- Three forms: (1) persistence of ostium secundum in midseptum (80% of cases); (2) persistent ostium primum (low septum); and (3) sinus venosus defect (upper septum)
- Oxygenated blood from higher-pressure left atrium passes into right atrium, increasing right ventricular output and pulmonary blood flow
- Prolonged high flow through pulmonary circulation often leads to severe pulmonary hypertension
- This can produce right-to-left shunting and cyanosis (Eisenmenger's syndrome)
- A patent foramen ovale (present in 20–30% of adults) is responsible for most paradoxical emboli

 CLINICAL FINDINGS

- Most small or moderate defects are asymptomatic
- Large shunts can produce exertional dyspnea or cardiac failure, usually after the fourth decade
- Moderately loud systolic ejection murmur in the second and third interspaces
- Prominent right ventricular and pulmonary artery pulsations are readily visible and palpable

 DIAGNOSIS

- ECG: incomplete or complete right bundle-branch block
- CXR: large pulmonary arteries, increased pulmonary vascularity, enlarged right atrium and ventricle
- Echocardiography usually diagnostic. Saline bubble contrast and Doppler flow can demonstrate shunting. Transesophageal echo has superior sensitivity for small shunts and patent foramen ovale
- Cardiac catheterization is definitive diagnostic procedure, can demonstrate increase in oxygen saturation between venae cava and right ventricle, quantify shunt, and measure pulmonary vascular resistance

 TREATMENT

- Patients with small shunts may live a normal life and do not require surgery
- Large shunts generally require surgery
- Withhold surgery in Eisenmenger's syndrome
- Surgical mortality rate <1% in patients younger than age 45 without cardiac failure and with systolic pulmonary artery pressures <60 mm Hg; otherwise, surgical mortality increases to 5–10%

Barry M. Massie, MD
Thomas M. Amidon, MD

Atropine & Anticholinergic Poisoning

 ### KEY FEATURES

- Atropine, scopolamine, belladonna, diphenoxylate with atropine, *Datura stramonium, Hyoscyamus niger,* some mushrooms, tricyclic antidepressants, and antihistamines are antimuscarinic agents with variable CNS effects

 ### CLINICAL FINDINGS

- Dryness of the mouth, thirst, difficulty swallowing, blurring of vision
- Dilated pupils, flushed skin, tachycardia, fever, delirium, myoclonus, ileus, flushed appearance
- Antidepressants and antihistamines may induce convulsions
- Diphenhydramine commonly causes delirium, tachycardia, and seizures. Massive overdose may mimic tricyclic antidepressant poisoning
- Terfenadine and astemizole cause QT interval prolongation and torsades de pointes and were removed from US market

 ### DIAGNOSIS

- Clinical or diagnosis by serum level

 ### TREATMENT

EMERGENCY AND SUPPORTIVE MEASURES

- Administer activated charcoal

SPECIFIC TREATMENT

- For pure atropine or related anticholinergic syndrome, if symptoms are severe (eg, hyperthermia or excessively rapid tachycardia), give physostigmine salicylate, 0.5–1 mg IV slowly over 5 min, with ECG monitoring, until symptoms are controlled. Bradyarrhythmias and convulsions are a hazard with physostigmine administration, and it should not be used in patients with tricyclic antidepressant overdose

Kent R. Olsen, MD

Avascular Necrosis of Bone

 ### KEY FEATURES

- A complication of corticosteroid use, trauma, systemic lupus erythematosus (SLE), pancreatitis, alcoholism, gout, sickle cell disease, and infiltrative diseases (eg, Gaucher's disease)
- Most commonly affected sites are the proximal and distal femoral heads
- The natural history is usually progression of the bony infarction to cortical collapse, resulting in significant joint dysfunction

 ### CLINICAL FINDINGS

- Hip or knee pain
- Many patients with hip disease first present with pain referred to the knee; however, internal rotation of the hip—not movement of the knee—is painful

 ### DIAGNOSIS

- Initially, radiographs are often normal; MRI, CT scan, and bone scan are all more sensitive techniques
- Differential diagnosis includes osteoarthritis or rheumatoid arthritis, fracture, joint pain resulting from other cause

 ### TREATMENT

- Avoidance of weight bearing on the affected joint for at least several weeks
- Surgical core decompression is controversial
- Total hip replacement is the usual outcome for all patients who are suitable candidates

David B. Hellmann, MD, FACP
John H. Stone, MD, MPH

Bacteremia, *Salmonella*

 ### KEY FEATURES

- This complication tends to occur in immunocompromised persons and is seen in HIV-infected individuals, who typically have bacteremia without an obvious source

 ### CLINICAL FINDINGS

- May be manifested by prolonged or recurrent fevers or local infection in bone, joints, pleura, pericardium, lungs, or other sites
- Mycotic abdominal aortic aneurysms may also be a complication

 ### DIAGNOSIS

- Serotypes other than *S typhi* usually are isolated in culture

 ### TREATMENT

- Treatment is the same as for typhoid fever (see enteric or typhoid fever) plus drainage of any abscesses
- In HIV-infected patients, relapse is common, and lifelong suppressive therapy may be needed
- Ciprofloxacin, 500 mg BID, is effective both for therapy of acute infection and for suppression of recurrence

Henry F. Chambers, MD

Bacteremia, Staphylococcal

 KEY FEATURES

- Although staphylococcal bacteremia commonly arises from skin lesions or IV catheters, whenever *S aureus* is recovered from blood cultures, the possibility of endocarditis, osteomyelitis, or other metastatic deep infections must be considered

 CLINICAL FINDINGS

- There may be symptoms and signs related to source of infection

 DIAGNOSIS

- Transesophageal echocardiography is a sensitive and cost-effective method for excluding underlying endocarditis and should be considered for patients for whom the pretest probability of endocarditis is 5% or higher and perhaps for all patients with unexplained *S aureus* bacteremia

 TREATMENT

- The appropriate duration of therapy for uncomplicated bacteremia arising from a removable source (eg, IV device) or drainable focus (eg, skin abscess) has not been well defined, but a 10- to 14-day course of therapy appears to be the minimum
- Nafcillin or oxacillin, 1.5 g IV q4–6h, cefazolin, 500–1000 mg q8h, or vancomycin, 1000 mg q12h, is recommended for uncomplicated staphylococcal bacteremia
- Vancomycin, which is less efficacious than beta-lactams, should be reserved for treatment of methicillin-resistant strains or for infection in patients with serious penicillin allergy
- Resistance to vancomycin remains rare and should not affect the choice of empirical therapy. Cases of vancomycin treatment failures in which the staphylococcal isolate exhibits a vancomycin MIC ≥ 4 mg/mL should be reported to CDC to help track this potentially serious and emerging problem

Henry F. Chambers, MD

Bacterial Overgrowth, Small Intestine

 KEY FEATURES

- Overgrowth of bacteria in normally sterile segments of small bowel; may result in malabsorption of fat with steatorrhea
- Causes include (1) gastric achlorhydria; (2) anatomic abnormalities of the small intestine with stagnation (afferent limb of Billroth II gastrojejunostomy, small intestine diverticula, obstruction, blind loop, radiation enteritis); (3) small intestine motility disorders (scleroderma, diabetic enteropathy, chronic intestinal pseudo-obstruction); (4) gastrocolic or coloenteric fistula (Crohn's disease, malignancy, surgical resection); and (5) miscellaneous disorders (AIDS, chronic pancreatitis)

 CLINICAL FINDINGS

- Many patients are asymptomatic
- Abdominal distension, weight loss, and steatorrhea
- Watery diarrhea

 DIAGNOSIS

- Qualitative or quantitative fecal fat assessment abnormal
- D-xylose absorption abnormal
- Aspirate and culture of proximal jejunal secretion demonstrate >10^5 organisms/mL
- ^{13}C- or ^{14}C-xylose breath test
- Megaloblastic anemia secondary to vitamin B_{12} deficiency
- Schilling test abnormal in phases I and II (without and with intrinsic factor) but normalizes after a course of antibiotics
- Small bowel barium radiography: helpful to document conditions predisposing to intestinal stasis
- Empirical antibiotic trial can be used as a diagnostic and therapeutic maneuver

 TREATMENT

- Correct the anatomic defect when possible
- Ciprofloxacin, 500 mg PO BID, norfloxacin, 400 mg PO BID, amoxicillin clavulanate, 875 mg PO BID, or combination of metronidazole, 250 mg PO TID, and trimethoprim-sulfamethoxazole (one double-strength tablet) PO BID, or cephalexin, 250 mg PO QID, for 1–2 weeks
- If symptoms recur off antibiotics, cyclic therapy (eg, 1 week of 4) may be sufficient
- Avoid continuous antibiotics to prevent development of bacterial antibiotic resistance
- Octreotide in small doses may be of benefit

Kenneth R. McQuaid, MD

Balantidiasis

 ### KEY FEATURES

- *Balantidium coli* is a large intestinal protozoan found worldwide but particularly in the tropics
- Pigs are the reservoir host, but the agent is found in other animals and insects
- The disease is rare in humans, occurring as an acute or chronic infection (sporadic or in outbreaks) resulting from ingestion of cysts passed in stools of humans or swine
- In properly treated mild to moderate symptomatic cases, the prognosis is good; in spite of treatment, fatalities have occurred in severe infections as a result of intestinal perforation or hemorrhage

 ### CLINICAL FINDINGS

- Many infections are asymptomatic and need not be treated
- Chronic recurrent diarrhea, alternating with constipation, is most common, but mild diarrhea to severe dysentery with bloody mucoid stools, tenesmus, and colic may occur
- Rarely, instances of infection in the lung, liver, and vagina can occur

 ### DIAGNOSIS

- Identify trophozoites in liquid stools, cysts in formed stools, or the trophozoite in scrapings or biopsy of ulcers of the large bowel. Specimens must be examined rapidly or placed in preservative

 ### TREATMENT

- The treatment of choice is tetracycline hydrochloride, 500 mg QID for 10 days. The alternative drug is iodoquinol (diiodohydroxyquin), 650 mg TID for 21 days
- Occasional success has also been reported with metronidazole (750 mg TID for 5 days) or paromomycin (25–30 mg/kg [base] in 3 divided doses for 5–10 days)

Bartholin's Duct Cyst and Abscess

 ### KEY FEATURES

- Trauma or infection may cause obstruction of the gland. Drainage of secretions is prevented, leading to pain, swelling, and abscess formation. The infection usually resolves and pain disappears, but stenosis of the duct outlet with distension often persists
- Reinfection causes recurrent tenderness and further enlargement of the duct

 ### CLINICAL FINDINGS

- Periodic painful swelling on either side of the introitus and dyspareunia
- A fluctuant swelling 1–4 cm in diameter in the inferior portion of either labium minus is a sign of occlusion of Bartholin's duct
- Tenderness is evidence of active infection

 ### DIAGNOSIS

- Pus or secretions from the gland should be cultured for gonococci, chlamydiae, and other pathogens

 ### TREATMENT

- Treat according to culture results
- Frequent warm soaks may be helpful
- If an abscess develops, aspiration or incision and drainage are the simplest forms of therapy, but the problem may recur
- Marsupialization, incision and drainage with the insertion of an indwelling Word catheter, or laser treatment will establish a new duct opening
- An asymptomatic cyst does not require therapy

H. Trent MacKay, MD, MPH

Behçet's Syndrome

 ### KEY FEATURES

- Causes recurrent attacks of oral apthous ulcers, genital ulcers, uveitis, and skin lesions
- Onset usually in young adults, aged 25–35 yr
- Blindness, CNS abnormalities, and thrombosis or rupture of large vessels are the most serious complications

 ### CLINICAL FINDINGS

- Recurrent oral and genital ulcers
- Eye: keratitis, retinal vasculitis, and anterior uveitis (often with hypopyon, or pus in the anterior chamber)
- Seronegative arthritis occurs in about two-thirds of patients, most commonly affecting the knees and ankles
- CNS abnormalities include cranial nerve palsies, convulsions, encephalitis, mental disturbances, and spinal cord lesions
- Clinical course may be chronic but is often characterized by remissions and exacerbations

 ### DIAGNOSIS

- Clinical diagnosis
- CNS lesions may mimic multiple sclerosis radiologically
- Differential diagnosis includes inflammatory bowel disease, systemic lupus erythematosus, recurrent aphthous ulcers, herpes simplex infection, ankylosing spondylitis, reactive arthritis (Reiter's syndrome), syphilis, sarcoidosis, HIV infection

 ### TREATMENT

- Corticosteroids, azathioprine, chlorambucil, pentoxifylline, and cyclosporine have been used with beneficial results

David B. Hellmann, MD, FACP
John H. Stone, MD, MPH

Bernard-Soulier Syndrome

 KEY FEATURES

- Rare autosomal recessive disorder. Platelets cannot adhere to subendothelium because of lack of receptors (composed of glycoprotein Ib) for von Willebrand factor

 CLINICAL FINDINGS

- Often severe mucosal and postoperative bleeding

 DIAGNOSIS

- Thrombocytopenia may be present. Bleeding time markedly prolonged. Platelet aggregation normal in response to standard agonists (collagen, adenosine 5'-diphosphate, thrombin), but platelets fail to aggregate in response to ristocetin. Normal plasma von Willebrand factor level

 TREATMENT

- Platelet transfusion when necessary

Charles A. Linker, MD

Berylliosis

 KEY FEATURES

- An acute or chronic pulmonary disorder related to beryllium exposure
- Beryllium is absorbed through the skin or lungs and widely disseminates
- Exposure occurs in machining and handling of beryllium products and alloys; beryllium miners are not at risk

 CLINICAL FINDINGS

- Acute berylliosis is a toxic, ulcerative tracheobronchitis and chemical pneumonitis after intense, severe exposure
- Chronic berylliosis is a more common, systemic disease resembling sarcoidosis

 DIAGNOSIS

- The beryllium lymphocyte proliferation test is a useful diagnostic test

 TREATMENT

- Avoid exposure to beryllium
- Corticosteroids are often prescribed despite lack of proven efficacy

Mark S. Chesnutt, MD
Thomas J. Prendergast, MD

β-Blocker Overdose

 KEY FEATURES

- The toxic β-blocker is propranolol, which competitively blocks β_1- and β_2- adrenoceptors and also has direct membrane-depressant and CNS effects

 CLINICAL FINDINGS

- Hypotension and bradycardia are common with mild or moderate intoxication
- Cardiac depression from more severe poisoning is often unresponsive to conventional β-adrenergic stimulants such as dopamine and norepinephrine
- With propranolol and other lipid-soluble drugs, seizures and coma may occur

 DIAGNOSIS

- Diagnosis is clinical
- Routine toxicology screening does not usually include β-blockers

 TREATMENT

- Initially, treat bradycardia or heart block with atropine (0.5–2 mg IV), isoproterenol (2–20 μg/min by IV infusion, titrated to desired heart rate)
- If the above measures are not successful in reversing bradycardia and hypotension, give glucagon, 5–10 mg IV, followed by infusion of 1–5 mg/h
- Administer activated charcoal, 60–100 g orally or via gastric tube, mixed in aqueous slurry. Repeated doses may be given

Kent R. Olsen, MD

Biliary Stricture

 ## KEY FEATURES

- Results from surgical anastomosis or injury in about 95% of cases
- Cholangitis is the most common complication
- Significant hepatocellular disease resulting from secondary biliary cirrhosis is inevitable if not treated

 ## CLINICAL FINDINGS

- Ductal injury may not be recognized in the immediate postoperative period
- If complete occlusion has occurred, jaundice develops rapidly; more often, a tear is accidentally made in the duct, with excessive or prolonged bile loss from the surgical drains as the earliest manifestation
- Typically, episodes of pain, fever, chills, and jaundice occur within a few weeks to months after cholecystectomy
- Right upper quadrant abdominal tenderness. There may be jaundice during an attack of cholangitis and right upper quadrant abdominal tenderness

 ## DIAGNOSIS

- Serum alkaline phosphatase is usually elevated. Hyperbilirubinemia is variable, fluctuating in the range of 5–10 mg/dL during exacerbations. Blood cultures may be positive during an episode of cholangitis
- Surgical exploration may be needed to differentiate from cholangiocarcinoma

 ## TREATMENT

- Endoscopic retrograde cholangiopancreatography or percutaneous transhepatic cholangiography can demonstrate the stricture, permit biopsy, and allow dilation and multiple stent placement
- Intraductal ultrasonography and cholangioscopy may help exclude malignancy
- Operative treatment frequently necessitates performance of an end-to-end ductal repair, choledochojejunostomy, or hepaticojejunostomy to reestablish bile flow into the intestine

Lawrence S. Friedman, MD

Bites, Snake & Lizard

 ## KEY FEATURES

- The venom may be neurotoxic (coral snake) or cytolytic (rattlesnakes, other pit vipers)
- Neurotoxins cause respiratory paralysis; cytolytic venoms cause tissue digestion and hemolysis with destruction of the endothelial lining of the blood vessels

 ## CLINICAL FINDINGS

- The manifestations of rattlesnake envenomation are mostly local pain, redness, swelling, and extravasation of blood
- Perioral tingling, metallic taste, nausea, vomiting, hypotension, ptosis, coagulopathy, dysphagia, diplopia, and respiratory arrest can occur
- Coagulopathy common and includes prolonged PT and thrombocytopenia (sometimes severe)

 ## TREATMENT

- Immobilize patient and bitten area in neutral position. Avoid manipulation of bitten area. Do *not* apply ice; do *not* apply a tourniquet. Incision and suction of the bite by unskilled persons are probably not useful. Transport patient to a medical facility
- Pit viper (eg, rattlesnake) envenomation: For local signs such as swelling, pain, and ecchymosis but no systemic symptoms, give 4–6 vials of crotalid antivenin (CroFab) by slow IV drip in 250–500 mL saline. Repeat doses of 2 vials q6h for up to 18 h. For more serious envenomation with marked local effects and systemic toxicity (eg, hypotension, coagulopathy), higher doses and additional vials may be required. Monitor vital signs and blood coagulation profile. Type and cross-match blood. Adequacy of venom neutralization is indicated by improvement in symptoms and signs and slowed rate of swelling
- Elapid (coral snake) envenomation: Give 1–2 vials of specific antivenom as soon as possible. To locate antisera, call a regional poison control center

Kent R. Olsen, MD

Bites, Spider & Scorpion

 ## CLINICAL FINDINGS

- Toxin of most species of spiders in the US causes only local pain, redness, swelling
- Venomous black widow spiders (*Latrodectus mactans*) cause generalized muscular pains, muscle spasms, rigidity
- Brown recluse spider (*Loxosceles reclusa*) causes progressive local necrosis as well as hemolytic reactions (rare)
- Stings by most scorpions in US cause only local pain. Stings by the more toxic *Centruroides* species (found in southwestern US) may cause muscle cramps, twitching and jerking, and occasionally hypertension, convulsions, and pulmonary edema

 ## TREATMENT

- Black widow spider bites: Relieve pain with parenteral narcotics or muscle relaxants (eg, methocarbamol, 15 mg/kg). Calcium gluconate 10%, 0.1–0.2 mL/kg IV, may relieve muscle rigidity. Antivenin is available, but because of concerns about acute hypersensitivity reactions it is often reserved for very young or elderly patients and those who do not respond to the above measures. Horse serum sensitivity testing is required. (Instruction and testing materials are in the antivenin kit)
- Brown recluse spider bites: Because bites occasionally progress to extensive local necrosis, some authorities recommend early excision of the bite site, whereas others use oral corticosteroids. Anecdotal reports claim success with dapsone and colchicine
- Scorpion stings: For *Centruroides* stings, some toxicologists use a specific antivenom developed in Arizona, but this is neither FDA-approved nor widely available

Kent R. Olsen, MD

Blastomycosis

 KEY FEATURES

- Blastomycosis occurs most often in men infected during occupational or recreational outdoor activities
- Geographically limited to south central and midwestern US and Canada
- A few cases have been found in Mexico and Africa

 CLINICAL FINDINGS

- Pulmonary infection most common and may be asymptomatic
- Cough, moderate fever, dyspnea, chest pain
- May resolve or progress, with bloody and purulent sputum, pleurisy, fever, chills, weight loss, prostration
- When disseminated, lesions most frequently affect skin, bones, urogenital system
- Verrucous cutaneous lesions with an abrupt downward sloping border. The border extends slowly, leaving a central atrophic scar. If left untreated, may mimic skin cancer
- Bone lesions often in ribs and vertebrae
- Epididymitis, prostatitis, and other involvement of the male urogenital system
- CNS involvement is uncommon
- In HIV-infected persons, disease may progress rapidly, with dissemination common

 DIAGNOSIS

- Leukocytosis and anemia
- CXR or CT usually reveals pulmonary infiltrates and enlarged regional lymph nodes, although less commonly than in histoplasmosis or coccidioidomycosis
- Bone lesions appear both destructive and proliferative on x-ray films
- Serological tests are not well standardized
- Clinical specimens demonstrate the organism as a thick-walled cell 5–20 μm in diameter that may have a single broad-based bud. *Blastomyces* grows readily on culture

 TREATMENT

- Itraconazole, 100–200 mg PO qd for at least 2–3 mo, for non-life-threatening, non-CNS disease achieves a response rate of > 80%
- Amphotericin B, 0.3–0.6 mg/kg/day IV for total dose of 1.5–2.5 g, for CNS disease or treatment failures
- Patients should be monitored for relapse for several years so that therapy may be resumed or another drug instituted

Richard J. Hamill, MD

Bone & Joint Mycotic Infections

 KEY FEATURES

CANDIDAL OSTEOMYELITIS

- Occurs in malnourished patients undergoing prolonged hospitalization for cancer, neutropenia, trauma, complicated abdominal surgical procedures, or IV drug use
- Infected IV catheters frequently serve as a hematogenous source

COCCIDIOIDOMYCOSIS

- Usually secondary to a primary pulmonary infection
- Arthralgia with periarticular swelling, especially in the knees and ankles, occurring as a nonspecific manifestation of systemic coccidioidomycosis, should be distinguished from actual bone or joint infection. Osseous lesions commonly occur in cancellous bone of the vertebrae or near the ends of long bones at tendinous insertions. These lesions are initially osteolytic and thus may mimic metastatic tumor or myeloma

 CLINICAL FINDINGS

- Joint and bone pain and swelling

 DIAGNOSIS

- Culture studies of synovial fluid
- Coccidiomycosis: recovery of *Coccidioides immitis* from the lesion or histological examination of tissue obtained by open biopsy; rising titers of complement-fixing antibodies also provide evidence of the disseminated nature of the disease

 TREATMENT

- Candidal: fluconazole, 200 mg PO BID, is probably as effective as amphotericin
- Coccidioidomycosis: itraconazole, 200 mg BID for 6–12 mo; may require operative excision of infected bone and soft tissue; amputation may be the only solution for stubbornly progressive infections

David B. Hellmann, MD, FACP
John H. Stone, MD, MPH

Bradycardias

 KEY FEATURES

- Bradycardia most commonly results from impaired sinus node function or from conduction abnormalities, which can occur between sinus node and atrium, within AV node, or within intraventricular conduction pathways
- Sick sinus syndrome occurs most commonly in the elderly and is often caused by drug therapy (digitalis, calcium channel blockers, β-blockers, sympatholytic agents, antiarrhythmics) and less often by sarcoidosis, amyloidosis, Chagas' disease, and various cardiomyopathies
- Atrioventricular block consists of several subtypes:
  - First-degree block and second-degree Mobitz type I block occur (1) with heightened vagal tone in normal individuals; (2) with drugs that block the AV node, often in individuals with organic heart disease; and (3) transiently or chronically with ischemia, infarction, inflammatory processes, fibrosis, calcification, or infiltration
  - Second-degree Mobitz type II block occurs with organic heart disease involving the infranodal conduction system
  - Third-degree (complete) block occurs with lesions distal to the His bundle and is associated with bilateral bundle branch block

 CLINICAL FINDINGS

- Sick sinus syndrome, first-degree block, and second-degree block: Most patients are asymptomatic; rarely, patients experience syncope, dizziness, confusion, palpitations, heart failure, or angina pectoris
- Such symptoms are nonspecific and can be due to other causes; thus, they must be shown to temporally coincide with arrhythmias
- In third-degree block, patients may be asymptomatic or may complain of weakness, dyspnea, or abrupt syncope if heart rate <35/min; slow ventricular rate, usually <50/min, that does not increase with exercise; S_1 varies in intensity; wide pulse pressure, and changing systolic blood pressure level; cannon venous pulsations in the neck

 DIAGNOSIS

- Sick sinus syndrome: ECG shows sinus arrest, sinoatrial exit block (a pause equal to a multiple of the underlying PP interval or progressive shortening of the PP interval before a pause), or persistent sinus bradycardia
- Prolonged ambulatory Holter monitoring or event recorder may be required to document correspondence of bradycardia with symptoms
- Atrioventricular block:
  - First-degree block: ECG shows PR interval >0.21 s with all atrial impulses conducted
  - Second-degree block: ECG shows intermittent blocked beats
  - Mobitz type I second-degree block: progressive lengthening of PR interval and shortening of RR interval before the blocked beat
  - Mobitz type II second-degree block: intermittent nonconducted atrial beats are not preceded by a lengthening PR interval
  - Third-degree (complete) block: ECG shows ventricular rate usually <50/min, wide QRS, and no supraventricular impulses being conducted to the ventricles
  - Narrow QRS complexes suggest nodal block and wide QRS complexes suggest infranodal block
- Electrophysiological studies may be necessary for accurate localization

 TREATMENT

- Discontinue offending medications
- Sick sinus syndrome: oral theophylline sometimes effective, especially for sinus bradycardia
- Most symptomatic patients require permanent (preferably dual-chamber) pacemaker implantation
- First-degree block and Mobitz type I block: After discontinuation of offending drugs, other therapy is not usually needed
- Mobitz type II block: Prophylactic ventricular pacemaker implantation is usually required because of the risk of progression to third-degree block
- Third-degree block: Permanent pacemaker implantation; temporary pacing if permanent pacing is delayed

Barry M. Massie, MD
Thomas M. Amidon, MD

Brain Mass, AIDS

 KEY FEATURES

- AIDS patients may present with primary cerebral lymphoma, cerebral toxoplasmosis, or cryptococcal meningitis
- PML or CMV meningoencephalitis can have occasionally similar clinical presentations and overlapping MRI findings

 CLINICAL FINDINGS

- Disturbances in cognition or consciousness, focal motor or sensory deficits, aphasia, seizures, and cranial neuropathies

 DIAGNOSIS

- Neither CT nor MRI findings distinguish primary cerebral lymphoma from toxoplasmosis
- Serological tests for toxoplasmosis are unreliable in AIDS patients; therefore, empiric treatment aids in diagnosis
- CT scans are usually normal in cryptococcal meningitis
- Diagnosis of cryptococcal meningitis is made with positive CSF India ink staining in 75–80% of cases and cryptococcal antigen tests in 95% of cases

 TREATMENT

- See *Lymphoma, Toxoplasmosis, Cryptococcal meningitis*

Michael J. Aminoff, DSc, MD, FRCP

Brain Metastases

 KEY FEATURES

- The most common source of intracranial metastasis is cancer of the lung followed by cancer of the breast, kidney, and GI tract
- 10–15% of brain metastases are of unknown primary source
- Most common metastatic carcinomas to the leptomeninges are breast, lymphomas, and leukemia

 CLINICAL FINDINGS

- Intracranial metastases and primary cerebral neoplasms present similarly
- Leptomeningeal metastases cause multifocal neurological deficits from infiltration of nerve roots, direct invasion of the brain or spinal cord, or obstructive hydrocephalus. Cranial nerve palsies are common

 DIAGNOSIS

- Laboratory and radiology studies are the same as for primary neoplasms
- Lumbar puncture is needed only if carcinomatous meningitis is suspected; elevated cerebrospinal fluid pressure, pleocytosis, increased protein levels, and decreased glucose concentration are seen. Malignant cells may be found
- In leptomeningeal metastases, CT scans show contrast enhancement in the basal cisterns or hydrocephalus without any evidence of mass lesions; gadolinium-enhanced MRI frequently shows leptomeningeal involvement; myelography may show deposits on multiple nerve roots

 TREATMENT

- A single cerebral metastasis may be irradiated, followed by surgical excision in some cases
- Leptomeningeal metastases receive irradiation and intrathecal methotrexate. Prognosis is poor, with only about a 10% 1-yr survival. Palliative care is important

Michael J. Aminoff, DSc, MD, FRCP

Breast Abscess

 KEY FEATURES

- In lactating women, common during nursing; infection is generally caused by *Staphylococcus aureus*
- In nonlactating young or middle-aged women, subareolar abscesses are rare
- In the nonlactating breast, consider inflammatory carcinoma

 CLINICAL FINDINGS

- Redness, tenderness, and induration in the breast

 DIAGNOSIS

- Differential diagnosis: breast cancer, especially inflammatory or Paget's disease of the breast, local irritation or trauma, fat necrosis, fibroadenoma
- In lactating women, diagnosis is generally clinical
- In nonlactating women, incision and biopsy of indurated breast tissue are indicated to rule out malignancy

 TREATMENT

LACTATING WOMEN

- In early stages, continue nursing and treat with antibiotics: dicloxacillin or oxacillin, 250 mg PO QID for 7–10 days
- If mass develops with local or systemic signs of infection, discontinue nursing and refer for surgical drainage

NONLACTATING WOMEN

- If abscess can be percutaneously drained and completely resolves, patient may be monitored conservatively
- However, an abscess will tend to recur after incision and drainage unless area is explored during a quiescent interval with excision of the involved ducts
- Biopsy is generally required to rule out malignancy

Armando E. Giuliano, MD

Breast Augmentation Disorders

 KEY FEATURES

- At least 4 million American women have had breast implants
- Silicone gel may be an immunological stimulant
- No increase in autoimmune disease associated with implants
- No increased risk of breast cancer associated with implants, but cancer can develop in implant patients

 CLINICAL FINDINGS

- Capsule contraction or scarring around the implant occurs in 15–25% of patients, leading to a firmness and distortion of the breast that can be painful
- Implant rupture may occur in as many as 5–10% of women, and bleeding of gel through the capsule is even more common

 DIAGNOSIS

- Breast cancer may be more difficult to diagnose because mammography is less able to detect early lesions if implants are present

 TREATMENT

- Women should consider removal of implants if they have significant pain or symptoms of autoimmune illnesses
- If a cancer develops, it should be treated in the same manner as in women without implants
- Radiotherapy of the augmented breast often results in marked capsular contracture

Armando E. Giuliano, MD

Breast Cancer, Male

KEY FEATURES

- Rare
- Average age, 60 yr
- Poorer prognosis than for female breast cancer (even stage I)
- Blood-borne metastases are usually present
- Hormonal influences likely play an important role

CLINICAL FINDINGS

- Painless lump beneath the areola, usually found after age 50
- Nipple discharge, retraction, or ulceration
- Gynecomastia not uncommonly precedes or accompanies male breast cancer
- Examination usually shows a hard, ill-defined, nontender mass beneath the nipple or areola
- Cancer staging is the same in men as in women

DIAGNOSIS

- Differential diagnosis: gynecomastia, metastatic cancer from another site (eg, prostate), fatty breast enlargement of obesity
- Biopsy is required to confirm diagnosis

TREATMENT

- Modified radical mastectomy in operable patients
- Irradiation for localized metastases to skin, lymph nodes, or skeleton that are causing symptoms
- Adjuvant chemotherapy is used for the same indications as in female breast cancer
- Tamoxifen, 20 mg PO qd, or castration should be tried for advanced-stage male breast cancer
- Castration produces regression in 60–70%, with average duration of remission of 30 mo and life prolongation; also relieves bone pain from metastases
- Medical adrenalectomy with aminoglutethimide, 250 mg PO QID, for relapse or resistant disease
- Estrogen therapy (diethylstilbestrol, 5 mg PO TID) may be effective as secondary hormonal manipulation after medical adrenalectomy

- For stage I disease, 5- and 10-yr survival rates are approximately 58% and 38%, respectively
- For stage II disease, 5- and 10-yr survival rates are 38% and 10%, respectively
- For all stages, 5- and 10-yr survival rates are approximately 36% and 17%, respectively

Armando E. Giuliano, MD

Breast Fat Necrosis

KEY FEATURES

- Rare
- Thought to be caused by trauma, but history of trauma present in only about half of patients
- Common after segmental resection, radiation therapy, or postmastectomy flap reconstruction of the breast

CLINICAL FINDINGS

- Breast mass
- Often associated with skin or nipple retraction
- Indistinguishable from cancer by exam
- Occasionally, ecchymosis present

DIAGNOSIS

- Differential diagnosis: breast cancer, fibroadenoma, breast abscess, fibrocystic disease or cyst, Paget's disease of the breast
- Needle biopsy often adequate for diagnosis
- Occasionally, mass must be excised to exclude carcinoma

TREATMENT

- If untreated, mass effect gradually disappears

Armando E. Giuliano, MD

Breast Fibroadenoma

KEY FEATURES

- Common benign neoplasm
- Most frequent in young women
- Occurs somewhat more frequently and at an earlier age in black women
- Multiple fibroadenomas in 10–15% of affected patients

CLINICAL FINDINGS

- Round or ovoid, rubbery, discrete, relatively mobile, nontender mass, 1–5 cm in diameter
- Usually discovered incidentally
- Does not occur after menopause unless on hormone replacement therapy

DIAGNOSIS

- Differential diagnosis: fibrocystic disease or cyst, breast cancer, lipoma, phyllodes tumor, breast abscess, intraductal papilloma, fat necrosis
- Breast ultrasonography useful in differentiating cystic from solid mass
- Needle biopsy or fine-needle aspiration generally adequate for diagnosis
- Excision with pathological examination if diagnosis remains uncertain

TREATMENT

- No treatment necessary

Armando E. Giuliano, MD

Bronchial Obstruction

 KEY FEATURES

- May be caused by retained secretions, aspiration, foreign bodies, bronchogenic carcinoma, extrinsic compression, or metastatic tumors
- Recurrent pneumonia in the same location or slow resolution (>3 mo) of a pneumonia suggests obstruction

 CLINICAL FINDINGS

- Dyspnea, cough, wheezing, and pulmonary infection may occur
- Prolonged expiration and localized wheezing may be found
- Complete obstruction of a main stem bronchus may manifest with asymmetric chest expansion, mediastinal shift, absent breath sounds, or dullness to percussion
- X-ray films may show atelectasis, postobstructive infiltrates, and air trapping
- CT scan may demonstrate the nature and exact location of obstruction

 DIAGNOSIS

- Bronchoscopy is required for definitive diagnosis

 TREATMENT

- Treatment of infection, if present
- Definitive treatment depends on the cause of the obstruction

Mark S. Chesnutt, MD
Thomas J. Prendergast, MD

Bursitis

 KEY FEATURES

- Inflammation may be secondary to trauma, infection, or arthritis (eg, gout, rheumatoid arthritis, or osteoarthritis)
- Subdeltoid, olecranon, ischial, trochanteric, semimembranous-gastrocnemius (Baker's cyst), and prepatellar bursae are common locations

 CLINICAL FINDINGS

- More likely than arthritis to begin abruptly and be tender and swollen
- Active and passive range of motion is usually much more limited in arthritis than in bursitis

 DIAGNOSIS

- Acute swelling and redness calls for aspiration to rule out infection
- A bursal fluid white blood cell count of greater than 1000/μL indicates inflammation from infection, rheumatoid arthritis, or gout
- In septic bursitis, the white cell count averages over 50,000/mL; most cases are caused by *Staphylococcus aureus*
- Chronic, stable olecranon bursa swelling without erythema or other signs of inflammation is unlikely to be infected and does not require aspiration
- A bursa can become symptomatic when it ruptures (eg, Baker's cyst, which, on rupture, can cause calf pain and swelling that mimic thrombophlebitis)
- Treatment of a ruptured cyst includes rest, leg elevation, and injection of triamcinolone, 20–40 mg, into the knee (which communicates with the cyst)

 TREATMENT

- Traumatic bursitis responds to local heat, rest, immobilization, NSAIDs, and local corticosteroid injections
- Bursectomy is indicated only when there are repeated infections
- Avoid repetitive minor trauma to the olecranon bursa by not resting the elbow on a hard surface or by wearing an elbow pad

David B. Hellmann, MD, FACP
John H. Stone, MD, MPH

Calcium Channel Blocker Overdose

 KEY FEATURES

- All calcium channel blockers (including verapamil, diltiazem, nifedipine, nicardipine, amlodipine, felodipine, isradipine, nisoldipine, nimodipine) share the ability to cause arteriolar vasodilation and depression of cardiac contractility after acute overdose

 CLINICAL FINDINGS

- Bradycardia, AV nodal block, hypotension, or a combination
- With severe poisoning, cardiac arrest may occur

 DIAGNOSIS

- Clinical
- Junctional bradycardia is a common finding with even moderate verapamil poisoning

 TREATMENT

- Administer activated charcoal
- In addition, perform whole-bowel irrigation as soon as possible if a sustained-release product has been ingested
- Treat hypotension and bradycardia with calcium chloride IV. Start with calcium chloride 10%, 10 mL, or calcium gluconate, 20 mL. Repeat the dose q3–5 min. The optimum (or maximum) dose has not been established, but there are reports of success after as much as 10–12 g of calcium chloride. Calcium is most useful in reversing negative inotropic effects and is less effective for AV nodal blockade and bradycardia
- Epinephrine infusion, 1–4 μg/min initially, and glucagon, 5–10 mg IV, have also been given with variable success
- A transcutaneous or internal cardiac pacemaker may be needed

Kent R. Olsen, MD

Calluses & Corns, Feet & Toes

 KEY FEATURES

- Callosities and corns are caused by pressure and friction resulting from faulty weight bearing, orthopedic deformities, improperly fitting shoes, neuropathies

 CLINICAL FINDINGS

- Tenderness on pressure and "after-pain" are the only symptoms
- The hyperkeratotic well-localized overgrowths always occur at pressure points
- Fingerprint lines are preserved over the surface (not so in warts)
- On paring, a glassy core is found (differentiating these disorders from plantar warts, which have multiple capillary bleeding points or black dots when pared)
- A soft corn often occurs laterally on the proximal portion of the fourth toe as a result of pressure against the bony structure of the interphalangeal joint of the fifth toe

 DIAGNOSIS

- Clinical

 TREATMENT

- Treatment consists of correcting mechanical abnormalities that cause friction and pressure
- Shoes must be properly fitted and orthopedic deformities corrected
- Callosities may be removed by careful paring of the callus after a warm-water soak or with keratolytic agents as found in various brands of corn pads
- Plantar hyperkeratosis of the heels can be treated successfully using 20% urea (Ureacin 20), urea/lactic acid combinations (Ulactin), or 12% lactic acid (Lac-Hydrin) nightly and a pumice stone after soaking in water

Timothy G. Berger, MD.

Campylobacter Infections

 KEY FEATURES

- Microaerophilic, motile, gram-negative rods
- Two species infect humans: *Campylobacter jejuni*, an important cause of diarrheal disease, and *Campylobacter fetus* subsp *fetus*, which typically causes systemic infection and not diarrhea
- Dairy cattle and poultry are important reservoirs

 CLINICAL FINDINGS

- *Campylobacter* gastroenteritis is associated with fever, abdominal pain, and diarrhea characterized by loose, watery, or bloody stools
- The disease is self-limited, but its duration can be shortened with antimicrobial therapy
- *C fetus* causes systemic infections that can be fatal, including primary bacteremia, endocarditis, meningitis, and focal abscesses. It infrequently causes gastroenteritis
- Patients infected with *C fetus* are often elderly, debilitated, or immunocompromised. Closely related species, collectively termed *Campylobacter*-like organisms, cause bacteremia in HIV-infected individuals

 DIAGNOSIS

- Blood culture
- Stool culture

 TREATMENT

- Both erythromycin, 250–500 mg QID for 5–7 days, and ciprofloxacin, 500 mg BID for 3–5 days, are effective regimens
- *C fetus*: Systemic infections respond to therapy with gentamicin, chloramphenicol, ceftriaxone, or ciprofloxacin. Ceftriaxone or chloramphenicol should be used to treat infections of the CNS because of their ability to penetrate the blood–brain barrier

Henry F. Chambers, MD

Cancer, Infectious Complications

 KEY FEATURES

- Increased susceptibility to bacterial and opportunistic infections
- Caused by impaired host defense mechanisms (breakdown of mucosal or other barriers) or myelosuppressive and immunosuppressive effects of chemotherapy
- At least 50% of infections in neutropenic patients are endogenous
- Incidence of bacteremia rises dramatically with WBC count <1000/µL or granulocytes <200/µL
- Common bacterial infections: *Enterobacteriaceae (Klebsiella, Enterobacter, Serratia, Escherichia coli), Pseudomonas, Staphylococcus,* and *Streptococcus, Corynebacterium, Clostridium difficile, Mycobacterium,* and *Legionella*
- With prolonged neutropenia or after bone marrow transplantation, there is an increased risk for fungal (*Candida, Aspergillus*), parasitic (pneumocystis), and viral (herpes zoster, cytomegalovirus, respiratory syncytial virus, influenza) infections

 CLINICAL FINDINGS

- Fever and neutropenia
- May not see fever in patients on corticosteroids; shaking chills, hypotension and breathing difficulties may be clues to acute infection

 DIAGNOSIS

- CBC with differential
- Urinalysis
- CXR
- Urine and blood cultures
- Symptom-directed evaluation

 TREATMENT

PROPHYLAXIS

- Oral antibiotics (eg, ciprofloxacin and amoxicillin/clavulanate) in low-risk patients; levofloxacin for higher-risk patients
- IV immunoglobulin for patients with B cell malignancies and acute infections

(chronic lymphocytic leukemia, multiple myeloma, bone marrow transplant)

- G-CSF and GM-CSF effective at reducing duration of neutropenia and frequency and severity of infection after myelosuppressive chemotherapy or bone marrow transplant for nonmyeloid malignancies

THERAPY

- Treat immediately before cultures positive
- Initial monotherapy with a third-generation cephalosporin (eg, ceftazidime or cefepime) or a combination β-lactam (eg, piperacillin)
- Add vancomycin or amphotericin B based on clinical suspicion, culture results, or prolonged fever in the absence of positive cultures
- For persistent fevers or clinical deterioration, change gram-negative coverage to an agent with a broader spectrum (eg, imipenem/meropenem)
- If *Stenotrophomonas* is suspected, add trimethoprim-sulfamethoxazole

Hope Rugo, MD

Candidiasis, Oral

 KEY FEATURES

- Commonly encountered among denture wearers, in debilitated states, diabetes, anemia, chemotherapy or local irradiation, corticosteroids or broad-spectrum antibiotics
- Often heralds HIV infection
- Angular cheilitis is a symptom, although it can be seen in nutritional deficiencies

 CLINICAL FINDINGS

- Painful creamy-white curd-like patches
- White patches can be easily rubbed off by a tongue depressor, unlike leukoplakia or lichen planus, revealing an underlying irregular erythema

 DIAGNOSIS

- Clinical
- A wet preparation using potassium hydroxide will reveal spores and may show nonseptate mycelia
- Biopsy will show intraepithelial pseudomycelia of *Candida albicans*

 TREATMENT

- Fluconazole (100 mg daily for 7–14 days), ketoconazole (200–400 mg with breakfast [requires acidic gastric environment for absorption] for 7–14 days), clotrimazole troches (10 mg dissolved orally 5 times daily), or nystatin vaginal troches (100,000 units dissolved PO 5 times daily) or mouth rinses (500,000 units [5 mL of 100,000 units/mL] held in the mouth before swallowing TID)
- Shorter duration therapy with fluconazole is effective
- In HIV infection, longer courses may be needed, and itraconazole (200 mg PO daily) may be indicated in fluconazole-refractory cases
- 0.12% chlorhexidine or half-strength hydrogen peroxide mouth rinses may provide local relief
- Nystatin powder (100,000 units/g) applied to dentures 3 or 4 times daily for several weeks may help denture wearers

Robert K. Jackler, MD
Michael J. Kaplan, MD

Carbon Monoxide Poisoning

 KEY FEATURES

- Avidly binds to hemoglobin, which results in reduced oxygen-carrying capacity and altered delivery of oxygen to cells

 CLINICAL FINDINGS

- At low carbon monoxide levels (carboxyhemoglobin < 25%) there may be headache, dizziness, nausea
- With higher levels, confusion, dyspnea, and syncope may occur
- Hypotension, coma, and seizures are common with levels >50–60%
- Survivors of acute severe poisoning may develop permanent neurological deficits

 DIAGNOSIS

- Suspect in the setting of severe headache or acutely altered mental status, especially if multiple victims
- Diagnosis depends on specific measurement of the arterial or venous carboxyhemoglobin saturation, although the level may have declined if high-flow oxygen therapy has already been administered
- Routine arterial blood gas testing and pulse oximetry are not useful because they may give falsely normal oxyhemoglobin saturation levels

 TREATMENT

- Remove victim from exposure
- Administer 100% oxygen by tight-fitting high-flow reservoir face mask or endotracheal tube
- Hyperbaric oxygen can provide 100% oxygen under higher than atmospheric pressures, further shortening the half-life; it may be useful if immediately available for patients with coma or seizures and in pregnant women

Kent R. Olsen, MD

Carcinoid Syndrome, Malignant

 ### KEY FEATURES

- Uncommon
- Caused by tumors of argentaffin cells such as carcinoid tumors of the small bowel metastatic to the liver; less commonly, primary carcinoid tumors of lung or stomach
- Related syndromes occur in patients with pancreatic tumors
- Caused by release of vasoactive substances: serotonin, histamine, catecholamines, prostaglandins, vasoactive intestinal peptide

 ### CLINICAL FINDINGS

- Facial flushing, telangiectasias
- Abdominal cramps and diarrhea
- Bronchospasm
- Edema of the head and neck (especially with bronchial carcinoid)
- Cardiac valvular lesions (tricuspid or pulmonary stenosis or regurgitation)

 ### DIAGNOSIS

- 24-h urine 5-hydroxyindoleacetic acid (5-HIAA) is increased to >25 mg/day

 ### TREATMENT

- Prednisone, 15–30 mg/day
- Hydration and diphenoxylate with atropine for diarrhea
- Cyproheptadine, 4 mg PO TID, or methysergide maleate, 2 mg PO TID (up to 16 mg) for severe diarrhea
- Cimetidine and phenothiazines also helpful
- Octreotide acetate, 100–600 µg/day SC in 2–4 divided doses, is the most effective agent for reducing symptoms and levels of urinary 5-HIAA
- Surgical resection of localized carcinoid tumors
- Chemotherapy is moderately effective in metastatic disease

Hope Rugo, MD

Carcinoid Tumors, Bronchial

 ### KEY FEATURES

- Diagnosis includes carcinoid and bronchial gland tumors, which are low-grade malignancies
- Most patients are younger than 60 yr; men and women are affected equally
- Tumors grow slowly and rarely metastasize

 ### CLINICAL FINDINGS

- Common symptoms are hemoptysis, cough, focal wheezing , recurrent pneumonia
- Carcinoid syndrome is rare
- Bronchoscopy may reveal a pink or purple tumor in a central airway
- Complications involve bleeding and airway obstruction rather than tumor invasion or spread

 ### DIAGNOSIS

- Biopsy may be complicated by significant bleeding
- CT is useful to localize lesions and follow their growth over time
- Octreotide scintigraphy may aid in tumor localization

 ### TREATMENT

- Surgical excision is necessary in some cases
- Prognosis is generally favorable
- Most bronchial carcinoid tumors are resistant to radiation or chemotherapy

Mark S. Chesnutt, MD
Thomas J. Prendergast, MD

Carcinoid Tumors, Gastric

 ### KEY FEATURES

- Gastric carcinoids are rare tumors, accounting for <1% of gastric neoplasms
- Occur sporadically (20%) or secondary to chronic hypergastrinemia (80%)
- Most sporadic carcinoids are solitary, >2 cm in size, and have strong propensity for metastatic spread and carcinoid syndrome
- Carcinoids secondary to chronic hypergastrinemia occur in association either with pernicious anemia (75%) or Zollinger-Ellison syndrome with multiple endocrine neoplasm type I (5%), tend to be multicentric, are <1 cm in size, and have a low potential for metastatic spread and carcinoid syndrome
- Metastatic disease has elevated serum levels of 5-hydroxytryptophan rather than serotonin or 5-hydroxyindoleacetic acid, as in small intestinal carcinoid

 ### CLINICAL FINDINGS

- Most asymptomatic; detected incidentally during endoscopy. May ulcerate, causing occult GI bleeding and anemia
- Metastatic gastric carcinoids may present with atypical carcinoid syndrome manifested by flushing and diarrhea

 ### DIAGNOSIS

- Endoscopy demonstrates solitary or multiple nodules, which may be umbilicated or ulcerated
- Diagnosis confirmed by biopsy showing small, round cells proved to be neuroendocrine cells by silver staining and immunohistochemical stains
- Staging included abdominal CT scan and nuclear somatostatin receptor scintography

 ### TREATMENT

- Small lesions treated with endoscopic resection followed by periodic endoscopic surveillance
- Alternatively, antrectomy reduces serum gastrin levels and may lead to regression in patients with multiple lesions
- Large or multiple carcinoids are treated with surgical tumor resection

- Symptomatic metastatic disease treated with resection, if possible. Somatostatin analog therapy (octreotide) or hepatic arterial chemoembolization

Kenneth R. McQuaid, MD

Cardiomyopathy, Hypertrophic

KEY FINDINGS

- Myocardial hypertrophy impinging on the left ventricular (LV) cavity, narrowing the LV outflow tract during systole, causes dynamic obstruction
- Obstruction is worsened by sympathetic stimulation, digoxin, postextrasystolic beats, Valsalva's maneuver, peripheral vasodilator drugs
- Inherited forms usually present in early adulthood
- Acquired forms in elderly patients with a long history of hypertension
- Atrial fibrillation is a long-term consequence and a poor prognostic sign
- Ventricular arrhythmias are common
- Sudden death may occur, often in athletes after extraordinary exertion

CLINICAL FINDINGS

- Often presents with dyspnea, chest pain, or syncope (typically postexertional)
- Physical examination: bisferiens carotid pulse, sustained or triple apical impulse, and loud S_4
- Loud systolic murmur that increases with upright posture or Valsalva's maneuver and decreases with squatting

DIAGNOSIS

- ECG: left ventricular hypertrophy and, occasionally, septal Q waves in the absence of myocardial infarction
- Echocardiogram: ventricular hypertrophy, which may be asymmetric; usually normal or enhanced contractility and signs of dynamic obstruction
- CXR: often unimpressive

TREATMENT

- β-blockers (Table 40, page 1233) indicated in symptomatic individuals, especially when dynamic outflow obstruction is noted on echocardiogram
- Calcium channel blockers, especially verapamil (Table 40, page 1233), also effective
- Excision of part of the myocardial septum in patients with severe symptoms
- Dual-chamber pacing may prevent the progression of hypertrophy and obstruction

- Nonsurgical septal ablation by injection of alcohol into septal branches of the left coronary artery
- Implantable defibrillator for malignant ventricular arrhythmias or unexplained syncope

Barry M. Massie, MD
Thomas M. Amidon, MD

Cardiomyopathy, Peripartum

KEY FEATURES

- Defined as heart failure during pregnancy or in the first 6 mo postpartum in a woman with no other cause
- Incidence from 1:4000 to 1:1000, higher in Africa; at risk are older women, mothers with twins, and patients with pregnancy-induced hypertension
- Cause unknown
- Mortality is 6% at 5 yr in patients with cardiomegaly 6 mo from symptom onset, with 50% recurrence rate in subsequent pregnancy and a 19% mortality rate

CLINICAL FINDINGS

- Congestive heart failure
- Sinus tachycardia and atrial or ventricular arrhythmias
- Death may result from a fatal arrhythmia or embolism

DIAGNOSIS

- Clinical presentation with echocardiographic findings of dilated cardiomyopathy and exclusion of other causes

TREATMENT

- Treat as for other causes of congestive heart failure (see *Congestive heart failure*)

William R. Crombleholme, MD

Cardiomyopathy, Primary Dilated

 KEY FEATURES

- Left ventricular (LV) dilation and systolic dysfunction
- Symptoms and signs of congestive heart failure (most commonly dyspnea)
- Causes: chronic alcohol abuse and unrecognized myocarditis, amyloidosis, sarcoidosis, hemochromatosis
- Often no cause can be identified
- Not associated with the major causes of cardiac disease, ischemic heart disease, hypertension, valvular disease, or congenital defects

 CLINICAL FINDINGS

- Symptoms of heart failure usually develop gradually
- The initial presentation may be severe biventricular failure
- Physical examination: cardiomegaly, S_3 gallop rhythm, and often a murmur of mitral regurgitation
- Arterial and pulmonary emboli occur more often in dilated cardiomyopathy than in ischemic cardiomyopathy

 DIAGNOSIS

- ECG: low QRS voltage, nonspecific repolarization abnormalities, intraventricular conduction delay
- CXR: cardiomegaly
- Echocardiogram: LV dilatation, thinning, and global dysfunction; can exclude valvular or other lesions
- Exercise scintigraphy: large reversible defect suggests underlying coronary disease, but false-positive tests are common
- Cardiac catheterization: seldom of value

 TREATMENT

- Few cases are amenable to specific therapy
- Discontinue alcohol use
- Treat endocrine causes (thyroid dysfunction, acromegaly, pheochromocytoma)
- Immunosuppressive therapy is not indicated
- Treat congestive heart failure (see *Congestive heart failure*)
- Chronic anticoagulation for emboli

Barry M. Massie, MD
Thomas M. Amidon, MD

Carotid Artery Aneurysm

 KEY FEATURES

- Much more common in the intracerebral than the cervical portion of carotid arteries
- Most often, cervical aneurysms arise in the common carotid artery, are fusiform, and are associated with atherosclerosis
- Traumatic aneurysms can be related to healing of an internal carotid dissection or to penetrating trauma
- Mycotic aneurysms can be caused by staphylococcal, *Escherichia coli*, or tuberculous infections
- Other causes: vasculitides, Behçet's disease, Takayasu's disease, fibromuscular dysplasia, and segmental arterial mediolysis

 CLINICAL FINDINGS

- Pulsatile mass in the neck
- Neck pain
- Cranial nerve dysfunction
- Transient ischemic attack or stroke

 DIAGNOSIS

- Diagnosis confirmed by angiography

 TREATMENT

- Surgery indicated for aneurysms resulting from penetrating trauma, aneurysms associated with neurological deficit, mycotic aneurysms, enlarging aneurysms, and aneurysms >2 cm diameter
- Primary repair of the artery indicated for most penetrating injuries
- Carotid resection and interposition grafting or simple carotid ligation indicated for most other aneurysms

Louis M. Messina, MD
Laura K. Pak, MD
Lawrence M. Tierney, Jr, MD

Carotid Body Tumor

 KEY FEATURES

- Carotid body tumors are also called paraganglionomas or chemodectomas
- Rare
- Usually present as painless neck masses
- Most are slow growing and benign, but lymph node metastases have been reported

 CLINICAL FINDINGS

- If untreated, they are locally invasive; a large tumor may cause vagus or hypoglossal nerve deficit from mass effect or may encircle the internal carotid artery to the skull base

 DIAGNOSIS

- Biopsy is contraindicated; diagnosis is made by angiography or MRA
- The tumor is hypervascular, splays the internal and external carotid arteries, and produces angiographic tumor blush in the center of a widened carotid bifurcation

 TREATMENT

- Preoperative angiography is performed for tumor embolization and test occlusion of the internal carotid artery for tumors >4 cm diameter
- Resection of large tumors is complicated by cranial nerve injury in 40%
- Excellent prognosis after complete resection; survival is equal to that of age-matched controls and long-term recurrence of only 6%

Louis M. Messina, MD
Laura K. Pak, MD
Lawrence M. Tierney, Jr, MD

Carotid Dissection

KEY FEATURES

- A false channel in the wall of the carotid artery produced by a tear in the intima
- May be spontaneous or traumatic (shearing of the internal carotid artery between the C2 and C3 transverse processes during deceleration injuries)

CLINICAL FINDINGS

- Classic triad of symptoms: unilateral neck pain or headache, stroke or transient ischemic attack, and incomplete Horner's syndrome (miosis and ptosis without anhidrosis)

DIAGNOSIS

- Diagnosis confirmed at angiography or CT angiography
- Noncontrast CT of the head to confirm no intracranial hemorrhage

TREATMENT

- Primary treatment is heparin followed by warfarin anticoagulation (to an INR of 2.0–3.0)
- With such treatment, 60–85% of carotid dissections will recannulate in 3–6 mo with complete or near-complete neurological recovery
- Recurrent dissection occurs in ~3% at 3 yr and ~12% at 10 yr
- Recurrent dissection most often involves a different cervical vessel, which justifies use of long-term aspirin
- Surgery (usually carotid interposition) or carotid stenting is indicated for ongoing symptoms with residual stenosis or aneurysm

Louis M. Messina, MD
Laura K. Pak, MD
Lawrence M. Tierney, Jr, MD

Carpal Tunnel Syndrome

KEY FEATURES

- An entrapment neuropathy from compression of the median nerve in the carpal tunnel, particularly from synovitis of the tendon sheaths or carpal joints and recent or poorly healed fractures
- Most frequently afflicts those who perform repetitive hand movements
- Associated with pregnancy, rheumatoid arthritis, myxedema, amyloidosis, sarcoidosis, leukemia (tissue infiltration), acromegaly, and hyperparathyroidism

CLINICAL FINDINGS

- Pain, burning, or tingling in the distribution of the median nerve
- Aching pain may radiate proximally into the forearm and occasionally to the shoulder
- Pain is exacerbated by manual activity, particularly by extremes of volar flexion or dorsiflexion of the wrist
- Impairment of sensation in the median nerve distribution may be demonstrable
- Tinel's or Phalen's sign may be positive. (Tinel's sign is shock-like pain on volar wrist percussion; Phalen's sign is pain in the distribution of the median nerve when both wrists are flexed 90° with the dorsal aspects of the hands held in apposition for 1 min)
- Muscle weakness or atrophy, especially of the thenar eminence, appears later than sensory disturbances

DIAGNOSIS

- Electromyography and determinations of segmental sensory and motor conduction delay

TREATMENT

- Change of manual activity (or ergonomic improvements); splinting of the hand and forearm at night
- NSAIDs and/or injection of corticosteroid by an experienced operator into the carpal tunnel
- Operative division of the volar carpal ligament gives lasting relief from pain

David B. Hellmann, MD, FACP
John H. Stone, MD, MPH

Cat Scratch Disease

KEY FEATURES

- Cat-scratch disease is an acute infection of children and young adults caused by *Bartonella henselae*
- It is transmitted from cats to humans as the result of a scratch or bite
- Disseminated forms of the disease—bacillary angiomatosis and peliosis hepatis—occur in HIV-infected persons

CLINICAL FINDINGS

- Within a few days, one third of patients will develop a papule or ulcer at the inoculation site
- One to 3 weeks later, fever, headache, and malaise occur
- The regional lymph nodes become enlarged, often tender, and may suppurate
- Lymphadenopathy resembles that resulting from neoplasm, tuberculosis, lymphogranuloma venereum, and bacterial lymphadenitis
- Encephalitis occurs rarely

DIAGNOSIS

- Clinical
- Special cultures for *Bartonella,* serology, or excisional biopsy, although rarely necessary, confirm the diagnosis
- The biopsy reveals necrotizing lymphadenitis and is itself not specific for cat scratch disease

TREATMENT

- Cat-scratch disease is usually self-limited, requiring no specific therapy
- Bacillary angiomatosis and endocarditis respond to treatment with a macrolide (eg, azithromycin, 500 mg QD) or doxycycline, 100 mg BID for 4–8 weeks

Henry F. Chambers, MD

Cataract

 KEY FEATURES

- Cataract means lens opacity
- Cataracts usually occur bilaterally
- Senile (age-related) cataract is the most common type
- Most persons older than 60 have some degree of lens opacity
- Other causes include congenital infections, diabetes mellitus, chronic corticosteroid use, uveitis, and ocular trauma

 CLINICAL FINDINGS

- Usually gradually progressive visual impairment

 DIAGNOSIS

- Ophthalmoscopy, particularly with a dilated pupil, shows opacities in the red reflex
- As the cataract progresses, retinal visualization becomes increasingly difficult

 TREATMENT

- When visual impairment significantly affects daily activities, surgical therapy is usually warranted
- Treatment involves surgical removal and insertion of an intraocular lens of appropriate refractive power

Paul Riordan-Eva, FRCOphth

Cellulitis

 KEY FEATURES

- A diffuse spreading infection of the skin
- Usually due to gram-positive cocci, though gram-negative rods such as *Escherichia coli* may be responsible
- The major portal of entry for lower leg cellulitis is toe web tinea pedis with fissuring of the skin at this site

 CLINICAL FINDINGS

- Usually on the lower leg
- The lesion is hot and red
- In cases of venous stasis, the only clue to cellulitis may be a new localized area of tenderness. Recurrent attacks may sometimes affect lymphatic vessels, producing a permanent swelling called "solid edema"
- Differential diagnosis
  - Deep vein thrombosis
  - Necrotizing fasciitis
  - Erysipelas
  - Venous stasis
  - Contact dermatitis
  - Candidiasis
  - Scarlet fever
  - Sclerosing panniculitis
  - Underlying osteomyelitis

 DIAGNOSIS

- Attempts to isolate the responsible organism by injecting and then aspirating saline are successful in 20% of cases

 TREATMENT

- Intravenous or parenteral antibiotics may be required for the first 24–72 h
- In mild cases or following the initial parenteral therapy, dicloxacillin or cephalexin, 250–500 mg four times daily for 7–10 days, is usually adequate
- In patients in whom intravenous treatment is not instituted, the first dose of oral antibiotic can be increased to 750–1000 mg to achieve rapid high blood levels

Timothy G. Berger, MD

Cerumen Impaction

 KEY FEATURES

- Cerumen is a protective secretion produced by the outer portion of the ear canal
- In most individuals, the ear canal is self-cleansing
- In most cases, cerumen impaction is self-induced through ill-advised attempts at cleaning the ear

 CLINICAL FINDINGS

- Fullness in ear
- Conductive hearing loss when accumulation blocks the canal

 DIAGNOSIS

- Made by otoscopic inspection

 TREATMENT

- Recommended hygiene consists of cleaning the external opening with a washcloth over the index finger without entering the canal itself
- May be relieved with detergent ear drops (eg, 3% hydrogen peroxide; 6.5% carbamide peroxide), mechanical removal, suction, or irrigation
- Irrigation is performed with water at body temperature to avoid a vestibular caloric response, which could produce nystagmus and nausea. The stream should be directed at the ear canal wall adjacent to the cerumen plug
- Irrigation should be performed only when the tympanic membrane is known to be intact
- Use of jet irrigators designed for cleaning teeth (eg, WaterPik) for wax removal should be avoided because they may result in tympanic membrane perforations
- After irrigation, the ear canal should be thoroughly dried (eg, by instilling isopropyl alcohol or using a hair blow-dryer on low-power setting) to reduce the likelihood of inducing external otitis
- Specialty referral for cleaning under microscopic guidance is indicated when the impaction has not responded to routine measures or if the patient has a history of chronic otitis media or tympanic membrane perforation

Robert K. Jackler, MD
Michael J. Kaplan, MD

Cervical Polyps

 KEY FEATURES

- Commonly occur after menarche and are occasionally noted in post-menopausal women
- The cause is not known, but inflammation may play an etiological role
- Must be differentiated from polypoid neoplastic disease of the endometrium, small submucous pedunculated myomas, and endometrial polyps
- Cervical polyps rarely contain malignant foci

 CLINICAL FINDINGS

- Discharge and abnormal vaginal bleeding
- Abnormal bleeding should not be ascribed to a cervical polyp without sampling the endocervix and endometrium

 DIAGNOSIS

- The polyps are visible in the cervical os on speculum examination

 TREATMENT

- Cervical polyps can generally be removed in the office by avulsion with a uterine packing forceps or ring forceps
- If the cervix is soft, patulous, or definitely dilated and the polyp is large, surgical D&C is required (especially if the pedicle is not readily visible)
- Because of the possibility of endometrial disease, cervical polypectomy should be accompanied by endometrial sampling, and all tissue removed should be submitted for microscopic examination

H. Trent MacKay, MD, MPH

Cervicitis

 KEY FEATURES

- Infection of the cervix must be distinguished from physiological ectopy of columnar epithelium, which is common in young women
- Infection may result from a sexually transmitted pathogen such as *Neisseria gonorrhoeae, Chlamydia,* or herpesvirus
- In most cases, none of these organisms can be isolated.

 CLINICAL FINDINGS

- Mucopurulent cervicitis is characterized by a red edematous cervix with a purulent yellow discharge
- Herpesvirus presents with vesicles and ulcers on the cervix during a primary herpetic infection

 DIAGNOSIS

- Mucopurulent cervicitis is an insensitive predictor of either gonorrheal or chlamydial infection and in addition has a low positive predictive value

 TREATMENT

- Treatment should be based on microbiological testing
- Presumptive antibiotic treatment is not indicated unless there is a high prevalence of either *N gonorrhoeae* or *Chlamydia* in the population or if the patient is unlikely to return for treatment
- Three months after treatment, approximately 20% of women will have persistent or recurrent mucopus in the cervix, not explained by relapse or reinfection

H. Trent MacKay, MD, MPH

Chancroid

 KEY FEATURES

- A sexually transmitted disease caused by the gram-negative bacillus *Haemophilus ducreyi*
- Incubation period is 3–5 days

 CLINICAL FINDINGS

- Initial lesion at the site of inoculation is a vesicopustule that breaks down to form a painful, soft ulcer with a necrotic base, surrounding erythema, and undermined edges
- Multiple lesions, started by autoinoculation, and inguinal adenitis often develop
- The adenitis is usually unilateral and consists of tender, matted nodes of moderate size with overlying erythema. These may become fluctuant and rupture spontaneously
- With lymph node involvement, fever, chills, and malaise may develop
- Balanitis and phimosis are frequent complications in men
- Women may have no external signs of infection

 DIAGNOSIS

- Culturing a swab of the lesion onto special medium

 TREATMENT

- A single dose of either azithromycin, 1 g PO, or ceftriaxone, 250 mg IM, is effective treatment
- Effective multiple-dose regimens are amoxicillin-potassium clavulanate, 500/125 mg, PO TID for 7 days; erythromycin, 500 mg PO QID for 7 days; or ciprofloxacin, 500 mg PO BID for 3 days

Henry F. Chambers, MD

Cholecystectomy, Pre- & Post-Syndrome

 KEY FEATURES

PRECHOLECYSTECTOMY

- In a small group of patients (mostly women) with biliary colic, conventional radiographic studies of the upper gastrointestinal tract and gallbladder, including cholangiography, are unremarkable. However, emptying of the gallbladder is markedly reduced on gallbladder scintigraphy after injection of cholecystokinin. This may occur from fibrotic stenosis, adhesions or kinking of the cystic duct, ampullary spasm, or biliary dyskinesia

POSTCHOLECYSTECTOMY

- After cholecystectomy, some continue to complain about right upper quadrant pain, flatulence, and fatty food intolerance
- Choledocholithiasis or common duct stricture should be ruled out as a cause of persistent symptoms
- Pain has been associated with dilation of the cystic duct remnant, neuroma formation in the ductal wall, foreign body granuloma, or traction on the common duct by a long cystic duct

 DIAGNOSIS

- Abdominal or endoscopic ultrasonography or retrograde cholangiography may be necessary to exclude biliary tract disease
- Biliary manometry may be useful in documenting elevated baseline sphincter of Oddi pressures typical of sphincter dysfunction
- Biliary scintigraphy shows promise as a screening test for sphincter dysfunction

 TREATMENT

- Cholecystectomy is usually curative for precholecystectomy symptoms
- Endoscopic sphincterotomy can relieve symptoms of postcholecystectomy syndrome, dilated common bile duct, and elevated liver tests or elevated sphincter pressure on manometry

Lawrence S. Friedman, MD

Chromoblastomycosis

 KEY FEATURES

- A chronic, principally tropical cutaneous infection
- Usually affects young men who are agricultural workers
- Caused by several species of closely related black molds (*Fonsecaea* species and *Phialophora* species)

 CLINICAL FINDINGS

- Cutaneous lesions usually occur on a lower extremity and begin as a papule or ulcer
- Over months to years, papules enlarge to become vegetating, papillomatous, verrucous, elevated nodules
- Satellite lesions may appear along lymphatics
- Secondary bacterial infection may occur
- Elephantiasis may result

 DIAGNOSIS

- Potassium hydroxide preparations of pus or skin scrapings are helpful, showing brown, thick-walled, spherical, sometimes septate cells
- The type of reproduction found in culture determines the species
- *Fonsecaea pedrosoi* is the pathogen in most cases

 TREATMENT

- Itraconazole, 200–400 mg PO qd for 6–18 mo, achieves response rate of 65%
- Addition of flucytosine to itraconazole may improve response rates
- Cryosurgery alone for smaller lesions
- Cryosurgery combined with itraconazole for larger lesions

Richard J. Hamill, MD

Churg-Strauss Syndrome

 KEY FEATURES

- Idiopathic vasculitis of small and medium-sized arteries seen in patients with symptoms of asthma
- Affects multiple organ systems, most commonly skin and lung, but heart, GI tract, and peripheral nerve involvement is also seen

 CLINICAL FINDINGS

- Marked peripheral eosinophilia
- CXR findings range from transient infiltrates to pulmonary nodules

 DIAGNOSIS

- Tissue biopsy demonstrating eosinophilic vasculitis is required to confirm the diagnosis and exclude other causes

 TREATMENT

- Combination therapy with corticosteroids (prednisone, 1 mg/kg/day, tapering over 3–6 mo) and cyclophosphamide (1–2 mg/kg/day, tapered 1 yr after remission is achieved)

Mark S. Chesnutt, MD

Thomas J. Prendergast, MD

Clonidine Overdose

 KEY FEATURES

- Symptoms usually resolve in 24 h
- Deaths are rare
- Similar symptoms may occur after ingestion of topical nasal decongestants chemically similar to clonidine (oxymetazoline, tetrahydrozoline, naphazoline, brimonidine)

 CLINICAL FINDINGS

- Bradycardia, hypotension, miosis, respiratory depression, and coma are caused by central α_2-adrenergic effects
- Hypertension occasionally occurs, a result of peripheral α_1-adrenergic effects

 DIAGNOSIS

- Clinical

 TREATMENT

- Symptomatic treatment is usually sufficient. Maintain blood pressure with IV fluids. Dopamine can also be used. Atropine is usually effective for bradycardia
- Administer activated charcoal, 60–100 g PO or via gastric tube, mixed in aqueous slurry. Do not use for comatose or convulsing patients unless it can be given by gastric tube and the airway is protected by a cuffed endotracheal tube
- There is no specific antidote. Tolazoline should not be used for clonidine overdose because its effects are unpredictable. Naloxone has had anectodal success

Kent R. Olsen, MD

Coagulopathy of Liver Disease

 KEY FEATURES

- All coagulation factors except factor VIII are synthesized in the liver
- With hepatic insufficiency, vitamin K–dependent factors (factors II, VII, IX, X) and factor V are first to be affected
- Because of rapid turnover (half-life 6 h), factor VII level declines first
- Conversely, decreased fibrinogen synthesis does not occur unless liver disease is severe
- Liver disease also increases fibrinolysis because liver synthesizes α_2-antiplasmin (main inhibitor of fibrinolysis)
- Biliary tract disease may lead to vitamin K malabsorption
- Congestive splenomegaly may cause thrombocytopenia

 CLINICAL FINDINGS

- Bleeding at any site from coagulopathy
- Oozing at venipuncture sites from excessive fibrinolysis
- Clinical signs of liver disease
- No response to vitamin K
- Disseminated intravascular coagulation (DIC) may occur in end-stage liver disease

 DIAGNOSIS

- PT more prolonged than PTT
- Early in course of liver disease, only PT affected
- Platelet count may be reduced by low levels of thrombopoietin, hypersplenism, bone marrow suppression by alcohol, and folic acid deficiency
- Fibrinogen levels and thrombin time normal unless dysfibrinogenemia present
- Peripheral blood smear may show target cells

 TREATMENT

- Long-term treatment with factor replacement is usually ineffective
- Fresh-frozen plasma is treatment of choice, but volume overload limits ability to maintain hemostatic factor levels
- Factor IX concentrates contraindicated because of tendency to cause DIC
- Platelet transfusion may help if thrombocytopenia is present, but platelet recovery usually disappointing because of hypersplenism

Charles A. Linker, MD

Coal Worker's Pneumoconiosis

 KEY FEATURES

- An occupational pulmonary disease resulting from macrophages ingesting inhaled coal dust
- Cigarette smoking may have an additive detrimental effect on ventilatory function

 CLINICAL FINDINGS

- Simple coal worker's pneumoconiosis is usually asymptomatic; pulmonary function tests are unimpressive
- Complicated disease, "progressive massive fibrosis," resembles complicated silicosis, with conglomeration and contraction in upper lung zones

 DIAGNOSIS

- CXR shows diffuse small opacities prominent in upper lungs

 TREATMENT

- No therapy has demonstrated efficacy in controlled trials
- As with many other progressive inflammatory disorders of the lung, steroids have been tried

Mark S. Chesnutt, MD
Thomas J. Prendergast, MD

Coarctation of the Aorta

 KEY FEATURES

- Narrowing of the aortic arch distal to the origin of the left subclavian artery
- Collateral circulation through intercostal arteries and branches of subclavian arteries
- One cause of secondary hypertension in young patients
- Bicuspid aortic valve in 25%

 CLINICAL FINDINGS

- Usually no symptoms until hypertension produces left ventricular (LV) failure or cerebral hemorrhage (sometimes associated with congenital cerebral aneurysms)
- Strong arterial pulsations in the neck and suprasternal notch
- Hypertension in the arms, but blood pressure is normal or low in the legs
- Delayed or weak femoral pulsations
- Harsh systolic murmur heard in the back

 DIAGNOSIS

- ECG: left ventricular hypertrophy (LVH)
- CXR: scalloping of the ribs as a result of enlarged collateral intercostal arteries
- Echo-Doppler is diagnostic and can estimate severity of obstruction
- Primary method of diagnosis: measurement of gradient across stenosis by catheterization and aortography

 TREATMENT

- Up to age 20: All coarctations should be resected
- Younger than age 40: Surgery is advisable if refractory hypertension or significant LVH
- Surgical mortality rate: 1–4%
- Older than age 50: considerable surgical mortality
- Balloon angioplasty may become procedure of choice, but there is risk of aortic tears
- Most untreated patients younger than 50 die from complications, LV failure, or cerebral hemorrhage
- About 25% of corrected patients develop complications of original condition

Barry M. Massie, MD
Thomas M. Amidon, MD

Cold Agglutinin Disease

 KEY FEATURES

- Acquired hemolytic anemia caused by IgM autoantibody against RBCs, which characteristically do not react with cells at 37°C but only at lower temperatures
- Because blood temperature rarely falls below 20°C, only antibodies active at higher temperatures than this produce clinical effects
- In cooler parts of the circulation (fingers, nose, ears), IgM binds RBC and fixes complement. When RBC returns to warmer temperature, IgM antibody dissociates, leaving complement on the cell. Lysis rarely occurs, but C3b present on RBC recognized by Kupffer cells in liver, resulting in RBC sequestration
- Most cases of chronic cold agglutinin disease idiopathic
- Occurs in mycoplasmal pneumonia, infectious mononucleosis, Waldenström's macroglobulinemia

 CLINICAL FINDINGS

- Mottled or numb fingers or toes on exposure to cold
- Hemolytic anemia, rarely severe
- Hemoglobinuria with exposure to cold

 DIAGNOSIS

- Mild anemia, with reticulocytosis and spherocytes
- Direct Coombs test positive for complement only
- Occasionally (in low-titer cold agglutinin disease), only the more sensitive micro-Coombs test is positive

 TREATMENT

- Mild disease: Avoid exposure to cold
- Severe disease: alkylating agents (eg, cyclophosphamide) or immunosuppressive agents (eg, cyclosporine)
- Splenectomy and prednisone usually ineffective
- High-dose IVIG (2 g/kg) may be effective temporarily
- Rituximab, 375 mg/m^2 IV every week for 4 weeks, may be effective

Charles A. Linker, MD

Colitis, Microscopic

 KEY FEATURES

- Chronic watery diarrhea with normal-appearing mucosa at endoscopy
- Much more common in women, especially in the fifth to sixth decades
- Associated with chronic NSAID use in up to half; idiopathic in the remainder

 CLINICAL FINDINGS

- Chronic or recurrent diarrhea; may remit spontaneously after many years

 DIAGNOSIS

- Sigmoidoscopy or colonoscopy with biopsy
- Histological evaluation of mucosal biopsies shows lymphocytic inflammation in the lamina propria

 TREATMENT

- Bulking agents or antidiarrheal agents (loperamide, cholestyramine) for mild disease
- Bismuth subsalicylate (2 tablets QID) for 2 mo may be effective
- 5-aminosalicylates (sulfasalazine, mesalamine) are of unproved benefit

Kenneth R. McQuaid, MD

Colorectal Cancer, Hereditary Nonpolyposis

 KEY FEATURES

- Markedly increased risk of colorectal cancer and other cancers, including endometrial, ovarian, renal or vesical, hepatobiliary, gastric, small intestine
- Accounts for 1–3% of all colorectal cancers
- Autosomal dominant
- Caused by a defect in 1 of several genes: *hMLH1, hMSH2, hMSH6, pPMS1,* and *hPMS2*
- Affected individuals have a 70–80% lifetime risk of colorectal carcinoma and a >30% lifetime risk of endometrial cancer
- HNPCC develops at an earlier age (mean, 44 yr) than sporadic colorectal cancers, and >66% arise proximal to the splenic flexure
- HNPCC cancers associated with markedly improved survival compared with sporadic colorectal cancers

 CLINICAL FINDINGS

- Few colonic adenomas, flat, and more often contain villous features or high-grade dysplasia
- Metachronous cancers within 10 yr occur in up to 45% of patients

 DIAGNOSIS

- Obtain thorough family history of cancer
- Offer genetic testing to patients whose families fulfill the Amsterdam criteria: ≥3 first-degree family members with colorectal cancer (or 1 of the other associated cancers); colon cancer involving at least 2 generations; (3) ≥1 colon cancer diagnosed before age 50
- Consider genetic testing also for individuals with colorectal cancer or endometrial cancer diagnosed before age 50 (especially if right sided, undifferentiated, or signet ring) or adenoma before age 40; those with colorectal cancer who have a first-degree relative with colorectal cancer or extracolonic cancer diagnosed before age 50; those with a personal history of 2 HNPCC-associated cancers

- Test tumor tissues of affected individuals or family members for microsatellite instability.

 TREATMENT

- If genetic testing documents HNPCC gene mutation, screen affected relatives with colonoscopy every 1–2 yr beginning at age 25 (or 5 yr younger than the earliest diagnosed family cancer)
- In families that fulfill the Amsterdam criteria or that have tumors with proved microsatellite instability but do not have a documented gene mutation, recommend colonoscopic screening for all family members
- Subtotal colectomy with ileorectal anastomosis if cancer is found (followed by annual surveillance of the rectal stump)
- Endometrial aspiration or transvaginal ultrasound screening for endometrial cancer in women beginning at age 25–35
- Prophylactic hysterectomy and oophorectomy considered in women of post–child-bearing age

Kenneth R. McQuaid, MD

Connective Tissue Disease, Mixed

 KEY FEATURES

- Features of more than one rheumatic disease; overlap connective tissue disease is the preferred designation for patients having features of different rheumatic diseases
- Special attention has been drawn to patients with overlapping features of systemic lupus erythematosus (SLE), systemic sclerosis, and polymyositis
- Initially, these patients were thought to have a distinct entity (mixed connective tissue disease) defined by a specific autoantibody to ribonuclear protein (RNP)
- With time, in many patients, the manifestations evolve to one predominant disease, such as scleroderma, and many patients with antibodies to RNP have clear-cut SLE

 CLINICAL FINDINGS

- Characteristics of multiple rheumatic diseases

 DIAGNOSIS

- Clinical
- Differential diagnosis includes SLE, scleroderma, polymyositis, Sjögren's syndrome, rheumatoid arthritis, eosinophilic fasciitis, graft-versus-host disease

 TREATMENT

- Symptom directed
- SLE, systemic sclerosis, or polymyositis features are treated the same way as the diseases

David B. Hellmann, MD, FACP
John H. Stone, MD, MPH

Contraception, Abstinence

 KEY FEATURES

- Contraception based on **abstinence during fertile periods** is most effective when intercourse is restricted to the postovular phase of the cycle or a barrier method is used at other times
- Women need to identify their fertile periods (see *Infertility*). Couples may achieve low pregnancy rates or as high as 20% with fertility awareness
- "**Symptothermal**" **natural family planning** is patient-observed increase in clear elastic cervical mucus, brief abdominal midcycle discomfort ("mittelschmerz"), and a sustained rise of the basal body temperature about 2 weeks after onset of menstruation
- Unprotected intercourse is avoided from shortly after the menstrual period, when fertile mucus is first identified, until 48 h after ovulation, as identified by a sustained rise in temperature and the disappearance of clear elastic mucus
- In the **calendar method,** after the length of the menstrual cycle has been observed for at least 8 mo, the following calculations are made: (1) The first fertile day is determined by subtracting 18 days from the shortest cycle; (2) the last fertile day is determined by subtracting 11 days from the longest cycle. For example, if the observed cycles run from 24 to 28 days, the fertile period would extend from the 6th day of the cycle (24–18) through the 17th day (28–11). Day 1 of the cycle is the first day of menses
- Basal body temperature method shows the safe time for intercourse after ovulation has passed
- The temperature must be taken immediately upon awakening, before any activity
- A slight drop in temperature often occurs 12–24 h before ovulation, and a rise of about 0.4°C occurs 1–2 days after ovulation
- The elevated temperature continues throughout the remainder of the cycle
- The risk of pregnancy increases starting 5 days before the day of ovulation, peaks on the day of ovulation, and then rapidly decreases to zero by the day after ovulation

H. Trent MacKay, MD, MPH

Contraception, Emergency

 KEY FEATURES

- Information on clinics or individual clinicians providing emergency contraception in the US may be obtained by calling 1-888-668-2528

 TREATMENT

MEDICATION

- The following methods should be started within 72 h after unprotected coitus:
  - Levonorgestrel, 0.75 mg given in 2 doses 12 h apart (available in the US prepackaged as Plan B), has a 1% failure rate and is associated with less nausea and vomiting than the following combination regimen
  - Ethinyl estradiol, 50 μg, with 0.5 mg norgestrel (available in the US prepackaged as Preven), given in a regimen of 2 tablets initially followed by 2 tablets 12 h later
  - A comparable regimen includes 4 pills 12 h apart of Lo/Ovral, Nordette, or Levlen or the same regimen with the yellow pills of Triphasil or Tri-Levlen. The failure rate is approximately 3%, and antinausea medication should be provided
  - Ethinyl estradiol, 2.5 mg BID for 5 days. This regimen is as efficacious as the others but is associated with a higher likelihood of nausea, vomiting, and breast tenderness
  - Mifepristone, 10 mg as a single dose, has been shown to have the same failure rate as the levonorgestrel regimen, with minimal side effects, and appears to be effective given up to 120 h after unprotected intercourse. It is not currently available at this dose in the US

INTRAUTERINE DEVICES

- Copper-bearing intrauterine devices (IUDs) inserted within 5 days after one episode of unprotected midcycle coitus will prevent pregnancy
- The disadvantage of this method is possible infection, especially in rape cases
- The advantage is ongoing contraceptive protection if this is desired in a patient for whom the IUD is a suitable choice

H. Trent MacKay, MD, MPH

Contraception, Sterilization

 KEY FEATURES

- In the US, sterilization is the most popular method of birth control for couples who want no more children
- Vasectomy is a safe, simple procedure in which the vas deferens is severed and sealed through a scrotal incision under local anesthesia
- Female sterilization is performed via laparoscopic bipolar electrocoagulation or plastic ring application on the uterine tubes or via minilaparotomy with tubal resection
- The cumulative 10-year failure rate for all methods combined is 1.85%, varying from 0.75% for postpartum partial salpingectomy and laparoscopic unipolar coagulation to 3.65% for spring clips

H. Trent MacKay, MD, MPH

Cor Pulmonale

 KEY FEATURES

- Right ventricular (RV) hypertrophy and failure from hypoxia-associated lung disease or pulmonary vascular disease
- Most common cause: chronic obstructive pulmonary disease (COPD)
- Less frequent causes: pneumoconiosis, pulmonary fibrosis, kyphoscoliosis, primary pulmonary hypertension, repeated pulmonary embolization, sleep apnea (Pickwickian syndrome)

 CLINICAL FINDINGS

- Predominant symptoms—intensified with RV failure—are related to the underlying pulmonary disorder: chronic productive cough, exertional dyspnea, wheezing, easy fatigability, and weakness
- Other possible findings: dependent edema, right upper quadrant pain (hepatic congestion), cyanosis, clubbing, distended neck veins, RV heave, gallop
- Polycythemia is often present
- The arterial oxygen saturation is often <85%

 DIAGNOSIS

- Symptoms and signs of COPD with elevated jugular venous pressure, parasternal lift, edema, hepatomegaly, ascites
- ECG: tall, peaked P waves (P pulmonale), right axis deviation, and RV hypertrophy. Q waves in leads II, III, and aVF may mimic myocardial infarction. Frequent, nonspecific supraventricular arrhythmias
- CXR: enlarged right ventricle and pulmonary artery. Possible signs of pulmonary parenchymal disease
- Pulmonary function tests to confirm underlying lung disease
- Echocardiogram or angiography to exclude primary left ventricular failure as a cause of right-sided heart failure

 TREATMENT

- Treat underlying lung disease
- Oxygen, salt and fluid restriction, and diuretics
- Compensated cor pulmonale has the same prognosis as the underlying lung disease
- The average life expectancy is 2–5 yr when congestive signs appear, but survival is significantly longer when uncomplicated emphysema is the cause

Barry M. Massie, MD
Thomas M. Amidon, MD

Coxsackievirus Infections

KEY FEATURES

- Named after a town in northern New York State, the Coxsackievirus causes several clinical syndromes
- Enterovirus occurs most often during the summer months
- More than 50 serotypes and 2 major subgroups: A and B

CLINICAL FINDINGS

- Herpangina (subtype A): sudden-onset fevers, headaches, myalgias, and petechiae on the soft palate that become shallow ulcers. Resolves in 3 days
- Epidemic pleurodynia (Bornholm disease, subtype B): pleuritic chest pain, systemic symptoms, including headache, malaise, pharyngitis
- Aseptic meningitis (subtypes A and B): fever, headache, stiff neck, and CSF lymphocytosis. Encephalitis and transverse myelitis may occur
- Acute pericarditis (subtype B): positional, pleuritic chest pain, fevers and myalgias. Clinical and echocardiographic signs of pericarditis
- Hand-foot-and-mouth disease (subtype A): stomatitis and vesicular rash on hands and feet
- Hepatitis, renal disease, and myocarditis are also caused by Coxsackievirus infections

DIAGNOSIS

- Clinical diagnosis
- No reliable laboratory abnormality
- Neutralizing antibodies appear during convalescence

TREATMENT

- Supportive measures
- In severe cases, immunoglobulin treatment is sometimes used (anecdotal evidence)

Wayne X. Shandera, MD
Samuel Shelburne, MD

Cyanide Poisoning

KEY FEATURES

- In its gaseous form, hydrogen cyanide is an important component of fire smoke
- Cyanide-generating glycosides are also found in the pits of apricots and other related plants
- Cyanide is generated by the breakdown of nitroprusside, and poisoning can result from rapid high-dose infusions
- Cyanide is also formed by metabolism of acetonitrile, found in some over-the-counter fingernail glue removers
- Cyanide is rapidly absorbed by inhalation, skin absorption, or ingestion

CLINICAL FINDINGS

- The onset of toxicity is nearly instantaneous after inhalation but may be delayed for minutes to hours after ingestion of cyanide salts or cyanogenic plants or chemicals. Effects include headache, dizziness, nausea, abdominal pain, and anxiety followed by confusion, syncope, shock, seizures, coma, and death. The odor of "bitter almonds" may be detected on the victim's breath or in vomitus, although this is not a reliable finding

DIAGNOSIS

- The venous oxygen saturation may be elevated (>90%) in severe poisonings because tissues have failed to take up arterial oxygen
- Obtain blood cyanide levels (not usually readily available)

TREATMENT

- Remove the victim from exposure, taking care to avoid exposure to rescuers. Administer activated charcoal. At the scene, induce emesis if charcoal is not immediately available
- Stop or slow the nitroprusside infusion rate for suspected cyanide toxicity
- In the US, there are prepackaged cyanide antidotes (Table 141, page 1324)

Kent R. Olsen, MD

Cytomegalovirus (CMV) Infection

KEY FEATURES

- Most CMV infections asymptomatic
- Age-related rise in seroprevalence
- Acute acquired CMV infection is similar to infectious mononucleosis; unusual to develop pharyngeal symptoms
- Most CMV-related diseases occur in immunocompromised individuals, especially the HIV infected: CMV retinitis, GI and hepatobiliary, pulmonary, and neurological disease
- Major pathogen in transplant recipients by both direct infection and increasing rates of transplant rejection

CLINICAL FINDINGS

- CMV inclusion disease among infants born to acutely infected mothers, with CNS and hepatic malfunction
- CMV retinitis occurs primarily in advanced AIDS
- Neovascular, proliferative retinal lesions are found with retinitis
- GI and hepatobiliary CMV occurs in AIDS or with high-dose chemotherapy
- Esophagitis, small bowel inflammation, colitis, or cholangiopathy occur
- Pneumonitis occurs in transplant recipients and HIV-infected patients
- Neurological manifestations include polyneuropathy, transverse myelitis, encephalitis

DIAGNOSIS

- Characteristic clinical symptoms in immunosuppressed patients
- Tzanck smear, CMV antibodies, and PCR helpful in the proper clinical context
- Tissue biopsy showing characteristic histology used to document invasive disease

TREATMENT

- Acute, severe infections: ganciclovir, valganciclovir, foscarnet, and cidofovir
- Improvement of immunosuppression especially important in AIDS patients
- Prophylactic therapy: IV ganciclovir, oral valganciclovir, or high-dose valacyclovir useful

- Antigen or PCR tests often used in transplant patients to guide pre-emptive therapy
- Prevention: no CMV vaccine currently available
- Use CMV-negative blood products in immunosuppressed patients

Wayne X. Shandera, MD
Samuel Shelburne, MD

Dengue

 KEY FEATURES

- Extremely common togavirus infection transmitted by the bite of the *Aedes* mosquito
- Incubation period is typically 7–10 days (can be longer)
- Found throughout the tropics
- In US, occurs in southern Texas and Puerto Rico

 CLINICAL FINDINGS

- Usually nonspecific; self-limited febrile illness that typically lasts 3–7 days followed by a remission
- Severe dengue associated with fevers, terrible body aches ("breakbone"), pharyngitis, hemorrhage, and shock
- Rash is very common in the remission period or early in a second febrile phase
- Rash has maculopapular, petechial, or other morphology, appears first on the hands and feet and spreads to the arms, legs, trunk, and neck, usually sparing the face
- Death seen in cases of dengue hemorrhagic fever and dengue shock syndrome

 DIAGNOSIS

- Leukopenia is characteristic
- Thrombocytopenia is common in the hemorrhagic form of the disease
- Rapid serological testing is available
- Must be considered in travelers recently returned from endemic areas

 TREATMENT

- No specific antiviral therapy
- Supportive measures, including analgesics (avoid aspirin) and hydration
- Prevention: A vaccine has been developed but is not yet available commercially
- Mosquito control measures

Wayne X. Shandera, MD
Samuel Shelburne, MD

Dermatitis Herpetiformis

 KEY FEATURES

- Highest prevalence in Scandinavia
- Is associated with HLA antigens -B8, -DR3, and -DQ2
- Associated with gluten-sensitive enteropathy, but in the great majority it is subclinical
- Ingestion of gluten plays a role in the exacerbation of skin lesions

 CLINICAL FINDINGS

- Uncommon disease manifested by pruritic papules, vesicles, and papulovesicles mainly on the elbows, knees, buttocks, posterior neck, scalp
- Patients with dermatitis herpetiformis are at increased risk for GI lymphoma, and this risk is reduced by a gluten-free diet

 DIAGNOSIS

- Diagnosis is made by light microscopy, which demonstrates neutrophils at the dermal papillary tips
- Direct immunofluorescence studies show granular deposits of IgA along the dermal papillae
- Circulating antiendomysium antibodies and antibodies to tissue transglutaminase are present in 70% of cases
- Differential diagnosis includes weeping or encrusted lesions (crusted lesions), impetigo, contact dermatitis (acute)
- Any vesicular dermatitis can become crusted
- See differential diagnosis for *Vesicular lesions*

 TREATMENT

- Strict long-term avoidance of dietary gluten has been shown to decrease the dose of dapsone (usually 100–200 mg/day) required to control the disease and may even eliminate the need for drug treatment

Timothy G. Berger, MD

Diverticulosis

 ### KEY FEATURES

- Incidence increases with age: 5% at age <40, 30% at age 60, 50% at age >80 in Western societies
- Uncommon in developing countries
- Most are asymptomatic, discovered incidentally at sigmoidoscopy or colonoscopy or on barium enema
- Causes: diet deficient in fiber, abnormal motility, hereditary factors, Ehlers-Danlos syndrome, Marfan's syndrome, and scleroderma

 ### CLINICAL FINDINGS

- Nonspecific complaints of chronic constipation, abdominal pain, fluctuating bowel habits
- Physical examination usually normal; may reveal mild left lower quadrant tenderness
- Complications occur in 33%, including lower GI bleeding and diverticulitis

 ### DIAGNOSIS

- Routine laboratory studies normal
- Barium enema best demonstrates diverticula
- Colonoscopy

 ### TREATMENT

- High-fiber diet or fiber supplements (bran powder, psyllium or methylcellulose 1–2 tbsp PO BID)

Kenneth R. McQuaid, MD

Down Syndrome

 ### KEY FEATURES

- Down syndrome is due to simple trisomy for chromosome 21 or unbalanced translocations involving the long arm of chromosome 21
- Risk of an affected fetus increases exponentially with the age of the mother at conception and begins a marked rise after age 35
- At maternal age 45, risk is 1 in 40

 ### CLINICAL FINDINGS

- Usually diagnosed at birth
- Typical facial features
- Hypotonia
- Single palmar crease
- Serious problems at birth or early in childhood, including duodenal atresia, congenital heart disease (especially atrioventricular canal defects), and leukemia
- Mental retardation, although intelligence varies across a wide spectrum
- Alzheimer-like dementia in the fourth or fifth decade
- For those who survive childhood, a reduced life expectancy

 ### DIAGNOSIS

- Cytogenetic analysis
- Most affected individuals have simple trisomy for chromosome 21
- Others have unbalanced translocations, usually resulting from a parent with a balanced translocation, incurring a substantial risk of Down syndrome in future offspring
- A fetus with Down syndrome can be detected in the early second trimester through screening maternal serum for alpha-fetoprotein and certain hormones (triple screen) and by observation of increased nuchal skin thickness on fetal ultrasonogram

 ### TREATMENT

- No treatment is effective for the mental impairment
- Congenital heart disease, duodenal atresia, and acute leukemia, if present, are treated by standard approaches

- Genetic counseling is essential for parents of a newly diagnosed child
- Prenatal diagnosis should be offered for subsequent pregnancies

Reed E. Pyeritz, MD, PhD

Dupuytren's Contracture

 ### KEY FEATURES

- Hyperplasia of the palmar fascia and related structures, with nodule formation and contracture
- Cause is unknown
- Occurs primarily in white men older than 50 yr. The incidence is higher among alcoholics and patients with chronic systemic disorders (especially cirrhosis)
- Also associated with systemic fibrosing syndrome, which includes Peyronie's disease, mediastinal and retroperitoneal fibrosis, and Riedel's struma

 ### CLINICAL FINDINGS

- Slowly progressive chronic disease
- Nodular or cord-like thickening of one or both hands, with the fourth and fifth fingers most commonly affected
- Tightness of the involved digits, with inability to satisfactorily extend the fingers
- The contracture is well tolerated because it exaggerates the normal position of function of the hand, although resulting cosmetic problems may be unappealing

 ### DIAGNOSIS

- Clinical findings outlined above

 ### TREATMENT

- If the palmar nodule is growing rapidly, injections of triamcinolone into the nodule may be of benefit
- Surgical intervention is indicated in patients with significant flexion contractures, depending on the location, but recurrence is not uncommon

David B. Hellmann, MD, FACP
John H. Stone, MD, MPH

Effusions, Malignant, Pleural, Pericardial, & Peritoneal

KEY FEATURES

- Half of undiagnosed effusions in patients not known to have cancer are malignant
- Occur in pleural, pericardial, and peritoneal spaces
- Caused by direct neoplastic involvement of serous surface or obstruction of lymphatic drainage

CLINICAL FINDINGS

- Chest pain
- Shortness of breath
- Cough
- Hypotension
- Muffled heart sounds
- Abdominal distension

DIAGNOSIS

- Thoracentesis, pericardiocentesis, or paracentesis; send fluid for cytology, cell count and differential, protein content, lactate dehydrogenase level
- Malignant effusions are generally bloody; chylous effusions occur with thoracic duct obstruction or enlarged mediastinal lymph nodes in lymphoma
- If pleural cytology is negative on two occasions but suspicion of tumor high, thoracoscopic pleural biopsy may be helpful
- Differential diagnosis: congestive heart failure, pulmonary embolism, trauma, infections. Effusions are a complication of some chemotherapeutic agents

TREATMENT

- Treatment of underlying malignancy is often ineffective in relieving effusions
- Pleural: Diuretics are used to minimize reexpansion pulmonary edema after thoracentesis
- Thoracentesis alone controls fewer than 10% of pleural effusions but may be useful in conjunction with systemic chemotherapy
- Pleural effusions managed acutely by closed water-seal drainage with a chest tube for 3–4 days, followed by chemosclerosis with talc, bleomycin, or mitoxantrone
- Pleuroperitoneal shunting occasionally helpful, but patient must pump shunt 100 times 5 times/day
- Pleurectomy is effective but has a high complication rate; is rarely indicated
- Pericardial: Pericardial window or stripping achieves good control (also useful for constrictive pericarditis after radiation therapy)
- Peritoneal: Diuretics are used in initial treatment of small to moderate peritoneal effusions and as adjunctive treatment after large-volume paracentesis

Hope Rugo, MD

Ehrlichiosis

KEY FEATURES

- Tick-borne gram-negative obligate intracellular bacteria
- Two main clinical entities: human granulocytic ehrlichiosis (typically *Ehrlichia phagocytophila*) and human monocytic ehrlichiosis (typically *E chaffeensis*)
- Bacteria form morulae, intracytoplasmic aggregates within leukocytes
- In US mainly found in mid-Atlantic, southeastern, and central states
- May see coinfection with other tick-borne illnesses (eg, Lyme disease)

CLINICAL FINDINGS

- Prodrome of malaise, rigors, and nausea followed by fever, headache, and rash
- Respiratory failure, renal failure, and encephalopathy may ensue in severe cases

DIAGNOSIS

- Leukopenia, lymphopenia, elevated liver function tests, and thrombocytopenia common
- May see morulae in cytoplasm of leukocytes
- PCR from whole blood useful
- Indirect fluorescent antibody test available from CDC

TREATMENT

- Doxycycline is treatment of choice, usually given for 7–10 days
- Attention to tick removal and acquisition is mainstay of prevention

Wayne X. Shandera, MD
Samuel Shelburne, MD

Enterococcal Infections

KEY FEATURES

- Two species—*Enterococcus faecalis* and *Enterococcus faecium*—are responsible for most human enterococcal infections

CLINICAL FINDINGS

- Wound infections
- Urinary tract infection
- Bacteremia
- Endocarditis
- Meningitis

DIAGNOSIS

- Cultures of affected fluids or tissue

TREATMENT

- Most enterococcal infections can still be treated with penicillin, 3 million units q4h; ampicillin (which is slightly more active than penicillin in vitro), 2 g q6h; or vancomycin, 1 g q12h
- Because these antibiotics are not bactericidal for enterococci, gentamicin, 1 mg/kg q8h, is added for treatment of endocarditis or other serious infection
- Quinupristin/dalfopristin and linezolid are FDA approved for treatment of infections caused by vancomycin-resistant strains of enterococci
- Quinupristin/dalfopristin is not active against strains of *E faecalis* and should be used only for infections caused by *E faecium*. Linezolid, an oxazolidinone, is active against both *E faecalis* and *E faecium*

Henry F. Chambers, MD

Enteropathy, Protein-Losing

 KEY FEATURES

- Defined as excessive loss of serum proteins into GI tract
- Essential diagnostic features are hypoalbuminemia and elevated fecal α_1-antitrypsin level
- Causes include mucosal disease with ulceration, lymphatic obstruction, idiopathic change in permeability of mucosal capillaries

 CLINICAL FINDINGS

- Hypoalbuminemia
- Edema
- Lymphocytopenia < 1000/μL, hypoglobulinemia, hypocholesterolemia in lymphatic obstruction

 DIAGNOSIS

- Obtain lymphocyte count, serum albumin, protein electrophoresis, cholesterol, ANA, and C3 levels
- Gut α_1-antitrypsin clearance (24-h volume of feces × stool concentration of α_1-antitrypsin/serum α_1-antitrypsin concentration) of >13 mL/24 h is diagnostic
- Stool samples ova and parasites
- Stool qualitative fecal fat determination
- Upper endoscopy with small bowel biopsy
- Small bowel barium series
- Barium enema or colonoscopy
- CT scan of the abdomen
- Lymphangiography (rarely needed)
- Laparotomy with full-thickness intestinal biopsy

 TREATMENT

- Treat underlying disease
- Low-fat diets supplemented with medium-chain triglycerides for cases caused by lymphatic obstruction
- Octreotide may benefit some patients

Kenneth R. McQuaid, MD

Eosinophilia-Myalgia Syndrome

 KEY FEATURES

- The eosinophilia-myalgia syndrome was first noted in patients who ingested tryptophan until it was banned by FDA

 CLINICAL FINDINGS

- Begins weeks to months after beginning ingestion of tryptophan
- Patients develop a syndrome of severe generalized myalgias and cutaneous abnormalities ranging from hives to generalized swelling and induration of the arms and legs
- Other common clinical manifestations include pulmonary symptoms, fever, myopathy, lymphadenopathy, and ascending polyneuropathy
- Death, especially from neurological involvement, can occur

 DIAGNOSIS

- Peripheral eosinophilia (>1000/μL) is characteristic
- Mild elevations of aldolase with normal creatine kinase levels and, frequently, positive ANA tests
- Full-thickness biopsies may reveal features of systemic sclerosis, evidence of fasciitis or myositis, or small-vessel vasculitis

 TREATMENT

- Although some patients improve after discontinuing tryptophan, others progress and require corticosteroid therapy, which is not always effective

David B. Hellmann, MD, FACP
John H. Stone, MD, MPH

Epicondylitis, Lateral & Medial

 KEY FEATURES

- Better known by their sports associations: tennis elbow and golf elbow, respectively
- The conditions are caused by overuse, and the pain results from minor tears in the tendons of the forearm's extensor and flexor muscles

 CLINICAL FINDINGS

- Pain and point tenderness at the site of tendon insertion
- Tasks that require grasping and squeezing, such as shaking hands or opening jars, are impaired and cause pain (ie, the pain may be reproduced by extension **(lateral epicondylitis)** or flexion **(medial epicondylitis)** of the wrist against pressure)

 DIAGNOSIS

- Clinical

 TREATMENT

- The use of "counterforce" straps (bands worn distal to the elbow, over the bulk of the forearm musculature), intended to decrease the forces transmitted to the elbow during activity, are inadequate substitutes for rest
- Symptoms that persist after 2 weeks of conservative therapy usually respond to infiltration of triamcinolone, 10–20 mg, mixed with 1% lidocaine, 1–2 mL, around the involved epicondyle

David B. Hellmann, MD, FACP
John H. Stone, MD, MPH

Epiglottitis

KEY FEATURES

- Suspect epiglottitis (or, more correctly, supraglottitis) when a patient presents with a rapidly developing sore throat or when odynophagia (pain on swallowing) is disproportional to apparently minimal oropharyngeal findings on examination
- May be viral or bacterial in origin

CLINICAL FINDINGS

- Swollen, erythematous epiglottis on laryngoscopy

DIAGNOSIS

- Unlike in children, indirect laryngoscopy is generally safe

TREATMENT

- Hospitalization and initial admission to ICU
- IV antibiotics (eg, ceftizoxime, 1–2 g IV q8–12 h; or cefuroxime, 750–1500 mg IV q8h)
- Dexamethasone, usually 4–10 mg as initial bolus and then 4 mg IV q6h, and observation of the airway
- Steroids may be tapered as signs and symptoms resolve. Similarly, substitution of oral antibiotics may be appropriate to complete a 10-day course
- When epiglottitis is recognized early in the adult, it is usually possible to avoid intubation
- Indications for intubation are dyspnea or rapid pace of sore throat (where progression to airway compromise may occur before the effects of steroids and antibiotics take hold)
- If the patient is not intubated, monitor oxygen saturation with continuous pulse oximetry

Robert K. Jackler, MD
Michael J. Kaplan, MD

Erythromelalgia

KEY FEATURES

- Paroxysmal bilateral vasodilatory disorder of unknown cause
- Idiopathic (primary) erythromelalgia occurs in otherwise healthy persons
- Affects men and women equally
- Secondary erythromelalgia occurs in patients with polycythemia vera, hypertension, gout, and neurological diseases

CLINICAL FINDINGS

- Erythema, warmth, and bilateral burning pain that lasts minutes to hours, at first involving circumscribed areas on the balls of the feet or palms and often progressing to involve the entire extremity
- Symptoms occur in response to vasodilation produced by exercise or heat (eg, at night when the extremities are warmed under bedclothes)
- Relief may be obtained by cooling and elevating the affected extremity

DIAGNOSIS

- No findings between attacks
- During attacks, skin temperature and arterial pulsations are increased, and involved areas are warm, erythematous, and sweaty

TREATMENT

PRIMARY ERYTHROMELALGIA

- Avoid warm environments
- Aspirin 650 mg q4—6h
- β-blockers, epidural corticosteroid injections, and lidocaine patches

SECONDARY ERYTHROMELALGIA

- Treatment of the primary disease process

Louis M. Messina, MD
Laura K. Pak, MD
Lawrence M. Tierney, Jr, MD

Esophageal Diverticula

KEY FEATURES

- Zenker's diverticulum is a protrusion of pharyngeal mucosa at the pharyngo-esophageal junction between the inferior pharyngeal constrictor and the cricopharyngeus
- Esophageal diverticula occur in the mid or distal esophagus secondary to motility disorders (diffuse esophageal spasm, achalasia) or may develop above esophageal strictures

CLINICAL FINDINGS

- Zenker's diverticulum: dysphagia and regurgitation, oropharyngeal dysphagia with coughing or throat discomfort
- Halitosis, spontaneous regurgitation of undigested food, nocturnal choking, gurgling in the throat, or protrusion in the neck may occur as the diverticulum enlarges and retains food
- Complications include aspiration pneumonia, bronchiectasis, and lung abscess
- Esophageal diverticula: seldom symptomatic
- Risk of perforation at endoscopy

DIAGNOSIS

- Diagnosis by barium esophagogram

TREATMENT

- Treatment directed at the underlying disorder
- Small asymptomatic diverticula may be observed
- Symptomatic upper esophageal myotomy and surgical diverticulectomy lead to improvement in >90%

Kenneth R. McQuaid, MD

Esophageal Injury, Caustic

KEY FEATURES

- Follows accidental or deliberate (suicidal) ingestion of alkali (drain cleaners, etc) or acid

CLINICAL FINDINGS

- Severe burning and chest pain, gagging, dysphagia, and drooling
- Aspiration results in stridor and wheezing

DIAGNOSIS

- Examine circulatory status
- Assess airway patency, including laryngoscopy
- Chest and abdominal radiographs
- Endoscopy

TREATMENT

- Supportive treatment, IV fluids, analgesics
- Nasogastric lavage and oral antidotes should not be administered
- Endoscopy within the first 24 h to assess extent and severity of mucosal damage
- Patients with mild damage (edema, erythema, exudates, or superficial ulcers) recover quickly, have low risk of stricture, and may be advanced from liquids to regular diet over 24–48 h
- Patients with severe injury (deep or circumferential ulcers or necrosis) have a high risk (up to 65%) of acute perforation with mediastinitis or peritonitis, bleeding, stricture, or esophageal-tracheal fistulas. Must be kept fasting and monitored closely for signs of deterioration that warrant emergency surgery
- Surgery: esophagectomy and colonic or jejunal interposition, nasoenteric feeding tube
- Neither steroids nor antibiotics are recommended
- Strictures develop in up to 70% of patients with serious esophageal injury weeks to months after initial injury, requiring recurrent dilations
- Esophageal squamous carcinoma occurs in 2–3%, warranting endoscopic surveillance 15–20 yr after the caustic ingestion

Kenneth R. McQuaid, MD

Esophageal Webs & Rings

KEY FEATURES

- Esophageal webs are thin, diaphragm-like membranes of squamous mucosa typically in the mid or upper esophagus
- Webs may be multiple congenital graft-versus-host disease, pemphigoid, epidermolysis bullosa, pemphigus vulgaris
- Web plus iron deficiency anemia is known as Plummer-Vinson syndrome
- Esophageal rings are smooth, circumferential, thin (<4 mm) mucosal structures in the distal esophagus at the squamo-columnar junction
- Rings are associated with hiatal hernia and may be related to gastroesophageal reflux disease

CLINICAL FINDINGS

- Solid-food dysphagia, characteristically intermittent and not progressive, with rings <13 mm in diameter

DIAGNOSIS

- Barium esophagogram with full esophageal distension
- Endoscopy is less sensitive for detection of subtle webs and rings

TREATMENT

- Passage of a large (>16-mm diameter) bougie dilator to disrupt the web or ring
- Single dilation, repeat dilations, graduated dilation for ringed esophagus
- Proton pump inhibitor chronic therapy for patients who have heartburn or who require repeated dilation

Kenneth R. McQuaid, MD

Esophagitis, Pill-Induced

KEY FEATURES

- Various medications may injure the esophagus, through direct, prolonged mucosal contact
- Most commonly implicated are alendronate, clindamycin, doxycycline, iron, NSAIDs, potassium chloride pills, quinidine, risedronate, tetracycline, trimethoprim-sulfamethoxazole, vitamin C, zalcitabine, and zidovudine
- Injury is most likely to occur if pills are swallowed without water or while supine
- Hospitalized or bed-bound patients at greater risk

CLINICAL FINDINGS

- Severe retrosternal chest pain
- Odynophagia
- Dysphagia

DIAGNOSIS

- Endoscopy reveals one or several discrete, shallow or deep ulcers
- Severe esophagitis with stricture, hemorrhage, or perforation

TREATMENT

- Prevention by instructing patients to take pills with 4 oz of water and to remain upright for 30 min after ingestion
- Known offending agents should not be given to patients with esophageal dysmotility, dysphagia, or strictures

Kenneth R. McQuaid, MD

Factitious Disorder

 KEY FINDINGS

- Characterized by self-induced symptoms or false physical and laboratory findings in an attempt to deceive clinicians
- Unlike the somatoform disorders, symptom production is intentional. There is no apparent external motivation for the deceptive behaviors other than achieving the sick role
- In Munchausen syndrome, the deception is carried out by the patient, whereas Munchausen by proxy is when a parent creates an illness in a child so that the parent can maintain a relationship with clinicians
- Patients are frequently connected in some way to the health professions and often are migratory

 CLINICAL FINDINGS

- Deceptions may involve fever, self-mutilation, hemorrhage, hypoglycemia, seizures, and many other symptoms
- False physical and/or laboratory findings may be present
- Presentations are often dramatic and exaggerated, but the duplicity may also be complex and difficult to recognize

 DIAGNOSIS

- Determining that physical or laboratory findings are false

 TREATMENT

- Early psychiatric consultation is indicated
- There are 2 main treatment strategies. One consists of a conjoint confrontation of the patient by both the primary clinician and the psychiatrist. The patient's disorder is portrayed as a cry for help, and psychiatric treatment is recommended. The second approach avoids direct confrontation and attempts to provide a face-saving way to relinquish the symptom without overt disclosure of the disorder's origin

Stuart J. Eisendrath, MD
Jonathan E. Lichtmacher, MD

Familial Adenomatous Polyposis

 KEY FEATURES

- Multiple (>100) colonic adenomatous polyps with extracolonic features
- Caused by inherited mutation in the adenomatous polyposis coli (*APC*) gene
- Autosomal dominant syndrome affecting 1:10,000 people
- Absence of a family history of inherited colon cancer in ~25%
- Polyps usually develop by a mean age of 15 years, almost always by age 35
- Colorectal cancer is inevitable by age 50 unless prophylactic colectomy is performed
- Adenomatous polyps of the duodenum and periampullary area develop in >90% of patients, resulting in a 5–8% lifetime risk of adenocarcinoma
- Gastric fundus polyps occur in >50% but have no malignant potential
- Extraintestinal manifestations vary among families depending on type or site of mutation in *APC* gene

 CLINICAL FINDINGS

- Multiple (>100) colonic adenomatous polyps
- Extraintestinal manifestations: soft tissue tumors of the skin, desmoid tumors, osteomas, congenital hypertrophy of the retinal pigment, malignancies of the CNS (Turcot's syndrome), tumors of the thyroid and liver (hepatoblastomas)

 DIAGNOSIS

- Genetic testing for *APC* mutation by protein truncation assay has a sensitivity of 80%; a negative result is considered a true negative only if an affected family member has a positive test result
- Annual sigmoidoscopy for family members beginning at age 12 yr if the assay cannot be done or is not informative
- Upper endoscopy of the stomach, duodenum, and periampullary area for affected patients every 1–3 yr

 TREATMENT

- Genetic counseling of patients and first-degree family members
- Complete proctocolectomy with ileoanal anastomosis or colectomy with ileorectal anastomosis is recommended, usually before age 20
- Ileorectal anastomosis affords superior bowel function but has a 10% risk of rectal cancer, requiring frequent sigmoidoscopy with fulguration of polyps
- Sulindac, aspirin, and COX-2 selective agents (celecoxib, rofecoxib) can decrease the number and size of polyps in the rectal stump
- Surgical resection for large (>2 cm) periampullary adenomas

Kenneth R. McQuaid, MD

Familial Mediterranean Fever

 KEY FEATURES

- Episodic bouts of acute peritonitis associated with serositis involving the joints and pleura
- Rare autosomal recessive disorder
- Almost exclusively affects people of Mediterranean ancestry, especially Sephardic Jews, Armenians, Turks, and Arabs
- Unknown pathogenesis
- Patients lack a protease in serosal fluids that normally inactivates interleukin-8 and complement factor 5A

 CLINICAL FINDINGS

- Symptom onset before the age of 20
- Fever
- Severe abdominal pain and abdominal tenderness with guarding or rebound tenderness
- Joint pain, inflammation
- Pleuritic chest pain, pleural effusion
- Secondary amyloidosis (renal, hepatic) occurs in 25% of cases and can lead to death

 DIAGNOSIS

- Usually a clinical diagnosis
- Gene responsible for familial Mediterranean fever (*MEFV*) has been identified
- Diagnosis can be established by genetic testing

 TREATMENT

- Patients may undergo unnecessary exploratory laparotomy
- Untreated, attacks resolve within 24–48 h
- Colchicine, 0.6 mg PO BID–TID, decreases the frequency and severity of attacks and can prevent or arrest amyloidosis

Kenneth R. McQuaid, MD

Fascioliasis

 KEY FEATURES

- Infection results from ingestion of encysted metacercariae on watercress or other aquatic vegetables or in water
- Eggs of the worm infect snails; the snails subsequently infect vegetation
- The disease is most prevalent in sheep-raising countries, particularly where raw salads are eaten

 CLINICAL FINDINGS

- A tender, enlarged liver, fever, leukocytosis, and marked eosinophilia (to 90%) are seen in the acute illness
- Right upper quadrant pain, headache, anorexia and vomiting, myalgia, urticaria, and other allergic reactions
- Jaundice, cachexia, and prostration may appear in severe illness
- The chronic latent phase may be asymptomatic or characterized by hepatomegaly and other acute findings
- The chronic obstructive phase produces a clinical picture similar to that of sclerosing cholangitis, biliary cirrhosis, or choledocholithiasis

 DIAGNOSIS

- Diagnosis is established by detecting eggs in the feces; sometimes eggs can only be found in biliary drainage
- Ultrasonography and cholangiography may show parasites in the gallbladder
- Eosinophilia is characteristic, and hypergammaglobulinemia and abnormal liver function tests may be present
- The ELISA is highly sensitive and specific in detection of both antibody and antigen, particularly in acute infections

 TREATMENT

- Triclabendazole (Novartis Agribusiness in US) is the drug of choice; 10 mg/kg given for 2 days with food achieves a cure rate of 80%. Bithionol (given as for paragonimiasis) is the alternative drug of choice

Fasciolopsiasis

 KEY FEATURES

- *Fasciolopsis buski* is a common parasite of humans and pigs in central and southern Asia
- When eggs shed in stools reach water, they hatch to produce free-swimming larvae that penetrate and develop in the flesh of snails. Cercariae escape from snails and infect various water plants, which are then eaten by humans (water chestnuts, bamboo shoots)

 CLINICAL FINDINGS

- After an incubation period of 2–3 mo, manifestations of GI irritation appear in all but light infections
- In severe infections there may be nausea, upper abdominal pain, diarrhea, sometimes alternating with constipation
- Ascites and edema of the face and lower extremities may occur late as well as intestinal obstruction, ileus, and cachexia

 DIAGNOSIS

- Diagnosis depends on finding characteristic eggs or, occasionally, flukes in the stools
- Leukocytosis with moderate eosinophilia is common
- No serological test is available
- The adult worms live for 6 mo; absence from the endemic area for a longer period makes the diagnosis unlikely

 TREATMENT

- The drug of first choice is praziquantel, 25 mg/kg 3 times in 1 day only
- The alternative drug is niclosamide (not available in US), given every other day for 3 doses. Taken in the morning before eating, the tablets must be chewed thoroughly and swallowed with water. Resume eating in 2 h
- In light infections—even without treatment—the prognosis is good; generally, spontaneous cure occurs within 1 yr

Fecal Incontinence

 KEY FEATURES

- Occurs in up to 10% of the elderly
- Minor incontinence is slight soilage of undergarments that tends to occur after bowel movements or with straining or coughing
- Causes: local anal problems such as hemorrhoids and skin tags, ulcerative proctitis, chronic diarrheal conditions, irritable bowel syndrome
- Major incontinence is complete uncontrolled loss of stool
- Causes: significant sphincteric or neurological damage resulting from obstetric trauma (especially forceps delivery, episiotomy, or pudendal nerve damage), prolapse, prior anal surgery, physical trauma, aging, diabetes mellitus, dementia, multiple sclerosis, spinal cord injury, cauda equina syndrome

 CLINICAL FINDINGS

- Incontinence of stool, minor or major

 DIAGNOSIS

- Confirm an intact anocutaneous reflex by stimulation of perianal skin
- Digital examination during relaxation and squeezing to assess resting tone and external sphincter function and to exclude fecal impaction
- Anoscopy to assess for prolapse of rectal mucosal hemorrhoids
- Proctosigmoidoscopy to exclude rectal neoplasm or proctitis
- Anal ultrasonography to assess integrity of sphincter
- Anal manometry and surface electromyography to assess rectal sensation, resting and voluntary squeeze pressures, and innervation

 TREATMENT

- Minor incontinence: fiber supplements, bulking agents, loose application of a cotton ball near the anal opening, Kegel perineal strengthening exercises
- Major incontinence: antidiarrheal drugs (eg, loperamide, 2 mg before meals and prophylactically before social engagements, shopping trips, etc), scheduled toilet use after glycerin suppositories or tap water enemas
- Provide elderly more time and assistance to reach toilet
- Prevent stool impaction and "overflow" incontinence
- Biofeedback training with anal sphincter exercises for patients with reduced sensation or poor voluntary squeeze pressures
- Surgical intervention in patients who have failed medical therapy, especially patients with traumatic disruption of sphincters

Kenneth R. McQuaid, MD

Femoral Aneurysm

 KEY FEATURES

- True aneurysms of the femoral artery are less common than popliteal or aortic aneurysms or femoral pseudoaneurysms
- Femoral pseudoaneurysms occur from injury produced by IV drug abuse, femoral artery puncture for angiography, previous surgery, or femoral catheter insertion

 CLINICAL FINDINGS

- Pulsatile groin mass
- Symptoms resulting from arterial thrombosis, peripheral embolization, or compression of adjacent structures with resultant venous thrombosis or neuropathy. Rupture is rare
- Arterial thrombosis leads to amputation in up to 30% of patients

 DIAGNOSIS

- Ultrasonography
- Conventional angiography

 TREATMENT

TRUE ANEURYSMS

- Incidence of complications is lower than with popliteal aneurysms
- Patients with combined disease undergo repair of aortoiliac and popliteal aneurysms before repair of the femoral aneurysm

PSEUDOANEURYSMS

- Uninfected, small (<5 cm) traumatic pseudoaneurysms can be treated by ultrasonogram-guided compression of the aneurysm neck or by thrombin injection, with reported 90% success rate
- If not successful, open repair is required. Open repair is also advised for any pseudoaneurysm after femoral bypass surgery
- Mycotic aneurysms should be widely débrided with proximal and distal ligation or interposition grafting using autologous vein

Louis M. Messina, MD
Laura K. Pak, MD
Lawrence M. Tierney, Jr, MD

Femoral Neuropathy

KEY FEATURES

- May occur in diabetics or from compression by retroperitoneal neoplasms or hematomas; may also result from pressure from the inguinal ligament when the thighs are markedly flexed and abducted, as in the lithotomy position
- The neuropathy may be asymptomatic, resolve rapidly and spontaneously, or become progressively more disabling

CLINICAL FINDINGS

- There is weakness of the quadriceps muscle, with sensory impairment over the anteromedian aspect of the thigh and sometimes also of the leg to the medial malleolus, and a depressed or absent knee jerk

DIAGNOSIS

- Electromyography and nerve conduction velocities are often indispensable for accurate localization of the focal lesion

TREATMENT

- Improvement may occur if any compression is relieved

Michael J. Aminoff, DSc, MD, FRCP

Fibromuscular Dysplasia

KEY FEATURES

- Nonatherosclerotic, noninflammatory disease of unknown cause characterized by segmental irregularity of small and medium-sized muscular arteries
- Occurs predominantly in women aged 30–50 yr
- Family history of disease often present
- Most frequently involved vessels are the renal, carotid, and common iliac arteries
- Four recognized histological types: medial fibrodysplasia (>80%), intimal fibroplasia, medial hyperplasia, and perimedial dysplasia

CLINICAL FINDINGS

- Renovascular hypertension
- Renal insufficiency
- Transient ischemic attacks
- Claudication
- Intracranial aneurysms present in as many as half of patients with internal carotid fibromuscular dysplasia

DIAGNOSIS

- Angiography: "string of beads" pattern of disease

TREATMENT

- Aspirin, 325 mg PO qd
- Percutaneous angioplasty for symptomatic patients
- Stents offer no any advantage over angioplasty alone
- More complex lesions require interposition grafting

Louis M. Messina, MD
Laura K. Pak, MD
Lawrence M. Tierney, Jr, MD

Fibromyalgia

KEY FEATURES

- One of the most common rheumatic syndromes in ambulatory medicine
- Although many of the clinical features of the 2 conditions overlap, musculoskeletal pain predominates in fibromyalgia and lassitude dominates chronic fatigue syndrome
- Cause is unknown

CLINICAL FINDINGS

- Chronic aching pain and stiffness, frequently involving the entire body but with prominence of pain around neck, shoulders, low back, and hips
- Fatigue, sleep disorders, subjective numbness, chronic headaches, and irritable bowel symptoms are common
- Physical examination is normal except for "trigger points" of pain produced by palpation of various areas such as the trapezius, the medial fat pad of the knee, and the lateral epicondyle of the elbow

DIAGNOSIS

- A diagnosis of exclusion
- Thyroid function tests are useful because hypothyroidism can produce a secondary fibromyalgia syndrome
- Polymyositis produces weakness rather than pain
- Polymyalgia rheumatica produces shoulder and girdle pain, is associated with an elevated sedimentation rate and anemia, and occurs after age 50

TREATMENT

- Patients can be comforted that they have a syndrome treatable by specific, though imperfect, therapies and that the course is not progressive
- Amitriptyline is initiated at a dosage of 10 mg at bedtime and gradually increased to 40–50 mg depending on efficacy and toxicity
- Exercise programs are also beneficial
- Opioids, NSAIDs, and steroids are ineffective

David B. Hellmann, MD, FACP
John H. Stone, MD, MPH

Focal Segmental Glomerular Sclerosis

 KEY FEATURES

- Idiopathic or secondary to heroin use, morbid obesity, HIV infection

 CLINICAL FINDINGS

- Nephrotic syndrome
- Microscopic hematuria in 80%
- Hypertension
- Decreased renal function at diagnosis in 25–50%

 DIAGNOSIS

- Renal biopsy: Light microscopy shows focal segmental glomerular sclerosis; immunofluorescence shows IgM and C3; electron microscopy shows fusion of epithelial foot processes

 TREATMENT

- Prednisone, 1–1.5 mg/kg/day PO for 2–3 mo followed by a slow steroid taper
- Remission in >50% of patients, most within 5–9 mo
- Cytotoxic drug therapy produces remission in <20%

Suzanne Watnick, MD
Gail Morrison, MD

Folic Acid Deficiency

 KEY FEATURES

- Folic acid present in most fruits and vegetables (especially citrus fruits and green leafy vegetables)
- Daily requirements of 50–100 µg/day usually met in the diet
- Total body stores of folate enough to supply requirements for 2–3 mo
- Most common cause of folate deficiency is inadequate dietary intake, which occurs in alcoholics, anorectic patients, persons who do not eat fresh fruits and vegetables, and those who overcook food
- Other causes: decreased absorption (tropical sprue, drugs, eg, phenytoin, sulfasalazine, trimethoprim-sulfamethoxazole); increased requirement (chronic hemolytic anemia, pregnancy, exfoliative skin disease); loss (dialysis); and inhibition of reduction to active form (methotrexate)

 CLINICAL FINDINGS

- Megaloblastic anemia, which may be severe
- Glossitis and vague GI disturbances (eg, anorexia, diarrhea)
- No neurological abnormalities, unlike vitamin B_{12} deficiency

 DIAGNOSIS

- Megaloblastic anemia identical to that in vitamin B_{12} deficiency (eg, macro-ovalocytes, hypersegmented neutrophils (see *Vitamin B_{12} deficiency*)
- Red blood cell folate level <150 ng/mL
- Serum vitamin B_{12} level normal
- Distinguish from anemia of liver disease (macrocytic anemia with target cells but no megaloblastic changes)

 TREATMENT

- Folic acid, 1 mg PO qd, for patients with folate deficiency or increased folate requirements
- Rapid improvement in sense of well-being, reticulocytosis in 5–7 days, and total correction of hematological abnormalities within 2 months

Charles A. Linker, MD

Fragile X Mental Retardation

 KEY FEATURES

- Fragile X mental retardation accounts for more cases of retardation in males than any condition except Down syndrome
- Inherited as an X-linked condition
- About 1 in 2000 males is affected

 CLINICAL FINDINGS

- Affected males show macro-orchidism (enlarged testes) after puberty, large ears and a prominent jaw, high-pitched voice, and mental retardation. Some show evidence of a mild connective tissue defect, with joint hypermobility and mitral valve prolapse
- Affected (heterozygous) women show no physical signs other than early menopause, but they may have learning difficulties or frank retardation

 DIAGNOSIS

- Cytogenetic studies demonstrate a small gap, or fragile site, near the tip of the long arm of the X chromosome
- Fragile site is due to expansion of a trinucleotide repeat (CGG) near a gene called *FMR1*
- One *FMR1* allele with ≥200 repeats results in mental retardation in virtually all men and about 60% of women
- Clinical DNA diagnosis for the number of CCG repeats can be performed for any male or female who has unexplained mental retardation
- Prenatal DNA diagnosis can be performed

 TREATMENT

- None

Reed E. Pyeritz, MD, PhD

Galactorrhea

 KEY FEATURES

- Defined as lactation that occurs in the absence of nursing
- Usually caused by hyperprolactinemia, either from overproduction of prolactin by a pituitary adenoma or loss of its inhibitory regulation by dopamine
- Nipple stimulation and nipple rings can increase prolactin and cause galactorrhea
- Idiopathic (benign) galactorrhea: Many parous (previously pregnant) women can express a small amount of breast milk; prolactin level is normal
- Normal breast milk may be various colors besides white, but bloody discharge raises suspicion of cancer

 CLINICAL FINDINGS

- Unilateral or bilateral milky nipple discharge
- Oligomenorrhea, amenorrhea, or infertility
- Large pituitary tumors may cause headaches, and visual field defects
- Pituitary prolactinomas may cosecrete growth hormone and cause acromegaly; large tumors may cause pituitary insufficiency (hypogonadism, hypothyroidism, adrenal insufficiency, growth hormone deficiency)

 DIAGNOSIS

- Galactorrhea requires evaluation if it is
  - Significant in amount
  - Occurring in a nulliparous woman
  - Associated with amenorrhea, headache, visual field abnormalities, or other symptoms implying endocrinopathy
- Serum prolactin level is elevated (Table 106, page 1289)
- Urine or serum hCG elevated if pregnancy is cause of galactorrhea
- TSH high if hypothyroidism is cause of hyperprolactinemia
- MRI of the pituitary and hypothalamus indicated for nonpregnant patients if persistently elevated prolactin with no discernible cause; nonpregnant patients if prolactin >200 ng/dL; if headaches or unusual visual field defects occur

 TREATMENT

- Reassure if normal prolactin in parous woman on no medication known to increase prolactin (Table 106, page 1289)
- Correct underlying cause of elevated prolactin
- Discontinue potentially offending medications and recheck in a few weeks
- Cabergoline or bromocriptine can reduce galactorrhea regardless of cause
- Treat prolactinoma using medication, surgery, or radiation (see *Hyperprolactinemia*)

Paul A. Fitzgerald, MD

Gamma Hydroxybutyrate Overdose

 KEY FEATURES

- A popular drug of abuse and for sexual assault; consumed as a liquid or powder added to a drink
- Other related chemicals with similar effects include butanediol and gamma-butyrolactone (GBL)
- A prolonged withdrawal syndrome has been described in some heavy chronic users

 CLINICAL FINDINGS

- Symptoms after ingestion include drowsiness and lethargy followed by coma with respiratory depression
- Muscle twitching and seizures are sometimes observed
- Recovery is usually rapid, with patients awakening within a few hours

 DIAGNOSIS

- Urine GHB analysis can be obtained from National Medical Labs and some forensic labs

 TREATMENT

- Administer activated charcoal, 60–100 g PO or via gastric tube, mixed in aqueous slurry for recent ingestions
- Do not use for comatose patients unless it can be given by gastric tube and the airway is first protected by a cuffed endotracheal tube
- There is no specific treatment
- GHB withdrawal syndrome may require very large doses of benzodiazepines over several days

Kent R. Olsen, MD

Gastritis, Atrophic

 KEY FEATURES

- An autoimmune disorder involving the fundic glands
- Results in achlorhydria and vitamin B_{12} malabsorption
- Fundic histology shows severe gland atrophy and intestinal metaplasia
- Inflammation and autoimmune destruction of the parietal cells lead to loss of intrinsic factor

 CLINICAL FINDINGS

- Hypergastrinemia may induce hyperplasia of gastric enterochromaffin-like cells, development of small, multicentric carcinoid tumors in 5%
- The risk of adenocarcinoma is increased threefold; prevalence of 1–3%

 DIAGNOSIS

- Endoscopy with biopsy
- Achlorhydria leads to pronounced hypergastrinemia (>1000 pg/mL)
- Parietal cell antibodies present in 90%
- Low serum vitamin B_{12} level
- Megaloblastic (macrocytic) anemia

 TREATMENT

- One-time endoscopic screening for adenocarcinoma or carcinoids recommended
- Patients with dysplasia or small carcinoids require periodic endoscopic surveillance

Kenneth R. McQuaid, MD

Gastroenteritis, *Escherichia coli*

 KEY FEATURES

- *E coli* causes gastroenteritis by organism growth in the gut with toxin production
- Enterotoxin causes hypersecretion in the small intestine

 CLINICAL FINDINGS

- Table 126, page 1308
- Enterotoxigenic *E coli* elaborates either a heat-stable or a heat-labile toxin that mediates diarrhea, including traveler's diarrhea
- Enteroinvasive *E coli* invades cells, causing bloody diarrhea and dysentery similar to infection with *Shigella* species
- Enterohemorrhagic *E coli* produces 2 Shiga-like toxins that mediate non-bloody diarrhea, hemorrhagic colitis, hemolytic-uremic syndrome, and thrombotic thrombocytopenic purpura. Serotype O157:H7 is responsible for most cases in the United States. Elderly individuals and young children are most severely affected; hemolytic-uremic syndrome is more common in the latter group

 DIAGNOSIS

- *E coli* O157:H7 is not identified by routine stool cultures. Isolation requires identification of sorbitol-negative colonies of *E coli* on sorbitol-MacConkey agar followed by serological testing to confirm serotype

 TREATMENT

- Antimicrobial therapy does not alter the course of the disease and may increase the risk of hemolytic-uremic syndrome. Treatment is primarily supportive

Henry F. Chambers, MD

Gastroenteritis, *Salmonella*

 KEY FEATURES

- The most common form of salmonellosis is acute enterocolitis
- Numerous *Salmonella* serotypes may cause enterocolitis
- The incubation period is 8–48 h after ingestion of contaminated food or liquid

 CLINICAL FINDINGS

- Fever (often with chills), nausea and vomiting, cramping abdominal pain, and diarrhea, which may be grossly bloody, lasting 3–5 days
- Usually self-limited, but bacteremia with localization in joints or bones may occur, especially in patients with sickle cell disease

 DIAGNOSIS

- Culturing the organism from the stool

 TREATMENT

- Mild to moderate disease can be treated symptomatically
- For severe diarrhea, either ciprofloxacin, 500 mg BID for 3 days, or levofloxacin, 500 mg once daily for 3 days, is effective; trimethoprim-sulfamethoxazole DS BID for 3 days is an effective alternative

Henry F. Chambers, MD

Gastroenteritis, Viral

 KEY FEATURES

- Viruses are major cause of infectious diarrhea
- Include rotaviruses, Norwalk and Norwalk-like caliciviruses, and enteric adenoviruses

 CLINICAL FINDINGS

- Usually include both vomiting and non-bloody diarrhea
- Often occur in an epidemic fashion in closed environments (eg, cruise ships, schools)

 DIAGNOSIS

- Generally restricted to outbreak investigations
- ELISA and PCR assays of stool

 TREATMENT

- Supportive with fluid and electrolyte replacement
- Environmental sanitation key to containing and preventing outbreaks
- Rotavirus vaccine suspended for fear it induced intussusception in infants (although data are controversial)

Wayne X. Shandera, MD
Samuel Shelburne, MD

Gastrointestinal Bleeding, Occult

 KEY FEATURES

- Presence of a positive fecal occult blood test (FOBT) or iron deficiency anemia in an adult in the absence of visible fecal blood loss
- 1–2.5% of patients in screening programs have a positive FOBT
- 2% of men and 5% of women have iron deficiency anemia
- In premenopausal women, most common cause is menstrual and pregnancy-associated iron loss; GI blood loss in 10%; no cause determined in 30–50%
- In men and postmenopausal women, blood loss in the colon in 15–30% and in the upper GI tract in 35–55%; malignancy in 10%
- Most common causes: neoplasms; vascular abnormalities (vascular ectasias, portal hypertensive gastropathy); acid-peptic lesions; infections (nematodes [especially hookworm], tuberculosis); medications (especially NSAIDs or aspirin); inflammatory bowel disorder or malabsorption (celiac sprue)

 CLINICAL FINDINGS

- Positive FOBT
- Iron deficiency anemia

 DIAGNOSIS

- Colonoscopy with or without upper endoscopy indicated for all adults older than 40–45 with positive FOBTs or iron deficiency anemia; for premenopausal women and younger men with GI symptoms; for those with family history of GI cancer; and for anemia that is disproportionate to the estimated menstrual blood loss
- Unless upper GI tract symptoms are present, colonoscopy should be done first
- Upper endoscopy indicated in patients with upper GI tract symptoms or iron deficiency anemia after nondiagnostic colonoscopy
- Small bowel enteroscopy, small bowel series or enteroclysis, video capsule device if persistent unexplained chronic GI blood loss or anemia that responds poorly to iron supplementation. Rarely, angiography or intraoperative endoscopy is indicated

 TREATMENT

- Colonoscopy detects >95% of colorectal polyps and cancer and permits polypectomy, tumor biopsy, or endoscopic cautery of vascular ectasias

Kenneth R. McQuaid, MD

Gastroparesis

 KEY FEATURES

- Chronic condition characterized by intermittent, waxing and waning symptoms of nausea, bloating, early satiety, and vomiting in the absence of any mechanical lesions
- Caused by endocrine disorders (diabetes mellitus, hypothyroidism, cortisol deficiency), postsurgical (vagotomy, partial gastric resection, fundoplication, gastric bypass, Whipple procedure), neurological (Parkinson's disease, muscular and myotonic dystrophy, autonomic dysfunction, multiple sclerosis, postpolio syndrome, porphyria), rheumatological (progressive systemic sclerosis), infections (postviral, Chagas' disease), amyloidosis, paraneoplastic syndromes, medications, and anorexia nervosa
- Cause may not always be identified

 CLINICAL FINDINGS

- Manifestations of gastroparesis may be chronic or intermittent
- Early satiety, bloating, nausea, and postprandial vomiting (1–3 h after meals)

 DIAGNOSIS

- Plain-film radiography shows dilatation of the esophagus and stomach
- Endoscopy or barium radiography (upper GI series) excludes mechanical obstruction
- Gastric scintigraphy with a low-fat solid meal assesses gastric emptying
- Gastric retention of 60% after 2 h or more than 10% after 4 h is abnormal

 TREATMENT

- No specific therapy
- Acute exacerbations treated with nasogastric suction and IV fluids, correction of electrolyte disturbance
- Chronic treatment includes small, frequent meals low in fiber, milk, gas-forming foods, and fat
- Jejunal feeding via external feeding tube or jejunostomy if oral feeding cannot meet nutritional needs
- Parenteral nutrition seldom required unless there is a diffuse gastric and intestinal motility disorder
- Avoid opioids, anticholinergics
- In diabetics, maintain glucose levels <200 mg/dL
- Metoclopramide, 5–20 mg PO QID or 5–10 mg IV or SC before meals, and erythromycin, 125–250 mg PO BID or 3 mg/kg IV q8h
- Tegaserod, 6 mg BID, enhances gastric emptying; however, its role in gastroparesis requires further study
- Gastric decompression: Patients with severe gastroparesis may require placement of a percutaneous endoscopic gastrostomy (PEG) to decompress the stomach
- Gastric pacing with internally implanted neurostimulators

Kenneth R. McQuaid, MD

Gaucher's Disease

 KEY FEATURES

- Gaucher's disease is caused by a deficiency of β-glucocerebrosidase, which leads to an accumulation of sphingolipid within phagocytic cells throughout the body
- Inherited as an autosomal recessive
- Over 200 mutations have been found to cause Gaucher's disease
- Two uncommon forms of Gaucher's disease, types II and III, involve neurological accumulation of sphingolipid and neurological problems
- Type II is of infantile onset and has a poor prognosis
- All forms are more common in people of Ashkenazi Jewish ancestry

 CLINICAL FINDINGS

- Episodes of bone pain
- Anemia and thrombocytopenia are common; are primarily due to hypersplenism and marrow infiltration with Gaucher cells
- Cortical erosions of bones, especially the vertebrae and femur, are due to local infarctions

 DIAGNOSIS

- Bone marrow aspirates reveal typical Gaucher cells, which have an eccentric nucleus and periodic acid–Schiff–positive inclusions, along with wrinkled cytoplasm and inclusion bodies of a fibrillar type
- Serum acid phosphatase elevated
- Deficient glucocerebrosidase activity in leukocytes

 TREATMENT

- Treatment of bone pain is supportive; risks for fracture should be reduced
- Splenectomy for thrombocytopenia

MEDICATIONS

- Imiglucerase, a recombinant form of the enzyme glucocerebrosidase, 30 units/kg/mo IV, reduces total body stores of glycolipid and improves orthopedic and hematological manifestations but not neurological manifestations

IMAGING

- During enzyme therapy, the platelet count should be monitored, and the size of the liver and spleen should be monitored by MRI
- An initial skeletal survey will detect occult bone involvement; new onset of bone pain requires evaluation for possible fracture

Reed E. Pyeritz, MD, PhD

Gender Identity Disorder

 KEY FEATURES

- Gender identity reflects a biological self-image and is usually well developed by age 3 or 4
- Gender dysphoria occurs when a sexual identity is developed that is opposite the biological identity

 CLINICAL FINDINGS

- Transsexuals assume a fixed role of attitudes, feelings, fantasies, and choices typical of the opposite sex. They typically lack interest in their genitals as evidence of their gender or as a focus for erotic behavior
- A desire for sex change starts early and may culminate in assumption of a feminine lifestyle, hormonal treatment, and use of surgical procedures such as castration and vaginoplasty

 DIAGNOSIS

- Clinical
- Aversion and operant condition are frequently tried but only occasionally result in a behavioral change
- Genital reconstructive surgeries are sometimes performed, but many patients are screened out by trial periods living as the intended sex

Stuart J. Eisendrath, MD
Jonathan E. Lichtmacher, MD

Genital Prolapse

 KEY FEATURES

- Cystocele, rectocele, and enterocele are vaginal hernias commonly seen in multiparous women
- Cystocele is a hernia of the bladder wall into the vagina, causing a soft anterior fullness
- Cystocele may be accompanied by urethrocele, which is not a hernia but a sagging of the urethra after its detachment from the pubic symphysis during childbirth
- Rectocele is a herniation of the terminal rectum into the posterior vagina, causing a collapsible pouch-like fullness
- Enterocele is a vaginal vault hernia containing small intestine, usually in the posterior vagina and resulting from a deepening of the pouch of Douglas
- Enterocele may also accompany uterine prolapse or follow hysterectomy, when weakened vault supports or a deep unobliterated cul-de-sac containing intestine protrudes into the vagina
- All 3 types of hernia may occur in combination

 TREATMENT

- Supportive measures include a high-fiber diet. Weight reduction in obese patients and limitation of straining and lifting are helpful
- Pessaries may reduce cystocele, rectocele, or enterocele temporarily and are helpful in women who do not wish surgery or are chronically ill
- The only cure for symptomatic cystocele, rectocele, or enterocele is corrective surgery. The prognosis after an uncomplicated procedure is good

H. Trent MacKay, MD, MPH

Gingivitis, Necrotizing Ulcerative

 KEY FEATURES

- Trench mouth, Vincent's infection
- Often caused by an infection of both spirochetes and fusiform bacilli
- Is common in young adults under stress (classically at examination time)
- Underlying systemic diseases may also predispose to this disorder

 CLINICAL FINDINGS

- Painful acute gingival inflammation and necrosis, often with bleeding
- Halitosis
- Fever
- Cervical lymphadenopathy

 DIAGNOSIS

- Clinical
- Culture

 TREATMENT

- Warm half-strength peroxide rinses and oral penicillin (250 mg TID daily for 10 days) may help
- Dental gingival curettage may prove necessary

Robert K. Jackler, MD
Michael J. Kaplan, MD

Glanzmann's Thrombasthenia

 KEY FEATURES

- Rare autosomal recessive disorder. Platelets are unable to aggregate because of lack of receptors (containing glycoproteins IIb and IIIa) for fibrinogen, which form bridges between platelets during aggregation

 CLINICAL FINDINGS

- Mucosal (epistaxis, gingival) bleeding, menorrhagia, and postoperative bleeding. Variable severity but may be severe

 DIAGNOSIS

- Platelet numbers and morphology normal, but bleeding time markedly prolonged. Platelets fail to aggregate in response to typical agonists (adenosine 5′-diphosphate, collagen, thrombin) but aggregate normally in response to ristocetin

 TREATMENT

- Platelet transfusions when necessary, but limited by tendency of patients to develop multiple alloantibodies

Charles A. Linker, MD

Glaucoma, Acute Angle-Closure

 KEY FEATURES

- Primary acute angle-closure glaucoma occurs in eyes with narrow anterior chamber angles, such as in the elderly, hyperopes, and Asians
- May be precipitated by pupillary dilation from sitting in the dark, from stress, rarely by pharmacological mydriasis for ophthalmological examination, or from medications with anticholinergic or sympathomimetic activity
- Secondary acute angle-closure glaucoma occurs in uveitis

 CLINICAL FINDINGS

- Extreme ocular pain
- Blurred vision, typically with halos around lights
- Nausea and vomiting
- The eye is red and the cornea is cloudy, usually with a moderately dilated, nonreactive pupil

 DIAGNOSIS

- Markedly elevated intraocular pressure confirmed by tonometry

 TREATMENT

- Immediate evaluation and treatment by an ophthalmologist are essential
- IV and oral acetazolamide and topical agents to lower intraocular pressure
- Topical pilocarpine is used after intraocular pressure is reduced to reverse the angle closure
- Definitive treatment is generally laser peripheral iridotomy, which is usually performed prophylactically on the fellow eye, or surgical peripheral iridectomy

Paul Riordan-Eva, FRCOphth

Glaucoma, Chronic Open-Angle

 KEY FEATURES

- Usually bilateral optic neuropathy characterized by optic disk cupping and progressive visual field loss, generally associated with elevated intraocular pressure
- In primary open-angle glaucoma, which is generally more severe in African-Americans, intraocular pressure is elevated because of abnormal drainage of aqueous
- In chronic angle-closure glaucoma, which is more common in Inuits and Asians, intraocular pressure is elevated as a result of obstruction to aqueous flow
- Secondary open-angle glaucoma occurs after ocular trauma, in uveitis, and with chronic topical or systemic steroid therapy
- In normal-tension glaucoma, which is common in Japanese, intraocular pressure is not elevated
- Ocular hypertension is elevated intraocular pressure without optic disk cupping or visual field loss

 CLINICAL FINDINGS

- Asymptomatic until severe visual loss has developed
- Visual fields progressively constrict, central vision (acuity) remaining good until late in the disease

 DIAGNOSIS

- Screening by tonometry, optic disk examination, and visual field testing are essential to early diagnosis
- All persons older than 40 should undergo tonometry and ophthalmoscopy every 2–5 y
- In diabetics and those with a family history of glaucoma, annual examinations are indicated

 TREATMENT

- See Table 10, page 1206: Topical Ophthalmic Agents
- Topical β-adrenergic blocking agents and prostaglandin analogs are the most commonly used agents to reduce intraocular pressure

- Other topical agents include α-adrenergic agonists, carbonic anhydrase inhibitors, and cholinergic agonists
- Surgical therapy, such as trabeculectomy or laser trabeculoplasty, may be undertaken if medical therapy is inadequate

Paul Riordan-Eva, FRCOphth

Glomerulonephritis, Cryoglobulin-Associated

 ## KEY FEATURES

- Essential (mixed) cryoglobulinemia is a disorder associated with cold-precipitable immunoglobulins (cryoglobulins)
- Glomerular disease occurs from the precipitation of cryoglobulins in glomerular capillaries
- Causes include underlying bacterial, fungal, and viral infections (eg, hepatitis B and C)

 ## CLINICAL FINDINGS

- Necrotizing skin lesions in dependent areas
- Arthralgias
- Fever
- Hepatosplenomegaly

 ## DIAGNOSIS

- Serum complement levels are low
- Renal biopsy: rapidly progressive glomerulonephritis with crescents

 ## TREATMENT

- Aggressive treatment of the underlying infection
- Pulse corticosteroids, plasma exchange, and cytotoxic agents
- α-Interferon for hepatitis C–related cryoglobulinemia

Suzanne Watnick, MD
Gail Morrison, MD

Glomerulonephritis, Membranopro-liferative

 ## KEY FEATURES

- Idiopathic or secondary to immune complex or paraprotein deposition and thrombotic microangiopathic glomerulonephritides
- Presents with nephritic or nephrotic features
- Most patients are older than 30 yr
- Two major subgroups: type I and type II; type II less common than type I

 ## CLINICAL FINDINGS

TYPE I

- History of recent upper respiratory tract infection in ~33%
- Nephrotic syndrome

TYPE II

- Glomerulonephritis findings

 ## DIAGNOSIS

TYPE I

- Serum complement levels are low
- Renal biopsy: light microscopy shows GBM is thickened by immune complex deposition, abnormal mesangial cell proliferation, "splitting" appearance to the capillary wall; immunofluorescence shows IgG, IgM, and granular deposits of C3, C1q, and C4

TYPE II

- Renal biopsy: light microscopy findings similar to type I, but electron microscopy shows dense deposit of homogeneous material replacing part of the glomerular basement membrane
- C3 nephritic factor, a circulating IgG antibody, found in serum

 ## TREATMENT

- Treatment is controversial
- Corticosteroid therapy
- Antiplatelet drugs: aspirin, 500–975 mg/day, plus dipyridamole, 225 mg/day
- In the past, 50% of patients progressed to end-stage renal disease in 10 yr; fewer

now with introduction of more aggressive therapy
- Prognosis less favorable with type II disease, early renal insufficiency, hypertension, and persistent nephrotic syndrome
- Renal transplantation, but both types may recur thereafter

Suzanne Watnick, MD
Gail Morrison, MD

Glomerulonephritis, Pauci-Immune

 KEY FEATURES

- Pauci-immune glomerular lesions are seen with small-vessel vasculitides, Wegener's granulomatosis, and microscopic polyangiitis
- Antineutrophil cytoplasmic antibody–associated glomerulonephritis can also present as a primary renal lesion

 CLINICAL FINDINGS

- Fever, malaise, weight loss
- Hematuria
- Proteinuria
- Purpura
- Mononeuritis multiplex
- In Wegener's, 90% have upper or lower respiratory tract lesions that bleed

 DIAGNOSIS

- A cytoplasmic pattern of ANCA is specific for antiproteinase 3 antibodies, whereas a perinuclear pattern (p-ANCA) is specific for antimyeloperoxidase antibodies
- 80–90% of patients with Wegener's syndrome have c-ANCA
- ~80% of patients with microscopic angiitis will have either a p-ANCA or c-ANCA
- Renal biopsy: necrotizing lesions and crescents signify a rapidly progressive glomerulonephritis

 TREATMENT

- Institute treatment early; prognosis depends mainly on extent of glomerular involvement before treatment is started
- High-dose corticosteroids (methylprednisolone, 1–2 g/day for 3 days, followed by prednisone, 1 mg/kg for 1 mo, with a slow taper over the next 6 mo) and cytotoxic agents (cyclophosphamide, 1.5–2 mg/kg PO for 3 mo, tapered over 1 yr)
- Monitor ANCA levels to help determine efficacy of treatment

Suzanne Watnick, MD
Gail Morrison, MD

Glomerulonephritis, Postinfectious

 KEY FEATURES

- Causes include infection from nephritogenic group A β-hemolytic streptococci, especially type 12; bacteremia (eg, *Staphylococcus aureus* sepsis); infective endocarditis; shunt infections; hepatitis B, cytomegalovirus infection, infectious mononucleosis, coccidioidomycosis, malaria, and toxoplasmosis

 CLINICAL FINDINGS

- Oliguria
- Edema
- Hypertension, variable

 DIAGNOSIS

- Serum complement levels are low
- Antistreptolysin O (ASO) titers sometimes high
- Urinalysis: cola-colored urine, with red blood cells, red cell casts, and proteinuria
- 24-h urine protein <3.5 g/day
- Renal biopsy: Light microscopy shows diffuse proliferative glomerulonephritis; immunofluorescence shows IgG and C3 in a granular pattern in the mesangium and along the capillary basement membrane; electron microscopy shows large, dense subepithelial deposits or "humps"

 TREATMENT

- Supportive measures
- Antibiotics, as indicated for infection
- Antihypertensive mediations
- Salt and water restriction
- Diuretics

Suzanne Watnick, MD
Gail Morrison, MD

Glossitis & Glossodynia

 KEY FEATURES

- Inflammation of the tongue with loss of filiform papillae leads to glossitis
- May be secondary to nutritional deficiencies (eg, niacin, riboflavin, iron, or vitamin E), drug reactions, dehydration, irritants, and possibly autoimmune reactions or psoriasis
- Glossodynia is burning and pain of the tongue; it may occur with or without glossitis
- It has been associated with diabetes, drugs (eg, diuretics), tobacco, xerostomia, and candidiasis as well as the causes of glossitis
- Periodontal disease is not a factor

 CLINICAL FINDINGS

- Rarely painful
- Glossitis: red, smooth-surfaced tongue

 DIAGNOSIS

- Clinical

 TREATMENT

GLOSSITIS

- If the primary cause cannot be treated, consider empirical nutritional replacement therapy

GLOSSODYNIA

- Reassurance that there is no infection or tumor
- Anxiolytic medications and evaluation of possible psychological status may be useful
- Treating possible underlying causes, changing chronic medications to alternative ones, and smoking cessation may resolve symptoms
- Consider an empiric trial of gabapentin for symptom control

Robert K. Jackler, MD
Michael J. Kaplan, MD

Glossopharyngeal Neuralgia

 KEY FEATURES

- An uncommon disorder with throat pain similar in quality to that in trigeminal neuralgia

 CLINICAL FINDINGS

- Pain occurs in the throat, about the tonsillar fossa, and sometimes deep in the ear and at the back of the tongue
- The pain may be precipitated by swallowing, chewing, talking, or yawning and is sometimes accompanied by syncope

 DIAGNOSIS

- In most instances, no underlying structural abnormality is present
- Microvascular compression of glossopharyngeal nerve may be underlying pathogenesis
- Multiple sclerosis or other brainstem lesions are sometimes responsible

 TREATMENT

- Carbamazepine is the treatment of choice and should be tried (in daily doses up to 1200 mg) before any surgical procedures are considered
- Microvascular decompression is generally preferred over destructive surgical procedures such as partial rhizotomy in medically refractory, idiopathic cases and is often effective without causing severe complications

Michael J. Aminoff, DSc, MD, FRCP

Glucose-6-Phosphate Dehydrogenase Deficiency

 KEY FEATURES

- Hereditary enzyme defect causing episodic hemolytic anemia because of decreased ability of RBCs to deal with oxidative stresses
- Hemoglobin may become oxidized, forming precipitants called Heinz bodies, which cause membrane damage, leading to removal of RBCs by spleen
- X-linked recessive disorder affecting 10–15% of black American males, who have a variant G6PD with 15% of normal enzyme activity; in addition, enzyme activity declines rapidly as RBC ages past 40 days
- Mediterranean variants have extremely low enzyme activity
- Female carriers are affected only when unusually high percentage of cells producing normal enzyme are inactivated (rare)

 CLINICAL FINDINGS

- Usually healthy, without chronic hemolytic anemia or splenomegaly
- Hemolysis occurs with oxidative stress resulting from either infection or exposure to certain drugs
- Common drugs initiating hemolysis: dapsone, primaquine, quinidine, quinine, sulfonamides, and nitrofurantoin
- Hemolytic episode self-limited, even with continued use of offending drug, because older RBCs (with low enzyme activity) removed and replaced with young RBCs with adequate functional levels of G6PD
- Chronic hemolytic anemia in severe G6PD deficiency (as in Mediterranean variants)

 DIAGNOSIS

- Coombs test is negative
- Blood is normal between hemolytic episodes
- Reticulocytosis and increased indirect bilirubin during hemolytic episodes
- G6PD enzyme assays low, especially in severe cases of G6PD deficiency
- G6PD enzyme assays may be misleadingly normal if performed shortly after hemolytic episode when enzyme-deficient RBCs have been removed
- RBC smear, although not diagnostic, may reveal "bite" cell
- Heinz bodies may be seen on peripheral blood smear with crystal violet stain

 TREATMENT

- Avoid known oxidant drugs
- Otherwise, no treatment necessary

Charles A. Linker, MD

Gnathostomiasis

KEY FEATURES

- Infection is usually caused by the larval stage of the nematode *Gnathostoma spinigerum*
- Infection is most common in southeast Asia, China, India, Ecuador, Israel, East Africa, and Mexico, where the infection is most commonly associated with eating of raw fresh-water fish, especially ceviche

CLINICAL FINDINGS

- Within 24–48 h, larval migration through the intestine can cause acute epigastric pain, vomiting, urticaria, and eosinophilia. The worm then migrates to subcutaneous and other tissues, causing pruritic subcutaneous swelling up to 25 cm across, occasionally accompanied by stabbing pain
- Over weeks to years, the swelling may remain constant or move continuously
- Occasionally the worm becomes visible under the skin
- Spontaneous pneumothorax, leukorrhea, hematemesis, hematuria, hemoptysis, coughing, edema of the pharynx, spinal cord invasion, eosinophilic meningoencephalitis, or subarachnoid hemorrhage can occur

DIAGNOSIS

- Diagnosis can be made by surgical removal of the worm when it appears close to the skin
- Marked eosinophilia is common, except for CNS involvement
- Serodiagnosis by immunoblot assay or ELISA is promising

TREATMENT

- Ivermectin, 200 µg/kg daily for 1 or 2 days, or albendazole, 400 mg twice daily for 21 days; larval death appears to occur slowly, and cure rates may reach 95%
- Courses of prednisolone provide temporary relief of symptoms

Goodpasture's Syndrome, Renal

KEY FEATURES

- Clinical constellation of glomerulonephritis and pulmonary hemorrhage
- Injury mediated by anti-glomerular basement membrane (anti-GBM) antibodies
- Up to one-third of patients with anti-GBM glomerulonephritis have no evidence of lung injury
- ~5% of patients with rapidly progressive acute glomerulonephritis have anti-GBM
- Incidence in males ~6 times that in females
- Occurs most commonly in the second and third decades
- Associated with influenza A infection, hydrocarbon solvent exposure, and HLA-DR2 and -B7 antigens

CLINICAL FINDINGS

- Upper respiratory tract infection precedes onset in 20–60% of cases
- Hemoptysis, dyspnea, and possible respiratory failure
- Hypertension
- Edema

DIAGNOSIS

- Iron deficiency anemia
- Complement levels are normal
- Sputum contains hemosiderin-laden macrophages
- Chest x-rays show shifting pulmonary infiltrates
- Diffusion capacity of carbon monoxide is markedly increased
- Circulating anti-GBM antibodies positive in >90%

TREATMENT

- Combination of plasma exchange therapy to remove circulating antibodies and administration of immunosuppressive drugs to prevent formation of new antibodies
- Corticosteroids: pulse doses of prednisone or methylprednisolone, 1–2 g/day for 3 days, then 1 mg/kg/day
- Cyclophosphamide, 2–3 mg/kg/day
- Plasmapheresis, performed daily for up to 2 weeks
- Prognosis poor in patients with oliguria and a serum creatinine >6–7 mg/dL

Suzanne Watnick, MD
Gail Morrison, MD

Granuloma Inguinale

KEY FEATURES

- A chronic, relapsing granulomatous anogenital infection caused by *Calymmatobacterium (Donovania) granulomatis*
- The incubation period is 8 days to 12 weeks

CLINICAL FINDINGS

- Onset is insidious
- Lesions occur on the skin or mucous membranes of the genitalia or perineal area
- Lesions are relatively painless, infiltrated nodules that soon slough. A shallow, sharply demarcated ulcer forms, with a beefy-red friable base of granulation tissue. The lesion spreads by contiguity. The advancing border has a characteristic rolled edge of granulation tissue
- Superinfection with spirochete-fusiform organisms is common. The ulcer then becomes purulent, painful, foul smelling, and extremely difficult to treat

DIAGNOSIS

- Culture

TREATMENT

- Doxycycline, 100 mg BID for 21 days
- Trimethoprim-sulfamethoxazole DS BID, azithromycin, 1g PO once weekly for 3 weeks

Henry F. Chambers, MD

Haemophilus Infections

 KEY FEATURES

- Cause sinusitis, otitis, bronchitis, epiglottitis, pneumonitis, cellulitis, arthritis, meningitis, and endocarditis
- Alcoholism, smoking, chronic lung disease, advanced age, and HIV infection are important risk factors

 CLINICAL FINDINGS

- Typical bacterial pneumonia, with purulent sputum containing a predominance of gram-negative, pleomorphic rods
- Epiglottitis is characterized by an abrupt onset of fever, drooling, and inability to handle secretions. The patient often has a severe sore throat despite an unimpressive examination of the pharynx. Stridor and respiratory distress result from laryngeal obstruction
- Meningitis with sinusitis or otitis

 DIAGNOSIS

- Culture: *Haemophilus* species frequently colonize the upper respiratory tract; in the absence of positive pleural fluid or blood cultures, distinguishing pneumonia from colonization or from bacterial bronchitis is difficult
- Epiglottitis: The diagnosis is best made by direct visualization of the cherry-red, swollen epiglottis at laryngoscopy

 TREATMENT

- For sinusitis, otitis, or respiratory tract infection, use oral amoxicillin, 750 mg, or amoxicillin, 875 mg, with clavulanate, 125 mg, BID for 10–14 days
- For penicillin allergy, use cefuroxime axetil, 250 mg BID, or trimethoprim-sulfamethoxazole, 800/160 mg PO BID for 10 days
- In the seriously ill patient, use cefuroxime, 750 mg q8h, or ceftriaxone, 1 g/day, pending organism susceptibilities
- *H influenzae* meningitis (Table 122, page 1303)

Henry F. Chambers, MD

Headache, Cluster

 KEY FEATURES

- Affects mainly middle-aged men
- May relate to a vascular headache or a disturbance of a serotonergic mechanism
- There is often no family history of headache or migraine

 CLINICAL FINDINGS

- Severe unilateral periorbital pain occurring daily for several weeks, often accompanied by ipsilateral nasal congestion, rhinorrhea, redness of the eye, lacrimation, or Horner's syndrome
- Episodes usually occur at night and last for less than 2 h
- During a bout, alcohol may trigger an attack; stress, glare, or specific foods may also precipitate attacks
- Spontaneous remission occurs, and the patient remains well for weeks or months before another bout occurs
- Typical attacks may occur without remission. This variant is chronic cluster headache

 TREATMENT

- Subcutaneous sumatriptan (6 mg), dihydroergotamine (1–2 mg), ergotamine tartrate aerosol or inhalation of 100% oxygen (7 L/min for 15 min) may be effective
- Butorphanol tartrate nasal spray, 1 mg (1 spray in 1 nostril), repeated after 60–90 min if necessary, may help
- For prophylaxis, give ergotamine tartrate as rectal suppositories (0.5–1 mg at night or BID), PO (2 mg daily), or by SC injection (0.25 mg TID for 5 days per week)
- Other potentially helpful prophylactic agents include propranolol, amitriptyline, valproate, cyproheptadine, lithium carbonate (monitored by plasma lithium determination), prednisone (20–40 mg daily or on alternate days for 2 weeks, followed by gradual withdrawal), verapamil (240–480 mg daily), and methysergide (4–6 mg daily)

Michael J. Aminoff, DSc, MD, FRCP

Headache, Tension

 KEY FEATURES

- Patients frequently complain of poor concentration and other vague nonspecific symptoms in addition to constant daily headaches that are often vise-like or tight in quality and may be exacerbated by emotional stress, fatigue, noise, or glare

 CLINICAL FINDINGS

- The headaches are usually generalized, may be most intense about the neck or back of the head, and are not associated with focal neurological symptoms

 DIAGNOSIS

- Diagnosis is made after exclusion of other causes of headache (see individual diagnoses, eg, *Sinusitis*)

 TREATMENT

- When treatment with simple analgesics is not effective, a trial of antimigrainous agents (see *Migraine headache*) is worthwhile
- Techniques to induce relaxation are also useful and include massage, hot baths, and biofeedback
- Exploration of underlying causes of chronic anxiety is often rewarding
- Anecdotal reports of beneficial responses to local injection of botulinum toxin type A have been published

Michael J. Aminoff, DSc, MD, FRCP

Heavy Chain Disease

 KEY FEATURES

- A rare gammopathy with excess production of a homogeneous α, γ, or μ heavy chain

 CLINICAL FINDINGS

- Clinical presentation is more typical of lymphoma than multiple myeloma
- Gamma chain disease presents as a lymphoproliferative disorder with autoimmune features
- Alpha chain disease is frequently associated with severe diarrhea and infiltration of the lamina propria of the small intestine with abnormal plasma cells
- Mu chain disease is associated with chronic lymphocytic leukemia

 DIAGNOSIS

- Immunofluorescence staining of biopsy tissue with anti-heavy chain antibodies

 TREATMENT

- Treat with chemotherapy as for a lymphoproliferative disorder
- If mu chain disease, treat underlying chronic lymphocytic leukemia
- Referral to medical oncologist is advised

Jeffrey L. Kishiyama, MD
Daniel C. Adelman, MD

Hemoglobinuria, Paroxysmal Nocturnal

 KEY FEATURES

- Acquired clonal stem cell disorder causing abnormal sensitivity of RBC membrane to lysis by complement
- Defect involves increased binding of C3b and increased vulnerability to lysis by complement
- Suspect diagnosis in confusing cases of hemolytic anemia or pancytopenia

 CLINICAL FINDINGS

- Hemoglobinuria (reddish-brown urine), particularly in first morning urine
- Anemia
- Increased susceptibility to thrombosis, especially of mesenteric and hepatic veins
- May progress to aplastic anemia, myelodysplasia, or acute myelogenous leukemia

 DIAGNOSIS

- Sucrose hemolysis test is best screening test
- Anemia of variable severity
- Reticulocytosis may or may not be present
- Blood smear abnormalities (eg, macro-ovalocytes) are nondiagnostic
- Urine hemosiderin test useful (indicates episodic intravascular hemolysis)
- Serum lactate dehydrogenase characteristically elevated
- Iron deficiency common because of chronic iron loss from hemoglobinuria
- WBC and platelet count may be low
- Bone marrow morphology variable; may show generalized hypoplasia or erythroid hyperplasia
- Flow cytometric assays may confirm diagnosis by demonstrating absence of CD59

 TREATMENT

- Iron replacement often indicated for iron deficiency; may improve anemia but also may cause transient increase in hemolysis
- Prednisone, including alternate-day regimens, may be effective in decreasing hemolysis
- Allogeneic bone marrow transplantation for severe cases and cases of transformation to myelodysplasia

Charles A. Linker, MD

Hemolytic Disease in Newborn

 KEY FEATURES

- Anti-Rho(D) antibody is responsible for most severe instances
- Occurs when a Rho(D)-negative woman carries a Rho(D)-positive fetus and develops antibodies against Rho(D)
- The antibody developed against Rho(D) persists and poses a threat of hemolytic disease in subsequent Rho(D)-positive fetuses
- Passive immunization of Rho(D)-negative mothers after delivery destroys fetal Rho(D)-positive cells and prevents formation of antibodies, which would cause disease in subsequent Rho(D)-positive gestations

 CLINICAL FINDINGS

- Routine antibody screen is positive

 DIAGNOSIS

- Because hemolytic disease may occur in association with Rh subgroups or other red blood cell antigens, atypical antibodies should be assessed in third trimester of all pregnancies

 TREATMENT

- Rho(D) immunoglobulin (Ig) is given to the mother within 72 h after delivery to prevent future erythroblastosis
- Additional protection is afforded by the routine administration of the Ig at week 28; the passive antibody titer is too low to harm the Rho(D)-positive fetus
- Rho(D) Ig should also be given after abortion, ectopic pregnancy, abruptio placenta, other antepartum bleeding, or amniocentesis or chorionic villus sampling

William R. Crombleholme, MD

Hemolytic Transfusion Reactions

 KEY FEATURES

- Most severe hemolytic transfusion reactions involve mismatches in ABO system resulting from clerical errors and mislabeled specimens
- Hemolysis is rapid and intravascular
- Severity depends on dose of RBCs given; the most severe reactions occur in surgical patients under anesthesia
- Hemolytic transfusion reactions caused by minor antigen systems are typically less severe
- Hemolysis is slower and extravascular and may be delayed for 5–10 days after transfusion. Most common antigens involved are Duffy, Kidd, Kell, and C and E loci of the Rh system
- Most transfusion reactions are not hemolytic but rather are reactions to antigens present on WBCs

 CLINICAL FINDINGS

- Fever, chills, backache, and headache in major hemolytic transfusion reactions
- Apprehension, dyspnea, hypotension, and vascular collapse. Disseminated intravascular coagulation (DIC) and acute renal failure from tubular necrosis may occur in severe cases
- Generalized bleeding and oliguria may be first indication in patients under general anesthesia

 DIAGNOSIS

- Hematocrit fails to rise as expected in major hemolytic reactions
- Renal failure may occur
- DIC (low fibrinogen, elevated fibrin degradation products, thrombocytopenia, prolonged PT)
- Hemoglobinemia turns plasma pink and eventually results in hemoglobinuria
- Hematocrit falls and indirect bilirubin rises in delayed hemolytic reactions
- New offending alloantibody easily detected in patient's serum

 TREATMENT

- Stop transfusion immediately
- Check identification of recipient and of blood. Return donor transfusion bag

with pilot tube to blood bank with fresh sample of recipient's blood for retyping and repeat of cross-match
- Centrifuge sample of anticoagulated blood from recipient; if free hemoglobin is present in plasma, hydrate patient vigorously to prevent acute tubular necrosis. Forced diuresis with mannitol may help prevent renal damage

Charles A. Linker, MD

Hemoptysis

 KEY FEATURES

- Expectoration of blood originating below the vocal cords
- Massive hemoptysis: >200–600 mL of blood/24 h, hemodynamic or airway compromise
- Causes can be classified anatomically: airway (bronchitis, bronchiectasis, malignancy), pulmonary vasculature (congestive heart failure, mitral stenosis, pulmonary emboli, arteriovenous malformation [AVM]), or parenchymal (pneumonia, crack use, autoimmune diseases, or iatrogenesis)

 CLINICAL FINDINGS

- Blood-tinged sputum to frank blood
- Dyspnea may be mild or severe

 DIAGNOSIS

- CXR may demonstrate the cause
- High-resolution CT of the chest can diagnose bronchiectasis and AVM as well as many malignancies
- Bronchoscopy is indicated when there is a suspicion of malignancy or a normal CXR

 TREATMENT

- In massive hemoptysis, airway protection and circulatory support are first steps
- Patients should be placed in decubitus position with affected lung down
- Rigid bronchoscopy and surgical consultation in uncontrollable hemorrhage
- Bronchoscopy and angiography can localize lesions
- Embolization is initially effective in 85% of cases, although 20% rebleed in 1 yr

Mark S. Chesnutt, MD
Thomas J. Prendergast, MD

Hemorrhagic Fever & Hantavirus

 KEY FEATURES

- Diverse group of illnesses associated with animal contact (eg, ticks, mosquitoes, rodents)
- Most prominent in tropics but have worldwide distribution
- Often named for area where they occur (eg, Omsk hemorrhagic fever)
- Includes Ebola, Lassa fever, and hantavirus pulmonary syndrome (Sin Nombre virus)

 CLINICAL FINDINGS

- Usually present with high fever, leukopenia, altered mental status; hemorrhagic diathesis not a feature of hantavirus
- Marked toxicity and death may occur; ARDS may develop as a manifestation of hantavirus pulmonary syndrome

 DIAGNOSIS

- Usually made by serological testing in proper clinical setting
- PCR testing becoming more widely available

 TREATMENT

- Supportive care key
- Patients must be isolated
- Hantavirus and Lassa fever infections treated with ribavarin
- Reduce the likelihood of vector contact (eg, rodents for Sin Nombre)

Wayne X. Shandera, MD
Samuel Shelburne, MD

Henoch-Schönlein Purpura

 KEY FEATURES

- The most common systemic vasculitis in children
- Occurs in adults as well

 CLINICAL FINDINGS

- Purpuric skin lesions typically located on the lower extremities; may also be seen on the hands, arms, trunk, and buttocks
- Joint symptoms are present in the majority of patients; the knees and ankles are most commonly involved
- Abdominal pain secondary to vasculitis of the intestinal tract is often associated with GI bleeding
- Hematuria signals the presence of a glomerular lesion that is usually reversible, although it occasionally may progress to renal insufficiency

 DIAGNOSIS

- Skin biopsy can demonstrate leukocytoclastic vasculitis with IgA deposition
- Kidney biopsy reveals segmental glomerulonephritis with crescents and mesangial deposition of IgA
- Differential diagnosis includes immune thrombocytopenic purpura, meningococcemia, Rocky Mountain spotted fever, rheumatoid arthritis (including juvenile form), polyarteritis nodosa, endocarditis, cryoglobulinemia

 TREATMENT

- Usually self-limited, lasting 1–6 weeks, and subsiding without sequelae if renal involvement is not severe
- Chronic courses with persistent or intermittent skin disease are more likely to occur in adults than children
- The efficacy of treatment is not well established

David B. Hellmann, MD, FACP
John H. Stone, MD, MPH

Hepatopathy, Ischemic

 KEY FEATURES

- Caused by an acute fall in cardiac output resulting from, for example, acute myocardial infarction or arrhythmia, usually in a patient with passive congestion of the liver

 CLINICAL FINDINGS

- Clinical hypotension may be absent
- In some cases, the precipitating event is arterial hypoxemia resulting from respiratory failure
- In severe cases, encephalopathy may develop
- The mortality rate resulting from the underlying disease is high; however, in patients who recover, the aminotransferase levels return to normal quickly, usually within 1 week, in contrast to viral hepatitis
- Hepatojugular reflux is present, and with tricuspid regurgitation the liver may be pulsatile
- Ascites may be out of proportion to peripheral edema

 DIAGNOSIS

- The hallmark is a rapid, striking elevation of serum aminotransferase levels (often >5000 units/L); an early rapid rise in the serum lactate dehydrogenase level is also typical, but elevations of serum alkaline phosphatase and bilirubin are usually mild. The prothrombin time may be prolonged
- In passive congestion of the liver caused by right-sided heart failure, the serum bilirubin level may be elevated, occasionally as high as 40 mg/dL, resulting partly from hypoxia of perivenular hepatocytes. Serum alkaline phosphatase levels are normal or slightly elevated
- Ascites generally has a high serum ascites–albumin gradient (>1.1) and a protein content of more than 2.5 g/dL

 TREATMENT

- Supportive. Treat underlying cardiac disease

Lawrence S. Friedman, MD

Hepatopulmonary Syndrome

 KEY FEATURES

- Triad of chronic liver disease, an increased alveolar–arterial gradient at room air, and intrapulmonary vascular dilations or arteriovenous communications that result in a right-to-left intrapulmonary shunt

 CLINICAL FINDINGS

- Dyspnea and arterial deoxygenation in the upright position (orthodeoxia) and relieved by recumbency
- The diagnosis should be suspected in a cirrhotic patient with a pulse oximetry level ≤92%

 DIAGNOSIS

- Contrast-enhanced echocardiography is a sensitive screening test for detecting pulmonary vascular dilations, whereas macroaggregated albumin lung perfusion scanning is more specific and is used to confirm the diagnosis
- High-resolution CT may be useful for detecting dilated pulmonary vessels

 TREATMENT

- Medical therapy has been disappointing; however, IV methylene blue may improve oxygenation by inhibiting nitric oxide-induced vasodilation
- The syndrome may reverse with liver transplantation, although postoperative mortality is increased when the preoperative arterial oxygen tension is ≤50 mm Hg or with substantial intrapulmonary shunting. Liver transplantation is contraindicated in moderate to severe pulmonary hypertension (mean pulmonary pressure >35 mm Hg), although in some cases treatment with epoprostenol may reduce pulmonary hypertension and thereby facilitate liver transplantation. TIPS may provide palliation in patients with hepatopulmonary syndrome awaiting transplantation

Lawrence S. Friedman, MD

Hepatorenal Syndrome

 ### KEY FEATURES

- Diagnosed when other causes of renal disease have been excluded in the setting of end-stage liver disease

 ### CLINICAL FINDINGS

- In type I hepatorenal syndrome, the serum creatinine doubles to a level >2.5 mg/dL or the creatinine clearance halves to <20 mL/min in fewer than 2 weeks
- Type II hepatorenal syndrome is chronic and slowly progressive
- The cause is unknown, but the pathogenesis involves intense renal vasoconstriction. Histologically, the kidneys are normal

 ### DIAGNOSIS

- Azotemia, hyponatremia, oliguria, unremarkable urinary sediment, no proteinuria
- 24-h urinary sodium <10 mEq
- Renal function fails to improve after IV infusion of 1.5 L of isotonic saline

 ### TREATMENT

- Treatment is generally ineffective
- Improvement may follow IV infusion of the long-acting vasoconstrictor ornipressin and albumin (but with a high rate of ischemic side effects), ornipressin and dopamine, terlipressin (a long-acting vasopressin analog) and albumin, or norepinephrine and albumin or administration of octreotide and midodrine, an α-adrenergic drug
- Survival benefit has occurred with the molecular adsorbent recirculating system (MARS), a modified dialysis method that selectively removes albumin-bound substances. Improvement may also follow TIPS placement
- Mortality is high without liver transplantation; death is due to complicating infection or hemorrhage

Lawrence S. Friedman, MD

Hiccups

 ### KEY FEATURES

- Usually benign and self-limited but may be persistent and a sign of serious underlying illness
- Causes of self-limited hiccups: gastric distension, sudden temperature changes, alcohol ingestion, and emotion
- Causes of recurrent or persistent hiccups
  1. CNS: neoplasms, infections, cerebrovascular accident, trauma
  2. Metabolic: uremia, hypocapnia (hyperventilation)
  3. Irritation of the vagus or phrenic nerve:
  – Head, neck: foreign body in ear, goiter, neoplasms
  – Thorax: pneumonia, empyema, neoplasms, myocardial infarction, pericarditis, aneurysm, esophageal obstruction, reflux esophagitis
  – Abdomen: subphrenic abscess, hepatomegaly, hepatitis, cholecystitis, gastric distension, gastric neoplasm, pancreatitis, pancreatic malignancy
  4. Surgical: general anesthesia, postoperative
  5. Psychogenic and idiopathic

 ### CLINICAL FINDINGS

- Detailed neurological examination

 ### DIAGNOSIS

- Serum creatinine, liver enzymes
- Chest radiograph, chest fluoroscopy
- CT of the head, chest, abdomen
- Echocardiography
- Bronchoscopy
- Upper endoscopy

 ### TREATMENT

ACUTE HICCUPS

- Irritation of the nasopharynx by tongue traction, lifting the uvula with a spoon, catheter stimulation of the nasopharynx, or eating 1 tsp dry granulated sugar
- Interruption of the respiratory cycle by breath holding, Valsalva's maneuver, sneezing, gasping, or rebreathing into a bag
- Stimulation of the vagus nerve by carotid massage
- Irritation of the diaphragm by holding knees to chest or by continuous positive airway pressure during mechanical ventilation
- Relief of gastric distention by belching or insertion of an NG tube

CHRONIC HICCUPS

- Chlorpromazine, 25–50 mg PO or IM TID–QID
- Anticonvulsants (phenytoin, carbamazepine), benzodiazepines (lorazepam, diazepam), metoclopramide, baclofen, and occasionally general anesthesia

Kenneth R. McQuaid, MD

Homocystinuria

 KEY FEATURES

- Caused by cystathionine β-synthase deficiency, which results in extreme elevations of plasma and urinary homocysteine levels
- Autosomal recessive pattern of inheritance

 CLINICAL FINDINGS

- Similar to Marfan's syndrome in body habitus and ectopia lentis
- Mental retardation often present
- Cardiovascular events caused by repeated arterial or venous thromboses
- Life expectancy is reduced, especially in untreated and pyridoxine-unresponsive patients
- Myocardial infarction, stroke, and pulmonary embolism are most common causes of death

 DIAGNOSIS

- Diagnosis suspected in patients in the second and third decades of life who have repeated arterial or venous thromboses and no other risk factors
- DNA analysis can detect mutations in the cystathionine β-synthase gene
- Amino acid analysis of plasma is helpful diagnostic test: elevated plasma methionine levels

 TREATMENT

- β-synthase deficiency improves biochemically and clinically with pharmacological doses of pyridoxine and folate
- Treatment from infancy can prevent retardation and the other clinical problems
- Pyridoxine nonresponders must be treated with dietary reduction in methionine and supplementation of cysteine
- Vitamin betaine useful in reducing plasma methionine levels
- Anticoagulation for documented venous thrombosis
- Prophylactic use of warfarin not recommended

Reed E. Pyeritz, MD, PhD

Human T Cell Lymphotrophic Virus (HTLV)

 KEY FEATURES

- Retroviruses including types 1 and 2
- HTLV-1 are the causative agents of adult T cell leukemia/lymphoma (ATL) and HTLV-associated myelopathy (HAM)
- Endemic in Caribbean, southern Japan, sub-Saharan Africa, and southeastern US

 CLINICAL FINDINGS

- ATL presents with diffuse lymphadenopathy, skin lesions, hypercalcemia, and lytic bone lesions
- HTLV predisposes to usual AIDS-associated opportunistic infections
- HAM characterized by progressive motor weakness, spastic paraparesis, and sensory disturbances

 DIAGNOSIS

- Serological testing for HTLV antibodies
- HTLV-associated ATL confirmed by proviral DNA integration

 TREATMENT

- ATL treated like other non-Hodgkin's lymphomas
- HAM treated with corticosteroids
- No benefit to antiretroviral therapy
- Blood supply is screened for HTLV-1 because transfusion is a recognized mode of transmission

Wayne X. Shandera, MD
Samuel Shelburne, MD

Hypercalcemia, Malignant

 KEY FEATURES

- Occurs in 10–20% of patients with cancer
- Common causes include cancers of breast, lung, kidney, and head and neck, and multiple myeloma and lymphoma
- Most result from bony metastases, but 20% are unrelated to bony lesions
- Parathyroid hormone–related protein identified in two-thirds of patients with malignant hypercalcemia

 CLINICAL FINDINGS

- Nausea and vomiting
- Constipation
- Polyuria
- Muscular weakness and hyporeflexia
- Confusion, psychosis, tremor, lethargy

 DIAGNOSIS

- Serum calcium increased
- ECG: shortening of the QT interval
- Renal insufficiency
- Be sure to adjust serum calcium level for low albumin or check ionized calcium level

 TREATMENT

- Emergency treatment: hydration (3–4 L/day of 0.9% saline) followed by furosemide, 10–40 mg IV. Aggressive hydration is critical
- Definitive treatment: bisphosphonate (eg, zoledronic acid, 4 mg IV over 15–min with adequate hydration, normalizes serum calcium in <3 days in 80–100%
- Gallium nitrate, 100–200 mg/m²/day continuous IV infusion for 5 days
- Calcitonin, 4-8 IU/kg IM, SC, or intranasally q12h, in conjunction with bisphosphonates, lowers calcium levels faster
- Plicamycin, 25 μg/kg/day IV for 3 or 4 days, is often effective but short lived and associated with hepatic, renal, and bone marrow toxicity
- Chemotherapy and prednisone effective in reducing serum calcium in lymphoid cancers
- Do not replace phosphate when calcium/phosphate product is high

Hope Rugo, MD

Hyperemesis Gravidarum

KEY FEATURES

- Persistent severe vomiting during pregnancy

CLINICAL FINDINGS

- Weight loss
- Dehydration
- Starvation ketosis
- Hypochloremic alkalosis
- Hypokalemia
- Mild elevation in liver enzymes

DIAGNOSIS

- TSH and free T_4 should be checked because thyroid dysfunction can be associated

TREATMENT

- Hospitalization with NPO and IV fluids and vitamins PRN
- TPN is rarely necessary
- As soon as possible, start a dry diet with 6 small daily feedings and clear liquids 1 h after meals
- Prochlorperazine rectal suppositories may be useful
- Once stabilized, patients may remain at home, even if IV fluids are required
- To limit the risk of teratogenicity, drug use in the first half of pregnancy should be limited to those of major importance to life and health (Table 68, page 1261, Table 71, page 1263)

William R. Crombleholme, MD

Hypermagnesemia

KEY FEATURES

- Almost always the result of renal insufficiency and excessive magnesium intake (eg, antacids, laxatives, IV administration)
- Suppresses secretion of parathyroid hormone with consequent hypocalcemia

CLINICAL FINDINGS

- Muscle weakness
- Decreased deep tendon reflexes
- Mental obtundation
- Confusion
- Weakness, even flaccid paralysis
- Hypotension
- There may be respiratory muscle paralysis or cardiac arrest
- In the common setting of renal failure, elevated BUN, serum creatinine, phosphate, and uric acid; serum K^+ may be elevated
- Serum Ca^{2+} is often low
- ECG may show increased PR interval, broadened QRS complexes, and peaked T waves, probably related to associated hyperkalemia

TREATMENT

- Treatment is directed toward therapy of renal insufficiency
- Calcium antagonizes Mg^{2+} and may be given IV as calcium chloride, 500 mg or more at a rate of 100 mg (4.5 mmol)/min
- Hemodialysis or peritoneal dialysis may be indicated

Masafumi Fukagawa, MD, PhD, FJSIM
Kiyoshi Kurokawa, MD, MACP
Maxine A. Papadakis, MD

Hyperphosphatemia

KEY FEATURES

- Renal failure is the most common cause
- Hyperphosphatemia in chronic renal failure leads to secondary hyperparathyroidism and renal osteodystrophy
- A serum calcium X serum phosphorus product >70 markedly increases the risk of nephrocalcinosis and soft tissue calcification

CLINICAL FINDINGS

- Clinical symptoms are those of the underlying disorders (eg, chronic renal failure, hypoparathyroidism)

DIAGNOSIS

- Other blood chemistry values are those of the underlying disease (renal failure, hypoparathyroidism)

TREATMENT

- Treatment is that of the underlying disease and of associated hypocalcemia if present
- In acute and chronic renal failure, dialysis will reduce serum phosphate
- Phosphate absorption can be reduced by calcium carbonate, 0.5–1.5 g TID with meals (500-mg tablets) (preferred to aluminum hydroxide because of concerns about aluminum toxicity)
- Another phosphate binder is sevelamer hydrochloride; does not contain calcium or aluminum and may be especially useful in hypercalcemia or uremia

Masafumi Fukagawa, MD, PhD, FJSIM
Kiyoshi Kurokawa, MD, MACP
Maxine A. Papadakis, MD

Hypersomnia

 KEY FEATURES

- Kleine-Levin syndrome
- A hypersomnia syndrome occurring mostly in young men
- Characterized by intermittent attacks of hypersomnia and other behavioral alterations
- Associated with antecedent neuralgic insults
- Nocturnal myoclonus is another presentation
- See *Obstructive sleep apnea*
- See *Narcolepsy*

 CLINICAL FINDINGS

KLEINE-LEVIN SYNDROME

- Hypersomnic attacks lasting up to 2 days and occurring 3–4 times/yr
- Awakening is accompanied by hyperphagia, hypersexuality, irritability, confusion
- Usually remits after age 40

NOCTURNAL MYOCLONUS

- Periodic lower leg movements occur during sleep with subsequent daytime sleepiness, anxiety, depression, cognitive impairment

 DIAGNOSIS

- Clinical or during a sleep study

 TREATMENT

KLEINE-LEVIN SYNDROME

- No treatment is known

NOCTURNAL MYOCLONUS

- Clonazepam can be used with variable results
- Dopaminergic agents (bromocriptine, carbodopa/levodopa) can be useful in some

Stuart J. Eisendrath, MD
Jonathan E. Lichtmacher, MD

Hyperthermia

 KEY FEATURES

- Hyperthermia is a rapidly life-threatening complication
- May be associated with poisoning by amphetamines (especially ecstasy), atropine and other anticholinergic drugs, cocaine, dinitrophenol and pentachlorophenol, phencyclidine (PCP), salicylates, strychnine, tricyclic antidepressants, and other medications
- Overdose of serotonin reuptake inhibitors (eg, fluoxetine, paroxetine, sertraline) or use in a patient taking a monoamine oxidase inhibitor may cause agitation, hyperactivity, and hyperthermia (serotonin syndrome)
- Haloperidol and other antipsychotic agents can cause rigidity and hyperthermia (neuroleptic malignant syndrome)
- Malignant hyperthermia is associated with general anesthetic agents (rare)

 CLINICAL FINDINGS

- Severe hyperthermia (temperature >40–41°C) may rapidly cause brain damage and multiorgan failure, including rhabdomyolysis, renal failure, and coagulopathy

 TREATMENT

- Remove all clothing, spraying with tepid water and fan the patient
- If a normal rectal temperature is not achieved within 30–60 min, or if there is significant muscle rigidity or hyperactivity, induce neuromuscular paralysis with a nondepolarizing neuromuscular blocker (eg, pancuronium, vecuronium)
- Once paralyzed, the patient must be intubated and mechanically ventilated
- In patients with seizures, absence of visible muscular convulsive movements may give the false impression that brain seizure activity has ceased; however, this must be confirmed by electroencephalography
- Dantrolene, 2–5 mg/kg IV, may be effective for muscle rigidity that does not respond to neuromuscular blockade (ie, malignant hyperthermia)
- Bromocriptine, 2.5–7.5 mg PO daily, can treat neuroleptic malignant syndrome
- Cyproheptadine, 4 mg PO qh for 3 or 4 doses, can treat serotonin syndrome

Kent R. Olsen, MD

Hyperuricemia

 KEY FEATURES

- Complication of rapidly proliferating malignancies as well as treatment-associated tumor lysis of hematological malignancies
- May be worsened by thiazide diuretic use
- Rapid increase in serum uric acid can result in acute urate nephropathy caused by uric acid crystallization in the distal tubules, collecting ducts, and renal parenchyma
- To prevent urate nephropathy, serum uric acid must be reduced before chemotherapy

 CLINICAL FINDINGS

- Acute renal failure
- Gouty arthritis (generally only with history of gout)

 DIAGNOSIS

- At-risk patients should have BID measurements of serum uric acid, phosphate, calcium, and creatinine for the first 2–3 days after initiation of chemotherapy
- Serum uric acid concentration >15 mg/dL imposes a high risk of uric acid nephropathy

 TREATMENT

PROPHYLAXIS

- Allopurinol, 600 mg PO 12–24 h before chemotherapy followed by 300 mg PO qd; higher doses (900–1200 mg/day) are used when severe hyperuricemia is anticipated
- Maintain adequate hydration
- Alkalinize urine with sodium bicarbonate, 6–8 g PO qd, or by infusion of 1 L of D_5W with 2–3 ampules of sodium bicarbonate; goal urine pH = 7.0

EMERGENCY TREATMENT

- Hydration with 2–4 L of fluid per day
- Alkalinization of the urine as above
- Allopurinol, 900–1200 mg/day
- In severe cases, emergency hemodialysis

Hope Rugo, MD

Hyperventilation Syndromes

KEY FEATURES

- Hyperventilation is an increase in alveolar ventilation leading to hypocapnia
- Causes include pregnancy, hypoxemia, obstructive and infiltrative lung disease, sepsis, liver failure, fever, and pain
- "Central neurogenic hyperventilation" describes monotonous, sustained deep breathing seen in comatose patients with brainstem injury

CLINICAL FINDINGS

- Acute hyperventilation: hyperpnea, paresthesias, carpopedal spasm, tetany, and anxiety
- Chronic hyperventilation presents non-specifically: fatigue, dyspnea, anxiety, palpitations, and dizziness

DIAGNOSIS

- Symptoms must be reproduced during voluntary hyperventilation

TREATMENT

- When organic causes have been excluded, rebreathing expired gas from a paper bag decreases respiratory alkalemia and its symptoms
- Anxiolytics may be helpful

Mark S. Chesnutt, MD
Thomas J. Prendergast, MD

Hypoventilation, Primary Alveolar

KEY FEATURES

- A rare syndrome ("Ondine's curse") of unknown cause
- Characterized by inadequate alveolar ventilation despite normal airways, lungs, chest wall, respiratory muscles, and neurological function
- Patients are usually nonobese males in their 40s and 50s

CLINICAL FINDINGS

- Lethargy, headache, and somnolence
- Dyspnea is not present
- Erythrocytosis may be present

DIAGNOSIS

- Arterial blood gas shows hypoxemia and hypercapnia, which improve with voluntary hyperventilation

TREATMENT

- Ventilatory stimulants are not effective
- Mechanical augmentation of ventilation via phrenic nerve stimulation, rocking bed, or ventilators may be helpful
- Supplemental oxygen should be given, with the caveat that nocturnal oxygen be given only if sleep study demonstrates that it is effective and safe

Mark S. Chesnutt, MD
Thomas J. Prendergast, MD

Immunoglobulin A Deficiency, Selective

KEY FEATURES

- The most common primary immunodeficiency disorder, estimated to affect 1 in 500 individuals

CLINICAL FINDINGS

- Most are asymptomatic
- Frequent and recurrent infections such as sinusitis, otitis, and bronchitis
- Can be associated with IgG subclass deficiency
- Increased atopic and autoimmune diseases
- Most severe consequence is serum sickness or anaphylaxis that develops after the infusion of IgA-containing plasma products (when the patient has anti-IgA antibodies)

DIAGNOSIS

- The absence of serum IgA with normal levels of total serum IgG and IgM

TREATMENT

- Treatment with commercial immune globulin is ineffective because IgA is present only in trace quantities in these preparations
- Antibiotics as needed for infections

Jeffrey L. Kishiyama, MD
Daniel C. Adelman, MD

Infertility, Assisted Reproductive Technologies

 KEY FEATURES

- Couples who have failed to respond to traditional infertility treatments may benefit from in vitro fertilization (IVF), gamete intrafallopian transfer (GIFT), and zygote intrafallopian transfer (ZIFT)
- Age is an important determinant of success: For couples younger than 35, the average rate of live birth is 32% per retrieval, whereas the rate for women older than 40 is 8%. More than one third of pregnancies have been multiple

 CLINICAL FINDINGS

- See *Infertility*

 DIAGNOSIS

- See *Infertility*

 TREATMENT

- All of the procedures involve ovarian stimulation to produce multiple oocytes, oocyte retrieval by transvaginal sector scan-guided needle aspiration, and handling of the oocytes outside the body
- With IVF, the eggs are fertilized in vitro and the embryos transferred to the uterine fundus. Extra embryos may be cryopreserved for subsequent cycles
- GIFT involves the placement of sperm and eggs in the uterine tube by laparoscopy or minilaparotomy and is more invasive than IVF
- GIFT is not appropriate for women with severe tubal diseases and is less successful than IVF with male factor infertility because fertilization cannot be documented
- With ZIFT, fertilization occurs in vitro, and the early development of the embryo occurs in the uterine tube after transfer by laparoscopy or minilaparotomy
- Intracytoplasmic sperm injection allows fertilization with a single sperm, which is helpful in the setting of severe oligospermia or obstructive azoospermia

H. Trent MacKay, MD, MPH

Interstititial Lung Disease, Respiratory Bronchiolitis–Associated

 KEY FEATURES

- Presentation similar to usual interstitial pneumonitis (UIP) but in younger patients
- Patients are invariably heavy smokers
- Prognosis is better than in UIP; median survival >10 yr

 CLINICAL FINDINGS

- Age 40–45 yr
- Insidious dry cough with exertional dyspnea over months to years
- Diffuse, fine, late inspiratory crackles on exam

 DIAGNOSIS

- Pulmonary function test shows restriction with decreased DLCO, usually less severe than that seen in UIP
- Biopsy shows increased numbers of macrophages localized within the peribronchiolar space; alveolar architecture is preserved, honeycomb change and fibrosis are minimal

 TREATMENT

- Spontaneous remission in up to 20% of patients
- Smoking cessation is crucial
- Corticosteroids are thought to be effective, although no randomized trial supports this

Mark S. Chesnutt, MD
Thomas J. Prendergast, MD

Intertrigo

 KEY FEATURES

- Caused by the macerating effect of heat, moisture, friction
- Especially likely to occur in obese persons and in humid climates

 CLINICAL FINDINGS

- Symptoms are itching, stinging, burning
- Body folds develop fissures, erythema, and sodden epidermis, with superficial denudation
- Candidiasis may complicate intertrigo

 DIAGNOSIS

- KOH prep and Wood's light to rule out *Candida,* tinea, and erythrasma
- Differential diagnosis includes candidiasis, tinea cruris (jock itch), psoriasis of body folds ("inverse psoriasis"), erythrasma, cellulitis, seborrheic dermatitis, tinea versicolor (pityriasis versicolor; rarely), scratching resulting from pediculosis (lice), contact dermatitis

 TREATMENT

- Maintain hygiene in the area, and keep it dry
- Compresses may be useful acutely
- Hydrocortisone 1% and an imidazole cream or nystatin cream are effective
- Recurrences are common

Timothy G. Berger, MD

Iron Poisoning

 KEY FEATURES

- Most children's preparations contain 12–15 mg of elemental iron per dose compared with 60–90 mg in most adult-strength preparations
- Iron is corrosive to the GI tract and has depressant effects on the myocardium and on peripheral vascular resistance

 CLINICAL FINDINGS

- Ingestion of <30 mg/kg of elemental iron usually produces only mild GI upset
- Ingestion of >40–60 mg/kg may cause vomiting, hematemesis, diarrhea, hypotension, and metabolic acidosis
- Death may occur from massive fluid losses and bleeding, metabolic acidosis, peritonitis from intestinal perforation, fulminant hepatic failure

 DIAGNOSIS

- Serum iron levels >350–500 µg/dL are potentially toxic, and levels >1000 µg/dL are usually associated with severe poisoning
- A plain abdominal x-ray film may reveal radiopaque tablets

 TREATMENT

- Treat hypotension aggressively with IV crystalloid solutions (0.9% saline or lactated Ringer's solution)
- Perform whole-bowel irrigation to remove unabsorbed pills, particularly when intact tablets are visible on abdominal x-ray film. Administer the balanced polyethylene glycol-electrolyte solution (CoLyte, GoLYTELY) into the stomach via gastric tube at a rate of 1–2 L/h until the rectal effluent is clear
- Activated charcoal is not effective
- For symptomatic toxicity, and particularly with markedly elevated serum iron levels (eg, greater than 800–1000 µg/dL), administer 10–15 mg/kg/h of deferoxamine by constant IV infusion; higher doses (up to 40–50 mg/kg/h) have been used in massive poisonings. Prolonged infusion (> 36–48 h) has been associated with development of acute respiratory distress syndrome

Kent R. Olsen, MD

Isoniazid Poisoning

 KEY FEATURES

- Acute ingestion of as little as 1.5–2 g can cause toxicity, and severe poisoning is likely to occur after ingestion of more than 80–100 mg/kg
- May cause hepatitis with chronic use

 CLINICAL FINDINGS

- Confusion, slurred speech, and seizures may occur abruptly after acute overdose
- Severe lactic acidosis—disproportional to the severity of seizures—is probably due to inhibited metabolism of lactate

 DIAGNOSIS

- Diagnosis is based on a history of ingestion and the presence of severe acidosis associated with seizures.
- Isoniazid is not usually included in routine toxicological screening, and serum levels are not readily available

 TREATMENT

- Seizures may require higher than usual doses of benzodiazepines (eg, lorazepam, 3–5 mg IV)
- Pyridoxine (vitamin B_6) is a specific antagonist of the acute toxic effects and is usually successful in controlling seizures that do not respond to benzodiazepines. Give 5 g IV over 1–2 min or, if the amount ingested is known, give a gram-for-gram equivalent amount of pyridoxine
- Administer activated charcoal, 60–100 g PO or via gastric tube, mixed in aqueous slurry. Do not use for comatose or convulsing patients unless it can be given by gastric tube and the airway is protected by a cuffed endotracheal tube

Kent R. Olsen, MD

Kawasaki Syndrome

 KEY FEATURES

- Mucocutaneous lymph node syndrome
- Usually affects children younger than 10, at times in an epidemic fashion
- No clear infectious cause identified

 CLINICAL FINDINGS

- Fever universal
- Bilateral nonexudative conjunctivitis
- Mucous membrane involvement
- Polymorphous rash
- Cervical lymphadenopathy

 DIAGNOSIS

- Clinical based on combination of above findings
- Potential for arteritis of coronary vessels leading to myocardial infarction

 TREATMENT

- High-dose aspirin
- IV immunoglobulin
- Warfarin for coronary artery aneurysms
- Role of steroids is controversial

Wayne X. Shandera, MD
Samuel Shelburne, MD

Klinefelter's Syndrome

 KEY FEATURES

- Males with 1 extra X chromosome (XXY)

 CLINICAL FINDINGS

- Boys are normal in appearance before puberty; after puberty, they have disproportionately long legs and arms, a female escutcheon, gynecomastia, and small testes
- Infertility resulting from azoospermia; the seminiferous tubules are hyalinized
- Mental retardation is somewhat more common than in the general population, and many have learning problems
- Higher risk of breast cancer
- Heightened risk of diabetes mellitus

 DIAGNOSIS

- Cytogenetic analysis

 TREATMENT

- Testosterone administration is advisable after puberty but will not restore fertility
- Intracytoplasmic sperm injection is possible using sperm obtained by testicular extraction

Reed E. Pyeritz, MD, PhD

Knee, Overuse Syndromes

 KEY FEATURES

- Runners, particularly those who overtrain, fail to stretch before running, or do not attain the proper level of conditioning before starting a running program, may develop a variety of painful overuse syndromes of the knee
- Most of these conditions are forms of tendinitis or bursitis that can be diagnosed on examination
- The most common conditions include anserine bursitis, iliotibial band syndrome, and popliteal and patellar tendinitis

 CLINICAL FINDINGS

- Symptoms worsen with continued running
- Anserine bursitis results in pain medial and inferior to the knee joint over the medial tibia
- The iliotibial band syndrome results in pain on the lateral side of the knee
- Patellar tendinitis, a cause of anterior knee discomfort, typically occurs at the tendon's insertion into the patella rather than at its more inferior insertion

 DIAGNOSIS

- Confirm the diagnoses by palpating the relevant sites around the knee
- Not associated with joint effusions or other signs of synovitis

 TREATMENT

- Rest and abstention from the associated physical activities for a period of days to weeks are essential
- Once the acute pain has subsided, a program of gentle stretching (particularly before resuming exercise) may prevent recurrence
- Corticosteroid with lidocaine injections may be useful when intense discomfort is present, but caution must be used when injecting corticosteroids into the region of a tendon since rupture may occur

David B. Hellmann, MD, FACP
John H. Stone, MD, MPH

Labor, Preterm

 KEY FEATURES

- Labor beginning before 37th week of pregnancy
- Responsible for 85% of neonatal illnesses and deaths

 CLINICAL FINDINGS

- Risk factors:
  - History of preterm labor
  - Premature rupture of membranes
  - Urinary tract infection
  - Diethylstilbestrol exposure
  - Multiple gestation
  - Abdominal or cervical surgery
  - Cervical length of <25 mm by second-trimester ultrasonogram

 DIAGNOSIS

- Fetal fibronectin measurement in cervicovaginal specimens can differentiate true from false labor
- A level <50 ng/mL has a negative predictive value of 93–97% for delivery in 7–14 days among women with a history of preterm labor currently having contractions

 TREATMENT

- Low rates of preterm delivery are associated with successful education of patients in identifying regular, frequent contractions
- Magnesium sulfate IV, 4–6-g bolus followed by infusion of 2–3 g/h titrated to blood levels of 6–8 mg/dL
- Terbutaline (2.5 μg/min IV titrated to a maximum 20 μg/min or 2.5–5 mg PO q2–4h) relaxes the myometrium via B_2-receptor activation
- Nifedipine, 10–20 mg PO q4–6h

William R. Crombleholme, MD

Lactase Deficiency

 KEY FEATURES

- Partial to complete lactose intolerance affects ~50 million people in US
- Occurs in 90% of Asian-Americans, 70% of African-Americans, 95% of Native Americans, 50% of Mexican-Americans, 60% of Jewish Americans, 25% of Caucasian adults
- Also occurs secondary to Crohn's disease, sprue, viral gastroenteritis, giardiasis, short bowel syndrome, malnutrition

 CLINICAL FINDINGS

- Bloating, abdominal cramps, and flatulence 1–3 h after ingesting milk products
- Diarrhea

 DIAGNOSIS

- Diarrheal specimens have an increased osmotic gap and pH < 6.0
- Hydrogen breath test: After ingestion of 50 g lactose, a rise in breath hydrogen of >20 ppm within 90 min is a positive test
- Empirical trial of a lactose-free diet for 2 weeks, leading to resolution of symptoms
- Differential diagnosis: inflammatory bowel disease, mucosal malabsorptive disorders, irritable bowel syndrome, pancreatic insufficiency

 TREATMENT

- Eliminate or restrict milk products
- Spread dairy product intake throughout the day
- Use lactase enzyme supplements (eg, nonprescription formulation [LactAid]) when ingesting dairy products
- Calcium supplementation

Kenneth R. McQuaid, MD

Larva Migrans, Cutaneous

 KEY FEATURES

- Caused by larvae of the dog and cat hookworms, *Ancylostoma braziliense* and *Ancylostoma caninum*
- Prevalent throughout the tropics and subtropics, including southeastern US
- Moist sandy soil (eg, beaches, children's sand piles) contaminated by dog or cat feces is a common site of infection

 CLINICAL FINDINGS

- At the site of larval entry, particularly on the hands or feet, up to several hundred minute, intensely pruritic erythematous papules appear. Two to 3 days later, serpiginous eruptions appear as the larvae migrate at a rate of several millimeters a day. The process may continue for weeks; the lesions may become severely pruritic, vesiculate, encrusted, or secondarily infected
- Without treatment, the larvae eventually die and are absorbed

 DIAGNOSIS

- Clinical and the frequent eosinophilia
- Biopsy is usually not indicated

 TREATMENT

- Mild transient cases may not require treatment
- For mild cases, use thiabendazole, applied topically TID for 5 or more days as a 15% cream, which can be formulated in a hygroscopic base using crushed 500-mg tablets
- For more severe cases, oral treatment is indicated. Give ivermectin, 200 µg/kg given for 1 or 2 days, and albendazole, 400 mg BID for 3–5 days or 400 mg daily for 7 days
- Thiabendazole, given PO as for strongyloidiasis, is less satisfactory because of its toxicity
- Antihistamines can help control pruritus
- Antibiotic (ointment or oral) may be necessary to treat secondary infections

Lead Poisoning

 KEY FEATURES

- Toxicity is usually from chronic exposure to contaminated dust or fumes
- Acute ingestion of lead fishing weights or curtain weights can cause poisoning

 CLINICAL FINDINGS

- Abdominal pain, constipation, headache, irritability
- Coma and convulsions in severe poisoning
- Chronic intoxication can cause learning disorders (in children) and motor neuropathy (eg, wrist drop)

 DIAGNOSIS

- Blood lead level
- Microcytic anemia with basophilic stippling and elevated free erythrocyte protoporphyrin may be seen
- Can be misdiagnosed as porphyria

 TREATMENT

- For recent ingestion, give activated charcoal, 60–100 g PO or via gastric tube, mixed in aqueous slurry
- If a large lead object remains visible on stomach x-ray film, repeated cathartics, whole-bowel irrigation, endoscopy, or surgical removal may be necessary
- Consult a medical toxicologist or regional poison control center for advice about chelation. For severe intoxication (encephalopathy or levels >70–100 µg/dL) give edetate calcium disodium (EDTA), 1500 mg/m^2/kg/day (approximately 50 mg/kg/day) in 4–6 divided doses or as a continuous IV infusion
- Dimercaprol, 4–5 mg/kg IM q4h for 5 days can be added
- Less severe symptoms with blood lead levels between 55 and 69 µg/dL may be treated with EDTA alone in dosages as above
- Succimer (dimercaptosuccinic acid), 10 mg/kg PO q8h for 5 days, then q12h for 2 weeks

Kent R. Olsen, MD

Leishmaniasis, Mucocutaneous

 KEY FEATURES

- Caused by the leishmania (viannia) group of organisms; most common is *L (V) brasiliensis* in Central and South America

 CLINICAL FINDINGS

- The initial lesion, single or multiple, is on exposed skin; at first it is papular, then nodular, and later may ulcerate or become wart-like or papillomatous. Local healing follows, with scarring within several months to a year
- Subsequent naso-oral involvement occurs in a few patients. It may appear concurrently with the initial lesion, shortly after healing, or after many years. Extensive destruction of the soft tissues and cartilage of the nose, oral cavity, and lips may follow and may extend to the larynx and pharynx
- Secondary bacterial infection is common
- Fever, keratitis, lymphangitis, weight loss, and anemia may be present

 DIAGNOSIS

- Diagnosis by detecting amastigotes in scrapings, biopsy impressions, or aspirated tissue fluid is difficult
- The organism grows with difficulty in culture or in hamster inoculation
- The skin test can be useful
- Standard serological tests are often not useful; a direct agglutination for IgM antibodies may become positive in 4–6 weeks and subsequently an IgG test may become positive, but at low titer

 TREATMENT

- See *Leishmaniasis*
- Failure rates are high in severe disease even when a full course (28 days) of sodium stibogluconate is used. If repeated and extended antimony treatment fails, amphotericin B desoxycholate or pentamidine is used
- Corticosteroids may control inflammation from release of antigens

Listeriosis

 KEY FEATURES

- *Listeria monocytogenes* is a motile, gram-positive rod that is a facultative intracellular organism
- Most cases of infection caused by *L monocytogenes* are sporadic, but outbreaks have been traced to eating contaminated food, especially unpasteurized dairy products

 CLINICAL FINDINGS

- Five types of infection are recognized:
  - Infection during pregnancy, usually in the last trimester, produces a mild febrile illness without an apparent primary focus. This is a relatively benign disease that may resolve without therapy
  - Granulomatosis infantisepticum is a neonatal infection characterized by disseminated abscesses and granulomas and a high mortality rate
  - Bacteremia with or without sepsis syndrome is an infection of neonates or immunocompromised adults. The presentation is that of a febrile illness without a recognized source
  - Meningitis affects infants younger than 2 mo and adults, ranking third and fourth, respectively, among the common causes of bacterial meningitis. Adults with meningitis are usually immunocompromised, and cases have been associated with HIV infection
  - Focal infections, including adenitis, brain abscess, endocarditis, osteomyelitis, and arthritis, occur rarely

 DIAGNOSIS

- Table 125, page 1307
- In meningitis, cerebrospinal fluid shows a neutrophilic pleocytosis

 TREATMENT

- Tables 122, page 1303, 128, page 1311
- The drug of choice is probably ampicillin, 8–12 g/day IV in 4–6 divided doses (the higher dose is recommended in cases of meningitis)
- Trimethoprim-sulfamethoxazole is an effective alternative

Henry F. Chambers, MD

Lithium Toxicity

 KEY FEATURES

- Occurs at serum lithium levels >2 mEq/L
- Sodium loss (diarrhea, diuretics, perspiration) results in elevated lithium levels
- Toxicity is more severe in the elderly

 CLINICAL FINDINGS

- Diarrhea, vomiting
- Tremors, marked weakness, confusion
- Dysarthria, ataxia, vertigo, choreoathetosis, hyperreflexia
- Myoclonus, seizures, opisthotonos, coma

 DIAGNOSIS

- Serum lithium levels confirm the diagnosis

 TREATMENT

- Induced emesis and gastric lavage for massive ingestions or levels > 2.5 mEq/L
- Osmotic or saline diuresis in patients with normal renal function
- Urinary alkalinization with sodium bicarbonate or acetazolamide

Stuart J. Eisendrath, MD
Jonathan E. Lichtmacher, MD

Livedo Reticularis

 KEY FEATURES

- An uncommon vasospastic disorder of unknown cause that results in a painless, mottled discoloration on large areas of the extremities in a fishnet pattern with reticulated cyanotic areas surrounding a paler central core
- Occurs in men and women of all ages
- In most instances, entirely benign
- Infrequently associated with an occult malignancy, polyarteritis nodosa, atherosclerotic microemboli, or antiphospholipid antibody syndrome

 CLINICAL FINDINGS

- Arteriolar vasoconstriction with capillary and venous dilation
- Most apparent on the thighs
- Can occur on the forearms or lower abdomen
- Most pronounced in cold weather
- Paresthesias, coldness, or numbness in a few patients
- Peripheral pulses are normal
- Affected regions may be cool
- Skin ulceration is rare

 DIAGNOSIS

- Clinical diagnosis

 TREATMENT

- Protection from exposure to cold
- Vasodilators seldom indicated
- If ulcerations or gangrene, exclude an underlying systemic disease

Louis M. Messina, MD
Laura K. Pak, MD
Lawrence M. Tierney, Jr, MD

Liver Neoplasms, Benign

 KEY FEATURES

- The most common benign hepatic neoplasm is the **cavernous hemangioma**, often an incidental finding on ultrasonography
- Two distinct benign entities have been described in women. **Focal nodular hyperplasia** occurs at all ages. **Liver cell adenoma** occurs most commonly in the third and fourth decades of life and is usually caused by oral contraceptives

 CLINICAL FINDINGS

- Focal nodular hyperplasia is often asymptomatic. Liver cell adenoma usually presents with acute abdominal pain because of necrosis of the tumor with hemorrhage. The only physical finding in both lesions is a palpable abdominal mass in a minority of cases

 DIAGNOSIS

- Cavernous hemangioma must be differentiated from other liver lesions, usually by MRI. Rarely, fine-needle biopsy is needed to differentiate these lesions and does not appear to carry an increased risk of bleeding
- Focal nodular hyperplasia appears as a hypervascular mass, occasionally with a central hypodense "stellate" scar on CT
- Liver cell adenoma is a hypovascular tumor and is a cold defect on liver scan
- In both focal nodular hyperplasia and liver cell adenoma, the liver function is usually normal. Arterial-phase helical CT and MRI can distinguish an adenoma from focal nodular hyperplasia in 80–90% of cases

 TREATMENT

- Cavernous hemangiomas rarely require treatment. Regression of benign hepatic tumors may follow cessation of oral contraceptives. Treatment of focal nodular hyperplasia is resection only in the symptomatic patient. The prognosis is excellent
- Liver cell adenoma often undergoes necrosis and rupture, and resection is advised, even in asymptomatic persons

Lawrence S. Friedman, MD

Locked-In Syndrome

 KEY FEATURES

- Acute destructive lesions (eg, infarction, hemorrhage, demyelination, encephalitis) involving the ventral pons and sparing the tegmentum
- Patient is mute and quadriparetic but conscious
- Such a patient can mistakenly be regarded as comatose
- Physicians should recognize that "locked-in" individuals are fully aware of their surroundings

 CLINICAL FINDINGS

- Mute, quadriplegic patient
- Conscious state
- Patient is capable of blinking and of voluntary eye movement in the vertical plane
- Preserved pupillary responses to light

 DIAGNOSIS

- Brain imaging with CT or MRI scan
- Obtain the expertise of a clinician familiar with this disorder to aid in the diagnosis

 TREATMENT

- The prognosis is variable, but recovery has occasionally been reported, in some cases including resumption of independent daily life, although this may take up to 2 or 3 yr

Michael J. Aminoff, DSc, MD, FRCP

LSD Overdose

 KEY FEATURES

- The mechanism of toxicity and the clinical effects vary for each substance

 CLINICAL FINDINGS

- Anticholinergic delirium: dilated pupils flushed skin, dry mucous membranes, tachycardia, and urinary retention
- LSD: marked visual hallucinations and perceptual distortion, widely dilated pupils, and mild tachycardia
- Phencyclidine (PCP) can produce fluctuating delirium and coma, often with vertical and horizontal nystagmus
- Toluene and other hydrocarbon solvents (eg, butane, trichloroethylene, "chemo") cause euphoria, delirium, and fatal dysrhythmias

 TREATMENT

- For recent ingestions, administer activated charcoal, 60–100 g PO or via gastric tube, mixed in aqueous slurry
- Treat anticholinergic delirium with physostigmine salicylate, 0.5–1 mg IV slowly over 5 min, with ECG monitoring, until symptoms are controlled. Bradyarrhythmias and convulsions can occur with physostigmine use, and it should be avoided in tricyclic antidepressant overdose
- Treat dysphoria, agitation, or psychosis from LSD or mescaline with lorazepam, 1–2 mg PO or IV, or haloperidol, 2–5 mg
- Monitor patients who have sniffed solvents for cardiac dysrhythmias; β-blockers (eg, propranolol, 1–5 mg IV, or esmolol, 250–500 µg/kg IV, then 50 µg/kg/min by infusion) may be used

Kent R. Olsen, MD

Lupus Anticoagulant

 KEY FEATURES

- IgM or IgG that produces prolonged PTT by binding to phospholipid used in PTT assay
- A laboratory artifact that does not cause clinical bleeding
- Occurs in 5–10% of patients with systemic lupus erythematosus; more common in patients without underlying disorder and in patients taking phenothiazines

 CLINICAL FINDINGS

- No bleeding unless a second disorder is present (eg, thrombocytopenia, hypoprothrombinemia, or prolonged bleeding time)
- Increased risk of thrombosis and recurrent spontaneous abortions

 DIAGNOSIS

- PTT prolonged, fails to correct when patient's plasma is mixed in 1:1 dilution with normal plasma because lupus anticoagulant acts as inhibitor
- PT normal or slightly prolonged
- Serum fibrinogen level and thrombin time normal
- Russell viper venom test is a sensitive assay designed to demonstrate presence of lupus anticoagulant
- False-positive VDRL test for syphilis
- A related autoantibody, anticardiolipin, can be detected by separate assays
- Factor VIIIc level, measured when acquired factor VIII inhibitor suspected, is normal in patients with lupus anticoagulant

 TREATMENT

- No specific treatment necessary
- Prednisone usually rapidly eliminates lupus anticoagulant, but it is unclear whether it affects thrombotic tendency
- Anticoagulation in standard doses for patients with thromboses
- Because of artificially prolonged PTT, heparin therapy is difficult to monitor; thus, low-molecular-weight heparin may be preferred
- Warfarin dose needs to be increased if baseline PT prolonged

Charles A. Linker, MD

Lymphocytic Choriomeningitis

 KEY FEATURES

- Arenavirus infection of CNS
- Main reservoir is house mouse, but other domestic animals may harbor virus
- Virus spread from animal to human by infected oronasal secretions, urine, or feces
- Person-to-person spread rare

 CLINICAL FINDINGS

- Symptoms are biphasic with a prodromal phase followed by a meningeal phase
- Fever, malaise, headache, and cough are common in prodromal phase
- Neck and back stiffness with a positive Kernig's sign are common in the meningeal phase
- Obstructive hydrocephalus is rare but serious complication

 DIAGNOSIS

- Leukocytosis or leukopenia
- CSF lymphocytic pleocytosis common
- CSF PCR for LCM virus is available, although rarely used
- Complement-fixing antibodies appear during second week of infection and may aid in diagnosis

 TREATMENT

- No specific antiviral therapy
- Supportive measures
- Attempt to prevent secondary complications

Wayne X. Shandera, MD
Samuel Shelburne, MD

Lymphogranuloma Venereum

 KEY FEATURES

- An acute and chronic sexually transmitted disease caused by *Chlamydia trachomatis* types L1–L3

 CLINICAL FINDINGS

- In men, the initial vesicular or ulcerative lesion (on the external genitalia) is evanescent and often goes unnoticed
- Inguinal buboes appear 1–4 weeks after exposure, are often bilateral, and have a tendency to fuse, soften, and break down to form multiple draining sinuses, with extensive scarring
- In women, the genital lymph drainage is to the perirectal glands. Early anorectal manifestations are proctitis with tenesmus and bloody purulent discharge; late manifestations are chronic cicatrizing inflammation of the rectal and perirectal tissue. These changes lead to obstipation and rectal stricture and, occasionally, rectovaginal and perianal fistulas. They are also seen in homosexual men

 DIAGNOSIS

- The complement fixation test may be positive, but cross-reaction with other chlamydiae occurs
- Specific immunofluorescence tests for IgM are more specific for acute infection

 TREATMENT

- Doxycycline, 0.1 g BID for 21 days Erythromycin, 500 mg QID, or trimethoprim-sulfamethoxazole, 160/800 mg BID for 21 days, also is effective

Henry F. Chambers, MD

Lymphoma, Gastric

 KEY FEATURES

- Second most common gastric malignancy, 3–6% of gastric cancers
- More than 95% are non-Hodgkin's B cell lymphomas
- May be primary (gastric mucosal lymphoma) or secondary (in patients with nodal lymphomas)
- ~60% of primary gastric lymphomas are mucosa-associated lymphoid tissue (MALT)
- B cells of nodal origin may be distinguished from B cells derived from MALT (CD19- and CD20-positive)
- Infection with *Helicobacter pylori* is an important risk factor for primary gastric lymphoma
- >85% of low-grade primary gastric lymphomas and 40% of high-grade lymphomas are associated with *H pylori*

 CLINICAL FINDINGS

- Abdominal pain
- Weight loss
- Upper GI bleeding

 DIAGNOSIS

- Endoscopy with biopsy useful in diagnosis
- Abdominal and chest CT and endoscopic ultrasonography useful in staging

 TREATMENT

- Primary low-grade gastric lymphomas are usually localized to the stomach wall (stage IE) or adjacent lymph nodes (stage IIE) and have an excellent prognosis
- Nodal lymphomas with secondary gastric involvement are usually at an advanced stage and thus seldom curable
- Complete lymphoma regression occurs in 75% of cases of stage IE low-grade lymphoma after successful *H pylori* eradication
- Patients with stage IE or IIE low-grade lymphomas who are not infected with *H pylori* or fail to respond to eradication therapy can be treated successfully with surgical resection, local radiation therapy, or combination therapy
- Stage IEE or 2EE high-grade lymphomas are treated with resection and CHOP chemotherapy (cyclophosphamide, hydroxydaunomycin, Oncovin, prednisone)
- Stage III or IV primary lymphomas are treated with combination chemotherapy; surgical resection is no longer recommended
- Long-term survival of primary gastric lymphoma for stage I is >85% and for stage II 35–65%

Kenneth R. McQuaid, MD

Macular Degeneration, Age-Related

 KEY FEATURES

- Age-related macular degeneration is the leading cause of permanent visual loss in the elderly
- Exact cause is unknown but a precursor is the development of macular drusen
- Two subtypes: atrophic and exudative

 CLINICAL FINDINGS

- Loss of central vision
- Atrophic subtype is characterized by progressive, bilateral visual loss of moderate severity resulting from atrophy and degeneration of the outer retina
- Exudative subtype is characterized by rapid and severe unilateral visual loss, with a high risk of subsequent involvement of the fellow eye
- Older patients developing sudden central visual loss, particularly paracentral distortion or scotoma with preservation of central acuity, should be referred urgently to an ophthalmologist for assessment

 DIAGNOSIS

- On ophthalmoscopic examination various abnormalities are visualized in the macula
- Fundal photography after IV fluorescein (fluorescein angiography) may be required

 TREATMENT

- No specific treatment is available for atrophic macular degeneration, but patients often benefit from low vision aids
- Retinal laser photocoagulation, including photodynamic therapy, or retinal surgery may be beneficial in exudative disease

Paul Riordan-Eva, FRCOphth

Measles

 KEY FEATURES

- Transmitted by inhalation of infected respiratory droplets
- Estimated 1 million deaths annually worldwide
- Declining incidence in US because of widespread vaccine use

 CLINICAL FINDINGS

- Initial prodrome of malaise and fever; rash 3–4 days later
- Fever persists through the early rash
- Koplik's spots, which appear as tiny "table crystals" on mucous membranes, are pathognomonic and appear 2 days before the rash
- Rash begins as pin-sized papules on face and behind ears, spreading to trunk and then extremities
- Pulmonary involvement occurs in up to 5% of cases and is the most common cause of death
- Encephalitis occurs in up to 0.1% of cases
- Subacute sclerosing panencephalitis (SSPE) is a rare, late CNS complication, largely among rural boys

 DIAGNOSIS

- Clinical symptoms often difficult to differentiate from other viral illnesses
- Koplik's spots clinch the diagnosis
- History of exposure to patients with measles helpful but not always present
- Leukopenia usually present
- Lymphocyte count <2000/μL is associated with poor prognosis
- Fourfold antibody rise diagnostic

 TREATMENT

- Supportive measures
- High-dose vitamin A recommended in children
- Antibiotics for bacterial pneumonia resulting from superinfection
- Prevention: measles vaccination of children and young adults
- Postexposure prophylaxis: Live virus vaccine may be effective in prevention up to 5 days postexposure in susceptible individuals
- Pregnant women and immunocompromised individuals should avoid vaccination, although adults HIV-infected appear to be safely vaccinated

Wayne X. Shandera, MD
Samuel Shelburne, MD

Meniscus Tears, Medial

 KEY FEATURES

- The most common knee injuries encountered in primary care; tears result from twisting on the knee joint while the foot is weight bearing

 CLINICAL FINDINGS

- There is usually a tearing or popping sensation followed by severe pain
- In contrast to ligamentous injuries, in which hemorrhage causes immediate swelling, effusions from meniscal injuries accumulate over hours and are typically worse the day after the injury
- Several days after resolution (full or partial), there may be joint locking or instability, recurrent swelling with activity, and pain

 DIAGNOSIS

- Joint effusion is usually present
- Tenderness may be localized to the medial joint line, and range of motion in the knee may be restricted
- In the absence of an acutely painful knee, perform a McMurray's test: With the patient supine with the hip and knee in full flexion, place one hand on the involved knee and the other on the ipsilateral foot. As the foot is externally rotated, extend the patient's knee. The presence of a "snap" (palpable or audible) suggests a medial meniscus lesion
- MRI confirms the diagnosis if plain films exclude other conditions

 TREATMENT

- Initial management is elevation, a compression dressing, and ice
- Weight bearing should be minimized for the first few days but may be resumed slowly thereafter
- Quadriceps-strengthening exercises by a physical therapist
- Surgery is reserved for patients with symptoms that recur on resumption of normal activities or for patients with irreducible locking caused by mechanical problems

David B. Hellmann, MD, FACP
John H. Stone, MD, MPH

Meralgia Paresthetica

 KEY FEATURES

- The lateral femoral cutaneous nerve, a sensory nerve arising from the L2 and L3 roots, may be compressed or stretched in obese or diabetic patients and during pregnancy
- Hyperextension of the hip or increased lumbar lordosis—as during pregnancy—leads to nerve compression by the posterior fascicle of the ligament. However, entrapment of the nerve at any point along its course may cause similar symptoms, and several other anatomical variations predispose the nerve to damage when it is stretched

 CLINICAL FINDINGS

- Pain, paresthesia, or numbness occurs about the outer aspect of the thigh, usually unilaterally, and is sometimes relieved by sitting

 DIAGNOSIS

- Examination shows no abnormalities except in severe cases when cutaneous sensation is impaired in the affected area

 TREATMENT

- Symptoms are usually mild and commonly settle spontaneously
- Hydrocortisone injections medial to the anterosuperior iliac spine often relieve symptoms temporarily, whereas nerve decompression by transposition may provide more lasting relief

Michael J. Aminoff, DSc, MD, FRCP

Mercury Poisoning

 KEY FEATURES

- Acute mercury poisoning usually occurs by ingestion of inorganic mercuric salts or inhalation of metallic mercury vapor

 CLINICAL FINDINGS

- Mercury salts: metallic taste, salivation, thirst, a burning sensation in the throat, discoloration and edema of oral mucous membranes, abdominal pain, vomiting, bloody diarrhea, and shock. Direct nephrotoxicity causes acute renal failure
- Inhalation of high concentrations of metallic mercury vapor may cause acute fulminant chemical pneumonia
- Chronic mercury poisoning causes weakness, ataxia, intention tremors, irritability, and depression
- Exposure to alkyl (organic) mercury derivatives from contaminated fish or fungicides used on seeds has caused ataxia, tremors, convulsions, and catastrophic birth defects

 TREATMENT

ACUTE POISONING

- There is no effective specific treatment for mercury vapor pneumonitis. Remove ingested mercuric salts by gastric lavage, and administer activated charcoal
- For acute ingestion of mercuric salts, administer chelation therapy with BAL (British Anti-Lewisite) or DMSA (succimer). Contact a poison control center or medical toxicologist for assistance

CHRONIC POISONING

- Remove from exposure
- Neurological toxicity is not considered reversible with chelation, although some recommend a trial of succimer

Kent R. Olsen, MD

Mesothelioma, Peritoneal

 KEY FEATURES

- Rare malignancy of peritoneum, pleura
- History of asbestos exposure in >70%

 CLINICAL FINDINGS

- Abdominal pain or bowel obstruction
- Increased abdominal girth, with small to moderate ascites

 DIAGNOSIS

- Chest radiograph shows pulmonary asbestosis in >50%
- Ascitic fluid is hemorrhagic, with low serum-ascites albumin gradient
- Ascitic fluid cytology is often negative
- Abdominal CT reveals sheet-like masses involving the mesentery and omentum
- Diagnosis at laparotomy or laparoscopy

 TREATMENT

- Prognosis is extremely poor, but long-term survivors have been described who received a combination of radiation therapy and systemic or intraperitoneal chemotherapy

Kenneth R. McQuaid, MD

Methanol and Ethylene Glycol Poisoning

 KEY FEATURES

- The toxicity of both agents is caused by metabolism to toxic organic acids—methanol to formic acid, ethylene glycol to glycolic and oxalic acids

 CLINICAL FINDINGS

- Shortly after ingestion of either agent, patients usually appear drunk
- After several hours, there is tachypnea, confusion, convulsions, and coma. Methanol intoxication frequently causes visual disturbances, whereas ethylene glycol often produces oxalate crystalluria and renal failure

 DIAGNOSIS

- Initially, the serum osmolality (and osmolar gap) is usually increased. After several hours, there is a severe anion gap metabolic acidosis
- Ethylene glycol often produces oxalate crystalluria
- Alcoholic ketoacidosis also can cause a combined anion gap acidosis and osmolar gap

 TREATMENT

- Empty stomach by gastric lavage and administer activated charcoal if ingestion is within 60 min. (However, charcoal is not very effective)
- Administer ethanol or fomepizole to block metabolism of methanol and ethylene glycol to their toxic metabolites. Contact a regional poison control center for indications and dosing
- For significant toxicity (manifested by severe metabolic acidosis, altered mental status, serum methanol, or ethylene glycol level >50 mg/dL, or osmolar gap >10 mOsm/L), perform hemodialysis as soon as possible

Kent R. Olsen, MD

Methemoglobinemia

 KEY FEATURES

- Agents include benzocaine, aniline, nitrites, nitrogen oxide gases, nitrobenzene, dapsone, phenazopyridine, and many other oxidants
- Dapsone has a long half-life and may produce prolonged or recurrent methemoglobinemia

 CLINICAL FINDINGS

- Dizziness, nausea, headache, dyspnea, confusion, seizures, coma
- Severity of symptoms depends on the percentage of hemoglobin oxidized to methemoglobin; severe poisoning is usually present when methemoglobin fractions are >40–50%. Even at low levels (15–20%), victims appear cyanotic because of the "chocolate brown" color of methemoglobin

 DIAGNOSIS

- PO_2 results are normal on arterial blood gas determinations. Pulse oximetry gives inaccurate oxygen saturation measurements
- Severe metabolic acidosis
- Hemolysis may occur, especially in with glucose-6-phosphate dehydrogenase deficiency

 TREATMENT

- Administer high-flow oxygen
- Administer activated charcoal, 60–100 g PO or via gastric tube, mixed in aqueous slurry for ingestions within 1 h. Repeat-dose activated charcoal may enhance dapsone elimination
- For symptomatic patients, administer methylene blue, 1–2 mg/kg (0.1–0.2 mL/kg of 1% solution) IV. The dose may be repeated once in 15–20 min if necessary. Patients with glucose-6-phosphate dehydrogenase deficiency may not respond to methylene blue

Kent R. Olsen, MD

Minimal Change Disease

 KEY FEATURES

- Most common in children; occurs occasionally in adults
- Equal distribution between men and women

 CLINICAL FINDINGS

- Nephrotic syndrome

 DIAGNOSIS

- Renal biopsy
  - Light microscopy and immunofluorescence: no changes
  - Electron microscopy: characteristic fusion of epithelial foot processes

 TREATMENT

- Prednisone, 1 mg/kg/day for up to 16 weeks, continued for several weeks after complete remission of proteinuria
- Cyclophosphamide or chlorambucil for patients with steroid resistance or relapses
- Progression to end-stage renal disease is rare but more common in adults
- Complications most often related to prolonged steroid use

Suzanne Watnick, MD
Gail Morrison, MD

Mitral Regurgitation

 KEY FEATURES

- In developed countries, the most common causes include myxomatous degeneration (eg, Marfan's syndrome), infective endocarditis, and subvalvular dysfunction resulting from papillary muscle dysfunction or ruptured chordae tendineae

 CLINICAL FINDINGS

- Pansystolic murmur at the apex, radiating into the axilla
- Often associated with an S_3
- Hyperdynamic left ventricular (LV) impulse
- Brisk carotid upstroke
- May be asymptomatic for many years (or life) or may cause left-sided heart failure
- When regurgitation develops acutely (eg, myocardial infarction [MI]–related papillary muscle dysfunction), left atrial pressure rises abruptly, leading to pulmonary edema if severe
- When regurgitation develops more slowly, exertional dyspnea and fatigue progress gradually over many years
- Left atrial enlargement may lead to atrial fibrillation
- Systemic embolization is more common than in other conditions causing atrial fibrillation
- Predisposition to infective endocarditis

 DIAGNOSIS

- ECG: left atrial abnormality or atrial fibrillation and LV hypertrophy
- CXR: left atrial and ventricular enlargement
- Echo-Doppler confirms the diagnosis and estimates severity
- Transesophageal echocardiography may reveal the cause and identify candidates for valvular repair
- Coronary angiography is often indicated to determine the presence of coronary artery disease before valve surgery

 TREATMENT

- Antibiotic prophylaxis for dental and other procedures
- Acute mitral regurgitation resulting from endocarditis, MI, and ruptured chordae tendineae often requires emergency surgery
- Temporary stabilization is often achieved with vasodilators or intra-aortic balloon counterpulsation
- Chronic regurgitation usually requires surgery when symptoms develop
- Because irreversible deterioration of LV function may occur before the onset of symptoms, surgery is indicated in asymptomatic patients with a declining ejection fraction (<55–60%) or marked LV dilation
- Surgical valve repair can avoid the complications of prosthetic valves
- Increasingly, surgery is done using the much less invasive thoracoscopic approach

Barry M. Massie, MD
Thomas M. Amidon, MD

Mitral Stenosis

 KEY FEATURES

- Underlying rheumatic heart disease in almost all patients (although history of rheumatic fever is often absent)

 CLINICAL FINDINGS

- Localized mid-diastolic, low-pitch murmur whose duration varies with the severity of stenosis and heart rate
- In severe stenosis, the murmur may be soft and difficult to find
- A sharp opening snap whose sound is widely distributed over the chest
- Initial phase: often long and asymptomatic
- Moderate stenosis: dyspnea and fatigue common, especially with tachycardia
- Severe stenosis: pulmonary congestion at rest, with dyspnea, fatigue, right-sided heart failure, orthopnea, paroxysmal nocturnal dyspnea, and occasional hemoptysis
- Severe pulmonary congestion may also be precipitated by an acute respiratory infection, excessive salt and fluid intake, endocarditis, and other conditions
- ~50–80% develop paroxysmal or chronic atrial fibrillation that may precipitate dyspnea or pulmonary edema

 DIAGNOSIS

- ECG typically shows left atrial abnormality and, often, atrial fibrillation
- Echo-Doppler confirms diagnosis and quantifies severity
- Cardiac catheterization to detect valve, coronary, or myocardial disease, usually only after a decision to intervene has been made

 TREATMENT

- Control heart rate
- Attempt conversion of atrial fibrillation
- Once atrial fibrillation occurs, provide lifelong anticoagulation with warfarin, even if sinus rhythm is restored
- Intervention to relieve stenosis indicated for (1) uncontrollable pulmonary edema; (2) limiting dyspnea and intermittent pulmonary edema; (3) evidence of pulmonary hypertension with right ventricular hypertrophy or hemoptysis; (4) limitation of activity despite ventricular rate control and medical therapy;

and (5) recurrent systemic emboli despite anticoagulation with moderate or severe stenosis
- Open mitral commissurotomy or balloon valvuloplasty when there is minimal mitral regurgitation
- Surgical valve replacement in combined stenosis and regurgitation or when the mitral valve is significantly distorted and calcified
- Operative mortality rate is ~1–3%

Barry M. Massie, MD
Thomas M. Amidon, MD

Mitral Valve Prolapse

 KEY FEATURES

- Usually asymptomatic
- When symptomatic, symptoms include nonspecific chest pain, dyspnea, fatigue, and ventricular or supraventricular arrhythmias
- Most patients are female, many are thin, and some have minor chest wall deformities
- The significance of mitral valve prolapse (MVP) is disputed because it is diagnosed frequently in healthy young women (up to 10%)
- In occasional patients, MVP is not benign
- Infective endocarditis may occur, chiefly in patients with murmurs

 CLINICAL FINDINGS

- One or more characteristic midsystolic clicks, often but not always followed by a late systolic murmur
- Findings are accentuated in the standing position
- A single midsystolic click is usually benign
- The late or pansystolic murmur may presage significant mitral regurgitation, often resulting from rupture of chordae tendineae

 DIAGNOSIS

- The diagnosis is primarily clinical but can be confirmed by echo-Doppler
- Echocardiography: Marked thickening or redundancy of the valve is associated with a higher incidence of complications

 TREATMENT

- Usually, no treatment is indicated
- In asymptomatic patients, serial clinical exams to rule out progression to mitral regurgitation
- In patients with murmurs, antibiotic prophylaxis before dental work and other procedures
- β-blockers for supraventricular arrhythmias
- A cardioverter-defibrillator for symptomatic ventricular tachycardia
- If regurgitation evolves, treat as indicated for mitral regurgitation (see *Mitral regurgitation*)

Barry Massie, MD
Thomas Amidon, MD

Molluscum Contagiosum

 KEY FEATURES

- Caused by a poxvirus
- The lesions are autoinoculable and spread by wet skin-to-skin contact
- In sexually active individuals, lesions may be confined to the penis, pubis, and inner thighs and are considered a sexually transmitted disease
- Common in AIDS, usually with a helper T cell count <100/μL. AIDS patients tend to develop extensive lesions over the face and neck as well as in the genital area
- Lesions are difficult to eradicate in AIDS unless immunity improves, in which case spontaneous clearing may occur
- Differential diagnosis includes warts, varicella (chickenpox), basal cell carcinoma, lichen planus, smallpox, cutaneous cryptococcosis (in AIDS)

 CLINICAL FINDINGS

- Presents as single or multiple rounded, dome-shaped, waxy papules 2–5 mm in diameter that are umbilicated
- Lesions at first are firm, solid, and flesh colored but on reaching maturity become softened, whitish, or pearly gray and may suppurate
- The principal sites are the face, lower abdomen, and genitals
- Individual lesions persist for ~2 mo

 DIAGNOSIS

- Clinical based on the distinctive central umbilication of the dome-shaped lesion

 TREATMENT

- The best treatment is by curettage or applications of liquid nitrogen as for warts but more briefly
- When lesions are frozen, the central umbilication often becomes more apparent
- Light electrosurgery with a fine needle is also effective

Timothy G. Berger, MD

Monoamide Oxidase Inhibitor Overdose

 KEY FEATURES

- Ingestion of tyramine-containing foods (eg, aged cheese and red wines) or any sympathomimetic drug may cause a severe hypertensive reaction
- Severe or fatal hyperthermia (serotonin syndrome) may occur when monoamine oxidase inhibitors are given with meperidine, fluoxetine, paroxetine, fluvoxamine, venlafaxine, tryptophan, dextromethorphan, moclobemide, or other serotonin-enhancing drugs
- The serotonin syndrome can also occur with serotonin reuptake inhibitors in large doses or in combination with other SSRIs, even in the absence of an MAO inhibitor or meperidine

 CLINICAL FINDINGS

- Acute overdose: agitation, hypertension, and tachycardia followed in several hours by hypotension, convulsions, and hyperthermia
- Food or drug hypertensive reaction: hypertension, tachycardia, headache, possible intracranial hemorrhage
- Serotonin syndrome: agitation, confusion, muscle hyperactivity, hyperthermia

 DIAGNOSIS

- Clinical

 TREATMENT

- Acute ingestion: Administer activated charcoal, 60–100 g PO or via gastric tube, mixed in aqueous slurry if ingestion is within 1 h
- Treat severe hypertension with nitroprusside, phentolamine, or other rapid-acting vasodilators
- Treat hypotension with fluids and positioning, but avoid use of pressor agents if possible
- Observe patients for at least 24 h because hyperthermia may be delayed (see *Hyperthermia*)
- Cyproheptadine, 4 mg PO (or by gastric tube) qh for 3 or 4 doses, can be effective

Kent R. Olsen, MD

Mononucleosis

 KEY FEATURES

- Acute infection can occur at any age but most common in those 10–35 yr
- Epstein-Barr Virus (EBV) is the causative agent, although similar syndromes are caused by cytomegalovirus (CMV), acute HIV infection, and toxoplasmosis
- EBV shows a strong serological association with several tumors, including lymphomas in the HIV infected, nasopharyngeal carcinoma, Burkitt's lymphoma, oral hairy leukoplakia, and posttransplant lymphoproliferative disorder

 CLINICAL FINDINGS

- Fever, sore throat common
- Lymphadenopathy very common
- Splenomegaly (50%)
- Maculopapular rash uncommon (15%) except in patients receiving ampicillin (90%)
- Exudative pharyngitis common
- Hepatitis, mononeuropathy, aseptic meningitis, hemolytic anemia uncommon
- Secondary bacterial infections of the throat
- Splenic rupture is rare but dramatic
- Nonspecific ECG changes (5%)

 DIAGNOSIS

- Combination of sore throat, fever, fatigue, adenopathy, and splenomegaly suggests the diagnosis
- Chronicity of pharyngitis makes infectious mononucleosis more likely than bacterial pharyngitis
- Granulocytopenia with lymphocytosis, especially large, atypical lymphocytes
- Hemolytic anemia and thrombocytopenia
- Heterophil antibody and Monospot tests usually positive
- Antibody (IgM) titers to early antigens including viral capsid antigen can be useful early in disease

 TREATMENT

- 95% of patients recover without antiviral therapy
- Acyclovir and other antiviral drugs are without verified clinical benefit

- Chronic EBV syndromes are increasingly recognized, especially in the immunodeficient (Duncan's syndrome)

Wayne X. Shandera, MD
Samuel Shelburne, MD

Moraxella catarrhalis Infection

 KEY FEATURES

- An infection caused by a gram-negative aerobic coccus, *Moraxella catarrhalis*, that is morphologically and biochemically similar to *Neisseria*

 CLINICAL FINDINGS

- Sinusitis, bronchitis, otitis, and pneumonia
- Bacteremia and meningitis have also been reported in immunocompromised patients

 DIAGNOSIS

- Culture
- The organism frequently colonizes the respiratory tract, and differentiation of colonization from infection can be difficult. If *M catarrhalis* is the predominant isolate, therapy should be directed against it

 TREATMENT

- Amoxicillin-clavulanate, ampicillin-sulbactam, trimethoprim-sulfamethoxazole, ciprofloxacin, and second- and third-generation cephalosporins
- Treatment is similar to that for *Haemophilus* infections (see *Haemophilus*)
- Typically produces beta-lactamase and, therefore, is usually resistant to ampicillin and amoxicillin

Henry F. Chambers, MD

Mucormycosis

 KEY FEATURES

- The term mucormycosis (zygomycosis, phycomycosis) applies to opportunistic infections caused by members of the genera *Rhizopus, Mucor, Absidia,* and *Cunninghamella*
- Predisposing conditions include diabetic ketoacidosis, chronic renal failure, use of corticosteroids or cytotoxic drugs

 CLINICAL FINDINGS

- Invasive disease of sinuses, orbits, lungs
- In acidotic diabetic patients, black necrotic lesions of nose or sinuses or new cranial nerve abnormalities
- Cerebral invasion may ensue without treatment
- Widely disseminated disease more common after aggressive chemotherapy

 DIAGNOSIS

- Cultures frequently negative
- Biopsy almost always required for diagnosis. Histology demonstrates organisms in tissues as broad, branching nonseptate hyphae

 TREATMENT

- High-dose amphotericin B, 1–1.5 mg/kg/day IV, for prolonged period
- Control of diabetes and other underlying conditions
- Extensive repeated surgical débridement of necrotic, nonperfused tissue
- Even with timely treatment, mortality is 30–50% for localized disease and higher for disseminated disease

Richard J. Hamill, MD

Multiple Endocrine Neoplasia, Type 1 (MEN 1)

 KEY FEATURES

- MEN 1 (Wermer's syndrome) consists of parathyroid (>80%), pancreatic (75%), pituitary (60%) tumors; occasionally adrenocortical adenoma, lipoma, carcinoid tumor, thyroid adenoma or papillary carcinoma
- MEN 1 is due to a mutation on long arm of chromosome 11 (11q13); autosomal dominant expression
- Most common pancreatic tumor in MEN 1 is gastrinoma; other tumor types include insulinomas, somatostatinomas, glucagonomas

 CLINICAL FINDINGS

- MEN 1 usually manifests by fourth decade but may present in childhood
- MEN 1: hypercalcemia (hyperparathyroidism); or peptic ulcer disease or diarrhea with Zollinger-Ellison syndrome (gastrinoma)
- Pituitary tumor may produce pressure effects (eg, visual field defects) or effects of hormone overproduction (eg, galactorrhea and amenorrhea [prolactin]), acromegaly or gigantism (growth hormone), or Cushing's syndrome (ACTH)

 DIAGNOSIS

- Genetic testing of index patient and other affected individuals to identify mutations and then family members (eg, siblings or children) to identify those at risk for MEN 1 syndrome
- Differential diagnosis includes sporadic or familial tumors of pituitary, parathyroids, or pancreatic islets or other cause of hypercalcemia, which may increase gastrin levels, simulating gastrinoma

 TREATMENT

- MEN 1: Surgical resection of multiple parathyroid adenomas can induce prolonged remissions, but resection of 3½ glands is often required, and relapse is typical because multiple glands are affected
- Genetic counseling: See *Acromegaly & gigantism; Cushing's syndrome; Hyperparathyroidism; Hyperprolactinemia; Islet cell tumors*

Paul A. Fitzgerald, MD

Multiple Endocrine Neoplasia, Type 2 (MEN 2)

 ### KEY FEATURES

- MEN 2a (Sipple's syndrome): medullary thyroid carcinoma (>50%): parathyroid adenoma (50%), pheochromocytoma (20%); also associated with Hirschsprung's disease
  - MEN 2a is due to *RET* proto-oncogene mutation on chromosome 10q11-2; autosomal dominant expression
- MEN 2b: medullary thyroid carcinoma (80%), pheochromocytoma (60%), mucosal and GI ganglioneuromas (> 90%)

 ### CLINICAL FINDINGS

- MEN 2a: thyroid mass, hypercalcemia, pheochromocytoma
- MEN 2b: mucosal neuromas (bumpy lips, enlarged tongue); Marfan-like habitus; pheochromocytoma; thyroid mass; intestinal abnormalities (75%), skeletal abnormalities (87%), delayed puberty (43%)

 ### DIAGNOSIS

- Genetic testing of affected individuals to identify mutations and then family members (eg, siblings or children) to identify those at risk for MEN 2 syndromes
- Screening serum calcitonin level, drawn after 3 days of omeprazole, 20 mg PO BID, is >80 pg/mL in women or >190 pg/mL in men with medullary thyroid carcinoma

 ### TREATMENT

- MEN 2a: prophylactic thyroidectomy, with timing indicated by specific mutation and case histories of family members
- MEN 2b: prophylactic thyroidectomy advisable if mucosal neuromas and family members with syndrome or *RET* proto-oncogene mutation
- Screen for pheochromocytoma in MEN 2 carriers before any surgery
- Genetic counseling
- See *Hyperparathyroidism, Hypoparathyroidism, Pheochromocytoma*

Paul A. Fitzgerald, MD

Mumps

 ### KEY FEATURES

- Spread by respiratory droplets
- Produces inflammation of salivary glands (eg, parotitis) and occasionally orchitis and meningitis

 ### CLINICAL FINDINGS

- Parotid tenderness and overlying facial edema common
- Fever and malaise variable
- Orchitis 7–10 days after parotitis; rarely leads to sterility
- Meningitis third most common manifestation
- Other complications include pancreatitis, oophoritis, thyroiditis, neuritis, hepatitis, myocarditis, encephalitis

 ### DIAGNOSIS

- Symptom onset occurs 14–21 days post-exposure
- Painful, swollen parotid and other salivary glands
- Orchitis, pancreatitis, or meningitis in setting of parotitis is usually diagnostic
- Lymphocytosis and elevated serum amylase are common
- Serological testing may be useful but not commonly done
- Serum neutralization titers best for determining immunity

 ### TREATMENT

- Supportive measures
- Febrile patients should be kept on bed rest and isolated while there is parotid swelling
- Orchitis can be managed with scrotal support and ice packs
- Prevention: mumps live virus vaccine is safe and highly effective
- Vaccine should be avoided in pregnant women and immunocompromised individuals
- Vaccine probably safe in patients with asymptomatic HIV infection

Wayne X. Shandera, MD
Samuel Shelburne, MD

Muscle Cramps

 ### KEY FEATURES

- Muscle cramps usually caused by sports or occupational muscle injury
- Causes include
  - Idiopathic (most common)
  - Electrolyte disorders (hypocalcemia, hypokalemia, hyponatremia, hypoglycemia, hyperkalemia, hypermagnasemia, alkalosis)
  - Systemic diseases (diabetes mellitus, Parkinson's disease, CNS or spinal cord lesions, peripheral neuropathy, hemodialysis, peripheral vascular disease, hyperthyroidism or hypothyroidism, pregnancy)
  - Drugs: cisplatin or vincristine
  - Hemodialysis

 ### CLINICAL FINDINGS

- Muscle cramping, often nocturnal
- Physical exam usually normal or shows signs of associated conditions listed above
- Exertional claudication and reduced pedal pulses suggest lower extremity arterial occlusive disease

 ### DIAGNOSIS

- Obtain serum calcium, potassium, sodium, glucose, magnesium levels
- Consider magnesium deficiency in tetany unresponsive to calcium
- If leg cramps during walking, consider serum TSH and Doppler ankle-brachial index evaluation for peripheral vascular disease
- Serum CK level is elevated in enzyme deficiencies such as McArdle's disease and carnitine palmitoyltransferase II deficiency

 ### TREATMENT

- Treat electrolyte disorders
- Gabapentin, 600–1200 mg/day divided PO BID–TID, is effective for recurrent, severe, or prolonged muscle cramping. May cause leukopenia or CNS effects
- Quinine, once commonly used to prevent nocturnal muscle cramps, can cause arrhythmias, dizziness, hemolytic-uremic syndrome, and agranulocytosis. Now used only for severe nocturnal cramping if patient accepts risks and need for clinical follow-up

- Calcium supplementation orally may reduce pregnancy-associated leg cramps
- Treat exertional claudication (caused by lower extremity arterial occlusive disease) with oral pentoxifylline, cilostazol, angioplasty, or arterial bypass (see *Peripheral vascular disease*)
- Botulinum toxin injections may be effective for recurrent cervicofacial dystonias, laryngeal dystonias, and hand cramps

Paul A. Fitzgerald, MD

Muscular Dystrophies

 ## KEY FEATURES

- Inherited myopathic disorders characterized by progressive muscle weakness and wasting
- They are subdivided by mode of inheritance, age at onset, and clinical features (Table 98, page 1280)
- A genetic defect on the short arm of the X chromosome occurs in Duchenne dystrophy. The affected gene codes for the protein dystrophin, which is almost absent from the diseased muscles
- Dystrophin levels are generally normal in the Becker variety, but the protein is qualitatively altered
- Duchenne muscular dystrophy is detectable in pregnancy

 ## CLINICAL FINDINGS

- Muscle weakness, often in a characteristic distribution
- Age at onset and inheritance pattern depend on the specific dystrophy
- In the Duchenne type, pseudohypertrophy of muscles frequently occurs at some stage; intellectual retardation is common; and there may be skeletal deformities, muscle contractures, and cardiac involvement

 ## DIAGNOSIS

- The serum creatine kinase level is increased, especially in the Duchenne and Becker varieties, and mildly increased in limb-girdle dystrophy
- Electromyography may confirm myopathic weakness rather than neurogenic
- Histopathological examination of a muscle biopsy specimen can distinguish between various muscle diseases

 ## TREATMENT

- There is no specific treatment for the muscular dystrophies, but it is important to encourage patients to lead as normal lives as possible
- Prolonged bed rest must be avoided because inactivity often leads to worsening of the underlying muscle disease
- Physical therapy and orthopedic procedures may help to counteract deformities or contractures

Michael J. Aminoff, DSc, MD, FRCP

Myasthenic Syndrome

 ## KEY FEATURES

- Clinical similarity to myasthenia gravis, but myasthenic syndrome occurs mainly as a paraneoplastic syndrome (Table 151, page 1340)
- There is defective release of acetylcholine in response to a nerve impulse, leading to weakness, especially of the proximal muscles of the limbs
- May be associated with small cell lung carcinoma, sometimes developing before the tumor is diagnosed, and occasionally occurs with certain autoimmune diseases

 ## CLINICAL FINDINGS

- Variable weakness, typically improving with activity
- Dysautonomic symptoms may also be present
- A history of malignant disease may be obtained
- Unlike myasthenia gravis, power steadily increases with sustained contraction

 ## DIAGNOSIS

- Electrophysiological diagnosis: the muscle response to stimulation of its motor nerve increases remarkably if the nerve is stimulated repetitively at high rates, even in muscles that are not clinically weak

 ## TREATMENT

- Plasmapheresis and immunosuppressive drug therapy (prednisone and azathioprine), in addition to any therapy directed at a tumor, if present, may lead to clinical and electrophysiological improvement
- Prednisone is usually initiated in a daily dose of 60–80 mg and azathioprine in a daily dose of 2 mg/kg
- Guanidine hydrochloride (25–50 mg/kg/day in divided doses) is occasionally helpful in seriously disabled patients, but adverse effects of the drug include marrow suppression
- The response to treatment with anticholinesterase drugs such as pyridostigmine or neostigmine, either alone or in combination with guanidine, is variable

Michael J. Aminoff, DSc, MD, FRCP

Mycetoma

 KEY FEATURES

- Mycetoma is a chronic local, slowly progressive destructive infection
- Begins in subcutaneous tissues, frequently after localized trauma, and spreads to contiguous structures
- Maduromycosis is mycetoma caused by true fungi
- Actinomycetoma is caused by *Nocardia* and *Actinomadura*

 CLINICAL FINDINGS

- Lesions begin as a papule, nodule, or abscess that, over months to years, forms multiple abscesses and sinus tracts ramifying deep into the tissue
- Secondary bacterial infection may occur in large open ulcers

 DIAGNOSIS

- X-ray films may show destructive changes in underlying bone
- Tissue Gram's stain reveals large hyphae with maduromycosis and fine branching hyphae with actinomycetoma
- The species is often identified by the color of characteristic grains within infected tissues

 TREATMENT

- For maduromycosis: ketoconazole or itraconazole for months
- For actinomycetoma: trimethoprim-sulfamethoxazole, 160/800 mg PO BID, or dapsone, 100 mg PO BID after meals, for months. Streptomycin, 14 mg/kg/d IM, may be useful during first month of therapy
- Oral medications must be continued for several months after clinical cure to prevent relapse
- Débridement assists healing
- The prognosis of maduromycosis is poor, although prolonged ketoconazole or itraconazole therapy combined with surgical débridement yields a response rate of 70%. Amputation is necessary in far-advanced cases
- Prognosis of actinomycetoma is good because it usually responds to sulfonamides and sulfones, especially if treated early

Richard J. Hamill, MD

Myocarditis, Acute

 KEY FEATURES

- Focal or diffuse inflammation of the myocardium
- Causes: infections, viral (most common), bacterial, rickettsial, spirochetal, fungal, or parasitic agents; toxins, drugs (especially cocaine), and immunological disorders
- Many cases resolve spontaneously
- In others, cardiac function deteriorates progressively and may lead to dilated cardiomyopathy

 CLINICAL FINDINGS

- Onset several days to a few weeks after onset of an acute febrile illness or respiratory infection
- Congestive heart failure, gradual or abrupt and fulminant
- Symptoms: chest pain (pleuritic or nonspecific), dyspnea
- Physical examination: tachycardia, gallop rhythm, edema or conduction defect

 DIAGNOSIS

- ECG: sinus tachycardia, ventricular ectopy, nonspecific repolarization changes, or intraventricular conduction delay
- CXR: nonspecific, cardiomegaly is common
- Echocardiogram: cardiomegaly and contractile dysfunction
- Myocardial biopsy, although not sensitive, may reveal a characteristic inflammatory pattern

 TREATMENT

- Specific antimicrobial therapy for any identified infectious agent
- Immunosuppressive therapy for acute (<6 mo) myocarditis only if myocardial biopsy suggests ongoing inflammation
- Otherwise, treat heart failure and arrhythmias

Barry M. Massie, MD
Thomas M. Amidon, MD

Myoclonus

 KEY FEATURES

- Myoclonic jerks are sudden, shock-like muscle contractions
- Occasional myoclonic jerks may occur in anyone, especially when drifting into sleep
- General or multifocal myoclonus: common in patients with idiopathic epilepsy and certain hereditary disorders
- Generalized myoclonic jerking may accompany metabolic encephalopathies, result from levodopa therapy, occur in alcohol or drug withdrawal states, or follow anoxic brain damage
- It is common in subacute sclerosing panencephalitis and Creutzfeldt-Jakob disease

 CLINICAL FINDINGS

- Myoclonus can be focal or generalized and can occur spontaneously or in response to certain stimuli (eg, noise)

 DIAGNOSIS

- Clinical
- An electroencephalogram is often helpful in clarifying an epileptic basis, and CT or MRI scan may reveal the causal lesion

 TREATMENT

- May respond to certain anticonvulsant drugs, especially valproic acid, or to one of the benzodiazepines, particularly clonazepam (Table 94, page 1278)
- It may also respond to piracetam (up to 16.8 g daily)
- Myoclonus after anoxic brain damage is often responsive to oxitriptan and sometimes to clonazepam
- Oxitriptan is given in gradually increasing doses up to 1–1.5 mg daily
- In patients with segmental myoclonus, a localized lesion (spinal or cerebral) should be searched for and treated appropriately

Michael J. Aminoff, DSc, MD, FRCP

Myotonic Dystrophy

 KEY FEATURES

- A slowly progressive, dominantly inherited myopathic disorder
- Usually manifests itself in the third or fourth decade but occasionally appears early in childhood
- The genetic defect has been localized to the long arm of chromosome 19

 CLINICAL FINDINGS

- Complaints of muscle stiffness
- Marked delay occurs before affected muscles can relax after a contraction; this can often be demonstrated clinically by delayed relaxation of the hand after sustained grip or by percussion of the belly of a muscle
- Weakness and wasting of the facial, sternocleidomastoid, and distal limb muscles
- Cataracts, frontal baldness, testicular atrophy, diabetes mellitus, cardiac abnormalities, and intellectual changes

 DIAGNOSIS

- Electromyographic sampling of affected muscles reveals myotonic discharges in addition to changes suggestive of myopathy

 TREATMENT

- Phenytoin, 100 mg TID; quinine sulfate, 300–400 mg TID; or procainamide, 0.5–1 g QID; phenytoin is preferred because the other drugs may have undesirable effects on cardiac conduction
- Tocainide and mexiletine have also been used
- Neither the weakness nor the course of the disorder is influenced by treatment

Michael J. Aminoff, DSc, MD, FRCP

Narcolepsy

 KEY FEATURES

- A disorder of excessive sleepiness, manifesting in "sleep attacks"
- Disorder begins in early adult life
- Affects both sexes equally
- Severity levels off at ~30 yr

 CLINICAL FINDINGS

- A tetrad of symptoms:
  - Sudden, brief sleep attacks during any type of activity
  - Cataplexy, a loss of specific or generalized muscle tone
  - Sleep paralysis: a flaccidity of muscles with full consciousness while falling or waking from sleep
  - Hypnagogic hallucinations, preceding sleep or occur during a sleep attack

 DIAGNOSIS

- Sleep study: Attacks are characterized by abrupt transition into REM sleep, a necessary criterion for diagnosis

 TREATMENT

- Dextroamphetamine, 10 mg PO qAM
- Modafinil, 200 mg PO qAM; mechanism of action is unknown, but risk of abuse is thought to be lower than with stimulants
- Imipramine, 75–100 mg qd, is effective in treatment of cataplexy but not narcolepsy

Stuart J. Eisendrath, MD
Jonathan E. Lichtmacher, MD

Nasal Trauma

 KEY FEATURES

- The nasal pyramid is the most frequently fractured bone in the body
- Epistaxis and pain are common, as are soft tissue hematomas ("black eye")
- Septal hematomas may become infected; *S aureus* is the predominant organism
- Persistent functional or cosmetic defects may be repaired by delayed reconstructive nasal surgery

 CLINICAL FINDINGS

- Fracture is suggested by crepitance or palpably mobile bony segments
- Intranasal examination should be performed in all cases to rule out septal hematoma, which appears as a widening of the anterior septum, visible just posterior to the columella. The septal cartilage receives its only nutrition from its closely adherent mucoperichondrium
- It is important to ensure that there is no palpable step-off of the infraorbital rim, which would indicate the presence of a zygomatic complex fracture

 DIAGNOSIS

- Radiological confirmation may be helpful but is not necessary in uncomplicated nasal fractures

 TREATMENT

- Treatment is aimed at maintaining long-term nasal airway patency and nasal aesthetics
- Closed reduction, using topical 4% cocaine and locally injected 1% lidocaine, should be attempted within 1 week of injury
- In the presence of marked nasal swelling, it is best to wait several days for the edema to subside before undertaking reduction
- An untreated subperichondrial hematoma will result in loss of the nasal cartilage with resultant saddle-nose deformity

Robert K. Jackler, MD
Michael J. Kaplan, MD

Nausea & Vomiting of Pregnancy

 KEY FEATURES

- "Morning sickness"
- Up to 75% of women complain of nausea and vomiting during early pregnancy
- Vast majority of symptomatic patients note nausea throughout the day
- Symptoms are particularly common with multiple pregnancy and hydatidiform mole
- High estrogen levels are believed to be responsible
- Exerts no adverse effects on the pregnancy and does not presage complications

 CLINICAL FINDINGS

- Morning or evening nausea and vomiting usually begin soon after the first missed period and ceases after the fifth month
- Persistent, severe vomiting is hyperemesis gravidarum, a distinct entity (see *Hyperemesis gravidarum*)

 DIAGNOSIS

- Clinical

 TREATMENT

- Reassurance and dietary advice are adequate in most cases
- Vitamin B_6, 50–100 mg PO qd, is nontoxic and may help some patients
- To limit the risk of teratogenicity, drug use in the first half of pregnancy should be limited to those of major importance to life and health (Tables 68, page 1261, 71, page 1263)

William R. Crombleholme, MD

Nephritis, Intersitial

 KEY FEATURES

- Fever
- Transient maculopapular rash
- Acute renal insufficiency
- Pyuria (including eosinophiluria), white blood cell casts, and hematuria
- Interstitial inflammatory response with edema and possible tubular cell damage, responsible for ~10–15% of cases of intrinsic renal failure
- Causes of acute interstitial nephritis: drugs (>70% of cases), infectious diseases, immunological disorders, idiopathic. Drug causes include penicillins, cephalosporins, sulfonamides, erythromycin, tetracycline, vancomycin, thiazides, furosemide, NSAIDs, rifampin, phenytoin, allopurinol, cimetidine. Infectious causes include streptococcal infections, leptospirosis, cytomegalovirus, Epstein-Barr virus, histoplasmosis, Rocky Mountain spotted fever, *Mycoplasma, Toxoplasma.* Immunological causes include systemic lupus erythematosus, Sjögren's syndrome, sarcoidosis, cryoglobulinemia
- Causes of chronic interstitial nephritis: obstructive uropathy, vesicoureteral reflux (reflux nephropathy), analgesic nephropathy, heavy metals (lead, cadmium, mercury, bismuth), multiple myeloma, gout

 CLINICAL FINDINGS

- Fever (>80%)
- Rash (25–50%)
- Arthralgias

 DIAGNOSIS

- Peripheral blood eosinophilia (80%)
- Urine often contains red cells (95%), white cells, and white cell casts
- Proteinuria usually modest
- Eosinophiluria
- Differential diagnosis: acute tubular necrosis, acute glomerulonephritis, prerenal azotemia, chronic glomerulopathy (eg, diabetes), hypertensive nephrosclerosis, obstructive uropathy

 TREATMENT

- Supportive measures
- Removal of inciting agent
- Methylprednisolone, 0.5–1 g/day for 1–4 days, or prednisone, 60 mg/day for 1–2 weeks, followed by a prednisone taper if renal failure persists after removal of the inciting agent
- Prognosis good; recovery occurs over weeks to months
- Dialysis may be necessary in up to 33%
- Patients rarely progress to end-stage renal disease
- Prognosis worse in those with prolonged courses of oliguric failure and advanced age

Suzanne Watnick, MD
Gail Morrison, MD

Nephritis, Lupus

KEY FEATURES

- Renal involvement is common in systemic lupus erythematosus (SLE), occurring in 35– 90% of SLE patients

CLINICAL FINDINGS

- Urinalysis: hematuria and proteinuria

DIAGNOSIS

- Renal biopsy shows 1 of 5 histological patterns: type I, normal; type II, mesangial proliferative; type III, focal and segmental proliferative; type IV, diffuse proliferative; type V, membranous nephropathy

TREATMENT

- No treatment required for types I and II
- Immunosuppressive therapy with corticosteroids and cytotoxic agents for extensive type III lesions and all type IV lesions
- Indications for treatment of type V disease are unclear
- Corticosteroids: methylprednisolone, 1 g IV qd for 3 days, followed by prednisone, 60 mg PO qd for 4–6 weeks
- Cytotoxic agents: cyclophosphamide, IV every month for 6 doses and then every 3 mo for 6 doses
- Cyclosporine useful
- Mycophenolate mofetil may be helpful
- Monitoring serum creatinine, dsDNA antibodies, C3, C4, and CH50, urinary protein, and sediment can be useful during treatment
- Renal transplantation, but recurrent renal disease occurs in 8% of cases

Suzanne Watnick, MD
Gail Morrison, MD

Nephropathy, Diabetic

KEY FEATURES

- Most common cause of end-stage renal disease in US
- Type 1 diabetes mellitus imposes a 30–40% risk of nephropathy after 20 yr
- Type 2 imposes a 15–20% risk after 20 yr
- Males, African-Americans, and Native Americans are at higher risk

CLINICAL FINDINGS

- Diabetic retinopathy is often present
- Microalbuminuria develops within 10–15 yr after onset of diabetes and progresses over the next 3–7 yr to overt proteinuria

DIAGNOSIS

- Increase in GFR at onset
- With the development of macroalbuminuria, GFR returns to normal and then to subnormal as nephropathy progresses
- Renal biopsy: Most common lesion is diffuse glomerulosclerosis, but nodular glomerulosclerosis (Kimmelstiel-Wilson nodules) is pathognomonic

TREATMENT

- Strict glycemic control and treatment of hypertension slow progression of diabetic nephropathy
- ACE inhibitors and angiotensin II receptor antagonists likely lower the rate of progression to clinical proteinuria and overt renal failure

Suzanne Watnick, MD
Gail Morrison, MD

Nephropathy, Immunoglobulin A

KEY FEATURES

- A primary renal disease of IgA deposition in the glomerular mesangium
- Inciting cause unknown
- Also associated with hepatic cirrhosis, celiac disease, and infections such as HIV and cytomegalovirus
- Most common form of acute glomerulonephritis in US
- Occurs most often in children and young adults
- Males affected 2–3 times more commonly than females

CLINICAL FINDINGS

- Gross hematuria frequently associated with an upper respiratory tract infection (50%), GI symptoms (10%), or flu-like illness (15%)
- Urine becomes red or cola-colored 1–2 days after onset
- Asymptomatic microscopic hematuria may occur as incidental finding
- Hypertension
- Nephrotic syndrome possible

DIAGNOSIS

- Persistent microscopic hematuria and proteinuria
- Serum creatinine and blood urea nitrogen sometimes elevated
- Serum IgA level is increased in ≤50% of patients
- Serum complement levels usually normal
- Renal biopsy: light microscopy shows focal glomerulonephritis with and proliferation of mesangial cells; immunofluorescence shows diffuse mesangial IgA, IgG, and C3 deposits
- Skin biopsy: granular deposits of IgA in dermal capillaries

TREATMENT

- ~33% of patients will experience clinical remission
- Chronic microscopic hematuria and stable serum creatinine in 50–60%; progressive renal insufficiency in 40–50%
- Prognosis worse if proteinuria >1 g/day

- ACE inhibitors or angiotensin II receptor-blocking drugs to reduce proteinuria and treat hypertension (Table 46, page 1241)
- Methylprednisolone, 1 g/day IV for 3 days during months 1, 3, and 5, plus prednisone, 0.5 mg/kg QOD for 6 mo in nephrotic patients
- Fish oil, 2–5 g/day, debatable
- Renal transplantation

Suzanne Watnick, MD
Gail Morrison, MD

Nephropathy, Membranous

 KEY FEATURES

- Most common cause of primary nephrotic syndrome in adults
- Caused by immune complex deposition in the subepithelial portion of glomerular capillary walls
- Associated with infections such as hepatitis B, endocarditis, syphilis; autoimmune disease such as systemic lupus erythematosus, mixed connective tissue disease, thyroiditis; carcinoma; certain drugs such as gold, penicillamine, captopril
- Occurs most commonly in adults in the fifth and sixth decades

 CLINICAL FINDINGS

- Nephrotic syndrome

 DIAGNOSIS

- Renal biopsy: light microscopy: increased capillary wall thickness; immunofluorescence: IgG and C3 along capillary loops; electron microscopy: discontinuous dense deposits along the subepithelial surface of the basement membrane

 TREATMENT

- Treatment is controversial
- Patients with proteinuria of <4 g/day: close monitoring, low-salt diet, strict blood pressure control, and ACE inhibitor
- Patients with proteinuria of 4–8 g/day and normal renal function: consider immunosuppressive regimens with corticosteroids and chlorambucil or cyclophosphamide (or cyclosporine) for 6 mo
- Patients with proteinuria of > 8 g/day and possible renal dysfunction: consider cyclosporine as a first-line immunosuppressant or corticosteroids with a cytotoxic agent
- Renal transplantation

Suzanne Watnick, MD
Gail Morrison, MD

Nephrotic Syndrome

 KEY FEATURES

- In adults, most commonly idiopathic; systemic renal disease such as diabetes mellitus, amyloidosis, or systemic lupus erythematosus in 33%

 CLINICAL FINDINGS

- Peripheral edema when serum albumin <3 g/dL
- Edema can become generalized
- Dyspnea caused by pulmonary edema, pleural effusions, and diaphragmatic compromise with ascites
- Abdominal distension with ascites
- Increased susceptibility to infection because of loss of immunoglobulins and complement in the urine
- Hypercoagulable state, with renal vein thrombosis and venous thromboemboli, particularly in membranous nephropathy

 DIAGNOSIS

- Urinalysis: proteinuria but few cellular elements or casts
- Oval fat bodies appear as "grape clusters" under light microscopy and "Maltese crosses" under polarized light
- Serum albumin decreased (<3 g/dL), serum protein decreased <6 g/dL
- Hyperlipidemia
- Elevated erythrocyte sedimentation rate
- Serum complement levels, serum and urine protein electrophoresis, ANA, and serological tests for hepatitis as indicated by clinical presentation
- Renal biopsy indicated in adults with new-onset idiopathic nephrotic syndrome if a primary renal disease that may require drug therapy is suspected
- Renal biopsy useful for prognosis and treatment decisions
- Four most common lesions: minimal change disease, focal glomerular sclerosis, membranous nephropathy, and membranoproliferative glomerulonephritis (Table 89, page 1272)

 TREATMENT

- Dietary protein intake should replace total daily urinary protein losses
- Dietary salt and water restriction for edema

- Loop and thiazide diuretics in combination
- Antilipidemic agents
- Corticosteroids, cytotoxic agents as indicated for primary renal lesion
- Warfarin anticoagulation for at least 3–6 mo in patients with thrombosis

Suzanne Watnick, MD
Gail Morrison, MD

Neurogenic Arthropathy (Charcot's Joint)

 ## KEY FEATURES

- Joint destruction resulting from loss or diminution of proprioception, pain, and temperature perception
- As normal muscle tone and protective reflexes are lost, secondary degenerative joint disease ensues
- Traditionally associated with tabes dorsalis; more frequently seen in diabetic neuropathy, syringomyelia, spinal cord injury, pernicious anemia, leprosy, and peripheral nerve injury

 ## CLINICAL FINDINGS

- An enlarged, boggy, painless joint with extensive cartilage erosion, osteophyte formation, and multiple loose-joint bodies

 ## DIAGNOSIS

- Radiographic changes may be degenerative or hypertrophic in the same patient
- Differential diagnosis includes repeated trauma (causing degenerative joint disease), rheumatoid arthritis, chronic hemarthrosis (bleed), chondrocalcinosis (eg, pseudogout, hemochromatosis, Wilson's disease)

 ## TREATMENT

- Directed against the primary disease
- Mechanical devices are used to assist in weight bearing and prevention of further trauma
- In some instances, amputation becomes unavoidable

David B. Hellmann, MD, FACP
John H. Stone, MD, MPH

Neuroleptic Malignant Syndrome

 ## KEY FEATURES

- A catatonia-like state manifested by extrapyramidal signs, blood pressure changes, altered consciousness, hyperpyrexia
- Uncommon complication of neuroleptic treatment
- Comorbid affective disorder as well as concomitant lithium use may increase risk
- In most cases, occurs within 2 weeks of starting neuroleptic agent

 ## CLINICAL FINDINGS

- Muscle rigidity, involuntary movements, confusion, dysarthria, dysphagia
- Pallor, cardiovascular instability, pulmonary congestion, diaphoresis
- Can result in stupor, coma, death

 ## DIAGNOSIS

- Elevated creatinine kinase and leukocytosis with left shift in 50% of cases

 ## TREATMENT

- Control of fever and IV fluid support
- Bromocriptine, 2.5–10 mg TID, and amantadine, 100–200 mg BID, are useful
- Dantrolene, 50 mg IV PRN to max of 10 mg/kg/day, can alleviate rigidity
- ECT has been used in resistant cases
- Clozapine has been used safely in patients with a history of NMS

Stuart J. Eisendrath, MD
Jonathan E. Lichtmacher, MD

Nevi, Congenital

 ## KEY FEATURES

- In contrast to the common nevi that appear after birth, congenital nevi by definition are present at birth
- The management of small congenital nevi—less than a few centimeters in diameter—is controversial. The vast majority will never become malignant, but some experts believe that the risk of melanoma in these lesions may be somewhat increased

 ## CLINICAL FINDINGS

- Most nevi are small and look like ordinary pigmented acquired nevi
- Giant congenital nevi may be quite large and involve the trunk, upper back, or shoulders
- The surface of the lesion may be smooth or irregular
- Color may range from pale tan to brown-black
- May be associated with an overgrowth of hair

 ## DIAGNOSIS

- Clinical or by biopsy

 ## TREATMENT

- Because 1% of whites are born with these lesions, management should be conservative and excision advised only for lesions in cosmetically nonsensitive areas where the patient cannot easily see the lesion and note any suspicious changes
- Excision should be considered for congenital nevi whose contour (bumpiness, nodularity) or color (different shades) makes it difficult for examiners to note early signs of malignant change
- Giant congenital melanocytic nevi (>5% BSA) are at greater risk for development of melanoma, and surgical removal in stages is often recommended

Timothy G. Berger, MD

Nevi, Dysplastic or Atypical

 KEY FEATURES

- The term *atypical nevus* or *atypical mole* has supplanted *dysplastic nevus*
- It is estimated that 5–10% of the US population have 1 or more atypical nevi
- There is an increased risk of melanoma in the following populations: patients with 50 or more nevi with 1 or more atypical moles and 1 mole at least 8 mm or larger, and patients with a few to many definitely atypical moles. These patients deserve education and regular (usually every 6–12 mo) follow-up. Kindreds with familial melanoma (numerous atypical nevi and a strong family history) deserve even closer attention because the risk of developing single or even multiple melanomas in these individuals approaches 50% by age 50

 CLINICAL FINDINGS

- The moles are large (>5 mm in diameter), with an ill-defined, irregular border and irregularly distributed pigmentation

 DIAGNOSIS

- The diagnosis is made clinically and not histologically

 TREATMENT

- Moles should be removed only if they are suspected to be melanomas

Timothy G. Berger, MD

Niacin Deficiency

 KEY FEATURES

- Most commonly results from alcoholism and nutrient–drug interactions
- Can also occur in inborn errors of metabolism
- Manifestations are nonspecific

 CLINICAL FINDINGS

- Common complaints include anorexia, weakness, irritability, mouth soreness, glossitis, stomatitis, weight loss
- More advanced deficiency results in the classic triad of pellagra: dermatitis, diarrhea, dementia
- Advanced pellagra can result in death

 DIAGNOSIS

- Diagnosis of pellagra is made clinically
- Measure niacin metabolites, particularly *N*-methylnicotinamide, in the urine
- Serum and red blood cell NAD and NADP levels are low

 TREATMENT

- Niacin, usually given as nicotinamide, 10–150 mg PO qd

Robert B. Baron, MD, MS

Nipple Discharge

 KEY FEATURES

- The most common causes of nipple discharge in the nonlactating breast, in order of decreasing frequency, are
  - Duct ectasia
  - Intraductal papilloma
  - Carcinoma
- Factors to be assessed by history and physical examination:
  - Nature of discharge (serous, bloody, or other)
  - Discharge associated with a mass
  - Unilateral or bilateral discharge
  - Single or multiple duct discharge
  - Discharge is spontaneous (persistent or intermittent) or must be expressed
  - Discharge is produced by pressure at a single site or by general pressure on breast
  - Relationship of discharge to menses
  - Premenopausal or postmenopausal patient
  - Patient taking oral contraceptives or estrogen

 CLINICAL FINDINGS

- Unilateral, spontaneous serous or serosanguineous discharge from a single duct usually caused by intraductal papilloma or, rarely, intraductal cancer
- Bloody discharge is worrisome for malignancy
- In premenopausal women, spontaneous brown or green discharge, from multiple ducts, unilaterally or bilaterally, most marked just before menstruation, is often due to mammary dysplasia
- In the nonlactating breast, milky discharge from multiple ducts occurs as a result of hyperprolactinemia in certain endocrine syndromes and from certain drugs (antipsychotics)
- A clear, serous, or milky discharge from single or multiple ducts can occur on oral contraceptives or estrogen replacement therapy. The discharge is more evident just before menstruation and disappears on stopping the medication
- Purulent discharge may originate in a subareolar abscess

 DIAGNOSIS

- Differential diagnosis: galactorrhea (eg, pregnancy, postpartum, hyperprolactinemia), mammary duct ectasia, intraductal papilloma, breast cancer, oral contraceptives or estrogen replacement therapy, fibrocystic disease, subareolar abscess

- If unilateral discharge present from single duct, involved duct can be identified by pressure at different sites around nipple at margin of areola
- Cytological examination of discharge may identify malignant cells, but if negative, does not rule out cancer
- Check serum prolactin and TSH levels if discharge is milky
- Mammography may be helpful if localization of lesion is not possible

 TREATMENT

- Any mass or, in the case of duct ectasia or intraductal papilloma, any involved duct should be excised
- Abscesses require drainage or removal along with the related lactiferous sinus
- When localization is not possible, no mass is palpable, and discharge is nonbloody, the patient should be reexamined every 2 or 3 mo for 1 yr, and mammography performed

Armando E. Giuliano, MD

Nocardiosis

 KEY FEATURES

- *Nocardia asteroides*, an aerobic filamentous soil bacterium, causes pulmonary and systemic nocardiosis
- Bronchopulmonary abnormalities (eg, alveolar proteinosis) predispose to colonization, but infection is unusual unless the patient is also receiving systemic corticosteroids or is otherwise immunosuppressed
- CNS involvement commonly accompanies pulmonary infection

 CLINICAL FINDINGS

- Pulmonary involvement usually begins with malaise, loss of weight, fever, and night sweats
- Cough and production of purulent sputum are the chief complaints
- Dissemination may involve any organ. Brain abscesses and subcutaneous nodules are most frequent. Dissemination is seen exclusively in immunocompromised patients

 DIAGNOSIS

- *N asteroides* is a branching, filamentous gram-positive bacterium that is weakly acid-fast
- Identification is made by culture
- CXR may show infiltrates accompanied by pleural effusion. The lesions may penetrate through the chest wall and invade the ribs

 TREATMENT

- IV trimethoprim-sulfamethoxazole is initially administered at a dosage of 5–10 mg/kg/day (trimethoprim) and continued with trimethoprim-sulfamethoxazole PO, one double-strength tablet BID
- Surgical procedures such as drainage and resection may be needed as adjunctive therapy
- Response may be slow, and therapy must be continued for at least 6 mo. The prognosis in systemic nocardiosis is poor when therapy is delayed

Henry F. Chambers, MD

Obesity-Hypoventilation Syndrome

 KEY FEATURES

- Massive obesity and alveolar hypoventilation while awake
- Hypoventilation resulting from blunted ventilatory drive and increased mechanical load imposed on the chest
- Most patients also have obstructive sleep apnea

 CLINICAL FINDINGS

- Obesity
- Lethargy, headache, hypersomnolence
- Loud snoring if accompanied by obstructive sleep apnea
- Dyspnea often absent
- Signs of cyanosis and cor pulmonale may be found
- Many patients have polycythemia

 DIAGNOSIS

- Arterial blood gas measurements confirm daytime hypoxemia and hypercapnia, which improve with voluntary hyperventilation
- Nocturnal sleep study to evaluate for obstructive sleep apnea

 TREATMENT

- Mainly consists of weight loss
- Noninvasive positive-pressure ventilation is helpful in some patients
- Respiratory stimulants (medroxyprogesterone acetate, 10–20 mg q8h, theophylline, acetazolamide) may help
- If present, obstructive sleep apnea must be treated aggressively
- Treatment of comorbid conditions

Mark S. Chesnutt, MD
Thomas J. Prendergast, MD

Opioid Poisoning

 KEY FEATURES

- Widely varying potencies and durations of action (eg, some of the illicit fentanyl derivatives are up to 2000 times more potent than morphine)

 CLINICAL FINDINGS

- Heroin's duration of action is usually 3–5 h; methadone may last for 48–72 h
- Euphoria, drowsiness, and constricted pupils can occur with mild intoxication
- Severe intoxication may cause hypotension, bradycardia, hypothermia, coma, pulmonary edema, and respiratory arrest. Death is usually due to apnea or pulmonary aspiration
- Propoxyphene may cause seizures and prolong the QRS interval. Tramadol, dextromethorphan, and meperidine also occasionally cause seizures. The meperidine metabolite normeperidine can cause seizures, particularly with repeated use in renal insufficiency
- Skin-popping, especially with "black tar" heroin, has been associated with wound botulism

 DIAGNOSIS

- Routine urine toxicology screening usually positive (except tramadol, methadone)

 TREATMENT

- Administer activated charcoal, 60–100 g PO or via gastric tube, mixed in aqueous slurry if ingestion is within 1 h. Do not use for comatose or convulsing patients unless the airway is protected by a cuffed endotracheal tube
- Give naloxone, 0.4–2 mg IV, and repeat to maintain airway reflexes and spontaneous breathing. The effect duration is about 2–3 h; repeated doses may be necessary for intoxication by methadone or other long-acting drugs. Large doses (10–20 mg) may be required for propoxyphene, codeine, and fentanyl derivatives. Continuous observation for at least 3 h after the last naloxone dose is mandatory

Kent R. Olsen, MD

Osmolar Gap

 KEY FEATURES

- Alcohol quickly equilibrates between intracellular and extracellular water, adding 22 mOsm/L for every 1000 mg/L
- When measured osmolality exceeds that calculated from values of serum Na⁺ and glucose and blood urea nitrogen, consider ethanol intoxication as an explanation of the discrepancy (osmolar gap)
- Toxic alcohol ingestion, particularly methanol or ethylene glycol, can produce an osmolar gap with an anion gap metabolic acidosis. However, the combination of anion gap metabolic acidosis and an osmolar gap exceeding 10 mOsm/kg is not specific for toxic alcohol ingestion. Nearly half of patients with alcoholic ketoacidosis or lactic acidosis have similar findings, caused in part by elevations of endogenous glycerol, acetone, and acetone metabolites

 DIAGNOSIS

- The following substances can produce an osmolar gap:
  - Methanol
  - Ethylene glycol
  - Isopropyl alcohol
  - Ethanol toxicity
  - Acetone
  - Propylene glycol
  - Severe alcoholic or diabetic ketoacidosis
  - Lactic acidosis

Masafumi Fukagawa, MD, PhD, FJSIM
Kiyoshi Kurokawa, MD, MACP
Maxine A. Papadakis, MD

Osteomyelitis, *Staphylococcus aureus*

 KEY FEATURES

- *S aureus* is the cause of approximately 60% of all cases of osteomyelitis
- Osteomyelitis may occur by direct inoculation (eg, from an open fracture or as a result of surgery), by extension from a contiguous focus of infection or open wound, or, more commonly, by hematogenous spread

 CLINICAL FINDINGS

- Acute, abrupt local symptoms and systemic toxicity; or insidious onset of vague pain over the site of infection, progressing to local tenderness
- Fever is absent in one third of cases

 DIAGNOSIS

- Isolation of *S aureus* from the blood (60%), bone, or a contiguous focus of a patient with signs and symptoms of focal bone infection
- Bone biopsy and culture should be considered if blood cultures are sterile
- Bone scan and gallium scan can identify the site of bone infection
- Spinal infection (unlike malignancy) traverses the disk space to involve the contiguous vertebral body
- MRI is slightly less sensitive than bone scan but has a specificity of 90%. MRI is indicated when epidural abscess is suspected in association with vertebral osteomyelitis

 TREATMENT

- Duration is 4–6 weeks or longer
- Parenteral regimens are advised during the acute phase:
  - Nafcillin or oxacillin, 9–12 g/day in 6 divided doses, is the drug of choice
  - Cefazolin, 1 g q6–8 h
- Vancomycin, 1 g q12h, may be used for penicillin-allergic patients
- Oral regimens are dicloxacillin or cephalexin, 1 g q6h, plus rifampin, 300 mg BID (prevents late relapse and is advised)

Henry F. Chambers, MD

Panbronchiolitis, Diffuse

 KEY FEATURES

- Idiopathic disorder of respiratory bronchioles
- Diagnosed frequently in Japan; under-recognized in US
- Slightly more prevalent in men, usually presenting between ages 30–70
- Approximately 66% of patients are non-smokers
- May progress to diffuse bronchiectasis and respiratory failure

 CLINICAL FINDINGS

- Marked dyspnea, cough, and sputum production
- Wheezing may occur
- Crackles and rhonchi are noted
- Most patients have history of chronic pansinusitis

 DIAGNOSIS

- Pulmonary function tests reveal obstructive airflow abnormalities
- CXR shows a distinct pattern of diffuse small nodular shadows and hyperinflation
- Open-lung biopsy is necessary for diagnosis

 TREATMENT

- Chronic low-dose macrolide antibiotics (eg, erythromycin, 200–600 mg/day for 2–6 mo)
- β_2-agonists or ipratropium bromide
- Treatment of sinus disease
- Corticosteroids have been used despite lack of evidence supporting their efficacy
- Treatment of bronchial infections is aided by sputum analysis

Mark S. Chesnutt, MD
Thomas J. Prendergast, MD

Paracoccidioido-mycosis

 KEY FEATURES

- *Paracoccidioides brasiliensis* infection, found only in patients who have resided in South or Central America or Mexico
- Long asymptomatic periods enable patients to travel far from endemic areas before symptoms occur

 CLINICAL FINDINGS

- Ulceration of oronasopharynx is usually first symptom
- Extensive coalescent ulcerations may result in destruction of epiglottis, vocal cords, uvula
- Extension to lips and face may occur
- Extensive ulceration of the upper GI tract may prevent caloric intake and cause cachexia
- Skin lesions, usually on face, are variable in appearance and may have necrotic central crater with hard hyperkeratotic border
- Papules ulcerate and enlarge peripherally and deeper into subcutaneous tissue
- Lymph node enlargement may follow mucocutaneous lesions, eventually ulcerating and forming draining sinuses
- Hepatosplenomegaly may be present
- Cough indicates pulmonary involvement, but symptoms are often mild despite radiographic findings
- Differential diagnosis: mucocutaneous leishmaniasis and syphilis

 DIAGNOSIS

- Laboratory tests are nonspecific
- CXR may show severe parenchymal changes in the lungs
- Serology by immunodiffusion is positive in 98%
- Complement fixation titers correlate with progressive disease and fall with effective therapy
- Biopsy with Gomori's stain may be helpful
- Clinical specimens demonstrate the fungus as a spherical cell with many buds arising from it

 TREATMENT

- Itraconazole, 100–200 mg PO qd, generally results in clinical response within 1 mo and effective control after 2–6 mo

Richard J. Hamill, MD

Paralysis, Periodic

 KEY FEATURES

- Episodes of flaccid weakness or paralysis occur, sometimes in association with abnormalities of the plasma potassium level
- May have a familial (dominant inheritance) basis
- The hypokalemic variety is commonly associated with hyperthyroidism in young Asian men
- The familial hyperkalemic periodic paralysis may have a defect in the sodium channel gene on the long arm of chromosome 17

 CLINICAL FINDINGS

- The hypokalemic variety is characterized by attacks that tend to occur on awakening, after exercise, or after a heavy meal and may last for several days. Strength is normal between attacks
- In hyperkalemic periodic paralysis, attacks also tend to occur after exercise but usually last for <1 h
- Normokalemic periodic paralysis is similar clinically to the hyperkalemic variety, but the plasma potassium level remains normal during attacks; treatment is with acetazolamide

 DIAGNOSIS

- Clinical and plasma potassium

 TREATMENT

- Patients should avoid excessive exertion in the hypokalemic variety. A low-carbohydrate, low-salt diet may help prevent attacks, as may acetazolamide, 250–750 mg/day. An ongoing attack may be aborted by potassium chloride given PO or by IV drip, provided the ECG can be monitored and renal function is satisfactory. Treatment of associated hyperthyroidism prevents recurrences
- In hyperkalemic periodic paralysis, attacks may be terminated by IV calcium gluconate (1–2 g) or by IV diuretics (furosemide, 20–40 mg), glucose, or glucose and insulin; daily acetazolamide or chlorothiazide may prevent recurrences
- Normokalemic periodic paralysis treatment is with acetazolamide

Michael J. Aminoff, DSc, MD, FRCP

Paraneoplastic Syndromes

 KEY FEATURES

- May affect up to 15% of patients with cancer
- The most common tumor associated with paraneoplastic syndromes is small cell cancer of the lung
- Can occur despite relatively limited neoplastic growth
- Provide an early clue to presence of certain types of cancer
- Course usually parallels course of the cancer: Effective cancer treatment should be accompanied by resolution of the syndrome; conversely, recurrence of the cancer is sometimes heralded by return of syndrome
- Metabolic or toxic effects of the syndrome (eg, hypercalcemia, hyponatremia) may be a more urgent hazard to life than the underlying cancer
- Caused by the secretion of proteins not normally associated with a cancer's normal tissue:
  - Effects caused by a tumor product such as ectopic hormone production (serotonin in carcinoid syndrome, PTH-related peptide in hypercalcemia, ACTH in Cushing's syndrome, ADH in the syndrome of inappropriate antidiuretic hormone secretion [SIADH])
  - Effects caused by destruction of normal tissues by tumor products (local secretion of cytokines leading to hypercalcemia)
  - Effects caused by unknown mechanisms such as circulating immune complexes stimulated by the tumor or unidentified tumor products (eg, certain neurological syndromes or osteoarthropathy resulting from bronchogenic carcinoma)

 CLINICAL FINDINGS

- Electrolytes: hypercalcemia, hyponatremia
- Endocrine: Cushing's syndrome, SIADH
- Neurological: neuropathy, encephalitis, cerebellar degeneration,
- Skin: dermatomyositis, Sweet's syndrome
- Hematological: polycythemia, thrombocytosis
- Renal disease
- GI: diarrhea
- Rheumatological: arthropathy

 DIAGNOSIS

- See Table 151, page 1340

 TREATMENT

- Treatment of underlying malignancy
- Bisphosphonates, steroids (depending on tumor type) for hypercalcemia
- Symptomatic measures

Hope Rugo, MD

Paraquat Poisoning

 KEY FEATURES

- Used as a herbicide

 CLINICAL FINDINGS

- Concentrated solutions are highly corrosive to oropharynx, esophagus, and stomach
- Fatal dose after absorption may be as small as 4 mg/kg. If ingestion of paraquat is not rapidly fatal because of its corrosive effects, the herbicide may cause progressive pulmonary fibrosis, with death ensuing after 2–3 weeks

 DIAGNOSIS

- Clinical
- Serum paraquat levels can be obtained through Syngenta (1-800-327-8633). Paraquat levels associated with a high likelihood of death are 2 mg/L at 4 h, 0.9 mg/L at 6 h, and 0.1 mg/L at 24 h after ingestion

 TREATMENT

- Administer 60 g of activated charcoal PO or by gastric tube. Results of charcoal hemoperfusion, 8 h/day for 2–3 weeks, are equivocal
- Supplemental oxygen should be withheld unless the P_{O_2} is <70 mm Hg because oxygen may contribute to the pulmonary damage

Kent R. Olsen, MD

Parasomnias

 KEY FEATURES

MOST COMMON DISORDERS

Sleep terror

- Distinct from sleep panic attacks
- Usually seen in preadolescent boys, although it may occur in adults

Nightmares

- Occur during REM sleep, unlike sleep terror, which occurs in stage 3 or 4

Sleepwalking

- Includes ambulation or other intricate behaviors while asleep
- Episodes can occur during stage 3 or 4 or REM sleep
- Causative factors include medical conditions and drugs of abuse

Enuresis

- Involuntary micturition during sleep occurring in a patient who usually has control
- Most common 3–4 h after bedtime, but not limited to a specific stage of sleep

 CLINICAL FINDINGS

- Sleep terror: fear, sweating, tachycardia, and confusion for several minutes
  - Abrupt, terrifying arousal in sleep
  - Patients have amnesia for the event
- Enuresis: Confusion during the event and amnesia after it are common

 DIAGNOSIS

- Sleep walking is confirmed by a sleep study

 TREATMENT

SLEEP TERROR AND NIGHTMARES

- Benzodiazepines (diazepam, 5–20 mg QHS, suppresses stage 3 and 4 sleep)

ENURESIS

- Desmopressin nasal spray is increasingly the treatment of choice; alternatively, imipramine, 50–100 mg QHS
- Behavioral approaches (eg, bells that ring when a pad is wet) have been successful

Stuart J. Eisendrath, MD
Jonathan E. Lichtmacher, MD

Patellofemoral Syndrome

 KEY FEATURES

- Anterior knee pain
- A variety of injuries or anatomic abnormalities predispose patients to irregular patellar movements, leading to the patellofemoral syndrome
- Predisposing conditions include imbalance of quadriceps strength, patella alta, recurrent patellar subluxation, direct trauma to the patella, and meniscal injuries

 CLINICAL FINDINGS

- Pain is in the front of the knee, around or underneath the patella
- Because of the flexion load, patients may have difficulty going up or down staircases
- May have crepitus, joint locking, or sensations of joint instability

 DIAGNOSIS

- The history is generally more useful than the physical examination in establishing the diagnosis, but a significant number of patients have characteristic physical findings
- When the knee is held in slight flexion, gentle pressure against the patella as the patient contracts the quadriceps muscles may reproduce the symptoms. In some cases, with the knee extended and the quadriceps relaxed, the typical pain may be reproduced by digital pressure under the medial or lateral border of the patella, with side-to-side movement of the bone

 TREATMENT

- Avoidance of flexion loads and strengthening of the quadriceps

David B. Hellmann, MD, FACP
John H. Stone, MD, MPH

Patent Ductus Arteriosus

 KEY FEATURES

- Embryonic ductus arteriosus fails to close, resulting in continuous (systolic and diastolic) shunt of blood from aorta to left pulmonary artery
- Usual location is near the origin of the left subclavian artery
- Increases work of left ventricle
- Obliterative changes in pulmonary arterioles cause pulmonary hypertension, with resultant bidirectional shunt or right-to-left (Eisenmenger's) shunt
- Small or moderately large patent ductus usually asymptomatic until middle age

 CLINICAL FINDINGS

- Symptoms only if left ventricular (LV) failure or pulmonary hypertension develops
- Heart typically normal size or slightly enlarged
- Hyperdynamic apical impulse
- Wide pulse pressure and low diastolic pressure
- Continuous rough "machinery" murmur
- Thrill common
- Advanced disease: cyanotic lower legs (especially toes) in contrast to normally pink fingers

 DIAGNOSIS

- ECG: Normal tracing or LV hypertrophy (LVH)
- CXR: normal-sized heart or LV and left atrial enlargement. Prominent pulmonary artery, aorta, and left atrium
- Echo-Doppler is helpful, but lesion best visualized by aortography
- Cardiac catheterization can assess severity of left-to-right shunt and pulmonary hypertension

 TREATMENT

- Large shunts: high mortality early in life
- Smaller shunts: compatible with long survival; congestive heart failure most common complication
- Antibiotic prophylaxis mandatory to prevent endocarditis
- Surgical ligation or transcatheter closure in uncomplicated patients with symptoms or large shunts

- Treatment controversial in asymptomatic adults with no LVH and small left-to-right shunts
- Treatment controversial in the presence of pulmonary hypertension

Barry M. Massie, MD
Thomas M. Amidon, MD

Penicillium marneffei Infection

 ## KEY FEATURES

- *Penicillium marneffei* is a dimorphic fungus, endemic in southeast Asia
- Causes systemic infection in both immunocompetent and immunocompromised hosts
- Disseminated infections occur in advanced AIDS, including in travelers returning from southeast Asia

 ## CLINICAL FINDINGS

- Fever
- Lymphadenopathy
- Generalized umbilicated papular rash
- Cough
- Diarrhea

 ## DIAGNOSIS

- Identification of the organism on smears, histopathological specimens, or culture; the fungus produces a characteristic red pigment
- Best sites for isolation include skin, blood, bone marrow, respiratory tract, lymph nodes

 ## TREATMENT

- Itraconazole, 400 mg PO qd for 8 weeks, for mild to moderate infection
- Amphotericin B, 0.5–0.7 mg/kg/day, for severe disease
- Because relapse rate after successful treatment is 30%, use maintenance therapy with itraconazole, 200–400 mg PO qd

Richard J. Hamill, MD

Perianal Abscess & Fistula

 ## KEY FEATURES

- Infection of anal glands located at the base of the anal crypts at the dentate line, leading to abscess formation
- Causes include anal fissure and Crohn's disease
- Fistula in ano arises in an anal crypt and is usually preceded by an anal abscess
- Causes of fistulas that connect to the rectum include Crohn's disease, lymphogranuloma venereum, rectal tuberculosis, cancer

 ## CLINICAL FINDINGS

- Perianal abscess: throbbing, continuous perianal pain
- Erythema, fluctuance, and swelling in the perianal region on external exam
- Swelling in the ischiorectal fossa on digital rectal exam
- Fistula in ano: purulent discharge itching, tenderness, and pain

 ## DIAGNOSIS

- Anorectal exam, anoscopy
- Fistulogram

 ## TREATMENT

- Perianal abscess treated by local surgical incision under anesthesia, ischiorectal abscess by drainage in the operating room
- Fistula in ano is treated by surgical excision under anesthesia
- Fistulas caused by Crohn's disease are frequently asymptomatic and may be treated initially with antibiotics (metronidazole, 250 mg PO TID, or ciprofloxacin, 500 mg PO BID)
- Patients with persistent or recurrent symptoms are treated with immunomodulators (6-mercaptopurine, 1-1.5 mg/kg/day) or the anti-TNF antibody infliximab (5 mg/kg IV at 2 and 6 weeks)

Kenneth R. McQuaid, MD

Pericardial Effusion

 ## KEY FEATURES

- Can develop from any form of pericarditis
- Slow development of large effusions may produce no hemodynamic effects
- Rapid appearance of smaller effusions can cause cardiac tamponade (elevated intrapericardial pressure that restricts venous return and ventricular filling), leading to shock and death

 ## CLINICAL FINDINGS

- Pain in acute inflammatory pericarditis; neoplastic and uremic effusions are often painless
- Dyspnea and cough, especially with tamponade
- Other symptoms reflect primary disease
- Pericardial friction rub may be present (even with large effusions)
- Pulsus paradoxus (>10 mm Hg decline in systolic pressure during inspiration)
- Tachycardia, tachypnea, narrow pulse pressure, and preserved systolic pressure are characteristic of tamponade
- Elevation of central venous pressure, edema, or ascites in chronic processes

 ## DIAGNOSIS

- ECG: often reveals nonspecific T wave changes and low QRS voltage. Electrical alternans is pathognomonic but uncommon
- CXR: normal or enlarged cardiac silhouette with a globular configuration
- Echocardiography is the primary mode of diagnosis and can distinguish effusion from congestive heart failure
- Diagnostic pericardiocentesis or biopsy is often indicated for microbiological and cytological studies

 ## TREATMENT

- Small effusions can be followed clinically and by echocardiogram
- Urgent pericardiocentesis is required for tamponade
- Partial pericardiectomy may be required for recurrent effusion in neoplastic disease and uremia
- Additional therapy (eg, dialysis) for the primary disease

Barry M. Massie, MD
Thomas M. Amidon, MD

Pericarditis, Acute

 KEY FEATURES

- Acute inflammation of the pericardium
- Causes: infections, autoimmune diseases, uremia, neoplasms, radiation, drug toxicity, hemopericardium, contiguous inflammatory processes of the heart or lung (eg, myocardial infarction, Dressler's syndrome, idiopathic)
- Viral infections are the most common cause; acute pericarditis often follows upper respiratory tract infection
- Males, usually younger than age 50, are most commonly affected

 CLINICAL FINDINGS

- Often associated with pleuritic chest pain, relieved by sitting, radiating to the neck, shoulders, back, or epigastrium
- Dyspnea and fever
- Pericardial friction rub with or without evidence of pericardial effusion or constriction
- Pericardial involvement
- Bacterial pericarditis: rare; patients appear toxic and are often critically ill
- Neoplastic pericarditis: often painless, hemodynamic compromise
- Dressler's syndrome (post-myocardial infarction [MI] pericarditis): occurs days to 3 mo post-MI, usually self-limited, treated with aspirin, NSAIDs, or corticosteroids

 DIAGNOSIS

- Diagnosis is usually clinical
- Leukocytosis
- ECG: generalized ST-T wave changes, characteristic progression beginning with diffuse ST elevations, followed by a return to baseline, then T wave inversions
- CXR: cardiac enlargement if pericardial effusion, signs of related pulmonary disease
- Echocardiogram: often normal in inflammatory pericarditis; otherwise, can demonstrate pericardial effusion, tamponade
- Rising titers in paired sera may confirm viral infection
- Cardiac enzymes slightly elevated if a myocarditic component
- Cytology of pericardial effusion or pericardial biopsy

- MRI and CT scan can visualize adjacent tumor when present

 TREATMENT

- Treat underlying causes (eg, antibiotics for bacterial infection, dialysis for uremia)
- Symptomatic treatment with NSAIDS or aspirin for pain
- Corticosteroids for unresponsive cases and Dressler's syndrome
- Symptoms usually subside in several days to weeks
- Constrictive pericarditis develops rarely but may require pericardial resection
- Partial pericardiectomy for tamponade
- Drainage of malignant effusion, instillation of chemotherapeutic agents or tetracycline to prevent recurrence
- Pericardial windows are rarely effective

Barry M. Massie, MD
Thomas M. Amidon, MD

Pericarditis, Restrictive

 KEY FEATURES

- Generally caused by inflammation leading to a thickened, fibrotic, adherent pericardium that restricts diastolic filling and produces chronically elevated venous pressures
- Most common causes: radiation therapy, cardiac surgery, viral pericarditis
- Less common causes: tuberculosis, histoplasmosis

 CLINICAL FINDINGS

- Slowly progressive dyspnea, fatigue, and weakness
- Chronic edema, hepatic congestion, and ascites are usually present
- Elevated jugular venous pressure with a rapid *y* descent
- Increased jugular venous pressure during inspiration (Kussmaul's sign)
- Atrial fibrillation is common
- Pulsus paradoxus is unusual

 DIAGNOSIS

- CXR: normal heart size or cardiomegaly. Pericardial calcification is common and best seen on lateral view
- Echocardiography: thick pericardium and small chambers
- CT and MRI may be more sensitive than echocardiography
- Exclude restrictive cardiomyopathy and cardiac tamponade

 TREATMENT

- Gentle diuresis
- Complete surgical pericardiectomy is usually required in symptomatic patients but carries relatively high mortality rate

Barry M. Massie, MD
Thomas A. Amidon, MD

Peritonitis, Tuberculous

KEY FEATURES

- Tuberculous involvement of the peritoneum
- Accounts for <2% of all causes of ascites in US
- Incidence higher among those with HIV disease, urban poor, nursing home residents, and immigrants from underdeveloped countries
- In US, half have underlying cirrhosis and ascites from portal hypertension

CLINICAL FINDINGS

- Low-grade fever
- Abdominal pain
- Anorexia, weight loss
- Abdominal swelling, clinically apparent ascites
- Abdominal examination shows doughy consistency

DIAGNOSIS

- Tuberculin skin tests positive in half (Table 22, page 1220)
- Chest radiographs abnormal in >70%
- Active pulmonary tuberculosis disease in <25%
- Ultrasound examination shows ascites in >95%
- Ascitic fluid total protein >3.5 g/dL, lactate dehydrogenase >90 units/L, or mononuclear cell-predominant leukocytosis >500/μL; each has a sensitivity of 70–80% but limited specificity
- Ascitic fluid smears for acid-fast bacilli are usually negative; cultures are positive in only 20%
- Ascitic fluid cultures of high-volume paracentesis fluid have increased sensitivity of ~85%
- Ascitic fluid adenosine deaminase activity has limited predictive value in cirrhotic ascites
- Laparoscopy establishes diagnosis
- Characteristic peritoneal nodules are visible in >90%
- Peritoneal biopsy reveals granulomas
- Peritoneal biopsy cultures are positive in <66% and require at least 4–6 weeks

TREATMENT

- Tuberculosis, initial treatment (Table 24, page 1221)
- Antituberculous drugs characteristic (Table 23, page 1221)

Kenneth R. McQuaid, MD

Pesticide Poisoning

KEY FEATURES

- Inhibit the enzyme acetylcholinesterase and increase acetylcholine activity at nicotinic and muscarinic receptors and in CNS
- Most are absorbed through intact skin
- Most chemical warfare "nerve agents" are organophosphates

CLINICAL FINDINGS

- Abdominal cramps, diarrhea, vomiting, excessive salivation, sweating, seizures, lacrimation, constricted pupils, wheezing, bronchorrhea, skeletal muscle weakness, respiratory arrest
- Initial tachycardia is usually followed by bradycardia
- Symptoms may persist or recur for days, especially with highly lipid-soluble agents such as fenthion or dimethoate

DIAGNOSIS

- Serum and red blood cell cholinesterase activity is usually at least 50% below baseline with severe intoxication

TREATMENT

- Empty stomach by gastric lavage and administer activated charcoal for ingestion within 1 h
- If the agent is on the victim's skin or hair, wash repeatedly with soap or shampoo and water. Dilute bleach solution may inactivate material on the skin. Care providers must avoid skin exposure by wearing gloves and waterproof aprons
- Administer atropine, 2 mg IV, and give repeated doses as needed (may need several hundred milligrams) to dry bronchial secretions and decrease wheezing
- Administer pralidoxime, 1–2 g IV, as soon as possible, and give a continuous infusion (200–400 mg/h) as long as there is any evidence of acetylcholine excess. Pralidoxime is of questionable benefit for carbamate poisoning

Kent R. Olsen, MD

Petroleum Distillate Poisoning

KEY FEATURES

- Toxicity may occur from inhalation of the vapor or as a result of pulmonary aspiration of the liquid during or after ingestion

CLINICAL FINDINGS

- Table 142, page 1324
- Aspiration pneumonitis
- With some hydrocarbons, severe systemic poisoning after oral ingestion
- Systemic intoxication can also occur by inhalation
- Vertigo, muscular incoordination, irregular pulse, myoclonus, and seizures occur with serious poisoning and may be due to hypoxemia or systemic effects of the agents
- Chlorinated and fluorinated hydrocarbons (eg, trichloroethylene, freons) and many other hydrocarbons can cause ventricular arrhythmias because of increased sensitivity of the myocardium to the effects of endogenous catecholamines

DIAGNOSIS

- Coughing or choking immediately after ingestion suggests pulmonary aspiration
- CXR findings may be delayed for several hours

TREATMENT

- Table 142, page 1324
- Remove the patient to fresh air
- Administration of activated charcoal may be helpful if the preparation contains toxic solutes (eg, an insecticide) or is an aromatic or halogenated product
- Observe the victim for 6–8 h for signs of aspiration pneumonitis
- Corticosteroids are not recommended
- If fever occurs, give a specific antibiotic only after identification of the bacterial pathogens
- Because of the risk of arrhythmias, use bronchodilators only with caution in patients with chlorinated or fluorinated solvent intoxication

Kent R. Olsen, MD

Plantar Fasciitis

KEY FEATURES

- The most common cause of foot pain in outpatient medicine is plantar fasciitis, which results from constant strain on the plantar fascia at its insertion into the medial tubercle of the calcaneus
- The majority of cases occur in patients with no associated disease. Most occur from excessive standing and improper footwear

CLINICAL FINDINGS

- Severe pain on the bottoms of the feet in the morning—the first steps out of bed in particular—but the pain subsides after a few minutes of ambulation

DIAGNOSIS

- Pain with palpation over the plantar fascia's insertion on the medial heel
- Radiographs have no role in the diagnosis of this condition; heel spurs frequently exist in patients without plantar fasciitis, and most symptomatic patients do not have heel spurs
- Differential diagnosis includes enthesopathy resulting from seronegative spondyloarthropathy, Achilles tendinitis, metatarsal stress fracture, genital herpes (referred pain from sacral ganglion), retrocalcaneal bursitis

TREATMENT

- An interval of days without prolonged standing and the use of arch supports
- NSAIDs may provide some relief
- In severe cases, a corticosteroid with lidocaine injection (small volume—no more than a total of 1.5 mL) directly into the most tender area on the sole of the foot is helpful

David B. Hellmann, MD, FACP
John H. Stone, MD, MPH

Pleuritis

KEY FEATURES

- Irritation of the parietal pleura causes the pain associated with pleuritis

CLINICAL FINDINGS

- Pain is localized, sharp, and fleeting and worsened by cough, sneeze, movement, or deep breathing
- Shoulder pain may be referred when there is irritation of the central portion of the ipsilateral diaphragmatic pleura

DIAGNOSIS

- The setting in which pain occurs can often narrow the broad list of potential causes
- In young, healthy individuals, pleuritis is usually due to a viral respiratory infection
- Presence of pleural effusion, pleural thickening, or pneumothorax requires additional diagnostic and therapeutic measures

TREATMENT

- Treatment is directed at the underlying disease
- NSAIDs (indocin, 25 mg BID–TID) may help pain relief
- Codeine (30–60 mg TID) may control cough
- Intercostal nerve blocks are occasionally helpful

Mark S. Chesnutt, MD
Thomas J. Prendergast, MD

Plexopathies

 KEY FEATURES

- Brachial plexus neuropathy may be idiopathic, follow trauma, or result from congenital anomalies, neoplastic involvement, or injury by various physical agents. In rare instances, the disorder occurs on a familial basis
- Cervical rib syndrome is the compression of the C8 and T1 roots or the lower trunk of the brachial plexus by a cervical rib or band arising from the seventh cervical vertebra
- Lumbosacral plexus lesions may develop in association with diabetes, cancer, or bleeding disorders, after injury, or occasionally without known cause

 CLINICAL FINDINGS

- Brachial plexus neuropathy begins with severe pain about the shoulder, followed within days by weakness, reflex changes, and sensory changes, especially involving C5 and C6. Symptoms are usually unilateral but may be bilateral. Wasting of affected muscles is sometimes profound
- Cervical rib syndrome results in weakness and wasting of intrinsic hand muscles, especially those in the thenar eminence. Pain and numbness is in the medial 2 fingers and the ulnar border of the hand and forearm. Compression of the subclavian artery may also occur
- Lumbosacral plexus lesions present with pain and weakness, which tend to be more pronounced than sensory symptoms; the distribution of symptoms depends on the level of neurological involvement

 DIAGNOSIS

- X-ray films can show the cervical rib or a large transverse process of the seventh cervical vertebra, but normal findings do not exclude the possibility of a cervical band. Adson's test for diagnosing compression of the subclavian artery is a diminished or obliterated radial pulse when the seated patient inhales deeply and turns the head to one side or the other
- Electrodiagnostic evaluation helps to localize a lesion to the plexus and is important for differential diagnosis

 TREATMENT

- Symptomatic or surgical excision of the rib or band in cervical rib syndrome
- Physical therapy is especially important in idiopathic cases
- Treat underlying cause

Michael J. Aminoff, DSc, MD, FRCP

Pneumonia, Chlamydial

 KEY FEATURES

- *Chlamydia pneumoniae* causes pneumonia and bronchitis
- *C pneumoniae* causes approximately 10% of community-acquired pneumonias
- *C pneumoniae* is second only to *Mycoplasma* as an agent of atypical pneumonia
- *C pneumoniae* has been associated seroepidemiologically with coronary artery disease

 CLINICAL FINDINGS

- The clinical presentation is that of an atypical pneumonia

 DIAGNOSIS

- Microimmunofluorescence or complement fixation test of acute and convalescent sera

 TREATMENT

- Doxycycline, 100 mg BID for 10–14 days
- Azithromycin, 500 mg once on day 1, then 250 mg QD for 4 days more
- Levofloxacin, 500 mg QD for 10–14 days

Henry F. Chambers, MD

Pneumonia, Eosinophilic

 KEY FEATURES

- One of a diverse group of eosinophilic pulmonary syndromes

 CLINICAL FINDINGS

- Fever, night sweats, weight loss, and dyspnea
- Pulmonary infiltrates on CXR are invariably peripheral
- Peripheral eosinophilia

 DIAGNOSIS

- CXR with peripheral airspace and interstitial infiltrates
- Peripheral eosinophilia
- Bronchoalveolar lavage to document eosinophils in the lung and exclude other causes
- Lung biopsy may be required

 TREATMENT

- Oral prednisone (1 mg/kg/day) for 1–2 weeks and tapered over many months usually results in dramatic improvement
- Most patients require 10–15 mg of prednisone every other day for 1 yr or longer to prevent relapses

Mark S. Chesnutt, MD
Thomas J. Prendergast, MD

Pneumonia, Usual Interstitial

 KEY FEATURES

- Clinical presentation is similar to that of other idiopathic fibrosing interstitial pneumonias
- Median survival is approximately 3 yr

 CLINICAL FINDINGS

- Age 55–60 with slight male predominance
- Insidious dry cough with months to years of exertional dyspnea
- Clubbing is present at diagnosis in 25–50%
- Pulmonary function tests: restriction and decreased diffusion capacity
- ANA and RF are positive in 25% of patients without documented collagen vascular disease

 DIAGNOSIS

- CXR findings: decreased lung volumes with linear or reticular bibasilar or subpleural opacities
- HRCT shows minimal ground-glass and variable honeycomb change
- Normal CXR findings in 2–10% at diagnosis
- Biopsy shows nonuniform distribution of fibrosis, with loss of type I pneumocytes and proliferation of alveolar type II cells
- Usual interstitial pneumonia can be diagnosed with 90% confidence in patients older than 65 with classic features, avoiding biopsy

 TREATMENT

- No randomized study has demonstrated a benefit to any treatment
- Response to corticosteroids and cytotoxic agents is 15% at best
- Recombinant interferon gamma-1b showed promise in a small, but well-designed study

Mark S. Chesnutt, MD
Thomas J. Prendergast, MD

Pneumonitis, Acute Interstitial

 KEY FEATURES

- Known clinically as Hamman-Rich syndrome

 CLINICAL FINDINGS

- Wide age range, including many young patients
- Acute onset of dyspnea followed by rapid development of respiratory failure
- Preceding viral syndrome is reported by half of patients
- Clinical course is indistinguishable from idiopathic ARDS

 DIAGNOSIS

- X-ray film shows diffuse bilateral airspace consolidation
- Areas of ground-glass attenuation are seen on HRCT
- Biopsy resembles the organizing phase of diffuse alveolar damage, with fibrosis and minimal collagen deposition
- Pathologically similar to usual interstitial pneumonitis but more homogenous, and honeycombing is typically absent

 TREATMENT

- Supportive care including mechanical ventilation is critical
- Benefit of specific therapies is unclear
- 50–90% of patients die within 2 mo
- Course is not progressive if patient survives
- Lung function may be permanently impaired in survivors

Mark S. Chesnutt, MD
Thomas J. Prendergast, MD

Pneumonitis, Nonspecific Interstitial

 KEY FEATURES

- Clinical presentation and features are similar to idiopathic fibrosing interstitial pneumonia (IFIP) but with distinct pathological findings and better prognosis
- The median survival is >10 yr

 CLINICAL FINDINGS

- Age 45–55 with slight female predominance
- Onset of dyspnea and cough over months; otherwise, presentation is similar to that of IFID

 DIAGNOSIS

- Radiographically, may be indistinguishable from UIP
- The most typical HRCT finding is bilateral areas of ground-glass attenuation and fibrosis with rare honeycombing
- Biopsy shows varying degrees of patchy inflammation and fibrosis, which are uniform in time. Honeycombing is scant
- See Table 28. page 1224, Table 29, page 1225

 TREATMENT

- Corticosteroids are thought to be effective, but no prospective clinical studies have been published
- Prognosis is good overall but depends on degree of fibrosis at diagnosis

Mark S. Chesnutt, MD
Thomas J. Prendergast, MD

Pneumonitis, Radiation

KEY FEATURES

- Usually presents 2–3 mo after completion of radiotherapy
- Radiographic findings correlate poorly with symptoms
- Resolution typically occurs after 2–3 weeks; death from ARDS is unusual

CLINICAL FINDINGS

- Insidious onset of dyspnea, dry cough, chest fullness or pain, weakness, and fever
- Inspiratory crackles may be heard
- In severe disease, respiratory distress and cyanosis may be present
- Leukocytosis and elevated ESR are common

DIAGNOSIS

- CXR usually shows alveolar or nodular infiltrate limited to the irradiated area; air bronchograms are common
- Pulmonary function tests: reduced volumes, compliance, and diffusion capacity
- Hypoxemia

TREATMENT

- Aspirin, cough suppression, and bed rest
- Corticosteroids have not been proven effective, but prednisone (1 mg/kg/day PO) is usually given for 1 week, reduced to 20–40 mg/day for several weeks before a slow taper

Mark S. Chesnutt, MD
Thomas J. Prendergast, MD

Poliomyelitis

KEY FEATURES

- Enteroviral infection of lower motor neurons
- Infection transmitted by fecal-oral route
- Rare in the developed world
- Targeted for global eradication by WHO

CLINICAL FINDINGS

- Fever, headache, stiff neck
- Lower motor neuron lesions lead to weakness, decreased deep tendon reflexes, muscle wasting
- 95% of infected patients are asymptomatic; the remainder have 1 of 3 types:
  - Minor (abortive) polio: fever, headache, diarrhea, sore throat
  - Nonparalytic polio: fever, headache, meningitis, and muscle spasms without paralysis
  - Paralytic polio (rare, 0.1%): Paralysis occurs any time during febrile period. Can be further subdivided into spinal polio, in which paralysis mainly affects muscles innervated by spinal nerves, and bulbar polio, which affects muscles supplied by the cranial nerves

DIAGNOSIS

- Diagnosis rarely made; majority of patients are asymptomatic
- CSF lymphocytosis
- Characteristic clinical symptoms and viral recovery from stools or neutralizing antibodies clinch diagnosis

TREATMENT

- Supportive measures, including bed rest and careful monitoring for bulbar symptoms
- Prevention: Inactive parenteral vaccine has replaced oral vaccine in developed world
- Adults not at high risk should not be routinely vaccinated
- IM injections should be avoided 1 mo after vaccination

Wayne X. Shandera, MD
Samuel Shelburne, MD

Polychondritis, Relapsing

KEY FEATURES

- Inflammatory destructive lesions of cartilaginous structures, principally the ears, nose, trachea, larynx, and chest wall cartilage
- Associated conditions include systemic lupus erythematosus, rheumatoid arthritis, Hashimoto's thyroiditis, cancer (especially multiple myeloma)

CLINICAL FINDINGS

- The cartilage is painful, swollen, and tender during an attack
- Subsequently becomes atrophic, resulting in permanent deformity
- Noncartilaginous manifestations of the disease include fever, episcleritis, uveitis, deafness, aortic insufficiency, and rarely glomerulonephritis
- In 85% of patients, a migratory, asymmetric, and seronegative arthropathy occurs, affecting both large and small joints and the costochondral junctions

DIAGNOSIS

- Clinical
- Differential diagnosis includes other causes of ear deformity (skin cancer, cauliflower ear [cartilage dissolution posttrauma], chondritis or perichondritis, chondrodermatitis nodularis helicis) and other causes of nose deformity (syphilis, rhinophyma [rosacea], Hansen's disease [leprosy], Wegener's granulomatosis)

TREATMENT

- Prednisone, 0.5–1 mg/kg/day, is often effective
- Dapsone, 100–200 mg/day, may also be effective, sparing the need for chronic high-dose corticosteroid treatment

David B. Hellmann, MD, FACP
John H. Stone, MD, MPH

Polycystic Kidney Disease

 KEY FEATURES

- Among the most common hereditary disease in US, affecting 1:1000 to 1:400 individuals
- 50% will have end-stage renal disease by age 60
- Variable penetrance
- Accounts for 10% of dialysis patients
- At least 2 genes account for disorder: *ADPKD1* on the short arm of chromosome 16 (86% of patients) and *ADPKD2* on chromosome 4
- Family history positive in 75%

 CLINICAL FINDINGS

- Abdominal or flank pain caused by infection, bleeding into cysts, nephrolithiasis, rupture of cyst, urinary tract infection, renal cell carcinoma
- Fever caused by infection
- Nephrolithiasis, primarily calcium oxalate stones, in up to 20%
- Hypertension in 50%
- Abdominal mass
- Arterial aneurysms in the circle of Willis in 10–15%
- Mitral valve prolapse in up to 25%
- Aortic aneurysms
- Aortic valve abnormalities

 DIAGNOSIS

- Can diagnose via ultrasonogram depending on age and number of cysts
- Urinalysis may be normal because the cyst does not communicate directly with the urinary tract, but blood cultures may be positive
- CT scan: Infected cyst has increased wall thickness
- Screening cerebral arteriography is not recommended unless patient has family history of aneurysms or is undergoing elective surgery with a high risk of developing hypertension

 TREATMENT

- Bed rest
- Analgesics
- Cyst decompression for pain
- Antibiotics: fluoroquinolones, trimethoprim-sulfamethoxazole, and chloramphenicol IV for 2 weeks followed by long-term PO therapy
- Hydration (2–3 L/day)
- Antihypertensive agents
- Diuretics used cautiously because their effect on renal cyst formation is unknown

Suzanne Watnick, MD
Gail Morrison, MD

Polyneuropathy, Chronic Inflammatory

 KEY FEATURES

- Clinically similar to Guillain-Barré syndrome except that it has a relapsing or steadily progressive course over months or years
- In the relapsing form, partial recovery may occur after some relapses, but in other instances no recovery occurs between exacerbations
- Although remission may occur spontaneously with time, the disorder frequently follows a progressive downhill course leading to severe functional disability
- Usually ascending, symmetric weakness
- Paresthesias are more variable

 CLINICAL FINDINGS

- A symmetric sensory, motor, or mixed deficit, which may be most marked distally or proximally
- See *Guillain-Barré syndrome*

 DIAGNOSIS

- Electrodiagnostic studies show marked slowing of motor and sensory conduction and focal conduction block. Signs of partial denervation may also be present owing to secondary axonal degeneration
- Nerve biopsy may show chronic perivascular inflammatory infiltrates in the endoneurium and epineurium without accompanying evidence of vasculitis. However, a normal nerve biopsy result or the presence of nonspecific abnormalities does not exclude the diagnosis

 TREATMENT

- Prednisone, 60 mg qd for 2–3 mo
- If no response has occurred despite 3 mo of treatment, a higher dose may be tried. In responsive cases, the dose is gradually tapered, but most patients become corticosteroid dependent, often requiring prednisone, 20 mg on alternate days, on a long-term basis
- Patients unresponsive to corticosteroids may benefit from a cytotoxic drug such as azathioprine
- Short-term benefit with plasmapheresis may occur

- High-dose IV immunoglobulin treatment (eg, 400 mg/kg/day) may produce clinical improvement lasting for weeks to months

Michael J. Aminoff, DSc, MD, FRCP

Popliteal Aneurysm

 ## KEY FEATURES

- 85% of all peripheral artery aneurysms

 ## CLINICAL FINDINGS

- Symptoms caused by arterial thrombosis, peripheral embolization, or compression of adjacent structures with resultant venous thrombosis or neuropathy; rarely caused by rupture
- Arterial thrombosis leads to amputation in up to 30% of patients

 ## DIAGNOSIS

- Ultrasonogram diagnostic to measure the diameter of the aneurysm and rule out aortic abdominal aneurysms
- MRA or conventional arteriography required before operative repair

 ## TREATMENT

- Surgery recommended for all asymptomatic aneurysms > 2 cm and all symptomatic aneurysms regardless of size
- Catheter-directed thrombolysis can be attempted if no patent distal vessels for bypass
- Saphenous vein bypass graft with proximal and distal ligation of the aneurysm if patent outflow vessel is identified for bypass
- Resection of the aneurysm in addition to grafting is required for large aneurysms producing popliteal vein or nerve compression

Louis M. Messina, MD
Laura K. Pak, MD
Lawrence M. Tierney, Jr, MD

Popliteal Artery Occlusion

 ## KEY FEATURES

- Causes athero-occlusive disease (most common), thrombosis of a popliteal aneurysm, popliteal entrapment syndrome, popliteal adventitial cystic disease, trauma (knee dislocation), or extrinsic compression by a Baker's cyst

POPLITEAL ENTRAPMENT SYNDROME

- Caused by anatomic anomalies that lead to arterial compression in the popliteal space
- Type 1 (20%): an abnormal course of the popliteal artery
- Type 2 (25%): medial insertion of the medial head of the gastrocnemius muscle
- Type 3 (30%): abnormal accessory slip of gastrocnemius muscle
- Type 4 (8%): abnormal accessory slip of popliteus muscle

POPLITEAL ADVENTITIAL DISEASE

- Rare formation of cysts within the wall of the popliteal artery, which compress the arterial lumen, causing stenosis or occlusion. It affects healthy men age 40–50

 ## CLINICAL FINDINGS

- Absent popliteal pulses with ankle-brachial index (ABI) <1.0
- History of claudication or rest pain
- Almost 30% of patients with entrapment have bilateral disease
- In patients with entrapment, claudication symptoms may be atypical, such as pain with walking but not with running

 ## DIAGNOSIS

- Diagnosis by MRA or positional angiography. Athero-occlusive disease is suggested with findings of bilateral multifocal lesions. With entrapment, the patent artery becomes impinged with passive dorsiflexion or active plantar flexion of the ankle
- Large adventitial cysts or Baker's cysts can sometimes be diagnosed by ultrasonography
- Most adventitial cysts are small and appear only as a thickening of the popliteal artery wall on MRA

- Any patient with history of knee dislocation and abnormal pulse exam or ABI should undergo conventional angiogram

 ## TREATMENT

- Angioplasty can be performed for short-segment athero-occlusive disease
- Bypass surgery is the preferred treatment for most patients with severe arterial insufficiency secondary to athero-occlusive disease
- Entrapment is treated by surgical transection of the abnormal muscle or short-segment bypass with greater or lesser saphenous vein if the artery is occluded
- Ultrasonogram-guided aspiration of adventitial cysts has been described, but the cyst frequently recurs. Interposition bypass grafting is curative

Louis M. Messina, MD
Laura K. Pak, MD
Lawrence M. Tierney, Jr, MD

Pregnancy, Third-Trimester Bleeding

KEY FEATURES

- Vaginal bleeding occurs in 5–10% of women in late pregnancy

CLINICAL FINDINGS

- Painless vaginal bleeding is characteristic of placenta previa
- Strong uterine contractions, continuous pain, and tenderness are more often associated with abruptio placentae

DIAGNOSIS

- Placental causes must be differentiated from nonplacental causes
- CBC should be ordered, with blood typed and cross-matched
- Coagulation studies may be indicated
- Ultrasonography can determine placental location
- Speculum and digital pelvic exams are avoided until placenta previa is excluded
- Amniocentesis may be performed to assess for fetal lung maturity in patients <36 weeks' gestational age

TREATMENT

- Approach should be conservative and expectant unless fetal distress or risk of severe maternal hemorrhage occurs
- Patients should be hospitalized and placed on bed rest with fetal monitoring
- Hospitalization and bed rest are continued if the patient is <36 weeks' gestation
- Home management may be considered in selected patients
- Betamethasone, 12 mg IM × 2 12–24 h apart, is indicated if fetal lung immaturity is present

William R. Crombleholme, MD

Pregnancy, Thyroid Disease

KEY FEATURES

THYROTOXICOSIS

- May result in fetal anomalies, late abortion, or preterm labor and fetal hyperthyroidism with goiter
- Thyroid storm in late pregnancy or labor is a life-threatening emergency
- Keep free T_4 in the high-normal range during pregnancy

RECURRENT POSTPARTUM THYROIDITIS

- A hyperthyroid state of 1–3-mo duration followed by hypothyroidism
- Occurs 3–6 mo after delivery
- Spontaneous recovery occurs in 90% after 3–6 mo

MATERNAL HYPOTHYROIDISM

- Even subclinical elevation of thyroid-stimulating hormone (TSH) may impact neuropsychological fetal development
- Check TSH level at the first prenatal visit in suspected hypothyroidism

CLINICAL FINDINGS

- Presentation is similar to that of the nonpregnant state. In first trimester persistent nausea, vomiting, and weight loss could be misdiagnosed as hyperemesis gravidarum

DIAGNOSIS

- Total T_4 and total T_3 normally elevated in pregnancy; free T_4 and free T_3 unchanged. Suppressed TSH can occur in up to 10% of normal pregnancy
- Thyroperoxidase antibodies and thryoglobulin antibodies are present in recurrent postpartum thryoiditis

TREATMENT

- Treat thyrotoxicosis with propylthiouracil. The initial dose is 100–150 mg TID qd. A maintenance dose of 100 mg/day minimizes the chance of fetal hypothyroidism
- Treat maternal hypothyroidism with T_4 to maintain normal TSH

William R. Crombleholme, MD

Prion Diseases

KEY FEATURES

- Proteinaceous infectious particles
- Transmissible agents that cause conversion of brain protein to abnormal isoform
- Cause disease in both humans (Creutzfeldt-Jakob) and animals (scrapie)
- Disease in human has sporadic, familial, iatrogenic, and new-variant forms

CLINICAL FINDINGS

- Classic Creutzfeldt-Jakob disease (CJD) occurs in late middle age
- Rapidly progressive dementia, myoclonic fasciculations, and ataxia
- New variant form occurs in younger individuals and associated with consumption of infected beef
- New variant with longer duration, more psychiatric and cerebellar symptoms versus classic form

DIAGNOSIS

- Combination of clinical findings, characteristic EEG, and MRI
- CSF can be analyzed for tau and 14-3-3 protein

TREATMENT

- No specific therapy available
- Disinfection of neurosurgical equipment key for prevention of iatrogenic transmission

Wayne X. Shandera, MD
Samuel Shelburne, MD

Pruritus

 KEY FEATURES

- Pruritus is a disagreeable sensation that provokes a desire to scratch
- Not all cases of pruritus are mediated by histamine
- Although many cases of generalized pruritus can be attributed to dry skin—whether naturally occurring and precipitated or aggravated by climatic conditions or arising from disease states—there are many other causes: scabies, dermatitis herpetiformis, atopic dermatitis, pruritus vulvae et ani, miliaria, insect bites, pediculosis, contact dermatitis, drug reactions, urticaria, urticarial eruptions of pregnancy, psoriasis, lichen planus, lichen simplex chronicus, exfoliative dermatitis, folliculitis, bullous pemphigoid, fiberglass dermatitis
- Persistent pruritus not explained by cutaneous disease should prompt a staged workup for systemic causes
- Perhaps the most common cause of pruritus associated with systemic disease is uremia in conjunction with hemodialysis
- Endocrine disorders such as hypo- or hyperthyroidism, psychiatric disturbances, lymphoma, leukemia, and other internal malignant disorders, iron deficiency anemia, and certain neurological disorders may also cause pruritus

 CLINICAL FINDINGS

- Bilirubin may be normal in patients with hepatic pruritus, and the severity of the liver disease may not correlate with the degree of itching
- Burning or itching involving the face, scalp, and genitalia may be manifestations of primary depression and treatable with drugs such as tricyclics (amitriptyline, imipramine, doxepin), SSRIs, and other antidepressants

TREATMENT

- Naltrexone and nalmefene have been shown to relieve the pruritus of liver disease
- Uremia in conjunction with hemodialysis and the pruritus of obstructive biliary disease may be helped by phototherapy with ultraviolet B or PUVA
- Danazol, 400–800 mg daily, may be tried for pruritus associated with myelo-

proliferative disorders and other systemic illnesses
- Idiopathic pruritus and that accompanying serious internal disease may not respond to any type of therapy
- Pruritus accompanying specific skin disease will subside when the disease is controlled
- Elimination of external factors and irritating agents may give complete relief from pruritus
- Naltrexone is not effective in pruritus associated with renal failure

Timothy G. Berger, MD

Pseudoallergic Reactions

 KEY FEATURES

- These reactions resemble immediate hypersensitivity reactions but are not mediated by allergen–IgE interaction; instead, direct mast cell activation occurs
- Examples of pseudoallergic or "anaphylactoid" reactions are the "red man syndrome" from rapid infusion of vancomycin, direct mast cell activation by opioids, and radiocontrast reactions
- If a patient has had an anaphylactoid reaction to conventional radiocontrast media, the risk for a second reaction on reexposure may be as high as 30%
- Unlike IgE-mediated reactions, these can often be prevented by prophylactic medical regimens

 CLINICAL FINDINGS

- Mimics allergic reactions, from urticaria/angioedema to anaphylaxis

 DIAGNOSIS

- Clinical

 TREATMENT

- Slow (vancomycin infusion) or stop (radiocontrast) exposure
- Antihistamines, bronchodilators, and steroids
- Prevention: low-osmolality contrast preparations
- Prevention: prophylactic administration of prednisone (50 mg PO q6h beginning 18 h before contrast) and diphenhydramine (25–50 mg IM 60 min before the contrast)
- The use of the lower-osmolality radiocontrast media in combination with the pretreatment regimen decreases the incidence of reactions to less than 1%

Jeffrey L. Kishiyama, MD
Daniel C. Adelman, MD

Pseudogout & Chondrocalcinosis

 KEY FEATURES

- Also known as calcium pyrophosphate dihydrate deposition disease (CPPD)
- Chondrocalcinosis is the presence of calcium-containing salts in articular cartilage
- May be familial and is associated with hemochromatosis, hyperparathyroidism, ochronosis, diabetes mellitus, true gout, hypothyroidism, Wilson's disease
- Usually seen in individuals 60 yr and older

 CLINICAL FINDINGS

- CPPD can be asymptomatic, cause recurrent, acute attacks of monoarthritis (pseudogout), or result in chronic arthritis resembling either osteoarthritis or rheumatoid arthritis
- Pseudogout, like gout, frequently develops 24–48 h after major surgery
- CPPD with osteoarthritic changes of second and third metacarpophalangeals suggests hemochromatosis

 DIAGNOSIS

- Identification of calcium pyrophosphate crystals in joint aspirates is diagnostic
- Rhomboid-shaped pseudogout crystals are blue when parallel and yellow when perpendicular to the axis of the compensator with polarized light microscopy. Needle-shaped gout crystals give the opposite color pattern
- X-ray examination shows not only calcification (usually symmetric) of cartilaginous structures but also signs of osteoarthritis
- Normal serum urate levels

 TREATMENT

- Treatment is directed at the primary disease, if present
- NSAIDs or COX-2 inhibitors are used for acute episodes. Colchicine is sometimes used for prophylaxis but is generally ineffective for acute episodes
- Intra-articular injection of triamcinolone, 10–40 mg

David B. Hellmann, MD, FACP
John H. Stone, MD, MPH

Pulmonary Alveolar Proteinosis

 KEY FEATURES

- Phospholipid accumulation within alveolar spaces
- May be primary (idiopathic) or secondary to immune deficiency, hematological malignancies, or inhalation of mineral dusts or may occur after lung infections

 CLINICAL FINDINGS

- Progressive dyspnea
- CXR shows bilateral pulmonary infiltrates suggestive of edema
- Spontaneous remission occurs in some; others develop progressive respiratory insufficiency
- Pulmonary infection with *Nocardia* or fungi may occur

 DIAGNOSIS

- Based on characteristic findings on alveolar lavage, a milky appearance and periodic acid–Schiff-positive lipoproteinaceous material, with typical clinical and radiographic features
- Biopsy is necessary in some cases

 TREATMENT

- Therapy consists of periodic whole-lung lavage

Mark S. Chesnutt, MD
Thomas J. Prendergast, MD

Pulmonary Edema, Acute

 KEY FINDINGS

- Acute onset or worsening of dyspnea at rest
- Tachycardia, diaphoresis, cyanosis
- Pulmonary rales, rhonchi; expiratory wheezing
- CXR shows interstitial and alveolar edema with or without cardiomegaly
- Arterial hypoxemia
- Cardiac causes include acute myocardial infarction (MI) or ischemia, congestive heart failure (CHF) exacerbation, valvular regurgitation, and mitral stenosis
- Noncardiac causes include IV narcotics, increased intracerebral pressure, high altitude, sepsis, medications, inhaled toxins, transfusion reactions, shock, and disseminated intravascular coagulation

 CLINICAL FINDINGS

- Severe dyspnea; pink, frothy sputum; diaphoresis; and cyanosis
- Rales, wheezing, or rhonchi in all lung fields
- Sudden onset in acute exacerbations of CHF or acute MI

 DIAGNOSIS

- Characteristic clinical findings
- CXR: pulmonary vascular congestion, increased interstitial markings, and characteristic butterfly pattern of alveolar edema; heart enlarged or normal in size
- Echocardiography: assesses ejection fraction, atrial pressure
- Pulmonary capillary wedge pressure is always elevated (usually >25 mm Hg) in cardiogenic pulmonary edema, normal or even low in noncardiogenic pulmonary edema

 TREATMENT

- Place patient in a sitting position with legs dangling over the side of the bed
- Give oxygen by mask for PaO_2 <60 mm Hg
- Noninvasive pressure support ventilation or endotracheal intubation and mechanical ventilation for respiratory distress
- Morphine, 4–8 mg IV or SC, repeated PRN after 2–4 h (avoid in patients with

narcotic-induced and neurogenic pulmonary edema)
- Diuretic IV (Table 44, page 1237)
- Nitrate SL, PO, or IV
- Inhaled β-adrenergic agonists or IV aminophylline for bronchospasm
- Parenteral vasodilator (eg, nitroprusside IV) for elevated arterial pressure
- Positive inotropic agents in low-output states, hypotension

Barry M. Massie, MD
Thomas M. Amidon, MD

Pulmonary Hemosiderosis, Idiopathic

 ## KEY FEATURES

- Recurrent pulmonary hemorrhage with hemoptysis
- Usually in children or young adults
- No known underlying cause
- Multiple episodes can result in interstitial fibrosis and pulmonary failure

 ## CLINICAL FINDINGS

- Hemoptysis, recurrent
- Dyspnea
- Alveolar infiltrates on CXR
- Anemia, often iron deficient

 ## DIAGNOSIS

- Exclusion of other causes of alveolar hemorrhage
- Hemoptysis, dyspnea, cough
- Chest radiograph opacities
- Iron-deficiency anemia
- Hemosiderin-laden macrophages on bronchoalveolar lavage and lung biopsy specimens

 ## TREATMENT

- Corticosteroids may be useful for acute episodes

Mark S. Chesnutt, MD
Thomas J. Prendergast, MD

Pulmonary Hypertension, Primary

 ## KEY FEATURES

- Elevated pulmonary vascular resistance and hypertension in the absence of other cardiac or pulmonary disease
- Pathological findings: diffuse narrowing of the pulmonary arterioles
- The diet pills fenfluramine, dexfenfluramine, and phentermine may cause a picture indistinguishable from primary pulmonary hypertension

 ## CLINICAL FINDINGS

- Clinical findings are similar to pulmonary hypertension from other causes
- Characteristically occurs in young women
- Weakness and fatigue from right-sided heart failure, low cardiac output
- Edema, ascites, peripheral cyanosis, and effort-related syncope as right-sided heart failure advances

 ## DIAGNOSIS

- ECG: right ventricular and atrial hypertrophy
- CXR: enlarged right ventricle, enlarged main pulmonary arteries with reduced peripheral branches
- Echocardiography, lung scanning, and (if necessary) pulmonary angiography are essential to exclude secondary causes

 ## TREATMENT

- Death usually occurs in 2–8 yr
- Chronic anticoagulation is recommended by some experts
- Vasodilator drugs are controversial because of possible life-threatening systemic hypotension
- Nifedipine and diltiazem (Table 47, page 1243) may be effective but only in early disease
- Epoprostenol (a potent pulmonary vasodilator) by continuous IV infusion may slow (but not halt) symptom progression in advanced disease
- Nitric oxide by inhalation is sometimes given for nonresponders to epoprostenol
- Bosentan (an oral endothelin antagonist) may become the treatment of choice for all stages of disease
- Heart–lung transplantation is definitive treatment

Barry M. Massie, MD
Thomas A. Amidon, MD

Pulmonary Radiation Fibrosis

 ## KEY FEATURES

- Occurs in nearly all patients who receive a full course of radiation therapy for breast or lung cancer
- Pulmonary fibrosis develops after a 6- to 12-week period of well-being
- Fibrosis may occur without preceding pneumonitis

 ## CLINICAL FINDINGS

- Most patients are asymptomatic; slowly progressive dyspnea may occur
- Cor pulmonale and chronic respiratory failure are rare

 ## DIAGNOSIS

- Radiographic findings include obliteration of normal lung markings, dense interstitial and pleural fibrosis, reduced lung volumes, tenting of the diaphragm, and sharp delineation of radiation margins

 ## TREATMENT

- No specific therapy is effective; corticosteroids are of no value

Mark S. Chesnutt, MD
Thomas J. Prendergast, MD

Pulmonary Stenosis

 KEY FEATURES

- Increased resistance to outflow, increased right ventricular (RV) pressure, decreased pulmonary blood flow
- Without shunting, arterial saturation normal, but severe stenosis causes peripheral cyanosis through decreased cardiac output
- Clubbing and polycythemia occur only with right-to-left shunting from patent foramen ovale or atrial septal defect

 CLINICAL FINDINGS

- Mild: asymptomatic
- Moderate: asymptomatic early, with symptoms of dyspnea, syncope, and chest pain evolving in adulthood
- Severe: right-sided congestive heart failure and sudden death in the 20s and 30s
- Palpable parasternal lift
- Loud, harsh systolic murmur and thrill in second and third left interspaces

 DIAGNOSIS

- High-pitched systolic ejection murmur and thrill in second left interspace
- ECG: right axis deviation or RV hypertrophy; peaked P waves
- CXR: heart size normal, RV and right atrium prominent, pulmonary artery dilatation
- Echocardiogram is diagnostic

TREATMENT

- Treatment indicated for symptomatic patients and those with RV hypertrophy and elevated pulmonary artery gradients
- Treatment of choice: percutaneous balloon valvuloplasty
- Surgery has excellent long-term results but a 2–4% operative mortality rate

Barry M. Massie, MD
Thomas A. Amidon, MD

Pulmonary Veno-Occlusive Disease

 KEY FEATURES

- A rare cause of postcapillary pulmonary hypertension
- Occurs in children and young adults
- Characterized by progressive fibrotic occlusion of pulmonary veins and venules with secondary hypertensive changes in the pulmonary arteriolar bed

 CLINICAL FINDINGS

- Difficult to recognize in early stages
- Progressive dyspnea
- Fatigue, exertional syncope
- Cardiac exam findings consistent with elevated right-sided pressures (see *Pulmonary hypertension, primary*)

 DIAGNOSIS

- CXR shows prominent symmetric interstitial markings, Kerley B lines, dilated pulmonary arteries, and normal left atrium and ventricle
- Premortem diagnosis is difficult but can be made with open-lung biopsy

 TREATMENT

- No effective therapy; most patients die within 2 yr

Mark S. Chesnutt, MD
Thomas J. Prendergast, MD

Q Fever

 KEY FEATURES

- Caused by *Coxiella burnetii*, a rickettsia that infects cows, goats, and sheep
- Transmission to humans occurs by inhalation of dry feces, milk, or dust contaminated by them
- Typical incubation period is 7–21 days

 CLINICAL FINDINGS

- Febrile illness with headache, myalgias, nonproductive cough
- Pneumonitis and granulomatous hepatitis commonly seen
- Endocarditis, usually of the aortic valve, can occur in chronic *Coxiella* infections
- Clinical course is variable, from acute to chronic and relapsing

 DIAGNOSIS

- Elevated liver enzymes
- Leukocytosis
- A rise in the complement-fixing antibodies is diagnostic
- A serum enzyme-linked immunoassay is also available and helpful

 TREATMENT

- Prevention: A vaccine is being developed for high-risk people who handle livestock or are laboratory workers
- Doxycycline and related medications are effective at treating most manifestations of the disease
- Endocarditis usually requires addition of a second agent, a sulfa, rifampin, or a fluoroquinolone, and therapy is usually needed for long periods, sometimes years
- In endocarditis, the rate of clinical failure with antibiotics is high, and surgical valve replacement is often necessary

Wayne X. Shandera, MD
Samuel Shelburne, MD

Rabies

KEY FEATURES

- A rhabdovirus infection causing encephalitis, transmitted by infected saliva after an animal bite
- Bats, raccoons, skunks, foxes, and coyotes are most common vectors in US
- Human cases rare in US
- Incubation period of 3–7 weeks is proportional to distance from wound to CNS
- Nearly always fatal unless patients receive postexposure prophylaxis

CLINICAL FINDINGS

- Prodrome includes pain at site of bite, fever, nausea
- CNS symptoms begin about 10 days later with encephalitis or paralysis
- Encephalitis associated with delirium and extremely painful laryngeal spasms that lead to hydrophobia
- Paralytic presentation less common; with ascending paralysis resembles Guillain-Barré syndrome
- Both paralytic and encephalitic forms progress to coma, autonomic dysfunction, death

DIAGNOSIS

- History of animal bite, initial viral prodrome followed by CNS symptoms should suggest diagnosis
- Diagnosis is confirmed with fluorescent antibody testing of the sacrificed animal brain
- Skin biopsy from the patient's posterior neck is up to 80% sensitive; PCR may play a role in future diagnosis

TREATMENT

- When an animal bite occurs, local wound cleansing, débridement and flushes are useful
- Animal bite wounds should not be sutured
- Decision to use postexposure immunization should be based on clinical guidelines when the disease is under serious consideration
- Treatment includes both passive antibody and vaccination
- Local health officials may aid in decision to treat
- Prevention: Immunization of household dogs is an effective strategy and avoidance of animals associated with rabies (bats, foxes, raccoons, skunks)

Wayne X. Shandera, MD
Samuel Shelburne, MD

Radial Neuropathy

KEY FEATURES

- Radial nerve is particularly liable to compression or injury in the axilla (eg, by crutches or by pressure when the arm hangs over the back of a chair)
- The neuropathy may be asymptomatic, resolve rapidly and spontaneously, or become progressively more disabling

CLINICAL FINDINGS

- Percussion of the nerve at the site of the lesion may lead to paresthesias in its distal distribution
- Leads to weakness or paralysis of muscles supplied by the nerve, including the triceps, except in cases involving injury near the spiral groove in which the triceps is spared (Saturday night palsy)
- Sensory changes may also occur in a small area on the back of the hand between the thumb and index finger
- If injured at or above the elbow, its purely motor posterior interosseous branch, supplying the extensors of the wrist and fingers, may be involved immediately below the elbow, but there is sparing of the extensor carpi radialis longus, so that the wrist can still be extended
- The superficial radial nerve may be compressed by handcuffs or a tight watch strap

DIAGNOSIS

- Electromyography and nerve conduction studies help to localize the focal lesion

TREATMENT

- If acute compression is the cause, then no treatment is needed in most cases
- If repetitive mechanical trauma is responsible, this is avoided by occupational adjustment

Michael J. Aminoff, DSc, MD, FRCP

Rat-Bite Fever

KEY FEATURES

- Rat-bite fever is an uncommon acute infectious disease caused by *Spirillum minus*. It is transmitted to humans by the bite of a rat
- Inhabitants of rat-infested slum dwellings and laboratory workers are at greatest risk

CLINICAL FINDINGS

- Rat bite heals promptly, but 1 to several weeks later the site becomes swollen, indurated, and painful; assumes a dusky purplish hue; and may ulcerate. Regional lymphangitis and lymphadenitis
- Fever, chills, malaise, myalgia, arthralgia, and headache
- Splenomegaly
- A sparse, dusky-red maculopapular rash on the trunk and extremities
- Arthritis
- After a few days, symptoms subside, only to reappear again in a few more days
- Relapsing fever for 3–4 days alternating with afebrile periods lasting 3–9 days; may persist for weeks

DIAGNOSIS

- Leukocytosis
- Nontreponemal test for syphilis often falsely positive
- Organism may be identified in dark-field examination of the ulcer exudate or an aspirated lymph node
- Differential diagnosis: streptobacillary fever, tularemia, rickettsial disease (eg, Rocky Mountain spotted fever, epidemic typhus), ehrlichiosis, *Pasteurella multocida* infection, relapsing fever

TREATMENT

- Procaine penicillin G, 600,000 units IM q12h, or tetracycline hydrochloride, 0.5 g PO q6h, for 10–14 days
- The usual mortality rate of about 10% can be markedly reduced by prompt diagnosis and antimicrobial treatment

Richard A. Jacobs, MD, PhD

Relapsing Fever

 KEY FEATURE

- Caused by *Borrelia recurrentis*
- Endemic in many parts of the world
- Both tick-borne and louse-borne disease occur
- For tick-borne disease, main reservoir is rodents, which serve as the source of infection for ticks
- In the US, infected ticks are found throughout the west, especially in mountainous areas
- Clinical cases are uncommon in humans
- Tick-borne relapsing fever is not transmitted from person to person
- In louse-borne disease, when an infected person harbors lice, the lice become infected with *Borrelia*
- Large epidemics may occur

 CLINICAL FINDINGS

- Abrupt onset of fever, chills, tachycardia, nausea and vomiting, arthralgia, and severe headache
- Hepatomegaly and splenomegaly, rashes
- Delirium, neurological and psychological abnormalities
- The attack terminates, usually abruptly, after 3–10 days. After an interval of 1–2 weeks, relapse occurs, and 3–10 relapses may occur before recovery

 DIAGNOSIS

- During episodes of fever, large spirochetes can be seen in blood smears stained with Wright's or Giemsa stain. Organisms can be cultured in special media
- Anti-*Borrelia* antibodies develop during the illness
- The Weil-Felix test for rickettsioses, nontreponemal serological tests for syphilis, and indirect fluorescent antibody and Western blot tests for *Borrelia burgdorferi* may be falsely positive
- Cerebrospinal fluid abnormalities occur in patients with meningeal involvement
- Mild anemia and thrombocytopenia are common
- Differential diagnosis: malaria, leptospirosis, meningococcemia, typhoid fever, yellow fever, epidemic typhus, rat-bite fever

 TREATMENT

- For louse-borne relapsing fever: tetracycline or erythromycin, 0.5 g PO once, or procaine penicillin G, 400,000–600,000 units IM once, constitutes adequate treatment
- For tick-borne relapsing fever: tetracycline or erythromycin, 0.5 g PO QID for 5–10 days
- Jarisch-Herxheimer reactions occur commonly and may be life threatening. Treatment with aspirin—but not hydrocortisone—may ameliorate this reaction
- With treatment, the initial attack is shortened and relapses are largely prevented
- Overall mortality rate is ~5%
- Fatalities most common in old, debilitated, or very young patients
- Prevention of relapsing fever is by prevention of tick bites and delousing procedures

Richard A. Jacobs, MD, PhD

Renal Artery Aneurysm

 KEY FEATURES

- Incidence: ~1% of adults
- Many affected patients are asymptomatic
- Causes: medial degeneration, trauma, and injury after renal biopsy or percutaneous nephrolithostomy

 CLINICAL FINDINGS

- Most are asymptomatic
- Rupture is initial presentation in 5%:
  - Hematuria/flank pain
  - Hypertension
  - Renal insufficiency

 DIAGNOSIS

- CT scan
- Conventional angiography is indicated if planning intervention

 TREATMENT

- Indications for treatment: size >2 cm, local symptoms, renovascular hypertension, distal embolization, growth on serial imaging, occurrence in women of child-bearing age
- Surgical treatment involves excision with interposition grafting; infrequently, ex vivo reconstruction may be required if the aneurysm extends into the branch vessels
- Interposition grafting of main renal arteries >5 mm in diameter yields 5-yr primary patency rate of ~70%
- Stent grafts for saccular aneurysms of the main renal artery
- Endovascular embolization with microcoils for interlobar artery aneurysms

Louis M. Messina, MD
Laura K. Pak, MD
Lawrence M. Tierney, Jr, MD

Retinal Detachment

 KEY FEATURES

- Retinal detachment is most commonly secondary to development of a hole or tear in the retina, which is usually spontaneous but may be secondary to trauma
- Spontaneous detachment most common in patients older than 50
- Cataract extraction and myopia are the 2 most common predisposing conditions

 CLINICAL FINDINGS

- Blurred vision in the involved eye, becoming progressively worse
- Often described as "a curtain coming down over the eye"
- Central vision remains intact until the macula becomes detached
- May be associated with "flashes" and "floaters"
- No pain or redness

 DIAGNOSIS

- On ophthalmoscopic examination, the retina may be seen hanging like a gray cloud

 TREATMENT

- Immediate referral to ophthalmologist is critical
- During transportation, patient's head should be positioned so that the detached portion of the retina will fall back with the aid of gravity
- Surgical therapy involves closing the retinal tears by creating a permanent adhesion between the neurosensory retina, retinal pigment epithelium, and choroid
- Laser photocoagulation or cryotherapy are the main tools used by the surgeon
- About 80% of uncomplicated cases are cured with 1 operation, 15% need further surgical therapy, and 5% never reattach

Paul Riordan-Eva, FRCOphth

Rheumatic Manifestations of Cancer

 KEY FEATURES

- Patients with malignancy-associated dermatomyositis tend to be older and have the type of cancer anticipated by their age and gender profiles
- Middle-aged or older patients with polyarthritis that mimics rheumatoid arthritis but is associated with new-onset clubbing and periosteal new bone formation should be suspected of having hypertrophic pulmonary osteoarthropathy
- Palmar fasciitis is characterized by bilateral palmar swelling and finger contraction and may be the first indication of cancer, particularly ovarian carcinoma
- Acute leukemia can produce joint pains that are disproportionately severe in comparison to the minimal swelling and heat that are present. Leukemic arthritis complicates approximately 5% of cases
- Rheumatic manifestations of myelodysplastic syndromes include cutaneous vasculitis, lupus-like syndromes, neuropathy, and episodic intense arthritis
- Erythromelalgia, a painful warmth and redness of the extremities that (unlike Raynaud's disease) improves with cold exposure or with elevation of the extremity, is often associated with myeloproliferative diseases

 CLINICAL FINDINGS

- Rheumatic symptoms tend to improve or resolve with treatment of the cancer, but may return with cancer recurrence

 DIAGNOSIS

- Malignancy workups should focus on screening tests appropriate to the patient's age (eg, colonoscopy in patients older than 50 yr). "Fishing expeditions" are not indicated

 TREATMENT

- Glucocorticoids are often helpful for arthritic symptoms
- Erythromelalgia may respond to ASA, 325 mg QD or BID

David B. Hellmann, MD, FACP
John H. Stone, MD, MPH

Rheumatic Manifestations of HIV

 KEY FEATURES

- Infection with HIV virus has been associated with various rheumatic disorders, most commonly arthralgias or Reiter's syndrome. More rarely, myositis, psoriatic arthritis, Sjögren's syndrome, or vasculitis occur
- It is possible that these disorders stem directly from HIV infection itself or from the many other infections that occur in immunodeficient patients
- The rheumatic syndromes may follow the diagnosis of AIDS or may precede it by several months

 CLINICAL FINDINGS

- Arthralgias
- Some rheumatic manifestations (eg, the arthritis of Reiter's syndrome or the cutaneous findings in psoriasis) tend to be accentuated in patients with HIV

 DIAGNOSIS

- Same criteria as for non–HIV-infected patients

 TREATMENT

- Many patients respond to NSAIDs, although a few are unresponsive and develop progressive deformities
- Immunosuppressive agents must be used with great caution. However, with the use of HAART, the paradoxical use of immunosuppression in HIV patients with inflammatory disease is sometimes required

David B. Hellmann, MD, FACP
John H. Stone, MD, MPH

Rheumatism, Palindromic

 KEY FEATURES

- Frequent recurring attacks at irregular intervals of acutely inflamed joints
- In some patients, palindromic rheumatism is a prodrome of rheumatoid arthritis

 CLINICAL FINDINGS

- Periarticular pain with swelling
- Attacks cease within several hours to several days
- Knee and fingers are most commonly affected, but any peripheral joint may be involved
- Systemic manifestations other than fever do not occur
- Although hundreds of attacks may take place over a period of years, there is no permanent articular damage

 DIAGNOSIS

- Clinical
- Laboratory findings are usually normal

 TREATMENT

- NSAIDs are usually all that is required during the attacks
- Hydroxychloroquine may be of value in preventing recurrences

David B. Hellmann, MD, FACP
John H. Stone, MD, MPH

Riboflavin Deficiency

 KEY FEATURES

- Almost always occurs in combination with deficiencies of other vitamins
- Caused by dietary inadequacy, interactions with a variety of medications, alcoholism, and other causes of protein-calorie undernutrition

 CLINICAL FINDINGS

- Cheilosis, angular stomatitis, glossitis, seborrheic dermatitis, weakness, corneal vascularization, anemia

 DIAGNOSIS

- Measure serum levels of the riboflavin-dependent enzyme erythrocyte glutathione reductase. Activity coefficients greater than 1.2–1.3 suggest riboflavin deficiency
- Less commonly measured: urinary riboflavin excretion and serum levels of plasma and red blood cell flavins

 TREATMENT

- Riboflavin, 5–15 mg PO qd, until clinical findings are resolved

Robert B. Baron, MD, MS

Right Middle Lobe Syndrome

 KEY FEATURES

- Recurrent or persistent atelectasis of the right middle lobe
- Related to the relatively long length and narrow diameter of the right middle lobe bronchus and the oval opening to the lobe
- Important to exclude obstructing lesion such as bronchogenic carcinoma

 CLINICAL FINDINGS

- Radiographic finding of recurrent atelectasis of right middle lobe
- Recurrent or slowly resolving pneumonia

 DIAGNOSIS

- CT scan or bronchoscopy is often necessary to rule out obstructing tumor
- Foreign body aspiration or other benign causes of atelectasis must be excluded

 TREATMENT

- Treatment is of the underlying condition

Mark S. Chesnutt, MD
Thomas J. Prendergast, MD

Rocky Mountain Spotted Fever

 ### KEY FEATURES

- Caused by *Rickettsia rickettsii*, a parasite of ticks, transmitted by tick bites
- Most cases occur in the middle and southern Atlantic seaboard and the central Mississippi River valley
- Most cases occur in late spring and summer
- Typical incubation period is 2–14 days (median, 7 days)

 ### CLINICAL FINDINGS

- Initial symptoms include fevers, chills, headache, nausea and vomiting
- Cough and pneumonitis often occur early in the disease
- Rash (not always found) begins as a faint macule that progresses to large maculopapules and often petechiae
- Rash begins on the wrists and ankles, characteristically involves palms and soles, and spreads to arms, legs, and trunk
- About 3–5% of recognized cases in US are fatal

 ### DIAGNOSIS

- Thrombocytopenia
- Hyponatremia
- Hepatitis
- CSF low glucose
- Immunohistological staining for *R rickettsi* in skin biopsy specimens and serological testing are the keys to a definitive diagnosis

 ### TREATMENT

- Doxycycline or chloramphenicol are usually highly effective
- Prevention: protective clothing and avoiding tick bites

Wayne X. Shandera, MD
Samuel Shelburne, MD

Rotator Cuff Injuries

 ### KEY FEATURES

- The majority of shoulder problems stem from disorders of the rotator cuff
- Rotator cuff tendinitis, subacromial bursitis, partial and complete rotator cuff tears, and calcific tendinitis frequently cause similar symptoms

 ### CLINICAL FINDINGS

- Nonspecific localized shoulder pain
- Locking sensations occur with motion (particularly abduction) of the shoulder
- Maximum tenderness is usually noted over the supraspinatus insertion
- Range of motion pain is worst between 60° and 120° of abduction, the site of greatest impingement of the rotator cuff tissues between the humerus and coracoacromial arch
- With rotator cuff tears, there may be an inability to abduct or flex the shoulder depending on the site of the tear, although full range of motion may be maintained by the shoulder's accessory rotator muscles
- Complete tears usually have positive "drop" signs: inability to sustain passive abduction of the arm to 90°

 ### DIAGNOSIS

- Clinical features; MRI may be of use

 ### TREATMENT

- Rest and abstention from inciting activities, along with NSAIDs
- For symptoms that persist after 2 weeks of conservative therapy, injection of 1 mL triamcinolone (40 mg/mL) with 2–3 mL of lidocaine hydrochloride (1–2%) may help. The procedure, along with continued rest, may be repeated after 2–3 weeks
- Physical therapy is valuable if the patient fails to maintain the shoulder's normal range of motion
- Aside from patients with complete rotator cuff tears, only those who fail to improve after months of conservative therapy are candidates for operation

David B. Hellmann, MD, FACP
John H. Stone, MD, MPH

Rubella

 ### KEY FEATURES

- Spread by respiratory droplets
- Rare disease in US
- Nonspecific features makes it difficult to distinguish from other viral infections

 ### CLINICAL FINDINGS

- Mild fever, malaise, and arthralgias, which are more common in women
- Cervical, postauricular lymphadenopathy common
- Fine, pink rash lasts 3 days in each area
- Rash typically starts on the face and spreads to trunk and extremities
- Exposure during pregnancy can lead to fetal infection and death
- Postinfectious encephalopathy is rare, few long-term sequelae
- Congenital rubella associated with CNS, cutaneous, ophthalmic (cataracts), otic (deafness), and cardiac disease

 ### DIAGNOSIS

- Exposure 14–21 days before symptom onset
- Leukopenia common
- Diagnosis established by clinical findings and rise in serum rubella antibody titers

 ### TREATMENT

- Symptomatic treatment and supportive measures
- Prevention: Live attenuated virus is safe and highly effective
- Women should be immunized when not pregnant

Wayne X. Shandera, MD
Samuel Shelburne, MD

Sciatic Nerve Palsy

 KEY FEATURES

- Misplaced deep intramuscular injections are probably the most common cause
- Trauma to the buttock, hip, or thigh may also be responsible
- The resulting clinical deficit depends on whether the whole nerve or only certain fibers have been affected
- In general, the peroneal fibers of the sciatic nerve are more susceptible to damage than those destined for the tibial nerve
- The common peroneal nerve itself may be compressed or injured in the region of the head and neck of the fibula (eg, by sitting with crossed legs or wearing high boots)

 CLINICAL FINDINGS

- There is weakness of dorsiflexion and eversion of the foot, accompanied by numbness or blunted sensation of the anterolateral aspect of the calf and dorsum of the foot

 DIAGNOSIS

- Suggested clinically and may be confirmed by electromyography
- A sciatic nerve lesion may be difficult to distinguish from peroneal neuropathy unless there is electromyographic evidence of involvement of the short head of the biceps femoris muscle

 TREATMENT

- Unless trauma has interrupted the continuity of the nerve, treatment is supportive
- Avoid pressure on the nerve

Michael J. Aminoff, DSc, MD, FRCP

Seafood Poisoning

 KEY FEATURES

- In the majority of cases, the seafood has a normal appearance and taste (scombroid may have a peppery taste)

 CLINICAL FINDINGS

- A variety of intoxications may occur. These include scombroid, ciguatera, paralytic shellfish, and puffer fish poisoning (Table 143, page 1325)
- Abrupt respiratory arrest may occur with acute paralytic shellfish and puffer fish poisoning

 DIAGNOSIS

- Table 143, page 1325

 TREATMENT

- Observe patients for at least 4–6 h. Replace fluid and electrolyte losses from gastroenteritis with IV saline or other crystalloid solution
- For recent ingestions, administer activated charcoal, 60–100 g PO or via gastric tube, mixed in aqueous slurry. Do not use for comatose or convulsing patients unless it can be given by gastric tube and the airway is first protected by a cuffed endotracheal tube
- There is no specific antidote for paralytic shellfish or puffer fish poisoning
- Ciguatera: Acute neurological symptoms may respond to mannitol, 1 g/kg IV (anecdotal)
- Scombroid: Antihistamines such as diphenhydramine, 25–50 mg IV, and the H_2 blocker cimetidine, 300 mg IV, are usually effective. For severe reactions, give also epinephrine, 0.3–0.5 mL of a 1:1000 solution SC

Kent R. Olsen, MD

Seborrheic Keratoses

 KEY FEATURES

- Seborrheic keratoses are common, especially in the elderly and may be mistaken for melanomas or other types of cutaneous neoplasms

 CLINICAL FINDINGS

- Seborrheic keratoses are benign plaques, beige to brown or even black, 3–20 mm in diameter, with a velvety or warty surface
- They appear to be stuck or pasted onto the skin

 DIAGNOSIS

- Clinical

 TREATMENT

- Although they may be frozen with liquid nitrogen or curetted if they itch or are inflamed, no treatment is needed

Timothy G. Berger, MD

Sedative-Hypnotic Agent Overdose

 ## KEY FEATURES

- Sedative-hypnotics depress the CNS reticular activating system, cerebral cortex, and cerebellum

 ## CLINICAL FINDINGS

- Mild intoxication produces euphoria, slurred speech, ataxia, and even hypoglycemia
- With severe intoxication, stupor, coma, bradycardia, hypotension, hypothermia, and respiratory arrest may occur
- Death is usually from respiratory arrest or pulmonary aspiration of gastric contents
- Massively intoxicated patients may appear dead, with no reflex responses or even electroencephalographic activity

 ## DIAGNOSIS

- Ethanol serum levels >300 mg/dL (0.3 g/dL; 65 mmol/L) usually produce coma in a novice user, but regular users may remain awake at much higher levels. Phenobarbital levels >80–100 mg/L usually cause coma

 ## TREATMENT

- Administer activated charcoal, 60–100 g PO or via gastric tube, mixed in aqueous slurry if given within 1 h of ingestion. Do not use for comatose patients unless it can be given by gastric tube and the airway is protected by a cuffed endotracheal tube
- Hemoperfusion may be necessary for severe phenobarbital intoxication but not for most other drugs in this group
- Flumazenil is a specific benzodiazepine antagonist and has no effect on other sedative-hypnotic agents. Give flumazenil, IV 0.2 mg over 30–60 s, repeated in 0.5-mg increments as needed up to a total dose of 3–5 mg. It may induce seizures in patients with preexisting seizures, benzodiazepine addiction, or concomitant overdose with tricyclic antidepressants

Kent R. Olsen, MD

Short Bowel Syndrome

 ## KEY FEATURES

- Malabsorptive condition secondary to removal of significant segments of the small intestine
- Causes: Crohn's disease, mesenteric infarction, radiation enteritis, trauma
- Type and degree of malabsorption depend on length and site of resection and degree of adaptation of remaining bowel

 ## CLINICAL FINDINGS

- Terminal ileal resection: watery diarrhea, malabsorption of bile salts and vitamin B_{12}, low serum vitamin B_{12} levels, abnormal Schilling test, steatorrhea and malabsorption of fat-soluble vitamins, cholesterol gallstones, calcium oxalate kidney stones
- Extensive small bowel resection: more than 40–50% of the total length of small intestine results in short bowel syndrome, characterized by weight loss and diarrhea, folate, iron, or calcium malabsorption

 ## DIAGNOSIS

- Clinical diagnosis based on presence of diarrhea and malabsorption with prior bowel resection

 ## TREATMENT

TERMINAL ILEAL RESECTION

- Vitamin B_{12} injections IM monthly
- If watery diarrhea, bile salt binding resins (eg, cholestyramine, 2–4 g PO TID with meals)
- If steatorrhea, low-fat diet and vitamins, medium-chain triglycerides
- Calcium supplements to bind oxalate

EXTENSIVE SMALL BOWEL RESECTION

- If the colon is preserved, 100 cm of proximal jejunum may be sufficient to maintain adequate oral nutrition with a low-fat, high–complex-carbohydrate diet
- If the colon has been removed, at least 200 cm of proximal jejunum is typically required to maintain oral nutrition
- Parenteral vitamin supplementation

- Monitor levels of zinc and magnesium should be monitored
- Antidiarrheal agents (eg, loperamide, 2–4 mg PO TID)
- Octreotide
- H_2 receptor antagonists to reduce acid hypersecretion
- TPN required if <100–200 cm of proximal jejunum intact
- TPN has an estimated annual mortality rate of 2–5% resulting from TPN-induced liver disease, sepsis, loss of venous access
- Small intestinal transplantation

Kenneth R. McQuaid, MD

Silicosis

 ## KEY FEATURES

- Extensive or prolonged inhalation of free silica results in small, rounded opacities (silicotic nodules) throughout the lung

 ## CLINICAL FINDINGS

- Calcification of peripheral hilar lymph nodes ("eggshell" calcification) strongly suggests silicosis
- Incidence of pulmonary tuberculosis is increased in patients with silicosis

 ## DIAGNOSIS

- Simple silicosis is usually asymptomatic without effect on pulmonary function tests
- Complicated silicosis presents with large conglomerate densities in the upper lung; dyspnea with restrictive, and obstructive dysfunction is common

 ## TREATMENT

- All patients require a tuberculin skin test and current CXR
- Patients with suspected old pulmonary tuberculosis should be treated with· multidrug regimens

Mark S. Chesnutt, MD
Thomas J. Prendergast, MD

Skin Infections, Streptococcal

 KEY FEATURES

- Group A β-hemolytic streptococci are not normal skin flora
- Usually result from colonization of normal skin by contact with other infected individuals or by preceding streptococcal respiratory infection

 CLINICAL FINDINGS

- Impetigo is a focal, vesicular, pustular lesion with a thick, amber-colored crust that has a "stuck-on" appearance
- Erysipelas is a painful superficial cellulitis that frequently involves the face. It is indurated, slightly elevated, and well demarcated from the surrounding normal skin

 DIAGNOSIS

- Cultures obtained from a wound or pustule are likely to grow group A β-hemolytic streptococci
- Blood cultures are occasionally positive

 TREATMENT

- Parenteral antibiotics are indicated for patients with facial erysipelas or evidence of systemic infection. Penicillin, 2 million units IV q4h, is the drug of choice, or cefazolin, 500 mg IV or IM q8h
- Initial therapy for severely ill patients or those who have risk factors for staphylococcal infection (eg, IV drug use, wound infection, diabetes) should include an agent, such as nafcillin, 1.5 g IV q6h, that also is active against *Staphylococcus aureus*
- Patients who do not require parenteral therapy may be treated with amoxicillin, 750 mg BID for 7–10 days
- Relatively high prevalence of resistance among strains makes macrolides a less attractive alternative for penicillin-allergic patients

Henry F. Chambers, MD

Smoke Inhalation

 KEY FEATURES

- 33% of patients treated for burn injuries also have pulmonary injury from smoke inhalation
- Injury occurs as a result of impaired oxygenation, thermal injury to the upper airway, and chemical injury to the lung

 CLINICAL FINDINGS

- Pulmonary edema, increased upper airway secretions, stridor, and respiratory failure may be present
- ARDS may develop 1–2 days after exposure
- Sloughing of the airway mucosa may occur in 2–3 days, leading to airway obstruction, atelectasis, and worsening hypoxemia
- Bacterial colonization and pneumonia are common 5–7 days after exposure

 DIAGNOSIS

- Typically, a history of smoke exposure is easily obtained or presumed
- Examination of the upper airway with a laryngoscope or bronchoscope is superior to physical exam
- Arterial blood gases are necessary to evaluate oxygenation and rule out carbon monoxide poisoning

 TREATMENT

- Supplemental oxygen, humidified air, bronchodilators, and suctioning of mucosal debris and secretions
- Positive end-expiratory pressure has been advocated when there is pulmonary edema
- Corticosteroids are unhelpful and may be harmful
- Monitoring for bacterial infection is important, but prophylactic antibiotics are not recommended

Mark S. Chesnutt, MD
Thomas J. Prendergast, MD

Spherocytosis, Hereditary

 KEY FEATURES

- Disorder of RBC membrane, leading to chronic hemolytic anemia
- Autosomal dominant disease of variable severity
- Membrane defect is in spectrin, an RBC skeleton protein, resulting in decreased surface–volume ratio and a spherical RBC shape, which is less deformable
- Hemolysis occurs because of trapping of RBCs within the spleen

 CLINICAL FINDINGS

- Often diagnosed in childhood, but milder cases discovered incidentally late in life. Family history often positive
- Anemia may or may not be present because bone marrow may be able to compensate for shortened RBC survival
- Severe anemia (aplastic crisis) may occur with folic acid deficiency or infection
- Jaundice and pigment (calcium bilirubinate) gallstones and cholecystitis in chronic hemolysis
- Palpable spleen

 DIAGNOSIS

- Microcytic, hyperchromic anemia of variable severity; hematocrit may be normal
- Increased mean corpuscular hemoglobin concentration, often >36 g/dL
- Reticulocytosis present
- Peripheral blood smear shows a small percentage of spherocytes, small cells that have lost their central pallor
- Indirect bilirubin often increased
- Coombs test negative
- Increased osmotic fragility (abnormally vulnerable to swelling induced by hypotonic media), although nonspecific

 TREATMENT

- Folic acid, 1 mg PO qd
- Splenectomy, which eliminates site of hemolysis
- Splenectomy may not be necessary in very mild cases discovered late in adult life

Charles A. Linker, MD

Spinal Cord Compression, Malignant

 ## KEY FEATURES

- Oncological emergency
- Complication of metastatic solid tumor, lymphoma, or myeloma

 ## CLINICAL FINDINGS

- Back pain (in >80%) aggravated by lying down, weight bearing, sneezing, coughing
- Progressive weakness of the lower extremities
- Sensory loss (usually in the lower extremities)
- Less commonly, chest or abdominal pain, signs of nerve root compression
- Late findings: bowel and bladder dysfunction
- Carcinomatous meningitis (leptomeningeal disease) is uncommon (3–8% of all cancers); presents with sequential cranial nerve abnormalities, stroke, hydrocephalus

 ## DIAGNOSIS

- MRI with and without contrast
- Bone radiographs and bone scans useful for detecting vertebral metastases but do not aid in assessing spinal cord or nerve root compromise
- Carcinomatous meningitis diagnosed by gadolinium-enhanced MRI scans showing enhancement of the meninges or by CSF cytology showing malignant cells

 ## TREATMENT

- Emergency surgery yields superior neurological outcomes for lesions involving a single vertebra with extension to only 1 superior or inferior vertebra compared with radiation alone with surgery for nonresponse
- Other indications for emergency surgery include spinal cord compression without a diagnosis of malignancy, already maximal doses of radiation to involved area, or progressive neurological deficits during radiation
- Radiation therapy either as primary therapy or after surgery
- High-dose glucocorticoids (eg, dexamethasone, 10–100 mg IV) as soon as possible followed by lower dose (eg, dexamethasone, 4–6 mg q6h IV PO) throughout course of radiation
- Chemotherapy for lymphomas and multiple myeloma in conjunction with or after radiation
- Carcinomatous meningitis treated with radiation, usually whole brain and spinal cord, or intrathecal chemotherapeutic agents, most commonly methotrexate and cytarabine

Hope Rugo, MD

Spinal Stenosis, Lumbar

 ## KEY FEATURES

- May be congenital or, more commonly, acquired
- Narrowing of the spinal canal most frequently results from enlarging osteophytes at the facet joints, hypertrophy of the ligamentum flavum, and protrusion or bulging of intervertebral disks
- Exactly how spinal stenosis results in pain is not defined
- Most patients with lumbar spinal stenosis are older than 60 yr

 ## CLINICAL FINDINGS

- When low back pain is the chief symptom, it is bilateral and often diffuse over the buttocks
- Gradual onset of pain, weakness, or unsteadiness in both legs precipitated by walking or prolonged standing and relieved by sitting
- The onset of symptoms with standing by itself, the location of the maximal discomfort to the thighs, and the preservation of pedal pulses help distinguish the "pseudoclaudication" of spinal stenosis from true claudication caused by vascular insufficiency
- May have fewer symptoms walking uphill than down

 ## DIAGNOSIS

- MRI
- Differential diagnosis includes claudication (arterial insufficiency), disk herniation, lumbar facet joint degenerative arthritis, sacroiliitis (eg, ankylosing spondylitis, epidural abscess or tumor, piriformis syndrome)

 ## TREATMENT

- Weight loss and exercises aimed at reducing lumbar lordosis, which aggravates symptoms of spinal stenosis
- When disabling symptoms persist, decompressive laminectomy can provide at least short-term relief in about 80% of patients

David B. Hellmann, MD, FACP
John H. Stone, MD, MPH

Sporotrichosis

 KEY FEATURES

- Sporotrichosis is a chronic fungal infection caused by *Sporothrix schenckii*
- Found worldwide; most patients have had contact with soil, sphagnum moss, or decaying wood
- Infection occurs via skin inoculation, usually on the hand, arm, or foot, especially during gardening
- Disseminated sporotrichosis is rare in immunocompetent patients but occurs in immunocompromised patients, especially those with AIDS and alcohol abuse

 CLINICAL FINDINGS

- Begins with a hard, nontender subcutaneous nodule, which later adheres to overlying skin and ulcerates
- Within days to weeks, similar nodules develop along lymphatics draining the area, and these may ulcerate. The lymphatics become indurated and are easily palpated
- Disseminated sporotrichosis presents with widespread cutaneous, lung, bone, joint, and CNS involvement

 DIAGNOSIS

- Cultures are needed to establish the diagnosis
- Antibody tests may be useful in disseminated disease, especially meningitis

 TREATMENT

- Itraconazole, 200–400 mg PO qd, for several months for localized disease and some milder cases of disseminated disease
- Saturated solution of potassium iodide, 5 drops TID, increasing to 40–50 drops TID for several months, is an alternative for localized lymphocutaneous disease
- Amphotericin B, 1–2 g IV, for meningeal and disseminated sporotrichosis
- Surgery usually contraindicated except for simple aspiration of secondary nodules
- Joint involvement may require arthrodesis
- Lymphocutaneous sporotrichosis has a good prognosis; pulmonary, joint, and disseminated disease respond less favorably

Richard J. Hamill, MD

Staphylococci Infections, Coagulase-Negative

 KEY FEATURES

- An important cause of infections of intravascular and prosthetic devices and of wound infection after cardiothoracic surgery
- Less virulent than *S aureus*, and infections tend to be more indolent
- Normal flora of human skin

 CLINICAL FINDINGS

- Often associated with a foreign body
- Fever, a new murmur, instability of the prosthesis, and signs of embolization are evidence of prosthetic valve infection

 DIAGNOSIS

- Infection (vs isolation as a contaminant) is more likely if the patient has a foreign body or an intravascular device in place
- Infection is more likely if the same strain is isolated from 2 or more blood cultures and from the foreign body site
- Contamination is more likely when a single blood culture is positive or if more than 1 strain is isolated from blood cultures. Antimicrobial susceptibility and speciation can help determine whether multiple strains have been isolated

 TREATMENT

- When possible, remove the foreign body or intravascular device. Treatment sometimes with antibiotics alone is preferable, understanding that surgical management may become necessary
- Vancomycin, 1 g IV q12h, is the treatment of choice
- Duration of therapy is not established for infections caused by foreign devices, which may be eliminated by simply removing the infected device
- Treat bone or a prosthetic valve infection for 6 weeks. Vancomycin plus rifampin, 300 mg PO BID, and gentamicin, 1 mg/kg IV q8h, is recommended for prosthetic valve endocarditis caused by methicillin-resistant strains

Henry F. Chambers, MD

Still's Disease, Adult

 KEY FEATURES

- A variant of rheumatoid arthritis
- High spiking fevers are much more prominent, especially at the outset, than in rheumatoid arthritis

 CLINICAL FINDINGS

- The fever is dramatic, often spiking to 40°C, associated with sweats and chills, and then plunging to several degrees below normal
- An evanescent salmon-colored nonpruritic rash, chiefly on the chest and abdomen, is a characteristic feature but is easily missed because it often appears only with the fever spike
- Sore throat
- Lymphadenopathy
- Joint symptoms are mild or absent in the beginning, but a destructive arthritis, especially of the wrists, may develop months later
- Anemia and leukocytosis, with white blood cell counts sometimes exceeding 40,000/mL, are the rule
- About one-third of patients have recurrent episodes

 DIAGNOSIS

- A diagnosis of exclusion (of other causes of fever and arthritis)
- Strongly suggested by the fever pattern, sore throat, and classic rash

 TREATMENT

- About half of the patients respond to high-dose aspirin (eg, 1 g TID) or other NSAIDs
- About half require prednisone, sometimes in doses >60 mg/day

David B. Hellmann, MD, FACP
John H. Stone, MD, MPH

Storage Pool Disease

 KEY FEATURES

- Group of mild bleeding disorders characterized by defective secretion of platelet granule contents (especially adenosine 5′-diphosphate) that stimulate platelet aggregation

 CLINICAL FINDINGS

- Mild increase in bruising and postoperative bleeding

 DIAGNOSIS

- Platelets normal in number and morphology, but bleeding time slightly prolonged, especially after aspirin. Variable abnormalities in platelet aggregation studies

 TREATMENT

- Most do not require treatment. Avoid aspirin. Platelet transfusions transiently correct bleeding tendency
- Desmopressin, 0.3 µg/kg IV q24h, may be helpful

Charles A. Linker, MD

Streptococcal, Group A Infections

 KEY FEATURES

- Arthritis, pneumonia, empyema, endocarditis, and necrotizing fasciitis are relatively uncommon infections that may be caused by group A streptococci

 CLINICAL FINDINGS

- Arthritis generally occurs in association with cellulitis
- Pneumonia and empyema often are characterized by extensive tissue destruction and an aggressive, rapidly progressive clinical course
- Endocarditis (rare) should be suspected when bacteremia accompanies pneumonia, particularly if the patient abuses parenteral drugs. The tricuspid valve is most commonly involved
- Necrotizing fasciitis is a rapidly spreading infection involving the fascia of deep muscle. The clinical findings at presentation range from severe cellulitis to systemic toxicity and severe pain
- Any streptococcal infection, especially necrotizing fasciitis, can be associated with streptococcal toxic shock syndrome, characterized by invasion of skin or soft tissues, acute respiratory distress syndrome, and renal failure

 DIAGNOSIS

- Culture of affected site or blood

 TREATMENT

- Arthritis: IV penicillin G, 2 million units q4h, and frequent percutaneous needle aspiration
- Pneumonia/empyema: high-dose penicillin and chest tube drainage for treatment of the empyema
- Endocarditis: 4 million units of penicillin G q4h for 4 weeks
- Necrotizing fasciitis: Early, extensive débridement is essential for survival
- Toxic shock syndrome: IV penicillin; consider the addition of clindamycin (600 mg IV q8h to halt toxin production) and IV immune globulin

Henry F. Chambers, MD

Stroke, Lacunar

 KEY FEATURES

- Small lesions (usually <5 mm in diameter) that occur in the distribution of short, penetrating arteries in the basal ganglia, pons, cerebellum, anterior limb of the internal capsule, and, less commonly, the deep cerebral white matter
- Risk factors include poorly controlled hypertension and diabetes
- Generally have a good prognosis, with partial or complete resolution often occurring over 4–6 weeks

 CLINICAL FINDINGS

- There are several clinical syndromes:
  - Contralateral pure motor or pure sensory deficit
  - Ipsilateral ataxia with crural paresis
  - Dysarthria with clumsiness of the hand
- Deficits may progress over 24–36 h before stabilizing

 DIAGNOSIS

- Sometimes visible on CT scans as small, punched-out, hypodense areas, but in other patients no abnormality is seen
- In some instances, patients with a clinical syndrome suggestive of lacunar infarction are found on CT scanning to have a severe hemispheric infarct

 TREATMENT

- Treat hypertension or diabetes
- Avoid tobacco use
- Anticoagulation is not indicated
- Aspirin, 325 mg daily, is of uncertain benefit

Michael J. Aminoff, DSc, MD, FRCP

Superior Vena Cava Obstruction

 KEY FEATURES

- A rare disorder caused by partial or complete obstruction of the superior vena cava
- Most frequent causes are (1) superior mediastinal tumors (eg, adenocarcinoma of the lung, lymphoma, thyroid carcinoma, thymoma, teratoma, synovial cell carcinoma, angiosarcoma); (2) chronic fibrotic mediastinitis, either idiopathic or secondary to tuberculosis, histoplasmosis, pyogenic infections, or drugs (eg, methysergide); (3) thrombophlebitis secondary to indwelling central venous catheters or pacemaker wires; (4) aneurysm of the aortic arch; and (5) constrictive pericarditis

 CLINICAL FINDINGS

- Swelling of the neck and face
- Headache
- Dizziness, stupor, syncope
- Visual disturbances
- Bending over or lying down accentuates symptoms
- Dilated anterior chest wall veins and/or collateral veins
- Facial flushing
- Brawny edema and cyanosis of the face and arms
- Cerebral and laryngeal edema

 DIAGNOSIS

- Usually suggested by the history and physical examination
- Duplex ultrasonogram offers limited view of central veins
- CT scan or MRA
- Contrast venography is reserved for patients undergoing surgical or endoscopic treatment

 TREATMENT

- Malignant tumors: endovascular stenting, chemotherapy, or external beam radiation
- Mediastinal fibrosis or constrictive pericarditis: surgical excision of the fibrous tissue or pericardial sac
- Thrombophlebitis: removal of central venous catheter, head elevation, and short-course warfarin anticoagulation or thrombolysis, and venous angioplasty or venous bypass

Louis M. Messina, MD
Laura K. Pak, MD
Lawrence M. Tierney, Jr, MD

Syncope

 KEY FEATURES

- Transient (few seconds to a few minutes) loss of consciousness and postural tone
- Abrupt onset
- Caused by inadequate cerebral blood flow
- Often leads to injury
- Prompt recovery without resuscitative measures
- Causes include cardiac, vascular, and neurological processes
- Most common in the elderly
- More likely in those with heart disease, older men, and young women prone to vasovagal episodes
- 30% of adults will experience ≥1 syncopal episode
- Accounts for ~3% of ER visits

 CLINICAL FINDINGS

VASOVAGAL SYNCOPE

- Caused by excessive vagal tone or impaired reflex control of the peripheral circulation
- The "common faint" occurs most often
- Often initiated by stressful, painful, or claustrophobic experiences
- Nausea, diaphoresis, tachycardia, and pallor are common premonitory symptoms
- Other varieties: carotid sinus hypersensitivity, postmicturition, or cough syncope

ORTHOSTATIC (POSTURAL) SYNCOPE

- Caused by impaired vasoconstrictive response to assuming upright posture, leading to abrupt decrease in venous return
- Occurs in those with advanced age, diabetes or other cause of autonomic neuropathy, blood loss or hypovolemia, and vasodilator, diuretic, or adrenergic-blocker drug therapy

CARDIOGENIC SYNCOPE

- Caused by rhythm disturbances (sick sinus syndrome, atrioventricular block, tachyarrhythmias) or mechanical causes (eg, aortic stenosis, pulmonary stenosis, hypertrophic obstructive cardiomyopathy, pulmonary hypertension, atrial myxoma)
- Episodes are often exertional

DIAGNOSIS

- Initial evaluation yields a specific cause in only 50% of cases
- Physical examination: orthostatic changes in blood pressure and pulse, carotid sinus massage, and cardiac exam
- Resting ECG: arrhythmias, accessory pathways, infarction, hypertrophy, and other abnormalities
- Do tilt-table testing before invasive studies unless clinical and ambulatory ECG evaluation suggests a cardiac cause

VASOVAGAL SYNCOPE

- Characteristic history. Carotid sinus massage under carefully monitored conditions or tilt-table testing may be diagnostic

ORTHOSTATIC SYNCOPE

- >20-mm Hg decline in blood pressure immediately on standing
- Tilt-table testing and Valsalva's maneuver diagnostic

CARDIOGENIC SYNCOPE

- Echocardiography to rule out mechanical causes
- If rhythm disturbance suspected, ambulatory ECG monitoring indicated. May need to repeat several times, up to 3 days
- Event recorder and transtelephone ECG monitoring indicated for more intermittent presyncopal episodes
- Electrophysiological studies indicated for recurrent episodes and nondiagnostic ambulatory ECGs

 TREATMENT

VASOMOTOR SYNCOPE

- Lying down or avoiding the inciting stimuli
- β-blockers may be helpful
- Permanent pacing for those with bradycardic responses to syncope

ORTHOSTATIC SYNCOPE

- Discontinue offending drugs; stand up slowly; fludrocortisone rarely

CARDIOGENIC SYNCOPE

- Treat the underlying disorder

Barry M. Massie, MD
Thomas M. Amidon, MD

Syringomyelia

 KEY FEATURES

- Destruction of gray and white matter adjacent to the central canal of the cervical spinal cord leads to cavitation and fluid collection within the cord
- Associated with Arnold-Chiari malformation, sometimes with accompanying meningomyelocele
- Cord cavitation may also occur with cord injury or neoplasm at any level of the cord

 CLINICAL FINDINGS

- With cervical lesions, there is segmental atrophy, areflexia, and loss of pain and temperature appreciation in a "cape" distribution owing to the destruction of fibers crossing in front of the central canal. Often there is thoracic kyphoscoliosis
- A pyramidal and sensory deficit may be present in the legs
- Upward extension of the cavitation (syringobulbia) leads to dysfunction of the lower brainstem and thus to bulbar palsy, nystagmus, and sensory loss over one or both sides of the face

 DIAGNOSIS

- Plain x-ray films of the skull and cervical spine may show skeletal abnormalities, and CT scans show caudal displacement of the fourth ventricle in Arnold-Chiari malformation. MRI or positive-contrast myelography may demonstrate the malformation itself
- Focal cord enlargement is found at myelography or by MRI in patients with cavitation related to past injury or intramedullary neoplasms

 TREATMENT

- Treatment of Arnold-Chiari malformation with associated syringomyelia is by suboccipital craniectomy and upper cervical laminectomy, with the aim of decompressing the malformation at the foramen magnum
- In cavitation associated with intramedullary tumor, treatment is surgical, but radiation therapy may be necessary if complete removal is not possible

- Posttraumatic syringomyelia is also treated surgically if it leads to increasing neurological deficits or to intolerable pain

Michael J. Aminoff, DSc, MD, FRCP

Tachycardia, Paroxysmal Supraventricular

 KEY FEATURES

- The most common paroxysmal tachycardia
- Often occurs in patients without structural heart disease
- Attacks begin and end abruptly and may last a few seconds to several hours or longer
- In the absence of heart disease, serious effects are rare
- Usually caused by AV nodal reentry tachycardia (AVNRT)
- Less commonly (one third of cases) caused by an AV accessory pathway (AVRT)

 CLINICAL FINDINGS

- Heart rate is 140–240 bpm (usually 160–220 bpm) and is perfectly regular (despite exercise or change in position)
- Patients may be asymptomatic except for awareness of rapid heartbeat
- Some patients have mild chest pain or shortness of breath, especially when episodes are prolonged, even in the absence of associated cardiac abnormalities
- May result from digitalis toxicity, in which case it is commonly associated with AV block

 DIAGNOSIS

- ECG or telemetry: perfectly regular rhythm with heart rate between 140–240 bpm (usually 160–220 bpm). P wave usually differs in contour from sinus beats. Accessory pathways (eg, Wolff-Parkinson-White syndrome) are often associated with a short PR interval and sometimes with an early delta wave at the onset of a wide, slurred QRS complex

 TREATMENT

- Effort should be made to terminate the attack quickly if congestive heart failure, syncope, or angina or if underlying cardiac or coronary disease
- Mechanical measures should be attempted first:
  – Episodes can be aborted with Valsalva's maneuver, stretching the arms and body, lowering the head between the knees, coughing, and breath holding
  – Carotid sinus massage unilaterally (do not perform if the patient has carotid bruits or a history of transient ischemic attacks) for 10–20 s
- Medications: If mechanical measures fail, give adenosine (initial 6 mg IV bolus; then, if no response after 1–2 min, a second 12-mg IV bolus, followed by a third if necessary; Table 40, page 1233)
- Alternative agents for narrow-complex supraventricular tachycardias include IV calcium channel blockers (diltiazem, verapamil), β-blockers (esmolol), and digoxin (Table 40, page 1233)
- Do not use digoxin, verapamil, or β-blockers if premature supraventricular tachycardia is associated with a known or suspected accessory pathway
- Electrical cardioversion: For patients who are hemodynamically unstable or if adenosine and verapamil are contraindicated or ineffective, synchronized electrical cardioversion (beginning at 100 J) is almost always successful
- Avoid electrical cardioversion if digitalis toxicity is suspected or documented
- Radiofrequency ablation is a preventive measure for patients with recurrent symptomatic reentry supraventricular tachycardia, whether from dual pathways within the atrial ventricular node or accessory pathways
- Medications as preventive measure: For narrow-complex supraventricular tachycardias, oral digoxin is the usual first choice. Verapamil, alone or in combination with digitalis, is a second choice. β-blockers are also effective (Table 40, page 1233). Use sotalol or amiodarone in patients with evidence of structural heart disease
- For wide-complex supraventricular tachycardias without atrial fibrillation or flutter (generally resulting from accessory pathways), use a combination of agents to increase refractoriness in the bypass tract (class Ia or Ic antiarrhythmic agents) and in the AV node (verapamil, digoxin, and β- blockers). Class III agents are also sometimes used (Table 40, page 1233)

Barry M. Massie, MD
Thomas M. Amidon, MD

Tachycardia, Ventricular

 KEY FEATURES

- Defined as 3 or more consecutive ventricular premature beats
- The usual rate is 160–240/min and is moderately regular
- Either nonsustained (lasting <30 s) or sustained (>30 s)
- Nonsustained ventricular tachycardia without underlying heart disease is not clearly associated with a poor prognosis
- Sustained ventricular tachycardia usually occurs with cardiac disease and is an unfavorable prognostic sign. When there is significant left ventricular dysfunction, sudden death is common

 CLINICAL FINDINGS

- Causes include acute myocardial infarction, dilated cardiomyopathy, coronary artery disease, hypertrophic cardiomyopathy, mitral valve prolapse, myocarditis, and other forms of myocardial disease
- May be asymptomatic or associated with syncope or milder symptoms of impaired cerebral perfusion

 DIAGNOSIS

- ECG: runs of ≥3 ventricular beats
- The distinction between ventricular tachycardia and aberrant conduction of supraventricular tachycardia may be difficult
- Torsades de pointes is a form of ventricular tachycardia in which QRS morphology twists around the baseline. It has a poor prognosis. It may occur with hypokalemia or hypomagnesemia or with use of drugs that prolong the QT interval

 TREATMENT

- Empiric magnesium replacement 1 g IV
- Nonsustained ventricular tachycardias in the presence of structural heart disease: β-blockers reduce the incidence of sudden death by 40–50%
- Avoid other antiarrhythmic agents (except, possibly, amiodarone)
- Acute sustained ventricular tachycardia:
  – In unstable patients (hypotension, heart failure, or myocardial ischemia),

immediate synchronized DC cardioversion with 100–360 J

- In stable patients, lidocaine 1 mg/kg IV bolus. Procainamide or amiodarone are alternative, second-line agents (Table 40, page 1233)
- Recurrent symptomatic or sustained ventricular tachycardia: implantable cardioverter-defibrillator device
- In patients with preserved left ventricular function: with amiodarone, optimally in combination with a β-blocker
- Electrophysiological studies may help identify candidates for radiofrequency ablation of a tachycardia focus

Barry M. Massie, MD
Thomas M. Amidon, MD

Tardive Dyskinesia

 ## KEY FEATURES

- A syndrome of involuntary stereotyped movements of the face, mouth, tongue, trunk, limbs
- Occurs after months or (typically) years of treatment in 20–35% of neuroleptic users
- Predisposing factors are older age, cigarette smoking, diabetes
- Atypical antipsychotics appear to be lower risk
- Symptoms do not necessarily worsen and may improve even when neuroleptics are continued

 ## CLINICAL FINDINGS

- Early signs: fine worm-like tongue movements, difficulty sticking out the tongue, facial tics, increased blink frequency, jaw movements
- Late signs: lip smacking, chewing motions, disturbed gag reflex, puffing of the cheeks, respiratory distress, disturbed speech, choreoathetoid movements

 ## DIAGNOSIS

- Differentiate early signs of TD from reversible side effects of meds such as tricyclic antidepressants and anti-parkinsonism agents

 ## TREATMENT

- Emphasis should be on prevention by using lowest effective dose
- Stop anticholinergic drugs and gradually discontinue neuroleptic dose
- Benzodiazepines, buspirone, phosphatidylcholine, clonidine, calcium channel blockers, vitamin E, and propranolol are of limited usefulness in treating symptoms

Stuart J. Eisendrath, MD
Jonathan E. Lichtmacher, MD

Theophylline Toxicity

 ## KEY FEATURES

- The usual serum half-life of theophylline is 4–6 h, but this may increase to >20 h after overdose

 ## CLINICAL FINDINGS

- Mild intoxication causes nausea, vomiting, tachycardia, tremulousness
- Ventricular and supraventricular tachyarrhythmias, hypotension, and seizures occur in severe intoxication (serum levels >100 mg/L). Status epilepticus is common and often intractable to usual anticonvulsants. Symptoms may be delayed for hours after acute ingestion, especially if a sustained-release preparation was taken
- Serious toxicity may develop at lower levels (ie, 40–60 mg/L) with chronic intoxication

 ## DIAGNOSIS

- Serum theophylline concentration
- Hypokalemia, hyperglycemia, and metabolic acidosis are common after acute overdose

 ## TREATMENT

- After acute ingestion, administer activated charcoal
- Repeated doses of activated charcoal may enhance gut decontamination and elimination by "gut dialysis"
- Whole-bowel irrigation should be considered for large ingestions involving sustained-release preparations
- Hemodialysis is indicated for status epilepticus or markedly elevated serum theophylline levels (eg, >100 mg/L after acute overdose or possibly for levels >60 mg/L with chronic intoxication)
- Treat seizures with benzodiazepines (lorazepam, 2–3 mg IV, or diazepam, 5–10 mg IV) or phenobarbital (10–15 mg/kg IV). Phenytoin is not effective
- Hypotension and tachycardia may respond to β-blocker therapy even in low doses: Administer esmolol, 25–50 µg/kg/min by IV infusion, or propranolol, 0.5–1 mg IV

Kent R. Olsen, MD

Thiamin Deficiency

 KEY FEATURES

- Most commonly caused by alcoholism
- Other causes are malabsorption, dialysis, chronic protein-calorie undernutrition
- Symptoms and signs can be precipitated by IV dextrose solutions in patients with marginal thiamin stores

 CLINICAL FINDINGS

- Early manifestations include anorexia, muscle cramps, paresthesias, and irritability
- Advanced deficiency affects chiefly the cardiovascular system (wet beriberi) or the nervous system (dry beriberi)
- Wet beriberi occurs with severe physical exertion and high carbohydrate intake and is characterized by marked peripheral vasodilation resulting in high-output heart failure with dyspnea, tachycardia, cardiomegaly, pulmonary and peripheral edema, and warm extremities
- Dry beriberi occurs with inactivity and low-calorie intake and involves both the peripheral and central nervous systems. Peripheral nerve involvement includes symmetric motor and sensory neuropathy with pain, paresthesias, and loss of reflexes in legs more than the arms. CNS involvement includes Wernicke-Korsakoff syndrome

 DIAGNOSIS

- Diagnosis can usually be established by clinical response to empiric thiamine therapy
- Biochemical tests: erythrocyte transketolase activity and urinary thiamin excretion coefficient greater than 15–20% suggest thiamin deficiency

 TREATMENT

- Thiamine, 50–100 mg IV or IM qd for the first few days, followed by 5–10 mg PO qd
- Therapeutic doses of other water-soluble vitamins
- Treatment results in complete resolution of symptoms and signs in 50% of patients (25% immediately and another 25% over days); the remaining 50% obtain only partial resolution or no benefit

Robert B. Baron, MD, MS

Tinnitus

 KEY FEATURES

- Tinnitus is the perception of abnormal ear or head noises. Persistent tinnitus usually indicates the presence of sensory hearing loss
- Intermittent periods of mild, high-pitched tinnitus lasting for several minutes are common in normal-hearing persons
- When severe and persistent, tinnitus may interfere with sleep and the ability to concentrate, resulting in considerable psychological distress

 CLINICAL FINDINGS

- Pulsatile tinnitus—often described by the patient as listening to one's own heartbeat—should be distinguished from tonal tinnitus. Although often caused by conductive hearing loss, this symptom may be far more serious and indicates a vascular abnormality such as glomus tumor, carotid vaso-occlusive disease, arteriovenous malformation, or aneurysm
- A staccato "clicking" tinnitus may result from middle-ear muscle spasm, sometimes associated with palatal myoclonus. The patient typically perceives a rapid series of popping noises, lasting seconds to a few minutes, accompanied by a fluttering feeling in the ear

 DIAGNOSIS

- MR angiography should be considered to establish the diagnosis in cases in which vascular abnormality suspected

 TREATMENT

- The most important treatment is avoidance of exposure to excessive noise, ototoxic agents, and other factors that may cause cochlear damage
- Masking the tinnitus with music or through amplification of normal sounds with a hearing aid may bring relief
- Oral antidepressants (eg, nortriptyline at an initial dosage of 50 mg PO at bedtime) often impact tinnitus-induced sleep disorder and depression

Robert K. Jackler, MD
Michael J. Kaplan, MD

Toxic Shock Syndrome, *Staphylococcus aureus*

 KEY FEATURES

- Strains of staphylococci may produce toxins that can cause 4 important entities: scalded skin syndrome, typically in children, or bullous impetigo in adults; necrotizing pneumonitis in children; toxic shock syndrome (TSS); and enterotoxin food poisoning
- Most cases (≥90%) of TSS have been reported in women of child-bearing age, especially common within 5 days of the onset of a menstrual period in women who have used tampons
- Nonmenstrual cases of toxic shock syndrome are now about as common as menstrual cases. Organisms from various sites, including the nasopharynx, bones, vagina, and rectum, or wounds have all been associated with the illness

 CLINICAL FINDINGS

- Abrupt onset of fever, vomiting, and watery diarrhea
- A diffuse macular erythematous rash and nonpurulent conjunctivitis are common, and desquamation, especially of the palms and soles, is typical during recovery

 DIAGNOSIS

- Blood cultures are negative because symptoms are due to the effects of the toxin and not to the invasive properties of the organism

 TREATMENT

- Rapid rehydration, antistaphylococcal drugs, management of renal or cardiac failure, and removal of sources of toxin, (eg, removal of tampon, drainage of abscess)

Henry F. Chambers, MD

Tracheal Stenosis

 KEY FEATURES

- As an acquired disorder, usually resulting from previous tracheotomy or endotracheal intubation
- Idiopathic cases occur, mostly in women
- Complications include recurrent pulmonary infection and respiratory failure

 CLINICAL FINDINGS

- Dyspnea, cough, and inability to clear pulmonary secretions occurring weeks to months after tracheal cannulation or intubation

 DIAGNOSIS

- Wheezing, a palpable tracheal thrill, or harsh breath sounds may be detected, but often not until tracheal diameter is decreased by 50%
- Diagnosis is confirmed by plain films or CT of the trachea

 TREATMENT

- Surgical reconstruction, endotracheal stent placement, or laser photoresection

Mark S. Chesnutt, MD
Thomas J. Prendergast, MD

Tremor, Essential

 KEY FEATURES

- The cause is uncertain, but it is sometimes inherited in an autosomal dominant manner
- Tremor may begin at any age and is enhanced by emotional stress

 CLINICAL FINDINGS

- Postural tremor usually involves 1 or both hands, the head, or the hands and head, whereas the legs tend to be spared
- Speech may also be affected if the laryngeal muscles are involved
- Examination reveals no other abnormalities
- Ingestion of a small quantity of alcohol commonly provides remarkable but short-lived relief by an unknown mechanism
- Although the tremor may become more conspicuous with time, it generally leads to little disability, and treatment is often unnecessary
- Occasionally, it interferes with manual skills and leads to impairment of handwriting

 TREATMENT

- Propranolol, either intermittently or indefinitely, in daily doses of 60–240 mg
- Primidone may be helpful, but patients are often very sensitive to it. They are, therefore, started on 50 mg daily, and the daily dose is increased by 50 mg every 2 weeks depending on the response; a maintenance dose of 125 mg TID is commonly effective
- Occasional patients fail to respond to these measures but are helped by alprazolam (up to 3 mg daily in divided doses), clozapine (30–50 mg twice daily), mirtazapine (15 or 30 mg at night), or topiramate (up to 400 mg daily titrated over 6–8 weeks)
- Disabling tremor unresponsive to medical treatment may be helped by unilateral or bilateral high-frequency thalamic stimulation

Michael J. Aminoff, DSc, MD, FRCP

Trench Fever

 KEY FEATURES

- A self-limited, louse-borne relapsing febrile disease caused by *Bartonella quintana*
- Epidemic infection in louse-infested troops and civilians during wars; endemic in scattered geographic areas (eg, Central America)
- An urban equivalent of trench fever has been described among the homeless
- Humans acquire infection when infected lice feces enter sites of skin breakdown

 CLINICAL FINDINGS

- Onset of symptoms is abrupt, and fever lasts 3–5 days with relapses
- The patient complains of weakness and severe pain behind the eyes and typically in the back and legs
- Lymphadenopathy, splenomegaly, and a transient maculopapular rash may appear
- Subclinical infection is frequent, and a carrier state is recognized
- The differential diagnosis includes other febrile, self-limited states such as dengue, leptospirosis, malaria, relapsing fever, and typhus

 DIAGNOSIS

- Blood cultures: *B quintana* will grow in standard BACTEC media, but growth may require incubation for 4–6 weeks
- Positive serology with a compatible clinical syndrome: either documented seroconversion or high titer of antibody (≥ 1:1600) in single ELISA or immunofluorescence test

 TREATMENT

- Doxycycline, 100 mg BID, or azithromycin, 500 mg, for 4–6 weeks for uncomplicated bacteremia, although recovery can occur in the absence of therapy
- Patients with endocarditis should be treated for 4–6 mo, with addition or a third-generation cephalosporin or aminoglycoside for the first 3 weeks

Henry F. Chambers, MD

Tricyclic Antidepressant Overdose

 KEY FEATURES

- TCAs contain both anticholinergic and cardiac depressant properties (quinidine-like sodium channel blockade)
- Newer antidepressants such as trazodone, fluoxetine, paroxetine, sertraline, bupropion, venlafaxine, and fluvoxamine are not chemically related to the TCAs and do not generally produce cardiotoxic effects. However, they may cause seizures and serotonin syndrome (see *Monoamine oxidase inhibitor poisoning/overdose*) in overdoses

 CLINICAL FINDINGS

- Severe symptoms may occur abruptly within 30–60 min after acute overdose. Anticholinergic effects include dilated pupils, tachycardia, dry mouth, flushed skin, muscle twitching, decreased peristalsis
- Quinidine-like cardiotoxic effects include QRS interval widening (>0.12 s), ventricular arrhythmias, atrioventricular block, and hypotension. Seizures and coma are common with severe intoxication. Life-threatening hyperthermia may result from status epilepticus and anticholinergic-induced impairment of sweating

 DIAGNOSIS

- QRS interval correlates with the severity of intoxication more reliably than the serum drug level

 TREATMENT

- Observe patients for at least 6 h, and admit if there are anticholinergic effects or signs of cardiotoxicity
- Administer activated charcoal and consider gastric lavage after recent large ingestions
- Treat cardiotoxic effects with boluses of sodium bicarbonate (50–100 mEq IV). Maintain the pH between 7.45 and 7.50. Alkalinization does not promote excretion of tricyclics

Kent R. Olsen, MD

Tuberculosis, Intestinal

 KEY FEATURES

- Common in developing nations; rare in US
- Incidence in US rising in immigrant groups and patients with AIDS
- Caused by *Mycobacterium tuberculosis* and *M bovis*

 CLINICAL FINDINGS

- Active pulmonary tuberculosis in <50%
- Most frequent involvement is ileocecal
- Chronic abdominal pain, obstructive symptoms, weight loss, diarrhea
- Abdominal mass palpable
- Complications include intestinal obstruction, hemorrhage, fistula formation

 DIAGNOSIS

- PPD skin test may be negative, especially in weight loss or AIDS
- Barium enema, small bowel follow-through
- Colonoscopy
- Differential diagnosis: Crohn's disease, carcinoma, intestinal amebiasis
- Definitive diagnosis by either endoscopic or surgical biopsy revealing acid-fast bacilli and caseating granuloma or by positive cultures
- Detection of tubercle bacilli in biopsy specimens by PCR

 TREATMENT

- Tuberculosis, initial treatment (Table 24, page 1221)
- Antituberculous drugs characteristics (Table 23, page 1221)

Kenneth R. McQuaid, MD

Turner's Syndrome (Gonadal Dysgenesis)

 KEY FEATURES

- Chromosomal disorder associated with primary hypogonadism, short stature, other phenotypic anomalies
- Common cause of primary amenorrhea and early ovarian failure
- Patients with classic syndrome lack 1 X chromosome (45,XO karyotype)
- <3% survive to term; incidence: about 1:10,000 female newborns
- May be diagnosed at birth: small newborns, often with lymphedema
- Often diagnosed in childhood during evaluation for short stature

 CLINICAL FINDINGS

- Features variable and may be subtle in girls with mosaicism
- Short stature, hypogonadism, webbed neck, high-arched palate, short fourth metacarpals, wide-spaced nipples, recurrent otitis media, hypertension, renal abnormalities, coarctation of aorta
- Hypogonadism presents as delayed adolescence (80%) or early ovarian failure (20%)
- Prone to keloid formation after ear piercing or surgery
- Prone to hypothyroidism, diabetes mellitus, dyslipidemia

 DIAGNOSIS

- Serum FSH and LH elevated (primary hypogonadism)
- Karyotype shows 45,XO (or X chromosome abnormalities, or mosaicism)
- Serum growth hormone and IGF-I levels normal (short stature evaluation)
- Yearly examinations and periodic thyroid, lipid, and glucose testing recommended
- Echocardiogram by age 16 yr

 TREATMENT

- Growth hormone, 0.1 unit/kg/day SC, plus an androgen (eg, oxandrolone) for ≥4 yr before epiphyseal fusion increases final height by ~10 cm over mean predicted height of 144.2 cm
- Estrogen therapy begun after age 12 (eg, conjugated estrogens, 0.3 mg PO on days 1–21/mo)

- Hormone replacement therapy begun with estrogen and progestin after growth stops
- Life expectancy is reduced due in part to increased risk for diabetes mellitus, hypertension, dyslipidemia, and osteoporosis

Paul A. Fitzgerald, MD

Typhus, Endemic

 ### KEY FEATURES

- Caused by *Rickettsia typhi* (ubiquitous) and *R felis* (southern US)
- Transmitted from rats (*R typhi*) or domestic animals (opossums, possibly cats) (*R felis*) to humans by fleas
- Less severe disease versus epidemic typhus

 ### CLINICAL FINDINGS

- Gradual onset of malaise, cough, fever, and headache
- Maculopapular rash concentrated on trunk with rapid fading

 ### DIAGNOSIS

- Thrombocytopenia and elevated liver function tests common
- Antibody testing establishes diagnosis

 ### TREATMENT

- Tetracycline, doxycyline, chorampheni-col given until more than 3 full days of defervescence

Wayne X. Shandera, MD
Samuel Shelburne, MD

Typhus, Epidemic Louse-Borne

 ### KEY FEATURES

- Infection with *Rickettsia prowazekii,* parasite of the body louse
- Transmission favored by famine, crowded living conditions, war
- Recrudescent typhus (Brill's disease) can occur years after initial exposure
- Ubiquitous with rare US cases associated with flying squirrels or travel

 ### CLINICAL FINDINGS

- Prodrome of malaise, cough, and headache followed by acute onset of fever, chills, and prostration
- Conjunctivitis, splenomegaly, and macular rash that starts in the axilla common

 ### DIAGNOSIS

- Diffuse symptoms with abrupt onset of fever, chills, and prostration
- Macular rash does not appear in all cases
- Antibodies usually appear within 1 week of symptom onset (IgM for acute disease, IgG for Brill's disease)

 ### TREATMENT

- Tetracycline and chloramphenicol effective when given for 4–10 days

Samuel Shelburne, MD
Wayne X. Shandera, MD

Typhus, Scrub

 ### KEY FEATURES

- Caused by *Orienta tsutsugamushi*, a parasite of rodents, and transmitted by mites
- Mites live on vegetation, but bite humans who contact infested vegetation
- Occurs most commonly in Southeast Asia, western Pacific, and Australia
- Typical incubation period is 7–21 days

 ### CLINICAL FINDINGS

- Malaise, chills, severe headache, backache
- Site of the bite turns from a papule to a flat black eschar with enlarged regional lymph nodes
- Gradual onset of fever with an accompanying macular rash
- Pneumonitis, myocarditis, encephalitis, granulomatous hepatitis, and GI hemorrhage are late complications

 ### DIAGNOSIS

- Fluorescein-labeled antirickettsial assays or enzyme-linked immunoassays are available to make the diagnosis
- PCR is an increasingly used and very sensitive way to confirm the diagnosis

 ### TREATMENT

- Doxycycline or chloramphenicol for 3–7 days
- Mortality rate for untreated patients may be as high as 30%
- Prevention: long-acting miticides and insecticides

Wayne X. Shandera, MD
Samuel Shelburne, MD

Ulnar Neuropathy

 KEY FEATURES

- Likely occur in the elbow region where the nerve runs behind the medial epicondyle and descends into the cubital tunnel
- In the condylar groove, the ulnar nerve is exposed to pressure or trauma. Moreover, any increase in the carrying angle of the elbow, whether congenital, degenerative, or traumatic, may cause excessive stretching of the nerve when the elbow is flexed
- May also result from thickening or distortion of the anatomical structures forming the cubital tunnel, and the resulting symptoms may also be aggravated by flexion of the elbow because the tunnel is then narrowed by tightening of its roof or inward bulging of its floor
- May also develop at the wrist or in the palm of the hand, usually owing to repetitive trauma or to compression from ganglia or benign tumors

 CLINICAL FINDINGS

- Sensory changes in the medial 1½ digits and along the medial border of the hand
- Weakness of the ulnar-innervated muscles in the forearm and hand, with lesions at the elbow
- With a cubital tunnel lesion there may be relative sparing of the flexor carpi ulnaris muscle
- Lesions at the wrist or palm cause weakness, sensory deficits, or both, restricted to the hand

 DIAGNOSIS

- Electrophysiological evaluation using nerve stimulation techniques allows precise localization of the lesion

 TREATMENT

- If repetitive mechanical trauma is responsible, this is avoided by occupational adjustment or job retraining
- If conservative measures are unsuccessful in relieving symptoms and preventing further progression, surgical treatment may be necessary. This consists of nerve transposition if the lesion is in the condylar groove or a release procedure if it is in the cubital tunnel

Michael J. Aminoff, DSc, MD, FRCP

Ureter & Renal Pelvis Cancer

 KEY FEATURES

- Most cancers of the ureter and renal pelvis are transitional cell carcinomas
- Rare; occur more commonly in smokers, those with Balkan nephropathy, those exposed to Thorotrast (a contrast agent with radioactive thorium in use until the 1960s), and those with a long history of analgesic abuse

 CLINICAL FINDINGS

- Gross or microscopic hematuria in most
- Flank pain secondary to bleeding and obstruction less common

 DIAGNOSIS

- Urinary cytology is often positive
- IV pyelography intraluminal filling defect, unilateral nonvisualization of the collecting system, and hydronephrosis
- Differential diagnosis: calculi, blood clots, papillary necrosis, or inflammatory or infectious lesions

 TREATMENT

- Direct biopsy, fulguration, or resection using a ureteroscope
- Treatment is based on the site, size, depth of penetration, and number of tumors present
- Most are excised with nephroureterectomy (renal pelvic and upper ureteral lesions) or segmental excision of the ureter (distal ureteral lesions)
- Endoscopic resection indicated in patients with limited renal function and in the management of focal, low-grade, upper tract cancers

Marshall L. Stoller, MD
Peter R. Carroll, MD, FACS

Urethritis & Cervicitis, Chlamydial

 KEY FEATURES

- *Chlamydia trachomatis* immunotypes D–K are isolated in about 50% of cases of nongonococcal urethritis and cervicitis by appropriate techniques
- Coinfection with gonococci is common
- Postgonococcal (ie, chlamydial) urethritis may persist after successful treatment of the gonococcus

 CLINICAL FINDINGS

- Urethritis and occasionally epididymitis, prostatitis, or proctitis
- Females may be asymptomatic or may have signs and symptoms of cervicitis, salpingitis, or pelvic inflammatory disease

 DIAGNOSIS

- The urethral or cervical discharge tends to be less painful and less purulent in chlamydial versus gonococcal infection
- Direct immunofluorescence assay, ELISA, and a DNA probe test, although less sensitive than culture, are sometimes used to confirm the diagnosis and for screening
- The ligase chain reaction (LCR) test has superior sensitivity compared with all other methods; LCR also has excellent specificity, approaching 100%, and it can be performed on urine. LCR will likely replace all other methods for diagnosis of chlamydial urethritis and cervicitis

 TREATMENT

- Sexual partners of infected patients should also be treated
- Therapy often must be given presumptively
- A single 1-g dose of azithromycin is effective for uncomplicated urethritis and cervicitis and has the advantage of improved patient compliance and minimal toxicity
- Doxycycline, 100 mg BID for 7 days

Henry F. Chambers, MD

Urticaria, Cold

KEY FEATURES

- Can be familial (autosomal dominant) or acquired
- Urticaria may develop on even limited exposure to cold (eg, wind, freezer compartments)
- Most cases of acquired cold urticaria are idiopathic but can be associated with medication (eg, griseofulvin), infection, cryoglobulinemia, or syphilis

CLINICAL FINDINGS

- Usually occurs only on exposed areas, but in markedly sensitive individuals can be generalized and fatal. Immersion in cold water may result in severe systemic reactions, including shock; histamine release occurs

DIAGNOSIS

- Apply ice cube to the forearm skin for 5 min, remove, and observe the area for 10 min. As the skin rewarms, an urticarial wheal appears at the site and may be accompanied by itching

TREATMENT

- Cyproheptadine, 16–32 mg/day in divided doses
- Alternatively, combination of terbutaline, 5 mg TID, and aminophylline, 150 mg TID

Richard Cohen, MD, MPH
Brent R. W. Moelleken, MD, FACS

Uterine Prolapse

KEY FEATURES

- Most commonly occurs as a delayed result of childbirth injury to the pelvic floor (particularly the transverse cervical and uterosacral ligaments). Unrepaired obstetric lacerations of the levator musculature and perineal body augment the weakness. Attenuation of the pelvic structures with aging can worsen the prolapse
- In slight prolapse, the uterus descends only partway down the vagina; in moderate prolapse, the corpus descends to the introitus and the cervix protrudes slightly beyond; and in marked prolapse (procidentia), the entire cervix and uterus protrude beyond the introitus and the vagina is inverted
- Inability to walk comfortably because of protrusion or discomfort from the presence of a vaginal mass is an indication that surgical treatment should be considered

TREATMENT

- The type of surgery depends on extent of prolapse, desire for menstruation, pregnancy, and coitus
- The simplest, most effective procedure is vaginal hysterectomy with appropriate repair of the cystocele and rectocele
- If pregnancy is desired, a partial resection of the cervix with plication of the cardinal ligaments can be attempted
- For older women who do not desire coitus, partial obliteration of the vagina is surgically simple and effective
- A well-fitted vaginal pessary (eg, inflatable doughnut type, Gellhorn pessary) may give relief if surgery is not an option

H. Trent MacKay, MD, MPH

Vasculitis, Cryoglobulinemic

KEY FEATURES

- Type I cryoglobulins (monoclonal proteins that lack rheumatoid factor activity) are more commonly seen in lymphoproliferative disease and usually cause hyperviscosity syndromes rather than vasculitis
- Type II (monoclonal antibody with rheumatoid factor activity) and type III (polyclonal antibody with rheumatoid factor activity) cryoglobulins cause vasculitis and are associated with hepatitis C and connective tissue diseases (eg, Sjögren's syndrome)

CLINICAL FINDINGS

- Palpable purpura
- Peripheral neuropathy
- Abnormal liver function tests
- Abdominal pain
- Pulmonary disease

DIAGNOSIS

- Compatible clinical picture and a positive serum test for cryoglobulins

DIFFERENTIAL DIAGNOSIS

- Other causes of palpable purpura and peripheral neuropathy (eg, polyarteritis nodosa, rheumatoid arthritis, sarcoidosis)

ASSOCIATED CONDITIONS

- Hepatitis C or B
- Lymphoproliferative disorders (eg, multiple myeloma, Waldenström's macroglobulinemia, chronic lymphocytic leukemia
- Sjögren's syndrome, systemic lupus erythematosus

TREATMENT

- Because 90% of cryoglobulinemia cases are associated with hepatitis C infections, the optimal approach to treatment is viral suppression with interferon-α with or without ribavirin
- Because immunosuppressive agents may facilitate viral replication, corticosteroids, cyclophosphamide, and other agents should be reserved for organ-threatening complications

David B. Hellmann, MD, FACP
John H. Stone, MD, MPH

Vegetative State, Persistent

 KEY FEATURES

- Patients with severe bilateral hemispheric disease may show some improvement from an initially comatose state, so that, after a variable interval, they appear to be awake but display no movement
- This persistent vegetative state has been variously referred to as akinetic mutism, apallic state, or coma vigil
- Most patients in a persistent vegetative state will die in months or years, but partial recovery has occasionally occurred and in rare instances has been sufficient to permit communication or even independent living

 CLINICAL FINDINGS

- Patients appear to be awake with open eyelids but lie motionless
- No evidence of awareness or higher mental activity
- Simulate coma
- Unresponsive

 DIAGNOSIS

- Obtain the expertise of a clinician familiar with this syndrome to aid in the diagnosis

Michael J. Aminoff, DSc, MD, FRCP

Venous Thrombosis, Intracranial

 KEY FEATURES

- May occur in association with intracranial or maxillofacial infections, hypercoagulable states, polycythemia, sickle cell disease, and cyanotic congenital heart disease and in pregnancy or during the puerperium

 CLINICAL FINDINGS

- Headache, focal or generalized convulsions, drowsiness, confusion, increased intracranial pressure, focal neurological deficits, and less commonly meningeal irritation

 DIAGNOSIS

- Confirmed by CT scanning and MRI, MR venography, or angiography

 TREATMENT

- Anticonvulsant drugs if seizures have occurred
- Antiedema agents (eg, dexamethasone, 4 mg QID and continued as necessary) to reduce intracranial pressure
- Anticoagulation with dose-adjusted IV heparin followed by oral anticoagulation for 6 mo reduces morbidity and mortality of venous sinus thrombosis

Michael J. Aminoff, DSc, MD, FRCP

Ventricular Septal Defect

 KEY FEATURES

- Persistent opening in upper interventricular septum permits blood to shunt from high-pressure left ventricle into low-pressure right ventricle
- Large shunts associated with early left ventricular failure; survival beyond age 40 unusual
- Shunt reversal occurs in ~25% of cases, producing Eisenmenger's syndrome
- Moderate shunts may lead to pulmonary vascular disease and right-sided failure
- Small to moderate shunts are often asymptomatic

 CLINICAL FINDINGS

- Large shunts: loud, harsh holosystolic murmur in third and fourth left interspaces along the sternum and, occasionally, mid-diastolic flow murmur
- Systolic thrill common
- Clinical evidence of pulmonary hypertension often more informative than murmur itself

 DIAGNOSIS

- ECG: left and/or right ventricular hypertrophy if shunt is reversed
- CXR: increased pulmonary vascularity
- Echo-Doppler is diagnostic and can assess magnitude of shunt and pulmonary artery pressure
- Cardiac catheterization permits definitive diagnosis and can measure pulmonary vascular resistance

 TREATMENT

- Endocarditis occurs more often with smaller shunts. Antibiotic prophylaxis is mandatory
- Small shunts in asymptomatic patients do not require closure
- Large shunts should be surgically or percutaneously repaired
- Surgical mortality is 2–3%, but ≥50% if pulmonary hypertension is present

- Surgery is contraindicated in Eisenmenger's syndrome
- Defer surgery until late childhood unless signs of heart failure or pulmonary hypertension

Barry Massie, MD
Thomas Amidon, MD

Vestibular Schwannoma (Acoustic Neuroma)

 KEY FEATURES

- Eighth nerve schwannomas are among the most common of intracranial tumors
- The lesions arise within the internal auditory canal and gradually grow to involve the cerebellopontine angle, eventually compressing the pons and resulting in hydrocephalus
- Any individual with a unilateral or asymmetric sensorineural hearing loss should be evaluated for an intracranial mass lesion
- Other lesions of the cerebellopontine angle such as meningioma and epidermoids may have similar audiovestibular manifestations

 CLINICAL FINDINGS

- Typical auditory symptoms are unilateral hearing loss with deterioration of speech discrimination exceeding that predicted by the degree of pure-tone loss
- Nonclassic presentations, such as sudden unilateral hearing loss, are fairly common
- Vestibular dysfunction more often takes the form of continuous dysequilibrium than episodic vertigo

 DIAGNOSIS

- Diagnosis is made by enhanced MRI, although auditory evoked responses may have a role in screening

 TREATMENT

- Microsurgical excision is most often indicated, although small tumors in older individuals may be managed with stereotactic radiotherapy or simply followed with serial imaging studies

Robert K. Jackler, MD
Michael J. Kaplan, MD

Vibrio Infections

 KEY FEATURES

- Vibrios other than *Vibrio cholerae* that cause human disease are *V parahaemolyticus*, *V vulnificus*, and *V alginolyticus*
- Infection is acquired by exposure to organisms in raw or undercooked crustaceans or shellfish and warm (>20°C) ocean waters and estuaries
- Oysters are implicated in up to 90% of food-related cases

 CLINICAL FINDINGS

- *V parahaemolyticus* causes acute watery diarrhea with fever, typically within 24 h after ingestion of contaminated shellfish. The disease is self-limited, and antimicrobial therapy is usually not necessary
- *V vulnificus* and *V alginolyticus*, neither of which cause diarrhea, cause cellulitis and primary bacteremia after ingestion of contaminated shellfish or exposure to seawater. Cellulitis with or without sepsis may occur with bulla formation, necrosis, and extensive soft tissue destruction, at times requiring débridement and amputation. The infection can progress rapidly and be severe in immunocompromised individuals, especially those with cirrhosis, with death rates of 50%

 DIAGNOSIS

- Culture

 TREATMENT

- Doxycycline, 100 mg BID for 7–10 days, is the drug of choice for cellulitis or bacteremia; fluoroquinolones and third-generation cephalosporins are also effective
- *V vulnificus* may be susceptible to penicillin, ampicillin, cephalosporins, chloramphenicol, aminoglycosides, and fluoroquinolones
- *V parahaemolyticus* and *V alginolyticus* are resistant to penicillin and ampicillin, but susceptibilities otherwise are similar to *V vulnificus*

Henry F. Chambers, MD

Visceral Artery Aneurysms

 KEY FEATURES

- Hepatic artery aneurysms are the most common
- Splenic artery aneurysms ~30%
- Superior mesenteric, celiac, gastric, and gastroepiploic artery aneurysms each represent about 5% of visceral aneurysms
- Aneurysms of mesenteric branch vessels are rare and often associated with connective tissue disease or vasculitis
- Historically, almost 10% mortality rate, resulting from rupture
- Causes of hepatic artery aneurysm: medial degeneration, injury during cholangiography, hepatic biopsy, blunt abdominal trauma
- Causes of splenic artery aneurysm: medial fibroplasia, portal hypertension, splenomegaly, pregnancy, amphetamine use, local inflammation
- Causes of superior mesenteric artery aneurysm: infective endocarditis, septic emboli, atherosclerosis
- Causes of celiac artery aneurysm: atherosclerosis

 CLINICAL FINDINGS

- Usually asymptomatic. If ruptured, patient presents with hypotension and abdominal pain

 DIAGNOSIS

- High-resolution CT scanning has increased detection of incidental mesenteric aneurysms

 TREATMENT

- Asymptomatic splenic aneurysms <2 cm rarely rupture
- No treatment unless patient is pregnant
- For symptomatic aneurysms and aneurysms >2 cm, surgical aneurysmectomy or aneurysmorrhaphy with ligation of branches, or endovascular (embolization) management

Louis M. Messina, MD
Laura K. Pak, MD
Lawrence M. Tierney, Jr, MD

Vitamin A Deficiency

 KEY FEATURES

- One of the most common vitamin deficiency syndromes in developing countries
- Most common cause of blindness
- Usually results from fat malabsorption syndromes or mineral oil laxative abuse
- Occurs most commonly in the elderly and urban poor

 CLINICAL FINDINGS

- Night blindness (early)
- Dryness (xerosis) of conjunctivae and small white patches on the conjunctivae (Bitot's spots) (early)
- Ulceration and necrosis of the cornea (keratomalacia), perforation, endophthalmitis, and blindness (late)
- Xerosis and hyperkeratinization of the skin
- Loss of taste

 DIAGNOSIS

- Abnormalities of dark adaptation
- Serum vitamin A levels below normal range of 30–65 mg/dL

 TREATMENT

- Early deficiency: 30,000 IU of vitamin A PO qd for 1 week
- Advanced deficiency: 20,000 units/kg PO qd for at least 5 days

Robert B. Baron, MD, MS

Vitamin B$_6$ Deficiency

 KEY FEATURES

- Vitamin B$_6$ deficiency most commonly occurs as a result of alcoholism or a variety of medications, especially isoniazid, cycloserine, penicillamine, and oral contraceptives
- Can also occur in a number of inborn errors of metabolism

 CLINICAL FINDINGS

- Mouth soreness, glossitis, cheilosis, weakness, irritability
- Severe deficiency can result in peripheral neuropathy, anemia, seizures

 DIAGNOSIS

- Serum pyridoxal phosphate levels are below normal levels of >50 ng/mL

 TREATMENT

- Vitamin B$_6$, 10–20 mg PO qd, is usually adequate
- Patients taking medications that interfere with pyridoxine metabolism may need doses as high as 100 mg/day. Inborn errors of metabolism require up to 600 mg/day
- Prophylaxis with vitamin B$_6$ should be routinely given to patients receiving medications (such as isoniazid) that interfere with pyridoxine metabolism and to elderly, urban poor, or alcoholic patients

Robert B. Baron, MD, MS

Vitamin C Deficiency

 KEY FEATURES

- Vitamin C deficiency is most commonly due to dietary inadequacy among urban poor, elderly, and chronic alcoholics and to chronic illnesses such as cancer and chronic renal failure

 CLINICAL FINDINGS

- Early: nonspecific malaise and weakness
- Late: scurvy, characterized initially by perifollicular hyperkeratotic papules, petechiae and purpura, splinter hemorrhages, bleeding gums, hemarthroses, and subperiosteal hemorrhages and in late stages by edema, oliguria, neuropathy, intracerebral hemorrhage, and death
- Anemia is common
- Wound healing is impaired

 DIAGNOSIS

- Characteristic skin lesions
- Atraumatic hemarthrosis
- Low plasma ascorbic acid levels, typically <0.1 mg/dL

TREATMENT

- Ascorbic acid (vitamin C), 300–1000 mg PO qd

Robert B. Baron, MD, MS

Vitamin E Deficiency

 KEY FEATURES

- Most commonly results from severe malabsorption (eg, cystic fibrosis), abetalipoproteinemia (genetic disorder), chronic cholestatic liver disease, including biliary atresia

 CLINICAL FINDINGS

- Areflexia, disturbances of gait, decreased proprioception and vibration, and ophthalmoplegia

 DIAGNOSIS

- Low plasma vitamin E levels, below 0.5–0.7 mg/dL

 TREATMENT

- Vitamin E, although optimum therapeutic dose has not been clearly defined

Robert B. Baron, MD, MS

Vitamin K Deficiency

 KEY FEATURES

- Vitamin K plays role in coagulation as a cofactor for the posttranslational carboxylation of factors II, VII, IX, and X. These modified factors are better able to participate in activation of factors X and II. Without this carboxylation, hemostasis is impaired
- Vitamin K is supplied exogenously in diet (primarily in leafy vegetables) and endogenously from synthesis by intestinal bacteria
- May be due to poor diet, malabsorption, and broad-spectrum antibiotics that suppress colonic flora
- Body stores of vitamin K are small; deficiency may develop in 1 week

 CLINICAL FINDINGS

- No specific clinical features
- Bleeding may occur at any site

 DIAGNOSIS

- PT prolonged to greater extent than PTT
- Only PT prolonged with mild vitamin K deficiency; fibrinogen level, thrombin time, and platelet count not affected
- Response to vitamin K therapy distinguishes it from hepatic coagulopathy
- Surreptitious warfarin use causes laboratory features indistinguishable from vitamin K deficiency

 TREATMENT

- Vitamin K, 15 mg SC once completely corrects laboratory abnormalities in 12–24 h
- Prognosis excellent; vitamin K deficiency is completely corrected with replacement

Charles A. Linker, MD

Vocal Cord Dysfunction

 KEY FEATURES

- A syndrome of acute and chronic upper airway obstruction characterized by paradoxical vocal cord adduction

 CLINICAL FINDINGS

- May present as dyspnea and wheezing and be confused with asthma
- Symptoms will not respond to a bronchodilator

 DIAGNOSIS

- Direct visualization of adduction of the vocal cords with both inspiration and expiration is diagnostic
- Spirometry will show evidence of upper airway obstruction but will be normal immediately after an attack
- Bronchial provocation test will be normal

 TREATMENT

- Speech therapy

Mark S. Chesnutt, MD
Thomas J. Prendergast, MD

Weakness & Paralysis

 KEY FEATURES

- Loss of muscle power may result from central disease involving the upper or lower motor neurons; from peripheral disease involving the roots, plexus, or peripheral nerves; from disorders of neuromuscular transmission; or from primary disorders of muscle

 CLINICAL FINDINGS

- Weakness resulting from upper motor neuron lesions is characterized by selective involvement of certain muscle groups and is associated with spasticity, increased tendon reflexes, and extensor plantar responses
- Lower motor neuron lesions lead to muscle wasting as well as weakness, with flaccidity and loss of tendon reflexes, but no change in the plantar responses unless the neurons subserving them are directly involved
- Fasciculations may be evident over affected muscles only in lower motor neuron or more peripheral neuropathic lesions
- In distinguishing between a root, plexus, or peripheral nerve lesion, the distribution of the motor deficit and of any sensory changes is of particular importance
- In disturbances of neuromuscular transmission, weakness is patchy in distribution, often fluctuates over short periods of time, and is not associated with sensory changes
- In myopathic disorders, weakness is usually most marked proximally in the limbs, is not associated with sensory loss or sphincter disturbance, and is not accompanied by muscle wasting or loss of tendon reflexes, at least not until an advanced stage

 DIAGNOSIS

- See individual disorders

 TREATMENT

- See individual disorders

Michael J. Aminoff, DSc, MD, FRCP

Wernicke's Encephalopathy

 KEY FEATURES

- Caused by thiamine deficiency
- In US, occurs most commonly in alcoholic patients
- It may also occur in patients with AIDS, in patients with hyperemesis gravidarum, or after surgery for morbid obesity

 CLINICAL FINDINGS

- Triad of confusion, ataxia, and nystagmus leading to ophthalmoplegia (lateral rectus muscle weakness, conjugate gaze palsies)
- Peripheral neuropathy may be present

 DIAGNOSIS

- The diagnosis is confirmed by the response to treatment within 1 or 2 days, which must not be delayed while laboratory confirmation is obtained

 TREATMENT

- In suspected cases, thiamine 50 mg, is given IV immediately and then IM on a daily basis until a satisfactory diet can be ensured
- IV glucose given before thiamine may precipitate the syndrome or worsen the symptoms

Michael J. Aminoff, DSc, MD, FRCP

Yellow Fever

 KEY FEATURES

- Zoonotic viral infection transmitted by the bite of the *Aedes* mosquito
- Found in South America and sub-Saharan Africa
- Incubation period is typically 3–6 days
- Adults and children equally susceptible

 CLINICAL FINDINGS

- Mild form (85%): fevers, malaise, retro-orbital pain, nausea, photophobia, bradycardia
- Severe form (15%): begins with the same symptoms as the mild form of the disease; then, after initial remission of symptoms, a toxic phase ensues with fever, bradycardia, hypotension, jaundice, delirium, hemorrhage

 DIAGNOSIS

- Leukopenia often but not always present
- Abnormal liver function tests, including prolonged PT
- Proteinuria, often in large quantities
- Serological diagnosis with rapid enzyme immunoassay

 TREATMENT

- Supportive measures, including analgesia and hydration
- No specific antiviral therapy
- Prevention: A highly effective and safe vaccine is available and should be used when living or traveling to endemic areas
- Mosquito control measures

Wayne X. Shandera, MD
Samuel Shelburne, MD

Reference
Tables

Table 1. Acetaminophen, COX-2 inhibitors, and useful nonsteroidal anti-inflammatory drugs.[1]

Drug	Usual Dose for Adults ≥ 50 kg	Usual Dose for Adults < 50 kg	Cost per Unit	Cost for 30 Days[2]	Comments[3]
Acetaminophen[4] (Tylenol, Datril, etc)	650 mg q4h or 975 mg q6h	10–15 mg/kg q4h (oral); 15–20 mg/kg q4h (rectal)	$0.04/325 mg (oral) OTC; $0.50/325 mg (rectal) OTC	$14.40 (oral); $180.00 (rectal)	Not an NSAID because it lacks peripheral anti-inflammatory effects. Equivalent to aspirin as analgesic and antipyretic agent.
Aspirin[5]	650 mg q4h or 975 mg q6h	10–15 mg/kg q4h (oral); 15–20 mg/kg q4h (rectal)	$0.03/325 mg OTC; $0.24/300 mg (rectal) OTC	$10.80 (oral); $86.40 (rectal)	Available also in enteric-coated form that is more expensive and more slowly absorbed but better tolerated.
Celecoxib[4] (Celebrex)	200 mg qd (osteoarthritis); 100–200 mg bid (rheumatoid arthritis)	100 mg qd–bid	$1.58/100 mg; $2.76/200 mg	$82.80 OA; $165.60 RA	Cyclooxygenase-2 inhibitors. No antiplatelet effects. Lower doses for elderly who weigh < 50 kg. Lower incidence of endoscopic gastrointestinal ulceration. Not known if true lower incidence of gastrointestinal bleeding. Can increase lithium levels. Celecoxib contraindicated in sulfonamide allergy.
Valdecoxib[4] (Bextra)	10 mg qd for OA or RA	10 mg qd	$2.92/10 mg or 20 mg	$87.60	
Rofecoxib[4] (Vioxx)	12.5–25 mg qd for OA	12.5 mg qd	$2.76/12.5 mg or $2.76/25 mg	$82.80 OA	
Choline magnesium salicylate[6] (Trilasate)	1000–1500 mg tid	25 mg/kg tid	$0.68/500 mg	$183.60	Salicylates cause less gastrointestinal distress and renal impairment than NSAIDs but are probably less effective in pain management than NSAIDs.
Choline salicylate[6] (Arthropan)	870 mg q3–4h		$48.93/480 mL; 174 mg/mL OTC	$98.00	Minimal antiplatelet effects.
Diclofenac (Voltaren, Cataflam, others)	50–75 mg bid–tid		$0.91/50 mg; $1.06/75 mg	$81.90; $95.40	May impose higher risk of hepatotoxicity. Low incidence of gastrointestinal side effects. Enteric-coated product; slow onset. Can increase lithium levels.
Diclofenac Sustained Release (Voltaren-XR)	100–200 mg qd		$4.20/100 mg	$252.00	
Diflunisal[7] (Dolobid)	500 mg q12h		$1.29/500 mg	$77.40	Fluorinated acetylsalicylic acid derivative.
Etodolac (Lodine)	200–400 mg q6–8h		$1.42/300 mg	$170.40	Perhaps less gastrointestinal toxicity.
Fenoprofen calcium (Nalfon)	300–600 mg q6h		$0.47/300 mg or 600 mg	$56.40	Perhaps more side effects than others, including tubulointerstitial nephritis.
Flurbiprofen (Ansaid)	50–100 mg tid–qid		$0.79/50 mg; $1.19/100 mg	$94.80; $142.80	Adverse gastrointestinal effects may be more common among elderly.
Ibuprofen (Motrin, Advil, Rufen, others)	400–800 mg q6h	10 mg/kg q6–8h	$0.20/400 mg Rx; $0.28/600 mg Rx; $0.05/200 mg OTC	$48.00; $33.60; $9.00	Relatively well tolerated. Less gastrointestinal toxicity. Can increase lithium levels.
Indomethacin (Indocin, Indometh, others)	25–50 mg bid–qid		$0.37/25 mg; $0.63/50 mg	$44.40; $75.60	Higher incidence of dose-related toxic effects, especially gastrointestinal and bone marrow effects. Can increase lithium levels.

(continued)

Table 1. Acetaminophen, COX-2 inhibitors, and useful nonsteroidal anti-inflammatory drugs.[1] (continued)

Drug	Usual Dose for Adults ≥ 50 kg	Usual Dose for Adults < 50 kg	Cost per Unit	Cost for 30 Days[2]	Comments[3]
Ketoprofen (Orudis, Oruvail, others)	25–75 mg q6–8h (max 300 mg/d)		$0.96/50 mg Rx; $1.07/ 75 mg Rx; $0.10/12.5 mg OTC	$172.80; $128.40; $18.00	Lower doses for elderly.
Ketorolac tromethamine (Toradol)	10 mg q4–6h to a maximum of 40 mg/d PO		$0.93/10 mg	Not recommended	Short-term use (< 5 days) only; otherwise, increased risk of gastrointestinal side effects.
Ketorolac tromethamine[8] (Toradol)	60 mg initially, then 30 mg q6h IM		$7.40/30 mg	Not recommended	Intramuscular NSAID as alternative to opioid. Lower doses for elderly. Short-term use (< 5 days) only.
Magnesium salicylate (various)	650 mg q4h		$0.17/325 mg OTC	$40.80	
Meclofenamate sodium[9] (Meclomen)	50–100 mg q6h		$3.40/100 mg	$408.00	Diarrhea more common.
Mefenamic acid (Ponstel)	250 mg q6h		$1.39/250 mg	$166.80	
Nabumetone (Relafen)	500–1000 mg once daily (max dose 2000 mg/d)		$1.30/500 mg; $1.53/750 mg	$137.70	May be less ulcerogenic than ibuprofen, but overall side effects may not be less.
Naproxen (Naprosyn, Anaprox, Aleve [OTC], others)	250–500 mg q6–8h	5 mg/kg q8h	$1.16/500 mg Rx; $0.10/ 220 mg OTC	$104.40 $9.00 OTC	Generally well tolerated. Lower doses for elderly. Can increase lithium levels.
Oxaprozin (Daypro)	600–1200 mg once daily		$1.51/600 mg	$90.60	Similar to ibuprofen. May cause rash, pruritus, photosensitivity.
Piroxicam (Feldene)	20 mg daily		$2.64/20 mg	$79.20	Single daily dose convenient. Long half-life. May cause higher rate of gastrointestinal bleeding and dermatologic side effects. Can increase lithium levels.
Sodium salicylate	325–650 q3–4h		$0.06/650 mg OTC	$14.40	
Sulindac (Clinoril)	150–200 mg bid		$0.98/150 mg; $1.21/200 mg	$58.80; $72.60	May cause higher rate of gastrointestinal bleeding. May have less nephrotoxic potential.
Tolmetin (Tolectin)	200–600 mg qid		$0.65/200 mg; $1.30/600 mg	$78.00; $156.00	Perhaps more side effects than others, including anaphylactic reactions.

OTC = over-the-counter; Rx = prescription; OA = osteoarthritis; RA = rheumatoid arthritis.

[1] Modified from Jacox AK et al: *Management of Cancer Pain: Quick Reference Guide for Clinicians No. 9.* AHCPR Publication No. 94–0593. Rockville, MD: Agency for Health Care Policy and Research, Public Health Service, U.S. Department of Health and Human Services. March 1994.

[2] Average wholesale price (AWP, for AB-rated generic when available) for quantity listed. Source: *Drug Topics Red Book,* May 2003; Vol. 22, No. 5. AWP may not accurately represent the actual pharmacy cost because wide contractual variations exist among institutions.

[3] The adverse effects of headache, tinnitus, dizziness, confusion, rashes, anorexia, nausea, vomiting, gastrointestinal bleeding, diarrhea, nephrotoxicity, visual disturbances, etc, can occur with any of these drugs. Tolerance and efficacy are subject to great individual variations among patients.

[4] Acetaminophen, celecoxib, rofecoxib, and valdecoxib lack the antiplatelet activities of most NSAIDs.

[5] May inhibit platelet aggregation for 1 week or more and may cause bleeding.

[6] May have minimal antiplatelet activity.

[7] Administration with antacids may decrease absorption.

[8] Has the same gastrointestinal toxicities as oral NSAIDs.

[9] Coombs-positive autoimmune hemolytic anemia has been associated with prolonged use.

Table 2. Useful opioid agonist analgesics.[1]

Drug	Approximate Equianalgesic Dose[2]		Usual Starting Dose				Potential Advantages	Potential Disadvantages
			Adults ≥ 50 kg Body Weight		Adults < 50 kg Body Weight			
	Oral	Parenteral	Oral	Parenteral	Oral	Parenteral		
OPIOID AGONISTS[3]								
Morphine[4]	30 mg q3–4h (repeat around-the-clock dosing); 60 mg q3–4h (single or intermittent dosing)	10 mg q3–4h	30 mg q3–4h; $0.18/15 mg	10 mg q3–4h; $0.65/10 mg	0.3 mg/kg q3–4h	0.1 mg/kg q3–4h	Standard of comparison; multiple dosage forms available.	No unique problems when compared with other opioids.
Morphine controlled-release[4] (MS Contin, Roxanol, Oramorph)	90–120 mg q12h	Not available	90–120 mg q12h; $1.69/30 mg	Not available	Not available	Not available		
Hydromorphone[4] (Dilaudid)	7.5 mg q3–4h	1.5 mg q3–4h	6 mg q 3–4h; $0.37/2 mg	1.5 mg q3–4h; $1.04/2 mg	0.06 mg/kg q3–4h	0.015 mg/kg q3–4h	Similar to morphine. Available in injectable high-potency preparation, rectal suppository.	Short duration.
Levorphanol (Levo-Dromoran)	4 mg q6–8h	2 mg q6–8h	4 mg q6–8h; $0.87/2 mg	2 mg q6–8h; $3.96/2 mg	0.04 mg/kg q6–8h	0.02 mg q6–8h	Longer-acting than morphine sulfate.	
Meperidine[5] (Demerol)	300 mg q2–3h; normal dose 50–150 mg q3–4h	100 mg q3h; $0.68/50	Not recommended; $0.68/50 mg	100 mg q3h; $1.09/100 mg	Not recommended	0.75 mg/kg q2–3h	May be useful for acute pain if the patient is intolerant to morphine.	Short duration. Metabolite in high concentrations may cause seizures.
Methadone (Dolophine, others)	20 mg q6–8h	10 mg q6–8h	20 mg q6–8h; $0.15/10 mg	10 mg q6–8h; $.80/10 mg	0.2 mg/kg q6–8h	0.1 mg/kg q6–8h	Somewhat longer-acting than morphine. Useful in cases of intolerance to morphine.	Analgesic duration shorter than plasma duration. May accumulate, requiring close monitoring during first weeks of treatment.
Oxymorphone[3] (Numorphan)	Not available	1 mg q3–4h	Not available	1 mg q3–4h; $2.95/1 mg				
Codeine[6,7] (with aspirin or acetaminophen)[8]	180–200 mg q3–4h; normal dose, 15–60 mg q4–6h	130 mg q3–4h	60 mg q4–6h; $0.46/60 mg	60 mg q2h (IM/SC); $1.06/60 mg	0.5–1 mg/kg q3–4h	Not recommended	Similar to morphine.	

(continued)

Table 2. Useful opioid agonist analgesics.[1] (continued)

| | Approximate Equianalgesic Dose[2] | | Usual Starting Dose | | | | Potential Advantages | Potential Disadvantages |
| | | | Adults ≥ 50 kg Body Weight | | Adults < 50 kg Body Weight | | | |
Drug	Oral	Parenteral	Oral	Parenteral	Oral	Parenteral		
COMBINATION OPIOID-NSAID OR ANTIDEPRESSANT PREPARATIONS								
Hydroco-done[6] (in Lorcet, Lortab, Vicodin, others)[8]	30 mg q3–4h	Not available	10 mg q3–4h; $0.32/ 5 mg	Not available	0.2 mg/kg q3–4h	Not available		Combination with acetaminophen limits dosage titration.
Oxycodone[6] (Roxico-done, Percocet, Percodan, Tylox, others)[8]	30 mg q3–4h	Not available	10 mg q3–4h; $0.26/ 5 mg	Not available	0.2 mg/kg q3–4h	Not available	Similar to morphine.	Combination with acetaminophen and aspirin limits dosage titration.
Oxycodone Con-trolled Release (Oxycon-tin)	40 mg q12h	Not available	20–40 mg q12h; $2.57/ 20 mg					

[1]Modified from Jacox AK et al: *Management of Cancer Pain: Quick Reference Guide for Clinicians No. 9.* AHCPR Publication No. 94–0593. Rockville, MD. Agency for Health Care Policy and Research, Public Health Service, U.S. Department of Health and Human Services. March 1994. Reproduced in part from Hosp Formul 1994;29(8 Part 2):586. (Erstad BL: A rational approach to the management of acute pain states.) Copyright by Advanstar Communications, Inc.

[2]Published tables vary in the suggested doses that are equianalgesic to morphine. Clinical response is the criterion that must be applied for each patient; titration to clinical efficacy is necessary. Because there is not complete cross-tolerance among these drugs, it is usually necessary to use a lower than equianalgesic dose initially when changing drugs and to retitrate to response.

[3]*Caution:* Recommended doses do not apply for adult patients with renal or hepatic insufficiency or other conditions affecting drug metabolism.

[4]*Caution:* For morphine, hydromorphone, and oxymorphone, rectal administration is an alternative route for patients unable to take oral medications. Equianalgesic doses may differ from oral and parenteral doses. A short-acting opioid should normally be used for initial therapy.

[5]Not recommended for chronic pain. Doses listed are for brief therapy of acute pain only. Switch to another opioid for long-term therapy.

[6]*Caution:* Doses of aspirin and acetaminophen in combination products must also be adjusted to the patient's body weight (Table 1).

[7]*Caution:* Doses of codeine above 60 mg often are not appropriate because of diminishing incremental analgesia with increasing doses but continually increasing nausea, constipation, and other side effects.

[8]*Caution:* Monitor total acetaminophen dose carefully, including any OTC use. Total acetaminophen dose maximum 4 g/d. If liver impairment or heavy alcohol use, maximum is 2 g/d.

Note: Average wholesale price (AWP, generic when available) for quantity listed. Source: *Drug Topics Red Book,* May 2003; Vol. 22, No. 5. AWP may not accurately represent the actual pharmacy because wide contractual variations exist among institutions.

Table 3. Simple geriatric screen.

Assessment Procedure	Abnormal	Action
Do you have difficulty with eyesight? Jaeger Card or Snellen chart Test each eye (with glasses)	Yes Can't read 20/40	Refer
Whisper short sentence from 6–12 inches (out of view) or audiometry	Unable to hear	Cerumen check Refer
"Touch the back of your head with your hands" "Pick up the pencil"	Unable to do either	Further examination Consider occupational therapy?
"Rise from your chair (do not use arms to get up), walk 10 feet, walk back to the chair, and sit down"	Observed problem, or unable to perform in < 15 seconds	Formal balance and gait evaluation; further examination; home evaluation and physical therapy
"Have you had any falls in the last year?" "Do you have trouble with stairs, lighting, bathroom, or other home hazards?"	Yes Yes to any	Formal balance and gait evaluation Home evaluation, physical therapy
Body mass index < 21 or weight loss exceeding 5%	Yes to either	Nutrition evaluation
"Do you have a problem with urine leaks or accidents?"	Yes	Incontinence evaluation
"Over the past month, have you often been bothered by feeling sad, depressed, or hopeless?" "During the last month, have you often been bothered by little interest or pleasure in doing things?"	Yes to either	Geriatric Depression Scale or other depression assessment
Name three objects: ask again in 3 minutes	Unable to recall	Mini-Mental State examination (Figure 1)

Do you have problems with any of the following areas? Who assists? Do you use devices to help you? (For "yes" answers, consider referral to occupational therapy, physical therapy, social services.)

–Strenuous activities (eg, fast walking, bicycling) –Cooking –Shopping –Heavy housework (eg, washing windows) –Doing laundry –Transportation by driving or bus –Managing finances	–Transferring out of bed –Dressing –Using the toilet –Eating –Walking –Bathing (sponge bath, tub, shower)

COMPLETE IF INDICATED CLINICALLY
(Ask general question and then ask specific questions to the right.)

Orientation *(Score 1 for each correct. max = 10)*

Where are you?   Name this place (building or hospital)
What floor are you on now?
What state are you in?
What country are you in?
(If not in a country, score correct if city is correct.)
What city are you in (or near) now?

What is the date today?   What year is it?
What season is it?
What month is it?
What is the day of the week?
What is the date today?

Registration *(Score 1 for each object correctly repeated. max = 3)*

Name three objects (ball, flag, and tree) and have patient repeat them.
(Say objects at about 1 word per second. If patient misses object, ask patient to repeat them after you until he/she learns them. Stop at 6 repeats.)

Attention and calculation *(Score 1 for each correct to 65. max = 5)*

Subtract 7s from 100 in a serial fashion to 65
(Alternatively, ask serial 3s from 20 or spell WORLD backwards.)

Recall *(Score 1 for each object recalled. max = 3)*

Do you recall the names of the three objects?

Language *(max = 8)*

Ask the patient to provide names of a watch and pen as you show them to him/her
(Score 1 for each object correct. max = 2)
Repeat "No ifs, ands, or buts."
(Only one trial. Score 1 if correct. max = 1)
Give the patient a piece of plain blank paper and say, "Take the paper in your right hand (1), fold it in half (2), and put it on the floor (3)."
(Score 1 for each part done correctly. max = 3)
Ask the patient to read and perform the following task written on paper: "Close your eyes."
(Score 1 if patient closes eyes. max = 1)
Ask the patient to write a sentence on a piece of paper.
(Score total of 1 if sentence has a subject, object and verb. max = 1)

Construction

Ask patient to copy the two interlocking pentagons.
(Score total of 1, if all 10 angles are present and the two angles intersect. Ignore tremor and rotation. max = 1)

Total Score *(Maximum = 30)*

Figure 1. Mini-mental State Exam. (Adapted from Folstein MF et al: Mini-mental state: a practical method for grading the cognitive state of patients for the clinician. J Psychiatr Res 1975;12:189.)

Table 4. Yesavage's Geriatric Depression Scale (short form).

1. Are you basically satisfied with your life? (no)
2. Have you dropped many of your activities and interests? (yes)
3. Do you feel that your life is empty? (yes)
4. Do you often get bored? (yes)
5. Are you in good spirits most of the time? (no)
6. Are you afraid that something bad is going to happen to you? (yes)
7. Do you feel happy most of the time? (no)
8. Do you often feel helpless? (yes)
9. Do you prefer to stay home at night, rather than go out and do new things? (yes)
10. Do you feel that you have more problems with memory than most? (yes)
11. Do you feel it is wonderful to be alive now? (no)
12. Do you feel pretty worthless the way you are now? (yes)
13. Do you feel full of energy? (no)
14. Do you feel that your situation is hopeless? (yes)
15. Do you think that most persons are better off than you are? (yes)

Score one point for each response that matches the yes-or-no answer after the question.
Scores: Normal 3 ± 2; Mildly depressed: 7 ± 3; Very depressed: 12 ± 2.

Table 5. Fall risk factors and targeted interventions.

Risk Factor	Targeted Intervention
Postural hypotension (> 20 mm Hg drop in systolic BP, or systolic BP < 90 mm Hg)	Behavioral recommendations, such as hand clenching, elevation of head of bed; discontinuation or substitution of high-risk medications
Use of benzodiazepine or sedative-hypnotic	Education about sleep hygiene; discontinuation or substitution of medications
Use of 3 prescription medications	Review of medications
Environmental hazards	Appropriate changes; installation of safety equipment (eg, grab bars)
Gait impairment	Gait training, assistive devices, balance or strengthening exercises
Impairment in transfer or balance	Balance exercises, training in transfers, environmental alterations (eg, grab bars)
Impairment in leg or arm muscle strength or limb range of motion	Exercise with resistance bands or putty, with graduated increases in resistance

Table 6. Useful topical dermatologic therapeutic agents.

Agent	Formulations, Strengths, and Prices[1]	Apply	Potency Class	Common Indications	Comments
Corticosteroids					
Hydrocortisone acetate	Cream 1%: $3.42/30 g Ointment 1%: $3.54/30 g Lotion 1%: $20.20/120 mL	bid	Low	Seborrheic dermatitis. Pruritus ani. Intertrigo.	Not the same as hydrocortisone butyrate or valerate! Not for poison oak! OTC lotion (Aquinil HC). OTC solution (Scalpicin, T Scalp).
	Cream 2.5%: $8.84/30 g Ointment 2.5%: $8.84/30 g Lotion 2.5%: $52.03/60 mL	bid	Low	As for 1% hydrocortisone.	Perhaps better for pruritus ani. Not clearly better than 1%. More expensive. Not OTC.
Alclometasone dipropionate (Aclovate)	Cream 0.05%: $19.71/15 g Ointment 0.05%: $41.09/45 g	bid	Low	As for hydrocortisone.	More efficacious than hydrocortisone. Perhaps causes less atrophy.
Desonide	Cream 0.05%: $18.17/15 g Ointment 0.05%: $45.92/60 g Lotion 0.05%: $36.69/60 mL	bid	Low	As for hydrocortisone. For lesions on face or body folds resistant to hydrocortisone.	More efficacious than hydrocortisone. Can cause rosacea or atrophy. Not fluorinated.
Prednicarbate (Dermatop)	Emollient cream 0.1%: $16.81/15 g Ointment 0.1%: $16.81/15g	bid	Medium	As for triamcinolone.	May cause less atrophy. No generic formulations. Preservative-free.
Triamcinolone acetonide	Cream 0.1%: $2.70/15 g Ointment 0.1%: $2.70/15 g Lotion 0.1%: $13.64/60 mL	bid	Medium	Eczema on extensor areas. Used for psoriasis with tar. Seborrheic dermatitis and psoriasis on scalp.	Caution in body folds, face. Economical in 0.5-lb and 1-lb sizes for treatment of large body surfaces. Economical as solution for scalp.
	Cream 0.025%: $1.82/15 g Ointment 0.025%: $4.26/80 g	bid	Medium	As for 0.1% strength.	Possibly less efficacy and few advantages over 0.1% formulation.
Fluocinolone acetonide	Cream 0.025%: $3.05/15 g Ointment 0.025%: $4.20/15 g	bid	Medium	As for triamcinolone.	
	Solution 0.01%: $11.00/60 mL	bid	Medium	As for triamcinolone solution.	
Mometasone furoate (Elocon)	Cream 0.1%: $25.08/15 g Ointment 0.1%: $25.08/15 g Lotion 0.1%: $51.92/60 mL	qd	Medium	As for triamcinolone.	Often used inappropriately on the face or in children. Not fluorinated.
Diflorasone diacetate	Cream 0.05%: $35.52/15 g Ointment 0.05%: $50.91/30 g	bid	High	Nummular dermatitis. Allergic contact dermatitis. Lichen simplex chronicus.	
Amcinonide (Cyclocort)	Cream 0.1%: $18.52/15 g Ointment 0.1%: $20.58/15 g	bid	High	As for betamethasone.	
Fluocinonide (Lidex)	Cream 0.05%: $9.00/15 g Gel 0.05%: $21.01/15 g Ointment 0.05%: $20.85/15 g Solution 0.05%: $26.08/60 mL	bid	High	As for betamethasone. Gel useful for poison oak.	Economical generics. Lidex cream can cause stinging on eczema. Lidex emollient cream preferred.

(continued)

Table 6. Useful topical dermatologic therapeutic agents. (continued)

Agent	Formulations, Strengths, and Prices[1]	Apply	Potency Class	Common Indications	Comments
Betamethasone dipropionate (Diprolene)	Cream 0.05%: $7.80/15 g Ointment 0.05%: $9.40/15 g Lotion 0.05%: $18.01/60 mL	bid	Ultra-high	For lesions resistant to high-potency steroids. Lichen planus. Insect bites.	Economical generics available.
Clobetasol propionate (Temovate)	Cream 0.05%: $23.99/15 g Ointment 0.05%: $23.99/15 g Lotion 0.05%: $53.10/50 mL	bid	Ultra-high	As for betamethasone dipropionate.	Somewhat more potent than diflorasone. Limited to 2 continuous weeks of use. Limited to 50 g or less per week. Cream may cause stinging; use "emollient cream" formulation. Generic available.
Halobetasol propionate (Ultravate)	Cream 0.05%: $32.16/15 g Ointment 0.05%: $32.16/15 g	bid	Ultra-high	As for clobetasol.	Same restrictions as clobetasol. Cream does not cause stinging. Compatible with calcipotriene (Dovonex).
Flurandrenolide (Cordran)	Tape: $18.84/80″ × 30″ roll	q12h	Ultra-high	Lichen simplex chronicus.	Protects the skin and prevents scratching.
Nonsteroidal anti-inflammatory agents					
Tacrolimus (Protopic)	Ointment 0.1%: $64.09/30 g Ointment 0.03%: $59.95/30 g	bid	N/A	Atopic dermatitis.	Steroid substitute not causing atrophy or striae. Burns in ≥ 40% of patients with eczema.
Pimecrolimus (Elidel)	Cream 1%: $47.52/30 g	bid	N/A	Atopic dermatitis.	Steroid substitute not causing atrophy or striae. Does not burn.
Antibiotics (for acne)					
Clindamycin phosphate	Solution 1%: $11.52/30 mL Gel 1%: $32.12/30 mL Lotion 1%: $44.68/60 mL Pledget 1%: $46.40/60	bid	N/A	Mild papular acne.	Lotion is less drying for patients with sensitive skin.
Erythromycin	Solution 2%: $7.53/60 mL Gel 2%: $24.73/30 g Pledget 2%: $25.34/60	bid	N/A	As for clindamycin.	Many different manufacturers. Economical.
Erythromycin/ Benzoyl peroxide (Benzamycin)	Gel: $58.94/23.3 g Gel: $124.05/46.6 g	bid	N/A	As for clindamycin. Can help treat comedonal acne.	No generics. More expensive. More effective than other topical antibiotics. Main jar requires refrigeration.
Clindamycin/ Benzoyl peroxide (Benzaclin)	Gel: $57.75/25 g Gel: $109.73/50 g	bid		As for benzamycin.	No generic. More effective than either agent alone.
Antibiotics (for impetigo)					
Mupirocin (Bactroban)	Ointment 2%: $43.85/22 g Cream 2%: $30.22/15 g	tid	N/A	Impetigo, folliculitis.	Because of cost, use limited to tiny areas of impetigo. Used in the nose twice daily for 5 days to reduce staphylococcal carriage.
Antifungals					
Clotrimazole	Cream 1%: $4.50/15 g OTC Solution 1%: $15.52/30 mL	bid	N/A	Dermatophyte and candida infections.	Available OTC. Inexpensive generic cream available.
Miconazole	Cream 2%: $3.20/30 g OTC	bid	N/A	As for clotrimazole.	As for clotrimazole.

(continued)

Table 6. Useful topical dermatologic therapeutic agents. (continued)

Agent	Formulations, Strengths, and Prices[1]	Apply	Potency Class	Common Indications	Comments
Other imidazoles					
Econazole (Spectazole)	Cream 1%: $18.78/15 g	qd	N/A	As for clotrimazole.	No generic. Somewhat more effective than clotrimazole and miconazole.
Ketoconazole	Cream 2%: $16.46/15 g	qd	N/A	As for clotrimazole.	No generic. Somewhat more effective than clotrimazole and miconazole.
Oxiconazole (Oxistat)	Cream 1%: $22.82/15 g Lotion 1%: $38.41/30 mL	bid	N/A		
Sulconazole (Exelderm)	Cream 1%: $12.56/15 g Solution 1%: $27.05/30 mL	bid	N/A	As for clotrimazole.	No generic. Somewhat more effective than clotrimazole and miconazole.
Other antifungals					
Butenafine (Mentax) (Lotrimin Ultra, OTC)	Cream 1%: $35.18/15 g Cream 1%: $8.28/12 g	qd	N/A	Dermatophytes.	Fast response; high cure rate; expensive. Available OTC.
Ciclopirox (Loprox) (Penlac)	Cream 0.77%: $40.71/30 g Lotion 0.77%: $82.81/60 mL Solution 8%: $126.26/6.6 mL	bid	N/A	As for clotrimazole.	No generic. Somewhat more effective than clotrimazole and miconazole.
Naftifine (Naftin)	Cream 1%: $41.62/30 g Gel 1%: $66.93/60 mL	qd	N/A	Dermatophytes.	No generic. Somewhat more effective than clotrimazole and miconazole.
Terbinafine (Lamisil)	Cream 1%: $6.79/12 g OTC	qd	N/A	Dermatophytes.	Fast clinical response. OTC.
Antipruritics					
Camphor/ menthol	Compounded lotion (0.5% of each)	bid–tid	N/A	Mild eczema, xerosis, mild contact dermatitis.	
Pramoxine hydrochloride (Prax)	Lotion 1%: $12.40/120 mL	qid	N/A	Dry skin, varicella, mild eczema, pruritus ani.	OTC formulations (Prax, Aveeno Anti-Itch Cream or Lotion; Itch-X Gel). By prescription mixed with 1% or 2% hydrocortisone.
Doxepin (Zonalon)	Cream 5%: $35.98/30 g	qid	N/A	Topical antipruritic, best used in combination with appropriate topical steroid to enhance efficacy.	Can cause sedation.
Emollients					
Aveeno	Cream, lotion, others	qd–tid	N/A	Xerosis, eczema.	Choice is most often based on personal preference by patient.
Aqua glycolic	Cream, lotion, shampoo, others	qd–tid	N/A	Xerosis, ichthyosis, keratosis pilaris. Mild facial wrinkles. Mild acne or seborrheic dermatitis.	Contains 8% glycolic acid. Available from other makers, eg, Alpha Hydrox, or generic 8% glycolic acid lotion. May cause stinging on eczematous skin.
Aquaphor	Ointment: $3.68/52.5 g	qd–tid	N/A	Xerosis, eczema. For protection of area in pruritus ani.	Not as greasy as petrolatum.
Carmol	Lotion 10%: $8.25/180 mL Cream 20%: $7.59/90 g	bid	N/A	Xerosis.	Contains urea as humectant. Nongreasy hydrating agent (10%); debrides keratin (20%).
Complex 15	Lotion: $6.48/240 mL Cream: $4.82/75 g	qd–tid	N/A	Xerosis. Lotion or cream recommended for split or dry nails.	Active ingredient is a phospholipid.

(continued)

Table 6. Useful topical dermatologic therapeutic agents. (continued)

Agent	Formulations, Strengths, and Prices[1]	Apply	Potency Class	Common Indications	Comments
DML	Cream, lotion, facial moisturizer	qd–tid	N/A	As for Complex 15.	Face cream has sunscreen.
Dermasil	Lotion, cream	qd–tid	N/A	Xerosis, eczema.	
Eucerin	Cream: $5.10/120 g Lotion: $5.10/240 mL	qd–tid	N/A	Xerosis, eczema.	Many formulations made. Eucerin Plus contains alpha-hydroxy acid and may cause stinging on eczematous skin. Facial moisturizer has SPF 25 sunscreen.
Lac-Hydrin-Five	Lotion: $10.12/240 mL OTC	bid	N/A	Xerosis, ichthyosis, keratosis pilaris.	Rx product is 12%.
Lubriderm	Lotion: $5.03/300 mL	qd–tid	N/A	Xerosis, eczema.	Unscented usually preferred.
Neutrogena	Cream, lotion, facial moisturizer: $7.39/240 mL	qd–tid	N/A	Xerosis, eczema.	Face cream has titanium-based sunscreen.
SBR Lipocream	Cream: $6.78/30 g	qd–tid	N/A	Xerosis, eczema.	Less greasy but effective moisturizer.
Triceram Cream	Cream: $30.00–$31.50/3.4 oz tube	bid	N/A	Xerosis, eczema.	Contains ceramide; antiinflammatory and nongreasy moisturizer.
U-Lactin	Lotion: $7.13/240 mL	qd	N/A	Hyperkeratotic heels.	Moisturizes and removes keratin.

[1]Average wholesale price (AWP, for AP-rated generic when available) for quantity listed. AWP may not acurately represent the actual pharmacy cost because wide contractual variations exist among institutions. Source: *Drug Topics Red Book,* May 2003; Vol. 22, No. 5.

Table 7. Morphologic categorization of skin lesions and diseases.

Pigmented	Freckle, lentigo, seborrheic keratosis, nevus, blue nevus, halo nevus, dysplastic nevus, melanoma
Scaly	Psoriasis, dermatitis (atopic, stasis, seborrheic, chronic allergic contact or irritant contact), xerosis (dry skin), lichen simplex chronicus, tinea, tinea versicolor, secondary syphilis, pityriasis rosea, discoid lupus erythematosus, exfoliative dermatitis, actinic keratoses, Bowen's disease, Paget's disease, intertrigo
Vesicular	Herpes simplex, varicella, herpes zoster, dyshidrosis (vesicular dermatitis of palms and soles), vesicular tinea, dermatophytid, dermatitis herpetiformis, miliaria, scabies, photosensitivity
Weepy or encrusted	Impetigo, acute contact allergic dermatitis, any vesicular dermatitis
Pustular	Acne vulgaris, acne rosacea, folliculitis, candidiasis, miliaria, any vesicular dermatitis
Figurate ("shaped") erythema	Urticaria, erythema multiforme, erythema migrans, cellulitis, erysipelas, erysipeloid, arthropod bites
Bullous	Impetigo, blistering dactylitis, pemphigus, pemphigoid, porphyria cutanea tarda, drug eruptions, erythema multiforme, toxic epidermal necrolysis
Papular	Hyperkeratotic: warts, corns, seborrheic keratoses Purple-violet: lichen planus, drug eruptions, Kaposi's sarcoma Flesh-colored, umbilicated: molluscum contagiosum Pearly: basal cell carcinoma, intradermal nevi Small, red, inflammatory: acne, miliaria, candidiasis, scabies, folliculitis
Pruritus[1]	Xerosis, scabies, pediculosis, bites, systemic causes, anogenital pruritus
Nodular, cystic	Erythema nodosum, furuncle, cystic acne, follicular (epidermal) inclusion cyst
Photodermatitis (photodistributed rashes)	Drug, polymorphic light eruption, lupus erythematosus
Morbilliform	Drug, viral infection, secondary syphilis
Erosive	Any vesicular dermatitis, impetigo, aphthae, lichen planus, erythema multiforme
Ulcerated	Decubiti, herpes simplex, skin cancers, parasitic infections, syphilis (chancre), chancroid, vasculitis, stasis, arterial disease

[1]Not a morphologic class but included because it is one of the most common dermatologic presentations.

Table 8. Skin reactions due to systemic drugs.

Reaction	Appearance	Distribution and Comments	Common Offenders
Toxic erythema	Morbilliform, maculo-papular, exanthematous reactions.	The commonest skin reaction to drugs. Often more pronounced on the trunk than on the extremities. In previously exposed patients, the rash may start in 2–3 days. In the first course of treatment, the eruption often appears about the seventh to ninth days. Fever may be present.	Antibiotics (especially ampicillin and trimethoprim-sulfamethoxazole), sulfonamides, and related compounds (including thiazide diuretics, furose-mide, and sulfonylurea hypoglycemic agents), and barbiturates.
Erythema multiforme major	Target-like lesions. Bullae may occur. Mucosal involvement.	Mainly on the extensor aspects of the limbs.	Sulfonamides, penicillamine, barbitu-rates, and NSAIDs.
Erythema nodosum	Inflammatory cutaneous nodules.	Usually limited to the extensor aspects of the legs. May be accompanied by fever, arthralgias, and pain.	Oral contraceptives.
Allergic vasculitis	Inflammatory changes may present as urticaria that lasts over 24 hours, hemorrhagic papules ("palpable purpura"), vesicles, bullae, or necrotic ulcers.	Most severe on the legs.	Sulfonamides, indomethacin, phenytoin, allopurinol, and ibuprofen.
Purpura	Itchy, petechial macular rash.	Dependent areas. Results most typically from thrombo-cytopenia.	Thiazides, sulfonamides, sulfonylureas, barbiturates, quinine, and sulindac.
Eczema	Similar to contact dermatitis.	A rare epidermal reaction in patients previously sensitized by external exposure who are given the same or a related substance systemically.	Penicillin, neomycin, phenothiazines, and local anesthetics.
Exfoliative dermatitis and erythroderma	Red and scaly.	Entire skin surface.	Allopurinol, sulfonamides, isoniazid, gold, or carbamazepine.
Photosensitivity: in-creased sensitivity to light, often of ultraviolet A wavelengths, but may be due to UVB or visible light as well	Sunburn, vesicles, papules in photodistrib-uted pattern.	Exposed skin of the face, the neck, and the backs of the hands and, in women, the lower legs. Exaggerated response to ultraviolet light. On occasion, ultraviolet emission from fluorescent lighting may be sufficient.	Sulfonamides and sulfonamide-related compounds (thiazide diuretics, furosemide, sulfonylureas), tetracyclines (especially demeclocy-cline), phenothiazines, sulindac, amiodarone, and NSAIDs.
Drug-related lupus erythematosus	May present with a photosensitive rash accompanied by fever, polyarthritis, myalgia, and serositis.	Less severe than systemic lupus erythematosus, sparing the kidneys and central nervous system. Recovery often follows drug withdrawal.	Hydralazine, procainamide; less often, isoniazid, phenytoin, lisinopril, hydrochlorothiazide; may cause subacute lupus erythematosus.
Lichenoid and lichen planus–like eruptions	Pruritic, erythematous to violaceous polygonal papules that coalesce or expand to form plaques.	May be in photo- or nonphotodistributed pattern.	Bismuth, carbamazepine, chlordiaze-poxide, chloroquine, chlorpropamide, dapsone, ethambutol, furosemide, gold salts, hydroxychloroquine, levamisole, meprobamate, methyl-dopa, paraphenylenediamine salts, penicillamine, phenothiazines, pin-dolol, propranolol, quinidine, quinine, quinacrine, streptomycin, sulfo-nylureas, tetracyclines, thiazides, and triprolidine.
Fixed drug eruptions	Single or multiple demar-cated, round, erythema-tous plaques that often become hyperpig-mented.	Recur at the same site when the drug is repeated. Hyperpigmentation, if present, remains after healing.	Numerous drugs, including antimicro-bials, analgesics, barbiturates, car-diovascular drugs, heavy metals, antiparasitic agents, antihistamines, phenolphthalein, ibuprofen, and naproxen.

(continued)

Table 8. Skin reactions due to systemic drugs. (continued)

Reaction	Appearance	Distribution and Comments	Common Offenders
Toxic epidermal necrolysis	Large sheets of erythema, followed by separation, which looks like scalded skin.	Rare.	In adults, the eruption has occurred after administration of many classes of drugs, particularly barbiturates, phenytoin, sulfonamides, and NSAIDs.
Urticaria	Red, itchy wheals that vary in size from <1 cm to many centimeters. May be accompanied by angioedema.	Chronic urticaria is rarely caused by drugs.	Acute urticaria: penicillins, NSAIDs, sulfonamides, opiates, and salicylates. Angioedema is common in patients receiving ACE inhibitors.
Pruritus	Itchy skin without rash.		Pruritus ani may be due to overgrowth of candida after systemic antibiotic treatment. NSAIDs may cause pruritus without a rash.
Hair loss		Hair loss most often involves the scalp, but other sites may be affected.	A predictable side effect of cytotoxic agents and oral contraceptives. Diffuse hair loss also occurs unpredictably with a wide variety of other drugs, including anticoagulants, antithyroid drugs, newer antimicrobials, cholesterol-lowering agents, heavy metals, corticosteroids, androgens, NSAIDs, retinoids (isotretinoin, etretinate), and beta-blockers.
Pigmentary changes	Flat hyperpigmented areas.	Forehead and cheeks (chloasma, melasma). The most common pigmentary disorder associated with drug ingestion. Improvement is slow despite stopping the drug.	Oral contraceptives are the usual cause.
	Blue-gray discoloration.	Light-exposed areas.	Chlorpromazine and related phenothiazines.
	Brown or blue-gray pigmentation.	Generalized.	Heavy metals (silver, gold, bismuth, and arsenic). Arsenic, silver, and bismuth are not used therapeutically, but patients who receive gold for rheumatoid arthritis may show this reaction.
Pigmentary changes (continued)	Yellow color.	Generalized.	Usually quinacrine.
	Blue-black patches on the shins.		Minocycline, chloroquine.
	Blue-black pigmentation of the nails and palate and depigmentation of the hair.		Chloroquine.
	Slate-gray color.	Primarily in photoexposed areas.	Amiodarone.
	Brown discoloration of the nails.	Especially in more darkly pigmented patients.	Zidovudine (azidothymidine; AZT), hydroxyurea.
Psoriasiform eruptions	Scaly red plaques.	May be located on trunk and extremities. Palms and soles may be hyperkeratotic. May cause psoriasiform eruption or worsen psoriasis.	Chloroquine, lithium, beta-blockers, and quinacrine.
Pityriasis rosea–like eruptions	Oval, red, slightly raised patches with central scale.	Mainly on the trunk.	Barbiturates, bismuth, captopril, clonidine, gold salts, methopromazine, metoprolol, metronidazole, and tripelennamine.

(continued)

Table 8. Skin reactions due to systemic drugs. (continued)

Reaction	Appearance	Distribution and Comments	Common Offenders
Seborrheic dermatitis–like eruptions	Diffuse redness and loose scale.	On scalp, face, mid-chest, axillae, groin.	Cimetidine, gold salts, and methyldopa.
Bullous eruptions	Tense blisters > 1 cm.	Hands, feet, genital areas common; other sites possible.	Aspirin, barbiturates, bromides, chlorpromazine, warfarin, phenytoin, sulfonamides and related compounds, and promethazine.

Table 9. The inflamed eye: Differential diagnosis of common causes.

	Acute Conjunctivitis	Acute Uveitis	Acute Glaucoma[1]	Corneal Trauma or Infection
Incidence	Extremely common	Common	Uncommon	Common
Discharge	Moderate to copious	None	None	Watery or purulent
Vision	No effect on vision	Often blurred	Markedly blurred	Usually blurred
Pain	Mild	Moderate	Severe	Moderate to severe
Conjunctival injection	Diffuse; more toward fornices	Mainly circumcorneal	Mainly circumcorneal	Mainly circumcorneal
Cornea	Clear	Usually clear	Steamy	Clarity change related to cause
Pupil size	Normal	Small	Moderately dilated and fixed	Normal
Pupillary light response	Normal	Poor	None	Normal
Intraocular pressure	Normal	Commonly low but may be elevated	Elevated	Normal
Smear	Causative organisms	No organisms	No organisms	Organisms found only in corneal ulcers due to infection

[1]Angle-closure glaucoma.

Table 10. Topical ophthalmic agents.

Agent	Representative Cost/Size[1]	Sig	Indications
AGENTS FOR GLAUCOMA AND INTRAOCULAR HYPERTENSION			
Sympathomimetics			
Apraclonidine HCl 0.5% solution (Iopidine)	$57.60/5 mL	1 drop three times daily	Reduction of intraocular pressure. Expensive. Reserve for treatment of resistant cases.
Apraclonidine HCl 1% solution (Iopidine)	$9.55/unit dose 0.1 mL	1 drop 1 hour before and immediately after anterior segment laser surgery	To control or prevent elevations of intraocular pressure after laser trabeculoplasty or iridotomy.
Brimonidine tartrate 0.2% solution (Alphagan)	$36.28/5 mL	1 drop two or three times daily	Reduction of intraocular pressure.
Dipivefrin HCl 0.1% solution (various)[2]	$14.07/5 mL	1 drop every 12 hours	Open-angle glaucoma.
Epinephrine HCl 0.25%, 0.5% (Epifrin), 1%, and 2% solution (various)[3]	1%: $49.69/15 mL 2%: $54.36/15 mL	1 drop twice daily	
Beta-adrenergic blocking agents			
Betaxolol HCl 0.5% solution (Betoptic) and 0.25% suspension (Betoptic S)[4]	0.5%: $50.64/10 mL	1 drop twice daily	Reduction of intraocular pressure.
Carteolol HCl 1% solution (Ocupress)[5]	$61.72/10 mL	1 drop twice daily	
Levobunolol HCl 0.25% and 0.5% solution (Betagan)[5]	0.5%: $32.29/10 mL	1 drop once or twice daily	
Metipranolol HCl 0.3% solution (OptiPranolol)[5]	$20.93/5 mL	1 drop twice daily	
Timolol 0.25% and 0.5% solution (Betimol)[5]	0.5%: $32.29/10 mL	1 drop once or twice daily	
Timolol maleate 0.25% and 0.5% solution (Timoptic) and 0.25% and 0.5% gel (Timoptic-XE)[5]	0.5% solution: $17.00/5 mL 0.5% gel: $31.50/5 mL	1 drop once or twice daily	
Miotics			
Pilocarpine HCl (various)[6] 1–4%, 6%, 8%, and 10%	2%: $11.80/15 mL	1 drop three or four times daily	Reduction of intraocular pressure, treatment of acute or chronic angle-closure glaucoma, and pupillary constriction.
Pilocarpine HCl 4% gel (Pilopine HS)	$37.86/4 g	Apply 0.5-inch ribbon in lower conjunctival sac at bedtime.	
Pilocarpine 20 μg/h for 7 days, and 40 μg/h for 7 days ocular therapeutic system (Ocusert Pilo-20 and Ocusert Pilo-40)[7]	40 μg/h: $52.65/8 each	Replace each unit every 7 days.	
Carbonic anhydrase inhibitors			
Dorzolamide HCl 2% solution (Trusopt)	$26.94/5 mL $53.91/10 mL	1 drop three times daily	Reduction of intraocular pressure.
Brinzolamide 1% suspension (Azopt)	$31.44/5 mL $62.94/10 mL	1 drop three times daily	

(continued)

Table 10. Topical ophthalmic agents. (continued)

Agent	Representative Cost/Size[1]	Sig	Indications
Prostaglandin analogs			
Bimatoprost 0.003% solution (Lumigan)	$55.79/2.5 mL	1 drop once daily in the evening	Reduction of intraocular pressure.
Latanoprost 0.005% solution (Xalatan)	$53.38/2.5 mL	1 drop once or twice daily in the evening	
Travoprost 0.004% solution (Travatan)	$55.75/2.5 mL	1 drop once daily in the evening	
Unoprostone 0.15% solution (Rescula)	$46.81/5 mL	1 drop twice daily	
ANTI-INFLAMMATORY AGENTS			
Nonsteroidal anti-inflammatory agents[8]			
Diclofenac sodium 0.1% solution (Voltaren)	$51.79/5 mL	1 drop to affected eye four times daily beginning 24 hours after cataract surgery and continuing through first 2 postoperative weeks	Treatment of postoperative inflammation following cataract extraction and laser corneal surgery.
Flurbiprofen sodium 0.03% solution (various)	$8.73/2.5 mL	1 drop every half hour beginning 2 hours before surgery	Inhibition of intraoperative miosis. Treatment of cystoid macular edema and inflammation after cataract surgery.
Ketorolac tromethamine 0.5% solution (Acular)	$56.26/5 mL	1 drop four times daily	Relief of ocular itching due to seasonal allergic conjunctivitis.
Corticosteroids[9]			
Dexamethasone sodium phosphate 0.1% solution (various)	$16.51/5 mL	1 or 2 drops as often as indicated by severity; use every hour during the day and every 2 hours during the night in severe inflammation; taper off as inflammation decreases	Treatment of steroid-responsive inflammatory conditions of anterior segment.
Dexamethasone sodium phosphate 0.05% ointment (various)	$6.34/3.5 g	Apply thin coating on lower conjunctival sac three or four times daily	
Fluorometholone 0.1% suspension (various)[10]	$26.20/10 mL	1 or 2 drops as often as indicated by severity; use every hour during the day and every 2 hours during the night in severe inflammation; taper off as inflammation decreases	
Fluorometholone 0.25% suspension (FML Forte)[10]	$37.60/10 mL		
Fluorometholone 0.1% ointment (FML S.O.P.)	$34.00/3.5 g	Apply thin coating on lower conjunctival sac three or four times daily	
Medrysone 1% suspension (HMS)	$33.24/10 mL	1 or 2 drops as often as indicated by severity of inflammation; use every hour during the day and every 2 hours during the night in severe inflammation; taper off as inflammation decreases	
Prednisolone acetate 0.12% suspension (Pred Mild)	$36.14/10 mL		
Prednisolone acetate 0.125% suspension (various)	$24.66/5 mL $36.96/10 mL		
Prednisolone sodium phosphate 0.125% solution (various)	$18.56/5 mL		

(continued)

Table 10. Topical ophthalmic agents. (continued)

Agent	Representative Cost/Size[1]	Sig	Indications
Corticosteroids[9] (continued)			
Prednisolone acetate 1% suspension (various)	$23.10/10 mL	1 or 2 drops as often as indicated by severity of inflammation; use every hour during the day and every 2 hours during the night in severe inflammation; taper off as inflammation decreases	Treatment of steroid-responsive inflammatory conditions of anterior segment.
Prednisolone sodium phosphate 1% solution (various)	$24.06/10 mL		
Rimexolone 1% suspension (Vexol)	$25.74/5 mL		
Mast cell stabilizers			
Cromolyn sodium 4% solution (Crolom)	$37.25/10 mL	1 drop four to six times daily	Allergic conjunctivitis.
Ketotifen fumarate 0.025% solution (Zaditor)	$46.51/5 mL	1 drop two to four times daily	Allergic conjunctivitis.
Lodoxamine tromethamine 0.1% solution (Alomide)	$58.02/10 mL	1 or 2 drops four times daily (up to 3 months)	Vernal keratoconjunctivitis.
Olopatadine hydrochloride 0.1% solution (Patanol)	$70.25/5 mL	1 drop twice daily	Allergic conjunctivitis.
ANTIBIOTIC OINTMENTS AND SOLUTIONS			
Bacitracin 500 units/g ointment (various)[11]	$4.28/3.5 g	Refer to package insert (instructions vary)	Infections involving lid, conjunctiva, or cornea.
Chloramphenicol 0.5% (5 mg/mL) solution (various)[12]	$23.26/7.5 mL		As above, with both gram-positive and gram-negative coverage.
Chloramphenicol 1% (10 mg/g) ointment (various)[12]	$21.55/3.5 g		
Ciprofloxacin HCl (various)	0.3% solution: $44.63/5 mL 0.3% ointment: $50.00/3.5 g		
Erythromycin 0.5% ointment (various)[13]	$5.62/3.5 g		
Gentamicin sulfate 0.3% solution (various)	$8.17/5 mL		
Gentamicin sulfate 0.3% ointment (various)	$19.67/3.5 g		
Ofloxacin 0.3% solution (Ocuflox)	$39.55/5 mL		
Polymyxin B sulfate 500,000 units, powder for solution (Polymyxin B Sulfate Sterile)[14]	$8.64/500,000 units		
Tobramycin 0.3% solution (various)	$15.00/5 mL		
Tobramycin 0.3% ointment (Tobrex)	$47.50/3.5 g		
SULFONAMIDES			
Sulfacetamide sodium 10% solution (various)	$5.08/15 mL	1 or 2 drops every 1–3 hours	Conjunctivitis, corneal ulcer, and other superficial ocular infections due to susceptible microorganisms. Used as adjunct to systemic sulfonamide therapy in treatment of trachoma.

(continued)

Table 10. Topical ophthalmic agents. (continued)

Agent	Representative Cost/Size[1]	Sig	Indications
SULFONAMIDES (continued)			
Sulfacetamide sodium 10% ointment (various)	$8.10/3.5 g	Apply small amount (0.5 inch) into lower conjunctival sac once to four times daily and at bedtime	Conjunctivitis, corneal ulcer, and other superficial ocular infections due to susceptible microorganisms. Used as adjunct to systemic sulfonamide therapy in treatment of trachoma.

Note: Many combination products containing antibiotics, antibiotics and steroids, or sulfonamides and steroids are available as solutions, suspensions, or ointment.

Agent	Representative Cost/Size[1]	Sig	Indications
TOPICAL ANTIFUNGAL AGENTS			
Natamycin 5% suspension (Natacyn)	$131.04/15 mL	1 drop every 1–2 hours	Fungal blepharitis, conjunctivitis, and keratitis caused by susceptible organisms. Drug of choice for *Fusarium solani* keratitis.
TOPICAL ANTIVIRAL AGENTS			
Ganciclovir 4.5 mg surgical insert (Vitrasert)	$5000.00 each	1 implant every 5–8 months	Treatment of CMV retinitis in patients with AIDS.
Trifluridine 1% solution (Viroptic)	$99.01/7.5 mL	1 drop onto cornea every 2 hours while awake for a maximum daily dose of 9 drops until resolution occurs; then an additional 7 days of 1 drop every 4 hours while awake (minimum five times daily)	Primary keratoconjunctivitis and recurrent epithelial keratitis due to HSV types 1 or 2.[15]
Vidarabine monohydrate 3% ointment (Vira-A)	$27.05/3.5 g	0.5 inch of ointment into the lower conjunctival sac five times daily at 3-hour intervals	Acute keratoconjunctivitis and recurrent epithelial keratitis due to HSV types 1 or 2.[15]
TOPICAL ANTIHISTAMINICS[16]			
Levocabastine HCl 0.05% ophthalmic solution (Livostin)	$81.29/10 mL	1 drop four times daily (up to 2 weeks)	Allergic conjunctivitis; temporary relief of seasonal allergic conjunctivitis.

[1] Average wholesale price (AWP, for AP-rated generic when available) for quantity listed. Source: *Drug Topics Red Book,* May 2003; Vol. 22, No. 5. AWP may not accurately represent the actual pharmacy cost because wide contractual variations exist among institutions.
[2] Macular edema occurs in 30% of patients.
[3] May (rarely) increase blood pressure. **Caution:** Avoid in patients with sulfite hypersensitivity (some brands contain sulfite).
[4] Cardioselective (β_1) β-blocker.
[5] Nonselective (β_1 and β_2) β-blocker. Monitor all patients for systemic side effects, particularly exacerbation of asthma.
[6] Decreased night vision, headaches possible.
[7] Sustained-release preparation. Refrigerate.
[8] Cross-sensitivity to aspirin and other NSAIDs.
[9] Long-term use may increase intraocular pressure or cause cataracts.
[10] May be less likely to elevate intraocular pressure.
[11] Little efficacy against gram-negative organisms (except *Neisseria*).
[12] Aplastic anemia has been reported with prolonged ophthalmic use. Use only in serious infections for which less toxic drugs are ineffective or contraindicated.
[13] Also indicated for prophylaxis of ophthalmia neonatorum due to *N gonorrhoeae* or *C trachomatis*. Increasing resistance of *S pneumoniae* and *P aeruginosa* has been noted.
[14] No gram-positive coverage.
[15] Recurrences are common and call for additional 7-day treatment
[16] Antihistamines (topical) are potential sensitizers and may produce local reactions.

Table 11. Common vestibular disorders: Differential diagnosis based on classic presentations.

Duration of Typical Vertiginous Episodes	Auditory Symptoms Present	Auditory Symptoms Absent
Seconds	Perilymphatic fistula	Positioning vertigo (cupulolithiasis), vertebrobasilar insufficiency, cervical vertigo
Hours	Endolymphatic hydrops (Ménière's syndrome, syphilis)	Recurrent vestibulopathy, vestibular migraine
Days	Labyrinthitis, labyrinthine concussion	Vestibular neuronitis
Months	Acoustic neuroma, ototoxicity	Multiple sclerosis, cerebellar degeneration

Table 12. Classification of severity of chronic stable asthma.[1]

	Symptoms	Nighttime Symptoms	Lung Function
Mild intermittent	Symptoms $\leq$ 2 times a week Asymptomatic and normal PEF between exacerbations Exacerbations brief (few hours to few days); intensity may vary	$\leq$ 2 times a month	FEV_1 or PEF $\geq$ 80% predicted PEF variability $\leq$ 20%
Mild persistent	Symptoms > 2 times a week but < 1 time a day Exacerbations may affect activity	> 2 times a month	FEV_1 or PEF > 80% predicted PEF variability 20–30%
Moderate persistent	Daily symptoms Daily use of inhaled short-acting β_2-agonist Exacerbations affect activity Exacerbations $\geq$ 2 times a week; may last days	> 1 time a week	FEV_1 or PEF > 60% to < 80% predicted PEF variability > 30%
Severe persistent	Continual symptoms Limited physical activity Frequent exacerbations	Frequent	FEV_1 or PEF $\leq$ 60% predicted PEF variability > 30%

[1]Adapted from National Asthma Education and Prevention Program. Expert Panel Report 2: Guidelines for the Diagnosis and Management of Asthma. National Institutes of Health Pub No. 97-4051. Bethesda, MD, 1997.

Table 13. Classification of severity of asthma exacerbations[1]

	Mild	Moderate	Severe	Impending Respiratory Failure
Symptoms				
Breathlessness	With activity	With talking	At rest	At rest
Speech	Sentences	Phrases	Words	Mute
Signs				
Body position	Able to recline	Prefers sitting	Unable to recline	Unable to recline
Respiratory rate	Increased	Increased	Often > 30/min	> 30/min
Use of accessory respiratory muscles	Usually not	Commonly	Usually	Paradoxical thoracoabdominal movement
Breath sounds	Moderate wheezing at mid- to end-expiration	Loud wheezes throughout expiration	Loud inspiratory and expiratory wheezes	Little air movement without wheezes
Heart rate (beats/min)	< 100	100–120	> 120	Relative bradycardia
Pulsus paradoxus (mm Hg)	< 10	10–25	Often > 25	Often absent
Mental status	May be agitated	Usually agitated	Usually agitated	Confused or drowsy
Functional assessment				
PEF (% predicted or personal best)	> 80	50–80	< 50 or response to therapy lasts < 2 hours	< 50
SaO_2 (%, room air)	> 95	91–95	< 91	< 91
PaO_2 (mm Hg, room air)	Normal	> 60	< 60	< 60
$PaCO_2$ (mm Hg)	< 42	< 42	≥ 42	≥ 42

[1]Adapted from National Asthma Education and Prevention Program. Expert Panel Report 2: Guidelines for the Diagnosis and Management of Asthma. National Institutes of Health Pub No. 97-4051. Bethesda, MD, 1997.

Table 14. Stepwise approach for managing asthma.[1,2]

	Long-Term Control	Quick Relief	Education
Step 1: Mild Inter-mittent	No daily medication needed.	Short-acting bronchodilator: **inhaled β_2-agonists** as needed for symptoms. Intensity of treatment will depend on severity of exacerbation. Use of short-acting **inhaled β_2-agonists** > 2 times a week may indicate the need for long-term control therapy.	Teach basic facts about asthma Teach inhaler/inhalation chamber technique Discuss roles of medications Develop self-management and action plans Discuss appropriate environmental control measures
Step 2: Mild Persistent	One daily medication: **Anti-inflammatory**: either **inhaled corticosteroid** (low doses) or **cromolyn** or **nedocromil** Less desirable alternatives: sustained-release **theophylline** or **leukotriene modifier**	Step 1 actions plus: Use of short-acting **inhaled β_2-agonists** on a daily basis, or increasing use, indicates the need for additional long-term control therapy.	Step 1 actions plus: Teach self-monitoring Refer to group education if available Review and update self-management plan
Step 3: Moderate Persistent	Daily medication: Either **Anti-inflammatory: inhaled corticosteroid** (medium dose) or Inhaled corticosteroid (low-medium dose) and a **long-acting bronchodilator** (long-acting **inhaled β_2-agonist,** sustained-release **theophylline** or long-acting **β_2-agonist tablets**) If needed: **Anti-inflammatory: inhaled corticosteroid** (medium-high dose) and **Long-acting bronchodilator** (long-acting **inhaled β_2-agonist,** sustained-release **theophylline** or long-acting **β_2-agonist tablets**)	As for step 2.	Step 1 actions plus: Teach self-monitoring Refer to group education if available Review and update self-management plan
Step 4: Severe Persistent	Daily medication: **Anti-inflammatory: inhaled corticosteroid** (high dose) and **Long-acting bronchodilator** (long-acting **inhaled β_2-agonist,** sustained release **theophylline** or long-acting **β_2-agonist tablets**) and **Corticosteroid tablets or syrup** (2 mg/kg/d, generally not to exceed 60 mg/d)	As for step 2.	Step 2 and 3 actions plus: Refer to individual education, counseling

Step down: Review treatment every 1–6 months; a gradual stepwise reduction in treatment may be possible.
Step up: If asthma control is not maintained, consider step up to next treatment level after reviewing medication technique, adherence, and environmental control.

[1]Modified from National Asthma Education and Prevention Program. Expert Panel Report 2: Guidelines for the Diagnosis and Management of Asthma. National Institutes of Health Pub. No. 97-4051. Bethesda, MD, 1997.
[2]Preferred treatments are in colored text; however, specific medication plans should be tailored to individual patients.

Table 15. Long-term control medications for asthma.[1]

Drug	Important Formulations	Usual Adult Dosage	Cost[2]	Comments
Inhaled corticosteroids[3]				
Beclomethasone dipropionate (QVAR)	40 µg/puff	Two or three puffs BID	$41.32/7.30 g	Chlorofluorocarbon-free; hydrofluoralkane propellant
	80 µg/puff	One to two puffs BID	$52.04/7.30 g	
Beclomethasone dipropionate (Vanceril)	MDI: 42 µg/puff; 200 puffs/inhaler	Two or three puffs four times a day, or four to six puffs twice daily	$46.52/16.80 g	Chlorofluorocarbon propellant
	84 µg/puff; 120 puffs/inhaler	Two puffs twice a day	$53.33/12.20 g	
Budesonide (Pulmicort Turbuhaler)	Dry powder delivery system: 200 µg/puff; 200 puffs/inhaler	One inhalation twice a day	$146.39/inhaler	Dry powder
Flunisolide (AeroBid)	MDI: 250 µg/puff; 100 puffs/inhaler	Two to four puffs twice a day	$71.03/7 g	Chlorofluorocarbon propellant
Fluticasone (Flovent)	MDI: 44, 110, or 220 µg/puff; 120 puffs/inhaler	Two or three puffs (of 110 µg) twice a day	$74.11/13 g	Chlorofluorocarbon propellant
(Flovent Rotadisk)	Dry powder delivery system: 44, 88, 220 µg/blister; 4 blisters/Rotadisk, 15 Rotadisks per tube	One or two puffs (of 88 µg) twice a day	$53.30/60 88 µg disks	Dry powder
Triamcinolone acetonide (Azmacort)	MDI: 100 µg/puff; 240 puffs/inhaler	Two or three puffs four times a day, or four to six puffs twice daily	$72.69/20 g	Chlorofluorocarbon propellant
Systemic corticosteroids				
Methylprednisolone (many)	Tablets: 4 mg	5–60 mg daily to every other day as needed	$0.54/4 mg	
Prednisolone (many)	Tablets: 5 mg	5–60 mg daily to every other day as needed	$0.04/5 mg	
Prednisone (many)	Tablets: 1, 2.5, 5, 10, 20, 50 mg	5–60 mg daily to every other day as needed	$0.04/5 mg	
Combination inhaled corticosteroid and long-acting β_2-agonist				
Fluticasone and salmeterol (Advair Diskus)	Dry powder delivery system: 100, 250, or 500 µg fluticasone per dose and 50 µg salmeterol per dose	One puff twice a day of 250/50; cannot use more than one puff twice a day due to salmeterol component.	$142.30/60 250/50 disks	Dry powder

(continued)

Table 15. Long-term control medications for asthma.[1] (continued)

Drug	Important Formulations	Usual Adult Dosage	Cost[2]	Comments
Cromolyn (Intal)	MDI: 800 μg per puff: 200 puffs/inhaler	2–4 puffs 4 times a day	$92.94/14.2 g	Chlorofluorocarbon propellant
	Nebulizer solution: 20 mg/2 mL ampule	20 mg (2 mL) four times a day	$1.12/2 mL	Administer with powered nebulizer
Nedocromil (Tilade)	MDI: 1.75 mg/puff; 112 puffs/inhaler	Two puffs four times a day	$46.58/16.2 g	Chlorofluorocarbon propellant
Long-acting β$_2$-agonists[4]				
Salmeterol (Serevent Diskus)	Dry powder: 50 μg/blister; 60 blisters per pack	One blister every 12 hours	$84.01/60	Dry powder
Formoterol (Foradil Aerolizer)	Dry powder: 12 μg/capsule; 60 capsules/Aerolizer	One capsule every 12 hours	$70.08/60	Dry powder
Sustained-release albuterol (Proventil Repetab)	Sustained-release tablet, 4 mg	One tablet every 12 hours	$0.88/4 mg	Usually reserved for nocturnal symptoms not improved with other therapies
Theophylline (many)	Sustained-release tablets and capsules	Initially 10 mg/kg/d up to 300 mg maximum; then 200–600 mg every 8–24 hours	$0.33/200 mg	Maintenance dose guided by serum drug level. Absorption and dosing vary with brand
Leukotriene modifiers Montelukast (Singulair)	Tablet, 10 mg	One tablet each evening	$2.93/10 mg $87.95/mo	
Zafirlukast (Accolate)	Tablet, 20 mg	One tablet twice a day	$1.26/20 mg $75.59/mo	Administration with meals decreases bioavailability; take at least 1 hour before or 2 hours after meals
Zileuton (Zyflo)	Tablet, 600 mg	One tablet four times a day	$0.86/600 mg $103.19/mo	Monitor hepatic enzymes

[1] Only drugs available in the United States are listed.
[2] Average wholesale price (AWP, for AB-rated generic when available) for quantity listed. Source: *Drug Topics Red Book*, May 2003;Vol. 22, No. 5. AWP may not accurately represent actual pharmacy cost because wide contractual variations exist among institutions.
[3] Dosing should be individualized. See text.
[4] Not for acute relief of symptoms.

Table 16. Quick-relief medications for asthma.[1]

Drug	Important Formulations	Usual Adult Dosage	Cost[2]	Comments
Short-acting Inhaled β₂-agonists				
Albuterol (Proventil, Ventolin)	MDI: 90 μg/puff, 200 puffs/canister	Two puffs 5 minutes before exercise Two puffs every 4–6 hours as needed	$29.79/17 g	Preferred formulation in most cases. Chlorofluorocarbon propellant.
	Nebulizer solutions: 5 mg/mL (0.5%)	1.25–5 mg (0.25–1 mL) in 2–3 mL of normal saline every 4–8 hours as needed	$16.71/20 mL	Administer with powered nebulizer. More frequent dosing is acceptable for acute or severe exacerbations.
	Unit dose: 0.083%, 3 mL	One dose every 4–8 hours as needed	$1.24/unit	May mix with cromolyn or ipratropium nebulizer solutions.
	Dry powder (Ventolin Rotocaps): 200 μg/capsule	One or two capsules every 4–6 hours as needed	$37.92/100 200-μg capsules	Rotohaler required for inhalation.
	Tablets: 2 mg, 4 mg	2–4 mg orally every 6–8 hours	$31.14/100 2-mg tablets	Extended-release 4-mg tablet (Proventil Repetab) available for use every 12 hours.
Albuterol HFA (Proventil HFA)	MDI: 90 μg/puff, 200 puffs/canister	Two puffs 5 minutes before exercise Two puffs every 4–6 hours as needed	$39.41/6.7 g	Nonchlorofluorocarbon propellant.
Bitolterol (Tornalate)	Nebulizer solution, 2 mg/mL (0.2%)	0.5–2 mg (0.25–1 mL) in 2–3 mL of normal saline every 4–8 hours as needed	$16.54/30 mL	Administer with powered nebulizer. May not mix with other nebulizer solutions.
Pirbuterol (Maxair)	MDI: 200 μg/puff, 300 puffs/canister	Two puffs every 4–6 hours as needed	$50.52/25 g	Chlorofluorocarbon propellant.
(Maxair Autoinhaler)	MDI 200 μg/puff, 400 puffs/canister	Two puffs every 4–6 hours as needed	$76.50/14 g	Breath-activated MDI system. Chlorofluorocarbon propellant.
Terbutaline (Brethine)	Tablets: 2.5 mg, 5 mg	2.5–5 mg orally three times a day	$49.79/100 5-mg tablets	Tremor, nervousness, palpitations common; therefore not recommended.
	Injection solution, 1 mg/mL	0.25 mg (0.25 mL) subcutaneously; may be repeated once in 30 minutes	$4.67/1 mg	Onset of action 30 minutes. Not limited to β₂-agonist effects.
Anticholinergics Ipratropium bromide (Atrovent)	MDI: 18 μg/puff, 200 puffs/canister	Two to four puffs every 6 hours	$54.91/14 g	Chlorofluorocarbon propellant.
	Unit dose nebulizer solution, 0.2 mg/mL (0.02%), 2.5 mL (0.5 mg)	0.25–0.5 mg (1–2 mL) every 6 hours	$1.76/unit	

(continued)

Table 16. Quick-relief medications for asthma.[1] (continued)

Drug	Important Formulations	Usual Adult Dosage	Cost[2]	Comments
Systemic corticosteroids				
Methylprednisolone (many)	Tablets: 4 mg	40–60 mg/d as single dose or in two divided doses for 3–10 days	$11.00/4 mg dose-pack	
Methylprednisolone sodium succinate (many)	Intravenous injection solution vials: 40, 125, 500 mg	0.5–1 mg/kg every 6 hours	$3.41/125 mg vial	
Prednisolone (many)	Tablets: 5 mg Syrup: 15 mg/5 mL	40–60 mg/d as single dose or in two divided doses for 3–10 days	$0.04/5 mg tablet $74.50/240 mL syrup	
Prednisone (many)	Tablets: 1, 2.5, 5, 10, 20, 50 mg	40–60 mg/d as single dose or in two divided doses for 3–10 days	$0.04/5 mg	

[1]Only drugs available in the United States are listed.
[2]Average wholesale price (AWP, for AB-rated generic when available) for quantity listed. Source: *Drug Topics Red Book,* May 2003; Vol. 22, No. 5. AWP may not accurately represent the actual pharmacy cost because wide contractual variations exist among institutions.

Table 17. Patterns of disease in advanced COPD.

	Type A: Pink Puffer (Emphysema Predominant)	Type B: Blue Bloater (Bronchitis Predominant)
History and physical examination	Major complaint is dyspnea, often severe, usually presenting after age 50. Cough is rare, with scant clear, mucoid sputum. Patients are thin, with recent weight loss common. They appear uncomfortable, with evident use of accessory muscles of respiration. Chest is very quiet without adventitious sounds. No peripheral edema.	Major complaint is chronic cough, productive of mucopurulent sputum, with frequent exacerbations due to chest infections. Often presents in late 30s and 40s. Dyspnea usually mild, though patients may note limitations to exercise. Patients frequently overweight and cyanotic but seem comfortable at rest. Peripheral edema is common. Chest is noisy, with rhonchi invariably present; wheezes are common.
Laboratory studies	Hemoglobin usually normal (12–15 g/dL). Pa_{O_2} normal to slightly reduced (65–75 mm Hg) but Sa_{O_2} normal at rest. Pa_{CO_2} normal to slightly reduced (35–40 mm Hg). Chest radiograph shows hyperinflation with flattened diaphragms. Vascular markings are diminished, particularly at the apices.	Hemoglobin usually elevated (15–18 g/dL). Pa_{O_2} reduced (45–60 mm Hg) and Pa_{CO_2} slightly to markedly elevated (50–60 mm Hg). Chest radiograph shows increased interstitial markings ("dirty lungs"), especially at bases. Diaphragms are not flattened.
Pulmonary function tests	Airflow obstruction ubiquitous. Total lung capacity increased, sometimes markedly so. $D_{L_{CO}}$ reduced. Static lung compliance increased.	Airflow obstruction ubiquitous. Total lung capacity generally normal but may be slightly increased. $D_{L_{CO}}$ normal. Static lung compliance normal.
Special evaluations V/Q matching	Increased ventilation to high V/Q areas, ie, high dead space ventilation.	Increased perfusion to low V/Q areas.
Hemodynamics	Cardiac output normal to slightly low. Pulmonary artery pressures mildly elevated and increase with exercise.	Cardiac output normal. Pulmonary artery pressures elevated, sometimes markedly so, and worsen with exercise.
Nocturnal ventilation	Mild to moderate degree of oxygen desaturation not usually associated with obstructive sleep apnea.	Severe oxygen desaturation, frequently associated with obstructive sleep apnea.
Exercise ventilation	Increased minute ventilation for level of oxygen consumption. Pa_{O_2} tends to fall, Pa_{CO_2} rises slightly.	Decreased minute ventilation for level of oxygen consumption. Pa_{O_2} may rise; Pa_{CO_2} may rise signficantly.

Table 18. Home oxygen therapy: requirements for Medicare coverage.[1]

Group I (any of the following):

1. $Pao_2 \leq 55$ mm Hg or $Sao_2 \leq 88\%$ taken at rest breathing room air, while awake.

2. During sleep (prescription for nocturnal oxygen use only):
   a. $Pao_2 \leq 55$ mm Hg or $Sao_2 \leq 88\%$ for a patient whose awake, resting, room air Pao_2 is ≥ 56 mm Hg or $Sao_2 \geq 89\%$,

   or

   b. Decrease in $Pao_2 > 10$ mm Hg or decrease in $Sao_2 > 5\%$ associated with symptoms or signs reasonably attributed to hypoxemia (eg, impaired cognitive processes, nocturnal restlessness, insomnia).

3. During exercise (prescription for oxygen use only during exercise):
   a. $Pao_2 \leq 55$ mg Hg or $Sao_2 \leq 88\%$ taken during exercise for a patient whose awake, resting, room air Pao_2 is ≥ 56 mm Hg or $Sao_2 \geq 89\%$,

   and

   b. There is evidence that the use of supplemental oxygen during exercise improves the hypoxemia that was demonstrated during exercise while breathing room air.

Group II:[2]

$Pao_2 = 56$–59 mm Hg or $Sao_2 = 89\%$ if there is evidence of any of the following:

1. Dependent edema suggesting congestive heart failure.
2. P pulmonale on ECG (P wave > 3 mm in standard leads II, III, or aVF).
3. Hematocrit > 56%.

---

[1]Health Care Financing Administration, 1989.
[2]Patients in this group must have a second oxygen test 3 months after the initial oxygen set-up.

Table 19. Characteristics and treatment of selected pneumonias.

Organism; Appearance on Smear of Sputum	Clinical Setting	Complications	Laboratory Studies	Antimicrobial Therapy[1,2]
Streptococcus pneumoniae (pneumococcus). Gram-positive diplococci.	Chronic cardiopulmonary disease; follows upper respiratory tract infection.	Bacteremia, meningitis, endocarditis, pericarditis, empyema.	Gram stain and culture of sputum, blood, pleural fluid	Preferred:[3] Penicillin G, amoxicillin. Alternative: Macrolides, cephalosporins, doxycycline, fluoroquinolones, clindamycin, vancomycin.
Haemophilus influenzae. Pleomorphic gram-negative coccobacilli.	Chronic cardiopulmonary disease; follows upper respiratory tract infection.	Empyema, endocarditis.	Gram stain and culture of sputum, blood, pleural fluid.	Preferred:[3] Cefotaxime, ceftriaxone, cefuroxime, doxycycline, azithromycin, TMP-SMZ.[4] Alternative: Fluoroquinolones, clarithromycin.
Staphylococcus aureus. Plump gram-positive cocci in clumps.	Residence in chronic care facility, nosocomial, influenza epidemics; cystic fibrosis, bronchiectasis, injection drug use.	Empyema, cavitation.	Gram stain and culture of sputum, blood, pleural fluid.	For methicillin-susceptible strains: Preferred: A penicillinase-resistant penicillin with or without rifampin, or gentamicin. Alternative: A cephalosporin; clindamycin, TMP-SMZ,[4] vancomycin. For methicillin-resistant strains: Vancomycin with or without gentamicin or rifampin.
Klebsiella pneumoniae. Plump gram-negative encapsulated rods.	Alcohol abuse, diabetes mellitus; nosocomial.	Cavitation, empyema.	Gram stain and culture of sputum, blood, pleural fluid.	Preferred: Third-generation cephalosporin. For severe infections, add an aminoglycoside. Alternative: Aztreonam, imipenem, β-lactam/β-lactamase inhibitor, or a fluoroquinolone.
Escherichia coli. Gram-negative rods.	Nosocomial; rarely, community-acquired.	Empyema.	Gram stain and culture of sputum, blood, pleural fluid.	Same as for *Klebsiella pneumoniae.*
Pseudomonas aeruginosa. Gram-negative rods.	Nosocomial; cystic fibrosis, bronchiectasis.	Cavitation.	Gram stain and culture of sputum, blood.	Preferred: An antipseudomonal β-lactam plus an aminoglycoside. Alternative: Ciprofloxacin plus an aminoglycoside or an antipseudomonal β-lactam.
Anaerobes. Mixed flora.	Aspiration, poor dental hygiene.	Necrotizing pneumonia, abscess, empyema.	Culture of pleural fluid or of material obtained by transtracheal or transthoracic aspiration.	Preferred: Clindamycin, β-lactam/β-lactamase inhibitor, imipenem.

Organism	Epidemiology/Clinical	Complications	Diagnosis	Treatment
Mycoplasma pneumoniae. PMNs and monocytes; no bacteria.	Young adults; summer and fall.	Skin rashes, bullous myringitis; hemolytic anemia.	PCR. Culture.[6] Complement fixation titer.[5] Cold agglutinin serum titers are not helpful as they lack sensitivity and specificity.	Preferred: Doxycycline or erythromycin. Alternative: Clarithromycin; azithromycin, or a fluoroquinolone.
Legionella species. Few PMNs; no bacteria.	Summer and fall; exposure to contaminated construction site, water source, air conditioner; community-acquired or nosocomial.	Empyema, cavitation, endocarditis, pericarditis.	Direct immunofluorescent examination or PCR of sputum or tissue; culture of sputum or tissue.[6] Urinary antigen assay for *L pneumophila* serogroup 1.	Preferred: A macrolide with or without rifampin; a fluoroquinolone. Alternative: Doxycycline with or without rifampin.
Chlamydia pneumoniae. Nonspecific.	Clinically similar to *M pneumoniae,* but prodromal symptoms last longer (up to 2 weeks). Sore throat with hoarseness common. Mild pneumonia in teenagers and young adults.	Reinfection in older adults with underlying COPD or heart failure may be severe or even fatal.	Isolation of the organism is very difficult. Serologic studies include microimmunofluorescence with TWAR antigen. PCR at selected laboratories.	Preferred: Doxycycline. Alternative: Erythromycin, clarithromycin, azithromycin, or a fluoroquinolone.
Moraxella catarrhalis. Gram-negative diplococci.	Preexisting lung disease; elderly; corticosteroid or immunosuppressive therapy.	Rarely, pleural effusions and bacteremia.	Gram stain and culture of sputum, blood, pleural fluid.	Preferred: TMP-SMZ,[4] a second- or third-generation cephalosporin, amoxicillin-clavulanic acid, or a macrolide. Alternative: A fluoroquinolone.
Pneumocystis jiroveci. Nonspecific.	AIDS, immunosuppressive or cytotoxic drug therapy, cancer.	Pneumothorax, respiratory failure, ARDS, death.	Methenamine silver, Giemsa, or DFA stains of sputum or bronchoalveolar lavage fluid.	Preferred: TMP-SMZ[4] or pentamidine isethionate plus prednisone. Alternative: Dapsone plus trimethoprim; clindamycin plus primaquine; trimetrexate plus folinic acid.

[1] Antimicrobial sensitivities should guide therapy when available. (Modified from: The choice of antibacterial drugs. Med Lett Drugs Ther 1999;41:95, and from Bartlett JG et al: Practice guidelines for the management of community-acquired pneumonia in adults. Clin Infect Dis 2000;31:347).
[2] For additional antimicrobial therapy information, see Tables 122 and 123.
[3] Consider penicillin resistance when choosing therapy.
[4] Trimethoprim-sulfamethoxazole.
[5] Fourfold rise in titer is diagnostic.
[6] Selective media are required.

Table 20. Scoring system for risk class assignment for PORT prediction rule.[1]

Patient Characteristic	Points Assigned[2]
Demographic factor	
Age: men	Number of years
Age: women	Number of years minus 10
Nursing home resident	10
Comorbid illnesses	
Neoplastic disease[3]	30
Liver disease[4]	20
Congestive heart failure[5]	10
Cerebrovascular disease[6]	10
Renal disease[7]	10
Physical examination finding	
Altered mental status[8]	20
Respiratory rate ≥ 30 breaths/min	20
Systolic blood pressure < 90 mm Hg	20
Temperature ≤ 35°C or ≥ 40°C	15
Pulse ≥ 125 beats/min	10
Laboratory or radiographic finding	
Arterial pH < 7.35	30
Urea nitrogen ≥ 30 mg/dL	20
Sodium < 130 mEq/L	20
Glucose > 250 mg/dL	10
Hematocrit < 30%	10
Arterial P_{O_2} < 60 mm Hg	10
Pleural effusion	10

[1]Modified and reproduced, with permission, from Fine MJ et al: A prediction rule to identify low-risk patients with community-acquired pneumonia. N Engl J Med 1997;336:243. Copyright © 1997 Massachusetts Medical Society. All rights reserved.
[2]A total point score for a given patient is obtained by summing the patient's age in years (age minus 10 for women) and the points for each applicable characteristic.
[3]Any cancer except basal or squamous cell of the skin that was active at the time of presentation or diagnosed within 1 year before presentation.
[4]Clinical or histologic diagnosis of cirrhosis or another form of chronic liver disease.
[5]Systolic or diastolic dysfunction documented by history, physical examination and chest radiograph, echocardiogram, MUGA scan, or left ventriculogram.
[6]Clinical diagnosis of stroke or transient ischemic attack or stroke documented by MRI or CT scan.
[7]History of chronic renal disease or abnormal blood urea nitrogen and creatinine concentration documented in the medical record.
[8]Disorientation (to person, place, or time, not known to be chronic), stupor, or coma.

Table 21. PORT risk class 30-day mortality rates and recommendations for site of care.[1]

Number of Points	Risk Class	Mortality at 30 days (%)	Recommended Site of Care
Absence of predictors	I	0.1–0.4	Outpatient
≤ 70	II	0.6–0.7	Outpatient
71–90	III	0.9–2.8	Outpatient or brief inpatient
91–130	IV	8.2–9.3	Inpatient
≥ 130	V	27.0–31.1	Inpatient

[1]Data from Fine MJ et al: A prediction rule to identify low-risk patients with community-acquired pneumonia. N Engl J Med 1997;336:243. Copyright © 1997 Massachusetts Medical Society. All rights reserved.

Table 22. Classification of positive tuberculin skin test reactions.[1,2]

Reaction Size	Group
≥ 5 mm	1. HIV-positive persons. 2. Recent contacts of individuals with active tuberculosis. 3. Persons with fibrotic changes on chest x-rays suggestive of prior tuberculosis. 4. Patients with organ transplants and other immunosuppressed patients (receiving the equivalent of > 15 mg/d of prednisone for 1 month or more).
≥ 10 mm	1. Recent immigrants (< 5 years) from countries with a high prevalence of tuberculosis (eg, Asia, Africa, Latin America). 2. HIV-negative injection drug users. 3. Mycobacteriology laboratory personnel. 4. Residents of and employees[3] in the following high-risk congregate settings: correctional institutions; nursing homes and other long-term facilities for the elderly; hospitals and other health care facilities; residential facilities for AIDS patients; and homeless shelters. 5. Persons with the following medical conditions that increase the risk of tuberculosis: gastrectomy, ≥ 10% below ideal body weight, jejunoileal bypass, diabetes mellitus, silicosis, chronic renal failure, some hematologic disorders, (eg leukemias, lymphomas), and other specific malignancies (eg, carcinoma of the head or neck and lung). 6. Children < 4 years of age or infants, children, and adolescents exposed to adults at high risk.
≥ 15 mm	1. Persons with no risk factors for tuberculosis.

[1]Adapted from: Screening for tuberculosis and tuberculosis infection in high-risk populations: recommendations of the Advisory Council for the Elimination of Tuberculosis. MMWR Morb Mortal Wkly Rep 1995;44(RR-11):19.
[2]A tuberculin skin test reaction is considered positive if the transverse diameter of the indurated area reaches the size required for the specific group. All other reactions are considered negative.
[3]For persons who are otherwise at low risk and are tested at entry into employment, a reaction of > 15 mm induration is considered positive.

Table 23. Characteristics of antituberculous drugs.

Drug	Most Common Side Effects	Tests for Side Effects	Drug Interactions	Remarks
Isoniazid	Peripheral neuropathy, hepatitis, rash, mild CNS effects.	AST and ALT; neurologic examination.	Phenytoin (synergistic); disulfiram.	Bactericidal to both extracellular and intracellular organisms. Pyridoxine, 10 mg orally daily as prophylaxis for neuritis; 50–100 mg orally daily as treatment.
Rifampin	Hepatitis, fever, rash, flu-like illness, gastrointestinal upset, bleeding problems, renal failure.	CBC, platelets, AST and ALT.	Rifampin inhibits the effect of oral contraceptives, quinidine, corticosteroids, warfarin, methadone, digoxin, oral hypoglycemics; aminosalicyclic acid may interfere with absorption of rifampin. Significant interactions with protease inhibitors and non-nucleoside reverse transcriptase inhibitors.	Bactericidal to all populations of organisms. Colors urine and other body secretions orange. Discoloring of contact lenses.
Pyrazinamide	Hyperuricemia, hepatotoxicity, rash, gastrointestinal upset, joint aches.	Uric acid, AST, ALT.	. . .	Bactericidal to intracellular organisms.
Ethambutol	Optic neuritis (reversible with discontinuance of drug; rare at 15 mg/kg); rash.	Red-green color discrimination and visual acuity (difficult to test in children under 3 years of age).	. . .	Bacteriostatic to both intracellular and extracellular organisms. Mainly used to inhibit development of resistant mutants. Use with caution in renal disease or when ophthalmologic testing is not feasible.
Streptomycin	Eighth nerve damage, nephrotoxicity.	Vestibular function (audiograms); BUN and creatinine.	Neuromuscular blocking agents may be potentiated and cause prolonged paralysis.	Bactericidal to extracellular organisms. Use with caution in older patients or those with renal disease.

Table 24. Recommended dosages for the initial treatment of tuberculosis.

Drugs	Daily	Cost[1]	Twice a Week[2]	Cost[1]/wk	Three Times a Week[2]	Cost[1]/wk
Isoniazid	5 mg/kg Max: 300 mg/dose	$0.08/300 mg	15 mg/kg Max: 900 mg/dose	$0.48	15 mg/kg Max: 900 mg/dose	$0.72
Rifampin	10 mg/kg Max: 600 mg/dose	$3.80/600 mg	10 mg/kg Max: 600 mg/dose	$7.60	10 mg/kg Max: 600 mg/dose	$11.40
Pyrazinamide	15–30 mg/kg Max: 2 g/dose	$3.68/2 g	50–70 mg/kg Max: 4 g/dose	$14.72	50–70 mg/kg Max: 3 g/dose	$16.56
Ethambutol	5–25 mg/kg Max: 2.5 g/dose	$11.27/2.5 g	50 mg/kg Max: 2.5 g/dose	$22.54	25–30 mg/kg Max: 2.5 g/dose	$33.81
Streptomycin	15 mg/kg Max: 1 g/dose	$6.90/1 g	25–30 mg/kg Max: 1.5 g/dose	$27.60	25–30 mg/kg Max: 1.5 g/dose	$41.40

[1]Average wholesale price (AWP, for AP-rated generic when available) for quantity listed. Source: *Drug Topics Red Book*, May 2003; Vol. 22, No. 5. AWP may not accurately represent the actual pharmacy cost because wide contractual variations exist among institutions.

[2]All intermittent dosing regimens should be used with directly observed therapy.

Table 25. TNM staging for lung cancer.[1]

Stage	T	N	M	Description
0	Tis			Carcinoma in situ
IA	T1	N0	M0	Limited local disease without nodal or distant metastases
IB	T2	N0	M0	
IIA	T1	N1	M0	Limited local disease with ipsilateral hilar or peribronchial nodal involvement but not distant metastases *or*
IIB	T2	N1	M0	Locally invasive disease without nodal or distant metastases
	T3	N0	M0	
IIIA	T3	N1	M0	Locally invasive disease with ipsilateral or peribronchial nodal involvement but not distant metastases *or*
	T1–3	N2	M0	Limited or locally invasive disease with ipsilateral mediastinal or subcarinal nodal involvement but not distant metastases
IIIB	Any T	N3	M0	Any primary with contralateral mediastinal or hilar nodes, or ipsilateral scalene or supraclavicular nodes *or*
	T4	Any N	M0	Unresectable local invasion with any degree of adenopathy but no distant metastases; malignant pleural effusion
IV	Any T	Any N	M1	Distant metastases

Primary Tumor (T)

TX	Primary tumor cannot be assessed; or tumor proved by the presence of malignant cells in sputum or bronchial washings but not visualized by imaging or bronchoscopy.
T0	No evidence of primary tumor.
Tis	Carcinoma in situ.
T1	A tumor ≤ 3 cm in greatest dimension, surrounded by lung or visceral pleura, and without evidence of invasion proximal to a lobar bronchus at bronchoscopy.
T2	A tumor > 3.0 cm in greatest dimension, or a tumor of any size that either involves a main bronchus (but is ≥ 2 cm distal to the carina), invades the visceral pleura, or has associated atelectasis or obstructive pneumonitis extending to the hilar region. Any associated atelectasis or obstructive pneumonitis must involve less than an entire lung.
T3	A tumor of any size with direct extension into the chest wall (including superior sulcus tumors), the diaphragm, the mediastinal pleura, or the parietal pericardium; or a tumor in the main bronchus < 2 cm distal to the carina without involving the carina; or associated atelectasis or obstructive pneumonitis of the entire lung.
T4	A tumor of any size with invasion of the mediastinum, heart, great vessels, trachea, esophagus, vertebral body, or carina; or with a malignant pleural or pericardial effusion; or with satellite tumor nodules within the ipsilateral lobe of the lung containing the primary tumor.

Regional Lymph Nodes (N)

NX	Regional lymph nodes cannot be assessed.
N0	No demonstrable metastasis to regional lymph nodes.
N1	Metastasis to lymph nodes in the peribronchial or the ipsilateral hilar region, or both, including direct extension.
N2	Metastasis to ipsilateral mediastinal lymph nodes and/or subcarinal lymph nodes.
N3	Metastasis to contralateral mediastinal lymph nodes, contralateral hilar lymph nodes, ipsilateral or contralateral scalene or supraclavicular lymph nodes.

Distant Metastases (M)

MX	Presence of distant metastasis cannot be assessed.
M0	No (known) distant metastasis.
M1	Distant metastasis present.

[1]Adapted from Mountain CF: Revisions in the international system for staging lung cancer. Chest 1997;111:1710.

Table 26. Approach to staging of patients with lung cancer.[1]

Part A: Recommended tests for all patients
   Complete blood cell count
   Electrolytes, calcium, alkaline phosphatase, albumin, AST, ALT, total bilirubin, creatinine
   Chest radiograph
   CT of chest through the adrenal glands[2,3]
   Pathologic confirmation of malignancy[4]

Part B: Recommended tests for selected but not all patients

Test	Indication
CT of liver with contrast or liver ultrasound	Elevated liver function tests; abnormal non–contrast-enhanced CT of liver or abnormal clinical evaluation
CT of brain with contrast or MRI brain	CNS symptoms or abnormal clinical evaluation
Radionuclide bone scan	Elevated alkaline phosphatase (bony fraction), elevated calcium, bone pain, or abnormal clinical evaluation
Pulmonary function tests	If lung resection or thoracic radiotherapy planned
Quantitative radionuclide perfusion lung scan or exercise testing to evaluate maximum oxygen consumption	Patients with borderline resectability due to limited cardiovascuar status

[1]Modified and reproduced, with permission, from: Pretreatment evaluation of non-small cell lung cancer. Consensus Statement of the American Thoracic Society and the European Respiratory Society. Am J Respir Crit Care Med 1997;156:320.
[2]May not be necessary if patient has obvious M1 disease on chest x-ray or physical examination.
[3]Intravenous iodine contrast enhancement is not essential but is recommended in probable mediastinal invasion.
[4]While optimal in most cases, tissue diagnosis may not be necessary prior to surgery in some cases where the lesion is enlarging or the patient will undergo surgical resection regardless of the outcome of a biopsy.

Table 27. Approximate survival rates following treatment for lung cancer.[1]

Non-Small Cell Lung Cancer: Mean 5-Year Survival Following Resection		
Stage	**Clinical Staging**	**Surgical Staging**
IA (T1N0M0)	60%	74%
IB (T2N0M0)	38%	61%
IIA (T1N1M0)	34%	55%
IIB (T2N1M0, T3N0M0)	23%	39%
IIIA	9–13%	22%
IIIB[2]	3–7%	
IV[2]	1%	

Small Cell Lung Cancer: 2-Year Survival Following Chemotherapy		
Stage	**Mean**	**Median**
Limited	15–20%	14–20 months
Extensive	< 3%	8–13 months

[1]Data from multiple sources. Modified and reproduced, with permission, from Reif MS et al: Evidence-based medicine in the treatment of non-small cell cancer. Clin Chest Med 2000;21:107.
[2]Independent of therapy, generally not surgical patients.

Table 28. Differential diagnosis of interstitial lung disease.

Drug-related
    Antiarrhythmic agents (amiodarone)
    Antibacterial agents (nitrofurantoin, sulfonamides)
    Antineoplastic agents (bleomycin, cyclophosphamide, methotrexate, nitrosoureas)
    Antirheumatic agents (gold salts, penicillamine)
    Phenytoin
Environmental and occupational (inhalation exposures)
    Dust, inorganic (asbestos, silica, hard metals, beryllium)
    Dust, organic (thermophilic actinomycetes, avian antigens, aspergillus species)
    Gases, fumes, and vapors (chlorine, isocyanates, paraquat, sulfur dioxide)
    Ionizing radiation
    Talc (injection drug users)
Infections
    Fungus, disseminated *(Coccidioides immitis, Blastomyces dermatitidis, Histoplasma capsulatum)*
    Mycobacteria, disseminated
    Pneumocystis jiroveci
    Viruses
Primary pulmonary disorders
    Bronchiolitis obliterans-organizing pneumonia (BOOP)
    Idiopathic fibrosing interstitial pneumonia: Acute interstitial pneumonitis, desquamative interstitial pneumonitis, nonspecific interstitial pneumonitis, usual interstitial pneumonitis, respiratory bronchiolitis-associated interstitial lung disease
    Pulmonary alveolar proteinosis
Systemic disorders
    Acute respiratory distress syndrome (ARDS)
    Amyloidosis
    Ankylosing spondylitis
    Autoimmune disease: Dermatomyositis, polymyositis, rheumatoid arthritis, systemic sclerosis (scleroderma), systemic lupus erythematosus
    Chronic eosinophilic pneumonia
    Goodpasture's syndrome
    Idiopathic pulmonary hemosiderosis
    Inflammatory bowel disease
    Langerhans cell histiocytosis (eosinophilic granuloma)
    Lymphangitic spread of cancer (lymphangitic carcinomatosis)
    Lymphangioleiomyomatosis
    Pulmonary edema
    Pulmonary venous hypertension, chronic
    Sarcoidosis
    Wegener's granulomatosis

Table 29. Idiopathic fibrosing interstitial pneumonias.

Name and Clinical Presentation	Histopathology	Radiographic Pattern	Response to Therapy and Prognosis
Usual interstitial pneumonia (UIP) Age 55–60, slight male predominance. Insidious dry cough and exertional dyspnea lasting months to years. Clubbing present at diagnosis in 25–50%. Diffuse fine late inspiratory crackles on lung auscultation. Restrictive ventilatory defect and reduced diffusing capacity on pulmonary function tests. ANA and RF positive in 25% in the absence of documented collagen-vascular disease.	Patchy, temporally and geographically nonuniform distribution of fibrosis, honeycomb change, and normal lung. Type I pneumocytes are lost, and there is proliferation of alveolar type II cells. "Fibroblast foci" of actively proliferating fibroblasts and myofibroblasts. Inflammation is generally mild and consists of small lymphocytes. Intra-alveolar macrophage accumulation is present but is not a prominent feature.	Diminished lung volume. Increased linear or reticular bibasilar and subpleural opacities. Unilateral disease is rare. HRCT shows minimal ground-glass and variable honeycomb change. Areas of normal lung may be adjacent to areas of advanced fibrosis. Between 2% and 10% have normal chest radiograph and HRCT scans on diagnosis.	No randomized study has demonstrated improved survival compared with untreated patients. Inexorably progressive. Response to corticosteroids and cytotoxic agents at best 15%, and these probably represent misclassification of histopathology. Median survival approximately 3 years, depending on stage at presentation. Current interest in antifibrotic agents.
Respiratory bronchiolitis–associated interstitial lung disease (RB-ILD)[1] Age 40–45. Presentation similar to that of UIP though in younger patients. Similar results on pulmonary function tests, but less severe abnormalities. Patients with respiratory bronchiolitis are invariably heavy smokers.	Increased numbers of macrophages evenly dispersed within the alveolar spaces. Rare fibroblast foci, little fibrosis, minimal honeycomb change. In RB-ILD the accumulation of macrophages is localized within the peribronchiolar air spaces; in DIP,[1] it is diffuse. Alveolar architecture is preserved.	May be indistinguishable from UIP. More often presents with a nodular or reticulonodular pattern. Honeycombing rare. HRCT more likely to reveal diffuse ground-glass opacities and upper lobe emphysema.	Spontaneous remission occurs in up to 20% of patients, so natural history unclear. Smoking cessation is essential. Prognosis clearly better than that of UIP: median survival greater than 10 years. Corticosteroids thought to be effective, but there are no randomized clinical trials to support this view.
Acute interstitial pneumonitis (AIP) Clinically known as Hamman-Rich syndrome. Wide age range, many young patients. Acute onset of dyspnea followed by rapid development of respiratory failure. Half of patients report a viral syndrome preceding lung disease. Clinical course indistinguishable from that of idiopathic ARDS.	Pathologic changes reflect acute response to injury within days to weeks. Resembles organizing phase of diffuse alveolar damage. Fibrosis and minimal collagen deposition. May appear similar to UIP but more homogeneous and there is no honeycomb change—though this may appear if the process persists for more than a month in a patient on mechanical ventilation.	Diffuse bilateral airspace consolidation with areas of ground-glass attenuation on HRCT scan.	Supportive care (mechanical ventilation) critical but effect of specific therapies unclear. High initial mortality: Fifty to 90 percent die within 2 months after diagnosis. Not progressive if patient survives. Lung function may return to normal or may be permanently impaired.
Nonspecific interstitial pneumonitis (NSIP) Age 45–55. Slight female predominance. Similar to UIP but onset of cough and dyspnea over months, not years.	Nonspecific in that histopathology does not fit into better-established categories. Varying degrees of inflammation and fibrosis, patchy in distribution but uniform in time, suggesting response to single injury. Most have lymphocytic and plasma cell inflammation without fibrosis. Honeycombing present but scant. Some have advocated division into cellular and fibrotic subtypes.	May be indistinguishable from UIP. Most typical picture is bilateral areas of ground-glass attenuation and fibrosis on HRCT. Honeycombing is rare.	Treatment thought to be effective, but no prospective clinical studies have been published. Prognosis overall good but depends on the extent of fibrosis at diagnosis. Median survival greater than 10 years.

(continued)

Table 29. Idiopathic fibrosing interstitial pneumonias. (continued)

Name and Clinical Presentation	Histopathology	Radiographic Pattern	Response to Therapy and Prognosis
Bronchiolitis obliterans-organizing pneumonia (BOOP) Typically age 50–60 but wide variation. Abrupt onset, frequently weeks to a few months following a flu-like illness. Dyspnea and dry cough prominent, but constitutional symptoms are common: fatigue, fever, and weight loss. Pulmonary function tests usually show restriction, but up to 25% show concomitant obstruction.	Included in the idiopathic interstitial pneumonias on clinical grounds. Buds of loose connective tissue (Masson bodies) and inflammatory cells fill alveoli and distal bronchioles.	Lung volumes normal. Chest radiograph typically shows interstitial and parenchymal disease with discrete, peripheral alveolar and ground-glass infiltrates. Nodular opacities common. HRCT shows subpleural consolidation and bronchial wall thickening and dilation.	Rapid response to corticosteroids in two-thirds of patients. Long-term prognosis generally good for those who respond. Relapses are common.

[1]Includes desquamative interstitial pneumonia (DIP).

Table 30. Frequency of specific symptoms and signs in patients at risk for pulmonary thromboembolism.

	UPET[1] PE+ (n = 327)	PIOPED[2] PE+ (n = 117)	PIOPED[2] PE− (n = 248)
Symptoms			
Dyspnea	84%	73%	72%
Respirophasic chest pain	74%	66%	59%
Cough	53%	37%	36%
Leg pain	nr	26%	24%
Hemoptysis	30%	13%	8%
Palpitations	nr	10%	18%
Wheezing	nr	9%	11%
Anginal pain	14%	4%	6%
Signs			
Respiratory rate ≥ 16 UPET, ≥ 20 PIOPED	92%	70%	68%
Crackles (rales)	58%	51%	40%[3]
Heart rate ≥ 100/min	44%	30%	24%
Fourth heart sound (S_4)	nr	24%	13%[3]
Accentuated pulmonary component of second heart sound (S_2P)	53%	23%	13%[3]
T ≥ 37.5°C UPET, ≥ 38.5°C PIOPED	43%	7%	12%
Homans' sign	nr	4%	2%
Pleural friction rub	nr	3%	2%
Third heart sound (S_3)	nr	3%	4%
Cyanosis	19%	1%	2%

[1]Data from the Urokinase-Streptokinase Pulmonary Embolism Trial, as reported in Bell WR, Simon TL, DeMets DL: The clinical features of submassive and massive pulmonary emboli. Am J Med 1977;62:355.

[2]Data from patients enrolled in the PIOPED Study, as reported in Stein PD et al: Clinical, laboratory, roentgenographic, and electrocardiographic findings in patients with acute pulmonary embolism and no preexisting cardiac or pulmonary disease. Chest 1991;100:598.

PE+ = confirmed diagnosis of pulmonary embolism; PE− = diagnosis of pulmonary embolism ruled out; nr = not reported.

[3]P < .05 comparing patients in the PIOPED Study.

Standard algorithm

Clinical suspicion of pulmonary thromboembolism
↓
Ventilation/perfusion lung scan

- Normal → Pulmonary thromboembolism excluded
- Low or indeterminate probability → Testing for deep venous thrombosis
  - Positive → Treatment
  - Negative → Pulmonary arteriogram or Serial noninvasive testing for deep venous thrombosis
    - Positive → Treatment
    - Negative → Pulmonary thromboembolism excluded
- High probability → Treatment

Emerging practice algorithm

D-Dimer by ELISA or other high-sensitivity assay

- < 500 ng/mL → **Clinical probability of pulmonary thromboembolism**
  - Low to medium → **STOP: Follow clinically. False-negative rate for clinically significant pulmonary thromboembolism probably <1%.**
  - High → **Chest helical CT**
- > 500 ng/mL → **Chest helical CT**

Chest helical CT
- Positive for pulmonary thromboembolism → **STOP: Treat with anticoagulation.**
- Negative for pulmonary thromboembolism but positive for alternative diagnosis → **STOP: Treat the alternative diagnosis. Rate of missed venous thromboembolism or pulmonary thromboembolism diagnoses is unknown. High (20%) mortality but clinically evident venous thromboembolism or pulmonary thromboembolism in ≤2% at 3 months.**
- Negative for pulmonary thromboembolism and negative for alternative diagnosis → **Lower extremity ultrasound**
  - Negative for venous thromboembolism → **STOP: Follow clinically. Overall mortality rate is approximately 4% at 12 weeks, but risk of death for undiagnosed pulmonary thromboembolism appears to be very low. If the prior probability of pulmonary thromboembolism is high, if there is no alternative diagnosis, or if there is a high risk of morbid event from undiagnosed pulmonary thromboembolism, then repeat lower extremity untrasound on day 4. In rare circumstances, with high-risk patients, consider pulmonary arteriogram.**
  - Positive for venous thromboembolism → **STOP: Treat with anticoagulation.**

Figure 2. Two simple algorithms to guide evaluation of suspected venous thromboembolism. The standard algorithm is based on the results of ventilation-perfusion lung scanning using PIOPED data. Management of patients with ventilation-perfusion lung scans of low and indeterminate probability must always be guided by clinical judgment based upon cumulative clinical information and the degree of suspicion of pulmonary thromboembolism. The second algorithm uses D-dimer, helical CT, and venous ultrasonography to describe an evidence-based, efficient evaluation that reflects emerging practice. This second algorithm is not based on the extensive experience of the standard ventilation-perfusion approach but anticipates a shift toward use of helical CT as the primary diagnostic test in pulmonary thromboembolism.

Table 31. Selected methods for the prevention of venous thromboembolism.[1]

Risk Group	Recommendations for Prophylaxis
Surgical patients	
General surgery	
Low-risk: Minor procedures, age under 40, and no clinical risk factors	Early ambulation
Moderate risk: Minor procedures with additional thrombosis risk factors; age 40–60, and no other clinical risk factors; or major operations with age under 40 without additional clinical risk factors	ES, or LDUH, or LMWH, or IPC; plus early ambulation if possible
Higher risk: Major operation, over age 40 or with additional risk factors	LDUH, or LMWH, or IPC
Higher risk plus increased risk of bleeding	ES or IPC
Very high risk: Multiple risk factors	LDUH, or higher-dose LMWH, plus ES or IPC
Selected very high risk	Consider ADPW, INR 2.0–3.0, or postdischarge LMWH
Orthopedic surgery	
Elective total hip replacement surgery	Subcutaneous LMWH, or ADPW, or adjusted-dose heparin started preoperatively; plus IPC or ES
Elective total knee replacement surgery	LMWH, or ADPW, or IPC
Hip fracture surgery	LMWH or ADPW
Neurosurgery	
Intracranial neurosurgery	IPC with or without ES; LDUH and postoperative LMWH are acceptable alternatives; IPC or ES plus LDUH or LMWH may be more effective than either modality alone in high-risk patients.
Acute spinal cord injury	LMWH; IPC and ES may have additional benefit when used with LMWH. In the rehabilitation phase, conversion to full-dose warfarin may provide ongoing protection.
Trauma	
With an identifiable risk factor for thromboembolism	LMWH; IPC or ES if there is a contraindication to LMWH; consider duplex ultrasound screening in very high-risk patients; IVC filter insertion if proximal DVT is identified and anticoagulation is contraindicated.
Medical patients	
Acute myocardial infarction	Subcutaneous LDUH, or full-dose heparin; if heparin is contraindicated, IPC and ES may provide some protection.
Ischemic stroke with impaired mobility	LMWH or LDUH or danaparoid; IPC or ES if anticoagulants are contraindicated.
General medical patients with clinical risk factors; especially patients with cancer, congestive heart failure, or severe pulmonary disease	Low-dose LMWH, or LDUH
Cancer patients with indwelling central venous catheters	Warfarin, 1 mg/d, or LMWH

[1]Recommendations assembled from Geerts WH et al: Prevention of venous thromboembolism. Chest 2001;119(Suppl):132.

Key:

ADPW = adjusted-dose perioperative warfarin: begin 5–10 mg the day of or the day following surgery; adjust dose to INR 2.0–3.0
DVT = deep venous thrombosis
ES = elastic stockings
IPC = intermittent pneumatic compression
IVC = inferior vena cava
LDUH = low-dose unfractionated heparin: 5000 units subcutaneously every 8–12 hours starting 1–2 hours before surgery.
LMWH = low-molecular weight heparin. See Table 32 for dosing regimens.

Table 32. Selected low-molecular-weight heparin and heparinoid regimens to prevent venous thromboembolism.[1]

Risk Group	Drug	Dose[2] Subcutaneous	Administration Regimen	Cost[3]
General surgery, moderate risk	Dalteparin (Fragmin)	2500 units	1–2 h preop and qd postop	$15.35/dose
	Enoxaparin (Lovenox)	20 mg	1–2 h preop and qd postop	$18.35/dose
	Nadroparin (Fraxiparin)	2850 units	2–4 h preop and qd postop	No price available: not available in USA.
	Tinzaparin (Innohep)	3500 units	2 h preop and qd postop	$29.40/dose
General surgery, high risk	Dalteparin (Fragmin)	5000 units	8–12 preop and qd postop	$24.90/dose
	Danaparoid (Orgaran)	750 units	1–4 h preop and q12h postop	$141.31/dose
	Enoxaparin (Lovenox)	40 mg	1–2 h preop and qd postop	$25.68/dose
	Enoxaparin (Lovenox)	30 mg	q12h starting 8–12 h postop	$1.27/dose
Orthopedic surgery	Dalteparin (Fragmin)	5000 units	8–12 h preop and qd starting 12–24 h postop	$24.90/dose
	Dalteparin (Fragmin)	2500 units	6–8 h postop then 5000 units qd	$15.35/dose
	Danaparoid (Orgaran)	750 units	1–4 preop and q 12 h postop	$141.31/dose
	Enoxaparin (Lovenox)	30 mg	q12h starting 12–24 h postop	$19.27/dose
	Enoxaparin (Lovenox)	40 mg	qd starting 10–12 h preop	$25.68/dose
	Nadroparin (Fraxiparin)	38 units/kg	12 h preop, 12 h postop, and qd on postop days 1, 2, 3; then increase to 57 units/kg qd	No price available: not available in USA.
	Tinzaparin (Innohep)	75 units/kg	qd starting 12–24 h postop	$37.80/dose (60 kg pt).
	Tinzaparin (Innohep)	4500 units	12 h preop and qd postop	$37.80/dose
Major trauma	Enoxaparin (Lovenox)	30 mg	q12h starting 12–36 h postinjury if hemostatically stable	$19.27/dose
Acute spinal cord injury	Enoxaparin (Lovenox)	30 mg	q12h	$19.27/dose
Medical conditions	Dalteparin (Fragmin)	2500 units	qd	$15.35/dose
	Danaparoid (Orgaran)	750 units	q12h	$141.31/dose
	Enoxparin (Lovenox)	40 mg	qd	$25.68/dose
	Nadroparin (Fraxiparin)	2850 units	qd	No price available: not available in USA.

[1]Modified and reproduced with permission, from Geerts WH et al: Prevention of venous thromboembolism. Chest 2001;119:132S.
[2]Dose expressed in anti-Xa units; for enoxaparin, 1 mg = 100 anti-Xa units.
[3]Average wholesale price (AWP, for AB-rated generic when available) for quantity listed. Source: *Drug Topics Red Book,* May 2003; Vol. 22, No. 5. AWP may not accurately represent the actual pharmacy cost because wide contractual variations exist among institutions.
Preop = preoperatively; Postop = postoperatively; qd = once daily.

Table 33. Intravenous heparin dosing based on body weight.[1]

Initial dosing
1. Load with 80 units/kg IV, then
2. Initiate a maintenance infusion at 18 units/kg/h
3. Check activated partial thromboplastin time (aPTT) in 6 hours

Dose adjustment schedule based on aPTT results

aPTT	Adjustment
< 35 s (< 1.2 × control)	Rebolus with 80 units/kg; increase infusion by 4 units/kg/h
35–45 s (1.2–1.5 × control)	Rebolus with 40 units/kg; increase infusion by 2 units/kg/h
46–70 s (1.5–2.3 × control)	No change
71–90 s (2.3–3 × control)	Decrease infusion rate by 2 units/kg/h
> 90 s (> 3 × control)	Stop infusion for 1 hour, then decrease infusion by 3 units/kg/h

Repeat aPTT every 6 hours for the first 24 hours. If the aPTT is 46–70 s after 24 hours, then recheck once daily every morning. If the aPTT is outside this therapeutic range at 24 hours, continue checking every 6 hours until it is 46–70 s. Once it has been in the therapeutic range on two consecutive measurements after 24 hours, check once daily every morning.

[1]Adapted from Raschke RA et al: The weight-based heparin dosing nomogram compared with a "standard care" nomogram. Ann Intern Med 1993;119:874.

Table 34. Selected low-molecular-weight heparin anticoagulation regimens.[1,2]

Drug	Suggested Subcutaneous Treatment Dose
Dalteparin	200 units/kg once daily (not to exceed 18,000 units/dose)
Enoxaparin	1.5 mg/kg once daily (single dose not to exceed 180 mg)
Nadroparin	86 units/kg twice daily for 10 days, or 171 units/kg once daily (single dose not to exceed 17,000 units)
Tinzaparin	175 units/kg once daily

[1]Modified and reproduced with permission, from Hyers TM et al: Antithrombotic therapy for venous thromboembolic disease. Chest 2001;119(Suppl):176S.
[2]Dose expressed in anti-Xa units; for enoxaparin, 1 mg = 100 anti-Xa units.

Table 35. Selected causes of hypersensitivity pneumonitis.

Disease	Antigen	Source
Farmer's lung	*Micropolyspora faeni, Thermoactinomyces vulgaris*	Moldy hay
"Humidifier" lung	Thermophilic actinomycetes	Contaminated humidifiers, heating systems, or air conditioners
Bird fancier's lung ("pigeon-breeder's disease")	Avian proteins	Bird serum and excreta
Bagassosis	*Thermoactinomyces sacchari* and *T vulgaris*	Moldy sugar cane fiber (bagasse)
Sequoiosis	*Graphium, aureobasidium,* and other fungi	Moldy redwood sawdust
Maple bark stripper's disease	*Cryptostroma (Coniosporium) corticale*	Rotting maple tree logs or bark
Mushroom picker's disease	Same as farmer's lung	Moldy compost
Suberosis	*Penicillium frequentans*	Moldy cork dust
Detergent worker's lung	*Bacillus subtilis* enzyme	Enzyme additives

Table 36. Causes of pleural fluid transudates and exudates.

Transudates	Exudates
Congestive heart failure (≈90% of cases)	Pneumonia (parapneumonic effusion)
Cirrhosis with ascites	Cancer
Nephrotic syndrome	Pulmonary embolism
Peritoneal dialysis	Bacterial infection
Myxedema	Tuberculosis
Acute atelectasis	Connective tissue disease
Constrictive pericarditis	Viral infection
Superior vena cava obstruction	Fungal infection
Pulmonary embolism	Rickettsial infection
	Parasitic infection
	Asbestos
	Meigs' syndrome
	Pancreatic disease
	Uremia
	Chronic atelectasis
	Trapped lung
	Chylothorax
	Sarcoidosis
	Drug reaction
	Post-myocardial infarction syndrome

Table 37. Characteristics of important exudative pleural effusions.

Etiology or Type of Effusion	Gross Appearance	White Blood Cell Count (cells/μL)	Red Blood Cell Count (cells/μL)	Glucose	Comments
Malignant effusion	Turbid to bloody; occasionally serous	1000 to < 100,000 M	100 to several hundred thousand	Equal to serum levels; < 60 mg/dL in 15% of cases	Eosinophilia uncommon; positive results on cytologic examination
Uncomplicated parapneumonic effusion	Clear to turbid	5000–25,000 P	< 5000	Equal to serum levels	Tube thoracostomy unnecessary
Empyema	Turbid to purulent	25,000–100,000 P	< 5000	Less than serum levels; often very low	Drainage necessary; putrid odor suggests anaerobic infection
Tuberculosis	Serous to serosanguineous	5000–10,000 M	< 10,000	Equal to serum levels; occasionally < 60 mg/dL	Protein 4.0 g/dL and may exceed 5 g/dL; eosinophils (> 10%) or mesothelial cells (> 5%) make diagnosis unlikely
Rheumatoid effusion	Turbid; greenish-yellow	1000–20,000 M or P	< 1000	< 40 mg/dL	Secondary empyema common; high LDH, low complement, high rheumatoid factor, cholesterol crystals are characteristic
Pulmonary infarction	Serous to grossly bloody	1000–50,000 M or P	100 to > 100,000	Equal to serum levels	Variable findings; no pathognomonic features
Esophageal rupture	Turbid to purulent; red-brown	< 5000 to > 50,000 P	1000–10,000	Usually low	High amylase level (salivary origin); pneumothorax in 25% of cases; effusion usually on left side; pH < 6.0 strongly suggests diagnosis
Pancreatitis	Turbid to serosanguineous	1000–50,000 P	1000–10,000	Equal to serum levels	Usually left-sided; high amylase level

M = mononuclear cell predominance; P = polymorphonuclear leukocyte predominance.

Table 38. Selected disorders associated with ARDS.

Systemic Insults	Pulmonary Insults
Trauma	Aspiration of gastric contents
Sepsis	Embolism of thrombus, fat, air, or amniotic fluid
Pancreatitis	
Shock	Miliary tuberculosis
Multiple transfusions	Diffuse pneumonia (eg, SARS)
Disseminated intravascular coagulation	Acute eosinophilic pneumonia
	Bronchiolitis obliterans-organizing pneumonia
Burns	
Drugs and drug overdose	Upper airway obstruction
Opioids	Free-base cocaine smoking
Aspirin	Near-drowning
Phenothiazines	Toxic gas inhalation
Tricyclic antidepressants	Nitrogen dioxide
Amiodarone	Chlorine
Chemotherapeutic agents	Sulfur dioxide
Nitrofurantoin	Ammonia
Protamine	Smoke
Thrombotic thrombocytopenic purpura	Oxygen toxicity
	Lung contusion
Cardiopulmonary bypass	Radiation exposure
Head injury	High-altitude exposure
Paraquat	Lung reexpansion or reperfusion
	Diffuse pneumonia (eg SARS)

Table 39. Thrombolytic therapy for acute myocardial infarction.

	Streptokinase	Alteplase; Tissue Plasminogen Activator (t-PA)	Reteplase	Anistreplase (APSAC)	Tenecteplase (TNK-t-PA)
Source	Group C streptococcus	Recombinant DNA	Recombinant DNA	Group C streptococcus	Recombinant DNA
Half-life	20 minutes	5 minutes	15 minutes	90 minutes	20 minutes
Usual dose	1.5 million units	100 mg	20 units	30 units	40 mg
Administration	750,000 units over 20 minutes followed by 750,000 units over 40 minutes	Initial bolus of 15 mg, followed by 50 mg infused over next 30 minutes and 35 mg over the following 60 minutes	10 units as a bolus over 2 minutes, repeated after 30 minutes	Infuse over 2–5 minutes	Single weight-adjusted bolus, 0.5 mg/kg
Anticoagulation after infusion	Aspirin, 325 mg daily; there is no evidence that adjunctive heparin improves outcome following streptokinase	Aspirin, 325 mg daily; heparin, 5000 units as bolus, followed by 1000 units per hour infusion, subsequently adjusted to maintain PTT 1½–2 times control	Aspirin, 325 mg; heparin as with t-PA	Aspirin, 325 mg daily	Aspirin, 325 mg daily
Clot selectivity	Low	High	High	Moderate	High
Fibrinogenolysis	+++	+	+	+	+
Bleeding	+	+	+	+	+
Hypotension	+++	+	+	+	+
Allergic reactions	++	0	0	+	+
Reocclusion	5–20%	10–30%	—	5–20%	5–20%
Approximate cost[1]	$594.50	$2974.13	$2872.50	$2835.58	$2832.50

[1]Average wholesale price (AWP, for AB-rated generic when available) for quantity listed. Source: *Drug Topics Red Book*, May 2003; Vol. 22, No. 5. AWP may not accurately represent the actual pharmacy cost because wide contractual variations exist among institutions.

Table 40. Antiarrhythmic drugs.

Agent	Intravenous Dosage	Oral Dosage	Therapeutic Plasma Level	Route of Elimination	Side Effects
Class Ia: Action: Sodium channel blockers: Depress phase 0 depolarization; slow conduction; prolong repolarization. **Indications:** Supraventricular tachycardia, ventricular tachycardia, prevention of ventricular fibrillation, symptomatic ventricular premature beats.					
Quinidine	6–10 mg/kg (IM or IV) over 20 min (rarely used parenterally)	200–400 mg every 4–6 h or every 8 h (long-acting)	2–5 mg/mL	Hepatic	GI, ↓LVF, ↑Dig
Procainamide	100 mg/1–3 min to 500–1000 mg; maintain at 2–6 mg/min	50 mg/kg/d in divided doses every 3–4 h or every 6 h (long-acting)	4–10 mg/mL; NAPA (active metabolite), 10–20 μg/mL	Renal	SLE, hypersensitivity, ↓LVF
Disopyramide		100–200 mg every 6–8 h	2–8 mg/mL	Renal	Urinary retention, dry mouth, markedly ↓LVF
Moricizine		200–300 mg every 8 h	*Note:* Active metabolites	Hepatic	Dizziness, nausea, headache, ↓theophylline level, ↓LVF
Class Ib: Action: Shorten repolarization. **Indications:** Ventricular tachycardia, prevention of ventricular fibrillation, symptomatic ventricular beats.					
Lidocaine	1–2 mg/kg at 50 mg/min; maintain at 1–4 mg/min		1–5 mg/mL	Hepatic	CNS, GI
Mexiletine		100–300 mg every 6–12 h; maximum: 1200 mg/d	0.5–2 mg/mL	Hepatic	CNS, GI, leukopenia
Phenytoin	50 mg/5 min to 1000 mg (12 mg/kg); maintain at 200–400 mg/d	200–400 mg every 12–24 h	5–20 mg/mL	Hepatic	CNS, GI
Class Ic: Action: Depress phase 0 repolarization; slow conduction. *Propafenone* is a weak calcium channel blocker and β-blocker and prolongs action potential and refractoriness. **Indications:** Life-threatening ventricular tachycardia or fibrillation, refractory supraventricular tachycardia.					
Flecainide		100–200 mg twice daily	0.2–1 mg/mL	Hepatic	CNS, GI, ↓↓LVF, incessant VT, sudden death
Propafenone		150–300 mg every 8–12 h	*Note:* Active metabolites	Hepatic	CNS, GI, ↓↓LVF, ↑Dig
Class II: Action: β-blocker, slows AV conduction. *Note:* Other β-blockers may also have antiarrhythmic effects but are not yet approved for this indication in the US. **Indications:** Supraventricular tachycardia; may prevent ventricular fibrillation.					
Esmolol	500 mg/kg over 1–2 min; maintain at 25–200 mg/kg/min	Other β-blockers may be used concomitantly	0.15–2 mg/mL	Hepatic	↓LVF, bronchospasm
Propranolol	1–5 mg at 1 mg/min	40–320 mg in 1–4 doses daily (depending on preparation)	Not established	Hepatic	↓LVF, bradycardia, AV block, bronchospasm
Metoprolol	2.5–5 mg	50–200 mg daily	Not established	Hepatic	↓LVF, bradycardia, AV block

(continued)

Table 40. Antiarrhythmic drugs. (continued)

Agent	Intravenous Dosage	Oral Dosage	Therapeutic Plasma Level	Route of Elimination	Side Effects
Class III: Action: Prolong action potential.					
Indications: *Amiodarone:* refractory ventricular tachycardia, supraventricular tachycardia, prevention of ventricular tachycardia, atrial fibrillation, ventricular fibrillation; *dofetilide:* atrial fibrillation and flutter; *sotalol:* ventricular tachycardia, atrial fibrillation; *bretylium:* ventricular fibrillation, ventricular tachycardia; *ibutilide:* conversion of atrial fibrillation and flutter.					
Amiodarone	150 mg infused rapidly, followed by 1-mg/min infusion for 6 hours (360 mg) and then 0.5 mg/min; additional 150 mg as needed	800–1600 mg/d for 7–21 days; maintain at 100–400 mg/d (higher doses may be needed)	1–5 mg/mL	Hepatic	Pulmonary fibrosis, hypothyroidism, hyperthyroidism, corneal and skin deposits, hepatitis, $\uparrow$ Dig, neurotoxicity, GI
Sotalol		80–160 mg every 12 h (higher doses may be used for life-threatening arrhythmias)		Renal (dosing interval should be extended if creatinine clearance is < 60 mL/min)	Early incidence of torsade de pointes, $\downarrow$LVF, bradycardia, fatigue (and other side effects associated with β-blockers)
Dofetilide		500 mg twice daily		Renal (dose must be reduced with renal dysfunction)	Torsade de pointes in 3%; interaction with cytochrome P450 inhibitors
Ibutilide	1 mg over 10 minutes, followed by a second infusion of 0.5–1 mg over 10 minutes			Hepatic and renal	Torsade de pointes in up to 5% of patients within 3 hours after administration; patients must be monitored with defibrillator nearby
Bretylium	5–10 mg/kg over 5–10 min; maintain at 0.5–2 mg/min; maximum: 30 mg/kg		0.5–1.5 mg/mL	Renal	Hypotension, nausea
Class IV: Action: Slow calcium channel blockers.					
Indications: Supraventricular tachycardia.					
Verapamil	10–20 mg over 2–20 min; maintain at 5 mg/kg/min	80–120 mg every 6–8 h; 240–360 mg once daily with sustained-release preparation	0.1–0.15 mg/mL	Hepatic	$\downarrow$LVF, constipation, $\uparrow$Dig, hypotension
Diltiazem	0.25 mg/kg over 2 min; second 0.35-mg/kg bolus after 15 min if response is inadequate; infusion rate, 5–15 mg/h	180–360 mg daily in 1–3 doses depending on preparation (oral forms not approved for arrhythmias)		Hepatic metabolism, renal excretion	Hypotension, $\downarrow$LVF
Miscellaneous: Indications: Supraventricular tachycardia.					
Adenosine	6 mg rapidly followed by 12 mg after 1–2 min if needed. Use half these doses if administered via central line.			Adenosine receptor stimulation, metabolized in blood	Transient flushing, dyspnea, chest pain, AV block, sinus bradycardia; effect $\downarrow$ by theophylline, $\uparrow$ by dipyridamole

Table 40. Antiarrhythmic drugs. (continued)

Agent	Intravenous Dosage	Oral Dosage	Therapeutic Plasma Level	Route of Elimination	Side Effects
Digoxin	0.5 mg over 20 min followed by increment of 0.25 or 0.125 mg to 1–1.5 mg over 24 hours	1–1.5 mg over 24–36 hours in 3 or 4 doses; maintenance, 0.125–0.5 mg/d	0.7–2 mg/mL	Renal	AV block, arrhythmias, GI, visual changes

Key: AV = atrioventricular; CNS = central nervous system; ↑Dig = elevation of serum digoxin level; GI = gastrointestinal (nausea, vomiting, diarrhea); ↓LVF = reduced left ventricular function; NAPA = N-acetylprocainamide; SLE = systemic lupus erythematosus; VT = ventricular tachycardia.

Table 41. Stages of heart failure.[1]

Stage	Description	Examples
A	Patients at high risk of developing heart failure because of the presence of conditions that are strongly associated with the development of heart failure. Such patients have no identified structural or functional abnormalities of the pericarcium, myocardium, or cardiac valves and have never shown symptoms or signs of heart failure.	Systemic hypertension; coronary artery disease; diabetes mellitus; history of cardiotoxic drug therapy or alcohol abuse; personal history of rheumatic fever; family history of cardiomyopathy.
B	Patients who have developed structural heart disease that is strongly associated with the development of heart failure but who have never shown symptoms or signs of heart failure.	Left ventricular hypertrophy or fibrosis; left ventricular dilatation or hypocontractility; asymptomatic valvular heart disease; previous myocardial infarction.
C	Patients who have current or prior symptoms of heart failure associated with underlying structural heart disease.	Dyspnea or fatigue due to left ventricular systolic dysfunction; asymptomatic patients who are undergoing treatment for prior symptoms of heart failure.
D	Patients with advanced structural heart disease and marked symptoms of heart failure at rest despite maximal medical therapy and who require specialized interventions.	Patients who are frequently hospitalized for heart failure and cannot be safely discharged from the hospital; patients in the hospital awaiting heart transplantation; patients at home receiving continuous intravenous support for symptom release or being supported with a mechanical circulatory assist device; patients in a hospice setting for the management of heart failure.

[1]Reproduced, with permission from www.acc.org/clinical/guidelines/failure/figures.htm.

Table 42. Lifestyle modifications for hypertension prevention and management.[1]

Lose weight if overweight

Limit alcohol intake to no more than 1 oz (30 mL) of ethanol (eg, 24 oz [720 mL] of beer, 10 oz [300 mL] of wine, or 2 oz [60 mL] of 100-proof whiskey) per day for men or 0.5 oz (15 mL) of ethanol per day for women and lighter-weight men

Increase aerobic physical activity (30–45 minutes most days of the week)

Reduce sodium intake to no more than 100 mmol/d (2.4 g of sodium or 6 g of sodium chloride)

Maintain adequate intake of dietary potassium (approximately 90 mmol/d)

Maintain adequate intake of dietary calcium and magnesium for general health

Stop smoking and reduce intake of dietary saturated fat and cholesterol for overall cardiovascular health

[1]From: The sixth report of the Joint National Committee on detection, education, and treatment of high blood pressure (JNC VI). Arch Intern Med 1997;157:2413.

Table 43. Risk stratification and treatment of hypertension.[1,2]

Blood Pressure Stages (mm Hg)	Risk Group A (No Risk Factors; No TOD/CCD[3])	Risk Group B (At Least 1 Risk Factor, Not Including Diabetes; No TOD/CCD)	Risk Group C (TOD/CCD and/or Diabetes, with or without Other Risk Factors)
High-normal (130–139/85–89)	Lifestyle modification	Lifestyle modification	Drug therapy[4]
Stage 1 (140–159/80–99)	Lifestyle modification (up to 12 mo)	Lifestyle modification[5] (up to 6 mo)	Drug therapy
Stages 2 and 3 (≥ 160/≥ 100)	Drug therapy	Drug therapy	Drug therapy

[1]From: The sixth report of the Joint National Committee on detection, education, and treatment of high blood pressure (JNC VI). Arch Intern Med 1997;157:2413.
[2]**Note:** For example, a patient with diabetes and blood pressure of 142/94 mm Hg plus left ventricular hypertrophy should be classified as having stage 1 hypertension with target organ disease (left ventricular hypertrophy) and with another major risk factor (diabetes). This patient would be categorized as "Stage 1, Risk Group C," and recommended for immediate initiation of pharmacologic treatment. Lifestyle modification should be adjunctive therapy for all patients recommended for pharmacologic therapy.
[3]TOD/CCD indicates target organ disease/clinical cardiovascular disease.
[4]For those with heart failure, renal insufficiency, or diabetes.
[5]For patients with multiple risk factors, clinicians should consider drugs as initial therapy plus lifestyle modifications.

Table 44. Antihypertensive drugs: Diuretics.

Drug	Proprietary Name	Initial Dosage	Dosage Range	Cost per Unit	Cost for 30 Days' Treatment[1] (Average Dosage)	Adverse Effects	Comments
THIAZIDES AND RELATED DIURETICS							
Hydrochlorothiazide	Esidrix, Hydro-Diuril	12.5 or 25 mg once daily	12.5–50 mg once daily	$0.08/25 mg	$2.40	$\downarrow K^+, \downarrow Mg^{2+}, \uparrow Ca^{2+}, \downarrow Na^+, \uparrow$ uric acid, $\uparrow$ glucose, $\uparrow$ LDL cholesterol, $\uparrow$ triglycerides; rash, erectile dysfunction.	Low dosages effective in many patients without associated metabolic abnormalities; metolazone more effective with concurrent renal insufficiency; indapamide does not alter serum lipid levels.
Chlorthalidone	Hygroton, Thalitone	12.5 or 25 mg once daily	12.5–50 mg once daily	$0.16/25 mg	$4.80		
Metolazone	Zaroxolyn	1.25 or 2.5 mg once daily	1.25–5 mg once daily	$1.24/5 mg	$37.20		
	Mykrox	0.5 mg once daily	0.5–1 mg once daily	$1.24/0.5 mg	$27.20		
Indapamide	Lozol	2.5 mg once daily	2.5–5 mg once daily	$0.83/2.5 mg	$24.90		
LOOP DIURETICS							
Furosemide	Lasix	20 mg bid	40–320 mg in 2 or 3 doses	$0.16/40 mg	$9.60	Same as thiazides, but higher risk of excessive diuresis and electrolyte imbalance. Increases calcium excretion.	**Furosemide:** Short duration of action a disadvantage; should be reserved for patients with renal insufficiency or fluid retention. Poor antihypertensive. **Torsemide:** Effective blood pressure medication at low dosage.
Bumetanide	Bumex	0.25 mg bid	0.5–10 mg in 2 or 3 doses	$0.45/1 mg	$27.00		
Torsemide	Demadex	2.5 mg once daily	5–10 mg once daily	$0.70/10 mg	$21.00		

(continued)

Table 44. Antihypertensive drugs: Diuretics. (continued)

Drug	Proprietary Name	Initial Dosage	Dosage Range	Cost per Unit	Cost for 30 Days' Treatment[1] (Average Dosage)	Adverse Effects	Comments
			COMBINATION PRODUCTS				
Hydrochlorothiazide and triamterene	Dyazide (25/50 mg) Maxzide (25/37.5 mg)	1 tab once daily	1 or 2 tabs once daily	$0.34	$10.20	Same as thiazides plus GI disturbances, hyperkalemia rather than hypokalemia, headache; triamterene can cause kidney stones and renal dysfunction; spironolactone causes gynecomastia. Hyperkalemia can occur if this combination is used in patients with renal failure or those taking ACE inhibitors.	Use should be limited to patients with demonstrable need for a potassium-sparing agent.
Hydrochlorothiazide and amiloride	Moduretic (50/5 mg)	½ tab once daily	1 or 2 tabs once daily	$0.33	$9.90		
Hydrochlorothiazide and spironolactone	Aldactazide (25/25 mg)	1 tab once daily	1 or 2 tabs once daily	$0.50	$15.00		

[1]Average wholesale price (AWP, for AB-rated generic when available) for quantity listed. Source: *Drug Topics Red Book*, May 2003; Vol. 22, No. 5. AWP may not accurately represent the actual pharmacy cost because wide contractual variations exist among institutions.

Table 45. Antihypertensive drugs: β-adrenergic blocking agents.

Drug	Proprietary Name	Initial Dosage	Dosage Range	Cost per Unit	Cost for 30 Days' Treatment (Based on Average Dosage)[1]	β₁ Selectivity[2]	ISA[3]	MSA[4]	Lipid Solubility	Renal vs Hepatic Elimination	Comments[5]
Acebutolol	Sectral	200 mg once daily	200–1200 mg in 1 or 2 doses	$1.34/400 mg	$40.20	+	+	+	+	H > R	Positive ANA; rare LE syndrome; also indicated for arrhythmias. Doses > 800 mg have β_1 and β_2 effects.
Atenolol	Tenormin	25 mg once daily	25–200 mg once daily	$0.83/50 mg	$24.90	+	0	0	0	R	Also indicated for angina pectoris and post-MI. Doses > 100 mg have β_1 and β_2 effects.
Betaxolol	Kerlone	10 mg once daily	10–40 mg once daily	$0.88/10 mg	$26.40	+	0	0	+	H > R	
Bisoprolol and hydrochlorothiazide	Ziac	5 mg/6.25 mg	2.5–10 mg plus 6.25 mg	$1.14/2.5/6.25 mg	$34.20	+	0	0	0	R = H	Low-dose combination approved for initial therapy. Bisoprolol also effective for heart failure.
Carteolol	Cartrol	2.5 mg once daily	2.5–10 mg once daily	$1.32/5 mg	$39.60	0	+	0	+	R > H	
Carvedilol	Coreg	6.25 mg	12.5–100 mg in 2 doses	$1.73/25 mg	$103.80 (25 mg bid)	0	0	0	+++	H > R	α:β-blocking activity 1:9; may cause orthostatic symptoms; effective for congestive heart failure.
Labetalol	Normodyne, Trandate	100 mg bid	200–1200 mg in 2 doses	$0.68/200 mg	$40.80	0	0/+	0	++	H	α:β-blocking activity 1:3; more orthostatic hypotension, fever, hepatotoxicity.

(continued)

Table 45. Antihypertensive drugs: β-adrenergic blocking agents. (continued)

Drug	Proprietary Name	Initial Dosage	Dosage Range	Cost per Unit	Cost for 30 Days' Treatment (Based on Average Dosage)[1]	Special Properties β₁ Selectivity[2]	ISA[3]	MSA[4]	Lipid Solubility	Renal vs Hepatic Elimination	Comments[5]
Metoprolol	Lopressor	50 mg in 1 or 2 doses	50–200 mg in 1 or 2 doses	$0.55/50 mg	$33.00	+	0	+	+++	H	Also indicated for angina pectoris and post-MI. Approved for heart failure. Doses > 100 mg have β₁ and β₂ effects.
	Toprol XL (SR preparation)	50 mg once daily	50–200 mg once daily	$1.14/100 mg	$34.20						
Nadolol	Corgard	20 mg once daily	20–160 mg once daily	$1.04/40 mg	$31.20	0	0	0	0	R	
Penbutolol	Levatol	20 mg once daily	20–80 mg once daily	$1.54/20 mg	$46.20	0	+	0	++	R > H	
Pindolol	Visken	5 mg bid	10–60 mg in 2 doses	$0.69/5 mg	$41.40	0	++	+	+	H > R	In adults, 35% renal clearance.
Propranolol	Inderal	20 mg bid	40–320 mg in 2 doses	$0.51/40 mg	$30.60	0	0	++	+++	H	Once-daily SR preparation also available. Also indicated for angina pectoris and post-MI.
Timolol	Blocadren	5 mg bid	10–40 mg in 2 doses	$0.38/10 mg	$22.80	0	0	0	++	H > R	Also indicated for post-MI. 80% hepatic clearance.

ISA = intrinsic sympathomimetic activity; MSA = membrane-stabilizing activity; 0 = no effect; +, ++, +++ = some, moderate, most effect.

[1] Average wholesale price (AWP, for AB-rated generic when available) for quantity listed. Source: Drug Topics Red Book, May 2003; Vol. 22, No. 5. AWP may not accurately represent the actual pharmacy cost because wide contractual variations exist among institutions.

[2] Agents with β₁ selectivity are less likely to precipitate bronchospasm and decreased peripheral blood flow in low doses, but selectivity is only relative.

[3] Agents with ISA cause less resting bradycardia and lipid changes.

[4] MSA generally occurs at concentrations greater than those necessary for β-adrenergic blockade. The clinical importance of MSA by β-blockers has not been defined.

[5] Adverse effects of all β-blockers: bronchospasm, fatigue, sleep disturbance and nightmares, bradycardia and atrioventricular block, worsening of congestive heart failure, cold extremities, gastrointestinal disturbances, impotence, ↑triglycerides, ↓HDL cholesterol, rare blood dyscrasias.

Table 46. Antihypertensive drugs: ACE inhibitors and angiotensin II receptor blockers.

Drug	Proprietary Name	Initial Dosage	Dosage Range	Cost per Unit	Cost of 30 Days' Treatment (Average Dosage)[1]	Adverse Effects	Comments
ACE INHIBITORS							
Benazepril	Lotensin	10 mg once daily	5–40 mg in 1 or 2 doses	$1.05/20 mg	$31.50	Cough, hypotension, dizziness, renal dysfunction, hyperkalemia, angioedema; taste alteration and rash (may be more frequent with captopril); rarely, proteinuria, blood dyscrasia. Contraindicated in pregnancy.	More fosinopril is excreted by the liver in patients with renal dysfunction (dose reduction may or may not be necessary). Captopril and lisinopril are active without metabolism. Captopril, enalapril, lisinopril, and quinapril are approved for congestive heart failure.
Captopril	Capoten	25 mg bid	50–300 mg in 2 or 3 doses	$0.65/25 mg	$39.00		
Enalapril	Vasotec	5 mg once daily	5–40 mg in 1 or 2 doses	$1.52/20 mg	$45.60		
Fosinopril	Monopril	10 mg once daily	10–80 mg in 1 or 2 doses	$1.19/20 mg	$35.70		
Lisinopril	Prinivil, Zestril	5–10 mg once daily	5–40 mg once daily	$1.06/20 mg	$31.80		
Moexipril	Univasc	7.5 mg once daily	7.5–30 mg in 1 or 2 doses	$0.98/7.5 mg	$29.40		
Perindopril	Aceon	4 mg once daily	4–16 mg in 1 or 2 doses	$1.86/8 mg	$55.80		
Quinapril	Accupril	10 mg once daily	10–80 mg in 1 or 2 doses	$1.19/20 mg	$35.70		
Ramipril	Altace	2.5 mg once daily	2.5–20 mg in 1 or 2 doses	$1.38/5 mg	$41.40		
Trandolapril	Mavik	1 mg once daily	1–8 mg once daily	$0.99/4 mg	$29.70		
ANGIOTENSIN II RECEPTOR BLOCKERS							
Candesartan cilexitil	Atacand	16 mg once daily	8–32 mg once daily	$1.45/16 mg	$43.40	Hyperkalemia, renal dysfunction, rare angioedema. Combinations have additional side effects. Contraindicated in pregnancy.	Losartan has a very flat dose-response curve. Valsartan and irbesartan have wider dose-response ranges and longer durations of action. Addition of low-dose diuretic (separately or as combination pills) increases the response.
Candesartan cilexitil/ HCTZ	Atacand HCT	16 mg/ 12.5 mg once daily	8–32 mg of candesartan once daily	$1.96/16 mg/12.5 mg	$58.80		
Eprosartan	Teveten	600 mg once daily	400–800 mg in 1–2 doses	$1.37/ 600 mg	$41.10		
Irbesartan	Avapro	150 mg once daily	150–300 mg once daily	$1.53/150 mg	$45.80		
Irbesartan and hydrochlorothiazide	Avalide	150 mg/ 12.5 mg once daily	150–300 mg irbesartan daily	$1.92/150 mg	$57.59		
Losartan	Cozaar	50 mg once daily	25–100 mg in 1 or 2 doses	$1.59/50 mg	$47.70		

(continued)

Table 46. Antihypertensive drugs: ACE inhibitors and angiotensin II receptor blockers. (continued)

Drug	Proprietary Name	Initial Dosage	Dosage Range	Cost per Unit	Cost of 30 Days' Treatment (Average Dosage)[1]	Adverse Effects	Comments
ANGIOTENSIN II RECEPTOR BLOCKERS (continued)							
Losartan and hydrochlorothiazide	Hyzaar	50 mg/12.5 mg once daily	One or 2 tablets once daily	$1.59/50 mg/12.5 mg/tablet	$47.70		
Telmisartan	Micardis	40 mg once daily	20–80 mg once daily	$1.54/40 mg	$46.20		
Telmisartan and HCTZ	Micardis HCT	40 mg/12.5 mg once daily	20–80 mg telmisartan daily	$1.67/40 mg/12.5 mg	$50.10		
Valsartan	Diovan	80 mg once daily	80–320 mg once daily	$1.67/160 mg	$50.10		
Valsartan and HCTZ	Diovan HCT	80 mg/12.5 mg once daily	80–320 mg valsartan daily	$1.95/160 mg/12.5 mg	$58.50		

[1]Average wholesale price (AWP, for AB-rated generic when available) for quantity listed. Source: *Drug Topics Red Book,* May 2003; Vol. 22, No. 5. AWP may not accurately represent the actual pharmacy cost because wide contractual variations exist among institutions.

Table 47. Antihypertensive drugs: Calcium channel-blocking agents.

Drug	Proprietary Name	Initial Dosage	Dosage Range	Cost for 30 Days' Treatment (Average Dosage)[1]	Special Properties				Adverse Effects	Comments
					Peripheral Vasodilation	Cardiac Automaticity and Conduction	Contractility			
				NONDIHYDROPYRIDINE AGENTS						
Diltiazem	Cardizem SR	90 mg bid	180–360 mg in 2 doses	$67.80 (120 mg bid)	++	↓↓	↓↓	Edema, headache, bradycardia, GI disturbances, dizziness, AV block, congestive heart failure, urinary frequency.	Also approved for angina.
	Cardizem CD Cartia XT	180 mg qd	180–360 mg qd	$61.53 (240 mg qd)						
	Dilacor XR	180 or 240 mg qd	180–480 mg daily	$34.50 (240 mg qd)						
	Tiazac SA	240 mg qd	180–540 mg qd	$62.84 (240 mg qd)						
Verapamil	Calan SR	180 mg qd	180–480 mg in 1 or 2 doses	$46.80	++	↓↓↓	↓↓↓	Same as diltiazem but more likely to cause constipation and congestive heart failure.	Also approved for angina and arrhythmias.
	Isoptin SR Verelan Covera-HS			$62.10 (240 mg qd)						

(continued)

Table 47. Antihypertensive drugs: Calcium channel-blocking agents. (continued)

Drug	Proprietary Name	Initial Dosage	Dosage Range	Cost for 30 Days' Treatment (Average Dosage)[1]	Special Properties Peripheral Vasodilation	Special Properties Cardiac Automaticity and Conduction	Special Properties Contractility	Adverse Effects	Comments
					DIHYDROPYRIDINES				
Amlodipine	Norvasc	5 mg qd	5–20 mg qd	$65.23 (10 mg qd)	+++	↓/0	↓/0	Edema, dizziness, palpitations, flushing, headache, hypotension, tachycardia, GI disturbances, urinary frequency, worsening of congestive heart failure (may be less common with felodipine, amlodipine).	Amlodipine, nicardipine, and nifedipine also approved for angina.
Felodipine	Plendil	5 mg qd	5–20 mg qd	$65.70 (10 mg qd)	+++	↓/0	↓/0		
Isradipine	DynaCirc	2.5 mg bid	2.5–5 mg bid	$120.95 (5 mg bid)	+++	↓/0	↓		
	DynaCirc CR	5 mg qd	5–10 mg qd	$68.34 (10 mg qd)					
Nicardipine	Cardene	20 mg tid	20–40 mg tid	$41.20 (20 mg tid)	+++	↓/0	↓		
	Cardene SR	30 mg bid	30–60 mg bid	$52.31 (30 mg bid)					
Nifedipine	Adalat CC	30 mg qd	30–120 mg qd	$65.10 (60 mg qd)	+++	↓	↓↓		
	Procardia XL	30 mg qd	30–120 mg qd	$68.70 (60 mg qd)					
Nisoldipine	Sular	20 mg/d	20–60 mg/d	$36.00 (40 mg qd)	+++	↓/0	↓		

[1]Average wholesale price (AWP, for AB-rated generic when available) for quantity listed. Source: *Drug Topics Red Book*, May 2003: Vol. 22, No. 5. AWP may not accurately represent the actual pharmacy cost because wide contractual variations exist among institutions.

Table 48. Alpha-adrenoceptor blocking agents, sympatholytics, and vasodilators.

Drug	Proprietary Name	Initial Dosage	Dosage Range	Cost per Unit	Cost for 30 Days' Treatment (Average Dosage)[1]	Adverse Effects	Comments
ALPHA-ADRENOCEPTOR BLOCKERS							
Prazosin	Minipress	1 mg hs	2–20 mg in 2 or 3 doses	$0.78/5 mg	$46.80 (5 mg bid)	Syncope with first dose; postural hypotension, dizziness, palpitations, headache, weakness, drowsiness, sexual dysfunction, anticholinergic effects; urinary incontinence; first-dose effects may be less with doxazosin.	May ↑HDL and ↓LDL cholesterol. May provide short-term relief of obstructive prostatic symptoms. Less effective in preventing cardiovascular events than diuretics.
Terazosin	Hytrin	1 mg hs	1–20 mg in 1 or 2 doses	$1.60/1, 2, 5, 10 mg	$48.00 (5 mg qd)		
Doxazosin	Cardura	1 mg hs	1–16 mg qd	$0.97/4 mg	$29.10 (4 mg qd)		
CENTRAL SYMPATHOLYTICS							
Clonidine	Catapres	0.1 mg bid	0.2–0.6 mg in 2 doses	$0.22/0.1 mg	$13.20 (0.1 mg bid)	Sedation, dry mouth, sexual dysfunction, headache, bradyarrhythmias; side effects may be less with guanfacine. Contact dermatitis with clonidine patch. Methyldopa also causes hepatitis, hemolytic anemia, fever.	"Rebound" hypertension may occur even after gradual withdrawal. Methyldopa should be avoided in favor of safer agents.
	Catapres TTS	0.1 mg/d patch weekly	0.1–0.3 mg/d patch weekly	$21.63/0.2 mg	$86.50 (0.2 mg weekly)		
Guanabenz	Wytensin	4 mg bid	8–64 mg in 2 doses	$0.66/4 mg	$39.60 (4 mg bid)		
Guanfacine	Tenex	1 mg once daily	1–3 mg qd	$0.87/1 mg	$26.10 (1 mg qd)		
Methyldopa	Aldomet	250 mg bid	500–2000 mg in 2 doses	$0.69/500 mg	$41.40 (500 mg bid)		
PERIPHERAL NEURONAL ANTAGONISTS							
Guanadrel	Hylorel	5 mg bid	10–70 mg in 2 doses	$2.00/10 mg	$120.00 (10 mg bid)	Orthostatic hypotension, diarrhea, exercise hypotension, sexual dysfunction, salt and water retention.	
Reserpine	Serpasil	0.05 mg once daily	0.05–0.25 mg qd	$0.32/0.1 mg	$9.60 (0.1 mg qd)	Depression (less likely at low dosages, ie, < 0.25 mg), night terrors, nasal stuffiness, drowsiness, peptic disease, gastrointestinal disturbances, bradycardia.	

(continued)

Table 48. Alpha-adrenoceptor blocking agents, sympatholytics, and vasodilators. (continued)

Drug	Proprietary Name	Initial Dosage	Dosage Range	Cost per Unit	Cost for 30 Days' Treatment (Average Dosage)[1]	Adverse Effects	Comments
DIRECT VASODILATORS							
Hydralazine	Apresoline	25 mg bid	50–300 mg in 2–4 doses	$0.05/25 mg	$3.00 (25 mg bid)	GI disturbances, tachycardia, headache, nasal congestion, rash, LE-like syndrome.	May worsen or precipitate angina.
Minoxidil	Loniten	5 mg once daily	5–40 mg qd	$1.29/10 mg	$38.70 (10 mg qd)	Tachycardia, fluid retention, headache, hirsutism, pericardial effusion, thrombocytopenia.	Should be used in combination with β-blocker and diuretic.

[1]Average wholesale price (AWP, for AB-rated generic when available) for quantity listed. Source: *Drug Topics Red Book*, May 2003; Vol. 22, No. 5. AWP may not accurately represent the actual pharmacy cost because wide contractual variations exist among institutions.

Table 49. Considerations for individualizing antihypertensive drug therapy.[1]

Indication	Drug Therapy
COMPELLING INDICATIONS UNLESS CONTRAINDICATED	
Diabetes mellitus (type 1) with proteinuria	ACE I
Diabetes mellitus (type 2)	ACE I or ARB
Heart failure	ACE I (ARB if intolerant), β-blockers, diuretics
Post-myocardial infarction	β-Blockers (non-ISA), ACE I (with systolic dysfunction)
Isolated systolic hypertension (older patients)	Diuretics (preferred), calcium antagonists
MAY HAVE FAVORABLE EFFECTS ON COMORBID CONDITIONS[2]	
Angina	β-Blockers, calcium antagonists
Atherosclerotic vascular disease	ACE inhibitors
Atrial tachycardia, fibrillation	β-Blockers, calcium antagonists (nondihydropyridine)
Cyclosporine-induced hypertension (caution with the dose of cyclosporine)	Calcium antagonists
Diabetes mellitus (type 2)	Low-dose diuretics
Essential tremor	β-Blockers (noncardioselective)
Migraine	β-Blockers (noncardioselective), calcium antagonists (nondihydropyridine)
Osteoporosis	Thiazides
Preoperative hypertension	β-Blockers
Prostatism (benign prostatic hyperplasia)	α-Blockers
Renal insufficiency (caution in renovascular hypertension and creatinine level ≥ 3 mg/dL [265.2 μmol/L])	ACE I, ARB
MAY HAVE UNFAVORABLE EFFECTS ON COMORBID CONDITIONS[2,3]	
Bronchospastic disease	β-Blockers[4]
Depression	β-Blockers, central α-agonists, reserpine[4]
Diabetes mellitus (with hyperglycosuria)	β-Blockers
Dyslipidemia	β-Blockers (non-ISA), diuretics (high-dose)
Gout	Diuretics
Heart block (2nd or 3rd degree)	β-Blockers,[4] calcium antagonists (nondihydropyridine)[4]
Heart failure	Calcium antagonists (except amlodipine), α–blockers, β-blockers[5]
Liver disease	Labetalol hydrochloride, methyldopa[4]
Peripheral vascular disease	β-Blockers
Pregnancy	ACE I,[4] ARB[4]
Renal insufficiency	Potassium-sparing agents
Renovascular disease	ACE I, ARB (contraindicated if bilateral renal artery stenosis)

ACE I, angiotensin-converting enzyme inhibitors; ARB, angiotensin II receptor blockers; ISA, intrinsic sympathomimetic activity.

[1]Modified from: The sixth report of the Joint National Committee on detection, education, and treatment of high blood pressure (JNC VI). Arch Intern Med 1997;157:2413.

[2]Conditions and drugs are listed in alphabetical order.

[3]These drugs may be used with special monitoring unless contraindicated.

[4]Contraindicated.

[5]β-Blockers may worsen heart failure initially but are indicated in stable patients.

Table 50. Drugs for hypertensive emergencies and urgencies.

Agent	Action	Dosage	Onset	Duration	Adverse Effects	Comments
PARENTERAL AGENTS (INTRAVENOUSLY UNLESS NOTED)						
Nitroprusside (Nipride)	Vasodilator	0.25–10 µg/kg/min	Seconds	3–5 minutes	GI, CNS; thiocyanate and cyanide toxicity, especially with renal and hepatic insufficiency; hypotension.	Most effective and easily titratable treatment. Use with β-blocker in aortic dissection.
Nitroglycerin	Vasodilator	0.25–5 µg/kg/min	2–5 minutes	3–5 minutes	Headache, nausea, hypotension, bradycardia.	Tolerance may develop. Useful primarily with myocardial ischemia.
Labetalol (Normodyne, Trandate)	β- and α-blocker	20–40 mg every 10 minutes to 300 mg; 2 mg/min infusion	5–10 minutes	3–6 hours	GI, hypotension, bronchospasm, bradycardia, heart block.	Avoid in congestive heart failure, asthma. May be continued orally.
Esmolol (Brevibloc)	β-blocker	Loading dose 500 µg/kg over 1 minute; maintenance, 25–200 µg/kg/min	1–2 minutes	10–30 minutes	Bradycardia, nausea.	Avoid in congestive heart failure, asthma. Weak antihypertensive.
Fenoldopam (Corlopam)	Dopamine receptor agonist	0.1–1.6 µg/kg/min	4–5 minutes	< 10 minutes	Reflex tachycardia, hypotension, ↑ intraocular pressure.	May protect renal function.
Nicardipine (Cardene)	Calcium channel blocker	5 mg/h; may increase by 1–2.5 mg/h every 15 minutes to 15 mg/h	1–5 minutes	3–6 hours	Hypotension, tachycardia, headache.	May precipitate myocardial ischemia.
Enalaprilat (Vasotec)	ACE inhibitor	1.25 mg every 6 hours	15 minutes	6 hours or more	Excessive hypotension.	Additive with diuretics; may be continued orally.
Furosemide (Lasix)	Diuretic	10–80 mg	15 minutes	4 hours	Hypokalemia, hypotension.	Adjunct to vasodilator.
Hydralazine (Apresoline)	Vasodilator	5–20 mg IV or IM (less desirable); may repeat after 20 minutes	10–30 minutes	2–6 hours	Tachycardia, headache, GI.	Avoid in coronary artery disease, dissection. Rarely used except in pregnancy.
Diazoxide (Hyperstat)	Vasodilator	50–150 mg repeated at intervals of 5–15 minutes, or 15–30 mg/min by IV infusion to a maximum of 600 mg	1–2 minutes	4–24 hours	Excessive hypotension, tachycardia, myocardial ischemia, headache, nausea, vomiting, hyperglycemia. Necrosis with extravasation.	Avoid in coronary artery disease and dissection. Use with β-blocker and diuretic. Mostly obsolete.
Trimethaphan (Arfonad)	Ganglionic blocker	0.5–5 mg/min	1–3 minutes	10 minutes	Hypotension, ileus, urinary retention, respiratory arrest. Liberates histamine; use caution in allergic individuals.	Useful in aortic dissection. Otherwise rarely used.
ORAL AGENTS						
Nifedipine (Adalat, Procardia)	Calcium channel blocker	10 mg initially; may be repeated after 30 minutes	15 minutes	2–6 hours	Excessive hypotension, tachycardia, headache, angina, myocardial infarction, stroke.	Response unpredictable.
Clonidine (Catapres)	Central sympatholytic	0.1–0.2 mg initially; then 0.1 mg every hour to 0.8 mg	30–60 minutes	6–8 hours	Sedation.	Rebound may occur.
Captopril (Capoten)	ACE inhibitor	12.5–25 mg	15–30 minutes	4–6 hours	Excessive hypotension.	

1248

Table 51. Causes of nausea and vomiting.

Visceral afferent stimulation	**Infections**
	Mechanical obstruction
	Gastric outlet obstruction: peptic ulcer disease, malignancy, gastric volvulus
	Small intestinal obstruction: adhesions, hernias, volvulus, Crohn's disease, carcinomatosis
	Dysmotility
	Gastroparesis: diabetic, medications, postviral, postvagotomy
	Small intestine: scleroderma, amyloidosis, chronic intestinal pseudo-obstruction, familial myoneuropathies
	Peritoneal irritation
	Peritonitis: perforated viscus, appendicitis, spontaneous bacterial peritonitis
	Viral gastroenteritis: Norwalk agent, rotavirus
	"Food poisoning": toxins from *B cereus, S aureus, C perfringens*
	Hepatitis A or B
	Acute systemic infections
	Hepatobiliary or pancreatic disorders
	Acute pancreatitis
	Cholecystitis or choledocholithiasis
	Topical gastrointestinal irritants
	Alcohol, NSAIDs, oral antibiotics
	Postoperative
	Other
	Cardiac disease: acute myocardial infarction, congestive heart failure
	Urologic disease: stones, pyelonephritis
Central nervous system disorders	**Vestibular disorders**
	Labyrinthitis, Ménière's syndrome, motion sickness, migraine
	Increased intracranial pressure
	CNS tumors, subdural or subarachnoid hemorrhage
	Migraine
	Infections
	Meningitis, encephalitis
	Psychogenic
	Anticipatory vomiting, bulimia, psychiatric disorders
Irritation of chemoreceptor trigger zone	**Antitumor chemotherapy**
	Drugs and medications
	Calcium channel blockers
	Opioids
	Anticonvulsants
	Antiparkinsonism drugs
	β-blockers, antiarrhythmics, digoxin
	Nicotine
	Radiation therapy
	Systemic disorders
	Diabetic ketoacidosis
	Uremia
	Adrenocortical crisis
	Parathyroid disease
	Hypothyroidism
	Pregnancy
	Paraneoplastic syndrome

Table 52. Common antiemetic dosing regimens.

	Dosage	Route
Serotonin 5-HT$_3$ antagonists		
Ondansetron	8 mg or 0.15 mg/kg once daily	IV
	8 mg twice daily	PO
Granisetron	1 mg or 0.01 mg/kg once daily	IV
	2 mg once daily	PO
Dolasetron	100 mg or 1.8 mg/kg once daily	IV
	100–200 mg once daily	PO
Corticosteroids		
Dexamethasone	8–20 mg once	IV
	4–20 mg once or twice daily	PO
Methylprednisolone	40–100 mg once	IV
Dopamine receptor antagonists		
Metoclopramide	10–30 mg or 0.5 mg/kg every 6–8 hours	IV
	10–20 mg every 6–8 hours	PO
Prochlorperazine	5–20 mg every 4–6 hours	PO, IM, IV
	25 mg suppository every 6 hours	PR
Promethazine	25 mg every 4–6 hours	PO, PR, IM
Trimethobenzamide	250 mg every 6–8 hours	PO
	200 mg every 6–8 hours	IM, PR
Sedatives		
Diazepam	2–5 mg every 4–6 hours	PO, IV
Lorazepam	1–2 mg every 4–6 hours	PO, IV

Table 53. Causes of ascites.

NORMAL PERITONEUM

Portal hypertension (SAAG ≥ 1.1 g/dL)
1. **Hepatic congestion[1]**
   Congestive heart failure
   Constrictive pericarditis
   Tricuspid insufficiency
   Budd-Chiari syndrome
   Veno-occlusive disease
2. **Liver disease[2]**
   Cirrhosis
   Alcoholic hepatitis
   Fulminant hepatic failure
   Massive hepatic metastases
   Hepatic fibrosis
   Acute fatty liver of pregnancy
3. **Portal vein occlusion**

Hypoalbuminemia (SAAG < 1.1 g/dL)
   Nephrotic syndrome
   Protein-losing enteropathy
   Severe malnutrition with anasarca

Miscellaneous conditions (SAAG < 1.1 g/dL)
   Chylous ascites
   Pancreatic ascites
   Bile ascites
   Nephrogenic ascites
   Urine ascites
   Myxedema (SAAG ≥ 1.1 g/dL)
   Ovarian disease

DISEASED PERITONEUM (SAAG < 1.1 g/dL)[2]

Infections
   Bacterial peritonitis
   Tuberculous peritonitis
   Fungal peritonitis
   HIV-associated peritonitis

Malignant conditions
   Peritoneal carcinomatosis
   Primary mesothelioma
   Pseudomyxoma peritonei
   Massive hepatic metastases
   Hepatocellular carcinoma

Other conditions
   Familial Mediterranean fever
   Vasculitis
   Granulomatous peritonitis
   Eosinophilic peritonitis

SAAG = serum-ascites albumin gradient.

[1]Hepatic congestion usually associated with SAAG ≥ 1.1 g/dL and ascitic fluid total protein > 2.5 g/dL.

[2]There may be cases of "mixed ascites" in which portal hypertensive ascites is complicated by a secondary process such as infection. In these cases, the SAAG is ≥ 1.1 g/dL.

Table 54. Treatment options for peptic ulcer disease.

Active *Helicobacter pylori*–associated ulcer:
1. Treat with anti–*H pylori* regimen for 10–14 days. Treatment options:

   Proton pump inhibitor twice daily[1]
   Clarithromycin 500 mg twice daily
   Amoxicillin 1 g twice daily (or metronidazole 500 mg twice daily, if penicillin allergic)

   Proton pump inhibitor twice daily[1]
   Bismuth subsalicylate two tablets four times daily
   Tetracycline 500 mg four times daily
   Metronidazole 250 mg four times daily

   Ranitidine bismuth citrate 400 mg twice daily (not available in US)
   Clarithromycin 500 mg twice daily
   Amoxicillin 1 g or tetracycline 500 mg or metronidazole 500 mg twice daily

   (Proton pump inhibitors administered before meals. Avoid metronidazole regimens in areas of known high resistance or in patients who have failed a course of treatment that included metronidazole.)

2. After completion of 10–14 day course of *H pylori* eradication therapy, continue treatment with proton pump inhibitor[1] once daily or H_2 receptor antagonist (as below) for 4–8 weeks to promote healing.

Active ulcer not attributable to *H pylori*:

1. Consider other causes: NSAIDs, Zollinger-Ellison syndrome, gastric malignancy. Treatment options:

   Proton pump inhibitors[1]:
      Uncomplicated duodenal ulcer: treat for 4 weeks
      Uncomplicated gastric ulcer: treat for 8 weeks
   H_2 receptor antagonists:
      Uncomplicated duodenal ulcer: cimetidine 800 mg, ranitidine or nizatidine 300 mg, famotidine 40 mg, once daily at bedtime for 6 weeks
      Uncomplicated gastric ulcer: cimetidine 400 mg, ranitidine or nizatidine 150 mg, famotidine 20 mg, twice daily for 8 weeks
      Complicated ulcers: proton pump inhibitors are preferred drugs

Prevention of ulcer relapse:

1. NSAID-induced ulcer: prophylactic therapy for high-risk patients (prior ulcer disease or ulcer complications, use of corticosteroids or anticoagulants, age > 70 with serious comorbid illnesses).
   Treatment options:

   Proton pump inhibitor once daily
   COX-2 selective NSAID (rofecoxib, celecoxib, valdecoxib)
   (In special circumstances: misoprostol 200 μg 3–4 times daily)

2. Chronic "maintenance" therapy indicated in patients with recurrent ulcers who either are *H pylori*–negative or who have failed attempts at eradication therapy: once-daily proton pump inhibitor[1] or H_2 receptor antagonist at bedtime (cimetidine 400–800 mg, nizatidine or ranitidine 150–300 mg, famotidine 20–40 mg)

---

[1] Proton pump inhibitors: omeprazole 20 mg, rabeprazole 20 mg, lansoprazole 30 mg, pantoprazole 40 mg, esomeprazole 40 mg.
All proton pump inhibitors are given twice daily except esomeprazole (once daily).

Table 55A. Staging of colorectal cancer.

American Joint Committee Classification	TNM			Dukes Class[1]
Stage 0				
Carcinoma in situ	Tis	N0	M0	
Stage I				
Tumor invades submucosa	T1	N0	M0	Dukes A
Tumor invades muscularis propria	T2	N0	M0	Dukes B_1
Stage II				
Tumor invades into subserosa or into nonperitonealized pericolic or perirectal tissues	T3	N0	M0	Dukes B_1 or B_2
Tumor perforates the visceral peritoneum or directly invades other organs or structures	T4	N0	M0	Dukes B_2
Stage III				
Any degree of bowel wall perforation with lymph node metastasis				
One to three pericolic or perirectal lymph nodes involved	Any T	N1	M0	Dukes C_1
Four or more pericolic or perirectal lymph nodes involved	Any T	N2	M0	Dukes C_2
Metastasis to lymph nodes along a vascular trunk	Any T	N3	M0	
Stage IV				
Presence of distant metastasis	Any T	Any N	M1	Dukes D

[1]Gastrointestinal Tumor Study Group modification of Dukes classification.

Table 55B. Recommendations for colorectal cancer screening.[1]

Average-risk individuals ≥ 50 years old[2]
  Annual fecal occult blood testing
  Flexible sigmoidoscopy every 5 years
  Annual fecal occult blood testing *and* flexible sigmoidoscopy every 5 years
  Colonoscopy every 10 years
  Barium enema every 5–10 years
Individuals with a family history of a first-degree member with colorectal neoplasia[3]
  Single first-degree relative with colorectal cancer diagnosed at age ≥ **60 years:**
    Begin screening at age 40. Screening guidelines same as average-risk individual; however, preferred method is colonoscopy every 10 years.
  Single first-degree relative with colorectal cancer diagnosed at age < **60 years,** or multiple first-degree relatives: Begin screening at age 40 or at age 10 years younger than age at diagnosis of the youngest affected relative, whichever is first in time. Recommended screening: colonoscopy every 3–5 years.

[1]For recommendations for families with inherited polyposis syndromes or hereditary nonpolyposis colon cancer, see separate section.
[2]Colorectal Cancer Screening and Rationale. Gastroenterology 1997; 112:5.
[3]Screening Recommendations of American College of Gastroenterology. Am J Gastroenterol 2000;95:868.

Table 56A. Classification of jaundice.

Type of Hyperbilirubinemia	Location and Cause
Unconjugated hyperbilirubinemia (predominant indirect-acting bilirubin)	Increased bilirubin production (eg, hemolytic anemias, hemolytic reactions, hematoma, pulmonary infarction)
	Impaired bilirubin uptake and storage (eg, posthepatitis hyperbilirubinemia, Gilbert's syndrome, Crigler-Najjar syndrome, drug reactions)
Conjugated hyperbilirubinemia (predominant direct-acting bilirubin)	**HEREDITARY CHOLESTATIC SYNDROMES** Faulty excretion of bilirubin conjugates (eg, Dubin-Johnson syndrome, Rotor's syndrome)
	HEPATOCELLULAR DYSFUNCTION Biliary epithelial damage (eg, hepatitis, hepatic cirrhosis)
	Intrahepatic cholestasis (eg, certain drugs, biliary cirrhosis, sepsis, postoperative jaundice)
	Hepatocellular damage or intrahepatic cholestasis resulting from miscellaneous causes (eg, spirochetal infections, infectious mononucleosis, cholangitis, sarcoidosis, lymphomas, industrial toxins)
	BILIARY OBSTRUCTION Choledocholithiasis, biliary atresia, carcinoma of biliary duct, sclerosing cholangitis, choledochal cyst, external pressure on common duct, pancreatitis, pancreatic neoplasms

Table 56B. Hyperbilirubinemic disorders.

	Nature of Defect	Type of Hyper-bilirubinemia	Clinical and Pathologic Characteristics
Gilbert's syndrome	Glucuronyl transferase deficiency	Unconjugated (indirect) bilirubin	Benign, asymptomatic hereditary jaundice. Hyperbilirubinemia increased by 24- to 36-hour fast. No treatment required. Prognosis excellent.
Dubin-Johnson syndrome (familial chronic idiopathic jaundice)[1]	Faulty excretory function of hepatocytes	Conjugated (direct) bilirubin	Benign, asymptomatic hereditary jaundice. Gallbladder does not visualize on oral cholecystography. Liver darkly pigmented on gross examination. Biopsy shows centrilobular brown pigment. Prognosis excellent.
Rotor's syndrome			Similar to Dubin-Johnson syndrome, but liver is not pigmented and the gallbladder is visualized on oral cholecystography. Prognosis excellent.
Benign recurrent intrahepatic cholestasis[2]	Cholestasis, often on a familial basis	Unconjugated plus conjugated (total) bilirubin	Episodic attacks of jaundice, itching, and malaise. Onset in early life and may persist for a lifetime. Alkaline phosphatase increased. Cholestasis found on liver biopsy. (Biopsy is normal during remission.) Prognosis excellent.
Recurrent jaundice of pregnancy			Benign cholestatic jaundice of unknown cause, usually occurring in the third trimester of pregnancy. Itching, gastrointestinal symptoms, and abnormal liver excretory function tests. Cholestasis noted on liver biopsy. Prognosis excellent, but recurrence with subsequent pregnancies or use of birth control pills is characteristic.

[1]The Dubin-Johnson syndrome is caused by a point mutation in the gene coding for an organic anion transporter in bile canaliculi on chromosome 10q23–24.
[2]Mutations in genes which control hepatocellular transport systems that are involved in the formation of bile and inherited as autosomal recessive traits are on chromosomes 18q21–22, 2q24, and 7q21 in families with progressive familial intrahepatic cholestasis. A gene mutation on chromosome 18q21–22 alters a P-type ATPase expressed in the small intestine and liver and causes benign recurrent intrahepatic cholestasis.

Table 57. Liver function tests: Normal values and changes in two types of jaundice.

Tests	Normal Values	Hepatocellular Jaundice	Uncomplicated Obstructive Jaundice
Bilirubin Direct Indirect	0.1–0.3 mg/dL 0.2–0.7 mg/dL	Increased Increased	Increased Increased
Urine bilirubin	None	Increased	Increased
Serum albumin/total protein	Albumin, 3.5–5.5 g/dL	Albumin decreased Total protein, 6.5–8.4 g/dL	Unchanged
Alkaline phosphatase	30–115 units/L	Increased (+)	Increased (++++)
Prothrombin time	INR[1] of 1.0–1.4. After vitamin K, 10% increase in 24 hours	Prolonged if damage severe and does not respond to parenteral vitamin K	Prolonged if obstruction marked, but responds to parenteral vitamin K
ALT, AST	ALT, 5–35 units/L; AST, 5–40 units/L	Increased in hepatocellular damage, viral hepatitis	Minimally increased

[1]INR = International Normalized Ratio.

Table 58. Common serologic patterns in hepatitis B virus infection and their interpretation.

HBsAg	Anti-HBs	Anti-HBc	HBeAg	Anti-HBe	Interpretation
+	–	IgM	+	–	Acute hepatitis B
+	–	IgG[1]	+	–	Chronic hepatitis B with active viral replication
+	–	IgG	–	+	Chronic hepatitis B with low viral replication
+	+	IgG	+ or –	+ or –	Chronic hepatitis B with heterotypic anti-HBs (about 10% of cases)
–	–	IgM	+ or –	–	Acute hepatitis B
–	+	IgG	–	+ or –	Recovery from hepatitis B (immunity)
–	+	–	–	–	Vaccination (immunity)
–	–	IgG	–	–	False-positive; less commonly, infection in remote past

[1]Low levels of IgM anti-HBc may also be detected.

Table 59. Modified Child-Pugh classification for cirrhosis.

Parameter	Numerical Score		
	1	2	3
Ascites	None	Slight	Moderate to severe
Encephalopathy	None	Slight to moderate	Moderate to severe
Bilirubin (mg/dL)	< 2.0	2–3	> 3.0
Albumin (g/dL)	> 3.5	2.8–3.5	< 2.8
Prothrombin time (seconds increased)	1–3	4–6	> 6.0

Total numerical score	Child-Pugh class
5–6	A
7–9	B
10–15	C

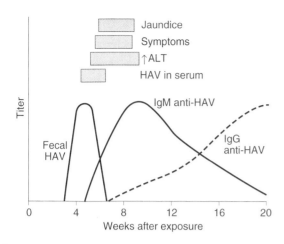

Figure 3. The typical course of acute type A hepatitis. (HAV, hepatitis A virus; anti-HAV, antibody to hepatitis A virus; ALT, alanine aminotransferase.) (Reproduced, with permission, from Koff RS: Acute viral hepatitis. In: *Handbook of Liver Disease.* Friedman LS, Keeffe EB [editors]. Churchill Livingstone, 1998.)

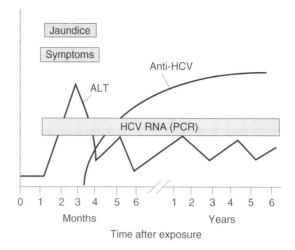

Figure 4. The typical course of acute and chronic hepatitis C. (ALT, alanine aminotransferase; Anti-HCV, antibody to hepatitis C virus by enzyme immunoassay; HCV RNA [PCR], hepatitis C viral RNA by polymerase chain reaction.)

Figure 5. The typical course of acute type B hepatitis. (HBsAg, hepatitis B surface antigen; anti-HBs, antibody to HBsAg; HBeAg, hepatitis Be antigen; anti-HBe, antibody to HBeAg; anti-HBc, antibody to hepatitis B core antigen; ALT, alanine aminotransferase.) (Reproduced, with permission, from Koff RS: Acute viral hepatitis. In: *Handbook of Liver Disease.* Friedman LS, Keeffe EB [editors]. Churchill Livingstone, 1998.)

Table 60. Diseases of the biliary tract.

	Clinical Features	Laboratory Features	Diagnosis	Treatment
Gallstones	Asymptomatic	Normal	Ultrasound	None
Gallstones	Biliary colic	Normal	Ultrasound	Laparoscopic cholecystectomy
Cholesterolosis of gallbladder	Usually asymptomatic	Normal	Oral cholecystography	None
Adenomyomatosis	May cause biliary colic	Normal	Oral cholecystography	Laparoscopic cholecystectomy if symptomatic
Porcelain gall-bladder	Usually asymptomatic, high risk of gallbladder cancer	Normal	X-ray or CT	Laparoscopic cholecystectomy
Acute cholecystitis	Epigastric or right upper quadrant pain, nausea, vomiting, fever, Murphy's sign	Leukocytosis	Ultrasound, HIDA scan	Antibiotics, laparoscopic chole-cystectomy
Chronic chole-cystitis	Biliary colic, constant epigastric or right upper quadrant pain, nausea	Normal	Ultrasound (stones), oral chole-cystography (nonfunctioning gallbladder)	Laparoscopic cholecystectomy
Choledocholithiasis	Asymptomatic or biliary colic, jaundice, fever; gallstone pancreatitis	Cholestatic liver function tests; leukocytosis and positive blood cultures in cholangitis; elevated amylase and lipase in pancreatitis	Ultrasound (dilated ducts), ERCP	Endoscopic sphincterotomy and stone extraction; antibiotics for cholangitis

ERCP = endoscopic retrograde cholangiopancreatography; HIDA = hepatic iminodiacetic acid.

Table 61. Severity index for acute pancreatitis.[1]

CT Grade		Points	Necrosis %	Necrosis Additional Point	Severity Index	Mortality Rate (%)
A	Normal pancreas	0	0	0	0	0
B	Pancreatic enlargement	1	0	0	1	0
C	Pancreatic inflammation and/or peripancreatic fat	2	< 30	2	4	0
D	Single peripancreatic fluid collection	3	30–50	4	7	> 17%
E	Two or more fluid collections or retroperitoneal air	4	> 50	6	10	

[1]Adapted from Balthazar EJ: Acute pancreatitis: assessment of severity with clinical and CT evaluation. Radiology 2002;223:603.

Table 62. Classification systems for Papanicolaou smears.

Numerical	Dysplasia	CIN	Bethesda System
1	Benign	Benign	Normal
2	Benign with inflammation	Benign with inflammation	Normal, ASC-US
3	Mild dysplasia	CIN I	Low-grade SIL
3	Moderate dysplasia	CIN II	High-grade SIL
3	Severe dysplasia	CIN III	High-grade SIL
4	Carcinoma in situ		
5	Invasive cancer	Invasive cancer	Invasive cancer

CIN = cervical intraepithelial neoplasia; SIL = squamous intraepithelial lesion; ASC-US = atypical squamous cells of undetermined significance.

Table 63. FIGO staging of cancer of the cervix.[1]

Preinvasive carcinoma

Stage 0 — Carcinoma in situ

Invasive carcinoma

Stage I — Carcinoma strictly confined to the cervix.

IA — Invasive cancer diagnosed only by microscopy. All gross lesions, even with superficial invasion, are stage IB.

- IA1 — Measured invasion of stroma no greater than 3 mm in depth and no wider than 7 mm.
- IA2 — Measured invasion of stroma greater than 3 mm in depth and no greater than 5 mm in depth and no wider than 7 mm.

IB — Clinical lesions confined to the cervix or preclinical lesions greater than 1A.

- IB1 — Clinical lesions no greater than 4 cm.
- IB2 — Clinical lesions greater than 4 cm.

Stage II — Carcinoma extends beyond the cervix but has not extended to the pelvic wall. The carcinoma involves the vagina but not as far as the lower third.

- IIA — No obvious parametrial involvement.
- IIB — Obvious parametrial involvement.

Stage III — Carcinoma has extended either to the lower third of the vagina or to the pelvic sidewall. All cases of hydronephrosis.

- IIIA — Involvement of lower third of vagina. No extension to pelvic sidewall.
- IIIB — Extension onto the pelvic wall and/or hydronephrosis or nonfunctioning kidney.

Stage IV — Carcinoma extended beyond the true pelvis or clinically involving the mucosa of the bladder or rectum.

- IVA — Spread of growth to adjacent organs.
- IVB — Spread of growth to distant organs.

[1]Shepherd JH: Staging announcement: FIGO staging of gynecologic cancers: cervical and vulva. Int J Gynecol Cancer 1995;5:319.

Table 64. Ovarian functional and neoplastic tumors.

Tumor	Incidence	Size	Consistency	Menstrual Irregularities	Endocrine Effects	Potential for Malignancy	Special Remarks
Follicle cysts	Rare in childhood; frequent in menstrual years; never in postmenopausal years.	< 6 cm, often bilateral.	Moderate	Occasional	Occasional anovulation with persistently proliferative endometrium	None	Often disappear after a 2-month regimen of oral contraceptives.
Corpus luteum cysts	Occasional, in menstrual years.	4–6 cm, unilateral.	Moderate	Occasional delayed period	Prolonged secretory phase	None	Functional cysts. Intraperitoneal bleeding occasionally.
Theca lutein cysts	Occurs with hydatidiform mole, choriocarcinoma; also with gonadotropin or clomiphene therapy.	To 4–5 cm, multiple, bilateral. (Ovaries may be ≥ 20 cm in diameter.)	Tense	Amenorrhea	hCG elevated as a result of trophoblastic proliferation	None	Functional cysts. Hematoperitoneum or torsion of ovary may occur. Surgery is to be avoided.
Inflammatory (tuboovarian abscess)	Concomitant with acute salpingitis.	To 15–20 cm, often bilateral.	Variable, painful	Menometrorrhagia	Anovulation usual	None	Unilateral removal indicated if possible.
Endometriotic cysts	Never in preadolescent or postmenopausal years. Most common in women aged 20–40 years.	To 10–12 cm, occasionally bilateral.	Moderate to softened	Rare	None	Very rare	Associated pelvic endometriosis. Medical treatment or conservative surgery recommended.
Teratoid tumors: Benign teratomas (dermoid cysts)	Childhood to postmenopause.	< 15 cm; 15% are bilateral.	Moderate to softened	None	None	Rare	Torsion can occur. Partial oophorectomy recommended.
Malignant teratomas	< 1% of ovarian tumors. Usually in infants and young adults.	> 20 cm, unilateral.	Irregularly firm	None	Occasionally, hCG elevated	All	Unresponsive to any therapy.

Tumor	Frequency	Size/Laterality	Consistency	Menstrual Effects	Hormones	Malignant	Comments
Cystadenoma, cystadenocarcinoma	Common in reproductive years.	Serous: < 25 cm, 33% bilateral; mucinous: up to 1 cm, 10% bilateral.	Moderate to softened	None	None	> 50% for serous, about 5% for mucinous	Peritoneal implants often occur with serous, rarely with mucinous. If mucinous tumor is ruptured, pseudomyxoma peritonei may occur.
Endometrioid carcinoma	15% of ovarian carcinomas.	Moderate, 13% bilateral.	Firm	None	None	All	Adenocarcinoma of endometrium coexists in 15–30% of cases.
Fibroma	< 5% of ovarian tumors.	Usually < 15 cm.	Very firm	None	None	Rare	Ascites in 20% (rarely, pleural fluid).
Arrhenoblastoma	Rare. Average age 30 years or more.	Often small (< 10 cm), unilateral.	Firm to softened	Amenorrhea	Androgens elevated	< 20%	Recurrences are moderately sensitive to irradiation.
Theca cell tumor (thecoma)	Uncommon.	< 10 cm, unilateral.	Firm	Occasional irregularity	Estrogens or androgens elevated	< 1%	
Granulosa cell tumor	Uncommon. Usually in prepubertal girls or women older than 50 years.	May be very small.	Firm to softened	Menometrorrhagia	Estrogens elevated	15–20%	Recurrences are moderately sensitive to irradiation.
Dysgerminoma	About 1–2% of ovarian tumors.	< 30 cm, bilateral in 33%.	Moderate to softened	None	—	All	Very radiosensitive.
Brenner tumor	About 1% of ovarian tumors.	< 30 cm, unilateral.	Firm	None	—	Very rare	> 50% occur in postmenopausal years.
Secondary ovarian tumors	10% of fatal malignant disease in women.	Varies; often bilateral.	Firm to softened	Occasional	Very rare (thyroid, adrenocortical origin)	All	Bowel or breast metastases to ovary common.

Table 65. Commonly used low-dose oral contraceptives.

Name	Type	Progestin	Estrogen (Ethinyl Estradiol)	Cost per Month[1]
Alesse	Combination	0.1 mg levonorgestrel	20 μg	$35.58
Cyclessa	Triphasic	0.1 mg desogestrel (days 1–7) 0.125 mg desogestrel (days 8–14) 0.15 mg desogestrel (days 15–21)	25 μg	$31.48
Mircette	Combination	0.5 mg desogestrel	20 μg	$35.81
Loestrin 1/20 Microgestin 1/20	Combination	1 mg norethindrone acetate	20 μg	$34.29 $28.66
Estrostep	Triphasic	1.0 mg norethindrone acetate (days 1–5)	20 μg	$33.17
		1.0 mg norethindrone acetate (days 6–12)	30 μg	
		1.0 mg norethindrone acetate (days 13–21)	35 μg	
Lo-Ovral Low-ogestrel	Combination	0.3 mg dL-norgestrel	30 μg	$36.03 $30.52
Nordette Levlen Levora	Combination	0.15 mg levonorgestrel	30 μg	$31.93 $34.33 $30.93
Norinyl 1/35 Ortho-Novum 1/35 Necon 1/35	Combination	1 mg norethindrone	35 μg	$36.62 $36.41 $29.47
Loestrin 1.5/30 Microgestin 1.5/30	Combination	1.5 mg norethindrone acetate	30 μg	$34.63 $28.94
Demulen 1/35 Zovia 1/35E	Combination	1 mg ethynodiol diacetate	35 μg	$33.31 $29.88
Brevicon Modicon Necon 0.5/35	Combination	0.5 mg norethindrone	35 μg	$27.63 $35.75 $32.14
Ovcon 35	Combination	0.4 mg norethindrone	35 μg	$35.09
Ortho-Cept Desogen	Combination	0.15 mg desogestrel	30 μg	$36.41 $32.45
Ortho-Cyclen	Combination	0.25 mg norgestimate	35 μg	$36.41
Ortho-Tricyclen	Triphasic	0.15 mg norgestimate (days 1–7) 0.215 mg norgestimate (days 8–14) 0.25 mg norgestimate (days 15–21)	35 μg	$35.38
Ortho-Novum 7/7/7	Triphasic	0.5 mg norethindrone (days 1–7) 0.75 mg norethindrone (days 8–14) 1 mg norethindrone (days 15–21)	35 μg	$36.41
Tri-Norinyl	Triphasic	0.5 mg norethindrone (days 1–7) 1 mg norethindrone (days 8–16) 0.5 mg norethindrone (days 17–21)	35 μg	$35.56
Triphasil Trivora	Triphasic	0.05 mg levonorgestrel (days 1–6) 0.0075 mg levonorgestrel (days 7–11) 0.125 mg levonorgestrel (days 12–21)	30 μg 40 μg 30 μg	$32.45 $27.47
Yasmin	Combination	3 mg drospirenone	30 μg	$33.00
Micronor Nor-QD	Progestin-only minipill	0.35 mg norethindrone to be taken continuously	(None)	$38.06 $44.05
Ovrette	Progestin-only minipill	0.075 mg/dL-norgestrel to be taken continuously	(None)	$33.63

[1]Average wholesale price (AWP, for AB-rated generic when available) for quantity listed. Source: *Drug Topics Red Book,* May 2003; Vol. 22, No. 5. AWP may not accurately represent the actual pharmacy cost because wide contractual variations exist among institutions.

Table 66. Contraindications to use of oral contraceptives.

Absolute contraindications
  Pregnancy
  Thrombophlebitis or thromboembolic disorders (past or present)
  Stroke or coronary artery disease (past or present)
  Cancer of the breast (known or suspected)
  Undiagnosed abnormal vaginal bleeding
  Estrogen-dependent cancer (known or suspected)
  Benign or malignant tumor of the liver (past or present)

Relative contraindications
  Age over 35 years and heavy cigarette smoking (> 15 cigarettes daily)
  Migraine or recurrent persistent severe headache
  Hypertension
  Cardiac or renal disease
  Diabetes
  Gallbladder disease
  Cholestasis during pregnancy
  Active hepatitis or infectious mononucleosis
  Sickle cell disease (S/S or S/C type)
  Surgery, fracture, or severe injury
  Lactation
  Significant psychologic depression

Table 68. Common drugs that are teratogenic or fetotoxic.[1]

ACE inhibitors	Estrogens
Alcohol	Griseofulvin
Amantadine	Hypoglycemics, oral
Aminopterin	Isotretinoin
Androgens	Lithium
Anticonvulsants	Methotrexate
Aminoglutethimide	Misoprostol
Carbamazepine	NSAIDs (third trimester)
Ethotoin	Opioids (prolonged use)
Phenytoin	Progestins
Valproic acid	Radioiodine (antithyroid)
Aspirin and other salicylates	Reserpine
(third trimester)	Ribavirin
Benzodiazepines	Sulfonamides (third trimester)
Carbarsone (amebicide)	Tetracycline (third trimester)
Chloramphenicol (third trimester)	Thalidomide
Cyclophosphamide	Tobacco smoking
Diazoxide	Trimethoprim (third trimester)
Diethylstilbestrol	Warfarin and other coumarin
Disulfiram	anticoagulants
Ergotamine	

[1]Many other drugs are also contraindicated during pregnancy. Evaluate any drug for its need versus its potential adverse effects. Further information can be obtained from the manufacturer or from any of several teratogenic registries around the country.

Table 67. Contraindications to IUD use.

Absolute contraindications
  Pregnancy
  Acute or subacute pelvic inflammatory disease or purulent cervicitis

Relative contraindications
  History of pelvic inflammatory disease since the last pregnancy
  Lack of available follow-up care
  Menorrhagia or severe dysmenorrhea (copper IUD)
  Cervical or uterine neoplasia
  Abnormal size or shape of uterus, including myomas distorting cavity

Table 69. Indicators of mild to moderate versus severe preeclampsia-eclampsia.

Site	Indicator	Mild to Moderate	Severe
Central nervous system	Symptoms and signs	Hyperreflexia Headache	Seizures Blurred vision Scotomas Headache Clonus Irritability
Kidney	Proteinuria	0.3–5 g/24 h	> 5 g/24 h or catheterized urine with 4+ protein
	Urine output	> 20–30 mL/h	< 20–30 mL/h
Liver	AST, ALT, LDH	Normal	Elevated LFTs Epigastric pain Ruptured liver
Hemato-logic	Platelets Hemoglobin	> 100,000/μL Normal range	< 100,000/mL Elevated
Vascular	Blood pressure Retina	< 160/110 mm Hg Arteriolar spasm	> 160/110 mm Hg Retinal hem-orrhages
Fetal-placen-tal unit	Growth retardation Oligohydramnios Fetal distress	Absent May be present Absent	Present Present Present

AST, aspartate aminotransferase; ALT, alanine aminotransferase; LDH, lactate dehydrogenase; LFTs, liver function tests.

Table 70. Screening and diagnostic criteria for gestational diabetes mellitus.

Screening for gestational diabetes mellitus
1. 50-g oral glucose load, administered between the 24th and 28th weeks, without regard to time of day or time of last meal. Recent recommendations suggest that universal blood glucose screening is appropriate for patients who are of Hispanic, African, Native American, South or East Asian, Pacific Island, or Indigenous Australian ancestry. Other patients who have no known diabetes in first-degree relatives, are under 25 years of age, have normal weight before pregnancy, and have no history of abnormal glucose metab-olism or poor obstetric outcome do not require routine screening.
2. Venous plasma glucose measure 1 hour later.
3. Value of 130 mg/dL (7.2 mmol/L) or above in venous plasma indi-cates the need for a full diagnostic glucose tolerance test.

Diagnosis of gestational diabetes mellitus
1. 100-g oral glucose load, administered in the morning after overnight fast lasting at least 8 hours but not more than 14 hours, and following at least 3 days of unrestricted diet (> 150 g carbohy-drate) and physical activity.
2. Venous plasma glucose is measured fasting and at 1, 2, and 3 hours. Subject should remain seated and should not smoke throughout the test.
3. Two or more of the following venous plasma concentrations must be equaled or exceeded for a diagnosis of gestational diabetes: fasting, 95 mg/dL (5.3 mmol/L); 1 hour, 180 mg/dL (10 mmol/L); 2 hours, 155 mg/dL (8.6 mmol/L); 3 hours, 140 mg/dL (7.8 mmol/L).

Table 71. Drugs and substances that require a careful assessment of risk before they are prescribed for breast-feeding women.[1]

Category	Specific Drugs or Compounds	Management Plan and Rationale
Analgesic drugs	Meperidine, oxycodone	Use alternatives to meperidine and oxycodone. Breast-fed infants whose mothers were receiving meperidine had a higher risk of neurobehavioral depression than breast-fed infants whose mothers were receiving morphine. In breast-fed infants, the level of exposure to oxycodone may reach 10% of the therapeutic dose. For potent analgesia, morphine may be given cautiously. Acetaminophen and nonsteroidal anti-inflammatory drugs are safe.
Antiarthritis drugs	Gold salts, methotrexate, high-dose aspirin	Consider alternatives to gold therapy. Although the bioavailability of elemental gold is unknown, a small amount is excreted in breast milk for a prolonged period. Therefore, the total amount of elemental gold that an infant could ingest may be substantial. No toxicity has been reported. Consider alternatives to methotrexate therapy, although low-dose methotrexate therapy for breast-feeding women with rheumatic diseases had lower risks of adverse effects in their infants than did anticancer chemotherapy. High-dose aspirin should be used with caution, since there is a case report of metabolic acidosis in a breast-fed infant whose mother was receiving high-dose therapy. Although the risk seems small, the infant's condition should be monitored clinically if the mother is receiving long-term therapy with high-dose aspirin.
Anticoagulant drugs	Phenindione[2]	Use alternatives to phenindione. Currently available vitamin K antagonists such as warfarin and acenocoumarol are considered safe, as is heparin.
Antidepressant drugs and lithium	Fluoxetine, doxepin, lithium[2]	Use fluoxetine, doxepin, and lithium with caution. Although the concentrations of these drugs in breast milk are low, colic (with fluoxetine) and sedation (with doxepin) have been reported in exposed infants. Near-therapeutic plasma concentrations of lithium were reported in an infant exposed to the drug in utero and through breast-feeding. The incidence of these adverse events is unknown.
Antiepileptic drugs	Phenobarbital, ethosuximide, primidone	In breast-fed infants, the level of exposure to phenobarbital, ethosuximide, and primidone may exceed 10% of the weight-adjusted therapeutic dose. Consider alternatives such as carbamazepine, phenytoin, and valproic acid.
Antimicrobial drugs	Chloramphenicol, tetracycline	Use alternatives to chloramphenicol and tetracycline. Idiosyncratic aplastic anemia is a possibility among breast-fed infants whose mothers are receiving chloramphenicol. Although tetracycline-induced discoloration of the teeth of breast-fed infants has not been reported, the potential risk of this event needs to be clearly communicated to lactating women.
Anticancer drugs	All (eg, cyclophosphamide,[2] methotrexate,[2] doxorubicin[2])	Because of their potent pharmacologic effects, cytotoxic drugs should not be given to breast-feeding women.
Anxiolytic drugs	Diazepam, alprazolam	Avoid long-term use of diazepam and alprazolam in breast-feeding women. Intermittent use poses little risk to their infants, but regular use may result in the accumulation of the drug and its metabolites in the infants. Lethargy and poor weight gain have been reported in an infant exposed to diazepam in breast milk, and the withdrawal syndrome was reported in a breast-fed infant after the mother discontinued alprazolam.
Cardiovascular and antihypertensive drugs	Acebutolol, amiodarone, atenolol, nadolol, sotalol	The use of acebutolol, amiodarone, atenolol, nadolol, and sotalol by breast-feeding women may cause relatively high levels of exposure among their infants, and these agents should therefore be used with caution. The two β-adrenergic antagonists propranolol and labetalol are considered safe.
Endocrine drugs and hormones	Estrogens, bromocriptine[2]	Estrogens and bromocriptine may suppress milk production. Oral contraceptives containing little or no estrogen have smaller risk than formulations with higher concentrations of estrogen. Nevertheless, caution should be exercised in their use.
Immunosuppressive drugs	Cyclosporine,[2] azathioprine	Maternal plasma concentrations of cyclosporine and azathioprine should be monitored. In nine reported cases in breast-fed infants who were exposed to azathioprine in breast milk, no obvious adverse effects were noted.
Respiratory drugs	Theophylline	Theophylline should be used with caution. When the mother's doses are high, the levels of exposure in the infant may be substantial (ie, 20% of the therapeutic dose).
Radioactive compounds	All	Breast feeding should be stopped for the length of the half-life of the radiolabeled compound used.

(continued)

Table 71. Drugs and substances that require a careful assessment of risk before they are prescribed for breast-feeding women. (continued)

Category	Specific Drugs or Compounds	Management Plan and Rationale
Drugs of abuse	All[1]	The use of drugs of abuse precludes breast feeding; cocaine-induced toxicity has been reported among breast-fed infants whose mothers abused cocaine. Methadone, used for the treatment of addiction, is safe for infants of breast-feeding women, at doses of up to 80 mg per day. Buprenorphine may be a safer alternative to methadone.
Nonmedicinal substances	Ethanol, caffeine, nicotine	In order to avoid exposure of the infant to ethanol, the mother should not consume alcohol or should consume no more than one drink 2 to 3 hours before breast feeding. The ingestion of moderate amounts of caffeine should be safe. Because of the effects of second-hand smoke and the fact that nicotine is excreted in breast milk, smoking is contraindicated in breast-feeding women.
Miscellaneous compounds	Iodides and iodine, ergotamine,[2] ergonovine	Use alternatives to iodine-containing antiseptic agents. Ergotamine and ergonovine may suppress prolactin secretion in breast-feeding women. However, the use of methylergonovine to stimulate uterine involution is considered safe in breast-feeding women.

[1]Data modified from Ito S: Drug therapy for breast-feeding women. N Engl J Med 2000;343:120. Drugs for which there is no information are not included, though a careful risk assessment is necessary before such drugs are prescribed.
[2]The use of this drug or these drugs by breast-feeding women is contraindicated according to the American Academy of Pediatrics.

Table 72. Effectiveness of agents used in treatment of allergic disorders.

Drug Class	Sneezing	Pruritus	Rhinorrhea	Congestion	Inflammation	Onset of Action
Antihistamines	++++	++++	+++	+	–	Rapid
Sympathomimetics	–	–	+	++++	–	Rapid
Glucocorticoids	+++	+++	+++	++++	++++	Slow (days)
Cromolyn-nedocromil sodium	++	+	+	+	++	Slow (weeks)
Anticholinergics	–	–	++++	–	–	Rapid
Immunotherapy	++++	++++	++++	++++	++++	Slow (months)

Table 73. Autoantibodies: Associations with connective tissue diseases.[1]

Suspected Disease State	Test	Primary Disease Association (Sensitivity, Specificity)	Other Disease Associations	Comments
CREST[2] syndrome	Anticentromere antibody	CREST (70–90%, high)	Scleroderma (10–15%), Raynaud's disease (10–30%).	Predictive value of a positive test is > 95% for scleroderma or related disease (CREST, Raynaud's). Diagnosis of CREST is made clinically.
Systemic lupus erythematosus (SLE)	Antinuclear antibody (ANA)	SLE (> 95%, low)	Rheumatoid arthritis (30–50%), discoid lupus, scleroderma (60%), drug-induced lupus (100%), Sjögren's syndrome (80%), miscellaneous inflammatory disorders.	Often used as a screening test; a negative test virtually excludes SLE; a positive test, while nonspecific, increases posttest probability of SLE. Titer does not correlate with disease activity.
	Anti-double-stranded-DNA (anti-ds-DNA)	SLE (60–70%, high)	Lupus nephritis, rarely rheumatoid arthritis, other connective tissue disease, usually in low titer.	Predictive value of a positive test is > 90% for SLE if present in high titer; a decreasing titer may correlate with worsening renal disease. Titer generally correlates with disease activity.
	Anti-Smith antibody (anti-Sm)	SLE (30–40%, high)		SLE-specific. A positive test substantially increases posttest probability of SLE. Test rarely indicated.
Mixed connective tissue disease (MCTD)	Anti-ribonucleoprotein antibody (RNP)	Scleroderma (20–30%, low), MCTD (95–100%, low)	SLE (30%), Sjögren's syndrome, rheumatoid arthritis (10%), discoid lupus (20–30%).	A negative test essentially excludes MCTD; a positive test in high titer, while nonspecific, increases posttest probability of MCTD.
Rheumatoid arthritis	Rheumatoid factor (RF)	Rheumatoid arthritis (50–90%)	Other rheumatic diseases, chronic infections, some malignancies, some healthy individuals, elderly patients.	Titer does not correlate with disease activity.
Scleroderma	Anti-Scl-70 antibody	Scleroderma (15–20%, low)		Predictive value of a positive test is > 95% for scleroderma.
Sjögren's syndrome	Anti-SS-A/Ro antibody	Sjögren's (60–70%, low)	SLE (30–40%), rheumatoid arthritis (10%), subacute cutaneous lupus, vasculitis.	Useful in counseling women of childbearing age with known connective tissue disease, since a positive test is associated with a small but real risk of neonatal SLE and congenital heart block.
Wegener's granulomatosis	Anti-neutrophil cytoplasmic antibody (ANCA)	Wegener's granulomatosis (systemic necrotizing vasculitis) (56–96%, high)	Crescentic glomerulonephritis or other systemic vasculitis (eg, polyarteritis nodosa).	Ability of this assay to reflect disease activity remains unclear.

[1]Modified, with permission, from Harvey AM et al (editors): *The Principles and Practice of Medicine,* 22nd ed. Appleton & Lange, 1988; White RH, Robbins DL: Clinical significance and interpretation of antinuclear antibodies. West J Med 1987;147:210; and Tan EM: Autoantibodies to nuclear antigens (ANA): their immunobiology and medicine. Adv Immunol 1982;33:167.

[2]CREST = calcinosis, Raynaud's phenomenon, esophageal dysmotility, sclerodactyly, and telangiectasia.

Table 74. Diagnostic value of the joint pattern.

Characteristic	Status	Representative Disease
Inflammation	Present	Rheumatoid arthritis, systemic lupus erythematosus, gout
	Absent	Osteoarthritis
Number of involved joints	Monarticular	Gout, trauma, septic arthritis, Lyme disease
	Oligoarticular (2–4 joints)	Reiter's disease, psoriatic arthritis, inflammatory bowel disease
	Polyarticular (≥ 5 joints)	Rheumatoid arthritis, systemic lupus erythematosus
Site of joint involvement	Distal inter-phalangeal	Osteoarthritis, psoriatic arthritis (not rheumatoid arthritis)
	Metacarpopha-langeal, wrists	Rheumatoid arthritis, systemic lupus erythematosus (not osteo-arthritis)
	First metatarsal phalangeal	Gout, osteoarthritis

Table 76. Neurologic testing of lumbosacral nerve disorders.

Nerve Root	Motor	Reflex	Sensory Area
L4	Dorsiflexion of foot	Knee jerk	Medial calf
L5	Dorsiflexion of great toe	None	Medial forefoot
S1	Eversion of foot	Ankle jerk	Lateral foot

Table 75. Examination of joint fluid.

Measure	Group I Normal	Group II (Noninflammatory)	Group III (Inflammatory)	(Purulent)
Volume (mL) (knee)	< 3.5	Often > 3.5	Often > 3.5	Often > 3.5
Clarity	Transparent	Transparent	Translucent to opaque	Opaque
Color	Clear	Yellow	Yellow to opalescent	Yellow to green
WBC (per μL)	< 200	200–300	3000–50,000	> 50,000[1]
Polymorphonuclear leukocytes	< 25%	< 25%	50% or more	75% or more[1]
Culture	Negative	Negative	Negative	Usually positive
Glucose (mg/dL)	Nearly equal to serum	Nearly equal to serum	> 25, lower than serum	< 25, much lower than serum

[1]Counts are lower with infections caused by organisms of low virulence or if antibiotic therapy has been started.

Table 77. Drugs associated with systemic lupus erythematosus.[1]

Definite association

Chlorpromazine	Methyldopa
Hydralazine	Procainamide
Isoniazid	Quinidine

Possible association

Beta-blockers	Methimazole
Captopril	Nitrofurantoin
Carbamazepine	Penicillamine
Cimetidine	Phenytoin
Ethosuximide	Propylthiouracil
Hydrazines	Sulfasalazine
Levodopa	Sulfonamides
Lithium	Trimethadione

Unlikely association

Allopurinol	Penicillin
Chlorthalidone	Phenylbutazone
Gold salts	Reserpine
Griseofulvin	Streptomycin
Methysergide	Tetracyclines
Oral contraceptives	

[1]Modified and reproduced, with permission, from Hess EV, Mongey AB: Drug-related lupus. Bull Rheum Dis 1991;40:1.

Table 78. Criteria for the classification of systemic lupus erythematosus.[1] (A patient is classified as having SLE if any four or more of eleven criteria are met.)

1. Malar rash
2. Discoid rash
3. Photosensitivity
4. Oral ulcers
5. Arthritis
6. Serositis
7. Renal disease
    a. > 0.5 g/d proteinuria, or—
    b. ≥ 3+ dipstick proteinuria, or—
    c. Cellular casts
8. Neurologic disease
    a. Seizures, or—
    b. Psychosis (without other cause)
9. Hematologic disorders
    a. Hemolytic anemia, or—
    b. Leukopenia (< 4000/μL), or—
    c. Lymphopenia (< 1500/μL), or—
    d. Thrombocytopenia (< 100,000/μL)
10. Immunologic abnormalities
    a. Positive LE cell preparation, or—
    b. Antibody to native DNA, or—
    c. Antibody to Sm, or—
    d. False-positive serologic test for syphilis
11. Positive antinuclear antibody (ANA)

[1]Modified and reproduced, with permission, from Tan EM et al: The 1982 revised criteria for the classification of systemic lupus erythematosus. Arthritis Rheum 1982;25:1271.

Table 79. Frequency (%) of autoantibodies in rheumatic diseases.

	ANA	Anti-Native DNA	Rheumatoid Factor	Anti-Sm	Anti-SS-A	Anti-SS-B	Anti-SCL-70	Anti-Centromere	Anti-Jo-1	ANCA
Rheumatoid arthritis	30–60	0–5	72–85	0	0–5	0–2	0	0	0	0
Systemic lupus erythematosus	95–100	60	20	10–25	15–20	5–20	0	0	0	0–1
Sjögren's syndrome	95	0	75	0	60–70	60–70	0	0	0	0
Diffuse scleroderma	80–95	0	25–33	0	0	0	33	1	0	0
Limited scleroderma (CREST syndrome)	80–95	0	25–33	0	0	0	20	50	0	0
Polymyositis/dermatomyositis	80–95	0	33	0	0	0	0	0	20–30	0
Wegener's granulomatosis	0–15	0	50	0	0	0	0	0	0	93–96[1]

ANA = antinuclear antibodies; ANCA = anti-neutrophil cytoplasmic antibody.
[1]Frequency for generalized, active disease.

Table 80. Frequency of laboratory abnormalities in systemic lupus erythematosus.[1]

Anemia	60%
Leukopenia	45%
Thrombocytopenia	30%
Biologic false-positive tests for syphilis	25%
Lupus anticoagulant	7%
Anti-cardiolipin antibody	25%
Direct Coombs-positive	30%
Proteinuria	30%
Hematuria	30%
Hypocomplementemia	60%
ANA	95–100%
Anti-native DNA	50%
Anti-Sm	20%

[1]Modified and reproduced, with permission, from Hochberg MC et al: Systemic lupus erythematosus: a review of clinicolaboratory features and immunologic matches in 150 patients with emphasis on demographic subsets. Medicine 1985;64:285.

Table 81. Treatment of hyperkalemia.[1]

EMERGENCY					
Modality	**Mechanism of Action**	**Onset**	**Duration**	**Prescription**	**K⁺ Removed from Body**
Calcium	Antagonizes cardiac conduction abnormalities	0–5 minutes	1 hour	Calcium gluconate 10%, 5–30 mL IV; or calcium chloride 5%, 5–30 mL IV	0
Bicarbonate	Distributes K⁺ into cells	15–30 minutes	1–2 hours	NaHCO₃, 44–88 mEq (1–2 ampules) IV	0
Insulin	Distributes K⁺ into cells	15–60 minutes	4–6 hours	Regular insulin, 5–10 units IV, plus glucose 50%, 25 g (1 ampule) IV	0
Albuterol	Distributes K⁺ into cells	15–30 minutes	2–4 hours	Nebulized albuterol, 10–20 mg in 4 mL normal saline, inhaled over 10 minutes	0

NONEMERGENCY				
Modality	**Mechanism of Action**	**Duration of Treatment**	**Prescription**	**K⁺ Removed from Body**
Loop diuretic	↑ Renal K⁺ excretion	0.5–2 hours	Furosemide, 40–160 mg IV or orally with or without NaHCO₃, 0.5–3 mEq/kg daily	Variable
Sodium polystyrene sulfonate (Kayexalate)	Ion exchange resin binds K⁺	1–3 hours	Oral: 15–30 g in 20% sorbitol (50–100 mL) Rectal: 50 g in 20% sorbitol	0.5–1 mEq/g
Hemodialysis	Extracorporeal K⁺ removal	48 hours	Blood flow ≥ 200–300 mL/min. Dialysate [K⁺] ~ 0	200–300 mEq
Peritoneal dialysis	Peritoneal K⁺ removal	48 hours	Fast exchange, 3–4 L/h	200–300 mEq

[1]Modified and reproduced, with permission, from Cogan MG: *Fluid and Electrolytes: Physiology and Pathophysiology.* McGraw-Hill, 1991.

Figure 6. Evaluation of hyponatremia using serum osmolality and extracellular fluid volume status. (Adapted, with permission, from Narins RG et al: Diagnostic strategies in disorders of fluid, electrolyte, and acid-base homeostasis. Am J Med 1982; 72:496.)

Table 82. Primary acid-base disorders and expected compensation.

Disorder	Primary Defect	Compensatory Response	Magnitude of Compensation
Respiratory acidosis			
Acute	$\uparrow P_{CO_2}$	$\uparrow HCO_3^-$	$\uparrow HCO_3^-$ 1 mEq/L per 10 mm Hg $\uparrow P_{CO_2}$
Chronic	$\uparrow P_{CO_2}$	$\uparrow HCO_3^-$	$\uparrow HCO_3^-$ 3.5 mEq/L per 10 mm Hg $\uparrow P_{CO_2}$
Respiratory alkalosis			
Acute	$\downarrow P_{CO_2}$	$\downarrow HCO_3^-$	$\downarrow HCO_3^-$ 2 mEq/L per 10 mm Hg $\downarrow P_{CO_2}$
Chronic	$\downarrow P_{CO_2}$	$\downarrow HCO_3^-$	$\downarrow HCO_3^-$ 5 mEq/L per 10 mm Hg $\downarrow P_{CO_2}$
Metabolic acidosis	$\downarrow HCO_3^-$	$\downarrow P_{CO_2}$	$\downarrow P_{CO_2}$ 1.3 mm Hg per 1 meq/L $\downarrow HCO_3^-$
Metabolic alkalosis	$\uparrow HCO_3^-$	$\uparrow P_{CO_2}$	$\uparrow P_{CO_2}$ 0.7 mm Hg per 1 mEq/L $\uparrow HCO_3^-$

Table 83. Hyperchloremic, normal anion gap metabolic acidoses.[1]

	Renal Defect	Serum [K+]	Distal H+ Secretion		Urinary Anion Gap	Treatment
			Urinary NH_4^+ Plus Minimal Urine pH	Titratable Acid		
Gastrointestinal HCO_3^- loss	None	↓	< 5.5	↑↑	Negative	Na^+, K^+, and HCO_3^- as required
Renal tubular acidosis I. Classic distal	Distal H+ secretion	↓	> 5.5	↓	Positive	$NaHCO_3$ (1–3 mEq/kg/d)
II. Proximal secretion	Proximal H+	↓	< 5.5	Normal	Positive	$NaHCO_3$ or $KHCO_3$ (10–15 mEq/kg/d), thiazide
III. Glomerular insufficiency	NH_3 production	Normal	< 5.5	↓	Positive	$NaHCO_3$ (1–3 mEq/kg/d)
IV. Hyporeninemic hypoaldosteronism	Distal Na^+ reabsorption, K^+ secretion, and H+ secretion	↑	< 5.5	↓	Positive	Fludrocortisone (0.1–0.5 mg/d), dietary K^+ restriction, furosemide (40–160 mg/d), $NaHCO_3$ (1–3 mEq/kg/d)

[1]Modified and reproduced, with permission, from Cogan MG: *Fluid and Electrolytes: Physiology and Pathophysiology.* McGraw-Hill, 1991.

Table 84. Metabolic alkalosis.[1]

Saline-Responsive (U_{Cl} < 10 mEq/d)	Saline-Unresponsive (U_{Cl} > 10 mEq/d)

Excessive body bicarbonate content
  Renal alkalosis
    Diuretic therapy
    Poorly reabsorbable anion therapy: carbenicillin, penicillin, sulfate, phosphate
    Posthypercapnia
  Gastrointestinal alkalosis
    Loss of HCl from vomiting or nasogastric suction
    Intestinal alkalosis: chloride diarrhea
  Exogenous alkali
    $NaHCO_3$ (baking soda)
    Sodium citrate, lactate, gluconate, acetate
    Transfusions
    Antacids
Normal body bicarbonate content
  "Contraction alkalosis"
	Excessive body bicarbonate content
	  Renal alkalosis
	    Normotensive
	      Bartter's syndrome (renal salt wasting and secondary hyperaldosteronism)
	      Severe potassium depletion
	      Refeeding alkalosis
	      Hypercalcemia and hypoparathyroidism
	    Hypertensive
	      Endogenous mineralocorticoids
	        Primary aldosteronism
	        Hyperreninism
	        Adrenal enzyme deficiency: 11- and 17-hydroxylase
	        Liddle's syndrome
	      Exogenous mineralocorticoids
	        Licorice

[1]Modified and reproduced, with permission, from Narins RG et al: Diagnostic strategies in disorders of fluid, electrolyte and acid-base homeostasis. Am J Med 1982;72:496.

Table 85. Vitamin D preparations used in the treatment of hypoparathyroidism.[1]

	Potency	How Supplied	Daily Dose (Range)	Time Required for Hypercalcemia to Subside
Ergocalciferol (ergosterol, vitamin D_2)	40,000 USP units/mg	Capsules of 25,000 and 50,000 units; solution, 8000 units/mL	25,000–200,000 units	6–18 weeks
Dihydrotachysterol (Hytakerol)	120,000 USP units/mg	Tablets of 0.125, 0.2, and 0.4 mg	0.2–1 mg	1–3 weeks
Calcifediol (Calderol)	...	Capsules of 20 and 50 µg	20–200 µg	3–6 weeks
Calcitriol (Rocaltrol)	...	Capsules of 0.25 and 0.5 µg	0.25–4 µg	1/2–2 weeks

[1]Reproduced, with permission, from Greenspan FS, Baxter JD (editors): *Basic & Clinical Endocrinology,* 4th ed. McGraw-Hill, 1994.

Table 86. Diagnostic criteria of different types of hypercalciuria.

	Absorptive Type I	Absorptive Type II	Absorptive Type III	Resorptive	Renal
Serum					
Calcium	N	N	N	↑	N
Phosphorus	N	N	↓	↓	N
PTH	N	N	N	↑	↑
Vitamin D	N	N	↑	↑	↑
Urinary calcium					
Fasting	N	N	↑	↑	↑
Restricted	↑	N	↑	↑	↑
After calcium load	↑	↑	↑	↑	↑

Key: ↑ = elevated; ↓ = low; N = normal.

Table 86A. American Urological Association symptom index for benign prostatic hyperplasia.[1,2]

Questions to Be Answered	Not at All	Less Than One Time in Five	Less Than Half the Time	About Half the Time	More Than Half the Time	Almost Always
1. Over the past month, how often have you had a sensation of not emptying your bladder completely after you finish urinating?	0	1	2	3	4	5
2. Over the past month, how often have you had to urinate again less than 2 hours after you finished urinating?	0	1	2	3	4	5
3. Over the past month, how often have you found you stopped and started again several times when you urinated?	0	1	2	3	4	5
4. Over the past month, how often have you found it difficult to postpone urination?	0	1	2	3	4	5
5. Over the past month, how often have you had a weak urinary stream?	0	1	2	3	4	5
6. Over the past month, how often have you had to push or strain to begin urination?						
7. Over the past month, how many times did you most typically get up to urinate from the time you went to bed at night until the time you got up in the morning?	0 (None)	1 (1 time)	2 (2 times)	3 (3 times)	4 (4 times)	5 (5 times)

[1]Sum of seven circled numbers equals the symptom score. See text for explanation.
[2]Reproduced, with permission, from Barry MJ et al: The American Urological Association symptoms index for benign prostatic hyperplasia. J Urol 1992;148:1549.

Table 87. Stages of chronic kidney disease: A clinical action plan.[1,2]

Stage	Description	GFR (mL/min/1.73 m^2)	Action[3]
1	Kidney damage with normal or ↑ GFR	≥ 90	Diagnosis and treatment. Treatment of comormid conditions. Slowing of progression. Cardiovascular disease risk reduction.
2	Kidney damage with mildly ↓ GFR	60–89	Estimating progression.
3	Moderately ↓ GFR	30–59	Evaluating and treating complications.
4	Severely ↓ GFR	15–29	Preparation for kidney replacement therapy.
5	Kidney failure	< 15 (or dialysis)	Replacement (if uremia is present).

[1]From National Kidney Foundation, KDOQI, chronic kidney disease guidelines.
[2]Chronic kidney disease is defined as either kidney damage or GFR < 60 mL/min add 1.73 m^2 for 3 or more months. Kidney damage is defined as pathologic abnormalities or markers of damage, including abnormalities in blood or urine tests or imaging studies.
[3]Includes actions from preceding stages.

Table 88. Major causes of chronic renal failure.

Glomerulopathies
  Primary glomerular diseases:
    1. Focal and segmental glomerulosclerosis
    2. Membranoproliferative glomerulonephritis
    3. IgA nephropathy
    4. Membranous nephropathy
  Secondary glomerular diseases:
    1. Diabetic nephropathy
    2. Amyloidosis
    3. Post-infectious glomerulonephritis
    4. HIV-associated nephropathy
    5. Collagen-vascular diseases
    6. Sickle cell nephropathy
    7. HIV-associated membranoproliferative glomerulonephritis
Tubulointerstitial nephritis
  Drug hypersensitivity
  Heavy metals
  Analgesic nephropathy
  Reflux/chronic pyelonephritis
  Idiopathic
Hereditary diseases
  Polycystic kidney disease
  Medullary cystic disease
  Alport's syndrome
Obstructive nephropathies
  Prostatic disease
  Nephrolithiasis
  Retroperitoneal fibrosis/tumor
  Congenital
Vascular diseases
  Hypertensive nephrosclerosis
  Renal artery stenosis

Table 89. Classification and findings in glomerulonephritis: Nephritic syndromes.

	Etiology	Histopathology	Pathogenesis
Acute (postinfectious) glomerulonephritis	Streptococci, other bacteria	Light: Diffuse proliferative glomerulonephritis Immunofluorescence: IgG; C3, granular pattern Electron microscopy: Subepithelial deposits or "humps"	Trapped immune complexes
IgA nephropathy (Berger's disease and Henoch-Schönlein purpura)	In association with viral upper respiratory tract infections; gastrointestinal infection or flu-like syndrome	Light: Mesangioproliferative glomerulonephritis Immunofluorescence: IgA (with or without IgG, C3) Electron microscopy: Mesangial deposits	Unknown
Rapidly progressive glomerulonephritis	Lupus erythematosus, mixed cryoglobulinemia, subacute infective endocarditis, shunt infections	Light: Crescentic glomerulonephritis Immunofluorescence: IgG, IgA; C3 granular pattern Electron microscopy: Deposits in subepithelium, subendothelium, or mesangium	Trapped immune complexes
	Goodpasture's syndrome or idiopathic	Light: Crescentic glomerulonephritis Immunofluorescence: IgG; C3, linear pattern Electron microscopy: Widening of basement membrane	Anti-GBM antibodies
	Wegener's granulomatosis, polyarteritis, idiopathic	Light: Crescentic glomerulonephritis Immunofluorescence: No immunoglobulins Electron microscopy: No deposits	Unknown

Peripheral nerve

Trigeminal
  Ophthalmic branch
  Maxillary branch
  Mandibular branch
Anterior cutaneous nerve of neck
Supraclavicular nerves
Axillary nerve
Medial cutaneous nerve of arm
Lateral cutaneous nerve of arm (branch of radial nerve)
Medial cutaneous nerve of forearm
Lateral cutaneous nerve of forearm
Radial
Median
Ulnar
Lateral femoral cutaneous
Obturator
Anterior femoral cutaneous
Lateral cutaneous nerve of calf
Saphenous
Superficial peroneal
Sural
Lateral and medial plantar
Deep peroneal

Nerve root

C3 C4 C5 T2 T3 T4 T5 T6 T7 T8 T9 T10 T11 T12 L1 L2 L3 L4 L5 S1 T2 T1 C6 C8 C7

Post. Mid. Ant.
Lateral thoracic rami
Anterior thoracic rami

x = Iliohypogastric
† = Ilioinguinal
★ = Genitofemoral
Dorsal nerve of penis
Perineal nerve of penis

Figure 7. Cutaneous innervation. The segmental or radicular (root) distribution is shown on the left side of the body and the peripheral nerve distribution on the right side. **Above:** anterior view; **facing page:** posterior view. (Reproduced, with permission, from Simon RP, Aminoff MJ, Greenberg DA: *Clinical Neurology*, 4th ed. McGraw-Hill, 1999.)

(continued)

Nerve root

Peripheral nerve

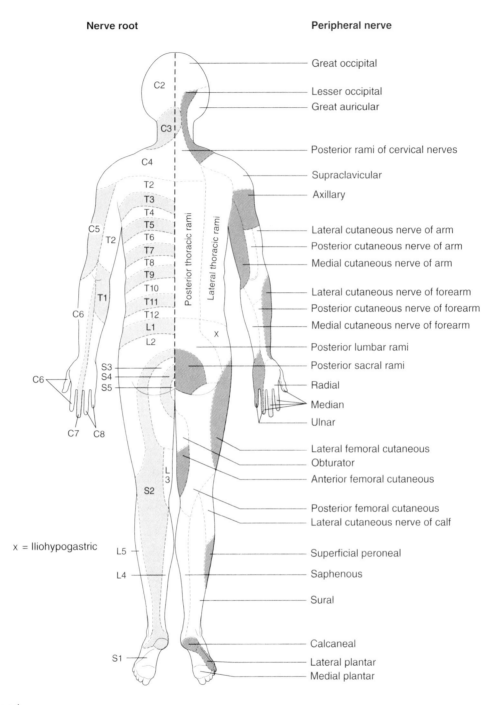

- Great occipital
- Lesser occipital
- Great auricular
- Posterior rami of cervical nerves
- Supraclavicular
- Axillary
- Lateral cutaneous nerve of arm
- Posterior cutaneous nerve of arm
- Medial cutaneous nerve of arm
- Lateral cutaneous nerve of forearm
- Posterior cutaneous nerve of forearm
- Medial cutaneous nerve of forearm
- Posterior lumbar rami
- Posterior sacral rami
- Radial
- Median
- Ulnar
- Lateral femoral cutaneous
- Obturator
- Anterior femoral cutaneous
- Posterior femoral cutaneous
- Lateral cutaneous nerve of calf
- Superficial peroneal
- Saphenous
- Sural
- Calcaneal
- Lateral plantar
- Medial plantar

C2
C3
C4
T2
T3
T4
T5
T6
T7
T8
T9
T10
T11
T12
L1
L2
C5
T2
C6
T1
C6
C7 C8
S3
S4
S5
L
3
S2
L5
L4
S1

Posterior thoracic rami

Lateral thoracic rami

x = Iliohypogastric

x

Figure 7. Continued

1304

Table 90. Clinical features associated with acute headache that warrant urgent or emergent neuroimaging.[1]

Prior to lumbar puncture
  Abnormal neurologic examination
  Abnormal mental status
  Abnormal funduscopic examination (papilledema; loss of venous pulsations)
  Meningeal signs

Emergent (conduct prior to leaving office or emergency department)
  Abnormal neurologic examination
  Abnormal mental status
  Thunderclap headache

Urgent (scheduled prior to leaving office or emergency department)
  HIV-positive patient[2]
  Age > 50 years (normal neurologic examination)

[1]Adapted from American College of Emergency Physicians. Clinical Policy: critical issues in the evaluation and management of patients presenting to the emergency department with acute headache. Ann Emerg Med 2002;39:108.
[2]Use CT with or without contrast or MRI if HIV-positive.

Table 91. Prophylactic treatment of migraine.

Drug	Usual Adult Daily Oral Dose	Common Side Effects
Aspirin	650–1950 mg	Dyspepsia, gastrointestinal bleeding.
Propranolol	80–240 mg	Fatigue, lassitude, depression, insomnia, nausea, vomiting, constipation.
Amitriptyline	10–150 mg	Sedation, dry mouth, constipation, weight gain, blurred vision, edema, hypotension, urinary retention.
Imipramine	10–150 mg	Similar to those of amitriptyline (above).
Sertraline	50–200 mg	Anxiety, insomnia, sweating, tremor, gastrointestinal disturbances.
Fluoxetine	20–60 mg	Similar to those of sertraline (above).
Ergonovine maleate	0.6–2 mg	Nausea, vomiting, abdominal pain, diarrhea.
Cyproheptadine	12–20 mg	Sedation, dry mouth, epigastric discomfort, gastrointestinal disturbances.
Clonidine	0.2–0.6 mg	Dry mouth, drowsiness, sedation, headache, constipation.
Methysergide	4–8 mg	Nausea, vomiting, diarrhea, abdominal pain, cramps, weight gain, insomnia, edema, peripheral vasoconstriction. Retroperitoneal and pleuropulmonary fibrosis and fibrous thickening of cardiac valves may occur.
Verapamil[1]	80–160 mg	Headache, hypotension, flushing, edema, constipation. May aggravate atrioventricular nodal heart block and congestive heart failure.

[1]Other calcium channel antagonists (eg, nimodipine, nifedipine, and diltiazem) may also be used.

Table 92. Features of major stroke subtypes.[1]

Stroke Type	Clinical Features	Diagnosis	Treatment
Ischemic Stroke			
Lacunar infarct	Small (< 5-mm) lesions in the basal ganglia, pons, cerebellum, or internal capsule; less often in deep cerebral white matter; prognosis generally good; clinical features depend on location, but may worsen over first 24–36 h	CT may reveal small hypodensity, but is often normal	Aspirin; long-term management is to control risk factors (hypertension and diabetes)
Carotid circulation obstruction	Signs vary depending on occluded vessel	Noncontrast CT to exclude hemorrhage; CT may be normal during first 6–24 h of an ischemic stroke, whereas diffusion-weighted MRI is more sensitive; ECG, blood glucose, complete blood count, and tests for hypercoaguable states, hyperlipidemia are indicated; echo-cardiography or Holter monitoring in selected instances	Select patients for intravenous thrombolytics; aspirin (325 mg PO/day) first-line therapy; if stroke occurs on aspirin, clopidogrel may be substituted for aspirin; antico-agulation with heparin for cardioembolic strokes and sometimes for evolving stroke when no contraindications exist
Vertebrobasilar occlusion	Signs vary based on location of occluded vessel	As for carotid circulation obstruction	As for carotid circulation obstruction
Hemorrhagic Stroke			
Spontaneous intracerebral hemorrhage	Commonly associated with hyper-tension; also with bleeding disorders, amyloid angiopathy; location: basal ganglia more common than pons, thalamus, cerebellum, or cerebral white matter	Noncontrast CT is superior to MRI for detecting bleeds < 48 h duration; lab-oratory tests to identify bleeding dis-order; angiography may be indicated to exclude aneurysm or AVM; do not per-form LP	Most managed supportively, but cerebellar bleeds or hematomas with gross mass effect benefit from urgent surgical evacuation
Subarachnoid hemorrhage	Presents with sudden onset or worst headache of life; may lead rapidly to loss of consciousness; signs of men-ingeal irritation often present; etiology usually aneurysm or AVM, but 20% have no source identified	CT to confirm diagnosis, but may be normal in rare instances; if CT is negative and suspicion high, perform LP to look for red blood cells or xanthochromia; angiography to determine source of bleed in candidates for treatment	See *Arteriovenous malformations; Aneurysm*
Intracranial aneurysm	Most located in the anterior circle of Willis and are typically asymptomatic until subarachnoid bleed occurs; 20% rebleed in first 2 weeks	CT indicates subarachnoid hemorrhage and angiography then demonstrates the aneurysms; angiography may not reveal aneurysm if vasospasm is present	Prevent further bleeding by clipping aneurysm or coil embolization; nimodipine helps pre-vent vasospasm; reverse vasospasm by intravenous fluids and induced hyperten-sion after aneurysm has been obliterated, if no other aneurysms are present; angio-plasty may also reverse symptomatic va-sospasm
AVMs	Focal deficit from hematoma or AVM itself	CT reveals bleed, and may reveal the AVM; may be seen by MRI; angiography demonstrates feeding vessels and vascular anatomy	Surgery indicated if AVM has bled or to pre-vent further progression of neurological deficit; other modalities to treat nonoperable AVMs are available at specialized centers

[1]CT, computed tomography; MRI, magnetic resonance imaging; ECG, electrocardiogram; LP, lumbar puncture; AVM, arteriovenous malformations.

Table 93. Seizure classification.

Seizure Type	Key Features	Other Associated Features
Partial seizures	Involve only restricted part of brain May become secondarily generalized	
Simple partial	Consciousness preserved	May be manifest by focal motor, sensory, or autonomic symptoms
Complex partial	Consciousness impaired	Above symptoms may precede, accompany, or follow
Generalized seizures	Diffuse involvement of brain at onset	
Absence (petit mal)	Consciousness impaired briefly Patient often unaware of attacks	May be clonic, tonic, or atonic components (ie, loss of postural tone); autonomic components (eg, enuresis); or accompanying automatisms Almost always begin in childhood and frequently cease by age 20
Atypical absences	May be more gradual onset and termination than typical absence	More marked changes in tone may occur
Myoclonic seizures	Single or multiple myoclonic jerks	
Tonic-clonic (grand mal)	*Tonic phase:* sudden loss of consciousness, with rigidity and arrest of respiration, lasting < 1 min *Clonic phase:* jerking occurs, usually for 2–3 min *Flaccid coma:* variable duration	May be accompanied by tongue biting, incontinence, or aspiration; commonly followed by postictal confusion of variable duration
Status epilepticus	Repeated seizures without recovery between them A fixed and enduring epileptic condition lasting 30 min	

Table 94. Drug treatment for seizures.

Drug	Usual Adult Daily Oral Dose	Minimum No. of Daily Doses	Time to Steady-State Drug Levels	Optimal Drug Level	Selected Side Effects and Idiosyncratic Reactions
Generalized tonic-clonic (grand mal) or partial (focal) seizures					
Phenytoin	200–400 mg	1	5–10 days	10–20 µg/mL	Nystagmus, ataxia, dysarthria, sedation, confusion, gingival hyperplasia, hirsutism, megaloblastic anemia, blood dyscrasias, skin rashes, fever, systemic lupus erythematosus, lymphadenopathy, peripheral neuropathy, dyskinesias.
Carbamazepine	600–1200 mg	2–3	3–4 days	4–8 µg/mL	Nystagmus, dysarthria, diplopia, ataxia, drowsiness, nausea, blood dyscrasias, hepatotoxicity, hyponatremia. May exacerbate myoclonic seizures.
(extended-release formulation)		(2)			
Valproic acid	1500–2000 mg	3	2–4 days	50–100 µg/mL	Nausea, vomiting, diarrhea, drowsiness, alopecia, weight gain, hepatotoxicity, thrombocytopenia, tremor.
Phenobarbital	100–200 mg	1	14–21 days	10–40 µg/mL	Drowsiness, nystagmus, ataxia, skin rashes, learning difficulties, hyperactivity.
Primidone	750–1500 mg	3	4–7 days	5–15 µg/mL	Sedation, nystagmus, ataxia, vertigo, nausea, skin rashes, megaloblastic anemia, irritability.
Felbamate[1,2]	1200–3600 mg	3	4–5 days	?	Anorexia, nausea, vomiting, headache, insomnia, weight loss, dizziness, hepatotoxicity, aplastic anemia.
Gabapentin[2]	900–1800 mg	3	1 day	?	Sedation, fatigue, ataxia, nystagmus, weight loss.
Lamotrigine	100–500 mg	2	4–5 days	?	Sedation, skin rash, visual disturbances, dyspepsia, ataxia.
Topiramate[2]	200–400 mg	2	4 days	?	Somnolence, nausea, dyspepsia, irritability, dizziness, ataxia, nystagmus, diplopia, renal calculi, weight loss.
Oxcarbazepine[4]	900–1800 mg	2	2–3 days	?	As for carbamazepine.
Levetiracetam[2]	1000–3000 mg	2	2 days	?	Somnolence, ataxia, headache.
Zonisamide[2]	200–600 mg	1–2	10 days	?	Somnolence, ataxia, anorexia, nausea, vomiting, rash, confusion, renal calculi. Do not use in patients with sulfonamide allergy.
Tiagabine[3]	32–56 mg	2	2 days	?	Somnolence, anxiety, dizziness, poor concentration, tremor, diarrhea.
Absence (petit mal) seizures					
Ethosuximide	100–1500 mg	2	5–10 days	40–100 µg/mL	Nausea, vomiting, anorexia, headache, lethargy, unsteadiness, blood dyscrasias, systemic lupus erythematosus, urticaria, pruritus.
Valproic acid	1500–2000 mg	3	2–4 days	50–100 µg/mL	See above.
Clonazepam	0.04–0.2 mg/kg	2	?	20–80 ng/mL	Drowsiness, ataxia, irritability, behavioral changes, exacerbation of tonic-clonic seizures.
Myoclonic seizures					
Valproic acid	1500–2000 mg	3	2–4 days	50–100 µg/mL	See above.
Clonazepam	0.04–0.2 mg/kg	2	?	20–80 ng/mL	See above.

[1]Not to be used as a first-line drug; when used, blood counts should be performed regularly (every 2–4 weeks). Should be used only in selected patients because of risk of aplastic anemia and hepatic failure.
[2]Approved as adjunctive therapy for partial and secondarily generalized seizures.
[3]Approved as adjunctive therapy for partial seizures.
[4]Approved as monotherapy for partial seizures.

Table 95. Primary intracranial tumors.

Tumor	Clinical Features	Treatment and Prognosis
Glioblastoma multiforme	Presents commonly with nonspecific complaints and increased intracranial pressure. As it grows, focal deficits develop.	Course is rapidly progressive, with poor prognosis. Total surgical removal is usually not possible. Radiation therapy and chemotherapy may prolong survival.
Astrocytoma	Presentation similar to glioblastoma multiforme but course more protracted, often over several years. Cerebellar astrocytoma may have a more benign course.	Prognosis is variable. By the time of diagnosis, total excision is usually impossible; tumor often is not radiosensitive. In cerebellar astrocytoma, total surgical removal is often possible.
Medulloblastoma	Seen most frequently in children. Generally arises from roof of fourth ventricle and leads to increased intracranial pressure accompanied by brainstem and cerebellar signs. May seed subarachnoid space.	Treatment consists of surgery combined with radiation therapy and chemotherapy.
Ependymoma	Glioma arising from the ependyma of a ventricle, especially the fourth ventricle; leads early to signs of increased intracranial pressure. Arises also from central canal of cord.	Tumor is not radiosensitive and is best treated surgically if possible.
Oligodendroglioma	Slow-growing. Usually arises in cerebral hemisphere in adults. Calcification may be visible on skull x-ray.	Treatment is surgical and usually successful.
Brainstem glioma	Presents during childhood with cranial nerve palsies and then with long tract signs in the limbs. Signs of increased intracranial pressure occur late.	Tumor is inoperable; treatment is by irradiation and shunt for increased intracranial pressure.
Cerebellar hemangioblastoma	Presents with dysequilibrium, ataxia of trunk or limbs, and signs of increased intracranial pressure. Sometimes familial. May be associated with retinal and spinal vascular lesions, polycythemia, and renal cell carcinoma.	Treatment is surgical.
Pineal tumor	Presents with increased intracranial pressure, sometimes associated with impaired upward gaze (Parinaud's syndrome) and other deficits indicative of midbrain lesion.	Ventricular decompression by shunting is followed by surgical approach to tumor; irradiation is indicated if tumor is malignant. Prognosis depends on histopathologic findings and extent of tumor.
Craniopharyngioma	Originates from remnants of Rathke's pouch above the sella, depressing the optic chiasm. May present at any age but usually in childhood, with endocrine dysfunction and bitemporal field defects.	Treatment is surgical, but total removal may not be possible.
Acoustic neurinoma	Ipsilateral hearing loss is most common initial symptom. Subsequent symptoms may include tinnitus, headache, vertigo, facial weakness or numbness, and long tract signs. (May be familial and bilateral when related to neurofibromatosis.) Most sensitive screening tests are MRI and brainstem auditory evoked potential.	Treatment is excision by translabyrinthine surgery, craniectomy, or a combined approach. Outcome is usually good.
Meningioma	Originates from the dura mater or arachnoid; compresses rather than invades adjacent neural structures. Increasingly common with advancing age. Tumor size varies greatly. Symptoms vary with tumor site—eg, unilateral exophthalmos (sphenoidal ridge); anosmia and optic nerve compression (olfactory groove). Tumor is usually benign and readily detected by CT scanning; may lead to calcification and bone erosion visible on plain x-rays of skull.	Treatment is surgical. Tumor may recur if removal is incomplete.
Primary cerebral lymphoma	Associated with AIDS and other immunodeficient states. Presentation may be with focal deficits or with disturbances of cognition and consciousness. May be indistinguishable from cerebral toxoplasmosis.	Treatment is by whole brain irradiation; chemotherapy may have an adjunctive role. Prognosis depends upon CD4 count at diagnosis.

Table 96. Some anticholinergic antiparkinsonian drugs.[1]

Drug	Usual Daily Dose
Benztropine mesylate (Cogentin)	1–6 mg
Biperiden (Akineton)	2–12 mg
Orphenadrine (Disipal, Norflex)	150–400 mg
Procyclidine (Kemadrin)	7.5–30 mg
Trihexyphenidyl (Artane)	6–20 mg

[1]Modified, with permission, from Aminoff MJ: Pharmacologic management of parkinsonism and other movement disorders. In: *Basic & Clinical Pharmacology*, 8th ed. Katzung BG (editor). McGraw-Hill, 2001.

Table 97. Acute cerebral sequelae of head injury.

Sequelae	Clinical Features	Pathology
Concussion	Transient loss of consciousness with bradycardia, hypotension, and respiratory arrest for a few seconds followed by retrograde and posttraumatic amnesia. Occasionally followed by transient neurologic deficit.	Bruising on side of impact (coup injury) or contralaterally (contrecoup injury).
Cerebral contusion or laceration	Loss of consciousness longer than with concussion. May lead to death or severe residual neurologic deficit.	Cerebral contusion, edema, hemorrhage, and necrosis. May have subarachnoid bleeding.
Acute epidural hemorrhage	Headache, confusion, somnolence, seizures, and focal deficits occur several hours after injury and lead to coma, respiratory depression, and death unless treated by surgical evacuation.	Tear in meningeal artery, vein, or dural sinus, leading to hematoma visible on CT scan.
Acute subdural hemorrhage	Similar to epidural hemorrhage, but interval before onset of symptoms is longer. Treatment is by surgical evacuation.	Hematoma from tear in veins from cortex to superior sagittal sinus or from cerebral laceration, visible on CT scan.
Cerebral hemorrhage	Generally develops immediately after injury. Clinically resembles hypertensive hemorrhage. Surgical evacuation is sometimes helpful.	Hematoma, visible on CT scan.

Table 98. The muscular dystrophies.

Disorder	Inheritance	Age at Onset (years)	Distribution	Prognosis	Genetic Locus
Duchenne type	X-linked recessive	1–5	Pelvic, then shoulder girdle; later, limb and respiratory muscles	Rapid progression. Death within about 15 years after onset.	Xp21
Becker's	X-linked recessive	5–25	Pelvic, then shoulder girdle	Slow progression. May have normal life span.	Xp21
Limb-girdle (Erb's)	Autosomal recessive (may be sporadic or dominant)	10–30	Pelvic or shoulder girdle initially, with later spread to the other	Variable severity and rate of progression. Possible severe disability in middle life.	Multiple
Facioscapulo-humeral	Autosomal dominant	Any age	Face and shoulder girdle initially; later, pelvic girdle and legs	Slow progression. Minor disability. Usually normal life span.	4q35
Emery-Dreifuss	X-linked recessive or autosomal dominant	5–10	Humeroperoneal or scapuloperoneal	Variable	Xq28, 1q11
Distal	Autosomal dominant or recessive	40–60	Onset distally in extremities; proximal involvement later	Slow progression.	2q13, 2p13
Ocular	Autosomal dominant (may be recessive)	Any age (usually 5–30)	External ocular muscles; may also be mild weakness of face, neck, and arms		
Oculopharyn-geal	Autosomal dominant	Any age	As in the ocular form but with dysphagia		14q11.2–q13

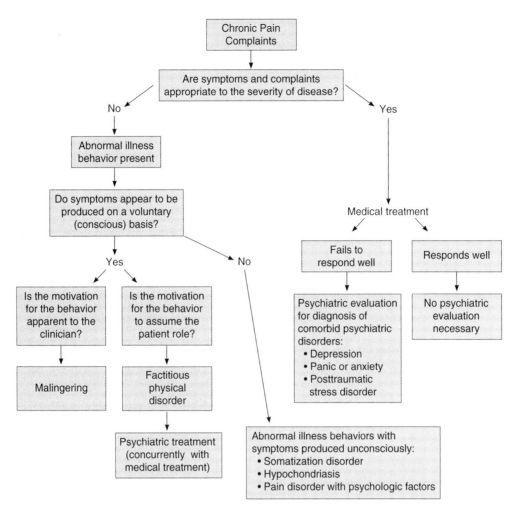

Figure 8. Algorithm for assessing psychiatric component of chronic pain. (Modified and reproduced, with permission, from Eisendrath SJ: Psychiatric aspects of chronic pain. Neurology 1995;45[Suppl 9]:S20.)

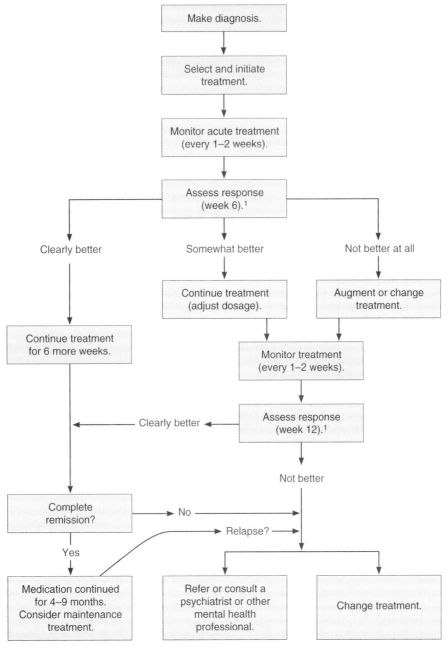

Figure 9. Overview of treatment for depression. (Reproduced, with permission, from Agency for Health Care Policy and Research: *Depression in Primary Care*. Vol. 2: *Treatment of Major Depression*. United States Department of Health and Human Services, 1993.)

Table 99. Screening for alcohol abuse.

1. CAGE screening test[1]

Have you ever felt the need to	Cut down on drinking?
Have you ever felt	Annoyed by criticism of your drinking?
Have you ever felt	Guilty about your drinking?
Have you ever taken a morning	Eye opener?

INTERPRETATION: Two "yes" answers are considered a positive screen. One "yes" answer should arouse a suspicion of alcohol abuse.

2. The Alcohol Use Disorder Identification Test (AUDIT).[2] (Scores for response categories are given in parentheses. Scores range from 0 to 40, with a cutoff score of ≥ 5 indicating hazardous drinking, harmful drinking, or alcohol dependence.)

1. How often do you have a drink containing alcohol?

(0) Never	(1) Monthly or less	(2) Two to four times a month	(3) Two or three times a week	(4) Four or more times a week

2. How many drinks containing alcohol do you have on a typical day when you are drinking?

(0) 1 or 2	(1) 3 or 4	(2) 5 or 6	(3) 7 to 9	(4) 10 or more

3. How often do you have six or more drinks on one occasion?

(0) Never	(1) Less than monthly	(2) Monthly	(3) Weekly	(4) Daily or almost daily

4. How often during the past year have you found that you were not able to stop drinking once you had started?

(0) Never	(1) Less than monthly	(2) Monthly	(3) Weekly	(4) Daily or almost daily

5. How often during the past year have you failed to do what was normally expected of you because of drinking?

(0) Never	(1) Less than monthly	(2) Monthly	(3) Weekly	(4) Daily or almost daily

6. How often during the past year have you needed a first drink in the morning to get yourself going after a heavy drinking session?

(0) Never	(1) Less than monthly	(2) Monthly	(3) Weekly	(4) Daily or almost daily

7. How often during the past year have you had a feeling of guilt or remorse after drinking?

(0) Never	(1) Less than monthly	(2) Monthly	(3) Weekly	(4) Daily or almost daily

8. How often during the past year have you been unable to remember what happened the night before because you had been drinking?

(0) Never	(1) Less than monthly	(2) Monthly	(3) Weekly	(4) Daily or almost daily

9. Have you or has someone else been injured as a result of your drinking?

(0) No	(2) Yes, but not in the past year	(4) Yes, during the past year

10. Has a relative or friend or a doctor or other health worker been concerned about your drinking or suggested you cut down?

(0) No	(2) Yes, but not in the past year	(4) Yes, during the past year

[1]Modified from Mayfield D et al: The CAGE questionnaire: validation of a new alcoholism screening instrument. Am J Psychiatry 1974;131:1121.
[2]From Piccinelli M et al: Efficacy of the alcohol use disorders identification test as a screening tool for hazardous alcohol intake and related disorders in primary care: a validity study. BMJ 1997;314:420.

Table 100. Personality disorders: Classification and clinical findings.

Personality Disorder	Clinical Findings
Paranoid	Defensive, oversensitive, secretive, suspicious, hyperalert, with limited emotional response.
Schizoid	Shy, introverted, withdrawn, avoids close relationships.
Obsessive-compulsive	Perfectionist, egocentric, indecisive, with rigid thought patterns and need for control.
Histrionic (hysterical)	Dependent, immature, seductive, egocentric, vain, emotionally labile.
Schizotypal	Superstitious, socially isolated, suspicious, with limited interpersonal ability, eccentric behaviors, and odd speech.
Narcissistic	Exhibitionist, grandiose, preoccupied with power, lacks interest in others, with excessive demands for attention.
Avoidant	Fears rejection, hyperreacts to rejection and failure, with poor social endeavors and low self-esteem.
Dependent	Passive, overaccepting, unable to make decisions, lacks confidence, with poor self-esteem.
Antisocial	Selfish, callous, promiscuous, impulsive, unable to learn from experience, has legal problems.
Borderline	Impulsive; has unstable and intense interpersonal relationships; is suffused with anger, fear, and guilt; lacks self-control and self-fulfillment; has identity problems and affective instability; is suicidal (a serious problem—up to 80% of hospitalized borderline patients make an attempt at some time during treatment, and the incidence of completed suicide is as high as 5%); aggressive behavior, feelings of emptiness, and occasional psychotic decompensation. This group has a high drug abuse rate, which plays a role in symptomatology. There is extensive overlap with other diagnostic categories, particularly mood disorders and posttraumatic stress disorder.

Table 101. Commonly used antianxiety and hypnotic agents.

Drug	Usual Daily Oral Dose	Usual Daily Maximum Dose	Cost for 30 Days' Treatment Based on Maximum Dosage[1]
Benzodiazepines (used for anxiety)			
Alprazolam (Xanax)[2]	0.5 mg	4 mg	$117.60
Chlordiazepoxide (Librium)[3]	10–20 mg	100 mg	$40.80
Clonazepam (Klonopin)[3]	1–2 mg	10 mg	$177.00
Clorazepate (Tranxene)[3]	15–30 mg	60 mg	$260.40
Diazepam (Valium)[3]	5–15 mg	30 mg	$28.80
Lorazepam (Ativan)[2]	2–4 mg	4 mg	$76.80
Oxazepam (Serax)[2]	10–30 mg	60 mg	$94.20
Benzodiazepines (used for sleep)			
Estazolam (Prosom)[2]	1 mg	2 mg	$29.70
Flurazepam (Dalmane)[3]	15 mg	30 mg	$10.50
Midazolam (Versed IV)[4]	5 mg IV		$1.56/dose
Quazepam (Doral)[3]	7.5 mg	15 mg	$92.70
Temazepam (Restoril)[2]	15 mg	30 mg	$26.40
Triazolam (Halcion)[5]	0.125 mg	0.25 mg	$21.60
Miscellaneous (used for anxiety)			
Buspirone (Buspar)[2]	10–30 mg	60 mg	$218.10
Phenobarbital[3]	15–30 mg	90 mg	$1.80
Miscellaneous (used for sleep)			
Chloral hydrate (Noctec)[2]	500 mg	1000 mg	$37.80
Hydroxyzine (Vistaril)[2]	50 mg	100 mg	$67.20
Zolpidem (Ambien)[5]	5–10 mg	10 mg	$80.70
Zaleplon (Sonata)[6]	5–10 mg	10 mg	$77.10

[1]Average wholesale price (AWP, for AB-rated generic when available) for quantity listed. Source: *Drug Topics Red Book,* May 2003; Vol. 22, No. 5. AWP may not accurately represent the actual pharmacy cost because wide contractual variations exist among institutions.
[2]Intermediate physical half-life (10–20 hours).
[3]Long physical half-life (> 20 hours).
[4]Intravenously for procedures.
[5]Short physical half-life (1–5 hours).
[6]Short physical half-life (about 1 hour).

Table 102. Commonly used antipsychotics.

Drug	Usual Daily Oral Dose	Usual Daily Maximum Oral Dose[1]	Cost per Unit	Cost for 30 Days' Treatment Based on Maximum Dosage[2]
Phenothiazines				
Chlorpromazine (Thorazine; others)	100–400 mg	1 g	$1.05/200 mg	$157.50
Thioridazine (Mellaril)	100–400 mg	600 mg	$1.10/200 mg	$99.00
Mesoridazine (Serentil)	50–200 mg	400 mg	$1.47/100 mg	$176.40
Perphenazine (Trilafon)[3]	16–32 mg	64 mg	$1.08/16 mg	$129.60
Trifluoperazine (Stelazine)	5–15 mg	60 mg	$1.58/10 mg	$284.40
Fluphenazine (Permitil, Prolixin)[3]	2–10 mg	60 mg	$1.15/10 mg	$207.00
Thioxanthenes				
Thiothixene (Navane)[3]	5–10 mg	80 mg	$0.65/10 mg	$156.00
Dihydroindolone				
Molindone (Moban)	30–100 mg	225 mg	$3.44/50 mg	$464.40
Dibenzoxazepine				
Loxapine (Loxitane)	20–60 mg	200 mg	$2.20/50 mg	$264.00
Dibenzodiazepine				
Clozapine (Clozaril)	300–450 mg	900 mg	$3.33/100 mg	$899.10
Butyrophenone				
Haloperidol (Haldol)	2–5 mg	60 mg	$2.52/20 mg	$226.80
Benzisoxazole				
Risperidone[4] (Risperdal)	2–6 mg	10 mg	$5.10/2 mg	$641.00
Thienbenzodiazepine				
Olanzapine (Zyprexa)	5–10 mg	10 mg	$9.63/10 mg	$288.90
Dibenzothiazepine				
Quetiapine (Seroquel)	200–400 mg	800 mg	$5.48/200 mg	$657.60
Benzothiazolyl piperazine				
Ziprasidone (Geodon)	40–160 mg	160 mg	$4.47/80 mg	$268.21
Dipiperazine				
Aripiprazole (Abilify)	10–15 mg	30 mg	$10.14/15 mg	$430.20

[1]Can be higher in some cases.
[2]Average wholesale price (AWP, for AB-rated generic when available) for quantity listed. Source: *Drug Topics Red Book,* May 2003; Vol. 22, No. 5. AWP may not accurately represent the actual pharmacy cost because wide contractual variations exist among institutions.
[3]Indicates piperazine structure.
[4]For risperidone, daily doses above 6 mg increase the risk of extrapyramidal syndrome. Risperidone 6 mg is approximately equivalent to haloperidol 20 mg.

Table 103. Relative potency and side effects of antipsychotics.

Drug	Chlorpromazine Potency Ratio	Anticholinergic Effects	Extrapyramidal Effects
Phenothiazines			
Chlorpromazine	1:1	4	1
Thioridazine	1:1	4	1
Mesoridazine	1:2	3	2
Perphenazine	1:10	2	3
Trifluoperazine	1:20	1	4
Fluphenazine	1:50	1	4
Thioxanthene			
Thiothixene	1:20	1	4
Dihydroindolone			
Molindone	1:10	2	3
Dibenzoxazepine			
Loxapine	1:10	2	3
Butyrophenone			
Haloperidol	1:50	1	4
Dibenzodiazepine			
Clozapine	1:1	4	—
Benzisoxazole			
Risperidone	1:50	1	1
Thienbenzodiazepine			
Olanzapine	1:20	1	1
Dibenzothiazepine			
Quetiapine	1:1	1	—
Benzisothiazolyl piperazine			
Ziprasidone	1:1	1	1
Dipiperazine			
Aripiprazole	1:20	1	0

Key: 4 = strong effect; 1 = weak effect.

Table 104. Commonly used antidepressants.

Drug	Usual Daily Oral Dose (mg)	Usual Daily Maximum Dose (mg)	Sedative Effects[1]	Anticho-linergic Effects[1]	Cost per Unit	Cost for 30 Days' Treatment Based on Maximum Dosage[2]
SSRIs AND OTHER NEW COMPOUNDS						
Fluoxetine (Prozac, Sarafem)	5–40	80	< 1	< 1	$2.67/20 mg	$320.40
Fluvoxamine (Luvox)	100–300	300	1	< 1	$2.64/100 mg	$237.60
Nefazodone (Serzone)	300–600	600	2	< 1	$1.62/200 mg	$146.05
Paroxetine (Paxil)	20–30	50	1	1	$2.82/20 mg	$171.71
Sertraline (Zoloft)	50–150	200	< 1	< 1	$2.65/100 mg	$159.00
Venlafaxine (Effexor)	150–225	375	1	< 1	$1.69/75 mg	$211.80
Venlafaxine XR (Effexor)	150–225	225	1	< 1	$2.85/75 mg	$178.80
Mirtazapine (Remeron)	15–45	45	4	2	$3.11/30 mg	$95.03
Citalopram (Celexa)	20	40	< 1	2	$2.52/40 mg	$75.60
Escitalopram (Lexapro)	10	20	< 1	1	$2.23/20 mg	$66.90
TRICYCLIC AND CLINICALLY SIMILAR COMPOUNDS						
Amitriptyline (Elavil)	150–250	300	4	4	$1.16/150 mg	$69.60
Amoxapine (Asendin)	150–200	400	2	2	$1.67/100 mg	$200.40
Clomipramine (Anafranil)	100	250	3	3	$1.40/75 mg	$126.00
Desipramine (Norpramin)	100–250	300	1	1	$1.50/100 mg	$135.00
Doxepin (Sinequan)	150–200	300	4	3	$1.00/100 mg	$90.00
Imipramine (Tofranil)	150–200	300	3	3	$1.22/50 mg	$219.60
Maprotiline (Ludiomil)	100–200	300	4	2	$0.93/75 mg	$111.60
Nortriptyline (Aventyl, Pamelor)	100–150	150	2	2	$1.46/50 mg	$131.40
Protriptyline (Vivactil)	15–40	60	1	3	$1.19/10 mg	$214.20
Trazodone (Desyrel)	100–300	400	4	< 1	$0.73/100 mg	$87.60
Trimipramine (Surmontil)	75–200	200	4	4	$2.24/100 mg	$134.40
Bupropion (Wellbutrin)	300[3]	450[3]		< 1	$0.96/100 mg	$129.60
Bupropion SR (Wellbutrin SR)	300	400[4]		< 1	$1.80/100 mg $1.93/150 mg	$216.00 $115.80
MONOAMINE OXIDASE INHIBITORS						
Phenelzine (Nardil)	45–60	90	...	...	$0.54/15 mg	$97.20
Tranylcypromine (Parnate)	20–30	50	...	...	$0.63/10 mg	$94.50

[1]**Key:** 4 = strong effect; 1 = weak effect.
[2]Average wholesale price (AWP, for AB-rated generic when available) for quantity listed. Source: *Drug Topics Red Book,* May 2003; Vol. 22, No. 5. AWP may not accurately represent the actual pharmacy cost because wide contractual variations exist among institutions.
[3]No single dose should exceed 150 mg.
[4]200 mg twice daily.

Table 105. Etiology of delirium and other cognitive disorders

Disorder	Possible Causes
Intoxication	Alcohol, sedatives, bromides, analgesics (eg, pentazocine), psychedelic drugs, stimulants, and household solvents.
Drug withdrawal	Withdrawal from alcohol, sedative-hypnotics, corticosteroids.
Long-term effects of alcohol	Wernicke-Korsakoff syndrome.
Infections	Septicemia; meningitis and encephalitis due to bacterial, viral, fungal, parasitic, or tuberculous organisms or to central nervous system syphilis; acute and chronic infections due to the entire range of microbiologic pathogens.
Endocrine disorders	Thyrotoxicosis, hypothyroidism, adrenocortical dysfunction (including Addison's disease and Cushing's syndrome), pheochromocytoma, insulinoma, hypoglycemia, hyperparathyroidism, hypoparathyroidism, panhypopituitarism, diabetic ketoacidosis.
Respiratory disorders	Hypoxia, hypercapnia.
Metabolic disturbances	Fluid and electrolyte disturbances (especially hyponatremia, hypomagnesemia, and hypercalcemia), acid-base disorders, hepatic disease (hepatic encephalopathy), renal failure, porphyria.
Nutritional deficiencies	Deficiency of vitamin B_1 (beriberi), vitamin B_{12} (pernicious anemia), folic acid, nicotinic acid (pellagra); protein-calorie malnutrition.
Trauma	Subdural hematoma, subarachnoid hemorrhage, intracerebral bleeding, concussion syndrome.
Cardiovascular disorders	Myocardial infarctions, cardiac arrhythmias, cerebrovascular spasms, hypertensive encephalopathy, hemorrhages, embolisms, and occlusions indirectly cause decreased cognitive function.
Neoplasms	Primary or metastatic lesions of the central nervous system, cancer-induced hypercalcemia.
Seizure disorders	Ictal, interictal, and postictal dysfunction.
Collagen-vascular and immunologic disorders	Autoimmune disorders, including systemic lupus erythematosus, Sjögren's syndrome, and AIDS.
Degenerative diseases	Alzheimer's disease, Pick's disease, multiple sclerosis, parkinsonism, Huntington's chorea, normal pressure hydrocephalus.
Medications	Anticholinergic drugs, antidepressants, H_2-blocking agents, digoxin, salicylates (chronic use), and a wide variety of other OTC and prescribed drugs.

Table 106. Causes of hyperprolactinemia.

Physiologic Causes	Pharmacologic Causes	Pathologic Causes
Exercise	Amoxapine	Acromegaly
Idiopathic	Amphetamines	Chronic chest wall stimulation (postthoracotomy, postmastectomy,
Macroprolactinemia	Anesthetic agents	herpes zoster, breast problems, nipple rings, etc)
("big prolactin")	Butyrophenones	Cirrhosis
Pregnancy	Cimetidine and ranitidine (not famotidine or nizatidine)	Hypothalamic disease
Puerperium	Estrogens	Hypothyroidism
Sleep (REM phase)	Hydroxyzine	Multiple sclerosis
Stress (trauma, surgery)	Methyldopa	Optic neuromyelitis
Suckling	Metoclopramide	Pituitary stalk section
	Narcotics	Prolactin-secreting tumors
	Nicotine	Pseudocyesis (false pregnancy)
	Phenothiazines	Renal failure (especially with zinc deficiency)
	Protease inhibitors	Spinal cord lesions
	Progestins	Systemic lupus erythematosus
	Reserpine	
	Risperidone	
	Selective serotonin reuptake inhibitors	
	Tricyclic antidepressants	
	Verapamil	

Table 107. The Diabetes Expert Committee criteria for evaluating the standard oral glucose tolerance test.[1]

	Normal Glucose Tolerance	Impaired Glucose Tolerance	Diabetes Mellitus[2]
Fasting plasma glucose (mg/dL)	< 110	110–125	≥ 126
Two hours after glucose load (mg/dL)	< 140	≥ 140 but < 200	≥ 200

[1]Give 75 g of glucose dissolved in 300 mL of water after an overnight fast in subjects who have been receiving at least 150–200 g of carbohydrate daily for 3 days before the test.
[2]A fasting plasma glucose ≥ 126 mg/dL is diagnostic of diabetes if confirmed on a subsequent day.

Table 108. Oral antidiabetic drugs that stimulate insulin secretion.

Drug	Tablet Size	Daily Dose	Duration of Action	Cost per Unit	Cost for 30 Days' Treatment Based on Maximum Dosage[1]
Sulfonylureas					
Tolbutamide (Orinase)	250 and 500 mg	0.5–2 g in 2 or 3 divided doses	6–12 hours	$0.28/500 mg	$33.60
Tolazamide (Tolinase)	100, 250, and 500 mg	0.1–1 g as single dose or in 2 divided doses	Up to 24 hours	$0.45/250 mg	$75.15
Acetohexamide (Dymelor)[2]	250 and 500 mg	0.25–1.5 g as single dose or in 2 divided doses	8–24 hours	$0.42/500 mg	$37.80
Chlorpropamide (Diabinese)[2]	100 and 250 mg	0.1–0.5 g as single dose	24–72 hours	$0.61/250 mg	$36.60
Glyburide					
(Diaβeta, Micronase)	1.25, 2.5, and 5 mg	1.25–20 mg as single dose or in 2 divided doses	Up to 24 hours	$0.78/5 mg	$93.60
(Glynase)	1.5, 3, and 6 mg	1.5–18 mg as single dose or in 2 divided doses	Up to 24 hours	$1.07/6 mg	$96.30
Glipizide					
(Glucotrol)	5 and 10 mg	2.5–40 mg as single dose or in 2 divided doses on an empty stomach	6–12 hours	$0.59/10 mg	$70.80
(Glucotrol XL)	5 and 10 mg	Up to 20 or 30 mg daily as a single dose	Up to 24 hours	$0.75/10 mg	$67.50
Glimeperide (Amaryl)	1, 2, and 4 mg	1–4 mg as single dose	Up to 24 hours	$1.02/4 mg	$30.60
Meglitinide analogs					
Repaglinide (Prandin)	0.5, 1, and 2 mg	4 mg in two divided doses given 15 minutes before breakfast and dinner	3 hours	$0.98/2 mg	$58.80
ᴅ-Phenylalanine derivative					
Nateglinide (Starlix)	60 mg and 120 mg	60 or 120 mg 3 times a day before meals	1.5 hours	$1.05/60 mg; $1.09/120 mg	$98.10

[1]Average wholesale price (AWP, for AB-rated generic when available) for quantity listed. Source: *Drug Topics Red Book,* May 2003; Vol. 22, No. 5. AWP may not accurately represent the actual pharmacy cost because wide contractual variations exist among institutions.
[2]There has been a decline in use of these formulations. In the case of chlorpropamide, the decline is due to its numerous side effects.

Table 109. Oral antidiabetic drugs that are insulin-sparing.

Drug	Tablet Size	Daily Dose	Duration of Action	Cost per Unit	Cost for 30 Days' Treatment Based on Maximum Dosage[1]
Biguanides					
Metformin (Glucophage)	500, 850, and 1000 mg	1–2.5 g; one tablet with meals 2 or 3 times daily	7–12 hours	$1.20/850 mg	$108.00
Extended-release metformin (Glucophage XR)	500 mg	500–2000 mg once a day	Up to 24 hours	$0.74/500 mg	$88.80
Thiazolidinediones					
Rosiglitazone (Avandia)	2, 4, and 8 mg	4–8 mg daily (can be divided)	Up to 24 hours	$5.12/8 mg	$153.60
Pioglitazone (Actos)	15, 30, and 45 mg	15–45 mg daily	Up to 24 hours	$5.12/30 mg	$153.60
Alpha-glucosidase inhibitors					
Acarbose (Precose)	50 and 100 mg	75–300 mg in 3 divided doses with first bite of food	4 hours	$0.83/100 mg	$74.70
Miglitol (Glyset)	25, 50, and 100 mg	75–300 mg in 3 divided doses with first bite of food	4 hours	$0.85/100 mg	$76.50

[1]Average wholesale price (AWP, for AB-rated generic when available) for quantity listed. Source: *Drug Topics Red Book,* May 2003; Vol. 22, No. 5. AWP may not accurately represent the actual pharmacy cost because wide contractual variations exist among institutions.

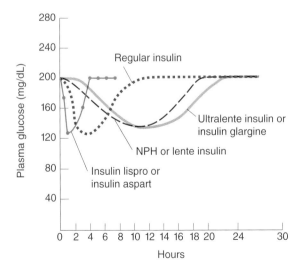

Figure 10. Extent and duration of action of various insulins (in a fasting diabetic). Duration is extended considerably when the dose of a given formulation increases above average therapeutic doses (except for insulin lispro).

Table 110. Some insulin preparations available in the United States.[1,2]

Preparation	Species Source	Concentration	Cost[2]
Ultra-short-acting insulins			
Insulin lispro (Humalog, Lilly)	Human analog (recombinant)	U100	$58.97
Insulin aspart (Novolog, Novo Nordisk)	Human analog (recombinant)	U100	$58.97
Short-acting insulins "Purified"[3]			
Regular Novolin (Novo Nordisk)[4]	Human	U100	$26.56
Regular Humulin (Lilly)	Human	U100, U500 20 mL	$26.56 $200.65
Regular Iletin II (Lilly)	Pork	U100	$47.98
Velosulin (Novo Nordisk)[5]	Human	U100	$39.00
Intermediate-acting insulins "Purified"[3]			
Lente Humulin (Lilly)	Human	U100	$26.56
Lente Iletin II (Lilly)	Pork	U100	$47.98
Lente Novolin (Novo Nordisk)	Human	U100	$26.56
NPH Humulin (Lilly)	Human	U100	$26.56
NPH Iletin II (Lilly)	Pork	U100	$47.98
NPH Novolin (Novo Nordisk)	Human	U100	$26.56
Premixed insulins % NPH/% regular			
Novolin 70/30 (Novo Nordisk)	Human	U100	$26.56
Humulin 70/30 and 50/50 (Lilly)	Human	U100	$26.56
% NPL/% insulin lispro Humalog Mix 75/25 (Lilly) 70% insulin aspart protamine/30% insulin aspart (Novolog Mix 70/30)	Human analog (recombinant)	U100 (insulin pen, prefilled syringes, 5×3-mL cartridges)	Pen $118.66 Vial $58.97
Long-acting insulins "Purified"[3]			
Ultralente Humulin (Lilly)	Human	U100	$26.56
Insulin glargine (Lantus, Aventis)	Human analog (recombinant)	U100	$51.21

[1]Modified and reproduced, with permission, from Katzung BG (editor): *Basic and Clinical Pharmacology,* 8th ed. McGraw-Hill, 2001.
[2]All of these agents (except insulin lispro and U500) are available without a prescription. Average wholesale price (AWP, for AB-rated generic when available) for 10-mL vial unless otherwise specified. Source: *Drug Topics Red Book,* May 2003; Vol. 22, No. 5. Wholesale prices for all human preparations (except insulin lispro and U500) are similar. AWP may not accurately represent the actual pharmacy cost because wide contractual variations exist among institutions.
[3]Less than 10 ppm proinsulin.
[4]Novo Nordisk human insulins are termed Novolin R, L, and N.
[5]Velosulin contains phosphate buffer, which favors its use to prevent insulin aggregation in pump tubing but precludes its being mixed with lente insulin. It is the only FDA-approved insulin for pump use.

Table 111. Combination oral antidiabetic drugs.

Drug	Tablet Size	Daily Dose	Duration of Action	Cost per Unit	Cost for 30 Days' Treatment Based on Maximum Dosage[1]
Glyburide/metformin (Glucovance)	1.25 mg/250 mg 2.5 mg/500 mg 5 mg/500 mg	Maximum daily dose of 20 mg glyburide/ 2000 mg metformin	See individual drugs[2]	$0.94/5/ 500 mg	$112.80
Rosiglitazone/metformin (Avandamet)	1 mg/500 mg 2 mg/500 mg 4 mg.500 mg	Maximum daily dose of 8 mg rosiglitazone/ 2000 mg metformin	See individual drugs[2]	$1.35/2/ 500 mg	$162.00

[1]Average wholesale price (AWP, for AB-rated generic when available) for quantity listed. Source: *Drug Topics Red Book,* May 2003; Vol. 22, No. 5. AWP may not accurately represent the actual pharmacy cost because wide contractual variations exist among institutions.
[2]Glyburide, Table 108; metformin, Table 109; and rosiglitazone, Table 109.

Table 112. Examples of intensive insulin regimens using insulin lispro or insulin aspart and ultralente, NPH, or insulin glargine in a 70-kg man with type 1 diabetes.[1,2,3]

	Pre-Breakfast	Pre-Lunch	Pre-Dinner	At Bedtime
Insulin lispro or aspart	5 units	4 units	6 units	—
Ultralente insulin	8 units	—	8 units	—
		OR		
Insulin lispro or aspart	5 units	4 units	6 units	—
NPH insulin	3 units	3 units	2 units	8–14 units
		OR		
Insulin lispro or aspart	5 units	4 units	6 units	
Insulin glargine	—	—	—	15–16 units

[1]Assumes that patient is consuming approximately 75 g carbohydrate at breakfast, 60 g at lunch, and 90 g at dinner.
[2]The dose of insulin lispro or insulin aspart can be raised by 1 or 2 units if extra carbohydrate (15–30 g) is ingested or if premeal blood glucose is > 170 mg/dL. Insulin lispro or insulin aspart can be mixed in the same syringe with ultralente or NPH insulin.
[3]Insulin glargine cannot be mixed with any of the available insulins and must be given as a separate injection.

Table 113. Secondary causes of lipid abnormalities.

Cause	Associated Lipid Abnormality
Obesity	Increased triglycerides, decreased HDL cholesterol
Sedentary lifestyle	Decreased HDL cholesterol
Diabetes mellitus	Increased triglycerides, increased total cholesterol
Alcohol use	Increased triglycerides, increased HDL cholesterol
Hypothyroidism	Increased total cholesterol
Hyperthyroidism	Decreased total cholesterol
Nephrotic syndrome	Increased total cholesterol
Chronic renal insufficiency	Increased total cholesterol, increased triglycerides
Hepatic disease (cirrhosis)	Decreased total cholesterol
Obstructive liver disease	Increased total cholesterol
Malignancy	Decreased total cholesterol
Cushing's disease (or steroid use)	Increased total cholesterol
Oral contraceptives	Increased triglycerides, increased total cholesterol
Diuretics[1]	Increased total cholesterol, increased triglycerides
β-blockers[1,2]	Increased total cholesterol, decreased HDL

[1]Short-term effects only.
[2]β-blockers with intrinsic sympathomimetic activity, such as pindolol and acebutolol, do not affect lipid levels.

Table 114. LDL goals and treatment cutpoints: Recommendations of the NCEP Adult Treatment Panel III Report.[1]

Risk Category	LDL Goal (mg/dL)	LDL at Which to Initiate Lifestyle Changes (mg/dL)	LDL Level at Which to Consider Drug Changes (mg/dL)
CHD or CHD risk equivalents	< 100	≥ 100	≥ 130
≥ 2 risk factors	< 130	≥ 130	10-year risk 10–20%: ≥ 130 10-year risk <10%: ≥ 160
0–1 risk factors	< 160	≥ 160	≥ 190

[1]Reproduced, with permission, from Executive Summary of The Third Report of The National Cholesterol Education Program (NCEP) Expert Panel on Detection, Evaluation, and Treatment of High Blood Cholesterol In Adults (Adult Treatment Panel III). JAMA 2001;285:2486. http://www.nhlbi.nih.gov/guidelines/cholesterol/index.htm.

Table 115. Effects of selected lipid-modifying drugs.

Drug Listed[1]	Lipid-Modifying Effects			Initial Daily Oral Dose	Maximum Daily Dose	Cost for 30 Days' Treatment with Dose
	LDL	HDL	Triglyceride			
Atorvastatin (Lipitor)	−25 to −40%	+5 to −10%	↓↓	10 mg once	80 mg once	$109.31 (20 mg once)
Cholestyramine (Questran, others)	−15 to −25%	+5%	±	4 g bid	24 g divided	$126.68 (8 g divided)
Colestipol (Colestid)	−15 to −25%	+5%	±	5 g bid	30 g divided	$106.45 (10 g divided)
Fluvastatin (Lescol)	−20 to −30%	+5 to −10%	↓	20 mg once	40 mg once	$53.42 (20 mg once)
Gemfibrozil (Lopid)	−10 to −15%	+15 to −20%	↓↓	600 mg once	1200 mg divided	$74.75 (600 mg bid)
Lovastatin (Mevacor)	−25 to −40%	+5 to −10%	↓	10 mg once	80 mg divided	$71.10 (20 mg once)
Niacin	−15 to −25%	+25 to −35%	↓↓	100 mg once	3–4.5 g divided	$7.20 (1.5 g bid)
Pravastatin (Pravachol)	−25 to −40%	+5 to −10%	↓	20 mg once	40 mg once	$92.41 (20 mg once)
Simvastatin (Zocor)	−25 to −40%	+5 to −10%	↓↓	5 mg once	80 mg once	$78.85 (10 mg once)

[1]Average wholesale price (AWP, for AB-rated generic when available) for quantity listed. Source: *Drug Topics Red Book,* May 2003; Vol. 22, No. 5. AWP may not accurately represent the actual pharmacy cost because wide contractual variations exist among institutions.
± = variable, if any.

Table 116. CDC AIDS case definition for surveillance of adults and adolescents.

Definitive AIDS diagnoses (with or without laboratory evidence of HIV infection)
1. Candidiasis of the esophagus, trachea, bronchi, or lungs.
2. Cryptococcosis, extrapulmonary.
3. Cryptosporidiosis with diarrhea persisting > 1 month.
4. Cytomegalovirus disease of an organ other than liver, spleen, or lymph nodes.
5. Herpes simplex virus infection causing a mucocutaneous ulcer that persists longer than 1 month; or bronchitis, pneumonitis, or esophagitis of any duration.
6. Kaposi's sarcoma in a patient < 60 years of age.
7. Lymphoma of the brain (primary) in a patient < 60 years of age.
8. *Mycobacterium avium* complex or *Mycobacterium kansasii* disease, disseminated (at a site other than or in addition to lungs, skin, or cervical or hilar lymph nodes).
9. *Pneumocystis jiroveci* pneumonia.
10. Progressive multifocal leukoencephalopathy.
11. Toxoplasmosis of the brain.

Definitive AIDS diagnoses (with laboratory evidence of HIV infection)
1. Coccidioidomycosis, disseminated (at a site other than or in addition to lungs or cervical or hilar lymph nodes).
2. HIV encephalopathy.
3. Histoplasmosis, disseminated (at a site other than or in addition to lungs or cervical or hilar lymph nodes).
4. Isosporiasis with diarrhea persisting > 1 month.
5. Kaposi's sarcoma at any age.
6. Lymphoma of the brain (primary) at any age.
7. Other non-Hodgkin's lymphoma of B cell or unknown immunologic phenotype.
8. Any mycobacterial disease caused by mycobacteria other than *Mycobacterium tuberculosis,* disseminated (at a site other than or in addition to lungs, skin, or cervical or hilar lymph nodes).
9. Disease caused by extrapulmonary *M tuberculosis.*
10. Salmonella (nontyphoid) septicemia, recurrent.
11. HIV wasting syndrome.
12. CD4 lymphocyte count below 200 cells/μL or a CD4 lymphocyte percentage below 14%.
13. Pulmonary tuberculosis.
14. Recurrent pneumonia.
15. Invasive cervical cancer.

Presumptive AIDS diagnoses (with laboratory evidence of HIV infection)
1. Candidiasis of esophagus: (a) recent onset of retrosternal pain on swallowing; and (b) oral candidiasis.
2. Cytomegalovirus retinitis. A characteristic appearance on serial ophthalmoscopic examinations.
3. Mycobacteriosis. Specimen from stool or normally sterile body fluids or tissue from a site other than lungs, skin, or cervical or hilar lymph nodes, showing acid-fast bacilli of a species not identified by culture.
4. Kaposi's sarcoma. Erythematous or violaceous plaque-like lesion on skin or mucous membrane.
5. *Pneumocystis jiroveci* pneumonia: (a) a history of dyspnea on exertion or nonproductive cough of recent onset (within the past 3 months); and (b) chest x-ray evidence of diffuse bilateral interstitial infiltrates or gallium scan evidence of diffuse bilateral pulmonary disease; and (c) arterial blood gas analysis showing an arterial oxygen partial pressure of < 70 mm Hg or a low respiratory diffusing capacity of < 80% of predicted values or an increase in the alveolar-arterial oxygen tension gradient; and (d) no evidence of a bacterial pneumonia.
6. Toxoplasmosis of the brain: (a) recent onset of a focal neurologic abnormality consistent with intracranial disease or a reduced level of consciousness; and (b) brain imaging evidence of a lesion having a mass effect or the radiographic appearance of which is enhanced by injection of contrast medium; and (c) serum antibody to toxoplasmosis or successful response to therapy for toxoplasmosis.
7. Recurrent pneumonia: (a) more than one episode in a 1-year period; and (b) acute pneumonia (new symptoms, signs, or radiologic evidence not present earlier) diagnosed on clinical or radiologic grounds by the patient's physician.
8. Pulmonary tuberculosis: (a) apical or miliary infiltrates and (b) radiographic and clinical response to antituberculous therapy.

Table 117. Laboratory findings with HIV infection.

Test	Significance
HIV enzyme-linked immuno-sorbent assay (ELISA)	Screening test for HIV infection. 50% of ELISA tests are positive within 22 days after HIV transmission; 95% are positive within 6 weeks after transmission. Sensitivity > 99.9%; to avoid false-positive results, repeatedly reactive results must be confirmed with Western blot.
Western blot	Confirmatory test for HIV. Specificity when combined with ELISA > 99.99%. Indeterminate results with early HIV infection, HIV-2 infection, autoimmune disease, pregnancy, and recent tetanus toxoid administration.
CBC	Anemia, neutropenia, and thrombocytopenia common with advanced HIV infection.
Absolute CD4 lymphocyte count	Most widely used predictor of HIV progression. Risk of progression to an AIDS opportunistic infection or malignancy is high with CD4 < 200 cells/μL.
CD4 lymphocyte percentage	Percentage may be more reliable than the CD4 count. Risk of progression to an AIDS opportunistic infection or malignancy is high with percentage < 20%.
HIV viral load tests	These tests measure the amount of actively replicating HIV virus. Correlate with disease progression and response to antiretroviral drugs. Treatment is recommended for HIV-infected patients with > 30,000 viral copies by branched-chain DNA or > 55,000 viral copies by PCR testing. Best tests available for diagnosis of acute HIV infection; however, false positives are common, especially when the viral load is low.
β_2-Microglobulin	Cell surface protein indicative of macrophage-monocyte stimulation. Levels > 3.5 mg/dL associated with rapid progression of disease. Not useful with intravenous drug users.
p24 antigen	Indicates active HIV replication. Tends to be positive prior to seroconversion and with advanced disease.

Table 118. Health care maintenance of HIV-infected individuals.

For all HIV-infected individuals:
  CD4 counts every 3–6 months
  Viral load tests every 3–6 months and 1 month following a change
    in therapy
  PPD
  INH for those with positive PPD and normal chest x-ray
  RPR or VDRL
  Toxoplasma IgG serology
  Cytomegalovirus IgG serology
  Pneumococcal vaccine
  Influenza vaccine in season
  Hepatitis B vaccine for those who are HBsAb-negative
  Haemophilus influenzae type b vaccination
  Papanicolaou smears every 6 months for women
  Consider anal swabs for cytologic evaluation yearly for patients with
    history of receptive anal intercourse
For HIV-infected individuals with CD4 < 500 cells/μL:
  Antiretroviral therapy (see Table 120)
For HIV-infected individuals with CD4 < 200 cells/μL:
  P jiroveci[1] prophylaxis (see Table 121)
For HIV-infected individuals with CD4 < 75 cells/μL:
  M avium complex prophylaxis
For HIV-infected individuals with CD4 < 50 cells/μL:
  Consider CMV prophylaxis

[1]Formerly known as *P carinii*.

Table 119. Treatment of AIDS-related opportunistic infections and malignancies.[1]

Infection or Malignancy	Treatment	Complications
P jiroveci infection[2]	Trimethoprim-sulfamethoxazole, 15 mg/kg/d (based on trimethoprim component) orally or IV for 14–21 days.	Nausea, neutropenia, anemia, hepatitis, drug rash, Stevens-Johnson syndrome.
	Pentamidine, 3–4 mg/kg/d IV for 14–21 days.	Hypotension, hypoglycemia, anemia, neutropenia, pancreatitis, hepatitis.
	Trimethoprim, 15 mg/kg/d orally, with dapsone, 100 mg/d orally, for 14–21 days.[3]	Nausea, rash, hemolytic anemia in G6PD-deficient patients. Methemoglobinemia (weekly levels should be < 10% of total hemoglobin).
	Primaquine, 15–30 mg/d orally, and clindamycin, 600 mg every 8 hours orally, for 14–21 days.	Hemolytic anemia in G6PD-deficient patients. Methemoglobinemia, neutropenia, colitis.
	Atovaquone, 750 mg orally 3 times daily for 14–21 days.	Rash, elevated aminotransferases, anemia, neutropenia.
	Trimetrexate, 45 mg/m^2 IV for 21 days (given with leucovorin calcium) if intolerant of all other regimens.	Leukopenia, rash, mucositis.
M avium complex infection	Clarithromycin, 500 mg orally twice daily with ethambutol, 15 mg/kg/d orally (maximum, 1 g). May also add:	Clarithromycin: hepatitis, nausea, diarrhea; ethambutol: hepatitis, optic neuritis.
	Rifabutin, 300 mg orally daily.	Rash, hepatitis, uveitis.
Toxoplasmosis	Pyrimethamine, 100–200 mg orally as loading dose, followed by 50–75 mg/d, combined with sulfadiazine, 4–6 g orally daily in 4 divided doses, and folinic acid, 10 mg daily for 4–8 weeks; then pyrimethamine, 25–50 mg/d, with clindamycin, 2 g/d, and folinic acid, 5 mg/d, until clinical and radiographic resolution is achieved.	Leukopenia, rash.
Lymphoma	Combination chemotherapy (eg, modified CHOP,[4] M-BACOD,[4] with or without G-CSF[5] or GM-CSF[5]). Central nervous system disease: radiation treatment with dexamethasone for edema.	Nausea, vomiting, anemia, leukopenia, cardiac toxicity (with doxorubicin).
Cryptococcal meningitis	Amphotericin B, 0.6 mg/kg/d IV, with or without flucytosine, 100 mg/kg/d orally in 4 divided doses for 2 weeks, followed by:	Fever, anemia, hypokalemia, azotemia.
	Fluconazole, 400 mg orally daily for 6 weeks, then 200 mg orally daily.	Hepatitis.
Cytomegalovirus infection	Valganciclovir, 900 mg orally twice a day for 21 days with food (induction), followed by 900 mg daily with food (maintenance).	Neutropenia, anemia, thrombocytopenia.
	Ganciclovir, 10 mg/kg/d IV in 2 divided doses for 10 days, followed by 6 mg/kg 5 days a week indefinitely. (Decrease dose for renal impairment.) May use ganciclovir as maintenance therapy (1 g orally with fatty foods 3 times a day).	Neutropenia (especially when used concurrently with zidovudine), anemia, thrombocytopenia.
	Foscarnet, 60 mg/kg IV every 8 hours for 10–14 days (induction), followed by 90 mg/kg once daily. (Adjust for changes in renal function.)	Nausea, hypokalemia, hypocalcemia, hyperphosphatemia, azotemia.
Esophageal candidiasis or recurrent vaginal candidiasis	Fluconazole, 100–200 mg daily for 10–14 days.	Hepatitis, development of imidazole resistance.
	Ketoconazole, 200 mg orally twice daily for 10–14 days.	Hepatitis, adrenal insufficiency.
Herpes simplex infection	Acyclovir, 200 mg 5 times daily for 7–10 days; or acyclovir, 5 mg/kg IV every 8 hours for severe cases.	Resistant herpes simplex with chronic therapy.
	Famciclovir, 500 mg orally twice daily for 7 days.	Nausea.
	Valacyclovir, 500 mg orally twice daily for 7 days	Nausea.
	Foscarnet, 40 mg/kg IV every 8 hours, for acyclovir-resistant cases. (Adjust for changes in renal function.)	See above.

(continued)

Table 119. Treatment of AIDS-related opportunistic infections and malignancies.[1] (continued)

Infection or Malignancy	Treatment	Complications
Herpes zoster	Acyclovir, 800 mg orally 4 or 5 times daily for 7 days. Intravenous therapy at 10 mg/kg every 8 hours for ocular involvement, disseminated disease.	See above.
	Famciclovir, 500 mg orally 3 times daily for 7 days.	Nausea.
	Valacyclovir, 500 mg orally 3 times daily for 7 days.	Nausea.
	Foscarnet, 40 mg/kg IV every 8 hours for acyclovir-resistant cases. (Adjust for changes in renal function.)	See above.
Kaposi's sarcoma Limited cutaneous disease	Observation, intralesional vinblastine.	Inflammation, pain at site of injection.
Extensive or aggressive cutaneous disease	Systemic chemotherapy (eg, liposomal doxorubicin). Alpha interferon (for patients with CD4 > 200 cells/μL and no constitutional symptoms). Radiation (amelioration of edema).	Bone marrow suppression, peripheral neuritis, flu-like syndrome.
Visceral disease (eg, pulmonary)	Combination chemotherapy (eg, daunorubicin, bleomycin, vinblastine).	Bone marrow suppression, cardiac toxicity, fever.

[1]For treatment of *Mycobacterium tuberculosis* infection, see Tables 23 and 24.

[2]For moderate to severe *P jiroveci* infection (oxygen saturation < 90%), corticosteroids should be given with specific treatment. The dose of prednisone is 40 mg twice daily for 5 days, then 40 mg daily for 5 days, and then 20 mg daily until therapy is complete.

[3]When considering use of dapsone, check G6PD level in African-American patients and those of Mediterranean origin.

[4]CHOP = cyclophosphamide, doxorubicin (hydroxydaunomycin), vincristine (Oncovin), and prednisone. Modified M-BACOD = methotrexate, bleomycin, doxorubicin (Adriamycin), cyclophosphamide, vincristine (Oncovin), and dexamethasone.

[5]G-CSF = granulocyte colony-stimulating factor (filgrastim); GM-CSF = granulocyte-macrophage colony-stimulating factor (sargramostim).

Table 120. Antiretroviral therapy.

Drug	Dose	Common Side Effects	Monitoring	Cost[1]	Cost/Month
Nucleoside analogs					
Zidovudine (AZT) (Retrovir)	500–600 mg orally daily in two divided doses	Anemia, neutropenia, nausea, malaise, headache, insomnia, myopathy	Complete blood count and differential (every 3 months once stable)	$5.90/300 mg	$354.50
Didanosine (ddl) (Videx)	400 mg orally daily or 200 mg orally twice daily (for pill formulation) for persons ≥60 kg	Peripheral neuropathy, pancreatitis, dry mouth, hepatitis	CBC and differential, aminotransferases, K+, amylase, triglycerides, bimonthly neurologic questionnaire for neuropathy	$4.43/200 mg chew tab $10.06/400 mg capsules	$266.26 $301.79
Zalcitabine (ddC) (Hivid)	0.375–0.75 mg orally 3 times daily	Peripheral neuropathy, aphthous ulcers, hepatitis	Monthly neurologic questionnaire for neuropathy, aminotransferases	$2.73/0.75 mg	$245.70
Stavudine (d4T) (Zerit)	40 mg orally twice daily for persons ≥60 kg	Peripheral neuropathy, hepatitis, pancreatitis	Monthly neurologic questionnaire for neuropathy, aminotransferases, amylase	$5.58/40 mg	$334.89
Lamivudine (3TC) (Epivir)	150 mg orally twice daily	Rash, peripheral neuropathy	No additional monitoring	$5.06/150 mg	$303.40
Abacavir (Ziagen)	300 mg orally twice daily	Rash, fever—if occur, rechallenge may be fatal	No special monitoring	$6.80/300 mg	$407.70
Nucleotide analog					
Tenofovir (Viread)	300 mg orally once daily	Gastrointestinal distress	Renal function	$13.60/300 mg	$408.00
Protease inhibitors					
Saquinavir soft gel (Fortovase)	1200 mg three times daily	Gastrointestinal distress, headache	Bimonthly aminotransferases, cholesterol, triglycerides	$1.34/200 mg	$720.96
Ritonavir (Norvir)	600 mg orally twice daily or 100–400 mg orally twice daily in combination with other protease inhibitors	Gastrointestinal distress, peripheral paresthesias	Bimonthly aminotransferases, CK, uric acid, triglycerides	$2.14/100 mg	$771.54
Indinavir (Crixivan)	800 mg orally three times daily	Kidney stones	Bimonthly aminotransferases, bilirubin level, cholesterol, triglycerides	$3.04/400 mg	$546.38
Nelfinavir (Viracept)	750 mg orally three times daily	Diarrhea	Cholesterol, triglycerides	$2.52/250 mg	$680.99

(continued)

Table 120. Antiretroviral therapy. (continued)

Drug	Dose	Common Side Effects	Monitoring	Cost[1]	Cost/Month
Protease inhibitors (cont.)					
Amprenavir (Agenerase)	1200 mg orally twice daily	Gastrointestinal, rash	Cholesterol, triglycerides	$1.47/150 mg	$706.12
Lopinavir/ritonavir (Kaletra)	400 mg/100 mg orally twice daily	Diarrhea	Cholesterol, triglycerides, every other month aminotransferases	$3.91/133 mg (lopinavir)	$703.50
Nonnucleoside reverse transcriptase inhibitors (NNRTIs)					
Nevirapine (Viramune)	200 mg orally daily for 2 weeks, then 200 mg orally twice daily	Rash	No additional monitoring	$6.12/200 mg	$366.94
Delavirdine (Rescriptor)	400 mg orally three times daily	Rash	No additional monitoring	$1.76/200 mg	$316.35
Efavirenz (Sustiva)	600 mg orally daily	Neurologic disturbances	No additional monitoring	$14.39/600 mg	$431.65

[1]Average wholesale price (AWP, for AB-rated generic when available) for quantity listed. Source: *Drug Topics Red Book,* May 2003; Vol. 22, No. 5. AWP may not accurately represent the actual pharmacy cost because wide contractual variations exist among institutions.

Table 121. *Pneumocystis jiroveci* prophylaxis.

Drug	Dose	Side Effects	Limitations
Trimethoprim-sulfamethoxazole	One double-strength tablet 3 times a week to one tablet daily	Rash, neutropenia, hepatitis, Stevens-Johnson syndrome	Hypersensitivity reaction is common but, if mild, it may be possible to treat through.
Dapsone	50–100 mg daily or 100 mg 2 or 3 times per week	Anemia, nausea, methemoglobinemia, hemolytic anemia	Less effective than above. G6PD level should be checked prior to therapy. Check methemoglobin level at 1 month.
Atovaquone	1500 mg daily with a meal	Rash, diarrhea, nausea	Less effective than suspension trimethoprim-sulfamethoxazole; equal efficacy to dapsone, but more expensive.
Aerosolized pentamidine	300 mg monthly	Bronchospasm (pretreat with bronchodilators); rare reports of pancreatitis	Apical *P jiroveci* pneumonia, extrapulmonary *P jiroveci* infections, pneumothorax.

Table 122. Drugs of choice for suspected or proved microbial pathogens.[1]

Suspected or Proved Etiologic Agent	Drug(s) of First Choice	Alternative Drug(s)
Gram-negative cocci		
Moraxella catarrhalis	TMP-SMZ,[2] a fluoroquinolone[3]	Cefuroxime, cefotaxime, ceftizoxime, ceftriaxone, cefepime, cefuroxime axetil, an erythromycin,[4] a tetracycline,[5] azithromycin, amoxicillin-clavulanic acid, clarithromycin
Neisseria gonorrhoeae (gonococcus)	Ciprofloxacin or ofloxacin	Ceftriaxone, spectinomycin, cefpodoxime proxetil
Neisseria meningitidis (meningococcus)	Penicillin[6]	Cefotaxime, ceftizoxime, ceftriaxone, ampicillin, chloramphenicol
Gram-positive cocci		
Streptococcus pneumoniae[8] (pneumococcus)	Penicillin[6]	An erythromycin,[4] a cephalosporin,[7] vancomycin, TMP-SMZ,[2] chloramphenicol, clindamycin, azithromycin, clarithromycin, a tetracycline,[5] imipenem, meropenem, quinupristin-dalfopristin, certain fluoroquinolones,[3] linezolid
Streptococcus, hemolytic, groups A, B, C, G	Penicillin[6]	An erythromycin,[4] a cephalosporin,[7] vancomycin, clindamycin, azithromycin, clarithromycin
Viridans streptococci	Penicillin[6] ± gentamicin	Cephalosporin,[7] vancomycin
Staphylococcus, methicillin-resistant	Vancomycin ± gentamicin ± rifampin	TMP-SMZ,[2] minocycline, a fluoroquinolone[3] linezolid, quinupristin-dalfopristin
Staphylococcus, non-penicillinase-producing	Penicillin[6]	A cephalosporin,[8] vancomycin, imipenem, meropenem, a fluoroquinolone,[3] clindamycin
Staphylococcus, penicillinase-producing	Penicillinase-resistant penicillin[9]	Vancomycin, a cephalosporin,[7] clindamycin, amoxicillin-clavulanic acid, ticarcillin-clavulanic acid, ampicillin-sulbactam, piperacillin-tazobactam, imipenem, meropenem, a fluoroquinolone,[3] TMP-SMZ[2]
Enterococcus faecalis	Ampicillin + gentamicin[10]	Vancomycin + gentamicin
Enterococcus faecium	Vancomycin + gentamicin[10]	Quinupristin-dalfopristin, linezolid
Gram-negative rods		
Acinetobacter	Imipenem or meropenem	Minocycline, TMP-SMZ,[2] doxycycline, aminoglycosides,[11] piperacillin, ceftazidime, a fluoroquinolone[3]
Prevotella, oropharyngeal strains	Clindamycin	Penicillin,[6] metronidazole, cefoxitin, cefotetan
Bacteroides, gastrointestinal strains	Metronidazole	Cefoxitin, chloramphenicol, clindamycin, cefotetan, cefmetazole, imipenem, meropenem, ticarcillin-clavulanic acid, ampicillin-sulbactam, piperacillin-tazobactam
Brucella	Tetracycline + rifampin[5]	TMP-SMZ[2] ± gentamicin; chloramphenicol ± gentamicin; doxycycline + gentamicin
Campylobacter jejuni	Erythromycin[4] or azithromycin	Tetracycline,[5] a fluoroquinolone,[3] gentamicin
Enterobacter	TMP-SMZ,[2] imipenem, meropenem	Aminoglycoside, a fluoroquinolone,[3] cefepime
Escherichia coli (sepsis)	Cefotaxime, ceftizoxime, ceftriaxone, ceftazidime, cefepime	Imipenem or meropenem, aminoglycosides,[11] a fluoroquinolone[3]
Escherichia coli (uncomplicated urinary infection)	Fluoroquinolones,[3] nitrofurantoin	TMP-SMZ,[2] oral cephalosporin, fosfomycin
Haemophilus (meningitis and other serious infections)	Cefotaxime, ceftizoxime, ceftriaxone, ceftazidime	Chloramphenicol, meropenem
Haemophilus (respiratory infections, otitis)	TMP-SMZ[2]	Ampicillin, amoxicillin, doxycycline, azithromycin, clarithromycin, cefotaxime, ceftizoxime, ceftriaxone, cefepime, cefuroxime, cefuroxime axetil, ampicillin-clavulanate

(continued)

Table 122. Drugs of choice for suspected or proved microbial pathogens, 2001.[1] (continued)

Suspected or Proved Etiologic Agent	Drug(s) of First Choice	Alternative Drug(s)
Gram-negative rods (continued)		
Helicobacter pylori proton pump inhibitor (PPI)	Amoxicillin + clarithromycin + or tetracycline[5] + metronidazole + bismuth subsalicylate + PPI	Clarithromycin + bismuth subsalicylate (Pepto-Bismol) + tetracycline; amoxicillin + metronidazole + bismuth subsalicylate; amoxicillin + clarithromycin + ranitidine bismuth subcitrate
Klebsiella	A cephalosporin	TMP-SMZ,[2] aminoglycoside,[11] imipenem or meropenem, a fluoroquinolone,[3] piperacillin, mezlocillin, aztreonam
Legionella species (pneumonia)	Erythromycin[4] or clarithromycin or azithromycin, or fluoroquinolones[3] ± rifampin	TMP-SMZ,[2] doxycycline ± rifampin
Proteus mirabilis	Ampicillin	An aminoglycoside,[11] TMP-SMZ,[2] a fluoroquinolone,[3] a cephalosporin[7]
Proteus vulgaris and other species (*morganella, providencia*)	Cefotaxime, ceftizoxime, ceftriaxone, ceftazidime, cefepime	Aminoglycoside,[11] imipenem, TMP-SMZ,[2] a fluoroquinolone[3]
Pseudomonas aeruginosa	Aminoglycoside[11] + antipseudomonal penicillin[12]	Ceftazidime ± aminoglycoside; imipenem or meropenem ± aminoglycoside; aztreonam ± aminoglycoside; ciprofloxacin ± piperacillin; ciprofloxacin ± ceftazidime; ciprofloxacin ± cefepime
Burkholderia pseudomallei (melioidosis)	Ceftazidime	Chloramphenicol, tetracycline,[5] TMP-SMZ,[2] amoxicillin-clavulanic acid, imipenem or meropenem
Burkholderia mallei (glanders)	Streptomycin + tetracycline[5]	Chloramphenicol + streptomycin
Salmonella (bacteremia)	Ceftriaxone, a fluoroquinolone[3]	TMP-SMZ,[2] ampicillin, chloramphenicol
Serratia	Cefotaxime, ceftizoxime, ceftriaxone, ceftazidime, cefepime	TMP-SMZ,[2] aminoglycosides,[11] imipenem or meropenem, a fluoroquinolone[3]
Shigella	A fluoroquinolone[3]	Ampicillin, TMP-SMZ,[2] ceftriaxone
Vibrio (cholera, sepsis)	Tetracycline[5]	TMP-SMZ,[2] a fluoroquinolone[3]
Yersinia pestis (plague, tularemia)	Streptomycin ± a tetracycline[5]	Chloramphenicol, TMP-SMZ[2]
Gram-positive rods		
Actinomyces	Penicillin[6]	Tetracycline,[5] clindamycin
Bacillus (including anthrax)	Penicillin[6] (ciprofloxacin or doxycycline for anthrax	Erythromycin,[4] tetracycline,[5] a fluoroquinolone[3]
Clostridium (eg, gas gangrene, tetanus)	Penicillin[6]	Metronidazole, chloramphenicol, clindamycin, imipenem or meropenem
Corynebacterium diphtheriae	Erythromycin[4]	Penicillin[6]
Corynebacterium jeikeium	Vancomycin	Ciprofloxacin, penicillin + gentamicin
Listeria	Ampicillin ± aminoglycoside[11]	TMP-SMZ[2]
Acid-fast rods		
Mycobacterium tuberculosis[13]	INH + rifampin + pyrazinamide ± ethambutol or streptomycin	Other antituberculous drugs (see Tables 23 and 24)
Mycobacterium leprae	Dapsone + rifampin ± clofazimine	Minocycline, ofloxacin, clarithromycin
Mycobacterium kansasii	INH + rifampin ± ethambutol	Ethionamide, cycloserine
Mycobacterium-avium complex	Clarithromycin or azithromycin + one or more of the following: ethambutol, rifampin or rifabutin, ciprofloxacin	Amikacin
Mycobacterium fortuitum-cheilonei	Amikacin + clarithromycin	Cefoxitin, sulfonamide, doxycycline, linezolid
Nocardia	TMP-SMZ[2]	Minocycline, imipenem or meropenem, sulfisoxazole, linezolid

(continued)

Table 122. Drugs of choice for suspected or proved microbial pathogen.[1] (continued)

Suspected or Proved Etiologic Agent	Drug(s) of First Choice	Alternative Drug(s)
Spirochetes		
Borrelia burgdorferi (Lyme disease)	Doxycycline, amoxicillin, cefuroxime axetil	Ceftriaxone, cefotaxime, penicillin, azithromycin, clarithromycin
Borrelia recurrentis (relapsing fever)	Doxycycline[5]	Penicillin[6]
Leptospira	Penicillin[6]	Doxycycline[5]
Treponema pallidum (syphilis)	Penicillin[6]	Doxycycline, ceftriaxone
Treponema pertenue (yaws)	Penicillin[6]	Doxycycline
Mycoplasmas	Erythromycin[4] or doxycycline	Clarithromycin, azithromycin, a fluoroquinolone[3]
Chlamydiae		
C psittaci	Doxycycline	Chloramphenicol
C trachomatis (urethritis or pelvic inflammatory disease)	Doxycycline or azithromycin	Ofloxacin
C pneumoniae	Doxycycline[5]	Erythromycin,[4] clarithromycin, azithromycin, a fluoroquinolone[3,14]
Rickettsiae	Doxycycline[5]	Chloramphenicol, a fluoroquinolone[3]

[1] Adapted from Med Lett Drugs Ther 2001;43:69.
[2] TMP-SMZ is a mixture of 1 part trimethoprim and 5 parts sulfamethoxazole.
[3] Fluoroquinolones include ciprofloxacin, ofloxacin, levofloxacin, moxifloxacin, gatifloxacin, and others. Gatifloxacin, levofloxacin, and moxifloxacin have the best activity against gram-positive organisms, including penicillin-resistant *S pneumoniae* and methicillin-sensitive *S aureus*. Activity against enterococci and *S epidermidis* is variable. Ciprofloxacin has the best activity against *P aeruginosa*.
[4] Erythromycin estolate is best absorbed orally but carries the highest risk of hepatitis; erythromycin stearate and erythromycin ethylsuccinate are also available.
[5] All tetracyclines have similar activity against most microorganisms. Minocycline and doxycycline have increased activity against *S aureus*. Dosage is determined by rates of absorption and excretion of various preparations.
[6] Penicillin G is preferred for parenteral injection; penicillin V for oral administration—to be used only in treating infections due to highly sensitive organisms.
[7] Most intravenous cephalosporins (with the exception of ceftazidime) have good activity against gram-positive cocci.
[8] Intermediate and high-level resistance to penicillin has been described. Infections caused by strains with intermediate resistance may respond to high doses of penicillin, cefotaxime, or ceftriaxone. Infections caused by highly resistant strains should be treated with vancomycin ± rifampin. Many strains of penicillin-resistant pneumococci are resistant to erythromycin, macrolides, TMP-SMZ, and chloramphenicol.
[9] Parenteral nafcillin or oxacillin; oral dicloxacillin, cloxacillin, or oxacillin.
[10] Addition of gentamicin indicated only for severe enterococcal infections (eg, endocarditis, meningitis).
[11] Aminoglycosides—gentamicin, tobramycin, amikacin, netilmicin—should be chosen on the basis of local patterns of susceptibility.
[12] Antipseudomonal penicillins: ticarcillin, piperacillin.
[13] Resistance may be a problem, and susceptibility testing should be done.
[14] Ciprofloxacin has inferior antichlamydial activity compared with newer fluoroquinolones.

Table 123. Examples of initial antimicrobial therapy for acutely ill adults pending identification of causative organism.

	Suspected Clinical Diagnosis	Likely Etiologic Diagnosis	Drugs of Choice
(A)	Meningitis, bacterial	Pneumococcus,[1] meningococcus	Cefotaxime,[2] 2–3 g IV every 6 hours, or ceftriaxone, 2 g IV every 12 hours plus vancomycin,10 mg/kg every 8 hours ± rifampin
(B)	Meningitis, bacterial, age > 50	Pneumococcus, meningococcus, *Listeria monocytogenes*,[3] gram-negative bacilli	Ampicillin, 2 g IV every 4 hours, plus cefotaxime or ceftriaxone and vancomycin as in (A)
(C)	Meningitis, postoperative (or posttraumatic)	*S aureus*, gram-negative bacilli (pneumococcus, in posttraumatic)	Vancomycin, 10 mg/kg every 8 hours, plus ceftazidime, 3 g IV every 8 hours
(D)	Brain abscess	Mixed anaerobes, pneumococci, streptococci	Penicillin G, 4 million units IV every 4 hours, + metronidazole, 500 mg PO every 8 hours, or cefotaxime or ceftriaxone as in (A) +metronidazole 500 mg PO every 8 hours
(E)	Pneumonia, acute, community-acquired, severe	Pneumococci, *M pneumoniae*, legionella, *C pneumoniae*	Erythromycin,[4] 0.5 g orally or IV four times daily, or doxycycline, 100 mg IV or orally every 12 hours, plus cefotaxime, 2 g IV every 8 hours (or ceftriaxone, 1 g IV every 24 hours); or a fluoroquinolone[6] alone
(F)	Pneumonia, postoperative or nosocomial	*S aureus*, mixed anaerobes, gram-negative bacilli	Cefotaxime or ceftriaxone or cefipime, 2 g IV every 8 hours, or piperacillin-tazobactam, 4–5 g IV every 6 hours, with or without tobramycin or ciprofloxacin
(G)	Endocarditis, acute (including IV drug user)	*S aureus*, *E faecalis*, gram-negative aerobic bacteria, viridans streptococci	Vancomycin, 15 mg/kg every 12 hours, plus gentamicin, 2 mg/kg every 8 hours
(H)	Septic thrombophlebitis (eg, IV tubing, IV shunts)	*S aureus*, gram-negative aerobic bacteria	Vancomycin, 15 mg/kg every 12 hours plus gentamicin,[5] 2 mg/kg every 8 hours
(I)	Osteomyelitis	*S aureus*	Nafcillin, 2 g IV every 4 hours, or cefazolin, 2 g IV every 8 hours
(J)	Septic arthritis	*S aureus*, *N gonorrhoeae*	Ceftriaxone, 1–2 g IV every 24 hours
(K)	Pyelonephritis with flank pain and fever (recurrent UTI)	*E coli*, klebsiella, enterobacter, pseudomonas	Ciprofloxacin, 400 mg IV every 12 hours, or levofloxacin, 500 mg IV once daily
(L)	Suspected sepsis in neutropenic patient receiving cancer chemotherapy	*S aureus*, pseudomonas, klebsiella, *E coli*	Ceftazidime, 2 g IV every 8 hours, or cefepime, 2 g IV every 8 hours
(M)	Intra-abdominal sepsis (eg, postoperative, peritonitis, cholecystitis)	Gram-negative bacteria, bacteroides, anaerobic bacteria, streptococci, clostridia	Ampicillin, 1–2 g every 6 hours, plus gentamicin, 2 mg/kg every 8 hours, plus metronidazole, 500 mg IV every 8 hours, or piperacillin-tazobactam as in (F) or ticarcillin-clavulanate, 3.1 g IV every 6 hours

[1]Some strains may be resistant to penicillin. Vancomycin should be used with or without rifampin.
[2]Cefotaxime, ceftriaxone, ceftazidime, or ceftizoxime can be used. Most studies on meningitis have been done with cefotaxime or ceftriaxone.
[3]TMP-SMZ can be used to treat *Listeria monocytogenes* in patients allergic to penicillin in a dosage of 15–20 mg/kg of TMP in three or four divided doses.
[4]Other macrolides such as azithromycin or clarithromycin can be used.
[5]Depending on local drug susceptibility pattern, use tobramycin, 5 mg/kg/d, or amikacin, 15 mg/kg/d, in place of gentamicin.
[6]Gatifloxacin, levofloxacin, moxifloxacin.

Table 124. Initial antimicrobial therapy for purulent meningitis of unknown cause.

Age Group	Common Microorganisms	Standard Therapy
18–50 years	*S pneumoniae*,[1] *N meningitidis*	Cefotaxime or ceftriaxone[2]
Over 50 years	*S pneumoniae*,[1] *N meningitidis*, *L monocytogenes*, gram-negative bacilli	Ampicillin,[3] cefotaxime, or ceftriaxone[2]
Impaired cellular immunity	*L monocytogenes*, gram-negative bacilli, *S pneumoniae*	Ampicillin[3] plus ceftazidime[4]
Postsurgical or posttraumatic	*S aureus*, *S pneumoniae*,[1] gram-negative bacilli	Vancomycin[5] plus ceftazidime[4]

[1]In areas where penicillin-resistant pneumococcus is prevalent, vancomycin, 10–15 mg/kg every 6 hours, should be included in the regimen.
[2]The usual dose of cefotaxime is 2 g every 6 hours and that of ceftriaxone is 2 g every 12 hours. If the organism is sensitive to penicillin, 3–4 million units IV every 4 hours is given.
[3]The dose of ampicillin is usually 2 g IV every 4 hours.
[4]Ceftazidime is given in a dose of 50–100 mg/kg every 8 hours up to 2 g every 8 hours.
[5]The dose of vancomycin is 10–15 mg/kg every 6 hours.

Table 125. Typical cerebrospinal fluid findings in various central nervous system diseases.

Diagnosis	Cells/μL	Glucose (mg/dL)	Protein (mg/dL)	OpeningPressure
Normal	0–5 lymphocytes	45–85[1]	15–45	70–180 mm H$_2$O
Purulent meningitis (bacterial)[2] community-acquired	200–20,000 polymorphonuclear neutrophils	Low (< 45)	High (> 50)	Markedly elevated
Granulomatous meningitis (mycobacterial, fungal)[3]	100–1000, mostly lymphocytes[3]	Low (< 45)	High (> 50)	Moderately elevated
Spirochetal meningitis	100–1000, mostly lymphocytes[3]	Normal	Moderately high (> 50)	Normal to slightly elevated
Aseptic meningitis, viral or meningoencephalitis[4]	25–2000, mostly lymphocytes[3]	Normal or low	High (> 50)	Slightly elevated
"Neighborhood reaction"[5]	Variably increased	Normal	Normal or high	Variable

[1]Cerebrospinal fluid glucose must be considered in relation to blood glucose level. Normally, cerebrospinal fluid glucose is 20–30 mg/dL lower than blood glucose, or 50–70% of the normal value of blood glucose.
[2]Organisms in smear or culture of cerebrospinal fluid; counterimmunoelectrophoresis or latex agglutination may be diagnostic.
[3]Polymorphonuclear neutrophils may predominate early.
[4]Viral isolation from cerebrospinal fluid early; antibody titer rise in paired specimens of serum; PCR for herpesvirus.
[5]May occur in mastoiditis, brain abscess, epidural abscess, sinusitis, septic thrombus, brain tumor. Cerebrospinal fluid culture results usually negative.

Table 126. Acute bacterial diarrheas and "food poisoning."

Organism	Incubation Period (hours)	Vomiting	Diarrhea	Fever	Microbiology	Pathogenesis	Clinical Features and Treatment
Staphylococcus	1–8, rarely up to 18	+++	+	–	Staphylococci grow in meats and in dairy and bakery products and produce enterotoxin.	Enterotoxin acts on receptors in gut that transmit impulses to medullary centers.	Abrupt onset, intense vomiting for up to 24 hours, regular recovery in 24–48 hours. Occurs in persons eating the same food. No treatment usually necessary except to restore fluids and electrolytes.
Bacillus cereus	1–8, rarely up to 18	+++	+	–	Reheated fried rice causes vomiting or diarrhea.	Enterotoxins formed in food or in gut from growth of *B cereus*.	After 1–6 hours, mainly vomiting. After 8–16 hours, mainly diarrhea. Both self-limited to less than 1 day.
Clostridium perfringens	8–16	±	+++	–	Clostridia grow in rewarmed meat dishes and produce an enterotoxin.	Enterotoxin produced in food and in gut causes hypersecretion in small intestine.	Abrupt onset of profuse diarrhea; vomiting occasionally. Recovery usual without treatment in 1–4 days. Many clostridia in cultures of food and feces of patients.
Clostridium botulinum	24–96	±	Rare	–	Clostridia grow in anaerobic foods and produce toxin.	Toxin absorbed from gut blocks acetylcholine at neuromuscular junction.	Diplopia, dysphagia, dysphonia, respiratory embarrassment. Treatment requires clear airway, ventilation, and intravenous polyvalent antitoxin. Toxin present in food and serum. Mortality rate high.
Clostridium difficile	?	–	+++	+	Associated with antimicrobial drugs, eg, clindamycin.	Enterotoxin causes epithelial necrosis in colon; pseudomembranous colitis.	Especially after abdominal surgery, abrupt bloody diarrhea and fever. Toxin in stool. Oral vancomycin or metronidazole useful in therapy.
Escherichia coli (some strains)	24–72	±	+	–	Organisms grow in gut and produce toxin. May also invade superficial epithelium.	Enterotoxin causes hypersecretion in small intestine.	Usually abrupt onset of diarrhea; vomiting rare. A serious infection in neonates. In adults, "traveler's diarrhea" is usually self-limited to 1–3 days and does respond to a fluoroquinolone.
Vibrio parahaemolyticus	6–96	+	+	±	Organisms grow in gut and produce toxin or invade.	Hypersecretion in small intestine; stools may be bloody.	Abrupt onset of diarrhea in groups consuming the same food, especially crabs and other seafood. Recovery is usually complete in 1–3 days. Food and stool cultures are positive.
Vibrio cholerae (mild cases)	24–72	+	+++	–	Organisms grow in gut and produce toxin.	Enterotoxin causes hypersecretion in small intestine. Infective dose: 10^7–10^9 organisms.	Abrupt onset of liquid diarrhea in endemic area. Needs prompt replacement of fluids and electrolytes intravenously or orally. Tetracyclines shorten excretion of vibrios. Stool cultures positive.

(continued)

Table 126. Acute bacterial diarrheas and "food poisoning." (continued)

Organism	Incubation Period (hours)	Vomiting	Diarrhea	Fever	Microbiology	Pathogenesis	Clinical Features and Treatment
Campylobacter jejuni	2–10 days	−	+++	+	Organisms grow in jejunum and ileum.	Invasion and enterotoxin production uncertain.	Fever, diarrhea; PMNs and fresh blood in stool, especially in children. Usually self-limited. Special media needed for culture at 43°C. Give a fluoroquinolone in severe cases with invasion. Recovery in 5–8 days is usual.
Shigella species (mild cases)	24–72	±	+	+	Organisms grow in superficial gut epithelium and gut lumen and produce toxin.	Organisms invade epithelial cells; blood, mucus, and PMNs in stools. Infective dose: 10^2–10^3 organisms.	Abrupt onset of diarrhea, often with blood and pus in stools, cramps, tenesmus, and lethargy. Stool cultures are positive. Therapy depends on sensitivity testing, but the fluoroquinolones are most effective. Do not give opioids. Often mild and self-limited.
Salmonella species	8–48	±	+	+	Organisms grow in gut. Do not produce toxin.	Superficial infection of gut, little invasion. Infective dose: 10^5 organisms.	Gradual or abrupt onset of diarrhea and low-grade fever. No antimicrobials unless systemic dissemination is suspected, in which case give a fluoroquinolone. Stool cultures are positive. Prolonged carriage is common.
Yersinia enterocolitica	?	±	+	+	Fecal-oral transmission (occasionally). Food-borne. In pets.	Gastroenteritis or mesenteric adenitis. Occasional bacteremia. Enterotoxin produced.	Severe abdominal pain, diarrhea, fever. PMNs and blood in stool; polyarthritis, erythema nodosum in children. If severe, give tetracycline or gentamicin. Keep stool at 4°C before culture.

Table 127. Recommended childhood immunization schedule[1]—United States, 2003.[1]

Vaccine	Range of recommended ages				Catch-up vaccination				Preadolescent assessment			
	Birth	1 mo	2 mos	4 mos	6 mos	12 mos	15 mos	18 mos	24 mos	4–6 yrs	11–12 yrs	13–18 yrs
Hepatitis B[2]	Hep B #1 only if mother HBsAg (*)										Hep B series	
		Hep B #2				Hep B #3						
Diphtheria,[3] Tetanus, Pertussis			DTaP	DTaP	DTaP		DTaP			DTaP	Td	
Haemophilus influenzae Type b[4]			Hib	Hib	Hib	Hib						
Inactivated Polio			IPV	IPV		IPV				IPV		
Measles, Mumps, Rubella[5]						MMR #1				MMR #2	MMR #2	
Varicella[6]						Varicella					Varicella	
Pneumococcal[7]			PCV	PCV	PCV	PCV				PCV	PPV	

Vaccines below this line are for selected populations

Hepatitis A[8]										Hepatitis A series		
Influenza[9]										Influenza (yearly)		

1. Indicates the recommended ages for routine administration of currently licensed childhood vaccines, as of December 1, 2002, for children through age 18 years. Any dose not given at the recommended age should be given at any subsequent visit when indicated and feasible. Indicates age groups that warrant special effort to administer those vaccines not given previously. Licensed combination vaccines may be used whenever any components of the combination are indicated and the vaccine's other components are not contraindicated. Providers should consult the manufacturers' package inserts for detailed recommendations.

2. **Hepatitis B vaccine (Hep B).** All infants should receive the first dose of HepB vaccine soon after birth and before hospital discharge; the first dose also may be given by age 2 months if the infant's mother is HBsAg-negative. Only monovalent HepB vaccine can be used for the birth dose. Monovalent or combination vaccine containing HepB may be used to complete the series; 4 doses of vaccine may be administered when a birth dose is given. The second dose should be given at least 4 weeks after the first dose except for combination vaccines, which cannot be administered before age 6 weeks. The third dose should be given at least 16 weeks after the first dose and at least 8 weeks after the second dose. The last dose in the vaccination series (third or fourth dose) should not be administered before age 6 months. *Infants born to HBsAg-positive mothers* should receive HepB vaccine and 0.5 mL hepatitis B immune globulin (HBIG) within 12 hours of birth at separate sites. The second dose is recommended at age 1–2 months. The last dose in the vaccination series should note be administered before age 6 months. These infants should be tested for HBsAg and anti-HBs at 9–15 months of age. *Infants born to mothers whose HBsAg status is unknown* should receive the first dose of the HepB vaccine series within 12 hours of birth. Maternal blood should be drawn as soon as possible to determine the mother's HBsAg status; if the HBsAg test is positive, the infant should receive HBIG as soon as possible (no later than age 1 week). The second dose is recommended at age 1–2 months. The last dose in the vaccination series should not be administered before age 6 months.

3. **Diphtheria and tetanus toxoids and acellular pertussis vaccine (DTaP).** The fourth dose of DTaP may be administered at age 12 months provided that 6 months have elapsed since the third dose and the child is un-likely to return at age 15–18 months. **Tetanus and diphtheria toxoids (Td)** are recommended at age 11–12 years if at least 5 years have elapsed since the last dose of the Td-containing vaccine. Subsequent routine Td boosters are recommended every 10 years.

4. *Haemophilus influenzae* **type b (Hib) conjugate vaccine.** Three Hib conjugate vaccines are licensed for infant use. If PRP-OMP (PedvaxHIB® or ComVax® [Merck]) is administered at age 2 and 4 months, a dose at age 6 months is not required. DTaP/Hib combination products should not be used for primary vaccination in infants at age 2, 4 or 6 months but can be used as boosters following any Hib vaccine.

5. **Measles, mumps, and rubella vaccine (MMR).** The second dose of MMR is recommended routinely at age 4–6 years but may be administered during any visit provided that at least 4 weeks have elapsed since the first dose and that both doses are administered beginning at or after age 12 months. Those who have not received the second dose previously should complete the schedule by the visit at age 11–12 years.

6. **Varicella vaccine.** Varicella vaccine is recommended at any visit at or after age 12 months for susceptible children (i.e., those who lack a reliable history of chickenpox). Susceptible persons aged ≥ 13 years should receive 2 doses given at least 4 weeks apart.

7. **Pneumococcal vaccine.** The heptavalent **pneumococcal conjugate vaccine (PCV)** is recommended for all children aged 2–23 months and for certain children aged 24–59 months. **Pneumococcal polysaccharide vaccine (PPV)** is recommended in addition to PCV for certain high-risk groups. See *MMWR* 2000;49(No. RR-9):1–37.

8. **Hepatitis A vaccine.** Hepatitis A vaccine is recommended for children and adolescents in selected states and regions, and for certain high-risk groups. Consult local public health authority and *MMWR* 1999;48(No. RR-12):1–37. Children and adolescents in these states, regions, and high-risk groups who have not been immunized against hepatitis A can begin the hepatitis A vaccination series during any visit. The two doses in the series should be administered at least 6 months apart.

Table 127. Recommended childhood immunization schedule*—United States, 2003[1]. (continued)

9. **Influenza vaccine**. Influenza vaccine is recommended annually for children aged ≥ 6 months with certain risk factors (including but not limited to asthma, cardiac disease, sickle cell disease, HIV, and diabetes, and household members of persons in groups at high risk (see *MMWR* 2002;51[No. RR-3]:1–31), and can be administered to all others wishing to obtain immunity. In addition, healthy children age 6–23 months are encouraged to receive influenza vaccine if feasible because children in this age group are at substantially increased risk for influenza-related hospitalizations. Children aged ≤ 12 years should receive vaccine in a dosage appropriate for their age (0.25 mL if 6–35 months or 0.5 mL if ≥ 3 years). Children aged ≤ 8 years who are receiving influenza vaccine for the first time should receive 2 doses separated by at least 4 weeks.

Additional information about vaccines, including precautions and contraindications for vaccine and vaccine shortages, is available at http://www.cdc.gov/nip or at the National Immunization hotline, 800-232-2522 (English) or 800-232-0233 (Spanish). Copies of the schedule can be obtained at http://www.cdc.gov/nip/recs/child-schedule.htm. Approved by the **Advisory Committee on Immunization Practices** (http://www. cdc.gov/nip/acip), the **American Academy of Pediatrics** (http://www.aap.org), and the **American Academy of Family Physicians** (http://www.aafp.org).

Table 128. Guide to tetanus prophylaxis in wound management.[1]

History of Absorbed Tetanus Toxoid	Clean, Minor Wounds		All Other Wounds[2]	
	Td[3]	TIG[4]	Td[3]	TIG[4]
Unknown or < 3 doses	Yes	No	Yes	Yes
3 or more doses	No[5]	No	No[6]	No

[1]From the Centers for Disease Control and Prevention. Recommended childhood immunization schedule—United States, 2002. JAMA 2002;287:707.
[2]Such as, but not limited to, wounds contaminated with dirt, feces, soil, saliva, etc; puncture wounds; avulsions; and wounds resulting from missiles, crushing, burns, and frostbite.
[3]Tetanus toxoid and diphtheria toxoid, adult form. Use only this preparation (Td-adult) in children older than 6 years.
[4]Tetanus immune globulin.
[5]Yes if more than 10 years have elapsed since last dose.
[6]Yes if more than 5 years have elapsed since last dose. (More frequent boosters are not needed and can enhance side effects.)

Table 129. Prevention regimens for infection in immunocompromised patients.

Etiology	Microorganism	Therapy	Dose/Duration

Transplant	*Pneumocystis jirovaci*	Trimethoprim-sulfamethoxazole (TMP-SMZ)
		
		In TMP-SMZ allergy
		  Aerosolized pentamidine
		  Dapsone (check glucose-6-phosphate dehydrogenase levels)
			One double-strength tablet three times a week *or* one double-strength tablet twice a day on weekends *or* one single-strength tablet daily for 3–6 months
			300 mg once a month
			50 mg daily or 100 mg three times a week

Solid organ or bone marrow herpes simplex seropositive patients	*Herpes simplex*	Acyclovir or ganciclovir	200 mg orally three times daily for 4 weeks (bone marrow transplants) or for 12 weeks (other solid organ transplants)
Cytomegalovirus (CMV)-seronegative solid organ transplant patients who receive transplants from seropositive donors	CMV	Ganciclovir	2.5–5 mg/kg intravenously twice daily during hospitalization (usually about 10 days) *then* oral ganciclovir, 1 g three times daily, for 3 months
CMV-seropositive solid organ transplant patients	CMV; herpesvirus	Ganciclovir	2.5–5 mg/kg intravenously twice daily during hospitalization (usually about 10 days) *then* oral acyclovir, 800 mg four times a day *or* oral ganciclovir, 1 g three times daily for 3 months
Periods of rejection	CMV	Ganciclovir	2.5–5 mg/kg intravenously twice daily during rejection therapy
Bone marrow transplant[1] Universal prophylaxis for all seropositive patients who receive allogeneic transplants	CMV	Ganciclovir	5 mg/kg intravenously every 12 h for a week *then* oral ganciclovir, 1 g three times daily to Day 100; alternatively, patients can be followed without specific therapy and have blood sampled weekly for the presence of CMV; if CMV is detected by an antigenemia assay, preemptive therapy
Preemptive therapy; less toxic than universal prophylaxis	CMV	Ganciclovir	5 mg/kg intravenously twice daily for 7–14 days *then* oral ganciclovir, 1 g three times daily to Day 100
CMV-seronegative recipients			Use of CMV-negative or leukocyte-depleted blood products
Severe hypogammaglobulinemia following bone marrow transplantation		Intravenous immunoglobulin	
Neutropenia[2–4]	Fungal	Amphotericin B Liposomal preparations of amphotericin B, aerosolized amphotericin B, itraconazole (capsules and solution), voriconazole	Moderate dose (0.5 mg/kg/day) and low dose (0.1–0.25 mg/kg/day)

[1]Whether universal prophylaxis or observation with preemptive therapy is the best approach has not been determined.
[2]Routine decontamination of the gastrointestinal tract to prevent bacteremia in the neutropenic patient is not recommended.
[3]Prophylactic administration of antibiotics in the afebrile, asymptomatic neutropenic patient is controversial, though many centers have adopted this strategy.
[4]Because voriconazole appears to be more effective than amphotericin for documented aspergillus infections, one approach to prophylaxis is to use fluconazole for patients at low risk for developing fungal infections (those who receive autologous bone marrow transplants) and voriconazole for those at high risk (allogeneic transplants).

Table 130. Antimicrobial agents for treatment of or for prophylaxis against anthrax.

First-line agents and recommended doses
    Ciprofloxacin, 500 mg twice daily orally or 400 mg every 12 hours intravenously
    Doxycycline, 100 mg every 12 hours orally or intravenously
Second-line agents and recommended doses
    Amoxicillin, 500 mg three times daily orally
    Penicillin G, 2 mU every 4 hours intravenously
Alternative agents with in vitro activity and suggested doses
    Rifampin, 10 mg/kg/d orally or intravenously
    Clindamycin, 450–600 mg every 8 hours orally or intravenously
    Clarithromycin, 500 mg twice daily
    Erythromycin, 500 mg every 6 hours intravenously
    Vancomycin, 1 g every 12 hours intravenously
    Imipenem, 500 mg every 6 hours intravenously

Table 131. Endocarditis prophylaxis.[1,2]

DENTAL, RESPIRATORY, OR ESOPHAGEAL PROCEDURES		
Oral	Amoxicillin	2 g 1 hour before procedure
Penicillin allergy	Clindamycin	600 mg 1 hour before procedure
	or	
	Cephalexin or cefadroxil[3]	2 g 1 hour before procedure
	or	
	Azithromycin or clarithromycin	500 mg 1 hour before procedure
Parenteral	Ampicillin	2 g IM or IV 30 minutes before procedure
Penicillin allergy	Clindamycin	600 mg IV 1 hour before procedure
	or	
	Cefazolin[3]	1 g IM or IV 30 minutes before procedure
GASTROINTESTINAL (EXCEPT ESOPHAGEAL) OR GENITOURINARY PROCEDURES		
High-risk patient (Table 132)	Ampicillin plus gentamicin	Ampicillin, 2 g IM or IV, plus gentamicin, 1.5 mg/kg (not to exceed 120 mg) 30 minutes before procedure; 6 hours later, ampicillin, 1 g IM or IV, or amoxicillin, 1 g orally
Penicillin allergy	Vancomycin plus gentamicin	Vancomycin, 1 g IV over 1–2 hours, plus gentamicin, 1.5 mg/kg (not to exceed 120 mg) IV or IM; complete infusion or injection 30 minutes before procedure
Moderate-risk patient	Amoxicillin or ampicillin	Amoxicillin, 2 g orally 1 hour before procedure, or ampicillin, 2 g IM or IV 30 minutes before starting procedure
Penicillin allergy	Vancomycin	Vancomycin, 1 g IV over 1–2 hours; complete infusion 30 minutes before procedure

[1]Modified and reproduced, with permission, from Dajani AS et al: Prevention of bacterial endocarditis. Recommendations by the American Heart Association. JAMA 1997;277:1794. Copyright © 1997 by American Medical Association.
[2]Viridans streptococci are the most common cause of endocarditis occurring after dental or upper respiratory procedures; enterococci are the most common cause after gastrointestinal or genitourinary procedures.
[3]Cephalosporins should not be used in individuals with immediate-type hypersensitivity reactions to penicillin.

Table 132. Cardiac lesions for which bacterial endocarditis prophylaxis is or is not recommended.[1,2]

Endocarditis prophylaxis recommended
1. High-risk category
    Prosthetic cardiac valves, including bioprosthetic and homograft valves
    Previous bacterial endocarditis, even in the absence of heart disease
    Complex cyanotic congenital heart disease (eg, single-ventricle states, transposition of the great arteries, tetralogy of Fallot)
    Surgically constructed systemic pulmonary shunts or conduits
2. Moderate-risk category
    Most congenital cardiac malformations (other than those listed above and below)
    Rheumatic and other acquired valvular dysfunction, even after valvular surgery
    Hypertrophic cardiomyopathy
    Mitral valve prolapse with valvular regurgitation[3,4]

Endocarditis prophylaxis not recommended[5]
    Isolated secundum septal defect
    Surgical repair of atrial septal defect, ventricular septal defect, or patent ductus arteriosus (without residua beyond 6 months)
    Previous coronary artery bypass graft surgery
    Mitral valve prolapse without valvular regurgitation[6]
    Physiologic, functional, or innocent heart murmurs
    Previous Kawasaki disease without valvular dysfunction
    Previous rheumatic fever without valvular dysfunction
    Cardiac pacemakers (intravascular and epicardial) and implanted defibrillators

[1]Modified and reproduced, with permission, from Dajani AS et al: Prevention of bacterial endocarditis. Recommendations by the American Heart Association. JAMA 1997;277:1794. Copyright © 1997 by American Medical Association.
[2]This table lists selected conditions and is not meant to be all-inclusive.
[3]Mitral regurgitation determined by the presence of a murmur or by echo-Doppler.
[4]Men older than 45 without a consistent systolic murmur may warrant prophylaxis even in the absence of resting regurgitation.
[5]Negligible risk category—no greater than in the general population.
[6]Individuals who have a mitral valve prolapse associated with thickening or redundancy of the valve leaflets may be at increased risk for bacterial endocarditis.

Table 133. Procedures for which bacterial endocarditis prophylaxis is or is not recommended.[1,2]

Endocarditis prophylaxis recommended[3]	Endocarditis prophylaxis not recommended

1. Dental
    Dental extractions
    Periodontal procedures
    Dental implant placement or reimplantation
    Endodontic (root canal) instrumentation or surgery only beyond the apex
    Subgingival placement of antibiotic fibers or strips
    Initial placement of orthodontic bands but not brackets
    Intraligamentary local anesthetic injections
    Prophylactic cleaning of teeth or implants where bleeding is anticipated
2. Respiratory tract
    Tonsillectomy, adenoidectomy
    Surgical operations that involve intestinal or respiratory mucosa
    Bronchoscopy with a rigid bronchoscope
3. Gastrointestinal tract[4]
    Sclerotherapy for esophageal varices
    Esophageal stricture dilation
    Endoscopic retrograde cholangiography with biliary obstruction
    Biliary tract surgery
    Surgical operations that involve intestinal mucosa
4. Genitourinary tract
    Prostatic surgery
    Cystoscopy
    Urethral dilation
	1. Dental
	    Restorative dentistry (filling cavities, operative and prosthodontic) with or without retraction cord[5]
	    Local anesthetic injections (nonintraligamentary)
	    Intracanal endodontic treatment; post placement and buildup
	    Placement of rubber dams, removable prosthodontic, or orthodontic appliances
	    Postoperative suture removal
	    Taking of oral impression
	    Fluoride treatments
	    Orthodontic appliance adjustment
	2. Respiratory tract
	    Endotracheal intubation
	    Bronchoscopy with a flexible bronchoscope, with or without biopsy[6]
	    Tympanostomy (insertion)
	3. Gastrointestinal tract
	    Transesophageal echocardiography[6]
	    Endoscopy with or without gastrointestinal biopsy[6]
	4. Genitourinary tract
	    Vaginal hysterectomy[6]
	    Vaginal delivery[6]
	    Cesarean section
	    In the absence of infection: urethral catheterization, uterine dilation and curettage, therapeutic abortion, sterilization procedures, insertion or removal of intrauterine devices
	5. Other
	    Cardiac catheterization, including balloon angioplasty; implanting cardiac pacemakers or defibrillators and coronary stents; incision or biopsy of surgically scrubbed skin; circumcision

[1]Reproduced, with permission, from Dajani AS et al: Prevention of bacterial endocarditis. Recommendation by the American Heart Association. JAMA 1997;277:1794. Copyright © 1997 by American Medical Association.

[2]This table lists selected procedures but is not meant to be all-inclusive.

[3]Recommended for individuals with high- and moderate-risk cardiac conditions (Table 132).

[4]Prophylaxis is recommended for high-risk patients, optional for moderate-risk patients.

[5]Clinical judgment may indicate antibiotic use in selected circumstances that may create significant bleeding.

[6]Prophylaxis is optional for high-risk patients.

Table 134. Treatment of infective endocarditis.

Microorganism	Standard Therapy	Remarks
Empirical regimens pending culture results	Nafcillin or oxacillin, 1.5 g intravenously every 4 h, plus penicillin, 2–3 million units every 4 h (or ampicillin, 1.5 g every 4 h), plus gentamicin, 1 mg/kg every 8 h	Should include agents active against staphylococci, streptococci, and enterococci
For penicillin allergy or if infection by methicillin-resistant staphylococci is suspected	Vancomycin, 15 mg/kg intravenously every 12 h	
Viridans streptococci		
Penicillin-susceptible viridans streptococci [ie, minimum inhibitory concentration (MIC) ≤ 0.1 µg/mL]	Penicillin G, 2–3 million units intravenously every 4 h for 4 weeks; the duration of therapy can be shortened to 2 weeks if gentamicin, 1 mg/kg every 8 h, is used with penicillin	
	Ceftriaxone, 2 g once daily intravenously or intramuscularly for 4 weeks	A convenient regimen for home therapy
For the penicillin-allergic patient	Vancomycin, 15 mg/kg intravenously every 12 h for 4 weeks	The 2-week regimen is not recommended for patients with symptoms of more than 3 months duration or patients with complications such as myocardial abscess or extracardiac infection; prosthetic valve endocarditis should be treated with a 6-week course of penicillin with at least 2 weeks of gentamicin
Viridans streptococci relatively resistant to penicillin (ie, MIC > 0.1 µg/mL but ≤ 0.5 µg/mL)	Penicillin G, 3 million units intravenously every 4 h for 4 weeks; combine with gentamicin, 1 mg/kg every 8 h for the first 2 weeks	
For the penicillin-allergic patient	Vancomycin, 15 mg/kg intravenously every 12 h for 4 weeks	
Enterococci	Ampicillin, 2 g intravenously every 4 h, or penicillin G, 3–4 million units every 4 h plus gentamicin, 1 mg/kg every 8 h for 4–6 weeks	The relapse rate is unacceptably high when penicillin is used alone; because aminoglycoside resistance occurs in enterococci, susceptibility should be documented; the longer duration of therapy is recommended for patients with symptoms for more than 3 months, relapse, or prosthetic valve endocarditis, though a recent retrospective study of native valve enterococcal endocarditis suggests that less than 4 weeks of an aminoglycoside may be sufficient
For the penicillin-allergic patient	Vancomycin, 15 mg/kg intravenously every 12 h, plus gentamicin, 1 mg/kg every 8 h, is recommended	
Enterococci that demonstrate high-level resistance to aminoglycosides (ie, not inhibited by 500 µg/mL of gentamicin)	Ampicillin, 2 g intravenously every 4 h, or penicillin G, 3–4 million units every 4 h for 4–6 weeks	The addition of an aminoglycoside will not be beneficial
Staphylococci		
For methicillin-susceptible *Staphylococcus aureus*	Nafcillin or oxacillin, 1.5 g intravenously every 4 h for 4–6 weeks	
For methicillin-resistant strain	Vancomycin, 15 mg/kg intravenously every 12 h for 4 weeks	Aminoglycoside combination regimens may be useful in shortening the duration of bacteremia; their maximum benefit is achieved at low doses (1 mg/kg every 8 h) and in the first 3–5 days of therapy, and they should not be continued beyond the early phase of therapy; for treatment of tricuspid valve endocarditis (with or without pulmonary involvement) in the injection drug user who does not have serious extrapulmonary sites of infection, the total duration of therapy can be shortened from 4 to 2 weeks if an aminoglycoside is added to an antistaphylococcal drug for the entire 2 weeks of therapy

(continued)

Table 134. Treatment of infective endocarditis. (continued)

Microorganism	Standard Therapy	Remarks
Coagulase-negative staphylococci	Vancomycin, 15 mg/kg intravenously for 6 weeks, rifampin, 300 mg orally every 8 h for 6 weeks, and gentamicin, 1 mg/kg intravenously every 8 h for the first 2 weeks	Routinely resistant to methicillin; β-lactam antibiotics should not be used until the isolate is known to be susceptible; if the organism is sensitive to methicillin, either nafcillin or oxacillin or cefazolin can be used in combination with rifampin and gentamicin
Prosthetic valve endocarditis	Combination therapy with nafcillin or oxacillin (vancomycin for methicillin-resistant strains or patients allergic to β-lactams), rifampin, and gentamicin	
HACEK organisms (*Haemophilus aphrophilus*, *Haemophilus parainfluenzae*, *Actinobacillus actinomycetemcomitans*, *Cardiobacterium hominis*, *Eikenella corrodens*, and *Kingella kingae*)	Ceftriaxone (or some other third-generation cephalosporin), 2 g intravenously or intramuscularly once daily for 4 weeks	These organisms can produce β-lactamase; prosthetic valve endocarditis should be treated for 6 weeks
In the penicillin-allergic patient	Trimethoprim-sulfamethoxazole, quinolones, and aztreonam have in vitro activity and should be considered	

Table 135. Treatment of anaerobic intra-abdominal infections.

Oral therapy
  Ciprofloxacin, 750 mg twice daily, plus metronidazole, 500 mg three times daily
Intravenous therapy
  Moderate to moderately severe infections:
    Ticarcillin/clavulanate, 3 g/0.1 g every 6 hours
                          or—
    Cefotetan, 2 g every 12 hours
                          or—
    Clindamycin, 600 mg every 8 hours, or metronidazole, 500 mg every 8 hours, plus gentamicin, 5 mg/kg/d
  Severe infections:
    Imipenem, 0.5 g every 6–8 hours, or ceftriaxone, 1 g every 24 hours, plus either clindamycin, 600 mg every 8 hours, or metronidazole, 500 mg every 8 hours

Table 136. Fecal leukocytes in intestinal disorders.

	Infectious		Noninfectious
Present	**Variable**	**Absent**	**Present**
Shigella	*Salmonella*	Norwalk virus	Ulcerative colitis
Campylobacter	*Yersinia*	Rotavirus	Crohn's disease
Enteroinvasive	*Vibrio parahaemolytica*		Radiation colitis
E coli (EIEC)	*Clostridium difficile*	*Giardia lamblia*	Ischemic colitis
	Aeromonas	*Entamoeba histolytica*	
		Cryptosporidium	
		"Food poisoning"	
		Staphylococcus aureus	
		Bacillus cereus	
		Clostridium perfringens	
		Escherichia coli	
		Enterotoxigenic (ETEC)	
		Enterohemorrhagic (EHEC)	

Table 137. Treatment of Lyme disease.

Manifestation	Drug and Dosage
Tick bite	No treatment in most circumstances; observe
Erythema migrans	Doxycycline, 100 mg twice daily, or amoxicillin, 500 mg three times daily, or cefuroxime axetil, 500 mg twice daily—all for 3–4 weeks
Neurologic disease Bell's palsy	Doxycycline, or amoxicillin as above for 2–3 weeks
Other central nervous system disease	Ceftriaxone, 2 g IV once daily, or penicillin G, 18–24 million units daily IV in 6 divided doses, or cefotaxime, 2 g IV every 8 hours—all for 2–4 weeks
Cardiac disease First-degree block (PR < 0.3 s)	Doxycycline or amoxicillin as above for 2–3 weeks
High-degree atrioventricular block	Ceftriaxone or penicillin G as above for 2–3 weeks
Arthritis Oral dosage	Doxycycline or amoxicillin as above for 4 weeks
Parenteral dosage	Ceftriaxone or penicillin G as above for 2–4 weeks
Acrodermatitis chronicum atrophicans	Doxycycline or amoxicillin as above for 4 weeks
"Chronic Lyme disease" or "post-Lyme disease syndrome"	Symptomatic therapy

Table 138. Treatment of amebiasis.

Clinical Presentation	Drug(s) of Choice	Alternative Drug(s)
Asymptomatic intestinal infection	Diloxanide furoate[1,2]	Iodoquinol (diiodohydroxyquin)[3] or paromomycin[4]
Mild to moderate intestinal disease (nondysenteric colitis)	(1) Metronidazole[5] or tinidazole[1,5] **plus** (2) Diloxanide furoate,[1,2] iodoquinol,[3] or paromomycin[4]	(1) Diloxanide furoate[1,2] or iodoquinol[3] **plus** (2) A tetracycline[6] **followed by** (3) Chloroquine[7] **or** (1) Paromomycin[4] **followed by** (2) Chloroquine[7]
Severe intestinal disease (dysentery)	(1) Metronidazole[5] or tinidazole[1,5] **plus** (2) Diloxanide furoate[1,2] or iodoquinol[3] **or, if parenteral therapy is needed initially:** (1) Intravenous metronidazole[8] until oral therapy can be started; (2) Then give oral metronidazole[5] plus diloxanide furoate[1,2] or iodoquinol[3]	(1) A tetracycline[6] **plus** (2) Diloxanide furoate[1,2] or iodoquinol[3] **followed by** (3) Chloroquine[9] **or, if parenteral therapy is needed initially:** (1) Dehydroemetine[10] or emetine[1,10] **followed by** (2) A tetracycline[6] plus diloxanide furoate[1,2] or iodoquinol[3] **followed by** (3) Chloroquine[9]
Hepatic abscess	(1) Metronidazole[5,8] or tinidazole[1,5] **plus** (2) Diloxanide furoate[1,2] or iodoquinol[3] **followed by** (3) Chloroquine[9]	(1) Dehydroemetine[11] or emetine[1,11] **followed by** (2) Chloroquine[12] **plus** (3) Diloxanide furoate[1,2] or iodoquinol[3]
Ameboma or extra-intestinal disease	As for hepatic abscess, but not including chloroquine	As for hepatic abscess, but not including chloroquine

[1]Not available in the USA.
[2]Diloxanide furoate, 500 mg three times daily with meals for 10 days.
[3]Iodoquinol (diiodohydroxyquin), 650 mg three times daily for 21 days.
[4]Paromomycin, 25–30 mg/kg (base) (maximum 3 g) in three divided doses after meals daily for 7 days.
[5]Metronidazole, 750 mg three times daily for 10 days. In countries where it is available (not in the USA), tinidazole is preferred over metronidazole as the nitroimidazole component in treatment; although the two drugs are equally effective, tinidazole is given in a shorter course of treatment and is better tolerated. The tinidazole dosage is 800 mg three times daily for 3 days; in severe intestinal disease and hepatic abscess, continue for 5 days.
[6]Tetracycline, 250 mg four times daily for 10 days; in severe dysentery, give 500 mg four times daily for the first 5 days, then 250 mg four times daily for 5 days. Tetracycline should not be used during pregnancy.
[7]Chloroquine, 500 mg (salt) daily for 7 days.
[8]An intravenous metronidazole formulation is available; change to oral medication as soon as possible. See manufacturer's recommendation for dosage and cautions.
[9]Chloroquine, 500 mg (salt) daily for 14 days.
[10]Dehydroemetine or emetine, 1 mg/kg subcutaneously (preferred) or intramuscularly daily for the least number of days necessary to control severe symptoms (usually 3–5 days) (maximum daily dose for dehydroemetine is 90 mg; for emetine, 65 mg).
[11]Use dosage recommended in footnote 10 for 8–10 days.
[12]Chloroquine, 500 mg (salt) orally twice daily for 2 days and then 500 mg orally daily for 19 days.

Table 139. Treatment of malaria in nonimmune adult populations.

Treatment[1] of Infection With All Species (Except Chloroquine-Resistant *P falciparum*)	Treatment[1] of Infection With Chloroquine-Resistant *P falciparum* Strains
Oral treatment of *P falciparum*[2] or *P malariae* infection Chloroquine phosphate, 1 g (salt)[3,4] as initial dose, then 0.5 g at 6, 24, and 48 hours. **Oral treatment of *P vivax*[5] or *P ovale* infection** Chloroquine[3,4] as above followed by 0.5 g on days 10 and 17 plus primaquine phosphate, 26.3 mg (salt)[3,4] daily for 14 days starting about day 4. **Parenteral treatment of severe attacks** Quinine dihydrochloride[6] or quinidine gluconate.[7] Start oral chloroquine therapy as soon as possible; follow with primaquine if needed.[4] or Parenteral artesunate,[13] artemether,[13] or chloroquine[14] until the patient can take oral chloroquine. Follow with primaquine if the infection is due to–or if there is concurrent infection with–*P vivax* or *P ovale*.	**Oral treatment** Quinine sulfate, 10 mg/kg 3 times daily for 3–7 days,[8] plus one of the following: (1) doxycycline,[9] 100 mg twice daily for 7 days; (2) clindamycin,[9] 900 mg 3 times daily for 5 days; (3) pyrimethamine, 25 mg twice daily for 3 days, plus sulfadiazine, 500 mg 4 times daily for 5 days; (4) tetracycline,[9] 250–500 mg 4 times daily for 7 days; (5) once only, pyrimethamine, 75 mg, and sulfadoxine, 1500 mg (= 3 tablets of Fansidar[10]). or Mefloquine,[11] 750 mg followed after 12 hours by 500 mg. or Malarone[9] two tablets twice daily with food for 3 days (each tablet contains atovaquone [250 mg] and proguanil [100 mg]) or Atovaquone/doxycycline, 500 mg/100 mg, twice daily for 3 days or Artesunate,[13] 4 mg/kg/d orally for 3 days followed by mefloquine[11] (750 mg followed by 500 mg 12 hours later) or Halofantrine[12] **Parenteral treatment of severe attacks** Quinine dihydrochloride[6] or quinidine gluconate[7] plus intravenous doxycycline or clindamycin. Start oral therapy with quinine sulfate plus the second drug as soon as possible to complete 7 days of treatment. or Artemether,[13] or artesunate[13]; followed by mefloquine[11] (750 mg followed by 500 mg 12 hours later)

[1]See text for cautions, contraindications, and side effects of each drug. For advice on management, call the Centers for Disease Control and Prevention (CDC), Atlanta, GA (770-488-7760).

[2]In falciparum malaria, if the patient has not shown a clinical response to chloroquine (48–72 hours for mild infections, 24 hours for severe ones), parasitic resistance to chloroquine should be considered. Chloroquine should be stopped and treatment started with oral quinine plus doxycycline, mefloquine, malarone, or halofantrine.

[3]500 mg chloroquine phosphate = 300 mg base; 26.3 mg of primaquine = 15 mg base.

[4]Chloroquine alone is curative for infection with sensitive strains of *P falciparum* and for *P malariae*, but primaquine is needed to eradicate the persistent liver stages of *P vivax* and *P ovale*. Start primaquine after the patient has recovered from the acute illness; continue chloroquine weekly during primaquine therapy. Patients should be screened for glucose-6-phosphate dehydrogenase deficiency before use of primaquine. An alternative mode for primaquine therapy is combined primaquine, 78.9 mg (salt), and chloroquine, 0.5 g (salt), weekly for 8 weeks.

[5]Strains of *P vivax* resistant to chloroquine have appeared in some regions. For their treatment, give quinine (plus doxycycline), mefloquine, Malarone or halofantrine as used to treat *P falciparum* resistant to chloroquine.

[6]Quinine dihydrochloride. As a loading dose, give 20 mg/kg (salt) in 500 mL of 5% glucose solution intravenously slowly over 4 hours; repeat using 10 mg/kg every 8 hours until oral therapy is possible (maximum, 1800 mg/d). If more than 48 hours of parenteral treatment is required, some authorities reduce the quinine dose by one-third to one-half. Blood pressure and ECG should be monitored constantly to detect arrhythmias or hypotension. As severe hypoglycemia may occur, blood glucose levels should be monitored. Extreme caution is required in treating patients with quinine who previously have been taking mefloquine as prophylaxis. In the USA, quinine dihydrochloride is no longer available.

(continued)

(Continuing footnotes (Table 139)

[7]When parenteral quinine is unavailable (as in the USA), quinidine gluconate can be used, administered as a continuous infusion. A loading dose of 10 mg/kg (salt) (maximum, 600 mg) is diluted in 300 mL of normal saline and administered over 1–2 hours, followed by 0.02 mg/kg/min (maximum, 10 mg/kg every 8 hours) by continuous infusion until oral quinine therapy is possible. If more than 48 hours of parenteral treatment is required, some authorities reduce the quinidine dose by one-third to one-half. Fluid status, glucose, blood pressure, and ECG should be closely monitored; widening of the QRS interval or lengthening of the QT interval requires discontinuation.

[8]Although quinine sulfate is usually given for 3 days, it should be continued for 7 days in patients who acquired infections in Southeast Asia and South America, where diminished responsiveness to quinine has been noted.

[9]Contraindicated in pregnant women.

[10]Fansidar should not be used for infections acquired in Southeast Asia, the Amazon Basin, Bangladesh, or Oceania.

[11]Serious side effects are rare. In the USA, a 250-mg tablet of mefloquine contains 228 mg of base; outside the USA, each 275-mg tablet contains 250 mg of base. Mefloquine is hazardous with quinine, quinidine, or halofantrine.

[12]The dosage is 500 mg (salt) every 6 hours for three doses and repeat in 1 week. A possible contraindication is the presence of cardiac conduction abnormalities. Do not use if mefloquine has been taken in previous 2–3 weeks or with recent use of quinine or quinidine. Not available in the USA.

[13]Not available in the USA. Give artesunate intravenously (2.4 mg/kg on the first day, followed by 1.2 mg/kg daily) or artemether intramuscularly (3.2 mg/kg on the first day, followed by 1.6 mg/kg daily); continue the drug for a minimum of 3 days until the patient can start oral artesunate. If parenteral treatment is not available, artemisinin rectal suppositories are being evaluated (40 mg/kg loading dose, then 20 mg/kg at 24, 48, and 72 hours) followed by oral medication. With all preparations of the artemisinin drugs, as soon as oral medication can be tolerated, treat concurrently with another effective blood schizonticide (mefloquine preferred).

[14]Give parenteral chloroquine (1) preferably intravenously, 10 mg base/kg in isotonic fluid by constant rate of infusion over 8 hours, followed by 15 mg/kg over the next 24 hours; or (2) intramuscularly or subcutaneously, 3.5 mg base/kg every 6 hours.

Table 140. Prevention of malaria in nonimmune travelers.[1]

**TO PREVENT ATTACKS OF ALL FORMS OF MALARIA
AND TO ERADICATE *P falciparum* AND *P malariae* INFECTIONS[2,3,4]**

REGIONS WITH CHLOROQUINE-SENSITIVE *P falciparum* malaria: Central America west of the Panama Canal, the Caribbean, Mexico, and parts of the Middle East and China.

Chloroquine[5]

Dose: Chloroquine phosphate, 500 mg salt (300 mg base) weekly. Give a single dose of chloroquine weekly starting 1 week before entering the endemic area, while there, and for 4 weeks after leaving.

REGIONS WITH CHLOROQUINE-RESISTANT *P falciparum* malaria: All other regions of the world; the frequency and intensity of resistance vary by region.

Malarone (atovaquone [250 mg] combined with proguanil [100 mg] [preferred method])[6]

Dose: One tablet daily. Give one tablet the day before entering the endemic area, daily while there, and daily for 1 week after leaving.

Mefloquine (preferred method)[7]

Dose: one 250-mg tablet salt (228 mg base) weekly. Give a single dose of mefloquine weekly starting 3 weeks before entering the endemic area, while there, and for 4 weeks after leaving.

Doxycycline (alternative method)[8]

Dose: 100 mg daily. Give the daily dose for 2 days before entering the endemic area, while there, and for 4 weeks after leaving.

TO ERADICATE *P vivax* AND *P ovale* INFECTIONS[2]

Primaquine[9]

Start primaquine only after returning home, during the last 2 weeks of chemoprophylaxis. Dose: 26.3 mg salt (15 mg base) daily for 14 days. An alternative regimen in regions where chloroquine is effective in prophylaxis is chloroquine phosphate, 500 mg (salt), plus primaquine phosphate 78.9 mg (salt), weekly for 8 weeks.

---

[1]For additional information on prophylaxis for specific countries, see the references or call the Centers for Disease Control and Prevention, Atlanta, GA at 770-488-7788 (for fax response: 888-232-3299). The information is also available on the Internet at http://www.cdc.gov (choose the Traveler's Health category).

[2]The blood schizonticides (chloroquine, mefloquine, Malarone, and doxycycline), when taken for 4 weeks (7 days for Malarone) after leaving the endemic area, are curative for sensitive *P falciparum* and *P malariae* infections; primaquine, however, is needed to eradicate the persistent liver stages of *P vivax* and *P ovale.*

[3]A test dose of the selected prophylactic drug should be given before departure to allow for changing to an alternative drug in the event of significant side effects: chloroquine (once weekly for 2 weeks), Malarone (daily for 2 days), doxycycline (daily for 2 days), mefloquine (weekly for 3 weeks). Side effects from mefloquine sometimes do not appear until after the third or later doses.

[4]See text for standby drugs for emergency self-treatment of presumptive malaria; such drugs should be used only when a physician is not immediately available. It is imperative, however, that medical follow-up be sought promptly.

[5]Chloroquine and proguanil can be used by pregnant women.

[6]Malarone recently became available in the USA. It eradicates falciparum infections after 1 week of postexposure treatment; its efficacy against *P malariae,* however, is undetermined. To eradicate *P vivax* and *P ovale* infections, a course of primaquine is needed, which should be started early in the final week of Malarone treatment. Malarone has not been shown to be safe in pregnancy. Malarone is more expensive than mefloquine.

[7]Because of the high frequency of resistance, mefloquine should not be used in Thailand or adjacent countries; it is now the preferred drug for sub-Saharan Africa. Mefloquine is generally not recommended in the first trimester of pregnancy or under some other condition.

[8]Doxycycline is used in Thailand and adjacent countries and in other regions by persons who cannot tolerate mefloquine or Malarone. It is contraindicated in pregnant women. Take with evening meals.

[9]Primaquine is indicated only for persons who have had a high probability of exposure to *P vivax* or *P ovale,* and who have not taken the drug for daily prophylaxis. The drug should be taken with food and is contraindicated in pregnancy. Before use, patients must be screened for glucose-6-phosphate dehydrogenase deficiency.

Figure 11. Hypothermia treatment algorithm. (VF, ventricular fibrillation; VT, ventricular tachycardia; J, joules.) (Reproduced, with permission, from American Heart Association. Circulation 2000;102[Suppl I]:I-229.)

Table 141. Currently available (prepackaged) cyanide antidotes.[1,2]

Antidote	How Supplied	Dose
Amyl nitrite	0.3 mL (aspirol inhalant)	Break one or two aspirols under patient's nose.
Sodium nitrite	3 g/dL (300 mg in 10 mL vials)	6 mg/kg IV (0.2 mL/kg)
Sodium thio-sulfate	25 g/dL (12.5 g in 50 mL vials)	250 mg/kg IV (1 mL/kg)

[1]Reproduced, with permission, from Saunders CE, Ho MT (editors): *Current Emergency Diagnosis & Treatment*, 4th ed. McGraw-Hill, 1992.
[2]In the United States, manufactured by Taylor Pharmaceuticals.

Table 142. Clinical features of hydrocarbon poisoning.[1]

Type	Examples	Risk of Pneumonia	Risk of Systemic Toxicity	Treatment
High-viscosity	Vaseline[2] Motor oil	Low	Low	None.
Low-viscosity, nontoxic	Furniture polish Mineral seal oil Kerosene Lighter fluid	High	Low	Observe for pneumonia. *Do not* induce emesis. *Do not* administer activated charcoal.
Low-viscosity, unknown systemic toxicity	Turpentine Pine oil	High	Variable	Observe for pneumonia. Consider activated charcoal.
Low-viscosity, known systemic toxicity	Camphor Phenol Chlorinated insecticides Aromatic hydrocarbons (benzene, toluene, etc)	High	High	Observe for pneumonia. Give activated charcoal.

[1]Reproduced, with permission, from Saunders CE, Ho MT (editors): *Current Emergency Diagnosis & Treatment*, 4th ed. McGraw-Hill, 1992.
[2]"Vaseline" is one of several proprietary names for petrolatum (petroleum jelly, paraffin jelly).

Table 143. Common seafood poisonings.

Type of Poisoning	Mechanism	Clinical Presentation
Ciguatera	Reef fish ingest toxic dinoflagellates, whose toxins accumulate in fish meat. Commonly implicated fish in the USA are barracuda, jack, snapper, and grouper.	1–6 hours after ingestion, victims develop abdominal pain, vomiting, and diarrhea accompanied by a variety of neurologic symptoms, including paresthesias, reversal of hot and cold sensation, vertigo, headache, and intense itching. Autonomic disturbances, including hypotension and bradycardia, may occur.
Scombroid	Improper preservation of large fish results in bacterial degradation of histidine to histamine. Commonly implicated fish include tuna, mahimahi, bonita, mackerel, and kingfish.	Allergic-like (anaphylactoid) symptoms are due to histamine, usually begin within 15–90 minutes, and include skin flushing, itching, urticaria, angioedema, bronchospasm, and hypotension as well as abdominal pain, vomiting, and diarrhea.
Paralytic shellfish poisoning	Dinoflagellates produce saxitoxin, which is concentrated by filter-feeding mussels and clams. Saxitoxin blocks sodium conductance and neuronal transmission in skeletal muscles.	Onset is usually within 30–60 minutes. Initial symptoms include perioral and intraoral paresthesias. Other symptoms include nausea and vomiting, headache, dizziness, dysphagia, dysarthria, ataxia, and rapidly progressive muscle weakness that may result in respiratory arrest.
Puffer fish poisoning	Tetrodotoxin is concentrated in liver, gonads, intestine, and skin. Toxic effects are similar to those of saxitoxin. Tetrodotoxin is also found in some North American newts and Central American frogs.	Onset is usually within 30–40 minutes but may be as short as 10 minutes. Initial perioral paresthesias are followed by headache, diaphoresis, nausea, vomiting, ataxia, and rapidly progressive muscle weakness that may result in respiratory arrest.

Table 144. Some of the "unsafe" and "probably safe" drugs used in the treatment of acute porphyrias.

Unsafe	Probably Safe
Alcohol	Acetaminophen
Alkylating agents	β-Adrenergic blockers
Barbiturates	Amitriptyline
Carbamazepine	Aspirin
Chlorpropamide	Atropine
Chloroquine	Chloral hydrate
Clonidine	Chlordiazepoxide
Dapsone	Diazepam
Ergots	Digoxin
Erythromycin	Diphenhydramine
Estrogens, synthetic	Guanethidine
Food additives	Glucocorticoids
Glutethimide	Hyoscine
Griseofulvin	Ibuprofen
Hydralazine	Imipramine
Ketamine	Insulin
Meprobamate	Lithium
Methyldopa	Naproxen
Metoclopramide	Nitrofurantoin
Nortriptyline	Opioid analgesics
Pentazocine	Penicillamine
Phenytoin	Penicillin and derivatives
Progestins	Phenothiazines
Pyrazinamide	Procaine
Rifampin	Streptomycin
Spironolactone	Succinylcholine
Succinimides	Tetracycline
Sulfonamides	Thiouracil
Theophylline	
Tolazamide	
Tolbutamide	
Valproic acid	

Table 145. Cancer screening recommendations for average-risk adults, 2003.

	Test	ACS[1]	CTF[2]	USPSTF[3]
Breast	Self-examination (BSE)	Monthly for women over age 20.	Fair evidence that BSE *should not* be used.	Insufficient evidence to recommend for or against.
	Clinical breast examination	Every 3 years age 20–40 and annually thereafter.	Every 1–2 years in age women 40–59.	Insufficient evidence to recommend for or against.
	Mammography	Annually age 40 and older.	Every 1–2 years in age women 40–59. Current evidence does not support the recommendation that screening mammography be included in or excluded from the periodic health examination of women aged 40–49.	Recommended every 1–2 years for women age 40 and over (B).
Cervix	Papanicolaou test	Annually beginning within 3 years after first vaginal intercourse or no later than age 21. After age 30, women with three normal tests may be screened every 2–3 years. Women may choose to stop screening after age 70 if they have had three normal (and no abnormal) results within the last 10 years.	Annually at age of first intercourse or by age 18; can move to every-2-year screening after two normal results.	Every 3 years beginning at onset of sexual activity.
Colon	Stool test for occult blood*	Screening recommended, with the combination of fecal occult blood test (FOBT) and sigmoidoscopy preferred over stool test or sigmoidoscopy alone. Barium enema and colonoscopy also considered reasonable alternatives.	Good evidence for screening every 1–2 years over age 50.	Screening strongly recommended (A), but insufficient evidence to determine best test.
	Sigmoidoscopy		Fair evidence for screening over age 50 (insufficient evidence about combining stool test and sigmoidoscopy).	
	Double-contrast barium enema		Not addressed.	
	Colonoscopy		Insufficient evidence for or against use in screening.	
	Digital rectal exam (DRE)	Not recommended.	No recommendation.	Not recommended.
Prostate	Digital rectal exam (DRE)	DRE and PSA should be offered annually to men age 50 and older who have at least a 10-year life expectancy. Information should be provided to men about the benefits and risks, and they should be allowed to participate in the decision. Men without a clear preference should be screened.	Insufficient evidence for or against including in routine care.	Insufficient evidence to recommend for or against.
	PSA blood test		Fair evidence *against* including in routine care.	
Other	Cancer-related checkup	Every 3 years for men 20–40 and annually thereafter; should include counseling and perhaps oral cavity, thyroid, lymph node, or testicular examinations.	Not assessed.	Not assessed.

*Home test with three samples.
[1]American Cancer Society recommendations, available at http://www.cancer.org
[2]Canadian Task Force on Preventive Health Care recommendations available at http://www.ctfphc.org
[3]United States Preventive Services Task Force recommendations available at http://www.ahrq.gov

Recommendation A: The USPSTF strongly recommends that clinicians routinely provide the service to eligible patients. (The USPTF found good evidence that the service improves important health outcomes and concludes that benefits substantially outweigh harms.)

Recommendation B: The USPSTF recommends that clinicians routinely provide the service to eligible patients. (The USPTF found at least fair evidence that the service improves important health outcomes and concludes that benefits substantially outweigh harms.)

Table 146. Incidence of and mortality from the ten most common cancers in the United States in males and females (all races).

Rank	Men	Incidence[1]	Mortality[1]	Women	Incidence[1]	Mortality[1]
1	Prostate	170	33	Breast	135	25
2	Lung	81	80	Lung	50	41
3	Colorectal	64	26	Colorectal	47	18
4	Bladder	36	8	Uterus[2]	34	7
5	Lymphoma[3]	27	10	Lymphoma[3]	18	7
6	Oropharyngeal[4]	23	7	Ovary	17	9
7	Melanoma	21	4	Melanoma	14	2
8	Leukemia[5]	16	10	Leukemia[5]	9	6
9	Kidney	15	6	Thyroid	10	0:5
10	Stomach	13	6	Pancreas	10	9

Data obtained from the NCI SEER Program. Ries LAG, Eisner MP, Kosary CL, Hankey BF, Miller BA, Clegg L, Edwards BK (editors): *SEER Cancer Statistics Review, 1973–1999,* National Cancer Institute, Bethesda, MD; http://seer.cancer.gov/csr/1973_1999/2002.
[1]Rates are per 100,000, 1996–2000, and are age-adjusted to the 2000 United States population by 5-year age groups.
[2]Uterus includes the cervix and corpus uteri.
[3]Both Hodgkin's disease and non-Hodgkin's lymphomas are included under lymphoma.
[4]Both oropharynx and larynx are included under oropharyngeal.
[5]All subtypes of leukemia are included.

Table 147. Lifetime risks for the most common cancers.[1]

Cancer	Risk of Diagnosis (%)	Risk of Death (%)
Prostate	16.0	3.1
Breast (women)	13.2	3.1
Lung		
(men)	7.9	7.5
(women)	5.8	4.9
Colorectal		
(men)	6.0	2.4
(women)	5.6	2.4
Bladder (men)	3.4	0.7
Uterus[2]	3.5	0.8
Any cancer		
(men)	43.4	23.9
(women)	38.0	20.4

[1]Data obtained from the NCI Seer Program. Ries LAG, Eisner MP, Kosary CL, Hankey BF, Miller BA, Clegg L, Edwards BK (editors): *SEER Cancer Statistics Review, 1973–1999,* National Cancer Institute, Bethesda, MD: http://seer.cancer.gov/csr/1973_1999/2002.
[2]Uterus includes the cervix and corpus uteri.

Table 148. Treatment choices for cancers responsive to systemic agents.

Diagnosis	Current Treatment of Choice	Other Valuable Agents and Procedures
Acute lymphocytic leukemia	**Induction:** Combination chemotherapy. *Adults:* Vincristine, prednisone, daunorubicin, and asparaginase (DVPLasp). **Consolidation:** Multiagent alternating chemotherapy. Allogeneic bone marrow transplant for young adults or high-risk disease or second remission. CNS prophylaxis with intrathecal methotrexate with or without whole brain radiation. **Remission maintenance:** Methotrexate, thioguanine.	Doxorubicin, cytarabine, cyclophospha-mide, etoposide, teniposide, allopurinol,[1] autologous bone marrow transplantation
Acute myelocytic and myelomonocytic leukemia	**Induction:** Combination chemotherapy with cytarabine and an anthracycline (daunorubicin, idarubicin). Tretinoin with idarubicin for acute promyelocytic leukemia. **Consolidation:** High-dose cytarabine. Autologous (with or without purging) or allogeneic bone marrow transplantation for high-risk disease or second remission.	Gemtuzumab ozogamicin (Mylotarg), mitoxantrone, idarubicin, etoposide, mercaptopurine, thioguanine, azacitidine,[2] amsacrine,[2] methotrexate, doxorubicin, tretinoin, allopurinol,[1] leukapheresis, prednisone, arsenic trioxide for acute promyelocytic leukemia
Chronic myelocytic leukemia	Imatinib mesylate (Gleevec), hydroxyurea, α-interferon. Allogeneic bone marrow transplantation for younger patients.	Busulfan, mercaptopurine, thioguanine, cytarabine, plicamycin, melphalan, auto-logous bone marrow transplantation,[2] allopurinol[1]
Chronic lymphocytic leukemia	Fludarabine, chlorambucil, and prednisone (if treatment is indicated). Second-line therapy: alemtuzumab (Campath-1H).	Vincristine, cyclophosphamide, doxoru-bicin, cladribine (2-chlorodeoxyadenosine; CdA), rituximab, allogeneic bone marrow transplant, androgens,[2] allopurinol[1]
Hairy cell leukemia	Cladribine (2-chlorodeoxyadenosine; CdA).	Pentostatin (deoxycoformycin), α-interferon
Hodgkin's disease (stages III and IV)	**Combination chemotherapy:** doxorubicin (Adriamycin), bleomycin, vinblastine, dacarbazine (ABVD) or alternative combination therapy without mechloretha-mine. Autologous bone marrow transplant for high-risk patients or relapsed disease.	Mechlorethamine, vincristine, prednisone, procarbazine (MOPP); carmustine, lomu-stine, etoposide, thiotepa, autologous bone marrow transplantation
Non-Hodgkin's lymphoma (intermediate to high grade)	**Combination therapy:** depending on histologic classification but usually in-cluding cyclophosphamide, vincristine, doxorubicin, and prednisone (CHOP) with or without rituximab in older patients. Autologous bone marrow transplan-tation in high-risk first remission or first relapse.	Bleomycin, methotrexate, etoposide, chlorambucil, fludarabine, lomustine, carmustine, cytarabine, thiotepa, am-sacrine, mitoxantrone, allogeneic bone marrow transplantation
Non-Hodgkin's lymphoma (low-grade)	Fludarabine, rituximab, if CD20 positive; ibritumomab tiuxetan or 1312 tositu-momab for relapsed or refractory disease.	**Combination chemotherapy:** cyclophosphamide, prednisone, doxoru-bicin, vincristine; chlorambucil, autologous or allogeneic transplantation
Cutaneous T cell lymphoma (my-cosis fungoides)	Topical carmustine, electron beam radiotherapy, photochemotherapy, targretin, denileukin diftitox (ONTAK) for refractory disease.	Interferon, combination chemotherapy, denileukin diftitox (ONTAK), targretin
Multiple myeloma	**Combination chemotherapy:** vincristine, doxorubicin, dexamethasone; mel-phalan and prednisone; melphalan, cyclosphosphamide, carmustine, vin-cristine, doxorubicin, prednisone, thalidomide. Autologous transplantation in first complete or partial remission, mini-allogeneic transplant for poor-prognosis disease. Bortezomib for relapsed or refractory disease.	Clarithromycin, etoposide, cytarabine, α-interferon, dexamethasone, autolo-gous bone marrow transplantation
Waldenström's macroglobulinemia	Fludarabine **or** chlorambucil **or** cyclophosphamide, vincristine, prednisone. Allogeneic bone marrow transplantation for high-risk young patients.	Cladribine, etoposide, α-interferon, doxorubicin, dexamethasone, plasma-pheresis, autologous bone marrow transplantation
Polycythemia vera, es-sential thrombocytosis	Hydroxyurea, phlebotomy for polycythemia. Anagrelide for thombocytosis.	Busulfan, chlorambucil, cyclophosphamide, alpha interferon, radiophosphorus ^{32}P

(continued)

Table 148. Treatment choices for cancers responsive to systemic agents. (continued)

Diagnosis	Current Treatment of Choice	Other Valuable Agents and Procedures
Carcinoma of the lung Small cell	**Combination chemotherapy:** cisplatin and etoposide. Palliative radiation therapy.	Cyclophosphamide, doxorubicin, vincristine
Non-small cell[3]	Localized disease: cisplatin or carboplatin, docetaxel Advanced disease: cisplatin or carboplatin, docetaxel, gemfitizib, etoposide, vinblastine, vinorelbine	Doxorubicin, etoposide, mitomycin, ifosfamide, paclitaxel, radiation therapy
Carcinoma of the head and neck[3]	**Combination chemotherapy:** cisplatin and fluorouracil, paclitaxel	Methotrexate, bleomycin, hydroxyurea, doxorubicin, vinblastine
Carcinoma of the esophagus[3]	**Combination chemotherapy:** fluorouracil, cisplatin, mitomycin	Methotrexate, bleomycin, doxorubicin, mitomycin
Carcinoma of the stomach and pancreas[3]	**Stomach:** etoposide, leucovorin,[1] fluorouracil (ELF) **Pancreas:** fluorouracil or ELF, gemcitabine	Carmustine, mitomycin, lomustine, doxorubicin, gemcitabine, doxorubicin, methotrexate, cisplatin, combinations for stomach.
Carcinoma of the colon and rectum[3]	**Colon:** leucovorin and irinotecan or oxaliplatin[2] (advanced) **Rectum:** fluorouracil with radiation therapy (adjuvant)	Capecitabine, methotrexate, mitomycin, carmustine, cisplatin, floxuridine.
Carcinoma of the kidney[3]	Floxuridine, vinblastine, IL-2, α-interferon; consider mini-allogeneic transplantation[2]	α-Interferon, progestins, infusional FUDR, fluorouracil
Carcinoma of the bladder[3]	Intravesical BCG or thiotepa. **Combination chemotherapy:** methotrexate, vinblastine, doxorubicin (Adriamycin), cisplatin (M-VAC) or CMV alone	Cyclophosphamide, fluorouracil, intravesical valrubicin, gemcitabine, cisplatin
Carcinoma of the testis[3]	**Combination chemotherapy:** etoposide and cisplatin. Autologous bone marrow transplantation for high-risk or relapsed disease.	Bleomycin, vinblastine, ifosfamide, mesna,[1] carmustine, carboplatin
Carcinoma of the prostate[3]	Estrogens or LHRH analog (leuprolide, goserelin, or triptorelin) plus an anti-androgen (flutamide)	Ketoconazole, doxorubicin, aminoglutethimide, progestins, cyclophosphamide, cisplatin, vinblastine, etoposide, suramin[2]; PC-SPES; estramustine phosphate
Carcinoma of the uterus[3]	Progestins or tamoxifen	Doxorubicin, cisplatin, fluorouracil, ifosfamide
Carcinoma of the ovary[3]	**Combination chemotherapy:** paclitaxel and cisplatin or carboplatin	Docetaxel, doxorubicin, topotecan, cyclophosphamide, doxorubicin, etoposide, liposomal doxorubicin
Carcinoma of the cervix[3]	**Combination chemotherapy:** methotrexate, doxorubicin, cisplatin, and vinblastine; or mitomycin, bleomycin, vincristine, and cisplatin with radiation therapy	Carboplatin, ifosfamide, lomustine
Carcinoma of the breast[3]	**Combination chemotherapy:** A variety of regimens are used for adjuvant therapy. For node-positive disease—combinations including doxorubicin or epirubicin and at least one of the following additional drugs: 5-FU, cyclophosphamide, docetaxel, paclitaxel. For node-negative disease—a combination of the drugs listed above or cyclophosphamide, methotrexate, and 5-FU (CMF). For estrogen- or progesterone-positive disease, tamoxifen is given for 5 years regardless of the use of adjuvant chemotherapy.	Trastuzumab (Herceptin) with chemotherapy, paclitaxel, docetaxel, epirubicin, mitoxantrone, topotecan, capecitabine, vinorelbine, thiotepa, vincristine, vinblastine, carboplatin or cisplatin, plicamycin, anastrozole, letrozole, exemestane, fulvestrant, toremifine, progestins
Choriocarcinoma (trophoblastic neoplasms)[3]	Methotrexate or dactinomycin (or both) plus chlorambucil	Vinblastine, cisplatin, mercaptopurine, doxorubicin, bleomycin, etoposide
Carcinoma of the thyroid gland[3]	Radioiodine (^{131}I)	Doxorubicin, cisplatin, bleomycin, melphalan
Carcinoma of the adrenal gland[3]	Mitotane	Doxorubicin, suramin[2]
Carcinoid[3]	Fluorouracil plus streptozocin with or without α-interferon	Doxorubicin, cyclophosphamide, octreotide, cyproheptadine,[1] methysergide[1]

(continued)

Table 148. Treatment choices for cancers responsive to systemic agents. (continued)

Diagnosis	Current Treatment of Choice	Other Valuable Agents and Procedures
Osteogenic sarcoma[3]	High-dose methotrexate, doxorubicin, vincristine	Cyclophosphamide, ifosfamide, bleomycin, dacarbazine, cisplatin, dactinomycin
Soft tissue sarcoma[3]	Doxorubicin, dacarbazine	Ifosfamide, cyclosphosphamide, etoposide, cisplatin, high-dose methotrexate, vincristine
Melanoma[3]	Dacarbazine, α-interferon, IL-2	Carmustine, lomustine, melphalan, thiotepa, cisplatin, paclitaxel, tamoxifen, vincristine, vaccine therapy (Melacine)[2]
Kaposi's sarcoma	Doxorubicin, vincristine alternating with vinblastine or vincristine alone. Palliative radiation therapy.	α-Interferon, bleomycin, etoposide, doxorubicin
Neuroblastoma[3]	**Combination chemotherapy:** variations of cyclophosphamide, cisplatin, vincristine, doxorubicin, dacarbazine	Melphalan, ifosfamide, autologous or allogeneic bone marrow transplantation

[1]Supportive agent; not oncolytic.

[2]Investigational agent or procedure. Treatment is available through qualified investigators and centers authorized by the National Cancer Institute and Cooperative Oncology Groups.

[3]These tumors are generally managed initially with surgery with or without radiation therapy with or without adjuvant chemotherapy. For metastatic disease, the role of palliative radiation therapy is as important as that of chemotherapy.

Table 149. Single-agent dosage and toxicity of anticancer drugs.

Drug	Dosage	Acute Toxicity	Delayed Toxicity
Alkylating agents			
Mechlorethamine	6–10 mg/m^2 IV every 3 weeks	Severe vesicant; severe nausea and vomiting	Moderate suppression of blood counts. Melphalan effect may be delayed 4–6 weeks. Excessive doses produce severe bone marrow suppression with leukopenia, thrombocytopenia, and bleeding. Alopecia and hemorrhagic cystitis occur with cyclophosphamide, while busulfan can cause hyperpigmentation, pulmonary fibrosis, and weakness. Ifosfamide is always given with mesna to prevent cystitis. Acute leukemia may develop in 5–10% of patients receiving prolonged therapy with melphalan, mechlorethamine, or chlorambucil; all alkylators probably increase the risk of secondary malignancies with prolonged use. Most cause either temporary or permanent aspermia or amenorrhea.
Chlorambucil	0.1–0.2 mg/kg/d orally (6–12 mg/d) or 0.4 mg/kg pulse every 4 weeks	None	
Cyclophosphamide	100 mg/m^2/d orally for 14 days; 400 mg/m^2 orally for 5 days; 1–1.5 g/m^2 IV every 3–4 weeks	Nausea and vomiting with higher doses	
Melphalan	0.25 mg/kg/d orally for 4 days every 6 weeks	None	
Busulfan	2–8 mg/d orally; 150–250 mg/course	None	
Estramustine	14 mg/kg orally in 3 or 4 divided doses	Nausea, vomiting, diarrhea	Thrombosis, thrombocytopenia, hypertension, gynecomastia, glucose intolerance, edema.
Carmustine (BCNU)	200 mg/m^2 IV every 6 weeks	Local irritant	Prolonged leukopenia and thrombocytopenia. Rarely hepatitis. Acute leukemia has been observed to occur in some patients receiving nitrosoureas. Nitrosoureas can cause delayed pulmonary fibrosis with prolonged use.
Lomustine (CCNU)	100–130 mg orally every 6–8 weeks	Nausea and vomiting	
Procarbazine	100 mg/m^2/d orally for 14 days every 4 weeks	Nausea and vomiting	Bone marrow suppression, mental suppression, MAO inhibition, disulfiram-like effect.
Dacarbazine	250 mg/m^2/d IV for 5 days every 3 weeks; 1500 mg/m^2 IV as single dose	Severe nausea and vomiting; anorexia	Bone marrow suppression; flu-like syndrome.
Cisplatin	50–100 mg/m^2 IV every 3 weeks; 20 mg/m^2 IV for 5 days every 4 weeks	Severe nausea and vomiting	Nephrotoxicity, mild otic and bone marrow toxicity, neurotoxicity.
Carboplatin	360 mg/m^2 IV every 4 weeks	Severe nausea and vomiting	Bone marrow suppression, prolonged anemia; same as cisplatin but milder.
Oxaliplatin	85 mg/m^2 IV in 250–500 mL D$_5$W over 2 hours, given with leucovorin, followed by fluorouracil on day 1. Leucovorin followed by fluorouracil without oxaliplatin is given on day 2.	Nausea, vomiting, diarrhea, fatigue, rare anaphylactic reactions	Peripheral neuropathy, cytopenias, pulmonary toxicity (rare)
Structural analogs or antimetabolites			
Methotrexate	2.5–5 mg/d orally; 20–25 mg IM twice weekly; high-dose: 500–1000 mg/m^2 IV every 2–3 weeks; 12–15 mg intrathecally every week for 4–6 doses	None	Bone marrow suppression, oral and gastrointestinal ulceration, acute renal failure; hepatotoxicity, rash, increased toxicity when effusions are present. **Note:** Citrovorum factor (leucovorin) rescue for doses over 100 mg/m^2.
Mercaptopurine	2.5 mg/kg/d orally; 100 mg/m^2/d orally for 5 days for induction	None	Well tolerated. Larger doses cause bone marrow suppression.
Thioguanine	2 mg/kg/d orally; 100 mg/m^2/d IV for 7 days for induction	Mild nausea, diarrhea	Well tolerated. Larger doses cause bone marrow suppression.

(continued)

Table 149. Single-agent dosage and toxicity of anticancer drugs. (continued)

Drug	Dosage	Acute Toxicity	Delayed Toxicity
Fluorouracil	15 mg/kg/d IV for 3–5 days every 3 weeks; 15 mg/kg weekly as tolerated; 500–1000 mg/m^2 IV every 4 weeks	None	Nausea, diarrhea, oral and gastrointestinal ulceration, bone marrow suppression, dacryocystitis.
Capecitabine	2500 mg/m^2 orally twice daily on days 1–14 every 3 weeks	Nausea, diarrhea	Hand and foot syndrome, mucositis.
Cytarabine	100–200 mg/m^2/d for 5–10 days by continuous IV infusion; 2–3 g/m^2 IV every 12 hours for 3–7 days; 20 mg/m^2 SC daily in divided doses	High-dose: nausea, vomiting, diarrhea, anorexia	Nausea and vomiting; cystitis; severe bone marrow suppression; megaloblastosis; CNS toxicity with high-dose cytarabine.
Temozolamide	150 mg /m^2 orally for 5 days; repeat every 4 weeks	Headache, nausea, vomiting	Unknown
Androgens and androgen antagonists			
Testosterone propionate	100 mg IM 3 times weekly	None	Fluid retention, masculinization, leg cramps. Cholestatic jaundice in some patients receiving fluoxymesterone.
Fluoxymesterone	20–40 mg/d orally	None	
Flutamide	250 mg 3 times a day orally	None	Gynecomastia, hot flushes, decreased libido, mild gastrointestinal side effects, hepatotoxicity.
Bicalutamide	50 mg/d orally		
Nilutamide	300 mg/d orally for 30 days, then 150 mg/d		
Ethinyl estradiol	3 mg/d orally	None	Fluid retention, feminization, uterine bleeding, exacerbation of cardiovascular disease, painful gynecomastia, thromboembolic disease.
Selective estrogen receptor modulators			
Tamoxifen	20 mg/d orally in 2 divided doses	Transient flare of bone pain; nausea, hot flushes, joint aching	Thromboembolic disease, anovulation, endometrial cancer, cataracts; vaginal bleeding, acne.
Toremifene	60 mg/d orally		
Aromatase inhibitors			
Anastrozole	1 mg orally daily	Hot flushes, joint aching	Thromboembolic disease, vaginal bleeding.
Letrozole	2.5 mg/d orally		
Exemestane	25 mg/d orally		
Pure estrogen receptor antagonist			
Fulvestrant	250 mg IM once a month	Transient injection site reactions	Nausea, vomiting, constipation, diarrhea, abdominal pain, headache, back pain, hot flushes.
Progestins			
Megestrol acetate	40 mg orally 4 times daily	Hot flushes	Fluid retention; rare thrombosis, weight gain.
Medroxyprogesterone	100–200 mg/d orally; 200–600 mg orally twice weekly	None	
GnRH analogs			
Leuprolide	7.5 mg IM (depot) once a month or 22.5 mg every 3 months as depot injection	Local irritation, transient flare of symptoms	Hot flushes, decreased libido, impotence, gynecomastia, mild gastrointestinal side effects, nausea, diarrhea, fatigue.

(continued)

Drug	Dosage	Acute Toxicity	Delayed Toxicity
Goserelin acetate	3.6 mg SC monthly or 10.8 mg every 3 months as depot injection		
Triptorelin pamoate	3.75 mg IM once a month (a 3-month depot formulation also exists)		
Adrenocorticosteroids			
Prednisone	20–100 mg/d orally or 50–100 mg every other day orally with systemic chemotherapy	Alteration in mood	Fluid retention, hypertension, diabetes, increased susceptibility to infection, "moon facies," osteoporosis, electrolyte abnormalities, gastritis.
Dexamethasone	5–10 mg orally daily or twice daily		
Ketoconazole	400 mg orally 3 times daily	Acute nausea	Gynecomastia, hepatotoxicity.
Biologic response modifiers			
Interferon alfa-2a Interferon alfa-2b	3–5 million units SC 3 times weekly or daily	Fever, chills, fatigue, anorexia	General malaise, weight loss, confusion, hypothyroidism, retinopathy, autoimmune disease.
Aldesleukin (IL-2)	600,000 units/kg IV over 15 minutes every 8 hours for 14 doses, repeated after 9-day rest period. Some doses may be withheld or interrupted because of toxicity. **Caution:** High doses must be administered in an ICU setting by experienced personnel.	Hypotension, fever, chills, rigors, diarrhea, nausea, vomiting, pruritus; liver, kidney, and CNS toxicity; capillary leak (primarily at high doses), pruritic skin rash, infections (can be severe)	Hypoglycemia, anemia.
Peptide hormone inhibitor			
Octreotide acetate	100–600 µg/d SC in 2 divided doses	Local irritant; nausea and vomiting	Diarrhea, abdominal pain, hypoglycemia.
Natural products and miscellaneous agents			
Vinblastine	0.1–0.2 mg/kg or 6 mg/m^2 IV weekly	Mild nausea and vomiting; severe vesicant	Alopecia, peripheral neuropathy, bone marrow suppression, constipation, SIADH, areflexia.
Vincristine	1.5 mg/m^2 (maximum: 2 mg weekly)	Severe vesicant	Areflexia, muscle weakness, peripheral neuropathy, paralytic ileus, alopecia (see text), SIADH.
Vinorelbine	30 mg/m^2 IV weekly	Mild nausea and vomiting, fatigue, severe vesicant	Granulocytopenia, constipation, peripheral neuropathy, alopecia.
Paclitaxel (Taxol)	135 mg/m^2 by continuous infusion over 24 hours every 3 weeks	Hypersensitivity reaction (premedicate with diphenhydramine and dexamethasone), mild nausea and vomiting	Peripheral neuropathy, bone marrow suppression, fluid retention.
Docetaxel (Taxotere)	60–100 mg/m^2 IV every 3 weeks		
Dactinomycin	0.04 mg/kg IV weekly	Nausea and vomiting; severe vesicant	Alopecia, stomatitis, diarrhea, bone marrow suppression.
Daunorubicin	30–60 mg/m^2 daily IV for 3 days, or 30–60 mg/m^2 IV weekly		Alopecia, stomatitis, bone marrow suppression, late cardiotoxicity. Risk of cardiotoxicity increases with radiation, cyclophosphamide.

(continued)

Table 149. Single-agent dosage and toxicity of anticancer drugs. (continued)

Drug	Dosage	Acute Toxicity	Delayed Toxicity
Idarubicin	12 mg/m^2 daily IV for 3 days		See Daunorubicin above
Doxorubicin	60 mg/m^2 IV every 3 weeks to a maximum total dose of 550 mg/m^2		
Epirubicin	60–100 mg/m^2 IV every 3 weeks		
Liposomal doxorubicin (Doxil)	20 mg/m^2 IV every 3 weeks	Mild nausea	Hand and foot syndrome; alopecia, stomatitis, and bone marrow suppression uncommon.
Liposomal daunorubicin (DaunoXome)	40 mg/m^2 IV every 2 weeks		
Etoposide	100 mg/m^2/d IV for 5 days or 50–150 mg/d orally	Nausea and vomiting; occasionally hypotension	Alopecia, bone marrow suppression, secondary leukemia.
Plicamycin (mithramycin)	25–50 µg/kg IV every other day for up to 8 doses	Nausea and vomiting	Thrombocytopenia, diarrhea, hepatotoxicity, nephrotoxicity, stomatitis.
Mitomycin	10–20 mg/m^2 every 6–8 weeks	Severe vesicant; nausea	Prolonged bone marrow suppression, rare hemolytic-uremic syndrome.
Mitoxantrone	12–15 mg/m^2/d IV for 3 days with cytarabine; 8–12 mg/m^2 IV every 3 weeks	Mild nausea and vomiting	Alopecia, mild mucositis, bone marrow suppression.
Bleomycin	Up to 15 units/m^2 IM, IV, or SC twice weekly to a total dose of 200 units/m^2	Allergic reactions, fever, hypotension	Fever, dermatitis, pulmonary fibrosis.
Hydroxyurea	500–1500 mg/d orally	Mild nausea and vomiting	Hyperpigmentation, bone marrow suppression.
Mitotane	6–12 g/d orally	Nausea and vomiting	Dermatitis, diarrhea, mental suppression, muscle tremors.
Fludarabine	25 mg/m^2/d IV for 5 days every 4 weeks	Nausea and vomiting	Bone marrow suppression, diarrhea, mild hepatotoxicity, immune suppression.
Cladribine (CdA)	0.09 mg/kg/d by continuous IV infusion for 7 days	Mild nausea, rash, fatigue	Bone marrow suppression, fever, immune suppression.
Topotecan	1.5 mg/m^2 IV daily for 5 days every 3 weeks	Nausea, vomiting, diarrhea, headache, dyspnea	Alopecia, bone marrow suppression.
Gemcitabine	1000 mg/m^2 every week up to 7 weeks, then 1 week off, then weekly for 3 out of 4 weeks	Nausea, vomiting, diarrhea, fever, dyspnea	Bone marrow suppression, rash, fluid retention, mouth sores, flu-like symptoms, paresthesias.
Irinotecan	125 mg/m^2 weekly for 4 weeks, then a 2-week rest, then repeat	Flushing, salivation, lacrimation, bradycardia, abdominal cramps, diarrhea	Bone marrow suppression, diarrhea.
Novel therapeutic agents			
Imatinib mesylate (STI571; Gleevec)	400–600 mg/d orally	Mild nausea	Myalgias, edema, bone marrow suppression, abnormal liver function tests.
Gemfinitib (Iressa)	250 mg by mouth daily	Nausea, vomiting	Diarrhea, rash, acne, dry skin, pruritus, anorexia, asthenia, interstitial lung disease (rare)

(continued)

Table 149. Single-agent dosage and toxicity of anticancer drugs. (continued)

Drug	Dosage	Acute Toxicity	Delayed Toxicity
Alemtuzumab (Campath-1H)	30 mg 3 times a week by SC injection for up to 12 weeks. (Use dose escalation to reduce infusion-related events.)	Severe infusion-related events, injection site irritation	Infections, short-term bone marrow suppression, autoimmune hemolytic anemia.
Gemtuzumab ozogamicin (Mylotarg)	9 mg/m² for 2 doses given 14 days apart	Infusion-related events	Profound bone marrow suppression.
Tretinoin	45 mg/m² by mouth daily until remission or for 90 days	Retinoic acid syndrome (fever, dyspnea, pleural or pericardial effusion) must be treated emergently with dexamethasone.	Headache, dry skin, rash, flushing.
Arsenic trioxide	Induction: 0.15 mg/kg IV daily until remission; maximum 60 doses Consolidation: 0.15 mg/kg IV daily for 25 doses	Same as tretinoin	Nausea, vomiting, diarrhea, edema.
Trastuzumab (Herceptin)	Load: 4 mg/kg IV followed by 2 mg/kg weekly	Low-grade fever, chills, fatigue, constitutional symptoms with first infusion	Cardiac toxicity, especially when given with anthracyclines.
Denileukin diftitox (ONTAK)	9–10 µg/kg/d IV for 5 days every 21 days	Hypersensitivity type reactions with first infusion	Vascular leak syndrome, low albumin, increased risk of infections, diarrhea, rash.
Rituximab	375 mg/m² IV weekly for 4–8 doses	Hypersensitivity type reactions with first infusion; fever, tumor lysis syndrome (can be life-threatening)	Mild cytopenias, rare red cell aplasia or aplastic anemia, severe mucocutaneous reactions.
Ibritumomab tiuxetan (Zevalin)	0.3–0.4 mCi/kg (not to exceed 32 mCi); dosing must follow rituximab	Rituximab infusion reaction symptom complex	Prolonged and severe myelosuppression, nausea, vomiting, abdominal pain, arthralgias.
Bortezomib (Velcade)	1.3 mg/m² by IV bolus twice a week for 2 weeks followed by a 10-day rest. Repeat every 3 weeks.	Low-grade nausea, diarrhea, low-grade fever, weakness	Peripheral neuropathy, thrombocytopenia, edema.
I 131 Tosotumomab (Bexxar)	I 131 tositumomab must be given with tosotumomab. Dosimetric step: 450 mg T over 60 min followed by I 131 T containing 35 mg T with 5 mCi I131. Therapeutic step: Calculated to deliver 75 cGy total body irradiation with 35 mg T.	Hypersensitivity reactions	Prolonged and severe myelosuppression, nausea, vomiting, abdominal pains, arthralgias.
Targretin	300 mg/m²/d/orally	Nausea	Hyperlipidemia, dry mouth, dry skin, constipation, leukopenia, edema.

(continued)

Table 149. Single-agent dosage and toxicity of anticancer drugs. (continued)

Drug	Dosage	Acute Toxicity	Delayed Toxicity
Supportive agents			
Allopurinol	300–900 mg/d orally for prevention or relief of hyperuricemia	None	Rash, Stevens-Johnson syndrome; enhances effects and toxicity of mercaptopurine when used in combination.
Mesna	20% of ifosfamide dosage at the time of ifosfamide administration, then 4 and 8 hours after each dose of chemotherapy to prevent hemorrhagic cystitis	Nausea, vomiting, diarrhea	None.
Leucovorin	10 mg/m^2 every 6 hours IV or orally until serum methotrexate levels are below 5×10^{-8} mol/L with hydration and urinary alkalinization (about 72 hours)	None	Enhances toxic effects of fluorouracil.
Amifostine	910 mg/m^2 IV daily, 30 minutes prior to chemotherapy	Hypotension, nausea, vomiting, flushing	Decrease in serum calcium.
Dexrazoxane	10:1 ratio of anthracycline IV, before (within 30 minutes of) chemotherapy infusion	Pain on injection	Increased bone marrow suppression.
Pilocarpine hydrochloride	5–10 mg orally 3 times daily	Sweating, headache, flushing; nausea, chills, rhinitis, dizziness, and urinary frequency at high dosage.	
Pamidronate	90 mg IV every month	Symptomatic hypoglycemia (rare), flare of bone pain, local irritation	None.
Zoledronic acid	4 mg IV every month		
Epoetin alfa (erythropoietin)	100–300 units/kg IV or SC 3 times a week	Skin irritation or pain at injection site	Hypertension, headache, seizures in patients on dialysis (rare).
Darbopoietin	200 µg SC q week[1]	Injection site pain	Hypertension, thromboses, headache, diarrhea.
Filgrastim (G-CSF)	5 µg/kg/d SC or IV	Mild to moderate bone pain, mild hypotension (rare), irritation at injection sites (rare)	Bone pain, hypoxia.
Pegfilgrastim	6 mg SC each 3-week cycle	Injection site reactions	Bone pain, hypoxia.
Sargramostim (GM-CSF)	250 µg/kg/d as a 2-hour IV infusion (can be given SC)	Fluid retention, dyspnea, capillary leak (rare), supraventricular tachycardia (rare), mild to moderate bone pain, irritation at injection sites	
Neumega (IL-11)	50 µg/kg/d SC	Fluid retention, arrhythmias, headache, arthralgias, myalgias	Unknown.
Samarium-153 lexidronam (Sm-153 EDTMP)	1 mCi/kg IV as single dose	None	Hematopoietic suppression.
Strontium-89	4 mCi every 3 months IV	None	Hematopoietic suppression.

[1]Off label.

Table 150. A common scheme for dose modification of cancer chemotherapeutic agents.[1]

Granulocyte Count	Platelet Count	Suggested Dosage (% of Full Dose)
> 2000/μL	> 100,000/μL	100%
1000–2000/μL	75,000–100,000/μL	50%
< 1000/μL	< 50,000/μL	0%

[1]In general, dose modification should be avoided to maintain therapeutic efficacy. The use of myeloid growth factors or a delay in the start of the next cycle of chemotherapy is usually effective.

Table 151. Paraneoplastic syndromes associated with common cancers.

Syndromes; Hormone Excess	Small Cell Lung Cancer	Non-Small Cell Lung Cancer	Breast Cancer	Multiple Myeloma	Gastro-intestinal Cancers	Hepato-cellular Cancer	Gestational Tropho-blastic Disease	Lympho-ma	Renal Cell Cancer	Carcinoid	Thymo-ma	Ovarian Cancer	Prostate Cancer	Myelo-prolifer-ative Disease	Adreno-cortical Tumors	Cerebel-lar Heman-gioblas-tomas
Endocrine																
Cushing's syndrome	XX	X														
SIADH	XX	X														
Hypercalcemia	XX	X	X	X				X				X				
Hypoglycemia					X	X										
Gonadotropin excess	XX	X			X		X		X	X						
Hyperthyroidism							X									
Neuromuscular																
Subacute cerebellar degeneration	XX	X			X			X				X				
Sensorimotor peripheral neuropathy	XX	X														
Lambert-Eaton syndrome	XX		X		X							X				
Stiff man syndrome			X									X				
Dermatomyo-sitis/poly-myositis	XX	X	X		XX							X		X		

(continued)

1339

Table 151. Paraneoplastic syndromes associated with common cancers. (continued)

Syndromes; Hormone Excess	Small Cell Lung Cancer	Non-Small Cell Lung Cancer	Breast Cancer	Multiple Myeloma	Gastrointestinal Cancers	Hepatocellular Cancer	Gestational Trophoblastic Disease	Lymphoma	Renal Cell Cancer	Carcinoid	Thymoma	Ovarian Cancer	Prostate Cancer	Myeloproliferative Disease	Adrenocortical Tumors	Cerebellar Hemangioblastomas
Skin																
Dermatomyositis	XX	X	X		XX							X		X		
Acanthosis nigricans		X	X		X					X			X	X		
Sweet's syndrome	X	X	X		X			XX	X			X	X	XX		
Hematologic																
Erythrocytosis						X			X			X			X	X
Pure red cell aplasia		X	X		X			X			XX					
Eosinophilia								XX								
Thrombocytosis	X	X	X	X	X	X	X	X	X	X	X	X	X	X	X	X
Coagulopathy			X					X	X				X	X		
Fever	X	X	X	X	X	X	X	X	X	X	X	X	X	X	X	X
Amyloidosis				X				X	X							

XX = strong association; X = reported association.